BRI

UNIT I Introduction to Pharmacology
1. The Clinical Judgment Measurement Model and the Nursing Process, 1
2. Drug Development and Ethical Considerations, 7
3. Pharmacokinetics and Pharmacodynamics, 19
4. Pharmacogenetics, 32
5. Complementary and Alternative Therapies, 39
6. Pediatric Considerations, 45
7. Drug Therapy in Older Adults, 52
8. Drugs in Substance Use Disorder, 58

UNIT II Pharmacotherapy and Drug Administration
9. Safety and Quality, 69
10. Drug Administration, 80
11. Drug Labels and Dosage Calculations, 92

UNIT III Maintenance of Homeostasis
12. Fluid Volume and Electrolytes, 133
13. Vitamin and Mineral Replacement, 154
14. Nutritional Support, 166

UNIT IV Autonomic Nervous System Drugs
15. Adrenergic Agonists and Antagonists, 175
16. Cholinergic Agonists and Antagonists, 187

UNIT V Central and Peripheral Nervous System Drugs
17. Stimulants, 199
18. Depressants, 206
19. Antiseizure Drugs, 220
20. Drugs for Parkinson and Alzheimer Disease, 229
21. Drugs for Neuromuscular Disorders and Muscle Spasms, 244

UNIT VI Mental and Behavioral Health Drugs
22. Antipsychotics and Anxiolytics, 259
23. Antidepressants and Mood Stabilizers, 274

UNIT VII Pain and Inflammation Management Drugs
24. Antiinflammatories, 287
25. Analgesics, 303

UNIT VIII Antimicrobial Drugs
26. Penicillins, Other Beta-Lactams, and Cephalosporins, 321
27. Macrolides, Oxazolidinones, Lincosamides, Glycopeptides, and Lipopeptides, 333
28. Tetracyclines, Glycylcyclines, Aminoglycosides, and Fluoroquinolones, 339
29. Sulfonamides and Nitroimidazoles Antibiotics, 348
30. Antituberculars, Antifungals, and Antivirals, 354
31. Antimalarials, Anthelmintics, and Peptides, 369

UNIT IX Immunologic Drugs
32. HIV- and AIDS-Related Drugs, 381
33. Transplant Drugs, 395
34. Vaccines, 407

UNIT X Antineoplastics and Biologic Response Modifiers
35. Anticancer Drugs, 421
36. Targeted Therapies to Treat Cancer, 446
37. Biologic Response Modifiers, 466

UNIT XI Respiratory Drugs
38. Upper Respiratory Disorders, 477
39. Lower Respiratory Disorders, 486

UNIT XII Cardiovascular Drugs
40. Cardiac Glycosides, Antianginals, and Antidysrhythmics, 501
41. Diuretics, 524
42. Antihypertensives, 536
43. Anticoagulants, Antiplatelets, and Thrombolytics, 551
44. Antihyperlipidemics and Drugs to Improve Peripheral Blood Flow, 563

UNIT XIII Gastrointestinal Drugs
45. Gastrointestinal Tract Disorders, 573
46. Antiulcer Drugs, 590

UNIT XIV Eye, Ear, and Skin Drugs
47. Eye and Ear Disorders, 603
48. Dermatologic Disorders, 620

UNIT XV Endocrine Drugs
49. Pituitary, Thyroid, Parathyroid, and Adrenal Disorders, 633
50. Antidiabetics, 649

UNIT XVI Renal and Urologic Drugs
51. Urinary Disorders, 665

UNIT XVII Reproductive and Gender-Related Drugs
52. Pregnancy and Preterm Labor, 673
53. Labor, Delivery, and Postpartum, 689
54. Neonatal and Newborn, 708
55. Female Reproductive Health, 713
56. Male Reproductive Health, 739
57. Sexually Transmitted Infections, 751

UNIT XVIII Emergency Drugs
58. Adult and Pediatric Emergency Drugs, 761

Appendix A: Answers to Review Questions, 777
Bibliography, 778
Glossary, 781

Sherpath® Vantage

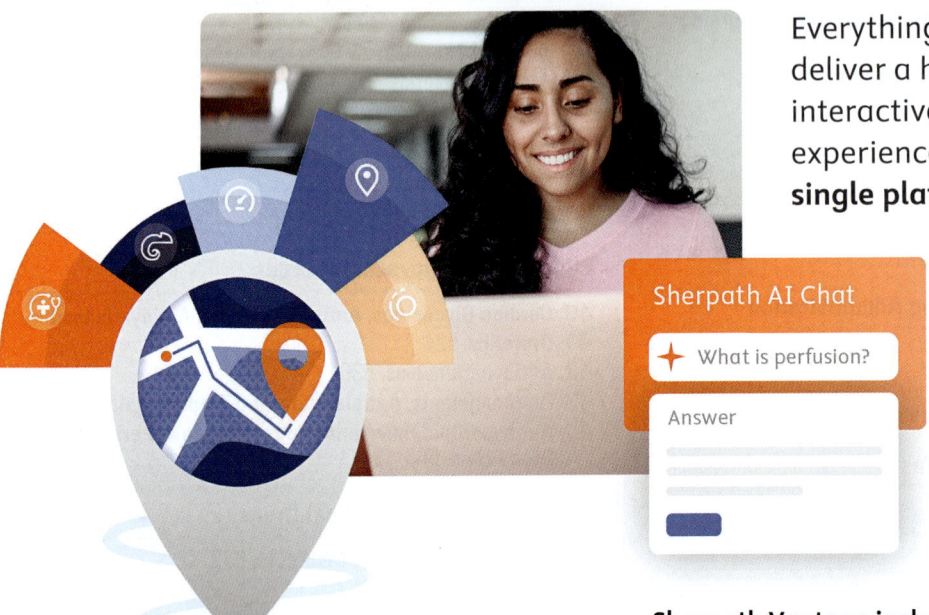

Everything you need to deliver a highly effective, interactive course experience — **all on a single platform**

Sherpath Vantage offers a variety of engaging assignment types, teaching resources, and learning tools — all on a single, integrated platform. It's everything needed to help students master key concepts and strengthen their skills competency and clinical judgment.

Plus, Sherpath Vantage's simple, seamless, and supportive environment saves instructors and students time and provides meaningful learning analytics to drive improved course outcomes.

*Available for select collections

Sherpath Vantage includes:

- Elsevier eBook
- Comprehensive digital lessons
- Assignment analytics
- Sherpath AI
- Elsevier Adaptive Quizzing (EAQ)
- Osmosis® videos*
- Shadow Health® Digital Clinical Experiences™
- Enhanced test banks (EAB)

STUDENTS — Ask your instructor about enhancing your course experience with Sherpath Vantage!

INSTRUCTORS — Scan code or visit myevolve.us/sv to learn more!

24-0482 TM/AF

Pharmacology

A PATIENT-CENTERED NURSING PROCESS APPROACH

EDITION 12

LINDA E. MCCUISTION, PhD, MSN, RN
Professor (Ret.), University of Holy Cross, New Orleans, Louisiana

KATHLEEN VULJOIN DIMAGGIO, MSN, RN
Professor Emerita, University of Holy Cross, New Orleans, Louisiana

MARY B. WINTON, PhD, MSN, RN
Associate Professor, Tarleton State University, Stephenville, Texas

JENNIFER J. YEAGER, PhD, MSN, RN
Associate Professor, Tarleton State University, Stephenville, Texas

Elsevier
3251 Riverport Lane
St. Louis, Missouri 63043

PHARMACOLOGY: A PATIENT-CENTERED NURSING PROCESS APPROACH,
TWELFTH EDITION

ISBN: 978-0-443-11525-7

Copyright © 2026 by Elsevier Inc. All rights are reserved, including those for text and data mining, AI training, and similar technologies.

Publisher's note: Elsevier takes a neutral position with respect to territorial disputes or jurisdictional claims in its published content, including in maps and institutional affiliations.

No part of this publication may be reproduced or transmitted in any form or by any means, electronic or mechanical, including photocopying, recording, or any information storage and retrieval system, without permission in writing from the publisher. Details on how to seek permission, further information about the Publisher's permissions policies and our arrangements with organizations such as the Copyright Clearance Center and the Copyright Licensing Agency, can be found at our website: www.elsevier.com/permissions.

This book and the individual contributions contained in it are protected under copyright by the Publisher (other than as may be noted herein).

Notice

Practitioners and researchers must always rely on their own experience and knowledge in evaluating and using any information, methods, compounds or experiments described herein. Because of rapid advances in the medical sciences, in particular, independent verification of diagnoses and drug dosages should be made. To the fullest extent of the law, no responsibility is assumed by Elsevier, authors, editors or contributors for any injury and/or damage to persons or property as a matter of products liability, negligence or otherwise, or from any use or operation of any methods, products, instructions, or ideas contained in the material herein.

Previous editions copyrighted 2023, 2021, 2018, 2015, 2012, 2009, 2003, 2000, 1997, 1993.

Executive Content Strategist: Lee Henderson
Senior Content Strategist: Yvonne Alexopoulos
Director, Content Development: Laurie Gower
Senior Content Development Specialist: Betsy McCormac
Production Services Managers: Julie Eddy; Catherine Jackson
Senior Project Manager: Jodi Willard
Design Direction: Brian Salisbury

Printed in India

Last digit is the print number: 9 8 7 6 5 4 3 2 1

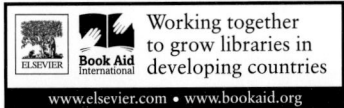

*To Joyce LeFever Kee, who originated this book;
to Evelyn R. Hayes for her previous contributions to the book;
to Dr. Gerald DeLuca and Sister Bernardino Hill for their expert guidance;
and in loving memory of my parents, Otto and Pauline Schmidt; my sisters,
Katrina Sue Benge and Christina Ann Milner; and my brother, Enno Schmidt.*

Linda E. McCuistion

*To my daughters, Christy, Maria, and Katie; my grandchildren,
Chloe, Sofia, Catherine, Mia, Jack, and Elaine; my great-granddaughter,
Gralynn; my dear friend, Linda; and the Department of Nursing at the University
of Holy Cross, New Orleans.*

Kathleen Vuljoin DiMaggio

*To my Lord and Savior for His gift of nursing and teaching;
to my husband, Dr. Richard A. Winton for his continual
love and support; to my daughters, Lin and Kristin, who will
always be my babies—may the Lord bless you and keep you.*

Mary B. Winton

*To Tracy L. Yeager, my husband, my soulmate, and support;
and to my boys, Jacob and Joshua, for putting
up with my hours on the computer; and I wouldn't be me without
thanking my dog, Xander, for being my constant companion.*

Jennifer J. Yeager

MEET THE AUTHORS

LINDA E. MCCUISTION

Dr. Linda E. McCuistion received a Diploma of Nursing from the Lutheran Hospital School of Nursing in Fort Wayne, Indiana; Bachelor of Science in Nursing from William Carey College in Hattiesburg, Mississippi; Master in Nursing from Louisiana State University Medical Center, New Orleans; and PhD in Curriculum and Instruction from the University of New Orleans. She was licensed as an advanced practice nurse in Louisiana and has many years of nursing experience that includes acute care and home health nursing. For 20 years, Linda was a nursing professor at the University of Holy Cross in New Orleans, Louisiana. She received an Endowed Professorship Award in 2000 and 2003. Linda also worked as a nursing professor at South University, Richmond, Virginia.

Linda has served as a president, vice president, and faculty advisor of the Sigma Theta Tau International Honor Society in Nursing, Xi Psi chapter-at-large. Moreover, she was an associate editor of the *NODNA Times*, a New Orleans District Nurses Association newsletter. She has been a member of Phi Delta Kappa and the American Society of Hypertension.

Linda was a coordinator for the Graduate Plus internship program, a preceptorship program for new nursing graduates in Louisiana. She has served as a legal nurse consultant; a member of a medical review panel; advisory board member, consultant, and reviewer of a software preparation company focused on the state licensure examination; advisory board member for a school for surgical technicians; and consultant to a local hospital to improve the quality of nursing care and assist acute care facilities in preparation for accreditation.

Linda was chosen as a "Great One-Hundred Nurse" by the New Orleans District Nurses Association in 1993. She is also listed in the 2005/2006 edition of the Empire Who's Who Executive and Professional Registry.

Linda has given numerous lectures and presentations regionally and nationally on many nursing topics. She has published articles in nursing journals and has authored many chapters in several nursing textbooks, including *Pharmacotherapeutics: Clinical Decision Making in Nursing* (1999), *Saunders Manual of Medical-Surgical Nursing: A Guide for Clinical Decision Making* (2002), and *Saunders Nursing Survival Guide: Pathophysiology* (2007). She is author and coauthor of many chapters and coeditor of *Saunders Nursing Survival Guide: Pharmacology* (2007).

Linda enjoys cruises, the beach, and other travel. When at home, she enjoys family, friends, golf, crafts, reading, writing, and her King Charles Cavalier Spaniel, Prince.

KATHLEEN VULJOIN DIMAGGIO

Kathleen Vuljoin DiMaggio received her Bachelor of Science in Nursing from Our Lady of Holy Cross College of New Orleans and her Master of Science in Nursing from Loyola University of New Orleans, with a focus on Healthcare Systems Management. She completed a preceptorship in palliative care at Ochsner Foundation Hospital through Loyola University. She received Level I designation from the National Hospice and Palliative Care Organization in hospice management and development. She is certified by the Louisiana Department of Health and Hospitals Developmental Disabilities as a registered nurse instructor in medication administration. Kathleen has more than 23 years of clinical nursing experience and more than 12 years of baccalaureate nursing education. Her professional practice experience includes medical-surgical nursing and home health and hospice nursing. She has experience in nursing management and has worked as director of nursing for a facility specializing in developmental disabilities. In addition, Kathleen has worked as director of nursing in home health and hospice care. She has worked in quality improvement, disease management, and case management.

Kathleen has served as a volunteer for Junior Achievement of New Orleans, has volunteered for a local hospice agency, has served in the homeless ministry, and teaches third-grade Sunday school classes through her church.

Kathleen is a member of the Sigma Theta Tau International Honor Society of Nursing, and Alpha Sigma Nu Jesuit Honor Society.

Kathleen is a recipient of the 2011 and 2015 Endowed Professorship from Eminent Eye, Ear, Nose and Throat Hospital. She has received the Order of St. Louis Award through the Archdiocese of New Orleans and has also received the Florence Nightingale Society Award for Nursing. Kathleen received the Outstanding Faculty of the Year Award in 2017 and the distinction of Professor Emerita in May 2018 from the University of Holy Cross, New Orleans.

Kathleen enjoys spending time with family and friends. She enjoys crocheting, quilting, cooking, and reading.

MARY B. WINTON

Dr. Mary B. Winton received her Associate Degree in Nursing from Tarleton State University in Stephenville, Texas, a member of the Texas A&M University System; her Bachelor and Master of Science in Nursing from the University of Texas at Arlington; and her PhD in Nursing from the University of Texas at Tyler. Additionally, she received board certification through the American Nurses Credentialing Center as an Acute Care Adult Nurse Practitioner. Mary has many years of hospital nursing experience in areas including critical care, emergency, and medical-surgical nursing both as a nurse and a nursing supervisor. She was employed with a hospitalist group as an Acute Care Nurse Practitioner for many years. Currently, she is an Associate Professor in the College of Health Sciences, School of Nursing, at Tarleton State University. Mary has experience in teaching graduate-level pharmacology, pathophysiology, health assessment, and nursing informatics, and she has vast experience teaching at all levels of the undergraduate nursing program, including nursing pathophysiology, pharmacology, and health assessment.

Mary has served as a faculty advisor for the Student Nurses Association at Tarleton. She has been a member of several organizations, including Sigma Theta Tau International Honor Society in Nursing, Tau Chi chapter; American Nurses Association/Texas Nurses Association; Critical Care Nursing Education; and Rural Nurse Organization. She is actively involved in various university, college, school, and departmental committees.

During her career as a nurse educator, Mary was the recipient of the Texas A&M Student Evaluation Teaching Excellence Award and the O.A. Grant Excellence in Teaching Award. She was also the recipient of the AACN 2020-2021 Scholarship of Teaching and Learning Excellence Award. She has also taught English as a second language at her church of membership.

Mary's research interests include health disparity among minorities, especially among Korean immigrants; student learning outcomes; and the use of technology in classrooms. She has presented at several conferences and has published on the health care of Korean immigrants.

During her spare time, Mary enjoys spending time with her husband, daughters, and grandchildren. She also enjoys traveling, reading, crocheting, and snow skiing.

JENNIFER J. YEAGER

Jennifer J. Yeager, PhD, MSN, RN was called to be a nurse during her senior year in high school. One morning, she woke up with the aim of becoming a nurse; until the day before, she had planned on becoming an English teacher. She is the only nurse in a large family of teachers and engineers.

She attended the University of Portland in Oregon on an Air Force ROTC nursing scholarship. After graduation, she moved to Texas to be an Air Force nurse at Wilford Hall Medical Center in San Antonio. After 6 years of service and earning the rank of Captain, she separated from the Air Force. She stayed in Texas, as she enjoys living in the state.

While in school in Portland, Jennifer looked at her instructors and knew that she would fill their shoes one day. In the back of her mind, she had set the goal to earn a doctoral degree before turning 50 and to become a nursing professor. In 1998 she earned her MSN as an Adult/Gerontological Nurse Practitioner with Educator Role from The University of Texas at Arlington; in 2013 she earned her PhD in Nursing at The University of Texas at Tyler. She achieved her goal through determination and hard work.

Since 2007, Jennifer has taught at Tarleton State University and will be retiring this year. For Jennifer, teaching students the art and science of nursing has been the most wonderful opportunity imaginable. Although her background has been working with older adults, she has taught various courses at all levels (undergraduate and graduate). She earned the O.A. Grant Excellence in Teaching Award in 2023; the Certificate in Effective College Instruction through the Association of College and University Educators and the American Council on Education in 2020; and the Faculty Excellence in Scholarship Award at Tarleton State University, College of Health Science and Human Services in 2018. In 2011 Jennifer was selected to participate in the Sigma Theta Tau International Nurse Faculty Leadership Academy.

Although Jennifer and her family made sacrifices to accomplish her goal, it has been worth it. Setting goals and reaching them through hard work, dedication, and learning through mistakes, and never quitting, has made reaching the goal all the sweeter.

IN RECOGNITION

Joyce LeFever Kee taught a pharmacology course to student nurses for 10 years from 1980 to 1990 at the University of Delaware. At the time, there were very few pharmacology texts available, and what was published was not appropriate for some BSN and ADN nursing programs. Daniel Ruth from W.B. Saunders approached Kee in 1990 to write a pharmacology book for nurses. With experience in teaching the subject, Kee developed the contents and format for a pharmacology text.

The chapter "Drug Action: Pharmaceutic, Pharmacokinetics, and Pharmacodynamics Phases" became the first chapter in the first edition. These drug phases appear both in the Prototype Drug Charts and within the contents in most of the current chapters. Kee developed many drug tables that have been updated by coauthors through the years. The important part that Kee established in the chapters was the five steps of the Nursing Process.

Dr. Evelyn R. Hayes joined Kee starting with the first edition. Hayes developed certain chapters and took the responsibility to work with contributors for the book such as the six chapters on Reproductive and Sex-Related Agents among others.

Linda E. McCuistion joined Kee and Hayes in 2005. McCuistion has updated many of Kee's chapters with new drugs and content.

CONTRIBUTORS AND REVIEWERS

CONTRIBUTORS

Christina DiMaggio Boudreaux, BSN, RN, IBCLC
Director of Nursing
Elba Medical Distributors
Metairie, Louisiana

Linda Laskowski-Jones, MS, APRN, ACNS-BC, CEN, NEA-BC, FAWM, FAAN
Clinical Nurse Specialist
Laskowski-Jones New Frontiers Health Consulting, LLC
Newark, Delaware;
Executive Director
Appalachian Center for Wilderness Medicine
Morganton, North Carolina

Jared Robertson III, MN, CRNA
Certified Registered Nurse Anesthesiologist, Anesthesia
U.S. Army
Pass Christian, Mississippi

REVIEWERS

Marci L. Dial, DNP, APRN, PMGT-BC CHSE, LNC
Professor of Nursing, Co-Clinical Coordinator
School of Nursing, Valencia College
Orlando, Florida

Denise E. King, MSN, RN-BC, CCM
Acting Executive Director and Senior Lecturer
Elizabeth T. MacNeil School of Nursing
Dominican University
River Forest, Illinois

Coleen Kumar, PhD, RN, CNE
Dean
HMH JFK Muhlenberg Harold B. and Dorothy A. Snyder
  School of Nursing and Medical Imaging
Plainfield, New Jersey

Meera Kiran Brown, PharmD, MBA
Senior Manager
Pharmacy Growth & Omnichannel
CVS Health
Austin, Texas

PREFACE

The 12th edition of *Pharmacology: A Patient-Centered Nursing Process Approach* is written for nursing students who can benefit from the straightforward, student-friendly presentation of the principles of pharmacology. It focuses on need-to-know content and helps students learn to administer drugs safely and eliminate medication errors through extensive practice of dosage calculations and evidence-based application of the nursing process.

ORGANIZATION

Pharmacology: A Patient-Centered Nursing Process Approach is organized into 18 units and 58 chapters. **Unit I** is an introduction to pharmacology and includes thoroughly updated chapters on drug action, the drug approval process, cultural and pharmacogenetic considerations, drug interactions, over-the-counter drugs, ethical considerations, pediatric and geriatric considerations, drugs for substance use disorder, complementary and alternative therapies, life span issues, patient collaboration in community settings, the nursing process, patient-centered care, and the role of the nurse in drug research. This unit introduces the Next-Generation NCLEX® Examination (NGN) Clinical Judgment Measurement Model (CJMM). Its focus is to develop clinical reasoning and clinical judgment skills in students' decision-making. This edition contains several unfolding and single-episode case studies presented using the six CJMM cognitive skills and contrasts these skills with the steps of the nursing process.

Unit II focuses on patient safety and quality in pharmacotherapy and medication administration, and it features a comprehensive review of drug dosage calculations for adults and children, which is a unique strength of this book. This unit includes systems of measurement with conversion factors, calculation methods: enteral and parenteral drug dosages, calculation methods: drugs that require reconstitution, calculation methods: insulin dosages, and calculation methods: intravenous flow rates. Five methods of dosage calculation are preceded by a ✳ for easy identification: basic formula, ratio and proportion/fractional equation, dimensional analysis, body weight, and body surface area. Integral to the sections on dosage calculations are clinical practice problems that feature actual drug labels in full color, which provide extensive practice in real-world dosage calculations. With this wide array of practice problems in a variety of healthcare settings, this unit eliminates the need to purchase a separate dosage calculation book.

Unit III addresses nutrition, fluids, and electrolytes with separate chapters that cover vitamin and mineral replacement, fluid and electrolyte replacement, and nutritional support.

Units IV through XVIII comprise the core of *Pharmacology: A Patient-Centered Nursing Process Approach* and cover the drug classifications students must understand to practice safely and effectively. Each drug family chapter includes a chapter outline, learning objectives, at least one prototype drug chart, a drug table, and an extensive Clinical Judgment [Nursing Process] section.

- The **prototype drug charts** are a unique tool that students can use to view the many facets of a prototype drug through the lens of the nursing process. Each prototype drug is one of the most common drugs in its class. The charts include drug class, contraindications, dosage, drug-lab-food interactions, pharmacokinetics, pharmacodynamics, therapeutic effects/uses, side effects, and adverse reactions. With these charts, students can see how the steps of the nursing process correlate with these key aspects of drug information and therapy.
- The **drug tables** provide a quick reference to routes, dosages, uses, and key considerations for the most prescribed drugs for a given class. They list the drug's generic name, dosages, uses and considerations, and specific information on half-life and protein binding.
- The **Clinical Judgment [Nursing Process] sections** provide a convenient summary of related concepts for concept-based curricula, patient assessments, patient problems, plan of care, and outcomes. These sections also include cultural content, nursing interventions, suggestions for patient teaching, and relevant herbal information.

ADDITIONAL FEATURES

Throughout this edition, we have retained, enhanced, and added a variety of features that teach students the fundamental principles of pharmacology and the role of the nurse in drug therapy:

- **Review questions** at the end of each chapter help prepare students for the NCLEX® Examination with its increasing emphasis on pharmacology; answers are provided in Appendix A at the end of the textbook.
- **Patient safety boxes** include information on medication safety, complementary and alternative therapies, and more.
- **Clinical judgment case studies**, **clinical judgment unfolding case studies**, and **clinical judgment single-episode case studies** have been added in many chapters of this edition. These case studies follow the new NGN CJMM and will challenge students to develop clinical judgment skills.
- **Complementary and Alternative Therapies** boxes appear throughout the text to provide students with a quick reference to information on popular herbs and their side effects, drug interactions, and more.
- **Anatomy and physiology** reviews are contained in all drug therapy chapters, including illustrated overviews of normal anatomy and physiology. These introductions provide a review of the foundation for understanding how drugs work in various body systems.
- **High-alert drugs** (❗) and **safety concerns** (⚡) are identified within the text with distinctive icons that make it easy to find crucial information.

TEACHING AND LEARNING RESOURCES

The 12th edition of *Pharmacology: A Patient-Centered Nursing Process Approach* is the core of a complete teaching and learning package for nursing pharmacology. Additional components of this package include resources designed specifically for students, resources designed specifically for faculty members, and resources designed for both students and faculty.

A comprehensive *Study Guide*, available for purchase separately, provides thousands of study questions and answers, including clinically based situational practice problems, drug calculation problems and questions (many with actual drug labels), and case studies to help students master textbook content. Answers are provided at the end of the *Study Guide*.

It is our hope that *Pharmacology: A Patient-Centered Nursing Process Approach* and its comprehensive ancillary package will serve as a dynamic resource for teaching students the basic principles of pharmacology as well as their vital role in drug therapy.

Linda E. McCuistion
Kathleen Vuljoin DiMaggio
Mary B. Winton
Jennifer J. Yeager

ACKNOWLEDGMENTS

We wish to extend our sincere appreciation to the many professionals who assisted in the preparation of the 12th edition of *Pharmacology: A Patient-Centered Nursing Process Approach* by reviewing chapters and offering suggestions.

We wish to especially thank Joyce LeFever Kee, who originated this pharmacology textbook, and her coauthor Evelyn R. Hayes, who worked tirelessly on many editions of this book.

We wish to thank the current contributors: Christina DiMaggio Boudreaux, Linda Laskowski-Jones, and Jared Robertson.

We wish to thank those who created and updated the previous established chapters: Margaret Barton-Burke, Joseph Boullata, Jacqueline Rosenjack Burchum, Katherine L. Byar, Michelle M. Byrne, Karen Carmody, Robin Webb Corbett, Sandy Elliott, Linda Goodwin, Janice Heinssen, Marilyn Herbert-Ashton, Judith W. Herrman, Kathleen J. Jones, Bettyrae Jordan, Robert J. Kizior, Paula R. Klemm, Anne E. Lara, Linda Laskowski-Jones, Ronald J. LeFever, Patricia S. Lincoln, Patricia O'Brien, Laura K. Williford Owens, Byron Peters, Lisa Ann Plowfield, Larry D. Purnell, Nancy C. Sharts-Hopko, Jane Purnell Taylor, Donald L. Taylor, Lynette M. Wachholz, Marcia Welsh, Gail Wilkes, and M. Linda Workman.

Of course, we are deeply indebted to the many patients and students we have had throughout our many years of professional nursing practice. From them we have learned many fine points about the role of therapeutic pharmacology in nursing practice.

Our deepest appreciation goes to pharmaceutical companies for use of their drug labels. Pharmaceutical companies that extended their courtesy to this book include the following:

- Abbott Laboratories
- AstraZeneca Pharmaceuticals
- Aventis
- Bayer Corporation
- Bristol-Myers Squibb (including Apothecon Laboratories and Mead Johnson Pharmaceuticals)
- DuPont/Merck Pharmaceuticals
- Eli Lilly and Company
- Elkins-Sinn, Inc.
- Glaxo-Wellcome
- Marion Merrell Dow, Inc.
- McNeill Laboratory, Inc.
- Merck and Co., Inc.
- Parke-Davis Co.
- Pfizer Inc.
- Rhone-Poulenc Rorer
- SmithKline Beecham Pharmaceutical
- Wyeth-Ayerst Laboratories

Thanks to Becton, Dickinson and Company for the syringe displays. Thanks to CareFusion Corporation for the photos of the infusion pumps.

Our sincere thanks to Elsevier, especially Yvonne Alexopoulos, Senior Content Strategist; Betsy McCormac, Senior Content Development Specialist; and Jodi Willard, Senior Project Manager, for their suggestions and wonderful assistance.

Linda E. McCuistion
Kathleen Vuljoin DiMaggio
Mary B. Winton
Jennifer J. Yeager

CONTENTS

UNIT I Introduction to Pharmacology

1. **The Clinical Judgment Measurement Model and the Nursing Process**, 1
   - Clinical Judgment and the Nursing Process, 1
   - Clinical Judgment Measurement Model, 2
2. **Drug Development and Ethical Considerations**, 7
   - Core Ethical Principles, 7
   - Objectives and Phases of Pharmaceutical Research, 10
   - American Nurses Association Code of Ethics, 11
   - Drug Standards and Legislation, 11
   - Drug Names and Resources, 14
3. **Pharmacokinetics and Pharmacodynamics**, 19
   - Pharmacokinetics, 19
   - Pharmacodynamics, 23
   - Drug Interactions, 26
4. **Pharmacogenetics**, 32
   - Foundations of Pharmacogenetics, 32
   - Key Considerations When Using Pharmacogenetics, 34
5. **Complementary and Alternative Therapies**, 39
   - Dietary Supplement Health and Education Act of 1994 and Current Good Manufacturing Practices, 40
   - Commonly Used Herbal Remedies, 41
   - Hazards, Tips, and Resources for Herbal Remedies, 42
6. **Pediatric Considerations**, 45
   - Pharmacokinetics and Pharmacodynamics, 46
   - Nursing Implications, 47
   - Considerations for the Adolescent Patient, 48
   - Family-Centered Collaborative Care, 49
7. **Drug Therapy in Older Adults**, 52
   - Physiologic Changes, 52
   - Nursing Implications: Older Adult Drug Dosing and Monitoring, 54
8. **Drugs in Substance Use Disorder**, 58
   - Substance Use Disorder, 58
   - Types of Substance Use Disorders, 59
   - Special Needs of Patients With Substance Use Disorder, 65
   - The Nurse With Substance Use Disorder, 66

UNIT II Pharmacotherapy and Drug Administration

9. **Safety and Quality**, 69
   - "Six Rights" of Medication Administration, 69
   - Promoting Safety in the Health Care Environment, 73
   - Safety Risks With Medication Administration, 75
   - Other Factors in the Prevention of Medication Errors, 77
10. **Drug Administration**, 80
    - Forms and Routes of Drug Administration, 80
    - Parenteral Medications, 84
11. **Drug Labels and Dosage Calculations**, 92
    - Overview of Dosage Calculations, 92
    - Calculation Methods, 98
    - Considerations for Enteral Administration, 107
    - Considerations for Parenteral Administration, 109
    - Answers to Practice Problems, 127

UNIT III Maintenance of Homeostasis

12. **Fluid Volume and Electrolytes**, 133
    - Fluid and Electrolyte, 133
    - Fluid Replacement, 134
    - Electrolytes, 138
13. **Vitamin and Mineral Replacement**, 154
    - Vitamins, 154
    - Minerals, 161
14. **Nutritional Support**, 166
    - Nutritional Support Therapy, 166
    - Enteral Nutrition, 166
    - Parenteral Nutrition, 170

UNIT IV Autonomic Nervous System Drugs

15. **Adrenergic Agonists and Antagonists**, 175
    - Nervous Systems of the Body, 175
    - Adrenergic Agonists, 175
    - Adrenergic Antagonists, 183
16. **Cholinergic Agonists and Antagonists**, 187
    - Parasympathetic Nervous System, 187
    - Cholinergic Agonists, 187
    - Cholinergic Antagonists, 191

UNIT V Central and Peripheral Nervous System Drugs

17. **Stimulants**, 199
    - Anatomy and Physiology of the Nervous System, 199
    - Central Nervous System Stimulants, 200
    - Amphetamines and Amphetamine-Like Drugs, 200
    - Anorexiants, 202
    - Analeptics, 203
18. **Depressants**, 206
    Jared Robertson
    - Sleep Disorders, 206
    - Sedative-Hypnotics, 207
    - Anesthetics, 214
19. **Antiseizure Drugs**, 220
    - Seizures, 220
    - Antiseizure Drugs, 220
    - Antiseizure Drugs in Selected Situations, 223
20. **Drugs for Parkinson and Alzheimer Disease**, 229
    - Parkinson Disease, 229
    - Drugs Used to Treat Parkinson Disease, 230
    - Alzheimer Disease, 238
21. **Drugs for Neuromuscular Disorders and Muscle Spasms**, 244
    - Myasthenia Gravis, 244
    - Multiple Sclerosis, 248
    - Skeletal Muscle Relaxants, 253

UNIT VI Mental and Behavioral Health Drugs

22 Antipsychotics and Anxiolytics, 259
- Pschopathology, 259
- Antipsychotics, 260
- Anxiety, 268
- Anxiolytics, 268

23 Antidepressants and Mood Stabilizers, 274
- Depression, 274
- Antidepressant Agents, 275
- Mood Stabilizers, 277

UNIT VII Pain and Inflammation Management Drugs

24 Antiinflammatories, 287
- Inflammation and Antiinflammatory Agents, 287
- Nonsteroidal Antiinflammatory Drugs and Corticosteroids, 288
- Disease-Modifying Antirheumatic Drugs, 295
- Antigout Drugs, 298

25 Analgesics, 303
- Pain, 303
- Nonopioid Analgesics, 305
- Opioid Analgesics, 306
- Adjuvants, Agonists, and Antagonists, 313
- Headaches: Migraine and Cluster, 314

UNIT VIII Antimicrobial Drugs

26 Penicillins, Other Beta-Lactams, and Cephalosporins, 321
- Pathophysiology, 321
- Antibacterials/Antibiotics, 322
- Penicillins and Other Beta-Lactam Antibacterials, 324
- Cephalosporins, 328

27 Macrolides, Oxazolidinones, Lincosamides, Glycopeptides, and Lipopeptides, 333
- Macrolides, 333
- Oxazolidinones, 336
- Lincosamides, 336
- Glycopeptides, 337
- Lipopeptides, 337

28 Tetracyclines, Glycylcyclines, Aminoglycosides, and Fluoroquinolones, 339
- Tetracyclines, 339
- Glycylcyclines, 340
- Aminoglycosides, 343
- Fluoroquinolones, 346

29 Sulfonamides and Nitroimidazoles Antibiotics, 348
- Sulfonamides, 348
- Trimethoprim-Sulfamethoxazole, 349
- Sulfonamides, Nitroimidazoles, Miscellaneous Antibacterials, 349
- Miscellaneous Antibacterial Drugs, 352

30 Antituberculars, Antifungals, and Antivirals, 354
- Tuberculosis, 354
- Antitubercular Drugs, 354
- Fungus: Pathophysiology, 358
- Viruses: Pathophysiology, 361

31 Antimalarials, Anthelmintics, and Peptides, 369
- Antimalarial Drugs, 369
- Anthelmintic Drugs, 372
- Peptides, 374

UNIT IX Immunologic Drugs

32 HIV- and AIDS-Related Drugs, 381
- Overview of HIV and AIDS, 382
- Antiretroviral Drugs, 383
- The Nurse's Role in Antiretroviral Therapy, 391

33 Transplant Drugs, 395
- Principles of Immunosuppression and Immunosuppressant Drugs, 395
- Drugs for Transplant Rejection, 402
- Drugs for Infection, 403
- Promoting Adherence, 403

34 Vaccines, 407
- Immunity, 408
- Vaccines, 408
- Vaccine-Preventable Diseases and Vaccine Recommendations, 409
- Vaccine Safety: Reporting Diseases and Adverse Reactions, 414
- Varicella Vaccine, 415
- Future Developments in Vaccines, 416

UNIT X Antineoplastics and Biologic Response Modifiers

35 Anticancer Drugs, 421
- Overview of Cancer, 421
- Cancer Chemotherapy, 423
- Alkylating Drugs, 427
- Antimetabolites, 429
- Antitumor Antibiotics, 433
- Plant Alkaloids, 436
- Other Drugs to Treat Cancer, 440

36 Targeted Therapies to Treat Cancer, 446
- Overview of Targeted Therapy, 446
- Angiogenesis Inhibitors/Vascular Endothelial Growth Factor Receptor Inhibitors, 447
- Epidermal Growth Factor Receptor Inhibitors, 448
- Tyrosine Kinase Inhibitors and Multikinase Inhibitors, 452
- mTOR Kinase Inhibitors and Proteasome Inhibitors, 455
- Monoclonal Antibodies, 459

37 Biologic Response Modifiers, 466
- Overview of Biologic Response Modifiers, 466
- Interferons, 467
- Colony-Stimulating Factors, 470
- Interleukin-2, 473

UNIT XI Respiratory Drugs

38 Upper Respiratory Disorders, 477
- Respiratory System, 477
- Common Cold, Acute Rhinitis, and Allergic Rhinitis, 477
- Other Upper Respiratory Disorders, 484

39 Lower Respiratory Disorders, 486
- Lower Respiratory System, 486
- Lower Respiratory System Disorders, 487
- Major Drug Categories That Treat Lower Respiratory Disorders, 489
- Asthma Drug Therapy for Special Populations, 498

UNIT XII Cardiovascular Drugs

40 Cardiac Glycosides, Antianginals, and Antidysrhythmics, 501
- Introduction, 501
- Cardiovascular System, 501
- Laboratory Tests to Diagnose Heart Failure, 503
- Agents Used to Treat Heart Failure, 503
- Angina Pectoris, 507
- Types of Antianginal Drugs, 507
- Cardiac Dysrhythmias, 512
- Types of Antidysrhythmic Drugs, 514

41 Diuretics, 524
- Diuretics, 524
- Thiazides and Thiazide-Like Diuretics, 525
- Loop Diuretics, 528
- Osmotic Diuretics and Carbonic Anhydrase Inhibitors, 532
- Potassium-Sparing Diuretics, 532

42 Antihypertensives, 536
- Hypertension, 536
- Pharmacologic Control of Hypertension, 537

43 Anticoagulants, Antiplatelets, and Thrombolytics, 551
- Pathophysiology, 551
- Anticoagulants, 551
- Antiplatelet Drugs, 556
- Thrombolytics, 559

44 Antihyperlipidemics and Drugs to Improve Peripheral Blood Flow, 563
- Lipoproteins, 563
- Antihyperlipidemics, 563
- Drugs to Improve Peripheral Blood Flow, 567

UNIT XIII Gastrointestinal Drugs

45 Gastrointestinal Tract Disorders, 573
- Overview of the Gastrointestinal System, 573
- Vomiting, 574
- Diarrhea, 580
- Constipation, 583

46 Antiulcer Drugs, 590
- Gastrointestinal Disorders and Nonpharmacologic Measures for Treatment, 590
- Antiulcer Drugs, 592

UNIT XIV Eye, Ear, and Skin Drugs

47 Eye and Ear Disorders, 603
- Overview of the Eye, 603
- Disorders of the Eye, 604
- Ophthalmic Drugs, 605
- Glaucoma and Ocular Hypertension Drugs, 610
- Overview and Disorders of the Ear, 614
- Drugs for the Ear, 615

48 Dermatologic Disorders, 620
- Anatomy and Physiology of the Skin, 620
- Acne Vulgaris, 621
- Psoriasis, 625
- Verruca Vulgaris and Drug-Induced Dermatitis, 628
- Contact Dermatitis, 628
- Impetigo, Rosacea, and Hair Loss, 628
- Burns and Burn Prevention, 629

UNIT XV Endocrine Drugs

49 Pituitary, Thyroid, Parathyroid, and Adrenal Disorders, 633
- Overview of the Pituitary Gland, 633
- Thyroid-Stimulating Hormone, 634
- Adrenocorticotropic Hormone, 634
- Prolactin, 634
- Pituitary Gland: Posterior Lobe, 636
- Drug Therapy for Anterior Pituitary Disorders: Growth Hormone Deficiency, 636
- Drug Therapy for Anterior Pituitary Disorders: Growth Hormone Excess, 636
- Other Drugs for Anterior Pituitary Disorders, 637
- Drug Therapy for Posterior Pituitary Disorders, 637
- Overview of the Thyroid Gland, 638
- Overview of the Parathyroid Glands, 642
- Overview of the Adrenal Glands, 644

50 Antidiabetics, 649
- Pathophysiology, 649
- Insulin, 650
- Oral Antidiabetic Drugs, 655
- Other Diabetic Drugs, 662

UNIT XVI Renal and Urologic Drugs

51 Urinary Disorders, 665
- Urinary Tract Disorders, 665
- Urinary Antiseptics/Antiinfectives and Antibiotics, 666
- Selective Urinary Agents, 670

UNIT XVII Reproductive and Gender-Related Drugs

52 Pregnancy and Preterm Labor, 673
Christina DiMaggio Boudreaux
- Physiology of Drug Use During Pregnancy, 673
- Therapeutic Drugs and Use of Herbs in Pregnancy, 674
- Drugs That Decrease Uterine Muscle Contractility, 681
- Corticosteroid Therapy in Preterm Labor, 683
- Drugs for Gestational Hypertension, 684

53 Labor, Delivery, and Postpartum, 689
Christina DiMaggio Boudreaux
- Drugs for Pain Control During Labor, 689
- Drugs That Enhance Uterine Muscle Contractility, 696
- Drugs Used During the Postpartum Period, 700
- Immunizations, 705

54 Neonatal and Newborn, 708
    Drugs Administered to Preterm Neonates, 708
    Drugs Administered to Full-Term, Healthy Neonates, 709

55 Female Reproductive Health, 713
Christina DiMaggio Boudreaux
    Drugs Used for Contraception, 713
    Drugs Used to Treat Disorders in Female Health, 722
    Drugs Used to Promote Fertility, 725
    Drugs Used in the Treatment of Menopause, 729
    Osteoporosis Disease, 732

56 Male Reproductive Health, 739
Jared Robertson
    Male Reproductive Processes, 739
    Disorders of the Male Reproductive System, 740
    Drugs Related to Male Reproductive Disorders, 741
    Other Male Reproductive Disorders, 746

57 Sexually Transmitted Infections, 751
    Sexually Transmitted Infections, 751
    Sexually Transmitted Pathogens, 752
    Prevention of Sexually Transmitted Infections, 756

UNIT XVIII Emergency Drugs

58 Adult and Pediatric Emergency Drugs, 761
Linda Laskowski-Jones
    Oxygen as an Emergency Drug, 762
    Emergency Drugs for Cardiac Disorders, 762
    For Intracranial Hypertension: Mannitol, 767
    Emergency Drugs for Drug Overdose, 767
    Emergency Drugs for Shock, 769
    Emergency Drugs for Hypertensive Crises, 772

Appendix A: Answers to Review Questions, 777
Bibliography, 778
Glossary, 781

UNIT I Introduction to Pharmacology

1

The Clinical Judgment Measurement Model and the Nursing Process

http://evolve.elsevier.com/McCuistion/pharmacology

OBJECTIVES

- Describe the role of clinical judgment in the nursing process.
- Summarize the six cognitive skills used in the Clinical Judgment Measurement Model.

OUTLINE

Clinical Judgment and the Nursing Process, 1
  Nursing Process, 1
  Components of the Nursing Process, 1
Clinical Judgment Measurement Model, 2
  Recognize Cues [Assessment], 2
  Analyze Cues [Analysis] and Prioritize Hypothesis [Analysis], 3
  Generate Solutions [Planning], 3

  Take Action [Nursing Implementation/Interventions], 4
  Important Nursing Considerations for Patient Education, 4
  Evaluate Outcomes [Evaluation], 6
  Comparison of the Nursing Process With the Clinical Judgment Measurement Model, 6
Clinical Judgment Case Study, 6
Review Questions, 6

In everyday practice, nurses have many important tasks, with drug administration at the top of their list. It is estimated that about 40% of the nurse's time is spent administering medication. Knowledge of medications is essential to patient safety. Nurses are often the first line of defense against drug errors in patient care. Federal, state, and local authorities issue regulations and guidelines for practice, and each state has a nurse practice act that defines the scope and function under which the nurse practices. Health care institutions also have policies that help nurses follow federal and state guidelines and regulations.

The National Council of State Boards of Nursing's (NCSBN) research has led to the development of the Next Generation NCLEX (NGN). The NGN is designed to measure new graduates' competence in clinical judgment. This chapter introduces the NCSBN's Clinical Judgment Measurement Model (CJMM) as it relates to the nursing process.

CLINICAL JUDGMENT AND THE NURSING PROCESS

Nursing Process

The NCSBN defines *clinical judgment* as the observed outcome of critical thinking and decision-making (NCSBN, 2022). This edition will offer students various case studies related to pharmacology that encourages the use of clinical judgment skills based on the NCSBN's CJMM (Fig. 1.1). The Unfolding Case Studies are somewhat complex and its encouraged students use clinical reasoning and clinical judgment skills to answer the questions.

The nursing process is used by nurses for the appropriate delivery of patient care. It is a systematic, rational method that addresses health needs and aids in developing a plan of care that includes drug administration. The nursing process supports the nurse in delivering prioritized patient care.

The NCSBN defines the nursing process as "a scientific, clinical reasoning approach to client care." Research by the NCSBN reveals that nurses use clinical judgment skills more than the nursing process. Good clinical judgment allows the nurse to recognize the patient's signs and symptoms and respond with knowledge and excellent judgment in addressing the patient's needs.

The steps in the nursing process include (1) assessment, (2) analysis, (3) planning, (4) implementation (intervention), and (5) evaluation (NCSBN, 2020). Analysis includes both defining and ranking the patient's problems according to priority.

Components of the Nursing Process

Patient Problems

Patient problems and needs are the basis for the patient plan of care. The problems presented in this chapter closely identify with the use of NANDA-1 language. However, nursing problems replace the use of nursing diagnoses. When using patient problem terminology, the language better defines nursing clinical practice. Patient problems

UNIT I Introduction to Pharmacology

Fig. 1.1 NCSBN Clinical Judgment Measurement Model.

BOX 1.1 Steps of the Clinical Judgment Measurement Model and the Nursing Process

Clinical Judgment Measurement Model	Nursing Process
Recognize Cues	Assessment
Analyze Cues	Analysis (Interpret problems)
Prioritize Hypothesis	Analysis (Rank problems)
Generate Solutions	Planning
Take Action	Implementation (Interventions)
Evaluate Outcomes	Evaluations

are in the Analyze Cues (interpret patient problems) and Prioritize Hypothesis (rank patient problems by priority) steps in the CJMM. In the nursing process, patient problems are in the Analysis phase (see Box 1.1).

Concept
The focus of *Concept* is on the patient-centered model of care instead of the disease-centered model of care. Concept influences the organization of patient information and the delivery of the patient's care using the nursing process according to the patient's problems. Nursing care plans use a nursing diagnosis to organize information according to the patient's medical diagnosis.

The Concept centers its focus on nursing care around the reason the care is being provided to the patient. It is a more holistic view of the patient rather than the disease model. The term *concept* includes health, illness, and health promotion of the patient. This involves preventive, primary, acute, and chronic health care for the ill patient.

Concepts are related to the patient's problems, the medications, or topics of care listed within the nursing process. A definition will immediately follow each concept (e.g., concept: safety—protecting the patient from possible injury by practicing safe medication administration).

By focusing on the concept, the nurse will provide patient education, restorative health needs, medication administration, and possibly emergency care. The nurse's attention is on promoting the patient's good health needs.

CLINICAL JUDGMENT MEASUREMENT MODEL

The student will use CJMM's six cognitive skills: (1) Recognize Cues, (2) Analyze Cues, (3) Prioritize Hypothesis, (4) Generate Solutions, (5) Take Action, and (6) Evaluate Outcomes (see Box 1.1, which compares the CJMM and the nursing process).

Recognize Cues [Assessment]
The nurse gathers cues (information) from the patient about their health and lifestyle practices. Cues are important facts about the patient that aid the nurse in making clinical care decisions. The nurse asks the patient direct questions about their illness. Data can be collected from many sources, including a systematic physical assessment of the patient's body systems and the medical record, which includes patient history, vital signs, and labs. With the patient's permission, information can be obtained from their family members. Also, other attending health care professionals can be consulted. The data collected

are both subjective and objective. Important cues are identified based on relevant (directly related) or irrelevant (unrelated) information concerning the patient's history, condition, and medical situation. The nurse must also review the patient's new drug orders and compare them to the drugs the patient has been taking at home. This is called "medication reconciliation". This step is important because it can help avoid drug errors such as omission, duplication, or interaction (see Chapter 9). It is vital to determine which data are most relevant to the patient's interventions and outcomes and which are of immediate concern for the delivery of priority care. The Recognize Cues [Assessment] phase is paramount because the nurse will use the information gathered to form the basis of the patient's plan of care, which includes drug administration.

Subjective Data

Subjective data include information provided verbally by the patient, family members, friends, or other sources. The patient must verbalize subjective data, which are imperceptible by the nurse's senses. Subjective data are based on what patients or family members communicate to the nurse. The nurse asks open-ended questions, allowing the patient to answer directly, such as, "Please tell me about your current medications." The nurse may help the patient explain or describe subjective data but must never speak for the patient. Subjective data comprise what the patient personally has to say about their medications, health problems, and lifestyle. Examples of pertinent information that the nurse can use to help solicit a response from the patient include the following:

- Inquire about the patient's current health history, including family history.
- Question whether or not the patient has problems swallowing (dysphagia).
- Have the patient verbalize signs and symptoms of their illness.
- Discuss the patient's current health concerns:
  - Knowledge of medications and side effects
  - Over-the-counter (OTC) remedies, nutritional supplements, herbal remedies, and contraceptives
  - Knowledge of side effects to report to the physician
  - Attitudes and beliefs about taking medications
  - Allergies
  - Financial barriers
  - Use of tobacco, alcohol, and caffeine
  - Cultural dietary barriers
  - The patient's home safety needs
  - Caregiver needs and support system

Enhancing the patient's medication adherence is an essential component of health teaching. The patient's attitudes and values about taking medication is an important consideration when determining readiness to learn. Attitudes and values should be considered when planning interventions to support the patient's decision to adopt healthy behaviors related to their medications. In addition, the patient's social support system should be emphasized. This special support system is unique to the individual and may be composed of persons who assist in preparing, organizing, and ordering medications. A support system can alert a patient to side effects, encourage actions that promote medication compliance, and notify the health care provider if a problem arises.

Objective Data

Objective data are what the nurse directly observes about the patient's health status. The process involves collecting the patient's health information by using personal senses: seeing, hearing, smelling, and touching. Objective data collection provides additional information about the patient's symptoms and also targets the organs most likely to be affected by drug therapy. For example, if a drug is nephrotoxic, the patient's creatinine clearance should be assessed.

The following are examples of objective data assessed by the nurse concerning medication administration:

- Physical health assessment
- Laboratory and diagnostic test results
- Data from the physician's notes (i.e., health history)
- Measurement of vital signs
- The patient's body language

Analyze Cues [Analysis] and Prioritize Hypothesis [Analysis]

Analyze Cues and Prioritize Hypothesis are part of the Analysis phase of the Nursing Process. This involves identifying, organizing, and prioritizing the patient's problems from the data collected. Analyze Cues (facts) interprets the patient's problem(s). Prioritize Hypothesis organizes and ranks the problem(s).

Analyze Cues [Analysis]

Consider the cues (facts) in the context of the patient's history and determine what kind of care the patient should receive. Ask yourself the following question, "How do these cues relate to the patient's condition or history?" Identify cues that support or contraindicate the problem or condition. Certain cues will be more concerning than others. This process will help identify potential complications as well as the patient's actual problems.

Prioritize Hypothesis [Analysis]

Once the cues (facts) are analyzed, the hypothesis (problem) is determined. The problems are organized, prioritized, and ranked according to acuity. There may be the need to collect additional patient assessment data.

When the cues show an abnormality, it serves as the defining characteristic of the patient's problem(s). Consider all possibilities about what is occurring in the patient's situation, including patient urgency and risk. Think about how the relevant cues relate to the patient's condition or history. Determine which cues are most likely serious and why. Rank the problems according to priority (urgency, likelihood, risk, difficulty, and time). More than one applicable patient problem may be generated.

Patient Problem(s)

Some common patient problems related to drug therapy include:
- Abdominal pain
- Confusion
- Decreased adherence
- Need for health teaching
- Cognitive decline
- Nonadherence

Use of the patient problem(s) is beneficial to the patient because its focus is on the individual patient's care as related to a problem derived from the patient's diagnostic illness. Its focus is patient centered and not disease oriented.

Generate Solutions [Planning]
Expected Outcomes

This phase identifies expected outcomes and uses the patient's problem(s) to define a set of interventions to achieve the most desirable outcomes. The interventions are specific, evidence-based actions related to the expected outcomes. Consider which actual or potential actions should be avoided or contraindicated, as certain actions may be harmful to the patient in some situations.

Outcomes are patient centered, describe a specific activity, and include a time frame for achievement and reevaluation. Generate Solutions [Planning] includes the development of nursing interventions that assist the patient in meeting medication outcomes. To develop patient-centered expected outcomes, collaboration with the patient and/or family is necessary.

Effective expected outcomes have the following qualities:
- The expected outcome is realistic, measurable, and includes reasonable deadlines.
- The expected outcome is acceptable to both the patient and nurse.
- The expected outcome is dependent on the patient's decision-making ability.
- The expected outcome is shared with the health care team.
- The expected outcome identifies components for evaluation.

Examples of well-written comprehensive expected outcomes include the following:
- The patient will independently administer the prescribed dose of 4 units of regular insulin by the end of the fourth session of instruction.
- The patient will prepare a 3-day medication recording sheet that correctly reflects the prescribed medication schedule by the end of the second session of instruction.

Take Action [Nursing Implementation/Interventions]

This phase provides nursing education, drug administration, patient care, and other interventions necessary to accomplish the expected outcomes. The nurse decides which actions will address the highest priority of care. Actions may include, but are not limited to, additional assessment, patient health teaching, documentation, requesting prescriptions from the provider, implementation of nursing skills, consultation with health care team members, and drug administration.

Patient Teaching

It is important for the nurse to keep in mind factors that help promote patient learning: the patient's *readiness* to learn and investment in their learning. If the patient buys into wanting to practice good health principles, learning can be successful. The nurse and patient together must become fully engaged in the learning process.

Timing is another important factor. What is the best time for the patient to learn? Is the patient a morning or night person? People seem to learn best if the time between the learning and implementation is short. The environment should be conducive to learning with a temperature that is comfortable and a setting that is quiet. It is important for the nurse to recognize that certain barriers to learning exist. Pain is an obstacle, and the patient's teaching should be postponed until pain is relieved. Be mindful of language barriers. If the patient does not speak the same language as the nurse, an interpreter may be needed.

Patient teaching is essential to the patient's recovery. It allows the patient to become informed about their health problems and to participate in creating interventions that can lead to good health outcomes. It is within the scope and practice of the nurse to embrace patient education and to use health-teaching strategies.

Nurses have a primary role in teaching both patients and families about drug administration. It is important that teachings are tailored to the patient's educational level and that the patient trusts the nurse for learning to begin. With the patient's consent, it is always important to include a family member or friend in the teaching to provide support to the patient with reminders and encouragement; they can also detect possible side effects that may occur in the patient.

The following are important principles to remember when teaching patients about their medications:
- Maintain the Health Insurance Portability and Accountability Act (HIPAA) when discussing the patient's medical records and personal health information with their family and friends.
- Prior to the teaching, assess the patient for health literacy skills such as the ability to read, write, listen, speak, communicate, and interact with others.
- Always allow the patient time to perform a repeat demonstration if they are taught a skill or allow a moment to teach back the information learned. This confirms learning has taken place.
- Instruct the patient to take the drug as prescribed. Consistency in adhering to the prescribed drug regimen is important.
- Provide simple written instructions with the doctor's and pharmacy's names and telephone numbers.
- Advise the patient to notify their health care provider if any of the following occur:
  - The dose, frequency, or time of the drug is adjusted.
  - A female patient becomes pregnant.
  - An OTC medication or supplement is added.

Side Effects

Give the patient instructions that will help minimize any side effects (e.g., avoid direct sunlight with drugs that can cause photosensitivity or sunburn). Advise patients of any expected changes in the color of urine or stool, and counsel the patient who has dizziness caused by orthostatic hypotension to rise slowly from a sitting to a standing position.

Self-Administration

Perform an ongoing health literacy assessment of the patient's motor skills and abilities. Remember that modifications may be necessary to the teaching plan based on the assessment.

Instruct the patient according to the prescribed route: eye or nose instillation, subcutaneous injection, suppository, oral/mucosal (e.g., swish-and-swallow suspensions), and inhaled via a metered-dose inhaler with or without a spacer. Include a return demonstration in the instructions when appropriate.

The use of drug cards is a helpful teaching tool (see Box 1.2). Drug cards can be obtained from the health care provider, pharmacy, or drug manufacturer, or simply designed by the patient or caregiver. They are helpful components for teaching. Drug cards may include the name of the drug, the reason for taking the drug, the drug dosage, times to take the drug, possible side effects, adverse effects, when to notify the care provider, and specific facts about what should or should not be done when taking the medication (e.g., take with food, do not crush tablets).

Diet

Advise the patient about foods to include in their diet and foods to avoid. Many foods interact with certain drugs. Depending on the nature of the interaction, certain foods have the ability to decrease drug absorption, increase the risk of drug toxicity, or create other problems that are important safety concerns.

Important Nursing Considerations for Patient Education

The nurse must keep in mind the patient's cultural needs to individualize the teaching plan. Begin by identifying their own cultural beliefs, practices, and values to keep them separate from those of the patient. If a language barrier exists, arrange for an interpreter who speaks the patient's language. Research shows that family members

BOX 1.2 Patient Teaching Card

Name of drug: Acetaminophen 325–650 mg
Reason for taking the drug: Minor aches, pains, and fever
Dosage: One or two tablets as needed every 4–6 hours; maximum dose is 3250 mg daily unless under health care provider supervision, then 4 g daily may be used.
Time to take the drug: 8:00 a.m./2:00 p.m./8:00 p.m.
Possible side effects: Nausea, upper stomach pain, itching, loss of appetite, dark urine, and jaundice
Possible adverse effects: Overdosage can affect the liver and cause hepatotoxicity.
Notify health care provider: If side effects occur
Health care provider's telephone #: _____
Warning:
Never take this medication with alcohol.
If pregnant or nursing, notify the health care provider before taking the medication.
Do not take this medication with other over-the-counter drugs or supplements without notifying the health care provider.

BOX 1.3 Important Points for Patients and Families to Remember

- Medications should be taken as prescribed by your health care provider. If problems arise with the dose or timing or if side effects occur, contact your medical provider.
- If drugs are placed in a drug box, keep the original labeled containers.
- Keep all drugs out of the reach of children.
- Before using any over-the-counter drugs, including vitamins and nutritional supplements, check with your health care provider. This includes the use of aspirin, ibuprofen, and laxatives. Consider consulting the pharmacist before buying or using a product.
- Bring all drugs with you when you visit the health care provider.
- Know the purpose of each medication and which side effect necessitates a call to the health care provider.
- Do not drink alcoholic beverages around the time you take your medications. Alcohol is absolutely contraindicated with certain medications, and it may alter the action and absorption of the medications.
- Be aware that smoking tobacco also can alter the absorption of some medications (e.g., theophylline-type drugs, antidepressants, pain medications). Consult your health care provider or pharmacist for specific information.
- Vaping (e-cigarettes) can damage a person's lungs and organs and cause breathing problems. Vaping is NOT safe and is habit forming.

are not recommended as an effective interpreter because they may hinder communication. Ask the patient if there is something special you should know concerning their cultural needs.
Additional suggestions include the following:

- Space instruction over several sessions, and be flexible in the timing of medication teaching as desired by the patient.
- Allow time for patients to respond to questions. Ask open-ended questions, and have patients demonstrate their understanding of treatments rather than verbalizing them.
- Review community resources related to the patient's plan of care including medications.
- Collaborate with the patient and family as well as other health care staff and agencies to meet the patient's health care needs.
- Identify patients at risk for noncompliance with their drug regimen. Alert the health care provider and pharmacist so they can develop a plan to minimize the number of drugs and the number of times drugs are administered.
- Evaluate the patient's understanding of the medication regimen on a regular basis.
- Empower the patient to take responsibility for their drug management. General points to remember and tips for successful patient education are presented in Box 1.3.

Many people take multiple drugs simultaneously several times each day, which presents a challenge to patients, their families, and nurses. This complex activity of taking several drugs can be segmented into several simple tasks that include the following:

- Drug boxes (Fig. 1.2) obtained from a local pharmacy may be used to prepare and organize medications. These boxes have labeled compartments for each day of the week and several rows of compartments for drugs taken multiple times a day. The boxes sort the drugs according to the time of day each pill is to be taken. They can simplify the task of taking medications. However, it is important to remember the pill boxes must be filled correctly. A trusted relative or friend can always assist the patient when filling the boxes.
- Multidose pill packets are available from many local pharmacies. The pharmacy will package the patient's prescription medications into easy-to-open packages. Many pharmacies can provide a 30-day supply of the patient's prescription medications, individually packaged and labeled according to dose, date, and time at no extra cost.

Fig. 1.2 Medication box and pill organizer. (Courtesy Apothecary Products, Inc., Burnsville, MN.)

BOX 1.4 Medication Recording Sheet

Medication	Dosage Daily	S	M	T	W	Th	F	S
Captopril	12.5 mg							
Digoxin	0.25 mg							
Furosemide	40 mg							

- A recording sheet may be helpful. When the drug is administered, the patient or family member marks the sheet. For example, the time can be noted by the patient after taking the medication, or it can be entered beforehand when the medication should be taken (Box 1.4).
- Alternatives to recording sheets are also available, and alarm reminder devices may be used.

> ### BOX 1.5 Checklist for Health Teaching in Drug Therapy
>
> - Assess the patient's health literacy skills to ensure that the patient has the capacity to obtain, process, and understand basic health information.
> - Reinforce the importance of drug adherence.
> - Always complete a health history and physical assessment on the patient.
> - Assess all of the drugs on the patient's profile for possible drug interactions.
> - Explain the reason the patient is taking the drug, the time it should be administered, and whether it should be taken with or without food.
> - Review the side effects and adverse reactions, and make sure the patient has the doctor's telephone number and knows when to notify the health care provider or pharmacist.
> - Distinguish whether the patient needs baseline or monthly laboratory work to monitor drug levels.
> - Keep in mind that patient validation of learning may include a return demonstration of psychomotor skills (insulin administration).
> - Show the patient how to record drug administration on a sheet of paper by indicating the day and time the drug is taken.
> - Discuss the patient's financial resources and, if needed, consult a social worker for resources.
> - Discuss the patient's support system such as family or friends as caregivers.
> - Provide the patient with a list of community resources.

Throughout the teaching plan, the nurse promotes patient independence (e.g., self-administering, safely storing, and ordering of the drug regimen). Always keep in mind patients' expected outcomes when teaching. Box 1.5 presents a checklist for health teaching in drug therapy.

Evaluate Outcomes [Evaluation]

The nurse evaluates whether the patient's interventions and outcomes have been met and compares the patient's response with the expected outcomes. What signs point to improvement, decline, or no change in the patient? Determine whether the nursing interventions were effective, ineffective, or made no difference. If the interventions and expected outcomes are unmet, the nurse will revise the interventions and expected outcomes to ensure success. If the interventions and expected outcomes are met, the nurse will document the successful attainment in the patient's plan of care.

Comparison of the Nursing Process With the Clinical Judgment Measurement Model

Compare each phase in the CJMM to the nursing process, as shown in Box 1.1, so you can understand how the two fit together.

CLINICAL JUDGMENT CASE STUDY

A 66-year-old man just arrived on the medical surgical unit after an emergency appendectomy. He is reporting incisional pain, nausea, and headache. His blood pressure is 150/80 mm Hg, his heart rate is 70 beats per minute, and his temperature is 100.8°F.

1. Identify the patient's highest priority assessment needs.
2. Formulate a nursing problem based on the patient's assessment data.
3. Name two nursing interventions that will achieve a positive outcome.
4. Evaluate the effectiveness of the interventions.
5. Have the expected outcomes been met?

REVIEW QUESTIONS

1. During a medication review session, a patient states, "I do not know why I am taking all of these pills." Based on this piece of subjective data, which problem will the nurse identify?
   a. Pain
   b. Knowledge
   c. Fatigue
   d. Anxiety

2. The nurse is developing a list of the patient's expected outcomes. Which is the best expected outcome for this patient?
   a. The patient will self-administer albuterol by taking a deep breath before inhaling.
   b. The patient will self-administer albuterol by the end of the second teaching session.
   c. The patient will independently self-administer the prescribed dose of albuterol by the end of the second teaching session.
   d. The patient will organize their medications according to the time each medication is due.

3. When developing an effective medication teaching plan, which component will the nurse identify as *most* essential?
   a. Written instructions
   b. The patient's readiness to learn
   c. Use of colorful charts
   d. A review of community resources

4. When developing an individualized medication teaching plan, which topics will the nurse include? Select all that apply.
   a. Adherence to the prescribed drug regimen
   b. Always using the prescribed drug route
   c. Knowing adverse side effects to report to the doctor
   d. Always doubling the next dose if the drug is missed
   e. Telling the doctor when taking over-the-counter (OTC) supplements

5. Which teaching strategy is most likely to succeed in health teaching with the patient and family?
   a. Know the reason why each drug was ordered.
   b. Have patients learn the generic name of each pill.
   c. A repeat demonstration should follow the nurse's teaching.
   d. Have the patient identify the number and color of the pills.

6. Prioritize the steps of the Clinical Judgment Measurement Model [Nursing Process]
   a. Generate Solutions [Planning]
   b. Analyze Cues [Analysis]
   c. Recognize Cues [Assessment]
   d. Prioritize Hypothesis [Analysis]
   e. Evaluate Outcomes [Evaluation]
   f. Take Action [Intervention]

Drug Development and Ethical Considerations

http://evolve.elsevier.com/McCuistion/pharmacology

OBJECTIVES

- Describe core ethical principles relevant to medical research using human subjects.
- Differentiate phases of pharmaceutical research using human subjects.
- Describe the American Nurses Association (ANA) Code of Ethics.
- Explain drug standards and legislation.
- Describe drug naming conventions and resources, including considerations for selecting brand name drugs versus generic drugs.

OUTLINE

Core Ethical Principles, 7
    Respect for Persons, 7
    Informed Consent, 8
    Beneficence, 10
    Justice, 10
Objectives and Phases of Pharmaceutical Research, 10
    Preclinical Trials, 10
    Human Clinical Experimentation, 10
    Clinical Research Study Design, 11
American Nurses Association Code of Ethics, 11
    The History of the American Nurses Association Code of Ethics, 11
    The Nurse's Role in Clinical Research, 11

Drug Standards and Legislation, 11
    Drug Standards, 11
    Federal Legislation, 12
    Nurse Practice Acts, 13
    Canadian Drug Regulation, 14
    Initiatives to Combat Drug Counterfeiting, 14
Drug Names and Resources, 14
    Over-the-Counter Drugs, 15
    Drug Resources, 16
Clinical Judgment Case Study, 17
Review Questions, 17

Approval of new drugs by the US Food and Drug Administration (FDA) has been steady since the early 2000s, with a peak of 59 new (novel) drugs approved in 2018; in 2022, 37 novel drugs were approved, and multiple drugs were approved for new indications and patient populations. To facilitate this increase, in 2004 the FDA established its Critical Path Initiative, a national strategy "to drive innovation in the scientific processes through which medical products are developed, evaluated, and manufactured" (FDA, 2018, Para 1). One focus of this initiative is on "improving the prevention, diagnosis, and treatment of rare and neglected disorders." In 2022, 54% of the novel drugs approved were for rare diseases, including generalized pustular psoriasis, obstructive hypertrophic cardiomyopathy, and hepatorenal syndrome.

The process of drug discovery and manufacturing takes 12 or more years, with costs ranging from $314 million to $2.8 billion for each drug. Ninety percent of clinical drugs fail to reach market, often due to lack of clinical efficacy and unmanageable toxicity. The steps of the process are shown in Fig. 2.1. Drug research and development is a complex process that is of particular interest and importance to professional nursing practice.

This chapter is devoted to a description of basic ethical principles that govern drug development and the nurse's role in this process.

CORE ETHICAL PRINCIPLES

Three core ethical principles are relevant to research involving human subjects: respect for persons, beneficence, and justice. Derived from the Belmont Report, the World Medical Association Declaration of Helsinki set out ethical principles for medical research that involves human subjects. These ethical principles are integral to the issues of informed consent and the risk-benefit ratio in such research.

Respect for Persons

Patients should be treated as independent people, who are capable of making decisions in their own best interests. Patients with diminished decision-making capacity are entitled to protection. When making health care decisions, patients should be made aware of alternatives available to them as well as the consequences that stem from those alternatives. The patient's choice should be honored whenever possible. It is imperative that nurses recognize when patients are not capable of making decisions in their own best interest and are therefore entitled to protection. The nurse can assist with the determination of decision-making capacity through frequent assessment of the patient's cognitive status.

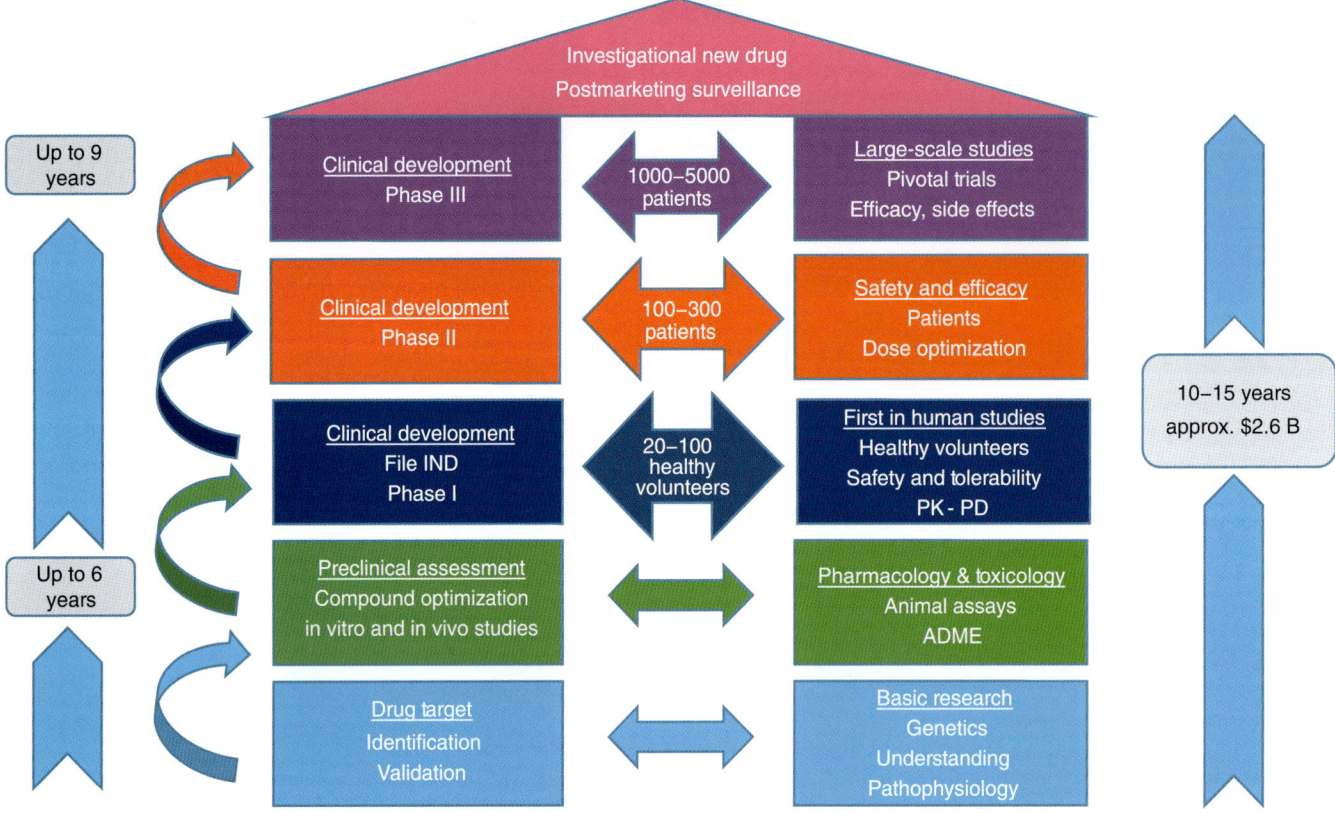

Fig. 2.1 The drug discovery and development process. *ADME*, Absorption, distribution, metabolism, and excretion; *FDA*, Food and Drug Administration; *IND*, investigational new drug; *PD*, pharmacodynamics; *PK*, pharmacokinetics. (From Wecker L, Taylor DA, Theobald RJ: *Brody's human pharmacology*, ed 6, 2019, Elsevier.)

Autonomy is an integral component of respect for persons. **Autonomy** is the right to self-determination. In health care settings, health care personnel must respect the patient's right to make decisions in their own best interest, even if the decision is not what the health care personnel want or think is best for the patient. Generally, patients can refuse all treatments (right of autonomy) except when the decision poses a threat to others—such as with tuberculosis, when taking medications is legally mandated. Autonomy is as relevant to the conduct of research as it is in health care decision-making; patients have the right to refuse to participate in a research study and may withdraw from studies at any time without penalty.

Informed Consent

Informed consent has its roots in the 1947 Nuremberg Code. The two most relevant aspects of the Code are the right to be informed and that participation is voluntary and without coercion. If coercion is suspected, the nurse is obligated to report this suspicion promptly. Informed consent has dimensions beyond the protection of the individual patient's choice:
- It is a mutual sharing of information, a process of communication.
- It expresses respect for the person.
- It gains the patient's active involvement in their care.
- It respects the patient's right to self-determination.

It is the role of the health care provider, *not* the nurse, to explain the study to the patient and what is expected of the patient and to respond to questions from the patient. When giving written consent, the patient must be alert and able to comprehend; consent forms should be written at or below the eighth-grade reading level, and words should be kept to fewer than three syllables.

BOX 2.1 Sample Inclusion and Exclusion Criteria

Inclusion
- Persons between the ages of 18 and 65
- Persons weighing between 50 and 100 kg
- Persons on a stable dose (i.e., no dose change in the previous 3 months) of cardiac medications (e.g., anticoagulants, angiotensin-converting enzyme inhibitors, angiotensin II receptor blockers, beta-blockers, and diuretics)
- Persons adhering to a no-added-salt diet

Exclusion
- Females who are pregnant or nursing
- Females of childbearing age who do not use oral contraceptives
- Persons with symptomatic cardiac disease, hepatic dysfunction, chronic kidney disease, neurologic disorders, or musculoskeletal disorders
- Persons with clinically significant abnormal laboratory values (chemistry and hematology)

Nurses are patient advocates. In collaboration with the health care provider and the pharmacist, the nurse must be knowledgeable about all aspects of a drug study—including all inclusion and exclusion criteria for participants (Box 2.1), study protocol, and study-related documentation—to promote participant safety and quality study results.

Fig. 2.2 shows a sample of an informed consent form for a clinical drug trial, and Box 2.2 shows an informed consent checklist.

Sample Informed Consent Form for Randomized Clinical Trial of a Drug

Title of study: Comparison of a new drug [A] with an existing drug [B} used in treatment of disease X

Principal investigator: Dr. ABC

Institute: Department of Pediatrics, Aga Khan University

Introduction:

I am Dr. [SAK] from Department of Pediatrics, the Aga Khan University and doing a research on treatment of disease [X, for example malaria]. There is a new drug [A] which is being recommended for its treatment. I want to see if the new drug [A] is as good as or better than the commonly used drug [B] for the treatment of disease [malaria]. Since you are a patient of (or suffering from) disease [malaria], I would like to invite you to join this research study.

Background information

Disease X (Malaria) is a common disease in Pakistan, Asia and Africa, caused by a germ (parasite) spread by mosquito. It causes high grade fever. Some patients may have complications and even die. The commonly used drugs are losing their effectiveness and germs are getting resistant to it. A new drug known as [A] is supposed to be effective in treatment of disease (malaria) but there is not enough evidence that it is as good as other drugs used for treatment of disease (malaria).

Purpose of this research study

The purpose of study is to find out if the new drug is as good as or better than other drugs used for treatment of malaria in our population and; also to see if germs are not resistant to it.

Procedures

In this study, all patients aged 15 to 50 years of age, presenting at the clinic with fever for less than one week duration and having no other diagnosis will be registered and screened for malaria. For diagnosis of disease (malaria), one ml of blood will be taken from the patients and checked for presence of germs (malarial parasite). Those patients having positive test for the disease (malaria), will be included in the study. They will be divided randomly in to two groups by a computer draw. One group will get the new drug (A) and the other group will get the commonly used drug (B). Neither the doctor nor the patient will know which drug he/she is getting for treatment of his/her disease. A record will be kept for the duration of fever and other symptoms including any other side effect. Other necessary treatment will also be provided if needed.

Possible risks or benefits

No significant side effects have been reported for this new drug (A). However, some patients may feel nausea or may have vomiting. Drawing of blood may cause some discomfort or blue discoloration at the site of bleeding. Lowering of white blood cells and platelet is a common feature of the disease.

There is no direct financial or other benefit for the participant of the study. However, all the investigations will be done free of cost to the patients and; the drugs (A) or (B) will be provided free. Treatment of any side effect will also be provided free of cost. Sponsor of the study will bear the cost of drugs, investigations and treatment of side effects related to the study drugs.

Right of refusal to participate and withdrawal

You are free to choose to participate in the study. You may refuse to participate without any loss of benefit which you are otherwise entitled to. You child will receive the same standard care and treatment which is considered best for him irrespective of your decision to participate in the study. You may also withdraw any time from the study without any adverse effect on management of your child or any loss of benefit which you are otherwise entitled to. You may also refuse to answer some or all the questions if you don't feel comfortable with those questions.

Confidentiality

The information provided by you will remain confidential. Nobody except principal investigator will have an access to it. Your name and identity will also not be disclosed at any time. However the data may be seen by Ethical review committee and may be published in journal and elsewhere without giving your name or disclosing your identity.

Available Sources of Information

If you have any further questions you may contact Principal Investigator (Dr. SAK), department of pediatrics at Aga Khan University on following phone number 486xxxx

Fig. 2.2 Sample informed consent for a clinical trial of a drug. (From Aga Khan University: *Sample informed consent for a randomized clinical trial of a drug,* n.d. http://www.aku.edu/research/urc/ethicalreviewcommittee/sampleconsentforms/Pages/sampleconsentforms.aspx.)

> **1. AUTHORIZATION**
>
> I have read and understand this consent form, and I volunteer to participate in this research study. I understand that I will receive a copy of this form. I voluntarily choose to participate, but I understand that my consent does not take away any legal rights in the case of negligence or other legal fault of anyone who is involved in this study. I further understand that nothing in this consent form is intended to replace any applicable Federal, state, or local laws.
>
> Participant's Name (Printed or Typed):
> Date:
>
> Participant's Signature or thumb impression:
> Date:
>
> Principal Investigator's Signature:
> Date:
>
> Signature of Person Obtaining Consent:
> Date:

Fig. 2.2, cont'd

Beneficence

Beneficence is the duty to protect research subjects from harm. It involves ensuring the risks and possible benefits from participating in a research study are clearly defined and ensuring the benefits are greater than the risk.

Risk-Benefit Ratio

The risk-benefit ratio is one of the most complex problems faced by the researcher. All possible consequences of a clinical study must be analyzed and balanced against the inherent risks and the anticipated benefits. Physical, psychological, and social risks must be identified and weighed against the benefits. A requirement of the Department of Health and Human Services is that institutional review boards (IRBs) determine that risks to subjects be reasonable in relation to the anticipated benefits, if any, for subjects. No matter how noble the intentions, the calculation of risks and benefits by the researcher cannot be totally accurate or comprehensive.

Justice

Justice requires that the selection of research subjects be fair. Research must be conducted so that the distribution of benefits and burdens is equitable (i.e., research subjects reflect all social classes and racial and ethnic groups).

OBJECTIVES AND PHASES OF PHARMACEUTICAL RESEARCH

The FDA requires clinical research to follow the Good Clinical Practice Consolidated Guideline, an international ethical and scientific quality standard for designing, conducting, monitoring, auditing, recording, analyzing, and reporting clinical research. It is the foundation of clinical trials that involve human subjects. Additional guidance and information sheets are available from the FDA on multiple topics related to clinical research.

Preclinical Trials

Before the implementation of clinical research, the FDA requires preclinical trials to determine a drug's toxic and pharmacologic effects through in vitro and in vivo animal testing in the laboratory. Through these trials, drug developers can determine genotoxicity, the ability of a compound to damage genetic information in a cell, in addition to drug absorption, distribution, metabolism, and excretion.

Human Clinical Experimentation

Historically, drug research was done only with White males, causing uncertainty as to the validity of research results for people of other ethnicities and for females and children. In 1993 Congress passed the National Institutes of Health Revitalization Act, which helped establish guidelines to include females and minorities in clinical research. In addition, the Best Pharmaceuticals for Children Act (BPCA) of 2002 and the Pediatric Research Equity Act of 2003 encourage pharmaceutical companies to study their drugs in children.

Clinical experimentation in drug research and development encompasses four phases, each with its own objectives (see Fig. 2.1). A multidisciplinary team approach that includes nurses, physicians, pharmacologists, statisticians, and research associates is required to ensure safety and quality in all phases of clinical research. A brief description of each phase follows.

Phase I: Researchers test a new drug or treatment in a small group of people for the first time to evaluate its safety, determine a safe dosage range, and identify side effects.

Phase II: The drug or treatment is given to a larger group of people to see whether it is effective and to further evaluate its safety.

Phase III: The drug or treatment is given to large groups of people to confirm its effectiveness, monitor side effects, compare it with commonly used treatments, and collect information that will allow the drug or treatment to be used safely.

Phase IV: Studies are done after the drug or treatment has been marketed to gather information on the drug's effects in various populations and to assess any side effects associated with long-term use.

Pharmaceutical companies are eager to bring new drugs to market. To reduce delays in the FDA approval process, in 1992 Congress passed the Prescription Drug User Fee Act, which provided the FDA with funds to expedite the review process. As a result, the average drug approval time has decreased from 30 months to 12 months.

Clinical Research Study Design

An appropriate experimental design is important to answer questions about drug safety and efficacy. Studies are designed to determine the effect of the independent variable (treatment, such as with a drug) on the dependent variable (outcome, such as clinical effect). Intervening (extraneous) variables are factors that may interfere with study results, and these may include age, sex, weight, disease state, diet, and the subject's social environment. It is important to control as many of the intervening variables as possible to increase study validity.

The *experimental group* in drug trials is the group that receives the drug being tested. The *control group* in drug trials may receive no drug; a different drug; a placebo (pharmacologically inert substance); or the same drug with a different dose, route, or frequency of administration.

AMERICAN NURSES ASSOCIATION CODE OF ETHICS

The History of the American Nurses Association Code of Ethics

The American Nurses Association (ANA) Code of Ethics "was developed as a guide for carrying out nursing responsibilities in a manner consistent with quality in nursing care and the ethical obligations of the profession." It was first adopted in 1950 and most recently was revised with interpretive statements in 2015. The ANA Code of Ethics is founded on the principles first identified by Florence Nightingale, who believed that a nurse's ethical duty was first and foremost to care for the patient. The 2015 update addresses advances in nursing leadership; social policy and global health; and the challenges nurses face related to social media, electronic health records, and the nurse's expanded role in clinical research.

The Nurse's Role in Clinical Research

Nurses are at the forefront of clinical research. Regardless of the setting (inpatient or outpatient), nurses are likely to encounter patients eligible to participate, considering participation, or actively participating in clinical research. As such, nurses are responsible for both the safety of the patient and the integrity of the research protocol.

DRUG STANDARDS AND LEGISLATION

Drug Standards

The set of drug standards used in the United States is the United States Pharmacopeia (USP). The *United States Pharmacopeia and the National Formulary* (USP-NF), the authoritative source for drug standards (dosage, forms, drug substances, excipients, biologics, compounded preparations, and dietary supplements), is published annually. Experts in nursing, pharmaceutics, pharmacology, chemistry, and microbiology all contribute. Drugs included in the USP-NF have met high standards for therapeutic use, patient safety, quality, purity, strength, packaging safety, and dosage form. Drugs that meet these standards have the initials "USP" following their official name, denoting global recognition of high quality.

CLINICAL JUDGMENT [NURSING PROCESS]
Clinical Research

Concept: Safety
- Protection of the patient from potential or actual harm; it is a basic human need.

Recognize Cues [Assessment]
- Identify patients who are eligible to participate in or who are participating in clinical research.
- Assess response to the study agent and identify adverse events (an unfavorable or unintended sign, symptom, or disease that was not present at the time of study enrollment and is associated with the treatment or procedure).

Analyze Cues and Prioritize Hypothesis [Patient Problems]
- Need for health teaching
- Potential for decreased adherence

Generate Solutions [Planning]
- Have a process in place to identify persons who are eligible to participate in clinical research or to identify participants actively participating in clinical research studies.
- Have a process in place to facilitate education and informed consent of eligible study participants.
- Plan educational programming for staff who provide direct care to study participants.
- Plan participant care to ensure integrity and compliance with study protocol.

Take Action [Nursing Interventions]
- Support the process of informed consent in a culturally competent manner.
  - Provide an interpreter when necessary.
  - Provide enough time for the person to read the consent and ask questions.
  - Serve as a witness to informed consent.
- After reviewing the study protocol, administer study agent(s).
- Accurately document all participant care, assessment findings, and study agent administration.
- Accurately and safely collect biospecimens.
- Act as advocate, educator, and collaborator in the research process.
  - Ensure safe care.
  - Ensure integrity of study data.
  - Communicate clearly.

Evaluate Outcomes [Evaluation]
- Determine whether the potential participant understands what it means to participate in the study by asking open-ended questions.
- Monitor response to the study agent or other interventions.
- Determine whether participants understand how to take their study agents, what to do if they miss a dose, how to store the study agent, and when to call their health care provider.

> **BOX 2.2 Informed Consent Checklist: Basic Elements**
>
> - A statement that the study involves research
> - An explanation of the purposes of the research
> - The expected duration of the subject's participation
> - A description of the procedures to be followed
> - Identification of any experimental procedures
> - A description of any reasonably foreseeable risks or discomforts to the subject
> - A description of any benefits to the subject or to others that may reasonably be expected from the research
> - A disclosure of appropriate alternative procedures or courses of treatment, if any, that might be advantageous to the subject
> - A statement describing the extent, if any, to which confidentiality of records identifying the subject will be maintained
> - For research that involves more than minimal risk, an explanation as to whether any compensation will be paid and whether any medical treatments are available if injury occurs, and if so, what the treatments consist of or where further information may be obtained
> - An explanation of whom to contact for answers to pertinent questions about the research and research subjects' rights and whom to contact in the event of a research-related injury to the subject
> - A statement that participation is voluntary, refusal to participate will involve no penalty or loss of benefits to which the subject is otherwise entitled, and the subject may discontinue participation at any time without penalty or loss of benefits to which the subject is otherwise entitled

From Office for Human Research Protections (OHRP): *Informed consent checklist (1998)*, 2014, U.S. Department of Health & Human Services. http://www.hhs.gov/ohrp/policy/consentckls.html.

The *International Pharmacopeia*, first published in 1951 by the World Health Organization (WHO), provides a basis for standards in strength and composition of drugs for use throughout the world. The book is published in English, Spanish, and French.

Federal Legislation

Federal legislation attempts to protect the public from drugs that are impure, toxic, ineffective, or not tested before public sale. The primary purpose of the legislation is to ensure safety. America's first law to regulate drugs was the Food and Drug Act of 1906, which prohibited the sale of misbranded and adulterated drugs but did not address drug effectiveness and safety.

1912: The Sherley Amendment

The Sherley Amendment prohibited labeling drugs with false therapeutic claims with the intent to defraud. However, the standard of intent was difficult to prove.

1914: The Harrison Narcotics Tax Act

The Harrison Narcotics Tax Act required prescriptions for drugs that exceeded set narcotic limits. It also mandated increased recordkeeping by physicians and pharmacists.

1938: The Federal Food, Drug, and Cosmetic Act

The Federal Food, Drug, and Cosmetic Act of 1938 empowered the FDA to ensure a drug was safe before marketing; it also required that drugs be labeled with accurate information and have detailed literature in the drug packaging that explained adverse effects. It eliminated the Sherley Amendment requirement to prove intent to defraud.

1941: Insulin Amendment

The Insulin Amendment required the FDA to test and certify the purity and potency of insulin.

1951: Durham-Humphrey Amendment

The Durham-Humphrey Amendment distinguished between drugs that could be sold with or without prescription by a licensed health care provider.

1962: Kefauver-Harris Amendment to the 1938 Act

The Kefauver-Harris Amendment resulted from the widely publicized thalidomide tragedy of the 1950s in which European patients who took the sedative-hypnotic thalidomide during the first trimester of pregnancy gave birth to infants with extreme limb deformities. The Kefauver-Harris amendment tightened controls on drug safety, especially experimental drugs, and required that adverse reactions and contraindications be labeled and included in the literature. The amendment also included provisions for the evaluation of testing methods used by manufacturers, the process for withdrawal of approved drugs when safety and effectiveness were in doubt, and the establishment of effectiveness of new drugs before marketing.

1965: Drug Abuse Control Amendments

Enacted in 1965, the Drug Abuse Control Amendments attempted to control the misuse of depressants, stimulants, and hallucinogens.

1970: The Comprehensive Drug Abuse Prevention and Control Act

In 1970 Congress passed the Comprehensive Drug Abuse Prevention and Control Act. This act, designed to remedy the escalating problem of substance use disorder, included several provisions: (1) promotion of drug education and research into the prevention and treatment of drug dependence; (2) strengthening of enforcement authority; (3) establishment of treatment and rehabilitation facilities; and (4) designation of schedules, or categories, for controlled substances according to misuse liability.

Based on their potential for misuse and acceptable medical use practices, **controlled substances** are categorized into five schedules, which are listed in Table 2.1. Schedule I drugs are not approved for medical use and have high potential for abuse; Schedule II through V drugs have acceptable medical use and decreasing potential for misuse leading to psychological and/or physiologic dependence.

Nurses are key to creating a culture of safety and accountability related to controlled substances. As such, nurses must:

- Verify orders before drug administration.
- Account for all controlled drugs.
- Maintain a controlled substance log that ensures all required information is documented accurately.
- Document all discarded or wasted medication; wastage must be witnessed by another nurse.
- Ensure timely documentation in the patient record after drug administration, including patient response to drug administration.
- Keep all controlled drugs in a locked storage area; keep narcotics under double lock. Be certain that only authorized persons have access to the keys, including keys for patient-controlled analgesia and epidural pumps. Medication may also be administered via an automated dispensing cabinet, with bioidentical identifiers used for access.
- The ANA recognizes the significant threat to patient safety and liability to health care organizations caused by nurse drug diversion and recommends that all states have a peer-to-peer assistance program for addicted nurses. Reporting is mandatory if suspected or known diversion occurs.

TABLE 2.1 Schedule Categories of Controlled Substances

Schedule	Examples	Description
I	Heroin, LSD, cannabis, peyote, methaqualone, and MDMA.	Substances in this schedule have no currently accepted medical use in the United States, a lack of accepted safety for use under medical supervision, and a high potential for abuse.
II	Combination products with less than 15 mg of hydrocodone per dosage unit, cocaine, methamphetamine, methadone, hydromorphone, meperidine, oxycodone, fentanyl, dextroamphetamine, dextroamphetamine/amphetamine, and methylphenidate.	Substances in this schedule have a high potential for misuse that may lead to severe psychological or physical dependence.
III	Products containing less than 90 mg of codeine per dosage unit (acetaminophen with codeine), ketamine, anabolic steroids, and testosterone.	Substances in this schedule have a lower potential for misuse than substances in Schedules I or II, and misuse may lead to moderate or low physical dependence or high psychological dependence.
IV	Alprazolam, carisoprodol, diazepam, lorazepam, zolpidem, and tramadol.	Substances in this schedule have a low potential for misuse relative to substances in Schedule III.
V	Cough preparations containing not more than 200 mg of codeine or per 100 mL (codeine/guaifenesin), diphenoxylate/atropine, difenoxin/atropine, and pregabalin.	Substances in this schedule have a low potential for misuse relative to substances listed in Schedule IV and consist primarily of preparations containing limited quantities of certain narcotics.

LSD, Lysergic acid diethylamide; *MDMA*, methylenedioxymethamphetamine.
From United States Drug Enforcement Administration: *Drug scheduling*, 2018. https://www.dea.gov/drug-scheduling.

1983: The Orphan Drug Act
The Orphan Drug Act was designed to promote the development and manufacture of drugs used in the treatment of rare diseases (orphan drugs).

1994: Dietary Supplement Health and Education Act
The Dietary Supplement Health and Education Act established labeling requirements for dietary supplements and authorized the FDA to promote safe manufacturing practices. It classified dietary supplements as food.

1996: Health Insurance Portability and Accountability Act
The Health Insurance Portability and Accountability Act (HIPAA) of 1996 protects health insurance coverage for workers who change or lose their jobs and sets the standard for the privacy of individually identifiable health information. The act provides patients with more control over their health information, including boundaries on the use and release of health records.

1997: The Food and Drug Administration Modernization Act
The five provisions in the Food and Drug Administration Modernization Act are (1) review and use of new drugs are accelerated, (2) drugs can be tested in children before marketing, (3) clinical trial data are necessary for experimental drug use for serious or life-threatening health conditions, (4) drug companies are required to give information on off-label (non–FDA approved) use of drugs and their costs, and (5) drug companies that plan to discontinue drugs must inform health professionals and patients at least 6 months before stopping drug production.

2002: Best Pharmaceuticals for Children Act
The BPCA gives manufacturers a 6-month extension of patents to evaluate drugs on the market for their safety and efficacy in children.

2003: Pediatric Research Equity Act
The Pediatric Research Equity Act authorizes the FDA to require that drug manufacturers test certain drugs and biologic products for their safety and effectiveness in children, noting that "children are not small adults." In addition, studies that involve children must be conducted with the same drug and in the same disease process as adults.

2007: Food and Drug Administration Amendments Act
The Food and Drug Administration Amendments Act allows the FDA to do more comprehensive reviews of potential new drugs, mandates postmarketing safety studies, and affects the distribution of drugs found to be not as safe as premarket studies indicated.

2010: Patient Protection and Affordable Care Act
The Patient Protection and Affordable Care Act was signed into law in 2010 and became effective January 1, 2014. Essential provisions of the reform include (1) quality, affordable health care for all Americans; (2) improved quality and efficiency of health care; (3) prevention of chronic disease and improved public health; (4) improved access to innovative medical therapies; and (5) community living services and supports.

2012: Food and Drug Administration Safety and Innovation Act
The Food and Drug Administration Safety and Innovation Act was signed into law on July 9, 2012. It strengthens the FDA's ability to safeguard and advance public health by:
- Collecting fees from industry to fund reviews of drugs with the "breakthrough therapy" designation, medical devices, generic drugs, and biosimilar biologic products
- Expediting development of innovative, safe, and effective products
- Increasing stakeholder engagement in FDA processes
- Enhancing the safety of the global drug supply chain

2020: Coronavirus Aid, Relief, and Economic Security Act
Enhanced the FDA's ability to identify, prevent, and mitigate possible drug shortages. Drug manufacturers must notify the FDA about permanent discontinuation of certain drugs and interruptions in manufacturing that can lead to supply disruption.

Nurse Practice Acts

All states and territories have rules and regulations in place to provide guidance and govern nursing practice, which includes drug

TABLE 2.2 Canadian Controlled Drugs and Substances Schedule

Schedule	Examples	Description
I	Codeine, hydrocodone, oxycodone, coca, cocaine, levomethorphan, ketamine, sufentanil, methamphetamine, amphetamine, GHB	Opium poppy, coca leaves, phenylpiperidines, phenazepines, amidones, methadols, phenalkoxams, thiambutenes, moramides, morphinans, benzazocines, ampromides, benzimidazoles, phencyclidine, fentanyls, tilidine, methamphetamine, amphetamine, flunitrazepam, and GHB and its derivatives, alkaloids, and salts
II	Nabilone	Synthetic cannabinoid receptor type 1 agonists
III	33 compounds including methylphenidate, LSD, psilocybin, and mescaline	
IV	26 parent compounds including chlorphentermine, butorphanol, nalbuphine, meprobamate, and zolpidem	Barbiturates, thiobarbiturates, benzodiazepines, and their salts and derivatives; anabolic steroids and their derivatives
V		Propylhexedrine and any of its salts
VI	Class A includes 23 compounds such as ephedrine, ergotamine, and pseudoephedrine. Class B includes six compounds such as acetone and sulfuric acid.	Part 1—Class A precursors Part 2—Class B precursors Part 3—Preparations and mixtures

GHB, Gamma hydroxybutyrate; *LSD*, lysergic acid diethylamide.
For more detailed information, see the Justice Laws Website at https://laws-lois.justice.gc.ca/eng/acts/c-38.8/page-14.html#h-95541.

administration by nurses. Generally, nurses cannot prescribe or administer drugs without a health care provider's order. Practicing nurses should be knowledgeable about the Nurse Practice Act in the state where they are licensed. (Information can be found through the National Council of State Boards of Nursing at www.ncsbn.org.) Nurses are responsible for knowing their state's law and administrative code. Nurses who administer a drug without a licensed health care provider's order are in violation of the Nurse Practice Act and can have their licenses revoked.

In a civil court, the nurse can be prosecuted for giving the wrong drug or dosage, omitting a drug dose, or giving the drug by the wrong route.

Canadian Drug Regulation

In Canada, before approval and becoming available to patients, drugs must be reviewed for safety, efficacy, and quality by the Health Products and Food Branch (HPFB) of Health Canada. Health Canada is a federal department tasked with the mission of improving the quality of life of all Canadians. (Further information can be found at www.hc-sc.gc.ca.)

In 1996 the Canadian government passed the Controlled Drugs and Substances Act. This act divided controlled drugs and substances into eight schedules and two classes of precursors (Table 2.2). In 2012 the Safe Streets and Communities Act was passed in Canada, which reclassified amphetamines—including methylenedioxyamphetamine (MDA) and methylenedioxymethamphetamine (MDMA)—and also flunitrazepam and gamma hydroxybutyrate (GHB) from Schedule III to Schedule I drugs. This change imposed stiffer penalties for dealers and those in possession of the drugs.

Initiatives to Combat Drug Counterfeiting

Distribution of counterfeit drugs is a worldwide problem; it is estimated that more than 10% of all drugs available are counterfeit. Counterfeit drugs may contain the incorrect ingredients, insufficient amounts of active ingredients, or no active ingredients. In addition, they may contain impurities and contaminants or may be distributed in fake packaging.

The most common drugs counterfeited are antibiotics, corticosteroids, drugs used to treat erectile dysfunction, cancer drugs, and antiretrovirals for HIV/AIDS. The high cost of drugs, combined with the need for prescription drugs to treat chronic diseases—as well as the desire by consumers to misuse drugs (e.g., steroid-containing drugs for bodybuilding)—generates a constant demand easily filled by criminals via rogue Internet drug sites. The FDA and consumer groups are working on strategies to combat this problem, including tougher oversight of distributors, a rapid alert system, and better-informed consumers.

The role of the nurse is critical in consumer education. The nurse must advise patients to report any differences in taste or appearance of a drug or in its packaging. Patients should be alert to slight variations in packaging or labeling (e.g., color, package seal), note any unexpected side effects, and buy drugs from reputable sources. Reputable online pharmacies carry the designation of Verified Internet Pharmacy Practice Site (VIPPS; a list of VIPPS-verified pharmacies can be found at https://nabp.pharmacy) and display an approval seal. If any suspicion of counterfeit arises, the patient, family, or nurse should contact the FDA at www.fda.gov/Safety/MedWatch/HowToReport.

DRUG NAMES AND RESOURCES

Drugs have several names. The **chemical name** describes the drug's chemical structure. The **generic name** is the official, *nonproprietary* name for the drug; this name is not owned by any drug company and is universally accepted. Nearly 80% of all prescription drugs in the United States are ordered by generic name. The **brand (trade) name**, also known as the *proprietary* name, is chosen by the drug company and is usually a registered trademark. Drug companies market a compound using its brand name. For example, Lunesta is the (proprietary) brand name of a drug whose generic name is eszopiclone.

Throughout this text, only generic names for each drug will be used because many brand names may exist for a single generic name—for example, the generic drug ibuprofen carries the brand names Advil, Medipren, Motrin, and Nuprin. Generic names are given in lowercase letters, whereas brand names always begin with a capital letter. An example of a generic and brand-name drug listing is *furosemide (Lasix)*.

Generic drugs must be approved by the FDA before they can be marketed. Generic drugs are tested by the FDA to ensure the safety, effectiveness, and strength of the generic drug are the same as the brand name. If the generic drug is found to be *bioequivalent* to the brand-name drug, the generic drug is considered *therapeutically equivalent* and is given an "A" rating. If there is less than a 20% variance in drug

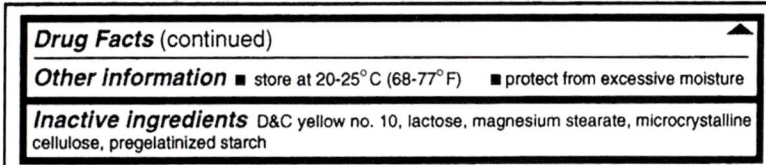

Fig. 2.3 Sample over-the-counter drug label. (From US Food and Drug Administration: *The over-the-counter medicine label: take a look*, 2017. https://www.fda.gov/drugs/resources-drugs/over-counter-medicine-label-take-look.)

absorption, distribution, metabolism, and excretion, a generic drug is considered *equivalent* to the brand-name drug. A list of FDA-approved drug products can be found at www.accessdata.fda.gov/scripts/cder/drugsatfda. The FDA also publishes a list of approved generic drugs that are bioequivalent to brand-name drugs.

Generic drugs have the same active ingredients as the brand-name product but are usually less expensive because manufacturers do not need to do extensive testing; these drugs were clinically tested for safety and efficacy by the pharmaceutical company that first formulated the drug. In addition, several pharmaceutical companies sell the same generic drugs, and market competition drives the prices lower. However, all drugs have varying inert fillers, binders, and excipients used to shape tablets and control how fast or slow the drug is released in the body, and these factors may result in variations in drug bioavailability.

Although the differences between the generic and brand name of the same product are usually not therapeutically significant, health care providers and patients must exercise care when choosing generic drugs because of possible variations in their action or in the patient's response to them. To maintain stable drug levels, patients should be cautioned *not* to change generic drug manufacturers; this is particularly true when patients are prescribed drugs with a narrow therapeutic index, such as blood thinners, thyroid drugs, and antiepileptics. Health care providers must note on prescriptions whether the pharmacist may substitute the generic drug when the brand name is prescribed. Nineteen states require pharmacists to substitute generic drugs when available; seven states and Washington, DC, require patient consent.

Over-the-Counter Drugs

Although all drugs carry risk, **over-the-counter (OTC)** drugs have been found to be safe and appropriate for use without the direct supervision of a health care provider. They are available for purchase without a prescription in many retail locations. Other OTC drugs (e.g., pseudoephedrine, emergency contraception) are available with some restrictions and must be kept behind the pharmacy counter; before dispensing, patient age and identification are verified, and education is provided.

More than $41 billion is spent annually on OTC drugs, which include vitamin supplements, cold remedies, analgesics, antacids, laxatives, antihistamines, sleep aids, nasal sprays, weight-control drugs, drugs for dermatitis and fungal infections, fluoride toothpaste, corn and callus removal products, and herbal products. Information related to OTC drugs available on the market can be found at http://www.drugs.com/otc.

In 2002 the FDA standardized OTC labeling to provide consumers with better information and to describe the benefits and risks associated with taking OTC drugs. It is an important nursing responsibility to ensure that patients can read and understand OTC labels. All OTC drugs must have labels that provide the following information in this specific order (Fig. 2.3):

- The product's active ingredients, including the amount in each dosage unit
- The purpose of the product
- The uses (indications) for the product
- Specific warnings, including when the product should not be used under any circumstances, substances or activities to avoid, side

> **BOX 2.3 Nursing Considerations Related to Over-the-Counter (OTC) Drugs**
>
> Nurses should advise patients of the following when they are considering taking OTC drugs:
> - Always read the instructions on the label.
> - Do not take OTC medicines in higher dosages or for a longer time than the label states.
> - If you do not get well, stop treating yourself and talk with a health care professional.
> - Side effects from OTCs are relatively uncommon, but it is your job to know what side effects might result from the medicines you are taking.
> - Because every person is different, your response to the medicine may be different from another person's response.
> - OTC medicines often interact with other medicines and with food or alcohol, or they might affect other health problems you may have.
> - If you do not understand the label, check with the pharmacist.
> - Do not take medicine if the package does not have a label on it.
> - Throw away medicines that have expired (are older than the date on the package).
> - Do not use medicine that belongs to a friend.
> - Buy products that treat only the symptoms you have.
> - If cost is an issue, generic OTC products may be cheaper than brand-name items.
> - Avoid buying these products online, outside of well-known Internet insurance company sites, because many OTC preparations sold through the Internet are counterfeit products. These may not be what you ordered and may be dangerous.
>
> Parents should know the following special information about using OTCs for children:
> - Parents should never guess the amount of medicine to give a child. Half an adult dose may be too much or not enough to be effective. This is very true of medicines such as acetaminophen (Tylenol) or ibuprofen (Advil), in which repeated overdoses may lead to poisoning of the child, liver destruction, or coma.
> - If the label says to take 2 teaspoons and the dosing cup is marked with ounces only, get another measuring device. Do not guess how much should be given.
> - Always follow the age limits listed. If the label says the product should not be given to a child younger than 2 years, do not give it.
> - Always use the child-resistant cap and relock the cap after use.
> - Throw away old, discolored, or expired medicine or medicine that has lost its label instructions.
> - Do not give medicine containing alcohol to children.

From Edmunds MW: *Introduction to clinical pharmacology*, ed 8, 2016, Mosby.

effects that could occur, and when it is appropriate to consult with a doctor or pharmacist
- Dosage instructions that include when, how, and how often to take the product
- The product's inactive ingredients and important information to help consumers avoid ingredients that may cause an allergic reaction

Nurses must be aware of OTC drugs and the implications of their use. OTC drugs provide both advantages and potential serious complications for the consumer. The nurse needs to emphasize that many of these drugs are potent and can cause moderate to severe side effects, especially when taken in combination with other drugs. In addition, many OTC drugs contain the same active ingredients, potentially leading to overdose. Self-diagnosis and self-prescribing OTC drugs may mask the seriousness of clinical conditions. See Box 2.3 for nursing considerations related to OTC drugs.

Many individuals routinely reach for aspirin, acetaminophen, and ibuprofen to relieve discomfort or pain without being aware of potential drug interactions and/or side effects. For example, ibuprofen is nephrotoxic and causes fluid retention. Daily use of ibuprofen may decrease the effectiveness of antihypertensive drugs. Ibuprofen carries a boxed warning for cardiovascular risk related to thrombotic events. Persons with aspirin allergy may also have a reaction to ibuprofen.

Acetaminophen has been associated with hepatotoxicity secondary to toxic metabolites, nephrotoxicity, and thrombocytopenia. Patients may also develop allergic reactions, including anaphylaxis, or potentially fatal skin reactions (Stevens-Johnson syndrome or toxic epidermal necrolysis) when taking acetaminophen. Because of the potential for harm caused with high doses or long-term use, since 2011 the FDA has limited the dose of acetaminophen to 325 mg when packaged in combination with other drugs.

Some OTC drugs, such as cough medicine, are a combination product of two to four drugs. It is conceivable that there could be a drug-drug interaction between a cough medicine and one of the drugs prescribed by the patient's health care provider.

Patients with asthma should be aware that aspirin can trigger an acute asthma episode. Patients may be allergic to aspirin, or aspirin may act as a deregulator of leukotrienes. Aspirin is also not recommended for children with viral infections such as influenza A and B, or varicella and gastroenteritis, due to its association with Reye syndrome, a rare condition affecting less than 0.1% of children who take aspirin.

Patients with kidney disease should avoid aspirin, acetaminophen, and ibuprofen as these drugs can further decrease kidney function, especially with long-term use. Patients taking moderate to high doses of aspirin, ibuprofen, or naproxen concurrently with an oral anticoagulant may be at increased risk for bleeding.

The previous examples are not all inclusive. Caution is advised before using any OTC preparation, including antacids, decongestants, and laxatives. Patients should check with their health care providers and read drug labels before taking OTC medications, so they are aware of possible contraindications and adverse reactions.

The acronym *SAFER* is a mnemonic for the instructions that the FDA recommends before taking any medicine: **s**peak up, **a**sk questions, **f**ind the facts, **e**valuate your choices, and **r**ead labels.

Drug Resources

Many drug references are available, including nursing texts that identify related nursing implications and areas for health teaching. Some recommended resources follow.

American Hospital Formulary Service (AHFS) Drug Information is published by the American Society of Health-System Pharmacists in Bethesda, Maryland. It provides accurate and complete drug information for both the health care provider and the consumer on nearly all prescription drugs marketed in the United States, for a fee. This text contains drugs listed according to therapeutic drug classification. The information given for each drug includes chemistry and stability, pharmacologic actions, pharmacokinetics, uses, cautions, contraindications, acute toxicity, drug interactions, dosage and administration, and preparations.

This reference is updated yearly with monthly supplements that provide information on new drugs such as dosage forms and strengths, uses, and cautions. The text is unbiased. Drug information from the AHFS is available online or in print format.

United States Pharmacopeia—Drug Information (USP-DI) is available in most hospitals and pharmacies either online or in print format. It provides drug information for the health care provider, including pharmacology, precautions to consider, side effects and adverse effects, patient consultation, general dosing information, and dosage forms. The USP-DI also contains patient information presented in a way that is easily understood. The topics include administration of drugs, drug effects, indications, adverse reactions, dosage guidelines, and what to do for missed doses.

The *Medical Letter* on drugs and therapeutics is a nonprofit publication for physicians, nurse practitioners, and other health professionals. Each biweekly issue provides reviews of new FDA-approved drugs and comparisons of drugs available for common diseases.

Prescriber's Letter is a newsletter published monthly by the Therapeutic Research Center in Stockton, California. It provides concise updates and advice concerning new FDA-approved drugs, various uses of older drugs, and FDA warnings.

MedlinePlus is a service of the US National Library of Medicine. Available at www.nlm.nih.gov/medlineplus/druginformation.html, it offers extensive information on prescribed drugs, as well as herbs and supplements, indexed by generic and brand names.

A good source for OTC drug information is *The Handbook of Nonprescription Drugs*, published by the American Pharmacists Association in Washington, DC. This resource is available online and in print format. The Internet can be another great resource, but only if credible websites are used.

CLINICAL JUDGMENT CASE STUDY

A patient is seen by their health care provider for chronic pain in the knees. They state the pain is a dull, constant ache in both knees that happens in the evenings after they've been working as a cashier all day.

1. What information is important for the nurse to gather about the patient's drugs?
2. The patient has taken ibuprofen for an extended time to control pain. What risk does this over-the-counter (OTC) drug pose?
3. What patient education should the nurse provide concerning OTC drugs?
4. The patient is advised by the health care provider to stop taking ibuprofen and begin taking acetaminophen. Before leaving the office, the patient asks the nurse how they will be able to remember the possible side effects of this drug. The nurse states they can read the label on the bottle. What is the standardized order of information on OTC drug labels?

REVIEW QUESTIONS

1. Which ethical principle related to clinical research is demonstrated by ensuring the patient's right to self-determination?
   a. Beneficence
   b. Respect for persons
   c. Justice
   d. Informed consent
2. The research nurse is meeting with a patient and determines the patient meets inclusion criteria for clinical research. The patient agrees to participate in the clinical trial. The nurse advises the patient that which member of the health care team has the responsibility to explain the study and respond to questions?
   a. Registered nurse
   b. Pharmacist
   c. Research associate
   d. Health care provider
3. Which percent of potential drugs is approved by the US Food and Drug Administration?
   a. 5%
   b. 10%
   c. 15%
   d. 20%
4. The nurse is interviewing a patient in a Phase I clinical trial. Which statement indicates the patient understands this trial phase?
   a. I am doing this to be sure this drug is safe.
   b. I am doing this to be sure this drug is effective.
   c. I hope this drug is better than the current treatment.
   d. I can be part of demonstrating a cure.
5. Good Clinical Practice is a reference for standards for clinical trials in which area? **Select all that apply.**
   a. Design
   b. Monitoring and auditing
   c. Analyses
   d. Reporting
   e. Outcomes evaluation
6. The nurse researcher reviews the proposed informed consent form for a future clinical trial. The nurse expects to find which information in the consent? **Select all that apply.**
   a. Description of benefits and risks
   b. Identification of related drugs, treatments, and techniques
   c. Description of outcomes
   d. Statement of compensation for participants
   e. Description of serious risks
7. Which ethical principle describes the risks and benefits related to clinical research?
   a. Respect for persons
   b. Justice
   c. Beneficence
   d. Informed consent
8. According to US standards, the highest potential for misuse of drugs with accepted medical uses is found in drugs included in which schedule?
   a. II
   b. III
   c. IV
   d. V
9. The nurse is reviewing the drug approval process in the United States and learns that the Food and Drug Administration Modernization Act of 1997 contains which provision? **Select all that apply.**
   a. Review of new drugs is accelerated.
   b. Drug companies must provide information on off-label use of drugs.
   c. Privacy of individually identifiable health information must be protected.
   d. Drug companies must offer advanced notice of plans to discontinue drugs.
   e. Drug labels must describe side effects and adverse effects.

10. Which factor alerts the individual that a drug is counterfeit or adulterated? **Select all that apply.**
    a. Variations in packaging
    b. Unexpected side effects
    c. Different taste
    d. Different chemical components
    e. Different odor
11. The nurse knows the importance of administering the right medication to the patient and that drugs have many names. It is therefore most important that drugs be ordered by which name?
    a. Generic
    b. Brand
    c. Trade
    d. Chemical
12. Which provision from the Controlled Substances Act of 1970 was designed to remedy drug misuse?
    a. Establishment of treatment and rehabilitation facilities
    b. Tightened controls on experimental drugs
    c. Required clinical trial data on drugs
    d. Required drug companies to give information on off-label use of drugs

Pharmacokinetics and Pharmacodynamics

http://evolve.elsevier.com/McCuistion/pharmacology

OBJECTIVES

- Describe key components of pharmacokinetics.
- Discuss pharmacodynamic principles influencing drug efficacy and safety.
- Discuss drug interactions in relationship to pharmacokinetic and pharmacodynamic processes.

OUTLINE

Pharmacokinetics, 19
  Drug Absorption, 19
  Drug Distribution, 21
  Drug Metabolism, 22
  Drug Excretion, 23
Pharmacodynamics, 23
  Dose-Response Relationship, 23
  Onset, Peak, and Duration of Action, 23
  Therapeutic Drug Monitoring, 24
  Receptor Theory, 24
  Agonists, Partial Agonists, and Antagonists, 25
  Nonspecific and Nonselective Drug Effects, 25
  Mechanisms of Drug Action, 26
  Side Effects, Adverse Drug Reactions, and Drug Toxicity, 26
  Drug Response Types, 26
Drug Interactions, 26
  Pharmacokinetic Interactions, 26
  Pharmacodynamic Interactions, 28
  Drug Interactions With Nutrients, Testing, and Light, 28
Clinical Judgment Case Study, 30
Review Questions, 30

Once a drug is administered, it goes through two phases, the pharmacokinetic phase and the pharmacodynamic phase. The *pharmacokinetic phase*, or what the body does to the drug, describes the movement of the drug through the body. It is composed of four processes: (1) absorption, (2) distribution, (3) metabolism (biotransformation), and (4) excretion (elimination). The *pharmacodynamic phase*, or what the drug does to the body, involves receptor binding, post-receptor effects, and chemical reactions. A biologic or physiologic response results from the pharmacodynamic phase.

PHARMACOKINETICS

Pharmacokinetics is the process of drug movement throughout the body necessary to achieve drug action. The four processes are (1) absorption, (2) distribution, (3) metabolism (or biotransformation), and (4) excretion (or elimination).

Drug Absorption

Drug absorption is the movement of the drug into the bloodstream after administration. Over 80% of drugs are taken by mouth (enteral). Dissolution is a process in which solid drug forms, like a tablet or capsule, disintegrate into small particles by combining with a liquid to form a solution absorbed by the gastrointestinal (GI) tract and bloodstream. Unlike drugs taken by mouth, eyedrops, eardrops, nasal sprays, respiratory inhalants, transdermal drugs, sublingual drugs, and parenteral drugs do not pass through the GI tract.

Tablets are not 100% drug. Fillers and inert substances—such as simple syrup, vegetable gums, aromatic powder, honey, and various elixirs—called *excipients* are used in drug preparation to allow the drug to take on a particular size and shape and to enhance drug dissolution. Some excipients, such as the ions potassium (K^+) in penicillin potassium and sodium (Na^+) in penicillin sodium, increase the absorbability of the drug. Penicillin is poorly absorbed by the GI tract because of gastric acid. However, by adding potassium or sodium salts, penicillin can be absorbed.

Disintegration is the breakdown of an oral drug into smaller particles. The rate of dissolution is the time it takes the drug to disintegrate and dissolve to become available for the body to absorb it. Drugs in liquid form are more rapidly available for GI absorption than are solids. Generally, drugs are both disintegrated and absorbed faster in acidic fluids with a pH of 1 or 2 rather than in alkaline fluids (those with a pH greater than 7). Both the very young and older adults have less gastric acidity; therefore drug absorption is generally slower for those drugs absorbed primarily in the stomach.

Enteric-coated (EC) drugs resist disintegration in the gastric acid of the stomach, so disintegration does not occur until the drug reaches the alkaline environment of the small intestine. EC tablets can remain in the stomach for a long time; therefore, their effect may be delayed in onset. EC tablets or capsules and sustained-release (beaded) capsules should not be crushed because crushing alters the place and time of absorption of the drug. Food in the GI tract may interfere with the dissolution of certain drugs. Some drugs irritate the gastric mucosa, so

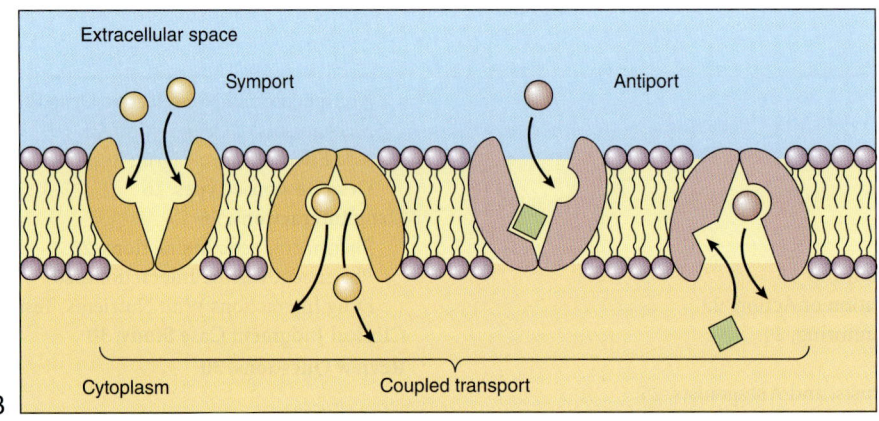

Fig. 3.1 (A) Passive and (B) active transport. (From Gartner LP. *Textbook of Histology*. 4th ed. Elsevier; 2017.)

fluids or food may be necessary to dilute the drug concentration and provide protection.

Most oral drugs enter the bloodstream after absorption across the mucosal lining of the small intestine. The epithelial lining of the small intestine is covered with villi, fingerlike protrusions that increase the surface area available for absorption. Absorption is reduced if the villi are decreased in number because of disease, drug effect, or the removal of some or all of the small intestine.

Absorption across the mucosal lining of the small intestine occurs through passive transport, active transport, or pinocytosis. **Passive transport** occurs through two processes, diffusion and facilitated diffusion. In **diffusion**, drugs move across the cell membrane from an area of higher concentration to one of lower concentration. **Facilitated diffusion** relies on a carrier protein to move the drug from an area of higher concentration to an area of lower concentration. Passive transport does not require energy to move drugs across the membrane. **Active transport** requires a carrier, such as an enzyme or protein, to move the drug against a concentration gradient. Energy is required for active absorption (Fig. 3.1). **Pinocytosis** is a process by which cells carry a drug across their membranes by engulfing the drug particles in a vesicle.

The mucous membrane that lines the GI tract is composed of lipids (fat) and protein such that lipid-soluble drugs can pass rapidly through the mucous membrane. Water-soluble drugs need a carrier, either an enzyme or a protein, to pass through the mucous membrane. Large particles can pass through the mucous membrane if they are nonionized (have no positive or negative charge). Drugs that are lipid soluble and nonionized are absorbed faster than water-soluble and ionized drugs.

Blood flow, pain, stress, hunger, fasting, food, and pH affect drug absorption. Poor circulation to the stomach because of shock, vasoconstrictor drugs, or disease hampers absorption. Pain, stress, and foods that are solid, hot, or high in fat can slow gastric emptying time, so drugs remain in the stomach longer. Exercise can decrease gastric blood flow by shunting blood flow to peripheral muscles, thereby decreasing blood circulation to the GI tract.

Drugs given intramuscularly are absorbed faster in muscles that have increased blood flow (e.g., deltoid) than in those that do not (e.g., gluteus maximus). Subcutaneous tissue has decreased blood flow compared with muscle, so absorption is slower when drugs are given subcutaneously. However, drugs that are given subcutaneously have a more rapid and predictable rate of absorption than those given by mouth.

Drugs given rectally are absorbed slower than drugs administered by the oral route. Absorption is slower because the surface area in the rectum is smaller than the stomach, and it has no villi. In addition, the composition of the suppository base (e.g., fatty bases or water-soluble bases) affects drug absorption.

After absorption of oral drugs from the GI tract, they pass from the intestinal lumen to the liver via the portal vein. In the liver, some drugs are metabolized to an inactive form and are excreted, thus reducing the amount of active drug available to exert a pharmacologic effect. This is referred to as the **first-pass effect** or **first-pass metabolism** (Fig. 3.2). Most oral drugs are affected to some degree by first-pass metabolism.

CHAPTER 3 Pharmacokinetics and Pharmacodynamics

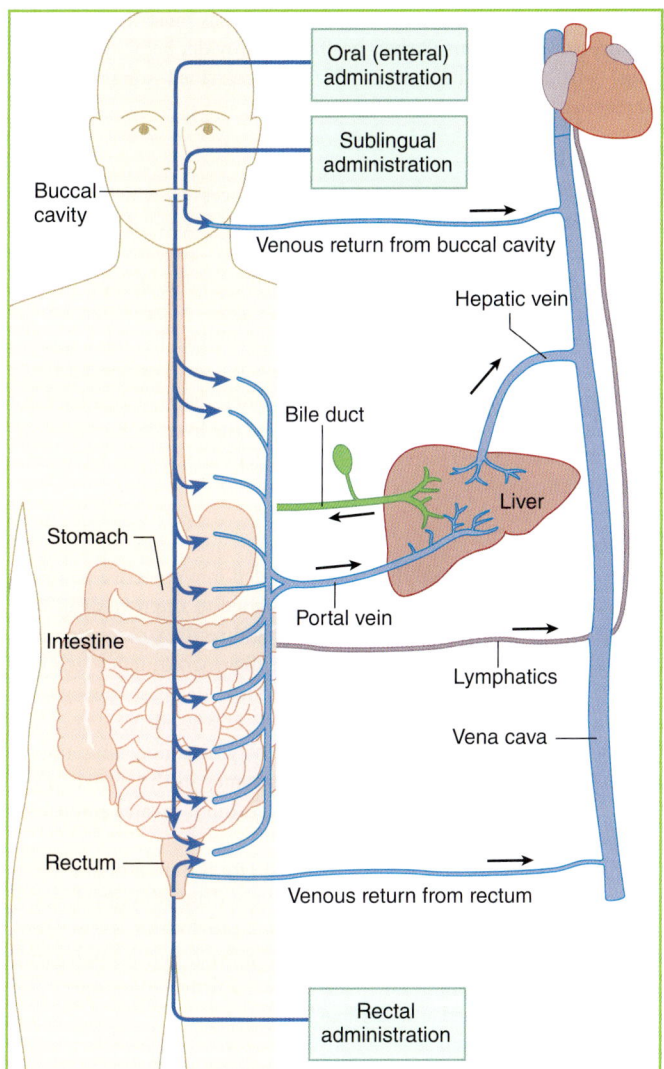

Fig. 3.2 First-pass metabolism. (From Kester M. *Elsevier's Integrated Review Pharmacology*. 2nd ed. Elsevier; 2012.)

Fig. 3.3 Protein binding. (A) Binding of drugs to albumin is reversible, (B) Protein bound drugs stay within the vasculature. *P*, Protein. (From Lilley LL, Rainform Collins S, Snyder JS. *Pharmacology and the Nursing Process*. 8th ed. Elsevier; 2016.)

Lidocaine and some nitroglycerines, for example, are not given orally because they have extensive first-pass metabolism and most of the drug is inactivated. Drugs that are delivered by other routes (intravenous [IV], intramuscular [IM], subcutaneous [SQ], nasal, sublingual, buccal) do not enter the portal circulation and are not subjected to first-pass metabolism.

Bioavailability refers to the percentage of administered drugs available for activity. For orally administered drugs, bioavailability is affected by absorption and first-pass metabolism. The bioavailability of oral drugs is always less than 100% and varies based on the rate of first-pass metabolism (i.e., the bioavailability of rosuvastatin is 20%, whereas the bioavailability of digoxin ranges from 75% to 95%). The bioavailability of IV drugs is 100%.

Factors that alter bioavailability include the (1) drug form, such as tablet, capsule, sustained-release beads, liquid, transdermal patch, suppository, or inhalation; (2) route of administration (e.g., enteral, topical, or parenteral); (3) gastric mucosa and motility; (4) administration with food and other drugs; and (5) changes in liver metabolism caused by liver dysfunction or inadequate hepatic blood flow. A decrease in liver function or a decrease in hepatic blood flow can increase the bioavailability of a drug, but only if the drug is metabolized by the liver. Less drug is destroyed by hepatic metabolism in the presence of a liver disorder.

Drug Distribution

Distribution is the movement of the drug from the circulation to body tissues. Drug distribution is influenced by vascular permeability and permeability of cell membranes, regional blood flow and pH, cardiac output, tissue perfusion, the ability of the drug to bind tissue and plasma proteins (Fig. 3.3), and the drug's lipid solubility. Drugs are easily distributed in highly perfused organs such as the liver, heart, and kidney. Tissues with decreased perfusion, such as muscle, fat, and peripheral organs, result in decreased drug distribution.

Protein Binding

As drugs are distributed in the plasma, many bind with plasma proteins (albumin, lipoproteins, and alpha-1-acid-glycoprotein [AGP]). Acidic drugs, such as aspirin and methotrexate, and neutral drugs, such as nortriptyline, bind with albumin or lipoproteins; however, basic drugs (morphine, amantadine) bind to AGP. Drugs that are more than 90% bound to protein are known as *highly protein-bound drugs* (e.g., diazepam, warfarin, glipizide, ibuprofen, and phenytoin); drugs that are less than 10% bound to protein are *weakly protein-bound drugs* (e.g., gentamicin, metformin, metoprolol, and lisinopril). The portion of the drug bound to protein is inactive because it is not available to interact with tissue receptors and therefore is unable to exert a pharmacologic effect. The portion that remains unbound is free, active drug. **Free drugs** can exit blood vessels and reach their site of action, causing a pharmacologic response.

When two highly protein-bound drugs are administered together, they compete for protein-binding sites, leading to an increase in free drug being released into the circulation. For example, if warfarin (99% protein bound) and furosemide (95% protein bound) were administered together, warfarin—the more highly bound drug—could displace furosemide from its binding site. In this situation, it is possible for drug accumulation to occur and for toxicity to result. Another factor that may alter protein binding is low plasma protein levels, which

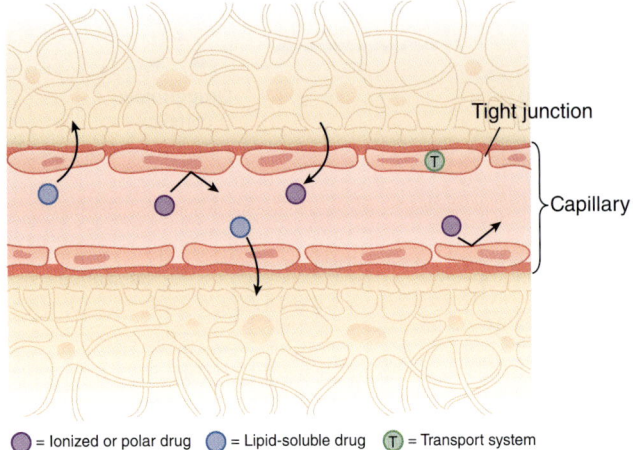

Fig. 3.4 Drug movement across the blood-brain barrier.

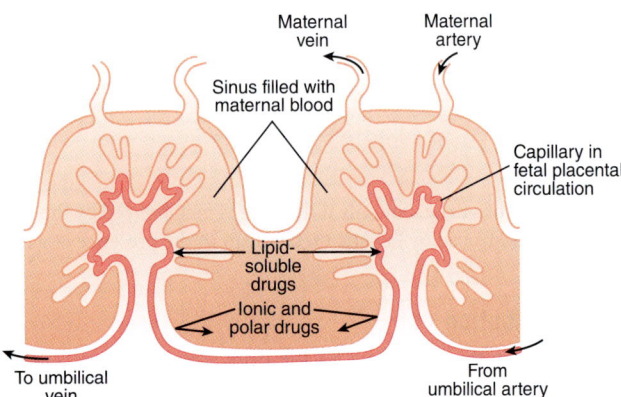

Fig. 3.5 Drug crossing the placenta.

potentially decrease the number of available binding sites and can lead to an increase in the amount of free drug available, resulting in drug accumulation and toxicity. Patients with liver or kidney disease and those who are malnourished may have significantly lower serum albumin levels. In addition, older adults are more likely to have hypoalbuminemia, particularly if they have multiple chronic illnesses. With these factors in mind, it is important for nurses to understand the concept of protein binding and check their patients' protein and albumin levels when administering drugs.

Blood vessels in the brain have a special endothelial lining where the cells are pressed tightly together (*tight junctions*); this lining is referred to as the blood-brain barrier (BBB). The BBB protects the brain from foreign substances, which includes about 98% of the drugs on the market. Some drugs that are highly lipid soluble and of low molecular weight (e.g., benzodiazepines) can cross the BBB through diffusion, and others cross via transport proteins. Water-soluble drugs (e.g., atenolol and penicillin) and drugs that are not bound to transport proteins (free drugs) are not able to cross the BBB, which makes it difficult for these drugs to reach the brain (Fig. 3.4).

During pregnancy, drugs can cross the placenta much as they do across other membranes, and this affects both the fetus and the mother (Fig. 3.5). Drugs taken during the first trimester can lead to spontaneous abortion. During the second trimester, drugs can lead to spontaneous abortion, teratogenesis, or other subtler defects. During the third trimester, drugs may alter fetal growth and development. The risk-benefit ratio should be considered before any drugs are given during pregnancy. During breast-feeding, drugs can pass into breast milk, which can affect the nursing infant. Nurses must teach females who breast-feed to consult their health care provider before taking any drug—whether over the counter (OTC) or prescribed—or any herb or supplement.

Drug Metabolism

Metabolism, or biotransformation, is the process by which the body chemically changes drugs into a form that can be excreted. The liver is the primary site of metabolism. Liver enzymes—collectively referred to as the *cytochrome P450 system*, or the *P450 system*, of drug-metabolizing enzymes—convert drugs to metabolites. A large percentage of drugs are lipid soluble; thus the liver metabolizes the lipid-soluble drug substance to a water-soluble substance for renal excretion. Liver diseases such as cirrhosis and hepatitis alter drug metabolism by inhibiting the drug-metabolizing enzymes in the liver. When the drug metabolism rate is decreased, excess drug accumulation can occur and can lead to toxicity.

Prodrugs

A prodrug is a compound that is metabolized into an active pharmacologic substance. Prodrugs are often designed to improve drug bioavailability; instead of administering a drug directly, a corresponding prodrug might be used instead to improve pharmacokinetics (absorption, distribution, metabolism, or excretion), decrease toxicity, or target a specific site of action. An example of a prodrug is codeine. Codeine itself has very little intrinsic activity at endogenous opioid receptors. However, drug-metabolizing enzymes in the liver convert codeine into morphine. Morphine, in turn, exhibits greater affinity for opioid receptors.

The drug half-life ($t½$) is the time it takes for the amount of drug in the body to be reduced by half. The amount of drug administered, the amount of drug remaining in the body from previous doses, metabolism, and elimination affect the half-life of a drug. For example, with liver or kidney dysfunction, the half-life of the drug is prolonged, and less drug is metabolized and eliminated.

A drug goes through several half-lives before complete elimination occurs, and drug half-life is used to determine the dosing interval. This is best understood with an example: ibuprofen has a half-life of about 2 hours. If a person takes 200 mg, in 2 hours, 50% of the drug will be gone, leaving 100 mg. Two hours later, another 50% of the drug will be gone, this time leaving 50 mg; in another 2 hours, 50% more will be gone, so only 25 mg will remain. This process continues such that 10 hours after 200 mg of ibuprofen has been taken, if no additional doses are administered, 6.25 mg of the drug remains.

Half-lives	% of Drug Eliminated From Body
1	50
2	75
3	87.5
4	93.75
5	96.875
6	98.474
7	99.25

From Medscape. *Space Out Drug Discontinuations prior to "Drug Holiday."* 2000. https://www.medscape.com/viewarticle/413306.

By knowing the half-life, the time it takes for a drug to reach a steady state (plateau drug level) can be determined. A steady state occurs when the amount of drug being administered is the same as the amount of drug being eliminated; a steady state of drug concentration is necessary to achieve optimal therapeutic benefit. This takes about four half-lives, if the size of all doses is the same. For example, digoxin—which has a half-life of 36 hours with normal renal function—takes approximately 6 days to reach a steady-state concentration.

Loading Dose

However, in the case of drugs with long half-lives, it may not be acceptable to wait for a steady state to be achieved. Take, for example, the case of a person with seizures receiving phenytoin. The half-life of phenytoin is approximately 22 hours; if all doses of the drug were the same, a steady state would not be achieved for about 3½ days. By giving a large initial dose, known as a **loading dose**, that is significantly higher than maintenance dosing, therapeutic effects can be obtained while a steady state is reached. It bears repeating that the loading dose is larger than the dose needed to maintain the drug at a steady state; it would produce toxic side effects if given in repeated doses. After the loading dose, maintenance dosing is begun; this is the dose needed to maintain drug concentration at a steady state when given repeatedly at a consistent dose and constant dosing interval.

Drug Excretion

The main route of drug **excretion**, elimination of drugs from the body, is through the kidneys. Drugs are also excreted through bile, the lungs, saliva, sweat, and breast milk. The kidneys filter free drugs (in healthy kidneys, drugs bound to protein are not filtered), water-soluble drugs, and drugs that are unchanged. The lungs eliminate volatile drug substances, and products metabolize to carbon dioxide (CO_2) and water (H_2O).

The urine pH influences drug excretion. Normal urine pH varies from 4.6 to 8.0. Acidic urine promotes the elimination of weak–base drugs, and alkaline urine promotes the elimination of weak-acid drugs. Salicylic acid (aspirin), a weak acid, is excreted rapidly in alkaline urine. Treatment of salicylate toxicity includes IV administration of sodium bicarbonate to increase urine pH to 8.0 or higher (alkaline); maintaining alkaline urine promotes the excretion of salicylate at 18 times the normal rate.

Prerenal, intrarenal, and postrenal conditions affect drug excretion. Prerenal conditions, such as dehydration or hemorrhage, reduce blood flow to the kidney and result in decreased glomerular filtration. Intrarenal conditions, such as glomerulonephritis and chronic kidney disease, affect glomerular filtration and tubular secretion and reabsorption. Postrenal conditions that obstruct urine flow—such as prostatic hypertrophy, stones, and neurogenic bladder—adversely affect glomerular filtration. With any of these situations, drug accumulation may occur, resulting in adverse drug reactions.

Common tests used to determine renal function include creatinine and blood urea nitrogen (BUN). Creatinine is a metabolic byproduct of muscle excreted by the kidneys; urea nitrogen is the metabolic breakdown product of protein metabolism. Based on National Kidney Foundation recommendations, the estimated glomerular filtration rate (eGFR) is now calculated as part of routine comprehensive metabolic panels and basic metabolic panels. The eGFR is calculated using the person's creatinine level, age, body size, and sex. Decreased eGFR is expected in older adult and female patients because of their decreased muscle mass. It is important for nurses to know their patient's kidney function to ensure correct drug dosage.

PHARMACODYNAMICS

Pharmacodynamics is the study of the effects of drugs on the body. Drugs act within the body to mimic the actions of the body's own chemical messengers. Drug response can cause a primary or secondary physiologic effect or both. A drug's primary effect is the desirable response, and the secondary effect may be desirable or undesirable. An example of a drug with a primary and secondary effect is diphenhydramine, an

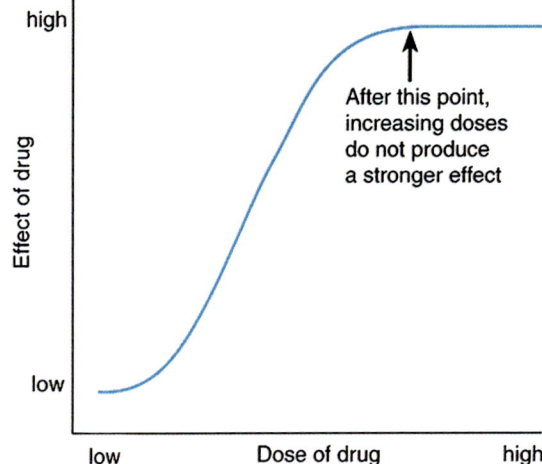

Fig. 3.6 Dose-response relationship. (From Carlson NR. *Foundations of Behavioral Neuroscience*. 8th ed. Pearson; 2010.)

antihistamine. The primary effect of diphenhydramine is to treat the symptoms of allergy; the secondary effect is a central nervous system (CNS) depression that causes drowsiness. The secondary effect is undesirable when the patient drives a car, but at bedtime it could be desirable because it causes mild sedation.

Dose-Response Relationship

The **dose-response relationship** is the body's physiologic response to changes in drug concentration at the site of action. Two concepts further describe this relationship. **Potency** refers to the amount of drug needed to elicit a specific physiologic response to a drug. A drug with high potency, such as fentanyl, produces significant therapeutic responses at low concentrations; a drug with low potency, such as codeine, produces minimal therapeutic responses at low concentrations. The point at which increasing a drug's dosage no longer increases the desired therapeutic response is referred to as **maximal efficacy** (Fig. 3.6).

Closely related to dose-response and efficacy is the **therapeutic index (TI)**, which describes the relationship between the *therapeutic dose* of a drug (ED_{50}) and the *toxic dose* of a drug (TD_{50}). ED_{50} is the dose of a drug that produces a therapeutic response in 50% of the population; TD_{50} is the dose of a drug that produces a toxic response in 50% of the population. The therapeutic index is the difference between these two points (Fig. 3.7). If the ED_{50} and TD_{50} are close, the drug is said to have a narrow therapeutic index. Drugs with a narrow therapeutic index—such as warfarin, digoxin, and phenytoin—require close monitoring to ensure patient safety. To be safe, plasma drug levels of drugs with a narrow therapeutic index must fall within the **therapeutic range** (also known as the therapeutic window). The therapeutic range is a range of doses that produce a therapeutic response without causing significant adverse effects in patients.

Onset, Peak, and Duration of Action

Other important aspects of pharmacodynamics to understand include a drug's onset, peak, and duration of action. **Onset** is the time it takes for a drug to reach the **minimum effective concentration** (MEC) after administration. The MEC is the minimum amount of drug required for drug effect. A drug's **peak** occurs when it reaches its highest concentration in the blood. **Duration of action** is the length of time the drug exerts a therapeutic effect. Fig. 3.8 illustrates the areas in which onset, peak, and duration of action occur.

It is necessary to understand this information in relation to drug administration. Some drugs produce effects in minutes, but others may take hours or days. If the drug plasma concentration decreases below the MEC, adequate drug dosing is not achieved; too high of a drug concentration can result in toxicity.

Therapeutic Drug Monitoring

Once a steady state has been achieved, drug concentration can be determined by measuring peak and trough drug levels. Peak and trough levels are requested for drugs that have a narrow therapeutic index and are considered toxic.

The **peak drug level** is the highest plasma concentration of drug at a specific time, and it indicates the rate of drug absorption. If the peak is too low, effective concentration has not been reached. If the drug is given orally, the peak time is usually 2 to 3 hours after drug administration. If the drug is given intravenously, the peak time is usually 30 to 60 minutes after the infusion is complete. If the drug is given intramuscularly, the peak time is usually 2 to 4 hours after injection. If a peak drug level is ordered, a blood sample should be drawn at the appropriate peak time based on the route of administration.

Most drugs only require trough concentration levels to be drawn (the exception is aminoglycoside antibiotics, which require both peak and trough levels). The **trough drug level** is the lowest plasma concentration of a drug, and it measures the rate at which the drug is eliminated. Trough levels are drawn just before the next dose of the drug regardless of route of administration.

Receptor Theory

Drugs act by binding to receptors. Binding of the drug may activate a receptor, producing a response, or it may inactivate a receptor, blocking a response. The activity of many drugs is determined by the ability of the drug to bind to a specific receptor. The better the drug fits at the receptor site, the more active the drug is. Drug-receptor interactions are like the fit of the right key in a lock. Fig. 3.9 illustrates drug-receptor binding.

Most **receptors**, which are protein in nature, are found on cell surface membranes or within the cell itself. Drug-binding sites are primarily on proteins, glycoproteins, proteolipids, and enzymes. The four receptor families (Fig. 3.10) include (1) cell membrane-embedded enzymes, (2) ligand-gated ion channels, (3) G protein-coupled receptor systems, and (4) transcription factors. The **ligand-binding domain** is the site on the receptor at which drugs bind.

- *Cell membrane-embedded enzymes.* The ligand-binding domain for drug binding is on the cell surface. The drug activates the enzyme inside the cell, and a response is initiated.
- *Ligand-gated ion channels.* The channel crosses the cell membrane. When the channel opens, ions flow into and out of the cells. This primarily affects sodium and calcium ions.
- *G protein-coupled receptor systems.* The three components to this receptor response are (1) the receptor, (2) the G protein that binds with guanosine triphosphate (GTP), and (3) the effector, which is either an enzyme or an ion channel. The system works as follows:

Drug $\xrightarrow{\text{Activates}}$ Receptors $\xrightarrow{\text{Activates}}$ G protein $\xrightarrow{\text{Activates}}$ Effect

Fig. 3.7 The therapeutic index. The therapeutic index is the ratio between the toxic dose of a drug and the therapeutic dose of a drug. (From Guzman F. *Pharmacology Corner.* n.d. http://pharmacologycorner.com/therapeutic-index/.)

Fig. 3.8 Onset, peak, and duration of action. (From McKenry LM, Tessier E, Hogan MA. *Mosby's Pharmacology in Nursing.* 22nd ed. Elsevier; 2006.)

- *Transcription factors.* Found in the cell nucleus on DNA, not on the surface. Activation of receptors through transcription factors regulates protein synthesis and is prolonged. With the first three receptor groups, activation of the receptors is rapid.

Agonists, Partial Agonists, and Antagonists

Drugs that activate receptors and produce a desired response are called **agonists**. **Partial agonists** are drugs that elicit only moderate activity when binding to receptors; partial agonists also prevent receptor activation by other drugs. Drugs that prevent receptor activation and block a response are called **antagonists**. Blocking receptor activation either increases or decreases cellular action, depending on the endogenous action of the chemical messenger that is blocked (see Fig. 3.9).

Nonspecific and Nonselective Drug Effects

Many agonists and antagonists lack specific and selective effects. Receptors produce a variety of physiologic responses, depending on where the receptor is located. Cholinergic receptors are in the bladder, heart, blood vessels, stomach, bronchi, and eyes. A drug that stimulates or blocks the cholinergic receptors affects all anatomic sites. Drugs that affect multiple receptor sites are considered **nonspecific**. For example, bethanechol may be prescribed for postoperative urinary retention to increase bladder contraction. This drug stimulates cholinergic receptors located in the bladder, and urination occurs by strengthening bladder contraction. However, because bethanechol is nonspecific, other cholinergic sites are also affected; the heart rate decreases, blood pressure decreases, gastric acid secretion increases, the bronchioles constrict, and the pupils of the eye constrict (Fig. 3.11). These other effects may be either desirable or harmful.

Some drugs affect multiple receptors, and these are considered **nonselective** drugs. For example, epinephrine, which is used for the treatment of anaphylaxis or severe asthma exacerbations, acts on the alpha$_1$, beta$_1$, and beta$_2$ receptors (Fig. 3.12), affecting multiple body systems.

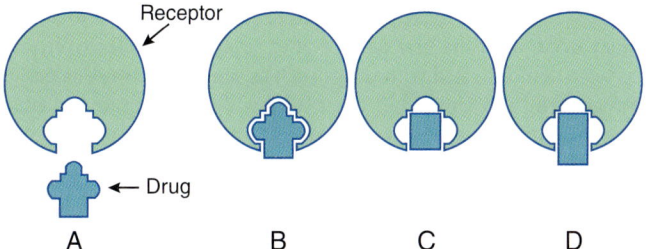

Fig. 3.9 (A) Drugs act by forming chemical bonds with specific receptor sites, similar to a key and lock. (B) The better the fit, the better the response. Drugs with complete attachment and response are called *agonists*. (C) Drugs that attach but do not elicit a response are called antagonists. (D) Drugs that attach and elicit a small response but also block other responses are called partial agonists. (From Clayton BD, Willihnganz MJ. *Basic Pharmacology for Nurses.* 17th ed. Elsevier; 2017.)

Fig. 3.10 The four receptor families: (1) cell membrane-embedded enzymes, (2) ligand-gated ion channels, (3) G protein-coupled receptor systems, and (4) transcription factors. (From Burchum J, Rosenthal L. *Lehne's Pharmacology for Nursing Care.* 9th ed. Elsevier; 2016.)

Fig. 3.11 Cholinergic receptors are located in the bladder, heart, blood vessels, stomach, bronchi, and eyes.

Fig. 3.12 Epinephrine affects three different receptors: alpha$_1$, beta$_1$, and beta$_2$.

Mechanisms of Drug Action

Mechanisms of drug action include (1) stimulation, (2) depression, (3) irritation, (4) replacement, (5) cytotoxic action, (6) antimicrobial action, and (7) modification of immune status. A drug that stimulates a receptor can enhance intrinsic activity (e.g., adrenergic drugs that increase heart rate, sweating, and respiratory rate during fight-or-flight response). Depressant drugs decrease neural activity and bodily functions (e.g., barbiturates and opiates). Drugs that irritate have a noxious effect, such as astringents. Replacement drugs such as insulins, thyroid drugs, and hormones replace essential body compounds. Cytotoxic drugs selectively kill invading parasites or cancers. Antimicrobial drugs prevent, inhibit, or kill infectious organisms. Drugs that modify immune status modify, enhance, or depress the immune system (e.g., interferons and methotrexate).

Side Effects, Adverse Drug Reactions, and Drug Toxicity

Side effects are secondary effects of drug therapy. All drugs have side effects. Even with correct drug dosage, side effects occur that can be predictable and range from inconvenient to severe or life-threatening. In some instances, the side effects may be desirable (e.g., using diphenhydramine at bedtime, when its side effect of drowsiness is beneficial). Chronic illness, age, weight, sex, and ethnicity all play a part in drug side effects.

It is important to know that the occurrence of side effects is one of the primary reasons patients stop taking their prescribed medications. An important role of the nurse includes teaching patients about a drug's side effects and encouraging them to report side effects. Many can be managed with dosage adjustments, changing to a different drug in the same class, or implementing other interventions.

Adverse drug reactions are unintentional, unexpected reactions to drug therapy that occur at normal drug dosages. The reactions may be mild to severe and include anaphylaxis (cardiovascular collapse). Adverse drug reactions are always undesirable, and the nurse must report and document them because they represent a variance from planned therapy.

Drug toxicity occurs when drug levels exceed the therapeutic range; toxicity may occur secondary to overdose (intentional or unintentional) or drug accumulation. Factors that influence drug toxicity include disease, genetics, and age.

Drug Response Types
Tolerance and Tachyphylaxis

Tolerance refers to a decreased responsiveness to a drug over the course of therapy; an individual with drug tolerance requires a higher dosage of drug to achieve the same therapeutic response. In contrast, tachyphylaxis refers to an acute, rapid decrease in response to a drug; it may occur after the first dose or after several doses. Tachyphylaxis has been demonstrated with drugs such as centrally acting analgesics, nitroglycerin, and ranitidine, to name a few. To provide safe and effective care, nurses must be aware of these potential reasons a patient may fail to respond therapeutically to drug administration.

Placebo Effect

Placebo effect is a drug response not attributed to the chemical properties of the drug. The response can be positive or negative and may be influenced by the beliefs, attitudes, and expectations of the patient. Although the placebo effect is psychological in origin, the response can be physiologic, resulting in changes in heart rate, blood pressure, and pain sensation.

DRUG INTERACTIONS

Seventy percent of Americans are taking one or more prescription drugs. Drug therapy is complex because of the great number of drugs available. Drug-drug, drug-nutrient (e.g., food, supplements, alcohol), drug-disease, and drug-laboratory interactions (when a drug interferes with laboratory testing) are an increasing problem. Because of the possibility of numerous interactions, the nurse must be knowledgeable about drug interactions and must closely monitor patient response to drug therapy. Thorough and timely communication among members of the health team is essential. Patients at high risk for interactions include those who have chronic health conditions, take multiple medications, see more than one healthcare provider, and use multiple pharmacies. Older adults are at especially high risk for drug interactions because 20% of older adults take five or more medications. Multiple drug interaction checker websites are available on the Internet for both health care personnel and consumer use, such as Drugs.com at www.drugs.com/drug_interactions.html or WebMD at www.webmd.com/interaction-checker.

A drug interaction is defined as an altered or modified action or effect of a drug because of interaction with one or multiple drugs. It should not be confused with drug incompatibility or an adverse drug reaction, an undesirable drug effect that ranges from mild untoward effects to severe toxic effects that include hypersensitivity reaction and anaphylaxis. Drug incompatibility is a chemical or physical reaction that occurs among two or more drugs in vitro. In other words, the reaction occurs between two or more drugs within a syringe, IV bag, or other artificial environment outside of the body.

Drug interactions can be divided into two categories, pharmacokinetic and pharmacodynamic interactions.

Pharmacokinetic Interactions

Pharmacokinetic interactions are changes that occur in the absorption, distribution, metabolism, and excretion of one or more drugs.

Absorption

When a person takes two drugs at the same time, the rate of absorption of one or both drugs can change. A drug can block, decrease, or increase the absorption of another drug. It can do this in one of three ways: (1) by increasing or decreasing gastric emptying time, (2) by changing the gastric pH, or (3) by forming drug complexes.

Drugs that increase the speed of gastric emptying, such as laxatives, may cause an increase in gastric and intestinal motility and a decrease in drug absorption. Most drugs are absorbed primarily in the small intestine; exceptions include barbiturates, salicylates, and theophylline, which undergo gastric absorption. Opioids and anticholinergic drugs such as atropine decrease gastric emptying time and GI motility, causing an increase in absorption rate. For drugs that undergo gastric absorption, the amount or extent of absorption increases the longer the drug remains in the stomach.

When the gastric pH is decreased, a weakly acidic drug such as aspirin is less ionized and is more rapidly absorbed. Drugs that increase the gastric pH decrease absorption of weak-acid drugs. Antacids such as magnesium hydroxide and aluminum hydroxide raise the gastric pH and block or slow absorption. Some drugs may react chemically. For example, tetracycline and the heavy metal ions calcium, magnesium, aluminum, and iron found in antacids or iron supplements may lead to the formation of a drug complex and thus prevent the absorption of tetracycline. This phenomenon may also be observed when products that contain calcium, magnesium, or iron are ingested with fluoroquinolone antibiotics such as ciprofloxacin. Consequently, dairy products, multivitamins, and antacids should be avoided 1 hour before and 2 hours after tetracycline or ciprofloxacin administration. The nonabsorbable cholesterol-lowering drug cholestyramine binds with multiple drugs and fat-soluble vitamins (e.g., vitamin K) in the GI tract, resulting in reduced absorption. Vitamin supplementation may be necessary when cholestyramine is prescribed.

At times, the formation of drug complexes is desired, for example, in the case of acute iron poisoning. In this situation, the chelating agent deferoxamine is administered; it binds to the excess iron in the blood so it can be excreted from the body via the kidneys.

GI bacteria account for 70% of the body's microbes. They play a major role in the absorption of drugs and nutrients and in the metabolism of bilirubin, bile acids, cholesterol, and steroid hormones as well as the synthesis of vitamins B and K. GI bacteria help maintain homeostasis and factor into the overall health and immune status of an individual. Alteration of bacteria normally found in the GI tract (caused by patient genotype, antibiotic treatment, diet, and environment) can affect drug pharmacokinetics. Orally administered drugs can be metabolized by intestinal microbial enzymes, resulting in toxic compounds or reduced drug absorption, which lead to decreased therapeutic response. For example, administration of antibiotics can alter the synthesis of vitamin K, interfering with therapeutic blood levels of the anticoagulant warfarin.

Metabolism

Many drug interactions of metabolism occur with the induction or inhibition of the hepatic microsomal system. A drug can increase the metabolism of another drug by stimulating liver enzymes. These enzymes produce a cascade effect in drug function. Drugs that promote induction of enzymes are called *enzyme inducers*. Some drugs—such as phenobarbital, carbamazepine, and rifampin—are enzyme inducers. Phenobarbital increases the metabolism of most antipsychotics and methylxanthine; phenobarbital, carbamazepine, and rifampin increase the metabolism of warfarin. Increased metabolism promotes drug elimination and decreases plasma concentration of the drug; the result is a decrease in therapeutic drug action. Care must be taken when enzyme inducers are discontinued because less drug is eliminated by hepatic metabolism, and toxicity can result.

Some drugs are enzyme inhibitors. The antiulcer drug cimetidine is an enzyme inhibitor that decreases metabolism of certain drugs (e.g., theophylline, warfarin, phenytoin) and causes an increase in the plasma concentration of these drugs. To avoid toxicity, dosage of these drugs must be reduced. If cimetidine or any enzyme drug inhibitor is discontinued, the dosage of other drugs affected by its administration should be adjusted, and blood levels should be closely monitored.

The use of tobacco has variable effects on drug metabolism. Polycyclic aromatic hydrocarbons found in cigarette smoke induce production of hepatic enzymes CYP1A2 and CYP2B6. CYP1A2 is involved in the metabolism of many drugs. The effect is dose-dependent on the number of cigarettes smoked per day, as well as genetic and ethnic individual variability. Smoking cessation results in a rapid reversal of enzyme induction. An example of smoking's effect on CYP1A2 enzyme production is seen with clozapine, where smoking cessation has led to drug toxicity. In addition to antipsychotics, the effects on enzyme activity can be found in antidepressants, benzodiazepines, methadone, anticoagulants, antiplatelet drugs and antihypertensives, as well as other classes of drugs.

Alcohol is metabolized by the CYP2E1 enzyme, the same enzyme used by acetaminophen. This enzyme reduces both drugs to their toxic metabolites. In low levels, the body can deactivate the metabolites; however, in instances of high intake of either drug, accumulation of toxic metabolites occurs, resulting in liver damage. Alcohol is a known inhibitor of CYP2C9, the same enzyme involved in the metabolization of warfarin. Inhibition of this enzyme increases the risk of bleeding. In addition, alcohol interacts with certain antibiotics, antihypertensives, antidiabetics, and analgesics, both narcotic and nonnarcotic.

Natural or herbal products can also affect drug metabolism. St. John's wort, an OTC herbal product used to manage symptoms of depression, induces CYP3A4 and CYP2C9. Induction of these enzymes can lead to lower levels of amitriptyline, cyclosporine, digoxin, methadone, theophylline, and many other drugs. This action potentially decreases the effectiveness of these drugs, possibly necessitating a dose increase to sustain efficacy. Flavonoids, a group of naturally occurring compounds

TABLE 3.1 Drugs: Enzyme Inducers and Enzyme Inhibitors

Drug Category	Drug Effect
Drug enzyme inducer	Onset and termination of drug effect is slow, approximately 1 week. Drug dosage may need to be increased with the use of drug inducer. Drug dosage should be adjusted after termination of drug inducer. Monitor serum drug levels, especially if the drug has a narrow therapeutic drug range.
Drug enzyme inhibitor	Onset of drug effect usually occurs rapidly. Half-life ($t\frac{1}{2}$) of the second drug may be increased, causing a prolonged drug effect. Interaction may occur related to the dosage prescribed. Disease entities affect drug dosing. Monitor serum drug levels, especially if the drug has a narrow therapeutic range.

found in the juice and pulp of citrus fruits, are potent inhibitors of the metabolism of certain drugs (e.g., carbamazepine, calcium channel blockers, and drugs for erectile dysfunction), due to the inhibition of the enzyme CYP3A4. Patients who are stabilized on therapeutic doses of these drugs may subject themselves to adverse effects from greater-than-expected drug levels if they eat or drink grapefruit products concurrently with the drug. Table 3.1 describes the effects of drug enzyme inducers and inhibitors.

Excretion

Most drugs are filtered through the glomeruli and are excreted in the urine. With some drugs, excretion occurs in the bile, which passes into the intestinal tract. Drugs can increase or decrease renal excretion and can influence the excretion of other drugs. Drugs that decrease cardiac output decrease blood flow to the kidneys; decreased blood flow results in decreased glomerular filtration rate, which can decrease or delay drug excretion.

Diuretics promote water and sodium excretion from the renal tubules. Furosemide acts on the loop of Henle, and hydrochlorothiazide acts on the distal tubules. Both diuretics decrease reabsorption of water, sodium, and potassium. The renal loss of potassium can result in *hypokalemia*, which can alter the action of some drugs; for example, it can enhance the action of digoxin and can lead to toxicity.

Two or more drugs that undergo the same route of excretion may compete with one another for elimination from the body. Probenecid, a drug for gout, decreases penicillin excretion by inhibiting the secretion of penicillin in the renal tubules of the kidneys. In some cases, this effect may be desirable to increase or maintain the plasma concentration of penicillin—which has a short half-life—for a prolonged period.

Changing urine pH affects drug excretion. The antacid sodium bicarbonate causes the urine to be alkaline. Alkaline urine promotes the excretion of drugs that are weak acids (e.g., aspirin, barbiturates). Drugs that acidify the urine, such as ascorbic acid, promote the excretion of drugs that are weak bases (e.g., amphetamine).

With decreased renal or hepatic function, there is usually an increase in free drug concentration. It is essential to closely monitor these patients for drug toxicity when they take multiple drugs. Checking serum drug levels, a practice known **as therapeutic drug monitoring (TDM)**, is especially important for drugs that have a narrow therapeutic range and are highly protein bound. Digoxin and phenytoin are two drugs that require TDM.

Pharmacodynamic Interactions

Pharmacodynamic interactions are those that result in additive, synergistic, or antagonistic drug effects.

Additive Drug Effects

When two drugs are administered in combination and the response is increased beyond what either could produce alone, the drug interaction is called an **additive effect**; it is the sum of the effects of the two drugs. Additive effects can be desirable or undesirable. For example, a desirable additive drug effect occurs when a diuretic and a beta blocker are administered for the treatment of hypertension. In combination, these two drugs use different mechanisms to have a more pronounced blood pressure–lowering effect. As another example, aspirin and codeine are two analgesics that work by different mechanisms but can be given together for increased pain relief.

An example of an undesirable additive effect is that from two vasodilators, hydralazine prescribed for hypertension and nitroglycerin prescribed for angina. The result could be a severe hypotensive response. Another example is the interaction of aspirin and alcohol. Aspirin is directly irritating to the stomach; it causes platelet dysfunction, and it inhibits prostaglandin-mediated mucus production of the gastric mucosa that protects the underlying tissues of the stomach. Alcohol disrupts the gastric mucosal barrier and suppresses platelet production. Both aspirin and alcohol can prolong bleeding time and, when taken together, may result in gastric bleeding.

Synergistic Drug Effects and Potentiation

When two or more drugs are given together, one drug can have a **synergistic effect** on another. In other words, the clinical effect of the two drugs given together is substantially greater than that of either drug alone. An example of this is the use of two cytotoxic drugs to reduce individual drug dosing, thereby decreasing side effects. An example of an undesirable effect occurs when alcohol and a sedative-hypnotic drug such as diazepam are combined. The resultant effect of this example is increased CNS depression.

Some antibiotics have an enzyme inhibitor added to the drug to potentiate the therapeutic effect. Examples are ampicillin with sulbactam and amoxicillin with clavulanate, in which sulbactam and clavulanate potassium are bacterial enzyme inhibitors. Ampicillin and amoxicillin can be given without these inhibitors; however, the desired therapeutic effect may not occur because of the bacterial beta-lactamase, which inactivates the drugs and causes bacterial resistance. The combination of the antibiotic with either sulbactam or clavulanate inhibits bacterial enzyme activity and enhances the effect, or broadens the spectrum of activity, of the antibacterial agent.

Antagonistic Drug Effects

When drugs with **antagonistic effects** are administered together, one drug reduces or blocks the effect of the other. In some situations, antagonistic effects are desirable. In morphine sulfate overdose, naloxone is given as an antagonist to block the narcotic effects of morphine sulfate. This is a beneficial drug interaction of an antagonist. Likewise, in the case of heparin overdose, protamine sulfate is administered to block the effects of heparin.

The most common symptoms of drug-drug interactions include drowsiness, dizziness, nausea or vomiting, diarrhea, aches and pains, depression, increased bruising or bleeding, rashes, and anxiety or restlessness. Patients should contact their pharmacist or health care provider if they experience any unusual reaction. The most feared interactions are those that result in a dramatic drop in blood pressure or cause a rapid or irregular heart rate. Also of concern are drug interactions that produce toxins capable of damaging vital organs such as the heart or liver. Fortunately, most interactions are not severe or life-threatening. Patients should be aware that prescription drugs, OTC drugs, and herbal products can interact with each other. It is a myth that interactions occur only with prescription medications. Severe adverse reactions are highlighted with a boxed warning in the product literature.

Drug Interactions With Nutrients, Testing, and Light

Drug-Nutrient Interactions

Food may increase, decrease, or delay the body's pharmacokinetic response to drugs. A classic drug-food interaction occurs when a monoamine oxidase inhibitor (MAOI) antidepressant (e.g., phenelzine) is taken with tyramine-rich foods such as cheese, wine, organ meats, beer, yogurt, sour cream, or bananas. MAOIs block monoamine oxidase, the enzyme that breaks down excess tyramine in the intestinal wall and liver. Tyramine is a potent vasoconstrictor, and when taken in conjunction with an MAOI, the result could be a hypertensive crisis. The patient must avoid these foods when taking MAOIs.

Nutritional deficiencies such as protein-energy malnutrition (PEM) may alter pharmacokinetic processes and drug responses, resulting in

CLINICAL JUDGMENT [NURSING PROCESS]
Pharmacokinetics and Pharmacodynamics

Concept: Caring Intervention
- Nursing intervention designed to meet the physical and emotional needs of the patient

Concept: Clinical Decision Making
- Process used by nurses to identify patient problems and intervene to achieve desired outcomes

Concept: Safety
- Protecting the patient from potential or actual harm; a basic human need

Recognize Cues [Assessment]
- Assess family patterns, economic concerns, and cultural patterns that influence adherence with the medical regimen.
- Assess language spoken, literacy level, preferred learning style, cognitive level, and use of glasses or other aids.
- Check peak levels and trough levels of drugs as appropriate.
- Detect possible interactions and cumulative or other adverse effects among prescribed drugs, self-administered over-the-counter (OTC) products, home remedies, herbal remedies, and foods.
- Determine whether the patient participates in traditional health practices or complementary and alternative medical practices.
- Determine kidney function by checking for adequate urine output; the guideline is 30 mL/h for adults; estimated glomerular filtration rate (eGFR; normal is 90–120 mL/min), and proteinuria (normal urine protein is up to 150 mg/day).
- Determine the potential for drug interactions related to increased or decreased absorption of drugs.
- Determine whether the patient smokes cigarettes or consumes alcohol.
- Identify all the patient's current drugs, including prescription and OTC drugs, supplements, herbs, and teas.
- Inquire about the patient's preferences regarding touch, modesty, and personal space.
- Perform a physical examination to identify problems that may affect pharmacokinetics and pharmacodynamics.
- Review all literature provided by drug companies and pharmacies; be sure to check the protein-binding percentage of the drug and any need for therapeutic monitoring.
- Take a thorough patient history to identify factors that may affect drug pharmacokinetics and pharmacodynamics.

Analyze Cues and Prioritize Hypothesis [Patient Problems]
- Anxiety
- Need for health teaching
- Potential for decreased adherence
- Coping

Generate Solutions [Planning]
- The patient will demonstrate behaviors that decrease the risk for injury.
- The patient will describe the rationale for the therapeutic regimen.
- The patient will discuss barriers to implementing a therapeutic regimen and/or related fears.
- Therapeutic communication techniques will be used.
- The patient will follow a mutually agreed-upon plan of care.
- The patient will be aware of drug interactions, will avoid drugs that may cause a severe reaction, and will know what to report immediately to the health care provider.
- The patient will effectively manage the therapeutic regimen.
- The patient will not take any OTC drugs without consultation with the health care provider.
- The patient's health care needs will be met within a culturally competent framework.
- The patient will express confidence in their personal ability to manage the health situation and remain in control of life.

Take Action [Nursing Interventions]
- Advise patients not to eat high-fat foods before ingesting an enteric-coated tablet; high-fat foods decrease the drug absorption rate.
- Incorporate traditional health practices with mainstream prescriptive therapies when appropriate.
- Anticipate unique responses to drugs based on social, cultural, and biologic influences.
- Determine drug-drug interactions utilizing a drug interaction program, such as the RxList Drug Interaction Checker (https://www.rxlist.com/drug-interaction-checker.htm).
- Contact the health care provider to assess the need for a drug dose adjustment if one has not been ordered after a drug enzyme inducer has been discontinued.
- If negative side effects of prescribed drugs are a problem, explain that many side effects can be controlled or eliminated.
- Include significant members of the social group in the planning and implementation of patient care, as desired by the patient.
- Monitor the therapeutic range of drugs that have a narrow therapeutic range.
- Notify the health care provider of drugs ordered that have antagonistic or opposite effects, such as beta stimulants and beta blockers.
- Recognize drugs of the same category that might have an additive effect. The additive drug effect might be undesirable and could cause a severe physiologic response.
- Recognize the need for patients to exercise control in their environment.
- Reconcile all drugs at discharge, and provide a list to the patient; ensure that accurate drug information is available to all health care personnel involved in patient care.
- Simplify therapy.
- Use appropriate translation resources per facility guidelines.
- Use therapeutic communication.
- Facilitate adherence to mainstream prescriptive therapies within the patient's social and cultural contexts.
- Provide health information written in the patient's primary language. Medline, an online service of the National Institutes of Health, offers a variety of patient education materials in a number of languages online at www.nlm.nih.gov/medlineplus/languages/languages.html.
- Advise patients not to take OTC drugs with prescribed drugs without first notifying the healthcare provider.
- Encourage the patient to use one pharmacy.
- Remind patients to be cautious about taking herbal products, especially if taking OTC or prescription medications; advise that they check with their healthcare provider first.
- Use illustrations to explain the drug regimen.

Evaluate Outcomes [Evaluation]
- Assess for signs and symptoms of drug interactions, side effects, and toxicity.
- Evaluate physical, social, and psychological outcomes of prescriptive therapies.
- Evaluate the effectiveness of the drugs.
- Monitor for patient adherence to prescriptive therapies.

toxicity. There are two forms of PEM, kwashiorkor and marasmus. Persons with either form of PEM may have altered pharmacokinetics, such as decreased drug absorption and decreased protein binding, altered volume of distribution and biotransformation, and decreased drug elimination. Because of the risk for toxicity, persons with PEM require careful monitoring and possible changes in drug dosing.

Drug-Laboratory Interactions

Drugs often interfere with clinical laboratory testing by cross-reaction with antibodies, interference with enzyme reactions, or alteration of chemical reactions. Drug-laboratory interactions may lead to misinterpretation or invalidation of test results, resulting in additional healthcare costs associated with unnecessary repeat laboratory testing or additional testing. Drug-laboratory interactions may also lead to missed or erroneous clinical diagnosis. Healthcare personnel and consumers can find information related to drug-laboratory interactions on several websites on the Internet, such as RxList at http://www.rxlist.com/script/main/hp.asp.

Drug-Induced Photosensitivity

A drug-induced photosensitivity reaction is a skin reaction caused by exposure to sunlight. It is caused most often by the interaction of a drug and exposure to ultraviolet A light, which can cause cellular damage; however, ultraviolet B light may also contribute to drug-induced photosensitivity reactions.

The two types of photosensitivity reactions are photoallergic and phototoxic. A *photoallergic reaction* occurs when a drug (e.g., sulfonamide) undergoes activation in the skin by ultraviolet light to a compound that is more allergenic than the parent compound. Because it takes time to develop antibodies, photoallergic reactions are a type of delayed hypersensitivity reaction. With a *phototoxic reaction*, a photosensitive drug undergoes photochemical reactions within the skin to cause damage. This type of reaction is not immune-mediated. The onset of a phototoxic reaction with erythema can be rapid, occurring within 2 to 6 hours of sunlight exposure.

Both types of reactions are the result of light exposure, but they differ according to the wavelength of light and the photosensitive drug. A phototoxic reaction may be the result of the drug dose, whereas a photoallergic reaction is not and only requires previous exposure, or sensitization, to the offending agent.

Most photosensitive reactions can be avoided by using sunscreen with a sun protection factor greater than 15; avoiding excessive sunlight, especially at the height of daylight hours; and wearing protective clothing. Decreasing the drug dose may decrease the risk of photosensitivity if treatment is required. It may be necessary, however, to discontinue the use of the offending drug.

CLINICAL JUDGMENT CASE STUDY

The nurse is caring for a patient who was admitted to the hospital with severe migraines. They have been taking warfarin, a highly protein-bound anticoagulant, for atrial fibrillation. After a thorough evaluation, the neurologist has ordered valproic acid, an antiseizure medication. Valproic acid is also highly protein bound.

1. What patient problem would be appropriate for this patient?
2. What information needs to be included in the interdisciplinary health/teaching plan for this patient?
3. During a teaching session, the patient shares that they plan to start taking over-the-counter products to boost energy. What is the nurse's best response to the patient's comment? Explain your answer.

REVIEW QUESTIONS

1. Which concept does the nurse need to understand before administering a drug? **Select all that apply.**
   a. Drugs with a smaller volume of drug distribution have a longer half-life.
   b. Oral drugs are dissolved through the process of pinocytosis.
   c. Patients with kidney disease may have fewer protein-binding sites.
   d. Rapid absorption decreases the bioavailability of the drug.
   e. When the drug metabolism rate is decreased, toxicity can occur.
2. The nurse will question the health care provider if a drug with a half-life ($t\frac{1}{2}$) of more than 24 hours is ordered to be administered at which interval?
   a. Once daily
   b. Every other day
   c. Twice weekly
   d. Once weekly
3. When explaining drug action, which statement is correct?
   a. Water-soluble and ionized drugs are quickly absorbed.
   b. A drug not bound to protein is an active drug.
   c. Most receptors are found under the cell membrane.
   d. Toxic effects can result if the trough level is low.
4. A patient newly diagnosed with type 2 diabetes mellitus is prescribed the antidiabetic drug metformin 500 mg by mouth with morning and evening meals. Which statement best indicates to the nurse that the patient will adhere to the therapeutic regimen?
   a. I will no longer put sugar on my cereal because that will help me be healthier.
   b. If I take this medicine, I will feel better soon and won't have to take it anymore.
   c. To reduce the possibility of damage to my body, I must take the medicine as scheduled.
   d. I have diabetes because of my ancestry, so there's not much I can do about it.
5. The nurse is aware that the rate of absorption can be changed by which action? **Select all that apply.**
   a. Modifying gastric emptying time
   b. Changing gastric pH
   c. Decreasing inflammation
   d. Forming drug complexes
   e. Eating too slowly

6. The nurse is meeting with a community group about drug safety. The nurse must emphasize that patients at high risk for drug interaction include which group? **Select all that apply.**
   a. Older patients
   b. Patients with chronic health conditions
   c. Patients taking three or more drugs
   d. Patients dealing with only one pharmacy
   e. Patients covered by private insurance
7. The nurse recognizes that when a patient takes a hepatic enzyme inducer, the dose of warfarin is usually modified in which way?
   a. It is increased.
   b. It is decreased.
   c. It remains the same.
   d. It is unpredictable.
8. Which statement is correct about synergistic drug effects?
   a. Two drugs have antagonistic effects on each other.
   b. The action of a drug is nullified by another drug.
   c. One drug acts as an antidote to the side effects of another drug.
   d. A greater effect is achieved when two drugs are combined.
9. A patient asks the nurse about drug interactions with over-the-counter preparations. Which response is best?
   a. Discuss this with the health care provider.
   b. There are not many interactions, so don't worry about it.
   c. Read the labels carefully, and check with your healthcare provider.
   d. Avoid over-the-counter preparations.
10. Codeine is an example of a(n) _____ as the cytochrome P450 system metabolizes the drug to facilitate receptor affinity.
    a. agonist
    b. prodrug
    c. antagonist
    d. enzyme

4

Pharmacogenetics

http://evolve.elsevier.com/McCuistion/pharmacology

OBJECTIVES

- Describe the history of pharmacogenetics and its clinical uses.
- Describe the role individual effects to drugs as well as legal and ethical issues play in clinical use of pharmacogenetics.

OUTLINE

Foundations of Pharmacogenetics, 32
    Brief History, 32
    Clinical Uses, 32
Key Considerations When Using Pharmacogentics, 34
    Individual Variation in Metabolism of Select Drugs, 34

Legal and Ethical Issues, 35
Clinical Judgment Case Study, 37
Review Questions, 38

FOUNDATIONS OF PHARMACOGENETICS

Each person responds to drugs differently; drugs are not "one size fits all" (Fig. 4.1). Most current drug prescribing occurs through trial and error (Fig. 4.2), typically based on age, weight, sex, and liver and kidney function. For drugs with established therapeutic monitoring parameters, dosing is also adjusted based on plasma drug levels.

Nearly 50% of persons stop taking their prescribed drugs due to side effects or failure of the drug to work as desired. Frequently, a person may try as many as four different drugs before finding one that works for them. Treatment failures result in an annual cost of more than $2500 to the patient. Clinically, treatment failures and adverse drug reactions result in over 125,000 deaths annually.

The Centers for Disease Control and Prevention (CDC) estimates nearly one million visits to the emergency department (ED) occur annually due to adverse drug reactions. A quarter of these visits result in hospitalization. Treatment of adverse drug reactions costs Americans more than $3.5 billion a year in health care expenditures. Anticoagulants, antibiotics, diabetes drugs, and opioid analgesics top the list of drugs leading to ED visits.

HR 6875, the Right Drug Dose Now Act, was introduced in 2022. The bill included funding to educate healthcare providers about pharmacogenomic testing and its ability to help reduce adverse drug reactions and funding to integrate pharmacogenomic information into electronic health records (EHRs) to ensure genotype information is available to providers. At this time, the bill has been referred to the Subcommittee on Health.

Pharmacogenetics is the study of how a patient's genetic factors influence their response to drugs (Table 4.1). Pharmacogenetics helps individualize drug treatment regimens to optimize therapy and decrease adverse drug reactions, thus promoting adherence and reducing overall healthcare costs. Nurses need to understand the issues related to pharmacogenetics, such as the role of genetic counseling and the legal and ethical questions surrounding genetic testing (Table 4.2). Nurses also need to have a basic understanding of pharmacogenetic technology to advocate and educate patients and their families so they can make the best decisions and pave the way for the best outcomes.

Brief History

For thousands of years, people have been breeding animals and growing plants to achieve specific characteristics. Genetic differences in humans have been recognized for centuries. In 1865 Gregor Mendel was the first to explain the difference between dominant and recessive genes in inheritance, using pea flowers as an example (Fig. 4.3). More recently, in 1953 James Watson and Francis Crick discovered that deoxyribonucleic acid (DNA), the main constituent of chromosomes and the carrier of genetic information, was composed of a double-stranded helix of nucleotides (Fig. 4.4). Advances in genetics came rapidly after this discovery. In 2003 the Human Genome Project completed mapping of the roughly 25,000 genes in human DNA (Box 4.1).

In 2015 the Precision Medicine Initiative launched (see https://allofus.nih.gov/). This initiative sought to expand the treatment and prevention of disease by considering a person's genes, environment, and lifestyle. The goal of the initiative is to expand the use of precision medicine, truly treating the right patient, with the right drug, at the right dose.

Clinical Uses

Mapping of the human genome has instilled hope for improving the diagnosis and treatment of disease, predicting disease potential based on genetic predisposition and personalizing medicine based on genetic profiles (Box 4.2). However, as with drugs not being "one size fits all," the use of pharmacogenetics is not appropriate for all patients (Table 4.3). Those who can benefit most are patients who are taking multiple prescription drugs or are on a complex treatment regimen,

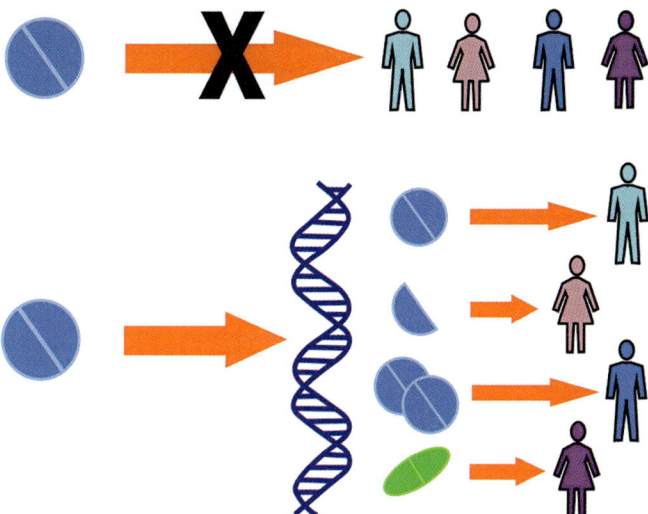

Fig. 4.1 One size does not fit all. The study of variability in drug response due to heredity. (From Pharmacogenomics Laboratory, Indiana University School of Medicine: Pharmacogenetics brochure, *Ignite* 2016. https://gmkb.org/?utm_source=ignite-genomics.org&utm_medium=referral.)

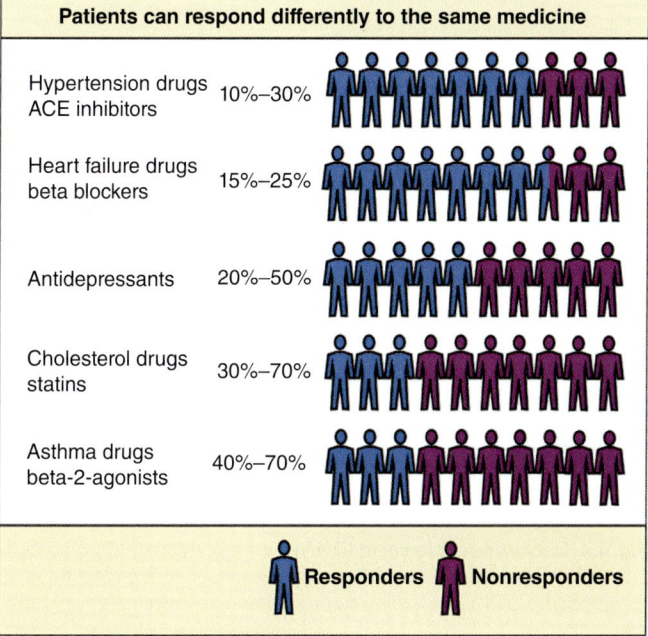

Fig. 4.2 Variable response to drugs. *ACE*, Angiotensin-converting enzyme. (From Pharmacogenomics Laboratory, Indiana University School of Medicine: Pharmacogenetics brochure, *Ignite* 2016. https://gmkb.org/?utm_source=ignite-genomics.org&utm_medium=referral.)

TABLE 4.1	Terminology
Pharmacogenetics[a]	The study of variability in drug response due to heredity.
Pharmacogenomics[a]	The study of the combination of pharmacology and genomics to develop effective and safe medications to compensate for genetic differences in patients that cause varied responses to a single therapeutic regimen.
Allele	One of two or more versions of a gene; an individual inherits two alleles for each gene, one from each parent; if the two alleles are the same (e.g., CYP2C19*1/*1), the individual is homozygous for that gene; if the alleles are different (e.g., CYP2C19*1/*2), the individual is heterozygous.
Extensive metabolizers	Individuals who have an ordinary response to drugs.
Gene	A region of DNA containing genetic information. It is the basic physical and functional unit of heredity.
Genome	The totality of genetic information found in an organism's DNA and/or RNA.
Genomics	The study of the combination of the environment, personal factors as well as all genetic variation.
Genotype	An individual's collection of genes.
Intermediate metabolizers	Decreased efficiency in drug metabolism and therefore an increased concentration of the parent drug with decreased formation of metabolites and a possible decrease in responsiveness.
Personalized medicine	The tailoring of medical treatment to the individual characteristics of each patient, which include genetic predisposition to disease, environmental and personal factors, and pharmacogenetics tailored to improve patient outcomes.
Phenotype	Clinical presentation or observable characteristics of an individual with a particular genotype.
Polymorphisms	Natural variations in a gene, DNA sequence, or chromosome that have no adverse effects on the individual and occur with high frequency in the general population.
Poor metabolizers	Significant decrease in drug metabolism, and as a result tend to have higher levels of the parent drug but with little to no therapeutic benefit and an increased risk for adverse drug responses.
Ultrarapid metabolizers	Increased efficiency in drug metabolism resulting in a possible decrease in effectiveness at established doses. Increased risk for adverse drug responses because of increased metabolite or active drug production.

[a]Often used interchangeably.
From Chang KL, Weitzel K, Schmidt S: Pharmacogenetics: using genetic information to guide drug therapy, *Am Fam Physician* 92(7):588–594, 2015; McClary LM: *Essentials of medical genetics for nursing and health professionals: an interprofessional approach*, 2020, Jones & Bartlett Learning; Montgomery S, Brouwer WA, Everett PC, Hassen E, Lowe T, McGral SB, Eggert J: Genetics in the clinical setting: what nurses need to know to provide the best patient care, *Am Nurse Today* 12(10):10–16, 2017.

patients who are not responding well to current therapy or have had previous adverse drug reactions, and patients taking any drug with pharmacogenetic information included in a boxed warning (e.g., abacavir, clopidogrel, lenalidomide, and succinylcholine) or in the prescribing information (e.g., aripiprazole, citalopram, propafenone, and warfarin). A process model has been developed to guide pharmacogenetic interventions (Fig. 4.5). Pharmacogenetic testing is not available for all drugs. One test cannot determine how a patient will respond to all drugs; if pharmacogenetic testing is appropriate, more than one test

TABLE 4.2 Available Pharmacogenetic Testing

Drug	Associated Diseases/Conditions	Gene(s) Tested
Warfarin	Excessive clotting disorder	VKORC1 and CYP2C9
Thiopurines (e.g., azathioprine, mercaptopurine, and thioguanine)	Autoimmune/childhood leukemia	TPMT
Clopidogrel	Cardiovascular	CYP2C19
Irinotecan	Cancer	UGT1A1
Abacavir	HIV	HLA-B*5701
Carbamazepine, phenytoin	Epilepsy	HLA-B*1502
Some antidepressants, some antiepileptics (e.g., phenytoin, phenobarbital, carbamazepine, valproic acid)	Psychiatric, epilepsy	CYP2D6, CYP2C9, CYP2C19, CYP1A2, SLC6A4, HTR2A/C
Tamoxifen	Cancer	CYP2D6
Some antipsychotics (e.g., haloperidol, mephobarbital, thioridazine)	Psychiatric	DRD3, CYP2D6, CYP2C19, CYP1A2
Methylphenidate	Attention deficit disorder	DRD4
Opioids	Pain management	OPRM1
5-Fluorouracil	Cancer	DPYD variants and TYMS gene mutations testing
SSRIs	Depression	5-HTT
Some statins (e.g., simvastatin)	High cholesterol	SLCO1B1

SSRIs, Selective serotonin reuptake inhibitors.

	X	Y
X^r	$X^r X$ Carrier Daughter; No Disease	$X^r Y$ Male; Has Disease
X	X X Normal Daughter; No Disease	X Y Male; No Disease

Fig. 4.3 Punnett square.

Fig. 4.4 Deoxyribonucleicacid (DNA). (From DNAdirect: *Chromosome analysis and fertility*, n.d. https://services.dnadirect.com/grc/patient-site/chromosome-analysis-infertility/chromosome-analysis-and-fertility.html.)

may be needed. Fig. 4.6 presents current challenges in the implementation of genetic testing.

KEY CONSIDERATIONS WHEN USING PHARMACOGENETICS

Individual Variation in Metabolism of Select Drugs

The US Food and Drug Administration (FDA) website provides updated information on multiple drugs related to clinical response variability, risk for adverse events, and genotype-specific dosing based on

BOX 4.1 Genes

- Each gene has a specific genetic code.
  - This code is a sequence of nucleotides (A, T, G, or C).
- For each nucleotide position in the gene, one of the four nucleotides is the predominant nucleotide in the general population.
  - This predominant nucleotide is usually referred to as *wild type*.
- If an individual has a nucleotide that is different from the wild type in one copy of their genes, that person is said to have a heterozygous variant.
- If an individual has the same variant nucleotide in both copies of their genes, that person is said to have a homozygous variant.

From American Association for Clinical Chemistry: Lab Tests Online: *Pharmacogenetic tests*, 2019. https://labtestsonline.org/tests/pharmacogenetic-tests.

BOX 4.2 Clinical Application of Pharmacogenetics

- Improve quality outcomes
- Customize patient plans of care
- Decrease adverse effects of drug therapy
- Predict patient response to drug therapy
- Save time and money by reducing "trial and error" in drug prescribing
- Decrease treatment failures

TABLE 4.3 Clinical Decision-Making Process for Integrating Pharmacogenomics in Practice

Factor	Questions
Patient or population	Is the variant likely relevant in the patient or population? How common is the variant?
Quality of evidence	What is the strength of the evidence for the use of data? Are clinical guidelines or FDA recommendations available?
Testing	Is testing available? Is the coverage appropriate? What is the turnaround time of results?
Data availability	Does pharmacogenomics data already exist? Is the data quality sufficient to use?
Drug factors	How important is the gene/variant for the pharmacokinetics or pharmacodynamics of the drug? Does the drug have a narrow therapeutic index? Is the drug a prodrug or active? Will the variant decrease efficacy and/or increase toxicity?
Clinical factors	Are there other factors relevant to the decision, like timing of drug start or previous use of the medication? How do comorbid clinical conditions affect expected phenotypes? Are there drug-drug interactions that affect expected phenotypes?

From Adams SM, Crisamore KR, Empey PE: Clinical pharmacogenomics, *Clin J Am Soc Nephrol* 13(10):1561–1571, 2018.

genetic biomarkers (https://www.fda.gov/drugs/science-and-research-drugs/table-pharmacogenomic-biomarkers-drug-labeling). As of 2020 nearly 300 drugs are included in these tables.

Mercaptopurine. The FDA recommends genetic testing before the administration of mercaptopurine to patients with acute lymphoblastic leukemia. Genetic variation in thiopurine *S*-methyltransferase (TPMT) and nudix hydrolase 15 (NUDT15) can interfere with the metabolism of the drug, leading to an increased severity in side effects and increased risk of myelosuppression and infection.

Irinotecan. Genetic testing is recommended for patients with colon cancer receiving irinotecan as part of their treatment protocol. Persons with variation in the *UGT1A1* gene may be unable to eliminate the drug, leading to severe diarrhea and severe neutropenia, resulting in life-threatening infections.

Abacavir. Between 6% and 10% of patients prescribed this drug for the treatment of human immunodeficiency virus develop potentially fatal multiorgan hypersensitivity. Genetic testing has identified the allele HLA-B*5701 in relation to hypersensitivity. The FDA now recommends genetic testing before initiating drug therapy or restarting the drug.

Warfarin. This drug is a vitamin K antagonist used for prophylaxis and treatment of venous thromboembolism and for persons with atrial fibrillation or heart valve replacement, among other uses. It has a narrow therapeutic range. From 10% to 16% of persons prescribed warfarin experience life-threatening bleeding. Alterations in CYP2C9 and vitamin K epoxide reductase (VKOR) enzymes result in decreased clearance and increased blood levels, thereby increasing the risk of bleeding. Warfarin labeling contains dosing information based on CYP2C9 and VKORC1 genotypes.

Clopidogrel. Persons with genetic variation in the CYP2C19 enzyme, which is necessary to convert the prodrug clopidogrel, an inhibitor of platelet aggregation, to the active metabolite, may be at risk for clot formation due to failure to convert the prodrug to an active drug. Point-of-care buccal swab genetic testing has been available since 2013 to help guide treatment. The test determines whether a person has the normal (also referred to as *wild type*) enzyme or a mutation in the CYP2C19 enzyme.

Opioids. Codeine and tramadol are prodrugs that do not exhibit analgesic properties until converted to an active drug by the CYP2D6 enzyme in the liver. Nearly 10% of the population lack this drug-metabolizing enzyme and therefore do not achieve pain relief with codeine or tramadol. In addition, this enzyme has several polymorphisms that alter drug metabolism. Persons with two variant alleles are considered poor metabolizers and will not achieve pain relief with codeine or tramadol. White individuals and people of Asian and Middle Eastern descent are most likely to have this variant. Persons with two *wild-type* alleles are designated ultrarapid metabolizers and are at risk for toxicity, sedation, and respiratory depression due to higher rates of conversion of codeine or tramadol to active drugs.

Mental health drugs. Many drugs used to treat depression (e.g., tricyclic antidepressants and selective serotonin reuptake inhibitors) and other psychiatric disorders (e.g., aripiprazole for use in bipolar disorder and schizophrenia, and atomoxetine for use in attention-deficit/hyperactivity disorder [ADHD]) are metabolized by the CYP2D6 enzyme. This enzyme has 90 known variants that slow drug metabolism, potentially leading to toxic drug concentrations (e.g., aripiprazole). In addition, a couple of known variants increase enzymatic activity, leading to subtherapeutic drug levels. Another variant results in an inactive form of the enzyme, resulting in severe adverse reactions to the drugs. Citalopram, metabolized by CYP2C19, also has dosing guidelines for persons who are considered poor metabolizers due to the increased risk for QT prolongation (maximum of 20 mg/day).

Carbamazepine. Persons with the human leukocyte antigen (HLA)–B*1502 variant should avoid using carbamazepine due to the increased risk of developing Stevens-Johnson syndrome or toxic epidermal necrolysis. Persons of Asian descent are most likely to carry this genetic variant.

Legal and Ethical Issues

Legal and ethical considerations encompass the principles of privacy, autonomy, and justice:
- Privacy
  - Who has access to patient genetic information?
  - Who owns the genetic information?
  - Concerns about patient "labeling" based on genetic code.

Fig. 4.5 General Pharmacogenomics (PGx) process model. (From O'Shea J, Ledwidge M, Gallagher J, Keenan C, Ryan C: Pharmacogenetic interventions to improve outcomes in patients with multimorbidity or prescribed polypharmacy: a systematic review, *Pharmacogenomics J* 22:89–99, 2022.)

Fig. 4.6 Challenges in the implementation of pharmacogenomics. *GINA*, Genetics Information Nondiscrimination Act. (From Adams SM, Crisamore KR, Empey PE: Clinical pharmacogenomics, *Clin J Am Soc Nephrol* 13(10):1561–1571, 2018.)

- Autonomy
  - A patient may consent to or refuse genetic testing.
  - Patients may change their minds about obtaining genetic testing.
- Justice
  - Equal and fair treatment of all.
  - Not everyone has access to the same level of care, nor can everyone afford care.

The healthcare community must not allow genetic profiling to occur. Within an ethnic group, not everyone shares the same genetic variations. Therefore the health care community must guard against denial of treatment based on race and ethnicity in the absence of available pharmacogenetic testing. It is vital to remember that medical conditions are not the result of genetics alone but the fusion of life choices and environment as well.

People have voiced concerns regarding the use of genetic information. Many decline to have genetic testing performed due to fears their employers or insurance companies will unfairly use the results. In response to these concerns, in 2008 the Genetic Information Nondiscrimination Act (GINA) was enacted, which prohibits insurance companies from requiring genetic testing to obtain health insurance and from using genetic information to determine coverage and premiums. The protections provided by GINA allow people to have genetic tests as recommended by their providers without fear that the results will adversely affect insurance or employment decisions. However, these protections do not extend to life insurance, disability insurance, and long-term care insurance, nor do they apply to military members, Indian Health Services, the Veterans Health Administration, or the Federal Employees Health Benefits Program.

Implementation of pharmacogenetics, in conjunction with other patient factors and clinical information, can improve patient safety, quality of care, morbidity, and mortality, as well as decrease cost. The hope for the future of pharmacogenetics is to ensure delivery of the right drug, at the right dose, to the right patient, via the right route, and administered at the right time.

CLINICAL JUDGMENT [NURSING PROCESS]
Pharmacogenetics

Concept: Safety
- Protection of the patient from potential or actual harm; it is a basic human need.

Recognize Cues [Assessment]
- Assess family history back three generations; does anyone in the family have a history of adverse reactions to drugs or treatment failures?
- Assess patient knowledge concerning genetics and genetic testing; explore concerns they may have.
- Determine patient ethnicity.
- Assess the patient for therapeutic response to the drug regimen.
- Determine side effects and adverse responses to drug therapy.

Analyze Cues and Prioritize Hypothesis [Patient Problems]
- Anxiety
- Coping
- Need for health teaching

Generate Solutions [Planning]
- Integrate patient preferences and family implications into developing evidence-based plans of care.
- Incorporate the patient's preferred language, values, traditions, religion, and health beliefs into plans of care.

Take Action [Nursing Interventions]
- Refer identified patients to genetic counseling as needed.
- Ensure patients know to report genetic findings to all of their healthcare providers to reduce duplicate testing and promote optimal prescribing.
- Encourage behavior change to reduce the environmental effect on a person's genetic makeup; refer to appropriate services as needed to facilitate positive treatment outcomes.
- Guide patients in the implications and uses of genetic results.
- Ensure the provision of holistic nursing care, and practice with compassion and respect for the inherent dignity, worth, and unique attributes of every person, regardless of genetic makeup.

Evaluate Outcomes [Evaluation]
- Evaluate the effectiveness of pharmacogenetic interventions and treatment on patient outcomes.

Additional Resources
Clinical Pharmacogenetics Implementation Consortium: https://cpicpgx.org/
Clinical Genome Resource: https://www.clinicalgenome.org/
Genetic Alliance: http://www.geneticalliance.org/
National Human Genome Research Institute: https://www.genome.gov/
Pharmacogenomics Knowledgebase: https://www.pharmgkb.org/

CLINICAL JUDGMENT CASE STUDY

The patient is prescribed tramadol 100 mg every 6 hours as needed for moderate to severe pain after a vertebral fracture. After routinely receiving the drug over 24 hours without relief, the prescriber increases the dose to 150 mg every 4 hours. The patient continues to complain of pain, rated at 8 out of 10, on routine dosing.

1. Which liver enzyme converts tramadol to its active metabolite?
2. Which polymorphism is suspected in this patient?
3. How do patients with this polymorphism metabolize their drugs? This leads to which potential side effects?

REVIEW QUESTIONS

1. Which class of drug is clopidogrel?
   a. Low-molecular-weight heparin
   b. Vitamin K antagonist
   c. Direct thrombin inhibitor
   d. Inhibitor of platelet aggregation
2. Patients with HIV should receive genetic testing for the allele HLA-B*5701 before being treated with which drug?
   a. Abacavir
   b. Tenofovir
   c. Lamivudine
   d. Rilpivirine
3. Which clinical applications are related to pharmacogenetics? **Select all that apply.**
   a. Improve quality outcomes.
   b. Customize patient plans of care.
   c. Decrease adverse effects of drug therapy.
   d. Reduce cost.
   e. Decrease treatment failures.
4. Which action should be taken with a patient prescribed mercaptopurine who has a deficiency of thiopurine S-methyltransferase (TPMT) or nudix hydrolase 15 (NUDT15)?
   a. The dose of mercaptopurine should be increased.
   b. The dose of mercaptopurine should be decreased.
   c. No change should be made to their dose of mercaptopurine.
   d. The dose of mercaptopurine should be decreased with TPMT deficiency and increased with NUDT15 deficiency.
5. Which factors are considered in personalized medicine? **Select all that apply.**
   a. Pharmacogenetic profile
   b. Lifestyle choices
   c. Environmental factors
   d. Provider decision-making
   e. Life expectancy

Complementary and Alternative Therapies

http://evolve.elsevier.com/McCuistion/pharmacology

OBJECTIVES

- Explain government regulation of dietary supplements, including current good manufacturing practices.
- Differentiate between the uses and effects of commonly used herbal remedies.
- Discuss the hazards, tips, and resources associated with the use and effects of herbal remedies for consumers and health care providers.

OUTLINE

Dietary Supplement Health and Education Act of 1994 and Current Good Manufacturing Practices, 40
  Dietary Supplement Health and Education Act of 1994, 40
  Current Good Manufacturing Practices, 40
Commonly Used Herbal Remedies, 41
  Herbal Remedies (A–G), 41
  Herbal Remedies (G–Z), 41

Hazards, Tips, and Resources for Herbal Remedies, 42
  Potential Hazards of Herbs, 42
  Tips for Consumers and Health Care Providers, 42
  Herbal Resources, 42
Clinical Judgment Case Study, 43
Review Questions, 43

Complementary and alternative medicine (CAM) is used by 40% of adults to either augment or replace traditional medical therapies. CAM practices include, but are not limited to, botanicals, nutritional products, and herbal supplements. It is critical for nurses to know about alternative medicine and to note its use in their assessment. CAM products can have both positive and negative effects, and they can interact with prescription and over-the-counter (OTC) medications. Nurses are in an excellent position to educate patients about these interactions.

Botanicals are additive substances that come from plants; an herb is any plant that is used for culinary or medicinal purposes. Plants have been the source of old and new drugs for some time: foxglove is the source of digitalis, snakeroot provides reserpine, willow bark is the source of aspirin, and paclitaxel comes from the Pacific yew tree, just to name a few. The therapeutic value of plants is the basis of phytomedicine. Research into the effects of CAM continues to grow.

Many Americans use botanical dietary supplements for therapeutic or preventive reasons, and herbal therapy has surged in popularity; marketing and media have fueled the demand, with advertisements and promotions on television, in magazines, and on the Internet. In the United States alone, sales have topped the $6 billion mark and are expected to continue to grow.

Few pharmacy schools in the United States offer courses in botanical remedies, but herbal therapy is being addressed in the professional literature with increasing frequency and seriousness. Healthcare providers and consumers are asking questions about herbal therapy's effectiveness, potential toxicity, and reactions with conventional medications. Consumers are right to question advertisements that imply that herbs will cure anything. Herbs can be useful, but they can also be ineffectual or even dangerous.

COMPLEMENTARY AND ALTERNATIVE THERAPIES
Patient Responsibility

To optimize the therapeutic regimen, the patient has the responsibility to (1) consult with the health care provider before taking any herbal preparation, (2) report all herbal preparations taken to all health care providers, (3) inform health care providers of any allergy or sensitivity to any herbal products, (4) use caution if pregnant or lactating, and (5) not take a greater dose than recommended.

In 1992 the US Congress instructed the National Institutes of Health (NIH) to develop an Office of Alternative Medicine to support studies of alternative therapies. This office is now called the *National Center for Complementary and Integrative Health* (NCCIH) and lists current clinical trials with herbal products on its website (www.nccam.nih.gov/research/clinicaltrials). The Natural Standard research collaboration also reviews global literature on herbal studies. These studies are important because CAM cannot be patented, so CAM manufacturers generally cannot justify the expenses associated with safety and efficacy testing in an already booming conventional medicine economy.

This chapter describes selected aspects of herbal therapy, including (1) the Dietary Supplement Health and Education Act of 1994, (2) varieties of herbal preparations, (3) the most commonly used herbs, (4) herbs used to treat selected common ailments, (5) potential hazards of herbs, (6) tips for consumers and health care providers, and (7) herbal resources.

DIETARY SUPPLEMENT HEALTH AND EDUCATION ACT OF 1994 AND CURRENT GOOD MANUFACTURING PRACTICES

Dietary Supplement Health and Education Act of 1994

In 1994 the US Congress enacted the **Dietary Supplement Health and Education Act (DSHEA)**, which defined a dietary supplement as the following:

- Is intended to supplement the diet
- Contains one or more dietary ingredients (including vitamins, minerals, herbs or other botanicals, amino acids, and certain other substances) or their constituents
- Is intended to be taken by mouth, in forms such as tablet, capsule, powder, softgel, gelcap, or liquid
- Is labeled as being a dietary supplement

Although dietary supplements are regulated through the US Food and Drug Administration (FDA), oversight is limited compared with prescription drugs (see http://www.fda.gov/Food/DietarySupplements/default.htm). Manufacturers are required to ensure that their products are safe and that the label information is truthful and not misleading; however, they are not required to demonstrate product safety before the product is sold. Packaging of all dietary supplements must bear the wording "This statement has not been evaluated by the US Food and Drug Administration (FDA). This product is not intended to diagnose, treat, cure, or prevent any disease."

In addition, all labels are required to have the following five components:

1. Name of the supplement
2. Amount of the supplement (net quantity)
3. Nutrition labeling
4. Ingredient list
5. Name and place of the manufacturer, packer, or distributor

Manufacturers of dietary supplements are allowed to make three types of claims: (1) health claims, (2) structure and function claims, and (3) nutrient content claims. To make these claims, manufacturers must have supporting data. The Federal Trade Commission (FTC) is responsible for regulating the truth in advertising related to dietary supplements. Herbal supplements can be marketed with suggested dosages. The physiologic effects of the product can be noted, but no claims can be made about preventing or curing specific conditions. For example, a product label cannot claim that the agent "prevents heart disease," but it can say that the agent "helps increase blood flow to the heart." Health maintenance claims (e.g., "maintains a healthy immune system") and claims for relief of minor symptoms related to life stages (e.g., "alleviates hot flashes") are acceptable because they do not relate to disease. Herbal products using a "may be beneficial" disclaimer, rather than claims of definite benefit, are appropriate legally. Dietary supplement manufacturers are still required to substantiate any claims they make. Consumers are reminded that premarket testing for safety and efficacy is not required, and manufacturing is not standardized.

Current Good Manufacturing Practices

The FDA proposed standards for marketing and labeling dietary supplements in 2003. Known as the **Current Good Manufacturing Practices (CGMPs)**, these standards are multifaceted and require that package labels give the quality and strength of all contents and that products be free of contaminants and impurities (Table 5.1). Manufacturing quality control procedures are part of the CGMPs.

In addition, a *seal of approval* is awarded to products that meet criteria similar to that of the CGMPs by four organizations: the US Pharmacopeial Convention (USP), ConsumerLab.com, National Products Association, and NSF International. The fee-based tests provide information on an herbal product's identity, potency, dissolution, purity, and labeling accuracy. However, the seal of approval is no indication of the product's safety or efficacy.

In November 2019 the Botanical Safety Consortium was established by the FDA, the National Institute of Environmental Health Sciences, and the Health and Environmental Sciences Institute with a mission "to provide a forum to generate a sound scientific basis for integrating existing safety data and the latest toxicology tools to evaluate safety in

TABLE 5.1 Definitions of Herbal Preparations

Preparation	Definition
Decoction	A tea made from boiling plant material—usually the bark, rhizomes, roots, or other woody parts—in water. May be used therapeutically. Natural dyes are often made this way.
Infusion	A tea made by pouring water over plant material (usually dried flowers, fruit, leaves, and other parts, although fresh plant material may also be used); the mixture is then allowed to steep. The water is usually boiling, but cold infusions are also an option. May be used therapeutically; hot tea is an excellent way to administer herbs.
Tincture	An extract of a plant made by soaking herbs in a dark place with a desired amount of either glycerin, alcohol, or vinegar for 2–6 weeks. The liquid is strained from the plant material and then may be used therapeutically.
Liniment	Extract of a plant added to either alcohol or vinegar and applied topically for therapeutic benefits.
Poultice	A therapeutic topical application of a soft, moist mass of plant material (e.g., bruised fresh herbs), usually wrapped in a fine woven cloth.
Essential oils	Aromatic volatile oils extracted from the leaves, stems, flowers, and other parts of plants. Therapeutic use generally includes dilution of the highly concentrated oil.
Herb-infused oils	A process of extraction in which the volatile oils of a plant substance are obtained by soaking the plant in a carrier oil for approximately 2 weeks and then straining the oil. The resulting oil is used therapeutically and may contain the plant's aromatic characteristics.
Percolation	A process to extract the soluble constituents of a plant with the assistance of gravity. The material is moistened and evenly packed into a tall, slightly conical vessel; the liquid (*menstruum*) is then poured onto the material and allowed to steep for a certain length of time. A small opening is then made in the bottom, which allows the extract to slowly flow out of the vessel. The remaining plant material (the *marc*) may be discarded. Many tinctures and liquid extracts are prepared this way.

botanical dietary supplements." More information on the consortium can be found at https://botanicalsafetyconsortium.org/.

COMMONLY USED HERBAL REMEDIES

Most herbal therapies are used to maintain or improve health (Fig. 5.1). This section discusses the most commonly used herbs. The NCCIH (https://nccih.nih.gov/) is an excellent resource for information on herbal therapies not discussed here.

Herbal Remedies (A–G)

Asian Ginseng (*Panax ginseng*)

Asian ginseng is used to increase resistance to environmental stress and improve well-being. It has also been used to improve physical stamina, concentration, and memory; stimulate immune function; and slow the aging process. A previous systematic review of 65 randomized controlled studies indicated that ginseng may improve glucose metabolism; however, the studies were not high quality, and the preparations of ginseng were diverse. Short-term use of the herb appears to be safe; insomnia is the most common side effect. There have also been reports of breast tenderness, menstrual irregularities, and high blood pressure, although it is not known whether it is the herb causing these effects or other components. Patients with diabetes should use caution when taking ginseng, especially if used in conjunction with other herbs or drugs, because hypoglycemia may result. Ginseng may interact with calcium channel blockers and other drugs used to treat high blood pressure, as well as statin drugs and some antidepressants. It may also interact with warfarin.

Chamomile (*Matricaria recutita* and *Chamomilla recutita*)

Chamomile is used primarily to treat sleeplessness, anxiety, and gastrointestinal conditions such as upset stomach, gas, and diarrhea. Little research has been conducted on chamomile; however, there is some evidence that it might be helpful for generalized anxiety disorder. In addition, when combined with other supplements, early evidence indicates there is some benefit for upset stomach and diarrhea in children and colic in infants. There is no evidence that chamomile is helpful in these conditions when taken alone. Side effects include nausea, dizziness, and allergic reactions, ranging from mild skin reactions to anaphylaxis. Allergic reactions are more likely to occur in persons who are allergic to ragweed or other members of the daisy family.

Fig. 5.1 Medicinal herbs. (Copyright © marilyna/iStock/Thinkstock.com.)

Echinacea (*Echinacea purpurea*)

Echinacea is commonly used for colds and upper respiratory conditions. It is thought to stimulate the immune system to fight infection. Research regarding the benefits of echinacea as a treatment for cold symptoms indicates it may slightly reduce the chance of "catching a cold." Short-term use of echinacea is most likely safe; the effects of long-term use are uncertain. The most common side effects are nausea and stomach pain. Some people may have allergic reactions, including rashes.

Garlic (*Allium sativum*)

Garlic is commonly used to help the heart and blood vessels, as well as to lower high blood cholesterol and high blood pressure. Research indicates there may be a slight benefit in the reduction of total cholesterol and low-density lipoprotein cholesterol levels in people with high levels of these blood lipids. There is also limited evidence that garlic may be beneficial for high blood pressure. Garlic is safe in the amounts eaten in foods. Garlic has few side effects but may cause heartburn and upset stomach; it has also been associated with body odor. Because it also reduces blood clotting, patients should be advised to notify their healthcare provider about taking garlic if they are having surgery or dental work. Patients should be cautioned not to take garlic if they have a bleeding disorder or if they are taking the drug saquinavir (a protease inhibitor used in the treatment of human immunodeficiency virus [HIV]). Garlic reduces the effectiveness of saquinavir.

Ginger (*Zingiber officinale*)

Ginger has been used to treat postoperative, pregnancy-related, and chemotherapy-related nausea as well as motion sickness and diarrhea. In addition, it may provide relief from pain, swelling, and stiffness of both osteoarthritis and rheumatoid arthritis. Available research suggests it is effective for the short-term treatment of nausea associated with pregnancy. Evidence is inconclusive concerning its use for motion sickness, as treatment of chemotherapy-induced or postoperative nausea, and in the treatment of arthritis. Side effects of ginger include gas, bloating, heartburn, and nausea.

Ginkgo (*Ginkgo biloba*)

Ginkgo has been used for anxiety, allergies, dementia, eye problems, peripheral artery disease, tinnitus, and other health problems. Although there have been many studies on ginkgo, studies have either been conflicting or unreliable. In a study involving 3000 older adults, it was determined that ginkgo neither prevented dementia nor cognitive decline. Although the evidence is inconclusive, there is some evidence for a slight benefit of taking ginkgo for anxiety, diabetic retinopathy, glaucoma, peripheral artery disease, premenstrual syndrome, schizophrenia, and vertigo. For most people, ginkgo is safe in moderate amounts. Side effects include headache, stomach upset, dizziness, palpitations, constipation, and allergic skin reactions. Ginkgo interacts with anticoagulants and increases the risk of bleeding.

Herbal Remedies (G–Z)

Lavender (*Lavandula angustifolia*)

Lavender has been used for anxiety, depression, and digestive symptoms. However, there have not been any high-quality studies demonstrating effectiveness. Studies do show it might be beneficial for anxiety, but the studies have been small and not generalizable. The use of lavender in the amount put in food is likely to be safe. Topical application may cause allergic skin reactions.

Saw Palmetto (*Serenoa repens*)

Saw palmetto has been used to treat urinary symptoms related to benign prostatic hypertrophy (BPH), chronic pelvic pain, and hair loss.

High-quality research indicates saw palmetto is no more effective than placebo in the treatment of BPH symptoms. Saw palmetto is well tolerated; side effects include digestive issues and headache. No drug interactions are reported.

St. John's Wort (*Hypericum perforatum*)

St. John's wort has been used to treat depression, menopausal symptoms, attention-deficit/hyperactivity disorder (ADHD), somatic symptom disorder, and obsessive-compulsive disorder. Topical use includes treatment of wounds, bruises, and muscle pain. The results of research concerning St. John's wort are mixed; there may be some benefit in patients with mild depression, but it has been reported to be no more effective than placebo in patients with moderate to severe depression. Evidence is insufficient to know if St. John's wort is useful for any other condition. Patients must be cautioned to see their healthcare provider before starting St. John's wort because it interacts with multiple drugs, sometimes in life-threatening ways. St. John's wort interacts in dangerous, sometimes life-threatening ways with a variety of medicines, including antidepressants (which can lead to serotonin syndrome), birth control pills, cyclosporine, digoxin, indinavir, irinotecan, drugs for seizure control, and anticoagulants. Side effects include sensitivity to sunlight, anxiety, dry mouth, dizziness, gastrointestinal problems, fatigue, headache, and sexual dysfunction.

Turmeric (*Curcuma longa*)

Turmeric has been used for arthritis, digestive disorders, respiratory infections, allergies, liver disease, and depression. However, little research has been conducted on the use of turmeric to treat health conditions as its active component, curcuminoids, is unstable and has low oral bioavailability. Turmeric is generally safe when taken in moderate amounts.

HAZARDS, TIPS, AND RESOURCES FOR HERBAL REMEDIES

Potential Hazards of Herbs

> Do not use herbs or other dietary supplements for prevention or treatment of COVID-19. They have not been shown to be effective.

Consumers and health care providers must be alert to potential hazards with herbal therapy; although herbs are natural substances, *natural* does not mean safe. Patients may not disclose the use of herbal products to health care providers for a variety of reasons, including the sense that the health care provider is biased against or not knowledgeable about herbal products or the belief that these products are not considered medications. However, it is essential that health care providers obtain a complete listing of all of the herbal preparations the patient takes in all forms—teas, infusions, tinctures, tablets, and dried herbs—the reason they are taken, and their perceived effectiveness to ensure that they do not interfere with the use and actions of prescribed medications (a 2022 listing of drug-herb interactions can be found at https://my.standardprocess.com/MediHerb-Document-Library/Catalog-Files/herb-drug-interaction-chart.pdf). This assessment should be updated regularly along with information on the patient's OTC and prescription drug use.

Healthcare providers must be alert for possible drug-herb interactions. For example, Asian ginseng induces the drug-metabolizing enzyme CYP3A; when taken in combination with other CYP3A substrates with a narrow therapeutic index, drug levels and therapeutic response should be monitored carefully. Goldenseal has a high potential for drug-herb interaction because it is a potent inhibitor of both CYP3A4 and CYP2D6. St. John's wort has significant documented interactions with cyclosporine, indinavir, oral contraceptives, warfarin, digoxin, and benzodiazepines, among other drugs; it is also a potent inducer of CYP-450 enzymes and intestinal p-glycoprotein.

Some herbal products can also directly affect laboratory test results. Two Chinese alternative therapies, Danshen and Chan Su, are known to interfere with tests to determine digoxin levels. It is *extremely important* that patients taking digoxin avoid these two products!

Not all compounds are safe via all routes. For example, comfrey has both internal and external preparations. Internal use is discouraged because hepatic damage may be fatal. For external use, comfrey is used as an ointment for relief of swelling associated with abrasions and sprains.

Many products have significance for patients facing surgery because they may interfere with the absorption, breakdown, and excretion of anesthetics, anticoagulants, and other surgery-related medications. The American Society of Anesthesiologists suggests patients discontinue herbal therapy beginning 2 to 3 weeks before surgery.

> **COMPLEMENTARY AND ALTERNATIVE THERAPIES**
>
> *Anticoagulants*
>
> The following commonly used herbal products have been reported to interfere with anticoagulants: bilberry, cat's claw, chamomile (German), Dong Quai, feverfew, garlic, ginseng, ginger, ginkgo, licorice, and St. John's wort.

Tips for Consumers and Healthcare Providers

The following are guidelines for prudent use of herbs:
- Do not take herbs without talking to your health care provider first if you are taking any prescription drugs.
- Do not take herbal supplements if you are pregnant, attempting to become pregnant, or are nursing.
- Do not give herbs to infants or young children.
- Follow the label instructions!
- If you experience any side effects that concern you, stop taking the herb and contact your health care provider.
- *Natural* does not mean safe!
- Herbal supplements may contain many compounds, and all of the ingredients may not be known; what is on the label may not be what is in the bottle.

Herbal Resources

It is the responsibility of consumers to educate themselves about herbs before use and to purchase products only from reputable dealers. Determination of the purity and concentration of a particular product can be done only through assays, a costly process; thus, most products have not had appropriate human toxicologic analysis. Many herbal resources are available on the Internet and from print sources, and the reader must evaluate each independently and decide whether the information is credible and appropriate.

CLINICAL JUDGMENT [NURSING PROCESS]
Complementary and Alternative Therapies

Concept: Culture
- Patient beliefs and healthcare practices exhibited by an identified group that are passed down through generations

Concept: Safety
- Protection of patients from potential or actual harm; a basic human need

Concept: Health, Wellness, and Illness
- A continuum of states that patients may experience throughout life. In the provision of holistic nursing care, it is important that nurses understand both conventional drug therapy and complementary and alternative practices.

Recognize Cues [Assessment]
- Assess for the influence of cultural beliefs, norms, and values in the patient's therapeutic regimen.
- Using culturally sensitive, nonjudgmental, and unbiased questioning, assess the following:
  - Which herbs are being used and how long ago were they started?
  - Why is the herb being used?
  - Who recommended the herb?
  - How often and how much of the herb is being taken?
- Assess use of other prescribed and over-the-counter (OTC) drugs and supplements, and include the reason for and duration of use.
- Assess for potential or actual side effects of any drug, herb, or supplement being used.
- Assess for potential or actual drug-drug, drug-herb, or drug-supplement interactions.
- Assess the patient's readiness to learn and literacy skills.

Analyze Cues and Prioritize Hypothesis [Patient Problems]
- Need for health teaching

Generate Solutions [Planning]
- The patient and family will verbalize understanding of herbal therapy, prescription and OTC drugs, interaction between herbal therapy and prescription and OTC drugs, and strategies for optimal participation in the therapeutic regimen.

Take Action [Nursing Interventions]
- Engage patients in the care planning process; provide information supportive of self-management and mutual goal setting; support patients and family choices.
- Consult a dietitian and other specialists as necessary.
- Use an individualized, culturally appropriate approach when discussing the therapeutic regimen.
- Use open-ended questions.
- Due to inconsistencies in manufacturing, advise patients to continue with the same brand of herbal therapy, and advise them to notify their healthcare provider if considering changing brands or preparations.
- Advise patients to first notify their health care provider before substituting any herbal product for a prescription or OTC medication.
- Encourage patients to read labels and heed the recommended information displayed on the label.
- Teach patients about foods that enhance or diminish the action of specific herbs.
- Advise patients about foods to avoid, if any, while taking herbs.
- Advise patients of potential side effects of herbal therapy.
- Counsel patients about symptoms that require prompt reporting to the health care provider.

Evaluate Outcomes [Evaluation]
- Evaluate the perceived effectiveness of herbal remedies for alleviating symptoms.
- Evaluate adherence to the therapeutic regimen.
- Evaluate drug-herb interactions or side effects.
- Evaluate the patient's use of resources.

CLINICAL JUDGMENT CASE STUDY

A 55-year-old is seen in follow-up after being diagnosed with type 2 diabetes. They were prescribed metformin 500 mg twice daily at the last visit. When talking to the patient, they admit they never filled their prescription but took their neighbor's advice instead and began taking cinnamon. The patient states they Googled the spice and found that it is effective at lowering blood sugar. Upon further questioning, they state they just grab a spoon from the drawer and use baking cinnamon and mix a heaping spoonful in their morning tea.

1. What additional information does the nurse need before developing a mutually agreed-upon plan of care?
2. What information should the nurse give the patient concerning the use of cinnamon to treat diabetes?

REVIEW QUESTIONS

1. Which provisions of the Dietary Supplement Health and Education Act (DSHEA) of 1994 are most important for the nurse to know related to patient health teaching? **Select all that apply.**
   a. Clarified marketing regulations
   b. Reclassified herbs as dietary supplements
   c. Stated that herbal products can be marketed with suggested dosages
   d. Required that package labels give quality and strength of all contents
   e. Stated that herbs can be used as drugs

2. The nurse discovers that a patient has recently decided to take four herbal preparations. Which action will the nurse take first?
   a. Discuss the cost of herbal products.
   b. Instruct the patient to inform the health care provider of all products taken.
   c. Instruct the patient to stop taking all herbal products immediately.
   d. Suggest that the patient taper off the use of herbal products over the next 2 weeks.

3. Labeling of herbal products is important. Which claim for an herbal product is appropriate?
   a. Prevents diabetes
   b. Helps increase blood flow to the extremities
   c. Cures Alzheimer disease
   d. Is safe for all
4. The nurse is reviewing a patient's current drug list. Which herbal product interferes with the action of anticoagulants? **Select all that apply.**
   a. Astragalus
   b. Garlic
   c. Ginger
   d. Licorice root
   e. Ginkgo
5. A patient being seen at a cardiovascular clinic mentions he takes garlic. Which statement indicates a need for further patient teaching? **Select all that apply.**
   a. I can just take garlic for my heart problems.
   b. Garlic may provide some decrease in blood pressure.
   c. Garlic is very effective in preventing depression.
   d. Garlic will not cure impotence.
   e. I will need to stop taking my garlic pills before dental work.

6

Pediatric Considerations

http://evolve.elsevier.com/McCuistion/pharmacology

OBJECTIVES

- Summarize the effects of developmental factors in the absorption, distribution, metabolism, and excretion of drugs in pediatric patients, and their impact on pharmacodynamics.
- Discuss nursing implications regarding the dosage and administration of drugs to children.
- Discuss considerations of drug administration in adolescents, including differences in physical, cognitive, and emotional development.
- Describe the role of the nurse in family-centered collaborative care.

OUTLINE

Pharmacokinetics and Pharmacodynamics, 46
   Absorption, 46
   Distribution, 46
   Metabolism, 47
   Excretion, 47
   Pharmacodynamics, 47
Nursing Implications, 47
   Pediatric Drug Dosing and Monitoring, 47
   Pediatric Drug Administration, 47

Considerations for the Adolescent Patient, 48
   Physical Development Considerations, 48
   Cognitive Development Considerations, 48
   Emotional Development Considerations, 49
Family-Centered Collaborative Care, 49
   Family and Patient Teaching, 49
   Over-the-Counter Drug Use, 49
Clinical Judgment Case Study, 50
Review Questions, 50

A nurse who is providing care to children must make certain adaptations in assessment, treatment, and evaluation of nursing care because of the physiologic, psychological, and developmental differences inherent in the pediatric population. This is especially true in the science of pharmacology, in both the administration of drugs to children and evaluation of the therapeutic and adverse effects of a drug. This chapter addresses pediatric nursing adaptations and discusses the effect of a child's growth and development on many aspects of pharmacology: pharmacokinetics, pharmacodynamics, dosing and monitoring, methods of drug administration, and nursing implications.

Pediatric pharmacology is limited to available research in the provision of dosing protocols, safe practices, key assessments, and important nursing implications. Most available information about drugs is derived from studies that use adult samples, small sample sizes, or samples with healthy children. Few studies have been conducted to determine the effectiveness of drugs in the pediatric population. Generalizing the results of studies using adult patients to pediatric populations may result in serious errors and ignores the effect of growth and development on pharmacology.

Research related to pediatric patients is limited because of several factors. Research risks and obtaining informed consent make it difficult to recruit a pediatric sample. Parents and guardians are reluctant to provide permission for children to participate in research studies because of the risk involved and the potentially invasive nature of data gathering. Pharmaceutical companies invest fewer resources in pediatric drug research because of the smaller market share afforded to pediatric drugs. However, many contend that lack of pediatric data reflects lack of due diligence, especially when drugs are administered to pediatric patients without supporting research data on which to base safe practices. As a result, less is known about the effects, uses, and dosages of pediatric drugs, and nurses must investigate pediatric drugs carefully to provide knowledgeable nursing care for children.

⚡ PATIENT SAFETY

Preventing Drug Administration Errors in Pediatric Pharmacology

- Owing to developmental factors and smaller body size, infants and young children may receive drug dosages much different from those of adults. Careful calculations, double-checking math, and checking with another registered nurse can prevent errors in drug administration.
- Ensure that families understand the units of measurement for a drug. Confusion may occur with the discussion of metric, household, and other measurement systems.
- For safety when administering injectable drugs to children, use the smallest syringe that ensures the most exact measurement of the drug.
- Use the correct drug and procedure to ensure safe dosing. Dilutions, different concentrations, and different solutions of a prescribed drug can complicate administration of appropriate pediatric dosages.
- Infants and children may not be able to confirm identity, allergies, or drugs. The nurse must be positive of such information before drug administration.
- Nurses must be vigilant for severe side effects or adverse reactions to drugs because information on pediatric drug response is limited.
- Regulatory agencies caution that drug administration errors are more common in pediatric patients, which warrants increased precautions in drug administration.

Closely aligned with the conflicts that affect pediatric pharmacologic research are those associated with drug labeling and dosing instructions. Because many drugs have not undergone the clinical trials required for federal approval, they have not been approved for pediatric use. Safe use for children may be guided by small studies or the judgment of the clinician and may be based on anecdotal evidence rather than scientific study. These conflicts have generated new legislation designed to protect pediatric patients and provide health care professionals with better information and resources.

Despite the permanent reauthorization of the Pediatric Research Equity Act (PREA) in 2012, which requires drug manufacturers to study pediatric drug use and offers incentives for pediatric pharmacology research, only half of all drugs carry federally approved indications for use in children. This means many drugs prescribed for children are being prescribed off-label, which means the drug is being used for some purpose for which it has not been approved. Current research agendas reinforce the need for pediatric drug research and establishment of safe guidelines for pediatric drug dosing, administration, and evaluation.

PHARMACOKINETICS AND PHARMACODYNAMICS

Significant differences exist in drug pharmacokinetics for pediatric patients versus adults. These distinctions stem from differences in body composition and organ maturity and appear to be more pronounced in neonates and infants but less significant in school-age and adolescent children. Pharmacokinetics may be defined as the study of the time course of drug absorption, distribution, metabolism, and excretion.

Absorption

The degree and rate of drug absorption are based on many factors such as age (Table 6.1), health status, weight, and route of administration. As children grow and develop, the absorption of drugs generally becomes more effective; therefore less-developed absorption in neonates and infants must be considered in dosage and administration. In contrast, poor nutritional habits, changes in physical maturity, and hormonal differences during the adolescent years may cause slowing of drug absorption. Hydration status, presence of underlying disease, and gastrointestinal (GI) disorders in the child may be significant factors in the absorption of drugs.

Drug absorption is initially influenced by the route of administration. For oral drugs, conditions in the stomach and intestine such as gastric acidity, gastric emptying, gastric motility, GI surface area, enzyme levels, and intestinal flora all mediate drug absorption. Lack of maturation of the GI tract is most pronounced in infancy, making the neonatal and infancy periods those most affected by changes in absorption physiology. Gastric pH is alkaline at birth; acid production begins in the neonatal period, and gastric acid secretion reaches adult levels around 2 to 3 years of age. A low pH, or acidic environment, favors acidic drug absorption, whereas a high pH, or alkaline environment, favors basic drug formulations; therefore, differences in pH may hinder or enhance drug absorption. Gastric emptying and GI motility are unpredictable in neonates and infants; however, it approaches that of adults between 6 and 8 months of age. Gastric emptying is affected by feeding, and breastfed infants have faster gastric emptying than formula-fed infants. Unpredictable GI motility may hinder or enhance absorption of oral drugs, depending on the usual site of chemical absorption.

Intestinal surface area in neonates does not reach that of adults until 20 weeks; before this, the reduced surface area leads to reduced drug absorption. Immature enzyme function may also affect drug absorption; neonates have inadequate production of bile salts and pancreatic enzymes, which leads to reduced absorption of lipid-soluble drugs. Intestinal microbial colonization begins in the first few hours after birth and is influenced by gestational age and whether the neonate is breast- or formula-fed; GI microbial colonization reaches adult levels in adolescence. All these factors must be considered when assessing the effectiveness of drugs administered by the oral route.

For drugs administered via the subcutaneous (subcut) or intramuscular (IM) routes, absorption occurs at the tissue level. The level of peripheral perfusion and effectiveness of circulation affects drug absorption. Conditions that alter perfusion—dehydration, cold temperatures, and alterations in cardiac status—may impede absorption of drugs in the tissues. Intravenous (IV) drugs are administered directly into the bloodstream and are immediately absorbed and distributed.

The skin of infants and young children is thinner than that of adults; in addition, the ratio of body surface area to body mass of infants and children is proportionately higher than for adults such that many drugs are more readily absorbed in children, and toxicity may result.

Distribution

Drug distribution is affected by factors such as body fluid composition, body tissue composition, protein-binding capability, and effectiveness of various barriers to drug transport. In neonates and infants, the body is about 75% water, compared with 60% in adults. This increased body fluid proportion allows for a greater volume of fluid in which to distribute drugs, which results in a lower drug concentration. Until about age 2 years, the pediatric patient requires higher doses of water-soluble drugs to achieve therapeutic levels. Younger patients also have higher levels of extracellular fluids, which increase the tendency for children to become dehydrated and changes the distribution of water-soluble drugs. Compared with older children, neonates and infants have fat stores with an increased ratio of water to lipids, which alters the distribution of some lipid-soluble drugs. Close monitoring of drug levels (e.g., antiepileptic drugs) can help ensure drug safety.

To varying degrees, drugs become bound to circulating plasma proteins in the body. Only drugs that are free, or unbound, are available to cross the cell membrane and exert their effect. Neonates and infants have decreased protein concentrations compared with adults, and they have fewer protein receptor sites with an affinity for drug binding in the first 12 months after birth; this results in higher levels of unbound drug and an increased risk of drug toxicity.

In neonates, high bilirubin levels may pose a health risk related to drug administration. Bilirubin molecules may bind with protein receptor sites, which makes the sites unavailable to drugs or displaces drugs from binding sites, allowing large amounts of drug to remain free and available for effect. When drugs are prescribed to neonates, dosages must be decreased and closely monitored to both avoid adverse effects and ensure therapeutic effectiveness.

Anatomic barriers to drug distribution, such as the blood-brain barrier (BBB), must be considered when drugs are administered to

TABLE 6.1	Pediatric Age Classification
Classification	**Age**
Neonate	Birth through 28 days
Infant/toddler	29 days to less than 2 years
Children	2 years to less than 12 years
Adolescent	Aged 12 through 21 (up to but not including the 22nd birthday)

From US Food and Drug Administration. *Pediatric Medical Devices.* Author; 2023. https://www.fda.gov/medical-devices/products-and-medical-procedures/pediatric-medical-devices.

pediatric patients. This barrier in neonates is relatively immature and allows drugs to pass easily into central nervous system (CNS) tissue, thereby increasing the likelihood for toxicity. As a child matures, the BBB becomes more impervious to drugs, and drug dosages must be titrated accordingly.

Metabolism

The metabolism of drugs depends greatly on the maturation level of the pediatric patient and varies from child to child. Metabolism is carried out primarily in the liver, with the kidneys and lungs playing a small part in metabolism. Infants have reduced hepatic blood flow and drug-metabolizing enzymes; however, by the time they reach 1 year of age, hepatic blood flow has reached that of an adult. Although drug-metabolizing enzymes reach an adult level at around 11 years of age, it is important to understand that the isoenzymes involved in the cytochrome P450 system—CYP1, CYP2, and CYP3—develop at different rates and demonstrate individual variation. Drug prescribing should be based on therapeutic effect and drug concentration. Such differences in drug metabolism, as with other pharmacokinetic factors, reinforce the importance of the nurse evaluating therapeutic effects and monitoring the adverse effects of drugs.

Excretion

Renal excretion is the predominant means of drug elimination. The glomerular filtration rate (GFR) in term neonates is roughly 30% that of adults. During infancy, the GFR rises, and by 12 months it reaches adult levels. Nurses must carefully monitor renal function, urine flow, and drug effectiveness to evaluate the effect of drug administration on patient status.

Pharmacodynamics

Pharmacodynamics refers to the mechanisms of action and effects of a drug on the body and includes the onset, peak, and duration of effect of a drug. It can also be described as the intensity and time course of therapeutic and adverse effects of drugs. The variables of pharmacokinetics—absorption, distribution, metabolism, and excretion—all affect the parameters of pharmacodynamics. These processes determine the time a drug begins to function, reaches its peak, and sustains its length of action. Variables such as organ function, developmental factors, and administration issues affect drug pharmacodynamics and drug half-life in pediatric patients, and these influence drug dosing.

NURSING IMPLICATIONS

Pediatric Drug Dosing and Monitoring

Because of the changes in pharmacokinetics and pharmacodynamics inherent in pediatric patients, a key nursing role is to monitor the patient for therapeutic effect and adverse reactions. The processes described earlier in the chapter may be measured using plasma or serum drug levels, which indicate the amount of drug in a patient's body. The therapeutic ranges established for many drug levels are based on adult studies; therefore, close monitoring of serum drug levels can assist in establishing appropriate dosages, schedules, and routes of administration. Monitoring can also assist in indicating when the dose is subtherapeutic or becomes toxic. Serum blood levels are not available for all drugs, so patient clinical responses to drugs are especially important when monitoring drug effects.

The calculation of pediatric dosages is based in part on US Food and Drug Administration (FDA) recommendations; however, only about 20% of drugs are labeled for pediatric use. For those drugs without pediatric dosing schedules, dosing is based on approved protocols, research studies, and provider experience. Drugs for pediatric patients are ordered based on either the child's weight in kilograms (mg/kg) or body surface area (BSA; or mg/m^2). Body surface is based on a percentage of adult surface area (1.73 m^2). Dosing must also consider the individual child's status, including age, organ function, health, and route of administration.

Pediatric Drug Administration

Developmental and cognitive differences must always be considered in pediatric drug administration. It is important for the nurse to differentiate the child's developmental age from chronologic age because this difference influences the child's response to drug administration. The pediatric patient's ability to understand the process, the reason for drug administration, and the need to cooperate with the procedure must always figure prominently in the nurse's plan of care. The child's temperament may influence understanding and level of cooperation. The concept of family-centered care is essential to ensure safety during and after health care interventions, especially drug administration. Teaching is directed toward both family members or caregivers and patients, commensurate with the cognitive level of the child. When possible, family members or caregivers should be asked to assist in drug administration. These significant people in the child's life, individuals who see the child on a day-to-day basis, are usually in the best position to evaluate the effectiveness of a drug and observe for adverse reactions. Some adverse drug reactions in children, such as ringing in the ears and nausea, may be difficult to evaluate; those closest to the child may be in the best position to assess for these reactions. However, family members or caregivers may request not to participate in invasive procedures such as injections. This request should be respected, and family members or caregivers should be encouraged to provide comfort to the child after drugs are administered. Family members or caregivers should always be supported in their caring function so that the child feels safe and secure.

Pediatric patients must be assessed for the ability to understand the reason for the drug, the need for the drug despite unpleasant taste or method of administration, and the need to complete all doses and courses of the drug. When the family is taught about pediatric drug administration, education for the child at a developmentally appropriate level must also be included. Communication with the child and family members or caregivers must always consider level of knowledge, developmental age, cultural factors, and anxiety levels. The nurse should use optimal interpersonal skills to ensure the best outcome in drug administration to pediatric patients.

The primary concerns in drug administration to infants are maintaining safety and providing care while ensuring as much comfort as possible. Family members or caregivers must be able to practice and repeat the psychomotor skills associated with drug administration. The following are tips to enhance safe drug administration and facilitate comfort:

- Toddlers may react violently and negatively to drug administration. Simple explanations, a firm approach, and enlisting the imagination of a toddler through play may enhance success.
- Preschoolers are cooperative and respond well to age-appropriate explanations. Allowing some level of choice and control may facilitate success with preschool children.
- School-age children, although often cooperative, may fear bodily injury and should be permitted even more control, involvement in the process, and information.
- Age-appropriate fears related to pain, changes in body image, and injury are prevalent among older school-age and adolescent patients. The nurse should establish a positive rapport with the patient, develop the plan of care in collaboration with the patient, and ensure privacy in all aspects of drug administration.

Atraumatic care principles should be used when possible. Donna Wong's **Principle of Atraumatic Care** is the philosophy of providing therapeutic care using interventions that eliminate or minimize the psychological and physical distress experienced by children and families. Atraumatic care is achieved by decreasing the separation of children from their family members or caregivers, identifying family and patient stressors, decreasing pain, and providing care within the framework of a collaborative partnership.

Most pediatric drugs are administered orally because this route is the least invasive and easiest to administer by family members or caregivers. Topical, rectal, and parenteral routes are also used to deliver drugs to pediatric patients for whom the oral route is contraindicated. Choice of route of administration is based on age, drug to be administered, and comorbidities. Because of tissue differences among children, the IV route is more predictable than other routes.

Most oral drugs administered to children younger than 6 years of age are given using an oral syringe. Oral syringes ensure more exact dosing and are relatively easy to use. Syringes may be marked to ensure correct dosages. The syringe is inserted into either side of the mouth and is pointed toward the buccal mucosa. Depositing the drug too close to the front of the mouth increases the likelihood that it will be spit out. Pointing the syringe directly toward the back of the mouth may increase the risk of gagging or choking. Infants may suck drugs from a bottle nipple into which the measured drug has been squirted from an oral syringe. Preschool and school-age children are usually able to inject oral drugs into their own mouths, enhancing their sense of control over what can be an anxiety-provoking situation.

Nurses may need to crush pills or dissolve the contents of capsules in fluid for administration to pediatric patients. The nurse should work closely with the pharmacist and in compliance with hospital policies to determine the advisability of crushing or dissolving a drug before administration; some drugs, particularly timed-release and enteric-coated drugs, should *not* be crushed or dissolved. Some drugs may be made more palatable by adding jam, yogurt, or honey (although infants younger than 1 year should not be given honey because of the risk of botulism). Small volumes (10 mL) should be used to dilute drugs, so the patient is ensured the full dose. For children who require tube feeding, oral drugs can be administered via nasogastric, orogastric, or gastrostomy tubes, if the drugs can be crushed or dissolved before administration.

When drug injection or venipuncture is necessary, topical anesthetic protocols may be followed to reduce the pain associated with the procedure. Agents such as eutectic mixture of local anesthetics (EMLA), topical liposomal 4% lidocaine cream (LMX4), or a vapocoolant spray may be effective in reducing the pain and fear associated with invasive procedures, such as injection or venipuncture, in children. However, current research into vapocoolants (a product which contains a liquified gas to rapidly cool the skin and provide some pain relief) indicates that while they are effective in adults, vapocoolants are ineffective in children.

Based on the cognitive level of the child, other nonpharmacologic methods of pain and anxiety control such as distraction, diversion, relaxation, and creative imagery can also be used to decrease the perception of pain. Injections should *never* be given to a sleeping child with the intent to surprise the child with a quick procedure. The child may subsequently experience a lack of trust and may be reluctant to sleep in the future.

IV infusion sites must be protected, especially in infants and toddlers, who do not understand the rationale or importance of maintaining the IV site. Commercial products are available to protect the IV site and maintain an intact IV infusion set. Stocking-like covers may hide the IV site from infants before they master the concept of object permanence. The patency of an IV site should be checked before each drug administration to avoid infiltration and extravasation. Any injection site on a preschooler should be covered with a bandage, preferably a decorated one, so that the child does not fear "leakage" from the area. Selection of injection and IV sites is made based on developmental variables, site of preference, and access to administration sites. The ventrogluteal or vastus lateralis are preferred sites for pediatric IM injections. The length of the needle depends on the child's muscle mass, their subcutaneous tissue, and the site of injection. Children may prefer subcutaneous injections in the leg or upper arm rather than in the abdomen. IV sites may be difficult to find in children. The amount of fatty tissue, hydration status of the child, and ability to isolate and immobilize veins are all mitigating factors.

When administering drugs to children, follow these basic principles: honesty, respect, age-appropriate teaching and explanations, attention to safety, atraumatic care, use of the least amount of restraint necessary (e.g., swaddling a neonate), providing positive reinforcement for age-appropriate cooperation, refraining from use of negative messages or behaviors, and upholding family-centered principles. These standards may be used throughout the pediatric life span and highlight the need for nursing interventions that are sensitive, individualized, and caring.

CONSIDERATIONS FOR THE ADOLESCENT PATIENT

Adolescent patients need individualized nursing care specific to their developmental stage. Age-oriented developmental considerations include physical changes, cognitive level and abilities, emotional factors, and effects of chronic illness.

Physical Development Considerations

Physically, adolescence is a highly diverse period of growth and development. Growth rates during these years may be affected by nutrition, factors within the environment, genetics and heredity, and sex. A group of adolescents of similar ages may manifest very different sizes, height-to-weight proportions, timing of secondary sex characteristics, and other indicators of physical maturity. These differences may warrant individualization of drug dosage based on weight or body surface area, even when the adolescent meets or exceeds the size of standard adults. For example, an adjustment may be required in the dosage of a lipid-soluble drug because of the changes in lean-to-fat body mass, especially in young adolescent males, which coincide with physical maturation. Hormonal changes and growth spurts may necessitate changes in drug dosages; many children with chronic illnesses require dosage adjustments in the early teen years because of these transitions. Sleep requirements and metabolic rates may greatly increase during the teen years, along with appetite and food consumption, which may affect the scheduling of and response to drugs. Although adolescents' physical appearance and organ structure and function resemble those of adults, their bodies continue to grow and change; this requires increased vigilance in monitoring therapeutic and toxic drug levels.

Cognitive Development Considerations

The cognitive level and abilities of adolescents may pose additional considerations. Cognitive theorists have posited that adolescents progress from concrete to abstract reasoning. Individuals who are still in the concrete operational stage may have difficulty comprehending how a drug exerts its effects on the body and the importance of meticulous dosing and administration. Adolescents may also have difficulty understanding such concepts as drug interactions, side effects, adverse reactions, and therapeutic levels. For example, the patient taking birth control pills may or may not be able to comprehend the reduced action of birth control pills caused by antibiotics taken during an acute infection and may fail to take extra precautions to prevent pregnancy.

An understanding of the adolescent brain and the ongoing development of social, reasoning, and decision-making skills can be used to guide nursing assessment and interventions with the pediatric patient. As adolescents learn to reason in an abstract manner, teaching may be based on more complex information. Potentially, adolescent perception of invulnerability and difficulty relating future consequences to current actions may dictate that the nurse adapts teaching to address specific adolescent thought processes. An adolescent who is told that an insulin injection schedule must be followed to avoid long-term complications may not understand the rationale for treatment if it is only substantiated by abstract, future-oriented risks. The same patient may find the relationship between using insulin to maintain normoglycemia and the ability to participate in sports more immediate and relevant. Allowing the adolescent to verbalize concerns about the drug and its regimen may offer opportunities for clarifying misconceptions and teaching new concepts.

Emotional Development Considerations

Emotional development of the adolescent also occurs on an individual basis. The adolescent years are characterized by sensation seeking, risk taking, questioning, formation of identity, and increasing influences exerted by peer groups. To avoid potential drug interactions, the nurse should assess for high-risk behaviors that include use of alcohol, tobacco, and recreational drugs. Other issues, including sexual practices and stressful family and social situations, may affect the patient's response to drugs. Nurses must be respectful of the emotional needs of adolescents while attending to the mental health issues that may surface during these years. A comprehensive history must be solicited from adolescent patients to ensure appropriate drug administration. The nurse must also be conscious of the need to exercise care in offering confidentiality if information needs to be divulged to other health care providers, family members, or caregivers to ensure patient safety.

As adolescents attain greater levels of independence from their parents, self-care behaviors increase. The nurse should assess the patient's abilities to self-administer drugs and monitor therapeutic and adverse reactions. Adolescents spend less time with family members and caregivers and may need increased instruction about their drug regimen and the key observations that are needed. Although adolescents frequently display "breaking away" behaviors in response to parental bonds, they often continue to use family members or caregiver drug habits as models for their own drug behaviors.

For the pediatric patient with a chronic illness, issues may change during adolescence. Engaging peers in the plan of care for drug administration, allowing the adolescent to make safe choices and have flexibility within that plan, setting up mutual drug contracts, and permitting the patient to design their own adult-monitored drug regimen may facilitate adherence. The nurse can facilitate required adaptations and support both the patient and family members during these times.

FAMILY-CENTERED COLLABORATIVE CARE

In working with pediatric patients, key developmental differences must be considered when administering and monitoring drugs. The nursing process provides the framework to guide nursing practice in administering drugs, planning and evaluating nursing care, providing patient and family teaching, and incorporating the family in all aspects of treatment.

Family and Patient Teaching

Family and patient teaching is a key role for the nurse. Issues such as indications for the drug, the side effects, the dose, how to measure the dose, how to administer the dose, the therapeutic effect, adverse effects to monitor for, the duration, and the frequency are all important information needed by the family or caregiver. Specifics such as the need for refrigeration, the need to shake the medicine, the difference between household and prescriptive measurements, and other issues should be addressed to ensure patient safety. Adherence to the drug regimen is of paramount importance with children and families; providing written instructions or a drug calendar may facilitate this through concrete reminders.

Over-the-Counter Drug Use

Nurses should also be aware of the tendency for parents to treat infants and children with over-the-counter (OTC) analgesics. Parents may provide frequent analgesia to their children and may be largely unaware of the potential for misuse and overuse in the pediatric population. Additional concern has arisen regarding the inappropriate use of OTC cough and cold remedies with children. Deaths and significant illness have been attributed to lack of label recommendations, misuse of adult drugs, poor drug instructions, and overdose, which warrants rigid restrictions on the use of these drugs in the pediatric population.

◎ CLINICAL JUDGMENT [NURSING PROCESS]
Pediatric Considerations

Concept: Safety
- Protection of the patient from potential or actual harm; a basic human need.

Concept: Health, Wellness, and Illness
- Health, wellness, and illness are a dynamic response to a continuum of biopsychosocial states experienced through all stages of life.

Concept: Illness
- Illness is an abnormal process where function is altered in comparison to previous status.

Recognize Cues [Assessment]
- Assess the context and meaning of illness.
- Assess the influence of cultural beliefs and values on the knowledge base.
- Assess developmental age, health status, nutritional status, and hydration status.
- Assess family members and caregiver health literacy level and the child's cognitive level.
- Assess family patterns, economic issues, and cultural patterns that influence adherence to a therapeutic regimen.
- Assess learning style.
- Assess readiness to learn.
- Assess the allergy history of the child, and determine family allergy history.
- Identify all of the patient's drugs (prescriptions, over-the-counter, and herbal).
- Record the age, weight, and height of the child. Drug calculations are based on these three factors.

Analyze Cues and Prioritize Hypothesis [Patient Problems]
- Need for health teaching
- Anxiety

Continued

CLINICAL JUDGMENT [NURSING PROCESS]—CONT'D

Pediatric Considerations

Generate Solutions [Planning]
- Family members and caregivers, as well as the pediatric patient, if appropriate, will recognize the need for drug administration.
- Family members and caregivers, as well as the pediatric patient if appropriate, will describe the rationale for drug therapy.
- Family members and caregivers, as well as the pediatric patient if appropriate, will incorporate the drug treatment regimen into their lifestyle.
- Family members and caregivers, as well as the pediatric patient, if appropriate, will demonstrate safe drug administration practices.
- Family members and caregivers, as well as the pediatric patient if appropriate, will state with confidence their ability to manage the treatment regimen and remain in control of their life.
- The pediatric patient will remain free of drug-related injuries.

Take Action [Nursing Interventions]
- Assist the patient, family members, and caregivers with appropriate follow-up resources and support.
- Avoid the use of restraints.
- Engage the patient, family members, and caregivers as partners in the educational process.
- Follow all rights of safe drug administration.
- Help patients, their family members, and caregivers manage complex drug schedules.
- Reconcile the drug list at discharge, and provide the list to the patient, family members, and caregivers as appropriate.
- Support patient, family member, and caregiver priorities, preferences, and choices.
- Use at least two methods of patient identification.
- Use open-ended questions, and encourage two-way communication.
- Consider the use of alternative settings for teaching the chronically ill pediatric patient, their family members, and caregivers.
- Provide a developmentally appropriate environment when addressing the health education needs of adolescents.
- Provide educational materials in the preferred language of patients, family members, and caregivers.
- Provide information to support self-efficacy, self-regulation, and self-management of the drug regimen.
- Use educational strategies that are interactive and engaging for younger children and toddlers.
- Use family-centered approaches when teaching children and adolescents.
- Use strategies to promote motivation and sustain learning.

Evaluate Outcomes [Evaluation]
- Evaluate the child's physiologic and psychological response to the drug regimen.
- Evaluate the family member's knowledge about the drug, the dosage, the schedule for administration, and the side effects.
- Evaluate the therapeutic and adverse effects of the drug(s).

CLINICAL JUDGMENT CASE STUDY

A 9-month-old infant weighing 20 pounds comes to the emergency department with a 3-day history of vomiting, fever greater than 102.5°F, and significant pain. Physical assessment reveals acute otitis media, for which the health care provider prescribed amoxicillin susp 400 mg twice a day for 10 days and ibuprofen 2.5 mL every 6 hours.

1. Which nursing assessments must take place before administration of amoxicillin?
2. How will the nurse instruct the family member to administer the drugs safely?

REVIEW QUESTIONS

1. A 4-year-old patient is discharged on an oral liquid drug suspension of 4 mL per dose. Which device will the nurse recommend ensuring the highest level of accuracy in home administration of the drug?
   a. Measuring spoon
   b. Graduated medicine cup
   c. Household teaspoon
   d. Oral syringe
2. Which pharmacokinetic principle does the nurse consider when administering drugs to children?
   a. Most children need a higher dose of drug, so the nurse will contact the physician for an increase in the ordered dose.
   b. Children excrete drugs rapidly, so the nurse must assess carefully for therapeutic effects of the drug.
   c. The most important assessment is to evaluate for drug accumulation because the excretion of drugs is slower in children.
   d. Excretion of most drugs is the same in children as in adults, but assessments are important to avoid side effects.
3. A parent is learning to administer drug to a school-age child. Which strategy will the nurse teach the parent to achieve cooperation in a child of this age?
   a. Enlisting physical restraint
   b. Establishing drug contracts
   c. Providing age-appropriate explanations
   d. Tolerating violent reactions
4. A nurse caring for a child with developmental delay prepares to teach the patient about their prescribed drugs. Which actions are essential to ensure patient safety? **Select all that apply.**
   a. Assess the child's developmental age.
   b. Assess for side effects the same as those experienced by adults.
   c. Consider the actions and uses of the drug.
   d. Focus on the child's chronologic age.
   e. Involve the family in teaching sessions.

5. Which components are part of the Principle of Atraumatic Care? **Select all that apply.**
   a. Reducing any pain associated with drug administration.
   b. Development of a collaborative partnership with the family during drug administration.
   c. Restraining infants during drug administration.
   d. Keeping the child apart from family members when administering drugs.
   e. Reducing the child's stress during drug administration.

6. Which strategies are helpful when working with adolescent patients to promote adherence? **Select all that apply.**
   a. Allow flexibility in the treatment plan.
   b. Use future-oriented examples and consequences to support the need for drug therapy.
   c. Guarantee the adolescent patient's privacy when obtaining history.
   d. Set up a mutually developed drug contract.
   e. Understanding the adolescent's sexual practices is not necessary to promote adherence.

7

Drug Therapy in Older Adults

http://evolve.elsevier.com/McCuistion/pharmacology

OBJECTIVES

- Describe the physiological changes in the older adult that influence pharmacokinetic processes and pharmacodynamic responses.
- Discuss nursing implications regarding the administration of drugs to older adults.

OUTLINE

Physiologic Changes, 52
    Pharmacokinetics, 52
    Pharmacodynamics, 54
Nursing Implications: Older Adult Drug Dosing and Monitoring, 54
    Polypharmacy, 54
    Beers Criteria for Potentially Inappropriate Medication Use in Older Adults, 54

Adverse Drug Events, 54
Adherence, 54
Health Teaching With the Older Adult, 55
Clinical Judgment Case Study, 56
Review Questions, 56

By 2030 all baby boomers will be older than 65 years of age. There are expected to be more than 82 million older adults by the year 2050. These numbers are staggering, considering 92% of older adults have at least one chronic illness, and more than 75% of older adults have two chronic illnesses. Typically, persons with two or more chronic conditions take five or more prescription drugs.

More than half of all older adults use at least one over-the-counter (OTC) drug, and nearly three-quarters of older adults use at least one supplement to augment their prescription drugs; however, older adults are more likely to experience adverse reactions or drug interactions related to OTC drugs and supplements, many times resulting in hospitalization.

Administration of drugs in the older adult population requires special attention to age-related factors that influence drug absorption, distribution, metabolism, and excretion. Drug dosages are often adjusted according to the older adult's weight, laboratory results (e.g., liver enzymes and glomerular filtration), and comorbid health problems. Because of altered organ function in the older adult, the effects of drug therapy must be closely monitored to prevent adverse reactions and possible toxicity.

Drug toxicity may develop in the older adult for drug doses within the therapeutic range for the younger adult. These therapeutic drug ranges are usually safe for young and middle-aged adults but are not always within the safe range for older adults. It has been suggested that drugs for older adults should initially be prescribed at low dosages with a gradual increase in dosage based on therapeutic response; this practice is commonly stated as *start low and go slow*. This approach to drug prescribing reduces the chance of drug toxicity.

Common characteristics in older adults that increase the risk for problems with drug administration include lack of coordinated care, recent discharge from the hospital, self-treatment, multiple diagnoses, sensory and physical changes associated with aging, multiple health care providers, and cognitive impairment.

PHYSIOLOGIC CHANGES

Physiologic changes associated with aging can influence absorption, distribution, metabolism, and excretion of drugs as well as pharmacodynamic responses at receptors and target organs. These physiologic changes include the following:

- A reduction in total body water and lean body mass, resulting in increased body fat, which alters the volume of distribution of drugs.
- A reduction in kidney mass and lower kidney blood flow, leading to a reduced glomerular filtration rate (GFR) and reduced clearance of drugs excreted by the kidneys.
- A reduction in liver size and blood flow, resulting in reduced hepatic clearance of drugs.

A decline in the physiologic processes that maintain equilibrium in the older adult may mean a higher incidence of adverse effects. Examples of this include:

- Postural hypotension in response to drugs that reduce blood pressure
- Volume depletion and electrolyte imbalance in response to diuretics
- Excessive bleeding with anticoagulant and antiplatelet drugs
- Altered glycemic response to antidiabetic drugs
- Gastrointestinal (GI) irritation with nonsteroidal antiinflammatory drugs (NSAIDs)

Physiologic changes with aging affect the determination of risk versus benefit underlying drug choice, dose, and frequency.

Pharmacokinetics

Pharmacologic processes have not received adequate study in the older adult; therefore a thorough understanding of pharmacokinetics is necessary for the safe administration of drugs in this population.

Absorption

Adults experience several GI changes with aging that may influence drug absorption. These include a decrease in small bowel surface area, slowed gastric emptying, reduced gastric blood flow, and a 5% to 10% decrease in gastric acid production. These changes are not always clinically relevant; however, calcium carbonate is affected by the decreased gastric acidity. Older adults should be prescribed calcium citrate, which requires a less acidic environment for dissolution. Other common problems that occur in older adults that can significantly influence drug absorption include swallowing difficulties, poor nutrition, and dependence on feeding tubes.

Distribution

Aging can significantly alter drug distribution. With aging, adults experience a decline in muscle mass and a 20% to 40% increase in fat. The increase in body fat means lipid-soluble drugs have a greater volume of distribution, increased drug storage, reduced elimination, and a prolonged period of action. Older adults have a 10% to 15% reduction in total body water, which affects water-soluble drugs, and a 10% reduction in albumin. Reduced albumin levels can result in decreased protein binding of drugs and increased free drug available to exert therapeutic effects, but it also increases the risk for drug toxicity.

Metabolism

Hepatic blood flow in the older adult may be decreased by 40%; aging also results in a 15% to 30% decrease in liver size and a reduction in cytochrome P450 (CYP450) enzyme activity, which is responsible for the breakdown of drugs. Drug clearance by hepatic metabolism can be reduced by these age-related changes. A reduction in hepatic metabolism can decrease first-pass metabolism and can prolong a drug's half-life, resulting in increased drug levels and potential drug toxicity. Nurses must be aware of these metabolic changes and must monitor response to drug therapy to avoid adverse reactions.

To assess liver function, liver enzymes must be checked. Elevated levels of alanine aminotransferase (ALT) and aspartate aminotransferase (AST) may indicate possible liver dysfunction, as well as elevated alkaline phosphatase (ALP), gamma-glutamyl transferase (GGT), L-lactate dehydrogenase (LD), and bilirubin. However, an older adult can have normal liver function test (LFT) results and still have impaired hepatic enzyme activity.

Excretion

Renal excretion of drugs decreases with age. Excretion is altered by age-related changes in kidney function, such as decreased renal size and volume, which differ for everyone. However, it is generally accepted that the GFR declines by 1 mL/min after 40 years of age (normal GFR is 100–125 mL/min). Despite a decline in kidney function, an individual's creatinine may remain normal as they age due to a decline in muscle mass and activity. Changes in kidney function affect many drugs, leading to a prolonged half-life and elevated drug levels. Changes in kidney function require dosage adjustment, especially if the drug has a narrow therapeutic range.

GFR can be calculated using the Cockcroft-Gault formula, which is the formula recommended by the US Food and Drug Administration and therefore used by pharmaceutical manufacturers when determining dosage adjustments:

$$C_{Cr} = \left[(140 - \text{Age}) \times \frac{\text{Weight}}{72 \times S_{Cr}} \times 0.85 (\text{If female})\right]$$

where

C_{Cr} (creatinine clearance) = mL/min
Age = years
Weight = kg
S_{Cr} (serum creatinine) = mg/dL

However, it can also be estimated by many calculators found on the Internet (www.globalrph.com/crcl.htm).

Nurses must have a general understanding of drug classifications that require dosage adjustment in patients with chronic kidney disease. The mnemonic *BANDD CAMP* (Table 7.1) may be helpful in remembering the drug classifications; however, nurses should not rely on their memory for drug administration. Package inserts, up-to-date drug reference books, and reputable websites (www.globalrph.com/index_renal.htm) maintain current dosing information.

TABLE 7.1 Drug Classes That Require Dosage Adjustment in Chronic Kidney Disease

	Drug Class	Adjust Dose	Avoid in Stages 4 and 5
B	Beta-blockers	Acebutolol, atenolol, bisoprolol, nadolol, sotalol	Sotalol
A	ACEIs/ARBs	All ACEIs	Olmesartan
N	NSAIDs, opioids	Codeine, morphine, oxycodone, tramadol	All NSAIDs, meperidine
D	Diuretics	Potassium-sparing diuretics, thiazide diuretics	Potassium-sparing diuretics, thiazide diuretics
D	Diabetic medications	Gliclazide, acarbose, insulin, gliptins	Glyburide, metformin, exenatide
C	Cholesterol medications	Pravastatin, rosuvastatin, fibrates	—
A	Antimicrobials (dose reductions are often delayed for 24–48 h to allow for aggressive dosing and for the drug to reach steady state)	Antibiotics: Most antibiotics except cloxacillin, clindamycin, metronidazole, erythromycin, azithromycin; Antifungals: Fluconazole, itraconazole; Antivirals: Acyclovir, famciclovir, valacyclovir	Nitrofurantoin
M	Miscellaneous	Allopurinol, colchicine, digoxin, H_2RAs	New anticoagulants
P	Psychotropics	Lithium, gabapentin, pregabalin, topiramate, vigabatrin, bupropion, duloxetine, paroxetine, venlafaxine	—

ACEI, Angiotensin-converting enzyme inhibitor; *ARB*, angiotensin II receptor blocker; *h*, hours; H_2RA, histamine-2 receptor antagonist; *NSAID*, nonsteroidal antiinflammatory drug.
From Meyer D, Damm T, Jensen K: *Drug dosage adjustments in chronic kidney disease: the pharmacist's role*, Saskatchewan Drug Information Services College of Pharmacy and Nutrition, 2012, University of Saskatchewan. www.rxfiles.ca/rxfiles/uploads/documents/ltc/HCPs/CKD/SDIS Renal_newsletter.pdf

Pharmacodynamics

Pharmacodynamic responses to drugs are altered with aging because of changes in the number of receptor sites, which affect the affinity of certain drugs. These changes are seen most clearly in the cardiovascular system and central nervous system (CNS).

Older adults experience a loss of sensitivity in adrenergic receptors, affecting both agonists and antagonists; this results in a reduced response to beta-blockers and $beta_2$ agonists. Older adults also experience a blunting in compensatory reflexes leading to orthostatic hypotension and falls.

With age, there is a reduction in dopaminergic and cholinergic receptors, neurons, and available neural connections in the brain. There is reduced blood flow to the brain, and the blood-brain barrier also becomes more permeable. This puts the older adult at risk for CNS drug side effects, which include dizziness, seizures, confusion, sedation, and extrapyramidal effects.

NURSING IMPLICATIONS: OLDER ADULT DRUG DOSING AND MONITORING

Polypharmacy

Polypharmacy refers to the use of more medications than is medically necessary. There is little agreement on the actual number of drugs that constitute polypharmacy, but researchers use five drugs because this number has been associated with increased incidence of adverse drug reactions, geriatric syndromes, and increased mortality.

Risk factors associated with polypharmacy include advanced age, female sex, multiple health care providers, use of herbal therapies and OTC drugs, multiple chronic diseases, and the number of hospitalizations and care transitions. Polypharmacy can cause an increase in geriatric syndromes (cognitive impairment, falls, decreased functional status, urinary incontinence, pressure injury, delirium, and weight loss) as well as an increased incidence of adverse drug reactions and poor adherence.

Pharmacotherapy in older adults is complex. To reduce the risk for and incidence of polypharmacy, nurses must be involved in the coordination of care for older adults. Older adults should be encouraged to use only one pharmacy and should give the pharmacist a list of all the drugs taken—prescribed, herbal, and OTC. A properly informed pharmacist will be able to conduct a clinical review of the patient's drugs to ensure the appropriateness of therapy. A pharmacist can also confirm patient understanding of individual therapy and can monitor responses to drug therapy. All of this is done to improve the overall quality of life of patients in their care.

Beers Criteria for Potentially Inappropriate Medication Use in Older Adults

The American Geriatrics Society Beers Criteria for Potentially Inappropriate Medication Use in Older Adults is a document developed by an interdisciplinary expert panel in geriatric care to aid healthcare providers in the safe prescription and administration of drugs to older adults (available free from https://agsjournals.onlinelibrary.wiley.com/doi/abs/10.1111/jgs.18372). First developed in 1991 it has been revised five times, most recently in 2023. The 2023 Beers Criteria added new criteria and modified existing criteria for drug administration in adults 65 years and older, in all settings except hospice and end-of-life care. As in previous editions, it continues to provide safety information based on best available evidence to use in decision-making for drug therapy. Although the document provides information on drugs to avoid in older adults and drugs to use with caution, it is not designed for use in isolation. All drug therapy decisions should be made taking into consideration an individual's preferences, values, and needs. It is very important that the nurse advocates for the patient in these areas to ensure safety and promote adherence.

Adverse Drug Events

No drug is safe. Every year, more than 450,000 emergency department visits occur due to older adults experiencing adverse drug events (ADEs); in addition, older adults are seven times more likely than younger adults to be hospitalized due to ADEs. Most visits and hospitalizations occur due to reactions to blood thinners, drugs used to treat diabetes and seizures, cardiac drugs, and drugs used for pain control.

According to the World Health Organization, ADEs are "unintended and undesired effects of a [drug] at the normal dose." There are five types of ADEs: (1) adverse drug reactions, (2) medication errors, (3) therapeutic failures, (4) adverse drug withdrawal events, and (5) overdoses. Older adults have multiple risk factors for ADEs, including frailty, multiple comorbidities, polypharmacy, and cognitive issues.

Adherence

Adherence to a drug regimen is a problem for all patient age groups, but it is especially troublesome in older adult patients. Older adults may fail to ask questions during interactions with healthcare providers, which leads to the drug regimen not being fully understood or precisely followed. Failure to adhere to a drug regimen can cause underdosing or overdosing that could be harmful to the patient's health. Table 7.2 lists barriers to effective drug use by older adults.

TABLE 7.2 Barriers to Effective Drug Use by Older Adults

Causes	Nursing Actions
Taking too many drugs at different times	Develop a chart indicating times to take drugs. Provide space to place a mark for each drug taken. Coordinate the drug regimen with activities of daily living (e.g., meals) and events. Use an organizer container (daily or weekly). Have the patient bring all drugs—including over-the-counter drugs and herbal, vitamin, and mineral supplements—to all health appointments.
Failure to understand the purpose or reason for a drug	Explain the purpose, drug action, and importance of the drug. Provide time for questions and reinforcement. Reinforce with written information.
Impaired memory	Encourage family members or friends to monitor the patient's drug regimen.
Decreased mobility and dexterity	Advise family members or friends to have drugs and water or other fluid accessible and to assist older adults as needed.
Visual and hearing disturbances	Suggest eye and ear examinations (glasses or hearing aids).
High cost of prescriptions	Contact the social services department of your institution and compassionate care programs as appropriate.
Childproof drug bottles	Suggest that the patient request nonchildproof bottle caps.
Side effects or adverse reactions from the drug	Educate the patient and family about side effects to report to the health care provider.

Failure to adhere to a drug regimen can lead to ADEs, resulting in hospital admission, readmission to healthcare institutions, and even death. Complex drug regimens may be difficult for older adults to follow. Education is the cornerstone of adherence, and this includes education of the patient, family, and formal and informal caregivers.

Working with older adult patients is an ongoing nursing responsibility. The nurse should plan strategies with the patient and family or friends to encourage adherence to prescribed regimens. Daily contact may be necessary at first. Simply ordering the drug does not mean that the patient is able to get the drug or take it correctly. Older adults should have their prescriptions filled at one pharmacy if possible, so a relationship can be established with a pharmacist and drug interactions can be identified and monitored closely.

The Medicare Modernization Act of 2003 made it possible for older adults to obtain prescription drug coverage through Medicare, with initial enrollment beginning in 2006. Older adults who are eligible for Medicare Part A or Part B are eligible for the optional Medicare Prescription Drug Plan (Part D) or coverage through a Medicare Advantage Plan (Part C). Each of these plans has its own formulary, copay rate, and in-network pharmacies. No plan is perfect for every older adult; the nurse, as advocate, must be able to assist the older adult to find the plan that is right for them and to make the most of the policy.

However, not all older adults have insurance that includes prescription drug coverage, nor are they able to afford their drugs even with insurance. Nurses need to assess the patient's ability to obtain prescriptions before sending the patient home. Options for assistance are available, and the nurse can assist patients in navigating the system to obtain their drugs for free or at a reduced cost (see Partnership for Prescription Assistance at www.pparx.org and Extra Help at www.ssa.gov/medicare/prescriptionhelp).

Health care professionals—nurses, pharmacists, and health care providers—need to work collaboratively to enhance safety and adherence of older adult patients and to avoid errors and unwarranted concerns. Nurses are in a unique position to educate patients and to monitor the effectiveness of therapeutic regimens. A handout of tips for patients on talking with their pharmacist is available at https://www.fda.gov/drugs/tips-seniors/stop-learn-go-tips-talking-your-pharmacist-learn-how-use-medicines-safely.

Health Teaching With the Older Adult

Specific factors that enhance educational readiness and promote adherence in the older adult include the following:

- Ensure that the patient is wearing eyeglasses and has working hearing aids in place if needed. Check sensory aids to be sure they are clean and working.
- Speak in a tone of voice that the patient can hear; sit facing the patient, and limit distractions.
- Treat the patient with respect; never infantilize (also referred to as "elderspeak"); expect that the patient can learn.
- Use large print and dark type against a light background; use a font with serifs, or "feet and tails" (like this font), which makes letters close together easier to read.
- Review all drugs at each patient visit; ask the patient to bring all drugs to each appointment, and advise the use of only one pharmacy.
- Advise the patient to complete the *vial of life* (medical information for emergency personnel to use in the provision of care; www.vialoflife.com) and keep it on the refrigerator door where safety personnel will know to look for it.
- Instruct the patient to keep a list of all drugs taken, bring it to all health appointments, and carry it when out of the house.
- Encourage a simple dosing schedule when possible.
- Suspect recently prescribed drug(s) if new confusion or disorientation occurs.
- Encourage the patient to report if a drug is not improving the condition for which it was prescribed.
- Consider the use of memory aids such as pill organizers or planners, alarms, blinking lights, or prerecorded messages.

The National Institutes of Health websites on aging are excellent resources for both healthcare providers and older adults and their families. The website for health care providers is www.nia.nih.gov; it has sections on health information, research, grants, training, news, and events. The website for older adults is https://www.nia.nih.gov/health.

CLINICAL JUDGMENT [NURSING PROCESS]

Older Adult

Concept: Communication
- A process by which information is exchanged using multiple methods

Concept: Safety
- Protecting the patient from potential or actual harm; a basic human need

Recognize Cues [Assessment]
- Assess for allergies.
- Assess for sensory and cognitive barriers.
  - Assess the patient's use of eyeglasses, and check the date of the last eye examination.
  - Is the patient confused or disoriented? If so, is this state transitory?
- Assess laboratory test results, and follow up as appropriate.
  - Decreased kidney and liver function can increase the half-life of drugs.
- Assess weight and vital signs.
- Determine all drugs the patient takes, including illicit, prescription, over-the-counter (OTC) drugs, and supplements.
  - Assess patient adherence to the drug regimen.
  - Assess patient knowledge of the purpose of each drug, how it works, and its possible side effects.
- Discern whether the patient has difficulty opening drug containers and whether the patient is experiencing side effects or adverse reactions.
- Discern whether the patient lives alone, with or without social support, and whether assistance is needed with drugs, including costs or the transportation to acquire them.
- Obtain a history of chronic conditions.

Analyze Cues and Prioritize Hypothesis [Patient Problems]
- Need for health teaching
- Changes in elimination
- Potential for decreased adherence

Generate Solutions [Planning]
- The patient will collaborate with health care providers to develop a therapeutic regimen that is congruent with health goals and lifestyle.
- The patient will describe why the drug is needed, how the drug is administered, common adverse reactions, and drug interactions.
- The patient will identify measures to prevent constipation.
- The patient will list resources that can be used for more information or support.
- The patient will verbalize the ability to manage the therapeutic regimen.

Continued

CLINICAL JUDGMENT [NURSING PROCESS]—CONT'D

Older Adult

Take Action [Nursing Interventions]
- Ascertain whether financial problems are preventing the patient from purchasing prescribed drugs. Assistance programs are available.
- Communicate with the pharmacist or health care provider when a drug dose is in question. Check drug references for recommended drug dosages for older adults.
- Establish a collaborative partnership with the patient to meet health-related goals.
- Monitor the patient's laboratory results to ensure that blood urea nitrogen, serum creatinine, estimated glomerular filtration rate, and liver enzymes are within normal range and that drug levels are within the therapeutic range. Discuss findings with the health care provider.
- Observe the patient for adverse reactions when multiple drugs are being taken.
- Recognize a change in usual behavior or an increase in confusion. One of the first signs of drug toxicity is a change in mental status. Report changes to the health care provider.
- Remind the patient and family to tell the pharmacist about OTC preparations the patient is taking when picking up prescriptions.
- Advise patients and family to request a nonchildproof cap from the pharmacy if the patient has arthritis in the hand joint or has difficulty opening childproof bottle caps. The patient may need to sign for this at the pharmacy, and the safety of children or pets in the environment must be ensured.
- Advise patients to keep a record of their drugs and when they are to be taken. Consider offering them a sample log for recording information. This removes barriers, increases drug adherence, and avoids drug errors.
- Advise patients to use one pharmacy to fill prescriptions, and instruct them to inform the pharmacist of all illicit, prescription, and OTC drugs and supplements taken.
- Be available to answer patient questions. Be supportive of the older adult and the family. Discuss problems related to the drugs.
- Counsel patients not to share prescribed drugs with others or to take drugs prescribed for another person.
- Explain to patients and family the importance of adherence to the drug regimen. Emphasize the importance of taking drugs as prescribed.
- To promote adherence, provide additional time for verbal and written explanations.
- Review drugs with patients and family, including the reason the drug was prescribed, route of administration, frequency, common side effects, and when to notify the health care provider.
- Recognize that language difficulties may interfere with older adults' understanding of the prescribed drug regimen; provide educational material in the patient's preferred language.

Evaluate Outcomes [Evaluation]
- Evaluate adherence to the drug regimen, and answer any questions the older adult may have.
- Evaluate therapeutic drug response, and ascertain side effects or adverse reactions.

CLINICAL JUDGMENT CASE STUDY

A 78-year-old female comes to the clinic for a new patient examination. She reports that she smokes *cannabis* several times a week and takes alprazolam 0.5 mg three times per day, a combination tablet of metoprolol tartrate 50 mg/hydrochlorothiazide 25 mg daily, aspirin 81 mg daily; garlic soft gels 1000 mg twice a day; and ibuprofen 400 mg four times a day.

1. Do any of these drugs appear on the 2019 American Geriatrics Society Beers Criteria for Potentially Inappropriate Medication Use in Older Adults? If so, what do the criteria say about them?
2. What interactions exist among the drugs and supplements this patient is taking?
3. What is the evidence for taking garlic to reduce cholesterol?

REVIEW QUESTIONS

1. Which factors negatively influence adherence to the prescribed drug regimen in an older adult? **Select all that apply.**
    a. Taking multiple drugs at one time
    b. Impaired memory
    c. Decreased dexterity
    d. Increased mobility
    e. Increased visual acuity
2. The nurse understands that the older adult's slower absorption of oral drugs is primarily because of which phenomenon?
    a. Decreased cardiac output
    b. Increased gastric emptying time
    c. Decreased gastric blood flow
    d. Increased gastric acid secretion
3. The older adult patient has questions about oral drug metabolism. Which information about drug metabolism is important to be included in an older adult's teaching plan?
    a. First-pass effect
    b. Enzyme function
    c. Glomerular filtration rate
    d. Motility
4. An older adult has just started on hydrochlorothiazide and is advised by the healthcare provider to eat foods rich in potassium. The older adult should be taught about which foods to consume?
    a. Cabbage and corn
    b. Bread and cheese
    c. Avocados and mushrooms
    d. Brown rice and fish

5. The nurse is developing teaching materials for an 82-year-old male with macular degeneration, who is being discharged on two new drugs. Which strategies would be best to use to impart the information? **Select all that apply.**
   a. Limit distractions in the room when teaching.
   b. Wait until discharge to teach so information is fresh in the memory.
   c. Augment teaching with audio material.
   d. Use "Honey" and other terms of familiarity when addressing him to promote trust.
   e. Use large, dark print on a light background for written material.
6. Which changes with aging alter drug distribution? **Select all that apply.**
   a. An increase in muscle mass and a decrease in fat
   b. A decrease in muscle mass and an increase in fat
   c. A decrease in serum albumin levels
   d. An increase in total body water
   e. A decrease in kidney mass
7. Which factors contribute to polypharmacy in older adults? **Select all that apply.**
   a. Multiple healthcare providers
   b. Multiple chronic diseases
   c. Use of a single pharmacy
   d. Care coordination by a nurse
   e. Few hospitalizations
8. Which measure is best for the nurse to use to determine a patient's kidney function?
   a. Creatinine clearance
   b. Estimated glomerular filtration rate
   c. Serum creatinine level
   d. Blood urea nitrogen level

8

Drugs in Substance Use Disorder

http://evolve.elsevier.com/McCuistion/pharmacology

OBJECTIVES

- Summarize the incidence of substance use disorders, terminology related to substance use disorder, and the neurobiological theory of addiction.
- Discuss the types of substance use disorder and the terminology associated with substance use disorder.
- Describe the special needs of patients with substance use disorder.
- Explain substance use disorder in nurses.

OUTLINE

Substance Use Disorder, 58
    Context, 58
    Definition, 58
    Neurobiology, 59
Types of Substance Use Disorders, 59
    Alcohol Use Disorder, 59
    Cannabis Use Disorder, 61
    Opioid Use Disorder, 62
    Tobacco Use Disorder, 63
    Other Substance Use Disorders, 64

Special Needs of Patients With Substance Use Disorder, 65
    Surgical Patients, 65
    Pain Management, 66
The Nurse With Substance Use Disorder, 66
    Contributing Factors and Characteristics, 66
    Management, 66
Clinical Judgment Case Study, 67
Review Questions, 67

Although most drugs are used safely and within prescribed guidelines, it is possible for all drugs to be misused. It has been reported that more than 40 million Americans 12 years of age and older use tobacco, alcohol, or illicit drugs. Drug use is a serious and complex social and health issue with negative consequences for both the individual and society that include family dysfunction, loss of employment, failure in school, domestic violence, and child abuse. The economic cost of drug use is staggering: $600 billion annually in costs related to lost productivity, health-related issues, and crime.

SUBSTANCE USE DISORDER

Context

Since 1975 the **Monitoring the Future project** has been tracking drug use in adolescents and young adults. Current data (2022) from the survey indicate that the percentage of 12th grade students who used cannabis in the past 12 months was 31%; who vaped nicotine was 27%; and who use alcohol was 52%. These numbers are stable from 2021. However, there were increases in the use of cocaine, hallucinogens, and heroin, as well as the use of prescription opioids. In addition, the use of anabolic steroids, creatine, and androstenedione has increased.

Many factors play into the decision to use drugs and whether an individual develops substance use disorder. Cognitive development at the time drugs are introduced plays a major role; adolescents are in a period of brain development where they are especially vulnerable to stress and risk-seeking behaviors. Other risk factors are also related to substance use disorder:

- *Family-related risk factors:* Between 16% and 29% of children who experience neglect or abuse—physical, sexual, and emotional—have tried or use drugs.
- *Social risk factors:* Deviant peer relationships (i.e., the adolescent associates with abusers and uses drugs to feel accepted), peer pressure, popularity, and bullying have all been correlated to drug use. Gang affiliation is associated with higher drug use and delinquent behavior.
- *Individual risk factors:* Individuals with attention-deficit/hyperactivity disorder (ADHD) are three times as likely as the general population to use drugs such as nicotine, alcohol, and drugs other than *cannabis*; depression is associated with alcohol use, particularly among young men.

It should be noted that positive family relationships are a protective factor that has been related to a decrease in drug use among adolescents.

Definition

According to the *Diagnostic and Statistical Manual of Mental Disorders* (5th edition [DSM-5]), **substance use disorder** occurs "when the recurrent use of alcohol and/or drugs causes clinically and functionally significant impairment, such as health problems, disability, and failure

TABLE 8.1 Substance Use Disorder Categories

Criteria	Subcomponents

• Mild substance use disorder (2–3 criteria required)
• Moderate substance use disorder (4–5 criteria required)
• Severe substance use disorder (6–7 criteria required)
	• The substance is often taken in larger amounts or over a longer period than was intended.
	• There is a persistent desire or unsuccessful effort to cut down on or control use of the substance.
	• A great deal of time is spent in activities necessary to obtain the substance, use the substance, or recover from its effects.
	• Craving, or a strong desire or urge to use the substance, is present.
	• Recurrent use of the substance results in a failure to fulfill major role obligations at work, school, or home.
	• Continued use of the substance occurs despite having persistent or recurrent social or interpersonal problems caused or exacerbated by the effects of its use.
	• Important social, occupational, or recreational activities are given up or reduced because of use of the substance.
	• Recurrent use of the substance occurs in situations in which it is physically hazardous.
	• Use of the substance is continued despite knowledge of having a persistent or recurrent physical or psychological problem that is likely to have been caused or exacerbated by the substance.
	• Tolerance[a] occurs, as defined by either of the following:
	  • A need for markedly increased amounts of the substance to achieve intoxication or desired effect
	  • A markedly diminished effect with continued use of the same amount of the substance
	• Withdrawal[a] occurs, as manifested by either of the following:
	  • The characteristic withdrawal syndrome for that substance is evident as specified in the DSM-5.
	  • The substance or a closely related substance is taken to relieve or avoid withdrawal symptoms.

DSM-5, *Diagnostic and Statistical Manual of Mental Disorders*, fifth edition.
[a]Does not apply when used appropriately under medical supervision.
Data from Horvath AT, Misra K, Epner AK, et al: *The diagnostic criteria for substance use disorders (addiction)*, n.d. www.amhc.org/1408-addictions/article/48502-the-diagnostic-criteria-for-substance-use-disorders-addiction; and National Institute on Drug Abuse: *The science of drug abuse and addiction: The basics*, 2014. www.drugabuse.gov/publications/media-guide/science-drug-abuse-addiction-basics.

to meet major responsibilities at work, school, or home." Substance use disorder is categorized along a continuum from mild to severe, based on the number of diagnostic criteria met (Table 8.1). The terms *abuse* and *dependence* are no longer used due to the violence and stigma associated with the term *abuse* and the ambiguity associated with the term *dependence*; gambling is the only condition in the category of behavioral addiction (continued involvement in an activity despite the substantial harm it causes). Excessive caffeine use is not considered a substance use disorder, even though there appears to be a withdrawal syndrome with cessation of use.

Neurobiology

Drugs that are misused typically increase the availability of dopamine and other neurotransmitters in the limbic system of the brain. This area contains the brain's **reward circuit**, a structure that regulates our ability to feel pleasure and other emotions, both positive and negative. The drugs interfere with the way neurons in the brain normally send, receive, and process information by mimicking the brain's own neurotransmitters; however, drugs do not copy neurotransmitters exactly, which results in faulty transmission or excessive stimulation. Most of the drugs facilitate an increase of dopamine in the system, leading to mood elevation or euphoria—factors that provide strong motivation to repeat the experience. Some drugs increase the availability of other neurotransmitters, such as serotonin and gamma-aminobutyric acid (GABA), but dopamine's effect on the reward system appears to be pivotal to substance use disorder.

Repeated use of drugs remodels the neural circuitry of the brain cells and reduces the responsiveness of receptors. This decreased responsiveness leads to **tolerance**, the need for a larger dose of a drug to obtain the original euphoria. Drug use results in levels of dopamine that do not naturally occur; tolerance also reduces the sense of pleasure from experiences that previously resulted in positive feelings, such as food, sex, or relationships. Without the drug, the individual may experience depression, anxiety, and/or irritability.

Current research is focused on **epigenetics**, the study of environmental influences on genetics. How a person responds to their social and cultural environment affects drug use. Altering environmental factors that increase the risk for drug use can discourage drug-seeking behavior. Studies have shown that drug use alters DNA proteins, those that affect both gene expression and function, and this influences drug-seeking behavior. Understanding these processes may lead to new treatments for substance use disorders.

TYPES OF SUBSTANCE USE DISORDERS

Alcohol Use Disorder

People drink for many reasons, including socializing, celebrating, and relaxing; people also drink to cope, because of low self-esteem and a need for approval, or because of peer pressure. Alcohol affects everyone differently, depending on the amount consumed, the frequency of consumption, age, health status, and family history.

Alcohol use inhibits the effects of GABA, thereby reducing neurotransmission in the brain. Short-term effects of alcohol use include nausea, vomiting, headaches, slurred speech, impaired judgment, memory loss, hangovers, and blackouts. Box 8.1 discusses **alcohol toxicity**.

Long-term problems associated with heavy drinking include stomach ailments, heart problems, cancer, brain damage, serious memory loss, immune system compromise, and liver cirrhosis. Persons with alcohol use disorder (AUD) increase their chances of dying from automobile accidents, homicide, and suicide. Spouses and children of persons with AUD may face family violence, and children may experience

> **BOX 8.1 Alcohol Toxicity**
>
> Alcohol toxicity is a life-threatening condition that can occur by drinking large amounts of alcohol over a short period of time. A standard drink contains 10 g of alcohol. This is equal to 10 ounces of beer with 5% alcohol, 3.25 ounces of wine with 12% alcohol, or 1 ounce of hard liquor with 40% alcohol (or 80 "proof"). Roughly 20% of alcohol is absorbed from the stomach, and the remainder is absorbed in the small intestine. Food intake slows absorption. Alcohol is metabolized in the liver and is excreted by the lungs and kidneys, and the average person can only metabolize 10 g of alcohol per hour.
>
> Complications of alcohol toxicity include aspiration of vomitus, asphyxiation, severe dehydration, seizures, hypothermia, brain damage, and death. Treatment involves airway management and supplemental oxygenation, correction of hypoglycemia if present, supportive care, and intravenous hydration. If the person chronically uses alcohol, thiamine 100 mg may be administered intramuscularly to prevent neurologic damage. Patients with impaired hepatic function may require hemodialysis to remove alcohol from the blood; however, this invasive treatment is only used in persons whose condition is rapidly deteriorating.

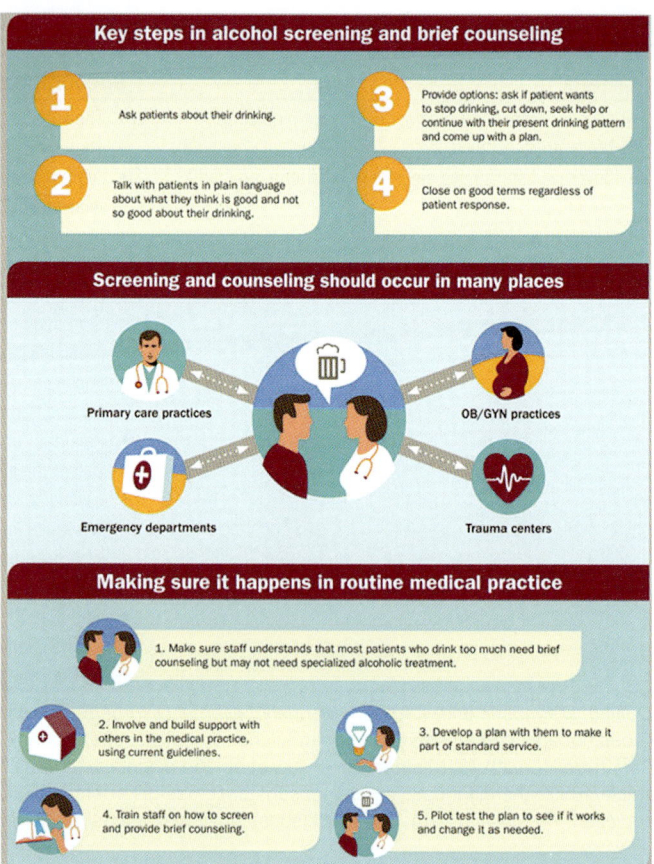

Fig. 8.1 Alcohol screening and brief counseling. (From National Center for Chronic Disease Prevention and Health Promotion, Division of Population Health. *Alcohol Screening and Counseling.* 2014. https://www.cdc.gov/vitalsigns/alcohol-screening-counseling/index.html.)

physical and sexual abuse and neglect and may develop psychological problems. Women who drink during pregnancy run a serious risk of their fetus developing fetal alcohol spectrum disorder. To intervene promptly and avoid long-term problems associated with AUD, nurses should question all patients about their drinking habits with every encounter, using plain language, without bias (Fig. 8.1).

Treatment

AUD can be treated through a variety of options. However, very few people with the disorder seek care. Alcohol treatment centers offer inpatient-type care, where the person undergoes stabilization in a controlled environment that includes group therapy. Persons with AUD are provided the tools they need to become abstinent and go into remission. Outpatient treatment is also available. People with AUD who participate in outpatient therapy, such as cognitive behavioral therapy, motivational interviewing, mindfulness, and contingency management, are given the tools to become abstinent and go into remission.

Drug-Assisted Treatment. Several drugs have been approved by the US Food and Drug Administration (FDA) to treat AUD. Disulfiram, acamprosate, and naltrexone are the most used (Table 8.2). Disulfiram inhibits aldehyde dehydrogenase, the enzyme involved in metabolizing alcohol. It is best used in people who are newly abstinent. Disulfiram is administered in tablet form; dosage ranges from 125 to 500 mg daily. It is contraindicated in persons who are intoxicated and should not be taken within 12 hours of alcohol consumption (including use of mouthwash, cough medicine, or eating desserts that contain alcohol or eating foods cooked in alcohol). Side effects occur within 10 minutes of alcohol consumption and can last for more than an hour. These side effects include nausea, headache, vomiting, chest pains, and difficulty breathing. Disulfiram keeps patients from drinking because of the unpleasant side effects that occur if alcohol is consumed while taking the drug. Patients who have recently been treated with metronidazole or paraldehyde should not take disulfiram because these same side effects will occur as if they had been drinking. Because of the risk for drug toxicity, disulfiram should *never* be used in combination with eliglustat or ritonavir.

Other side effects of disulfiram include rash, drowsiness, impotence, acne, and a metallic aftertaste. Serious reactions include psychosis, hepatotoxicity, peripheral neuropathy, and optic neuritis. Patients taking disulfiram should have baseline liver function studies obtained; liver function studies should be repeated after 2 weeks of therapy. For disulfiram to be effective, persons with AUD also need to participate in behavior modification, psychotherapy, and counseling. Whether disulfiram will harm the fetus is unknown; however, it is excreted into breast milk. Therefore, a decision should be made to either discontinue breast-feeding or discontinue the drug, considering the importance of the drug to the mother.

Acamprosate is a GABA analogue thought to work in the brain to restore the balance between neuronal excitation and inhibition via GABA and glutamate. It should only be used in persons who are abstinent; however, acamprosate may be continued through a relapse. Usual dosing is 666 mg orally three times per day. Dosing is adjusted in kidney disease, and a serum creatinine level should be obtained at baseline. Persons with a creatinine clearance of 30 to 50 mL/min should only take 333 mg three times per day. Acamprosate is contraindicated in people with a creatinine clearance less than 30 mL/min. Common side effects include pain, loss of appetite, nausea, diarrhea, dizziness, anxiety, pruritus, depression, insomnia, xerostomia, and paresthesia. Patients should be assessed for suicidal ideation before beginning treatment. This drug is used in conjunction with behavior modification and counseling. Naltrexone increases acamprosate levels. No dosage adjustment is needed, but patients should be monitored closely. It is not known if acamprosate will harm the fetus or if it is excreted into breast milk. Therefore, a decision should be made to either discontinue

TABLE 8.2 Pharmacokinetics of Drug-Assisted Treatments

Drug Name	Absorption	Distribution	Metabolism	Excretion
Acamprosate	Peak plasma time: 3–8 h Bioavailability: 11%, decreased by food but not clinically important	Protein binding: Negligible	Not metabolized	In urine as unchanged drug Half-life: 20–33 h
Buprenorphine	Extensive first-pass effect if taken orally; 31% bioavailability (SL) Time to peak plasma varies from 40 min to 3.5 h	Highly lipophilic Highly protein bound (96%)	Extensive hepatic	In bile and feces, 70%; urine, 30% Half-life: SL, 37 h
Disulfiram	Absorbed from the GI tract (80%–90%), onset is 3–12 h after administration Effects may persist up to 14 d after the last dose	Highly lipophilic	Hepatic	In urine primarily but also in feces (5%–20% unchanged) and lungs
Methadone	Oral administration: Bioavailability ranges from 36%–100%, and peak plasma concentrations are achieved between 1 and 7.5 h	Lipophilic; 85%–90% protein bound	Hepatic, into inactive metabolite	Renal and fecal Half-life is highly variable
Naloxone	Onset: Administered IV, 2 min; subcut and IM, 5 min; Intranasal route: 1 mg in each nostril × 1 Duration of action is 30–60 min	Plasma protein binding occurs but is relatively weak	Hepatic	In urine Half-life is 1–1.5 h
Naltrexone	96% absorbed from the GI tract; extensive first-pass metabolism; 5%–40% reaches the systemic circulation Onset is 15–30 min; duration is 24 h and is dose dependent	Protein bound: 21%–28%	Hepatic, into active metabolite	In urine
Varenicline	Well absorbed from the GI tract and unaffected by food Time to peak plasma: 3–4 h	Less than 20% protein binding	Minimal hepatic (<10%)	In urine, 92% unchanged Half-life: 24 h

d, Day; *GI*, gastrointestinal; *h*, hours; *IM*, intramuscular; *IV*, intravenous; *min*, minutes; *SL*, sublingual; *subcut*, subcutaneous.
From Drugs.com. For Healthcare Professionals. n.d. www.drugs.com/professionals.html; Medscape.com. Drugs, OTCs & Herbals. n.d. http://reference.medscape.com/drugs.

breast-feeding or discontinue the drug, considering the importance of the drug to the mother.

Naltrexone is a competitive opioid antagonist with a high affinity for mu receptors. Oral forms absorbed through the gastrointestinal (GI) tract undergo up to 40% first-pass metabolism. Onset occurs in 15 to 30 minutes with peak occurring in 1 hour. Naltrexone is used in persons who are abstinent. If there is concern about comorbid opioid use disorder (OUD), a naloxone challenge test may be done before initiating treatment, in which a test dose of 25 mg is administered orally, and the patient is observed for 1 hour. If no withdrawal is observed, dosing may begin the next day at 50 mg per day for 12 weeks or less. Dosing using 380 mg intramuscularly (IM) once every 4 weeks can be used for maintenance therapy. Common side effects include insomnia, nausea, vomiting, anxiety, headache, abdominal pain, myalgia, arthralgia, rash, dizziness, fatigue, constipation, and increased creatine phosphokinase. Serious reactions include suicidality, depression, hepatotoxicity, and hypersensitivity reaction. Patients should be assessed for suicidal ideation before beginning treatment. This drug should *not* be taken in conjunction with any drugs that bind to opioid receptors because withdrawal may be precipitated in persons with OUD. It is not known if naltrexone will harm the fetus, and it is excreted into breast milk. Therefore, a decision should be made to either discontinue breast-feeding or discontinue the drug, considering the importance of the drug to the mother.

Cannabis Use Disorder

Cannabis is the most used recreational drug in the United States. Users report feeling an alteration in their senses and an altered sense of time as well as changes in mood. *Cannabis* goes by many street names, including Marijuana, Blunt, Bud, Dope, Ganja, Grass, Green, Herb, Joint, Mary Jane, Pot, Reefer, Sinsemilla, Skunk, Smoke, Trees, and Weed; names for various forms of hashish include Boom, Gangster, Hash, and Hemp. *Cannabis* contains more than 60 related psychoactive chemicals known as *cannabinoids*; however, the most abundant of these is delta-9-tetrahydrocannabinol (THC).

When smoked, THC rapidly crosses the blood-brain barrier and binds to cannabinoid receptors in many areas of the brain, overwhelming the endocannabinoid system and making it difficult for the user to respond appropriately to incoming stimuli. The drug impairs short-term memory, learning, and ability to focus, and it can cause problems with balance and coordination. In addition, *cannabis* increases heart rate and may cause hallucinations, anxiety, panic attacks, and psychosis in some people. When smoked, *cannabis* may harm the lungs, and concurrent use of alcohol increases blood pressure in addition to heart rate and further slows mental processes and reaction times. Box 8.2 discusses issues associated with **vaping** *cannabis*.

Long-term use of *cannabis* is associated with chronic cough, frequent respiratory infections, and exposure to cancer-causing compounds because the smoke has many of the same irritating and lung-damaging properties as tobacco. Ingestion of the drug increases the heart rate for hours, increasing the risk for heart attack and stroke. When repeated use begins in adolescence, there is an association with decreased motivation and decreased performance on memory-related tasks. The drug has also been linked to mental health problems and increased symptoms in persons with schizophrenia. Babies born to

> **BOX 8.2 Vaping Cannabis**
>
> Use of *cannabis* in e-cigarettes is a public health concern. Recent reports indicate 8.9% of middle- and high-schoolers have vaped *cannabis*. Johns Hopkins School of Medicine researchers note that "compared with smoking *cannabis*, vaping it increased the rate of short-term anxiety, paranoia, memory loss and distraction when doses were the same" in infrequent users. Persons who vape the drug may also experience nausea, vomiting, and hallucination for hours after use (McMains, 2018).
>
> Additional concerns surround the farming and manufacturing processes of *cannabis* oil. Not only is there little oversight of *Cannabis* farmers and the chemicals used to eliminate mites, mold, and mildew on the plants and to make the buds denser, but there is also no oversight on the process and chemicals used to extract the substance, referred to as butane hash oil, that is often made in "the basement or backyard." Although California and Oregon are trying to regulate the industry, "black market" cartridges show up in dispensaries. Lewis (2017) stated, "You don't know what's in the oil you're vaping, and you don't know how it's going to affect your health."
>
> E-cigarettes with *cannabis* oil in the cartridge heat the liquid until it vaporizes. They generate very little odor, and the cartridges look like a flash drive, making it nearly impossible to tell if the user is vaping tobacco or *cannabis*. Nurses who work with children and adolescents must be diligent in asking about the use of *cannabis* oil in e-cigarettes and providing counseling concerning the dangers of using them.

Excerpts from McMains V. Vaping Marijuana Might Be Too Much for First-timers. 2018. https://www.futurity.org/vaping-cannabis-anxiety-1925032-2/; Lewis, A. C. Are Weed Vape Pens Safe? 2017. https://www.rollingstone.com/culture/culture-features/are-weed-vape-pens-safe-202125/.

> **BOX 8.3 Medical Marijuana**
>
> In 38 states and Washington DC there are comprehensive medical marijuana use programs; in 24 states and Washington, DC, adult recreational use of marijuana is legal. However, a recent meta-analysis of randomized controlled trials and observational studies concluded "Convincing or converging evidence supports avoidance of cannabis during adolescence and early adulthood, in people prone to or with mental health disorders, in pregnancy and before and while driving. Cannabidiol is effective in people with epilepsy. Cannabis-based medicines are effective in people with multiple sclerosis, chronic pain, inflammatory bowel disease, and in palliative medicine but not without adverse events."

From Solmi M, De Toffol M, Kim J Y, Choi M J, Stubbs B, Thompson T, et al. Balancing risks and benefits of cannabis use: umbrella review of meta-analyses of randomised controlled trials and observational studies BMJ. 2023;382:e072348.

women who use *cannabis* have behavioral issues and problems with attention, memory, and problem solving.

Many have supported the nationwide legalization of *cannabis* to treat medical conditions. See Box 8.3 concerning the use of medical marijuana.

Cognitive behavioral therapy (CBT), contingency management, and motivational enhancement therapy may be effective in the treatment of *cannabis* use disorder; however, no medications are currently approved or indicated for this use.

Opioid Use Disorder

Opioids (e.g., oxycodone, hydrocodone, morphine, methadone, and fentanyl) are controlled substances legally prescribed to treat moderate to severe pain. These drugs interact with opioid receptors in the brain and nervous system to reduce pain. In addition to reducing pain, this receptor interaction floods the brain's reward system with dopamine, producing a sense of euphoria and tranquility.

Short-term effects of opioid use include drowsiness, mental confusion, nausea, constipation, and dose-dependent respiratory depression. When taken with alcohol, users may experience dangerous slowing of heart rate and breathing, leading to coma or death. When taken with serotonergic drugs (e.g., selective serotonin reuptake inhibitors, serotonin-norepinephrine reuptake inhibitors, and antimigraine agents), serotonin syndrome may occur. Symptoms of serotonin syndrome include agitation, hallucinations, coma, tachycardia, hypertension, hyperthermia, and rigidity.

In addition to the oral route, when misused, opioids are smoked, snorted, or administered parenterally. Prescription opioids are also known by numerous street names, including Vikes, Cody, China White, Fizzies, M, Demmies, Blue Heavens, Juice, Smack, Hillbilly Heroin, and Roxy.

Nonmedical use of prescription opioid drugs is considered a public health emergency; 75% of drug overdose deaths in 2021 involved an opioid. Over 10 million people misused prescription opioids in the past year, and over 1.5 million met criteria for OUD.

With repeated use, tolerance to the euphoric effects of the drug increase, and users may not be able to obtain the drug from friends, relatives, or any doctor; this causes them to turn to the street for drugs. Some users switch from prescription drugs to cheaper and riskier substitutes, like heroin.

⚡ The FDA has toughened the safety warnings on opioids, including adding a boxed warning about the potentially lethal risks associated with misuse. The safety warning includes a caution regarding the use of opioids during pregnancy and the risk of neonatal opioid withdrawal syndrome, which can be life-threatening.

Contingency management therapy or 12-step facilitation therapy may be useful in treating prescription opioid addiction. Treatment approaches are tailored to each patient and are often combined with medication therapy.

Drug-Assisted Treatment

Naloxone (see Table 8.2) is the drug of choice in the treatment of respiratory depression associated with opioid overdose. Naloxone is a short-acting opioid antagonist that competitively attaches to opioid receptors in the central nervous system (CNS), thereby blocking activation by opioid drugs. In emergency situations, it is administered intravenously (IV); however, it may also be administered IM or subcutaneously (subcut). In persons with suspected OUD, dosing begins at 0.1 to 0.2 mg every 2 to 3 minutes until the patient responds. Properly equipped non–health care professionals can also potentially reverse opioid mortality (Box 8.4 and Fig. 8.2). Careful monitoring is required to prevent opioid withdrawal. Symptoms of withdrawal include nausea and vomiting, abdominal cramps, hyperthermia, hypertension, and restlessness.

Naltrexone is approved by the FDA to treat OUD. (See the previous discussion under "Alcohol Use Disorder.") Dosing begins at 50 mg daily after the patient has been opioid free for 7 to 10 days. It is also available in an injectable, extended-release form, with dosing at 380 mg each month. Once treated with naltrexone, patients may have reduced tolerance to opioids; if they relapse after a period of abstinence and resume opioid use at previous doses, they may experience life-threatening consequences, including respiratory arrest and circulatory collapse.

Since the 1950s, methadone has been prescribed to treat persons with OUD. When taken as prescribed and combined with counseling and behavioral therapies, administration of this long-acting opioid

BOX 8.4 Naloxone Use by Non–Health Care Professionals

When administered by non–health care professionals trained to recognize opioid overdose, the use of intranasal naloxone can reverse the symptoms of overdose, thereby reducing mortality.

Naloxone distribution programs provide kits to opioid users and their friends and family. This practice is endorsed by the American Medical Association, the American Public Health Association, the United Nations Office on Drugs and Crime, and the World Health Organization.

The overdose kits contain naloxone, gloves, a breathing shield, and instructions. Fig. 8.2 shows proper use of intranasal naloxone. When an overdose is identified, the non–health care professionals should call 911 and give naloxone. Once the drug is administered, it acts in 2 to 3 minutes. Rescue breathing should be performed while waiting for the drug to take effect.

There are minimal risks associated with the use of naloxone by non–health care professionals. If the recipient is not using opiates, it may make them uncomfortable, but it will not harm them (unless pregnant, nursing, or allergic to naloxone). It only works to reverse the effects of opioids, not other drugs such as benzodiazepines, bath salts, cocaine, methamphetamine, or alcohol.

Bar-Ilan University. Properly Equipped Laypersons Can Potentially Reverse Opioid Overdose Mortality. EurekAlert! 2020. https://www.eurekalert.org/pub_releases/2020-08/bu-plc073020.php; NIDA. Naloxone for Opioid Overdose: Life-Saving Science. 2017.https://www.drugabuse.gov/publications/naloxone-opioid-overdose-life-saving-science.

Fig. 8.2 Properly equipped non–health care professionals can potentially reverse opioid overdose mortality.

drug is safe and effective. Methadone has a boxed warning concerning the risk of cardiac and respiratory-related deaths due to QT prolongation and cardiac arrhythmias. Methadone used for stabilization and maintenance of persons with OUD may only be administered by programs certified by the Substance Abuse and Mental Health Services Administration and approved by state authority. Opioid treatment programs must follow federal guidelines and standards for medically monitored withdrawal and treatment.

Methadone works by changing the way a person's brain responds to pain; it is an opioid receptor agonist at the mu receptor and an antagonist at the N-methyl-D-aspartate receptor. Taken daily, it blocks the sense of euphoria and tranquility caused by opioid use and prevents opioid withdrawal and craving. Concurrent administration of rifampin, phenytoin, St. John's wort, phenobarbital, and carbamazepine can reduce serum methadone levels and precipitate withdrawal. Administration with zidovudine may lead to toxicity.

Initial dosing ranges from 20 to 30 mg, followed by 5 to 10 mg, adjusting the methadone dose to suppress withdrawal and block the euphoric effects of opioids. The maximum dosage is 40 mg on the first day of stabilization. Maintenance therapy is based on patient assessment and ranges from 80 to 120 mg a day. Tapering methadone should only be done under medical supervision, with dose reductions of less than 10% every 14 days.

Common methadone side effects include lightheadedness, constipation, dizziness, sedation, nausea, and vomiting. Patients should be educated to prevent theft and misuse of methadone by friends, family, and others. Whether methadone will harm the fetus is unknown, but it is excreted into breast milk; therefore, a decision should be made to either discontinue breast-feeding or discontinue the drug, considering the importance of the drug to the mother.

Buprenorphine is a long-acting, mixed narcotic agonist-antagonist. It binds to various opioid receptors in the brain, producing partial antagonism at mu receptors and antagonism at kappa receptors, resulting in decreased withdrawal symptoms and cravings. Although it does produce some euphoria, there is a ceiling effect; increasing the dose beyond a moderate level (8–16 mg) does not increase euphoria, so it has a low potential for misuse. To further deter people from misusing buprenorphine, naloxone is added. Because of the almost complete first-pass metabolism of naloxone, it has minimal pharmacologic activity when the drug is used appropriately as a sublingual tablet. However, if the tablet is crushed and injected, the effects of naloxone lead to opioid withdrawal.

This drug may be administered in qualified outpatient settings (e.g., office, health department, or correctional facility) after providers have received training. When taken as prescribed and used in combination with counseling and behavioral therapies, it is safe and effective. Initial dosing begins when the person with OUD has been opioid free for at least 12 hours and is beginning to experience withdrawal. Dosing starts at 2 to 4 mg sublingual (SL) for the first day and then is raised to 8 to 16 mg SL for 1 to 2 days. Once the patient is stable and is not experiencing cravings or significant side effects, dosing is tailored to the individual. Although the maximum daily dose of buprenorphine is 44 mg, doses higher than 24 mg/day do not provide any clinical advantage.

Side effects of buprenorphine include nausea, vomiting, and constipation; muscle aches and cramps; and cravings, sedation, headache, depression, anxiety, and withdrawal symptoms. Whether buprenorphine will harm the fetus is unknown, but it is excreted into breast milk. Therefore, a decision should be made to either discontinue breast-feeding or discontinue the drug, considering the importance of the drug to the mother.

Tobacco Use Disorder

In 2021, 11.5% of adults used tobacco products; 12.6% of high school students and 6.6% of middle school students report using tobacco products. Tobacco comes in many forms, including e-cigarettes, cigarettes, cigars, smokeless tobacco, pipe tobacco, bidis, hookah, heated tobacco products, and nicotine pouches.

When smoked, nicotine is absorbed from the lungs into the pulmonary venous circulation. It then enters arterial circulation and moves quickly to the brain. Once across the blood-brain barrier, nicotine stimulates the release of dopamine, norepinephrine, GABA, glutamate, and endorphins, resulting in stimulation and pleasure and a reduction in stress and anxiety. These sensations fuel the brain's reward circuit.

Short-term effects of tobacco use include increased blood pressure, breathing, and heart rate. Tobacco use does long-term damage to nearly every organ in the human body, often leading to a variety of cancers, respiratory disorders, heart disease, stroke, immune dysfunction, and type 2 diabetes. Women who smoke while pregnant may experience miscarriage, premature delivery, and stillbirth and may have infants of lower birth weight. Children born to women who used tobacco while pregnant may be born with learning and behavior problems. Persons with tobacco use disorder (TUD) have increased health care utilization and higher health care costs compared with nonusers, and they are frequently absent from work.

Within 1 to 2 years of quitting, persons with TUD significantly reduce their risk for cancer, heart disease, stroke, and respiratory illness. Quitting is difficult. Persons attempting to quit experience irritability, anger, anxiousness, difficulty thinking, cravings, and increased hunger. Support is a very important part of the process and is often combined with pharmacological measures.

CBT is a goal-directed and problem-focused therapy designed to help the person with TUD identify negative thought patterns and inaccurate beliefs to learn new ways of coping and develop new ways of thinking. It helps the person increase their self-confidence in the ability to quit. CBT helps people identify their triggers and learn to either avoid them or respond differently to them. It also helps with any ambivalence people may feel about quitting.

Self-help materials in the form of Internet-based aids or cell phone apps are available to assist the person with TUD. For example, the American Lung Association offers *Freedom from Smoking Online* (https://www.freedomfromsmoking.org/), which offers modules with lessons and activities that reinforce the person's commitment to quit. Phone apps are available as well. Some require a small fee, such as *Butt Out—Quit Smoking Forever*, which monitors progress and helps the person stay focused on the goal to quit by providing motivational pictures and messages. Other apps are free, such as *Get Rich or Die Smoking*, which shows the person how much money they are saving each day by not smoking. It also monitors their health progress and shows what the person could buy with the money they have saved, and it rewards the app user with trophies.

Telephone-based resources link persons with TUD with counselors trained to assist the caller in developing an individualized plan to quit smoking. Telephone-based counseling is easy to use because it does not require the person to drive or find childcare to attend a meeting in person; in addition, it is available nights and weekends.

Combining a nonpharmacologic support measure, such as CBT, motivational interviewing, mindfulness, and contingency management, with drug-assisted treatment is the most effective means to quit smoking.

Drug-Assisted Treatment

Nicotine replacement drugs—sold as a gum, patch, spray, inhaler, or lozenge—mimic the nicotine effects of tobacco by binding to nicotine receptors in the CNS (see Table 8.2). They are used to relieve the withdrawal symptoms associated with smoking cessation and provide some of the stimulation and stress-relief effects the user gained from smoking. Those who choose to use nicotine replacement gums, sprays, inhalers, or lozenges dose themselves when they feel the urge to smoke; those who use the patch have a sustained nicotine level throughout the day (see Nursing Process: Patient-Centered Collaborative Care—Tobacco Use Disorder). Side effects include hypertension, tachycardia, dizziness, insomnia, irritability, anorexia, dyspepsia, nausea, vomiting, hiccups, and cough. Nicotine should be used during pregnancy only if the benefit outweighs the risk to the fetus. Nicotine has been shown to cause adverse fetal outcomes in animals; however, nicotine replacement is believed to be safer during pregnancy than smoking. Nicotine is excreted into breast milk and may increase infant heart rate; therefore, a decision should be made to discontinue breast-feeding or discontinue the drug, considering the importance of the drug to the mother.

Bupropion, an antidepressant drug, increases levels of dopamine and norepinephrine in the brain, mimicking the effects of nicotine. It also has some neuronal nicotinic receptor–blocking activity, reducing reinforcement from the brain's reward circuit. When used for smoking cessation, the dosage is 150 mg ER once daily for 3 days; increase to 150 mg ER twice daily (maximum dose 300 mg ER/day) if tolerated. Treatment should continue for 7 to 12 weeks; however, ongoing treatment for a year has shown benefit.

When starting the drug, smokers continue to smoke for the first week but have a stop date set for the second week. If patients have not quit smoking by week 7, providers may add a nicotine replacement drug. Bupropion should not be used by those who have seizures or eating disorders. In addition, it should not be taken within 14 days of taking a monoamine oxidase inhibitor. Bupropion should not be stopped suddenly; instead, the patient should be weaned off the drug to avoid withdrawal symptoms. The drug can cause a false-positive drug screen; when providing urine for a drug screen, laboratory personnel should be told of bupropion use. Whether bupropion will harm the fetus is unknown, but it is excreted into breast milk; therefore, a decision should be made to either discontinue breast-feeding or discontinue the drug, considering the importance of the drug to the mother.

Varenicline is a partial alpha-4–beta-2 nicotinic receptor agonist that stimulates dopamine activity in the brain but not to the extent of nicotine, thereby reducing cravings and withdrawal. Dosing begins 1 week before an identified quit date at 0.5 mg daily for 3 days, then 0.5 mg is taken twice daily for 4 days, then maintenance therapy begins at 1 mg twice daily for 11 weeks. Dosage is adjusted for patients with a creatinine clearance (CrCl) less than 30 mL/min (maximum dosage, 0.5 mg twice daily). Common side effects include nausea and vomiting, insomnia, headache, abnormal dreams, constipation or diarrhea, fatigue and malaise, upper respiratory tract infection, dyspnea, chest pain, abdominal pain, xerostomia, appetite changes, rash, and emotional disturbances. ⚡ Varenicline carries a black-box warning for serious neuropsychiatric symptoms including behavior changes, hostility, agitation, depression, and suicidality. Nurses must caution patients and their families about this warning and advise them to contact their provider immediately if suicidal thoughts or actions occur. It is unknown whether varenicline will harm the fetus or if it is excreted in breast milk; therefore, a decision should be made to either discontinue breast-feeding or discontinue the drug, considering the importance of the drug to the mother.

To advocate for their patients, nurses must keep in mind that 80% of those with TUD who attempt to quit relapse in the first month; only 3% remain abstinent at 6 months. Patients with TUD require multiple attempts at quitting before they achieve sustained remission.

Box 8.5 discusses **e-cigarettes** (electronic cigarettes).

Other Substance Use Disorders

Cough and Cold Products

Cough and cold products contain ingredients that are psychoactive when taken in higher-than-recommended amounts (sometimes up

> **BOX 8.5 Electronic Cigarettes (e-Cigarettes)**
>
> Electronic cigarettes are a tobacco product often marketed as a tool to stop smoking; however, marketing is also aimed at children and adolescents. A reported 2.4 million middle and high school students use e-cigarettes, also known as *Hookah Pens*, *e-Hookahs*, and *Vape Pipes*. E-cigarettes aerosolize "e-juice," a mixture of flavorings, propylene glycol (a toxic component of antifreeze), glycerin, and nicotine. The vapor from e-cigarettes contains heavy metals and formaldehyde, a breakdown product of propylene glycol. Because of this, the secondhand aerosol from e-cigarettes is also potentially harmful. Some of the flavors used in e-cigarettes contain carcinogens and other harmful chemicals. For example, the butter flavoring may contain diacetyl, the chemical used to give popcorn a buttery flavor and that causes irreversible lung disease when inhaled, a disease referred to as *popcorn lung*.
>
> According to the Centers for Disease Control and Prevention (CDC), e-cigarettes are no safer than traditional tobacco cigarettes, nor are they a more effective method of quitting smoking than counseling and drug-assisted treatments. When users try to quit e-cigarettes, they experience the same withdrawal symptoms as users of traditional tobacco cigarettes, including irritability, depression, restlessness, and anxiousness. E-cigarettes increase the risk for myocardial infarction due to hypertension, tachycardia, and hardening of the arteries secondary to nicotine. Nicotine has been shown to adversely affect adolescent brain development, leading to cognitive and behavioral issues. There are more than 500 brands of e-cigarettes, each of which contains *some* level of nicotine—even those that claim they do not. E-juice refill cartridges often contain more nicotine than is indicated on the label.
>
> In August 2016 the US Food and Drug Administration (FDA) began regulation of all tobacco products, including e-cigarettes, cigars, hookah tobacco, and pipe tobacco. The sale of all tobacco products, including e-cigarettes, will be prohibited to those younger than 18 years of age; packaging and marketing of all tobacco products, including e-cigarettes, will require the display of health warnings; and the FDA will be able to stop manufacturers from making statements about their products that have not been proven by research.
>
> In 2019 the CDC released information identifying the additive vitamin E acetate in vaping products as the presumed causative agent in persons presenting with e-cigarette product use lung injury (EVALI). However, the CDC cautioned it was too soon to rule out other chemicals as additional causative agents. By November 2019, nearly 2300 cases of EVALI had been reported to the CDC from 49 states, including 47 deaths. Please refer to https://www.cdc.gov/tobacco/basic_information/e-cigarettes/severe-lung-disease.html for further information and updates.
>
> Nurses who work with children and adolescents must be diligent in asking about the use of e-cigarettes and providing counseling concerning the dangers of using them. Related to this, they must ask about media and Internet usage and teach young people critical viewing skills; that is, they must help young people understand that what appears in the media does not always represent reality; often, it is a representation of someone's or something's special interest. Nurses must urge children and adolescents who use e-cigarettes to quit, and they must provide the help needed to achieve sustained remission.

to 25 times the recommended dose). Dextromethorphan (DXM), an antitussive that can be purchased without a prescription, and promethazine-codeine cough syrup, available by prescription only, are the products most frequently misused. Using DXM is known on the street as "robotripping" or "skittling"; when taken in higher-than-recommended amounts, users may experience euphoria, dissociative effects, or hallucinations. Side effects of DXM include nausea and vomiting, stomach pain, confusion, dizziness, double or blurred vision, slurred speech, impaired coordination, tachycardia, drowsiness, numbness, and disorientation. Many of the DXM-containing products used to get high also contain other drugs, such as antihistamines, analgesics, or decongestants. High doses of these drugs can lead to hepatic damage or failure, cardiovascular effects, and coma.

Promethazine-codeine cough syrup can result in relaxation and euphoria when taken in higher-than-recommended amounts; when combined with soda, it is referred to as Syrup, Sizzurp, Purple drank, Barre, or Lean. Hard candy may be added for flavor. (See the previous section on OUD for information concerning codeine, an opioid drug.)

Teens may also misuse antihistamines, wherein they may take up to 40 tablets of dimenhydrinate or diphenhydramine. Apparently, such excessive doses induce feelings like a narcotic high, complete with hallucinations. Misusing these over-the-counter drugs is not without danger. The FDA reports teenagers ending up in emergency departments or dying after participating in the "Benadryl Challenge" encouraged in videos posted on the social media application TikTok.

There are no FDA-approved drugs to treat substance use disorders related to cough and cold products. More research is needed to find out if behavioral therapies can be used to treat such misuse.

Anabolic-Androgenic Steroids

An anabolic-androgenic steroid (AAS) is a synthetic agent used to treat conditions caused by low levels of testosterone in the body, such as delayed puberty, hypogonadism, and cachexia related to chronic disease states. By binding to androgen receptors, these prescription drugs (e.g., danazol, fluoxymesterone, nandrolone, and oxandrolone) exert *anabolic effects*, such as growth of muscle and bone and red blood cell production, and *androgenic effects*, such as production of primary and secondary sexual characteristics. AASs have been used to enhance athletic and sexual performance and physical appearance in all age groups. Street names of these drugs include Juice, Gym Candy, Pumpers, Stackers, and Roids. The drug may be taken orally or may be administered IM in doses 10 to 100 times higher than what would be recommended for medical conditions.

Short-term effects of AAS use include headache, acne, fluid retention in the hands and feet, oily skin, yellowing of the skin and whites of the eyes, aggression, extreme mood swings, anger, paranoid jealousy, extreme irritability, delusions, impaired judgment, and infection at the injection site. Long-term effects include kidney damage or failure, liver damage, high blood pressure, enlarged heart, or changes in cholesterol leading to increased risk of stroke or heart attack. In addition, men may experience shrunken testicles, infertility, baldness, development of breasts, and an increased risk for prostate cancer. Women may experience excess facial and body hair, male-pattern baldness, menstrual cycle changes, enlargement of the clitoris, and deepened voice. Adolescents who use anabolic steroids may experience stunted bone growth and height.

Withdrawal from AAS use may lead to mood swings, fatigue, restlessness, loss of appetite, and decreased sex drive. ⚡ Nurses must be alert when caring for persons withdrawing from AAS use because withdrawal may cause depression lasting up to a year, which can result in suicide attempts. Antidepressants and behavioral therapy may be helpful.

Box 8.6 discusses dehydroepiandrosterone and its risks and benefits.

SPECIAL NEEDS OF PATIENTS WITH SUBSTANCE USE DISORDER

Surgical Patients

Patients with substance use disorder are at high risk for drug interactions, postoperative complications, and death when surgery is required. An assessment of drug use and application of the CAGE questionnaire, a screening tool for alcohol misuse, should be part of all patient histories. Respiratory changes in persons with TUD make introduction of endotracheal and suction tubes more difficult and increase the risk for

> **BOX 8.6 Dehydroepiandrosterone**
>
> Dehydroepiandrosterone (DHEA), a precursor to testosterone and estrogen, can be found in many dietary supplements. Many people take supplements that contain DHEA in the belief that it will slow aging, increase energy levels, and build bone and muscle strength. However, there is no evidence to support these claims. Small studies have noted that DHEA may be effective in the relief of mild depression and skin changes associated with aging. Side effects include oily skin and acne, hair loss, nausea, hypertension, menstrual changes, deepening of the voice in women, fatigue, headache, irregular heartbeat, insomnia, and hypercholesterolemia. Long-term effects include stunting of growth, aggressive behavior, mood swings, and hepatic toxicity. Nurses who care for patients who take dietary supplements containing DHEA should be sure to counsel them about the risks and benefits associated with DHEA use.

postoperative respiratory problems. During the postoperative period, nurses should be alert for signs and symptoms of drug interactions with pain medications or anesthesia and for signs of withdrawal.

Special precautions must be taken for the patient with AUD who requires surgery. Alcohol use may be overlooked in an accident victim if there are injuries that cause CNS depression. In addition, many persons are undiagnosed as persons with AUD at the time of admission for elective surgery. The patient with AUD may require an increased level of anesthesia, which can increase the risk for cardiovascular instability in susceptible patients. Delirium may be triggered by surgery and abstinence. After surgery, patients with AUD may develop withdrawal syndrome, indicated by tremors, mild anxiety, gastric distress, and headache; left untreated, withdrawal may progress to withdrawal seizures or delirium tremens, manifested by hallucinations, disorientation, tachycardia, hypertension, hyperthermia, agitation, and diaphoresis. Symptoms may develop anywhere from 6 hours to 5 days after the last drink; left untreated, alcohol withdrawal syndrome can be fatal. Use of tools, such as the Clinical Institute Withdrawal Assessment of Alcohol Scale, Revised, can improve recognition and treatment of alcohol withdrawal. A copy of this tool can be found at https://www.ci2i.research.va.gov/paws/pdfs/ciwa-ar.pdf. The goal of treatment is the alleviation of symptoms and the provision of supportive care with fluids and nutrition.

Pain Management

Although health care personnel may be reluctant to administer narcotic analgesics to persons with substance use disorders, there is no evidence that providing narcotic analgesia to these patients in any way worsens their disease. *When patients experience pain, the goal is to treat the pain.* All patients should be treated with dignity and respect. Withholding adequate analgesia due to misconceptions leads to unnecessary suffering and harm and is a breach of the ethical principles central to nursing care. Addressing substance use disorder is *not* a priority when a patient is in pain.

When patients acknowledge substance use disorder, it is important to determine which drug is used and the amount taken each day. If the patient misuses opioids, it is often best to avoid further exposure to the drug of choice because recommended opioid doses do not provide adequate pain relief due to tolerance. Paradoxically, significantly increasing the dose of opioid to achieve pain control can induce hyperalgesia, where patients become abnormally sensitive to pain. Effective doses of other analgesics can be determined if daily doses of the drug of choice are known. Nonopioid and adjuvant analgesics and nonpharmacologic pain relief measures may also be used, particularly when the person with OUD is on drug-assisted treatment with buprenorphine or naltrexone.

THE NURSE WITH SUBSTANCE USE DISORDER

Substance use disorder is no more prevalent among nurses than it is among the rest of the population. However, nurses care for others during the most vulnerable times of their life; nurses have the lives of others in their hands and are therefore held to a higher standard than other professionals. Drug use is a serious concern in health care professions. It is estimated that 1 in 10 nurses misuse drugs or alcohol, including benzodiazepines and opioids such as fentanyl and hydrocodone.

Contributing Factors and Characteristics

Factors

Factors that contribute to drug use among nurses have been identified as job stress, the emotional demands of nursing, long hours and shift rotations, and easy access to drugs. In addition, nurses internalize their feelings to stay in control during crisis and have little to no time to decompress. Nurses take care of others before themselves.

Characteristics

Signs and symptoms of substance use disorder may be indicated by changes in personality and behavior, including alterations in job performance, unexplained absence from the unit, arriving to work late and leaving early poor judgment and errors (e.g., medication errors), alteration of verbal and telephone orders, and illogical documentation.

Signs and symptoms of substance use disorder also include physical changes. Behaviors related to influence of the drug or signs of withdrawal may also be present, such as subtle changes in appearance, self-imposed isolation, inappropriate responses to situations (i.e., both verbal and emotional), confusion, lapses in memory, and decreased levels of alertness.

Discrepancies in controlled-drug handling and records may indicate drug diversion, the deliberate redirecting of a drug from a patient or facility to the employee for personal use. Indications of drug diversion include frequent narcotic wastage, multiple corrections to medication records and other documentation, and frequent reports of uncontrolled pain from patients.

Nurses often enable drug use among coworkers by covering up their mistakes or tardiness, excusing their behavior, or simply ignoring obvious signs and symptoms. When it is recognized that a nurse is impaired, help for the nurse requires sharing observations and concerns with the nurse and supervisor to provide the means for rehabilitation. For more information related to substance use disorder among nurses, please go to the National Council of State Boards of Nursing website at www.ncsbn.org.

Management

In most states, nurses may enter nondisciplinary programs designed for evaluation and treatment. These programs include compliance monitoring during treatment and recovery as well as abstinence monitoring upon the nurse's return to work. These programs allow nurses to maintain their licenses. The goals of these programs are to protect the safety of the public, to maintain the integrity of the profession, and to ensure that the nurse is offered the possibility of treatment and rehabilitation before the license to practice is revoked or the job is terminated. Further information can be found at www.ncsbn.org/substance-use-in-nursing.htm.

Given the prevalence of drug use, all nurses care for patients who use drugs, regardless of whether the use has been identified as substance use disorder. Therefore, it is important for nurses to identify patients who misuse drugs and to intervene. Knowledge of the most misused drugs and their treatments is critical to sustained remission and promotion of healthy lifestyles.

CHAPTER 8 Drugs in Substance Use Disorder

CLINICAL JUDGMENT [NURSING PROCESS]
Tobacco Use Disorder

Concept: Coping
- Coping is a process involving cognitive and behavioral actions designed to manage internal or external situations that are perceived as difficult and/or beyond the individual's current resources.

Concept: Safety
- Protecting the patient from potential or actual harm; a basic human need.

Recognize Cues [Assessment]
- Ask the patient to identify any barriers or impediments to quitting.
- Assess current smoking status and smoking history.
- Assess for feelings of hopelessness, depression, and apathy.
- Assess health history.
- Assess the patient's decision-making capacity.
- Determine the willingness of the patient to attempt to quit.
- Have the patient identify negative consequences of smoking and the potential benefits of quitting.
- Identify the cultural context of the patient's smoking pattern.
- Identify the patient's locus of control.
- Identify what rewards for quitting are most important to the patient.

Analyze Cues and Prioritize Hypothesis [Patient Problems]
- Potential for nonadherence
- Coping/decreased ability to cope
- Need for health teaching

Generate Solutions [Planning]
- The patient begins to identify ways to achieve control over nicotine use.

- The patient demonstrates positive health maintenance behaviors as evidenced by keeping scheduled appointments and participating in a tobacco cessation program.
- The patient identifies and uses available resources.

Take Action [Nursing Interventions]
- Advise the patient to keep a list of "slips" and "near-slips" to learn to avoid their causes.
- Assist the patient with problem solving.
- Define your role as the patient's advocate.
- Encourage the patient to avoid environments and activities previously associated with smoking.
- Enhance the patient's sense of autonomy by involving the patient in decision making.
- Help the patient choose the best method to quit smoking based on patient preferences and anticipated benefits.
- Refer the patient to support groups or programs available in the community.
- Schedule frequent follow-up contacts with the patient to offer encouragement and help the patient deal with relapses.
- Set a quit date with the patient, ideally within 1 to 2 weeks.
- Teach the patient about drug-assisted treatment available to assist in smoking cessation.
- Teach the patient to anticipate the withdrawal symptoms and challenges of quitting.

Evaluate Outcomes [Evaluation]
- To avoid relapse, evaluate the effectiveness of the cessation plan, including the use of drug-assisted treatment and support systems.

CLINICAL JUDGMENT CASE STUDY

A 57-year-old is admitted to the surgical unit in preparation for back surgery after conservative treatment for a recent back injury failed to relieve his pain. The patient's partner tells the nurse they hope the surgery will be successful, and confides that the patient has just been sitting around the house drinking more beer than usual because they have not been able to work. The patient appears relaxed and unconcerned about the anticipated surgery.

1. What assessments of the patient's alcohol use should the nurse make and communicate to the surgeon and anesthesiologist before the patient is further prepared for surgery?
2. During the patient's postoperative period, when will the nurse expect signs of withdrawal syndrome to occur?
3. What early signs and symptoms would alert the nurse to the development of withdrawal syndrome?
4. What goal of treatment during the patient's postoperative period is related to alcohol withdrawal syndrome?

REVIEW QUESTIONS

1. When caring for a patient recovering from an episode of opioid toxicity, the nurse determines that the patient has opioid use disorder based on which finding?
   a. Withdrawal symptoms
   b. A history of daily use
   c. Craving that results in drug-seeking behaviors
   d. Intravenous, rather than oral, use of the drug

2. A patient hospitalized with a fractured femur after an automobile accident develops nausea and vomiting, abdominal cramps, and restlessness. The nurse suspects that the patient is experiencing which reaction?
   a. Opioid withdrawal
   b. Alcohol toxicity
   c. Flashbacks from LSD use
   d. Nicotine withdrawal

3. Which treatments will the nurse anticipate administering to a patient who has been admitted with alcohol toxicity? **Select all that apply.**
   a. Naloxone
   b. Thiamine
   c. Intravenous fluids
   d. Naltrexone
   e. Intravenous glucose solution
   f. Flumazenil
4. The nurse observes another nurse taking oral opioids from the medication room at the hospital. Which action is appropriate for the nurse who observes drug diversion to take?
   a. Report the finding to the nursing supervisor to enable the nurse's participation in a nondisciplinary program.
   b. Ignore the situation to protect the nurse from dismissal and possible loss of licensure.
   c. Confront the nurse and demand that the drugs be returned before someone notices their absence.
   d. Ask the nurse to request pain medications from a physician rather than stealing them from the hospital.
5. A patient is to start disulfiram to help with alcohol use disorder. The nurse providing medication education about the drug will include which topics in the education plan? **Select all that apply.**
   a. Importance of taking the medication every day
   b. That better results are experienced when a support group helps with treatment adherence
   c. Common food and hygiene products that contain alcohol
   d. That disulfiram treatment should be stopped 1 day before alcohol consumption
   e. That disulfiram works by disrupting the metabolism of alcohol
   f. That use of alcohol with disulfiram may cause nausea and vomiting and may even be fatal

UNIT II Pharmacotherapy and Drug Administration

9

Safety and Quality

http://evolve.elsevier.com/McCuistion/pharmacology

OBJECTIVES

- Describe the "Six Rights" of medication administration.
- Discuss the actions and guidelines of various regulatory bodies to promote safety in health care.
- Describe the key risks to safety in medication administration, including the prevention of medication errors.
- Describe other actions and resources for ensuring safe medication administration.

OUTLINE

"Six Rights" of Medication Administration, 69
    Right Patient, 70
    Right Drug, 70
    Right Dose, 71
    Right Time, 72
    Right Route, 73
    Right Documentation, 73
Promoting Safety in the Health Care Environment, 73
    Just and Safe Culture, 73
    The Joint Commission's "Do Not Use List" and the Institute for Safe Medication Practices' "List of Error-Prone Abbreviations", 74
    US Food and Drug Administration, 74
    Drug Reconciliation, 75

Disposal of Medications, 75
Sharps Safety, 75
Safety Risks With Medication Administration, 75
    Counterfeit Drugs, 76
    Dosage Forms: To Crush or Not to Crush, 76
    High-Alert Medications, 76
    Look-Alike and Sound-Alike Drug Names, 77
Other Factors in the Prevention of Medication Errors, 77
    Resources for Preventing Errors in Medication Administration, 78
    Pregnancy Categories and Subsections, 78
    Guidelines for Medication Administration, 78
Clinical Judgment Case Study, 79
Review Questions, 79

According to the IQVIA Institute for Human Data Science (2023), total net spending on medicine is expected to reach $380–400 billion in 2025, up from $329 billion in 2020. In 2022, it is estimated that medication errors resulted in 1.5 million injuries and deaths in the United States. Medication errors are responsible for 7000 deaths annually in the United States (https://www.iqvia.com/insights/the-iqvia-institute/reports/the-global-use-of-medicines-2023).

The focus of this chapter is quality and safety in medication administration. It involves a discussion of safety initiatives and interventions that include the "Six Rights" of medication administration, the Nurse's Bill of Rights, the Culture of Safety, and The Joint Commission (TJC) National Patient Safety Goals. Also included are high-alert drugs, look-alike and sound-alike drugs, and dosage forms to crush or not to crush.

"SIX RIGHTS" OF MEDICATION ADMINISTRATION

The "Six Rights" of medication administration are important goals for medication safety. The nurse following these guidelines will verify the following: (1) the right patient, (2) the right drug, (3) the right dose, (4) the right time, (5) the right route, and (6) the right documentation. The original six rights have included subsequent additions throughout the years in an attempt to maintain safety (e.g., the right assessment, the right education, the right evaluation, and the right of the patient to refuse). All interventions are designed to ensure safe medication practices. It is important to remember the nurse collaborates with other health care providers (HCPs), such as the physician, the pharmacist, and the nurse practitioner, to provide safe medication administration. The nurse relays the patient's response to

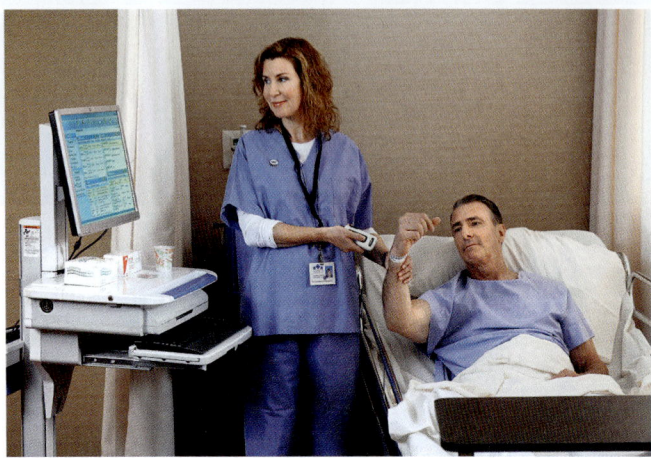

Fig. 9.1 Bar code scanner used to access the patient's medical record. (From Ignatavicius DD, Workman LM, Rebar CR, et al. *Medical-Surgical Nursing.* 9th ed. Elsevier; 2018.)

the entire health care team (https://www.chop.edu/health-resources/sixrights-medication-administration).

Right Patient

The **right patient** determination is essential. TJC requires at least two forms of identification before drug administration (http://www.jointcommission.org):

- Ask the patient to state their full name and birth date, and compare these with the patient's identification (ID) band and the medication administration record (MAR).
- Many facilities have electronic health records (EHRs) that allow the nurse to directly scan the bar code from the patient's ID band. Once the band is scanned, the patient's medication record appears for the nurse to view (Fig. 9.1). Additional nursing implications include the following:
  - Most hospitals have color-coded ID bands that include bands coded for allergy, do not resuscitate (DNR), fall risk, and restricted extremity. Always check facility policies for the use of color-coded bands and their meanings.
  - Verify the patient's identification by using two methods of identification each time a medication is administered.
  - If the patient is an adult with a cognitive disorder or a child, verify the patient's name with a family member. In the event a family member is unavailable and the patient is unable to self-identify, follow the facility's policy. Many facilities have policies that include a photo ID on the band with the patient's name and birth date affixed to the band.
  - Distinguish between two patients with the same first or last name by placing "name-alert" stickers as warnings on the medical records.

Right Drug

The nurse must accurately determine the **right drug** before administration. When working with an EHR, after scanning the wristband, the patient's drug profile appears on the computer screen. The nurse's next step is to scan the medication label, and it will automatically validate the time, date, and nurse administering the patient's medication. If it is not the correct medication, the nurse will receive an alert and will be unable to proceed in the MAR until the correct medication is scanned.

Both federal and state legislation governs who may write a prescription order. Medication orders are prescribed by a licensed HCP under authority from the state to prescribe drugs. The disciplines that have prescriptive authority are the medical doctor (MD), dentist (doctor of dental surgery [DDS]), podiatrist (doctor of podiatric medicine [DPM]), certified nurse practitioner (CNP), advanced practice registered nurse (APRN), physician assistant (PA), veterinarian (DVM), chiropractor (DC), and optometrist (OD). In addition, medical clinical psychiatrists and pharmacists have prescriptive authority with strict guidelines set by the state. Prescriptions may be handwritten by the HCP, delivered as a telephone order (T/O) or verbal order (V/O), or directly entered into the patient's EHR. Handwritten prescriptions are written on a provider's legal prescription pad and are filled by a pharmacist.

Sometimes providers order medications by directly speaking to the nurse. All telephone orders or verbal orders for medications are either handwritten by the nurse taking the order or entered directly into a computer and "read back" to ensure accuracy. The nurse will write the name of the prescribing provider and add a notation that the order was verified. The order will be completed when the doctor affixes their signature onto the order. After dictating a verbal order, the provider must sign it within 24 hours. If the order is a controlled medication, most facilities require two licensed nurses to listen to the order and sign it. Nursing students are not allowed to accept or take provider orders, but they may administer the medication after a registered nurse (RN) has verified it.

Many hospitals are implementing computerized physician order entry (CPOE) systems to handle HCP medication orders. This method of ordering medications can help decrease drug errors by decreasing transcription errors. HCPs using a CPOE will directly input the prescription into the patient's EHR; the order is electronically signed by the HCP and is sent directly to the pharmacy, and it is recorded as part of the patient's MAR. A strong safety feature is the ability to identify drug interactions with the patient's current drugs and any newly prescribed medications.

The use of computerized ordering systems has added speed and a measure of safety to the ordering process. Orders can be written from virtually any location and sent electronically, but the computer will not process the order until all necessary information is provided. Because the order is computerized, illegible orders or signatures are prevented. Before the nurse can administer the medication, both the pharmacy and the nurse must validate the accuracy of the patient's prescription order in the EHR.

The components of a drug order are as follows (Fig. 9.2):

- Patient name and birth date
- Date the order is written
- Provider signature or name if an electronic order, T/O, or V/O
- Signature of licensed staff who took the T/O or V/O, if applicable
- HCPs who wish to prescribe controlled drugs must register with the US Federal Drug Enforcement Agency (DEA); when prescribing controlled substances, the HCP's DEA number must be on the prescription
- Drug name and strength
- Drug frequency or dose (e.g., once daily)
- Route of administration
- Duration of administration (e.g., ×7 days, ×3 doses, when applicable)
- Number of patient refills
- Number of pills to be dispensed
- Any special instructions for withholding or adjusting dosage based on nursing assessment, drug effectiveness, or laboratory results

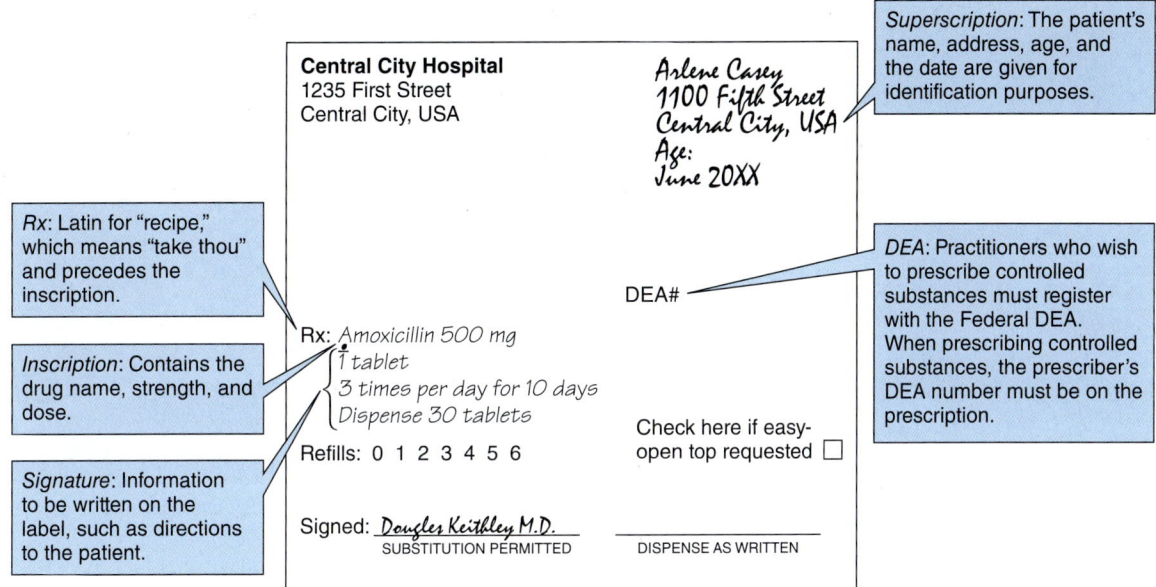

Fig. 9.2 Example of a drug order. *DEA*, Drug Enforcement Agency. (From Medical School Headquarters. *Prescription Writing 101*. n.d. http://medicalschoolhq.net/prescription-writing-101.)

It is the nurse's responsibility to administer the drug, as ordered, by the provider, and if the drug order is incomplete, the drug should not be administered. Verification of a questionable order must be done in a timely manner. The HCP is usually contacted, and the conversation is documented. Nurses must become familiar with the components of a drug order and question any incomplete or unclear orders. Nurses are legally liable if they give a prescribed drug and the dosage is incorrect, or if the drug is contraindicated for the patient's health status. Once the drug has been administered, the nurse becomes liable for the predicted effects of that drug.

Medication administration is never considered just a process of "passing" drugs. Nurses must use critical thinking skills and sound clinical judgment when assessing the patient's correct medication for their particular diagnosis. The nurse must ask critical questions: Is the dose appropriate? What is the patient's expected response? Also, the nurse must teach the patient about the drug's side effects and when it is necessary for the patient to notify the HCP.

To avoid drug errors, the drug label should be read three times: (1) when the nurse picks up the drug and removes it from the automatic dispensing cabinet (ADC), (2) as the nurse prepares the drug for administration, and (3) when the nurse administers the drug.

Nursing interventions related to drug orders can ensure correct administration of medications:
- The nurse should verify the identity of the patient by comparing the name on the wristband with the name on the MAR for accuracy.
- Always use two patient identifiers, such as having patients repeat their name and date of birth.
- The nurse must become familiar with the patient's health history and always perform a head-to-toe assessment on the patient, including a complete set of vital signs.
- Always review the patient's laboratory work before the administration of drugs.
- Read the drug order carefully. If the order is unclear, verify it with the HCP before administering the drug.
- Know the patient's allergies.
- Know the reason the patient is to receive the medication.
- Check the drug label by identifying the drug name, the amount of the drug (tablet or volume), and its suitability for administration by the intended route.
- Check dosage calculations.
- Know the date the medication was ordered and the ending date. Some agencies have automatic stop orders that are generally facility specific. Examples of such orders include controlled drugs that need to be renewed every 48 hours, antibiotics usually renewed every 7 to 14 days, and cancellation of all medications when the patient goes to surgery.
- All orders—including first-dose, one-time, and as-needed (prn) medication orders—should be checked against the original orders.

Right Dose

The **right dose** refers to verification by the nurse that the dose administered is the amount ordered and that it is safe for the patient for whom it is prescribed. The right dose is based on the patient's physical status. Many medications require the patient's weight to determine the right dose. Usually pediatrics, medical-surgical, and critical care situations require weight to complete the drug calculation and determine the correct dose (heparin and digoxin drips are examples of medications calculated according to weight). The nurse determines whether the drug is safe to administer according to the drug's pharmacodynamics (action) and the patient's vital signs.

Before administration, it is important the nurse carefully review the patient's current laboratory results. A chemistry panel includes renal and liver function and sodium and potassium levels. Renal and hepatic functions are important considerations because many drugs are cleared through the kidneys and metabolized by the liver. Also, the nurse should review the hematology laboratory reports, which include a complete blood count, red blood cells, hemoglobin, hematocrit, and platelets. It is most important that the nurse check the drug's correct dose range in a reliable drug resource book or by consulting with a pharmacist. In most cases, the right dose for a specific patient is within the recommended range for the drug.

Nurses use dimensional analysis or ratio and proportion when calculating a drug dose (see Chapter 11). Always recheck the drug

Fig. 9.3 Automated dispensing cabinet used to hold patients' medications for dispensing. (From Potter PA, Perry AG. *Fundamentals of Nursing*. 7th ed. Elsevier; 2009.)

Fig. 9.4 Unit dose sheets. Courtesy Omnicell, Inc.

calculation, especially if the dose is within a fraction or an extremely large dose. Consult another nurse or the pharmacist when in doubt.

Today, most drugs are dispensed through ADCs (Fig. 9.3), which are computerized drug storage cabinets that store and dispense medications near the point of care while controlling and tracking drug distribution. The patient's drugs are stocked in the cabinet by the pharmacist and are accessed under the patient's name. The nurse can select and pull the patient's drugs from the cabinet. This technology improves patient care by promoting accurate and quick access to medications, locked storage for all medications, and electronic tracking for controlled substances. Automation of drug administration saves time and decreases costs associated with drug administration.

Another method of dispensing drugs is the unit dose method, in which drugs are individually wrapped and labeled for single-dose use for each patient. The unit dose method has reduced dosage errors because no calculations are required. Some facilities still use a multidose vial from the ADC. If this occurs, the nurse must complete a calculation to retrieve the correct amount ordered by the physician from the vial. If there is any medication left in the vial, it is disposed of according to the facility's policy for disposal of drugs.

Long-term care, day care, and assisted living facilities use punch cards to organize medications. This special packaging is obtained from the facility's pharmacy. The pharmacy sends a 30-day supply of medication for each prescription in a punch card, and the nurse administers the medication from the card (Fig. 9.4).

An important nursing intervention related to the right dose includes calculating the drug dose correctly. If in doubt about the amount to be administered, consult with a nurse peer to validate the correct amount. In some settings, two RNs are required to check the dosage for certain medications, such as insulin and heparin.

Right Time

The right time refers to the time the prescribed dose is ordered for administration. Daily drug dosages are given at specified intervals, such as twice a day (bid), three times a day (tid), four times a day (qid), or every 6 hours. This is so the plasma level of the drug is maintained at a therapeutic level. Every drug cannot be given exactly when ordered; therefore health care agencies have policies that specify a range of times within which drugs can be administered (check your agency's policy). When a drug has a long half-life, it is usually given once a day. Drugs with a short half-life are given several times a day at specified intervals. Some drugs are given before meals, whereas others must be given with meals.

Fig. 9.5 Military time.

Use of military time, which is based on a 24-hour clock (Fig. 9.5), reduces administration errors and decreases documentation. Many nursing facilities use military time rather than standard time. Nursing interventions related to the right time include the following:
- Administer drugs at the specified times (refer to agency policy).
- Administer drugs that are affected by food, such as tetracycline, 1 hour before or 2 hours after meals.
- Give food with drugs that can irritate the stomach (gastric mucosa)—for example, potassium and aspirin. Some medications are absorbed better after eating.
- Adjust the medication schedule to fit the patient's lifestyle, activities, tolerances, or preferences as much as possible.
- Check whether the patient is scheduled for any diagnostic procedures that contraindicate the administration of medications, such as endoscopy or fasting blood tests. Determine whether the medication should be given before or after the test based on the policy.
- Check the expiration date. If the date has passed, discard the medication or return it to the pharmacy, depending on the policy.

- Administer antibiotics at even intervals (e.g., every 8 hours rather than three times daily) throughout the 24-hour period to maintain therapeutic blood levels.
- Patients who require dialysis usually have blood pressure medications stopped before dialysis because dialysis can decrease blood pressure. However, some doctors order the medications to be given before dialysis. If any questions arise, check with the HCP before proceeding.

Right Route

The right route is necessary for adequate or appropriate absorption. The **right route** is ordered by the HCP and indicates the mechanism by which the medication enters the body. The more common routes of **absorption** include the following: oral (drug in the form of a liquid, elixir, or suspension); pill (tablet or capsule); sublingual (under the tongue for venous absorption); buccal (between the cheek and gum); feeding tube (enteral); topical (applied to the skin); inhalation (aerosol sprays); otic (ear); ophthalmic (eye); nasal (spray instillation); suppository (rectal or vaginal); and through the parenteral routes: (1) intradermal, (2) subcutaneous (subcut or SQ), (3) intramuscular (IM), or (4) intravenous (IV).

Nursing interventions related to the right route include the following:
- Assess the patient's ability to swallow before administering oral medications; ensure the patient does not have an order requiring nothing by mouth (NPO).
- Do not crush or mix medications in other substances without consulting a pharmacist or a reliable drug reference. Do not mix medications in an infant's formula feeding.
- If the medication must be mixed with another substance, explain this to the patient. For example, elderly patients may use applesauce or yogurt to mix their medications to make them easier to swallow. Medications should be administered one at a time in the substance.
- Best Practice Guidelines and TJC state that drugs must be identifiable up until the point of delivery. When administering many drugs at one time, it is *not* recommended to mix drugs together. The correct practice is to administer one pill at a time. When a patient has an enteral tube, it is important to follow these guidelines; this allows the nurse to flush the tube before and after each pill or liquid is administered to prevent the tube from clogging. In the event the patient's drug inadvertently falls to the ground, the nurse will be able to identify, discard, and replace the pill.
- Instruct the patient that medications must be swallowed with water. Juice can interfere with the absorption of certain medications; however, it is recommended that iron be taken with orange juice or vitamin C supplements to aid in its absorption.
- Use aseptic technique when administering drugs. Sterile technique is required with the parenteral routes.
- Administer drugs at the appropriate sites for the route.
- Stay with the patient until oral drugs have been swallowed.

Right Documentation

The **right documentation** requires the nurse to immediately record the appropriate information about the drug administered. Many systems are available for documenting drug administration. Both paper and computerized MAR systems include information about the drug to be administered, including (1) the name of the drug, (2) the dose, (3) the route, (4) the time and date, and (5) the nurse's initials or signature.

One of the oldest documentation methods is the paper MAR. This method is usually found in clinics, nursing homes, and assisted living facilities. The pharmacy furnishes a written MAR record. Using this method, the nurse initials next to the patient's name and drug, verifying administration of the drug.

Most large facilities have computerized charting, in which the nurse provides a personal identification and password to enter the system. By scanning the patient's identification band, which includes the patient's bar code information, the nurse accesses the patient's personal MAR within the EHR system. Once the nurse scans the bar code on the patient's medication package, the administration is validated in the computerized MAR. The computerized system interfaces with other departments, including the pharmacy, laboratory, and sometimes the physician's office.

Documentation of the patient's response to the medication is required with a variety of medications such as (1) opioid and nonopioid analgesics (How effective was pain relief?); (2) sedatives (How effective was relaxation?); and (3) antiemetics (Was nausea/vomiting decreased or eliminated?). The nurse continues to assess and evaluate the patient's response to the medication (e.g., Is there any gastrointestinal upset or skin sensitivity?). All information obtained is documented into the patient's medical record. Keep in mind that patient responses are not necessarily verbal; they may be physiologic (e.g., blood pressure decreasing in response to an antihypertensive).

Delay in scanning/charting may result in forgetting to chart the medication, and another nurse can inadvertently readminister the drug, assuming it was not given because it was not charted. Therefore it is important to remember that drugs *must* be charted when the drug is administered. Graphic formats or computerized systems (Fig. 9.6) assist in the accurate and timely recording of drugs administered.

The American Nurses Association (ANA) published a Bill of Rights for nurses containing seven premises concerning workplace expectations and environments that nurses from across the United States recognize as necessary for safe nursing practice. The Bill of Rights supports nurses in workplace situations and includes issues such as unsafe staffing, mandatory overtime, and health and safety issues in the workplace. These issues are essential to meet the responsibilities of patient care, including safe drug administration and the responsibility nurses have to themselves (https://www.nursingworld.org/practice-policy/workenvironment/healthsafety/bill-of-rights).

Facilities have an obligation to both nurses and patients to educate and provide guidelines and policies concerning patient safety in all aspects of patient care. Many disciplines are involved in medication administration, and the different departments must work together to provide a method of drug delivery and administration in a safe environment for the patient and the nurse. This can be done by having modern equipment, staff education opportunities, policies and procedures, and communication among the different departments involved in drug administration.

PROMOTING SAFETY IN THE HEALTH CARE ENVIRONMENT

Just and Safe Culture

The National Coordinating Council for Medication Error Reporting (NCCMERP 2023) defines medication error as "any preventable event that may cause or lead to inappropriate medication use or harm to a patient while the medication is in the control of the health care professional" (http://www.nccmerp.org).

Much progress has been made concerning the area of patient safety to embrace change in the medical culture so reporting of errors does not result in personal blame but a failure of the system. The landmark decision of the National Academy of Medicine (previously known as the

TABLE 9.1 "Do Not Use" Abbreviations

The Joint Commission's "Do Not Use List" of abbreviations is shown below. These abbreviations must be written out to avoid misinterpretation. Please visit http://www.thejointcommission.org and http://www.ismp.org for detailed safety information concerning "Do Not Use" abbreviations.

Do Not Use Abbreviation	Use Instead
q.d., Q.D., QD, qd	Write "daily."
q.o.d., Q.O.D., QOD, qod	Write "every other day."
U, u	Write "unit."
IU	Write "International Unit."
MS	Write "morphine sulfate."
$MgSO_4$, MSO_4	Write "magnesium sulfate."
Lack of leading zero (.X mg)	Use a zero before a decimal point when the dose is less than a whole unit (e.g., write 0.X mg).
Trailing zero (X.0 mg)	Do not use a decimal point or zero **after** a whole number (write X mg or write 0.X mg).

Copyright © 2023 Do Not Use List of Abbreviations/The Joint Commission.

Fig. 9.6 Medication administration record. (A) Computerized format. (B) Written format. Labeling for Human Prescription Drug & Biological Products.

Institute of Medicine) report, *To Err Is Human: Building a Safer Health Care System*, has certainly effected a positive change in the development of a "Culture of Safety." The report serves as a basis for creating an awareness of patient safety systems in health care and has led to the development of safety tools instrumental in decreasing the number of drug errors. Over the years, drug administration and the margin of error have shown some improvements with the development of bar coding, CPOE systems, EHRs, and ADCs. However, there is still much work ahead. The ANA's position statement titled "Just Culture" encourages individuals to report drug errors, so the system can be repaired and the problems fixed. "Just Culture" does not hold individual practitioners responsible for a failing system, although it does not tolerate disregard for a patient or gross misconduct (https://nursingworld.org/practtice-policy/nursing-excellence/officialposition-statements/id/just-culture).

In a true culture of safety, everyone in the organization is committed and driven to keep patients safe from harm. Risk management is a process that identifies weaknesses in the system. It then allows changes to be made to minimize the effects of adverse patient outcomes. Most organizations have a risk management department staffed with nurse managers and risk managers who conduct **root cause analysis**, a method of problem solving used to identify potential workplace errors. Such analysis presents opportunities for learning and focuses on strategies that can be put in place to correct problems.

Drug administration is a vulnerable area where the possibility for error is high. If a patient is injured or dies as the result of a drug error, a **sentinel event occurs**. This is an unanticipated event in a health care setting that results in death or serious harm to a patient unrelated to the natural course of the patient's illness. TJC tracks sentinel events in a database to ensure they are adequately analyzed and that unsafe processes are caught and resolved. The most common occurrence of sentinel events is medication errors, and of those, the most frequently implicated drug was potassium chloride (KCl). Most often, KCl was mistaken for sodium chloride, heparin, or furosemide.

The Joint Commission's "Do Not Use List" and the Institute for Safe Medication Practices' "List of Error-Prone Abbreviations"

In addition, TJC has taken steps to support safety and quality care in the workplace. TJC has developed National Patient Safety Goals, which focus on problems in health care safety and how to solve them. These goals are updated and published annually. Once a goal becomes a standard, the goal number is retired and is not used again, and the standard must be adopted by all TJC-accredited agencies. An important goal that has already become a standard for TJC-accredited organizations is the "do not use list" of abbreviations (Table 9.1).

The list of acceptable abbreviations is no longer provided because abbreviations have been found to contribute to drug errors. Table 9.2 contains a list of Error Prone Abbreviations. This provides the user with caution and discretion prior to use. The items contained in the list are frequently used for handwritten, preprinted, and electronic forms of communication.

US Food and Drug Administration

Another safety feature is the US Food and Drug Administration's (FDA) black-box warning system. When a prescription drug is known to be effective for some patients, but may cause serious side effects in others, the FDA will require the drug's printed materials to carry a

TABLE 9.2 Error Prone Abbreviations

Abbreviation/Meaning	Best Practice
Drug Doses and Measurement Unit	
cc (cubic centimeters)	Use mL
l (liter)	Use L (UPPERCASE) for liter
ml (milliliter)	Use mL (lowercase m, UPPERCASE L) for milliliter
Ug (microgram)	Use mcg
Abbreviations for Route of Administration	
AD, AS, AU	Use right ear, left ear, or each ear
OD, OS, OU	Use right eye, left eye, or each eye
Per os	Use PO, by mouth, or orally
SC, SQ, sq, or sub q	Use SUBQ (all UPPERCASE letters, without spaces or periods between letters) or subcutaneous(ly)
Abbreviations for Frequency/Instructions for Use	
HS	Use the word half-strength
hs	Use HS (all UPPERCASE letters) for bedtime
o.d. or OD (once daily)	Use daily
Qhs (nightly at bedtime)	Use nightly or HS for bedtime
Qn (nightly or at bedtime)	Use nightly or HS for bedtime
Q1day (daily)	Use daily
Q6PM, etc.	Use daily at 6PM or 6PM daily
SSRI	Use sliding scale (insulin)
SSI	Use sliding scale insulin
TIW or tiw	Use 3 times weekly
BIW or biw	Use 2 times weekly
UD	Use as directed
D/C	Use discharge and discontinue or stop
Ij	Use injection
OJ	Use orange juice
Period following abbreviations (e.g., mg., mL.)	Use mg, mL, etc., without a terminal period

Copyright ISMP 2024. Reproduction is prohibited without written permission from ISMP. For a complete list of Error Prone Abbreviations, please visit www.errorproneabbreviations/ismp.org.

warning about the adverse effects surrounded by a black box. A black-box warning is the strongest form of warning issued by the FDA about a drug (http://fda.gov).

Drug Reconciliation

Drug reconciliation is an important component of the culture of safety. It is defined as the process of identifying the most accurate list of all medications that the patient is taking at transitions in care. This includes admission and discharge from a hospital to another health care setting such as a long-term care facility. Correct drug reconciliation is important because it prevents discrepancies that can cause a drug error. One in five patients experience an adverse event when transitioning from hospital to home.

Drug reconciliation was created to provide drug continuity during care transitions, thereby promoting patient safety. For this reason, the nurse should advise patients to do the following:
- Always carry a list of personal drug information in case of an emergency.
- Update this list of drugs whenever a change occurs.
- Bring a list of medications to each HCP appointment.

Disposal of Medications

The FDA and DEA issue guidelines for appropriate disposal of prescription drugs based on the Secure and Responsible Disposal Act issued by Congress. This encourages both public and private entities to develop secure, convenient, and responsible methods for collecting and destroying medications and controlled substances. It also recommends a decrease in the amount of controlled substances released into the environment, especially into water and sewage systems.

General guidelines include drug take-back events, mail-back programs, and collection receptacles provided by authorized DEA collection companies for facilities to dispose of unwanted controlled substances. Facilities may contract with an independent or local collection program authorized by the state and the DEA to dispose of medical waste and hazardous materials. The drugs are disposed of in a receptacle that must comply with strict security and record-keeping requirements as established by the FDA and DEA. The company then incinerates the waste.

Consumers who do not have available DEA-authorized collectors or medicine take-back programs can follow these simple steps:
1. Remove medications from the original packaging and mix them (do not crush tablets or capsules) with an unpalatable substance such as dirt, kitty litter, or used coffee grounds. This method is intended to make medications less attractive to people and animals.
2. Place the mixture in a container such as a sealed plastic bag.
3. Throw the container in the household trash.
4. Scratch out all personal information on the prescription label before disposing of the empty container.

Unless specifically instructed, individuals should not flush drugs down the toilet, where they will pollute the environment and pose a danger to humans and animals. (Exceptions to this rule are listed in Box 9.1.) Nurses and patients can consult a pharmacist with questions related to medication disposal. Pharmacists are always available to answer questions on how to properly dispose of unused medications (https://www.fda.gov/drugs/disposal-unused-medicines-what-you-shouldknow/drug-disposal-fdas-flush-list-certain-medicines).

Sharps Safety

US hospital-based health care professionals experience more than 600,000 needlestick injuries each year (http://www.osha.gov). The ANA's campaign for "Safe Needles Save Lives" prompted the Occupational Safety and Health Administration (OSHA) to enforce a Needlestick Safety and Prevention Act (NSPA). The act requires that employers implement safer medical devices for their employees, provide a safe and secure workplace environment with educational opportunities, and develop written policies to help prevent sharps injuries.

SAFETY RISKS WITH MEDICATION ADMINISTRATION

Every year the FDA receives more than 100,000 reports that are related to hospital medication errors. Data support that a hospitalized patient is subject to one medication administration error per day. Most medication errors occur in the transcription stage (56%), followed by the

BOX 9.1 Medications Recommended for Disposal by Flushing

Active Ingredient	Found in Brand Names
Benzhydrocodone/acetaminophen	Apadaz
Buprenorphine hydrochloride	Belbuca, Bunavail, Butrans, Cassipa, Suboxone, Subutex, Zubsolv, Naloxone
Fentanyl	Abstral, Actiq, Duragesic, Fentora, Onsolis
Diazepam	Diastat/Diastat AcuDial rectal gel
Hydrocodone	Anexsia, Hysingla ER, Lortab, Norco, Reprexain, Vicodin, Vicoprofen, Zohydro ER
Hydromorphone	Dilaudid, Exalgo
Meperidine	Demerol
Methadone	Dolophine, Methadose
Methylphenidate	Daytrana transdermal patch system
Morphine	Arymo ER, Embeda, Kadian, Morphabond ER, MS Contin, Avinza
Oxycodone	Combunox, Oxaydo (formerly Oxecta), OxyContin, Percocet, Percodan, Roxicet, Roxicodone, Roxybond, Targiniq ER, Xartemis XR, Xtampza ER
Oxymorphone	Opana, Opana ER
Tapentadol	Nucynta, Nucynta ER
Sodium oxybate	Xyrem oral solution

From US Food and Drug Administration. *Medications Recommended for Disposal by Flushing: Listed by Medicine and Active Ingredient.* https://www.fda.gov.

TABLE 9.3 Abbreviations for Sustained- or Extended-Release Medications

Abbreviation	Meaning
CD	Controlled delivery
CR	Controlled release
ER	Extended release
IR	Immediate release
LA	Long-acting
MR	Modified release
SA	Sustained action (ambiguous, can also mean short acting)
SR	Sustained release
TR	Timed release
XR	Extended release
XT	Extended time

From http://www.pharmacytimes.com/medicationacronyms.

---

nurse administration stage (41%), and finally the doctor prescribing stage (39%) (www.drugerrorstatistics/fda.gov and www.drugerrorstatistics/singlecare.com).

Examples of risks to safety include the following:

- *Tablet splitting.* In an effort to counteract steeply rising drug costs, some patients are cutting their pills in half. However, this is not recommended by the FDA. The only time tablet splitting is advisable is when it is specified by the pharmacist on the label. Splitting tablets is risky because the patient may not receive an equal distribution of the medication with each dose. Some tablets are not recommended for splitting and are difficult to split. The FDA recommends that a patient receive advice directly from the pharmacist to determine whether tablet splitting is appropriate for a particular drug.
- *Buying drugs over the Internet.* Consumers may find it convenient to order drugs over the Internet, but precautions must be taken because drugs sold online may be too old, too strong, or too weak to be effective. Online sources may sell expired medications without the consumer knowing. The FDA suggests drugs obtained from these sites may not be made using safe standards, are unsafe to use with other medications, and may be expired. Patients should look for websites that (1) require a prescription from an HCP; (2) have a licensed pharmacist to answer questions and a contact person to consult if problems arise; (3) are in the United States; and (4) are licensed by the state board of pharmacy. Some sites may sell counterfeit drugs.

Counterfeit Drugs

Counterfeit drugs look like the desired drug but may have no active ingredient, the wrong active ingredient, or the wrong amount of active ingredient. Improper packaging and contamination are also problems. Counterfeit drugs may look remarkably like the real thing. To report suspected counterfeit products, nurses should call the FDA Office of Counterfeit Issues at 1-800-551-3989. To reduce the risk of exposure to counterfeit drugs, patients should purchase drugs only from licensed pharmacies.

Dosage Forms: To Crush or Not to Crush

Although some drugs can be crushed, there are many that shouldn't be crushed. Always consult with the pharmacist or, when possible, the HCP before crushing a patient's drug. Also, consult a reliable drug guide to confirm the medication is crushable. Do not crush any extended- or sustained-release drugs because this will change the pharmacokinetic phase of the drug. There is no industry standard for sustained- or extended-release abbreviations, which can cause confusion and drug errors. For a current complete listing of drugs that **should not** be crushed, see http://www.ismp.org/do-not-crush. Table 9.3 includes abbreviations for sustained- and extended-release drugs. It is important to remember when using drug acronyms there is a lack of standardization in the process of naming an acronym, so use with great caution to avoid errors. See http://www.pharmacytimes.com/medicationacronyms.

⚡ High-Alert Medications

High-alert drugs can cause significant harm to the patient. If a high-alert medication is given in error, it can have a major effect on the patient's organs; this includes cardiac, respiratory, vascular, and neurologic systems. A high-alert drug can also affect the sympathetic and parasympathetic nervous systems. Specific high-alert medications as listed by the Institute for Safe Medication Practices (ISMP) include epinephrine (SQ and IM); epoprostenol (IV); insulin U-500 (SQ and IV); magnesium sulfate injection; methotrexate (oral nononcologic use); opium tincture; oxytocin (IV); nitroprusside sodium for injection; potassium chloride concentrate for injection; potassium phosphate injection; promethazine (IV); and vasopressin (IV). Please note that all forms of insulin, subcutaneous and IV, are considered high-alert medications. For additional classes and categories of high-alert medications, visit the Institute for Safe Medication Practice's website at (www.highalertdrugs/ismp.org). Lists are provided to reduce the risk of errors, but specific strategies can optimize safety when dealing with high-alert drugs:

1. Simplify the storage, preparation, and administration of high-alert drugs.
2. All high-alert medications must be confirmed and documented by two nurses before administering.
3. Write policies concerning safe administration.
4. Improve information and education.
5. Limit access to high-alert medications.
6. Use labels and automated alerts.
7. Use redundancies (automated or independent double-checks).
8. Closely monitor the patient's response to the medication (possibly the most important step).

⚡ Look-Alike and Sound-Alike Drug Names

Nurses should be aware that certain drug names sound alike and are spelled similarly. Examples of drugs involved in medication errors and recognized as confusing drug names include *CeleXA* with *CeleBREX*; *diazePAM* with *dilTIAZem*; *ePHEDrine* with *EPINEPHrine*; *glipiZIDE* with *glyBURIDE*; *HumaLOG* with *HumuLIN*; *SOLU-Medrol* with *Solu-CORTEF*; *SOLU-Medrol* with *DEPO-Medrol*; *ZyrTEC* with *ZyPREXA*. The FDA, ISMP, and TJC advocate the use of "tall-man" letters as a safety strategy to reduce confusion between similar-sounding drugs. For example, *risperiDONE* and *rOPINIRole* to call attention to differences in spelling. Tall-man letters should be used for computer listing and storage labeling for look-alike and sound-alike drug names. This is now the standard; the complete list may be found at (www.ismp list of confused drug names 2023). Nursing students must become familiar with this list.

OTHER FACTORS IN THE PREVENTION OF MEDICATION ERRORS

Creating a distraction-free environment is critical to safe administration of medications. Data show that interruptions are responsible for 45% of medication errors (www.ismp/safemedicationadministrationpractices/). To avoid drug errors, many facilities are creating medication safety zones by implementing policies that provide for a medication room or safety area. When a nurse enters this safety zone, they are not to be disturbed. The zone offers a quiet atmosphere in which nurses can dispense medications from an ADC system and prepare the medication for administration. The patient's medical record is available to the nurse in the safety zone, which has proper lighting and a design conducive to safe preparation of medications. Overall, the nurse's role is best achieved by the application of the nursing process.

◎ CLINICAL JUDGMENT [NURSING PROCESS]
Medication Safety

Concept: Safety
- Protecting the patient from possible injury by practicing safe medication administration

Recognize Cues [Assessment]
- Assess the patient's vital signs and perform a head-to-toe physical assessment.
- Assess the patient's current laboratory results such as hematology laboratories, chemistry panel, and other pertinent laboratory tests pertaining to the patient's diagnosis and designated medication profile.
- Assess the patient's history, including current diagnostics and ability of the patient to swallow oral medications.
- Assess medication orders for completeness. Know the purpose and the expected effect of the medications and possible interactions, including any over-the-counter (OTC) and herbal preparations. Question the health care provider (HCP) if the prescription is unclear or seems inappropriate for the client's condition.
- ⚡ Use critical thinking skills by applying the assessment data and laboratory values to determine whether it is safe to administer the patient's medications.
- Report any abnormal findings to the provider.
- ⚡ Refuse to give a medication if you believe it to be unsafe, and notify the patient's HCP and the nurse manager.

Analyze Cues and Prioritize Hypothesis [Patient Problems]
- Need for health teaching
- Pain (surgical)
- Decreased adherence

Generate Solutions [Planning]
- ⚡ Calculate doses accurately, and if necessary, verify dosages with a colleague or pharmacist.
- Measure doses accurately and double-check high-alert medications.
- Avoid distractions during drug preparation.

Take Action [Nursing Interventions]
- ⚡ Use relevant resources and calculate doses correctly.
- Avoid skin contamination or inhalation of substances to minimize exposure.
- Always use hand hygiene before administering drugs.
- ⚡ Never administer medications that another nurse has prepared.
- ⚡ Use two forms of identification when identifying the patient.
- ⚡ Administer medications according to the Six Rights: right patient, right drug, right dose, right time, right route, and right documentation.
- Stay with the patient until the medication is taken.
- Discard needles and syringes in appropriate containers; be alert to sharps safety.
- Use aseptic/sterile technique appropriate for the route of administration.
- Thoroughly document drug administration in a timely manner.
- Document a patient's refusal to take a medication, and notify the HCP.

Patient Teaching
- Counsel patients and families on anticipated effects of the medications.
- Counsel patients on side effects and adverse reactions.
- Advise patients what foods to eat or avoid.
- Advise patients whether to take medications before, with, or after meals to promote optimal absorption.

Evaluate Outcomes [Evaluation]
- Evaluate the patient's response to the medication.
- Assess the patient for side effects. Document and report them appropriately.
- Evaluate the patient's understanding of the expected results from the medication and what to report to the HCP.
- Omit or delay doses, as indicated by the patient's condition, and if not administered, report this to the provider.

Resources for Preventing Errors in Medication Administration

Several resources address medication errors and their prevention:
- The ISMP provides accurate medication safety information. Also, the ISMP provides knowledge and understanding of the system-based causes of medication errors based largely on interdisciplinary reviews of thousands of reports to its national Medication Error Reporting Program (MERP) as well as hundreds of visits to health care organizations nationwide.
- The FDA database of medication errors and "near misses" assists all health care personnel to identify, implement, and evaluate strategies to prevent medication errors. It is strongly suggested that health care workers report errors and near misses to the FDA. Reports are confidential.
- When the nurse is unsure about a dosage, potential side effects, expected therapeutic effects, contraindications, or adverse reactions, an external resource—a drug reference book, a pharmacist, or an acceptable technology resource—should be consulted to determine the correct answer (e.g., Micromedex, Epocrates).

Pregnancy Categories and Subsections

The FDA pregnancy categories and subsection labeling system provides a broad explanation based on current available information of the benefits and risks medications can have to the mother, the fetus, and the breastfeeding child. The subsections are listed as Pregnancy (includes Labor and Delivery); Lactation (includes Nursing Mothers); and Females and Males of Reproductive Potential (Table 9.4). The Pregnancy subsection provides information relevant to the use of the drug in pregnant females, such as dosing, potential risks to the fetus, information about whether a registry collects and maintains data on how pregnant females are affected when they use a medication, and relevant information to help HCPs make prescribing and counseling decisions. The Lactation subsection provides information about using the drug while breastfeeding, such as the amount of the drug in breast milk and potential effects on the breastfed child. The Females and Males of Reproductive Potential subsection includes information about pregnancy testing, contraception, and infertility as it relates to the drug. For more information, see www.drugs/labeling/pregnancy-and-lactation-labeling-drugs-final-rule/fda.

Guidelines for Medication Administration

General guidelines for correct administration of medications are listed in Box 9.2. Nurses should follow these guidelines to enhance safety when administering medications. Application of the Clinical Judgment Measurement Model [Nursing Process] to medication administration is presented in Chapter 1.

TABLE 9.4 US Food and Drug Administration Pregnancy Categories

8.1 Pregnancy (Includes Labor and Delivery)	8.2 Lactation (Includes Nursing Mothers)	8.3 Females and Males of Reproductive Potential
Information Included in Subsection		
Pregnancy Exposure Registry	Risk Summary	Pregnancy Testing
Risk Summary	Clinical Considerations	Contraception Recommendations
Clinical Considerations	Data	Infertility Information
Data		

From www.fda.gov/drugs/labeling/pregnancy-and-lactation-labeling-drugs-final-rule/

BOX 9.2 Guidelines for Correct Administration of Medications

Preparation
1. Perform hand hygiene.
2. Access the patient's medication administration record (MAR) or electronic health record (EHR).
3. Check the patient's drugs with the health care provider's order for accuracy.
4. Obtain the patient's drugs from the automatic dispensing cabinet (ADC), remote stock, or pharmacy while checking the drug label with the patient's drug order for accuracy.
5. Check drug allergies.
6. Prepare drugs for only one patient at a time.
7. Calculate the drug dose, and perform a double-check of the calculation.
8. Check the expiration date on the drug label, and use the drug only if the date is current.
9. While preparing the drug, check the label against the MAR for accuracy.
10. If a unit dose is prescribed, open the packet at the patient's bedside.
11. If a liquid is prescribed, measure it in a calibrated syringe and put it into a drug cup (see Chapter 10; Fig. 10.2).
12. Never leave medications unattended.

Administration
13. Only administer drugs that have been personally prepared.
14. Identify patients by using at least two patient identifiers (e.g., name and birth date). Compare the patient's name and birth date from the MAR, computer printout, or EHR with the information on the patient's identification (ID) bracelet. If possible, ask the patient to state their name and birth date.
15. Assist the patient into an appropriate position, depending on the route of administration.
16. Before administering compare the label on the medication with the MAR to complete the three checks.
17. Explain each drug and its action to the patient.
18. For patients who cannot hold the drug, place the cup to their lips. Introduce one drug at a time, and do not rush the patient.
19. Stay with the patient until all drugs have been taken.
20. Dispose of used supplies, and perform hand hygiene.
21. Evaluate the patient's response to the drugs.
22. Educate patients and family members about drug actions and side effects.

Documentation
23. Report any drug errors immediately to the patient's health care provider and to the nurse manager; complete an incident report per your facility's policy.
24. Record effectiveness and results of drugs administered, especially medications administered as needed (prn).
25. Record drugs that were refused, and report refusal to the patient's health care provider along with the reason given for the refusal.
26. Record the amount of fluid taken with medications on an input and output chart.

CLINICAL JUDGMENT CASE STUDY

A 70-year-old female patient was admitted to the medical-surgical unit with a diagnosis of heart failure. This morning her blood pressure was elevated. She denies chest pain but complains of shortness of breath. Her morning weight indicated a 4-lb increase from the previous day. The nurse notified the health care provider, who ordered a diuretic of furosemide 40 mg PO immediately.

1. How will the nurse identify the patient before administering the drug?
2. What safety measures will the nurse implement to ensure accuracy?
3. The nurse scans the patient's armband and then attempts to scan the drug into the electronic health record (EHR). However, the EHR will not accept the drug scan. When the nurse compares the label with the order, the nurse realizes two 20 mg tablets should have been pulled from the automatic dispensing cabinet (ADC) to complete the order of 40 mg. The nurse only pulled one 20 mg tablet. What is the nurse's next step?
4. Explain the necessary steps when retrieving medications from the ADC and the steps prior to patient administration to avoid drug errors.

REVIEW QUESTIONS

1. The patient asks the nurse how to dispose of old medications. What should the nurse tell the patient? Select all that apply.
   a. Mix old drugs with cat litter before disposing.
   b. Flush the medications down the toilet.
   c. Remove personal information from the bottle.
   d. Add water and crush drugs before disposing of them.
   e. Throw the bottle of medication into the trashcan.
2. The nurse educator on the unit receives a list of high-alert drugs. Which strategy is recommended to decrease the risk of errors? Select all that apply.
   a. Store drugs on a shelf for quick retrieval.
   b. Limit access to high-alert drugs.
   c. Use special labels for high-alert drugs.
   d. Provide increased training to staff.
   e. Prior to administration, have two nurses confirm and document the correct drug and dose.
3. The Joint Commission recommends which of the following abbreviations for the "Do Not Use List"?
   a. qd
   b. NPO
   c. qid
   d. bid
4. A patient refuses to take the prescribed medication. Which is the nurse's best response to this patient?
   a. Leave the medication at the patient's bedside.
   b. Persuade the patient to take the medication.
   c. Tell the patient there is no choice in the matter.
   d. Explain the benefits and side effects of the drug.
5. What information is essential for the nurse to document when giving drugs? Select all that apply.
   a. Document all drugs given by the end of a shift.
   b. Document the correct site of an injectable drug.
   c. Document the patient's response to the drug.
   d. Document the blood pressure before giving a drug.
   e. Document the date, time, and dose of the drug that is given.
6. The nurse prepares to administer medications. Which drug orders are complete? Select all that apply.
   a. Aspirin 81 mg PO daily
   b. Multivitamin sustained
   c. Vitamin D PO
   d. Ciprofloxacin 500 mg PO tid
   e. Promethazine 25 mg STAT
7. A medication error occurred on the medical-surgical floor with a high alert drug. The payient was rushed to the Intensive Care Unit (ICU). In the true culture of safety, the risk manager was called to the unit. Choose the risk manager's first and most important decision in the investigation of this occurrence.
   a. Reprimand those involvede
   b. Maintain privacy of the event
   c. Notify the FDA
   d. Perform a root cause analysis

10

Drug Administration

http://evolve.elsevier.com/McCuistion/pharmacology

OBJECTIVES

- Relate the principles of nursing care to drug administration.
- Discuss guidelines for administration of parenteral medications.

OUTLINE

Forms and Routes of Drug Administration, 80
    Tablets and Capsules, 80
    Liquids, 81
    Transdermals, 81
    Topicals, 81
    Instillations, 81
    Inhalations, 81
    Nasogastric and Gastrostomy Tubes, 84
    Suppositories, 84
Parenteral Medications, 84
    Intradermal, 85

    Subcutaneous, 85
    Intramuscular, 87
    Preferred Intramuscular Injection Sites, 87
    Z-track Injection Technique, 88
    Intravenous, 88
    Nursing Implications for Administration of Parenteral Medications, 89
    Developmental Needs of a Pediatric Patient, 90
Clinical Judgment Case Study, 90
Review Questions, 90

Administration of medications is a complex but routine nursing activity practiced by nurses daily. Nurses have a significant responsibility in preparing, administering, teaching, and evaluating patients' responses to the medications they administer. Whether in an acute care, clinic, long-term care, or home setting, nurses work closely with patients and their family members. Patients must receive adequate training from the nurse to self-administer medications upon discharge. Nurses share their knowledge about the many aspects of drug administration, including drug interactions, safety practices, side effects, and dosage calculations. This chapter will explain drug administration routes and procedures.

FORMS AND ROUTES OF DRUG ADMINISTRATION

A variety of forms and routes are used for the administration of drugs. These include sublingual, buccal, oral (tablets, capsules, liquids, suspensions, and elixirs), transdermal, topical, instillation (drops and sprays), inhalation, nasogastric and gastrostomy tubes, suppositories, and parenteral forms (Fig. 10.1).

Tablets and Capsules

- Tablets and capsules are the most common drug forms; they are convenient and less expensive and do not require additional supplies for administration.
- ⚡ Oral drugs are not given to patients who are vomiting, who lack a gag reflex, or who are comatose.

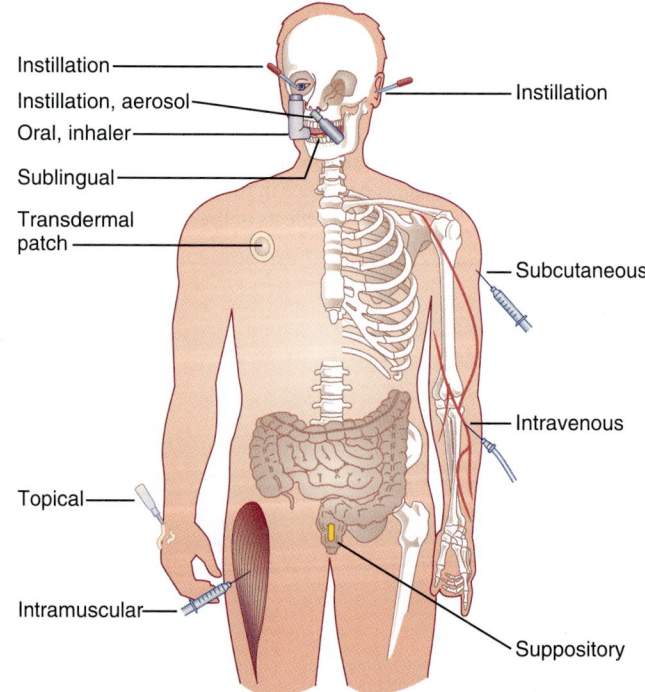

Fig. 10.1 Routes for medication administration.

- Do not mix a drug with large amounts of food or beverage. Patients may not be able to consume it and will not get the full dose of medication. Do not mix drugs in infant formula.
- Enteric-coated and timed-release capsules must be swallowed whole to maintain a therapeutic drug level, so the drug is released gradually. If crushed, the initial excessive drug release poses a risk of toxicity such that it could lead to a potentially fatal ⚡ overdose. Crushing can increase the rate of absorption, and it can cause oropharyngeal irritation. Advise the patient or family member to notify the health care provider (HCP) or pharmacist if the patient is having difficulty swallowing the medication. Instruct the patient to never cut or crush medications unless advised by the HCP or pharmacist that cutting or crushing is safe. In acute care settings, the nurse should follow the agency's policy for changing or altering drugs. Most policies indicate to notify the HCP or pharmacist if the patient is unable to swallow the drug. Many drugs can be given in liquid or intravenous (IV) form, or in a non–extended-release form.
- ⚡ Extended release medications should never be cut in half or crushed. They are intended to be released slowly over time. Cutting in half or crushing can lead to the entire dose being released at once. This can be fatal to the patient. If the patient has difficulty swallowing, inquire whether a liquid form is available.
- Administer irritating drugs with food to decrease gastrointestinal (GI) discomfort.
- Administer drugs on an empty stomach if food interferes with medication absorption.
- Drugs given via **sublingual** (under the tongue) or **buccal** (between the cheek and gum) routes remain in place until fully absorbed; therefore no food or fluid should be taken while the medication is in place.
- If patients have difficulty opening child-resistant caps, tell them to request non–child-resistant caps from the pharmacist.

Liquids
- Forms of liquid medication include elixirs, emulsions, and suspensions. *Elixirs* are sweetened, hydro-alcoholic liquids used in the preparation of oral liquid medications. *Emulsions* are a mixture of two liquids that are not mutually soluble. *Suspensions* are liquids in which particles are mixed but not dissolved.
- Read the labels to determine whether diluting or shaking is required.
- ⚡ Parents must be advised to never add drugs to the infant's formula as the drug might interact with the milk or other liquids.
- Make sure your facility has plastic dosing cups that measure in milliliters (mL) and not in archaic drams. One dram is equivalent to 3.7 mL. To avoid mix-ups, it is always best to measure the prescribed dose of liquid medication in a syringe calibrated for milliliters and to then squirt the medication into the oral measuring cup. According to the US Pharmacopeia Convention, a proposed change is required for all facilities to supply dosing cups with legible markings in metric units (Fig. 10.2).

Transdermals
- **Transdermal** medication is stored in a patch placed on the skin and is absorbed through the skin to produce a systemic effect. A patch may be left in place for as little as 12 hours or as long as 7 days depending on the drug. Transdermal drugs provide more consistent blood levels than oral and injectable forms, and they avoid GI absorption problems associated with oral products. To prevent skin breakdown, transdermal patches should be rotated to different sites and should not be reapplied over the exact same area every time. In addition, the area should be thoroughly cleansed before administration of a new transdermal patch. ⚡ The patch should never be cut

Fig. 10.2 (A) Liquid medication in a unit-dose package. (B) Liquid measured into a medicine cup from a multidose container. (C) Liquid medication in an oral-dosing syringe. (From Lilley LL, et al. *Pharmacology and The Nursing Process*. 8th ed. Elsevier; 2017.)

in half because the drug in each half of the patch will be released too quickly and could be fatal to the patient.
- Perform hand hygiene and apply gloves when administering medicated patches to prevent transfer of medication; advise the patient to do the same for self-administration. Never cut the patch in half.
- Advise patients to secure the patch with tape, being careful not to apply the tape too tightly, which could alter the drug delivery.

Topicals
- **Topical** medications are most frequently applied to the skin by painting or spreading the medication over an area and applying a moist dressing or leaving the area exposed to air. Such medications can be applied to the skin in several ways, such as with a glove, tongue blade, or cotton-tipped applicator. ⚡ Never apply a patient's topical medication without first putting on gloves.
- Use the appropriate technique to remove the medication from the container, and apply it to clean, dry skin when possible. Do not contaminate the drug in a container; instead, use gloves or an applicator.
- Gloves and applicators that come in contact with a patient should not be reinserted into the container. Estimate the amount of medication needed, and remove it from the container, or use a fresh sterile applicator each time the container is entered.

Instillations
Instillations are liquid medications usually administered as drops, ointments, or sprays in the following forms:
Eyedrops (Box 10.1 and Fig. 10.3)
Eye ointments (Box 10.2 and Fig. 10.4)
Eardrops (Box 10.3 and Fig. 10.5)
Nose drops and sprays (Box 10.4 and Figs. 10.6 and 10.7)

Inhalations
- **Metered-dose inhalers (MDIs)** are handheld devices used to deliver a number of commonly prescribed asthma and bronchitis drugs to the lower respiratory tract (Box 10.5) via **inhalation**. When the airway becomes constricted, the drug is needed quickly. When properly used, MDIs get up to 12% to 14% of the drug deep into the lungs with each puff. MDIs act faster than drugs taken by mouth, and fewer side effects occur because the drug goes right to the lungs and not to other parts of the body. Some MDIs have a counter to indicate the number of inhalations used. For those that

BOX 10.1 Administration of Eyedrops

1. Perform hand hygiene, and wear gloves.
2. Instruct the patient to lie down or sit back in a chair, and have them look at the ceiling.
3. Remove any discharge by gently wiping from the inner to outer canthus. ⚡ Use a separate cloth for each eye.
4. Gently draw the skin down below the affected eye to expose the conjunctival sac (see Fig. 10.3).
5. Notify the patient immediately before administering drops so they are prepared to avoid blinking when the drops hit the conjunctiva.
6. Administer the prescribed number of drops into the center of the sac. If the drug is placed directly on the cornea, it can cause discomfort or damage. ⚡ Avoid touching eyelids or eyelashes with the dropper.
    a. Gently press on the lacrimal duct with a sterile cotton ball or tissue for 1 to 2 minutes after instillation to prevent systemic absorption through the lacrimal canal.
    b. Instruct the patient to keep their eyes closed for 1 to 2 minutes after application to promote absorption.

Fig. 10.4 Administering eye ointment. Squeeze a ¼-inch-wide strip of ointment into the conjunctival sac.

BOX 10.3 Administration of Eardrops

1. Perform hand hygiene, and wear gloves.
2. Ensure the medication is at room temperature.
3. Instruct the patient to sit up with the head tilted slightly toward the unaffected side. This position straightens the external ear canal for better visualization. Maintain this position for 2 to 3 minutes to facilitate drops reaching the affected area (see Fig. 10.5).
4. Pull down and back on the auricle for a child younger than 3 years of age. For a child older than 3 years or an adult, pull upward and outward on the auricle.
5. Instill the prescribed number of drops. Take measures to avoid allowing drops to fall directly on the tympanic membrane. Drops should be aimed at the side of the ear canal and should be allowed to run down into the ear.
6. ⚡ Do not contaminate the dropper.

Fig. 10.3 Administering eyedrops. Gently pull down on the skin below the eye to expose the conjunctival sac. Apply drops to the middle third of the sac, and apply gentle pressure over the lacrimal duct after administration.

BOX 10.2 Administration of Eye Ointment

1. Perform hand hygiene, and wear gloves.
2. Instruct the patient to lie down or sit, and have them look at the ceiling.
3. Remove any discharge by gently wiping outward from the inner canthus. ⚡ Use a separate cloth for each eye.
4. Gently draw the skin down below the affected eye to expose the conjunctival sac.
5. Prepare the patient by explaining that ointment will be placed in the eye, so they can help by not blinking.
6. Squeeze a strip of ointment (about ¼ inch unless stated otherwise) onto the conjunctival sac (see Fig. 10.4). ⚡ Medication placed directly on the cornea can cause discomfort or damage. Avoid touching eyelids or eyelashes with the applicator tip.
7. Instruct the patient to close their eyes for 2 to 3 minutes.
8. Instruct the patient to expect blurred vision for a short time. If possible, apply at bedtime.

A

B

Fig. 10.5 Administering eardrops. (A) Straighten the external ear canal by pulling the auricle down and back in children under 3 years of age. (B) In patients older than 3 years of age, including adults, pull the auricle upward and outward.

BOX 10.4 Administration of Nose Drops and Sprays

1. Perform hand hygiene, and wear gloves.
2. Advise the patient to blow their nose.
3. Advise the patient to tilt the head back for drops to reach the frontal sinus and to tilt the head to the affected side to reach the ethmoid sinus (see Figs. 10.6 and 10.7).
4. ⚡ Administer the prescribed number of drops or sprays without touching the tip of the medication applicator to the nasal passages.
5. Some sprays have instructions to close one nostril, tilt the head to the closed side, and hold the breath or breathe through the nose for 1 minute.
6. If a patient is using a nasal spray to reach the sinuses, proper head position is with the patient looking down at the feet with the spray tip aimed toward the eye.
7. Advise the patient to keep the head tilted back for 5 minutes after instillation of drops.

BOX 10.5 Correct Use of a Metered-Dose Inhaler

1. Explain what a metered dose is, and warn the patient about overuse and side effects of the drug.
2. Explain the steps for administering the drug using a squeeze-and-breathe metered-dose inhaler (MDI), and demonstrate the steps when possible. Consult a pharmacist for details if necessary.
3. Insert the medication canister into the plastic holder.
4. If a spacer is used, insert the MDI into the end of the spacer.
5. Shake the inhaler vigorously five or six times before using. Remove the cap from the mouthpiece.
6. Have the patient breathe out through the mouth and exhale.
7. An MDI may be positioned in one of two ways:
    a. With the mouth closed around the MDI with the opening toward the back of the throat
    b. With the device positioned 1 to 2 inches from the mouth
    c. If a spacer is used, the patient closes the mouth around the mouthpiece of the spacer. ⚡ Avoid covering the small exhalation slots with the lips.
8. With the inhaler properly positioned, have the patient hold the inhaler with the thumb at the mouthpiece and the index finger and middle finger at the top (see Fig. 10.8).
9. Instruct the patient to take a slow, deep breath through the mouth and during inspiration, to push the top of the medication canister once.
10. Have the patient hold the breath for 10 seconds and then exhale slowly through pursed lips.
11. If a second dose is required, wait 1 to 2 minutes, and repeat the procedure by first shaking the canister in the plastic holder with the cap on.
12. When it is first used or if it has not been used recently, test the inhaler by spraying it into the air before administering the metered dose.
13. If a glucocorticoid inhalant is to be used with a bronchodilator, wait 5 minutes before using an inhaler that contains a steroid.
14. Teach the patient to self-monitor their pulse rate.
15. Caution against overuse because side effects and tolerance may result.
16. Teach the patient to monitor the amount of medication remaining in the canister. Advise the patient to ask an HCP or pharmacist to estimate when a new inhaler will be needed based on the dosing schedule.
17. ⚡ Teach the patient to rinse their mouth after using an MDI. This is especially important when using a steroid drug. Rinsing the mouth helps prevent irritation and secondary infection to oral mucosa.
18. ⚡ Advise the patient to avoid smoking.
19. Teach the patient to do daily cleaning of equipment; this should include (1) performing hand hygiene; (2) taking apart all the washable parts of the equipment and washing them with warm water; (3) rinsing; (4) placing the parts on a clean towel and covering them with another clean towel to air dry; and (5) storing the parts in a clean plastic bag once completely dry. Alternate two sets of washable equipment to make this process easier.

Fig. 10.6 Administering nose drops.

Fig. 10.7 Administering nasal spray.

do not, ask the pharmacist the number of inhalations the inhaler will provide and then count the number of inhalations used. Every effort should be made to have the patient know how much medication is in the canister and to anticipate and obtain refills in a timely manner.

- ⚡ Take special measures when handling the capsules used in some MDIs to prevent the transfer of medication (e.g., powder from a punctured capsule can get on the hands and transfer to the eyes or absorb into the skin).
- Spacers are devices used to enhance the delivery of medications from the MDI (see Fig. 10.8). A *nebulizer* is a device that changes a

Fig. 10.8 Metered-dose inhaler with spacer. (From Potter PA, Perry AG, Stockert PA, Hall AM. *Fundamentals of Nursing*. 9th ed. Elsevier; 2017.)

Fig. 10.9 Inserting a rectal suppository.

liquid medication into a fine mist or aerosol and has the ability to reach the lower, smaller airways. Handheld nebulizers deliver a very fine particle in a spray of medication.
- When administering drugs via an MDI or nebulizer, the preferred patient position is the semi-Fowler or high-Fowler position.
- Instruct the patient on the correct use and cleaning of MDIs or nebulizers.

Nasogastric and Gastrostomy Tubes
- ⚡ Before administering drugs, always check for proper tube placement of any feeding tube that enters the mouth, nose, or abdomen, and always assess the gastric residual. Return any aspirated gastric fluid to the stomach. (Check the agency's policy for tube placement and residual; see Chapter 14.)
- ⚡ Place the patient in a high-Fowler position or elevate the head of the bed at least 30 degrees to avoid aspiration.
- Make sure the drug is crushable. If it is a capsule, assess whether it can be opened and administered through the tube. The crushed drug should be placed into a plastic dosing cup. A small amount of water is added to liquefy the dry medication.
- Remove the plunger from the syringe, and attach it to the feeding tube, pour liquefied medication into the syringe, release the clamp, and allow the medication to flow in properly by gravity.
- ⚡ Ensure proper identification of each drug up until the time of administration. Do this by administering one drug at a time. Flush with 10 to 15 mL of water between each administration to maintain patency of the tubing.
- When finished with drug administration, flush tubing with 30 mL of water or whichever amount is recommended by the agency's policy. Always record the amount of water used with the administration of drugs on the patient's input sheet.
- Clamp the tube, and remove the syringe.
- If the patient has a nasogastric tube to suction, clamp the tube for 30 minutes to allow medication to be absorbed before placing the patient back on suction.

Suppositories
A suppository is a solid medical preparation that is cone- or spindle-shaped for insertion into the rectum, globular or egg-shaped for use in the vagina, or pencil-shaped for insertion into the urethra. Suppositories are made from glycerinated gelatin or high-molecular-weight polyethylene glycols and are common vehicles for a variety of drugs. A suppository is a useful route in babies, in uncooperative patients, and in cases of vomiting or certain digestive disorders.

Rectal Suppositories
- Medications administered as suppositories or enemas can be given rectally for local and systemic absorption. The numerous small capillaries in the rectal area promote medication absorption.
- The foil around the suppository is removed, and the suppository may be lubricated before insertion.
- During insertion, place the suppository past the internal anal sphincter; otherwise, the suppository will be expelled before it can dissolve and absorb into the mucosa.
- Some suppositories tend to soften at room temperature and therefore may be refrigerated before use.
- Explain administration procedures to the patient, and provide for privacy.
- Use gloves for insertion.
- Instruct the patient to lie in the modified left lateral recumbent position and to breathe slowly through the mouth to relax the anal sphincter.
- Apply a small amount of water-soluble lubricant to the tip of the unwrapped suppository, and gently insert the suppository beyond the internal sphincter (Fig. 10.9).
- Ask the patient to remain flat or on one side for at least 30 minutes to prevent expulsion of the suppository.
- Observe for effects of the suppository that correlate with the medication's onset, peak, and duration.

Vaginal Medications
Vaginal drugs are available as suppositories, foams, jellies, or creams. They are individually packaged in foil wrappers and are sometimes stored in the refrigerator to prevent the solid, oval-shaped suppositories from melting. Foams, jellies, creams, and suppositories are generally inserted into the vagina with an applicator supplied with the medication (Fig. 10.10). Gloves should be worn, and the patient should be in the lithotomy position. Advise patients to remain lying for a time sufficient to allow medication absorption; times vary depending on the medication. After insertion, provide the patient with a sanitary pad. If the patient is able, they may want to personally insert the vaginal drug.

PARENTERAL MEDICATIONS

⚡ Safety is a special concern with **parenteral** drugs, which are administered via injection. Manufacturers have responded with safety features to help decrease or eliminate needlestick injuries and possible transfer of blood-borne diseases such as hepatitis and human immunodeficiency virus; Fig. 10.11 shows examples of safety needles. Methods of parenteral administration include **intradermal, subcutaneous, intramuscular, Z-track technique**, and **IV** administration. A description of each follows with special considerations noted for the pediatric patient.

Intradermal

Action.
- Local effect
- Administered for skin testing (e.g., tuberculin screening, allergy testing, and testing for other drug sensitivities; some immunotherapy for cancer)

Sites.
- Locations are chosen so an inflammatory reaction can be observed. Preferred areas are lightly pigmented, free of lesions, and hairless, such as the ventral midforearm, clavicular area of the chest, or scapular area of the back (Fig. 10.12).

Equipment.
- Needle: 25- to 27-gauge, ¼ to ½ inch long, tuberculin syringe.
- Syringe: 1 mL calibrated in increments of (0.01) hundredth mL represented on syringe as 0.1 to 1 mL. Syringe holds up to 1 mL of solution; however, tuberculin skin tests require injection of a small amount of solution (usually 0.01–0.1 mL) to ensure formation of bleb.

Technique.
- Perform hand hygiene, and wear gloves.
- Cleanse the area with a circular motion using aseptic technique.
- Hold the skin taut.
- Insert the needle, bevel up, at a 10- to 15-degree angle; the tip of the needle should be visible under the skin (Fig. 10.13).
- Inject the medication slowly to form a bleb (or wheal). A small amount is injected so the volume will not interfere with bleb formation or cause a systemic reaction. If the bleb does not appear, the needle has been injected subcutaneously. Document according to facility policy, and inform the HCP. The nurse may need to obtain orders to repeat the procedure.
- Remove the needle slowly, and do not recap it.
- Do *not* massage the area, and instruct the patient not to do so.
- Mark the area with a pen, and ask the patient not to wash it off until the response can be "read" by an HCP.
- ⚡ It is not recommended to put an adhesive bandage over the intradermal tuberculin testing site because it can alter the results of the test.
- Assess for allergic reaction in 24 to 72 hours; measure the diameter of any local reaction. For tuberculin testing, measure only the indurated area; do not include the area of erythema in the measurement.

Subcutaneous

Action.
- Systemic effect
- Sustained effect; absorbed mainly through capillaries; usually slower in onset than with the intramuscular (IM) route.

Sites.
- Locations for subcutaneous injections are chosen for adequate fat-pad size. Areas such as the upper outer aspect of the arms; the abdomen, at least 2 inches from the umbilicus; and the anterior thighs are important subcutaneous sites (Fig. 10.14). Sites should be rotated with subcutaneous injections, such as with insulin and heparin.

Fig. 10.10 Inserting a vaginal suppository.

Fig. 10.11 Safety needles.

Fig. 10.12 Common sites for intradermal injection.

Fig. 10.14 Common sites for subcutaneous injections.

Fig. 10.13 Needle angles for intradermal, subcutaneous, and intramuscular injections.

- Usually, 0.5 to 1 mL of solution is given subcutaneously. A larger amount (2 mL) of medication may have to be divided and administered at two sites. Larger amounts add to the patient's discomfort and predispose to poor absorption. Refer to agency policy for the maximum amount of medication to be administered via this route.

Equipment.
- Needle: 25- to 27-gauge; ⅜ to ⅝ inch long.
- The length of the needle and the angle of the needle insertion are based on the amount of subcutaneous tissue present. The shorter, ⅜-inch needle should be inserted at 90-degree angle, and the longer, ⅝-inch needle is inserted at a 45-degree angle (see Fig. 10.13).
- Syringe: 1 to 3 mL (injection of solution is usually 0.5–1 mL).
- Insulin syringe measured in units for use with only insulin.

Technique.
- Perform hand hygiene, and wear gloves.
- Cleanse the area with a circular motion using aseptic technique.
- Grasp or gently pinch the area of the patient's loose fatty tissue with the fingers of your nondominant hand.
- Insert the needle quickly.
- Release the pinch, and use the hand to stabilize the syringe.
- Do not aspirate.
- Inject the medication slowly.
- Remove the needle quickly; do not recap.
- Apply gentle pressure to the injection site to prevent bleeding or oozing into the tissue with subsequent bruising and tissue damage, especially if the patient is on anticoagulant therapy.
- Apply a bandage if needed.

CHAPTER 10 Drug Administration

TABLE 10.1 Intramuscular Injection Sites: Patient Position, Advantages, and Disadvantages

Site	Patient Position	Anatomic Landmark
Ventrogluteal	Supine, lateral	Locate the ventrogluteal muscle by placing the heel of the hand over the greater trochanter of the patient's hip with the wrists perpendicular to the femur. Use the right hand for the patient's left hip and the left hand for the right hip. Point the thumb toward the patient's groin and the index finger toward the anterior superior iliac spine, and extend the middle finger back along the iliac crest toward the buttock. The index finger, the middle finger, and the iliac crest form a V-shaped triangle; the injection site is the center of the triangle (see Fig. 10.15). ⚡ The ventrogluteal is the preferred site for most injections given to adults and all children, including infants of any age.
Deltoid	Lateral, prone, sitting, supine	Palpate the lower edge of the patient's acromion process, which forms the base of a triangle in line with the midpoint of the lateral aspect of the upper arm. The injection site is in the center of the triangle, about 1–2 inches below the acromion process. Or locate the site by placing four fingers across the deltoid muscle with the top finger along the acromion process. The injection site is then three finger widths below the acromion process (see Fig. 10.16).
Vastus lateralis	Sitting, supine flex knee to help relax muscle if supine	Located on the anterior lateral aspect of the thigh, it extends in an adult from a handbreadth above the knee to a handbreadth below the greater trochanter of the femur. Use the middle third of the muscle for injection. ⚡ With young children or cachectic patients, it helps to grasp the body of the muscle during injection to ensure delivery of the drug into the muscle. Vastus lateralis is frequently used in infants (less than 12 months) receiving immunizations and is often used in older children and toddlers receiving immunizations (see Fig. 10.17).

Intramuscular

Action.
- Systemic effect.
- Usually a more rapid effect of drug than with a subcutaneous route.
- Used for solutions that are more viscous and irritating for adults, children, and infants.
- ⚡ IM injections are associated with many risks, so the nurse should use accurate, careful technique when administering an IM injection and should check the agency's policy.

Sites.
Locations are chosen for adequate muscle size and minimal major nerves and blood vessels in the area. Other considerations include the volume of drug administered, needle size, angle of injection, patient position, site location, and advantages and disadvantages of the site. Underweight patients should be evaluated for sites with adequate muscle.

Equipment.
- Needle: 18- to 25-gauge; ⅝ to 1½ inches long. Patient's weight, age, and the amount of adipose tissue influence needle length.

Technique.
- Perform hand hygiene, and apply gloves.
- Same as for subcutaneous injection with two exceptions: Flatten the skin area using the thumb and index finger and inject between them, and insert the needle at a 90-degree angle into the muscle (see Fig. 10.13).
- Syringe: 1 to 3 mL, although this varies based on the intended site, the age of the patient, and the developed muscle site. (Check the agency's policy.)

Preferred Intramuscular Injection Sites

Table 10.1 shows the three sites along with the patient positioning and advantages and disadvantages of each injection site.
- *Ventrogluteal* (Fig. 10.15). Located near the gluteus medius, a deep muscle, away from major nerves, this site is well suited for Z-track injections. It is administered with an 18- to 25-gauge, 1½-inch needle. The gauge and length of the needle depend on the medication to be administered and the size of the patient. Slightly angle

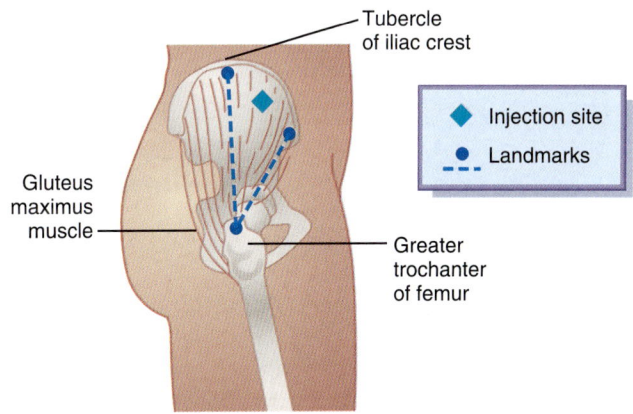

Fig. 10.15 Ventrogluteal injection site.

the needle toward the iliac crest. The ventrogluteal is the preferred site for most injections given to adults and all children, including infants of any age.
- *Deltoid* (Fig. 10.16). This muscle is easy to find, but it is not well developed in many adults. The volume of drug administered is 0.5 to 1 mL, with a 23- to 25-gauge, ⅝- to 1½-inch needle. Place the needle at a 90-degree angle to the skin or slightly toward the acromion. ⚡ Choose the site carefully; there is risk for injury because of the nerves and arteries that lie within the upper arm along the humerus. Use this site for small medication volumes or when other sites are inaccessible. ⚡ This site is not used in infants or children due to underdeveloped muscles.
- *Vastus lateralis* (Fig. 10.17). The vastus lateralis is a good site for multiple injections. It is frequently used in infants (less than 12 months) and is often used in older children and toddlers receiving immunizations. ⚡ If a long needle is used, insert it with caution to avoid sciatic nerve or femoral structures. The volume of drug administered is 0.5 mL in infants (maximum [max] 1 mL), 1 mL in pediatric patients, and 1 to 1.5 mL in adults (max 2 mL).

Z-track Injection Technique

The Z-track injection technique shown in Fig. 10.18 is recommended when administering IM injections to help minimize local skin irritation by sealing the medication in the muscle tissue. The ventrogluteal site is preferred. Using aseptic technique, draw up the medication. Replace the first needle with a second needle of appropriate gauge and length to ensure the needle will penetrate the muscle. Holding the skin taut, inject the needle at a 90-degree angle deep into the muscle, and if there is no blood return on aspiration, slowly inject the medication. Allow the needle to remain inserted for 10 seconds for the medication to disperse evenly.

Intravenous

Action.
- Systemic effect
- More rapid than IM or subcutaneous routes

Sites. Accessible peripheral veins are preferred (e.g., cephalic or cubital vein of arm, dorsal vein of hand; Fig. 10.19). When possible, ask the patient about their preference, and avoid needless body restriction. In newborns, the veins of the feet, lower legs, and head may also be used after other sites have been exhausted.

Equipment.
- Needle
  - Adults: 20- to 21-gauge, 1 to 1½ inches
  - Infants: 24-gauge, 1 inch
  - Children: 22-gauge, 1 inch
- Larger bore for viscous drugs and whole blood and a large volume for rapid infusion
- Electronic IV delivery device, an infusion controller, or pump
- May use a mixture of lidocaine/prilocaine anesthetic before starting IV site

Technique.
- Perform hand hygiene, and apply gloves.
- Apply a tourniquet.
- Apply anesthetic 30 minutes before the procedure on unbroken skin.
- Cleanse the area using aseptic technique with an appropriate solution.
- Insert catheter, and feed it up into the vein until blood returns. Remove the tourniquet.
- Stabilize the needle or IV catheter, and apply dressing to site.
- Flush the catheter with sodium chloride or sterile water to check for site patency.
- Monitor flow rate, distal pulses, skin color and temperature, and insertion site.
- Consult agency policy regarding IV fluids, intermittent IV (IVPB), and direct IV (IV push) drugs. ⚡ The pharmacy adds medications to the IV bag to avoid error; except in specialty areas such as critical care, nurses should *never* add medications to the IV bag.

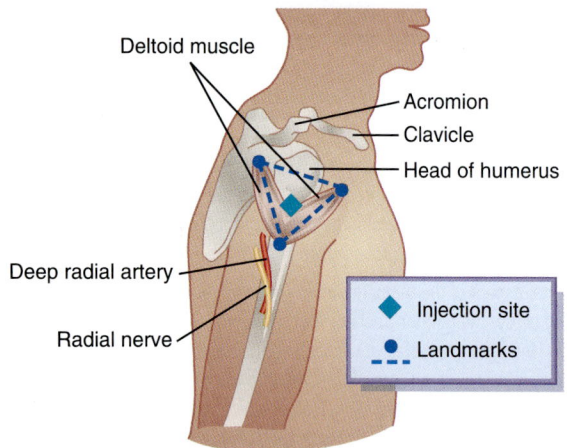

Fig. 10.16 Deltoid injection site.

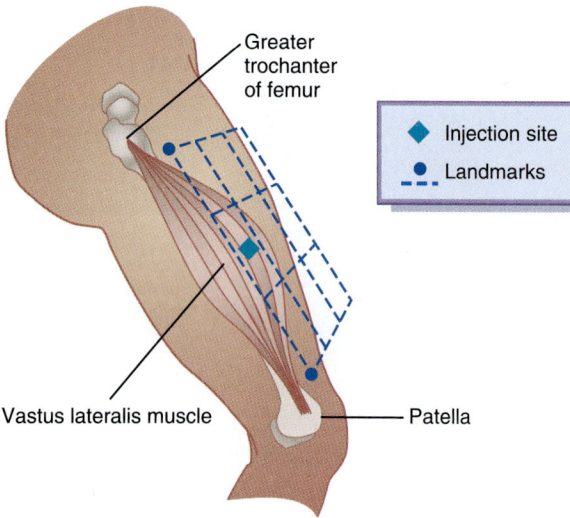

Fig. 10.17 Vastus lateralis injection site in children.

Fig. 10.18 Z-track injection. (A) Use a deep muscle, such as in the ventrogluteal injection, and pull skin approximately 1–1½ inches laterally to one side and hold it taut with the nondominant hand. (B) Inject the needle at a 90-degree angle deep into the muscle, and if no blood returns on aspiration, slowly inject the medication. (C) Wait 10 s before withdrawing the needle and releasing the skin. This technique prevents medication from entering subcutaneous tissue.

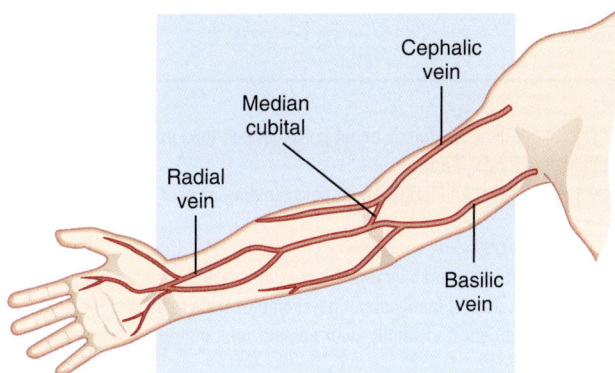

Fig. 10.19 Common sites for intravenous administration.

Nursing Implications for Administration of Parenteral Medications

Sites
- The ventrogluteal site is preferred for IM injections in adults and children, including infants of any age. The gluteal muscle is a deep muscle, situated away from major nerves and blood vessels.
- For infants younger than 12 months and toddlers not walking alone, the vastus lateralis is the preferred site for immunizations.

Equipment
- The syringe size should approximate the volume of medication to be administered.
- Use the tuberculin syringe for amounts less than 1 mL.
- Use the filter needle to draw up drugs taken from a glass vial or ampule. Change the needle before administration to prevent tissue irritation.

Technique
- Perform hand hygiene, and apply gloves.
- Correctly identify the patient.
- Explain the procedure to the patient.
- Position the patient.
- Follow the rights of medication administration (see Chapter 9).
- Inspect the site, choose the correct anatomic markers, and assess skin for breakdown.
- Inject the drug slowly to minimize tissue damage.
- Stabilize the skin during needle removal to reduce pain.
- ⚡ Do not administer injections if sites are inflamed, edematous, or lesioned (e.g., moles, scars).
- Rotate the injection site to enhance absorption of the drug.
- Document the injection site.
- Observe the patient to evaluate drug effectiveness.
- Report any adverse reactions immediately.
- Multiple products are available to reduce the pain of parenteral drug administration (e.g., lidocaine, prilocaine, and benzocaine/tetracaine).

CLINICAL JUDGMENT [NURSING PROCESS]
Overview Drug Administration

Concept: Caring Interventions
- The nurse performs caring interventions during medication administration. These interventions ensure safe practice outcomes. The interventions are the result of scientific research and best practice guidelines composed by the professional body of nursing for quality care and safe practice.

Recognize Cues [Assessment]
- Obtain appropriate vital signs and relevant laboratory test results for future comparisons and to evaluate therapeutic response.
- Determine the patient's level of consciousness, risk for aspiration, and ability to take medications.
- Obtain a drug history that includes drug allergies.
- Identify patients at high risk for reactions.
- Assess the patient's capability to follow the therapeutic regimen.
- Assess possible contraindications to certain medication regimens.

Analyze Cues and Prioritize Hypothesis [Patient Problems]
- Potential for injury
- Need for health teaching
- Acute pain
- Decreased mobility

Generate Solutions [Planning]
- Identify patient goals.
- Promote therapeutic response, and prevent or minimize adverse reactions.
- Identify strategies to promote adherence to the drug regimen.
- Identify interventions that foster patient independence and safety.

Take Action [Nursing Interventions]
- Prepare the equipment and environment, and perform hand hygiene.
- Evaluate for allergies and other assessment data.
- View the drug label three times; check the expiration date and apply the rights of medication administration.
- Verify the calculated dose with another registered nurse, licensed personnel, or pharmacy as necessary.
- Measure liquids in a milliliter syringe, and squirt the medication into a plastic measuring cup calibrated in milliliters.
- Avoid contact with topical and inhalation preparations by wearing gloves.
- Verify the patient by using two patient identifiers.
- Only administer drugs personally prepared.
- Assist the patient into the appropriate position.
- Discard needles and syringes in a sharps container. Do not recap needles.
- Store all drugs properly, especially regarding temperature, light, and moisture.
- The drug must be identifiable up until the time of patient administration.
- Follow agency policy related to discarding drugs and controlled substances.
- Report drug errors immediately.
- Document all appropriate information in a timely manner.
- Record effectiveness of administered drugs, side effects, adverse effects, and if a drug is refused, document the patient's reason for refusing the drug. Depending on the drug refused, notify the HCP.
- Assess the patient for pain control.
- If a language barrier exists, request a professional translator.
- Communicate respect for the culture and practices of the patient and family.

Patient Teaching
General
- Emphasize safety.
- Monitor the patient's physical abilities regularly as needed.
- Store medications in original, labeled containers with child-resistant caps when needed.

Continued

CLINICAL JUDGMENT [NURSING PROCESS]—CONT'D

Overview Drug Administration

- Provide the patient and family with written instructions about the drug regimen; provide audio instructions if the patient or family is visually impaired or unable to read.
- Advise the patient and family about expected therapeutic effects, anticipated onset of action, and expected duration of treatment.
- Educate the patient and family on possible side effects or signs of an adverse reaction.
- Instruct the patient and family about possible laboratory tests that may be required.
- Advise the patient of nonpharmacologic measures to promote therapeutic response.
- Encourage the patient and family to have an adequate supply of medications available.
- Caution against the use of over-the-counter preparations, including herbal remedies, without first contacting the HCP.
- Reinforce the importance of follow-up appointments with the HCP.
- Encourage the patient to wear a medical alert band with drugs or allergies indicated.
- As needed, encourage lifestyle changes associated with drug administration (e.g., smoking cessation, exercise, limiting salt or fat intake).
- Encourage use of community resources to assist with patient and family needs.

Diet
- Advise the patient and family about possible drug-food interactions and contraindicated foods, if any.
- Advise the patient and family about possible drug-alcohol interactions.

Self-Administration
- Advise the patient and family regarding drug dose and dosing schedule.
- Teach the patient and family about psychomotor skills related to the drug.
- Provide the patient and family with contact information for questions and concerns.

Side Effects
- Counsel the patient and family about general side effects and adverse reactions of the medications.
- Instruct the patient and family to monitor drug effects as appropriate (e.g., check blood pressure if the drug is to treat hypertension).
- Advise the patient and family when and how to notify the HCP.

Evaluate Outcomes [Evaluation]
- Evaluate the effectiveness of the drugs administered.
- Identify the expected time frame of the desired response from the drug.
- Determine the patient's satisfaction with the therapeutic regimen.

Developmental Needs of a Pediatric Patient

Anticipate patients' developmental needs. Examples of needs associated with administration of medications include the following (see Chapter 6):

- Stranger anxiety (infant): Act to instill a sense of safety and security in the infant.
- Hospitalization, illness, or injury is viewed as punishment (3–6 years of age): Allow control when appropriate; obtain the child's view of the situation; encourage activities, positive relationships, and expression of feelings in an acceptable manner. Include a family member or support person, if appropriate.
- Fear of the procedure (3–6 years of age): Explain procedures carefully; use less intrusive routes, such as the oral route, whenever possible; allow children to give "play" injections to a doll or stuffed animal.

Safety

Developmental factors and young children's body size determine reasons children receive drug doses different from adults. Always ensure families understand the correct dose to be administered to the child. When using injectables always choose the smallest syringe that ensures the correct measurement of the drug.

CLINICAL JUDGMENT CASE STUDY

A 66-year-old female newly diagnosed with diabetes is planning to be discharged from the hospital on long-acting insulin. The nurse is planning the first teaching on how to inject subcutaneous insulin. Please answer the important questions the nurse will include in this patient's teaching.

1. Name three subcutaneous injection sites.
2. How is the skin held when administering a subcutaneous injection prior to inserting the needle?
3. With what measurement is an insulin syringe calibrated?
4. What happens after the medication is injected into the site?
5. How will the nurse evaluate the effectiveness of the teaching?

REVIEW QUESTIONS

1. The nurse is administering oral medications to a patient. Which considerations are important? **Select all that apply.**
   a. Always administer gastrointestinal-irritating drugs with food.
   b. Avoid mixing medications into infant formula.
   c. Enteric-coated capsules may be chewed.
   d. Stop oral medications for nausea and vomiting.
   e. Cut all transdermal patches to the correct dose.

2. The clinic nurse is preparing to administer an intradermal injection. Which needle and gauge are most appropriate for this procedure?
   a. ¾- to ⅝-inch needle, 25- to 27-gauge
   b. ⅝- to 1½-inch needle, 18- to 25-gauge
   c. 1- to 1½-inch needle, 20- to 21-gauge
   d. ¼- to ½-inch needle, tuberculin syringe

3. The nurse is administering an intramuscular injection to a 5-year-old child. Choose the correct site the nurse will use.
   a. Ventral forearm
   b. Dorsogluteal
   c. Deltoid muscle
   d. Ventrogluteal
4. The nurse administers a variety of drugs to a patient. Which statement by the patient indicates a need for further teaching?
   a. "I do not eat or drink when I have sublingual nitroglycerin in place."
   b. "I mix the drugs in my dessert and hope I am not too full to finish."
   c. "I keep the drugs in the original containers with the label attached to the bottle."
   d. "I store drugs in the medicine cabinet away from children and pets."
5. The nurse is teaching a patient to use an inhaler. What common teaching point is essential for the nurse to include?
   a. Cleaning the metered-dose inhaler is not recommended.
   b. The semi-Fowler or high-Fowler position is recommended.
   c. Spacers decrease delivery of medication and are not used.
   d. Nebulizers change the drug to a large-particle powder mist.
6. A 3-year-old patient has an intramuscular medication ordered. What is the most appropriate approach to gain the child's cooperation?
   a. Engage a second nurse to hold the child's body down.
   b. Have the child give a pretend injection to a toy animal.
   c. Restrain the child's lower extremities, and give the injection.
   d. Request that all family members wait outside of the room.
7. As the nurse prepares to administer oral medications, which nursing intervention is of "most importance" to ensure the patient's safety?
   a. Perform an assessment on the patient for risk of aspiration.
   b. Crush and mix the medications into the patient's meal.
   c. Administer drugs on a full stomach to avoid gastrointestinal upset.
   d. Administer unpleasant-tasting drugs with a glass of water.
8. A patient is to start on a lidocaine transdermal patch. What is essential for the nurse to include in the patient's teaching? **Select all that apply.**
   a. Wear gloves when applying the patch.
   b. Cut the patch in half to decrease the dose.
   c. Wear gloves when removing the patch.
   d. Rotate placement of the patch to different sites.
   e. Remove the patch if it becomes loose.

11

Drug Labels and Dosage Calculations

http://evolve.elsevier.com/McCuistion/pharmacology

OBJECTIVES

- Explain the requirements for dosage calculations.
- Examine the methods of math computations commonly used for dosage calculations.
- Explain the routes for enteral administration.
- Discuss the considerations for parenteral drug administration.

OUTLINE

Overview of Dosage Calculations, 92
 Systems of Measurement and Conversion Factors, 92
 Interpreting Drug Labels, 94
 Rounding Rules, 98
Calculation Methods, 98
 Basic Formula, 99
 Ratio and Proportion: Linear Method and Fractional Equation, 99
 Dimensional Analysis, 100
 Calculations Based on Body Weight and Body Surface Area, 101
Considerations for Enteral Administration, 107
 Tablets, Capsules, and Liquids, 108
 Drugs Administered via Nasogastric Tube, 109
Considerations for Parenteral Administration, 109
 Injectable Preparations, 109

 Intravenous Routes, 110
 Calculating Intravenous Flow Rate, 116
Answers to Practice Problems, 127
 Metric System Conversions, 127
 English System Conversions, 128
 Interpreting Drug Labels, 128
 Drug Reconstitution, 128
 Calculating Dosages Based on Body Weight, 128
 Calculating Dosages Based on Body Surface Area—Square Root Method, 128
 Enteral Administration, 128
 Subcutaneous and Intramuscular Administration, 129
 Calculating Intravenous Administration, 130

OVERVIEW OF DOSAGE CALCULATIONS

Nurses perform basic mathematical operations on a regular basis when preparing drugs for administration. To accurately calculate drug dosages, a systematic process is used. The same process should be used for every drug calculation so a step is not missed. Missed steps could lead to errors that can cause serious harm or even death to a patient.

This chapter explains three common methods for dosage calculation. The three methods generally used are (1) the basic formula, (2) a ratio and proportion/fractional equation, and (3) dimensional analysis. The nurse should select one of these methods for the calculation of drug dosages. When dosage calculations need to be individualized, body weight (BW) and body surface area (BSA) are included for proper dosing. This chapter uses numerous drug labels in dosage calculation problems to familiarize the reader with the information on a typical drug label. Answers to the practice problems can be found at the end of this chapter.

Keeping in mind that the goal is to prepare and administer drugs in a safe and correct manner, the following recommendations are offered:
- Think. Focus on each step of the problem. This applies to both simple and difficult problems.
- Read accurately. Be attentive to the location of the decimal point and to the operation to be performed, such as conversion from one system of measurement to another.
- Picture the problem.
- Identify an expected range for the answer. The dose should be *reasonable*.
- Seek to understand the problem. Do not merely master the mechanics of the mathematical operations. Seek a second opinion to ensure that the calculation is correct.
- To decrease drug errors, always perform *three checks* before administering a drug: (1) when retrieving the drug from a dispensing system, (2) when preparing the drug, and (3) just before administering the drug to the patient.

Systems of Measurement and Conversion Factors

To calculate correct dosages, knowing how to convert from one unit to another is essential because this is the basis for most drug calculations. Metric and English (household) measurements are shown. However, to calculate dosages, the metric system, also known as the *International System of Units* (SI), is the internationally accepted system of measure. Even though the English system is more widely used in the United States, it is not the considered form when determining dosages for drug administration. Chapter 9 lists and discusses currently approved abbreviations used in drug dosages.

Metric System

The metric system is a decimal system based on the power of 10. The basic units of measure used in dosage calculations include the gram (g, gm, G, Gm) for weight, **liter** (L) for volume, and **meter** (m, M) for linear measurement or length. Prefixes such as *nano, micro, milli, centi,* and *kilo* indicate the size of the units in powers of 10 of the base unit and stand for a specific degree of magnitude: for instance, *kilo* stands for thousands, *milli* for one-thousandth, and *centi* for one-hundredth. To convert a quantity, one of the values must be known, such as a gram (g, G), liter (l, L), meter (m), milligram (mg), milliliter (mL), millimeter (mm), or microgram (mcg). Grams, liters, and meters are larger units, whereas milligrams, milliliters, millimeters, and micrograms are smaller units. Because the conversion between degrees of magnitude always involves multiplying by a power of 10, converting from one magnitude to another is relatively easy. Common conversions used to calculate drug dosages using the metric and English systems are listed in Table 11.1.

Grams and milligrams are related by three factors of 10 according to this relationship. In the first illustration that follows, the larger unit (gram) is converted to the smaller unit (milligram). In the second illustration, the smaller unit is converted to the larger unit.

$$1\,g = 1\,mg \times 10^3 = 1000\,mg$$

and

$$1000\,mg = 1\,g \times 10^{-3} = 1\,g$$

The easiest way to convert larger units to smaller units is to move the decimal point the appropriate number of spaces to the *right*. In the next illustration, grams have been converted to milligrams by moving the decimal point three spaces to the right:

$$1\,g = 1.000 = 1000\,mg$$

To convert smaller units to larger units, move the decimal point the appropriate number of spaces to the *left*. In the next illustration, milligrams have been converted to grams by moving the decimal point three spaces to the left (thousandths):

$$1000\,mg = 1.000 = 1\,g$$

Remember: When changing larger units to smaller units, move the decimal point to the *right;* when changing smaller units to larger units, move the decimal point to the *left*. There should always be a zero (0) placed before the decimal point, called a *leading zero*, to alert the reader that the number is less than 1. For example, *0.5* clearly indicates a value of ½. If the number was written as .5, the reader could mistake the number for *5*. Do not leave extraneous zeroes after a decimal point (trailing zeroes). The reader may perceive a number many times larger than the desired dose. For example, *1.0* could be misread as *10*.

(100,000)	(10,000)	(1000)	(100)	(10)	(1)	Decimal point	(0.1)	(0.01)	(0.001)	(0.0001)	(0.00001)
Hundred-thousands	Ten-thousands	Thousands	Hundreds	Tens	Ones (Units)	↓	Tenths	Hundredths	Thousandths	Ten-thousandths	Hundred-thousandths
6	5	4	3	2	1	.	1	2	3	4	5

Whole Numbers to the Left — **Decimal Numbers to the Right**

PRACTICE PROBLEMS
Metric System Conversions

Larger to Smaller Units	Smaller to Larger Units
1. Change 2 g to mg	4. Change 1500 mg to g
2. Change 0.5 g to mg	5. Change 3000 mcg to mg
3. Change 2.5 L to mL	6. Change 500 mL to L

TABLE 11.1 Equivalent Units of Measurement

Units	Metric				English
Weight	1 kilogram (kg, Kg)	=	1000 g	=	2.2 lb
	1 gram (g, gm, G, Gm)	=	1000 mg		
	1 milligram (mg)	=	1000 mcg		
	1 microgram (mcg)	=	1000 ng (nanograms)		
Fluid Volume	1 liter (L)	=	1000 mL (milliliters)	=	
	240 mL			=	1 c (cup)
	30 mL			=	1 oz (ounce)
	15 mL			=	1 T (tablespoon)
	5 mL			=	1 t (teaspoon)
	60 gtt (drop)			=	1 t
Length	1 kilometer (km)	=	1000 m		
	1 meter (m, M)	=	100 cm		
	1 centimeter (cm)	=	10 mm		
	2.54 cm	=	1 inch		
	25.4 millimeters (mm)	=	1 inch		

English System

In the United States, English measurements are still widely used for powders and liquids. However, the English measurement is not as accurate as the metric system. Converting English measurements to the metric system will be necessary when calculating dosages. Table 11.1 provides the equivalents of the English measurement to the metric system.

When converting larger units to smaller units within the English system, multiply the requested number by the basic equivalent value. When converting smaller units to larger units in the English system, divide the requested number of units by the basic equivalent value.

Examples
Larger to Smaller Units
1. Convert 2T to t.
   The equivalent value of 1T is 3t (1T = 3t).
   To solve the problem, multiply 2T with 3t to get 6t (2T × 3t = 6t).
2. Convert 2T to milliliters (mL).
   The equivalent value of 1T is 15mL (1T = 15mL).
   To solve the problem, multiply 2T with 15mL to get 30mL (2T × 15mL = 30mL).

Smaller to Larger Units
1. Convert 6 t to T.
   The equivalent value of 3 t is 1T (3 t = 1T).
   To solve the problem, divide 6t by 3t to get 2T (6t ÷ 3t = 2T).
2. Convert 30mL to T.
   The equivalent value of 15mL is 1T (15mL = 1T).
   To solve the problem, divide 30mL by 15mL to get 2T (30mL ÷ 15mL = 2T).

Because English measurements are not as accurate as metric measurements, instruct patients and caregivers to obtain an approved drug-measuring device to dispense liquid medicine, such as the following:

PRACTICE PROBLEMS
English System Conversions

Remember: To change larger units to smaller units, *multiply* the requested number of units by the basic equivalent value. To change smaller units to larger units, *divide* the requested number of units by the basic equivalent value.

Larger to Smaller Units	Smaller to Larger Units
1. Change 3 oz to T	4. Change 3T to oz
2. Change 5T to t	5. Change 12 t to T
3. Change 2T to mL	6. Change 45 mL to t

Other Measuring Systems

Drugs are most commonly measured in grams, milligrams, or micrograms. However, some are measured in **units**. This includes insulin and heparin. Typically, units are not converted to any other measure.

Insulin is prescribed and measured in US Pharmacopeia (USP) units. Most insulins are produced in concentrations of 100 units/mL. Insulin should be administered with an insulin syringe, which is calibrated to correspond with the concentration of 100 units of insulin per mL in the vial. If the prescribed insulin dosage is 30 units, using an insulin syringe calibrated to 100 units/mL, withdraw insulin from the vial to the 30-unit mark (Fig. 11.1). ❗ *Note that 30 units are not interchangeable with 30 mL or 0.3 mL.*

U-100 insulin syringes are available in various sizes, such as low-dose insulin syringes that hold a total of 0.3 mL or 0.5 mL. The size of the insulin syringe does not alter the calibration of 100 units/mL. The US Food and Drug Administration (FDA) has now approved a U-500 insulin syringe specifically dedicated to be used with regular U-500 insulin. The U-100 and U-500 insulin syringes are *not* interchangeable. Some insulin is available in insulin pen injectors and insulin pumps. These are further illustrated in Chapter 50.

Administering insulin with a tuberculin syringe is to be *avoided*. Although both syringes have 1-mL capacities, the **tuberculin syringe** is calibrated in milliliters rather than units. It is critical that the correct type and dose of insulin is administered to avoid severe aberrations of the patient's blood glucose. Chapter 50 provides information on the different types of insulin.

Interpreting Drug Labels

Pharmaceutical companies usually label their drugs with the brand name, also called the **trade name**, and the generic name. Labels for generic drugs may have only the generic name of the drug listed. The formulation or the drug amount per tablet, capsule, or unit of liquid (for oral and parenteral doses) is printed on the drug label. Other information found on drug labels includes lot number, expiration date, proper storage of the drug, and whether it is a controlled substance. Examples of drug labels are given as follows.

Fig. 11.1 Vial U-100 insulin and U-100 syringe. (From Kee JL, Marshall SM: *Clinical calculations*, ed 7, St. Louis, 2013, Elsevier.)

Examples

1. *Tylenol* is the brand (trade) name, *acetaminophen* is the generic name, and the formulation is 500 mg per caplet.

2. This label lists the generic name only (folic acid). The formulation is 5 mg/mL. There are 10 mL in the vial.

3. This label lists the drug (heparin) and its purpose (heparin lock flush). Note: It is not intended for anticoagulant therapy.

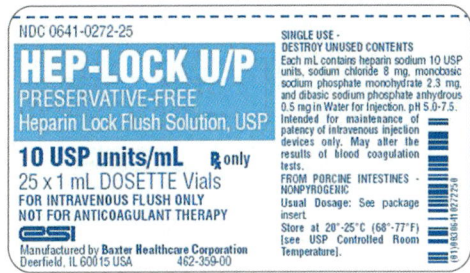

4. The following provides additional information provided on drug labels. Kadian[1] is the brand (trade) name and *morphine sulfate*[2] is the generic name. The formulation[3] (unit or form) is 60 mg per capsule, and the container holds 100[4] capsules. It is a Schedule II[5] drug, which is a **controlled substance** because of its potential for abuse. The label indicates how the drug is to be stored,[6] and the lot number[7] also appears.

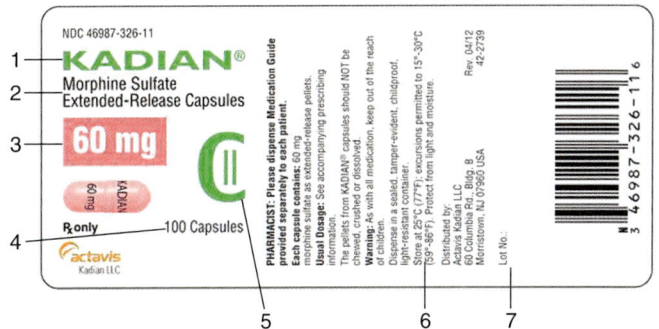

Precautions When Reading Drug Labels

Be aware of drug names that sound or look alike; for example, note the similarity between the trade names *Percodan* and *Percocet*. Percocet, which contains oxycodone and acetaminophen, is the preparation most commonly prescribed.

Percodan contains oxycodone and aspirin, and a patient may be allergic to aspirin or should not take aspirin because of a stomach ulcer. Acetaminophen can cause liver toxicity; in persons with normal liver function, the maximum dosage of acetaminophen is 3000 mg per 24 hours.

Note the similarity between *quinine sulfate* and *quinidine gluconate*. These drugs differ greatly. Quinine is prescribed for malaria, whereas quinidine is prescribed for cardiac arrhythmias.

To decrease medication errors, the nurse administering the drug should perform a minimum of three label checks with the patient's medication administration record (MAR).

PRACTICE PROBLEMS

Interpreting Drug Labels

1.
   a. What are the generic names? _____
   b. What are the trade names? _____
   c. Is this drug a controlled substance? _____
   d. What is the amount of the drug and the form? _____
   e. How many tablets are in the package? _____
   f. How should this drug be stored? _____

2.
   a. What is the generic name? _____
   b. What is the trade name? _____
   c. Is this drug a controlled substance? _____
   d. What is the amount of the drug and the form? _____
   e. How many tablets are in the package? _____
   f. How should this drug be stored? _____

CHAPTER 11 Drug Labels and Dosage Calculations

PRACTICE PROBLEMS—CONT'D
Interpreting Drug Labels

3.

a. What is the generic name? _____
b. What is the trade name? _____
c. Is this drug a controlled substance? _____
d. What is the concentration of the drug? _____
e. What is the total volume? _____
f. How should this drug be stored? _____

4.

a. What is the generic name? _____
b. What is the concentration of the drug? _____
c. Is the purpose of the drug for heparin locks? _____
d. What route can the drug be given? _____
e. Is the vial for single use or multiple use? _____

Reading Drug Labels for Drug Reconstitution

Drugs that come in powder or liquid form may need reconstitution. The liquid used to reconstitute the drug is called a **diluent**. Diluents can be nonsterile water for enteral administration, sterile water intended for injection, 0.9% saline solution, or a special liquid supplied by the manufacturer. The nurse must follow manufacturer's directions for reconstitution.

1. The following is a label for reconstituting oral cefadroxil.

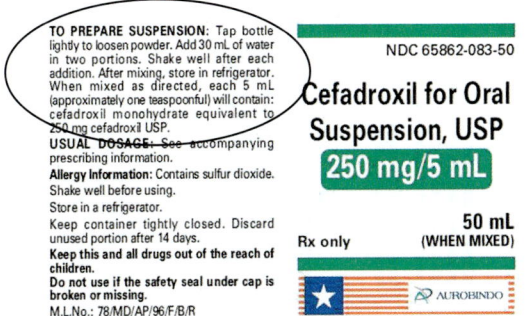

Read the left side of the label that says *To Prepare Suspension*. Note that 30 mL of water in two portions is needed to liquefy the powder. This is an oral drug, so drinking water can be used. The nurse is instructed to shake the powder loose to prevent clumping. Add 15 mL of water and shake well. Add another 15 mL of water and shake well. The powder has now been reconstituted into a **suspension**, and each 5 mL of liquid contains 250 mg of cefadroxil. The entire bottle has 50 mL when mixed, a number that is irrelevant when calculating a dose. Now the equation can be set up for calculation of a dosage.

2. The following is a label of a parenteral drug that requires reconstitution.

Read the left side of the label. For intramuscular (IM) injection, it states to reconstitute with 1 mL of 1% lidocaine hydrochloride (this diluent is sometimes used when a medication is very painful when given IM) *or* 1 mL sterile water for injection. After this preparation is reconstituted and shaken, each milliliter contains 350 mg. The figure

500 mg in the center of the label is the dose contained in the *whole vial*. If the medication is to be given intravenously, the instructions are written in the package insert. The nurse will need to read the drug insert to determine proper reconstitution for the intravenous (IV) route.

Rounding Rules

Notice when to round. Tablets and caplets can be rounded to the nearest half if they are scored (see the image for citalopram). Some tablets are scored in fourths. In this case the dosage can be rounded to the nearest fourth or quarter tablet. However, tablets and caplets that are extended release, sustained release, controlled release, or enteric coated should not be split because splitting or crushing these preparations destroys the properties that render the drug long-lasting. For this reason, these preparations in addition to capsules are rounded to the nearest whole number. Liquid drugs can be rounded to the nearest tenth; the exception to this rule is when calculating dosages of drops, which are rounded to the nearest whole number.

When rounding, determine how many places beyond the decimal point are appropriate. The general rounding rules are:
1. If a number to the right of the digit that needs to be rounded is less than 5, round down. For example, when rounding 1.343 to the hundredth place, the number becomes 1.34. Rounding 1.343 to the tenth place, it becomes 1.3. Rounding 1.343 to a whole number, it becomes 1.
2. If a number to the right of the digit that needs to be rounded is 5 or greater, round up. For example, when rounding 1.745 to the hundredth place, the number becomes 1.75. Rounding 1.745 to the tenth place, it becomes 1.7. Rounding 1.745 to a whole number, it becomes 2.

CALCULATION METHODS

Drug calculations are usually made for one dose. For example, if the prescription states that a patient is to be given 500 mg of a drug three times a day, the nurse would calculate the amount of drug equivalent to 500 mg. Occasionally, nurses calculate the full daily dose, which in this case would be 1500 mg (500 mg times three doses).

The three general methods for dosage calculations are the (1) basic formula (BF), (2) ratio and proportion/fractional equation (RP/FE), and (3) dimensional analysis (DA). These methods are used to calculate most enteral and parenteral drug dosages. The nurse should select one of the methods to calculate drug dosages and use that method consistently. All but the DA require using the same units of measure. It is most helpful to convert to the system used on the **drug label**. If the drug is prescribed in grams (g, G) and the drug label gives the dose in milligrams (mg), convert grams to milligrams (the measurement on the drug label) and proceed with the drug calculation. If conversion factors are needed during calculation, BF and RP/FE become a multistep process, which increases the risk of miscalculation.

PRACTICE PROBLEMS
Drug Reconstitution

1. Erythromycin label

a. How many milliliters of diluent are needed? _____
b. What is the final concentration? _____
c. How many mL would the nurse administer for 500 mg? _____

2. Amoxicillin/clavulanate label

a. How many total milliliters of diluent are used? _____
b. How many milliliters of diluent are needed for initial mixing? _____
c. What is the final concentration for each drug? _____
d. How many mL would the nurse administer for amoxicillin/clavulanate 500 mg/125 mg? _____

Basic Formula

The basic formula (BF) is easy to recall:

$$\frac{D}{H} \times V = A$$

where D is the desired dose (as prescribed), H is the drug on hand (available), V is the *vehicle* or *volume* of a drug form (tablet, capsule, liquid [mL]), and A is the *amount* calculated to be given to the patient.

Examples Using the Basic Formula
1. **Prescribed:** Cefaclor 0.5 g PO bid
   Available:

   How many capsules would the patient receive per dose? (This is a two-step process.)
   a. The unit of measure that is prescribed (grams) and the unit of measure on the label (milligrams) are from the same system of measurement—the metric system. Conversion to the same unit as on the label is necessary to solve the problem. Because the label is in milligrams, convert grams to milligrams. To convert grams (large value) to milligrams (smaller value), move the decimal point three spaces to the right as discussed earlier:

   $\frac{D}{H} \times V$; where $D = 500$ mg, $H = 500$ mg,
   and $V = 1$ capsule; then

   $\frac{D}{H} \times V = \frac{500 \text{ mg}}{500 \text{ mg}} \times 1 \text{ capsule} = 1 \text{ capsule}$

   Answer: 500 mg, or 1 capsule
   The patient would receive 1 capsule per dose.

2. **Prescribed:** Phenobarbital 30 mg PO STAT
   Available:

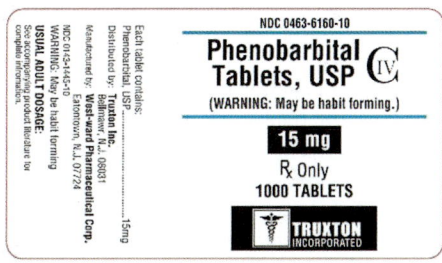

   How many tablets would the patient receive per dose?
   The dosage is prescribed in milligrams, and the unit of measure on the label is also expressed in milligrams. There is no need for conversion.

   $\frac{D}{H} \times V$; then

   $\frac{30 \text{ mg}}{15 \text{ mg}} \times 1 \text{ tablet} = 2 \text{ tablets}$

   Answer: 30 mg = 2 tablets
   The patient would receive 2 tablets per dose.

Ratio and Proportion: Linear Method and Fractional Equation

The ratio and proportion (RP) method can be expressed linearly or as a fraction (a fractional equation). The linear setup is as follows:

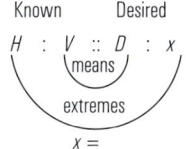

where D is the *desired* dose (as prescribed),
H is the drug on *hand* (available),
V is the *vehicle* or *volume* of a drug form (tablet, capsule, liquid [mL]),
x is the *unknown* amount to give to the patient.
The double colon symbol (::) stands for "as" or "equal to."

Multiply the extremes and the means (Hx: : VD). Solve for x $\left(\frac{Hx}{H} :: \frac{VD}{H}\right)$; H is the divisor $\left(x = \frac{VD}{H}\right)$.

The **fractional equation (FE)** setup is written as a fraction and is more commonly used than the linear setup.

Cross-multiply and solve for x, where $Hx = VD$; then $x = \frac{VD}{H}$.

Examples Using Ratio and Proportion: Linear Method
1. **Prescribed:** Amoxicillin 100 mg PO qid
   Available:

   How many milliliters would the patient receive per dose?
   Conversion is not needed because both are expressed in the same unit of measure.

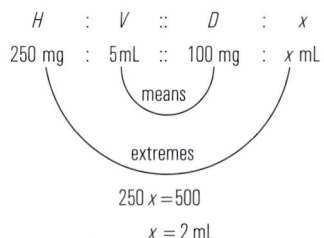

   $250 x = 500$
   $x = 2$ mL

   Answer: Amoxicillin 100 mg = 2 mL
   The patient would receive 2 mL per dose.

2. **Prescribed:** Aspirin 162 mg PO once daily
   Available:

How many tablets would the patient receive per dose?

$$H : V :: D : x$$
$$81\,\text{mg} : 1\,\text{tab} :: 162\,\text{mg} : x$$

means
extremes

$$81x = 162\,\text{mg}$$
$$x = 2\,\text{tablets}$$

Answer: Aspirin 162 mg = 2 tablets
The patient would receive 2 tablets per dose.

Examples Using Fractional Equation

1. **Prescribed:** Ciprofloxacin 500 mg PO q12h
   Available:

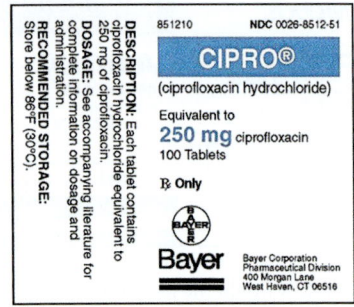

How many tablet(s) should the patient receive per dose?

$$\frac{H}{V} = \frac{D}{x}$$

where:
$H = 250\,\text{mg}$
$V = \text{tablet (tab)}$
$D = 500\,\text{mg}$
$x = \text{unknown number of tablets}$

$$\frac{250\,\text{mg}}{1\,\text{tab}} = \frac{500\,\text{mg}}{x\,\text{tab}}$$

Cross-multiply and solve for x.

$$250x = 500$$
$$x = 2$$

Answer: 500 mg = 2 tablets
The nurse would administer 2 tablets per dose.

2. **Prescribed:** Citalopram 10 mg PO once daily
   Available:

How many tablets would the nurse administer per dose?

$$\left(\frac{H}{V} = \frac{D}{x}\right)$$

$$\frac{20\,\text{mg}}{1\,\text{tab}} = \frac{10\,\text{mg}}{x\,\text{tab}}$$

Cross-multiply and solve for x.

$$20x = 10$$
$$x = 0.5\,\text{tablet}\left(\frac{1}{2}\,\text{tab}\right)$$

(Note that this tablet is scored to allow it to be split in half.)
Answer: $x = 0.5$ tablet
The nurse would administer 0.5 tablet per dose.
(For the duration of this chapter, any RP or FE calculation will be shown using the FE method.)

✦ Dimensional Analysis

Dimensional analysis (DA) is a calculation method known as *units and conversions*. The *D*, *H*, and *V* are still used in DA. The advantage of DA is that all steps for calculating drug dosages are conducted in one equation without having to remember various formulas. However, conversion factors (CFs) still need to be memorized.

Steps for Dimensional Analysis

1. Identify the unit/form (tablet, capsule, mL) of the drug to be calculated. Place this unit/form to the left side of the equal sign (=). This is your desired unit/form.
2. From the drug label, determine the *known* dose and unit/form that matches the *desired unit/form*, and place it as the first numerator on the other side of the equal sign.
3. Continue with additional fractions, including conversion factors, using a multiplication operation between each fraction to cancel out the matching unit/form in the denominator and numerator until all but the desired *unit/form* is eliminated.
4. Multiply the numerators, and multiply the denominators.
5. Divide the denominator into the numerator.
6. Solve for x (the unknown unit/form).

Examples Using Dimensional Analysis

1. **Prescribed:** Amoxicillin 500 mg PO q8h
   Available: 250 mg per capsule
   How many capsules (cap) would the nurse administer per dose?

   $$\text{cap} = \frac{1 \text{ cap}}{250 \text{ mg}} \left(H = \text{on hand} \right)$$

   a. Note that the drug form "cap" to the left of the equal sign is the same as the "cap" in the numerator to the right of the equal sign. (We must determine how many capsules need to be administered for the dose to be 500 mg.) The available capsule is 250 mg; this is placed in the denominator.
   b. The available strength (250 mg) is the denominator, and the unit/form "mg" must match the next numerator, which is the ordered dose of 500 mg (*desired dose*). The next *denominator* would be *x cap* (*unknown*) or it would be left blank.

   $$\text{cap} = \frac{1 \text{ cap}}{250 \text{ mg}} \times \frac{500 \text{ mg}}{x \text{ cap}}$$

   c. Cancel out the *mg*, multiply the numerators, then multiply the denominators.
   d. Solve for *x* by isolating *x*; reduce the resulting fraction. (Reducing fractions could be done earlier.) What remain are *cap* and 2.

   $$\frac{500}{250 \, x}; \text{ then } x = 2 \text{cap}$$

   Answer: 2 capsules

When conversions are needed (e.g., between milligrams and grams) a CF is needed to calculate dosages using the BF or RP/FE, requiring a multistep process. When using DA, there should *only* be the one unknown value in the equation (*x*). This will be especially important when calculating dosages that involve milligrams per kilogram (mg/kg) or milligrams per meters squared (mg/m²).

2. **Prescribed:** Amoxicillin 0.5 g PO q8h
   Available: 250 mg per capsule
   How many capsules would the nurse administer?
   A conversion is needed between grams and milligrams. Following the steps for DA, the equation looks like this:

   $$H \times CF \times \frac{D}{\text{unknown}}$$

   $$\text{cap} = \frac{1 \text{cap}}{250 \text{ mg}} \times \frac{1000 \text{ mg}}{1 \text{ g}} \times \frac{0.5 \text{g}}{x \text{ cap}} = \frac{1000 \times 0.5}{250}$$

   $$= \frac{500}{250} = 2 \text{ capsules of amoxicillin}$$

   As with other methods of calculation, the three components are *D*, *H*, and *V* as indicated in the previous problem. With DA, the CF is built into the equation and is included when the ordered drug's unit of measurement and the drug available differ. If the same units of measurement are used, the CF is eliminated from the equation, as shown in the first example.

3. **Prescribed:** Acetaminophen 1 g PO q6h PRN for headache
   Available: Acetaminophen 325 mg per tablet

   Conversion factor: 1000 mg = 1 g
   How many tablet(s) would be given?

   $$\text{tap} = \frac{1 \text{ tap}}{325) \overline{\text{mg}}} \times \frac{1000) \overline{\text{mg}}}{1) \overline{g}} \times \frac{1) \overline{g}}{x \text{ tap}} = \frac{1000}{325} = 3.07$$

   Answer: 1000 mg [1 G] = 3 tablets
   The nurse would administer 3 tablets per dose.

Calculations Based on Body Weight and Body Surface Area

For drugs that require individualized dosing, calculation by body weight (BW) or body surface area (BSA) may be necessary. If the child's BSA and the average or normal adult dose are known, then a more precise child's dose can be determined. These methods are mostly used for the calculation of pediatric dosages and for drugs used in the treatment of cancer (antineoplastic drugs). BW and BSA methods of calculation are also useful for individuals whose BW is low, who are obese, or who are older adults.

✳ Body Weight

The **body weight (BW)** method of calculation allows for individualization of the drug dosage and involves the following three steps:
1. Convert pounds to kilograms; 2.2 lb is equivalent to 1 kg.
2. Determine the drug dose for the body weight by multiplying as follows:

   $$\text{Drug dose} \times \text{Body weight} = \text{Patient's dose}$$

3. Follow the BF, RP/FE, or DA method to calculate the drug dosage.

Examples of Using Body Weight

1. **Prescribed:** Fluorouracil 12 mg/kg per day IV for a patient who weighs 176 lb
   Available:

   How many milliliters would the nurse administer per day?

Basic Formula
a. The first step is to convert pounds to kilograms by dividing the number of pounds the patient weighs by 2.2 (1 kg = 2.2 lb).

$$\frac{176 \text{ lb}}{2.2 \text{ lb}} \times 80 \text{ kg}$$

b. The second step is to multiply the ordered dose by the patient's weight in kilograms.

$$\text{mg} \times \text{kg} = \text{patient dose}$$

$$12 \text{ mg} \times 80 \text{ kg} = 960 \text{ mg per day}$$

c. The third step is to determine the volume in milliliters to administer 960 mg.

$$\frac{D}{H} \times V = \frac{960 \text{ mg}}{50 \text{ mg}} \times 1 \text{ mL}$$

$$= 19.2 \text{ mL}$$

Dimensional Analysis
(Note that the CFs are included in this one equation.)

$$\text{mL} = \frac{1 \text{ mL}}{50 \text{ mg}} \times \frac{12 \text{ mg}}{1 \text{ kg}} \times \frac{1 \text{ kg}}{2.21 \text{ lb}} \times \frac{176 \text{ lb}}{x \text{ mL}}$$

$$= \frac{2112 \text{ mL}}{110}$$

$$= 19.2 \text{ mL}$$

(Since liquid medications can be given in partial amounts, round to the nearest tenth.)

2. **Prescribed:** Cefaclor oral suspension 20 mg/kg per day in three divided doses for a pediatric patient who weighs 66 lb
   Available: Cefaclor oral suspension 125 mg/5 mL

How many milliliters would the nurse administer per dose? _____

Basic Formula
a. Convert pounds to kilograms.

$$\frac{66 \text{ lb}}{2.2 \text{ lb}} = 30 \text{ kg}$$

b. Multiply the desired dosage with the patient's weight in kg.

$$20 \text{ mg} \times 30 \text{ kg} = 600 \text{ mg per day}$$

c. Divide by the number of doses needed for the day.

$$\frac{600 \text{ mg}}{3 \text{ doses}} = 200 \text{ mg per dose}$$

d. Using the BF, determine the mL per dose.

$$\frac{D}{H} \times V = \frac{200 \text{ mg}}{125 \text{ mg}} \times 5 \text{ mL} = 8 \text{ mL}$$

Dimensional Analysis

$$\text{mL} = \frac{5 \text{ mL}}{125 \text{ mg}} \times \frac{20 \text{ mg}}{1 \text{ kg}} \times \frac{1 \text{ kg}}{2.2 \text{ lb}} \times \frac{66 \text{ lb}}{3 \text{ doses}}$$

$$= \frac{6600 \text{ mL}}{825 \text{ mg}}$$

$$= 8 \text{ mL per dose}$$

Body Surface Area

The measurement of **body surface area (BSA)** is the most precise method for calculating drug dosages. BSA can be measured using the West nomogram or the square root method.

The BSA by the West nomogram (Fig. 11.2A) is measured in square meters (m^2) and is determined by the patient's height and weight. Determine where the height and weight intersect on the nomogram scale; the height and weight can be in inches and pounds or centimeters and kilograms depending on the column used, but the systems of measurement must match. Centimeters and kilograms are both within the metric system and are most commonly used for the calculation of BSA. To calculate a drug dosage, multiply the dose ordered with the patient's BSA.

The Square Root Method is the most precise way to determine BSA. The height and weight must be known. When calculating the BSA in household measurement (inches and pounds), the following formula applies:

$$\text{BSA} = \sqrt{\frac{\text{Height (in)} \times \text{Weight (lb)}}{3131 \text{ (constant)}}}$$

When calculating the BSA using the metric system (centimeters and kilograms), the following formula applies:

$$\text{BSA} = \sqrt{\frac{\text{Height (cm)} \times \text{Weight (km)}}{3600 \text{ (constant)}}}$$

When calculating a child's dose and the child's BSA and the *average/normal* adult dose are known, the following formula applies:
Child's BSA/1.73 m^2 × Average adult dose

Examples of Using Body Surface Area
1. Drug dosage will be determined using the West nomogram and the square root calculations for a patient who is 70 inches tall and weighs 160 lb.
   a. Determining body surface area using the west nomogram (using inches and pounds): Draw a straight line from *70* in the *inches* column to *160* in the *pounds* column (Fig. 11.2B). Note that the line intersects between 1.9 and 2 m^2.
   b. Determining body surface area using the west nomogram (using centimeters and kilograms): The patient is 178 cm tall (1 in = 2.54 cm) and weighs 73 kg (2.2 lb = 1 kg). The height and the weight were rounded to whole numbers. Draw a straight line from 178 in the *centimeters* column to 73 in the *kilograms* column (Fig. 11.2C). Note that the line also intersects between 1.9 and 2. For the purposes of calculation, 1.95 can be used.

Fig. 11.2A West nomogram. The outside columns are used to calculate the meters squared (m²) of adults. The middle column is used to calculate the meters squared of children. (Modified from data by Boyd E, West CD: In Kliegman RM, Stanton BF, St. Geme III, JW, et al., editors: *Nelson textbook of pediatrics*, ed 19, Philadelphia, 2011, Saunders.)

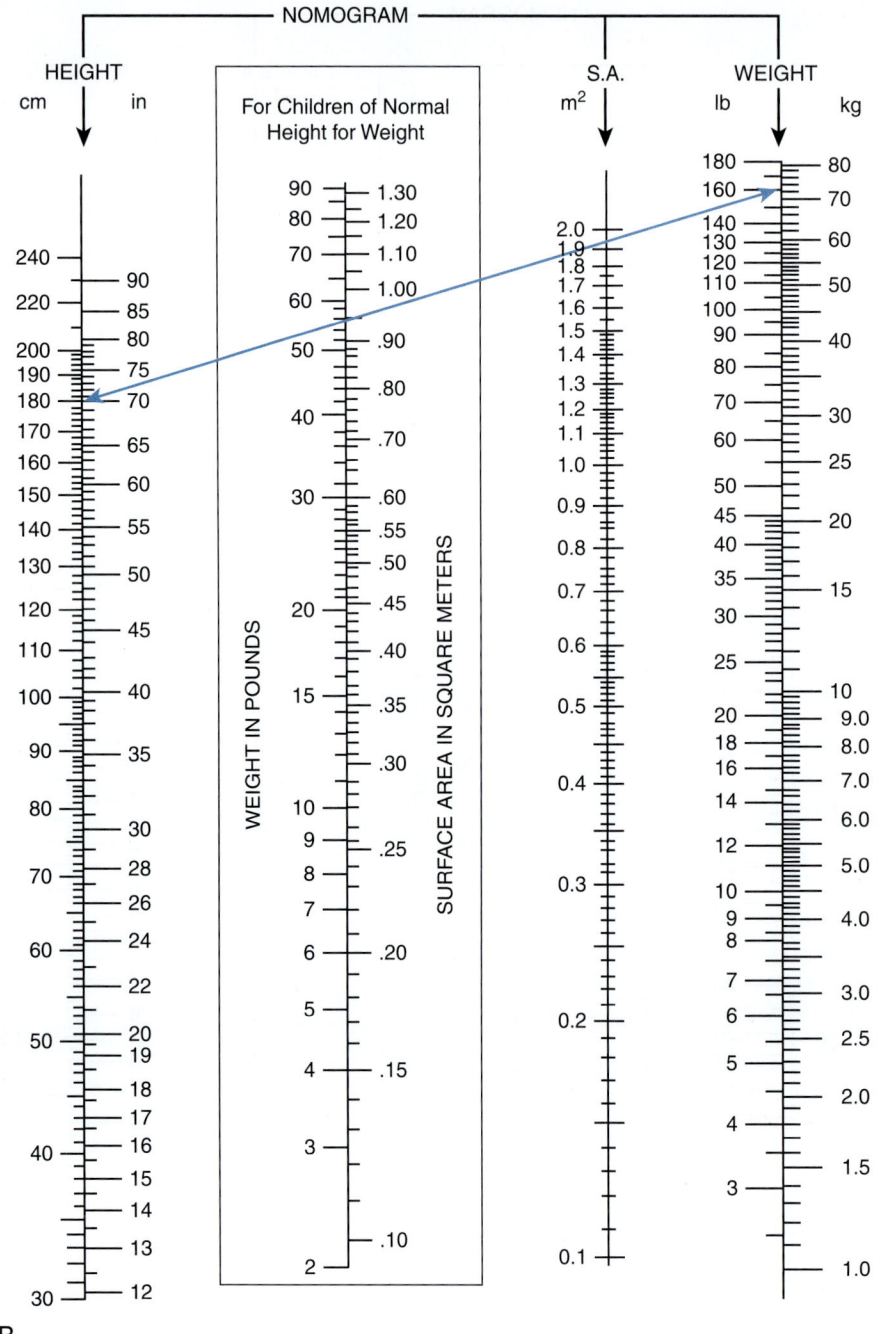

Fig. 11.2B West nomogram using inches and pounds. (Modified from Boyd E, West CD: In Kliegman RM, Stanton BF, St. Geme III, JW, et al., editors: *Nelson textbook of pediatrics*, ed 19, Philadelphia, 2011, Saunders.)

c. Determining body surface area using the square root method.

$$BSA = \sqrt{\frac{Height\ (in) \times Weight\ (lb)}{3131\ (constant)}}$$

$$= \sqrt{\frac{70\ in \times 160\ lb}{3131}}$$

$$= \sqrt{\frac{11,200}{3131}}$$

$$= \sqrt{3.6}$$

$$= \sqrt{3.6} = 1.9\ m^2$$

Calculating the BSA using the metric system (centimeters and kilograms).

$$BSA = \sqrt{\frac{Height\ (cm) \times weight\ (km)}{3600\ (constant)}}$$

$$= \sqrt{\frac{178\ cm \times 73\ kg}{3600}} = \sqrt{\frac{12,994}{3600}} = \sqrt{3.6}$$

$$= \sqrt{3.6} = 1.9\ m^2$$

CHAPTER 11 Drug Labels and Dosage Calculations

C

Fig. 11.2C West nomogram using centimeters and kilograms. (Modified from Boyd E, West CD: In Kliegman RM, Stanton BF, St. Geme III JW, et al., eds., *Nelson textbook of pediatrics*, ed 19, Philadelphia, 2011, Saunders.)

(Numbers have been rounded to the nearest tenth, which is common for adults.)

Note that both results using the square root method agree and are more precise than using the West nomogram. The variance of 0.05 from the lowest calculated BSA to the highest calculated BSA is negligible.

2. The following drug dosage for this patient is calculated using a BSA of 1.9 m².
   Prescribed: CISplatin 20 mg/m² IV today

Available:

(Note that the label also states 100 mg/100 mL and 1 mg/mL. These two expressions are equivalent since they have the same numerical value. Using the lowest numbers listed on a drug label helps prevent errors by eliminating extraneous zeroes.)
a. How many milligrams are prescribed?
b. To calculate the child's dose, multiply 20 mg with 1.9 m² to get 38 mg.
c. How many milliliters would the nurse administer?

Basic Formula

$$\frac{D}{H} \times V$$
$$= \frac{38 \text{ mg}}{1 \text{ mg}} \times 1 \text{ mL}$$
$$= 38 \text{ mL}$$

Ratio and Proportion/Fractional Equation

$$\frac{H}{V} = \frac{D}{x}$$
$$\frac{1 \text{ mg}}{1 \text{ mL}} = \frac{38 \text{ mg}}{x}$$
$$x = 38 \text{ mL}$$

Dimensional Analysis

$$\text{mL} = \frac{1 \text{ mL}}{1 \text{ mg}} \times \frac{1000 \text{ mg}}{1 \text{ g}} \times \frac{38 \text{ mg}}{x}$$
$$x = 38 \text{ mL}$$

Answer: The nurse would administer 38 mL of CISplatin intravenously.

3. Calculating a pediatric dose based on BSA using the West nomogram and the square root method is illustrated in the following:
Prescribed: Vincristine 2 mg/m² today
Available: Vincristine 1 mg/mL

How many milliliters would the nurse administer?
This pediatric patient's height and weight fall within the normal percentile. The child weighs 44 lb (20 kg).
a. Using the center column on the West nomogram, the child's BSA is 0.8 m².
b. Use the square root method to calculate BSA using inches and pounds if the child is 36 inches tall.

$$\text{BSA} = \sqrt{\frac{36 \text{ in} \times 44 \text{ lb}}{3131}} = \sqrt{\frac{1584}{3131}} = \sqrt{0.51} = 0.71 \text{ m}^2$$

(Rounding numbers to the hundredth place is common when calculating pediatric dosages.)
c. Use the square root method to calculate BSA using centimeters and kilograms.

$$\text{BSA} = \sqrt{\frac{91.4 \text{ cm} \times 20 \text{ kg}}{3600}} = \sqrt{\frac{1828}{3600}} = \sqrt{0.51} = 0.71 \text{ m}^2$$

d. The more precise number, 0.71 m², will be used to calculate the drug dosage.

Basic Formula
a. Determine the desired dose based on the previous BSA.
b. Determine the mg by multiplying with the BSA.

$$\frac{D}{H} \times V;$$
$$\text{mg} = \frac{2 \text{ mg}}{\text{m}^2} \times 0.71 \text{ m}^2 = 1.42 \text{ mg}$$

c. Solve for the desired unit of measure.

$$\frac{D}{H} \times V$$
$$\frac{1.42 \text{ mg}}{1 \text{ mg}} \times 1 \text{ mL} = 1.4 \text{ mL}$$

The dose was rounded to the tenth place to accommodate the calibrations on a syringe.

Dimensional Analysis
a. Determine BSA (we will use the calculated BSA from earlier, 0.71 m²).
b. Solve for the desired unit of measure.

$$\text{mL} = \frac{1 \text{ mL}}{1 \text{ mg}} \times \frac{2 \text{ mg}}{\text{m}^2} \times \frac{1.71 \text{ m}^2}{x} = 1.4 \text{ mL}$$

The dose was rounded to the tenth place to accommodate the calibrations on a syringe.

4. Calculating a pediatric dose when given the *average/normal* adult dose are illustrated in the following:
Prescribed: Cefaclor for a child whose BSA is 0.72 m²
Available: *Average* adult dose is 250 mg tid

a. How many mg would the nurse administer? Determine the mg using the basic formula and dimensional analysis
b. How many mL would the nurse administer? Determine the numbers of mL using basic formula and dimensional analysis.

Basic Formula
a. BSA is provided (0.72 m²)
b. The "*Average* Adult Dose" of cefaclor is 250 mg tid. Since the usual adult dose is provided, divide the child's BSA by 1.73 m².
a. How many mg?

$$\frac{D}{H} \times V = A$$
$$= \frac{0.72 \text{ m}^2}{1.73 \text{ m}^2} \times 250 = 104.0462 \text{ mg; round to the nearest whole number} = 104 \text{ mg}$$

Since one is unable to administer partial mg, the dose is rounded to the nearest whole number.

PRACTICE PROBLEMS

Calculating Dosages Based on Body Weight

1. **Prescribed:** Valproic acid oral solution PO 15 mg/kg per day in two divided doses for a pediatric patient who weighs 66 lb
   Available:

   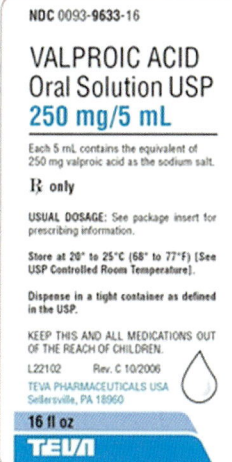

   a. How many kilograms does the child weigh? _____
   b. How many milligrams per *day* would the child receive? _____
   c. How many milligrams per *dose* would the child receive? _____
   d. How many *milliliters* per dose would the child receive? _____

2. **Prescribed:** Gentamicin 2.5 mg/kg q8h IM for a pediatric patient who weighs 33 lb
   Available:

   a. How many kilograms does the child weigh? _____
   b. How many milligrams per dose would the child receive? _____
   c. How many milliliters per dose would the child receive? _____

b. How many mL?

$$\frac{D}{H} \times V = A$$

There is 125 mg/5 mL

$$\frac{104\ mg}{125\ mg} \times 5\ mL = 4.16\ mL;\ \text{round to the nearest tenth} = 4.2\ mL$$

Dimensional Analysis

a. $mg = \dfrac{125\ mg}{1.73\ m^2} \times \dfrac{0.72\ m^2}{x} = 104.0462 = 104\ mg$

b. $mL = \dfrac{5\ mL}{125\ mg} \times \dfrac{104\ mg}{x} = 4.16 = 4.2\ mL$

CONSIDERATIONS FOR ENTERAL ADMINISTRATION

Most drugs are administered orally. Oral drugs are available in tablet, caplet, capsule, powder, and liquid forms. Oral medications are absorbed by the gastrointestinal (GI) tract, mainly from the small intestine.

Oral medications have several advantages: (1) the patient can often take oral medications without assistance, (2) the cost of oral medications is usually less than that of parenteral preparations, and (3) oral medications are easy to store. The disadvantages include (1) variation in absorption because of food in the GI tract and pH variation of GI secretions, (2) irritation of the gastric mucosa by certain drugs (e.g., potassium chloride), and (3) destruction or partial inactivation of the drugs by liver enzymes. Oral drugs (tablets, capsules, liquids) that may irritate the gastric mucosa should be taken with 6 to 8 ounces of fluids or should be taken with food.

PRACTICE PROBLEMS

Calculating Dosages Based on Body Surface Area—Square Root Method

1. **Prescribed:** Carboplatin 300 mg/m² per IV infusion today for a patient 66 inches tall who weighs 176 lb
   Available:

   a. Use the square root method to determine the patient's square meters (BSA) based on inches and pounds.
   b. What is the dosage in milligrams? _____
   c. How many milliliters would the patient receive? _____

2. **Prescribed:** Fluorouracil 350 mg/m² per day IV for a patient 164 cm tall who weighs 66.8 kg.

   a. Use the square root method to determine the patient's square meters (BSA) based on centimeters and kilograms.
   b. How many milligrams would the patient receive? _____

Nursing considerations when administering enteral drugs are further illustrated in Chapter 10.

Tablets, Capsules, and Liquids

Tablets come in different forms and drug strengths. Many tablets are scored and thus can be readily broken when half of the drug amount is needed. **Capsules** are gelatin shells that contain powder or timed-release pellets (beads). Capsules that are **sustained release** (pellet) or controlled release *should not* be crushed and diluted because the medication will be absorbed at a much faster rate than indicated by the manufacturer. Many medications sold in tablet form are also available in liquid form. When the patient has difficulty taking tablets, the oral liquid form of the medication is given. The liquid form can be in a suspension, syrup, elixir, or tincture. Some liquid medications that irritate the stomach, such as potassium chloride, are diluted. The tincture form is always diluted.

Tablets that are **enteric coated** (with a hard shell) must *not* be crushed because the medication could irritate the gastric mucosa. Enteric-coated drugs pass through the stomach into the small intestine where the drug's enteric coating dissolves, and then absorption occurs. Fig. 11.3 shows the different forms of tablets and capsules.

Liquid medications are poured into a medicine cup that is calibrated (i.e., ounces, teaspoons, tablespoons, and milliliters). Fig. 11.4 shows the markings on a medicine cup.

Fig. 11.3 Shapes of tablets and capsules. (A) Nonscored tablets. (B) Scored tablets. (C) Nonextended-release capsule. (D) Extended-release capsule.

Fig. 11.4 Medicine cup for liquid measurement. (From Kee JL, Marshall SM: *Clinical calculations*, ed 7, St. Louis, 2013, Elsevier.)

PRACTICE PROBLEMS

Enteral Administration

1. **Prescribed:** Acetaminophen 360 mg PO q4h PRN pain or fever
   Available:

   Administer how many tablets per dose? _____

2. **Prescribed:** Doxycycline 100 mg PO q12h
   Available:

   Administer how many capsules per dose? _____

3. **Order:** Warfarin 2 mg PO once daily
   Available:

   Administer how many tablets per dose? _____

4. **Prescribed:** Hydrochlorothiazide 12.5 mg PO every morning
   Available:

   Administer how many tablets per dose? _____

CHAPTER 11 Drug Labels and Dosage Calculations

PRACTICE PROBLEMS—CONT'D

Enteral Administration

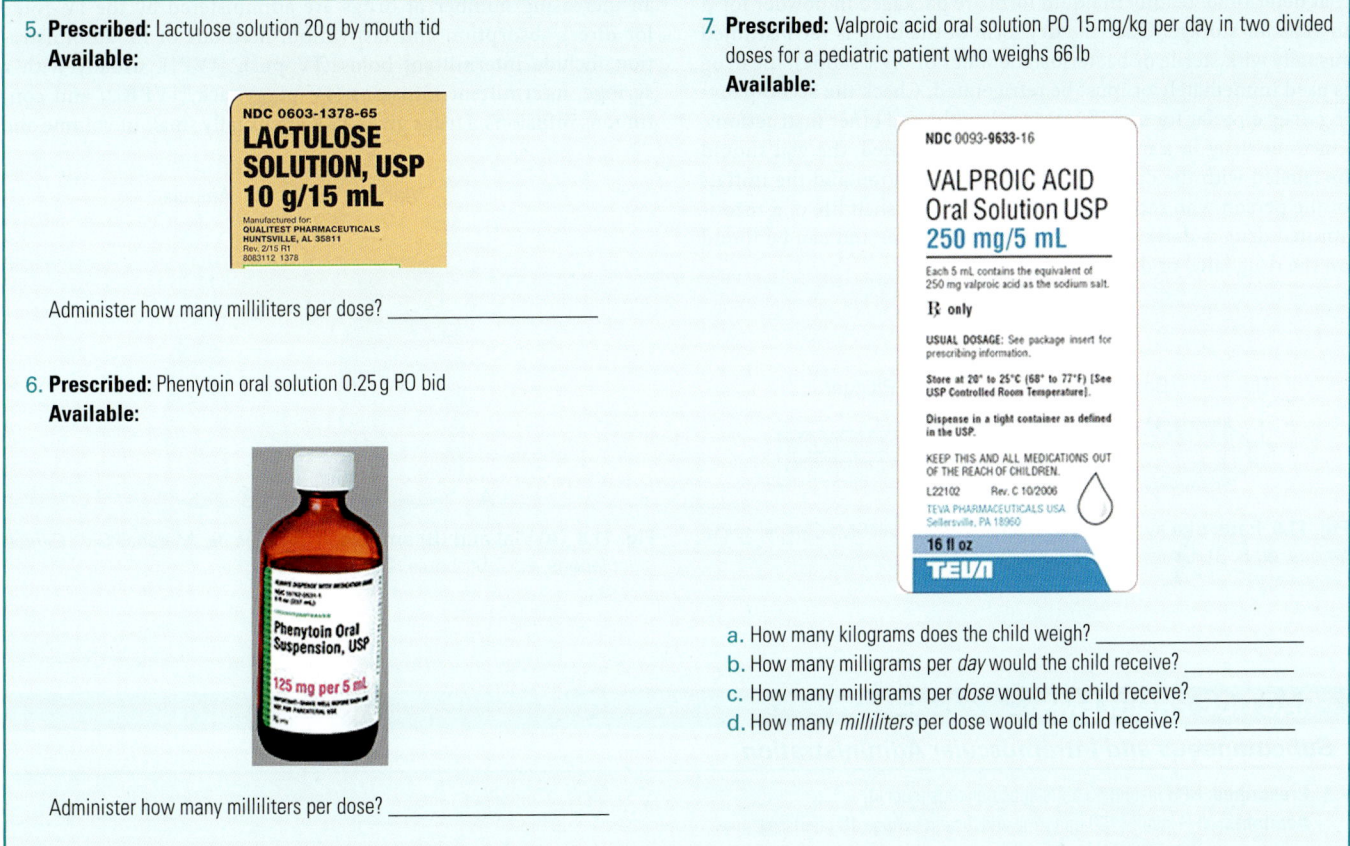

5. **Prescribed:** Lactulose solution 20 g by mouth tid
   Available:

   Administer how many milliliters per dose? _____

6. **Prescribed:** Phenytoin oral solution 0.25 g PO bid
   Available:

   Administer how many milliliters per dose? _____

7. **Prescribed:** Valproic acid oral solution PO 15 mg/kg per day in two divided doses for a pediatric patient who weighs 66 lb
   Available:

   a. How many kilograms does the child weigh? _____
   b. How many milligrams per *day* would the child receive? _____
   c. How many milligrams per *dose* would the child receive? _____
   d. How many *milliliters* per dose would the child receive? _____

Drugs Administered via Nasogastric Tube

Oral medications can be administered through a nasogastric (NG) or other feeding tube for enteral administration. If the patient is receiving a **tube feeding**, the drug should *not* be mixed with the feeding solution. Mixing the medications in a large volume of tube feeding solution decreases the amount of drug the patient receives for a specific time. The medication (but *not* timed-release or sustained-release capsules and psyllium hydrophilic mucilloid) should be diluted in 15 to 30 mL of water or other desired fluid unless otherwise instructed. The medication is administered through the tube via a syringe, followed by another 15 to 30 mL of water to ensure that the drug reaches the stomach and is not left in the tube. Nurses should be familiar with the institution's policy prior to administering medications through a feeding tube.

CONSIDERATIONS FOR PARENTERAL ADMINISTRATION

When medications cannot be taken by mouth because of (1) an inability to swallow, (2) a decreased level of consciousness, (3) an inactivation of the drug by gastric juices, or (4) a desire to increase the effectiveness of the drug, the parenteral route may be the route of choice. **Parenteral** medications are administered under the skin (intradermally [ID]), into the fatty tissue (subcutaneously [subcut]), within the muscle (intramuscularly [IM]), or in the vein (intravenously [IV]). Nursing considerations when administering parenteral drugs are further discussed in Chapter 10.

Injectable Preparations

The appropriate drug container (vial or ampule) and the correct selection of needle and syringe are essential in the preparation of the prescribed drug dose. The route of administration is part of the medication order.

Syringes

The **syringe** is composed of a barrel (outer shell), plunger (inner part), and the tip where the needle joins the syringe (Fig. 11.5). Syringes are available in various types and sizes, including tuberculin and insulin syringes. Syringes prefilled with drugs may be glass, plastic, or metal. The tip of the syringe, inside of the barrel, and the plunger should remain sterile.

Vials and Ampules

A **vial** is usually a small glass vacuum container with a self-sealing rubber top. Some are multiple-dose vials, and when properly stored, they can be used over time. An **ampule** is a glass container with a tapered neck for snapping open and using only once. Caution is advised when snapping an ampule to prevent skin laceration. Also, glass fragments can occur; therefore a filter needle must be used to withdraw medication. Fig. 11.6 shows a vial and an ampule. Drugs that deteriorate readily in liquid form are packaged in powder form in vials for storage. Once the dry form of the drug is reconstituted (usually with sterile or bacteriostatic water or 0.9% saline), the drug is used immediately or must be refrigerated. Check the accompanying drug circular for specific storage lengths and other instructions. Once the drug in a multidose vial is reconstituted, the vial should be labeled with the date and time of reconstitution and the initials of the person who reconstituted the drug. The shelf life of a reconstituted drug is determined by the manufacturer and can be found on the drug label or drug circular.

Intravenous Routes

Intravenous (IV) therapy is used to administer fluids that contain water, dextrose, vitamins, electrolytes, and other drugs. Today an increasing number of drugs are administered by the IV route for direct absorption and fast action. Methods of IV administration include intermittent bolus **(IV push [IVP])**, usually with a syringe; intermittent infusions **(IV piggyback [IVPB])**; and continuous infusions. Drugs given IVP are usually small in volume and

Fig. 11.5 Parts of a syringe. (From Kee JL, Marshall SM: *Clinical calculations*, ed 8, St. Louis, 2015, Elsevier.)

Fig. 11.6 (A) Vial and (B) ampule. (From Kee JL, Marshall SM: *Clinical calculations*, ed 7, St. Louis, 2013, Elsevier.)

PRACTICE PROBLEMS

Subcutaneous and Intramuscular Administration

1. **Prescribed:** NPH insulin 45 units subcutaneous (subcut)
   Available: NPH insulin 100 units/mL and insulin syringe 100 units/mL
   Indicate on the insulin syringe the amount of insulin that should be withdrawn.

2. **Prescribed:** Regular insulin 23 units subcut
   Available: Regular insulin 100 units/mL and insulin syringes 100 units/mL as 1-mL and 0.5-mL syringes
   Specify which insulin syringe is best to use, and indicate on the appropriate syringe the amount of insulin to be withdrawn.

CHAPTER 11 Drug Labels and Dosage Calculations

PRACTICE PROBLEMS—CONT'D

Subcutaneous and Intramuscular Administration

3. **Prescribed:** Furosemide 20 mg IM STAT
   Available:

   Administer how many milliliters per dose? _____
   (Note that this label can be confusing to the reader. The concentration is 10 mg/mL, and it is a 4-mL vial, so the vial contains 40 mg.)

4. **Prescribed:** Atropine sulfate 0.4 mg subcut STAT
   Available:

   Administer how many milliliters for the STAT dose? _____
   (There could be a point of confusion with this label. The concentration is 1 mg/mL in each vial, and there are 25 vials in the package.)

5. **Prescribed:** Heparin 7500 units subcut now; 3500 units subcut daily
   Available:

   a. Administer how many milliliters for the now dose? _____
   b. Administer how many milliliters for the daily dose? _____
   c. How many vial(s) of heparin are needed? _____

6. **Prescribed:** Ceftriaxone 1.5 g IM now
   Available:

   1. How many milliliters of diluent are needed for reconstitution? _____
   2. What is the final drug concentration? _____
   3. How many milliliters would the nurse administer for the now dose? _____
   _____

---

are administered over a few seconds to a few minutes. Medications administered by this route have a rapid onset of action, and calculation errors can have serious and even fatal consequences. The nurse must read drug inserts carefully to obtain administration information and must give attention to the amount of drug that can be given per minute. If the drug is pushed into the bloodstream at a rate faster than that specified in the drug literature, adverse reactions can occur.

IVPBs contain a larger volume of diluent and are administered over a longer period (e.g., 30 minutes, 1 hour, 3 hours). Continuous infusions, such as 0.9% saline solution or insulin drip, flow continuously until the container of solution is changed or the order for the infusion is stopped.

Many IV drugs irritate the veins; therefore they are diluted before administration. The amount of diluent used depends on the drug; drugs given by IVP can be diluted in small amounts of diluent, whereas other drugs are diluted in a large volume of fluid given over a specific period, such as 4 to 8 hours. Continuous IV infusion replaces fluid loss, maintains fluid balance, and serves as a vehicle for IV drugs.

The current trend in IV medication administration is the use of premixed IV drugs in 50- to 500-mL containers. These premixed IV medications are prepared by the manufacturer or by the hospital pharmacy. The problems of contamination and drug errors are decreased with the use of premixed IV medications. Each IV solution container has separate tubing to prevent admixture. With the use of premixed IV solution containers, the cost is higher, but the risk of medication error is lower. Because not all medication can be premixed in the solution, nurses will continue to prepare some drugs for IV administration.

Nurses have an important role in the preparation and administration of IV solutions such as 0.9% sodium chloride (normal saline, [NS]), 0.45% sodium chloride (½NS), 5% dextrose in water (D_5W), and lactated Ringer's solution (LR) and also IV drugs. Chapter 12 further discusses different types of IV solutions. The nursing functions and responsibilities during IV preparation include the following:

- Gathering equipment
- Knowing IV sets, including drop factors
- Calculating appropriate IV flow rates
- Mixing and diluting drugs in compatible IV fluids
- Knowing the pharmacotherapeutics, pharmacokinetics, and pharmacodynamics of drugs and their side and adverse effects

Nursing responsibilities continue with an assessment of the patient for expected outcomes and adverse effects of the therapy in addition to assessment of the IV site. The nurse calculates the **IV flow rate** according to the IV tubing's drop factor, the volume of fluids to be administered, the length of time for infusion, and whether an electronic infusion device will be used. IV infusions are ordered to be delivered in some unit of measure over time (e.g., mL/h, mcg/

kg per min, unit/h, and drops per minute [gtt/min]). Nurses calculate the rate of infusion in mL/h when using an electronic infusion device. If no infusion device is available, the IV medication must be infused by gravity. The nurse will need to manually regulate the flow rate by calculating the infusion rate in drops per minute. The type and size of IV administration tubing must be known when calculating gtt/min.

Intravenous Administration Sets

IV administration sets (Fig. 11.7) include printed information on the packaging cover, such as the **drop factor** or the number of drops per milliliter (Fig. 11.8). A set that delivers large drops (10–20 gtt/mL) is a **macrodrip set**, and one that delivers small drops (60 gtt/mL) is a **microdrip (minidrip) set**. A macrodrip IV set is commonly used for adults, and a microdrip IV set is used when small amounts of drug or more precise administration is warranted.

At times, primary IV fluids are given at a slow rate, ordered to **keep vein open (KVO)**, also called **to keep open (TKO)**. The reasons for KVO include a suspected or potential emergency situation for rapid administration of fluids and drugs and the need for an open line to give IV drugs at specified hours. For KVO, a microdrip set (60 gtt/mL) and a 250-mL IV solution bag may be used. KVO is usually regulated to deliver 10 to 30 mL/h.

Drugs prescribed as IVPB (Fig. 11.9) are administered via separate tubing for IV drugs, the **secondary IV line set**, which is connected into an access port on the continuous or **primary IV line set**; the port should be above the IV pump.

Fig. 11.7 Intravenous infusion sets. (From Morris DG: *Calculate with confidence*, ed 6, St. Louis, 2014, Elsevier.)

Secondary Intravenous Administration Sets

Two secondary IV administration sets available to administer IV drugs are the calibrated cylinder (volume-controlled chamber) with tubing (Fig. 11.10)—such as the Buretrol, Volutrol, and Soluset—and the secondary IV set, which is similar to a regular IV set except the tubing is shorter. The cylinder can be used with a primary or secondary line and when measurement of small-volume IV therapy needs to be more accurate, such as in pediatric or critical care settings. The volume-controlled chamber holds up to 150 mL of solution. The secondary IV line set is primarily used to **piggyback** onto a primary line (IVPB). The cylinder and some secondary IV tubing contain a port to inject medications.

When using a calibrated cylinder, such as the Buretrol, add 15 mL of IV solution, such as 0.9% sodium chloride, to flush the drug out of the IV line after the drug infusion is completed. The flush volume is added to the patient's intake. Check hospital policy for guidance.

Intermittent Infusion Adapters and Devices

When continuous IV infusion is to be discontinued but the patient still requires IV access, the IV tubing is removed and a saline lock is attached. Saline locks have ports (stoppers) where needles and needleless or IV tubing can be inserted as needed to continue drug therapy. The use of a saline lock increases the patient's mobility by not having an IV line tagging along, and it is cost effective because less IV tubing, solution, and equipment are needed. Fig. 11.11 shows examples of needleless infusion devices.

Electronic Infusion Devices

Pumps are **electronic intravenous devices** used in hospitals and some community settings. Such IV pumps are set to deliver a prescribed rate of volume. IV pumps deliver IV solution against resistance. If the flow is obstructed, an alarm sounds; however, the alarm does not sound until the pump has exerted its maximum pressure to overcome resistance. Pumps do not recognize infiltration; therefore the nurse must frequently assess the IV site. When an electronic IV device is used, the flow rate is set in milliliters per hour (mL/h).

IV pumps are recommended for use with all IV therapy; however, some noncritical IV solutions and drugs can be administered using gravity by manually calculating drops per minute. Ongoing nursing assessment is essential with any IV therapy to ensure proper duration of administration.

Several electronic infusion devices are available that include electronic volumetric pumps (IV pumps), syringe pumps, and **patient-controlled analgesia (PCA)** devices. Fig. 11.12 shows a variety of electronic IV regulators for the administration of IV solutions and drugs.

The objective of PCA is to provide a uniform serum concentration of the medication, thus avoiding drug peaks and valleys. This method is designed to meet the needs of patients who require at least 24 to 48 hours of frequent IM or IV narcotic injections.

Several reasons for the use of PCA include (1) effective pain control without the patient feeling oversedated, (2) considerable reduction in the amount of narcotic used (approximately one-half that of IM delivery), and (3) patients' feelings of having greater control over their pain.

Choices are available in the delivery of PCA. The pump can be programmed to administer the prescribed medication (1) at patient demand, (2) continuously, or (3) continuously and supplemented by patient demand (see Chapter 25).

The health care provider's order must include the following:
- Drug prescribed
- Loading dose to obtain a baseline serum concentration of analgesic

Fig. 11.8 (A) Macrodrip and (B) microdrip intravenous sets. (From Morris DG: *Calculate with confidence,* ed 6, St. Louis, 2014, Elsevier.)

- PCA dose, administered each time the patient activates the button
- Lockout interval, the time during which the drug cannot be administered
- Dose limit, the maximum amount the patient can receive during a specified time

Patient Teaching
- Inform the patient that the pain should be tolerable but not necessarily absent.
- Advise the patient of the pump's safety features, including the alarms.
- Instruct the patient in the use of the control button (medication is administered when the button is *released*).
- Instruct the patient to report any side effects or adverse reactions to the drug.
- Have naloxone, the reversal agent for opioids, easily accessible.
- Instruct patients, family members, and caregivers that the PCA button is to be depressed only by the patient.

UNIT II Pharmacotherapy and Drug Administration

Fig. 11.9 Intravenous piggyback setup. (From Morris DG: *Calculate with confidence*, ed 6, St. Louis, 2014, Elsevier.)

Fig. 11.10 Volume-controlled chamber. (From Morris DG: *Calculate with confidence*, ed 6, St. Louis, 2014, Elsevier.)

Fig. 11.11 Needleless infusion devices. (From Kee JL, Marshall SM: *Clinical Calculations*, ed 7, St. Louis, 2013, Elsevier.)

Fig. 11.12 Electronic infusion devices. (A) Alaris system with two channels. (B) Alaris system with patient-controlled analgesia module. (Modified from Kee JL, Marshall SM: *Clinical Calculations*, ed 7, St. Louis, 2013, Elsevier.)

Safety Considerations for Intravenous Infusions

All IV infusions and sites should be checked frequently. Common problems associated with IV infusions are kinked tubing, infiltration, and so-called free-flow IV rates. If IV tubing kinks, the flow is interrupted and the prescribed amount of fluid will not be given. The access site can also become obstructed, which prevents the flow. When **infiltration** occurs, IV fluid extravasates into the tissues and not into the vascular space. Trauma occurs to the tissues around the IV site. A **free-flow** IV rate refers to a rapid infusion of IV fluids that is faster than prescribed, which can cause fluid overload due to rapid infusion. Because of the possibility of a free-flow IV rate, electronic infusion pumps with multiple safety features are commonly used today.

Electronic infusion pumps are not without flaws, and mechanical problems can occur. Also, incorrectly programming an infusion pump can result in an incorrect infusion rate. Frequent monitoring of IV infusions can prevent complications of IV therapy such as fluid overload, thrombus formation, and infiltration.

Safety Considerations When Administering Heparin Sodium

Like insulin, heparin sodium is prescribed in unit dosages. Heparin is a high-alert drug that is available in multiple concentrations from 10 to 50,000 units/mL. It is important for the nurse to identify the label dosage strength and verify the patient's MAR; significant risk of causing serious injury or death can occur with errors. Heparin labels must be read carefully to ensure the correct drug is being administered. The following four heparin labels are examples of available strengths. Note that *only one* is indicated for heparin flush (100 units/mL). All other labels indicate "NOT for Lock Flush."

Heparin can be given as a direct IV injection and as a continuous infusion. IV infusion is calculated in units per hour.

Calculating Intravenous Flow Rate

Calculating Drops per Minute (gtt/min)

1. **Prescribed:** 500 mL of 0.45% sodium chloride (½NS) to be infused over 8 hours. IV tubing reads 10 gtt/mL.
   What is the flow rate in drops per minute?
   (The question is asking for flow rate with a given drop factor. When the drop factor is involved in computing flow rate, solve for drops per minute.)

Basic Formula

$$\frac{gtt}{min} = \frac{\text{amount of solution in mL} \times \text{gtt factor}}{\text{Time in h} \times 60 \text{ min}}$$

$$= \frac{500 \text{ mL} \times 10 \text{ gtt/mL}}{8 \text{ h} \times 60 \text{ min}}$$

$$= \frac{10 \text{ gtt}}{\text{min}} \text{(A partial drop cannot be administered.)}$$

Ratio and Proportion/Fractional Equation
This will take two steps to solve for gtt/min.
a. Determine milliliters per hour.
b. Determine drops per minute.

$$\frac{500 \text{ mL}}{8 \text{ h}} = \frac{x}{1 \text{ h}}, \text{ then cross multiply and divide}$$

$$\frac{62.5 \text{ mL}}{h}; \text{ then}$$

$$\frac{62.5 \frac{mL}{h}}{60 \text{ min}} = \frac{x}{10 \text{ gtt/mL}}, \text{ then cross multiply and divide}$$

$$62.5 \times 10 = 60x; \text{ then solve for } x$$

$$x = 10.4 \text{ gtt/min} = 10 \text{ gtt/min per the rounding rule}$$

Dimensional Analysis

$$\frac{gtt}{min} = \frac{10 \text{ gtt}}{mL} \times \frac{500 \text{ mL}}{8 \text{ h}} \times \frac{1 \text{ h}}{60 \text{ min}}$$

$$= \frac{10 \text{ gtt}}{8} \times \frac{500}{60 \text{ min}}; \text{ divide the product of the}$$

denominator into the product of the numerator

$$= \frac{5000 \text{ gtt}}{480 \text{ min}}$$

$$x = 10.41 \text{ gtt/min} = \frac{10 \text{ gtt}}{\text{min}}$$

2. **Prescribed:** A client is to receive D_5 ½NS at 75 mL/h. The drop factor is 20 gtt/mL.
   Calculate the flow rate.
   (The question is asking for flow rate with a given drop factor. When the drop factor is involved in computing flow rate, solve for drops per minute.)

Dimensional Analysis

$$\frac{gtt}{min} = \frac{20 \text{ gtt}}{mL} \times \frac{75 \text{ mL}}{1 \text{ h}} \times \frac{1 \text{ h}}{60 \text{ min}}$$

$$= \frac{25 \text{ gtt}}{\text{min}}$$

3. **Prescribed:** 1 L of 0.9% sodium chloride (NS) to be infused over 12 hours.
   What is the flow rate with the pictured IV tubing?

$$gtt/min = \frac{15 \text{ gtt}}{1 \text{ mL}} \times \frac{1000 \text{ mL}}{12 \text{ h}} \times \frac{1 \text{ h}}{60 \text{ min}} = 20.8$$

$$\text{Answer} = \frac{21 \text{ gtt}}{\text{min}} \text{(per the rounding rule)}$$

When an electronic device is not used and the nurse manually regulates the IV rate to administer IV medications by gravity, the nurse must calculate the number of drops per minute (gtt/min). The flow rate in drops per minute is determined by the size of the IV tubing (gtt/mL) as discussed earlier in this chapter. To convert hours to minutes, multiply the hours with 60 minutes. The drops will always be rounded to a whole number because a partial drop is not deliverable.

When delivering IV drugs via electronic devices, the flow rate is calculated for milliliters per hour (mL/h). Most IV pumps can be programmed to deliver partial milliliters.

Regardless of the method used to determine the rate, the nurse should have the following information before calculating the flow rate: (1) the volume to be infused, (2) the drop factor of the infusion set, and (3) the time frame or how long to infuse the fluid. As with previous drug calculations, the nurse should select one method, be familiar with it, and consistently use it to calculate IV flow rate.

Calculating Milliliters Per Hour

Example
1. **Prescribed:** 500 mL of 0.45% sodium chloride (½NS) to be infused over 8 hours.
   Calculate the flow rate.

Basic Formula

$$\frac{\text{Amount of solution}}{\text{Hours to administer}} = \text{milliliters per hour(mL/h)}$$

$$\frac{x \text{ mL}}{h} = \frac{500 \text{ mL}}{8 \text{ h}}$$

$$= 62.5 \text{ mL/h}$$

Ratio and Proportion/Fractional Equation

$$\frac{\text{Total volume}}{\text{Time(h)}} = \frac{x\ \text{mL}}{1\ \text{h}}\ \frac{500\ \text{mL}}{8\ \text{h}}$$

$$= \frac{x\ \text{mL}}{1\ \text{h}} 8\ x$$

$$= 500x$$

$$= 62.5\ \text{mL/h}$$

Dimensional Analysis

$$\text{mL/h} = \frac{500\ \text{mL}}{8\ \text{h}} = 62.5\ \text{mL/h}$$

(DA for this particular problem is set up similar to the BF.)

2. **Prescribed:** 1000 mL of 0.9% sodium chloride (NS) to infuse at 75 mL/h
   What is the total infusion time in hours and minutes?

Dimensional Analysis

$$\text{Time(h and min)} = \frac{1\ \text{h}}{75\ \text{mL}} \times \frac{1000\ \text{mL}}{x\ \text{time}}$$

$$\frac{1000}{75} = 13.33\ \text{h; and}$$

$$0.33\ \text{h} \times 60\ \text{min} = 19.8\ \text{min} = 20\ \text{min}$$

Answer: Total infusion time is 13 h and 20 min.

3. Using the total time in Example 2, what time will the infusion complete if the initial infusion was started at 2:00 p.m.?
   Convert 2:00 p.m. to military time (1400 h), then add 13 h and 20 min.
   1400 + 1320 = 2720 = 3:20 p.m. the next day

4. Infuse lactated Ringer's solution (LR) 1000 milliliters over 12 hours.
   Calculate the flow rate.

Answer:

$$\text{mL/h} = \frac{1000\ \text{mL}}{12\ \text{h}} = 83.3\ \text{mL/h}$$

5. D_5 ½NS has been infusing at 125 mL/h.
   After 5½ hours, the IV infiltrated, and the infusion had to be stopped. How many milliliters are left in the IV bag?

Dimensional Analysis
Answer:

$$1000\ \text{mL} - \left(\frac{125\ \text{mL}}{1\ \text{h}} \times \frac{5.5\ \text{h}}{x\ \text{mL}}\right) = 312.5\ \text{mL}$$

Solve the equation remembering the order of operation.

CLINICAL JUDGMENT UNFOLDING CASE STUDY

Phase 1
Question 1
SLO: Applying the nursing process in preparing medications.
NGN Item Type: Enhanced SATA.
Cognitive Skills: Recognize cues.

The nurse received morning report at 0700 on C.J., a 34-year-old female who weighs 243 pounds and has left leg pain and swelling, in room 18. At 0830, the nurse reviews C.J.'s medication administration record (MAR):

- Enoxaparin 1 mg/kg twice daily subcutaneously
- Warfarin 7.5 mg orally every night at bedtime.

While reviewing the patient's information in preparing to administer 0900 medications, the nurse considers the following:

- Name on the MAR is C.J.
- C.J. is in room 18
- Dose of enoxaparin is 110 mg at 0900
- Warfarin 7.5 mg at 2100
- Enoxaparin is given subcutaneously
- Warfarin is given orally
- Medication cup is needed for warfarin
- The right medication
- C.J.'s ethnicity is White

Highlight the information above that the nurse recognizes as part of the six rights of medication administration.

Answers
- **Name on the MAR is C.J.**
- C.J. is in room 18
- **Dose of enoxaparin is 110 milligrams at 0900**
- Warfarin 7.5 mg at 2100
- **Enoxaparin is given subcutaneously**
- Warfarin is given orally
- Medication cup is needed for warfarin
- **The right medication**
- C.J.'s ethnicity is White

Rationale
Nurses have the duty to ensure patients are safe while administering medications. The six rights of medication administration include (1) the right patient, (2) the right medication, (3) the right dose, (4) the right time, (5) the right route, and (6) the right documentation. C.J. is the right patient. The nurse is preparing to administer 0900 medications; therefore right medication, dose, route, and time is enoxaparin 110 milligrams subcutaneously at 0900. C.J. weighs 243 pounds, which is equal to 110 kg; therefore the dose is 110 milligrams. Although knowing

Continued

CLINICAL JUDGMENT UNFOLDING CASE STUDY—CONT'D

the room number is needed, it is not part of the six rights of medication administration. Patients can be reassigned to a different room. Warfarin would not be correct because it is ordered for 2100. The nurse would gather all the necessary supplies needed to administer subcutaneous medications, such as alcohol swabs and the appropriate syringe and needle. The medication cup is not needed for this patient. Ethnicity can affect the drug's pharmacokinetic and pharmacodynamic profile, but it is not considered as one of the six rights to medication administration.

Question 2
SLO: Applying nursing process in preparing medications.
NGN Item Type: Cloze.
Cognitive Skills: Analyze cues.

C.J., a 34-year-old female, presented to the emergency department with left leg pain and swelling. C.J. is diagnosed with a deep vein thrombosis and was started on enoxaparin 1 mg/kg subcutaneously bid and warfarin 7.5 mg PO daily at 2100.

Choose the most likely options for the missing information in the following statements by selecting from the lists of options provided.

Before administering the medications, the nurse will assess patient's _____1_____ for warfarin and determine the patient's _____2_____ for the proper dose of enoxaparin.

Options for 1	Options for 2
Partial thromboplastin time (PTT)	Blood pressure
Weight	Heart rate
International normalized ratio (INR)	INR
Hemoglobin level	Weight
Blood pressure	PTT

Answers

Options for 1	Options for 2
Partial thromboplastin time (PTT)	Blood pressure
Weight	Heart rate
International normalized ratio (INR)	INR
Hemoglobin level	*Weight*
Blood pressure	PTT

Rationale
Warfarin is an anticoagulant prescribed for persons with blood clots, such as deep vein thrombosis. Warfarin affects the coagulation profile, more specifically the prothrombin time (PT) and the international normalized ratio (INR). Warfarin's therapeutic level in patients without mechanical heart valve is an INR value of 2 to 3 seconds. If the INR value is higher than 3 seconds, the warfarin should be held, and it should be documented in the patient's chart that warfarin was held and why. Prior to administering warfarin, the nurse must assess the INR. PTT is a coagulation profile for intravenous heparin. Weight is needed to determine the correct amount of enoxaparin, not warfarin. Hemoglobin level should be monitored on a regular basis to assess for anemia due to blood loss; however, it does not need to be assessed before administering warfarin. Blood pressure should be measured on a regular basis because hypotension can be a sign of decreased fluid volume due to blood loss, but it does not need to be checked just before administering warfarin.

Enoxaparin is also an anticoagulant prescribed for persons with blood clots. Enoxaparin is a low-molecular-weight heparin and is administered subcutaneously. Since the dose of enoxaparin is based on weight, the patient's weight in kilograms is needed. Blood pressure and heart rate are important to obtain but are not required to determine proper dosing. INR is required prior to warfarin, not enoxaparin. PTT is needed when patients are on intravenous heparin, not enoxaparin.

Reference
Hull RD, Garcia DA, Vasquez SR: *Patient education: warfarin (beyond the basics)*, UpToDate, 2019. https://www.uptodate.com/contents/warfarin-beyond-the-basics#topicContent

Question 3
SLO: Calculating correct dosages.
NGN Item Type: Extended drag and drop.
Cognitive Skills: Generate solutions.

C.J. was diagnosed with a deep vein thrombosis and was prescribed enoxaparin 1 mg/kg subcutaneously bid and warfarin 7.5 mg PO daily at 2100. C.J. weighs 243 lb. The nurse retrieves the packages from the medication dispensing system. **Indicate in the third column which medication label in the first column is appropriate for each calculation in the second column**. Note: You will use the labels in the first column more than once.

CLINICAL JUDGMENT UNFOLDING CASE STUDY—CONT'D

Medication Label	Dosage Calculation	Appropriate Medication Label
CAMBER NDC 31722-329-01 Warfarin Sodium Tablets, USP Crystalline 2.5 mg PHARMACIST: Dispense the Medication Guide provided separately to each patient. HIGHLY POTENT ANTICOAGULANT WARNING: Serious bleeding results from overdosage. Do not use or dispense before reading directions and warnings in accompanying product information. Rx Only 100 Tablets	mg = 1 mg/kg × 1 kg/2.2 lb × 243 lb/x = 110 mg	
NDC 63323-586-21 Enoxaparin Sodium Injection, USP 100 mg per mL One 1 mL Sterile Single-Dose Syringe with Automatic Safety Device For Subcutaneous Injection Rx only	tab = 1 tab/2.5 mg × 7.5 mg/x = 3 tabs	
NDC 65162-762-10 Warfarin Sodium Tablets, USP 2 mg PHARMACIST: Dispense the enclosed Medication Guide to each patient. HIGHLY POTENT ANTICOAGULANT WARNING: Serious bleeding results from over dosage. Do not use or dispense before reading directions and warnings in accompanying product information. Rx only 100 Tablets amneal	mL = 1 mL/100 mg × 100 mg/x = 1.1 mL	
Amerinet Choice OPEN Remove syringe by peeling lid completely off. Then gently lift syringe straight up by grasping middle of syringe. Do not remove syringe by pulling on plunger. See www.amphastar.com ENOXAPARIN SODIUM INJECTION 40 mg/0.4 mL	mL = 1 mL/100 mg × 1 mg/kg × 1 kg/2.2 lb × 243 lb/x = 1.1 mL	

Continued

CLINICAL JUDGMENT UNFOLDING CASE STUDY—CONT'D

Answers

Medication Label	Dosage Calculation	Appropriate Medication Label
Warfarin Sodium Tablets, USP 2.5 mg (Camber, NDC 31722-329-01, 100 Tablets)	mg = 1 mg/kg × 1 kg/2.2 lb × 243 lb/x = 110 mg	No label is needed.
Enoxaparin Sodium Injection, USP 100 mg per mL (NDC 63323-586-21)	tab = 1 tab/2.5 mg × 7.5 mg/x = 3 tabs	Warfarin Sodium Tablets, USP 2.5 mg (Camber, NDC 31722-329-01, 100 Tablets)
Warfarin Sodium Tablets, USP 2 mg (NDC 65162-762-10, Amneal, 100 Tablets)	mL = 1 mL/100 mg × 100 mg/x = 1.1 mL	Enoxaparin Sodium Injection, USP 100 mg per mL (NDC 63323-586-21)
Enoxaparin Sodium Injection 40 mg/0.4 mL (Amerinet Choice)	mL = 1 mL/100 mg × 1 mg/kg × 1 kg/2.2 lb × 243 lb/x = 1.1 mL	Enoxaparin Sodium Injection, USP 100 mg per mL (NDC 63323-586-21)

CHAPTER 11 Drug Labels and Dosage Calculations

CLINICAL JUDGMENT UNFOLDING CASE STUDY—CONT'D

Rationale
The nurse would correctly read the medication label to determine the amount of the available drug and administer the prescribed amount. To correctly calculate the volume of enoxaparin, the dosage based on the patient's weight must be determined. The calculation mg = 1 mg/kg × 1 kg/2.2 lb × 243 lb/x = 110 mg does not require a drug label. The calculation tab = 1 tab/2.5 mg × 7.5 mg/x = 3 tabs requires the warfarin label with 2.5 mg/1 tab, not warfarin 2 mg/tablet label. The calculation mL = 1 mL/100 mg × 110 mg/x = 1.1 mL requires the enoxaparin label with 100 mg/1 mL, not the 40 mg/0.4 mL. However, a nurse could still use the label with 40 mg/0.4 mL; the calculation would then be mL = 0.4 mL/40 mg × 110 mg = 1.1 mL. The last calculation uses dimensional analysis with conversion factors: mL = 1 mL/100 mg × 1 mg/kg × 1 kg/2.2 lb × 243 lb/x = 1.1 mL.

Phase 2
Question 4
SLO: Assessing the actions of the anticoagulants.
NGN Item Type: Extended drag and drop.
Cognitive Skills: Prioritize hypotheses.

C.J., a 34-year-old female, was admitted to the medical-surgical floor for a diagnosis of deep vein thrombosis to the left leg. She has been receiving enoxaparin 81 mg subcutaneously bid and warfarin 7.5 mg PO daily at 2100 without complications. Her international normalized ratio (INR) has been between 2 and 3 for the last 3 days. C.J. weighs 243 lb. On day 5 of hospitalization, C.J. reported shortness of breath and chest pain. A computed tomography (CT) scan revealed a large pulmonary embolus. Enoxaparin and warfarin were discontinued, and the patient was started on heparin intravenously according to the following heparin protocol:

aPTT (s)	Bolus Dose (units/kg)	Stop Infusion (h)	Rate Change (units/kg/h)
Initial dose	80	–	Initial rate: 18
Less than 35	80	–	Increase by 4
35–54	40	–	Increase by 2
55–90	–	–	No change
91–100	–	–	Decrease by 2
101–139	–	1	Decrease by 3
Greater than 139	–	2	Decrease by 4

Indicate at which aPTT value a rate change is needed by placing an "X" in the appropriate space and indicate by how much by identifying the amount of rate change.

	Rate Change Warranted	Amount of Rate Change
aPTT = 40		
aPTT = 150		
aPTT = 34		
aPTT = 58		
Increase by 2 units/kg/h		
No change		
Increase by 4 units/kg/h		

	Rate Change Warranted	Amount of Rate Change
Decrease by 4 units/kg/h		

Answer

	Rate Change Warranted	Amount of Rate Change
aPTT = 40	X	Increase by 2 units/kg/h
aPTT = 150	X	Decrease by 4 units/kg/h
aPTT = 34	X	Increase by 4 units/kg/h
aPTT = 58		No change

Rationale
The therapeutic range for heparin is between 55 and 90 seconds. When aPTT is below the therapeutic range, patients are at an increased risk for further thrombus formation. When aPTT is higher than the therapeutic range, the patient is at risk for bleeding. According to the heparin protocol, an aPTT of 40 is between 35 and 54, which warrants a rate change by 2 units/kg/h; an aPTT of 150 is greater than 139, so the infusion should be stopped for 2 hours and then decreased by 4 units/kg/h upon resuming; an aPTT of 34 seconds is less than 35, so a bolus of 80 units/kg would be administered, followed by an increase in the infusion by 4 units/kg/h; and an aPTT of 58 is appropriate according to the protocol, so the nurse would continue the infusion at the current rate.

Reference
Warnock LB, Huang D: *Heparin*, 2020, StatPearls. https://www.ncbi.nlm.nih.gov/books/NBK538247/

Question 5
SLO: Adjusting heparin dose.
NGN Item Type: Cloze.
Cognitive Skills: Generate solutions.

C.J., a 34-year-old female, was admitted to the medical-surgical floor for a diagnosis of deep vein thrombosis to the left leg complicated by a pulmonary embolism. C.J. weighs 243 lb. The patient has been on heparin intravenously according to the following heparin protocol at 18 units/kg/h:

aPTT (s)	Bolus Dose (units/kg)	Stop Infusion (h)	Rate Change (units/kg/h)
Initial dose	80	–	Initial rate: 18
Less than 35	80	–	Increase by 4
35–54	40	–	Increase by 2
55–90	–	–	No change
91–100	–	–	Decrease by 2
101–139	–	1	Decrease by 3
Greater than 139	–	2	Decrease by 4

After 12 hours of receiving intravenous heparin on the following heparin solution, aPTT was 30 seconds.

Continued

CLINICAL JUDGMENT UNFOLDING CASE STUDY—CONT'D

**Label:**
250 mL SINGLE-DOSE CONTAINER NDC 0409-7793-52
HEPARIN
25,000 USP Units/250 mL
(100 USP Units/mL)
HEPARIN SODIUM IN 5% DEXTROSE INJECTION
WARNING: CONTAINS SULFITES
EACH 100 mL CONTAINS
50

Choose the most likely option for the missing information in the following statement by selecting from the list of options provided.

Based on the data provided, the nurse would ___Option A___ heparin with ___Option B___ and infuse heparin at ___Option C___.

Option A	Option B	Option C
Continue	0 units	18 units/kg/h
Rebolus	8836 units	24.3 mL/h
Increase	2 units/kg/h	22.1 mL/h
Decrease	4 units/kg/h	15.5 mL/h
Stop	1 h	16.6 mL/h

Answer
Based on the data provided, the nurse would ___rebolus___ heparin with ___8836 units___ and infuse heparin at ___24.3 mL/h___.

Rationale
A nurse caring for a patient who is receiving intravenous heparin would monitor their aPTT. C.J. has an aPTT of 30 seconds after 12 hours of receiving heparin, which is subtherapeutic. Based on the heparin protocol, the nurse would *rebolus* heparin at 80 units/kg, which is 8836 units followed by increasing heparin infusion by *4 units/kg/h* for a total of 22 units/kg/h. The heparin infusion would resume at *24.3 mL/h*.

Phase 3
Question 6
SLO: Teaching about side effects of heparin.
NGN Item Type: Matrix.
Cognitive Skills: Take action.

C.J. has been receiving intravenous heparin for a pulmonary embolus and is being prepared to transition to an oral anticoagulant. **In the proper column, mark an X indicating whether the teaching is appropriate (correct) or inappropriate (incorrect).**

Health Teaching	Appropriate	Inappropriate
"You will be discharged with intravenous heparin and oral medicine."		
"You will need to continue to monitor for blood in your urine or stool."		
"Notify a health care member for any dizziness."		
"You will need more frequent blood work with the oral medicine."		
"Blood oozing from previous puncture sites is normal."		
"Do not take any over-the-counter medications without talking with your health care provider first."		

Answers

Health Teaching	Appropriate	Incorrect
"You will be discharged with intravenous heparin and oral medicine."		X
"You will need to continue to monitor for blood in your urine or stool."	X	
"Notify a health care member for any dizziness."	X	
"You will need more frequent blood work with the oral medicine."		X
"Blood oozing from previous puncture sites is normal."		X
"Do not take any over-the-counter medications without talking with your health care provider first."	X	

Rationale
Intravenous and oral anticoagulants can injure a patient. Ensuring patients understand the benefits and risks and the need for regular monitoring while on anticoagulants is important. Health teaching that is appropriate for C.J. includes the *need to continue to monitor for blood in your urine or stool*. Common side effects of anticoagulants include bleeding in urine or stool or when brushing teeth or uncontrolled bleeding from wounds. Also, nurses would teach patients to *notify a health care member for any dizziness*. Dizziness can be an indication of internal bleeding. Patients who are on anticoagulants should *not take any over-the-counter medications without talking with their health care provider first*. A number of medications, such as aspirin, ibuprofen, and cimetidine, among others, as well as herbal products, can interact with anticoagulants. One of the incorrect responses includes *You will be discharged with intravenous heparin and oral medicine*. Usually, the parenteral anticoagulant (e.g., heparin) is discontinued after 2 to 10 days of starting oral anticoagulant. The number of days for bridging parenteral with oral anticoagulants is dependent on the type of oral anticoagulant and the patient's renal function. Another incorrect response is *You will need more frequent blood work with the oral medicine*. The patient is at risk for bleeding, so a CBC will be periodically monitored rather than every 6 hours. If the patient is prescribed warfarin, then an international normalized ratio (INR) will need periodic monitoring to adjust warfarin dose. *Blood oozing from previous puncture sites is normal* is incorrect. Patients should notify their health care provider if they develop oozing of blood from previous puncture sites or bleeding from gums when brushing teeth.

Reference
Hull RD, Garcia DA, Vasquez SR: *Patient education: warfarin (beyond the basics)*, 2019, UpToDate. https://www.uptodate.com/contents/warfarin-beyond-the-basics#topicContent

CLINICAL JUDGMENT UNFOLDING CASE STUDY—CONT'D

Question 7
SLO: Evaluate patient's assessment findings to determine effectiveness of anticoagulation for pulmonary embolus.
NGN Item Type: Matrix.
Cognitive Skills: Evaluate outcomes.

C.J. has been on parenteral heparin and dabigatran for 4 days for venous thromboembolism (VTE). **For each assessment finding, use an X to indicate whether nursing and collaborative interventions were effective (helped meet expected outcomes), ineffective (did not help meet expected outcomes), or unrelated (not related to expected outcomes).**

Assessment Finding	Effective	Ineffective	Unrelated
Spontaneous oxygen saturation at 95%			
The infusion pump is frequently alarming			
Reports increased swelling to left leg			
aPTT has been 62 seconds for the last 24 hours			
INR is 2.7 seconds			
Reports no evidence of blood in urine or stool			
Denies chest pain			
Multiple petechiae to trunk and arms			

Answers

Assessment Finding	Effective	Ineffective	Unrelated
Spontaneous oxygen saturation at 95%	X		
The infusion pump is frequently alarming			X
Reports increased swelling to left leg		X	
aPTT has been 62 seconds for the last 24 hours	X		
INR is 2.7 seconds			X
Reports no evidence of blood in urine or stool	X		
Denies chest pain	X		
Multiple petechiae to trunk and arms		X	

Rationale
Effective outcome includes spontaneous oxygen saturation (SpO$_2$) of 90% or greater, aPTT between 50 and 90 seconds, patient denying blood in urine or stool, and denying chest pain. If the SpO$_2$ was less than 90%, the nurse would be concerned about worsening pulmonary embolus. An activated partial thromboplastin time (aPTT) of 62 seconds is within the therapeutic range according to the heparin protocol. Patient would be at an increased risk of blood clots or pulmonary embolus with lower aPTT level. If the aPTT was supratherapeutic, the patient would be at an increased risk of bleeding, and patient may develop blood in urine or stool. Ineffective outcomes include increased swelling to the left leg. This could indicate the thrombus to the leg is worsening. Reports of chest pain could indicate worsening pulmonary embolus, an ineffective outcome. Another ineffective outcome includes the presence of multiple petechiae to the trunk and arms. Petechiae could be an indication of bleeding if the patient is receiving too much anticoagulation. The infusion pump frequently alarming and an INR of 2.7 seconds are unrelated to the expected outcomes of anticoagulant therapy with heparin and dabigatran. INR would be appropriate if the patient was on warfarin.

References
Hull RD, Garcia DA, Vasquez SR: *Patient education: warfarin (beyond the basics)*, 2019, UpToDate. https://www.uptodate.com/contents/warfarin-beyond-the-basics#topicContent

Kang H.G, Lee SJ, Chung JY, Cheong JS: Thrombocytopenia induced by dabigatran: two case reports, *BMC Neurol 17*(1):124, 2017. https://doi.org/10.1186/s12883-017-0900-8

Leung LLK: *Direct oral anticoagulants (DOACs) and parenteral direct-acting anticoagulants: dosing and adverse effects*, 2020, UpToDate. https://www.uptodate.com/contents/direct-oral-anticoagulants-doacs-and-parenteral-direct-acting-anticoagulants-dosing-and-adverse-effects?search=dabigatran&source=search_result&selectedTitle=1~110&usage_type=default&display_rank=1#H27804459

PRACTICE PROBLEMS

Intravenous Administration

1. **Prescribed:** 1000 mL of D$_5$ ½NS to infuse over 12 hours
   Available: Microdrip set with a drop factor of 60 gtt/mL
   a. Calculate the IV flow rate in drops per minute. _____

2. **Prescribed:** 3 L of IV solution to infuse over 24 hours: with 1 L of D$_5$W and 2 L of D$_5$ ½NS
   a. One liter is equal to how many milliliters? _____
   b. Each liter should infuse for how many hours? _____
   c. The institution uses a set with a drop factor of 15 gtt/mL. How many drops per minute should the patient receive per liter of fluid? _____

3. **Prescribed:** 250 mL of D$_5$W over 3 hours
   a. Determine the flow rate. _____

Continued

PRACTICE PROBLEMS—CONT'D

Intravenous Administration

4. **Prescribed:** 1000 mL of D_5 ½NS, 1 vial of multiple vitamin (MVI), and 10 mEq of potassium chloride (KCl) to be infused over 10 hours
   Available: 1000 mL of D_5 ½NS; MVI 1 vial = 10 mL; KCl 20 mEq/20 mL vial; macrodrip set, 15 gtt/mL; microdrip set, 60 gtt/mL
   a. What is the total volume of the solution? _____
   b. How many drops per minute should the patient receive using the macrodrip set? _____ The microdrip set? _____
   c. The IV pump is set at how many milliliters per hour? _____

5. **Prescribed:** Protamine sulfate 40 mg IV STAT; IV infusion not to exceed 5 mg/min
   Available:

   a. How many milliliters should the patient receive? _____
   b. Over how many minutes should protamine be administered? _____

6. **Prescribed:** Morphine sulfate 5 mg IV q3h PRN
   Available:

   Instructions are to dilute the dose with 5 mL of NS and to administer 2.5–15 mg over 5 minutes.
   a. How many milliliters of morphine should the patient receive? _____
   b. For how many minutes should morphine be administered? _____

7. **Prescribed:** Furosemide 80 mg IV now
   Available:

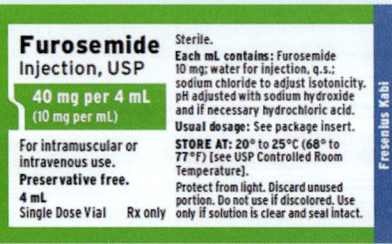

   Drug insert states rate of administration is 20 mg/min.
   a. How many milliliters will the nurse administer? _____
   b. How long should furosemide be given? _____

CHAPTER 11 Drug Labels and Dosage Calculations

PRACTICE PROBLEMS—CONT'D

Intravenous Administration

8. **Prescribed:** Regular insulin 20 units IV for blood glucose over 600
   Available:

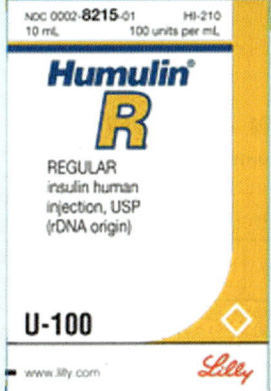

Indicate by shading the appropriate syringe to show the amount of insulin to give.

9. **Prescribed:** Digoxin 0.375 mg IV over 5 min
   Available: Digoxin 0.25 mg/mL
   How many milliliters will the nurse administer? _____
   (When giving drugs by IV, always verify the compatibility of the IV solution and the drug; otherwise, precipitation can result. Incompatibility can be avoided if the IV tubing is flushed with a compatible solution of either normal saline or sterile water before and after administration.)

10. **Prescribed:** 1000 mL D_5W with heparin sodium 20,000 units to infuse at 30 mL/h.
    Calculate the units per hour.

11. **Prescribed:** Heparin sodium 750 units/h.
    Available: Heparin sodium 25,000 units in 500 mL D_5W.
    Calculate the milliliters per hour.

12. **Prescribed:** Heparin sodium 80 units/kg IV bolus is ordered followed by heparin sodium infusion at 15 units/kg/h for a patient who weighs 175 lb.
    Available:

Continued

PRACTICE PROBLEMS—CONT'D

Intravenous Administration

    a. Calculate the amount of bolus in units and milliliters to administer.
    b. Calculate flow rate in units per hour.
    c. Calculate flow rate in milliliters per hour.

13. **Prescribed:** Heparin sodium 800 units/h
    Available: Heparin sodium 40 units/mL

    Calculate the flow rate. _____

14. **Prescribed:** 250 mL 0.9% sodium chloride (NS) with heparin sodium 25000 units to infuse at 35 mL/h.
    Calculate units per hour. _____

15. **Prescribed:** Heparin flush Mediport every 3 days.
    Which heparin product is appropriate?

16. **Prescribed:** Bolus with heparin at 80 units/kg, then initiate heparin infusion at 20 units/kg/h for a patient who weighs 150 lb
    Available: Heparin sodium 25,000 units in 500 mL 5% dextrose in water (D_5W)
        a. Calculate bolus dose in units. _____
        b. Calculate bolus dose in milliliters. _____
        c. What is the flow rate of the heparin infusion? _____

17. **Prescribed:** Infuse heparin sodium 25000 units in 1000 mL of NS at 30 mL/h
    Calculate units per hour. _____

Calculating Critical Care Drugs

Most drugs administered in critical care are *titrated* (adjusted) according to the patient's response to the drug therapy. The patient is monitored closely for therapeutic effects and any adverse events. When calculating critical care drugs, any method previously discussed is effective; however, DA is the best method because units and CFs are calculated in one equation.

1. **Prescribed:** Infuse dopamine at 5 mcg/kg/min to maintain systolic blood pressure above 110 mm Hg. The patient weighs 130 lb.
   Available: Dopamine hydrochloride (HCl) 200 mg in 250 mL of 5% dextrose in water (D_5W).
   Calculate milliliters per hour.
   Answer:

   $$mL/h = \frac{250 \text{ mL}}{200 \text{ mg}} \times \frac{1 \text{ mg}}{1000 \text{ mcg}} \times \frac{5 \text{ mcg}}{1 \text{ kg}} \times \frac{1 \text{ kg}}{2.2 \text{ lb}} \times \frac{130 \text{ lb}}{1 \text{ min}} \times \frac{60 \text{ min}}{1 \text{ h}} = 22.2 \text{ mL/h}$$

   (All the CFs for milligrams per microgram, pounds per kilogram, and units are eliminated except for milliliters and hours.)

2. **Prescribed:** Dobutamine HCl 2 mcg/kg/min, titrated to maintain hemodynamic goals in a patient who weighs 180 lb.
   Available: Dobutamine HCl 250 mg in 500 mL of D_5W
   Calculate micrograms per kilograms per minute.
   Calculate milliliters per hour.
   Answer:

   $$mcg/kg/min = \frac{2 \text{ mcg}}{1 \text{ kg}} \times \frac{1 \text{ kg}}{2.2 \text{ lb}} \times \frac{180 \text{ lb}}{x \text{ min}} = 163.6 \text{ mcg/kg/min}$$

   $$mL/h = \frac{500 \text{ mL}}{250 \text{ mg}} \times \frac{1 \text{ mg}}{1000 \text{ mcg}} \times \frac{2 \text{ mcg}}{1 \text{ kg}} \times \frac{1 \text{ kg}}{2.2 \text{ lb}} \times \frac{180 \text{ lb}}{1 \text{ min}} \times \frac{60 \text{ min}}{1 \text{ h}} = 19.6 \text{ mL/h}$$

   ⚡ (Be aware of sound-alike drugs, dopamine and dobutamine. *Dopamine* is an adrenergic agonist that affects dopamine receptors. *Dobutamine* is a beta$_1$-adrenergic agonist and does *not* affect dopamine receptors. They both have inotropic properties and are used as vasopressors.)

3. **Prescribed:** Isoproterenol 2 mg in 250 mL of D_5W to infuse at 8 mcg/min
   Calculate milliliters per hour.
   Answer:

   $$mL/h = \frac{250 \text{ mL}}{2 \text{ mg}} \times \frac{1 \text{ mg}}{1000 \text{ mcg}} \times \frac{8 \text{ mcg}}{1 \text{ min}} \times \frac{60 \text{ min}}{1 \text{ h}} = 60 \text{ mL/h}$$

Additional practice problems for all drug calculations are available in the Study Guide and on the Evolve website.

ANSWERS TO PRACTICE PROBLEMS

Metric System Conversions

Converting From Larger Units to Smaller Units
The gram is three factors of 10 greater than the milligram, so the decimal point is moved three spaces to the right.

1. If 1 g = 1000 mg, then
   2 g = 2.000 = 2000 mg

2. If 1 g = 1000 mg, then
   0.5 g = 0.500 = 500 mg

3. If 1 L = 1000 mL, then
   2.5 L = 2.500 = 2500 mL

Converting From Smaller Units to Larger Units
The milligram is three factors of 10 smaller (less) than the gram, so the decimal point is moved three spaces to the left.

4. If 1000 mg = 1 g, then
   1500 mg = 1500. = 1.5 g

   (Note there are no trailing zeroes [no 00] after the decimal.)

5. If 1000 mcg = 1 mg, then
   3000 mcg = 3.000 = 3 mg

   (Note there are no trailing zeroes [no 000] after the decimal.)

6. If 1000 mL = 1 L, then
   500 mL = 0.500 = 0.5 L

   (Note that a leading zero was placed before the decimal.)

English System Conversions
Converting From Larger Units to Smaller Units
1. If 1 oz = 2 T, then
   3 oz = 3 × 2 T = 6 T
2. If 1 T = 3 t, then
   5 T = 5 × 3 t = 15 t
3. If 1 T = 15 mL, then
   2 T = 2 × 15 mL = 30 mL

Converting From Smaller Units to Larger Units
4. If 2 T = 1 oz, then
   3 T = 3 ÷ 2 T = 1.5 oz
5. If 3 t = 1 T, then
   12 t = 12 ÷ 3 t = 4 T
6. If 15 mL = 1 T and 1 T = 3 t, then
   15 mL = 3 t, so
   (45 mL ÷ 15 mL) × 3 t = 3 × 3 t = 9 t

Interpreting Drug Labels
1. a. Lisinopril and hydrochlorothiazide
   b. There is no trade name
   c. No
   d. Lisinopril 10 mg; hydrochlorothiazide 12.5 mg per tablet
   e. 30 tablets
   f. At room temperature (68°F–77°F)
2. a. Furosemide
   b. Lasix
   c. No
   d. 40 mg per tablet
   e. 100 tablets
   f. Room temperature (59°F–86°F)
3. a. Hydromorphone
   b. Dilaudid
   c. Yes, Schedule II
   d. 1 mg/mL (oral)
   e. 473 mL = 473 mg
   f. Room temperature (59°F–86°F)
4. a. Heparin sodium
   b. 1000 units/mL
   c. No
   d. IV or subcut
   e. Multiple use

Drug Reconstitution
1. a. 77 mL
   b. 200 mg per 5 mL
   c. $mL = \dfrac{5\ mL}{200\ mg} \times \dfrac{500\ mg}{x} = 12.5\ mL$
2. a. 65 mL
   b. 65 ÷ 3 = 21.6 × 2 = 43.3 mL ($\frac{2}{3}$ of 65 mL)
   c. Amoxicillin 250 mg and Clavulanic acid 62.5 mg per 5 mL
   d. Amoxicillin: $mL = \dfrac{5\ mL}{250\ mg} \times \dfrac{500\ mg}{x\ mL} = 10\ mL$

   Clavulanic acid: $mL = \dfrac{5\ mL}{62.5\ mg} \times \dfrac{125\ mg}{x\ mL} = 10\ mL$

   (Note that the amoxicillin and clavulanic acid were both 10 mL; therefore a total of 10 mL will be given for a 500 mg/250 mg dose.)

Calculating Dosages Based on Body Weight
1. a. kg = 66 lb/2.2 lb = 30 kg
   b. 15 mg × 30 kg = 450 mg/day
   c. 450 mg ÷ 2 = 225 mg/dose
   d. $mL = \dfrac{5\ mL}{250\ mg} \times \dfrac{225\ mg}{x} = 4.5\ mL$

Dimensional Analysis

$$mL = \dfrac{5\ mL}{250\ mg} \times \dfrac{15\ mg}{1\ kg} \times \dfrac{1\ kg}{2.2\ lb} \times \dfrac{66\ lb}{2\ dose} = 4.5\ mL/dose$$

2. a. kg = 33 lb/2.2 lb = 15 kg
   b. mg = 2.5 mg × 15 kg = 37.5 mg
   c. $mL = \dfrac{1\ mL}{10\ mg} \times \dfrac{37.5\ mg}{x} = 3.8\ mL$

Dimensional Analysis

$$mL = \dfrac{1\ mL}{10\ mg} \times \dfrac{2.5\ mg}{1\ kg} \times \dfrac{1\ kg}{2.2\ lb} \times \dfrac{33\ lb}{x} = 3.8\ mL$$

Calculating Dosages Based on Body Surface Area—Square Root Method
1. a. $BSA(m^2) = \sqrt{\dfrac{66\ in \times 176\ lb}{3131}} = \sqrt{\dfrac{11616}{3131}} = 1.93\ m^2$
   b. mg = 300 mg × 1.93 m² = 579 mg

Dimensional Analysis

$$mL = \dfrac{1\ mL}{10\ mg} \times \dfrac{300\ mg}{m^2} \times \dfrac{\sqrt{\dfrac{66\ in \times 176\ lb}{3131}}\ m^2}{x} = 57.8\ mL$$

Note that the volume to administer is less since the BSA was not rounded up. Instead, rounding was performed on the final answer.

2. a. $\sqrt{\dfrac{164\ cm \times 66.8\ kg}{3600}}\ m^2 = 1.74\ m^2$
   b. mg = 350 mg × 1.74 m² = 609 mg

Dimensional Analysis

$$mg = \dfrac{350\ mg}{m^2} \times \dfrac{\sqrt{\dfrac{66.8\ kg \times 164\ cm}{3600}}\ m^2}{x} = 611\ mg$$

Note that the mg to administer is more since the BSA was not rounded down. Instead, rounding was performed on the final answer.

Enteral Administration
All answers will be shown using dimensional analysis.

1. $tab = \dfrac{1\ tab}{160\ mg} \times \dfrac{360\ mg}{x} = 2\ tabs$
2. $cap = \dfrac{1\ cap}{100\ mg} \times \dfrac{100\ mg}{x} = 1\ cap$
3. $tab = \dfrac{1\ tab}{2\ mg} \times \dfrac{2\ mg}{x} = 1\ tab$

4. $\text{tab} = \dfrac{1 \text{ tab}}{25 \cancel{\text{ mg}}} \times \dfrac{12.5 \cancel{\text{ mg}}}{x} = 0.5 \text{ tab}$

5. $\text{mL} = \dfrac{15 \text{ mL}}{10 \cancel{\text{ g}}} \times \dfrac{20 \cancel{\text{ g}}}{x} = 30 \text{ mL}$

6. $\text{mL} = \dfrac{5 \text{ mL}}{125 \cancel{\text{ mg}}} \times \dfrac{1000 \cancel{\text{ mg}}}{1 \cancel{\text{ g}}} \times \dfrac{0.25 \cancel{\text{ g}}}{x} = 10 \text{ mL}$

7. a. $\dfrac{66 \text{ lb}}{2.2} = 30 \text{ kg}$

   b. $\dfrac{\text{mg}}{\text{day}} = \dfrac{15 \text{ mg}}{\cancel{\text{kg}}} \times \dfrac{1 \cancel{\text{kg}}}{2.2 \cancel{\text{ lb}}} \times \dfrac{66 \cancel{\text{ lb}}}{\text{day}} = 450 \text{ mg/day}$

   c. $\text{mg/dose} = 450 \text{ mg} \div 2 \text{ doses} = 225 \text{ mg/dose}$

Dimensional Analysis

$\dfrac{\text{mg}}{\text{dose}} = \dfrac{15 \text{ mg}}{\cancel{\text{kg}}} \times \dfrac{1 \cancel{\text{kg}}}{2.2 \cancel{\text{ lb}}} \times \dfrac{66 \cancel{\text{ lb}}}{2 \text{ doses}} = 225 \text{ mg/day}$

Dimensional Analysis

d. $\dfrac{\text{mL}}{\text{dose}} = \dfrac{\text{mL}}{250 \cancel{\text{ mg}}} \times \dfrac{15 \cancel{\text{ mg}}}{\cancel{\text{kg}}} \times \dfrac{1 \cancel{\text{kg}}}{2.2 \cancel{\text{ lb}}} \times \dfrac{66 \cancel{\text{ lb}}}{2 \text{ doses}} = 4.5 \text{ mL/dose}$

Subcutaneous and Intramuscular Administration

1. Answer:

2. Answer: The best syringe is the 50-unit syringe. It is marked in 1-unit increments to withdraw a more precise dose. The 100-unit syringe has 2-unit increments.

3. $\text{mL} = \dfrac{1 \text{ mL}}{10 \cancel{\text{ mg}}} \times \dfrac{20 \cancel{\text{ mg}}}{x} = 2 \text{ mL}$

4. $\text{mL} = \dfrac{1 \text{ mL}}{1 \cancel{\text{ mg}}} \times \dfrac{0.4 \cancel{\text{ mg}}}{x} = 0.4 \text{ mL}$

5.
   a. $\text{mL} = \dfrac{1 \text{ mL}}{5000 \cancel{\text{ mg}}} \times \dfrac{7500 \cancel{\text{ units}}}{x} = 1.5 \text{ mL}$

(Note that units are spelled out rather than using only U, which could be mistaken for a zero.)

b. $mL = \dfrac{1\,mL}{5000\,\text{units}} \times \dfrac{3500\,\text{units}}{x} = 0.7\,mL$

(Note "units" is spelled out rather than using "U," which could be mistaken for a zero.)

c. 1.5 mL + 0.7 mL = 2.2 mL, so 2 vials are needed

6.
   a. 4.2 mL
   b. 350 mg/mL
   c. $mL = \dfrac{1\,mL}{350\,mg} \times \dfrac{1000\,mg}{1\,g} \times \dfrac{1.5\,g}{x} = 4.28\,mL = 4.3\,mL$ per rounding rule (since the total volume is greater than 3 mL, administer in two seperate injections)

Calculating Intravenous Administration

All answers are provided using dimensional analysis.

1. $gtt/min = \dfrac{60\,gtt}{1\,mL} \times \dfrac{1000\,mL}{12\,h} \times \dfrac{1\,h}{60\,min} = 83\,gtt/min$

2.
   a. 1000 mL
   b. $\left(\dfrac{24\,h}{3\,L} = 8\,h/L\right)$
   c. $gtt/min = \dfrac{15\,gtt}{1\,mL} \times \dfrac{1000\,mL}{8\,h} \times \dfrac{1\,h}{60\,min} = \dfrac{15000\,gtt}{480\,min} = 31\,gtt/min$

3. $\dfrac{mL}{h} = \dfrac{250\,mL}{3\,h} = \dfrac{83.3\,mL}{h}$

4.
   a. 1030 mL; 10 mL of MVI and 20 mL of KCl is added to 1000 mL of IV fluid.
   b. Macro drip set: $gtt/min = \dfrac{15\,gtt}{1\,mL} \times \dfrac{1030\,mL}{10\,h} \times \dfrac{1\,h}{60\,min} = \dfrac{15450\,gtt}{600\,min} = 25.75\,gtt/min = 26\,gtt/min$ after rounding to the nearest whole number

   Micro drop set: $gtt/min = \dfrac{60\,gtt}{1\,mL} \times \dfrac{1030\,mL}{10\,h} \times \dfrac{1\,h}{60\,min} = \dfrac{61800\,gtt}{60\,min} = 103\,gtt/min$

   c. $\dfrac{mL}{h} = \dfrac{1030\,mL}{10\,h} = \dfrac{103\,mL}{h}$

5.
   a. 4 mL
   b. $\dfrac{1\,min}{5\,mg} \times \dfrac{40\,mg}{x} = 8\,min$ or 0.5 mL/min

6.
   a. $\dfrac{1\,mL}{10\,mg} \times \dfrac{5\,mg}{x} = 0.5\,mL$
   b. Because 2.5 to 5 mg can be given over 5 minutes, 5 mg is given over 5 minutes.

7.
   a. $\dfrac{1\,mL}{10\,mg} \times \dfrac{80\,mg}{x} = 8\,mL$
   b. $\dfrac{1\,min}{20\,mg} \times \dfrac{80\,mg}{x} = 4\,min$ or 2 mL/min

8.

(The top syringe is calibrated in units; the bottom syringe is in milliliters.)

9. $\text{mL} = \dfrac{1\,\text{mL}}{0.25\,\cancel{\text{mg}}} \times \dfrac{0.375\,\cancel{\text{mg}}}{x} = 1.5\,\text{mL}$

10. $\text{units/h} = \dfrac{20000\,\text{units}}{1000\,\cancel{\text{mL}}} \times \dfrac{30\,\cancel{\text{mL}}}{1\,\text{h}} = 600\,\text{units/h}$

11. $\text{mL/h} = \dfrac{500\,\text{mL}}{25000\,\cancel{\text{units}}} \times \dfrac{750\,\cancel{\text{units}}}{1\,\text{h}} = 15\,\text{mL/h}$

12. a. $\text{units} = \dfrac{80\,\text{units}}{1\,\cancel{\text{kg}}} \times \dfrac{1\,\cancel{\text{kg}}}{2.2\,\cancel{\text{lb}}} \times \dfrac{175\,\cancel{\text{lb}}}{x} = 6364\,\text{units bolus}$

$\text{mL} = \dfrac{1\,\text{mL}}{100\,\cancel{\text{units}}} \times \dfrac{6364\,\cancel{\text{units}}}{x} = 63.6\,\text{mL bolus}$

b. $\text{units/h} = \dfrac{15\,\text{units}}{1\,\cancel{\text{kg}}} \times \dfrac{1\,\cancel{\text{kg}}}{2.2\,\cancel{\text{lb}}} \times \dfrac{175\,\cancel{\text{lb}}}{x} = 1193\,\text{units/h}$

c. $\text{mL/h} = \dfrac{1\,\text{mL}}{100\,\cancel{\text{units}}} \times \dfrac{15\,\cancel{\text{units}}}{1\,\cancel{\text{kg}}} \times \dfrac{1\,\cancel{\text{kg}}}{2.2\,\cancel{\text{lb}}} \times \dfrac{175\,\cancel{\text{lb}}}{x} = 11.9\,\text{mL/h}$

13. $\text{mL/h} = \dfrac{1\,\text{mL}}{40\,\cancel{\text{units}}} \times \dfrac{800\,\cancel{\text{units}}}{1\,\text{h}} = 20\,\text{mL/h}$

14. $\text{units/h} = \dfrac{25000\,\text{units}}{250\,\cancel{\text{mL}}} \times \dfrac{35\,\cancel{\text{mL}}}{1\,\text{h}} = 3500\,\text{units/h}$

15.

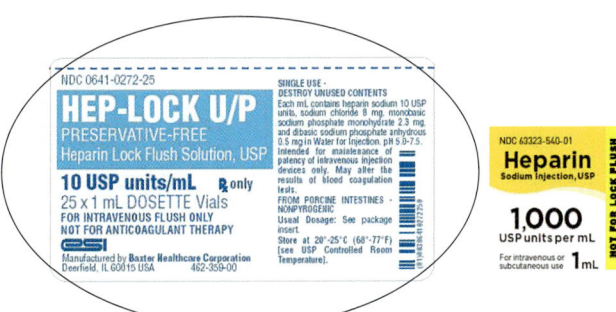

16. a. $\text{Bolus in units} = \dfrac{80\,\text{units}}{1\,\cancel{\text{kg}}} \times \dfrac{1\,\cancel{\text{kg}}}{2.2\,\cancel{\text{lb}}} \times \dfrac{150\,\cancel{\text{lb}}}{x} = 5454.5\,\text{units; round to the nearest whole number} = 5455\,\text{units}$

b. $\text{Bolus in milliliters} = \dfrac{500\,\text{mL}}{25000\,\cancel{\text{units}}} \times \dfrac{80\,\cancel{\text{units}}}{1\,\cancel{\text{kg}}} \times \dfrac{1\,\cancel{\text{kg}}}{2.2\,\cancel{\text{lb}}} \times \dfrac{150\,\cancel{\text{lb}}}{x} = 109.1\,\text{mL}$

c. $\text{Flow rate in mL/h} = \dfrac{500\,\text{mL}}{25000\,\cancel{\text{units}}} \times \dfrac{20\,\cancel{\text{units}}}{1\,\cancel{\text{kg}}} \times \dfrac{1\,\cancel{\text{kg}}}{2.2\,\cancel{\text{lb}}} \times \dfrac{150\,\cancel{\text{lb}}}{h} = 27.3\,\text{mL/h}$

17. $\text{units/h} = \dfrac{25000\,\text{units}}{100\,\cancel{\text{mL}}} \times \dfrac{30\,\cancel{\text{mL}}}{1\,\text{h}} = 750\,\text{units/h}$

UNIT III Maintenance of Homeostasis

12

Fluid Volume and Electrolytes

http://evolve.elsevier.com/McCuistion/pharmacology

OBJECTIVES

- Relate principles of nursing care to disturbances in fluid volume and electrolytes.
- Interpret the restoration choices related to replacement therapy.
- Determine the principles of nursing care related to improving patient's fluid balance and electrolyte levels.

OUTLINE

Fluid and Electrolyte, 133
    Homeostasis, 134
    Osmolality, 134
Fluid Replacement, 134
    Fluid Intake and Loss, 134
    Intravenous Solutions, 134
Electrolytes, 138
    Potassium, 138

Sodium, 139
Calcium, 144
Magnesium, 147
Chloride, 148
Phosphorus, 149
Clinical Judgment Unfolding Case Study, 149
Review Questions, 153

FLUID AND ELECTROLYTE

Fluid and electrolyte balance is necessary to maintain homeostasis. An equal balance of intake and output helps the human body maintain proper equilibrium within all body systems. Intake and output of water are regulated by the kidneys, the pulmonary system, and hormonal and neural functions. Fluid and electrolyte balance is the foundation on which nurses make important decisions concerning patient care.

To function normally, body cells must have fluid and electrolytes in the right compartments and in the right amounts. Total body fluid is contained in two major compartments: the **intracellular fluid** (ICF) is contained within the body's cells, and the **extracellular fluid** (ECF) comprises the fluid outside of the cells. The ECF is further divided into three subcompartments: the **interstitial compartment** bathes and surrounds the tissue cells; the **intravascular compartment** contains the plasma and blood vessels; and the **transcellular compartment**, also known as the **third space**, contains mucus and gastrointestinal (GI), cerebrospinal, pericardial, synovial, and ocular fluids. Table 12.1 shows the sum of fluids within all compartments, which constitutes the total body water (TBW). Fluids move freely between the intracellular and extracellular compartments to maintain balance and homeostasis.

The TBW of a 70-kg (154-lb) male is approximately 60% (40 L) of fluid volume. This percentage varies with age, sex, and percentage of body fat. Neonates are 75% to 80% water, whereas older adults are 45% to 55% water. Females tend to have less body water than males because of hormones and higher amounts of adipose tissue, which contains very little water.

Water that moves through the compartments of the body contains electrolytes. **Electrolytes** are substances that separate or dissociate into ions (charged particles) in solution, and they are abundant in both ICF and ECF. Ions carry either a positive charge **(cation)** or a negative charge **(anion)**. Major cations and anions are listed in Table 12.2. Electrolyte balance is essential for normal physiologic functioning and is closely linked with fluid balance. In addition, most electrolytes interact with hydrogen ions to maintain an acid-base balance. Electrolyte balance must be kept within a narrow range to maintain homeostasis. Many illnesses and body system alterations cause electrolyte imbalances. Electrolytes are important because they carry electrical impulses to other cells in the body.

The major electrolytes in body fluids are sodium, potassium, calcium, magnesium, chloride, phosphorus, sulfate, hydrogen, and bicarbonate ions and many proteins. Electrolyte concentrations differ in ICF and ECF. Table 12.3 lists the major cations and anions found in body fluids.

Administering intravenous (IV) fluids and electrolyte replacements may be thought of as routine nursing care; however, both require as much diligence and critical thinking as administration of any medication. This chapter describes fluid replacement strategies, pharmacologic management of specific electrolyte imbalances, and nursing care of patients with fluid and electrolyte imbalances.

TABLE 12.1 Adult Body Fluid Volume

Fluid Compartment	Percentage
Intracellular fluid	40%
Extracellular fluid	20%
Interstitial fluid	15%
Intravascular fluid	5%
Transcellular fluid	Approximately 1–2 L total (generally not included in calculations)
Total body fluid	60%

TABLE 12.2 Cations and Anions

Cations	Anions
Potassium (K^+)	Chloride (Cl^-)
Sodium (Na^+)	Bicarbonate (HCO_3^-)
Calcium (Ca^{2+})	Phosphate (PO_4^-)
Magnesium (Mg^{2+})	Sulfate (SO_4^-)

TABLE 12.3 Electrolyte Concentration in Body Fluids

Intracellular Fluid	Extracellular Fluid
Major Cations	**Major Cations**
Potassium	Sodium
Magnesium	Potassium
Sodium	Calcium
	Magnesium
Major Anions	**Major Anions**
Phosphorus	Chloride
	Phosphorus

Homeostasis

Homeostasis maintains a constant internal balance within the body despite the effects of a constantly changing external environment. Two principles stand out when considering homeostasis and fluid and electrolyte balance. The first principle is that anions and cations must be balanced within each compartment and remain electrically neutral. The amount of fluid within each compartment remains constant, and compartments work continuously to maintain fluid balance and replace and exchange ions to maintain neutrality. The second principle is that the fluid compartments remain in osmotic equilibrium except for transient changes.

Movement of fluid and particles between and within compartments is controlled by a number of processes, including *osmosis*, the movement of water across a semipermeable membrane from areas of low solute concentration to those of high solute concentration; *diffusion*, movement of molecules from an area of high concentration to one of low concentration; *hydrostatic pressure*, the force within a fluid compartment; *osmolality*, which describes the concentration of fluids; and *active transport*, which requires metabolic activity and expenditure of energy to move a substance across a cell membrane. The number of solutes in a solution is expressed as a unit of measurement called the *osmole*, which is particularly useful when referencing osmotic solutions.

Osmolality

Osmolality refers to the number of particles dissolved in the serum, primarily sodium, urea (blood urea nitrogen [BUN]), and glucose. It also is a measure of the concentration of solutes per kilogram in urine. Normal serum osmolality ranges from 275 to 295 mOsm/kg. As the number of particles increases, the concentration of the solution also increases. The change in the concentration of particles will affect chemical behavior and movement of water. Sodium is the primary electrolyte in the ECF and keeps water in this compartment.

The following three types of fluid concentration are based on the osmolality of body fluids:
1. *Iso-osmolar* fluid has the same weight proportion of particles (e.g., sodium, glucose) and water.
2. *Hypo-osmolar* fluid contains fewer particles than water.
3. *Hyperosmolar* fluid contains more particles than water.

Hypo-osmolality of body fluid may be the result of excess water intake or fluid overload (edema) caused by an inability to excrete excess water. *Hyper-osmolality* of body fluid may be caused by severe diarrhea, increased salt and solute (protein) intake, inadequate water intake, diabetes, ketoacidosis, or sweating.

The terms *osmolality* and *tonicity* are similar but not identical. *Osmolality* refers to the concentration of particles in a solution. *Tonicity* is used primarily as a measurement of the concentration of IV solutions compared with the osmolality of body fluids.

FLUID REPLACEMENT

Fluid Intake and Loss

All routes of fluid intake and loss must be considered when assessing fluid balance. General guidelines can be used as the basis for establishing fluid needs. The recommended water intake for a healthy adult is about 2300 to 2900 mL per day; oral intake accounts for 1200 to 1500 mL, solid foods about 800 to 1100 mL, and oxidative metabolism about 300 mL daily.

Patients lose water daily through various routes: kidneys, skin, lungs, and GI tract. The kidneys, the major organ regulating fluid loss, produce 1200 to 1500 mL of urine daily. *Insensible water loss* is continuous and occurs daily through the skin and lungs without awareness and is not measurable. *Sensible water loss* occurs through the lungs/respiration (500 mL/day), perspiration/skin (500–600 mL/day), and the GI tract/feces (200 mL/day) and is measurable. The minimum urinary output for an adult is 0.5 to 1 mL/kg/h or 35 to 70 mL/h for a 70-kg patient.

Daily water requirements differ according to the patient's age and medical problems. Intravenous fluids (IVFs) are ordered based on an evaluation of the patient's fluid and electrolyte balance, fluid requirements, and fluid needs. Several questions must be addressed: is the purpose of IV therapy replacement or maintenance? What are the patient's water, electrolyte, and protein requirements? The patient's weight, caloric needs, and body surface area are other important considerations. Illness and surgery increase the amount of fluids lost and affect fluid and electrolyte needs. Ongoing assessment and monitoring of the patient's responses to fluid and electrolyte therapy are vital for patients with fluid and electrolyte imbalances.

Intravenous Solutions

With fluid volume deficit (FVD) from the extracellular body compartment, fluid is lost from the interstitial and vascular spaces. Different types and concentrations of IVFs are available to replace body fluid losses.

Types of Intravenous Solutions

The three general classifications of IV solutions used for fluid replacement are crystalloids (with and without added electrolytes), colloids, and blood and blood products.

TABLE 12.4 Crystalloids Intravenous Solutions

Classifications of Crystalloids	Examples of IVF[a]	General Indications and Cautions for Use
Isotonic	LR 0.9% NaCl 5% Dextrose in water (D₅W)	LR provides electrolytes and is used for rehydration in all types of dehydration and FVD. ⚡ Use cautiously in patients with renal failure (contains K+). Use cautiously in alkalosis and liver disease; liver converts LR to bicarbonate. **Hydration** Corrects dehydration and sodium depletion. Replaces GI losses. Dextrose provides some calories. ⚡ Use with caution in patients with cardiac or renal disease due to risk for FVE. ⚡ Do not administer isotonic solutions to patients with known or suspected increased intracranial pressure.
Hypotonic	0.45% NaCl (½ NS) 0.33% NaCl (⅓ NS) 0.225% NaCl (¼ NS)	Replaces cellular fluid by treating intracellular dehydration (diabetic ketoacidosis, hyperosmolar hyperglycemic state). Provides free water to allow excretion of body wastes. Dextrose provides some calories. ⚡ Do not administer hypotonic solutions to patients with known or suspected increased ICP or patients with liver disease, shock, trauma, or burns (risk of depleting intravascular volume). ⚡ Monitor for signs of FVD and worsening hypovolemia due to a decrease in vascular volume.
Hypertonic	3% NaCl 5% NaCl 5% Dextrose in 0.45% NaCl 5% Dextrose and 0.9% NaCl 5% Dextrose in LR 10% Dextrose in water (D₁₀W)	Increases serum osmolality. Corrects severe hyponatremia. Decreases ICP in patients with cerebral edema. Dextrose provides some calories. ⚡ Use with caution; may cause intravascular volume overload and pulmonary edema. ⚡ Administer slowly and carefully with infusion control pump and constant monitoring; monitor electrolytes and monitor for signs of FVE. Avoid prolonged use. ⚡ Contraindicated for patients with cardiac or renal disease and for those with dehydration or diabetic ketoacidosis. Higher concentrations of dextrose (>10%) must be given through a central venous access device; may be added to amino acid solutions as total parenteral nutrition.

>, Greater than; <, less than; *FVD*, fluid volume depletion; *FVE*, fluid volume excess; *GI*, gastrointestinal; *ICP*, intracranial pressure; *IVF*, intravenous fluids; *K*, potassium; *LR*, lactated Ringer's solution; *NaCl*, sodium chloride; *NS*, normal saline.
[a]Examples of IV fluids: Refer to manufacturer's label on individual bags of intravenous fluids (IVFs) for exact osmolarity.

Crystalloids. Crystalloid solutions contain fluids and electrolytes and freely cross capillary walls. They do not contain any proteins, which are necessary to maintain the colloidal oncotic pressure that prevents water from leaving the intravascular space. Crystalloids are used as short-term maintenance fluids and to treat dehydration and electrolyte imbalances. Crystalloids cause early plasma expansion but have a shorter duration of action than colloid solutions.

The three major classifications of crystalloid IVFs are hypotonic, isotonic, and hypertonic (Table 12.4 and Fig. 12.1):

- **Hypotonic** solutions exert less osmotic pressure than ECF, which allows water to move into the cell. IV infusions of hypotonic solutions result in an increased solute concentration in the intravascular space, causing fluid to move into the intracellular and interstitial spaces. ⚡ Excessive infusion of hypotonic solutions may cause hemolysis, decreased blood pressure, and decreased IVF volume.
- **Isotonic** solutions have the same approximate osmolality as ECF or plasma. Because of the osmotic equilibrium, water does not enter or leave the cell; therefore there is no effect on red blood cells (RBCs). Isotonic solutions are primarily used for hydration and to expand ECF volume, because the fluid remains in the intravascular space.
- **Hypertonic** solutions exert greater osmotic pressure than ECF, resulting in a higher solute concentration than the serum. When

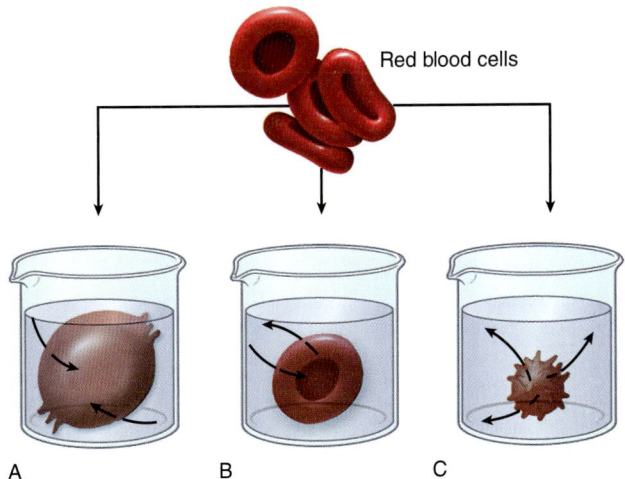

Fig. 12.1 Effects of water on red blood cells (RBCs). (A) Hypotonic solution (H2O excess) results in cellular swelling. (B) Isotonic solution (normal H2O balance) results in no change. (C) Hypertonic solution (H2O deficit), results in cellular shrinking. (From Harding MM. *Lewis's Medical-Surgical Nursing: Assessment and Management of Clinical Problems*, 11th ed, Elsevier Inc; 2020.)

administered, hypertonic IVF fluids pull water from the interstitial space to the ECF via osmosis and cause cell shrinkage. ⚡ Patients receiving hypertonic solutions must be monitored carefully for signs of circulatory overload (because of the increase in ECF volume).

Parenteral solutions containing dextrose are available in different concentrations and in combination with other solutions, such as normal saline and lactated Ringer's solution. Dextrose solutions provide hydration and some calories and increase glucose levels in the blood. The pharmacist will use dextrose solutions to dilute IV medications for administration. The addition of dextrose to an IV solution affects the tonicity of the solution after it is infused. Five-percent dextrose solutions are hypertonic when added to normal saline or lactated Ringer's solution, but the remaining solution is isotonic because the dextrose is quickly metabolized to carbon dioxide and water.

⚡ The Infusion Nursing Society's Practice Guidelines recommend that dextrose solutions higher than 10% should be given via a central vein. An exception is 50% dextrose, which may be given in small amounts via a peripheral vein to correct hypoglycemia. Dextrose can be irritating to veins because of the pH of the solution (3.4–4). If hypertonic solutions are not diluted and are given peripherally, there is a risk of vein irritation, damage, and thrombosis. Long-term use of hypertonic solutions may result in electrolyte depletion, increased intravascular volume, fluid overload, water intoxication, and pulmonary edema. Rapid infusions of dextrose solutions may cause hyperglycemia, which can lead to osmotic diuresis and fluid and electrolyte imbalance.

Sodium solutions are available in various concentrations and tonicities. Isotonic solutions are primarily used for hydration to expand the ECF and during blood product transfusions. Rapid infusion of isotonic saline solutions may lead to hypernatremia, fluid volume excess (FVE), and electrolyte depletion. Long-term use should also be avoided because normal saline provides no calories. Hypotonic solutions are also used for hydration and to treat hyperosmolar diabetes. Hypertonic saline solutions are used to treat severe hyponatremia or hypochloremia; careful monitoring of electrolyte levels is important to avoid excess replacement.

Balanced electrolyte solutions, such as lactated Ringer's solution and Ringer's solution, contain electrolytes (no magnesium) and minimal calories with the addition of dextrose. Their primary use is hydration and electrolyte replacement. However, they do not provide adequate electrolytes for maintenance therapy for patients with limited or no oral intake. Lactated Ringer's solution is similar to plasma in electrolyte content. Lactate is added as a buffering agent and is metabolized to bicarbonate. ⚡ Complications of infusions of Ringer's and lactated Ringer's include fluid overload, excess electrolytes, and metabolic acidosis with long-term therapy. Because lactate is metabolized in the liver, lactated Ringer's is contraindicated for patients with liver disease.

Colloids. Colloid solutions contain protein or other large molecular substances that increase *osmolarity* without dissolving in the solution. Because of their size, the particles are unable to pass through the semipermeable membranes of the capillary walls and stay within the intravascular compartment; thus colloids are also known as *plasma expanders*. They act by increasing the colloidal oncotic pressure and pulling fluids from the interstitial space into the plasma, increasing blood volume. The composition of colloid solutions includes proteins, carbohydrates, and lipids. Colloids typically have small and large particles, except albumin, whose particles are all one size. Commonly used colloids are shown in Table 12.5.

TABLE 12.5 Common Colloid Solutions

Common Solutions[a]	Indications	Nursing Implications	Adverse Effects and Contraindications
High-molecular-weight dextran 75 Dextran 70 6% in 5% dextrose	Treatment of shock caused by hemorrhage, burns, or trauma Maximum volume expansion effect 1 h after administration with normal renal functioning Increased volume is excreted within 24 h	Administer colloid solutions with an 18-g or larger needle. Dextran solutions are not a substitute for blood products and have no oxygen-carrying capacity but may be used emergently if cross-matching or blood products are unavailable. Monitor pulse, BP, CVP, and urine output every 5–15 min for the first hour, and hourly thereafter Increased volume may cause dilution of Hgb and Hct. Assess fluid volume status; may cause circulatory overload. Monitor for signs and symptoms of FVE.	Bleeding; hypotension; wheezing; urticaria; chest tightness; nausea and vomiting may occur ⚡ Severe anaphylaxis reactions, leading to death ⚡ Contraindicated for patients with impaired hepatic or renal disease, heart failure, and bleeding disorders ⚡ May interfere with laboratory testing for typing and cross-matching; draw necessary blood samples before administration.
Hydroxyethyl starch 6% (hetastarch) A synthetic polymer closely related to human albumin	Early fluid replacement and treatment of hypovolemic shock and burns Maximum volume expansion occurs shortly after infusion is completed Duration of action is 24–36 h	Hetastarch 6% with 0.9% NaCl is isotonic Hetastarch 6% with 7.2% NaCl is hypertonic Does not interfere with blood typing and cross-matching Assess fluid volume status; may cause circulatory overload.	⚡ May cause severe anaphylactic reaction Interferes with platelet function by increasing bleeding time ⚡ Contraindicated for patients with bleeding disorders and renal, cardiac, or liver disease
Albumin 5% Albumin 25% Prepared from human blood and blood products Considered a blood product	Regulates plasma volume and tissue–fluid balance 5% solution is isotonic and is used to treat hypovolemia 25% solution is hypertonic and is generally used for patients with fluid and sodium restrictions	Assess fluid volume status Can cause circulatory overload.	⚡ Contraindicated in patients with heart failure or severe anemia ⚡ Hold ACEIs at least 24 h before administering albumin due to the risk of adverse reactions, including hypotension and flushing.

ACEI, Angiotensin-converting enzyme inhibitor; *BP*, blood pressure; *CVP*, central venous pressure; *FVE*, fluid volume excess; *g*, gauge; *h*, hour; *Hct*, hematocrit; *Hgb*, hemoglobin; *min*, minute; *NaCl*, sodium chloride.
[a]Common solutions: Refer to manufacturer's label on individual bags of intravenous fluids (IVFs) for exact osmolarity.

CHAPTER 12 Fluid Volume and Electrolytes

Blood and Blood Products. Nurses complete a thorough patient assessment before, during, and after administration of blood products. Each facility has a policy and procedure for blood transfusions, and each registered nurse is oriented in the correct procedure. Blood products include packed red blood cells (PRBCs), plasma, platelets, and cryoprecipitate. A unit of PRBCs contains concentrated RBCs with most of the plasma and platelets removed; the approximate volume is 350 mL/unit. The approximate volume of a unit of whole blood is 500 mL/unit. Infusing PRBCs over whole blood offers an advantage because packed cells allow an increase in oxygen-carrying capacity with a smaller volume. One unit of whole blood elevates the hemoglobin by approximately 0.5 to 1 g/dL, and one unit of PRBCs elevates the hematocrit by three points.

It is important for nurses to understand the specific blood components before beginning the infusion. ⚡ Proper product-to-patient identification is paramount in preventing transfusion reactions. Reducing errors during blood administration is a focus of The Joint Commission's 2018 National Patient Safety Goals (http://www.joint-commission.org). Also, the National Healthcare Safety Network's Hemovigilance Module was developed to increase patient safety and decrease costs associated with transfusion-related adverse events (http://www.cdc.gov/nhsn/pdfs/biovigilance/bv-hv-protocol-current.pdf).

The maximum rate of an infusion is 4 hours per unit, beginning with removal of the unit from the refrigerator. ⚡ If the transfusion is not finished by the 4-hour mark, the transfusion bag must be returned to the blood bank, and a new bag issued to complete the transfusion. ⚡ *Never* add medications to the unit of blood.

Loop diuretics are often prescribed to patients receiving whole blood or PRBCs to prevent circulatory overload, particularly in patients who are at risk for developing pulmonary edema and FVE. For patients receiving multiple blood transfusions, the serum ionized calcium level should be monitored. Both PRBCs and whole blood products are processed using sodium citrate and citric acid for anticoagulation; multiple blood transfusions can result in a decrease in the plasma calcium levels. Practice guidelines are available from The Joint Commission (see http://www.jointcommission.org/bloodmanagement). ⚡ Always confirm with the patient any ethical or legal issues preventing the administration of blood or blood products that might conflict with the patient's personal belief system.

IV fat emulsion, also known as *lipid emulsion*, is a component of parenteral nutrition for patients who are unable to get nutrition through an oral diet (see Chapter 14). Fat emulsion can supply up to 30% of the patient's caloric intake and is usually recommended for patients who are unable to tolerate oral or enteral feedings for 7 days or more. The contents of fat emulsion are primarily soybean or safflower and triglycerides with egg phospholipids added as an emulsifier. Parenteral nutrition provides essential nutrients intravenously, including proteins, carbohydrates, electrolytes, trace minerals, and vitamins. Fat emulsion is often added to parenteral nutrition formulas by the pharmacist. ⚡ The patient must have a centrally or peripherally inserted vascular access device to receive parenteral nutrition formulas. Nausea, vomiting, and elevated temperature have been reported when fat emulsion is infused too quickly. It is used cautiously in patients at risk for fat embolism, such as with a fractured femur, and in patients with an allergy to eggs or soybeans and those with pancreatitis, bleeding disorders, liver failure, and respiratory disease.

⊙ CLINICAL JUDGMENT [NURSING PROCESS]

Fluid Imbalances (Fluid Volume Deficit and Fluid Volume Excess)

Concept: Fluid and Electrolytes
- Patients require the regulation of fluid and electrolytes to maintain homeostasis. Nurses will encounter potential and actual alterations of fluid and electrolyte balance when caring for patients. Nursing assessments and interventions ensure the intake of fluid and electrolytes remains balanced by closely monitoring the patient's intake and output and careful assessment of laboratory values.

Recognize Cues [Assessment]
- Identify patients at risk for fluid volume deficit (FVD) and fluid volume excess (FVE).
- ⚡ Contributing factors for FVD include prolonged inadequate intake, excessive losses due to bleeding or trauma, and gastrointestinal (GI) losses. Contributing factors for FVE include heart failure, liver disease, kidney failure, excessive sodium intake, and excessive or too rapid infusion of intravenous fluids (IVFs).
- Assess the patient's history to identify factors that may contribute to FVD and FVE.
- ⚡ Differentiate between causes of FVD, including hypovolemia and dehydration, and causes of FVE, including heart failure and kidney and liver diseases.
- Assess the patient's vital signs, and note usual baseline values. Report abnormal findings.
- Assess the patient's laboratory values. A complete blood count, basic metabolic profile, and serum osmolality are good indicators of the patient's hydration status.
- Determine the patient's input and output.
- Obtain urine specific gravity. The normal range is 1.005 to 1.030 g/mL.
- Check the types of IVF ordered per day, including the amount to be infused, the hourly rate, and the solution for tonicity and electrolyte content. Consider if fluid ordered is appropriate for the patient's history and clinical condition. If any questions arise, collaborate with the health care provider (HCP) to determine appropriate fluid replacement for the patient. ⚡ Excessive administration of IVF containing sodium to patients with altered regulatory mechanisms may precipitate FVE.
- Assess the patient's current weight and baseline weight.

Analyze Cues and Prioritize Hypothesis [Patient Problems]
- Dehydration
- Fluid overload
- Disrupted fluid and electrolyte balance

Generate Solutions [Planning]
- The patient will exhibit balanced fluid volume within 24 hours as evidenced by normal electrolyte panel.
- The patient will have balanced intake and output over a 24-hour period.
- The patient will experience hydration as evidenced by moist mucous membranes, elastic skin turgor, and vital signs within normal limits; adequate urine output; urine specific gravity between 1.005 and 1.010 g/mL; stable weight; and no changes in mental status.
- With FVE, the patient will not exhibit signs of circulatory overload as evidenced by absence of signs and symptoms of edema or anasarca, having clear lung sounds, being free of jugular venous distension, and vital signs within normal limits.

Continued

CLINICAL JUDGMENT [NURSING PROCESS]—CONT'D
Fluid Imbalances (Fluid Volume Deficit and Fluid Volume Excess)

- Patient and family will verbalize an understanding of teaching related to FVD and FVE as evidenced by notifying the doctor of signs and symptoms:
  - ⚡ FVD signs to notify provider are excessive thirst, confusion, decreased urine output, nausea, vomiting, diarrhea, and weakness.
  - ⚡ FVE signs to notify provider include weight gain, swelling in body including feet, difficulty breathing, anxiety, and changes in urine output.

Take Action [Nursing Interventions]
General
- Monitor and record vital signs; assess trends and deviation from baseline and document findings. Report significant changes to the HCP.
- Measure and record intake and output every 4 hours. Identify sources of excessive intake or fluid losses.
- Measure urine specific gravity. Readings greater than 1.025 g/mL indicate concentrated urine, whereas those less than 1.010 g/mL indicate dilute urine.
- ⚡ Implement strict aseptic technique when inserting intravenous (IV) access devices. Check IV site for patency and signs of complications such as phlebitis and infiltration. Adhere to agency policy regarding site rotation and dressing and tubing changes.
- Avoid contamination when administering IV medications. Follow evidence-based practice guidelines, and implement interventions to decrease central line–associated infections.
- ⚡ Monitor IV infusions at least hourly, and ensure that the prescribed amount infuses hourly. Set the IV pump correctly, and validate the correct drip rate.
- Measure the patient's weight daily, and compare it with the baseline measurement. A gain of 1 kg (2.2 lb) is equivalent to 1 L of fluid.
- Use an interpreter if appropriate.
- With the patient's permission, involve the extended family in health teaching and support.

Fluid Volume Deficit
- Administer isotonic IVF as ordered.
- Monitor strict intake and output hourly. Encourage frequent oral intake if the patient can drink liquids. Provide oral care if the patient is unable to perform independently. Moisturize skin to prevent dryness, and reposition the patient every 2 hours, padding bony prominences; monitor frequently for skin breakdown and pressure.
- ⚡ Monitor for signs and symptoms of FVD because of hypovolemia, including thirst (usually the first sign of dehydration), restlessness, headaches, inability to concentrate, dry mucous membranes, poor skin turgor, tachycardia, changes in mental status, and slightly decreased systolic blood pressure.
- ⚡ Recognize late symptoms of hypovolemia, which include cyanosis; cold, clammy skin; weak thready pulse; confusion; and oliguria.
- ⚡ Monitor vital signs for indications of FVD, including increased temperature, weak pulse, tachycardia (early sign), hypotension, and tachypnea.
- ⚡ Assess for orthostatic hypotension, and use safety precautions when transferring the patient from bed to chair, avoiding abrupt changes in position. Other signs and symptoms of FVD include flattened neck veins; weight loss; decreased skin turgor; dry mucous membranes; decreased capillary refill; pale, cool, clammy skin; and muscle weakness.
- ⚡ Monitor laboratory values associated with FVD daily, including increased hemoglobin and hematocrit; urine specific gravity greater than 1.030 g/mL; and increased sodium, BUN, creatinine, electrolyte levels, and serum osmolality.

Fluid Volume Excess
- ⚡ Monitor and record vital signs that indicate FVE, including tachycardia, bounding pulse, tachypnea, increased blood pressure, and increased pulse pressure. Other signs and symptoms of FVE include altered mental status; generalized edema (use +1 to +4 scale to quantify edema); anasarca; constant, irritated cough; dyspnea; orthopnea; crackles; pulmonary congestion; muffled heart sounds; fatigue; increased central venous pressure; jugular vein distension; and increased urine output. Listen to lung sounds for crackles, and monitor respirations. The most consistent sign of FVE is increased body weight.
- ⚡ Monitor laboratory results associated with FVE daily, including BUN, hemoglobin, hematocrit, sodium, potassium, creatinine, albumin, and urine specific gravity below 1.010. Chest radiography may reveal pulmonary congestion. Monitor intake and output, and note trends that reflect urine output.
- ⚡ Monitor daily weight for sudden increases.
- ⚡ Administer diuretics as ordered; implement fluid and sodium restrictions. Recommend a nutritionist consult if warranted. Position the patient with the head of bed elevated 30 to 45 degrees to facilitate respiration. Monitor edematous areas for signs of pressure and altered skin integrity, and provide meticulous skin care; reposition the patient at least every 2 hours.

Patient Teaching
General
- ⚡ Instruct patients that thirst means a mild fluid deficit. Oral fluid intake is the best means of fluid replacement for a patient with FVD.
- ⚡ Advise patients to report vomiting or diarrhea. When these occur constantly or over several days, severe fluid volume and electrolyte imbalance can result.
- If a patient has FVE, fluid may be restricted. Instruct patients on limited intake of fluids around the clock.
- Assist patients in planning a typical 24-hour fluid intake based on individual fluid needs. ⚡ Encourage patients to monitor fluid intake and output, and advise them to report to their HCP any abnormal findings such as changes in urination patterns, fatigue, shortness of breath, weight gain (>3 lb in 2 days or 1.4 kg), peripheral edema, or tight shoes and rings.
- Provide (if ordered) and instruct patient in a low-sodium diet: Fresh fruits and vegetables, sodium-free herbs and spices, frozen vegetables, broiled meats and chicken. Avoid canned foods, sausage, or deli meats.

Evaluate Outcomes [Evaluation]
- The patient's vital signs should remain within normal limits.
- Fluid intake is balanced with output.
- Urine output is adequate for age, weight, and history.
- The patient and family understand the treatments and are able to verbalize the treatment plan and expected outcomes.
- IVFs are administered as ordered without complications or harm to the patient.

ELECTROLYTES

Potassium

Potassium (K^+) is the primary intracellular cation, and 98% of the body's potassium is found within the cells. Its concentration inside the cell is roughly 150 to 160 mEq/L, which is 25 to 35 times greater than extracellular concentration. Only 2% of potassium is found in the extracellular concentration. Potassium is essential for neuromuscular activity and cellular metabolism. Potassium levels affect cardiac and skeletal muscle activity and play a major role in muscle and nerve cell electrodynamics.

Potassium moves in and out of the cells under the influence of the potassium-sodium pump. It maintains the concentration difference in the cells by pumping potassium into the cells and pumping sodium out. Acid-base balance also influences potassium levels. *Acidotic* conditions tend to pull potassium out of cells, whereas *alkalotic* conditions tend to put potassium back into cells. The kidneys are the primary route for potassium loss, eliminating about 90% of the daily potassium intake. An inverse relationship exists between sodium and potassium reabsorption in the kidneys. Aldosterone also plays a role in the excretion of potassium.

Daily dietary intake is necessary because potassium is poorly stored in the body. Recommended daily potassium intake is 40 to 80 mEq/day in 1 or 2 divided doses within 24 hours in either potassium-rich foods or a potassium supplement. Foods rich in potassium include tuna, fruits, and vegetables such as mangoes, oranges, avocados, tomatoes, cucumbers, spinach, strawberries, and bananas.

Functions

Potassium is necessary for transmission and conduction of nerve impulses and for contraction of skeletal, cardiac, and smooth muscles. It is also necessary for normal kidney function and for the enzyme action used to change carbohydrates to energy (glycolysis) and amino acids to protein. Potassium promotes glycogen storage in hepatic cells, regulates the osmolality of cellular fluids, and plays a role in acid-base balance.

Hypokalemia

Hypokalemia, or potassium deficit, is generally defined as a serum potassium concentration of less than 3.5 mEq/L. Most cases of hypokalemia are caused by excessive loss rather than deficient intake. Whenever cells are damaged from trauma, injury, surgery, or shock, potassium leaks from the cells into the intravascular fluid and is excreted by the kidneys. With cellular loss of potassium, potassium shifts from the blood plasma into the cells to restore the cellular potassium balance; hypokalemia usually results. GI sources of potassium loss include vomiting, diarrhea, suctioning, recent ileostomy formation, draining fistulae, and diuretic therapy. Between 80% and 90% of potassium in the body is excreted in the urine; another 8% is excreted in the feces. Other causes of potassium loss include burns, total parenteral nutrition therapy, alkalosis, prolonged laxative use, excessive licorice consumption, corticosteroid use, increased aldosterone levels, and decreased magnesium levels.

It is important to recognize the signs and symptoms of hypokalemia. Hypokalemia may not be symptomatic until potassium levels fall below 3.0 mEq/L. Muscle weakness does not usually occur until potassium levels fall below 2.5 mEq/L. Quadricep weakness is one of the earliest signs of hypokalemia. Other early signs include fatigue, muscle weakness, anorexia, nausea, and vomiting. Severe signs and symptoms include paresthesia, leg cramps, decreased bowel motility and paralytic ileus, confusion, rhabdomyolysis and myoglobinuria, atrial and ventricular dysrhythmias, and cardiac arrest. Electrocardiogram (ECG) changes include flattened or inverted T waves and depressed ST segments. ⚡ If severe enough, hypokalemia can result in cardiac arrest, paralysis, respiratory arrest, and death.

Certain drugs, such as potassium-wasting diuretics and cortisone preparations, promote potassium loss. Patients receiving these drugs should increase their potassium intake by consuming foods rich in potassium or by taking potassium supplements as prescribed by their health care provider (HCP). Keep in mind that potassium-sparing diuretics do not deplete potassium stores, so patients would not be requested to increase potassium intake or to take supplements. Serum potassium levels should be monitored periodically for abnormalities.

Treatment for hypokalemia due to excessive potassium loss depends on the severity of the deficit. Patients with low-normal serum potassium levels may be advised to consume additional foods high in potassium. Management goals for patients with hypokalemia include preventing and treating life-threatening complications, replacing potassium and returning levels to normal, and diagnosing and correcting the cause of the deficiency.

Potassium replacements can be given orally or intravenously (Box 12.1). Table 12.6 lists the potassium preparations used to treat hypokalemia, and see the Prototype Drug Chart: Potassium Chloride, which compares the pharmacokinetics and pharmacodynamics of oral and IV potassium preparations.

Pharmacodynamics

Potassium maintains neuromuscular activity. It is vital for every cell in the human body. Onset of action of oral potassium depends on the formulation and the patient's condition; with IV potassium, onset is rapid. Duration of action of potassium is also unknown; however, it may vary according to the dose taken. ⚡ Continuous cardiac monitoring and serum potassium levels should be closely monitored when large doses are administered. To raise the serum potassium level by 1 mEq, the patient should receive 100 to 200 mEq of IV potassium.

Hyperkalemia

Hyperkalemia is defined as a serum potassium level above 5.0 mEq/L. Causes include excessive intake, impaired renal excretion, or a shift from intracellular to extracellular spaces. The most common causes are renal failure and medications that interfere with potassium excretion. Renal disease or kidney failure results in potassium accumulating in the intravascular fluid, which results in hyperkalemia. ⚡ Persons at risk for developing hyperkalemia include premature infants, older adults, and those with a history of genitourinary disease, adrenal insufficiency, cancer, poorly controlled diabetes, or polypharmacy. Hyperkalemia manifests primarily as cardiac and neuromuscular symptoms. ⚡ Signs and symptoms include cardiac dysrhythmias that include characteristic changes on the ECG, such as early tachycardia followed by bradycardia; paresthesia of the face, tongue, hands, and feet; and GI hyperactivity, including nausea, diarrhea, and abdominal cramping. Metabolic acidosis may also be present.

Management goals are to eliminate the cause of the excess potassium, shift potassium back into the cells, increase potassium excretion, decrease potassium intake, and prevent further episodes of hyperkalemia. For mild hyperkalemia, foods rich in potassium are usually restricted. Treatment strategies for hyperkalemia are outlined in Box 12.2.

Effect of Drugs on Potassium Balance

Potassium-wasting diuretics are a major cause of hypokalemia. Diuretics are divided into two categories: potassium-wasting and potassium-sparing drugs. Potassium-wasting diuretics cause excretion of potassium and other electrolytes, such as sodium and chloride, in the urine. Potassium-sparing diuretics cause retention of potassium, but sodium and chloride are excreted in the urine (see Chapter 41).

Laxatives, corticosteroids, antibiotics, and potassium-wasting diuretics are the major drug classifications that can cause hypokalemia. Other drug classifications that may cause hyperkalemia include oral and IV potassium salts, central nervous system (CNS) agents, and potassium-sparing diuretics. Tables 12.7 and 12.8 identify drugs that affect potassium balance.

Sodium

Sodium is the major cation in the ECF. The normal serum sodium level is 135 to 145 mEq/L. A serum sodium level below 135 mEq/L is called hyponatremia, and a serum sodium level above 145 mEq/L is called

CLINICAL JUDGMENT [NURSING PROCESS]

Potassium

Concept: Fluid and Electrolyte Balance
- Patients require the regulation of fluid and electrolytes to maintain homeostasis. Nurses will encounter potential and actual alterations of fluid and electrolyte balance when caring for patients. Nursing assessments and interventions ensure the intake of fluid and electrolytes remains balanced by closely monitoring the patient's intake and output and careful assessment of laboratory values.

Recognize Cues [Assessment]
- ⚡ Assess for signs and symptoms of potassium imbalance. Symptoms of **hypokalemia** include nausea and vomiting; polyuria; cardiac dysrhythmias; abdominal distension; and soft, flabby muscles. Symptoms of **hyperkalemia** include oliguria, nausea, abdominal cramps, tachycardia and later bradycardia, weakness, and numbness or tingling in the extremities.
- Assess serum potassium level; a normal level is 3.5 to 5.0 mEq/L. Report serum potassium deficits or excesses to the health care provider (HCP).
- ⚡ Obtain baseline vital signs and electrocardiogram (ECG) readings and report abnormal findings. Vital signs and ECG results can be compared with future readings.
- ⚡ Check for signs and symptoms of digitalis toxicity when the patient is receiving a digitalis preparation and a potassium-wasting diuretic or a cortisone preparation. A decreased serum potassium level enhances the action of digitalis and increases the likelihood of digitalis toxicity. Signs and symptoms of digitalis toxicity are nausea, vomiting, anorexia, bradycardia (pulse rate <60 or markedly decreased), cardiac dysrhythmias, and visual disturbances.

Analyze Cues and Prioritize Hypothesis [Patient Problems]
- Hypokalemia
- Hyperkalemia
- Dehydration
- Fluid overload

Generate Solutions [Planning]
- The patient's serum potassium level will remain within normal ranges (K+ 3.5–5.0 mEq/L).
- The patient will verbalize understanding of the potassium imbalance and state methods to decrease recurrence.
  - Patients with hypokalemia will eat potassium-rich foods.
  - Patients with hyperkalemia will avoid potassium-rich foods.
- At the end of the first teaching, the patient will name four signs and symptoms of hypokalemia and four signs and symptoms of hyperkalemia.
- At the end of the second teaching, the patient will name four signs and symptoms of fluid overload and four signs and symptoms of fluid deficit.

Take Action [Nursing Interventions]
- ⚡ Administer oral potassium with enough water or orange juice (at least 8 oz) and with meals. Potassium is extremely irritating to the gastric mucosa.
- ⚡ Administer potassium-containing intravenous (IV) solutions with a calibrated infusion pump. Potassium IV solutions should always be diluted and thoroughly mixed in 100 to 1000 mL of IV solution and must be infused slowly (generally no faster than 10 mEq/h).
- ⚡ Never administer potassium intramuscularly or as an IV bolus or push. Giving IV potassium directly into the vein causes cardiac dysrhythmias, cardiac arrest, and death. (Potassium chloride is one of the agents used in lethal injection because rapid infusion results in immediate cardiac arrest.)
- Evaluate the amount of urine output. Potassium accumulation occurs if a patient is receiving potassium and urine output is below 25 mL/h or below 600 mL/d. Remember that 80% to 90% of potassium is excreted in the urine. Report results to the health care provider.
- ⚡ Monitor serum potassium levels frequently in addition to serum creatinine, blood urea nitrogen (BUN), glucose, electrolytes, and arterial blood gases. Report abnormal results to the health care provider (HCP).
- ⚡ Monitor ECG. With **hypokalemia**, there is a flat or inverted T wave, a depressed ST segment, and a prolonged QT interval. With **hyperkalemia**, there is a narrow and peaked T wave, a widened QRS complex, a prolonged PR interval, flattened or absent T waves, and a depressed ST segment.
- Monitor the patient's response to activity, and plan frequent rest periods due to muscle weakness associated with potassium imbalances.
- ⚡ Evaluate the IV site for infiltration if a patient is receiving IV potassium. Potassium can cause extravasation and tissue necrosis if it infiltrates into subcutaneous tissue. Discontinue IV fluids immediately if infiltration occurs.
- Monitor patients receiving medications for hyperkalemia for signs and symptoms of continuing hyperkalemia or iatrogenic hypokalemia.
- Use an interpreter as appropriate.
- Involve the extended family in health teaching and support.

Patient Teaching
General
- Advise patients to have the serum potassium level checked at regular intervals as prescribed by the HCP when taking medications that affect potassium levels.
- Instruct patients to drink a full glass of water when taking oral potassium supplements. Potassium preparations can be taken during or after a meal. Explain to patients that potassium is very irritating to the stomach.
- Encourage patients to comply with the prescribed potassium dose, regular laboratory tests, and medical follow-up related to the health problem and drug regimen.
- Instruct patients on the signs and symptoms of hypokalemia and hyperkalemia to report to their physician.

Diet
- Instruct patients who are taking medications that promote potassium loss to eat potassium-rich foods.
- Instruct patients at risk for potassium imbalances regarding dietary sources of potassium and the potassium content of foods.

Evaluate Outcomes [Evaluation]
- ⚡ Evaluate the patient's serum potassium level and ECG.
  - The cardiac rhythm is normal baseline without dysrhythmias.
  - The serum potassium level is within normal range.
  - Report to the HCP if the level does not return to normal, in which case the potassium replacements and diet may need modification.

BOX 12.1 Oral and Intravenous Potassium Preparations

⚡ Potassium (K⁺) Preparations

Potassium preparations are individualized according to the needs of the patient. Requirement estimation is based on clinical condition, which includes electrocardiogram (ECG), plasma concentrations, and patient's response.

- *Potassium Acetate:* Available for intravenous (IV) administration. ⚡ NOTE: Potassium chloride is typically used for the acute treatment of hypokalemia; however, potassium acetate may be used if correction of acidemia is needed.
- *Potassium Bicarbonate:* Available in oral/granule dosing. NOTE: Potassium chloride is typically used for replacement; however, bicarbonate is recommended when potassium depletion occurs in the setting of metabolic acidosis (pH less than 7.4).
- *Potassium Phosphate:* Available in oral dose and solution for injection. NOTE: Guidelines generally recommend the use of potassium phosphate for potassium serum concentration less than 4 mg/dL and sodium phosphate for potassium serum concentration more than 4 mg/dL. Potassium phosphate is usually appropriate as most conditions associated with hypophosphatemia are also associated with hypokalemia.
- *Potassium Gluconate:* Available as elixir or tablet. Potassium gluconate is a dietary supplement used to maintain potassium balance (i.e., hypokalemia prevention).
- *Potassium Chloride:* Available as a liquid, powder, tablet, capsule, controlled-release microencapsulated tablet, enteric-coated tablet, and effervescent tablet and parenteral use.
  - Potassium chloride is used for the treatment of hypokalemia and to maintain acid-base balance.

Nursing Implications for Oral Preparations

- Tablets and capsules should be administered with or after meals followed by a large glass of water while the patient is sitting up to decrease gastrointestinal irritation. The patient should remain upright at least 30 minutes after administration. Use of tablets and capsules should be reserved for patients who cannot tolerate liquid preparations.
  - Dissolve effervescent tablets in 3 to 8 oz of cold water. Ensure the tablet is fully dissolved.
  - Powders and liquid solutions should be diluted in 3 to 8 oz of cold water or juice.
  - Dilute liquid forms before administering via an enteral feeding tube.
- ⚡ Do not chew or crush enteric-coated or extended-release tablets or capsules. They must be swallowed.
- ⚡ Advise patients not to suck on tablets to avoid oral ulceration.
- ⚡ Advise patients to avoid salt substitutes.
- ⚡ Patients on K⁺ therapy should have levels drawn to monitor progress.
- ⚡ Explain to patients the need to take medications as directed, especially when concurrent digoxin or diuretics are taken.

Nursing Implications for Intravenous Potassium Administration

- ⚡ IV therapy is indicated for patients who are unable to tolerate oral therapy or, in addition to oral therapy, for patients with severe hypokalemia.
- ⚡ Medication errors involving too rapid infusion or bolus of IV administration of K⁺ chloride or K⁺ acetate have resulted in fatalities.
- ⚡ *Never* administer potassium via IV push or bolus.
  - ⚡ The Joint Commission recommends special storage requirements for intravenous K+ salts that have been administered IVP in error, leading to fatal outcomes. Access should not be available in patient care areas.

Potassium Acetate (Continuous IV)ᵃ

- ⚡ Do not administer undiluted. Each single dose *must* be diluted and thoroughly mixed in 100 to 1000 mL normal saline (preferred), Ringer's, or lactated Ringer's solutions. Usually limited to 10 mEq/100 mL or 40 mEq/1000 mL via a peripheral line. Pain is associated with peripheral infusion; administer central vein when possible.
- ⚡ Rate: Infuse slowly at a rate up to 10 mEq/h in adults. Check hospital policy for maximum infusion rates. (The maximum rate in a monitored setting is 40 mEq/h in adults.)

Potassium Chloride (Continuous IV)ᵃ

- ⚡ Do not administer undiluted; fatalities have occurred. Concentrated products have black caps on vials or black stripes above the constriction on ampules and are labeled with a warning about dilution requirements. Each single dose must be diluted and thoroughly mixed in 100 to 1000 mL of IV solution and is usually limited to 10 to 20 mEq/L via a peripheral line. Administer central vein when possible.
- ⚡ Rate: Infuse slowly at a rate up to 10 mEq/h in adults. Check the hospital policy for maximum infusion rates (maximum rate in a monitored setting is 40 mEq/h in adults). Always use an infusion pump.
- ⚡ Monitor the IV site and infusion carefully to avoid extravasation and infiltration.
- ⚡ Too rapid an infusion may cause fatal hyperkalemia.
- ⚡ Symptoms of toxicity: Slow, irregular heartbeat; fatigue; muscle weakness; paresthesia; confusion; dyspnea; peaked T waves; depressed ST segments; prolonged QT segments; widened QRS complexes; loss of P waves; and cardiac arrhythmias.

ᵃ ⚡ The Institute for Safe Medication Practices (ISMP) includes Potassium (IV formulation) among its list of drugs that have a heightened risk of causing significant patient harm when used in error.

TABLE 12.6 Potassium ❗ Chloride

Preparation	Drug
Capsules, tablets, oral solution	Normal dose: 40–80 mEq/d Hypokalemia: 40–100 mEq/d Divide larger doses 2–3/d
Powder for oral solution	40–100 mEq/d in 2–5 divided doses; limit single doses to 40 mEq/dose; *max:* 200 mEq/24 h
Intravenous (IV) potassium	IV: Infusion rate 10 mEq/h. Never administer undiluted (Na + Cl is preferred diluent). Doses >10 mEq/h: ECG monitoring and repeat serum lab values necessary. ⚡ It is preferable to administer all concentrations of potassium chloride infusions via a central line when possible. Higher concentrations 400 mEq/L **MUST** be administered via central line. **High Risk**: Burning and phlebitis.

d, Daily; *g*, grams; *h*, hour; *L*, liter; *max*, maximum; *mL*, milliliters; *mEq*, milliequivalent.

CLINICAL JUDGMENT [NURSING PROCESS]

Sodium

Concept: Fluid and Electrolyte Balance
- Patients require the regulation of fluid and electrolytes to maintain homeostasis. ⚡ Nurses will encounter potential and actual alterations of fluid and electrolyte balance when caring for patients. Nursing assessments and interventions ensure the intake of fluid and electrolytes remains balanced by closely monitoring the patient's intake and output, and careful assessment of laboratory values.

Recognize Cues [Assessment]
- ⚡ Assess the patient for signs and symptoms of sodium imbalance. Symptoms of *hyponatremia* are muscle weakness, headaches, lethargy, confusion, seizures, abdominal cramps, nausea and vomiting, tachycardia and hypotension, pale skin, and dry mucous membranes. Symptoms of *hypernatremia* are flushed, dry skin; agitation; elevated body temperature; rough, dry tongue; nausea and vomiting; anorexia; tachycardia; hypertension; muscle twitching; and hyperreflexia.
- ⚡ Check the serum sodium level. Report critically low sodium levels (<125 mEq/L) to the health care provider (HCP) because prompt medical care is required.
- Obtain a history of health problems that may lead to sodium loss or excess.

Analyze Cues and Prioritize Hypothesis [Patient Problems]
- Hypernatremia
- Hyponatremia
- Confusion
- Dehydration
- Disrupted fluid and electrolyte balance

Generate Solutions [Planning]
- The patient's serum sodium level will reach normal range (135–145 mEq/L in 3–5 days).

Take Action [Nursing Interventions]
- Monitor the prescribed medical regimen for correction of hyponatremia or hypernatremia.
- ⚡ Instruct patients on the signs and symptoms of hyponatremia and hypernatremia, and instruct them to notify their HCP if any of these occur.
- ⚡ Monitor serum sodium levels and report abnormal levels.
- Use an interpreter if the patient has a language barrier.
- Involve the extended family in health teaching and support.

Patient Teaching
- Instruct patients with hypernatremia to avoid foods high in sodium, to avoid using salt when cooking, and to refrain from adding extra salt to their food at the table.
- Emphasize the importance of reading labels on food products.

Evaluate Outcomes [Evaluation]
- Evaluate the patient's serum sodium level. Report if the sodium imbalance continues.
- Monitor fluid intake and output carefully; monitor daily weights.
- ⚡ Assess patients for signs of circulatory overload and deficit.

---

hypernatremia. Sodium and chloride imbalances typically occur together. The most serious problems associated with serum sodium deficit (hyponatremia) are cerebral edema, altered mental status, confusion, and seizure. In sodium excess imbalances (hypernatremia), a rapid decrease occurs in intracellular water to the brain, which results in cerebral dehydration, seizure, and coma.

The dietary requirement for sodium is 2000 to 4000 mg daily. Sodium-rich foods include bacon, luncheon meats, corned beef, decaffeinated coffee, ham, tomato juice, pickles, and soda crackers.

Functions

Sodium is found in most body fluids; it plays a major role in fluid volume balance and is the primary determinant of plasma osmolality. Sodium combines readily with chloride (Cl^-) or bicarbonate (HCO_3^-) to promote acid-base balance. Sodium is important for the maintenance of neuromuscular irritability and for conduction of nerve impulses. In conjunction with neural and hormonal mediators, the kidney maintains normal serum sodium concentrations through renal tubular reabsorption. The serum sodium level reflects the ratio of sodium to water, not necessarily the loss or gain of sodium.

Hyponatremia

Hyponatremia is caused by a loss of sodium-containing fluids, deficient intake, or water gain. Sodium loss can result from vomiting, diarrhea, nasogastric suctioning, burns, wound drainage, trauma, renal failure, heart failure, third spacing, syndrome of inappropriate antidiuretic hormone (SIADH), excessive hypertonic IVF, surgery, and thiazide diuretics.

Hyponatremia may occur with hypovolemia and hypervolemia symptoms will depend on the onset and degree of deficit. ⚡ Signs and symptoms of hyponatremia due to water shifting into cells are primarily neuromuscular and GI and include muscle weakness, decreased deep tendon reflexes, headaches, lethargy, confusion, seizures, coma, abdominal cramps, nausea and vomiting, pale skin, and dry mucous membranes.

Oral sodium replacement is the preferred treatment if the patient can tolerate oral intake or if the deficit is mild. Sodium may also be replaced via enteral feeding tubes. For a serum sodium level between 125 and 135 mEq/L, IV normal saline (0.9% sodium chloride) may increase sodium content in vascular fluid. For a serum sodium level below 120 mEq/L, a hypertonic 3% or 5% saline solution may be necessary.

Hypernatremia

⚡ Hypernatremia can be caused by sodium gain, sodium retention, or water loss. Causes include excessive oral sodium intake, deficient water intake, hypertonic tube feedings, hypertonic IVF, hyperaldosteronism, Cushing syndrome, corticosteroid use, and acute kidney failure. Other causes include vomiting, diarrhea, burns, diabetes insipidus, and mineralocorticoid excess.

⚡ Signs of fluid imbalance depend on the cause; water loss presents with symptoms of FVD, whereas sodium gain presents with symptoms of FVE. Signs and symptoms of hypernatremia are dry, sticky mucous membranes; flushed, dry skin; agitation; elevated body temperature; rough, edematous, dry tongue; nausea and vomiting; anorexia; tachycardia; hypertension; muscle twitching; hyperreflexia; seizures; and coma.

Management of hypernatremia depends on the cause and severity of the deficit. Frequent monitoring of sodium levels is necessary while the underlying cause is being treated. When the serum sodium level is elevated above 145 mEq/L, sodium restriction is indicated. Treatments include administration of IVF and diuretics.

PROTOTYPE DRUG CHART

Potassium Chloride

Drug Class	Dosage
Electrolyte replacement	Treatment of hypokalemia (serum K+ level of <3.5 mEq/L) ADULTS: PO: Capsules/tablets/oral solution: 40–100 mEq/day in 2–5 divided doses/with meal not to exceed 200 mEq/day ⚡ IV: K+ level 2.5–3.5 mEq/L, use 10 mEq/h not to exceed 200 mEq/in 24 h; K+ level <2.5 with ECG changes evident of symptomatic hypokalemia, use 40 mEq/h (with central line, continuous ECG, and lab monitoring) not to exceed 400 mEq in 24 h ⚡ IV: **DO NOT** administer IV push. **MUST** be diluted before administration. Peripheral line: Infusion may cause burning pain and phlebitis at site. Recommend 100 mEq/L not to exceed 200 mEq/L. Central line: It is preferable to administer all concentrations via central line when possible. Highest concentration 400 mEq/L in adults have been safely administered via central line.
Contraindications	**Drug-Lab-Food Interactions**
Renal insufficiency or failure, Addison disease, hyperkalemia, severe dehydration, acidosis, potassium-sparing diuretics, in patients with known hypersensitivity ⚡ Caution: Cardiac and renal disease, burns, hypomagnesemia, and cirrhosis	Drug: Any disease or condition in which high potassium levels may occur through potassium retention or other processes. Food: Excessive intake of licorice may cause hypokalemia and sodium retention; salt substitutes contain potassium.
Pharmacokinetics	**Pharmacodynamics**
Absorption: Well absorbed after oral administration Distribution: Enters extracellular fluid and is then actively transported into cells Metabolism: Excreted 80%–90% in urine by the kidneys and 10% in feces Half-life: UK Protein binding: UK	PO: Onset: 15–30 min Peak: 1–2 h Duration: 2–3 h IV: Onset: Rapid Peak: End of infusion Duration: UK
Therapeutic Effects/Uses	
To correct potassium deficit and treat hypokalemic alkalosis, strengthen cardiac and muscular activities, and prevent hypokalemia in at-risk patients Mechanism of Action: Transmits and conducts nerve impulses; contracts skeletal, smooth, and cardiac muscles	
Side Effects	**Adverse Reactions**
Nausea, vomiting, diarrhea, abdominal cramps, irritability, rash (rare); phlebitis with IV administration	⚡ Hyperkalemia (older adults with renal impairment); oliguria, ECG changes (peaked T waves, widened QRS complex, prolonged PR interval), GI ulceration ⚡ *Life-threatening:* Cardiac dysrhythmias, respiratory distress, ventricular fibrillation, cardiac arrest

A, Adult; *d*, day; *ECG*, electrocardiography; *GI*, gastrointestinal; *h*, hour; *IV*, intravenous; *max*, maximum; *PO*, by mouth; *UK*, unknown; *meq*, milliequivalent; *L*, liter; *K+*, potassium.

BOX 12.2 Hyperkalemia: Treatments and Rationales

Potassium Restriction
- Restriction of potassium intake will slowly lower the serum level.
- For mild hyperkalemia (slightly elevated K+ levels [5.4–5.6 mEq/L]), potassium restriction is normally effective.

Intravenous Sodium Bicarbonate
- Sodium bicarbonate elevates the pH level, potassium moves back into cells and lowers the serum level.
- This is a temporary treatment.

Calcium Gluconate 10%
- 10% IV solution contains 1 g Ca+ gluconate/10 mL and 90 mg (4.5 mEq) of elemental Ca+
- Decreases irritability of myocardium resulting from hyperkalemia
- A temporary treatment that does not promote K+ loss
- ⚡ Caution: Administering 10% calcium gluconate to a patient on digitalis can cause digitalis toxicity.

Insulin and Glucose
- Administering insulin and glucose will move the potassium back into cells.
- A temporary treatment effective for approximately 6 hours, and not always as effective when repeated.

Sodium Polystyrene Sulfonate
- Sodium polystyrene sulfonate is used to treat high levels of potassium in the blood for severe hyperkalemia; may cause hypocalcemia, hypomagnesemia, and sodium retention.
- Can be administered orally or rectally.

Oral Administration
- Sodium polystyrene sulfonate: PO (adults) 15 g one to four times daily in water (up to 40 g four times daily).
- The oral route is the preferred route and is more effective than the rectal route.

Rectal Administration
- Sodium polystyrene sulfonate: (Adults) 30 to 50 g as a retention enema; repeat as needed every 6 hours. Constipation is a common adverse effect. Assess bowel function daily, and monitor for fecal impaction. A mild laxative may be prescribed.

TABLE 12.7 Drugs That Cause Hypokalemia

Substances	Rationale
Acetylsalicylic acid/acetaminophen	Causes changes in acid-base balance.
Antibiotic I: Amphotericin B; polymyxin B; gentamicin; neomycin; amikacin; tobramycin	These have a toxic effect on renal tubules and thus decrease potassium reabsorption.
Antibiotic II: Penicillin; ampicillin; carbenicillin; ticarcillin; nafcillin; piperacillin	These enhance potassium excretion by the presence of nonabsorbable anions.
Alpha-adrenergic blockers Insulin Glucose	These promote movement of potassium into cells, thus lowering the serum potassium level.
Beta$_2$ agonists: terbutaline, albuterol	These promote potassium loss.
Cardiac glycoside: digoxin	Used with caution in patients with electrolyte imbalances; can result in toxicity.
Corticosteroids	Absorption of calcium is reduced.
Cortisone	Cortisone causes electrolyte disturbances.
Dextrose intravenous (IV) solution	Can worsen hypokalemia by stimulating insulin release, which will cause intracellular shifting of potassium.
Diuretics LOOP: furosemide, torsemide THIAZIDE: hydrochlorothiazide	Diuretics deplete potassium through urination.
Laxatives Enemas (hyperosmolar)	Abuse can cause potassium depletion.
Prednisone	Steroids promote potassium loss and sodium retention.
Sodium polystyrene sulfonate enema	Exchanges a potassium ion for a sodium ion.

TABLE 12.8 Drugs That Cause Hyperkalemia

Substances	Rationale
Angiotensin-converting enzyme inhibitors (ACE inhibitors)	ACEs increase the state of hypo-aldosterone (decrease sodium and increase potassium) and impair renal potassium excretion.
Angiotensin receptor blockers (ARBs)	ARBs decrease adrenal synthesis of aldosterone; potassium is retained, and sodium is excreted.
Antifungals	Elevate serum potassium levels.
Beta-adrenergic blockers	Beta-blockers decrease cellular uptake of potassium and decrease Na-K-ATPase function.
CNS agents: Barbiturates; sedatives; opioids; heroin, amphetamines	CNS substances are usually characterized by muscle necrosis and cellular shift of potassium from cells to serum.
Digoxin	The therapeutic dose is not affected; however, with overdose, potassium excess may occur.
Heparin	Heparin inhibits adrenal aldosterone production.
LMWH (Fractionated Heparin)	LMWHs suppress aldosterone and decrease potassium homeostasis; renal excretion of potassium is reduced.
Immunosuppressive drugs: cyclosporine; tacrolimus, cyclophosphamide	Reduce potassium excretion by induction of hypo-aldosterone and loss of potassium from cells.
Nonsteroidal antiinflammatory drugs	NSAIDs impair potassium homeostasis and block cellular potassium uptake.
Potassium chloride (oral or IV); potassium salt substitutes; potassium penicillin; potassium phosphate (KPO$_4$) enema; potassium-sparing diuretics	Excess ingestion or infusion can cause potassium excess.
Succinylcholine	Succinylcholine allows for leakage of potassium out of the cells.
Transfusion of packed red blood cells (PRBCs)	There is evidence that transfusion of PRBCs can lead to increased potassium levels, especially in cases of large volume transfusions

ATPase, Adenosine triphosphates; *CNS*, central nervous system; *IV*, intravenous; *K*, potassium; *LMWH*, low-molecular-weight heparin; *Na*, sodium; *NSAID*, nonsteroidal antiinflammatory drug.

Calcium

Calcium is the most abundant mineral in the body, accounting for approximately 40% of all body minerals and 2% of body weight. The total serum calcium range is 8.6 to 10.2 mg/dL. A calcium deficit (<8.6 mg/dL) is called **hypocalcemia**, and a calcium excess (>10.2 mg/dL) is called **hypercalcemia**. More than 90% of the body's calcium is found in bones and teeth. Of the remaining calcium found in the blood, about 50% is bound to protein, primarily albumin, a serum protein. Another 50% is free and not bound to protein and is called the *ionized form* of calcium; it can leave the vascular space and be active in cellular functions. Normal ionized calcium levels are reported separately (4.64–5.28 mg/dL).

Calcium levels are affected by acid-base balance and plasma albumin levels. When an individual is acidotic (decreased plasma pH), there is a decrease in calcium binding to the albumin, which leads to more ionized calcium. During alkalosis (increased plasma pH), increases in calcium binding lead to decreased ionized calcium. Alterations in serum albumin levels affect the interpretation of total calcium levels. Low albumin levels result in a drop in the total calcium level, although the level of ionized calcium is not affected.

Functions

Calcium is necessary for the transmission of nerve impulses and normal contraction of skeletal and heart muscles, regulation of the heart and blood pressure, hormone secretion, maintenance of muscle tone. This cation also maintains normal cellular permeability and promotes blood clotting by converting prothrombin into thrombin. Calcium is also needed for formation of bone and teeth. Two hormones, parathyroid hormone (PTH) and thyrocalcitonin (TCT), along with vitamin D and the blood pH, play an important role in maintaining the balance of serum calcium. Calcium functions are closely related to magnesium and phosphorus. Calcium and phosphorus have an inverse relationship; that is, increased calcium levels result in decreased phosphorus levels.

PROTOTYPE DRUG CHART

⚡ Calcium

Drug Class	Dosage
Electrolyte Calcium carbonate (chewable) Calcium citrate (capsule/tablet) Calcium gluconate (IV) Calcium chloride (IV) ⚡ IV form is a high-alert drug.	Calcium carbonate: 250 mg/400 mg/500 mg/750 mg in 1–3 divided doses Calcium citrate: 200 mg/d to 1 g/d divided doses Calcium gluconate: 1–2 g IV q6h (**Note:** 500 mg calcium gluconate is equal to 45 mg [2.25 mEq] elemental calcium) Calcium chloride IV: 1000 mg over 10 min; repeat every 60 min until s/s resolved; 1 g is equal to 270 mg of elemental calcium

Contraindications	Drug-Lab-Food Interactions
⚡ Hypercalcemia, patients receiving digitalis glycosides and patients with renal calculi, severe respiratory insufficiency, and cardiac disease	⚡ Drug: Increased risk of digoxin toxicity with calcium channel blockers, tetracyclines, fluoroquinolones, phenytoin, iron salts, thiazides, sodium polystyrene sulfonate Food: Cereals, spinach, rhubarb Lab: May affect serum calcium or ionized calcium, sodium, potassium, magnesium, albumin, and parathyroid hormone.

Pharmacokinetics	Pharmacodynamics
Absorption: From GI tract, requires vitamin D Distribution: Readily enters ECF Metabolism and excretion: Excreted mostly in the feces; 20% eliminated by the kidneys Half-life: UK	PO: Onset: UK Peak: UK Duration: UK IV: Onset: Immediate Peak: Immediate Duration: 0.5–2 h

⚡ Safety alert from the Institute for Safe Medication Practices: Errors with IV calcium gluconate (CaGl) and calcium chloride (CaCl) have occurred secondary to confusion over which salt is ordered. Clarify incomplete orders. Confusion has occurred with milligram doses of CaCl and CaGl, which are not equal. Calcium chloride and calcium gluconate IV forms are routinely available on most hospital crash carts; physicians should specify the form of calcium desired, and doses should be expressed in milliequivalents.

⚡ CONCERN: Extravasation: Parenteral calcium is a vesicant; ensure proper catheter or needle position prior to and during infusion. Avoid extravasation; adverse events from extravasation can be devasting. Monitor IV site closely.

Therapeutic Effects/Uses
To correct calcium deficit or tetany symptoms, prevent osteoporosis.
Mechanism of Action: Transmits nerve impulses, contracts skeletal and cardiac muscles, maintains cellular permeability, and promotes strong bones and teeth

Side Effects	Adverse Reactions
PO: Nausea, vomiting, constipation, pain, drowsiness, headache, muscle weakness	⚡ Hypercalcemia, ECG changes, metabolic alkalosis, heart block, rebound hyperacidity ⚡ *Life-threatening:* Renal failure, cardiac dysrhythmias, cardiac arrest

A, Adult; *d*, day; *ECF*, extracellular fluid; *ECG*, electrocardiogram; *GI*, gastrointestinal; *g*, gram; *h*, hour; *IV*, intravenous; *mg*, milligram; *mEq*, milliequivalent; *PO*, by mouth; *s/s*, signs and symptoms; *UK*, unknown.

Vitamin D is needed for calcium absorption from the GI tract. Aspirin and anticonvulsants can alter vitamin D, affecting calcium absorption. Loop or high-ceiling diuretics (see Chapter 41), steroids (cortisone), magnesium preparations, and phosphate preparations promote calcium loss. Conversely, thiazide diuretics increase serum calcium levels.

Hypocalcemia

Inadequate calcium intake causes calcium to leave bone to maintain a normal serum calcium level. Because of calcium loss from bones (bone demineralization), pathologic fractures may occur if calcium deficit persists. Common causes of hypocalcemia include hyperphosphatemia, acute pancreatitis, widespread bony metastases, hypoparathyroidism, alkalosis, diarrhea, alcoholism, malnutrition, use of loop diuretics, vitamin D deficiency, and multiple blood transfusions.

⚡ Signs and symptoms of hypocalcemia reflect calcium's role in nerve transmission and heart and muscle function. Neurologic and neuromuscular symptoms include anxiety, irritability, and tetany; twitching; hyperactive deep tendon reflexes; spasms of hands, wrist, feet, and ankles; spasmodic contractions; laryngeal spasm; and seizures. Cardiovascular manifestations include decreased cardiac output, dysrhythmias, and ECG changes.

Calcium preparations can be administered orally or intravenously. The treatment depends on the cause, degree of deficit, and clinical condition of the patient. IV calcium replacement should be administered only to acutely symptomatic patients. Calcium preparations are combined with various salts such as chloride, carbonate, citrate, and gluconate. The two main forms of oral calcium supplements are calcium carbonate, which contains 40% elemental calcium, and calcium citrate, which contains 21% elemental calcium. There is a threefold difference in the primary cation between calcium gluconate, which contains 4.65 mEq Ca^{++}/g, and calcium chloride, which contains 13.6 mEq Ca^{++}/g. When ordering IV calcium, this difference has important implications.

⚡ Calcium chloride is more irritating when given intravenously.

CLINICAL JUDGMENT [NURSING PROCESS]

Calcium

Concept: Fluid and Electrolyte Balance
- Patients require the regulation of fluid and electrolytes to maintain homeostasis. Nurses will encounter potential and actual alterations of fluid and electrolyte balance when caring for patients. Nursing assessments and interventions ensure the intake of fluid and electrolytes remains balanced by closely monitoring the patient's intake and output and careful assessment of laboratory values.

Recognize Cues [Assessment]
- ⚡ Assess the patient for signs and symptoms of calcium imbalance. Signs and symptoms of *hypocalcemia* are tetany, muscle cramps, bleeding tendencies, and cardiac contractions. Signs and symptoms of *hypercalcemia* are flabby muscles, pain over bony areas, and kidney stones of calcium composition.
- ⚡ Check serum calcium levels; a normal total calcium level is 8.6 to 10.2 mg/dL. Report abnormal test results.
- ⚡ Assess albumin levels; a normal albumin level is 3.4 to 5.4 g/dL. Low levels of albumin decrease total calcium levels.
- ⚡ Obtain baseline vital signs and electrocardiogram (ECG) readings. Report abnormal findings.
- ⚡ Gather a current patient drug history. If the patient is receiving digoxin, calcium enhances the effect of digoxin. An elevated serum calcium level can cause digitalis toxicity, signs and symptoms of which include nausea, vomiting, anorexia, bradycardia (pulse rate <60 or markedly decreased), cardiac dysrhythmias, and visual disturbances. Thiazide diuretics can increase serum calcium levels. Drugs that decrease the effect of calcium are calcium channel blockers, tetracycline, and sodium chloride.

Analyze Cues and Prioritize Hypothesis [Patient Problems]
- Weight loss
- Decreased sensation in upper extremities
- Reduction in motor function
- Hypercalcemia

Generate Solutions [Planning]
- The patient's serum calcium level remains within normal range.
- Tetany symptoms will cease.
- The patient will eat calcium-rich foods or take calcium supplements as ordered.
- Patients with hypercalcemia will avoid calcium-rich foods.

Take Action [Nursing Interventions]
- ⚡ Monitor vital signs and report abnormal findings. Compare with baseline vital signs.
- ⚡ Assess patients on digitalis for digitalis toxicity (e.g., bradycardia).
- ⚡ Administer intravenous fluids slowly with 10% calcium gluconate or chloride. The pharmacist will add or decrease calcium to the solutions as ordered by the provider and will dilute in compatible solutions (e.g., normal saline [NS], 5% dextrose in water [D_5W], 10% dextrose in water [$D_{10}W$]).
- ⚡ Assess the intravenous site for infiltration. Calcium can cause tissue necrosis and sloughing if it infiltrates into subcutaneous tissue. Concentrations of calcium chloride (CaCl) of 20 mg/mL are usually recommended for central lines; concentrations of no more than 1 mg/mL given over 10 minutes have been recommended for peripheral lines.
- ⚡ Monitor serum total calcium and ionized calcium levels.
- ⚡ Monitor ECGs. In hypocalcemia, the ST segment is lengthened, and the QT interval is prolonged. In hypercalcemia, the ST segment is decreased, and the QT interval is shortened.
- If a language barrier exists, use an interpreter if appropriate.
- Involve the extended family in health teaching and support.

Patient Teaching
General
- ⚡ Instruct patients to avoid overuse of antacids and chronic use of laxatives. Overuse of certain antacids may cause alkalosis, decreasing calcium ionization. Chronic use of laxatives decreases calcium absorption from the gastrointestinal tract. Suggest high-fiber foods for improving bowel elimination.
- ⚡ Encourage patients taking calcium supplements to check with the pharmacist to ensure that the calcium tablet is absorbable.
- ⚡ Advise patients to take oral calcium supplements with meals or after meals to increase absorption.
- ⚡ Instruct patients to report symptoms of hypercalcemia, including muscle weakness and pain over bony areas. Remind patients to report any chest pain or urinary problems because calcium can cause ECG changes and renal stones.
- ⚡ Instruct patients to report symptoms of hypocalcemia, including neuromuscular signs such as numbness, tingling sensations in fingers and toes, and muscle cramps. Wheezing may develop from bronchospasm, dysphagia, voice changes, fatigue, and seizures.

Diet
- Instruct the patient to consume high-calcium foods such as milk and dairy products.
- Remind the patient that foods rich in protein and vitamin D enhance calcium absorption.

Evaluate Outcomes [Evaluation]
- ⚡ Evaluate the patient's serum calcium and electrolyte levels. Report if the calcium imbalance continues.
- ⚡ Monitor patients for neuromuscular and cardiac manifestations of calcium imbalance.

Both calcium chloride 10% (CaCl) and calcium gluconate 10% (CaGl) can be used for acute hypocalcemia and during cardiac resuscitation. Calcium gluconate has the same action on the heart as digitalis; it increases the force of systolic contractions. Prototype Drug Chart: Calcium describes the pharmacokinetics and pharmacodynamics of calcium preparations.

⚡ The patient's renal functioning should be assessed before administering IV calcium chloride; this solution contains aluminum, which can be toxic if renal insufficiency exists. IV calcium should be administered cautiously in patients who take digitalis because an increase in serum calcium increases the risk of digitalis toxicity. Calcium chloride 10% solution should be administered slowly via an infusion control pump, and the patient should be monitored frequently. ⚡ Care should be taken to prevent extravasation; local extravasation may cause tissue necrosis and sloughing. Nurses should refer to the agency's policy if infiltration occurs. Too rapid an infusion may cause cardiac syncope and decreased blood pressure from peripheral vasodilation. Oral calcium preparations are available in tablets, capsules, gelcaps, and powders.

Patients with hypocalcemia should be assessed for hypomagnesemia, hypokalemia, and acid-base imbalances, and any abnormalities should be corrected. Hypomagnesemia should be corrected first; low magnesium levels may prevent the patient from responding to treatment for hypocalcemia.

Pharmacokinetics

Vitamin D promotes calcium absorption from the GI tract; phosphorus inhibits calcium absorption. The pH affects the amount of ionized calcium. When pH is decreased (acidic), there is more free ionized calcium because it has been released from protein-binding sites. With an increased pH (alkalosis), more calcium is bound to protein.

Hypercalcemia

Elevated serum calcium may be a result of hyperparathyroidism, malignancy, hypophosphatemia, excessive calcium intake, prolonged immobilization, multiple fractures, drugs such as thiazide diuretics, and steroids. Signs and symptoms of hypercalcemia are fatigue, muscle weakness, depressed deep tendon reflexes, confusion, impaired memory, anorexia, nausea, vomiting, constipation, and kidney stones of calcium composition. ⚡ The patient may experience ECG changes and exhibit decreased heart rate and dysrhythmias.

Effect of Drugs on Calcium Balance

Phosphate preparations, corticosteroids, loop diuretics, aspirin, anticonvulsants, magnesium sulfate, and plicamycin (an antineoplastic antibiotic) are a few of the drugs that can lower serum calcium levels. Excess calcium salt ingestion or infusion and thiazide diuretics can all contribute to an increased serum calcium level. Table 12.9 lists some drugs that affect calcium balance.

Clinical Management of Calcium Imbalance

Clinical management of hypocalcemia consists of oral supplements and IV calcium. Table 12.10 lists oral and IV preparations of calcium salts, their dosages, and drug forms. Calcium carbonate can cause GI upset because it produces carbon dioxide. For better calcium absorption, calcium supplements should contain vitamin D, and oral calcium should be taken 30 minutes before meals.

The goal for managing hypercalcemia is to correct the underlying cause of serum calcium excess. IV saline solution and drugs such as calcitonin and loop diuretics can be used to promote rapid urinary excretion of calcium.

Magnesium

Magnesium is most plentiful in the ICF, and it plays a role in maintaining normal calcium and potassium balance. Magnesium deficit often occurs with hypokalemia and hypocalcemia. The normal serum magnesium level is 1.5 to 2.5 mEq/L. Magnesium deficit is called **hypomagnesemia**, and magnesium excess is called **hypermagnesemia**. The daily magnesium requirement is 8 to 20 mEq/day.

Functions

Magnesium promotes transmission of neuromuscular activity and is an important mediator of neural transmission in the CNS. ⚡ Alterations in serum magnesium levels profoundly affect neuromuscular excitability and contractility. Like potassium, magnesium promotes contraction of the myocardium. Magnesium activates many enzymes for metabolism of carbohydrates and protein and is responsible for transportation of sodium and potassium across cell membranes.

⚡ Serum magnesium deficit increases the release of acetylcholine from the presynaptic membrane of the nerve fiber, which increases

TABLE 12.9 Drugs Affecting Calcium Balance

Substances	Rationale
Drugs That Cause Hypocalcemia	
Bisphosphonates	Used in the treatment of osteoporosis. Prevents bones from leaking calcium, which means less calcium in the bloodstream.
Cinacalcet	Used to decrease parathyroid hormone levels in chronic kidney disease and decrease risk of kidney stones. Decreases calcium levels.
Cisplatin	Chemo medication used to treat cancer. Known to cause low blood calcium levels.
Corticosteroids and mineralocorticoids	Decreases calcium mobilization and inhibits calcium absorption.
Denosumab	A human monoclonal antibody used in the treatment of osteoporosis. Decreases blood calcium levels.
Diuretics: loop	Decreases calcium mobilization and inhibits calcium absorption decreasing calcium.
Estrogen	Can alter vitamin D metabolism needed for calcium absorption decreasing calcium.
Magnesium sulfate	Inhibits parathyroid hormone secretion and decreases serum calcium level.
Phenytoin	Decreases vitamin D levels that decrease calcium absorption and lowers calcium levels.
Phosphate preparations: oral, enema, intravenous; sodium phosphate, potassium phosphate	Can increase serum phosphorus level and decrease serum calcium level.
Drugs That Cause Hypercalcemia	
Aminoglycosides	
Calcium acetate Calcium carbonate Calcium salts Vitamin D (calcitriol)	Excess ingestion of calcium and vitamin D and infusion of calcium can increase serum calcium level.
Intravenous fat emulsion	Can increase serum calcium level.
Diuretics: thiazides (chlorthalidone)	Can induce hypercalcemia by preventing calcium release in the urine. Can lead to kidney stones.
Lithium	Increases parathyroid hormone secretion.

TABLE 12.10 Calcium Oral Preparations

Calcium Name	Drug Form	Drug Dose
Calcium carbonate	Chewable	250 mg/400 mg/500 mg/750 mg
Calcium citrate	Caplet Tablet	200 mg/950 mg
Calcium gluconate	Tablet	500 mg

neuromuscular excitability. Serum magnesium excess has a sedative effect on the neuromuscular system, which can result in loss of deep tendon reflexes. Cardiac (ventricular) dysrhythmias, hypotension, and heart block can occur because of hypomagnesemia.

⚡ Hypomagnesemia is probably the most undiagnosed electrolyte deficiency. This is most likely because it is asymptomatic until the serum magnesium level approaches 1 mEq/L. To correct severe hypomagnesemia, IV magnesium sulfate is usually given. For hypermagnesemia, calcium gluconate may be given to decrease the serum magnesium level.

Causes of Magnesium Imbalance

Prolonged parenteral nutrition without magnesium supplements can decrease magnesium levels. Also, diuretics, certain antibiotics, laxatives, and steroids are drug groups that promote magnesium loss. Like hypokalemia, hypomagnesemia enhances the action of digitalis and can cause digitalis toxicity. Chronic alcoholism, prolonged fasting, starvation, or increased renal losses can promote hypomagnesemia.

⚡ Magnesium sulfate corrects hypomagnesemia and symptoms of digitalis toxicity. It is common practice after bypass surgery or myocardial infarction for patients to be given magnesium sulfate orally, even when blood levels are normal, to prevent ventricular arrhythmias in the perioperative period.

Excess intake of magnesium salts is the major cause of serum magnesium excess. Commonly used medications that may cause hypermagnesemia include laxatives and antacids. A patient with chronic kidney disease who ingests products that contain magnesium will have a problem with excess magnesium. Patient teaching regarding prolonged or frequent use of laxatives, particularly in older adults, is an important intervention in preventing electrolyte imbalance. Table 12.11 lists some drugs that affect magnesium balance.

Chloride

Chloride is the principal anion of ECF. The chloride ion is a major contributor to acid-base balance, gastric juice acidity, and the osmolality of ECF. A normal serum chloride level is 96 to 106 mEq/L. **Hypochloremia** is a decreased serum chloride level, and **hyperchloremia** is an elevated level. With increased serum osmolality (>300 mOsm per kg of water), there are more sodium and chloride ions proportional to the water. Sodium and chloride frequently work in combination. For example, during sodium retention, chloride is also frequently retained, resulting in increased water retention. ⚡ Clinical manifestations of

---

⊚ CLINICAL JUDGMENT [NURSING PROCESS]
Magnesium

Concept: Fluid and Electrolyte Balance
- Patients require the regulation of fluid and electrolytes to maintain homeostasis. Nurses will encounter potential and actual alterations of fluid and electrolyte balance when caring for patients. Nursing assessments and interventions ensure the intake of fluid and electrolytes remains balanced by closely monitoring the patient's intake and output and careful assessment of laboratory values.

Recognize Cues [Assessment]
- ⚡ Assess the patient for signs and symptoms of magnesium imbalance. Signs and symptoms of *hypomagne*semia are tetany-like symptoms caused by hyperexcitability (tremors, twitching of the face) and ventricular tachycardia that leads to ventricular fibrillation and hypertension. Signs and symptoms of *hypermagnesemia* are lethargy, drowsiness, weakness and paralysis, loss of deep tendon reflexes, hypotension, and heart block.
- ⚡ Check serum magnesium levels for magnesium imbalance. Symptoms of magnesium deficiency may not be seen until the serum level is below 1 mEq/L.
- ⚡ Observe patients taking digitalis preparations for digitalis toxicity. Like potassium deficit, magnesium deficit enhances the action of digitalis, causing digitalis toxicity.
- ⚡ Use with caution in patients with renal impairment; accumulation of magnesium may lead to magnesium intoxication.

Analyze Cues and Prioritize Hypothesis [Patient Problems]
- Dysrhythmias
- Hypomagnesemia
- Hypermagnesemia

Generate Solutions [Planning]
- The patient's serum magnesium level is within normal range (1.5–2.5 mEq/L).
- The patient will not experience life-threatening symptoms of magnesium imbalance such as central nervous symptoms (confusion, coma) and cardiac dysrhythmias (premature ventricular contractions and ventricular fibrillation).

Take Action [Nursing Interventions]
- ⚡ Communicate to the health care provider (HCP) if a patient is ordered nothing by mouth (NPO) and is receiving intravenous fluids (IVFs) without magnesium salts for a prolonged period.
- Monitor urinary output. Most of the body's magnesium is excreted by the kidneys. Report if urine output falls below 600 mL/day.
- ⚡ Monitor for digitalis toxicity (e.g., nausea, vomiting, bradycardia) in patients who have hypomagnesemia and are taking digoxin. Magnesium deficit enhances the action of digitalis preparations.
- ⚡ Monitor vital signs and compare with baseline values. Report abnormal findings to the health care provider.
- ⚡ Monitor serum electrolyte results. Report low serum potassium or calcium levels because low serum magnesium levels may be attributed to hypokalemia or hypocalcemia. When correcting a potassium deficit, potassium is not replaced in cells until magnesium is replaced. A serum magnesium level of 1 mEq/L or less can cause cardiac arrest.
- ⚡ Prepare for emergency reversal of hypomagnesemia deficit by having available intravenous (IV) calcium gluconate.
- Use an interpreter as needed.
- Involve the extended family in health teaching and support.

Patient Teaching
- Advise patients with hypomagnesemia to eat foods rich in magnesium (green vegetables, fruits, fish, grains, and nuts).
- Instruct patients with hypermagnesemia to avoid routine use of laxatives and antacids that contain magnesium. Suggest that patients check drug labels and speak with a pharmacist.
- Instruct patients on signs and symptoms of hypomagnesemia and hypermagnesemia.

Evaluate Outcomes [Evaluation]
- Evaluate the patient's serum magnesium level. Report if the magnesium imbalance continues.
- Have the patient verbalize the signs and symptoms of hypomagnesemia and hypermagnesemia, and instruct them to report these to their health care provider.

TABLE 12.11 Drugs That Affect Magnesium Balance

Drugs	Rationale
Drugs That Cause Hypomagnesemia	
Diuretics: loop and thiazide	Promote urinary loss of magnesium
Antibiotics: gentamicin, tobramycin, aminoglycosides, amphotericin B	Can cause magnesium loss via kidneys
Laxatives, cisplatin	Abuse can cause magnesium loss via the gastrointestinal tract
Drugs That Cause Hypermagnesemia	
Magnesium salts (oral and enema); magnesium hydroxide; magnesium sulfate; magnesium citrate	Excessive use can increase serum magnesium level. Use of excessive magnesium sulfate in treatment of toxemia can cause hypermagnesemia

hypochloremia include tremors, twitching, and slow, shallow breathing. With severe chloride loss, decreased blood pressure is seen. Clinical manifestations of hyperchloremia include weakness; lethargy; deep, rapid breathing; and eventual unconsciousness.

Phosphorus

Phosphorus is the primary anion in ICF and is the second most abundant element in the body. The majority of the body's phosphorus is found as phosphate; therefore these two terms are used interchangeably.

Both phosphorus and calcium levels are regulated by PTH and need vitamin D for absorption from the GI tract. ⚡ A reciprocal relationship exists between phosphorus and calcium. High serum phosphate levels cause low calcium levels; low calcium levels stimulate the release of PTH, which decreases reabsorption of phosphorus.

A normal serum phosphorus level is 2.4 to 4.4 mEq/L. Regulation of phosphate balance requires adequate renal functioning because the kidneys are the major route of phosphate excretion.

Phosphorus is essential in bone and teeth formation and for neuromuscular activity. Phosphorus is an important component of nucleic acids (DNA and RNA) and assists in energy transfer in cells, helps maintain cellular osmotic pressure, and supports the acid-base balance of body fluids. ⚡ Clinical manifestations of hypophosphatemia include muscle weakness, tremors, paresthesia, bone pain, hyporeflexia, seizures, hyperventilation, anorexia, and dysphagia. Symptoms of hyperphosphatemia are like those of hypocalcemia and include hyperreflexia, tetany, flaccid paralysis, muscular weakness, tachycardia, nausea, diarrhea, and abdominal cramps. Phosphorus-rich foods include whole-grain cereals, nuts, milk, and meat. Phosphorus deficiency can result from decreased intestinal absorption, malnutrition, alcoholism, vomiting, diarrhea, use of concentrated glucose solutions, respiratory alkalosis, glycosuria, hypokalemia, hypomagnesemia, or use of thiazide diuretics. Hypophosphatemia may lead to hemolytic anemia, platelet dysfunction, and reduced oxygen transport. Hyperphosphatemia is most often related to chronic kidney disease. Increased intake in the form of laxatives may also increase serum levels.

Treatment of phosphorus imbalance is aimed at eliminating or reducing the cause. Monitoring phosphorus, calcium, and magnesium levels and assessing the patient for signs of electrolyte and acid-base imbalance are important nursing interventions. Phosphorus replacement is guided by the degree of deficit, onset, and patient presentation. Oral intake is the preferred route of replacement. IV phosphorus is available for treatment of patients who are unable to tolerate oral replacements or those with severe deficits. ❗ Potassium phosphate is an Institute for Safe Medication Practices (ISMP) high-alert medication used for IV phosphorus replacement. Potassium phosphate must be diluted before use and must be infused slowly using an infusion control pump. Too rapid an infusion may cause potassium toxicity in patients with severe renal or adrenal insufficiency. The IV insertion site must be monitored for infiltration; potassium phosphate may cause tissue necrosis and sloughing if infiltration occurs. Phosphorus, potassium, and calcium levels as well as renal function should be monitored during and after infusion. Use of potassium phosphate is contraindicated in patients with hyperkalemia or hypocalcemia.

Hyperphosphatemia in patients with chronic kidney disease is treated with restriction of dietary phosphorus, phosphorus-binding medications such as calcium acetate, or dialysis. Hyperphosphatemia can lead to secondary hyperparathyroidism and osteodystrophy.

CLINICAL JUDGMENT UNFOLDING CASE STUDY

Cognitive Skill: Recognize cues (enhanced hot spot)

Question 1

A 70-year-old active male is admitted to the emergency department from home. The patient's wife tells the nurse he appears to have gained weight (normal weight is 175) and is feeling short of breath (SOB). The nurse takes his vitals and performs a complete physical assessment. His medication profile includes 25 mg thiazide daily. His wife indicates he has refused to take his prescribed medication because it makes him tired. The nurse documents the following assessment findings.
- Blood pressure 180/90 mm Hg and heart rate of 100 bpm
- Pain rated 1 on a scale of 0 to 10
- Tachypnea (28 breaths per minute [bpm])
- Bilateral crackles base of lungs
- Patient reports tiredness and fatigue
- Bowel sounds present ×4
- Bilateral pedal edema +3
- Oriented to person, place, and time
- Weight gain of 10 lbs (185 lb)
- Oxygen saturation 96% (room air)

Highlight or place a check mark next to the assessment findings that require follow-up by the nurse.

Answers
Blood pressure 180/90 mm Hg and heart rate of 100 bpm
- Tachypnea (28 bpm)
- Bilateral crackles base of lungs
- Patient reports tiredness and fatigue
- Bilateral pedal edema +3
- Weight gain of 10 lbs (185 lb)
- Oxygen saturation 96% (room air)

Rationale
The previous signs are indicative of a patient with fluid overload. The patient stopped taking his prescribed diuretic. This caused increased bodily fluids to build up in his body. This results in an excessive amount of fluid circulating around the heart and lungs. Increased bodily fluids can cause weight gain, increased blood pressure, and increased heart rate. As fluid enters the lungs, the patient can develop crackles at the lung base, increased respiratory rate, shortness of

Continued

CLINICAL JUDGMENT UNFOLDING CASE STUDY—CONT'D

breath, and decreased oxygen saturation as they struggle to breathe. The most consistent sign of fluid overload is increased body weight.

References
Lewis, et al: Fluid & electrolyte imbalances. In: *Medical surgical nursing*, ed 10, St. Louis, 2017, Elsevier, pp 270–299.
  McCuistion, et al: Fluid volume and electrolytes. In: *Pharmacology: a patient-centered nursing process approach*, ed 11, St. Louis, 2023, Elsevier, pp 135–155.

Cognitive Skill: Analyze cues (cloze).

Question 2
A 70-year-old active male is admitted to the emergency department from home. The patient's wife tells the nurse he appears to have gained weight (normal weight is 175) and is feeling short of breath (SOB). His vitals are taken, and a complete physical assessment is performed. His medication profile includes 25 mg thiazide daily. His wife indicates he has refused to take his prescribed medication because it makes him tired. The nurse documents the following assessment findings.

- Blood pressure 180/90 mm Hg and heart rate of 100 bpm
- Pain rated 1 on a scale of 0 to 10
- Tachypnea (28 bpm)
- Bilateral crackles base of lungs
- Patient reports tiredness and fatigue
- Bowel sounds present ×4
- Bilateral pedal edema +3
- Oriented to person, place, and time
- Weight gain of 10 lb (185 lb)
- Oxygen saturation 96% (room air)

Choose the most likely information missing from the statements below by selecting the information from the list of options provided.

Based on the patient's assessment data, the nurse determines that the patient's vital sign findings are due to _____(1)_____. Bilateral crackles at the base of the lungs and oxygen saturation of 96% indicate the need for _____(2)_____. The provider orders the following blood tests to evaluate the patient's health status: _____(3)_____, _____(3)_____, and _____(3)_____.

Option 1	Option 2	Option 3
a. Bradycardia	a. Chest x-ray	a. Complete blood count
b. Respiratory failure	b. Fasting blood glucose	b. Urine specific gravity
c. COVID-19	c. Kidney function test	c. Basic metabolic panel
d. Fluid volume excess	d. CPAP	d. Lipid panel
e. Fluid volume deficit	e. Oxygen at 8 L/NC	c. Hepatitis level
f. Weight loss	f. Barium swallow test	d. Calcium level

Answers
Based on the patient's assessment data, it is determined that the patient's vital sign findings are due to fluid volume excess (d). Bilateral crackles at the base of the lungs and oxygen saturation of 96% indicate the need for chest x-ray (a). The following blood tests are ordered to evaluate the patient's health status: complete blood count (a), basic metabolic panel (c), and urine specific gravity level (b).

Rationale
Excess body fluids can dilute (and lower) the hemoglobin and hematocrit levels found in the complete blood count. Excess body fluids can dilute (and lower) the potassium and sodium levels found in the basic metabolic panel. Fluid excess can dilute (and lower) the urine-specific gravity levels as well. These tests can help identify the patient's problem of fluid volume excess. When a patient has bilateral crackles at the base of the lungs and an oxygen saturation of 96% (room air), and is experiencing tachypnea with a rate of 28 bpm, standard protocol is for the provider to order a chest x-ray. This will indicate if there is fluid in the patient's lungs from fluid overload.

References
Lewis, et al: Fluid & electrolyte imbalances. In: *Medical surgical nursing*, ed 10, St. Louis, 2017, Elsevier, pp 270–299.
  McCuistion, et al: Fluid volume and electrolytes. In: *Pharmacology: a patient-centered nursing process approach*, ed 11, St. Louis, 2023, Elsevier, pp 135–155.

Cognitive Skill: Prioritize hypothesis (extended multiple response).

Question 3
The health care provider admits a 70-year-old active patient to the telemetry unit for monitoring. The patient has a weight gain of 10 pounds with bilateral crackles at the base of the lungs. The provider orders oxygen 2 L NC, and the patient's oxygen saturation has increased to 99%. He is now resting comfortably.

Circle or place a check mark next to the serum lab result that supports the diagnosis of fluid volume overload.

a. Urine specific gravity 1.000 g/mL
b. Hemoglobin 15.5 gd/L
c. Hematocrit 30.5%
d. Potassium 3.2 mEq/L
e. Sodium 120.0 mEq/L
f. Chloride (blood) 85 mEq/L
g. Calcium (total) 9.0 mg/dL
h. Platelet 200,000/μL
i. Creatinine (blood) 0.8 mg/dL
j. Total red blood count $5.0 \times 10^6/\mu L$
k. Answers:

a. Urine specific gravity 1.000 g/mL	✓
b. Hemoglobin 15.5 gd/L	
c. Hematocrit 30.5%	✓
d. Potassium 3.2 mEq/L	✓
e. Sodium 120.0 mEq/L	✓
f. Chloride (blood) 85 mEq/L	✓
g. Calcium (total) 9.0 mg/dL	
h. Platelet 200,000/μL	
i. Creatinine (blood) 0.8 mg/dL	
j. Total red blood count $5.0 \times 10^6/\mu L$	

Rationale
Increased body fluids will dilute (and lower) the hemoglobin and hematocrit (normal range: 42%–52%) (complete blood count) as well as the potassium (normal range 3.5–5.0 mEq/L), sodium (normal range: 135–145 mEq/L), and chloride (normal range 96–106 mEq/L) (basic metabolic panel) in the patient's body. It can also dilute (and lower) the urine specific gravity (normal range: 1.005–1.030 g/mL). This can help identify the patient's fluid volume excess.

References
McCuistion, et al: Fluid volume and electrolytes. In: *Pharmacology: a patient-centered nursing process approach*, ed 11, St. Louis, 2023, Elsevier, pp 135–155.
  Lewis, et al: Fluid & electrolyte imbalances. In: *Medical surgical nursing*, ed. 10, St. Louis, 2017, Elsevier, Appendix C.

Cognitive Skill: Generate solutions (drag & drop)

CLINICAL JUDGMENT UNFOLDING CASE STUDY—CONT'D

Question 4

The health care provider admits a 70-year-old active patient to the telemetry unit for monitoring. The patient has a weight gain of 10 pounds with bilateral crackles at the base of the lungs. The provider orders oxygen 2 L NC, and the patient's oxygen saturation has increased to 99%. He is now resting comfortably. In addition, the provider has changed his medication from 25 mg of thiazide to furosemide 20 mg and has added potassium 20 mEq daily.

Indicate which patient teaching is appropriate by placing the appropriate response in the column to the far right.

Nurse's Teaching	Patient Question	Which teaching response is appropriate for each patient question?
1. While in the hospital your provider has placed you on fluid restriction of 1000 mL/day. You must record your intake and output daily.	"I will forget. Can you show me how to record?"	
2. The provider has placed you on a low-sodium diet.	"What is a low-sodium diet?"	
3. You must weigh yourself every day and notify your provider for a weight gain >3 lbs in 2 days.	"Why every day?"	
4. Your provider has stopped thiazide 25 mg and has started you on furosemide 20 mg/d and potassium 20 mEq/d.	"Why have my medications been changed?"	
5. Do not add extra salt to your food. Make low-sodium choices.		
6. Use this list to record your fluid intake (remember 237 mL = 1 cup). This container is used to measure your urine output daily. Record the output on this list.		
7. Furosemide is a loop diuretic. It will decrease the amount of fluid in your body and lower your blood pressure. It also depletes the level of potassium (K^+) in your blood so a K^+ supplement is necessary. You must take this medication as prescribed by the provider.		
8. If a weight gain occurs, it is important to notify your provider immediately to avoid fluid volume overload.		

Answers

Nurse's Teaching	Patient Question	Which teaching response is appropriate for each patient question?
1. While in the hospital your provider has placed you on fluid restriction of 1000 mL/day. You must record your intake and output daily.	"I will forget. Can you show me how to record?"	6. Use this list to record your fluid intake (remember 237 mL = 1 cup). This container is used to measure your urine output daily. Record the output on this list.
2. The provider has placed you on a low-sodium diet.	"What is a low-sodium diet?"	5. Do not add extra salt to your food. Make low-sodium choices.
3. You must weigh yourself every day and notify your provider for a weight gain >3 lb in 2 days.	"Why every day?"	8. If a weight gain occurs, it is important to notify your provider immediately to avoid fluid volume overload.
4. Your provider has stopped thiazide 25 mg and has started you on furosemide 20 mg/d and potassium 20 mEq/d.	"Why have my medications been changed?"	7. Furosemide is a loop diuretic. It will decrease the amount of fluid in your body and lower your blood pressure. It also depletes the level of potassium (K^+) in your blood so a K^+ supplement is necessary. You must take this medication as prescribed by the provider.

Rationale

These questions are important for the nurse to validate the patient's understanding of care for fluid volume excess. Intake and output records provide valuable information about fluid and electrolyte problems. They reveal sources of excess fluid intake and/or fluid losses. Sodium is an essential mineral important to fluid and electrolyte balance and blood pressure maintenance. Limiting sodium through a low-sodium diet will prevent the buildup of excessive fluid in the body. Daily weigh-ins serve as the most authentic measure of volume status. If a weight gain occurs of greater than 3 lbs in 2 days, it is necessary to notify the provider immediately to avoid hospitalization. Furosemide is a loop diuretic that decreases the amount of fluid buildup in the body. It can also deplete potassium supply, which is why the doctor ordered a potassium supplement.

References

Lewis, et al: Fluid & electrolyte imbalances. In: *Medical surgical nursing*, ed 10, St. Louis, 2017, Elsevier, pp 270–299.

McCuistion, et al: Fluid volume and electrolytes. In: *Pharmacology: a patient-centered nursing process approach*, ed 11, St. Louis, 2023, Elsevier, pp 135–155.

McCuistion, et al: Diurecs. In: *Pharmacology: a patient centered nursing process approach*, ed 11, St. Louis, 2023, Elsevier, pp 507–517.

Cognitive Skill: Take action (extended multiple response).

Continued

CLINICAL JUDGMENT UNFOLDING CASE STUDY—CONT'D

Question 5
This 70-year-old male patient is resting comfortably. His oxygen saturation on room air is 99%. His blood pressure is 140/80 mm Hg and heart rate 60 bpm. On auscultation his lungs are bilaterally clear. The nurse is preparing the patient for possible morning discharge. More patient instruction is needed concerning the low-sodium diet. When presented with this list, the patient is asked to check off the best food choices for a low-sodium diet.

Circle or place a check mark next to the best low-sodium food choice. Select all that apply.
a. Canned vegetables
b. Fresh fruit
c. Sausage and deli meats
d. Sodium-free herbs and spices
e. Frozen vegetables (nothing added)
f. Canned meat or fish
g. Frozen dinners
h. Broiled chicken and meats (plain)
i. Breaded meats

Answers

a. Canned vegetables	
b. Fresh fruit	✓
c. Sausage and deli meats	
d. Sodium-free herbs and spices	✓
e. Frozen vegetables (nothing added)	✓
f. Canned meat or fish	
g. Frozen dinners	
h. Broiled chicken and meats (plain)	✓
i. Breaded meats	

Rationale
The nurse is validating that the patient understands what is contained in a low-sodium diet. Sodium is an essential mineral important to fluid and electrolyte balance and blood pressure maintenance. Limiting sodium intake through a low-sodium diet will prevent the buildup of excessive fluid in the body.

References
Lewis, et al: Fluid & electrolyte imbalances. In: *Medical surgical nursing*, ed 10, St. Louis, 2017, Elsevier, pp 270–299.
McCuistion, et al: Fluid volume and electrolytes. In: *Pharmacology: a patient-centered nursing process approach*, ed 11, St. Louis, 2023, Elsevier, pp 135–155.
McCuistion, et al: Diurecs. In: *Pharmacology: a patient centered nursing process approach*, ed 11, St. Louis, 2023, Elsevier, pp 507–517.

Cognitive Skill: Evaluate outcomes (matrix).

Question 6
After the patient experiences a stable and restful night, the nurse performs a careful morning assessment for possible discharge. The assessment includes information for a health teaching plan for this patient prior to discharge.

For each assessment finding, use an X to indicate whether the nurse's teaching was "Effective" (helped to meet expected outcomes), **"Ineffective"** (did not help to meet expected outcomes), or **"Unrelated"** (not related to the expected outcomes).

Assessment Finding	Effective	Ineffective	Unrelated
The patient's lungs are clear (bilaterally), no SOB, oxygen saturation is 100% on room air.			
Patient states, "I will weigh each morning and call the health care provider if I gain more than 3 pounds in 2 days."			
Patient's vital signs are 120/80 mm Hg, pulse 60, and weight 175 lb.			
Patient states, "I cannot wait to get home to have bacon and ham with my morning breakfast."			
Patientt states, "My provider says I should exercise by walking. Should I walk in the morning or the evening with my neighborhood friends?"			
Patient states, "I will take my medication as ordered by my provider every morning."			

Answers

Assessment Finding	Effective	Ineffective	Unrelated
The patient's lungs are clear (bilaterally), no SOB, oxygen saturation is 100% on room air.	X		
Patient states, "I will weigh each morning and call the health care provider if I gain more than 3 pounds in 2 days."	X		
Patient's vital signs are 120/80 mm Hg, pulse 60, and weight 175 lbs.	X		
Patient states, "I cannot wait to get home to have bacon and ham with my morning breakfast."		X	
Patient states, "My provider says I should exercise by walking. Should I walk in the morning or the evening with my neighborhood friends?"			X
Patient states, "I will take my medication as ordered by my provider every morning."	X		

CLINICAL JUDGMENT UNFOLDING CASE STUDY—CONT'D

Rationale
The nurse evaluates the patient's expected outcomes to validate their effectiveness prior to discharge. The patient's lungs are clear (bilaterally), no SOB, and oxygen saturation is 100% (effective). The patient validates knowledge of the importance of daily weigh-ins (effective). The patient's vital signs are within normal range, and his weight has returned to normal (effective). The patient validates taking his medications as ordered by the provider (effective). The nurse will document the effectiveness of these expected outcomes in the nursing notes. When the patient expresses his desire to eat bacon and ham with breakfast, this is an ineffective outcome. The nurse must provide more teaching on making better low-sodium choices. After additional teaching, the nurse will document the outcome in the nursing notes. It is good that the provider has given permission for the patient to exercise by walking. The time of day the patient chooses to walk is up to the patient and is unrelated.

References
Lewis, et al: Fluid & electrolyte imbalances. In: *Medical surgical nursing*, ed 10, St. Louis, 2017, Elsevier, pp 270–299.

McCuistion, et al: Fluid volume and electrolytes. In: *Pharmacology: a patient-centered nursing process approach*, ed 11, St. Louis, 2023, Elsevier, pp 135–155.

REVIEW QUESTIONS

1. Three days after a patient's total colectomy and ileostomy, he has a nasogastric tube for continuous suction and a Foley catheter for continuous drainage. The night nurse reports a high output from the ileostomy. The patient's pulse is irregular, and he reports muscle weakness and leg cramping. Based on this situation, the nurse would correctly suspect what type of imbalance?
   a. Hypokalemia
   b. Hyperkalemia
   c. Hypomagnesemia
   d. Hypochloremia

2. A patient is receiving intravenous (IV) potassium supplements. What is the most important nursing implication when administering this drug?
   a. It is administered via a central vascular access device.
   b. It is diluted with IV fluids and delivered by infusion pump.
   c. IV potassium must be chilled before administration.
   d. IV potassium preparations should not contain preservatives.

3. A patient is receiving 10 mEq of potassium chloride in 100 mL of normal saline intravenously (IV) to infuse over 1 hour via infusion pump. The patient has a 22-gauge peripheral IV in his right forearm and reports pain at the insertion site; the nurse notes that the site is reddened, warm, and tender to the touch. Which action would the nurse take?
   a. Aspirate and check for blood return, and then slow the IV rate.
   b. Discontinue the IV, and then have a central line inserted.
   c. Stop the infusion, and discontinue the IV immediately.
   d. Apply warm compresses to the IV site and elevate extremity.

4. The health care provider orders a hypertonic crystalloid IV solution for a 70-year-old patient. Which solution will the nurse hang?
   a. Lactated Ringer's
   b. 0.45% sodium chloride (NaCl)
   c. 0.9% sodium chloride (NaCl)
   d. 5% dextrose in 0.9% sodium chloride (NaCl)

5. A patient is receiving fluid replacement. The nurse's primary Clinical Judgment [Nursing Process] plan of care and Take Action [Nursing Interventions] include which of the following statements? **Select all that apply.**
   a. Measure the patient's weight every morning.
   b. Know that thirst means a mild fluid deficit.
   c. Monitor fluid intake and fluid output daily.
   d. Avoid using calcium and chloride supplements.
   e. Review the patient's daily electrolyte labs for changes.

6. A patient gained 4.4 lb (2 kg), and it has been determined that the weight gain is caused by fluid retention. The nurse correctly estimates that the weight gain may be equivalent to approximately how much fluid?
   a. 1 L
   b. 2 L
   c. 6 L
   d. 8 L

7. A patient has hypernatremia. Which components are appropriate to include in the Clinical Judgment [Nursing Process] plan of care? **Select all that apply.**
   a. Instruct the patient on seizure precautions.
   b. Keep appointments for laboratory tests.
   c. A sign of hypernatremia is hypotension.
   d. Explain the meaning of fluid restriction.
   e. Instruct the patient on how to read food labels.

8. The nurse is reviewing the medication list of a patient with hypokalemia. Which products may contribute to the cause of this imbalance? **Select all that apply.**
   a. Cortisone
   b. Licorice
   c. Azithromycin
   d. Estrogen
   e. Digoxin

13 Vitamin and Mineral Replacement

http://evolve.elsevier.com/McCuistion/pharmacology

OBJECTIVES

- Relate the principles of nursing care to the patient's health and use of vitamins.
- Relate the principles of nursing care to the patient's health and use of minerals.

OUTLINE

Vitamins, 154
    Dietary Reference Intakes, 154
    Fat-Soluble Vitamins, 155
    Water-Soluble Vitamins, 158
Minerals, 161
    Iron, 161

    Copper, 162
    Zinc, 162
    Chromium, 162
    Selenium, 163
Clinical Judgment Case Study, 164
Review Questions, 165

Vitamins and minerals are needed in the correct portions for normal body function. Most vitamin and mineral nutrients can be safely obtained through the diet. Overuse of vitamins and minerals occurs easily, especially if the nutrients are coming from pills instead of food. It is important to check all supplements with the patient's health care provider (HCP).

VITAMINS

Vitamins are organic substances necessary for normal metabolic functions and for tissue growth and healing. The body needs only a small number of vitamins daily, which are obtained through the diet. A well-balanced diet has all of the vitamins and minerals needed for body functioning. The intake of vitamins should be increased by people experiencing periods of rapid body growth; those who are pregnant or breast-feeding; patients with debilitating illnesses; those with malabsorptive issues, such as Crohn's disease; and those with inadequate diets, which includes alcoholics and some geriatric patients. Children who have poor nutrient intake and are malnourished may need vitamin replacement. People on "fad" or restrictive diets may have vitamin deficiencies, as may those who are unable to afford or do not select a wide variety of foods.

The sale of vitamins in the United States is a multibillion-dollar business. About 80% of US adults use a variety of nutritional supplements (http://www.crnusa.org). Older females and people with higher education are typical users of nutritional supplements. Numerous vitamins and herbal medications are available for specialized needs such as cholesterol, memory, menopause, and prostate support. Before purchasing these agents, the patient should discuss with their HCP the use and health benefits of multiple vitamins and herbal medications. Vitamin supplements are not necessary if the individual is healthy and consumes a well-balanced daily diet on a regular basis.

Dietary Reference Intakes

The Food and Nutrition Board of the National Academy of Medicine has established the Dietary Reference Intakes (DRIs). https://ods.od.nih.gov/Healthinformation/nutrienttrecommendations.aspx. The DRI nutrient recommendations include these components:

1. **Adequate intake (AI)** is the consumption and absorption of sufficient food, vitamins, and essential minerals necessary to maintain health.
2. **Estimated average requirement (EAR)** is the daily intake of a specific nutrient estimated to meet the requirement in 50% of healthy people in an age- and sex-specific group.
3. **Recommended dietary allowance (RDA)** is the amount of vitamins, minerals, or other essential nutrients that should be ingested every day by a normal person engaged in average activities. RDAs are increased for patients who are experiencing increased activity, children who are growing, and females who are pregnant and lactating. RDAs assume a state of wellness and are of little use in patients who are ill.
4. **Tolerable upper intake level (UL)** is the maximum level of continuing daily nutrient intake that is likely to pose no risk to the health of most of those in the age group for which it has been established. Vitamin deficiencies can cause cellular and organ dysfunction that may result in slow recovery from illness. Vitamin supplements are necessary for the vitamin deficiencies described in Table 13.1, but vitamins are frequently taken prophylactically rather than therapeutically.

With the goal of facilitating better nutrition, the US Department of Agriculture has developed http://www.choosemyplate.gov. "Choose My Plate" is an interactive tool that helps Americans eat more healthy foods (Fig. 13.1). The website offers a variety of features, including both consumer and professional information.

TABLE 13.1 Vitamin Deficiencies That Require Use of Vitamin Supplements

Categories	Deficiencies
Inability to metabolize and absorb vitamins	Malabsorption disorders: Diarrhea, infectious and inflammatory diseases (e.g., Crohn's disease, celiac disease); liver disease, kidney disease
Inability to use vitamins	Liver disease (cirrhosis, hepatitis), renal disease, certain hereditary deficiencies (cystic fibrosis)
Increased vitamin losses	Fever from infectious processes, hyperthyroidism, hemodialysis, cancer, starvation, crash diets
Increased vitamin requirements	Early childhood, pregnancy, debilitating disease (cancer, alcoholism), gastrointestinal surgery, special diets

Fig. 13.1 The US Department of Agriculture's Choose My Plate.

The Food and Nutrition Board of the National Academy of Medicine publishes the US RDA for daily dose requirements of each vitamin. The US Food and Drug Administration (FDA) requires all vitamin products to be labeled according to the vitamin content and the proportion of the RDA provided by the vitamin product. Individuals should be encouraged to check the RDA listed on the vitamin label to determine whether the product provides the RDA dose requirements. The RDA may need to be modified for patients who are ill.

Megadoses of vitamins are available and are advertised for specific health conditions, but high doses of some vitamins can be toxic. Patients should be advised to contact their HCP before taking any of these products. Megadoses of fat-soluble vitamins (A, D, E, and K) may cause toxic effects, whereas megadoses of water-soluble vitamins are eliminated via the urine and thus are generally not toxic. Adverse reactions—kidney stones and nerve damage, respectively—have been reported from vitamins C and B_6. However, it is also claimed that B vitamins may positively influence metabolism in older adults.

Table 13.2 lists fat- and water-soluble vitamins, their functions, suggested food sources, and related deficiency conditions.

Fat-Soluble Vitamins

Vitamins fall into two general categories: fat-soluble and water-soluble. The **fat-soluble vitamins** are A, D, E, and K. They are metabolized slowly; can be stored in fatty tissue, liver, and muscle in significant amounts; and are excreted in the urine at a slow rate. Vitamins A and D are toxic if taken in excessive amounts over time. Current research shows that vitamin D toxicity is quite rare, and its symptoms are nonspecific. Given that many people are found to be vitamin D deficient, it is not uncommon to see high-dose vitamin D therapy (e.g., 50,000 units/week).

Foods rich in vitamins A, D, E, and K are shown in Table 13.2.

Vitamin A

Vitamin A is a fat-soluble vitamin that is available from both plant and animal sources. Animal sources of vitamin A are referred to as retinoids, while carotenoids refer to vitamin A precursors, such as beta-carotene, derived from plants. Vitamin A is essential for bone growth and for maintenance of epithelial tissues, skin, eyes, and hair. Vitamin A has antioxidant properties. Excessive doses can become toxic. During pregnancy, the female should maintain an RDA of 770 mcg/day because excessive amounts of vitamin A can cause fetal harm. Prototype Drug Chart: Vitamin A describes the pharmacologic data on vitamin A.

Pharmacokinetics. Vitamin A is absorbed in the gastrointestinal (GI) tract, and 90% is stored in the liver; however, this function can be inhibited with liver disease. Massive doses of vitamin A can cause hypervitaminosis. Signs and symptoms include hair loss, peeling skin, anorexia, abdominal pain, lethargy, nausea, and vomiting. Retinol esters are hydrolyzed by pancreatic enzymes in the GI lumen. Carotenoids are absorbed in the small intestines by passive diffusion.

The RDA for adult males is 900 mcg/day (3000 international units [IU]) by mouth daily. The RDA for adult females is 700 mcg/day (2300 IU) by mouth daily. The UL for adults is 10,000 IU/day by mouth. Vitamin A toxicity affects multiple organs, especially the liver. Mineral oil, cholestyramine, alcohol, and antihyperlipidemic drugs decrease the absorption of vitamin A. Vitamin A is excreted through the kidneys and feces.

Pharmacodynamics. Vitamin A is necessary for many biochemical processes. It aids in the formation of the visual pigment needed for night vision. This vitamin is needed in bone growth and development, and it promotes the integrity of the mucosal and epithelial tissues. An early sign of vitamin A deficiency (hypovitaminosis A) is night blindness. This may progress to dryness and ulceration of the cornea and cause blindness.

Vitamin A taken orally is readily absorbed from the GI tract, resulting in 70% to 90% of the dose absorbed, and peaks in 3 to 5 hours. Its duration of action is unknown. Because vitamin A is stored in the liver, the vitamin may be available to the body for days, weeks, or months.

Vitamin D

Vitamin D has a major role in regulating calcium and phosphorus metabolism, and it is needed for calcium absorption from the intestines. Dietary vitamin D is absorbed in the small intestine and requires bile salts for absorption. There are two compounds of vitamin D: vitamin D_2, *ergocalciferol*, a synthetic fortified vitamin D, and vitamin D_3, *cholecalciferol*, a natural form of vitamin D influenced by ultraviolet sunlight on the skin. Over-the-counter vitamin D supplements usually contain vitamin D_3. Once absorbed, vitamin D is converted to calcifediol (also known as *25-hydroxycholecalciferol*) in the liver. Calcifediol is

TABLE 13.2 Vitamins: Functions, Suggested Food Sources, and Deficiency Conditions

Vitamin	Function	Food Sources	Deficiency Conditions
A (retinol) (fat-soluble)	Required for development and maintenance of healthy eyes, gums, teeth, skin, hair, glands, and immune function.	Darkly colored fruits and vegetables including carrots, cantaloupe, mangoes, spinach, pumpkin, and sweet potatoes. Natural vitamin A is found only in foods of animal origin: Dairy products, meat, fish oil, and fish.	Night blindness is often the first indication of deficiency. Skin lesions and dysfunction of mucous membranes also occur.
B-Complex Vitamin			
B_1 (Thiamine) (water-soluble/B-complex group)	Promotes carbohydrate metabolism (energy) and is required for good function of the nervous system and as a replacement in deficiency.	Enriched, fortified whole-grain products; legumes; cereal grains; pork is the richest source of the natural vitamin.	Beriberi; metabolic disorders; necrotizing encephalomyelopathy; cardiovascular complications; neurologic disorders; ataxia; diplopia; Wernicke encephalopathy and Korsakoff syndrome, significant CNS disorders, and alcoholism.
B_2 (Riboflavin) (water-soluble/in B-complex group)	Promotes body's use of carbohydrates, proteins, and fats; is required for tissue integrity; necessary for normal RBC function.	Milk, enriched flour, green vegetables, yogurt, eggs, nuts, cheese, and meats, especially organ meats (liver and kidney).	Sore throat, dry/cracked skin at the corners of the mouth can signal deficiency, pellagra (dermatitis/mental disturbance), microcytic anemia, and alcoholism.
B_3 (Niacin or nicotinic acid) (water-soluble in B-complex group)	In all body tissues; necessary for energy-producing reactions (lipid metabolism, glycogenolysis, and tissue respiration) and assists nervous system. Large doses decrease lipoprotein and triglyceride synthesis by inhibiting the release of free fatty acids from adipose tissue and decreasing hepatic lipoprotein synthesis.	In many foods: animal and plant protein, liver, peanuts, mushrooms, whole wheat, enriched grains, green vegetables, and unpolished rice.	Pellagra (rough skin), flushing of the face and neck, pruritus, abdominal pain, hepatotoxicity, headache, dizziness, blurred vision, orthostatic hypertension, memory loss, anorexia, insomnia, and alcoholism.
B_6 (pyridoxine) (water-soluble/in B-complex group)	Required for amino acid, carbohydrate, and lipid metabolism, protein synthesis, and formation of RBCs.	Cereal grains, meat, fish, vegetables, legumes, white potatoes, and organ meats.	Neuritis, convulsions, seborrheic dermatitis, anemia, depression, confusion, and alcoholism.
B_{12} (cobalamin) (water-soluble)	Functions as nucleic acid to help RBCs; aids in functioning of the nervous system; assists in the making of DNA in our cells.	Liver, kidney, fish, dairy products, eggs, chicken, and meat.	Low levels can cause GI disorders, poor growth, neurologic damage from anemia, and pernicious anemias. Deficiency may be found in strict vegans. Receive laboratory work before treatment: Iron, reticulocyte, Hct, folate, and B_{12} concentrations.
Folic acid (vitamin B_9) (folate) (water-soluble, in B-complex group)	Essential in the synthesis of DNA; assists with intestinal functioning and prevents certain anemias.	Leafy green vegetables, yellow fruits and vegetables, yeast, organ meats, black-eyed peas, and lentils.	Decreases occur in WBC count and clotting factors, along with anemias (pernicious, thalassemia, megaloblastic, macrocytic), intestinal disturbances, depression, and alcoholism.
Pantothenic acid (vitamin B_5) (folate) (water-soluble)	Essential nutrient in multiple biochemical processes: gluconeogenesis, carbohydrate metabolism, fatty acid synthesis, biosynthesis of steroid hormones, and acetylcholine.	Present in peas, beans, lean meat, fish, poultry, eggs, milk, and whole-grain cereals (most foods).	Unlike other vitamins, pantothenic acid has no RDA. It is questionable whether a true deficiency state can be produced in the absence of other deficiencies, perhaps due to the widespread availability of pantothenic acid in foods. Deficiency states have been observed in conjunction with other B-complex vitamin deficiencies.
Biotin (vitamin H; coenzyme R; classified as a B vitamin) (water-soluble)	Responsible for metabolism and synthesis of fats, carbohydrates, and amino acids in energy production.	Eggs (egg yolk), milk, liver, kidney, nuts, soybean, and oat bran.	Natural deficiency is unknown in humans. There is a risk of hypersensitivity as with all medications: Chest pain, shortness of breath, hives, and skin rash.
C (ascorbic acid) (water-soluble)	Free radical antioxidant, essential for tissue repair and growth, required for formation of collagen.	Citrus fruits, cantaloupe, tomatoes, leafy green vegetables, green peppers, potatoes, strawberries, and kiwi fruit.	Deficiency leads to poor wound healing, bleeding gums, scurvy, and faulty bone and tooth development. Deficiency is prevalent in critical illness. High doses of vitamin C used in treatment of sepsis, trauma, and burns with beneficial effects and no adverse reactions.

TABLE 13.2 Vitamins: Functions, Suggested Food Sources, and Deficiency Conditions—cont'd

Vitamin	Function	Food Sources	Deficiency Conditions
D (cholecalciferol—vitamin D_3 and ergocalciferol, vitamin D_2) (fat-soluble)	Promotes phosphorus and calcium balance, important for strong teeth and bones.	Vitamin D–fortified milk, cereal, eggs, fatty fish, and liver.	Rickets can occur in children; osteomalacia in adults.
E (alpha-tocopherol) (fat-soluble)	Promotes formation and functioning of RBCs, muscles, and other tissues. Acts as an antioxidant and plays a role in antiinflammatory processes, inhibition of platelet aggregation, and immune enhancement.	Whole-grain cereals, wheat germ, sunflower seeds, milk, eggs, meat, avocados, asparagus, broccoli, spinach, and vegetable oils.	Breakdown of RBCs can occur with deficiency. Also, peripheral neuropathies, ataxia, retinopathy, and impairment of the immune response.
K (phytonadione) (fat-soluble)	Essential for blood clotting (the "coagulations vitamin").	Leafy green vegetables (broccoli, brussel sprouts, collard greens, lettuce, spinach), liver, cheese, egg yolk, and vegetable oil (soybean and canola).	Increased clotting time leads to increased bleeding and hemorrhage.

CNS, Central nervous system; *GI*, gastrointestinal; *Hct*, hematocrit; *RBC*, red blood cell; *RDA*, required dietary allowance, *WBC*, white blood cell.

PROTOTYPE DRUG CHART

Vitamin A

Drug Class	Dosage
Vitamin A (retinol) Fat-soluble vitamin	Daily requirements[a]: A: 700 mcg/day (females); 900 mcg/day (males) NOTE: Pregnancy: 770 mcg/day RDA Vitamin A in excess of RDA can cause fetal harm. Tolerable upper limit (UL) of vitamin A 3000 mcg/d Severe deficiency: A: IM 30,000 mcg/day × 3 days; then 15,000 mcg/day IM × 14 days, then follow-up with oral supplement

Contraindications	Drug-Lab-Food Interactions
Presence of cases of Hypervitaminosis A; Vitamin A in pregnancy avoid amounts > RDA (770 mcg/day) requirement in excess can result in fetal abnormalities. Hypersensitivity to ingredients in parenteral preparations (Polysorbate-80).	Drugs that decrease absorption of vitamin A: Castor oil (toxic effect), mineral oil, cholestyramine, colestipol, colesevelam, orlistat. Moderate risk of phototoxicity reaction: St John's Wort; veteporfin. Porfimer has a major risk of photosensitivity. Moderate risk of dryness of skin: Salicylic acid, sodium thiosulfate. Lab: May increase BUN, calcium, cholesterol, and triglycerides; may lower erythrocyte and leukocyte counts. Food: None known

Pharmacokinetics	Pharmacodynamics
Absorption: PO: 1 h (GI absorption requires bile acids, fat, lipase, and protein) Distribution: PB: Large amounts concentrate in liver for storage. Metabolism: Mostly through the liver; t½: UK Excretion: Excreted in urine and feces	PO: Onset: quickly Peak: 3–5 h Duration: UK

Therapeutic Effects/Uses

Treatment of vitamin A deficiency, biliary tract or pancreatic disease, colitis, cirrhosis, celiac disease, skin disorders, prevention of night blindness, and promotion of bone development
Mechanism of Action: Essential for developmental growth, bone and teeth development, vision, integrity of skin and mucous membranes, and reproduction

Side Effects	Adverse Reactions
Headache, fatigue, drowsiness, irritability, anorexia, vomiting, diarrhea, dry skin, visual changes	Anaphylactic shock and anaphylactoid reactions, increased intracranial pressure, hypervitaminosis A, thrombocytopenia, cholestasis, hepatomegaly, metabolic acidosis, hypotension

A, Adult; *BUN*, blood urea nitrogen; *C*, child; *GI*, gastrointestinal; *IM*, intramuscular; *PB*, protein binding; *PO*, by mouth; *t½*, half-life; *UK*, unknown; *RDA*, recommended dietary allowance.
[a]For daily requirements, see https://www.nal.usda.gov/programs/fnic and https://www.ods.od.nih.gov

then converted to an active form, calcitriol, in the kidneys. Studies have suggested that vitamin D taken with calcium can reduce the incidence of fractures. Vitamin D deficiency can cause rickets in children and osteomalacia in adults as well as bone fractures.

Calcitriol, the active form of vitamin D, functions as a hormone, and along with parathyroid hormone (PTH) and calcitonin, it regulates calcium and phosphorus metabolism. Calcitriol and PTH stimulate bone reabsorption of calcium and phosphorus. Excretion of vitamin D is primarily in bile; only a small amount is excreted in the urine. If serum calcium levels are low, more vitamin D is activated; when serum calcium levels are normal, activation of vitamin D is decreased. The normal adult RDA of vitamin D is 15 mcg/day (600 IU/day) by mouth a day.

Tolerable upper intake level is 4000 International units/day (100 mcg/day). Excess vitamin D ingestion (>4000 IU/day) results in hypervitaminosis D and may cause hypercalcemia (an elevated serum calcium level). Anorexia, nausea, and vomiting are early symptoms of vitamin D toxicity.

Vitamin E

Vitamin E has antioxidant properties that protect cellular components from being oxidized and protect red blood cells (RBCs) from hemolysis. Vitamin E depends on bile salts, pancreatic secretion, and fat for its absorption. Vitamin E is stored in all tissues, especially the liver, muscle, and fatty tissue. About 75% of vitamin E is excreted in bile.

Although early evidence had suggested the potential for vitamin E to reduce cardiovascular disease (CVD), more recent outcome studies have not shown CVD benefits with vitamin E. Currently, the American Heart Association guidelines do not recommend vitamin E therapy as a preventative measure for CVD. Vitamin E has been of interest for its antioxidant properties, and it has been used off-label for various conditions, including Alzheimer disease.

The RDA of vitamin E in adults is 22.4 IU/day (15 mg/day) and should not exceed the UL of 1000 mg/day (1500 IU/day) in oral intake. The dosage is determined by nutritional intake or degree of deficiency by the HCP. The RDA for lactating persons is 19 mg (28.4 IU) by mouth daily. Vitamin E deficiency is rare, and supplementation of vitamin E during lactation is not necessary for people with normal fat absorption.

Side effects of large doses of vitamin E may include fatigue, weakness, nausea, GI upset, headache, bleeding, and breast tenderness. Vitamin E may prolong the prothrombin time (PT), and patients taking warfarin should have their PT monitored closely. Iron and vitamin E should not be taken together because iron can interfere with the body's absorption and use of vitamin E.

Vitamin K

Vitamin K received its name in 1935 when it was called "Koagulationsvitamin," which means "clotting vitamin." Vitamin K occurs in three forms. Vitamin K_1 (phytonadione) is the most active form and is a synthetic type of vitamin K made by plants, and it represents the bulk of dietary vitamin K. Vitamin K_2 (menaquinone) is synthesized by probiotic bacteria in the digestive tract. Vitamin K_3 (menadione) is another synthetic form of vitamin K. After vitamin K is absorbed, it is stored primarily in the liver and in other tissues. Half of vitamin K comes from the intestinal flora, and the remaining portion comes from the diet. The RDA for an adult male is 120 mcg/day, and for an adult female the RDA is 90 mcg/day. The National Academy of Medicine has not been able to determine a tolerable upper level for vitamin K, so always speak to an HCP before increasing the dose of vitamin K.

Vitamin K is needed for the synthesis of prothrombin and clotting factors VII, IX, and X. For oral anticoagulant overdose, vitamin K_1 (phytonadione) is the only vitamin K form available for therapeutic use and is most effective in preventing hemorrhage. Vitamin K is used for two purposes: as an antidote for oral anticoagulant overdose and to prevent and treat the hypoprothrombinemia of vitamin K deficiency. Spontaneous hemorrhage may occur with vitamin K deficiency due to lack of bile salts and malabsorption syndromes that interfere with vitamin K uptake (e.g., celiac disease). Vitamin K deficiency is uncommon in adults, but certain people are at increased risk: those taking anticoagulant therapy such as warfarin, people receiving antibiotic therapy, and those who have fat malabsorption syndrome. Some of the side effects of vitamin K deficiency are increased bruising, bleeding from mucous membranes, and dark, tarry stools. When vitamin K levels are too high, people can form excessive blood clots quickly, which can cause stroke, heart attack, and blocked blood flow anywhere in the body. Vitamin K (Phytonadione) carries the FDA Blackbox Warning.

Newborns are vitamin K deficient, oral administration of vitamin K for prophylaxis of vitamin K deficiency bleeding (VKDB) is common in other countries; however, intramuscular (IM) administration of vitamin K is standard practice in the United States due to its superior efficacy for preventing late VKDB. The controversy in other countries is because it can elevate the bilirubin level and can cause hyperbilirubinemia with a risk of kernicterus. Oral and parenteral forms of phytonadione are available; intravenous (IV) administration is dangerous and may cause death.

Water-Soluble Vitamins

Water-soluble vitamins are the B-complex vitamins and vitamin C. This group of vitamins is not usually toxic unless taken in extremely excessive amounts. Water-soluble vitamins are not stored by the body, so consistent, steady supplementation is required. Water-soluble vitamins are readily excreted in the urine. Protein binding of water-soluble vitamins is minimal. Foods that are high in vitamin B are grains, cereals, breads, and meats. There are reports that B vitamins may promote a sense of well-being and increased energy as well as decreased anger, tension, and irritability. Citrus fruits and green vegetables are high in vitamin C. If the fruits and vegetables are cut or cooked, a large amount of vitamin C is lost.

Vitamin B Complex

Vitamin B_1 (thiamine), vitamin B_2 (riboflavin), vitamin B_3 (nicotinic acid or niacin), and vitamin B_6 (pyridoxine) are four vitamins in the vitamin B–complex group that are water-soluble. Vitamin B complex is a common group of vitamins administered in the clinical setting, especially to patients with alcoholism.

Thiamine deficiency can lead to the polyneuritis and cardiac pathology seen in Beriberi or Wernicke encephalopathy that progresses to Korsakoff syndrome, conditions most commonly associated with alcohol abuse. Wernicke-Korsakoff syndrome is a significant central nervous system (CNS) disorder characterized by confusion, nystagmus, diplopia, ataxia, and loss of recent memory. If not treated, it can cause irreversible brain damage. IV administration of thiamine is recommended for treatment of Wernicke-Korsakoff syndrome. Thiamine must be given before giving any glucose to avoid aggravation of symptoms.

Riboflavin may be given to manage dermatologic problems such as scaly dermatitis, cracked corners of the mouth, and inflammation of the skin and tongue. To treat migraine headaches, riboflavin is given in larger doses than for dermatologic concerns.

Niacin is given to alleviate pellagra and hyperlipidemia, for which large doses are required. Chapter 44 offers a discussion of niacin use to reduce cholesterol levels. However, large doses may cause GI irritation and vasodilation, resulting in a flushing sensation.

Pyridoxine is administered to correct vitamin B_6 deficiency. It may also help alleviate the symptoms of neuritis caused by isoniazid (INH) therapy for tuberculosis. Vitamin B_6 is essential as a building block of nucleic acids, in RBC formation, and in synthesis of hemoglobin. Pyridoxine is used to treat vitamin B_6 deficiency caused by lack of adequate diet, inborn errors of metabolism, or drug-induced deficiencies secondary to INH, penicillamine, or cyclosporine (or hydralazine) therapy. It is also used to treat neonates with seizures refractory to traditional therapy. Vitamin B_6 deficiencies may occur in patients with alcoholism along with deficiencies of other B-complex vitamins. Patients with diabetes or alcoholism may benefit from daily supplementation. Pyridoxine is readily absorbed in the jejunum and is stored in the liver, muscle, and brain. It is metabolized in the liver and excreted in the urine.

Vitamin C

Vitamin C (ascorbic acid) is absorbed from the small intestine. Vitamin C aids in the absorption of iron and in the conversion of folic acid. Vitamin C is not stored in the body and is excreted readily in the urine. A high serum vitamin C level that results from excessive dosing of vitamin C is excreted by the kidneys unchanged. Vitamin C is used in the treatment of scurvy, which is rare in developed countries but seen in individuals who consume few fruits and vegetables. Also, scurvy is seen in people who are on restricted diets or who abuse alcohol or drugs.

The RDA of vitamin C (adult dose) is 75 mg/day for females and 90 mg/day for males to prevent deficiency. Some individuals take greater amounts. Massive doses of vitamin C can cause GI upset.

PROTOTYPE DRUG CHART

Vitamin C

Drug Class	Dosage
Water-soluble vitamin	Daily requirements[a]: A: PO 75 mg/d (female); 90 mg/d (males); (male smokers PO 125 mg/d, female smokers PO 110 mg/d) Severe deficit: Scurvy A: PO: 500 mg to 1000 mg/d 2–4 weeks. IV: 200 mg/day × 1 week; if treatment unresolved may continue dose until symptoms resolve
Contraindications	**Drug-Lab-Food Interactions**
Caution: Acute and chronic oxalate nephropathy has been reported with prolonged administration of high doses of ascorbic acid. Acidification of the urine by ascorbic acid may lead to precipitation of cysteine, urate, or oxalate stones. Use cautiously in recurrent kidney stones. Patients with renal disease, renal impairment, or renal failure may be at increased risk. Can increase risk of iron toxicity in patients with hemochromatosis; patients should limit intake to no more than 500 mg/day. Ascorbic acid is a strong reducing agent and can lead to lab test interference based on oxidation-reduction reactions.	Decreases ascorbic acid uptake when taken with salicylates; may decrease effect of oral anticoagulants (warfarin); may decrease elimination of aspirins Lab: May decrease bilirubin and urinary pH; may increase uric acid and uric oxalate Food: None known
Pharmacokinetics	**Pharmacodynamics**
Absorption: PO: Quickly absorbed in the intestines (70–90%) Distribution: PB: 25% Metabolism: t½: 8–40 days related to body stores Excretion: In the urine; unchanged with high doses	PO: Absorbed orally through active transport Onset: >2 days–3 wks Peak: UK Duration: UK
Therapeutic Effects/Uses	
To prevent and treat vitamin C deficiency (scurvy), to increase wound healing, and for burns; preserves integrity of blood vessels. Mechanism of Action: A water-soluble vitamin, it is essential for collagen formation and tissue repair (bones, skin, blood vessels) and for synthesis of lipids, protein, and carnitine.	
Side Effects	**Adverse Reactions**
Oral: Nausea, vomiting, diarrhea, heartburn, headache Parenteral: Flushing, headache, dizziness, soreness at injection site	Kidney stones, crystalluria, hyperuricemia, hemolytic anemia Life-threatening: Sickle cell crisis, deep venous thrombosis

A, Adult; *bid*, twice a day; *C*, child; *d*, day; *IM*, intramuscular; *IV*, intravenous; *PB*, protein binding; *PO*, by mouth; *RDA*, recommended dietary allowance; *t½*, half-life; *UK*, unknown; *wks*, weeks.

[a]For daily requirements, see https://www.nal.usda.gov/program/fnic and https://www.ods.od.nih.gov

Prototype Drug Chart: Vitamin C details pharmacologic data on vitamin C.

Pharmacokinetics. Vitamin C is absorbed readily through the GI tract and is distributed throughout the body fluids. Approximately 70% to 90% of the usual dietary intake of ascorbic acid (30 to 180 mg/day) is absorbed, although absorption falls to 50% or less with doses above 1 g/day or in patients with GI disease. The half-life of ascorbic acid varies widely from 8 to 40 days and is inversely related to body stores.

Intravenous doses can produce plasma concentrations 30- to 70-fold higher than the maximum tolerated oral doses. Peak concentrations after IV infusion are reached at the end of 30 minutes. The elimination half-life of ascorbic acid after IV administration is approximately 7 hrs.

The kidneys completely excrete vitamin C mostly unchanged.

Pharmacodynamics. Vitamin C is needed for carbohydrate metabolism and protein and lipid synthesis. Collagen synthesis also requires vitamin C because it is part of the intercellular matrix that binds cells together and aids in wound healing. Smoking decreases serum vitamin C levels. Vitamin C in doses greater than 500 mg aids iron absorption; however, it may decrease the effect of oral anticoagulants.

The use of large doses of vitamin C is questionable. Large doses of any vitamin can cause toxicity. Most authorities believe that vitamin C does not prevent the common cold, cure advanced cancer, or treat schizophrenia. Moreover, large doses of vitamin C can cause nausea, abdominal cramps, and diarrhea. If taken with aspirin or sulfonamides, it may cause crystal formation in the urine. Vitamin C directly irritates the intestinal mucosa in the GI tract. This is why the Food and Nutrition Board has set 2 g/day as the adult UL for vitamin C. Large doses of vitamin C can decrease the effect of oral anticoagulants. If large doses of any vitamin are to be discontinued, a gradual reduction of the dosage is necessary to avoid vitamin deficiency.

Folic Acid (Folate)

Folic acid is a water-soluble, B-complex vitamin that is available orally and parenterally. This vitamin is found in a variety of foods including liver, kidneys, yeast, and leafy, green vegetables. A deficiency in folic acid can cause a variety of hematologic complications including megaloblastic and macrocytic anemias. Folic acid is absorbed from the small intestine, and the active form of folic acid—folate—is circulated to all tissues. One-third of folate is stored in the liver, and the rest is stored in the tissues. It is excreted 80% in bile and 20% in urine. The peak activity of folic acid occurs within one hour of administration.

Folic acid is essential for body growth. It is needed for DNA synthesis, and without folic acid, cellular division is disrupted. Adults' (oral dose) RDA is 0.4 mg/day. The adult tolerable UL for folic acid (oral) is 1 mg/day. Chronic alcoholism, poor nutritional intake, malabsorption syndromes, pregnancy, and drugs that cause inadequate absorption (phenytoin, barbiturates) or folic acid antagonism (methotrexate, triamterene, trimethoprim) are causes of folic acid deficiencies. Symptoms of folic acid deficiencies include anorexia, nausea, stomatitis, diarrhea, fatigue, alopecia, and blood dyscrasias (megaloblastic anemia, leukopenia, thrombocytopenia). These symptoms are usually not noted until 2 to 4 months after folic acid storage is depleted.

Folic acid **deficiency** during the first trimester of pregnancy can affect the development of the CNS of the fetus. This may cause neural tube defects such as spina bifida, defective closure of the bony structure of the spinal cord, or anencephaly, which is lack of brain mass formation. The US Public Health Services recommends that all females who may become pregnant consume 600 mcg (0.6 mg) of supplemental folic acid each day in addition to the folate they get with food. Synthetic folate is more stable than folic acid obtained from food: bioavailability is greater than 85% with synthetic folate and less than 59% for food-sourced folic acid.

Excessive doses of folic acid may mask signs of vitamin B_{12} deficiency, which is a risk in older adults. Patients taking phenytoin to control seizures should be cautious about taking folic acid. This vitamin can lower the serum phenytoin level, which could increase the risk of seizures; the phenytoin dose would need to be adjusted in such patients. This is a complex interaction that is not fully understood, but it is thought that 1 mg or less per day of folic acid is safe in patients with controlled epilepsy.

Vitamin B_{12}

Vitamin B_{12} (Cyanocobalamin), like folic acid, is essential for DNA synthesis. Vitamin B_{12} aids in the conversion of folic acid to its active form. With active folic acid, vitamin B_{12} promotes cellular division. It is also needed for normal hematopoiesis (development of RBCs in bone marrow) and to maintain nervous system integrity, especially of the myelin. The RDA for adults and adolescents >14 years of age is 2.4 mcg/day. Adults older than 50 years are advised to meet their RDA mainly by taking B_{12}-containing supplements or through foods fortified with B_{12} due to malabsorption of food-bound vitamin B_{12}. For pregnant adults and adolescents, their RDA is 2.6 mcg orally/day. For adults and adolescents who are lactating, their RDA is 2.8 mcg orally/day.

The gastric parietal cells produce an intrinsic factor that is necessary for the absorption of vitamin B_{12} through the intestinal wall. Without the intrinsic factor, little or no vitamin B_{12} is absorbed. After absorption, vitamin B_{12} binds to the protein transcobalamin II and is transferred to the tissues. Most vitamin B_{12} is stored in the liver and is slowly excreted, and it can take 2 to 3 years for stored vitamin B_{12} to be depleted and for a deficit to be noticed. After oral administration peak plasma levels are attained in 8–12 hours.

Adults who are deficient in vitamin B_{12} may receive it orally 1000 to 2000 mcg/day for 1–2 weeks, followed by 500 to 100 mcg/day. Vitamin B_{12} deficiency is uncommon unless there is a disturbance of the intrinsic factor and intestinal absorption. Pernicious anemia (lack of the intrinsic factor) is the major cause of vitamin B_{12} deficiency, but deficiency can also develop in strict vegetarians who do not consume meat, fish, or dairy products. Other possible causes of vitamin B_{12} deficiency include malabsorption syndromes (cancer, celiac disease, and certain drugs), gastrectomy, Crohn's disease, and liver and kidney diseases. Vitamin B_{12} deficiency is commonly seen with the use of metformin and proton pump inhibitors (e.g., omeprazole). Symptoms may include numbness and tingling in the lower extremities, weakness, fatigue, anorexia, loss of taste, diarrhea, memory loss, mood changes, dementia, psychosis, megaloblastic anemia with macrocytes (overenlarged erythrocytes [RBCs]) in the blood, and megaloblasts (overenlarged erythroblasts) in the bone marrow.

To correct vitamin B_{12} deficiency, cyanocobalamin in crystalline form can be given intramuscularly for severe deficits. A dose of 1000 mcg IM can be given daily or every other day for 1 week, then weekly for 4 to 8 weeks, then monthly until recovery. It cannot be given intravenously because of possible hypersensitivity reactions. Cyanocobalamin can be given orally and is commonly found in multivitamin preparations. It can also be given as a subcutaneous.

CHAPTER 13   Vitamin and Mineral Replacement

CLINICAL JUDGMENT [NURSING PROCESS]

Vitamins

Concept: Health, Wellness, and Illness

Health, wellness, and illness reflect the many stages of a person's life. Health looks at the absence of illness. Wellness is a balance of well-being throughout the life span. Illness refers to disease, disorder, morbidity, or sickness that impairs a person's normal body functioning. This may apply to physical problems experienced by the patient.

Recognize Cues [Assessment]
- Check the patient for vitamin deficiency before the start of therapy and regularly thereafter. Explore such areas as inadequate nutrient intake, debilitating disease, and gastrointestinal (GI) disorders.
- Obtain a 24- and 48-hour diet history analysis.
- When possible, obtain laboratory results to assess serum blood levels.

Analyze Cues and Prioritize Hypothesis [Patient Problems]
- Weight loss
- Hypokalemia
- Need for health teaching

Generate Solutions [Planning]
- The patient will verbalize the food groups included in ChooseMyPlate.gov at the end of the teaching session.
- The patient will explain the importance of vitamin C supplements before discharge.
- The patient will verbalize which foods contain fat-soluble vitamins A, D, E, and K before the next teaching.
- The patient will verbalize which foods contain water-soluble vitamins B, C, folic acid, and B_{12} before discharge.

Take Action [Nursing Interventions]
- Administer vitamins with food to promote absorption.
- Store vitamins in light-resistant containers.
- Use the supplied calibrated dropper for accurate dosing when administering vitamins in drop form. Solutions may be administered mixed with food or drink.
- Administer vitamins intramuscularly for patients who are unable to take vitamins by the oral route (e.g., those with GI malabsorption syndrome).
- Monitor serum blood levels of patient's suspected vitamin or mineral deficiency.
- Determine the patient's preferred and meaningful foods, and incorporate them into the food and supplement plan.
- Use interpreters as appropriate if the patient has a language barrier.

Patient Teaching

General
- Advise patients to take the prescribed amount of vitamins.
- Counsel patients to read vitamin labels carefully and discuss with a health care provider (HCP) before taking any vitamin or supplement.
- Advise patients to consult with an HCP or pharmacist regarding interactions with prescription and over-the-counter medications.
- Discourage patients from taking large-dose vitamins over a long period of time.
- Instruct patients to only take supplements prescribed by HCP.
- Instruct patients when stopping long-term use of high-dose vitamin therapy, a gradual decrease in vitamin intake is advised to avoid vitamin deficiency and always notify HCP.
- Instruct patients that skipping vitamins for short-term use is not a cause of concern because deficiencies occur over long-term omissions.
- Advise patients to check expiration dates on vitamin containers before purchasing. Potency of vitamins is reduced after the expiration date.
- Counsel patients to avoid taking mineral oil with vitamin A on a regular basis because it interferes with absorption of the vitamin; mineral oil also interferes with vitamin K absorption. If needed, take mineral oil at bedtime and vitamins in the morning.
- Instruct patients that there is no scientific evidence that large doses of vitamin C will cure a cold.
- Alert patients not to take large doses of vitamin C with aspirin or sulfonamides because crystals may form in the kidneys and urine.
- Alert patients to avoid excessive intake of alcoholic beverages. Alcohol can cause vitamin B–complex deficiencies.

Diet
- Advise patients to eat a well-balanced diet. Vitamin supplements are not necessary if the person is healthy and receives proper nutrition on a regular basis.
- Educate patients about foods rich in vitamin A, including milk, butter, eggs, and leafy green and yellow vegetables. Foods rich in various vitamins are listed in Table 13.2.
- Have the patient keep a diet chart for a full week to determine typical nutrition.
- Have the patient verbalize important foods that contain fat- and water-soluble vitamins.

Side Effects
- Advise patients that nausea, vomiting, headache, loss of hair, and cracked lips (symptoms of hypervitaminosis for vitamin A) should be reported to the HCP. Early symptoms of hypervitaminosis vitamin D are anorexia, nausea, and vomiting.

Evaluate Outcomes [Evaluation]
- Evaluate the patient's understanding of the purpose and use of vitamins.
- Evaluate the effectiveness of the patient's diet.
- Determine whether the patient with malnutrition is receiving appropriate vitamin therapy.

MINERALS

Various minerals—such as iron, copper, zinc, chromium, and selenium—are needed for body function.

 ## Iron

Iron is used in the treatment and prevention of iron-deficiency anemia and for nutritional supplementation when iron intake in the diet is inadequate to meet body needs. Iron is an essential mineral and is a component of hemoglobin, myoglobin, and multiple enzymes. A normal diet contains 5 to 20 mg of iron per day. Foods rich in iron include liver, lean meats, egg yolks, dried beans, green vegetables (e.g., spinach), and fruit. Food and antacids slow the absorption of iron, and vitamin C increases iron absorption.

During pregnancy, iron requirements increase due to the expansion of maternal blood volume and production of RBCs by the fetus. The iron needs of pregnancy are too great to be met through diet alone;

therefore supplementation is needed. In pregnancy, adults are recommended 27 mg daily.

The required iron dose for males is 8 mg/day. The dose for females ages 19–50 is 18 mg/day or 8 mg/day for those older than 51 years. Maximum Dose Limit: Dosage with iron must be individualized according to the patient's age, dietary intake requirements, and the degree of iron deficiency. Excess accumulation may occur if iron therapy is continued after the correction of the dietary deficiency. Prototype Drug Chart: Iron describes the pharmacologic data on iron.

Pharmacokinetics

Iron is absorbed by the intestines and enters the plasma as hemoglobin, or it may be stored as ferritin. Although food decreases absorption by 25% to 50%, it may be necessary to take iron preparations with food to avoid GI discomfort. Vitamin C at doses greater than 500 mg may slightly increase iron absorption, whereas tetracycline, quinolone antibiotics (ciprofloxacin, levofloxacin, etc.), and antacids can decrease absorption.

> **COMPLEMENTARY AND ALTERNATIVE THERAPIES**
>
> *Iron*
>
> Chamomile, feverfew, peppermint, and St. John's wort interfere with the absorption of iron and other minerals.

Pharmacodynamics

Iron replacement is given primarily to correct or control iron-deficiency anemias, which are diagnosed by a laboratory blood smear. Clinical signs and symptoms for deficiency include fatigue, weakness, shortness of breath, pallor, and, in cases of severe anemia, increased GI bleeding.

The onset of action for iron therapy takes days, and its peak action does not occur for days or weeks; therefore the patient's symptoms are slow to improve. Increased hemoglobin and hematocrit levels occur within 3 to 7 days.

About 30% to 50% of adults on parenteral nutrition have been shown to have iron deficiency.

 Iron toxicity is a serious cause of poisoning in children and carries a black-box warning from the FDA. As few as 10 tablets of ferrous sulfate (3 g) taken at one time can be fatal within 12 to 48 hours; hemorrhage from the ulcerogenic effects of unbound iron leads to shock. Therefore parents should be strongly cautioned against leaving iron tablets that look like candy within a child's reach. (Most iron products are distributed in bubble packs.) There is also danger of children and adults overdosing on multivitamins that contain iron.

Copper

Copper is needed for the formation of RBCs and connective tissues. Copper is a cofactor of many enzymes, and its function is in the production of the neurotransmitters, norepinephrine, and dopamine. Excess serum copper levels may be associated with Wilson disease, an inborn error of metabolism that allows for large amounts of copper to accumulate in the liver, kidneys, brain, and cornea (brown or green Kayser-Fleischer rings).

A prolonged copper deficiency may result in anemia that cannot be corrected by taking iron supplements. Abnormal blood and skin changes caused by a copper deficiency include a decrease in white blood cell count, glucose intolerance, and a decrease in skin and hair pigmentation. Intellectual disability may also occur in the young. Copper deficiency in patients receiving parenteral nutrition ranges from 30% to 56% and includes both adults and children.

The RDA for copper in adults 19 yrs and older is 900 mcg/day. Most adults consume about 1 mg/day. Foods rich in copper are shellfish (crab, oysters), liver, nuts, seeds (sunflower, sesame), legumes, and cocoa.

Zinc

Zinc is a trace element and important to many enzymatic reactions. It is essential for biologic functions and, in animals, is important in growth, appetite, testicular maturation, skin integrity, mental activity, wound healing, and immunocompetence. Zinc deficiency is associated with diets high in unrefined cereal and unleavened bread, total parenteral nutrition (TPN), intestinal disease (i.e., Crohn's disease, pancreatic insufficiency), alcoholism, pregnancy, or acrodermatitis enteropathy, an autosomal recessive disease characterized by zinc malabsorption. Some believe zinc can alleviate symptoms of the common cold and shorten its duration, although studies have disputed this claim. Large amounts of zinc can be toxic. Zinc in lozenge form can cause nausea and can leave an unpleasant taste, and zinc in nasal sprays has caused patients to lose their sense of smell. Patients should always check with an HCP before taking zinc. The adult RDA for adults older than 19 years of age for females is 8 mg/day/PO and males 11 mg/day/PO. Foods rich in zinc include beef, lamb, eggs, and leafy and root vegetables.

Large doses, more than 150 mg, may cause a copper deficiency, a decrease in high-density lipoprotein (HDL) cholesterol ("good" cholesterol), and a weakened immune response. Zinc can inhibit tetracycline absorption. Patients taking zinc and an antibiotic should not take them together; zinc should be taken at least 2 hours after taking an antibiotic. About 10% of adults on long-term parenteral nutrition develop a zinc deficiency. Zinc is the most common deficiency likely to occur in parenteral nutrition because zinc is lost in the patient's stool.

Chromium

Chromium, in its trivalent state (i.e., Cr^{3+}), is an essential trace element required for proper carbohydrate, lipid, and nucleic acid metabolism in the human body. Overt signs and symptoms of chromium deficiency are usually only observed in adult patients eating diets high in refined foods or who are receiving long-term TPN without chromium supplementation. Chromium supplementation should only be expected to improve disorders that are due to chromium deficiency.

Limited studies have reported that chromium helps normalize blood glucose by increasing the effects of insulin on the cells. However, the importance of chromium deficiency in the average patient with type 2 diabetes has not been established. In addition, there are claims that chromium weight loss and muscle building. Multiple studies have concluded that there is no evidence that chromium supplementation increases muscle mass to a level greater than that which is produced with a healthy diet and exercise alone. Multivitamin and mineral preparations contain chloride salt of chromium. Some signs and symptoms of chromium deficiency are low blood sugar, dizziness, a need for frequent meals, sleepiness at odd times, a craving for sweet food, and excessive thirst. In chromium excess or toxicity, patients may experience GI bleeding, coagulopathy, seizures, and pulmonary dysfunction.

PROTOTYPE DRUG CHART

Iron

Drug Class	Dosage
Ferrous sulfate (20% elemental iron), ferrous gluconate (12% elemental iron), ferrous fumarate (33% elemental iron). Mineral to decrease anemia Note: Various iron products are not exchangeable on a milligram-to-milligram basis because each contains different amounts of elemental iron.	*Daily oral requirements*[a]: A: 18 mg/d (females 19–50 yrs old); A: 8 mg/d (females 51 or older); A: Males 8 mg/d; Pregnant persons 27 mg/d; Lactating Adults 9 mg/d. *Iron Deficiency Anemia:* 60 mg of elemental iron 1–3 times/d × 4 wk (repeat labs)
Contraindications	**Drug-Lab-Food Interactions**
⚠ High Alert Drug Black-Box Warning: Absolute contraindications: Hemosiderosis (excessive iron deposits in tissues); Hemochromatosis (iron overload); Sideroblastic anemia and Thalassemia (iron-loading anemias). Caution: Hemolytic anemia, peptic ulcer disease, and colitis. Caution: Bronchial asthma, iron hypersensitivity.	Increased effect of iron with vitamin C; decreased effect of tetracycline, antacids, aspirin, proton pump inhibitors, and (major) penicillamine Lab: May increase bilirubin; may decrease calcium. Monitor: Iron or ferritin levels, periodic CBC or hematocrit/hemoglobin levels. Food: None known
Pharmacokinetics	**Pharmacodynamics**
Absorption: PO: 10%–30% intestines Distribution: PB: UK Metabolism: t½: 6–8 h Excretion: In urine, feces, and sweat	PO: Onset: 4 d Peak: 7–14 d Duration: 3–4 mo
Therapeutic Effects/Uses	
To prevent and treat iron-deficiency anemia Mechanism of Action: Enables RBC development and oxygen transport via hemoglobin	
Side Effects	**Adverse Reactions**
Nausea, vomiting, diarrhea, constipation, epigastric pain; elixir may stain teeth.	May aggravate existing GI conditions and may cause pallor or drowsiness *Life-threatening:* Iron poisoning (mostly in children) may result in cardiovascular collapse, metabolic acidosis Toxicity: Nausea, vomiting, diarrhea (green then tarry stools), hematemesis, pallor, cyanosis, shock, coma

A, Adult; *bid*, two times a day; *C*, child; *GI*, gastrointestinal; *PB*, protein binding; *PO*, by mouth; *RBC*, red blood cell; *t½*, half-life; *UK*, unknown; mo, month; h, hours.
[a]For daily requirements, see https://www.nal.usda.gov/programs/fnic and https://www.ods.od.nih.gov.

There is no RDA for chromium. For adults, adolescents, and pregnant females, suggested intake is 29 to 30 mcg/PO/d; for adult and adolescent lactating females, it is 44 to 45 mg/PO/d. For adult males >50 years, it is 30 mcg/PO/d, and for adult females > 50 years, it is 20 mcg/PO/d.

Foods rich in chromium include meats, whole-grain cereals, and brewer's yeast.

Selenium

Selenium is an essential nonmetallic element chemically related to sulfur. It is nutritionally essential for humans and is a constituent of more than two dozen selenoproteins (a protein that includes selenocysteine amino acid residue) that play critical roles in reproduction, thyroid hormone metabolism, DNA synthesis, and protection from oxidative damage and infection. Symptoms of selenium deficiency include hypothyroidism, muscle weakness, myalgia, myositis, increased erythrocyte fragility, pancreatic degeneration, macrocytosis, and pseudoalbinism. Selenium works with vitamin E.

It is thought that selenium has an anticarcinogenic effect, and doses lower than 200 mcg may reduce the risk of lung, prostate, and colorectal cancer. However, research has never proven selenium's anticarcinogenic properties. Excess doses of more than 200 mcg might cause weakness, hair loss, dermatitis, nausea, diarrhea, and abdominal pain. Also, there may be a garlic-like odor from the skin and breath.

The adult RDA for selenium is 55 mcg/PO/d. The maximum adult dosage including geriatric adults is 400 mcg/d/PO; 60 mcg/day IV per FDA approved labeling. Foods rich in selenium include meats, especially liver, seafood, poultry, and grains.

CLINICAL JUDGMENT [NURSING PROCESS]

Antianemia Mineral: Iron

Concept: Health, Wellness, and Illness
Health, wellness, and illness reflect the many stages of a person's life. Health looks at the absence of illness. Wellness is a balance of well-being throughout the life span. Illness refers to disease, disorder, morbidity, or sickness that impairs a person's normal body functioning. This may apply to physical problems experienced by the patient.

Recognize Cues [Assessment]
- Obtain a history of current drugs and herbs the patient is taking.
- Obtain a medical history of health problems such as anemia.
- Assess the patient for signs and symptoms of iron-deficiency anemia, such as fatigue, malaise, pallor, shortness of breath, tachycardia, and cardiac dysrhythmia.
- Assess the patient's red blood cell (RBC) count, hemoglobin, hematocrit, iron level, and reticulocyte count before the start of and throughout therapy.

Analyze Cues and Prioritize Hypothesis [Patient Problems]
- Weight loss
- Confusion
- Fatigue
- Constipation

Generate Solutions [Planning]
- The patient will name at least six foods high in iron content.
- The patient will consume foods rich in iron.
- The patient will explain the importance of iron supplements.
- The patient will explain the significance of the red blood count, hemoglobin, and hematocrit labs related to anemia prior to discharge.

Take Action [Nursing Interventions]
- Encourage patients to eat a nutritious diet to obtain sufficient iron. Iron supplements are not needed unless a person is malnourished or pregnant or has abnormal menses.
- Store vitamins in light-resistant containers.
- Administer iron intramuscularly by the Z-track method to avoid leakage of iron into the subcutaneous tissue and skin, resulting in irritation and stains to the skin.
- Discuss the importance of keeping appointments with the health care provider (HCP) and receiving the required laboratory work before each visit with the HCP.
- Use an interpreter if needed.

Patient Teaching
General
- Advise patients to take the tablet or capsule between meals with at least 8 ounces of juice or water to promote absorption. If gastric irritation occurs, instruct the patient to take supplements with food.
- Advise patients to swallow the tablet or capsule whole.
- Encourage patients to maintain an upright position for 30 minutes after taking oral iron preparations to prevent esophageal corrosion from reflux.
- Do not administer the iron tablet within 1 hour of ingesting antacids, milk, or milk products, such as ice cream or yogurt.
- Counsel patients that certain herbal supplements can decrease absorption of iron and other minerals (see Complementary and Alternative Therapies: Iron).
- Advise patients to increase fluids, activity, and dietary bulk to avoid or relieve constipation. Slow-release iron capsules decrease constipation and gastric irritation.
- Instruct adults not to leave iron tablets within reach of children. Iron has a black-box warning and is high risk to overdose in children. If a child swallows many tablets, induce vomiting and immediately call the local poison control center.
- Encourage patients to take only the prescribed amount of drug to avoid iron poisoning. Be alert to the iron in multivitamin preparations.
- Be alert that iron content varies among iron salts; therefore do not substitute one for another.
- Advise patients that drug treatment for anemia is generally less than 6 months.

Diet
- Counsel patients to include iron-rich foods in their diet, such as lean meats, egg yolk, dried beans, green vegetables, and fruit.

Side Effects
- Advise patients taking a liquid iron preparation to use a straw to prevent discoloration of tooth enamel.
- Alert patients that the drug turns stools a harmless black or dark green.
- Instruct patients about signs and symptoms of toxicity, including nausea, vomiting, diarrhea, pallor, hematemesis, shock, and coma, and report these occurrences to the HCP.

Evaluation Outcomes [Evaluation]
- Evaluate the effectiveness of iron therapy by determining that the patient is not fatigued or short of breath and that the hemoglobin level is within the desired range.

CLINICAL JUDGMENT CASE STUDY

The patient is a 60-year-old female who has been prescribed ferrous sulfate 325 mg/day for anemia. During the nursing assessment, the patient expressed desire to feel better so she can babysit her 2-year-old grandchild.

1. What precautions should the patient take regarding the container of ferrous sulfate? Explain your answer.
2. The patient asks whether she can take iron in the morning before breakfast. How should the nurse respond?
3. The patient asks the nurse whether any side effects are associated with taking iron. What is an appropriate response?
4. The patient asks whether she should include foods high in iron in her daily diet. How should the nurse respond?

REVIEW QUESTIONS

1. The nurse is reviewing a patient's laboratory test results and current medications and notes that the patient's prothrombin time is prolonged. The nurse checks the patient's medication list. What vitamin or mineral might be contributing to this?
   a. Vitamin A
   b. Selenium
   c. Vitamin D
   d. Vitamin E

2. A patient comes to the office with a chief complaint of hair loss and peeling skin. The nurse notes many vitamins and minerals are on the medication list. The patient reports using vitamins to treat liver disease. The patient's complaint may be caused by an excess of which vitamin or mineral?
   a. Vitamin A
   b. Zinc
   c. Vitamin C
   d. Vitamin D

3. The nurse routinely includes health teaching about vitamins to patients. Vitamin D has a major role in which process?
   a. Prevents night blindness and improves vision
   b. Regulates calcium and phosphorous metabolism
   c. Important for growth and development in children
   d. Responsible for DNA and prothrombin synthesis

4. The nurse is doing preconception counseling with a patient. The patient asks why she must take folic acid (folate) during pregnancy. What is the nurse's response?
   a. Folic acid prevents neural tube defects in the developing fetus.
   b. Folic acid is known to lower blood glucose in diabetic patients.
   c. Folic acid in the gastrointestinal system prevents celiac disease.
   d. Folic acid will prevent migraine headaches in pregnant females.

5. A prenatal patient tells the nurse that she is not taking vitamins because she heard that vitamins may cause damage to the fetus. What is the nurse's best response?
   a. Vitamins are beneficial to the pregnant mother and baby.
   b. Take extra vitamins now to make up for missed doses.
   c. Megadose of vitamins can be harmful in the first trimester.
   d. Taking vitamin doses above the recommended dietary allowance is not advised.

6. A patient asks the nurse for information about fat-soluble vitamins. What is the nurse's best response?
   a. Fat-soluble vitamins are metabolized rapidly.
   b. Fat-soluble vitamins cannot be stored in the liver.
   c. Fat-soluble vitamins are excreted slowly in urine.
   d. Fat-soluble vitamins can never be toxic.

7. A patient complains of night blindness. The nurse correctly recommends which foods?
   a. Skim milk and peas
   b. Fortified milk and eggs
   c. Nuts and yeast
   d. Enriched breads and cereals

8. A patient diagnosed with alcoholism has questions about his medications. The nurse correctly explains that alcoholism can be associated with deficiency of which vitamin?
   a. A (beta-carotene)
   b. B (B complex)
   c. D (ergocalciferol)
   d. K (phytonadione)

9. Which vitamin plays a major role in regulating calcium and phosphorus absorption?
   a. A
   b. B
   c. C
   d. D

10. A patient takes iron on a daily basis. Which comment from the patient suggests the need for health teaching related to iron?
    a. I will swallow the tablet whole.
    b. I will take the tablet before I go to bed.
    c. I will drink a cup of water after swallowing the iron tablet.
    d. I will keep the tablets out of children's reach.

11. A patient asks the nurse, "What does copper do for me? I think it must be bad for me." What is the nurse's "best" response?
    a. Copper is needed for red blood cell formation.
    b. Be sure to include nuts and seeds in your diet.
    c. Why do you think copper is bad for you?
    d. Only take your prescribed dose of copper 5 mg/d.

14

Nutritional Support

http://evolve.elsevier.com/McCuistion/pharmacology

OBJECTIVES

- Discuss the importance of adequate nutrition and hydration for maintenance of good health.
- Describe the recommended usage of preparations for enteral feeding.
- Describe the recommended usage of preparations for parenteral nutrition.

OUTLINE

Nutritional Support Therapy, 166
    Benefits of Nutrition, 166
    Oral Feeding, 166
Enteral Nutrition, 166
    Enteral Feedings: Routes, Solutions, and Delivery Methods, 167
    Enteral Feedings: Complications, Safety, and Medications, 168

Parenteral Nutrition, 170
    Patient Need, 170
    Parenteral Solutions, 170
Clinical Judgment Single-Episode Case Study, 172
Review Questions, 173

Nutrients are substances that nourish and aid in the development of the body. Nutrients provide energy, promote growth and development, and regulate body processes. Inadequate nutrient intake can cause malnutrition. Patients experiencing chronic or critical illnesses that result in surgery are at risk for malnutrition. Without adequate nutritional support, the body's metabolic processes slow down or stop. This can greatly diminish the body's organ functioning and cause a poor immune response. There are two routes for administering nutritional support: enteral nutrition (EN), which involves the gastrointestinal (GI) tract and can be given orally or by tube feeding; and total parenteral nutrition (TPN), which administers high-caloric nutrients through large veins.

NUTRITIONAL SUPPORT THERAPY

Benefits of Nutrition

The length of time a person may survive without nutrients is influenced by body weight, composition, genetics, health, and hydration. Patients who are critically ill may only tolerate a lack of nutrient support for a short period before organ failure occurs. Recovery is more rapidly needed for patients who have experienced trauma or burns so nutrition is started within 24 to 48 hours of admission to the hospital. Early administration of EN restores intestinal motility, maintains GI function, reduces the movement of bacteria and other organisms, improves wound healing, decreases the incidence of infection, and ultimately decreases the length of the hospital stay. Early nutritional support improves the patient's general health and produces favorable outcomes. In addition to nutrients, both hydration and electrolyte balance must be considered. If all three are not addressed, preventable complications like constipation, urinary tract infection, and pressure ulcers can occur. The requirements for fluid balance are usually between 30 and 35 mL/kg per day. A healthy person requires 2000 calories per day; critically ill patients require 50% more than the normal energy requirement (approximately 3000 calories per day). If a patient has a 10% weight loss within the past 3 to 6 months, and has had little or no nutrition for more than 5 days, nutritional supplementation should be considered. Nutrition and hydration are essential components necessary for everyday life.

Oral Feeding

Many patients require nutritional supplementation due to malnutrition or anorexia (e.g., a deficiency of certain nutrients, vitamins, or minerals). Many factors may affect a patient's appetite: psychological stress about their illness, family problems, finances, and employment issues are just a few of the many challenges a patient may experience. If the patient can swallow and has a working GI tract, oral nutritional supplementation between meals can help increase caloric intake. Many commercially available products may be used to supplement intake. These are marketed as puddings, bars, and supplemental nutritional drinks.

ENTERAL NUTRITION

EN involves the delivery of nutrition or fluid via a tube into the GI tract, which requires a functional, accessible GI tract. Depending on the different pathologies present, EN may be used for short-term nutritional supplementation, such as with reduced appetite or swallowing difficulties. It can also be used for long-term nutritional supplementation for malabsorption disorders or increased catabolism.

Enteral Feedings: Routes, Solutions, and Delivery Methods

Enteral Routes

A multidisciplinary team approach is used when a decision is required regarding which feeding route to use. Many factors are considered: the patient's condition, preferences, the length of the feeding, physiologic conditions, tolerance, and the integrity of the patient's GI tract.

The GI routes used for enteral tube feedings are the nasogastric, nasoduodenal/nasojejunal, gastrostomy, or jejunostomy routes (Fig. 14.1). The nasogastric and gastrostomy routes deliver food directly to the stomach. The nasoduodenal/nasojejunal and the jejunostomy routes deliver food after the stomach or below the pyloric sphincter and are used for patients at risk for aspiration. These GI routes deliver food by a tube inserted through the nose (nasogastric, nasoduodenal/nasojejunal) or directly into the GI tract (gastrostomy or jejunostomy) through the abdominal wall. The nasogastric, nasoduodenal, and nasojejunal routes are for short-term nutrition of less than 4 weeks' duration. If long-term nutrition is required, the patient may receive a gastrostomy or a jejunostomy tube placed in the stomach or small bowel by a surgical, endoscopic, or fluoroscopic procedure.

The gastrointestinal tubes are small in diameter, are made of urethane or silicone, and are flexible and long. They are radiopaque, which makes their position easy to identify by x-ray. These tubes easily clog, especially when using thick feedings and when the patient's medications are crushed and put down the tube. Always flush the tube before and after medication administration and when determining residual volume, so the tube remains patent and does not clog. If the tube becomes clogged, a new tube may have to be placed, which results in extra discomfort to the patient. It is important to note that these tubes can become dislodged, knotted, or kinked during patient coughing or vomiting. The gastrostomy tube, also known as the *percutaneous endoscopic gastrostomy* (PEG) tube, and the jejunostomy (J) tube are placed surgically, endoscopically, or radiologically. With the PEG tube, the patient must have an intact GI system. For patients with chronic reflux, a J-tube is placed either endoscopically or with laparoscopic surgery. Usually, the doctor orders intravenous (IV) antibiotics to decrease the risk of infection. After placement, always check your facility's policy before initiating the tube feeding, and use correct nursing procedure when putting medication and food through the tubes. Before the initial feeding, the policy in most facilities is to confirm correct placement of the tube with an x-ray.

Enteral Solutions

Many different types of enteral formulas are used for enteral feedings. These solutions differ according to their various nutrients, caloric values, and osmolality. The four groups of enteral solutions are (1) polymeric, (2) modular components, (3) semielemental or elemental, and (4) specialty formulas designed to meet specific nutritional needs in certain illnesses such as diabetes, renal, respiratory, and oncology (Table 14.1). Some of the modular components of enteral solutions include (1) carbohydrates in the form of dextrose, sucrose, lactose, starch, or dextrin (the first three are simple sugars that are absorbed quickly); (2) protein in the form of intact or hydrolyzed proteins or free amino acids; and (3) lipids in the form of corn, soybean, or safflower oil (some have a higher oil content than others). With all EN, sufficient water is needed to maintain hydration.

Methods for Delivery

Enteral feedings are given by continuous infusion pump, intermittent infusion by gravity, intermittent bolus by syringe, and cyclic feedings by infusion pump. Continuous feedings are prescribed for the critically ill and for those who receive feedings into the small intestine. The enteral feedings are given by an infusion pump, which is set to control the flow at a slow rate over 24 hours. Intermittent enteral feedings are administered every 3 to 6 hours over 30 to 60 minutes by gravity drip or infusion pump. At each feeding, 300 to 400 mL of solution is administered. Intermittent infusion is considered an inexpensive method for administering EN. The bolus method was the first method used to deliver enteral feedings, and with this method, 250 to 400 mL of solution is rapidly administered through a syringe into the tube four to six times a day. This method takes about 15 minutes each feeding, but it may not be tolerated well by the patient because a massive volume of solution is given in a short period. The bolus method may cause nausea, vomiting, aspiration, abdominal cramping, and diarrhea. This method is usually reserved for ambulatory individuals. The cyclic method is another type of continuous feeding infused over 8 to 16 hours daily (day or night). Administration during daytime hours is suggested for patients who are restless or for those who have a greater risk for aspiration. The nighttime schedule allows more freedom during the day for patients who are ambulatory.

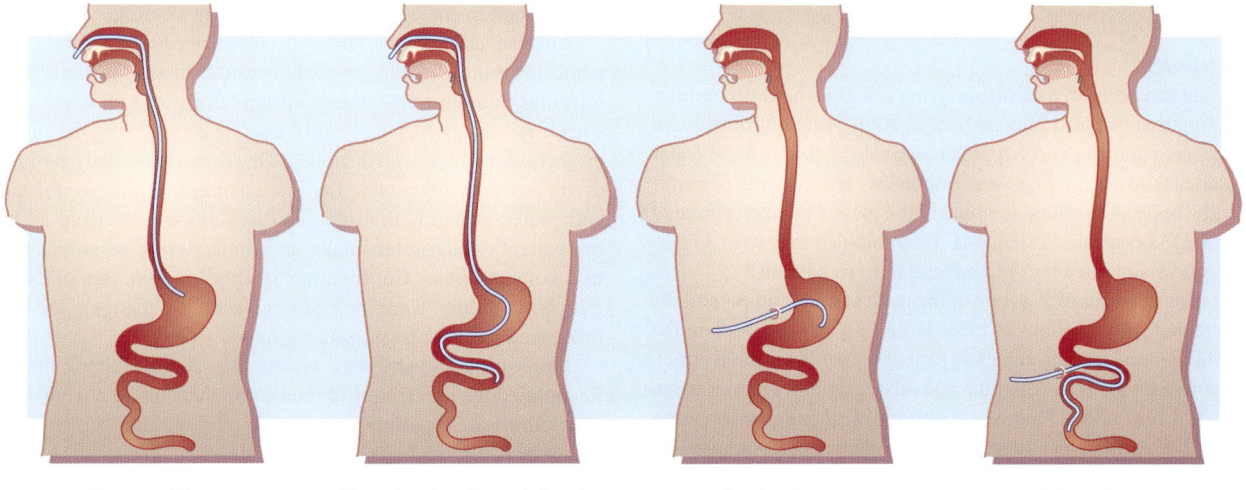

Nasogastric   Nasoduodenal/nasojejunal   Gastrostomy   Jejunostomy

Fig. 14.1 Types of gastrointestinal tubes used for enteral feedings. A *nasogastric* tube is passed from the nose into the stomach. A weighted *nasoduodenal/nasojejunal* tube is passed through the nose into the duodenum/jejunum. A *gastrostomy* tube is introduced through a temporary or permanent opening on the abdominal wall (stoma) into the stomach. A *jejunostomy* tube is passed through a stoma directly into the jejunum.

TABLE 14.1 Preparations for Enteral Feeding

Category	Characteristics	Recommended Usage
Polymeric • Isotonic • High protein • High energy • Fiber content	Mimics macronutrients as found in whole food Available with different protein contents, energy densities, and fiber Meets RDA or micronutrients in 1–1.5 L/day	Isotonic, polymeric formula is regarded as a safe option when initiating enteral feeding Supplements prescribed for patients without malabsorptive disorders Fiber can be added to decrease incidence of diarrhea May be used as tube feeding, meal replacement, or oral supplement Blenderized forms are infrequently used because they are more likely to clog the feeding tubes because of their high viscosity
Modular	Carbohydrates Protein Lipid	Contains specific nutrients, usually a single macronutrient (carbohydrates, proteins, or lipids) Tailored to the individual's needs
Semielemental or elemental	Macronutrients are hydrolyzed to aid in absorption Available in different energy and protein densities	Patients with impaired GI functioning/malabsorption Patients post GI surgery with reduced nutrient absorption capability and/or prolonged bowel rest Patients with pancreatic dysfunction
Specialty formulas • Diabetes • Renal (low sodium) • Respiratory • Oncology/immune modulating	Modified macronutrient composition to promote glycemic control Available in different energy and protein products Polymeric formula with reduced sodium content Higher energy and protein content to limit excessive fluid administration Modified macronutrient content to reduce CO_2 production Contains omega-3-fatty acids for antiinflammatory properties Contains pharmacologically active substances aimed at modulating the immune response and improving outcome	Used for patients with diabetes mellitus, if adequate blood glucose control cannot be achieved through polymeric formula Uses high fiber and fat content products in patients with gastroparesis For use in patients with persistent hypernatremia Patients with renal impairment can be managed with polymeric products with added protein content Should be used with caution in critically ill, septic patients, due to immune-nutritional components Used in patients with excess CO_2 production Potential benefit of patients undergoing elective surgery; however, cannot be recommended for routine use among critically ill patients

CO_2, Carbon dioxide; *GI*, gastrointestinal; *L*, liter; *RDA*, recommended dietary allowance.
From http://www.nutritioncare/aspen.org and http://www.saspen.com/Websites/saspen/files/Content/6280465/1252-8445-1-PB.pdf.

Enteral Feedings: Complications, Safety, and Medications

Complications

Dehydration can occur in patients receiving EN. Diarrhea is a common complication that can lead to dehydration. High-protein formulas can also cause dehydration, and hyperosmolar solutions can draw water out of the cells to maintain serum osmolality. Fluid intake is monitored, and if appropriate, fluid is added to the patient's daily regimen of feedings. Unless contraindicated, it is recommended that 30 to 35 mL/kg per day be maintained for fluid balance in most patients.

Aspiration pneumonitis is one of the most serious and potentially life-threatening complications of tube feedings. It can occur when the contents of the tube feeding enter the patient's lungs from the GI tract. Consequences range from coughing and wheezing to infection, tissue necrosis, and respiratory failure. An important nursing intervention is to check the agency's policy for specific guidelines before initiating EN. It is imperative that the nurse check for gastric residual by gently aspirating the stomach contents before initiating enteral feeding and thereafter every 4 hours between feedings. Usually, if the residual is greater than 150 mL (check the agency policy), the nurse will hold the feeding, and the residual is checked again in 1 hour. If the residual still exceeds this amount, the provider is notified. Large residuals mean the patient may have an obstruction and is not digesting the feeding. This is important to correct before continuing the feeding.

Another common problem of enteral feeding is diarrhea. Rapid administration of feedings, contamination of the formula, low-fiber formulas, tube movement, and various drugs can all cause diarrhea. Check for drugs that can cause diarrhea; these may be antibiotics or sorbitol in liquid medications. Diarrhea can usually be managed or corrected by decreasing the rate of infusion, diluting the solution with water, changing the solution, discontinuing the drug, increasing the patient's daily water intake, or administering an enteral solution that contains fiber. Constipation is another common problem that frequently occurs. It can be easily corrected by changing the formula, increasing water, or requesting a laxative.

Monitoring is essential when the patient is receiving EN. Recommended parameters to monitor include blood chemistry, blood urea nitrogen, creatinine, and electrolytes; glucose; triglycerides; serum proteins; intake and output; and weight. Frequency of monitoring is patient dependent and should be implemented during the entire EN process.

Enteral Safety

The nurse has an important role in administering tube feedings safely. Some of the important safety concerns are patient position, aspiration

risk, residual volumes, and tube position. Following are important safety pointers for patients receiving EN:
- The head of the bed should be elevated to 30 to 45 degrees during the feeding, and if intermittent, keep the head of the bed elevated for 30 to 60 minutes after the feeding. By elevating the head of the bed, the risk of aspiration is decreased.
- Ensure the patient has audible bowel sounds by performing a GI assessment with auscultation. This ensures a working GI tract.
- Always check the gastric residual volume before initiating tube feedings and every 4 to 6 hours if the feedings are continuous.
- Confirm the position of the newly inserted tubing before beginning the initial feeding. This is a required policy for most agencies.
- Initially, after the tube is placed, most agencies require an x-ray to confirm placement. Always follow the agency's policy and procedure for initial confirmation of placement.
- Before each enteral feeding, the nurse should check placement to confirm the tubing has not moved or shifted from the GI tract. Some agencies require pH testing of gastric secretions, whereas others recommend listening for gurgling sounds after inserting air into the tubing. Each of these measures has limitations, so more than one bedside test may be used for confirmation. Check the agency's guidelines.

The American Society for Parenteral and Enteral Nutrition (ASPEN) works to improve the quality of nutrition through its guidelines and standards. ASPEN advocates for high-priority issues about nutrition. They work in conjunction with the National Institutes of Health and the Center for Medicare and Medicaid Services to improve funding and education in the field of enteral and parenteral nutrition (PN). ASPEN was first to issue guidelines for the use of parenteral and enteral nutrition in adults and pediatric populations, and it continues to update, educate, and monitor use of safe practices. Another agency that advocates for safety in both EN and PN is the National Institute for Health and Care Excellence (NICE), which dedicates itself to the practice of health care in society and provides guidance and quality standards for public health care issues that include but are not limited to EN and PN. NICE set the standard that all patients should be screened for malnutrition and treated by a multidisciplinary team of health care professionals. It also stipulates that patients and caregivers should be given adequate training for self-care if they so desire.

The Joint Commission issued an alert on the seriousness of tube misconnections, which can result in severe injury or death to the patient. One situation involved a feeding administration tube that was inadvertently connected to a tracheostomy tube, which caused serious harm to the patient. It is most important to trace all lines from the site of origin back to the patient to avoid dislodgement and misconnection errors.

◎ CLINICAL JUDGMENT [NURSING PROCESS]
Enteral Nutrition

Concept: Caring Intervention
- Caring interventions are interventions performed by the nurse, so the nurse can perform care for the physical and emotional needs of the clients and families. These interventions help the nurse achieve specific patient outcomes, and they are based on the professional guidelines of nursing practice.

Recognize Cues [Assessment]
- Confirm the feeding tube is securely in place.
- Assess the patient's tolerance of enteral feeding, including possible gastrointestinal (GI) disturbance (nausea, cramping, diarrhea).
- Determine urine output, and record it for future comparisons.
- Obtain the patient's weight, and use it for future comparisons.
- Listen for bowel sounds. Report diminished or absent bowel sounds immediately to the health care provider. Also palpate the abdomen for distension.
- Assess baseline laboratory values, and compare these with future laboratory results.

Analyze Cues and Prioritize Hypothesis [Patient Problems]
- Dysphagia
- Dehydration
- Diarrhea
- Constipation

Generate Solutions [Planning]
- The patient will not aspirate during enteral feedings, especially those given via GI route.
- The patient will receive adequate nutritional support through enteral feedings.
- The patient will be free from complications of diarrhea.

Take Action [Nursing Interventions]
- Perform hand hygiene and apply clean gloves.
- Check the tube placement by aspirating gastric secretions or by injecting air into the tube to listen by stethoscope for air movement in the stomach. (Follow agency guidelines.)
- Determine gastric residual before the enteral feeding. When the residual is more than 100 to 150 mL, hold the feeding for 1 hour and recheck the residual. If it is still more than 100 to 150 mL, notify the health care provider. (Always check your agency's policy.)
- Check the continuous route for gastric residual every 4 to 6 hours.
- Always raise the head of the bed to a 30- to 45-degree angle during infusion of feedings. If elevating the head of the bed is contraindicated, position the patient on the right side.
- Deliver enteral feedings according to the method ordered: bolus, continuous, intermittent, or cyclic.
- Flush the feeding tube as appropriate: for intermittent feeding, flush with 30 mL before and after; for continuous feeding, flush with 30 mL every 4 hours. When administering drugs through the tube, use a 30-mL flush of water at the beginning and end of administration; flush with 15 mL of water between administration of each drug.
- Monitor for adverse effects of enteral feedings, such as diarrhea. To manage or correct diarrhea, decrease the enteral feeding flow rate, and as diarrhea lessens, slowly increase the feeding rate. The enteral solution may be diluted, with the provider's order, and then gradually increased to full strength. Determine whether side effects of drugs could be causing diarrhea.
- Monitor vital signs and report abnormal findings.
- Give additional water during the day to prevent dehydration. Consult with the health care provider.
- Weigh the patient to determine weight gain or loss. Compare with the patient's baseline weight. Patients should be weighed at the same time each day with the same scale and the same amount of clothing.
- Change the feeding bag daily. Do not add the new solution to the old solution in the feeding bag. The nutritional solution should be at room temperature.
- Use an interpreter if the patient has a language barrier.

Patient Teaching
- Instruct patients to report any problems related to enteral feedings, such as diarrhea, sore throat, and abdominal cramping.

Evaluate Outcomes [Evaluation]
- Determine that the patient is receiving the prescribed nutrients daily and is free of complications associated with enteral feedings.

Enteral Medications

Many mistakes can occur during enteral tube feedings. These mistakes are often the result of administering drugs that are incompatible with administration through a tube, failure to prepare the drug properly, and use of faulty techniques. These problems can result in an occluded feeding tube, reduced drug effect, or drug toxicity and can cause patient harm or death.

When administering nonliquid drugs through an enteral tube, the nurse should always ensure that the drug is crushable. (For a current and complete listing of drugs that should not be crushed, see http://www.ismp.org/tools/donotcrush.pdf or consult with a pharmacist.) Also, validate with the pharmacist that the drug will dissolve in water and that it can be absorbed through the enteral route. Drugs that cannot be dissolved are timed-release, enteric-coated, and sublingual forms and bulk-forming laxatives; these medications should *not* be crushed. Prepare each medication separately so that the medication is identifiable up until the time of delivery. Open capsules separately, and check with the pharmacist about whether the capsule contents can be crushed. Crush the solid dosage forms after ensuring the medications are crushable, and dissolve each medication separately in about 15 mL of water. The drug must be in liquid form or dissolved in water before administration through enteral tubing. Properly dilute liquid medication with water when administering it through the feeding tube. *Never mix medications with feeding formulas.* Before and after the drug is administered, flush with about 15 mL of water. Proper flushing ensures that the drug has been delivered and the tube is clear. Once the tube has been flushed, the feeding can be restarted after the drug is given.

Many drugs can be given to patients who require tube feeding to aid in absorption and digestion and to promote gastric emptying; these include pancreatic enzymes, probiotics, antiemetics, proton pump inhibitors, and drugs to prevent gastric ulcers.

It is essential to know the importance of temporarily stopping the infusion when certain types of drugs are administered. Some medications require that the feeding is stopped for as long as 30 minutes to allow for adequate absorption.

PARENTERAL NUTRITION

Patient Need

The terms **parenteral nutrition, total parenteral nutrition, and hyperalimentation (HA)** are used synonymously. PN is the administration of nutrients by a route other than the GI tract (e.g., the bloodstream). If a patient is not eligible for EN because of a nonfunctioning GI tract or intestinal failure, PN is delivered intravenously. The word "total" suggests that the patient is receiving all of the required nutrients, fluid, and electrolyte requirements in the bag. In some circumstances, PN and EN may be given concurrently. The delivery of both EN and PN is used when the GI tract is partially functioning or if the patient is being weaned off of PN. PN has many risks, so the option of EN should be fully explored before starting PN. Suggested indications for patients who require PN are those with bowel obstruction, prolonged paralytic ileus, inflammatory bowel disease, or severe pancreatitis, and those who require bowel rest after complex GI surgery. Also, patients with greater nutritional needs sometimes require PN, such as those who have sustained severe trauma or burns and the severely malnourished.

Parenteral Solutions

Solutions

Solutions for PN include amino acids, carbohydrates, electrolytes, fats, trace elements, vitamins, and water. PN is individualized according to the patient's general health. Each element of the prescription can be manipulated according to changes in the patient's clinical requirements. The entire process requires a multidisciplinary team approach that involves the nurse, nutritionist, and pharmacist with the patient's provider leading the care team. Commercially prepared PN base solutions are available and contain dextrose and protein in the form of amino acids. The pharmacist can add prescribed electrolytes, vitamins, and trace elements to customize the solution to meet the patient's needs. Calories are provided by carbohydrates in the form of dextrose and by fat in the form of fat emulsion. Carbohydrates provide 60% to 70% of calorie (energy) needs. Amino acids (proteins) provide about 3.5% to 20% of energy needs. PN has a high glucose concentration. Fat emulsion (lipid) therapy provides an increased number of calories, usually 30%, and is a carrier of fat-soluble vitamins. The recommended energy intake is 25 to 35 cal/kg per day in a nonobese patient. Solutions differ for pediatric patients, who have varied fluid needs and require more energy per kilogram.

High glucose concentrations are irritating to peripheral veins, so PN is administered through either a peripherally inserted central catheter (PICC) via the cephalic or basilica vein, or a central venous catheter via the subclavian or internal jugular vein; this depends on the tonicity of the concentration. The rapid blood flow of the central veins allows placement of the catheter in the vena cava, which has the greatest blood flow of any vein in the body and reduces the risk of thrombophlebitis. If the treatment is used for short-term therapy (<4 weeks), a PICC line is inserted. If the treatment will last longer than 4 weeks, a central line catheter is placed. PN must always be administered by an infusion pump to allow for an accurate flow rate. PN enhances wound healing and provides the necessary nutrients to prevent cellular catabolism. Policies and procedures for PN therapy may vary by region and facility and must be researched and followed accordingly.

Complications

Complications associated with PN can result from catheter insertion and PN infusion. See Table 14.2 for a list of PN complications.

Air embolism occurs when air enters into the central line catheter system. To prevent air embolism during dressing, cap, and tubing changes, ask the patient to turn their head in the opposite direction of the insertion site and to take a deep breath, hold it, and bear down. This is called the **Valsalva maneuver**, and it will increase intrathoracic venous pressure while preventing the risk of air embolism. Always keep the clamp on the central line tubing closed except when in use.

Use strict aseptic technique when changing IV tubing and dressings at the insertion site. PN solution has a high concentration of glucose and is an excellent medium for bacterial growth. Monitor the patient's temperature closely, and if fever occurs, suspect sepsis. Always follow the facility's policy for the correct protocol in changing the PN solutions (12–24 hours), IV tubing (24 hours), and central line dressing (48 hours). Keep the prepared PN solutions refrigerated, and administer the full amount within the designated time according to the agency's policy.

Hyperglycemia occurs primarily because of the hypertonic dextrose solution, but it also occurs when the infusion rate for PN is too rapid. In some cases the pharmacist can add insulin to the PN solution if ordered by the provider. Assess the patient carefully for glucose intolerance. The infusion is started at a slow rate of 40 to 60 mL/h as prescribed. Monitor the patient's blood glucose level every 4 to 6 hours until stable and then every 24 hours or according to the facility's policy. Many providers will order sliding-scale insulin for their patients receiving PN.

The sudden interruption of PN therapy can cause **hypoglycemia**; therefore it is wise to keep a bag of 10% dextrose in the patient's room. If the next bag of PN is late in arriving from the pharmacy, the bag of dextrose can be hung to avoid hypoglycemia. Gradually decrease the infusion rate when PN is discontinued, and monitor the patient's blood glucose level.

TABLE 14.2 Complications of Total Parenteral Nutrition

Complication	Explanation/Cause	Symptoms
Catheter Insertion		
Pneumothorax	An abnormal collection of air or gas in the pleural space that causes the lung to collapse **Cause:** Punctured lung or lung injury during procedure or trauma	Sharp chest pain, decreased breath sounds, tachycardia, absence of breath sounds on the affected side
Hemothorax	A collection of blood in the space between the chest wall and the lung (the pleural cavity) **Cause:** Trauma is the most common cause	Anxiety; chest pain; low blood pressure; pale, cool, and clammy skin; rapid heart rate; rapid, shallow breathing; restlessness; shortness of breath
Total Parenteral Nutrition Infusion		
Air embolism	A pathologic condition caused by a gas bubble in the vascular system **Cause:** Disconnected IV tubing; the catheter system opens, and air enters IV tubing during changes	Coughing, shortness of breath, chest pain, cyanosis, hypotension, apprehension
Infection	The result of the body's inability to fight off foreign microorganisms that may cause damage or disease if left untreated **Cause:** Poor aseptic technique or catheter or solution contamination	Fever/temperature greater than 100°F (37.7°C), chills, increased WBC, redness or drainage
Hyperglycemia	High blood glucose **Cause:** Fluid infused too rapidly, insufficient insulin coverage, infection	Nausea, headache, weakness, thirst, elevated blood glucose (>200 mg/dL), restlessness, confusion, Kussmaul respirations
Hypoglycemia	Low blood glucose **Cause:** Fluids discontinued abruptly, too much insulin being administered	Diaphoresis, shakiness, weakness, low blood glucose level (<70 mg/dL), hunger, anxiety
Hypervolemia	Condition characterized by excessive fluid volume **Cause:** Increased IV rate, renal dysfunction, heart failure, hepatic failure	Weight gain greater than desired; jugular venous distension; full, bounding pulse; lung crackles; headache; hypertension

C, Centigrade; *F*, Fahrenheit; *IV*, intravenous; *mg/dL*, milligrams per deciliter; *WBC*, white blood cell.

CLINICAL JUDGMENT [NURSING PROCESS]
Total Parenteral Nutrition

Concept: Caring Intervention
- Caring interventions are interventions performed by the nurse, so the nurse can perform care for the physical and emotional needs of the clients and families. These interventions help the nurse achieve specific patient outcomes, and they are based on the professional guidelines of nursing practice.

Recognize Cues [Assessment]
- Obtain baseline vital signs for future comparisons.
- Confirm baseline weight.
- Determine laboratory results (electrolytes, glucose, protein [prealbumin], and white blood cell levels frequently change during parenteral [PN] therapy). Early laboratory results are useful for future comparisons.
- Check urine output and report abnormal findings.
- Carefully read the label on the bag of PN solution. Compare the ingredients with the health care provider's order.
- Assess the PN insertion site for erythema, edema, swelling, tenderness, and drainage.

Analyze Cues and Prioritize Hypothesis [Patient Problems]
- Decreased gas exchange
- Disrupted fluid and electrolyte balance
- Dehydration
- Wound infection
- Need for health teaching

Generate Solutions [Planning]
- The patient's nutrient needs will be met via PN by patient achieving a weight gain of 3 to 5 lb.
- Refrigerate PN solution that is not in use. Because of its high glucose concentration, the formula is an excellent medium for bacterial growth. Always check your agency's policy concerning storing of PN.
  - Avoid infection by closely monitoring the patient's temperature and ensuring a normal temperature is maintained (98.6°F [37°C]).
  - Do not draw blood from or administer medications through the central line, and do not check central venous pressure via the PN line. Results could be invalid.

Take Action [Nursing Interventions]
- Maintain sterile technique when accessing central line.
- Perform a full set of vital signs, and report changes.
- Determine body weight, and compare it with the baseline weight.
- Monitor lab results—especially hematology labs, electrolytes, protein, and glucose—and report abnormal findings.
- Compare laboratory results with baseline findings to assess any changes.
- Measure fluid intake and output. Volume deficit or excess may occur due to the hyperosmolar content of the PN solution.
- Monitor temperature changes for possible infection or a febrile state. Use aseptic technique when changing dressings and solution bags.

Continued

CLINICAL JUDGMENT [NURSING PROCESS]—CONT'D
Total Parenteral Nutrition

- Check the blood glucose level according to your agency's policy. Initially, glucose levels may be high.
- Monitor the flow rate of PN. Start with 60 to 80 mL/h, and increase slowly to the ordered level to avoid hyperglycemia.
- If PN finishes before the next time it is due to be administered, hang a bag of dextrose 10% to avoid hypoglycemia.
- During tubing and dressing changes, have the patient perform a Valsalva maneuver (taking a deep breath, holding it, and bearing down). Always clamp tubing during bag and tubing changes to prevent air embolus.
- Check for signs and symptoms of overhydration—coughing, dyspnea, engorged neck veins, or chest rhonchi—and report any findings.
- Follow your agency's policy for dressing and tubing changes.
- Respect the patient's beliefs about refusing PN.
- Explain reasons for adequate nutrition, and find ways to meet nutritional needs.
- Use an interpreter as appropriate if a language barrier exists.

Patient Teaching
- Provide emotional support to patients and family before and during PN therapy.
- Be available to discuss the patient's concerns or refer the patient to the appropriate health care provider.
- Instruct patients to notify their health care provider immediately if they experience discomfort or reactions.
- Keep the patient informed of the progress and effectiveness of PN.

Evaluate Outcomes [Evaluation]
- Evaluate the patient's positive and negative response to PN therapy.
- Determine periodically whether the patient's serum electrolytes, protein, and glucose levels are within desired ranges.
- Evaluate nutritional status by weight changes, energy level, feelings of well-being, symptom control, and healing.
- Evaluate patient and family understanding of the purpose and possible complications of PN therapy.

CLINICAL JUDGMENT SINGLE-EPISODE CASE STUDY

Cognitive Skill: Prioritize hypothesis (Cloze)
Objective: Prioritize care for a patient with a central line receiving parenteral nutrition (PN).

A 50-year-old female patient who hasn't eaten in 5 days after complex GI surgery has received a central line and an order for parenteral nutrition. The nurse reviews the patient's morning labs and notes the patient has a potassium level of 3.2 mEq/L. Choose the priority nursing interventions for the information missing from the statements below by selecting from the list of options provided.

Upon receipt of the PN order, the nurse reviews the label of contents to confirm ___(1)___ is included in the bag. Next, a full set of vital signs is performed including ___(1)___ and ___(1)___. The nurse assesses the central line for patency while maintaining ___(1)___. The nurse instructs the patient on how to perform the ___(2)___ and explains this is always done when accessing the central line prior to hanging the PN and when tubing is changed because it prevents the risk of ___(2)___. Finally, the patient is instructed to notify the nurse if they begin to experience ___(2)___, ___(2)___, or ___(2)___.

OPTIONS FOR 1	OPTIONS FOR 2
Sodium	Coughing
Aseptic technique	Valsalva maneuver
Potassium	Fatigue
Weight	Air embolism
Temperature	Dry skin
Vitamin B complex	Shortness of breath
Clean technique	Nausea
Apical pulse	Chest pain
Magnesium	Increase in mucous secretion

Answers
Upon receipt of parenteral nutrition, the nurse reviews the label of contents to confirm potassium is included in the bag of PN. Next, a full set of vital signs is performed including temperature and weight. The nurse assesses the central line for patency while maintaining aseptic technique. The nurse instructs the patient on how to perform the Valsalva maneuver and explains this is always done when accessing the central line prior to hanging the PN and when tubing is changed because it prevents the risk of air embolism. Finally, the patient is instructed to notify the nurse if they begin to experience coughing, shortness of breath, or chest pain.

Rationale
The nurse should carefully read the label on the bag of PN solution and compare the electrolyte ingredients to the patient's most current laboratory results. This patient has a low potassium level of 3.2 mEq/L. The nurse would expect to see potassium included on the PN label. Sodium, vitamin B complex, and magnesium are not indicated for this patient. Always maintain excellent aseptic technique when changing IV tubing and dressings at the insertion site. PN solution has a high concentration of glucose and is a medium for bacterial growth, which can result in infection. Instruct the patient in the Valsalva maneuver, which can prevent air embolism. The patient is asked to turn their head in the opposite direction of the insertion site and take a deep breath, hold it, and bear down. This increases intrathoracic venous pressure while preventing the risk of air embolism. Air embolism is a condition caused by a gas bubble that enters the vascular system. This can easily occur when the catheter system is open to hang a new bag of PN or change the tubing. Symptoms of air embolism include coughing, shortness of breath, and chest pain. Fatigue, dry skin, nausea, and increase in mucous secretions are not symptoms related to air embolism.

References
McCuistion, et al. Nutritional support. In: *Pharmacology: A Patient-Centered Nursing Process Approach*. 11th ed. Missouri: Elsevier; 2023:167–174.
Lewis, et al. Nutritional problems. In: *Medical Surgical Nursing*. 11th ed. Missouri: Elsevier; 2020:849–867.

REVIEW QUESTIONS

1. The nurse is determining a patient's gastric residual before administering an enteral feeding; the last feeding was 240 mL. The patient will be discharged on enteral feedings. It is important to include in the teaching plan that a residual of more than which amount would indicate delayed gastric emptying (based on the last feeding)?
   a. 60 mL
   b. 125 mL
   c. 150 mL
   d. 75 mL
2. The nurse is reviewing the plan of care for a patient receiving enteral therapy. What is the most common complication of enteral therapy?
   a. Aspiration
   b. Constipation
   c. Diarrhea
   d. Muscle weakness
3. Which is appropriate nursing care for a patient receiving total parenteral nutrition (TPN) in an acute care setting? **Select all that apply.**
   a. Monitor patient's blood glucose level.
   b. Measure patient's fluid intake and output closely.
   c. Administer blood through the TPN line.
   d. Monitor the TPN insertion site for erythema.
   e. Monitor the patient's monthly weight.
   f. Sterile technique isn't necessary when accessing the patient's central TPN line.
   g. Determining a baseline weight of the patient prior to TPN is not important.
4. A patient has been on TPN for 1 month, and there is an order to discontinue TPN tomorrow. The nurse contacts the health care provider because sudden interruption of TPN therapy may cause which condition?
   a. Dehydration
   b. Tremors
   c. Urinary retention
   d. Hypoglycemia
5. A patient is receiving TPN at home. The visiting nurse assists the family with the care plan, which includes changing the TPN solution and tubing. What is the recommended initial frequency for changing the tubing?
   a. Every 24 hours
   b. Every 36 hours
   c. Every 48 hours
   d. Every 72 hours
6. The nurse is reviewing the care plan with a patient using enteral nutrition (EN). Which interventions by the nurse are appropriate for this strategy? **Select all that apply.**
   a. Check the continuous route for gastric residual every 2 to 4 hours.
   b. Elevate the bed to a 30- to 45-degree angle before administering EN.
   c. Change the enteral feeding bag and tubing every 3 to 4 days.
   d. Report absent bowel sounds to the health care provider.
   e. Explain that diarrhea is never a result of the EN therapy.
   f. Assessing patient's blood pressure is unnecessary.
   g. Additional water administration is not required.
7. The nurse is to administer enteral medications to a patient who cannot swallow and is receiving continuous enteral feedings. Which is correct concerning administration of the enteral medications?
   a. All ordered medications are added to the enteral feeding solution.
   b. Dilute liquid medications before administering through the feeding tube.
   c. Extra amounts of water are used to dissolve timed-release medications.
   d. Undiluted hyperosmolar medications may be given to patients on fluid restriction.

UNIT IV Autonomic Nervous System Drugs

15

Adrenergic Agonists and Antagonists

http://evolve.elsevier.com/McCuistion/pharmacology

OBJECTIVES

- Describe the structures and functions of each nervous system in the body.
- Explain the action of adrenergic agonists.
- Explain the action of adrenergic antagonists.

OUTLINE

Nervous Systems of the Body, 175
    Autonomic Nervous System, 175
    Neurons, 175
    Sympathetic and Parasympathetic Nervous Systems, 175
Adrenergic Agonists, 175
    Inactivation of Neurotransmitters, 177
    Classification of Sympathomimetics, 177
    Epinephrine, 180

    Central-Acting Alpha-Adrenergic Agonists, 180
Adrenergic Antagonists, 183
    Alpha-Adrenergic Antagonists, 183
    Beta-Adrenergic Antagonists, 183
    Adrenergic Neuron Antagonists, 186
Clinical Judgment Case Study, 186
Review Questions, 186

This chapter discusses two groups of drugs that affect the sympathetic nervous system—adrenergic agonists, or **sympathomimetics**, and *adrenergic antagonists*, also called *adrenergic blockers* or **sympatholytics**—along with their dosages and uses.

NERVOUS SYSTEMS OF THE BODY

The *central nervous system* (CNS) is the body's primary nervous system and consists of the brain and spinal cord. The *peripheral nervous system* (PNS), located outside the brain and spinal cord, is made up of two divisions: the autonomic and the somatic. After interpretation by the CNS, the PNS receives stimuli and initiates responses to these stimuli.

Autonomic Nervous System

The *autonomic nervous system* (ANS), also called the *visceral system*, acts on smooth muscles and glands. Its functions include control and regulation of the heart, respiratory system, gastrointestinal (GI) tract, bladder, eyes, and glands. The ANS is an involuntary nervous system, over which we have little or no control: we breathe, our hearts beat, and peristalsis continues without our realizing it. However, unlike the ANS, the *somatic nervous system* is a voluntary system that innervates skeletal muscles, over which there is control.

Neurons

The two sets of neurons in the autonomic component of the PNS are the (1) afferent, or *sensory*, neurons and the (2) efferent, or *motor*, neurons. The *afferent neurons* send impulses to the CNS, where they are interpreted. The *efferent neurons* receive the impulses (information) from the brain and transmit these impulses through the spinal cord to the effector organ cells.

Sympathetic and Parasympathetic Nervous Systems

The efferent pathways in the ANS are divided into two branches: the sympathetic and the parasympathetic nerves. Collectively, these two branches are called the *sympathetic nervous system* and the *parasympathetic nervous system* (Fig. 15.1).

The sympathetic and parasympathetic nervous systems act on the same organs but produce opposite responses to provide homeostasis (balance; Fig. 15.2). Drugs act on the sympathetic and parasympathetic nervous systems by either stimulating or depressing responses.

The sympathetic nervous system is also called the *adrenergic system*. Norepinephrine is the neurotransmitter that innervates smooth muscle. The adrenergic receptor organ cells are of four types: $alpha_1$, $alpha_2$, $beta_1$, and $beta_2$ (Fig. 15.3). Norepinephrine is released from the terminal nerve ending and stimulates the cell receptors to produce a response.

ADRENERGIC AGONISTS

Drugs that stimulate the sympathetic nervous system are called *adrenergic agonists*, *adrenergics*, or *sympathomimetics* because they mimic the sympathetic neurotransmitters norepinephrine and epinephrine.

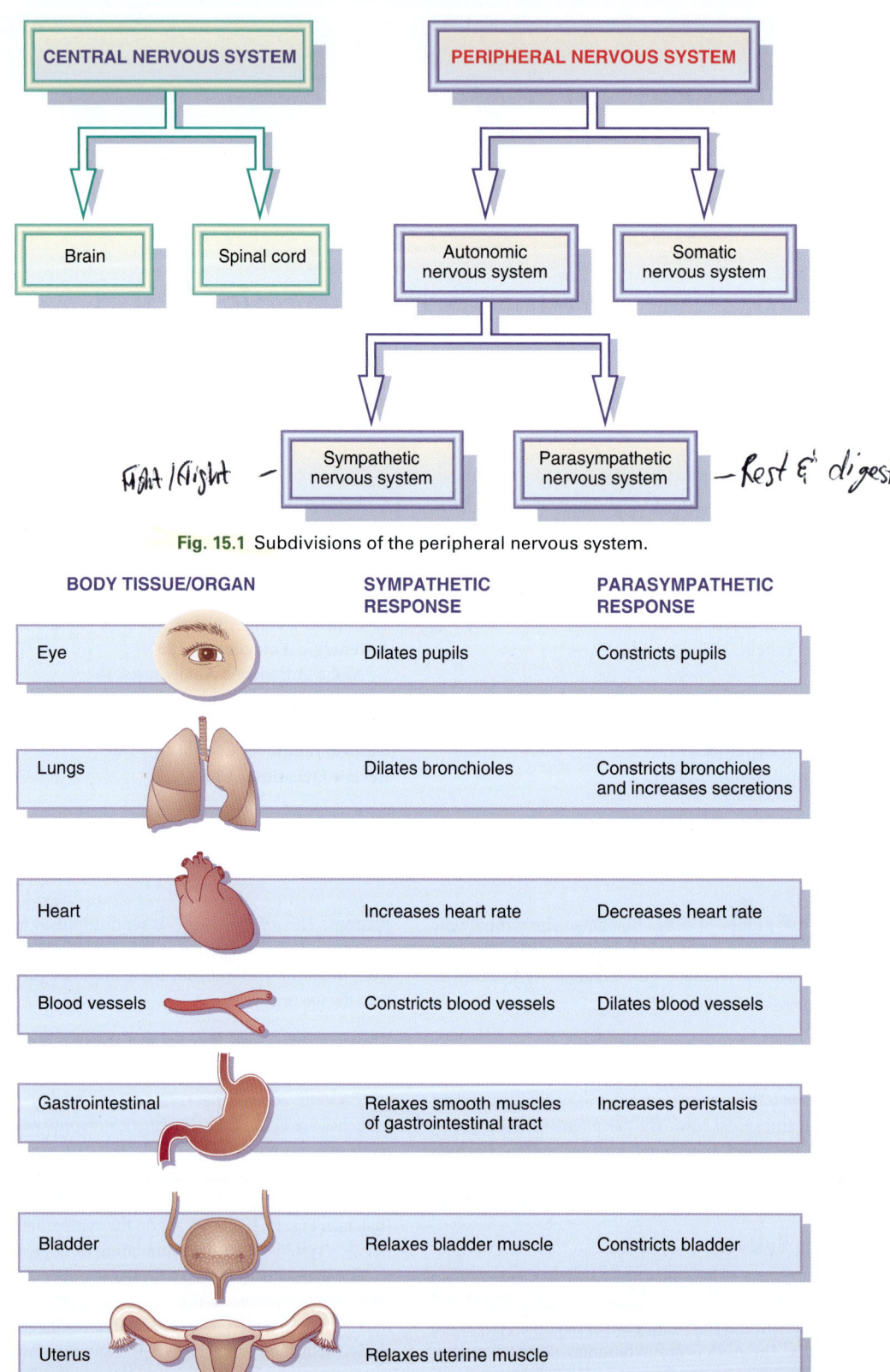

Fig. 15.1 Subdivisions of the peripheral nervous system.

Fight/flight — Sympathetic nervous system
Parasympathetic nervous system — Rest & digest

Fig. 15.2 **Sympathetic and parasympathetic effects on body tissues.** The sympathetic and parasympathetic nervous systems have opposite responses on body tissues and organs.

Fig. 15.3 Sympathetic transmitters and receptors. *NE,* Norepinephrine.

TABLE 15.1	Effects of Adrenergic Agonists at Receptors
Receptor	Physiologic Responses
Alpha$_1$	Increases force of heart contraction; vasoconstriction increases blood pressure; mydriasis (dilation of pupils) occurs; secretion in salivary glands decreases; urinary bladder relaxation and urinary sphincter contraction increases
Alpha$_2$	Inhibits release of norepinephrine; dilates blood vessels; produces hypotension; decreases gastrointestinal motility and tone
Beta$_1$	Increases heart rate and force of contraction; increases renin secretion, which increases blood pressure
Beta$_2$	Dilates bronchioles; promotes gastrointestinal and uterine relaxation; promotes increase in blood glucose through glycogenolysis in the liver; increases blood flow in skeletal muscles

They act on one or more **adrenergic receptor** sites located in the effector cells of muscles such as the heart, bronchiole walls, GI tract, urinary bladder, and ciliary muscles of the eye. There are many adrenergic receptors. The four main receptors are alpha$_1$, alpha$_2$, beta$_1$, and beta$_2$, which mediate the major responses described in Table 15.1 and illustrated in Fig. 15.4.

> ⚡ **PATIENT SAFETY**
>
> Intravenous (IV) adrenergic agonists and antagonists are high-alert medications because they can cause significant harm to a patient in the event of a medication error.

The alpha-adrenergic receptors are located in the blood vessels, eyes, bladder, and prostate. When the alpha$_1$ receptors in vascular tissues (vessels) of muscles are stimulated, the arterioles and venules constrict; this increases peripheral resistance and blood return to the heart, circulation improves, and blood pressure is increased. When too much stimulation occurs, blood flow is decreased to the vital organs.

The alpha$_2$ receptors are located in the postganglionic sympathetic nerve endings. When stimulated, they inhibit the release of norepinephrine, which leads to a decrease in vasoconstriction. This results in vasodilation and a decrease in blood pressure.

The beta$_1$ receptors are located primarily in the heart but are also found in the kidneys. Stimulation of the beta$_1$ receptors increases myocardial contractility and heart rate.

The beta$_2$ receptors are found mostly in the smooth muscles of the lung and GI tract, the liver, and the uterine muscle. Stimulation of the beta$_2$ receptor causes (1) relaxation of the smooth muscles of the lungs, which results in bronchodilation; (2) a decrease in GI tone and motility; (3) activation of glycogenolysis in the liver and increased blood glucose; and (4) relaxation of the uterine muscle, which results in a decrease in uterine contraction (Fig. 15.5; see also Table 15.1).

Other adrenergic receptors are dopaminergic and are located in the renal, mesenteric, coronary, and cerebral arteries. When these receptors are stimulated, the vessels dilate, and blood flow increases. Only dopamine can activate these receptors.

Inactivation of Neurotransmitters

After the neurotransmitter (e.g., norepinephrine) has performed its function, the action must be stopped to prevent prolonging the effect. Transmitters are inactivated by (1) *reuptake* of the transmitter back into the neuron (nerve cell terminal), (2) enzymatic *transformation* or degradation, and (3) *diffusion* away from the receptor. The mechanism of norepinephrine reuptake plays a more important role in inactivation than does the enzymatic action. After the reuptake of the transmitter in the neuron, the transmitter may be degraded or reused. The two enzymes that inactivate norepinephrine are monoamine oxidase (MAO), which is *inside* the neuron, and catechol-*O*-methyltransferase, which is *outside* the neuron.

Drugs can prolong the action of the neurotransmitter (e.g., norepinephrine) by either inhibiting reuptake, which prolongs the action of the transmitter, or inhibiting the degradation by enzymatic action.

Classification of Sympathomimetics

The sympathomimetic (adrenergic agonist) drugs that stimulate adrenergic receptors are classified into three categories according to their effects on organ cells. Categories include (1) direct-acting sympathomimetics, which directly stimulate the adrenergic receptor (e.g., epinephrine or norepinephrine); (2) indirect-acting sympathomimetics, which stimulate the release of norepinephrine from the terminal nerve endings (e.g., amphetamine); and (3) mixed-acting (both direct- and indirect-acting) sympathomimetics, which stimulate the adrenergic receptor sites and stimulate the release of norepinephrine from the terminal nerve endings (e.g., ephedrine; Fig. 15.6).

Pseudoephedrine is an example of a mixed-acting sympathomimetic. It acts indirectly by stimulating the release of norepinephrine from the nerve terminals, and it acts directly on the alpha$_1$ and beta$_1$ receptors. Pseudoephedrine, like epinephrine, increases heart rate. It is not as potent a vasoconstrictor as epinephrine, and the risk of hemorrhagic stroke and hypertensive crisis is less. Pseudoephedrine, an over-the-counter (OTC) drug but controlled, is helpful to relieve nasal and sinus congestion without rebound congestion. This drug is contraindicated in hypertension, closed-angle glaucoma, bronchitis, emphysema, and urinary retention, and should be used with caution in diabetes mellitus.

Catecholamines are the chemical structures of a substance, either endogenous or synthetic, that can produce a sympathomimetic response. Examples of endogenous catecholamines are epinephrine, norepinephrine, and dopamine. The synthetic catecholamines are isoproterenol and dobutamine. Noncatecholamines such as phenylephrine, metaproterenol, and albuterol stimulate the adrenergic receptors. Most noncatecholamines have a longer duration of action than the endogenous or synthetic catecholamines.

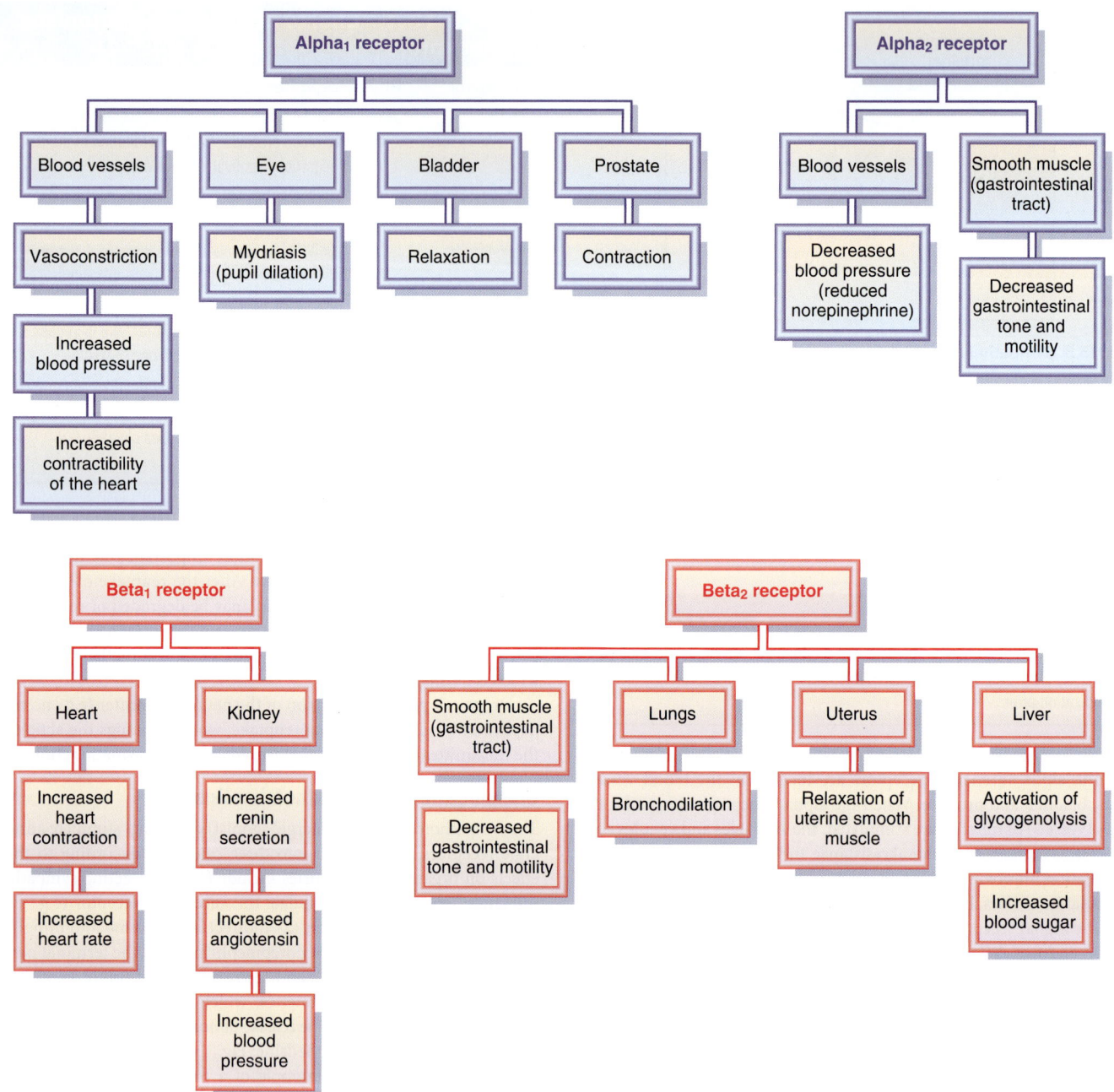

Fig. 15.4 Effects of activation of alpha$_1$, alpha$_2$, beta$_1$, and beta$_2$ receptors.

Many of the adrenergic agonists stimulate more than one of the adrenergic receptor sites. An example is epinephrine, which acts on alpha$_1$-, beta$_1$-, and beta$_2$-adrenergic receptor sites. The responses from these receptor sites include increase in blood pressure, pupil dilation, increase in heart rate (tachycardia), and bronchodilation. In anaphylactic shock, epinephrine is useful because it increases blood pressure, heart rate, and airflow through the lungs. Because epinephrine affects different adrenergic receptors, it is **nonselective**. Additional side effects result when more responses occur than are desired. Pseudoephedrine is commonly used for illegal production of amphetamine and methamphetamine. National regulatory measures control pseudoephedrine drug sales with individual limits of 3.6 g/day and 9 g within 30 days. Identifications are scanned with each purchase. The database is linked nationally and keeps a 2-year tally. **Prototype Drug Chart: Epinephrine** lists the pharmacologic behavior of epinephrine.

Albuterol sulfate, a beta$_2$-adrenergic agonist, is **selective** for beta$_2$-adrenergic receptors, so the response is relaxation of bronchial smooth muscle and bronchodilation to prevent and treat bronchospasm. A patient with asthma may tolerate albuterol better than isoproterenol, which activates beta$_1$ and beta$_2$ receptors, because albuterol's action is more selective; it activates only the beta$_2$ receptors of smooth muscle in the lungs and uterus, as well as in the vasculature that supplies the skeletal muscles. By using selective sympathomimetics, fewer undesired adverse effects will occur. However, high dosages of albuterol may affect beta$_1$ receptors, causing an increase in heart rate.

Tremors, headache, and nervousness are the most common side effects of oral or inhalation albuterol. Other side effects include tachycardia, palpitations, dizziness, dysrhythmia, nausea, and vomiting. **Beta antagonists (beta-blockers)** may inhibit the action of albuterol.

CHAPTER 15 Adrenergic Agonists and Antagonists

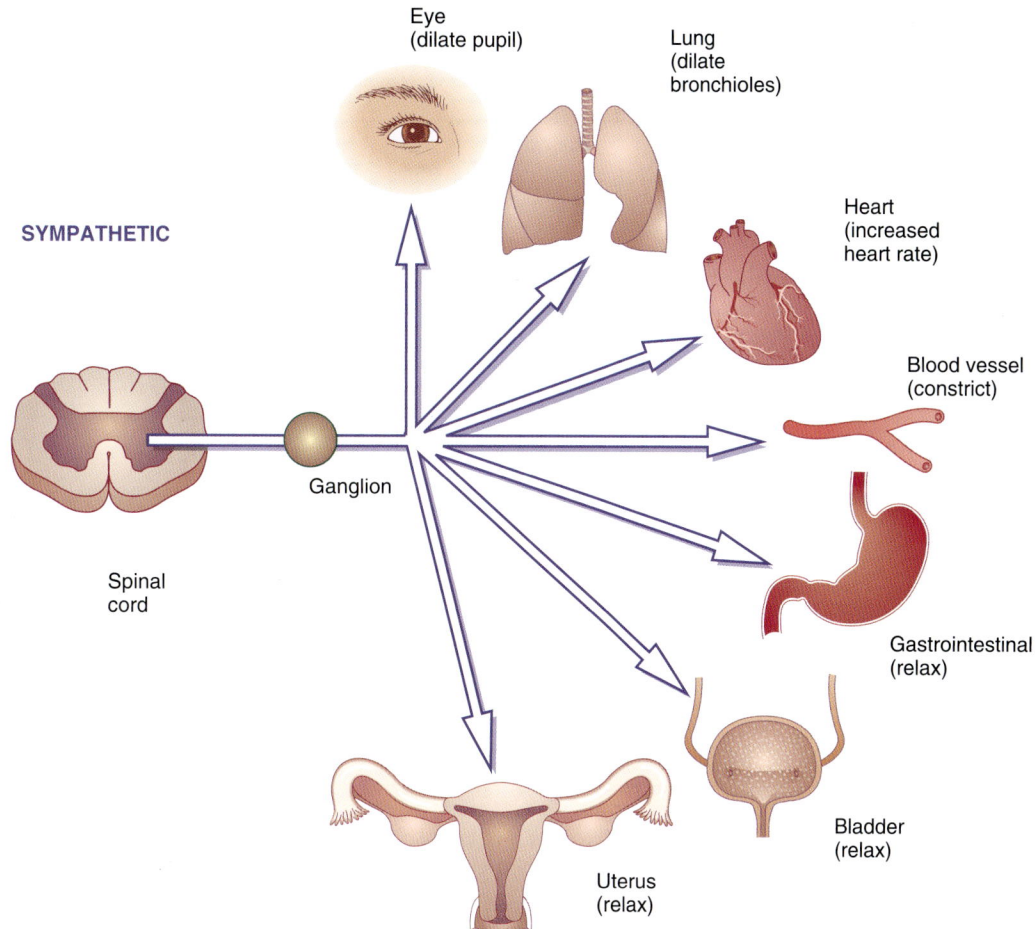

Fig. 15.5 **Sympathetic responses.** Stimulation of the sympathetic nervous system or use of sympathomimetic (adrenergic agonist) drugs can cause the pupils and bronchioles to dilate, heart rate to increase, blood vessels to constrict, and muscles of the gastrointestinal tract, bladder, and uterus to relax, thereby decreasing contractions.

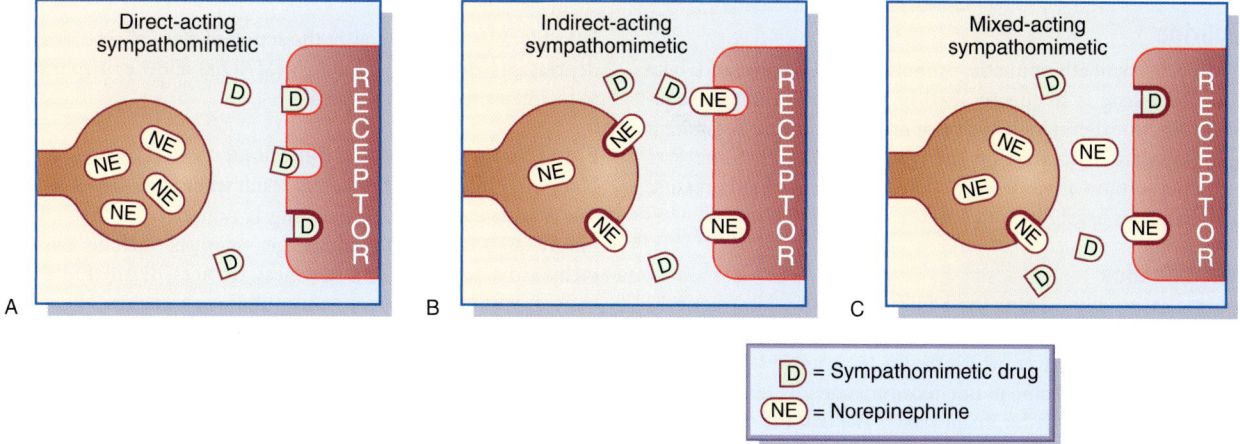

Fig. 15.6 (A) Direct-acting sympathomimetics. (B) Indirect-acting sympathomimetics. (C) Mixed-acting sympathomimetics.

PROTOTYPE DRUG CHART

Epinephrine

Drug Class	Dosage
Sympathomimetic: adrenergic agonist	Anaphylaxis: A: IM/subcut: 0.2–0.5 mg EpiPen autoinjector, may repeat in 5–15 min; *max*: 3 doses IV: 0.05–0.1 mg of 0.1 mg/mL solution, may repeat q5–15 min PRN
Contraindications: Closed-angle glaucoma	**Drug-Lab-Food Interactions**
Caution: Parkinsonism, closed-angle glaucoma, cerebrovascular disease, labor, hypertension, cardiac disease, hyperthyroidism, diabetes mellitus, hypovolemia, renal disease, older adult, children, breastfeeding, pregnancy	Drug: Increased effects with TCAs and MAOIs; methyldopa and beta-blockers antagonize epinephrine effects; digoxin may cause dysrhythmias with epinephrine Lab: Increased blood glucose, serum lactic acid
Pharmacokinetics	**Pharmacodynamics**
Absorption: Subcut/IM/IV: Rapidly; inactivated in GI tract Distribution: PB: UK Metabolism: t½: <5 min IV Excretion: In urine and feces	Subcut: Onset: 5–10 min Peak: 20 min Duration: 1–4 h IM: Onset: variable Duration: 1–4 h IV: Onset: Immediate Peak: 2–5 min Duration: 5–10 min Inhaled: Onset: 1 min Peak: 3–5 min Duration: 1–3 h
Therapeutic Effects/Uses	
To treat nasal congestion, allergic reaction, anaphylaxis, asthma exacerbation, bronchospasm, angioedema, status asthmaticus, cardiac arrest, cardiac resuscitation Mechanism of Action: Acts on alpha and beta receptors; promotion of CNS and cardiac stimulation and bronchodilation; strengthens cardiac contraction, increases cardiac rate and cardiac output; reduces mucosal congestion by inhibiting histamine release; reverses anaphylactic reactions	
Side Effects	**Adverse Reactions**
Nausea, vomiting, restlessness, tremor, agitation, memory impairment, headache, pallor, diaphoresis, oliguria, weakness, fatigue, dizziness, throat irritation, rhinorrhea, sneezing, hypo/hyperglycemia, paresthesia	Palpitations, tachycardia, hypertension, injection site reaction *Life threatening:* Dysrhythmias, pulmonary edema

<, Less than; *A*, adult; *CNS*, central nervous system; *h*, hours; *IM*, intramuscular; *IV*, intravenous; *MAOI*, monoamine oxidase inhibitor; *max*, maximum; *min*, minute; *PB*, protein binding; *PRN*, as needed; *q5–15 min*, every 5–15 minutes; *subcut*, subcutaneous; *t½*, half-life; *TCA*, tricyclic antidepressant; *UK*, unknown.

Epinephrine

Epinephrine, a sympathomimetic, stimulates both alpha and beta receptors. This drug is frequently used in emergencies to treat anaphylaxis, a life-threatening allergic response. Epinephrine is a potent inotropic (myocardial contraction-strengthening) drug that increases cardiac output, promotes vasoconstriction and systolic blood pressure elevation, increases heart rate, and produces bronchodilation.

Pharmacokinetics

Epinephrine is usually administered intramuscularly, intravenously, or endotracheally. It is not given orally because it is rapidly metabolized in the GI tract and liver, which results in unstable serum levels. Subcutaneous administration is not recommended as absorption is slower and less dependable for anaphylaxis. The half-life of epinephrine is less than 5 minutes intravenously (IV), and the percentage by which the drug is protein bound is unknown. Epinephrine is metabolized by the liver and is excreted in the urine.

Pharmacodynamics

The onset of action and peak concentration times are rapid. The use of decongestants with epinephrine has an additive effect. When epinephrine is administered with digoxin, cardiac dysrhythmia may occur. Beta-blockers can antagonize the action of epinephrine. Tricyclic antidepressants and MAO inhibitors (MAOIs) allow epinephrine's effects to be intensified and prolonged.

Side Effects and Adverse Reactions

Undesired side effects frequently result when the adrenergic drug dosage is increased or when the drug is nonselective. Side effects commonly associated with adrenergic agonists include hypertension, tachycardia, palpitations, restlessness, tremors, dysrhythmia, dizziness, nausea, vomiting, dyspnea, and pulmonary edema. High doses can result in cardiac dysrhythmia, which necessitates electrocardiogram (ECG) monitoring.

Names of adrenergic drugs, the receptors they activate, dosage information, and common uses are listed in Table 15.2. Epinephrine is also discussed in Chapter 55 as one of the drugs used during emergencies.

Central-Acting Alpha-Adrenergic Agonists

Alpha$_2$ drugs are central acting and produce vasodilation by stimulating alpha$_2$ receptors in the CNS, leading to a decrease in blood pressure (see Chapter 42). Alpha$_2$ drugs act by decreasing the release of norepinephrine from sympathetic nerves and by decreasing peripheral adrenergic receptor activation.

TABLE 15.2 Adrenergic Agonists: Alpha$_1$, Beta$_1$, and Beta$_2$

Drug	Route and Dosage	Uses and Considerations
Epinephrine; alpha$_1$, beta$_1$, and beta$_2$	See Prototype Drug Chart: Epinephrine	
Ephedrine hydrochloride, ephedrine sulfate; alpha$_1$, beta$_1$, and beta$_2$	Hypotension: A: IV: 5–10 mg, may repeat PRN; *max:* 50 mg/dose	For hypotension. May cause restlessness, headache, dizziness, dysrhythmia, bradycardia, tachycardia, hypertension, nausea, vomiting, tolerance, and palpitations. PB: UK; t½: 3–6 h
Norepinephrine bitartrate; alpha$_1$ and beta$_1$	Acute hypotension: A: IV: Initially 8–12 mcg/min inf, titrate to maintain adequate BP; *max:* 3.3 mcg/kg/min continuous infusion	For acute hypotension and cardiogenic and septic shock. Monitor blood pressure and rhythm every 2–5 min during infusion. May cause anxiety, headache, bradycardia, hypertension, pulmonary edema, and tissue necrosis. PB: 25%; t½: 2.4 min
Dopamine hydrochloride; alpha$_1$ and beta$_1$	A: IV/inf: Initially 2–5 mcg/kg/min; gradually increase; *maint:* 2–20 mcg/kg/min; *max:* 50 mcg/kg/min	For hypotension, heart failure, septic shock, and cardiogenic shock. May cause anxiety, hypo/hypertension, bradycardia, tachycardia, dysrhythmia, palpitations, headache, angina, dyspnea, nausea, vomiting, and tissue necrosis. PB: UK; t½: 2 min
Midodrine hydrochloride; alpha$_1$	A: PO: 10 mg tid; *max:* 30 mg/d	For orthostatic hypotension. Do not administer within 4 h of bedtime. May cause anxiety, headache, hypertension, bradycardia, paresthesias, pruritus, abdominal pain, urinary retention/urgency/frequency, dysuria, and piloerection. PB: insignificant; t½: 25 min
Phenylephrine hydrochloride; alpha$_1$	Nasal decongestion: A: PO: 10–20 mg q4–6 h PRN; *max:* 60 mg/d Intranasal: A: 2–3 sprays each nostril q4h PRN; *max:* 3 sprays each nostril within 4-h period	For sinus and nasal congestion, hypotension or shock, pupillary dilation. Have patient blow nose before drug is administered intranasally. May cause anxiety, headache, blurred vision, nasal irritation, nausea, tachycardia, bradycardia, hypertension, paresthesias, dysrhythmias, and tissue necrosis. PB: UK; t½: 2.1–3.4 h
Pseudoephedrine hydrochloride; alpha$_1$, alpha$_2$, and beta$_1$	Regular release: A: PO: 60 mg q4–6 h; *max:* 240 mg/d 12 h Extended release: A: PO: 120 mg q12h; *max:* 240 mg/d 24 h Extended release: A: PO: 240 mg qd; *max:* 240 mg/d	For nasal congestion. May cause anxiety, hypertension, tachycardia, palpitations, dizziness, headache, seizure, nausea, urinary retention, restlessness, insomnia, and dysrhythmias. PB: UK; t½: 9–16 h
Albuterol; beta$_2$	Bronchospasm prophylaxis: Immediate release: A: PO: 2–4 mg q6–8 h; *max:* 32 mg/d Extended release: A: PO: 4–8 mg q12h; *max:* 32 mg/d Inhalation: A: 180 mcg (2 actuations of 90 mcg/actuation) inhaled by mouth 15–30 min before exercise	For prophylaxis and treatment of bronchospasm. May cause headache, anxiety, pharyngitis, tremor, dizziness, nausea, vomiting, muscle cramps, infection, palpitations, tachycardia, and hypo/hypertension. PB: 10%; t½: 2.7–6 h
Dobutamine hydrochloride; beta$_1$	A: IV: Initially 0.5–1 mcg/kg/min continuous inf; titrate dose gradually; *max:* 20 mcg/kg/min	For heart failure, cardiogenic shock, and for cardiac surgery. May cause dysrhythmia, tachycardia, angina, palpitations, headache, nausea, hypo/hypertension, hypokalemia, and dyspnea. PB: UK; t½: 2 min
Terbutaline sulfate; beta$_2$	Asthma: A: PO: 2.5–5 mg tid; *max:* 15 mg/d Bronchospasm: A: subcut: Initially 0.25 mg, may repeat in 15–30 min PRN; *max:* 0.5 mg in 4 h	For asthma and acute bronchospasm. May cause tremors, dizziness, drowsiness, headache, hyperhidrosis, nausea, vomiting, hyperglycemia, palpitations, tachycardia, weakness, and hypokalemia. PB: 25%; t½: 2.9–14 h
Central-Acting Alpha Agonists Clonidine hydrochloride Alpha$_2$	Immediate-release tablets: A: PO: Initially 0.1 mg bid; *maint:* 0.1–0.8 mg/d; *max:* 2.4 mg/d A: Transdermal: 1 patch q7d	For hypertension. May cause dizziness, anxiety, drowsiness, confusion, headache, fatigue, nightmares, pruritus, nausea, abdominal pain, constipation, dry mouth, orthostatic hypotension, and bradycardia. PB: 20%–40%; t½: 12–16 h, transdermal 20 h

A, adult; *BP*, blood pressure; *d*, day; *h*, hour; *inf*, infusion; *IV*, intravenously; *maint*, maintenance; *max*, maximum; *min*, minute; *PB*, protein binding; *PO*, by mouth; *PRN*, as needed; *q4h*, every 4 hours; *subcut*, subcutaneous; *t½*, half-life; *tid*, three times a day; *UK*, unknown.

Clonidine

Clonidine, as a selective alpha$_2$-adrenergic agonist, suppresses sympathetic stimulation of nerves to the heart and blood vessels. By promoting cardiac suppression and vasodilation, this drug is used primarily to treat hypertension.

Clonidine may produce bradycardia, decrease in cardiac output, and hypotension. It can also cause drowsiness and dry mouth at very low doses. Abrupt discontinuation of clonicine may cause rebound hypertension.

Side Effects and Adverse Reactions

Additional undesired side effects of central-acting alpha-adrenergic agonists include headache, nasal congestion, nightmares, constipation, and edema. Anxiety, fatigue, and nausea may also occur.

CLINICAL JUDGMENT [NURSING PROCESS]
Adrenergic Agonists

Concept: Perfusion
- The passage of blood flow through arteries and capillaries, which deliver oxygen and nutrients to body cells

Recognize Cues [Assessment]
- Record baseline vital signs for future comparisons.
- Assess the patient's drug history.
- Determine patient's health history. Most adrenergic agonists are contraindicated if the patient has a cardiac dysrhythmia, narrow-angle glaucoma, or cardiogenic shock.
- Determine baseline glucose level.

Analyze Cues and Prioritize Hypothesis [Patient Problems]
- Dyspnea
- Decreased gas exchange
- Hypotension
- Decreased tissue perfusion
- Hypoxemia

Generate Solutions [Planning]
- Patient's vital signs will be within acceptable ranges.
- Patient will experience therapeutic effects by improved blood pressure, breathing pattern, and cardiac output.

Take Action [Nursing Interventions]
- Administer intravenous (IV) epinephrine 1 mg (10 mL of a 1:10,000 concentration per American Heart Association [AHA] guidelines) for cardiac resuscitation; may repeat every 3 to 5 minutes. Follow each dose with a 20-mL saline flush to ensure proper delivery. Normally, epinephrine is administered 1 mg IV over 1 minute or more.
- ⚡ Monitor IV site frequently when administering norepinephrine bitartrate or dopamine because extravasation of these drugs causes tissue damage and necrosis within 12 hours. These drugs should be diluted sufficiently in IV fluids.
- Administer antidote, phentolamine mesylate 5 to 10 mg, diluted in 10 to 15 mL of normal saline infiltrated into the area for IV extravasation of norepinephrine and dopamine.
- Record patient's vital signs. Report signs of increasing blood pressure and increasing heart rate. If the patient receives an alpha-adrenergic agonist intravenously for shock, check the blood pressure every 3 to 5 minutes or as indicated to avoid severe hypertension.
- Monitor ECG for dysrhythmia when adrenergic agonists are given intravenously.
- Report side effects of adrenergic drugs such as tachycardia, palpitations, dysrhythmias, tremors, dizziness, and increased blood pressure.
- Offer food to the patient when giving adrenergic agonists to avoid nausea and vomiting.
- Evaluate blood glucose levels in patients with diabetes mellitus for potential elevation.

Patient Teaching
General
- Advise the patient to read labels on all over-the-counter (OTC) drugs for cold symptoms and diet pills. Many of these have properties of sympathetic drugs (adrenergic agonists, sympathomimetics) and should not be taken if a patient has hypertension, diabetes mellitus, cardiac dysrhythmia, or coronary artery disease.
- Explain that continuous use of nasal sprays or drops that contain adrenergic agonists may result in rebound nasal congestion (inflamed and congested tissue).

Self-Administration
- Encourage the patient to take medication as prescribed.
- Advise the patient and family on proper administration of the drug and allow a return demonstration. Cold medications by spray or drops in the nostrils should be used with the head in an upright position. Use of nasal spray while lying down can cause systemic absorption. Coloration of nasal spray or drops might indicate deterioration.
- Notify the health care provider if an EpiPen is needed more than twice a week.
- Encourage the patient to have an EpiPen readily available at all times and to store additional medication in a cool, dark place. Refrigeration is not recommended.
- ⚡ Teach the patient and family that the EpiPen must be used immediately upon the initial occurrence of difficulty breathing, wheezing, hoarseness, hives, itching, or swelling of the lips and tongue.
- Teach the patient to administer the EpiPen properly. Inspect the solution for particles or discoloration before administration. Do not use if particles are pink to brown in color. Take care to inject subcutaneously and not intradermally, and be sure to apply sufficient pressure to activate the EpiPen while holding the device in place for 5 to 10 seconds. The EpiPen should be inserted into the outer thigh. After administration, massage the injection site for 10 seconds to promote absorption and reduce vasoconstriction and tissue irritation.

Side Effects
- ⚡ Encourage the patient to report side effects such as rapid heart rate, palpitations, rash, itching, flushing, chest pain, irregular heartbeat, vomiting, or numbness of fingers and toes to a health care provider because the dose may require adjustment.

Evaluate Outcomes [Evaluation]
- Evaluate the patient's response to the adrenergic agonist.
- Evaluate vital signs and report abnormal findings. Epinephrine stimulates alpha$_1$ (increases blood pressure), beta$_1$ (increases heart rate), and beta$_2$ (dilates bronchial tubes) receptors. Albuterol stimulates beta$_2$ receptors.
- Report possible drug-drug interactions. Beta-blockers decrease the effect of epinephrine and albuterol. OTC cold and allergy drugs, caffeine, alcohol, herbs, and dietary supplements may lead to interactions.

ADRENERGIC ANTAGONISTS

Drugs that block the effects of adrenergic neurotransmitters are called *adrenergic antagonists, adrenergic blockers,* or *sympatholytics*. They act as antagonists to adrenergic agonists by blocking the alpha- and beta-receptor sites. Most adrenergic antagonists (adrenergic blockers) block either the alpha receptor or the beta-receptor. They block the effects of the neurotransmitter either directly by occupying the receptors or indirectly by inhibiting the release of the neurotransmitters norepinephrine and epinephrine. Table 15.3 lists the effects of alpha-blockers and beta-blockers at receptors.

Alpha-Adrenergic Antagonists

Drugs that block or inhibit a response at the alpha-adrenergic receptor site are called *alpha-adrenergic antagonists, adrenergic blockers,* or *alpha-blockers*. Alpha-blocking agents are divided into two groups: *selective* alpha-blockers block $alpha_1$, and *nonselective* alpha blockers block $alpha_1$ and $alpha_2$. Because alpha-adrenergic antagonists can cause orthostatic hypotension and reflex tachycardia, many of these drugs are not as frequently prescribed as beta antagonists.

Alpha antagonists (alpha-blockers) promote vasodilation, causing a decrease in blood pressure. If vasodilation is long-standing, orthostatic hypotension can result. Dizziness may also be a symptom of a decrease in blood pressure. As blood pressure decreases, pulse rate usually increases to compensate for the low blood pressure and inadequate blood flow. Alpha antagonists can be used to treat peripheral vascular disease such as Raynaud disease. Vasodilation occurs, permitting more blood flow to the extremities. These drugs are also helpful in decreasing symptoms of benign prostatic hyperplasia. Alpha antagonists are also discussed in Chapter 39.

Beta-Adrenergic Antagonists

Beta-adrenergic antagonists, more commonly called *beta-blockers*, decrease heart rate, and a decrease in blood pressure usually follows. Some beta-blockers are nonselective, blocking both $beta_1$ and $beta_2$ receptors. Not only does the heart rate decrease because of $beta_1$ blocking, but bronchoconstriction also occurs. Nonselective beta-blockers block both $beta_1$ and $beta_2$ and should be used with extreme caution in any patient who has chronic obstructive pulmonary disease (COPD) or asthma.

Propranolol hydrochloride was the first beta blocker prescribed to treat angina, cardiac dysrhythmia, hypertension, and heart failure. Propranolol has many side effects, partly because of its nonselective response in blocking both $beta_1$ and $beta_2$ receptors.

A selective adrenergic antagonist has a greater affinity for certain receptors. If the desired effect is to decrease pulse rate and blood pressure, a selective $beta_1$ blocker such as atenolol or metoprolol tartrate may be ordered.

Intrinsic sympathomimetic activity (ISA) is a term used to describe the ability of certain beta-blockers to bind with a beta-receptor to prevent strong agonists from binding to that receptor, producing complete activation. Nonselective beta-blockers that have ISA include carvedilol, penbutolol, and pindolol. The selective blocker (blocks $beta_1$ only) that has ISA is acebutolol, and such an agent may be recommended for hypertensive patients who are experiencing bradycardia.

Atenolol, a selective $beta_1$ blocker, decreases sympathetic outflow to the periphery and suppresses the renin-angiotensin-aldosterone system response. It is contraindicated in bradycardia, heart block, cardiogenic shock, acute heart failure, asthma, and sick sinus syndrome. Beta-blockers should be used with caution in patients with COPD. Prototype Drug Chart: Atenolol describes the pharmacologic behavior of atenolol.

Beta-blockers are useful in treating mild to moderate hypertension, angina, heart failure, and myocardial infarction (MI). Beta-blockers should not be abruptly discontinued but rather should be tapered off over 1 to 2 weeks to avoid tachycardia, hypertension, severe angina, dysrhythmia, and MI. The use of beta-blockers as antihypertensives, antidysrhythmics, and drugs for angina is discussed in Chapters 37 and 39. Table 15.4 lists the alpha and beta-blockers and their dosages, uses, and considerations.

PROTOTYPE DRUG CHART

Atenolol

Drug Class	Dosage
$Beta_1$-adrenergic blocker	Hypertension: A: PO: Initially 25–50 mg/d; may increase to 100 mg/d after 7–14 d; *max:* 100 mg/d

Contraindications	Drug-Lab-Food Interactions
Hypersensitivity, bradycardia, heart block greater than first degree, cardiogenic shock, uncompensated cardiac failure *Caution:* Renal dysfunction, diabetes mellitus, depression, thyroid disease, COPD, bronchospasm, asthma, cardiovascular disease, PVD, myasthenia gravis, pheochromocytoma, pulmonary edema, pregnancy, lactation, breastfeeding, older adult, children, abrupt discontinuation	Drug: Increased absorption with anticholinergics, decreased effects with NSAIDs, increased risk of hypoglycemia with insulin and sulfonylureas, increased hypotension with prazosin and terazosin, increased lidocaine and verapamil levels with toxicity

Pharmacokinetics	Pharmacodynamics
Absorption: 50% absorbed in GI tract Distribution: PB: 10% Metabolism: $t^{1/2}$: 6–7 h Excretion: Urine and feces	PO: Onset: 1 h Peak: 2–4 h Duration: 24 h

Therapeutic Effects/Uses

To treat hypertension, angina, and prophylaxis and treatment of acute myocardial infarction
Mechanism of action: Selectively blocks $beta_1$-adrenergic receptor sites, decreases sympathetic outflow to the periphery, suppresses renin-angiotensin-aldosterone system

Side Effects	Adverse Reactions
Drowsiness, dizziness, headache, depression, fatigue, nausea, diarrhea, erectile dysfunction	Bradycardia, tachycardia, hypotension, chest pain, heart failure, dyspnea *Life threatening:* Bronchospasm, renal failure, dysrhythmia, thrombocytopenia

A, Adult; *COPD*, chronic obstructive pulmonary disease; *d*, day; *GI*, gastrointestinal; *h*, hour; *max*, maximum; *NSAID*, nonsteroidal antiinflammatory drug; *PB*, protein binding; *PO*, by mouth; *PVD*, peripheral vascular disease; $t^{1/2}$, half-life.

TABLE 15.3 Effects of Adrenergic Blockers at Receptors

Receptor	Responses
$Alpha_1$	Vasodilation: decreases blood pressure; reflex tachycardia might result; mydriasis (constriction of pupil) occurs; suppresses ejaculation; reduces contraction of smooth muscle in bladder neck and prostate gland
$Beta_1$	Decreases heart rate; reduces force of contractions
$Beta_2$	Constricts bronchioles; contracts uterus; inhibits glycogenolysis, which can decrease blood glucose

TABLE 15.4 Adrenergic Antagonists

Drug	Route and Dosage	Uses and Considerations
Phentolamine mesylate; alpha₁	A: Subcut: 5–10 mg in 10 mL NS injected into extravasation area to prevent dermal necrosis	Antidote for dopamine, dobutamine, phenylephrine, epinephrine, norepinephrine, and necrosis from extravasation. May cause ocular/dental/abdominal pain, dysgeusia, tachycardia, injection site reaction. PB: UK; t½: 19 min
Doxazosin mesylate; alpha₁	Hypertension: A: PO: Initially 1 mg/d; *max:* 16 mg/d	For hypertension and BPH. May cause anxiety, dizziness, headache, asthenia, fatigue, edema, visual impairment, erectile dysfunction, and orthostatic hypotension. PB: 98%; t½: 22 h
Prazosin hydrochloride; alpha₁	Hypertension: A: PO: Initially 1 mg bid/tid; *maint:* 2–20 mg/d in divided doses; *max:* 40 mg/d	For hypertension. May cause headache, dizziness, drowsiness, fatigue, weakness, orthostatic hypotension, dyspnea, peripheral edema, nausea, and palpitations. PB: 97%; t½: 2–4 h
Terazosin hydrochloride; alpha₁	Hypertension: A: PO capsules: Initially 1 mg at bedtime; *maint:* 1–20 mg/d; *max:* 20 mg/d	For hypertension and BPH. May cause nasal congestion, dizziness, drowsiness, headache, peripheral edema, orthostatic hypotension, nausea, myalgia, weakness, palpitations, dyspnea, and erectile dysfunction. PB: 90%–94%; t½: 12 h
Carvedilol; alpha₁, beta₁, and beta₂	Heart failure: Immediate release: A >85 kg: PO: 3.125 mg bid for 2 weeks; *maint:* 50 mg bid; *max:* 50 mg/bid A 85 kg or <: 3.125 mg for 2 weeks, *maint:* 25 mg bid Extended release: A: Initially 10 mg/d; *max:* 80 mg/d	For hypertension and HF. May cause drowsiness, dizziness, orthostatic hypotension, bradycardia, weight gain, dyspnea, fatigue, headache, peripheral edema, hyperglycemia, diarrhea, erectile dysfunction, and weakness. PB: 98%; t½: 7–11 h
Labetalol; alpha₁, beta₁, and beta₂	Hypertension: A: PO: Initially 100 mg bid; dose may be increased q2–3d; *maint:* 200–400 mg bid; *max:* 2400 mg/d	For hypertension. May cause drowsiness, orthostatic hypotension, nasal congestion, dizziness, fatigue, headache, nausea, paresthesia, erectile/ejaculation dysfunction, hyperhidrosis, and dyspnea. PB: 50%; t½: 6–8 h
Propranolol hydrochloride; beta₁ and beta₂	Hypertension: Immediate release: A: PO: Initially: 40 mg bid; may increase q3–7d; *maint:* 160–480 mg/d in 2–3 divided doses; *max:* 640 mg/d Extended release capsules: A: PO: Initially 80 mg/d, may increase q3–7d; *maint:* 120–160 mg/d; *max:* 640 mg/d	For hypertension, angina, MI, and dysrhythmia. May cause agitation, fatigue, dizziness, visual impairment, erectile dysfunction, bradycardia, hypo/hypertension, hyperkalemia, and dyspnea. PB: 90%; t½: 2–6 h
Nadolol; beta₁ and beta₂	A: PO: Initially 40 mg/d; *maint:* 40–80 mg/d; *max:* 320 mg/d for hypertension and 240 mg/d for angina	For hypertension and angina. May cause dizziness, drowsiness, fatigue, bradycardia, hypotension, palpitations, dyspnea, and erectile dysfunction. PB: 30%; t½: 10–24 h
Pindolol; beta₁ and beta₂	A: PO: Initially 5 mg bid; *maint:* 10–30 mg in 2–3 divided doses; *max:* 60 mg/d	For hypertension. May cause bradycardia, tachycardia, bradycardia, hypotension, edema, anxiety, fatigue, myalgia, dizziness, palpitations, visual impairment, weight gain, erectile dysfunction, and dyspnea. PB: 40%–60%; t½: 3–4 h
Sotalol; beta₁ and beta₂	Atrial flutter/fibrillation: A: PO: 80 mg bid; may increase gradually; *max:* 320 mg/d	For ventricular dysrhythmias, atrial flutter, and atrial fibrillation. May cause headache, dizziness, dyspnea, asthenia, bradycardia, palpitations, hypotension, HF, hyperhidrosis, nausea, vomiting, fatigue, and dysrhythmia exacerbation. PB: 0%; t½: 12 h
Timolol maleate; beta₁ and beta₂	Hypertension: A: PO: Initially 10 mg bid; *maint:* 10–20 mg bid; *max:* 60 mg/d in 2 doses	For hypertension and glaucoma treatment and for migraine prophylaxis. May cause blurred vision, conjunctivitis, ocular irritation, weakness, dizziness, fatigue, nausea, bradycardia, dyspnea, HF, pulmonary edema, and dysrhythmias. PB: 10%; t½: 4 h
Selective Beta-Adrenergic Blockers		
Metoprolol tartrate; beta₁	Angina: Immediate release: A: PO: Initially 50 mg bid; *maint:* 100–400 mg/d in 2 divided doses; *max:* 450 mg/d Extended release: A: PO: Initially 100 mg/d; *maint:* 100–400 mg/d; *max:* 400 mg/d	For hypertension, angina, HF, and acute MI. May cause bradycardia, dizziness, drowsiness, fatigue, nightmares, diarrhea, depression, insomnia, palpitations, erectile dysfunction, hypo/hypertension, dyspnea, peripheral edema, HF, and dysrhythmias. Decrease gradually over 1–2 weeks when discontinuing. PB: 10%–12%; t½: 3–7 h
Atenolol; beta₁	See Prototype Drug Chart: Atenolol	
Acebutolol hydrochloride; beta₁	Hypertension: A: PO: Initially: 400 mg/d; *maint:* 400–800 mg/d; *max:* 1200 mg/d Older adults: Initially 200–400 mg/d; *max:* 800 mg/d	For hypertension and dysrhythmias. May cause bradycardia, hypotension, dizziness, fatigue, headache, nausea, diarrhea, constipation, visual impairment, edema, and dyspnea. PB: 26%; t½: 3–4 h

TABLE 15.4 Adrenergic Antagonists—cont'd

Drug	Route and Dosage	Uses and Considerations
Betaxolol; beta$_1$	Hypertension: A: PO: Initially 10 mg/d; After 7–14 days, may titrate up to 20 mg/d; *max:* 20 mg/d Older adult: Initially 5 mg/d; May then titrate up to 20 mg/d; *max:* 20 mg/d	For hypertension and glaucoma. May cause bradycardia, headache, dizziness, insomnia, fatigue, nausea, diarrhea, arthralgia, edema, palpitations, and chest pain. PB: 50%; t½: 15 h
Bisoprolol fumarate; beta$_1$	A: PO: Initially: 2.5–5 mg/d; *max:* 20 mg/d	For hypertension. May cause dizziness, bradycardia, headache, fatigue, arthralgia, diarrhea, orthostatic hypotension, weakness, and peripheral edema. PB: 30%; t½: 9–12 h
Esmolol hydrochloride; Nebivolol; beta$_1$	Paroxysmal supraventricular tachycardia: A: IV: LD: Initially 50 mcg/kg/min continuous infusion; *max:* 500 mcg/kg/ dose or 300 mcg/kg/min continuous infusion A: PO: Initially 5 mg/d, may increase at 2 weeks intervals; *max:* 40 mg/d	For paroxysmal supraventricular tachydysrhythmia and hypertension. May cause headache, hypotension, dizziness, drowsiness, bradycardia, nausea, and injection site reaction. PB: 55%; t½: 9 min For hypertension. May cause dizziness, drowsiness, headache, dyspnea, fatigue, weakness, bradycardia, tachycardia, and erectile dysfunction. PB: 98%; t½: 12 h

A, adult; *bid*, two times a day; *BPH*, benign prostatic hyperplasia; *d*, day; *h*, hour; *HF*, heart failure; *IV*, intravenous; *maint*, maintenance; *max*, maximum; *MI*, myocardial infarction; *min*, minute; *NS*, normal saline; *PB*, protein binding; *PO*, by mouth; *q2–3d*, every 2–3 days; *subcut*, subcutaneously; *t½*, half-life; *tid*, three times a day; *UK*, unknown.

CLINICAL JUDGMENT [NURSING PROCESS]
Adrenergic Neuron Antagonists

Concept: Perfusion
- The passage of blood flow through arteries and capillaries, which deliver oxygen and nutrients to body cells

Recognize Cues [Assessment]
- Obtain baseline vital signs and ECG for future comparisons. Bradycardia and a decrease in blood pressure are common cardiac effects of adrenergic neuron blockers.
- Determine what drugs the patient currently takes. Report if any are diuretics, nonsteroidal antiinflammatory drugs (NSAIDs), digoxin, monoamine oxidase inhibitors (MAOIs), or central nervous system (CNS) depressants.
- Obtain a health history. Depression, dysrhythmias, and heart failure may result from taking an adrenergic neuron blocker, and these drugs could potentiate preexisting conditions.

Analyze Cues and Prioritize Hypothesis [Patient Problems]
- Hypertension
- Reduced sexual expression

Generate Solutions [Planning]
- Patient will verbalize that they will adhere to the drug regimen.
- Patient's vital signs will be within the desired range.

Take Action [Nursing Interventions]
- Monitor blood pressure. Report marked decreases in blood pressure.
- Monitor apical pulse. Withhold and report if less than 60 beats/min.
- Report any complaints of excessive dizziness, lightheadedness, early morning insomnia, mental depression, or chest pain.
- Assist patient with ambulation to avoid falls from orthostatic hypotension, which is more common with high doses.
- Note any complaint of stuffy nose because vasodilation may result, and nasal congestion can occur.

Patient Teaching
General
- Encourage the patient to adhere to the drug regimen.
- Advise the patient that the therapeutic effects of adrenergic neuron antagonists may not occur for 2 to 3 weeks after initiation of therapy.

Self-Administration
- Teach the patient and family how to take pulse and blood pressure.
- Encourage the patient to take the adrenergic neuron antagonist at the same time every day and not to discontinue it without permission from the health care provider.

Side Effects
- ⚡ Encourage the patient to avoid orthostatic (postural) hypotension by slowly rising from supine or sitting positions to standing.
- Inform patients and family of possible psychological changes when taking adrenergic neuron antagonists, which occur because of catecholamine depletion. Psychological changes can include depression, sleep disorders, emotional lability, memory impairment, confusion, nightmares, and hallucinations.
- Warn patients that adrenergic neuron antagonists may cause erectile or ejaculation dysfunction, which is usually dose-related.
- ⚡ Advise patients not to drive or operate dangerous equipment until the drug response is known.

Evaluate Outcomes [Evaluation]
- Evaluate the effectiveness of the adrenergic neuron blocker. Vital signs must be stable within the desired range.

Pharmacokinetics
Atenolol distribution into the CNS by crossing the blood-brain barrier is minimal and is 50% to 60% absorbed by the GI tract. The protein-binding capacity is 10%. Atenolol has a half-life of 6 to 7 hours and is eliminated in urine.

Pharmacodynamics
By blocking beta$_1$ receptors, atenolol decreases the heart rate, peripheral vascular resistance, force of cardiac contractions, and cardiac output and reduces both systolic and diastolic blood pressure. It is available in tablets and for IV administration. The onset of action of the oral preparation is 1 hour; peak time is 2 to 4 hours, and duration of action is 24 hours. This drug is effective for once-daily dosing, especially for patients who do not adhere to drug dose schedules that require dosing several times a day.

Drug Interactions
Many drugs interact with atenolol. NSAIDs decrease the hypotensive effect of atenolol. Hypotension can be potentiated if atenolol is taken with another antihypertensive, although this may be the desired result. When atenolol is given concurrently with atropine and other anticholinergics, absorption is increased.

Side Effects and Adverse Reactions
The side effects commonly associated with beta-blockers are bradycardia, hypotension, headache, dizziness, cold extremities, and bronchospasm. Other side effects of beta-adrenergic blockers include cardiac dysrhythmia, fatigue, erectile dysfunction, and depression. Usually the side effects are dose related.

Adrenergic Neuron Antagonists
Drugs that block the release of norepinephrine from the sympathetic terminal neurons are called adrenergic neuron antagonists (adrenergic neuron blockers). The clinical use is to decrease blood pressure. For example, reserpine is an antihypertensive agent that closely resembles alpha- and beta-adrenergic blockers; it also reduces the serotonin and catecholamine transmitters, depletion of which may lead to severe mental depression.

CLINICAL JUDGMENT CASE STUDY

An older adult patient has asthma, and an adrenergic agonist is selected for treatment.
1. What are the drug advantages and disadvantages associated with the use of an adrenergic agonist, such as metaproterenol or albuterol, for this patient? Explain your answer.
2. Is age a factor in drug selection? Explain your answer.

An older adult patient has hypertension and asthma. An adrenergic blocker is selected for treatment.
1. What are the drug advantages and disadvantages associated with the use of doxazosin, prazosin, propranolol, metoprolol, and atenolol for this patient? Explain your answer.
2. What needs to be included when teaching this patient about the use of an adrenergic blocker?

REVIEW QUESTIONS

1. The nurse will monitor the patient taking albuterol for which conditions? **Select all that apply.**
   a. Palpitations
   b. Hypertension
   c. Hypoglycemia
   d. Bronchospasm
   e. Uterine contractions
   f. Hypotension
   g. Blurred vision
2. Nadolol is prescribed for a patient. The nurse realizes that this drug is a beta-adrenergic blocker and is contraindicated for patients with which condition?
   a. Hypothyroidism
   b. Angina pectoris
   c. Bronchial asthma
   d. Liver dysfunction
3. The nurse realizes that beta$_1$ receptor stimulation is differentiated from beta$_2$ stimulation in that stimulation of beta$_1$ receptors leads to which condition?
   a. Increased bronchodilation
   b. Decreased uterine contractility
   c. Increased myocardial contractility
   d. Decreased blood flow to skeletal muscles
4. A patient is given epinephrine, an adrenergic agonist (sympathomimetic). The nurse should monitor the patient for which condition?
   a. Decreased pulse
   b. Pupil constriction
   c. Bronchial constriction
   d. Increased blood pressure
5. A patient who is taking epinephrine is also taking several other medications. The nurse should realize that there is a possible drug interaction with which drugs? **Select all that apply.**
   a. Albuterol
   b. Metoprolol
   c. Propranolol
   d. Digoxin
   e. Methyldopa
6. A patient is prescribed metoprolol to treat hypertension. It is important for the nurse to monitor the patient for which condition? **Select all that apply.**
   a. Bradycardia
   b. Hypotension
   c. Diaphoresis
   d. Agitation
   e. Erythema
7. The nurse is administering atenolol to a patient. Which concurrent drugs does the nurse expect to most likely cause an interaction? **Select all that apply.**
   a. Ginseng
   b. Insulin
   c. Atropine
   d. Haloperidol
   e. Methyldopa

16

Cholinergic Agonists and Antagonists

http://evolve.elsevier.com/McCuistion/pharmacology

OBJECTIVES

- Describe the two types of cholinergic receptors at organ cells.
- Explain the action of the parasympathetic neurotransmitter acetylcholine.
- Describe major responses of the body to cholinergic antagonists.

OUTLINE

Parasympathetic Nervous System, 187
  Overview, 187
  Parasympathetic Nervous System Stimulants, 187
Cholinergic Agonists, 187
  Direct-Acting Cholinergic Agonists, 188
  Indirect-Acting Cholinergic Agonists, 190
  Reversible Cholinesterase Inhibitors, 190
  Irreversible Cholinesterase Inhibitors, 191

Cholinergic Antagonists, 191
  Atropine, 193
  Antiparkinson Anticholinergic Drugs, 194
  Anticholinergics for Treating Motion Sickness, 195
Clinical Judgment Case Study, 197
Review Questions, 197

The two groups of drugs discussed in this chapter affect the parasympathetic nervous system. They include cholinergic agonists—muscarinic agonists or parasympathomimetics—and the cholinergic antagonists (blocking agents)—muscarinic antagonists, parasympatholytics, or more commonly called anticholinergics.

PARASYMPATHETIC NERVOUS SYSTEM

Overview

The parasympathetic nervous system is called the *cholinergic system* because the neurotransmitter at the end of the neuron that innervates the muscle is acetylcholine.

The cholinergic receptors at organ cells are either nicotinic or muscarinic, meaning that they are stimulated by the alkaloids, nicotine, and muscarine, respectively (Fig. 16.1).

Parasympathetic Nervous System Stimulants

Acetylcholine stimulates the receptor cells to produce a response, but the enzyme acetylcholinesterase may inactivate acetylcholine before it reaches the receptor cell.

Drugs that mimic the neurotransmitters norepinephrine and acetylcholine produce responses opposite to each other in the same organ. For example, an *adrenergic drug* (sympathomimetic) *increases* the heart rate, whereas a *cholinergic drug* (parasympathomimetic) *decreases* the heart rate (see Fig. 15.2 in Chapter 15). However, a drug that mimics the sympathetic nervous system and a drug that blocks the parasympathetic nervous system can cause similar responses in the organ. For instance, the sympathomimetic and the parasympatholytic (blocks impulses from PNS) drugs both *increase* heart rate; the adrenergic blockers and the cholinergic drugs both *decrease* heart rate.

Many name classifications are given to drugs that mimic or block both the sympathetic and the parasympathetic nervous systems (Table 16.1).

CHOLINERGIC AGONISTS

Drugs that stimulate the parasympathetic nervous system are called *cholinergic agonists*, or *parasympathomimetics*, because they mimic the parasympathetic neurotransmitter acetylcholine. The neurotransmitter located at the ganglions and the parasympathetic terminal nerve endings is acetylcholine (ACh). It innervates cholinergic receptors in organs, tissues, and glands. The two types of cholinergic receptors are muscarinic receptors, which stimulate smooth muscle and slow the heart rate, and nicotinic receptors (neuromuscular), which affect the skeletal muscles. Many cholinergic agonists are nonselective because they can affect both the muscarinic and the nicotinic receptors. However, there are selective cholinergic agonists for the muscarinic receptors that do *not* affect the nicotinic receptors. Fig. 16.2 illustrates the effects of parasympathetic, or cholinergic, stimulation.

There are two types of cholinergic agonists: direct-acting cholinergic agonists act on receptors to activate a tissue response (Fig. 16.3A), and indirect-acting cholinergic agonists inhibit the action of the enzyme cholinesterase (ChE), also called acetylcholinesterase (AChE), by forming a chemical complex that allows acetylcholine to persist and attach to the receptor (Fig. 16.3B). Drugs that inhibit ChE are called *cholinesterase inhibitors, acetylcholinesterase inhibitors*, or *anticholinesterases*. ChE may destroy acetylcholine before it reaches the

187

receptor or after it has attached to the site. By inhibiting or destroying the ChE, more acetylcholine is available to stimulate the receptor and to remain in contact with it longer.

Cholinesterase inhibitors can be separated into reversible and irreversible inhibitors. The *reversible inhibitors* bind the ChE for several minutes to hours, and the *irreversible inhibitors* bind the enzyme permanently. The resulting effects vary with how long the ChE is bound.

The major responses of cholinergic agonists are to stimulate bladder and gastrointestinal (GI) tone; constrict the pupils of the eyes, known as **miosis**; and increase neuromuscular transmission. Other effects of cholinergic agonists include decreased heart rate and blood pressure and increased salivary, GI, and bronchial secretions. Table 16.2 lists the responses of direct- and indirect-acting cholinergic agonists.

Direct-Acting Cholinergic Agonists

Many drugs classified as direct-acting cholinergic agonists are primarily selective to the muscarinic receptors but are nonspecific because the muscarinic receptors are located in the smooth muscle of the GI and genitourinary tracts, glands, and heart. Bethanechol chloride, a direct-acting cholinergic agonist, acts on the muscarinic (cholinergic) receptor and is used primarily to increase urination in the treatment of urinary retention and neurogenic bladder. Metoclopramide hydrochloride (HCl) is a direct-acting cholinergic agonist that is usually prescribed to treat gastroparesis, nausea, and gastroesophageal reflux disease (GERD). In low doses, metoclopramide enhances gastric motility and thus accelerates gastric emptying time. Prototype Drug Chart: Bethanechol Chloride details the pharmacologic behavior of bethanechol, a classic cholinergic agonist.

Pharmacokinetics

Bethanechol chloride is poorly absorbed in the GI tract. The percentage of protein binding and the half-life are unknown. The drug is most likely excreted in the urine.

Fig. 16.1 Parasympathetic transmitters and receptors. *ACh*, Acetylcholine; *AChE*, acetylcholinesterase.

PROTOTYPE DRUG CHART
Bethanechol Chloride

Drug Class	Dosage
Cholinergic: Parasympathomimetic	Urinary retention A: PO: Initially 5–10 mg q1h until effective response or 50 mg given; *maint*: 10–50 mg tid/qid; *max*: 200 mg/d
Contraindications	**Drug-Lab-Food Interactions**
Contraindicated: Intestinal or urinary tract obstruction, IBS, bradycardia, hypotension, hypertension, asthma, peptic ulcer, hyperthyroidism, seizures, parkinsonism *Caution:* COPD, syncope, ileus, children, pregnancy, breastfeeding	Drug: Decreases bethanechol effect with antidysrhythmics (e.g., procainamide); ganglionic blocking agents (e.g., mecamylamine) cause significant hypotension after severe abdominal symptoms. False test results (amylase, lipase) may result. Atropine, flavoxate, and opiates counteract bethanechol action. Lab: Increases AST, bilirubin, amylase, lipase
Pharmacokinetics	**Pharmacodynamics**
Absorption: Poorly absorbed PO Distribution: PB: UK Metabolism: t½: UK Excretion: In urine	PO: Onset: 0.5–1.5 h Peak: 1–2 h Duration: 1 h Subcut: Onset: 5–15 min Peak: 15–30 min Duration: 2 h
Therapeutic Effects/Uses	
To treat urinary retention and neurogenic bladder Mechanism of action: Stimulates the cholinergic (muscarinic) receptors; promotes contraction of the bladder; increases GI secretions and peristalsis, pupillary constriction, and bronchoconstriction	
Side Effects	**Adverse Reactions**
Nausea, vomiting, diarrhea, abdominal cramps, hypersalivation, diaphoresis, headache, dizziness, flushing, urinary urgency and frequency, miosis, lacrimation	Tachycardia, hypotension *Life-threatening:* Bronchospasm, wheezing, seizures

A, Adult; *AST*, aspartate aminotransferase; *COPD*, chronic obstructive pulmonary disease; *d*, day; *GI*, gastrointestinal; *h*, hour; *IBS*, irritable bowel syndrome; *maint*, maintenance; *max*, maximum; *min*, minute; *PB*, protein binding; *PO*, by mouth; *q1h*, every 1 hour; *qid*, four times a day; *subcut*, subcutaneous; *t½*, half-life; *tid*, three times a day; *UK*, unknown.

TABLE 16.1 Autonomic Nervous System Stimulants: Sympathetic and Parasympathetic

Sympathetic Stimulants
Sympathomimetics (Adrenergics, Adrenomimetics, or Adrenergic Agonists)
Action:
- Increase blood pressure
- Increase pulse rate
- Relax bronchioles
- Dilate pupils of eyes
- Relax uterine muscles
- Increase blood glucose

Sympathetic Depressants
Sympatholytics (Adrenergic Blockers, Adrenolytics, or Adrenergic Antagonists)
Action:
- Decrease pulse rate
- Decrease blood pressure
- Constrict bronchioles

Direct-Acting Parasympathetic Stimulants
Parasympathomimetics (Cholinergics or Cholinergic Agonists)
Action:
- Decrease blood pressure
- Decrease pulse rate
- Constrict bronchioles
- Constrict pupils of eyes
- Increase urinary contraction
- Increase peristalsis

Indirect-Acting Cholinesterase Inhibitors (Anticholinesterase)
Action:
- Increase muscle tone

Parasympathetic Depressants
Parasympatholytics (Anticholinergics, Cholinergic Antagonists, or Antispasmodics)
Action:
- Increase pulse rate
- Decrease mucous secretions
- Decrease gastrointestinal motility
- Increase urinary retention
- Dilate pupils of eyes

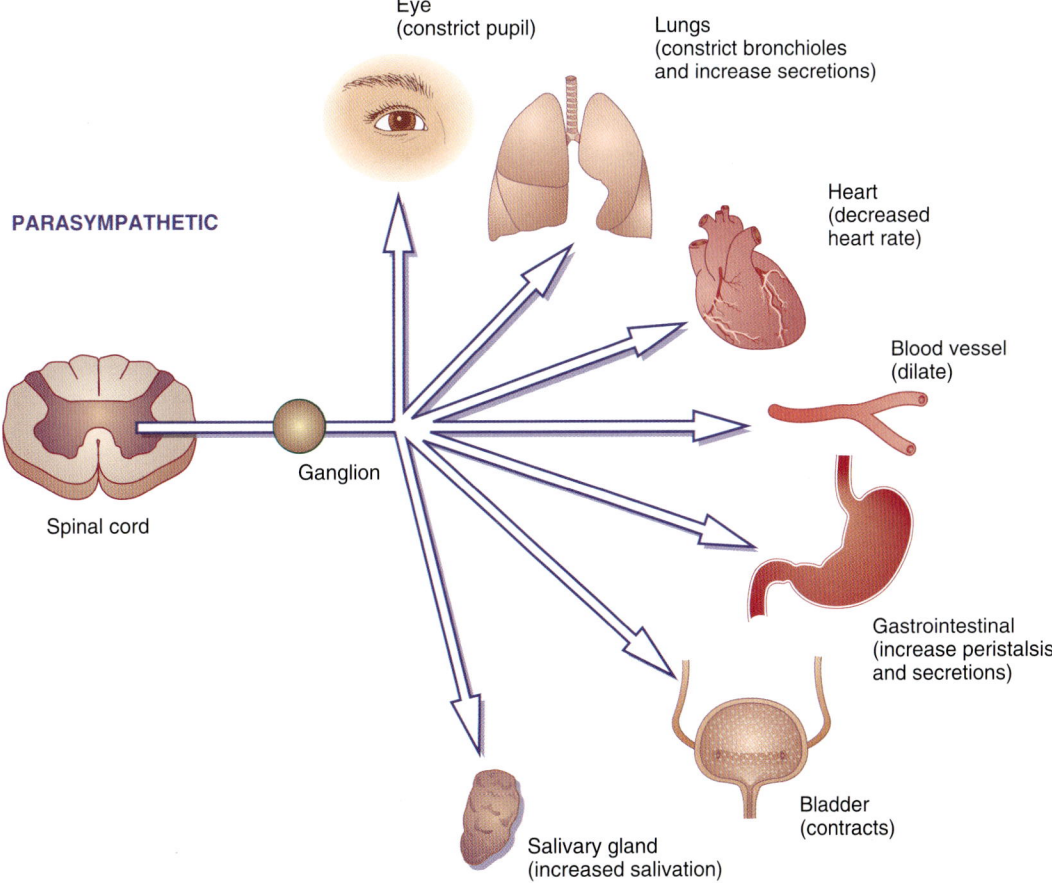

Fig. 16.2 Parasympathetic responses. Stimulation of the parasympathetic nervous system or use of parasympathomimetic drugs will cause the pupils to constrict, bronchioles to constrict and bronchial secretions to increase, heart rate to decrease, blood vessels to dilate, peristalsis and gastric secretions to increase, the bladder muscle to contract, and salivary glands to increase salivation.

Fig. 16.3 (A) Direct-acting parasympathomimetic (cholinergic agonist). Cholinergic agonists resemble acetylcholine and act directly on the receptor. (B) Indirect-acting parasympathomimetic (cholinesterase inhibitor). Cholinesterase inhibitors inactivate the enzyme acetylcholinesterase (cholinesterase), thus permitting acetylcholine to react to the receptor. *ACh*, Acetylcholine; *AChE*, acetylcholinesterase or cholinesterase; *D*, cholinergic agonist; *DD*, cholinesterase inhibitor (anticholinesterase).

TABLE 16.2	Effects of Cholinergic Agonists
Body Tissue	Response
Cardiovascular[a]	Decreased heart rate, lowered blood pressure because of vasodilation, and slowed conduction of atrioventricular node
Gastrointestinal[b]	Increased tone and motility of smooth muscle of stomach and intestine, increased peristalsis, and relaxed sphincter muscles
Genitourinary	Contraction of muscles of the urinary bladder, increased tone of ureters, relaxed bladder sphincter muscles, and stimulated urination
Ocular[b]	Increased pupillary constriction or miosis (pupil becomes smaller) and increased accommodation (flattening or thickening of eye lens for distant or near vision)
Glandular[a]	Increased salivation, perspiration, and tears
Bronchial (lung)[a]	Stimulation of bronchial smooth muscle contraction and increased bronchial secretions
Striated muscle[b]	Increased neuromuscular transmission and maintenance of muscle strength and tone

[a]Tissue responses to large doses of cholinergic agonists.
[b]Major tissue responses to normal doses of cholinergic agonists.

Pharmacodynamics

The principal use of bethanechol is to promote urination by stimulating the muscarinic cholinergic receptors in the detrusor muscle to contract the bladder and produce urine output. Because of the increased tone of the detrusor muscle, the onset of action is 30 minutes after taking an oral dose of bethanechol, and the duration is 1 hours. Bethanechol also increases peristalsis in the GI tract and gastric emptying time, and the drug should be taken 1 before or 2 hours after meals.

Side Effects and Adverse Reactions

Mild to severe side effects of most muscarinic agonists, such as bethanechol, include hypotension, tachycardia, excessive salivation, increased gastric acid secretion, abdominal cramps, diarrhea, and bronchospasm. This group of agents should be prescribed cautiously for patients with low blood pressure and chronic obstructive pulmonary disease (COPD). Muscarinic agonists are contraindicated for patients with intestinal or urinary tract obstruction, severe bradycardia, or active asthma.

Direct-Acting Cholinergic Agonists: Eye

Pilocarpine is a direct-acting cholinergic agonist that constricts the pupils of the eyes, thus opening the Schlemm canal to promote drainage of aqueous humor (fluid). This drug is used to treat glaucoma by relieving (intraocular) fluid pressure in the eye and to promote miosis in eye surgery and examinations. Pilocarpine also acts on the nicotinic receptor, as does carbachol. Both agents are discussed in more detail in Chapter 44. An oral form of pilocarpine is used to relieve xerostomia (dry mouth).

Indirect-Acting Cholinergic Agonists

The indirect-acting cholinergic agonists do not act on receptors; instead, they inhibit or inactivate the enzyme cholinesterase, permitting acetylcholine to accumulate at the receptor sites (see Fig. 16.3B). This action gives them the name *cholinesterase inhibitors, acetylcholinesterase inhibitors*, or *anticholinesterases*, of which there are two types: reversible and irreversible.

The function of the enzyme cholinesterase is to break down acetylcholine into choline and acetic acid. A small amount of cholinesterase can break down a large amount of acetylcholine in a short period. A cholinesterase inhibitor drug binds with cholinesterase, allowing acetylcholine to activate the muscarinic and nicotinic cholinergic receptors. This action permits skeletal muscle stimulation, which increases the force of muscular contraction. Because of this action, cholinesterase inhibitors are useful to increase muscle tone for patients with myasthenia gravis (a neuromuscular disorder). By increasing acetylcholine, additional effects occur, such as increases in GI motility, bradycardia, miosis, bronchial constriction, and increased micturition.

The primary use of *reversible* cholinesterase inhibitors is to treat myasthenia gravis; another use is to treat Alzheimer disease. The primary clinical indication for *irreversible* cholinesterase inhibitors is glaucoma.

Reversible Cholinesterase Inhibitors

Reversible cholinesterase inhibitors are used to produce pupillary constriction in the treatment of glaucoma and to increase muscle strength in patients with myasthenia gravis. Drug effects persist for several

CLINICAL JUDGMENT [NURSING PROCESS]
Cholinergic Agonist, Direct Acting: Bethanechol

Concept: Elimination
- The excretion of metabolic waste products from the body, such as urination

Recognize Cues [Assessment]
- Assess baseline vital signs for future comparisons.
- Assess urine output (should be >1500 mL/day).
- Obtain patient history of health problems such as peptic ulcer, urinary obstruction, or asthma. Cholinergic agonists can aggravate symptoms of these conditions.

Analyze Cues and Prioritize Hypothesis [Patient Problems]
- Hypotension
- Urinary retention
- Potential for falls
- Fatigue

Generate Solutions [Planning]
- Patient will void with more frequency after taking cholinergic agonists.

Take Action [Nursing Interventions]
- Monitor vital signs. Heart rate and blood pressure decrease when large doses of cholinergics are taken. Orthostatic hypotension is a side effect of cholinergic agonists, such as bethanechol.
- Record fluid intake and output. Decreased urinary output should be reported because it may be related to urinary obstruction.
- Give cholinergic agonists 1 hour before or 2 hours after meals to minimize nausea and vomiting. If a patient complains of gastric pain, the drug may be given with meals.
- Check serum amylase, lipase, aspartate aminotransferase (AST), and bilirubin levels. These laboratory values may increase slightly in a patient taking cholinergic agonists.
- Observe the patient for side effects such as gastric pain or cramping, diarrhea, increased salivary or bronchial secretions, tachycardia, and orthostatic hypotension.
- Auscultate breath sounds for rales, crackling sounds from fluid congestion in the lungs, or rhonchi, rough sounds resulting from mucous secretions in the lungs. Cholinergic agonists can increase bronchial secretions.
- ⚡ Have intravenous (IV) atropine sulfate (0.6–1.2 mg) available as an antidote for cholinergic overdose. Early signs of overdosing include flushing, salivation, sweating, nausea, and abdominal cramps.
- Increase bathing frequency and linen change when needed. Diaphoresis (excessive perspiration) may occur.
- ⚡ Monitor for possible cholinergic crisis (overdose), including symptoms of muscular weakness and increased salivation.

Patient Teaching
- Teach patients to take the cholinergic agonist as prescribed. Compliance with the drug regimen is essential.
- Direct patients to report severe side effects, such as profound dizziness or a decrease in heart rate below 60 beats/min.
- ⚡ Teach patients to arise from a lying position slowly to avoid dizziness. This is most likely a result of orthostatic hypotension.
- Encourage patients to maintain effective oral hygiene if excess salivation occurs.
- Advise patients to report any difficulty in breathing as a result of respiratory distress.

Evaluate Outcomes [Evaluation]
- Determine the effectiveness of the cholinergic agonist or anticholinesterase drug.
- Evaluate the stability of patient vital signs, and note the presence of side effects or adverse reactions.

---

hours. Drugs used to increase muscular strength in myasthenia gravis include neostigmine (short acting), pyridostigmine bromide (moderate acting), ambenonium chloride (long acting), and edrophonium chloride (short acting, for diagnostic purposes). These drugs are discussed in more detail in Chapter 21. A reversible anticholinesterase drug is physostigmine, which is used as an antidote for atropine to reverse anticholinergic toxicity. Ophthalmic agents are further discussed in Chapter 44.

Side Effects
Common side effects from reversible cholinesterase inhibitors are hypotension, bradycardia, sweating, hypersalivation, and GI distress, which includes anorexia, nausea, vomiting, abdominal pain, and diarrhea. Reversible cholinesterase inhibitors are contraindicated for patients with asthma, diabetes, cardiovascular disease, and GI or genitourinary obstruction. Caution is required for patients who have bradycardia, peptic ulcers, seizures, or dysrhythmia. Cholinesterase inhibitors are contraindicated for patients with intestinal or urinary obstruction.

Irreversible Cholinesterase Inhibitors
Irreversible cholinesterase inhibitors are potent agents because of their long-lasting effects. The enzyme cholinesterase must be regenerated before the drug effect diminishes, a process that may take days or weeks. These drugs are used to produce pupillary constriction.

Table 16.3 lists examples of cholinergic drugs and their standard dosages and common uses.

CHOLINERGIC ANTAGONISTS

Drugs that inhibit the actions of acetylcholine by occupying the acetylcholine receptors are called cholinergic antagonists (blocking agents), muscarinic antagonists, anticholinergics, cholinergic blocking agents, antispasmodics, or parasympatholytics. The major body tissues and organs affected by the anticholinergic group of drugs are the heart, respiratory tract, GI tract, urinary bladder, eyes, and exocrine glands. By blocking the parasympathetic nerves, the sympathetic (adrenergic) nervous system dominates. Anticholinergics and adrenergic agonists produce many of the same responses.

Anticholinergic and cholinergic agonists have opposite effects. The major responses to anticholinergics are a decrease in GI motility, a decrease in salivation, dilation of pupils—also called mydriasis—and an increase in pulse rate. Other effects of anticholinergics include decreased bladder contraction, which can result in urinary retention, and decreased rigidity and tremors related to neuromuscular excitement. An anticholinergic can act as an antidote to the toxicity caused by cholinesterase inhibitors and organophosphate ingestion. The various effects of anticholinergics are described in Table 16.4.

TABLE 16.3 Cholinergic Agonists

Drug	Route and Dosage	Uses and Considerations
Direct-Acting Cholinergic Agonists		
Bethanechol chloride	See Prototype Drug Chart: Bethanechol Chloride	
Metoclopramide hydrochloride	Postoperative nausea/vomiting: A: IM/IV: 10 mg near end of procedure, then may repeat q4–6 h PRN; *max:* 20 mg single dose	For GERD, gastroparesis, nausea and vomiting. May cause drowsiness, dizziness, fatigue, restlessness, headache, dysgeusia, nausea, vomiting, edema, bradycardia, tachycardia, hypo/hypertension, and EPS. PB: 30%; t½: 2.5–6 h
Carbachol	See Chapter 44	See Chapter 44
Pilocarpine hydrochloride	See Chapter 44	See Chapter 44
Cholinesterase Inhibitor		
Donepezil hydrochloride	See Chapter 20	See Chapter 20
Rivastigmine	See Chapter 20	See Chapter 20
Indirect-Acting Cholinergics or Cholinesterase Inhibitors for the Eye		
Echothiophate iodide	See Chapter 44	See Chapter 44
Reversible Cholinergics or Cholinesterase Inhibitors		
Neostigmine methylsulfate	Myasthenia gravis: A: PO: Initially 15 mg tid, may gradually increase to *maint:* 15–375 mg/d in divided doses A: Subcut/IM: 0.5 mg; *max:* 0.5 mg/dose	For myasthenia gravis, urinary retention, and ileus and for neuromuscular blockade reversal. May cause dizziness, headache, nausea, vomiting, bradycardia, hypotension, tachycardia, muscle cramps, seizures, and dyspnea. PB: 15%–25%; t½: 42–60 min
Physostigmine salicylate	Anticholinergic toxicity: A: IV/IM: 0.5–2 mg/dose slow IV, repeat q10–30 min PRN	For anticholinergic syndrome, neuromuscular blockade reversal, and glaucoma. May cause diaphoresis, hypersalivation, nausea, vomiting, bradycardia, hypotension, seizures, confusion, muscle weakness/paralysis, dyspnea, and bronchospasm. PB: UK; t½: 1–2 h
Pyridostigmine bromide	Neuromuscular blockade reversal: A: IV: 0.1–0.25 mg/kg simultaneously or immediately preceded by atropine 0.6–1.2 mg IV	For myasthenia gravis, neuromuscular blockade reversal, and nerve gas exposure prophylaxis. May cause nausea, vomiting, abdominal cramps, diarrhea, headache, bronchospasm, diaphoresis, hypersalivation, and urinary frequency/incontinence. PB: None; t½: 3 h
Antidote for Irreversible and Reversible Cholinesterase Inhibitors		
Pralidoxime chloride	Cholinesterase inhibitor overdose: A: IV: 1–2 g infused over 15–30 min; follow with 250 mg q5min PRN; *max:* 2 g/dose	For cholinesterase inhibitor overdose and organophosphate pesticide poisoning. May cause dizziness, blurred vision, headache, drowsiness, tachycardia, hypertension, muscle weakness/paralysis, and hypertonia. PB: None; t½: 74–77 min

A, Adult; *d*, day; *GERD*, gastroesophageal reflux disease; *h*, hour; *IM*, intramuscular; *IV*, intravenous; *maint*, maintenance; *max*, maximum; *min*, minute; *PB*, protein binding; *PO*, by mouth; *PRN*, as needed; *q4–6h*, every 4–6 hours; *q5min*, every 5 minutes; *q10–30 min*, every 10–30 minutes; *subcut*, subcutaneous; *t½*, half-life; *tid*, three times a day; *UK*, unknown.

TABLE 16.4 Effects of Anticholinergic Drugs

Body Tissues	Responses
Cardiovascular	Heart rate increases with large doses; small doses can decrease heart rate.
GI	Relaxed smooth muscle tone of GI tract, decreased GI motility and peristalsis; gastric and intestinal secretions are decreased.
Urinary tract	Relaxed bladder detrusor muscle and increased constriction of internal sphincter; urinary retention can result.
Ocular	Dilated pupils (mydriasis) and paralyzed ciliary muscles (cycloplegia) cause a decrease in accommodation.
Glandular	Salivation, perspiration, and bronchial secretions are decreased.
Bronchial	Bronchi are dilated, and bronchial secretions decrease.
Central nervous system	Tremors and rigidity of muscles are decreased; drowsiness, disorientation, and hallucinations can result from large doses.

GI, Gastrointestinal.

Muscarinic receptors are a type of cholinergic receptor involved in tissue and organ responses to anticholinergics because anticholinergics inhibit the actions of acetylcholine by occupying these receptor sites. Fig. 16.4 illustrates this action of anticholinergic drugs; these drugs may also block the effect of direct-acting parasympathomimetics, such as bethanechol and pilocarpine, and of indirect-acting parasympathomimetics, such as physostigmine and neostigmine.

Atropine

Atropine sulfate, first derived from the belladonna plant (*Atropa belladonna*) and purified in 1831, is a classic anticholinergic—or muscarinic antagonist—drug. Scopolamine was the second belladonna alkaloid produced. Atropine and scopolamine act on muscarinic receptors, but they have little effect on nicotinic receptors except in high doses. Atropine is useful primarily as a preoperative medication to decrease salivary secretions and as an agent to increase heart rate when bradycardia is present. Atropine can also be used as an antidote for muscarinic agonist poisoning caused by an overdose of a cholinesterase inhibitor or a muscarinic drug such as bethanechol and for neuromuscular blockade reversal. However, if a patient takes atropine or an atropine-like drug (e.g., an antihistamine), side effects can occur. Prototype Drug Chart: Atropine details the pharmacologic behavior of atropine.

Synthetic anticholinergic drugs are also used as antispasmodics to treat peptic ulcers and intestinal spasticity. One example is propantheline bromide, which has been available for several decades. It decreases gastric secretions and GI spasms in duodenal ulcers. Since the introduction of the histamine (H_2) blockers, anticholinergic agents such as propantheline are rarely used to decrease gastric secretions.

Fig. 16.4 Anticholinergic Response. The anticholinergic drug occupies the receptor sites, blocking acetylcholine. *ACh*, Acetylcholine; *D*, anticholinergic drug.

PROTOTYPE DRUG CHART
Atropine

Drug Class	Dosage
Anticholinergic: Parasympatholytic	Bradycardia: A: IV: 0.5–1 mg, repeat q3–5 min PRN up to 3 mg

Contraindications	Drug-Lab-Food Interactions
Hypersensitivity, glaucoma *Caution:* Renal, hepatic, or respiratory impairment, COPD, cardiovascular disease, myocardial ischemia, tachycardia, GI obstruction, ileus, ulcerative colitis, GI disease, hyperthyroidism, urinary retention, dysrhythmias, hypertension, diarrhea, myasthenia gravis, older adults, pregnancy, breastfeeding	Drug: Increases anticholinergic effect with phenothiazines, antihistamines, TCAs, amantadine, quinidine; high-dose anticholinergics may decrease effects of carbidopa/levodopa by delaying GI absorption; anticholinergics may enhance therapeutic effects at therapeutic doses.

Pharmacokinetics	Pharmacodynamics
Absorption: PO/IM: Well absorbed Distribution: PB: 14%–22% Metabolism: t½: 2–4 h Excretion: 13%–57% Excreted in urine	IM: Onset: 10–30 min Peak: 0.5–1 h Duration: 4 h IV: Onset: Immediate Peak: 5 min Duration: UK

Therapeutic Effects/Uses

Preoperative medication to reduce salivation, increase heart rate for bradycardia, for neuromuscular blockade reversal, for cholinergic crisis, and to dilate pupils for ocular diagnostic examinations
Mechanism of action: Inhibits acetylcholine by occupying the receptors; increases heart rate by blocking vagus stimulation; promotes pupil dilation by blocking iris sphincter muscle

Side Effects	Adverse Reactions
Drowsiness, dizziness, nausea, dry mouth, headache, confusion, insomnia, amnesia, constipation, flushing, restlessness, blurred vision, mydriasis, anxiety, photophobia, palpitations, urinary retention, erectile dysfunction, hypo/hyperreflexia, ataxia, weakness, anhidrosis, impaired body temperature regulation, dehydration, injection site reaction	Tachycardia, paradoxical bradycardia, angina, hypertension, hypotension, pulmonary edema, respiratory depression, ileus, seizures, hypo/hyperglycemia, hypokalemia, hyponatremia *Life-threatening:* Dysrhythmias, laryngospasm, coma

A, Adult; *COPD*, chronic obstructive pulmonary disease; *GI*, gastrointestinal; *h*, hour; *IM*, intramuscular; *IV*, intravenous; *PB*, protein binding; *PO*, by mouth; *PRN*, as needed; *q3–5min*, every 3–5 minutes; *t½*, half-life; *TCA*, tricyclic antidepressant.

Pharmacokinetics
Atropine sulfate is well absorbed orally and parenterally. It crosses the blood-brain barrier and exerts its effect on the central nervous system (CNS). The protein binding is unknown. It crosses the placenta. Atropine has a short half-life of 2 to 4 hours, so there is little cumulative effect. Most of the absorbed atropine is excreted in the urine (15%–57%).

Pharmacodynamics
Atropine sulfate blocks acetylcholine by occupying the muscarinic receptor. It increases the heart rate by blocking vagus stimulation and promotes dilation of the pupils by paralyzing the iris sphincter. The two most frequent uses of atropine are to decrease salivation and respiratory secretions preoperatively and to treat sinus bradycardia by increasing the heart rate. Atropine also is used ophthalmically for mydriasis and cycloplegia before eye examinations and to treat inflammation of the iris (iritis) and uveal tract.

Its onset of action for the intramuscular (IM) route is 10 to 30 minutes, and it peaks at 30 minutes to 1 hour. The duration is 4 hours. The onset of action for the IV route is immediate, and peak action occurs in 5 minutes.

Side Effects and Adverse Reactions
The common side effects of atropine and atropine-like drugs include xerostomia (dry mouth), nasal dryness, blurred vision, tachycardia, constipation, and urinary retention. Other side effects and adverse reactions are nausea, headache, dehydration, seizures, hypotension or hypertension, photophobia (intolerance of bright light), and coma.

Antiparkinson Anticholinergic Drugs
Studies indicate that anticholinergics affect the CNS as well as the parasympathetic nervous system. Anticholinergics affect the CNS by suppressing the tremors and muscular rigidity of parkinsonism, but they have little effect on mobility and muscle weakness. As a result of these findings, several anticholinergic drugs were developed for the treatment of parkinsonism (e.g., trihexyphenidyl hydrochloride, biperiden, and benztropine). These drugs can be used alone in the early stages of parkinsonism; they may be used in combination with levodopa/carbidopa to control parkinsonism, or they can be used alone to treat pseudoparkinsonism, which results from the side effects of the phenothiazines in antipsychotic drugs. Drugs used to treat parkinsonism are described in more detail in Chapter 20. Prototype Drug Chart: Benztropine lists the drug data related to benztropine, which is used for parkinsonism.

Pharmacokinetics
Benztropine is well absorbed from the GI tract. Its protein-binding percentage and half-life are unknown. It is excreted in the urine.

Pharmacodynamics
Benztropine decreases involuntary movement and diminishes the signs and symptoms of tremors and muscle rigidity that occur with

---

PROTOTYPE DRUG CHART
Benztropine

Drug Class	Dosage
Antiparkinson: anticholinergic agent	Parkinsonism: A: PO/IM: Initially 0.5-1 mg/d at bedtime; *maint*: 1–2 mg/d; *max*: 6 mg/d Drug-induced extrapyramidal symptoms: A: PO/IM/IV: Initially 1–4 mg qd/bid; *max*: 8 mg/d

Contraindications	Drug-Lab-Food Interactions
Hypersensitivity, dementia, children *Caution:* Tachycardia, cardiac disease, autonomic neuropathy, prostatic hypertrophy, psychosis, glaucoma, myasthenia gravis, hyperthermia, alcohol use disorder, urinary retention/obstruction, ambient temperature increase, older adults, pregnancy, breastfeeding	Drug: Increases anticholinergic effect with phenothiazines, tricyclic antidepressants, and other anticholinergics

Pharmacokinetics	Pharmacodynamics
Absorption: PO: Well absorbed Distribution: PB: UK Metabolism: t½: UK Excretion: In urine	PO: Onset: 1 h Peak: 7 h Duration: 6–10 h

Therapeutic Effects/Uses	
To decrease involuntary symptoms of parkinsonism or drug-induced parkinsonism Mechanism of action: Blocks cholinergic (muscarinic) receptors, thus decreasing acetylcholine to reduce excess cholinergic activity (involuntary movements); also blocks dopamine reuptake to prolong dopamine effects and decrease involuntary movement	

Side Effects	Adverse Reactions
Nausea, vomiting, dry mouth, constipation, anhidrosis, dizziness, headache, drowsiness, blurred vision, confusion, depression, psychosis, hallucinations, weakness, hyperthermia, paresthesia, mydriasis, urinary retention	Tachycardia, ocular hypertension, heat stroke *Life-threatening:* Ileus, coma

A, Adult; *bid*, two times a day; *d*, day; *h*, hour; *IM*, intramuscular; *IV*, intravenous; *max*, maximum; *PB*, protein binding; *PO*, by mouth; *qd*, once daily; *t½*, half-life; *UK*, unknown.

CLINICAL JUDGMENT [NURSING PROCESS]
Anticholinergic Drugs: Atropine

Concept: Perfusion
- The passage of blood flow through arteries and capillaries, which deliver oxygen and nutrients to body cells

Recognize Cues [Assessment]
- Obtain baseline vital signs for future comparisons. Tachycardia is a side effect that occurs with large doses of anticholinergics such as atropine sulfate.
- Assess urine output. Urinary retention may occur.
- Check the patient's medical history. Atropine and atropine-like drugs are contraindicated in patients with narrow-angle glaucoma, obstructive gastrointestinal (GI) disorders, paralytic ileus, ulcerative colitis, benign prostatic hypertrophy, or myasthenia gravis.
- Obtain the patient's drug history. Phenothiazines and antidepressants increase the effect of anticholinergics.

Analyze Cues and Prioritize Hypothesis [Patient Problems]
- Hypertension
- Urinary retention
- Decreased visual acuity
- Constipation

Generate Solutions [Planning]
- Patient secretions will be decreased before surgery.
- Patient's heart rate will be increased.

Take Action [Nursing Interventions]
- Monitor patient vital signs. Report if tachycardia occurs.
- Determine fluid intake and output. Encourage patients to void before taking the medication, and report decreased urine output; anticholinergics can cause urinary retention. Maintain adequate fluid intake.
- Assess bowel sounds. Absence of bowel sounds may indicate paralytic ileus resulting from a decrease in GI motility (peristalsis).
- Examine for constipation caused by a decrease in GI motility. Encourage ingestion of foods that are high in fiber, intake of adequate amounts of fluids, and exercise if possible.
- Use bed alarms for patients who are confused and debilitated. Atropine could cause central nervous system stimulation (excitement, confusion) or drowsiness.
- Provide mouth care. Atropine decreases oral secretions and can cause dryness.
- Administer intravenous atropine undiluted or diluted in 10 mL of sterile water. Rate of administration is 1 mg or some fraction thereof per minute.

Patient Teaching
General
- Direct patients to avoid hot environments and excessive physical exertion. Elevations in body temperature can result from diminished sweat gland activity.
- ⚡ Teach patients with narrow-angle glaucoma to avoid atropine-like drugs. Anticholinergics cause mydriasis and increase intraocular pressure. Instruct patients to check labels on over-the-counter drugs to determine whether they are contraindicated for glaucoma.
- ⚡ Instruct patients not to drive a motor vehicle or participate in activities that require alertness. Drowsiness is common.
- Tell patients with mydriasis after an eye examination to use sunglasses in bright light because of photophobia.

Side Effects
- Advise patients of common side effects such as dry mouth, decreased urination, and constipation that can occur as a result of anticholinergic use.
- Direct patients to increase fluid intake and consumption of high-fiber foods to prevent constipation when taking anticholinergics for a prolonged period.
- Instruct patients to urinate before taking the anticholinergic because urinary retention can be a problem.
- Advise patients to report any marked decrease in urine output.
- Suggest that patients use hard candy, ice chips, or chewing gum. Maintain effective oral hygiene if a patient's mouth is dry. Anticholinergics decrease salivation.
- Encourage patients to use eye drops to moisten dry eyes that result from decreased lacrimation (tearing).

Evaluate Outcomes [Evaluation]
- Evaluate patient response to the anticholinergic.
- Determine whether constipation, urinary retention, or increased pulse rate is a problem.

---

parkinsonism. It is available as an oral tablet and as parenteral IM and IV injections. Alcohol and other CNS depressants potentiate sedation. Anticholinergics, phenothiazines, and tricyclic antidepressants (TCAs) may increase the anticholinergic effects of benztropine. The side effects are similar to those of other anticholinergic drugs.

Anticholinergics for Treating Motion Sickness
The effects of anticholinergics on the CNS benefit patients who are prone to motion sickness. An example of such an anticholinergic, classified as an antihistamine for motion sickness, is scopolamine. It is available topically as a skin patch placed behind the ear. Prevention of motion sickness is also provided via wristbands and ginger, including ginger gum or candy. Transdermal scopolamine is delivered over 3 days and is frequently prescribed for activities such as flying, cruising on the water, and bus or automobile trips. Other drugs classified as antihistamines for motion sickness are dimenhydrinate, cyclizine, and meclizine hydrochloride. Most of these drugs can be purchased over the counter with the exception of scopolamine.

Examples of anticholinergic drugs and their dosages and common uses are found in Table 16.5. Dosages may vary according to age, sex, and weight. Because anticholinergic drugs can increase intraocular pressure, they should not be administered to patients diagnosed with glaucoma.

Side Effects and Adverse Reactions
Side effects of antihistamines used as anticholinergics include xerostomia, drowsiness, visual disturbances (especially blurred vision resulting from pupillary dilation), constipation secondary to decreased GI peristalsis, urinary retention related to decreased bladder tone, tachycardia (when taken in large doses), hypotension, dysphagia, anhidrosis, heat stroke, and flushing.

TABLE 16.5 Anticholinergics

Drug	Route and Dosage	Uses and Considerations
Anticholinergics: Gastrointestinal or Cholinergic Blockers		
Atropine sulfate	See Prototype Drug Chart: Atropine	
Dicyclomine hydrochloride	A: PO: Initially 20 mg qid for 7 d; *maint:* 20–40 mg qid for 2 wk; *max:* 40 mg qid A: IM: 10–20 mg q6h for 1–2 d; *max:* 80 mg/d	For IBS. May cause dry mouth, agitation, confusion, dizziness, drowsiness, blurred vision, weakness, constipation, and nausea. PB: UK; t½: 9–10 h
Glycopyrrolate	Preoperative: aspiration prophylaxis A: IM: 4 mcg/kg 30 min to 1 h before anesthesia induction	For duodenal/peptic ulcer, aspiration prophylaxis, and neuromuscular blockade reversal. May cause flushing, dry mouth, headache, palpitations, hypo/hypertension, tachycardia, blurred vision, sinusitis, dyspnea, nausea, vomiting, constipation, infection, and urinary retention. PB: UK; t½: 0.55–1.25 h
Hyoscyamine SO$_4$	IBS: Immediate release: A: PO/SL: 0.125–0.25 mg q4h PRN; *max:* 1.5 mg/d Extended release: A: 0.375–0.75 mg q12h; *max:* 1.5 mg/d A: subcut/IM/IV: 0.25–0.5 mg as a single dose or bid/qid	Treatment of aspiration prophylaxis, neuromuscular blockade reversal, and IBS. May cause flushing, confusion, blurred vision, dizziness, drowsiness, photophobia, dysphagia, anhidrosis, constipation, palpitations, tachycardia, urinary retention, and erectile dysfunction. PB: 50%; t½: Immediate release 2–3.5 h, Extended release 7.5 h
Methscopolamine bromide	A: PO: 2.5 mg tid ac and 2.5–5 mg at bedtime; *max:* 12.5 mg/d	For peptic ulcer. May cause dizziness, drowsiness, confusion, blurred vision, anhidrosis, dry mouth, constipation, palpitations, tachycardia, urinary retention, and erectile dysfunction. PB: UK; t½: UK
Cholinergic Antagonists: Eye		
Cyclopentolate hydrochloride	See Chapter 44	See Chapter 44
Homatropine	See Chapter 44	See Chapter 44
Tropicamide	See Chapter 44	See Chapter 44
Anticholinergic-Antiparkinson Drugs		
Benztropine mesylate	See Prototype Drug Chart: Benztropine	
Trihexyphenidyl hydrochloride	Parkinsonism: A: PO: Initially 1 mg, may increase by 2 mg q3–5d; *maint:* 6–10 mg/d, divided in 3 doses with meals; *max:* 15 mg/d	For parkinsonism and drug-induced EPS. May cause dizziness, blurred vision, anxiety, insomnia, nausea, vomiting, constipation, dry mouth, restlessness, and urinary retention. PB: UK; t½: 33 h
Anticholinergic–Antimuscarinic Drugs		
Tolterodine tartrate	See Prototype Drug Chart: Tolterodine Tartrate	
Others		
Ipratropium bromide	A: MDI: 2 inhal 4–6 times daily PRN; *max:* 12 inhal/d	For bronchospasm associated with asthma and COPD, and rhinorrhea associated with allergy and common cold. May cause headache, dyspnea, back pain, epistaxis, nasopharyngitis, sinusitis, dry mouth, nasal dryness, nausea, and chest pain. PB: Minimal; t½: 2 h

A, Adult; *ac*, before meals; *bid*, two times a day; *COPD*, chronic obstructive pulmonary disease; *d*, day; *EPS*, extrapyramidal syndrome; *h*, hours; *IBS*, irritable bowel syndrome; *IM*, intramuscular; *inhal*, inhalation; *IV*, intravenous; *maint:* maintenance; *max*, maximum; *MDI*, metered-dose inhaler; *min*, minute; *PB*, protein binding; *PO*, by mouth; *PRN*, as needed; *q4h*, every 4 hours; *q6h*, every 6 hours; *q12h*, every 12 hours; *q3–5d*, every 3–5 days; *qid*, four times a day; *SL*, sublingual; *subcut*, subcutaneous; *t½*, half-life; *tid*, three times a day; *UK*, unknown; *wk*, weeks.

PROTOTYPE DRUG CHART

Tolterodine Tartrate

Drug Class	Dosage
Antimuscarinic agent: anticholinergic	Immediate release: A: PO: 1–2 mg bid; *max:* 4 mg/d Extended release: A: PO: 2–4 mg/d; *max:* 4 mg/d
Contraindications	**Drug-Lab-Food Interactions**
Hypersensitivity, urinary retention, gastric paresis, GI obstruction, and glaucoma *Caution:* Hypothyroidism, cardiovascular disease, bradycardia, heart failure, GERD, ulcerative colitis, myasthenia gravis, prostatic hypertrophy, renal or hepatic dysfunction, hypokalemia, hypocalcemia, hypomagnesemia, autonomic neuropathy, urinary obstruction, dysrhythmias, contact lenses, older adults, children, pregnancy, breastfeeding	Drug: Increased effects with amantadine, amoxapine, bupropion, clozapine, cyclobenzaprine, disopyramide, maprotiline, olanzapine, orphenadrine, H_1 blockers, phenothiazines, and TCAs; decreased effects with azole antifungals (e.g., ketoconazole) or macrolide antibiotics (e.g., erythromycin), and fluoxetine Food: Grapefruit juice may increase drug levels
Pharmacokinetics	**Pharmacodynamics**
Absorption: GI absorption is decreased with food intake. Distribution: PB: 96% Metabolism: t½: IR, 2–4 h; ER, 7–18 h Excretion: Urine and feces	PO: Onset: UK Peak: IR, 1–2 h; ER, 2–6 h Duration: UK
Therapeutic Effects/Uses	
To decrease urinary frequency, urgency, and incontinence Mechanism of action: Blocks cholinergic (muscarinic) receptors selectively in the urinary bladder	
Side Effects	**Adverse Reactions**
Drowsiness, dizziness, dry mouth and eyes, headache, blurred vision, confusion, diarrhea, abdominal pain, constipation, dyspepsia, dysuria, fatigue, weight gain, arthralgia, hallucinations, and urinary retention	Angioedema, chest pain, tachycardia, peripheral edema *Life-threatening:* Stevens-Johnson syndrome

A, Adult; *bid*, two times a day; *d*, day; *ER*, extended release; *GERD*, gastroesophageal reflux disease; *GI*, gastrointestinal; H_1, histamine 1; *h*, hours; *IR*, immediate release; *max*, maximum; *PB*, protein binding; *PO*, by mouth; *t½*, half-life; *TCA*, tricyclic antidepressant; *UK*, unknown.

CLINICAL JUDGMENT CASE STUDY

A 70-year-old male is scheduled for surgery to remove gallstones. He has been in fairly good health. His only other clinical problem is a slight tremor in his hands. His health care provider would like him to start on benztropine after surgery for his tremor. Preoperative medications, meperidine 75 mg and atropine sulfate 0.4 mg, were given intramuscularly 1 hour before surgery.

1. What are the advantages of giving atropine sulfate before surgery?
2. What are some contraindications of atropine sulfate?
3. If a patient received an atropine-like drug for several months, what assessments should the nurse make related to its effects?
4. How does atropine sulfate differ from bethanechol chloride?
5. What classification of drug is benztropine, and how does it work? Explain your answer.
6. What patient teaching should the nurse include related to the use of benztropine?

REVIEW QUESTIONS

1. A patient is receiving bethanechol. The nurse realizes that the action of this drug is to treat which condition?
   a. Glaucoma
   b. Urinary retention
   c. Delayed gastric emptying
   d. Gastroesophageal reflux disease
   e. Gastroparesis
   f. Parkinsonism
   g. Myasthenia gravis

2. The nurse teaches the patient receiving atropine to expect which side effect?
   a. Diarrhea
   b. Sweating
   c. Blurred vision
   d. Frequent urination

3. When benztropine is ordered for a patient, the nurse acknowledges that this drug is an effective treatment for which condition?
   a. Parkinsonism
   b. Paralytic ileus
   c. Motion sickness
   d. Urinary retention

4. Dicyclomine is an anticholinergic, which the nurse realizes is given to treat which condition?
   a. Mydriasis
   b. Constipation
   c. Urinary retention
   d. Irritable bowel syndrome
5. The nurse realizes that cholinergic agonists mimic which parasympathetic neurotransmitter?
   a. Dopamine
   b. Acetylcholine
   c. Cholinesterase
   d. Monoamine oxidase
6. The nurse is administering bethanechol, a cholinergic agonist, and should know that the expected cholinergic effects include which of the following?
   a. Increased heart rate
   b. Decreased peristalsis
   c. Decreased salivation
   d. Increased pupil constriction
7. When a patient has a cholinergic overdose from excessive dosing of bethanechol, the nurse anticipates administration of which drug as the antidote?
   a. Atropine
   b. Tolterodine
   c. Benztropine
   d. Metoclopramide

UNIT V   Central and Peripheral Nervous System Drugs

17

Stimulants

http://evolve.elsevier.com/McCuistion/pharmacology

OBJECTIVES

- Explain the purpose and type of nervous system in the body.
- Describe the major drug groups used for central nervous system stimulants, their actions, and conditions they treat.
- Summarize the pharmacology of amphetamines and amphetamine-like drugs.
- Describe the action and contraindications of anorexiants.
- Explain the action and use of analeptics.

OUTLINE

Anatomy and Physiology of the Nervous System, 199
    Central Nervous System, 199
    Peripheral Nervous System, 199
Central Nervous System Stimulants, 200
    Types of Stimulants, 200
    Conditions Treated With Central Nervous System Stimulants, 200
Amphetamines and Amphetamine-Like Drugs, 200
    Amphetamine Actions, Side Effects, and Adverse Reactions, 200
    Amphetamine-Like Drugs Used in the Treatment of Attention-Deficit/Hyperactivity Disorder and Narcolepsy, 200

Anorexiants, 202
    Action of Anorexiants, 202
    Side Effects and Adverse Reactions of Anorexiants, 203
Analeptics, 203
    Action of Analeptics, 203
    Side Effects and Adverse Reactions of Analeptics, 203
Clinical Judgment Case Study, 205
Review Questions, 205

ANATOMY AND PHYSIOLOGY OF THE NERVOUS SYSTEM

The nervous system is composed of all nerve tissues: brain, spinal cord, nerves, and ganglia. The purpose of the nervous system is to receive stimuli and transmit information to nerve centers for an appropriate response. There are two types of nervous systems: the central nervous system and the peripheral nervous system.

Central Nervous System

The central nervous system (CNS), composed of the brain and spinal cord, regulates body functions (Fig. 17.1). The CNS interprets information sent by impulses from the peripheral nervous system (PNS) and returns the instruction through the PNS for appropriate cellular actions. Stimulation of the CNS may either increase nerve cell (neuron) activity or block nerve cell activity.

Peripheral Nervous System

The PNS consists of two divisions: the somatic nervous system (SNS) and the autonomic nervous system (ANS). The SNS is voluntary and acts on skeletal muscles to produce locomotion and respiration. The ANS, also called the *visceral system*, is involuntary; it controls and regulates the functioning of the heart, respiratory system, gastrointestinal (GI) system, and glands. The ANS, a large nervous system that functions without our conscious control, has two subdivisions: the sympathetic and the parasympathetic nervous systems.

Sympathetic and Parasympathetic Nervous Systems

The sympathetic nervous system of the ANS is called the *adrenergic system* because its neurotransmitter is norepinephrine. The parasympathetic nervous system is called the *cholinergic system* because its neurotransmitter is acetylcholine. Because organs are innervated by both the sympathetic and the parasympathetic systems, they can produce opposite responses. The sympathetic response is excitability, and the parasympathetic response is inhibition.

The sympathetic and the parasympathetic nerve pathways originate from different locations in the spinal cord. These nervous systems send information by two types of nerve fibers, preganglionic and postganglionic, and by the ganglion between these fibers. The preganglionic nerve fiber carries messages from the CNS to the ganglion, and the postganglionic fiber transmits impulses from the ganglion to body tissues and organs.

Fig. 17.1 Brain and spinal cord.

CENTRAL NERVOUS SYSTEM STIMULANTS

Types of Stimulants

Numerous drugs can stimulate the CNS. Medically approved use of CNS stimulants is limited to the treatment of attention-deficit/hyperactivity disorder (ADHD) in children, narcolepsy, and the reversal of respiratory distress. The major groups of CNS stimulants include amphetamines, which stimulate the cerebral cortex of the brain; analeptics, which act on the brain stem and medulla to stimulate respiration; and anorexiants, which are thought to suppress appetite by stimulating the satiety center in the hypothalamic and limbic areas of the brain. Amphetamines and related anorexiants are greatly abused. Long-term use of amphetamines can produce psychological dependence or tolerance, conditions in which larger and larger doses of a drug are needed to reproduce the initial response. These medications are recommended for short-term use only (up to 12 weeks). Gradually increasing a drug dose and then abruptly stopping the drug may result in depression and withdrawal symptoms.

Conditions Treated With Central Nervous System Stimulants

Attention-Deficit/Hyperactivity Disorder

ADHD might be caused by a dysregulation of the transmitters: serotonin, norepinephrine, and dopamine. ADHD occurs primarily in children, usually before 7 years of age, and may continue through the teenage years. In some cases, it may not be identified until early adulthood. The incidence of ADHD is three to seven times more common in boys than in girls. Characteristic behaviors of the various types of ADHD include inattentiveness, inability to concentrate, restlessness (fidgety), hyperactivity (excessive and purposeless activity), inability to complete tasks, and impulsivity.

The child with ADHD may display poor coordination, and there may be abnormal electroencephalograph findings. Intelligence is usually not affected, but learning disabilities are often present. This disorder has also been called *minimal brain dysfunction, hyperactivity in children, hyperkinesis,* and *hyperkinetic syndrome with learning disorder.* Some professionals state that ADHD is often incorrectly diagnosed and results in many children receiving unnecessary treatment for months or years.

Narcolepsy

Narcolepsy is characterized by falling asleep during normal waking activities, such as driving a car or talking with someone. Sleep paralysis, the condition of muscle paralysis that is normal during sleep, usually accompanies narcolepsy and affects the voluntary muscles. The patient with narcolepsy is unable to move and may collapse.

AMPHETAMINES AND AMPHETAMINE-LIKE DRUGS

Amphetamine Actions, Side Effects, and Adverse Reactions

Amphetamines stimulate the release of the neurotransmitters norepinephrine and dopamine from the brain and sympathetic nervous system (peripheral nerve terminals) and block the reuptake of these transmitters. Amphetamines ordinarily cause euphoria and increased alertness, but they can also cause xerostomia (dry mouth), insomnia, restlessness, tremors, irritability, and weight loss. Cardiovascular problems such as increased heart rate, palpitations, cardiac dysrhythmia, and increased blood pressure can result from cardiac stimulation and vasoconstriction with continuous use of amphetamines. These drugs have a high potential for abuse, tolerance, and dependence. Excessive use may lead to psychosis.

The half-life of amphetamines usually varies from 9 to 15 hours. Amphetamines and dextroamphetamine are prescribed for narcolepsy and ADHD when amphetamine-like drugs are ineffective.

Amphetamines can cause adverse effects in the CNS and the cardiovascular, GI, and endocrine systems. Side effects and adverse reactions include dizziness, headache, euphoria, insomnia, tachycardia, hypertension, palpitations, dry mouth, anorexia, diarrhea, and erectile dysfunction.

Amphetamine-Like Drugs Used in the Treatment of Attention-Deficit/Hyperactivity Disorder and Narcolepsy

Methylphenidate and dexmethylphenidate, classed as amphetamine-like drugs, are given to increase a child's attention span and cognitive performance (e.g., memory, reading) and to decrease impulsiveness, hyperactivity, and restlessness. Dosage should be minimal in controlling ADHD symptoms. Methylphenidate is also used to treat narcolepsy. Because of the potential for abuse of methylphenidate, it is classified as a Controlled Substance Schedule (CSS) II drug. Prototype Drug Chart: Methylphenidate illustrates the pharmacokinetics, pharmacodynamics, and therapeutic effects of methylphenidate in the treatment of ADHD and narcolepsy. Amphetamine and amphetamine-like drugs should not be taken in the evening or before bedtime because insomnia may result. These drugs should be taken upon awakening.

Modafinil is an amphetamine-like stimulant that increases wakefulness in patients with sleep disorders such as narcolepsy. Its mechanism of action is not fully known.

Methylphenidate is the most frequently prescribed drug used to treat ADHD. Table 17.1 lists the amphetamines and amphetamine-like drugs and their dosages, uses, and considerations, including common side effects and a few serious adverse effects.

Pharmacokinetics

Methylphenidate is well absorbed from the GI mucosa and is usually administered to children twice a day before breakfast and lunch. Because food affects its absorption rate, this drug should be given upon awakening or 30 to 45 minutes before meals. Methylphenidate should be given 6 hours or more before sleep because it can cause insomnia. This drug is excreted in the urine, and 40% of methylphenidate is excreted unchanged.

TABLE 17.1 Amphetamines and Amphetamine-Like Drugs

Drug	Route and Dosage	Uses and Considerations
Amphetamines		
Amphetamine sulfate CSS II	ADHD: Immediate-release tab: A: PO: Initially 5–10 mg/d in morning; *max:* 60 mg/d Adol 6–17 y: PO: Initially 5 mg qd/bid; *max:* 60 mg/d C 3–5 y: PO: Initially 2.5 mg/d; *max:* 40 mg/d Extended release: A: PO: 12.5 mg/d in morning; *max:* 12.5 mg/d Adol/C 6–12 y PO: Initially 6.3 mg/d; *max:* 12.5 mg/d	For narcolepsy, ADHD, obesity. May cause growth suppression, dizziness, restlessness, insomnia, headache, weakness, dyspnea, confusion, anorexia, abdominal pain, dry mouth, weight loss, palpitations, tachycardia, hypertension, dysrhythmias, anxiety, fatigue, irritability, tremors, tolerance, constipation, diarrhea, and erectile dysfunction. PB: 16%; t½: 10–13 h
Dextroamphetamine sulfate CSS II	ADHD: Immediate release: A: PO: 5 mg qd/bid; *max:* 40 mg/d Adol/C >6 y: PO: 5 mg qd/bid; *max:* 40 mg/d C 3–5 y: PO: 2.5 mg/d; *max:* 40 mg/d Extended release: A/Adol/C >6 y: PO: Initially 5 mg qd/bid; *max:* 40 mg/d	For ADHD and narcolepsy. May cause headache, euphoria, anorexia, abdominal pain, constipation, diarrhea, weight loss, growth suppression, insomnia, irritability, restlessness, tremor, palpitations, tachycardia, hypertension, tolerance, erectile dysfunction, and blurred vision. PB: UK; t½: 10–12 h
Lisdexamfetamine dimesylate CSS II	ADHD: A: PO: Initially 30 mg/d; *max:* 70 mg/d Adol/C >6 y: PO: Initially 20–30 mg/d; *max:* 70 mg/d	For binge-eating disorder and ADHD. May cause growth suppression, insomnia, irritability, anxiety, dizziness, weight loss, anorexia, nausea, vomiting, constipation, diarrhea, abdominal pain, dry mouth, tachycardia, and bradycardia. PB: UK; t½: <1 h
Combinations of Amphetamines		
Amphetamine and dextroamphetamine	Narcolepsy: A/Adol/C >12 y: PO: Initially 10 mg/d in the morning; *max:* 60 mg/d C 6–11 y: PO: Initially 5 mg/d in the morning; *max:* 60 mg/d	For ADHD and narcolepsy. May cause abdominal pain, anorexia, dry mouth, insomnia, headache, weight loss, anxiety, agitation, exaggerated mood changes, dizziness, nausea, vomiting, and diarrhea. PB: 16% amphetamine, UK dextroamphetamine; t½: 10–13 h amphetamine, 10–12 h dextroamphetamine
Amphetamine-Like Drugs		
Methylphenidate hydrochloride CSS II	See Prototype Drug Chart: Methylphenidate.	
Modafinil CSS IV	Narcolepsy: A: PO: 200 mg/d in the morning; *max:* 400 mg/d	For narcolepsy, ADHD, shift work sleep disorder, and sleep apnea. May cause headache, dizziness, anxiety, anorexia, nausea, diarrhea, dry mouth, insomnia, rhinitis, back pain. PB: 60%; t½: 15 h
Dexmethylphenidate hydrochloride	Immediate release: A: PO: Initially 2.5 mg bid; *maint:* 2.5–10 mg bid; *max:* 20 mg/d Extended release: A: PO: Initially 10 mg/d in the morning; *maint:* 10–40 mg q am; *max:* 40 mg/d	For ADHD. May cause headache, dizziness, restlessness, irritability, anxiety, insomnia, anorexia, nausea, vomiting, dry mouth, abdominal pain, dyspepsia, weight loss, nasal congestion, and palpitations. PB: 12%–15%; t½: 2–4.5 h
Armodafinil	Narcolepsy: A: PO: 150–250 mg/d in the morning; *max:* 250 mg/d	For narcolepsy, shift work sleep disorder, and sleep apnea. May cause headache, anxiety, dizziness, insomnia, nausea, dyspepsia, dry mouth, diarrhea, depression, and suicidal ideation. PB: 60%; t½: 15 h
Selective Norepinephrine Reuptake Inhibitor		
Viloxazine	A/C 12–17 y: PO: 200 mg/d; *max:* A 600 mg/d, C 12–17 y 400 mg/d C >6 y: PO: 100 mg/d; *max:* 400 mg/d	For ADHD. May cause drowsiness, headache, fatigue, irritability, insomnia, abdominal pain, dry mouth, anorexia, nausea, vomiting, constipation, suicidal ideation, and infection. PB: 76%–82%; t½: 2–12 h
CNS Stimulant		
Serdexmethylphenidate and dexmethylphenidate	A/Adol/C 6–12 y: Initially 39.2 mg serdexmethylphenidate, 7.8 mg dexmethylphenidate/d in morning for 1 wk; *max:* 52.3 mg serdexmethylphenidate, 10.4 mg dexmethylphenidate/d	For ADHD. May cause drowsiness, abdominal pain, dry mouth, anorexia, nausea, vomiting, weight loss, agitation, anxiety, arthralgia, blurred vision, dizziness, headache, insomnia, bradycardia/tachycardia, and irritability. PB: 56% serdexmethylphenidate, 47% dexmethylphenidate; t½: 5.7 h serdexmethylphenidate, 11.7 h dexmethylphenidate
Other Narcolepsy Agents		
Histamine-3 Receptor Antagonists		
Pitolisant	A: PO: Initially 8.9 mg/d upon awakening for 1 wk, then 17.8 mg/d for 1 wk; *max:* 35.6 mg/d	For excessive daytime sleepiness associated with narcolepsy. May cause headache, anxiety, nausea, insomnia, infection, and musculoskeletal pain. PB: 91%–96%; t½: 7.5–24.2 h
Dopamine and Norepinephrine Inhibitors		
Solriamfetol	Excess drowsiness: A: PO: Initially 75 mg/d upon awakening; for 3 days, then may give 150 mg/d; *max:* 150 mg/d	For excessive daytime drowsiness associated with narcolepsy and obstructive sleep apnea. May cause headache, anxiety, irritability, xerostomia, insomnia, hypertension, palpitations, nausea, constipation, and diarrhea. PB: <20%; t½: 7.1 h

>, Greater than; <, less than; *A*, adult; *ADHD*, attention-deficit/hyperactivity disorder; *Adol*, adolescent; *bid*, twice a day; *C*, child; *CSS*, Controlled Substances Schedule; *d*, day; *h*, hour; *maint.*, maintenance; *max*, maximum; *PB*, protein binding; *PO*, by mouth; *q*, every; *t½*, half-life; *UK*, unknown; *wk*, week; *y*, year.

Pharmacodynamics

Methylphenidate inhibits the reuptake of dopamine and norepinephrine, resulting in CNS stimulation and an augmentation of serotonin action. This action helps correct ADHD by decreasing hyperactivity and improving attention span. This drug may also be prescribed for treating narcolepsy. Amphetamine-like drugs are considered generally more effective in treating ADHD than are amphetamines, which are generally avoided because they have a higher potential for abuse, habituation, and tolerance. Sympathomimetics (e.g., pseudoephedrine) and psychostimulants (e.g., caffeine) taken concurrently with methylphenidate increase stimulatory effects of irritability, nervousness, tremors, and insomnia. Concurrent use within 14 days of monoamine oxidase inhibitors (MAOIs) may cause hypertensive crisis. Methylphenidate potentiates the action of CNS stimulants, such as caffeine, and inhibits the metabolism of some barbiturates, such as phenobarbital, which can lead to increased blood levels and potential toxicity.

ANOREXIANTS

Action of Anorexiants

Anorexiants cause a stimulant effect on the hypothalamic and limbic regions of the brain to suppress appetite. Most of the anorexiants used to suppress appetite (Table 17.2) do not have serious side effects.

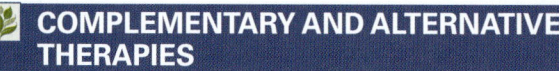

COMPLEMENTARY AND ALTERNATIVE THERAPIES

CNS Stimulants

> Korean ginseng may potentiate drug effects of central nervous system (CNS) stimulants.

Associated with amphetamines. For weight loss attempts, emphasis should be placed on a nutritious diet, exercise, and behavior modification. Reliance on appetite suppressants should be discouraged. Individuals who take anorexiants should be under the care of a health care provider. Anorexiants are contraindicated in hypertension, hyperthyroidism, glaucoma, and within 14 days of MAOI therapy and should be given with caution in patients with diabetes mellitus, seizures, Tourette syndrome, and bipolar disorder.

PROTOTYPE DRUG CHART

Methylphenidate

Drug Class	Dosage
Amphetamine-like drug: CNS stimulant CSS II	ADHD: Immediate release: A: PO: 20–30 mg/d in 2–3 divided doses, 30–45 min before meals, take last dose before 6 pm; *max:* 60 mg/d Adol/C 6–17 y: PO: Initially 5 mg bid before breakfast and lunch; *max:* 60 mg/d Extended release: A: PO: Initially 25 mg/d in the morning; *max:* 100 mg/d Adol/C 6–17 y: PO: Initially 25 mg/d in the morning; *max:* 100 mg/d
Contraindications	**Drug-Lab-Food Interactions**
MAOI therapy, and hereditary fructose intolerance *Caution:* Glaucoma, dysrhythmias, peripheral vascular disease, psychosis, depression, alcohol abuse, bipolar disorder, hyperthyroidism, hypertension, cardiovascular disease, seizures, GI obstruction, suicidal ideation, Tourette syndrome, older adult, pregnancy, breastfeeding	Drug: May increase stimulatory effects of sympathomimetics and psychostimulants; may reduce effect of antihypertensives; increases effects of oral anticoagulants, barbiturates, anticonvulsants, and TCAs; increases hypertensive crisis with MAOIs Food: Caffeine, chocolate, tea, colas may increase effects. Herbs: St. John's wort may decrease drug efficacy
Pharmacokinetics	**Pharmacodynamics**
Absorption: Well absorbed from GI tract Distribution: PB: 10%–33% Metabolism: $t\frac{1}{2}$: 1.3–7.7 h Excretion: 90% excreted unchanged in urine	PO: Onset: 0.5–1 h release: Peak 1.9 h Duration: 3–6 h Extended release: Peak 4.7 h Duration: 8 h
Therapeutic Effects/Uses	
To correct hyperactivity caused by ADHD, increase attention span, and control narcolepsy Mechanism of action: Research suggests modulation of serotonergic pathways occurs by blocking dopamine transport and increasing sympathomimetic activity	
Side Effects	**Adverse Reactions**
Anorexia, dry mouth, nausea, vomiting, dizziness, insomnia, irritability, restlessness, anxiety, confusion, depression, euphoria, hyperhidrosis, tremors, blurred vision, headache, abdominal pain, weight loss, constipation, diarrhea, paresthesia	Tachycardia, hypertension, bradycardia, growth suppression, palpitations, seizures, psychosis, Tourette syndrome, MI, stroke *Life-threatening:* Blood dyscrasias, dysrhythmias, hepatotoxicity, and ocular hypertension

>, Greater than; *<*, less than; *A*, adult; *ADHD*, attention-deficit/hyperactivity disorder; *Adol*, adolescent; *bid*, twice a day; *CNS*, central nervous system; *CSS*, Controlled Substances Schedule; *d*, day; *GI*, gastrointestinal; *h*, hour; *MAOI*, monoamine oxidase inhibitor; *max*, maximum; *MI*, myocardial infarction; *min*, minute; *PB*, protein binding; *PO*, by mouth; *tid*, three times a day; $t\frac{1}{2}$, half-life; *TCA*, tricyclic antidepressant; *y*, year.

Side Effects and Adverse Reactions of Anorexiants

Children younger than 12 years should not be given anorexiants, and self-medication with anorexiants should be discouraged. Long-term use of these drugs frequently results in severe side effects such as euphoria, restlessness, insomnia, palpitations, tachycardia, hypertension, and erectile dysfunction.

ANALEPTICS

Action of Analeptics

Analeptics, which are CNS stimulants, mostly affect the brain stem and spinal cord but also affect the cerebral cortex. The primary use of an analeptic is to stimulate respiration. One subgroup of analeptics is the xanthines (methylxanthines). Depending on the dose, caffeine stimulates the CNS, and large doses stimulate respiration. Newborns with respiratory distress might be given caffeine to increase respiration. Table 17.2 lists the analeptics and their dosages, uses, and considerations, including common side effects and a few serious adverse effects.

Side Effects and Adverse Reactions of Analeptics

Side effects from caffeine are similar to those from anorexiants: restlessness, tremors, palpitations, tachycardia, and insomnia. Other side effects include headache, GI irritation (e.g., nausea), and urinary frequency. Excess caffeine affects the CNS and heart and can cause dysrhythmias and seizures. High doses of caffeine in coffee, chocolate, and cold relief medications can cause psychological dependence. The half-life of caffeine is approximately 4 hours; however, the half-life is prolonged in patients with liver disease and in patients who are taking oral contraceptives or are pregnant. Caffeine is contraindicated during pregnancy because its effect on the fetus is unknown.

CLINICAL JUDGMENT [NURSING PROCESS]
Central Nervous System Stimulant: Methylphenidate Hydrochloride

Concept: Cognition
- The process of attaining knowledge through the mental processes of thinking, learning, and memory

Recognize Cues [Assessment]
- Determine whether the patient has a history of heart disease, hypertension, hyperthyroidism, parkinsonism, or glaucoma; in such cases, this drug is usually contraindicated.
- Assess vital signs to be used for future comparisons. Closely monitor patients with cardiac disease because this drug may cause tachycardia, hypertension, and stroke.
- Assess patient mental status, such as mood, affect, and aggressiveness.
- Evaluate height, weight, and growth of children.
- Assess complete blood count, differential white blood cells, and platelets before and during therapy.

Analyze Cues and Prioritize Hypothesis [Patient Problems]
- Hypertension
- Diarrhea
- Reduced functional ability

Generate Solutions [Planning]
- Patient will display less hyperactivity.
- Patient will demonstrate increased attention span.
- Patient's blood pressure and heart rate will be within normal limits.
- Patient will behave in a calm manner.

Take Action [Nursing Interventions]
- Monitor vital signs, and report irregularities.
- Evaluate height, weight, and growth of children.
- Observe patients for withdrawal symptoms such as nausea, vomiting, weakness, and headache.
- Monitor patients for side effects such as insomnia, restlessness, nervousness, tremors, irritability, tachycardia, and elevated blood pressure. Report findings.

Patient Teaching
General
- Teach patients to take the drug before meals.
- ⚡ Advise patients to avoid alcohol consumption.
- Encourage use of sugarless gum to relieve dry mouth.
- Teach patients to monitor weight twice a week and report weight loss.
- ⚡ Advise patients to avoid driving and using hazardous equipment when experiencing tremors, nervousness, or increased heart rate.
- ⚡ Teach patients not to abruptly discontinue the drug; the dose must be tapered to avoid withdrawal symptoms. Consult a health care provider before modifying doses.
- ⚡ Encourage patients to read labels on over-the-counter (OTC) products because many contain caffeine. A high plasma caffeine level could be fatal.
- Teach nursing mothers to avoid taking all central nervous system (CNS) stimulants (e.g., caffeine). These drugs are excreted in breast milk and can cause hyperactivity or restlessness in infants.
- Direct families to seek counseling for children with ADHD. Drug therapy alone is not an appropriate therapy program. Notify school nurse of drug therapy regimen.
- Explain to patients and family that long-term use may lead to drug abuse.

Diet
- Advise patients to avoid foods that contain caffeine (e.g., coffee, tea, chocolate, soft drinks, and energy drinks).
- Encourage parents to provide children with a nutritious breakfast because the drug may have anorexic effects.

Side Effects
- Teach patients about drug side effects and the need to report tachycardia and palpitations.
- Monitor children for onset of Tourette syndrome.

Evaluate Outcomes [Evaluation]
- Evaluate effectiveness of drug therapy, level of hyperactivity, and presence of adverse effects.
- Monitor weight, sleep patterns, and mental status.
- Evaluate patient knowledge of methylphenidate therapy.

TABLE 17.2 Anorexiants and Analeptics

Drug	Route and Dosage	Uses and Considerations
Anorexiants		
Benzphetamine hydrochloride CSS III	A: PO: 25–50 mg daily; *max:* 150 mg/d	Short-term treatment for obesity. May cause restlessness, dizziness, headache, insomnia, nausea, dry mouth, dysgeusia, anorexia, diarrhea, erectile dysfunction, palpitations, tachycardia, and hypertension. PB: UK, $t\frac{1}{2}$: UK
Diethylpropion hydrochloride CSS IV	Immediate release: A: PO: 25 mg tid 1 h before meals; *max:* 75 mg/d Extended release: A: PO: 75 mg/d mid morning; *max:* 75 mg/d	Short-term use for obesity. May cause headache, blurred vision, dizziness, anxiety, insomnia, dry mouth, abdominal pain, dysgeusia, nausea, vomiting, constipation, diarrhea, palpitations, tachycardia, hypertension, restlessness, erectile dysfunction, tremor, seizures, dependence, and tolerance. PB: UK; $t\frac{1}{2}$: 4–8 h
Phentermine hydrochloride CSS IV	A: PO: 15–37.5 mg/d in the morning; *max:* 37.5 mg/d	Short-term use for obesity. May cause restlessness, dizziness, headache, insomnia, euphoria, dysphoria, dry mouth, dysgeusia, nausea, constipation, diarrhea, hypertension, tachycardia, palpitations, tremors, and tolerance. PB: 17.5%; $t\frac{1}{2}$: 20 h
Phentermine-topiramate	Extended release: A: PO: 3.75 mg phentermine/23 mg topiramate/d for 14 d in the morning, then 7.5 mg phentermine/46 mg topiramate/d; *max:* 15 mg phentermine/92 mg topiramate/d	Used short term for obesity. May cause blurred vision, headache, dizziness, impaired cognition, pharyngitis, dry mouth, nausea, diarrhea, constipation, dysgeusia, tachycardia, hypertension, paresthesia, suicidal ideation, insomnia, infection, and hypokalemia. Evaluate weight loss in 12 wk. PB: 17.5% phentermine, 15%–41% topiramate; $t\frac{1}{2}$: 20 h phentermine, 65 h topiramate
Phendimetrazine	Immediate release: A: PO: 35 mg bid/tid, 1 h before meals; *max:* 70 mg tid Extended release: A: PO: 105 mg/d 30–60 min before breakfast; *max:* 105 mg/d	Used short term for obesity. May cause headache, insomnia, dizziness, dry mouth, restlessness, blurred vision, constipation, tachycardia, palpitations, hypertension, diarrhea, erectile dysfunction, tremor, dysuria, and tolerance. PB: UK; $t\frac{1}{2}$: Immediate release 1.9 h, Extended release 9.8 h
Liraglutide	Obesity: A: Subcut: Initially 0.6 mg/d for 1 wk; *max:* 3 mg/d	Used short term for obesity and type 2 diabetes mellitus. May cause headache, fever, dizziness, fatigue, nausea, vomiting, constipation, diarrhea, tachycardia, palpitations, suicidal ideation, injection site reaction, and hypoglycemia. PB: >98%; $t\frac{1}{2}$: 13 h
Naltrexone hydrochloride/ bupropion hydrochloride	Extended release: A: PO: Initially 8 mg naltrexone/90 mg bupropion/d in the morning; *max:* 32 mg naltrexone/360 mg bupropion/d	Used short term for obesity. May cause headache, anxiety, dizziness, insomnia, abdominal pain, nausea, vomiting, constipation, suicidal ideation, hypertension, elevated hepatic enzymes, and erectile dysfunction. PB: 21% naltrexone, 84% bupropion; $t\frac{1}{2}$: 5 h naltrexone, 21 h bupropion
Setmelanotide	A: Subcut: Initially 2 mg/d for 2 wk; *max:* 3 mg/d	Used for chronic weight management for those with monogenic or syndromic obesity. May cause abdominal pain, arthralgia, weakness, back pain, fatigue, depression, headache, insomnia, injection site reaction, dry mouth, nausea, vomiting, diarrhea, constipation, infection, and skin hyperpigmentation. PB: 79.1%; $t\frac{1}{2}$: 11 h
Semaglutide	A: Subcut: Wk 1–4: 0.25 mg once weekly, Wk 5–8: 0.5 mg once weekly, Wk 9–12: 1 mg once weekly, Wk 13–16: 1.7 mg once weekly, Wk 17 onward: 1.7 mg or 2.4 mg once weekly	Used for obesity/weight loss and diabetes mellitus. May cause headache, dizziness, fatigue, pharyngitis, nausea, vomiting, abdominal pain, diarrhea, constipation, hypoglycemia, dyspepsia, eructation, and flatulence. PB: 99%; $t\frac{1}{2}$: 1 wk
Tirzepatide	A: Subcut: Initially 2.5 mg every week for 4 wk, then 5 mg/wk, may increase 2.5 mg increments q4wk; *max:* 15 mg/wk	Used for obesity/weight loss and diabetes mellitus. May cause dizziness, fatigue, antibody development, tachycardia, abdominal pain, decreased appetite, vomiting, diarrhea, constipation, and dyspepsia. PB: 99%; $t\frac{1}{2}$: 5 days
Analeptics		
Methylxanthines		
Caffeine citrate	Mental alertness: A: PO: 100–200 mg q3–4h PRN; *max:* 1200 mg/d	For neonatal apnea and mental alertness. May cause headache, insomnia, irritability, gastritis, dyspepsia, nausea, tachycardia, palpitations, urinary frequency, hypo/hyperglycemia, tremors, and withdrawal. PB: 36%; $t\frac{1}{2}$: 3–7 h

>, Greater than; *A*, adult; *bid*, twice a day; *CSS*, Controlled Substances Schedule; *d*, day; *h*, hour; *max*, maximum; *PB*, protein binding; *PO*, by mouth; *PRN*, as needed; *q*, every; *subcut*, subcutaneous; $t\frac{1}{2}$, half-life; *tid*, three times a day; *UK*, unknown; *wk*, week.

CLINICAL JUDGMENT CASE STUDY

A 7-year-old child has been diagnosed with attention-deficit/hyperactivity disorder. The physician is considering putting the child on medication.
1. What symptoms does a child with attention-deficit/hyperactivity disorder display?
2. What medication might be prescribed? What class of drugs does the medication fall under?
3. What behavioral improvements might be seen after medication administration?
4. What physical assessment should be completed before medication administration?
5. What teaching should the nurse include related to the use of methylphenidate?

REVIEW QUESTIONS

1. When a 12-year-old child is prescribed methylphenidate, which is most important for the nurse to monitor?
   a. Temperature
   b. Respirations
   c. Intake and output
   d. Height and weight
2. Several children are admitted for diagnosis with possible attention-deficit/hyperactivity disorder. Which is most important for the nurse to observe?
   a. A girl who is lethargic
   b. A girl who lacks impulsivity
   c. A boy with smooth coordination
   d. A boy with an inability to complete tasks
3. The nurse monitoring a patient for methylphenidate withdrawal should observe the patient for which condition?
   a. Tremors
   b. Insomnia
   c. Weakness
   d. Tachycardia
4. The nurse is teaching a patient to self-administer medications. The nurse knows that which drug is used to treat narcolepsy?
   a. Modafinil
   b. Atomoxetine
   c. Lisdexamfetamine
   d. Phendimetrazine
5. The nurse is monitoring a patient who is taking phentermine. Which is important for the nurse to observe? **Select all that apply.**
   a. Euphoria
   b. Dry mouth
   c. Insomnia
   d. Hypotension
   e. Bradycardia
   f. Palpitations

18
Depressants
Jared Robertson III, MN, CRNA

http://evolve.elsevier.com/McCuistion/pharmacology

OBJECTIVES

- Describe nonpharmacologic methods to respond to problems associated with sleep disorders.
- Summarize the effect of different doses of sedative-hypnotics.
- Summarize the classifications and mechanism of action of anesthetics.

OUTLINE

Sleep Disorders, 206
    Stages of Sleep, 206
    Nonpharmacologic Methods to Promote Sleep, 206
Sedative-Hypnotics, 207
    Sedatives, 207
    Hypnotics, 207
    Barbiturates, 208
    Benzodiazepines, 208
    Nonbenzodiazepines, 212
    Melatonin Agonists, 212
    Sedatives and Hypnotics for Older Adults, 212

Anesthetics, 214
    Balanced Anesthesia, 214
    Stages of General Anesthesia, 214
    Assessment Before Surgery, 214
    Inhalation Anesthetics, 214
    Intravenous Anesthetics, 215
    Topical Anesthetics, 216
    Local Anesthetics, 216
    Spinal Anesthesia, 216
Clinical Judgment Case Study, 218
Review Questions, 218

Drugs that are central nervous system (CNS) depressants cause varying degrees of depression (reduction in functional activity) within the CNS. The degree of depression depends primarily on the drug and the amount of drug taken. The broad classification of CNS depressants includes sedative-hypnotics, general anesthetics, analgesics, opioid and nonopioid analgesics, anticonvulsants, antipsychotics, and antidepressants. The last five groups of depressant drugs are presented in separate chapters. Sedative-hypnotics and general anesthetics are discussed in this chapter.

SLEEP DISORDERS

Sleep disorders such as **insomnia**, the inability to fall asleep or remain asleep, occur in 10% to 30% of Americans. Insomnia occurs more frequently in females, and the incidence increases with age.

The Centers for Disease Control and Prevention cite that approximately 70 million Americans have chronic sleep problems and experience sleep deprivation. The cost is billions of dollars in lost productivity, and millions of dollars are spent each year on over-the-counter (OTC) sleep aids. The primary ingredient in OTC sleep aids is an antihistamine such as diphenhydramine.

Stages of Sleep

People spend approximately one-third of their lives, or as much as 25 years, sleeping. Normal sleep is composed of two definite phases: **rapid eye movement (REM)** and **non–rapid eye movement (NREM) sleep**. Both REM and NREM sleep occur cyclically at about 90-minute intervals during sleep (Fig. 18.1). The four succeedingly deeper stages of NREM sleep end with an episode of REM sleep, and the cycle begins again. If sleep is interrupted, the cycle begins again with stage 1 of NREM sleep. Individuals perform better during their waking hours if they experience all types and stages of sleep.

During REM sleep, individuals experience most of their recallable dreams. Children have few REM sleep periods and have longer periods of stage 3 and 4 NREM sleep. Older adults experience a decrease in stage 3 and 4 NREM sleep and have frequent waking periods.

It is difficult to rouse a person during REM sleep, and the period of REM sleep episodes becomes longer during the sleep process. Frequently, if a person is roused from REM sleep, a vivid, bizarre dream may be recalled. If these dreams are unpleasant, they may be called *nightmares*. Sleepwalking or nightmares that occur in children take place during NREM sleep.

Nonpharmacologic Methods to Promote Sleep

Before using sedative-hypnotics or OTC sleep aids, various nonpharmacologic methods should be used to promote sleep. Once the nurse discovers why the patient cannot sleep, the following ways to promote sleep may be suggested:

1. Arise at a specific time in the morning.
2. Take few or no daytime naps.
3. Avoid drinks that contain caffeine and alcohol 6 hours before bedtime. Also avoid smoking nicotine products for 6 hours before bedtime.
4. Avoid heavy meals or strenuous exercise before bedtime.
5. Take a warm bath, listen to quiet music, or perform other soothing activities before bedtime.
6. Decrease exposure to loud noises.

7. Avoid drinking copious amounts of fluids before sleep.
8. Drink warm milk before bedtime.

SEDATIVE-HYPNOTICS

Sedative-hypnotics are commonly ordered for treatment of sleep disorders. The mildest form of CNS depression is sedation, which diminishes physical and mental responses at lower dosages of certain CNS depressants but does not affect consciousness. Sedatives are used mostly during the daytime. Increasing the drug dose can produce a hypnotic effect—not hypnosis but a form of "natural" sleep. Sedative-hypnotic drugs are sometimes the same drug; however, certain drugs are used more often for their hypnotic effect. With very high doses of sedative-hypnotic drugs, anesthesia may be achieved.

Sedatives

Sedatives were first prescribed to reduce tension and anxiety. Barbiturates, which stimulate the inhibitory gamma-aminobutyric acid (GABA) system in the brain, were initially used for their antianxiety effect until the early 1960s, when benzodiazepines were introduced. Because of the many side effects of barbiturates and their potential for physical and mental dependency, they are now less frequently prescribed for this purpose.

Hypnotics

Hypnotics may be short or intermediate acting. Short-acting hypnotics are useful in achieving sleep because they allow the patient to awaken early in the morning without experiencing lingering side effects. Intermediate-acting hypnotics are useful for sustaining sleep; however, after using one, the patient may experience residual drowsiness, or hangover, in the morning. This may be undesirable if the patient is active and requires mental alertness. The ideal hypnotic promotes natural sleep without disrupting normal patterns of sleep and produces no hangover or undesirable effect. Table 18.1 lists the common side effects and adverse reactions associated with sedative-hypnotic use and abuse.

Hypnotic drug therapy should usually be short term to prevent drug dependence and tolerance. Interrupting hypnotic therapy can decrease drug tolerance, but abruptly discontinuing a high dose of hypnotic taken over a long period can cause withdrawal symptoms. In such cases the dose should be tapered to avoid withdrawal symptoms. As a general rule, the lowest dose should be taken to achieve sleep. Patients with severe respiratory disorders should avoid hypnotics, which could cause an increase in respiratory depression. Usually,

Fig. 18.1 Types and stages of sleep. *NREM*, Non–rapid eye movement (four stages); *REM*, rapid eye movement (dreaming).

TABLE 18.1	Common Side Effects and Adverse Reactions of Sedative-Hypnotics
Side Effects and Adverse Reactions	**Explanation of the Effects**
Hangover	A hangover is residual drowsiness resulting in impaired reaction time. The intermediate- and long-acting hypnotics are frequently the cause of drug hangover. The liver biotransforms these drugs into active metabolites that persist in the body, causing drowsiness.
REM rebound	REM rebound, which results in vivid dreams and nightmares, frequently occurs after taking a hypnotic for a prolonged period then abruptly stopping. However, it may occur after taking only one hypnotic dose.
Dependence	Dependence is the result of chronic hypnotic use. Physical and psychological dependence can result. Physical dependence results in the appearance of specific withdrawal symptoms when a drug is discontinued after prolonged use. The severity of withdrawal symptoms depends on the drug and dosage. Symptoms may include muscular twitching and tremors, dizziness, orthostatic hypotension, delusions, hallucinations, delirium, and seizures. Withdrawal symptoms start within 24 hours and can last for several days.
Tolerance	Tolerance results when there is a need to increase the dosage over time to obtain the desired effect. It is mostly caused by an increase in drug metabolism by liver enzymes. The barbiturate drug category can cause tolerance after prolonged use. Tolerance is reversible when the drug is discontinued.
Excessive depression	Long-term use of a hypnotic may result in CNS depression, which is characterized by lethargy, sleepiness, lack of concentration, confusion, and psychological depression.
Respiratory depression	High doses of sedative-hypnotics can suppress the respiratory center in the medulla.
Hypersensitivity	Skin rashes and urticaria can result when taking barbiturates. Such reactions are rare.

CNS, Central nervous system; *REM*, rapid eye movement.

hypnotics are contraindicated during pregnancy. Ramelteon is the only major sedative-hypnotic approved for long-term use. This drug may be used for treating chronic insomnia.

The category of sedative-hypnotics includes barbiturates, benzodiazepines, and nonbenzodiazepines, among others. Each category is discussed separately. Prototype drug charts are included for benzodiazepines and nonbenzodiazepines.

Barbiturates

Barbiturates were introduced as a sedative in the early 1900s. They are classified as long, intermediate, or short acting.
- The *long-acting* group includes phenobarbital, which is used to control seizures in epilepsy.
- The *intermediate-acting* barbiturates, such as butabarbital (no longer available in the United States), are useful as sleep sustainers for maintaining long periods of sleep. Because these drugs take approximately 1 hour for the onset of sleep, they are not prescribed for those who have trouble getting to sleep. Vital signs should be closely monitored in persons who take intermediate-acting barbiturates.
- The *short-acting* barbiturate pentobarbital may be used for procedure sedation. Vital signs should be closely monitored in persons who take short-acting barbiturates.
- Methohexital, an *ultra short-acting barbiturate*, is useful as an anesthetic or induction of general anesthesia

Barbiturates should be restricted to short-term use (2 weeks or less) because of their numerous side effects, including tolerance to the drug. In the United States barbiturates are classified under the Controlled Substances Act as Schedule II for short acting, Schedule III for intermediate-acting, and Schedule IV for long-acting hypnotics. In Canada barbiturates are classified as Schedule G. Barbiturates are listed in Table 18.2.

Pharmacokinetics

Pentobarbital has been available for nearly half a century and was the hypnotic of choice until the introduction of benzodiazepines in the 1960s. It has a slow absorption rate and is moderately protein bound. The long half-life is mainly because of the formation of active metabolites resulting from liver metabolism.

Pharmacodynamics

Pentobarbital may be used for short-term treatment of insomnia. Other uses include emergency control of seizures, preoperative anxiety, sedation induction, and lowering intracranial pressure in a critical care setting. It has a rapid onset with a short duration of action and is considered a short-acting barbiturate.

Many drug interactions are associated with barbiturates. Alcohol, opioids, and other sedative-hypnotics used in combination with barbiturates may further depress the CNS. Pentobarbital increases hepatic enzyme action, causing an increased metabolism and decreased effect of drugs such as oral anticoagulants, glucocorticoids, tricyclic antidepressants, and quinidine. Pentobarbital may cause hepatotoxicity if taken with large doses of acetaminophen.

> ⚡ **PATIENT SAFETY**
>
> **Do Not Confuse**
> - **Phenobarbital**, a long-acting barbiturate used to control seizures, with **pentobarbital**, a short-acting barbiturate used as a procedural anesthetic or induction of general anesthesia.

❗ Benzodiazepines

Selected benzodiazepines, minor tranquilizers and anxiolytics, were introduced with chlordiazepoxide in the 1960s as antianxiety agents. This drug group is ordered as sedative-hypnotics for inducing sleep. Several benzodiazepines marketed as hypnotics include flurazepam, alprazolam (Prototype Drug Chart: Alprazolam), temazepam, triazolam, estazolam, and quazepam (Table 18.3). Increased anxiety might be the cause of insomnia for some patients, so lorazepam and diazepam can be used to alleviate the anxiety. These drugs are classified

TABLE 18.2 Sedative-Hypnotics: Barbiturates and Other Drugs

Drug	Route and Dosage	Uses and Considerations
Barbiturates: Short-Acting		
Pentobarbital CSS II	Sedation induction: A: IM: 150–200 mg before procedure A: IV: Initially 100 mg; after 1 min assessment, may repeat up to 200–500 mg	For sedation induction, seizures. May cause hypotension, bradycardia, drowsiness, dizziness, ataxia, agitation, confusion, constipation, impaired cognition, erectile dysfunction, and respiratory depression. PB: 35%–45%; t½: approximately 22 hours in adults; range of 15 to 50 h
Methohexital CSS IV	General anesthesia induction: A: IV: 1–1.5 mg/kg of a 1% solution given at a rate of about 1 ml per 5 seconds (range 50–120 mg)	General anesthesia induction and maintenance; Must be administered by someone trained in general anesthetic administration. PB: 80–84.5%; t½: 3.9 h
Barbiturates: Long Acting		
Phenobarbital CSS IV	Sedation induction: A: IM/IV: 100–200 mg 60–90 min before procedure 15–20 mg/kg/dose IV as a single dose; may administer 5–10 mg/kg/dose IV after 10 min if needed for treatment of status epilepticus	Used for seizure control, sedation induction, and insomnia. May cause ataxia, depression, bradycardia, hypotension, dizziness, confusion, drowsiness, headache, impaired judgment, nightmares, constipation, and erectile dysfunction. Monitor for respiratory depression. PB: 15–55%; t½: 53–118 h for adults, 37–69 h for children, 47–63 h for infants

<, Less than; *A*, adult; *CSS*, Controlled Substances Schedule; *d*, day; *h*, hour; *IM*, intramuscular; *IV*, intravenous; *min*, minutes; *PB*, protein binding; *PO*, by mouth; *qid*, four times a day; *t½*, half-life; *tid*, three times a day.

TABLE 18.3 Sedative-Hypnotics: Benzodiazepines, Nonbenzodiazepines, and Opioid Agonists

Drug	Route and Dosage	Uses and Considerations
Benzodiazepines		
Alprazolam CSS IV	See Prototype Drug Chart: Alprazolam	
Estazolam CSS IV	A: PO: 1–2 mg at bedtime; *max:* 2 mg/d Older A: PO: 0.5–1 mg at bedtime; *max:* 2 mg/d	For treatment of insomnia. Should not be used longer than 6 weeks. May cause tolerance, dizziness, drowsiness, anterograde amnesia, confusion, ataxia, edema, dependence, withdrawal, weakness, and sleep-related behaviors. PB: 93%; *t½*: 10–24 h
Lorazepam CSS IV	Insomnia: A: PO: 2–4 mg at bedtime; *max:* 10 mg/d Older A: PO: Initially 1–2 mg at bedtime; *maint:* 2–4 mg at bedtime; *max:* 10 mg/d	Used for sedation induction and to reduce anxiety, insomnia, and seizures. May cause tolerance, drowsiness, dizziness, hypotension, blurred vision, anterograde amnesia, memory impairment, agitation, nightmares, dependence, injection site reaction, and suicidal ideation. PB: 85%; *t½*: 12–14 h
Temazepam CSS IV	Insomnia: A: PO: 15–30 mg at bedtime; *max:* 30 mg/d Older A: PO: 7.5 mg at bedtime; *max:* 30 mg/d	To treat insomnia. May cause tolerance, drowsiness, dizziness, confusion, palpitations, hypotension, dependence, withdrawal, anterograde amnesia, and sleep-related behavior. PB: 98%; *t½*: 8–15 h
Triazolam CSS IV	Insomnia: A: PO: 0.125–0.25 mg at bedtime; *max:* 0.5 mg/d Older A: PO: 0.125 mg at bedtime; *max:* 0.25 mg/d	For management of insomnia. Should not be used longer than 7–10 d at a time to avoid tolerance. Avoid alcohol and smoking when taking triazolam. May cause tolerance, drowsiness, dizziness, nausea, ataxia, confusion, visual impairment, headache, tachycardia, depression, dependence, withdrawal, anterograde amnesia, and sleep-related behaviors. PB: 90%; *t½*: 1.5–5.5 h
Remimazolam CSS IV	A: IV: 2.5–5 mg over 1 min, may repeat at least 2 min later with 1.25–2.5 mg over 15 s	Used for induction and maintenance of sedation for procedures, such as cardioversion, bronchoscopy, TEE, EGD, colonoscopy, or other procedures lasting 30 minutes or less. Concomitant administration with opioid analgesics or sedative-hypnotics may result in profound sedation, respiratory depression, coma, and death. Do not give to patients with known hypersensitive reactions to benzodiazepines and/or Dextran 40. PB: 91%; *t½*: 37–53 min
Benzodiazepine Antagonists		
Flumazenil	A: IV: 0.2 mg over 30 s; may repeat after 45 s, then repeat q1min PRN; *max:* 4 doses	For management of benzodiazepine toxicity and sedation reversal. May cause drowsiness, dizziness, blurred vision, ataxia, seizures, hyperacusis, palpitations, vomiting, and dry mouth. PB: 50%; *t½*: 40–80 min
Nonbenzodiazepines		
Zolpidem tartrate CSS IV	See Prototype Drug Chart: Zolpidem Tartrate	
Eszopiclone CSS IV	Insomnia: A: PO: Initially 1 mg at bedtime; *maint:* 2–3 mg at bedtime; *max:* 3 mg/d Older A: PO: 1–2 mg at bedtime; *max:* 2 mg/d	To treat insomnia. May cause headache, dizziness, drowsiness, unpleasant taste, sleep-related behaviors, infection, depression, and suicidal ideation. PB: 52%–59%; *t½*: 6 h
Zaleplon CSS IV	Insomnia: A: PO: 10 mg at bedtime; *max:* 20 mg Older A: PO: 5 mg at bedtime; *max:* 10 mg/d	For ultra short–term treatment of insomnia. May cause headache, dizziness, drowsiness, nausea, abdominal pain, weakness, and sleep-related behaviors. PB: 45%–75%; *t½*: 1 h
Melatonin Agonist		
Ramelteon	A: PO: 8 mg within 30 min of bedtime; *max:* 8 mg/d	For treatment of insomnia. May cause dizziness, nausea, drowsiness, fatigue, depression, suicidal ideation, and sleep-related behaviors. PB: 82%; *t½*: 1–2.6 h
Tasimelteon	A: PO: 20 mg without food 1 h before bedtime; *max:* 20 mg/d	For treatment of insomnia in non–24 hour sleep-wake disorder and nighttime sleep disturbances in patient with Smith-Magenis Syndrome. May cause headache, nightmares, upper respiratory infections, urinary tract infections, and elevated hepatic enzymes or increased alanine aminotransferase. PB: 90%; *t½*: 1.3 h

Continued

TABLE 18.3 Sedative-Hypnotics: Benzodiazepines, Nonbenzodiazepines, and Opioid Agonists—cont'd

Drug	Route and Dosage	Uses and Considerations
Orexin Antagonist		
Daridorexant	A: PO: 25–50 mg/d 30 min before bedtime with at least 7 hours before planned awakening; Max: 50 mg	For the treatment of insomnia characterized by difficulties with sleep onset and/or sleep maintenance in adults. May cause headache, fatigue, dizziness, nightmares, sleep paralysis, complex sleep-related behaviors such as sleepwalking, sleep driving, etc. PB: 99.7%; t½: 8 h
Sufentanil	A: PO: 10–20 mg/d 30 min before bedtime with at least 7 hours before planned awakening; Max. 20 mg	For the treatment of insomnia characterized by difficulties with sleep onset and/or sleep maintenance in adults. May cause headache, fatigue, dizziness, nightmares, sleep paralysis, complex sleep-related behaviors such as sleepwalking, sleep driving, etc. PB: >99%; t½: 12 h
Opioid Agonists		
Alfentanil CSS II	A: IV: 130–245 mcg/kg over 3 min as induction; maint: 0.5–1.5 mcg/kg/min; max: dependent on procedure duration	For general anesthesia induction and maintenance and sedation maintenance. Must be administered by someone trained in general anesthetic administration. May cause dizziness, confusion, dysrhythmias, hypotension or hypertension, respiratory depression, bronchospasm, tachycardia, bradycardia, chest wall rigidity, nausea, and vomiting. Use caution in patients with head trauma and liver dysfunction. PB: 88%–92%; t½: 90–111 min
Sufentanil CSS II	A: IV: 8–30 mcg/kg increments or infusion for induction; maint: 0.5–10 mcg/kg intermittent or continuous IV; max: dependent on procedure duration Sublingual: 30 mcg sublingually every 1 h as needed for up to 72 h. Max: 360 mcg/24 h.	For general anesthesia induction and maintenance, obstetric anesthesia, and severe pain. Must be administered by someone trained in general anesthetic administration. May cause drowsiness, pruritus, bradycardia, hypertension or hypotension, dysrhythmia, chest wall rigidity, bronchospasm, respiratory depression, urinary retention, headache, dizziness, nausea, and vomiting. PB: 93%; t½: 164 min
Remifentanil	A: IV: 0.1–1 mcg/kg/min continuous infusion	For general anesthesia induction and maintenance and moderate to severe pain. Must be administered by someone trained in general anesthetic administration. May cause dizziness, pruritus, confusion, chest wall rigidity, hypotension, bradycardia, dysrhythmias, fever, headache, nausea, and vomiting. PB: 70%; t½: 10–20 min

A, Adult; *CSS*, Controlled Substances Schedule; *d*, day; *EGD*, esophagogastroduodenoscopy; *h*, hour; *IV*, intravenous; *maint*, maintenance; *max*, maximum; *min*, minute; *PB*, protein binding; *PO*, by mouth; *PRN*, as needed; *q1min*, once per minute; *s*, second; *t½*, half-life; *TEE*, transesophageal echocardiogram.

PROTOTYPE DRUG CHART
Alprazolam

Drug Class	Dosage
Sedative-hypnotic: benzodiazepine CSS IV	Immediate release: A: PO: Initially 0.25–0.5 mg tid, may increase q3–4d by no >1 mg/day; max: 4 mg/d Older A: PO: Initially 0.25 mg bid/tid, may increase q3–4d; max: 4 mg/d Extended release: A: PO: Initially 0.5–1 mg/d in the morning, may increase q3–4d by no >1mg/day; max: 10 mg/d Older A: PO: Initially 0.5 mg/d, may increase q3–4d; max: 10 mg/d; use the lowest effective dose All Patients: If discontinuation becomes necessary, decrease the daily dose by no more than 0.5mg/day

Contraindications	Drug-Lab-Food Interactions
Respiratory depression, acute alcohol intoxication, psychotic reactions, recent respiratory depressants, hypersensitivity Caution: Older adults, sleep apnea, renal or liver dysfunction, depression, suicidal ideation, substance abuse, alcohol abuse, psychosis, respiratory depression	Drug: Decreases respiration with alcohol, CNS depressants; azole antifungals (ketoconazole), antibiotics (erythromycin), aprepitant, cimetidine, diltiazem, and verapamil increase blood levels of alprazolam; rifabutin, rifampin, cortisone, and phenytoin decrease blood levels; alprazolam increases digoxin and lithium levels Food: Grapefruit increases alprazolam levels; green tea decreases alprazolam effects

Pharmacokinetics	Pharmacodynamics
Absorption: PO: 90% absorbed from GI tract Distribution: PB: 80% Metabolism: t½: IR, 6.3–26.9 h; ER, 11–16 h Excretion: In urine as metabolites	PO: Onset: 15–30 min Peak: IR, 1–2 h; ER, 9 h Duration: UK

PROTOTYPE DRUG CHART—CONT'D

Alprazolam

Therapeutic Effects/Uses

To treat anxiety and panic disorders

Mechanism of Action: CNS depression, binds receptors in limbic system and reticular formation, increases GABA to GABA receptors; shift of chloride ions leads to less excitability and stabilizes neuronal membranes

Side Effects	Adverse Reactions
Lethargy, drowsiness, dizziness, headache, constipation, anterograde amnesia, memory impairment, fatigue, agitation, ataxia, increased appetite, blurred vision, decreased libido, dry mouth, nausea, edema, weight gain/loss, nasal congestion, rash, irritability	Depression, tolerance, dependence, withdrawal, hypotension, tachycardia, seizures *Life-threatening:* Hepatic failure, Stevens-Johnson syndrome

A, Adult; *bid*, twice daily; *CNS*, central nervous system; *CSS*, Controlled Substances Schedule; *d*, day; *Dtab*, disintegrating tablet; *ER*, extended release; *GABA*, gamma-aminobutyric acid; *GI*, gastrointestinal; *h*, hour; *IR*, immediate release; *max*, maximum; *min*, minute; *PB*, protein binding; *PO*, by mouth; *q*, every; *t½*, half-life; *tid*, three times a day; *UK*, unknown.

CLINICAL JUDGMENT [NURSING PROCESS]

Sedative-Hypnotics: Benzodiazepines

Concept: Sleep
- A phase of our daily life cycle when the brain and body rest and rejuvenate; the eyes are closed, metabolism slows, and postural muscles are relaxed.

Recognize Cues [Assessment]
- Obtain a drug history of current drugs and complementary and alternative therapies that the patient is taking, especially central nervous system (CNS) depressants, which would potentiate respiratory depression and hypotensive effects.
- Assess baseline vital signs for future comparisons.
- Determine whether the patient has a history of insomnia or anxiety disorders.
- Assess renal function. Urine output should be 1500 mL/day. Renal impairment could prolong drug action by increasing the half-life of the drug.

Analyze Cues and Prioritize Hypothesis [Patient Problems]
- Decreased functional ability
- Reduced stamina
- Decreased level of consciousness
- Decreased ability to cope

Generate Solutions [Planning]
- Patient will receive adequate sleep when taking benzodiazepines.

Take Action [Nursing Interventions]
- Monitor vital signs, especially respirations and blood pressure.
- Use a bed alarm for older adults and for patients receiving a hypnotic for the first time. Confusion can occur, and injury could result.
- Observe the patient for adverse reactions, especially an older adult or a debilitated patient.
- Examine the patient's skin for rashes. Skin eruptions may occur in patients taking benzodiazepines.

Patient Teaching

General
- Teach patients to use nonpharmacologic methods to induce sleep such as taking a warm bath, listening to quiet music, drinking warm fluids, and avoiding drinks with caffeine for 6 hours before bedtime.
- Encourage patients to avoid alcohol and antidepressant, antipsychotic, and opioid drugs while taking benzodiazepines. Respiratory depression can occur when these drugs are combined.
- Warn patients that certain complementary and alternative therapy products may interact with benzodiazepines (see Complementary and Alternative Therapies). These products may need to be discontinued or the prescription drug dose may need to be modified.
- Advise patients not to drive a motor vehicle or operate machinery when using benzodiazepines. Caution is always encouraged.
- Encourage patients to check with a health care provider about over-the-counter (OTC) sleeping aids. Drowsiness may result from taking these drugs; therefore caution while driving is advised.

Side Effects
- Advise patients to report adverse reactions such as cognitive changes and paradoxical reactions to their health care provider. Drug selection or dosage might need to be changed.
- Teach patients that benzodiazepines should be gradually withdrawn, especially if they have been taken for several weeks. Abrupt cessation may result in withdrawal symptoms such as tremors and muscle twitching.

Evaluate Outcomes [Evaluation]
- Assess the effectiveness of benzodiazepines.
- Evaluate respiratory status to ensure that respiratory depression has not occurred.

COMPLEMENTARY AND ALTERNATIVE THERAPIES

Sedatives

- Kava kava should not be taken in combination with central nervous system (CNS) depressants such as barbiturates and opioids. This product may increase the sedative effect.
- Valerian, when taken with alcohol and other CNS depressants such as barbiturates, may increase the sedative effects of the prescribed drug.

PATIENT SAFETY

Do Not Confuse
- **Lorazepam**, a benzodiazepine used to reduce anxiety, with **alprazolam**, a benzodiazepine used to treat anxiety and insomnia.

as Schedule IV according to the Controlled Substances Act. The benzodiazepines increase the action of the inhibitory neurotransmitter GABA to the GABA receptors. Neuron excitability is reduced.

Benzodiazepines (except for temazepam) can suppress stage 4 of NREM sleep, which may result in vivid dreams or nightmares and can delay REM sleep. Benzodiazepines are effective for sleep disorders for several weeks longer than other sedative-hypnotics; to prevent REM rebound, however, they should not be used for longer than 3 to 4 weeks.

Triazolam is a short-acting hypnotic with a half-life of 2 to 5 hours. It does not produce any active metabolites. Adverse effects of anterograde amnesia or memory impairment occur more frequently with triazolam than with other benzodiazepines, and the risk increases with higher doses and with concurrent alcohol or opioid ingestion. Currently, it is seldom prescribed and should not be taken longer than 7 to 10 days.

One adverse effect closely associated with benzodiazepines is anterograde amnesia, an impaired ability to recall events that occur after dosing. Associated with anterograde amnesia are sleep-related behaviors, such as preparing and eating meals, sleep driving, engaging in sex, or making phone calls during sleep without any memory of the event. Alcohol and CNS depressants increase the risk of sleep-related behaviors.

Small doses of benzodiazepines are recommended for patients with renal or hepatic dysfunction. For benzodiazepine overdose, the benzodiazepine antagonist flumazenil may be administered. Benzodiazepines prescribed as antianxiety drugs are discussed in Chapter 22.

Pharmacokinetics

Benzodiazepines are well absorbed through the gastrointestinal (GI) mucosa. They are rapidly metabolized in the liver to active metabolites. Benzodiazepines usually have an intermediate half-life of usually 8 to 24 hours and are highly protein bound. When taken with other highly protein-bound drugs, more free (or unbound) drug is available, resulting in an increased risk for adverse effects.

Pharmacodynamics

Benzodiazepines are used to treat insomnia by inducing and sustaining sleep. They have a rapid onset of action and intermediate- to long-acting effects. The normal recommended dose of a benzodiazepine may be too much for the older adult, so half the dose is recommended initially to prevent overdosing.

Nonbenzodiazepines

Zolpidem is a nonbenzodiazepine that differs in chemical structure from benzodiazepines. It is used for short-term treatment (<10 days) of insomnia and affects sleep through the GABA system. Its duration of action is 6 to 8 hours with a short half-life of 1.4 to 8.4 hours. Zolpidem is metabolized in the liver to three inactive metabolites and is excreted in bile, urine, and feces. When zolpidem is prescribed for older adults, the dose should be decreased. Table 18.3 lists the benzodiazepines and nonbenzodiazepines used as sedative-hypnotics and their dosages, uses, and considerations, including common side effects and a few serious adverse effects. Zolpidem is described in the Prototype Drug Chart: Zolpidem Tartrate.

Daridorexant is a dual orexin (orexin A and orexin B) receptor antagonist (DORA) indicated for the treatment of insomnia characterized by difficulty with onset of sleep and/or sleep maintenance in adults. It functions to block awake-promoting neuropeptides orexin A and orexin B from binding to orexin receptors type 1 and type 2, which promote wakefulness. Peak plasma levels are achieved within 1 to 2 hours after oral intake and is dose proportional in doses from 25 to 50 mg. The half-life of daridorexant is 8 hours. It is metabolized by CYP3A4 found mainly in the liver and intestines. Age does not have a clinically significant effect on dosing. Daridorexant may cause worsening of depression and/or suicidal tendencies.

Suvorexant is another DORA with indications similar to that of daridorexant; however, it is indicated for patients with mild to moderate Alzheimer's. Peak plasma levels are reached at a median time of 2 hours (range of 30 minutes to 6 hours), with delays experienced when taken soon after a high fat-content meal. Its mean half-life is approximately 12 hours and is metabolized primarily by CYP3A4.

Melatonin Agonists

Ramelteon is in the newest category of sedative-hypnotics called *melatonin agonists*. Ramelteon is the first hypnotic approved by the US Food and Drug Administration (FDA) that is *not* classified as a controlled substance. This drug acts by selectively targeting melatonin receptors to regulate circadian rhythms in the treatment of insomnia. Ramelteon has not been shown to decrease REM sleep. This new drug has a half-life of 1 to 2.6 hours. Adverse effects of ramelteon include drowsiness, dizziness, fatigue, headache, nausea, and suicidal ideation.

Tasimelteon is a melatonin receptor agonist used for treatment of non-24-hour sleep-wake disorder and nighttime sleep disturbances in patients with Smith-Magenis syndrome. The mean elimination half-life is 1.3 hours. Adverse effects of tasimelteon include headache, nightmares, upper respiratory tract infections, and urinary tract infections.

Sedatives and Hypnotics for Older Adults

Identifying the cause of insomnia in an older adult should be the first diagnostic consideration, and nonpharmacologic methods should be

---

📋 PROTOTYPE DRUG CHART
Zolpidem Tartrate

Drug Class	Dosage
Sedative-hypnotic: Nonbenzodiazepine CSS IV	Immediate release: A males: PO: 5–10 mg at bedtime with at least 7–8 hours remaining before planned time to awake; *max:* 10 mg/d A females/older A: PO: 5 mg at bedtime with at least 7–8 hours remaining before planned time to awake; *max:* 10 mg/d for females, 5 mg/d for older adults SL tabs/oral spray: A: PO: 5–10 mg at bedtime; *max:* 10 mg/d Older A: PO: 5 mg at bedtime; *max:* 5 mg/d Extended release: A: PO: 6.25–12.5 mg at bedtime; *max:* 12.5 mg/d Older A: PO: 6.25 mg at bedtime, *max:* 6.25 mg/d

PROTOTYPE DRUG CHART—CONT'D

Zolpidem Tartrate

Contraindications	Drug-Lab-Food Interactions
Hypersensitivity to benzodiazepine, drug-induced complex sleep-related behaviors *Caution:* Renal or liver dysfunction; mental depression, suicidal ideation; pregnancy; children, older adults, pulmonary disease, alcohol/substance abuse, breastfeeding	Drug: Decreases CNS function with alcohol, CNS depressants, anticonvulsants, and phenothiazines; increased levels with azole antifungals; decreased levels with rifampin Food: Decreases absorption

Pharmacokinetics	Pharmacodynamics
Absorption: PO: well absorbed Distribution: PB: 92% Metabolism: t½: 1.2–8.3 h Excretion: In bile, urine, and feces	PO: Immediate release: Onset: 30 min Peak: 90 min Duration: 6–8 h SL/spray mist: Onset: UK Peak: 35–82 min Duration: UK Extended release: Onset: UK Peak: UK Duration: UK

Therapeutic Effects/Uses
To treat insomnia
Mechanism of Action: CNS depression, neurotransmitter inhibition

Side Effects	Adverse Reactions
Drowsiness, lethargy, headache, hot flashes, hangover (residual sedation), irritability, dizziness, ataxia, visual impairment, anxiety, nausea and vomiting, edema, erectile dysfunction, anterograde amnesia, memory impairment, nightmares, binge eating	Tolerance, psychological or physical dependence, withdrawal; sleep-related behaviors, hypotension, angioedema, dysrhythmias, depression, suicidal ideation *Life-threatening:* Pulmonary edema, renal failure

A, Adult; *CNS*, central nervous system; *CSS*, Controlled Substances Schedule; *d*, day; *h*, hour; *max*, maximum; *min*, minute; *PB*, protein binding; *PO*, by mouth; *SL*, sublingual; *t½*, half-life; *UK*, unknown.

CLINICAL JUDGMENT [NURSING PROCESS]

Sedative-Hypnotics: Nonbenzodiazepines

Concept: Sleep
- A phase of our daily life cycle when the brain and body rest and rejuvenate; the eyes are closed, metabolism slows, and postural muscles are relaxed.

Recognize Cues [Assessment]
- Assess baseline vital signs and laboratory tests (e.g., aspartate aminotransferase [AST], alanine aminotransferase [ALT], bilirubin) for future comparisons.
- Obtain a drug history. Taking central nervous system (CNS) depressants with nonbenzodiazepine hypnotics can depress respirations.
- Ascertain the patient's problem with sleep disturbance.

Analyze Cues and Prioritize Hypothesis [Patient Problems]
- Decreased functional ability
- Reduced stamina
- Decreased level of consciousness
- Decreased ability to cope

Generate Solutions [Planning]
- Patient will remain asleep for 6 to 8 hours.

Take Action [Nursing Intervention]
- Monitor vital signs. Check for signs of respiratory depression (slow, irregular breathing patterns).
- Use a bed alarm for older adults or patients receiving nonbenzodiazepines for the first time. Confusion may occur, and injury may result.
- Observe the patient for side effects of nonbenzodiazepines such as hangover (residual sedation), lightheadedness, dizziness, or confusion.

Patient Teaching
General
- Teach patients to use nonpharmacologic methods to induce sleep (taking a warm bath, listening to music, drinking warm fluids such as milk, avoiding drinks with caffeine after dinner).
- Encourage patients to avoid alcohol, antidepressants, antipsychotics, and narcotic drugs while taking nonbenzodiazepines. Severe respiratory depression may occur when these drugs are combined.
- Advise patients to take nonbenzodiazepines before bedtime. Alprazolam takes effect within 15 to 30 minutes.
- Suggest that patients urinate before taking nonbenzodiazepines to prevent sleep disruption.
- Encourage patients to check with a health care provider about over-the-counter (OTC) sleeping aids.
- Warn the patient to use caution while driving because drowsiness may occur.

Side Effects
- Advise patients to report adverse reactions such as hangover to a health care provider. Drug selection or dosage may need to be changed if hangover occurs.

Evaluate Outcomes [Evaluation]
- Evaluate effectiveness of sedative-hypnotics in promoting sleep.
- Determine whether side effects such as hangover occur after several days of taking a sedative-hypnotic. Another hypnotic may be prescribed if side effects persist.

used before sleep medications are prescribed. Because of physiologic changes in older adults, the use of hypnotics can cause a variety of side effects.

Barbiturates increase CNS depression and confusion in older adults and should *not* be taken for sleep. The short- to intermediate-acting benzodiazepines—such as estazolam, temazepam, and triazolam—are considered to be safer than barbiturates. Long-acting hypnotic benzodiazepines such as flurazepam, quazepam, and diazepam should be avoided. In many cases, older adults should be instructed to take the prescribed benzodiazepine no more than four times a week to avoid side effects and drug dependency. They can choose selected nights to take the hypnotic.

The main sleep problem experienced by older adults is frequent nighttime awakening. Reports have shown that older females experience more troublesome sleep patterns than males. Sleep disturbance may be caused by discomfort or pain. Occasionally a nonsteroidal antiinflammatory drug (NSAID) such as ibuprofen may alleviate the discomfort that prevents sleep.

ANESTHETICS

Anesthetics are classified as *general* and *local*. General anesthetics depress the CNS, alleviate pain, and cause a loss of consciousness. The first anesthetic, nitrous oxide ("laughing gas"), was used for surgery in the early 1800s. It is still an effective anesthetic and is frequently used in dental procedures and surgery. Nitrous oxide is sometimes used to dull pain and lessen anxiety during labor and delivery.

Several theories exist regarding how inhalation anesthetics cause CNS depression and a loss of consciousness. The differing theories suggest the following about inhalation anesthetics:
1. The lipid structure of cell membranes is altered, resulting in impaired physiologic functions.
2. The inhibitory neurotransmitter GABA is activated to the GABA receptor that pushes chloride ions into the neurons. This greatly decreases the action potentials of the neurons.
3. The ascending reticular activating system is altered, and the neurons cease to transmit information (stimuli) to the brain.

Balanced Anesthesia

Balanced anesthesia is a combination of drugs frequently used in general anesthesia. Balanced anesthesia may include the following:
1. A hypnotic given the night before
2. Premedication with an opioid analgesic or benzodiazepine (e.g., midazolam) plus an anticholinergic (e.g., glycopyrrolate) given about 1 hour before surgery to decrease oral secretions
3. A short-acting nonbarbiturate such as propofol
4. An inhaled gas, often a combination of an inhalation anesthetic, nitrous oxide, and oxygen
5. A muscle relaxant given as needed

Balanced anesthesia minimizes cardiovascular problems, decreases the amount of general anesthetic needed, reduces possible postanesthesia nausea and vomiting, minimizes the disturbance of organ function, and decreases pain. Because the patient does not receive large doses of general anesthetics, fewer adverse reactions occur, and recovery is enhanced by allowing quicker mobility.

Stages of General Anesthesia

General anesthesia proceeds through four stages; analgesia, excitement or delirium, surgical, and medullary paralysis (Table 18.4). The surgical procedure is usually performed during the third stage. If an anesthetic agent is given immediately before inhalation anesthesia, the third stage can occur without the early stages of anesthesia being observed. However, if the drug is given slowly, all stages of anesthesia are usually observed.

TABLE 18.4 Stages of Anesthesia

Stage	Name	Description
1	Analgesia	Begins with consciousness and ends with loss of consciousness; speech is difficult, sensations of smell and pain are lost, dreams and auditory and visual hallucinations may occur; this stage may be called the *induction stage*.
2	Excitement or delirium	Produces a loss of consciousness caused by depression of the cerebral cortex; confusion, excitement, or delirium occur, and induction time is short.
3	Surgical	Surgical procedure is performed during this stage. As anesthesia deepens, respirations become shallower, and the respiratory rate is increased.
4	Medullary paralysis	Toxic stage of anesthesia in which respirations are lost and circulatory collapse occurs; ventilatory assistance is necessary.

Assessment Before Surgery

The patient's response to anesthesia may differ according to variables related to the health status of the individual. These variables include age (young and older adults), a current health disorder (e.g., cardiovascular, pulmonary, renal, liver), pregnancy, history of heavy smoking, and frequent use of alcohol and drugs. These problems must be identified *before* surgery because the type and amount of anesthetic required may need to be adjusted.

Inhalation Anesthetics

During the third stage of anesthesia, inhalation anesthetics—that is, gas or volatile liquids administered as gas—are used to deliver general anesthesia. Certain gases, notably nitrous oxide, are absorbed quickly, have a rapid action, and are eliminated rapidly. Cyclopropane was a popular inhalation anesthetic from 1930 to 1960, but because of its highly flammable state as ether, it is no longer used. In the late 1950s, halothane was introduced as a nonflammable alternative. Other inhalation drugs used as anesthetics include enflurane, isoflurane, desflurane, and sevoflurane.

Inhalation anesthetics typically provide smooth induction. Upon discontinuing administration of halothane or isoflurane, full recovery of consciousness usually occurs in approximately 1 hour. Recovery from desflurane and sevoflurane is within minutes. Inhalation anesthetics are usually combined with a nonbarbiturate, such as propofol; a strong analgesic, such as morphine; and a muscle relaxant, such as rocuronium, for surgical procedures.

Adverse effects from inhalation anesthetics include respiratory depression, hypotension, dysrhythmias, and hepatic dysfunction. In patients at risk, these drugs may trigger malignant hyperthermia. The newer drugs primarily cause less nausea and vomiting than the older anesthetics.

TABLE 18.5 Inhalation and Intravenous Anesthetics

Drug	Induction Time	Considerations
Inhalation: Volatile Liquids		
Halothane (no longer available in the United States)	Rapid	Highly potent anesthetic; recovery is rapid; could decrease blood pressure, has a bronchodilator effect, and is contraindicated in obstetrics.
Enflurane (no longer available in the United States)	Rapid	Can depress respiratory function; ventilatory support may be necessary. This drug should not be used during labor because it could suppress uterine contractions; avoid use in patients with seizure disorders.
Isoflurane	Rapid	Frequently used in inhalation therapy; has a smooth and rapid induction of anesthesia and rapid recovery; could cause hypotension and respiratory depression. This drug should not be used during labor because it suppresses uterine contractions. Cardiovascular effect is minimal.
Desflurane	Rapid	Volatile liquid anesthetic; recovery is rapid after anesthetic administration has ceased; could cause hypotension and respiratory depression.
Sevoflurane	Rapid	For induction and maintenance during surgery; sevoflurane may be given alone or combined with nitrous oxide.
Inhalation: Gas		
Nitrous oxide ("laughing gas")	Very rapid	Must be administered at no less than a mixture of 21% oxygen; potency is low. Recovery is rapid with minimal cardiovascular effect.
Intravenous (Ultra Short-Acting Barbiturates)		
Methohexital sodium	Rapid	Has short duration; frequently used for induction and with other drugs as part of balanced anesthesia; an inhalation anesthesia usually follows.
Benzodiazepines		
Diazepam	Moderate to rapid	For induction of anesthesia; no analgesic effect.
Midazolam	Rapid	For induction of anesthesia and for endoscopic procedures; IV drug can cause conscious sedation and should be avoided if a cardiopulmonary disorder is present.
Others		
Droperidol and fentanyl	Moderate to rapid	A neuroleptic analgesic when combined with fentanyl (potent opiate narcotic); frequently used with a general anesthetic, can also be used as a preanesthetic drug and is also used for diagnostic procedures; may cause hypotension and respiratory depression.
Etomidate	Rapid	Etomidate is used for short-term surgery, for induction of anesthesia, or with a general anesthetic to maintain the anesthetic state.
Ketamine hydrochloride	Rapid	Used for short-term surgery or for induction of anesthesia; increases salivation, blood pressure, and heart rate; may be used for diagnostic procedures; avoid use in patients with a history of psychiatric disorders.
Propofol	Rapid	For induction of anesthesia; may be used with general anesthesia; duration of action is short; may cause hypotension and respiratory depression. Pain can occur at the injection site, so a local anesthetic (lidocaine) may be administered intravenously before injection of propofol to decrease pain.
Fospropofol	Rapid	For induction and maintenance of anesthesia; may cause hypotension and respiratory depression.

Intravenous Anesthetics

Intravenous (IV) anesthetics may be used for general anesthesia or for the induction stage of anesthesia. For outpatient surgery of short duration, an IV anesthetic might be the preferred form of anesthesia. Propofol, droperidol, etomidate, and ketamine hydrochloride are commonly used to provide a total intravenous anesthetic (TIVA). IV anesthetics have a rapid onset and short duration of action. Table 18.5 describes the inhalation and IV anesthetics used for general anesthesia.

Midazolam and propofol are commonly administered for the induction and maintenance of anesthesia or for conscious sedation for minor surgery or procedures like intubation and mechanical ventilation. Patients are sedated and relaxed but, depending on the dose, they are responsive to commands.

Adverse effects from IV anesthetics include respiratory and cardiovascular depression. Propofol supports microbial growth and may increase the risk for bacterial infection. Discarding opened vials within 6 hours is a necessary precaution in the prevention of sepsis. If propofol is administered from its original container, the IV tubing and unused portion must be discarded within 12 hours of initiation.

Topical Anesthetics

Use of topical anesthetic agents is limited to mucous membranes, broken or unbroken skin surfaces, and burns. Topical anesthetics come in different forms: solutions, liquid sprays, ointments, creams, gels, and powders. Topical anesthetics decrease the sensitivity of nerve endings in the affected area.

Local Anesthetics

Local anesthetics block pain at the site where the drug is administered by preventing conduction of nerve impulses. Local anesthetics are useful in dental procedures, suturing skin lacerations, short-term (minor) surgery at a localized area, blocking nerve impulses (nerve block) below the insertion of a spinal anesthetic, and diagnostic procedures such as lumbar puncture and thoracentesis. Local anesthetics may also be used to perform regional blocks—such as brachial plexus, axillary, femoral, or sciatic blocks—to provide analgesia for surgery of the upper or lower extremities.

Most local anesthetics are divided into two groups, the esters and the amides, according to their basic structures. The amides have a very low incidence of allergic reaction.

The first local anesthetic used was cocaine hydrochloride in the late 1800s. Procaine hydrochloride, a synthetic of cocaine, was discovered in the early 1900s. Lidocaine hydrochloride was developed in the mid-1950s to replace procaine except in dental procedures. Lidocaine has a rapid onset and a long duration of action, is more stable in solution, and causes fewer hypersensitivity reactions than procaine. Since the introduction of lidocaine, many local anesthetics have been marketed. Table 18.6 describes the various types of local anesthetics according to short-, moderate-, and long-acting effects.

Orthopedic joint surgeries, mastectomy, cesarean delivery, hysterectomy, hernia repair, and cholecystectomy frequently use the postoperative pain control provided by an anesthetic pump. For example, the patient who has a bilateral hernia repair has a catheter inserted into the deep fascia of the lower abdomen. A continuous flow of bupivacaine, a local anesthetic, is delivered via a Y-connector to both sides. By controlling pain with this delivery method, the patient is allowed increased mobility; reduced opioid use, which reduces associated drowsiness and nausea; and a reduced hospital stay. Yet another use of local the anesthetic, bupivacaine liposome, offers prolonged pain relief of 3 to 5 days when infiltrated in specific approved nerve or field blocks.

Spinal Anesthesia

Spinal anesthesia requires that a local anesthetic be injected into the subarachnoid space below the first lumbar space (L1) in adults and the third lumbar space (L3) in children. If the local anesthetic is given or spreads too high in the spinal column, the respiratory muscles could be affected, and respiratory distress or respiratory failure could result. A postdural puncture headache might result after spinal anesthesia (a "spinal"), possibly because of a decrease in cerebrospinal fluid pressure caused by a leak of fluid at the needle insertion point. Encouraging the patient to remain flat after surgery with spinal anesthesia and to take increased fluids usually decreases the likelihood of leaking spinal fluid. Postdural puncture headaches occur most frequently in females and in younger patients, with the highest incidence occurring in obstetric patients. Hypotension also can result after spinal anesthesia due to the ensuing sympathetic blockade and predisposing factors that include sensory block location, history of hypertension, and chronic alcohol intake.

Various sites of the spinal column can be used for a nerve block with a local anesthetic (Fig. 18.2). A spinal block results from the penetration of the anesthetic into the subarachnoid space, which is the space between the pia mater membrane and the arachnoid membrane. An epidural block is the placement of the local anesthetic in the epidural space just posterior to the spinal cord or the dura mater. The epidural space is located between the posterior longitudinal ligament on the anterior side and the ligamentum flavum posteriorly. A caudal block is an epidural block placed by administering a local anesthetic through the sacral hiatus. A saddle block is given at the lower end of the spinal column to block the perineal area. Blood pressure should be monitored during administration of these types of anesthesia because

TABLE 18.6 Local Anesthetics

Anesthetics	Type	Uses and Considerations
Short Acting (30 min to 1 h)		
Chloroprocaine hydrochloride	Ester	For infiltration, caudal, and epidural anesthesia; onset of action is 6–12 min
Procaine hydrochloride	Ester	For nerve block, infiltration, epidural, and spinal anesthesia; useful in dentistry; use with caution in patients allergic to ester-type anesthetics
Moderate Acting (1–3 h)		
Lidocaine hydrochloride	Amide	For nerve block, infiltration, epidural, and spinal anesthesia; allergic reaction is rare. Lidocaine is used to treat cardiac dysrhythmias (see Chapter 37)
Mepivacaine hydrochloride	Amide	For nerve block, infiltration, caudal, and epidural anesthesia; may be used in dentistry
Prilocaine hydrochloride	Amide	For peripheral nerve block, infiltration, caudal, and epidural anesthesia; may be used in dentistry
Long Acting (3–10 h)		
Bupivacaine hydrochloride	Amide	For peripheral nerve block, infiltration, caudal, and epidural anesthesia
Dibucaine hydrochloride	Amide	For topical use (creams and ointment) to affected areas
Tetracaine hydrochloride	Ester	For spinal anesthesia (high and low saddle block); also for topical use to affected areas, such as the eye to anesthetize the cornea, the nose and throat for bronchoscopy, and the skin for relief of pain and pruritus (itching)

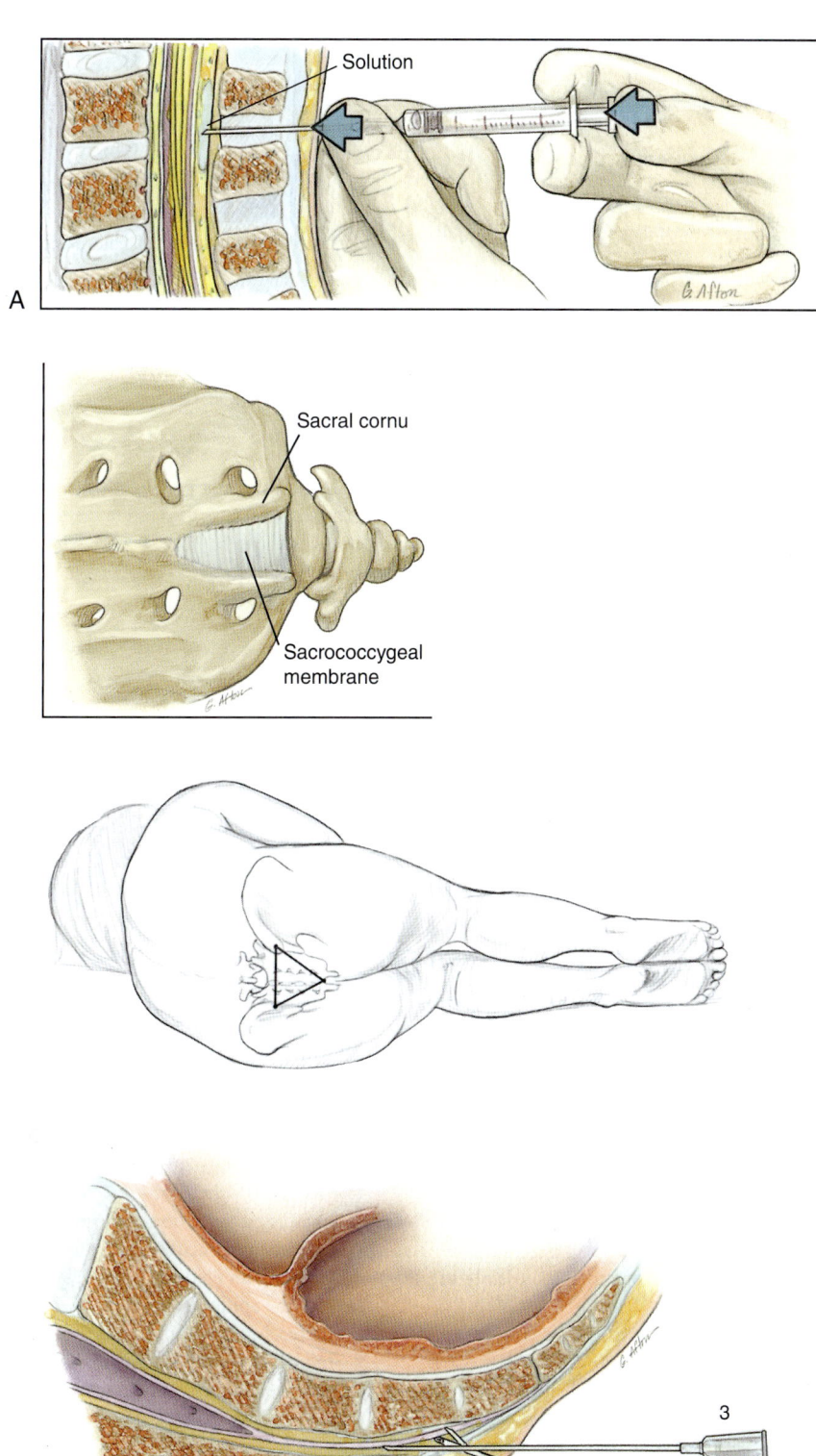

Fig. 18.2 (A) Administration of solution for epidural placement. (B) Caudal anesthesia.

CLINICAL JUDGMENT [NURSING PROCESS]
Anesthetics

Concept: Intraoperative Care
- Monitoring of the patient and the surgical environment throughout a surgical procedure to ensure patient safety

Recognize Cues [Assessment]
- Assess baseline vital signs.
- Obtain a drug and health history, noting drugs that affect the cardiopulmonary system.

Analyze Cues and Prioritize Hypothesis [Patient Problems]
- Airway obstruction
- Acute pain

Generate Solutions [Planning]
- Patient will participate in preoperative preparation and will verbalize understanding of postoperative care.
- Patient's vital signs will remain stable after surgery.

Take Action [Nursing Interventions]
- Monitor the postoperative state of sensorium. Report if a patient remains excessively nonresponsive or confused.
- Observe preoperative and postoperative urine output. Report deficit of hourly or 8-hour urine output.
- ⚡ Monitor vital signs after general and local anesthesia; hypotension and respiratory depression may result.
- Administer an analgesic or a narcotic-analgesic with caution until the patient fully recovers from the anesthetic. To prevent adverse reactions, the dosage might need to be adjusted if the patient is under the influence of an anesthetic.

Patient Teaching
- Explain to patients the preoperative preparation and postoperative nursing assessment and interventions.

Evaluate Outcomes [Evaluation]
- Evaluate the patient's response to the anesthetics. Continue to monitor for adverse reactions.

---

a decrease in blood pressure resulting from the drug and procedure might occur. Further discussion of labor and delivery drugs can be found in Chapter 50. Nurses play an important role in patient assessment before and after general and local anesthesia is administered.

Preparing the patient for surgery by explaining the preparations and completing the preoperative orders, including premedications, is necessary to enhance the safety and effectiveness of anesthesia and surgery.

CLINICAL JUDGMENT CASE STUDY

J.Z., a 72-year-old female, has difficulty staying asleep. She asks the nurse whether she should take a sleeping medication, such as lorazepam, before bedtime.

1. Before J.Z. takes any sleep aid or hypnotic, what nursing assessments should be made?
2. Describe a nursing plan that may help alleviate J.Z.'s sleep disturbance.
3. Would J.Z. be a candidate for taking a benzodiazepine? Explain your answer.
4. What follow-up plan should the nurse have related to J.Z.'s sleep problem?

REVIEW QUESTIONS

1. It is important for the nurse teaching the patient regarding secobarbital to include which information about the drug?
   a. It is a short-acting drug that may cause one to awaken early in the morning.
   b. It is an intermediate-acting drug that frequently causes rapid eye movement rebound.
   c. It is an intermediate-acting drug that frequently causes a hangover effect.
   d. It is a long-acting drug that is frequently associated with dependence.
   e. It is an ultra short-acting central nervous system depressant that induces hypnosis.
   f. It may cause seizures after prolonged use.
2. A patient taking lorazepam asks the nurse how this drug works. The nurse should respond by stating that it is a benzodiazepine that acts by which mechanism?
   a. Depressing the central nervous system, leading to a loss of consciousness
   b. Depressing the central nervous system, including the motor and sensory activities
   c. Increasing the action of the inhibitory neurotransmitter gamma-aminobutyric acid (GABA) to GABA receptors
   d. Creating an epidural block by placement of the local anesthetic into the epidural space
   e. Increasing melatonin, thus inducing sleep
   f. Increasing cortisol, allowing for natural sleep
3. A patient is taking ramelteon for insomnia. The nurse prepares a care plan that includes monitoring of the patient for side effects/adverse reactions of this drug. Which is a side effect of ramelteon?
   a. Insomnia
   b. Bradycardia
   c. Laryngospasm
   d. Sleep-related behaviors
   e. Increased salivation
   f. Pupillary constriction
4. A patient received spinal anesthesia. Which is most important for the nurse to monitor?
   a. Loss of consciousness
   b. Hangover effects and dependence
   c. Hypotension and headaches

d. Excitement or delirium
   e. Venous dilation
   f. Increased respiratory rate
5. A nurse is teaching a patient about zolpidem. Which is important for the nurse to include in the teaching of this drug?
   a. The maximum dose is 20 mg/day.
   b. It is used for short-term treatment less than 10 days.
   c. For older adults, the dose is 15 mg at bedtime.
   d. The drug should only be used for 21 days or less.
   e. The drug may cause increased salivation.
   f. The drug may cause excitation.
6. A patient is taking triazolam. Which instructions about this drug are important for the nurse to include?
   a. It may be used as a barbiturate for only 4 weeks.
   b. Use as a nonbenzodiazepine to reduce anxiety.
   c. It may cause agranulocytosis and thrombocytopenia.
   d. Avoid alcohol and smoking while taking this drug.
   e. It is an ultra-short-acting medication.
   f. Long-term use is encouraged.
7. A patient is to receive conscious sedation for a minor surgical procedure. Which drug administration should the nurse expect? **Select all that apply.**
   a. Propofol to reduce anxiety
   b. Lidocaine to provide local anesthesia
   c. Midazolam to promote sedation and following of commands
   d. Ketamine for rapid induction and prolonged duration of action
   e. Phenobarbital for short-acting duration of sleep
   f. Fentanyl for pain control
   g. Intravenous bupivacaine for prolonged analgesia

19

Antiseizure Drugs

http://evolve.elsevier.com/McCuistion/pharmacology

OBJECTIVES

- Explain the characteristics of a seizure.
- Explain the purpose and types of antiseizure drugs.
- Explain antiseizure drug use in pregnancy, febrile seizures, and status epilepticus.

OUTLINE

Seizures, 220
    International Classification of Seizures, 220
    Pharmacophysiology: Action of Antiseizure Drugs, 220
Antiseizure Drugs, 220
    Hydantoins, 221
    Barbiturates, 223
    Succinimides, 223
    Benzodiazepines, 223

    Iminostilbenes, 223
    Valproic Acid, 223
Antiseizure Drugs in Selected Situations, 223
    Antiseizure Drugs and Pregnancy, 223
    Antiseizure Drugs and Febrile Seizures, 223
    Antiseizure Drugs and Status Epilepticus, 223
Clinical Judgment Case Study, 227
Review Questions, 228

SEIZURES

Approximately 3.4 million people in the United States have active epilepsy, a **seizure** disorder that results from abnormal electric discharges from the cerebral neurons characterized by a loss or disturbance of consciousness and usually involuntary, uncontrolled movements. Seizures occur when there is a disruption in the electrical functioning of the brain due to an imbalance in the excitation and inhibition of electrical impulses. An excessive amount of excitation discharges could be due to several reasons, such as a defect in the neuronal membrane, the degree of sodium influx, or a decrease in the gamma-aminobutyric acid (GABA) inhibitory action. The **electroencephalogram (EEG)**, computed tomography, and magnetic resonance imaging are useful in diagnosing epilepsy. The EEG records abnormal electric discharges of the cerebral cortex. Of all seizure cases, 75% are considered to be primary, or **idiopathic** (of unknown cause), and the remainder are secondary to brain trauma, brain **anoxia** (absence of oxygen), infection, or cerebrovascular disorders (e.g., cerebrovascular accident, stroke). Epilepsy is a chronic, usually lifelong disorder. The majority of persons with seizure disorder had their first seizure before 20 years of age.

Seizures that are not associated with epilepsy could result from fever, stress, hypoglycemic reaction, electrolyte imbalance (hyponatremia), metabolic imbalance (acidosis or alkalosis), and alcohol or drug use disorders. When these conditions are corrected, the seizures cease. Recurrent seizures may result from birth and perinatal injuries, head trauma, congenital malformations, neoplasms (tumors), or idiopathic, or unknown causes.

International Classification of Seizures

There are various types of seizures, such as **tonic-clonic** (formerly known as *grand mal*), **absence** (formerly known as *petit mal*), and **psychomotor**. The International Classification of Seizures (Table 19.1) describes two seizure categories: generalized and partial. A person may also have mixed seizures that comprise more than one type.

Pharmacophysiology: Action of Antiseizure Drugs

Antiseizure drugs work in one of three ways: (1) by suppressing sodium influx through the drug binding to the sodium channel when it is inactivated, which prolongs the channel inactivation and thereby prevents neuron firing; (2) by suppressing the calcium influx, which prevents the electric current generated by the calcium ions to the T-type calcium channel; or (3) by increasing the action of GABA, which inhibits neurotransmitters throughout the brain. The drugs that suppress sodium influx are phenytoin, fosphenytoin, carbamazepine, oxcarbazepine, valproic acid, topiramate, zonisamide, and lamotrigine. Valproic acid and ethosuximide are examples of drugs that suppress calcium influx. Examples of drug groups that enhance the action of GABA are barbiturates, benzodiazepines, and tiagabine. Gabapentin promotes GABA release.

ANTISEIZURE DRUGS

Drugs used for epileptic seizures are called **antiseizure drugs**, *anticonvulsants*, or *antiepileptic drugs*. Antiseizure drugs stabilize nerve cell membranes and suppress the abnormal electric impulses in the cerebral cortex. These drugs prevent seizures but do not eliminate the cause or provide a cure. Antiseizure drugs are classified as central nervous system depressants.

With the use of antiseizure drugs, seizures are controlled in approximately 70% of patients. These drugs are usually taken throughout the person's lifetime; however, the health care provider might discontinue the medication if no seizures have occurred after 3 to 5 years in some cases.

TABLE 19.1 International Classification of Seizures

Category	Characteristics
Generalized seizure	Seizures involve both cerebral hemispheres of the brain
Tonic-clonic seizure	Also called *grand mal seizure*, the most common form; in the *tonic phase*, skeletal muscles contract or tighten in a spasm that lasts 3–5 s; in the *clonic phase*, a dysrhythmic muscular contraction occurs with a jerkiness of legs and arms that lasts 2–4 min
Tonic seizure	Sustained muscle contraction
Clonic seizure	Dysrhythmic muscle contraction
Absence seizure	Also called *petit mal seizure*; brief loss of consciousness lasts less than 10 s with fewer than three spike waves on the electroencephalogram printout. This type usually occurs in children
Myoclonic seizure	Isolated clonic contraction or jerks that last 3–10 s may be limited to one limb (focal myoclonic) or may involve the entire body (massive myoclonic); may be secondary to a neurologic disorder such as encephalitis or Tay-Sachs disease
Atonic seizure	Head drop, loss of posture, and sudden loss of muscle tone occur. If lower limbs are involved, the patient could collapse
Infantile spasms	Muscle spasm
Partial seizure	Involves one hemisphere of the brain; no loss of consciousness occurs in simple partial seizures, but there is a loss of consciousness in complex partial seizures.
Simple seizure	Occurs in motor, sensory, autonomic, and psychic forms; no loss of consciousness occurs.
Motor	Formerly called the *Jacksonian seizure*, this type involves spontaneous movement that spreads; it can develop into a generalized seizure.
Sensory	Visual, auditory, or taste hallucinations
Autonomic response	Paleness, flushing, sweating, or vomiting
Psychological	Personality changes
Complex seizure	Loss of consciousness occurs, and the patient does not recall behavior immediately before, during, and immediately after the seizure.
Psychomotor	Complex symptoms include automatisms (repetitive behavior such as chewing or swallowing motions), behavioral changes, and motor seizures.
Cognitive	Confusion or memory impairment
Affective	Bizarre behavior
Compound	May lead to generalized seizures such as tonic or tonic-clonic

Many types of antiseizure drugs are used to treat seizures, including hydantoins (phenytoin), long-acting barbiturates (phenobarbital, primidone), succinimides (ethosuximide), benzodiazepines (diazepam, clonazepam), iminostilbanes (carbamazepine), and valproate (valproic acid). Antiseizure drugs are not indicated for all types of seizures. For example, phenytoin is effective in treating tonic-clonic and partial seizures but is not effective in treating absence seizures.

Hydantoins

The first antiseizure drug used to treat seizures was phenytoin, a hydantoin discovered in 1938 and still commonly used for controlling seizures. Hydantoins inhibit sodium influx, stabilize cell membranes, reduce repetitive neuronal firing, and limit seizures. By increasing the electrical stimulation threshold in cardiac tissue, it also acts as an antidysrhythmic. It has a slight effect on general sedation, and it is nonaddicting. However, this drug should *not* be used during pregnancy because it can have a teratogenic effect on the fetus.

> ⚡ **PATIENT SAFETY**
>
> **Do Not Confuse**
> - **Cerebyx**, a hydantoin antiseizure drug, with **Celebrex**, a nonsteroidal antiinflammatory drug. The names of these drugs look and sound alike, but the drugs are different in their pharmacology.

Drug dosage for phenytoin and other antiseizure drugs is age-related. Newborns, persons with liver disease, and older adults require a lower dosage because of a decrease in metabolism that results in more available drugs. Conversely, individuals with an increased metabolic rate, such as children, may require an increased dosage. The drug dosage is adjusted according to the therapeutic plasma or serum level. Phenytoin has a narrow therapeutic range of 10 to 20 mcg/mL, which is generally considered equivalent to 1 to 2 mcg/mL unbound or free phenytoin. The benefits of an antiseizure drug become apparent when the serum drug level is within the therapeutic range. Typically, if the drug level is below the desired range, the patient is not receiving the required drug dosage to control seizure activity. If the drug level is above the desired range, drug toxicity may result. Monitoring the therapeutic serum drug range is of utmost importance to ensure drug effectiveness. Prototype Drug Chart: Phenytoin lists the pharmacologic data associated with phenytoin.

Pharmacokinetics

Phenytoin is slowly absorbed from the small intestine. It is a highly protein-bound (90%–95%) drug; therefore a decrease in serum protein or albumin can increase the free phenytoin serum level. With a small to average drug dose, the half-life of phenytoin averages approximately 22 hours, but the range can be from 7 to 60 hours. Phenytoin is metabolized to inactive metabolites and excreted in the urine.

PROTOTYPE DRUG CHART

Phenytoin

Drug Class	Dosage
Anticonvulsant: Hydantoin	Status epilepticus: A: IV: LD: 20 mg/kg/dose not to exceed 50 mg/min, then in 10 min may give 5–10 mg/kg as a single dose if needed to control seizures; *max.* 1500 mg/dose Therapeutic serum range: 10–20 mcg/mL Toxic level: >20 mcg/mL
Contraindications	**Drug-Lab-Food Interactions**
Hypersensitivity, AV heart block, bradycardia, Adams-Stokes syndrome *Caution:* Hyponatremia, hypotension, heart failure, vitamin K deficiency, hypoglycemia, psychosis, suicidal ideation, myasthenia gravis, hypothyroidism, alcohol abuse, cardiovascular disease, diabetes mellitus, renal and hepatic impairment, porphyria, older adults, Asian ethnicity, depression, osteoporosis, abrupt discontinuation, dysrhythmias, pregnancy, breastfeeding	Drug: Increased effects with cimetidine, isoniazid; decreased effects with folic acid, calcium, antacids, sucralfate, cisplatin Decreases effects of anticoagulants, oral contraceptives, antineoplastics, theophylline, cyclosporine, quinidine, dopamine, and rifampin Food: Decreases effects of folic acid, calcium, and vitamin D because absorption is decreased by phenytoin
Pharmacokinetics	**Pharmacodynamics**
Absorption: PO: Slowly absorbed; IM: Erratic rate of absorption Distribution: PB: 90%–95% Metabolism: t½: 7–60 h Excretion: In bile and urine	PO: Onset: 0.5–2 h Peak: 1.5–3 h Duration: 6–12 h IV: Onset: Within minutes Peak: 10–30 min Duration: >12 h
Therapeutic Effects/Uses	
Treatment of tonic-clonic and partial seizures and status epilepticus Mechanism of action: Reduces motor cortex activity and alters ion transport by acting on sodium channels on neuronal cell membranes	
Side Effects	**Adverse Reactions**
Headache, confusion, dizziness, drowsiness, tinnitus, insomnia, nystagmus, asthenia, ataxia, paresthesia, hyporeflexia, tremor, gingival hyperplasia, abdominal pain, dysgeusia, nausea, vomiting, constipation, amblyopia, erectile dysfunction	Hypotension, bradycardia, tachycardia, hyperglycemia, depression, peripheral neuropathy, injection site reaction (purple glove syndrome), cerebral edema, hypothyroidism *Life-threatening:* Agranulocytosis, leukopenia, thrombocytopenia, hepatic/renal failure, coma, Stevens-Johnson syndrome, ventricular fibrillation, suicidal ideation

>, Greater than; *A*, adult; *h*, hour; *IV*, intravenous; *LD*, loading dose; *max*, maximum; *min*, minute; *PB*, protein binding; *PO*, by mouth; *t½*, half-life.

Pharmacodynamics

The pharmacodynamics of orally administered phenytoin include onset of action within 30 minutes to 2 hours, peak serum concentration in 1.5 to 3 hours, and a duration of 6 to 12 hours. The onset of action for intravenous (IV) administration is with minutes, peak action is 10 to 30 minutes, and the duration is up to 12 hours.

IV infusion of phenytoin should be administered by direct injection into a large vein via a central line or peripherally inserted central catheter (PICC). The drug may be diluted in saline solution; however, dextrose solution should be avoided because of drug precipitation. The manufacturer recommends use of an in-line filter when the drug is administered as an infusion. IV phenytoin, 50 mg or a fraction thereof, should be administered over 1 minute for adults and at a rate of 25 mg/min for older adults. Infusion rates of more than 50 mg/min may cause severe hypotension or cardiac dysrhythmias, especially for older and debilitated patients. Local irritation at the injection site may be noted, and **sloughing**—formation of dead tissue that separates from living tissue—may occur. The IV line should always be flushed with saline before and after each dose to reduce venous irritation. Intramuscular (IM) injection of phenytoin irritates tissues and may cause damage. For this reason, and because of its erratic absorption rate, phenytoin is *not* given by the IM route.

Side Effects and Adverse Reactions

The adverse effects of hydantoins include psychiatric effects such as depression, suicidal ideation, Stevens-Johnson syndrome, ventricular fibrillation, and blood dyscrasias such as thrombocytopenia (low platelet count) and leukopenia (low white blood cell count). Injection site reactions, such as purple glove syndrome (swollen, discolored, and painful extremities that may require amputation), may occur. Patients on hydantoins for long periods might have elevated blood glucose (hyperglycemia) that results from the drug inhibiting the release of insulin. Less severe side effects include nausea, vomiting, **gingival hyperplasia** (overgrowth of gums or reddened gums that bleed easily), constipation, drowsiness, headaches, slurred speech, confusion, and **nystagmus** (constant, involuntary, cyclical movement of the eyeball).

Drug-Drug Interactions

Drug interaction is common with hydantoins because they are highly protein bound. Hydantoins compete with other drugs (e.g., anticoagulants, aspirin) for plasma protein-binding sites. The hydantoins displace anticoagulants and aspirin, causing more free-drug availability and increasing their activity. Barbiturates, rifampin, and chronic ingestion of ethanol increase hydantoin metabolism. Drugs like sulfonamides and cimetidine can increase the action of hydantoins by inhibiting liver metabolism, which is necessary for drug excretion. Antacids, calcium preparations, sucralfate, and antineoplastic drugs also decrease the absorption of hydantoins. Antipsychotics and certain herbs can lower the seizure threshold, the level at which seizure may be induced, and they increase seizure activity. The patient should be closely monitored for seizure occurrence.

COMPLEMENTARY AND ALTERNATIVE THERAPIES

Antiseizure Drugs

- Evening primrose and borage may lower the seizure threshold when taken with antiseizure drugs. The antiseizure dose may need modification.
- Ginkgo may decrease phenytoin, carbamazepine, and valproate effectiveness.

Barbiturates

Phenobarbital, a long-acting barbiturate, is prescribed to treat tonic-clonic, partial, and myoclonic seizures and status epilepticus, a rapid succession of epileptic seizures. Barbiturates reduce seizures by enhancing the activity of GABA, an inhibitory neurotransmitter. Possible teratogenic effects and other side effects related to phenytoin are less pronounced with phenobarbital. The therapeutic serum range of phenobarbital is 10 to 40 mcg/mL. Risks associated with the use of phenobarbital include sedation and tolerance to the drug. High doses may lead to respiratory depression and coma. Discontinuance of phenobarbital should be gradual to avoid recurrence of seizures. Barbiturates may be taken with food to minimize gastrointestinal (GI) irritation.

Succinimides

The succinimide drug group is used to treat absence seizures. Succinimides act by decreasing calcium influx through the T-type calcium channels. The therapeutic serum range of ethosuximide is 40 to 100 mcg/mL. Adverse reactions include blood dyscrasias, psychosis, systemic lupus erythematosus, and suicidal ideation.

Benzodiazepines

The benzodiazepines that have antiseizure effects are clonazepam, clorazepate, lorazepam, and diazepam. Clonazepam is effective in controlling absence and myoclonic seizures, but tolerance may occur 6 months after drug therapy starts; consequently, clonazepam dosage must be adjusted. Clorazepate is administered for treating partial seizures.

Diazepam is administered by IV to treat status epilepticus. The drug has a short-term effect; thus, other antiseizure drugs, such as phenytoin or phenobarbital, must be given during or immediately after administration of diazepam.

Iminostilbenes

Carbamazepine, an iminostilbene, is used to control tonic-clonic and partial seizures. Carbamazepine is also used for psychiatric disorders (e.g., bipolar disorder), and trigeminal neuralgia (as an analgesic). The therapeutic serum range of carbamazepine is 4 to 12 mcg/mL.

A potentially toxic interaction can occur when grapefruit juice is taken with carbamazepine, and drug concentrations must be carefully monitored.

Valproic Acid

Valproic acid is prescribed for tonic-clonic, absence, and partial seizures, although the safety and efficacy of this drug have not been established for children younger than 2 years. Care should be taken when giving this drug to very young children and to patients with liver disorders because hepatotoxicity is one of the possible adverse reactions. Liver enzymes should be monitored. The therapeutic serum range for a patient with seizures is 50 to 100 mcg/mL. Valproic acid may be taken with food to avoid GI distress.

Table 19.2 lists the various antiseizure drugs and their dosages, uses, and considerations, including common side effects and a few serious adverse effects. Table 19.3 lists selected antiseizure drugs frequently prescribed to treat seizure disorders.

Antiseizure drug dosages usually start low and gradually increase over a period of weeks until the serum drug level is within therapeutic range or the seizures cease. Serum antiseizure drug levels should be closely monitored to prevent toxicity.

ANTISEIZURE DRUGS IN SELECTED SITUATIONS

Antiseizure Drugs and Pregnancy

Approximately one-third of females with a seizure disorder are at greater risk for an increase in seizures, usually due to preeclampsia, fetal growth restriction, and stillbirth during pregnancy. Hypoxia that may occur during seizures places both the pregnant female and her fetus at risk. A neurologist consultation is recommended to control seizures before pregnancy.

Many antiseizure drugs have teratogenic properties that increase the risk for fetal malformations. Phenytoin and carbamazepine have been linked to fetal anomalies, such as cardiac defects and cleft lip and palate. It has been reported that valproic acid is known to cause major congenital malformations in infants in pregnant females who take the drug. As expected, the highest incidence of birth defects occurs when the female takes combinations of antiseizure drugs.

Antiseizure drugs, such as phenytoin, carbamazepine, and phenobarbital tend to act as inhibitors of vitamin K, contributing to hemorrhage in infants shortly after birth. Frequently, pregnant females taking antiseizure drugs are given vitamin D and K prenatal vitamins, and vitamin K is administered to the infant soon after birth.

Antiseizure drugs also increase the loss of folate (folic acid) in pregnant females; thus pregnant individuals should ideally take daily folate supplements started before conception.

Antiseizure Drugs and Febrile Seizures

Seizures associated with fever usually occur in children between 3 months and 5 years of age. Epilepsy develops in approximately 2.5% of children who have had one or more febrile seizures. Prophylactic antiseizure drug treatment, such as phenobarbital or diazepam, may be indicated for high-risk patients. Valproic acid should not be given to children younger than 2 years because of its possible hepatotoxic effect.

Antiseizure Drugs and Status Epilepticus

Status epilepticus, a continuous seizure state, is considered a medical emergency. If treatment is not begun immediately, death could result. The choices of pharmacologic agents are diazepam administered by IV or lorazepam followed by IV administration of phenytoin. For continued seizures, midazolam or propofol and then high-dose barbiturates are used. These drugs should be administered slowly to avoid respiratory depression.

The pharmacologic behavior of specific anticonvulsants, including a few common side effects and severe adverse effects, is summarized in Table 19.2.

CLINICAL JUDGMENT [NURSING PROCESS]
Antiseizure Drugs: Phenytoin

Concept: Intracranial Regulation
- The process of regulating the function of the brain and nervous system

Recognize Cues [Assessment]
- Obtain a health history that includes current drugs and herbs the patient uses. Report and document any probable drug-drug or drug-herb interactions.
- Assess the patient's knowledge regarding the medication regimen.
- Check urinary output to determine whether it is adequate (>1500 mL/d).
- Determine laboratory values related to renal and liver function. If both blood urea nitrogen (BUN) and creatinine levels are elevated, a renal disorder should be suspected. Elevated serum liver enzymes (alkaline phosphatase, alanine aminotransferase, gamma-glutamyl transferase, 59-nucleotidase) indicate a hepatic disorder.

Analyze Cues and Prioritize Hypothesis [Patient Problems]
- Potential for falls
- Potential for injury
- Need for patient teaching

Generate Solutions [Planning]
- Patient's seizure frequency will diminish.
- Patient will adhere to antiseizure drug therapy.
- Patient's side effects from phenytoin will be minimal.

Take Action [Nursing Interventions]
- Monitor serum drug levels of antiseizure medication to determine therapeutic range (10–20 mcg/mL).
- Encourage the patient's compliance with the medication regimen.
- Monitor the patient's complete blood count (CBC) levels for early detection of blood dyscrasias.
- ⚡ Use seizure precautions (environmental protection from sharp objects, such as table corners) for patients at risk for seizures.
- Determine whether the patient is receiving adequate nutrients; phenytoin may cause anorexia, nausea, and vomiting.
- Advise female patients who are taking oral contraceptives and antiseizure drugs to use an additional contraceptive method.

Patient Teaching
General
- Teach patients to shake suspension-form medications thoroughly before use to adequately mix the medication to ensure accurate dosage.
- ⚡ Advise patients not to drive or perform other hazardous activities when initiating antiseizure therapy because drowsiness may occur.
- Counsel female patients contemplating pregnancy to consult with a health care provider because phenytoin and valproic acid may have a teratogenic effect.
- Monitor serum phenytoin levels closely during pregnancy because seizures tend to become more frequent due to increased metabolic rates.
- Warn patients to avoid alcohol and other central nervous system (CNS) depressants because they can cause an added depressive effect on the body.
- Explain to patients that certain herbs can interact with antiseizure drugs (see Complementary and Alternative Therapy), and dose adjustment may be required.
- Encourage patients to obtain a medical alert identification card, medical alert bracelet, or tag that indicates their diagnosis and drug regimen.
- ⚡ Teach patients not to abruptly stop drug therapy but rather to withdraw the prescribed drug gradually under medical supervision to prevent seizure rebound (recurrence of seizures) and status epilepticus.
- Counsel patients about the need for preventive dental checkups.
- Warn patients to take their prescribed antiseizure drug, get laboratory tests as ordered, and keep follow-up visits with health care providers.
- Teach patients not to self-medicate with over-the-counter (OTC) drugs without first consulting a health care provider.
- Advise patients with diabetes to monitor serum glucose levels more closely than usual because phenytoin may inhibit insulin release, causing an increase in glucose level.
- Inform patients of the existence of national, state, and local associations that provide resources, current information, and support for people with epilepsy.

Diet
- Coach patients to take antiseizure drugs at the same time every day with food or milk.

Side Effects
- Tell patients that urine may be a harmless pinkish-red or reddish-brown color.
- Advise patients to maintain good oral hygiene and to use a soft toothbrush to prevent gum irritation and bleeding.
- Teach patients to report symptoms of sore throat, bruising, and nosebleeds, which may indicate a blood dyscrasia.
- Encourage patients to inform health care providers of adverse reactions such as gingivitis, nystagmus, rash, and dizziness. (Stevens-Johnson syndrome begins with a rash.)

Evaluate Outcomes [Evaluation]
- Evaluate the effectiveness of drugs in controlling seizures.
- Monitor serum phenytoin levels to determine whether they are within the desired range. High serum levels of phenytoin are frequently indicators of phenytoin toxicity.
- Monitor patients for hydantoin overdose. Initial symptoms are nystagmus and ataxia (impaired coordination). Later symptoms are hypotension, unresponsive pupils, and coma. Respiratory and circulatory support, as well as hemodialysis, are usually used in the treatment of phenytoin overdose.

TABLE 19.2 Anticonvulsants

Drug	Route and Dosage	Uses and Considerations
Barbiturates		
Phenobarbital CSS IV	Status epilepticus: A: IV: 15–20 mg/kg as a single dose, after 10 minutes may give 5–10 mg/kg/dose if needed, maintenance dose should be given 8–12 h after loading dose Seizure prophylaxis: A: PO/IM/IV: 30–100 mg qd–tid Therapeutic serum range: 10–40 mcg/mL	For tonic-clonic, myoclonic, and partial seizures; status epilepticus; sedation induction and maintenance; anxiety and insomnia. May cause dizziness, drowsiness, weakness, headache, confusion, ataxia, hypotension, bradycardia, nausea, vomiting, constipation, and nightmares. PB: 15–55%; t½: 53–118 h
Primidone	Seizures: A: PO: Initially 100–125 mg/d at h.s. for 3 d, then bid for 3 d, then tid for 3 d; *maint:* 250 tid-qid; *max:* 2 g/d Therapeutic serum range: 10–40 mcg/mL	For tonic-clonic and partial seizures. May cause dizziness, drowsiness, irritability, diplopia, ataxia, confusion, nightmares, weakness, depression, suicidal ideation, fatigue, nystagmus, anorexia, nausea, vomiting, erectile dysfunction, vitamin D deficiency, tolerance, and respiratory depression. PB: 20%–45%; t½: 10–12 h
Benzodiazepines (Anxiolytics)		
Clonazepam CSS IV	Seizure prophylaxis: A: PO: Initially 1.5 mg/d in 3 divided doses; increase dose by 0.5–1 mg q3d until seizures are controlled; *maint:* 2–8 mg/d; *max:* 20 mg/d	For absence and myoclonic seizures and panic disorder. May cause dizziness, drowsiness, anorexia, blurred vision, ataxia, fatigue, dependence, depression, memory impairment, erectile dysfunction, constipation, infection, and dysmenorrhea. PB: 85%; t½: 30–40 h
Clorazepate CSS IV	Partial seizures: A: PO: 7.5 mg bid/tid, may increase by 7.5 mg/d; *max:* 90 mg/d	May be used for partial seizures, generalized anxiety disorder, and alcohol withdrawal. May cause blurred vision, ataxia, confusion, dizziness, drowsiness, headache, fatigue, dry mouth, tremor, tolerance, dependence, withdrawal, hypotension, depression, suicidal ideation, and respiratory depression. PB: 97%–98%; t½: 40–50 h
Diazepam CSS IV	Tonic-clonic Seizures: A: PO: 2–10 mg bid-qid: *max:* 40 mg/d	For status epilepticus (drug of choice), partial and tonic-clonic seizures, muscle spasms, anxiety, sedation induction, and alcohol withdrawal. May cause fatigue, dizziness, drowsiness, euphoria, confusion, ataxia, nasal irritation, headache, hypotension, memory impairment, diarrhea, dependence, and respiratory depression. Administer IV slowly to avoid respiratory depression and hypotension; PB: 95%–98%; t½: 48–86 h
Lorazepam CSS IV	Status epilepticus: A: IV/IM: 0.1 mg/kg/dose as a single dose, may repeat once in 5–15 min	To control status epilepticus, anxiety, and insomnia and for sedation induction. May cause drowsiness, dizziness, memory impairment, ataxia, confusion, weakness, restlessness, constipation, hypotension, injection site reaction, tolerance, and dependence. PB: 85%; t½: 9–27 h
Midazolam	Repetitive seizures: A: Intranasal: 1 spray (5 mg) into 1 nostril; If no response in 10 min, may give 1 spray in opposite nostril; *max:* 2 doses/single episode	For acute repetitive seizures, anesthesia and procedural sedation, and status epilepticus. May cause headache, hiccups, drowsiness, agitation, erythema, throat irritation, hypotension, rhinorrhea, nausea, vomiting, tolerance, dependence, respiratory depression, and apnea. PB: 97%; t½: 2–6 h
Hydantoins		
Fosphenytoin	Status epilepticus: A: IV: Initially 20 mg PE/kg as a single dose; after 10 min may give additional 5–10 mg as a single dose; Therapeutic serum range: 10–20 mcg/mL	For tonic-clonic and partial seizures, status epilepticus, and prophylaxis during neurosurgery. Dilute in D_5W or 0.9% NaCl to a concentration of 1.5–25 mg PE/mL. Administer at 150 mg PE/min to avoid hypotension or cardiac disease. Monitor ECG, blood pressure and respiratory functioning during infusion until 10–20 min post-infusion. May cause dizziness, drowsiness, nystagmus, gingival hyperplasia, ataxia, tinnitus, headache, pruritus, nausea, vomiting, purple glove syndrome, hypo/hypertension, and tremor. PB: 95%–99%; t½: 7–60 h
Phenytoin	See Prototype Drug Chart: Phenytoin	
Iminostilbene		
Carbamazepine	Seizure prophylaxis: A: PO: Initially 200 mg bid; may increase by 200 mg/d weekly as needed; *max:* 1600 mg/d in 3–4 divided doses for immediate-release tablets and in 2 divided doses for extended-release tablets; Therapeutic serum range: 4–12 mcg/mL	For tonic-clonic and partial seizures, neuropathic pain, and bipolar disorder. May cause rash, pruritus, dizziness, drowsiness, blurred vision, ataxia, dry mouth, nausea, vomiting, constipation, oligospermia, and weakness. PB: 76%; t½: Initially 25–65 h, then 12–17 h with repeated dosing
Oxcarbazepine	Immediate release: A: PO: Initially 300 mg bid; increase dose by 300 mg/d q3d to a 1200 mg/d dose; *max:* 2400 mg/d Extended release: A 18–64 y: PO: Initially 600 mg/d; increase by 600 mg/d weekly to 1200–2400 mg/d Older A: PO: Initially 300–450 mg/d increase by 300–450 mg/d weekly to 1200–2400 mg/d	For partial seizures. May cause dizziness, drowsiness, confusion, headache, dyspepsia, nausea, vomiting, diarrhea, abdominal pain, insomnia, fatigue, weakness, tremor, ataxia, anxiety, hyponatremia, diplopia, and visual impairment. PB: 40%; t½: 2 h immediate release, 7–11 h extended release
Eslicarbazepine	A: PO: Initially 400 mg/d, may increase weekly by 400–600 mg; *max:* 1600 mg/d	For partial seizures. May cause dizziness, drowsiness, ataxia, headache, impaired cognition, fatigue, diplopia, blurred vision, tremor, nausea, vomiting, diarrhea, depression, suicidal ideation. PB: 40%; t½: 13–20 h
Succinimides		
Ethosuximide	A: PO: Initially 250 mg bid; may increase dose by 250 mg/d q4-7d until seizures are controlled; *max:* 1.5 g/d in divided doses	For absence seizures. May cause dizziness, drowsiness, headache, ataxia, nightmares, impaired cognition, gingival hyperplasia, anorexia, dyspepsia, nausea, vomiting, diarrhea, depression, and suicidal ideation. PB: UK; t½: 30–60 h

Continued

TABLE 19.2 Anticonvulsants—cont'd

Drug	Route and Dosage	Uses and Considerations
Valproate Valproic acid	Partial seizure prophylaxis: A: PO: Initially 10–15 mg/kg/d in 2–3 divided doses, increase by 5–10 mg/kg/d weekly until seizures controlled; *max:* 60 mg/kg/d Therapeutic serum range: 50–100 mcg/mL	For partial, myoclonic, absence, and tonic-clonic seizures; bipolar disorder; and migraine prophylaxis. May cause dizziness, drowsiness, weakness, diplopia, insomnia, anorexia, oligomenorrhea, suicidal ideation, thrombocytopenia, abdominal pain, dyspepsia, nausea, vomiting, and diarrhea. PB: 90%; t½: 9–16 h
Miscellaneous Acetazolamide	Seizure prophylaxis: A: PO/IV: 8–30 mg/kg/d in up to 4 divided doses; *maint:* 375–1000 mg/d; *max:* 1 g/d	For absence, partial, and tonic-clonic seizures; altitude sickness, glaucoma, and edema. May cause dizziness, drowsiness, confusion, depression, headache, ataxia, fatigue, flushing, dysgeusia, nausea, vomiting, diarrhea, electrolyte disorders, hypo/hyperglycemia, renal failure, and crystalluria. PB: 90%; t½: 10–15 h
Gabapentin	Seizure prophylaxis: Immediate-release: A: PO: Initially 300 mg tid; *maint:* 900–1800 mg/d in 3 divided doses; *max:* 3600 mg/d and max time between doses 12 h	For partial, tonic-clonic seizures, restless leg syndrome, and neuropathic pain. May cause dizziness, drowsiness, headache, nystagmus, blurred vision, fatigue, peripheral edema, tremor, ataxia, weakness, hostility, depression, suicidal ideation, nausea, vomiting, and diarrhea. PB: <3%; t½: 5–7 h
Lamotrigine	Partial seizures: Immediate release: A: PO: Initially 50 mg/d for 2 wks; *maint:* 250 mg bid Extended release: A: PO: Initially 50 mg/d for 2 wks; *maint:* 250–300 mg/d	For partial and tonic-clonic seizures, Lennox-Gastaut syndrome, and bipolar disorder. May cause dizziness, drowsiness, blurred vision, diplopia, fatigue, abdominal/back pain, asthenia, nausea, vomiting, diarrhea, ataxia, tremor, fever, pharyngitis, and rash. PB: 55%; t½: 14–59 h
Levetiracetam	Partial seizures: Immediate release: A: PO: Initially 500 mg bid; may increase dose by 1000 mg/d q2wk; *max:* 3 g/d Extended release: A: PO: Initially 1 g/d, may increase dose by 1000 mg/d q2wk; *max:* 3 g/d	For partial, tonic-clonic, and myoclonic seizures. May cause drowsiness, dizziness, irritability, rhinitis, headache, cough, fatigue, anorexia, nausea, vomiting, diarrhea, weakness, infection, hallucinations, psychosis, and hypertension. PB: <10%; t½: 6–8 h
Brivaracetam	A: PO/IV: Initially 50 mg bid; *max:* 200 mg/d	For partial seizures. May cause dizziness, drowsiness, ataxia, fatigue, nausea, vomiting, dysgeusia, euphoria, psychosis, suicidal ideation, irritability, and nystagmus. PB: <20%; t½: 9 h
Tiagabine	A: PO: Initially 4 mg/d for 1 wk may increase by 4–8 mg/d weekly; *maint:* 32–56 mg/d in 2–4 divided doses; *max:* 56 mg/d in 2–4 divided doses	For partial seizures. May cause dizziness, drowsiness, tremor, weakness, ataxia, nausea, vomiting, diarrhea, pharyngitis, amblyopia, influenza, and infection. PB: 96%; t½: 7–9 h
Topiramate	Seizures: Immediate release: A: PO: Initially 25 mg bid; maint: 200 mg/d; *max:* 400 mg/d Extended release: A: PO: Initially 50 mg/d; *max:* 400 mg/d	For partial and tonic-clonic seizures, Lennox-Gastaut syndrome, and migraine prophylaxis. May cause dizziness, drowsiness, memory impairment, fever, diplopia, nystagmus, ataxia, infection, fatigue, dysgeusia, anorexia, nausea, abdominal pain, diarrhea, weight loss, depression, hyperammonemia, metabolic acidosis, and paresthesia. PB: 15%–41%; t½: 21 h immediate release, 31 h extended release
Zonisamide	A: PO: Initially 100 mg/d in 1–2 divided doses; may increase 100 mg/d q2wk; *max:* 600 mg/d	For partial seizures. May cause dizziness, drowsiness, headache, confusion, insomnia, agitation, memory impairment, depression, fatigue, ataxia, diplopia, irritability, abdominal pain, anorexia, and nausea. PB: 40%; t½: 63–105 h
Pregabalin	Partial seizures: A: PO: Initially 150 mg/d in 2–3 divided doses; *max:* 600 mg/d	For partial seizures, neuropathic pain, and fibromyalgia. May cause confusion, drowsiness, dizziness, euphoria, headache, tremor, infection, blurred vision, amblyopia, peripheral edema, fatigue, weakness, xerostomia, appetite stimulation, constipation, weight gain, and ataxia. PB: 0%; t½: 6 h
Lacosamide	Partial seizures: Immediate release: A: PO/IV: Initially 100 mg bid or 200 mg qd; *maint:* 150–200 mg bid; *max:* 400 mg/d Extended release: Initially 200 mg/d; *maint:* 300–400 qd	For partial and tonic-clonic seizures. May cause dizziness, drowsiness, euphoria, confusion, blurred vision, nystagmus, diplopia, headache, ataxia, tremor, fatigue, nausea, and vomiting. PB: 15%; t½: 13 h
Felbamate	Partial seizures: A: PO: Initially 1200 mg/d in 3–4 divided doses; *max:* 3600 mg/d	For partial seizures and Lennox-Gastaut syndrome. May cause drowsiness, dizziness, headache, fatigue, anxiety, paresthesia, diplopia, dyspepsia, nausea, diarrhea, vomiting, and constipation. PB: 25%–35%; t½: 13–23 h
Perampanel	Partial seizures: A: PO: Initially 2 mg/d at bedtime; *maint:* 8–12 mg/d; *max:* 12 mg/d	For partial and tonic-clonic seizures. May cause dizziness, drowsiness, ataxia, headache, fatigue, nausea, vomiting, weight gain, irritability, and hostility. PB: 95%–96%; t½: 105 h
Cenobamate Ganaxolone	A: PO: Initially 12.5 mg/d for 2 wk, then 25 mg/d for 2 wk, then 50 mg/d for 2 wk, then 100 mg/d for 2 wk, then 150 mg/d for 2 wk, then 200 mg/d; *max:* 400 mg/d A: Initially 150 mg tid for 7 d, gradually titrate up; max: 1800 mg/d	For partial seizures. May cause dizziness, drowsiness, fatigue, diplopia, headache, blurred vision, nystagmus, ataxia, nausea, vomiting, constipation, dysarthria, dysrhythmias, and hyperkalemia. PB: 60%; t½: 50–60 h For seizures associated with cyclin-dependent kinase-like 5 deficiency disorder. May cause drowsiness, fever, infection, nasal congestion, influenza, gait disturbance, depression, and suicidal thoughts. PB: 99%; t1/2: 34 h

<, less than; *A*, adult; *bid*, twice a day; *CSS*, Controlled Substances Schedule; *d*, day; *D5W1*, Dextrose 5% in Water; *h*, hour; *h.s.*, at bedtime; *IM*, intramuscular; *IV*, intravenous; *maint*, maintenance; *max*, maximum; *min*, minute; *NaCl*, sodium chloride; *PB*, protein binding; *PE*, phenytoin equivalents; *PO*, by mouth; *q3d*, every 3 days; *q4–7d*, every 4–7 days; *q2wks*, every 2 weeks; *qid*, four times a day; *t½*, half-life; *tid*, three times a day; *UK*, unknown; *wk*, weeks.

TABLE 19.3 Selected Anticonvulsants for Seizure Disorders

	Drug Therapy
Tonic-clonic	Phenytoin Carbamazepine Fosphenytoin Valproic acid Lamotrigine Primidone Phenobarbital Diazepam Levetiracetam Topiramate
Partial (complex secondarily generalized)	Phenytoin Carbamazepine Oxcarbazepine Levetiracetam Primidone Phenobarbital Tiagabine Topiramate Zonisamide Gabapentin Valproic acid Diazepam Fosphenytoin Lamotrigine Eslicarbazepine Clorazepate Pregabalin Lacosamide Felbamate
Absence (petit mal)	Ethosuximide Valproic acid Clonazepam
Myoclonic, atonic, atypical absence	Valproic acid Levetiracetam Clonazepam
Status epilepticus	Diazepam Fosphenytoin Lorazepam Phenytoin Phenobarbital

CLINICAL JUDGMENT CASE STUDY

A 26-year-old female takes phenytoin 100 mg three times daily to control tonic-clonic seizures. She and her husband are contemplating starting a family.

1. What action should the nurse take in regard to the patient's family planning?

    The patient complains of frequent upset stomach and bleeding gums when brushing her teeth.

2. To decrease gastrointestinal distress, what can be suggested?
3. To alleviate bleeding gums, what patient teaching may be included?
4. The nurse checks the patient's serum phenytoin level. What are the indications of an abnormal serum level? What appropriate actions should be taken?

REVIEW QUESTIONS

1. The nurse witnesses a patient's seizure involving generalized contraction of the body followed by jerkiness of the arms and legs. The nurse reports this as which type of seizure?
   a. Myoclonic
   b. Absence
   c. Tonic-clonic
   d. Psychomotor

2. Phenytoin has been prescribed for a patient with seizures. The nurse should include which appropriate nursing intervention in the plan of care?
   a. Report an abnormal phenytoin level of 18 mcg/mL.
   b. Monitor complete blood count levels for early detection of blood dyscrasias.
   c. Encourage the patient to brush teeth vigorously to prevent plaque buildup.
   d. Teach the patient to stop the drug immediately when passing pinkish-red or reddish-brown urine.

3. When administering phenytoin, the nurse realizes more teaching is needed if the patient makes which statement?
   a. "I must shake the oral suspension very well before pouring it in the dose cup."
   b. "I cannot drink alcoholic beverages when taking phenytoin."
   c. "I should take phenytoin 1 hour before meals."
   d. "I will need to get periodic dental checkups."

4. A patient is having absence seizures. Which of the following does the nurse expect to be prescribed for this type of seizure? **Select all that apply.**
   a. Phenytoin
   b. Phenobarbital
   c. Valproic acid
   d. Clonazepam
   e. Ethosuximide

5. A patient is admitted to the emergency department with status epilepticus. Which drug should the nurse most likely prepare to administer to this patient? **Select all that apply.**
   a. Diazepam
   b. Midazolam
   c. Gabapentin
   d. Levetiracetam
   e. Topiramate

6. The nurse should monitor the patient receiving phenytoin for which adverse effect?
   a. Psychosis
   b. Nosebleeds
   c. Hypertension
   d. Gum erosion

7. A nurse administering valproic acid to a patient checks the laboratory values and finds a serum range for valproic acid of 150 mcg/mL. What should the nurse do?
   a. Increase the daily dose to get the patient's level into the therapeutic range.
   b. Hold the morning dose, but give the other scheduled dosages for the day.
   c. Ask the patient if they are having any adverse effects from the medication.
   d. Hold the medication, and notify the health care provider.

20

Drugs for Parkinson and Alzheimer Disease

http://evolve.elsevier.com/McCuistion/pharmacology

OBJECTIVES

- Describe principles of nursing care for the use of drugs for Parkinson disease.
- Differentiate among the drugs that treat Parkinson disease.
- Describe principles of nursing care for the use of drugs for Alzheimer disease.

OUTLINE

Parkinson Disease, 229
    Parkinsonism and Extrapyramidal Symptoms, 229
    Nonpharmacologic Measures, 230
    Pathophysiology, 230
Drugs Used to Treat Parkinson Disease, 230
    Anticholinergics, 230
    Dopaminergics, 232
    Dopamine Agonists, 233
    Monoamine Oxidase B Inhibitors, 233

    Catechol-*O*-Methyltransferase Inhibitors, 233
    Dopamine Receptor Antagonists, 233
    Precautions for Drugs Used to Treat Parkinson Disease, 238
Alzheimer Disease, 238
    Pathophysiology, 238
    Acetylcholinesterase/Cholinesterase Inhibitors, 239
    Amyloid Monoclonal Antibody (IgG1), 239
Clinical Judgment Case Study, 242
Review Questions, 243

Parkinson disease (PD) is a chronic, progressive neurologic disorder that affects the extrapyramidal motor tract, which controls posture, balance, and locomotion. PD is the most common form of parkinsonism, which is considered a syndrome, or a combination of similar symptoms, because of its major features: rigidity (abnormal increased muscle tone), bradykinesia (slow movement), gait disturbances, and tremors. Rigidity increases with movement. Postural changes caused by rigidity and bradykinesia include the chest and head thrust forward with the knees and hips flexed, a shuffling gait, and the absence of arm swing. Other characteristic symptoms are masked facies (no facial expression), involuntary tremors of the head and neck, and pill-rolling motions of the hands. The tremors may be more prevalent at rest.

Alzheimer disease (AD) is a chronic, progressive, neurodegenerative disorder with marked cognitive dysfunction, such as impairment of memory, reasoning, language, and perception. Various theories exist as to the cause of AD, such as neuritic plaques (i.e., senile plaques), degeneration of the cholinergic neurons, and deficiency in acetylcholine (ACh) among them.

PARKINSON DISEASE

PD was first medically described as a neurologic syndrome by James Parkinson in 1817, although fragments of parkinsonism can be found in earlier descriptions. Dr. James Parkinson described PD as having "shaking palsy." Three symptoms were described: (1) involuntary tremors of the limbs, (2) rigidity of muscles, and (3) slowness of movement with a propensity to bend the trunk forward and to pass from a walking to a running pace. In the United States approximately 1 million people have PD, and 60,000 new cases are diagnosed each year. It is expected by 2030 to rise to 1.2 million. PD generally affects patients 50 to 60 years of age and older, males are more likely to have PD than females, and the number of those diagnosed with PD increases with age, regardless of sex.

PD is a long-term (chronic) condition that gets worse over time (is progressive). PD results from a loss of neurons in a specific part of the brain called the *substantia nigra*. Some chemicals in the substantia nigra make an important brain chemical called dopamine (DA), which is needed to control movement. As PD worsens, neurons make less DA. This makes it hard to control movement. The cardinal symptoms of PD are rigidity, tremors, gait disturbance, and bradykinesia. Normally the symptoms have a gradual onset and are usually mild and unilateral in the beginning but worsen over time.

Parkinsonism and Extrapyramidal Symptoms

Certain drugs may cause parkinsonism and lead to extrapyramidal symptoms: neuroleptics (antipsychotics and DA receptor blockers). The lack of DA often mimics idiopathic pathologies of the extrapyramidal system.

These include acute dyskinesias (involuntary movement) and dystonic reactions (sustained involuntary contractions of muscles), tardive dyskinesia (repetitive movements), parkinsonism (a condition that causes a combination of the movement abnormalities seen in PD), akinesia (loss of ability to move muscles voluntarily), akathisia (feeling of muscle quivering, restlessness, and inability to sit still), and neuroleptic malignant syndrome (an adverse reaction to medications with dopamine receptor antagonist [DRA] properties).

229

Nonpharmacologic Measures

Symptoms of PD can be lessened using nonpharmacologic measures such as patient teaching, exercise, nutrition, and group support. Exercise can improve mobility and flexibility; the patient with PD should enroll in a therapeutic exercise program tailored to this disorder. A balanced diet with fiber and fluids helps prevent constipation and weight loss. Patients with PD and their family members should be encouraged to attend a support group to help cope with and understand this disorder.

Medical marijuana (cannabis) is legalized in many states, and there is strong interest in its therapeutic properties for PD. Despite several clinical studies, it has not been demonstrated that cannabis can directly benefit people with PD. Researchers issue caution for people with PD who use cannabis because of its effect on thinking. PD can impair executive function—the ability to make plans and limit risky behavior. People with a medical condition that impairs executive function should be cautious about using any medication that can compound this effect.

Pathophysiology

PD is caused by an imbalance of the neurotransmitters **Dopamine(DA)** and **Acetylcholine (ACh)**, and it is marked by degeneration of neurons of the extrapyramidal (motor) tract in the substantia nigra of the midbrain. The reason for the degeneration of neurons is unknown, but there is some evidence for the role of genetics and environmental factors.

The two neurotransmitters within the neurons of the striatum of the brain are DA, an inhibitory neurotransmitter, and ACh, an excitatory neurotransmitter. DA is released from the dopaminergic neurons, and ACh is released from the cholinergic neurons. DA normally maintains control of ACh and inhibits its excitatory response. In PD, an unexplained degeneration of the dopaminergic neurons occurs, and an imbalance between DA and ACh results. With less DA production, the excitatory response of ACh exceeds the inhibitory response of DA. An excessive amount of ACh stimulates neurons that release gamma-aminobutyric acid (GABA). With increased stimulation of GABA, the symptomatic movement disorders of PD occur. The striatal neurons synthesize DA from levodopa and release DA as needed. Before the next dose of levodopa, symptoms such as slow walking and loss of dexterity return or worsen, but within 30 to 60 minutes of receiving a dose, the patient's functioning is much improved.

DRUGS USED TO TREAT PARKINSON DISEASE

Drugs used to treat PD replace the DA deficit and reduce the symptoms. These drugs fall into five categories: (1) anticholinergics, which increase the effects of DA in the brain by reducing the effects of ACh; (2) dopaminergic replacement therapy, which stimulates the production of DA in the brain; (3) dopamine agonists, which mimic the effects of DA in the brain by directly stimulating DA receptors; (4) monoamine oxidase B (MAO-B) inhibitors, which inhibit the inactivation of DA in the brain; (5) catechol-*O*-methyltransferase (COMT) inhibitors, which inhibit the COMT enzyme that inactivates DA; and (6) dopamine antagonists, which disrupt the activity of DA by blocking DA receptor sites without activating them.

Table 20.1 compares the various drugs for PD.

Anticholinergics

Anticholinergic drugs increase the effects of DA in the brain by reducing the effects of ACh. This reduces the rigidity and some of the tremors characteristic of PD but has a minimal effect on bradykinesia. The anticholinergics are parasympatholytics that inhibit the release of ACh. Anticholinergics are still used to treat drug-induced parkinsonism, or pseudoparkinsonism, a side effect of the antipsychotic phenothiazine drug group. Examples of anticholinergics used for PD include trihexyphenidyl and benztropine.

Table 20.2 lists the anticholinergics and their dosages, uses, and considerations. Anticholinergics, also referred to as cholinergic antagonists, are discussed in Chapter 16.

TABLE 20.1 Comparison of Drugs Used to Treat Parkinson Disease (PD)

Drug	Purpose
Anticholinergics	
Benztropine	*Benztropine* is a synthetic muscarinic receptor antagonist.
Trihexyphenidyl	*Trihexyphenidyl* is a synthetic tertiary antimuscarinic.
	Both drugs have an anticholinergic action similar to atropine. They were listed as the first group of drugs to treat Parkinson disease (PD) before levodopa and dopamine agonists were introduced, and they are useful in decreasing tremors related to Parkinson disease (PD). The major use of these agents currently is to treat drug-induced parkinsonism. Treatment starts with a low dosage that is gradually increased. Older adults are more susceptible to the many side effects of anticholinergics, and patients with memory loss or dementia should *not* be on anticholinergic therapy (see Table 20.2).
Dopaminergics	
Levodopa inhalation	*Levodopa inhalation* is administered via an inhalation pump directly into the lungs. It is a dopamine precursor. It is used "as needed" for patients with PD who are affected by an "off" period. These periods may come on slowly between regularly scheduled carbidopa/levodopa doses or abruptly at unpredictable times.
Carbidopa-levodopa	*Carbidopa-levodopa* is used to decrease symptoms of Parkinson disease (PD) and parkinsonism. Carbidopa, carbidopa, a decarboxylase inhibitor which permits more levodopa to reach the striatum nerve terminals, where levodopa is converted to dopamine. With the use of carbidopa, less levodopa is needed (see Prototype Drug Chart: Carbidopa-Levodopa).
Dopamine Agonist	
Apomorphine	*Apomorphine* is a nonnarcotic derivative of morphine. It was approved as a sublingual film for treatment of acute, intermittent "off" episodes of PD and as a subcutaneous injection in advanced PD. Coadministration with antiemetic is suggested due to high incidence of nausea. It is also used as a diagnostic test for dopaminergic responsiveness.
Bromocriptine	*Bromocriptine* is a synthetic dopamine agonist and an ergot derivative, bromocriptine can be used for early treatment of PD. With increasing motor symptoms, it can be given with levodopa therapy. It was the first dopamine agonist marketed for the treatment of PD in adults as monotherapy or as an adjunct to levodopa-based treatment; however, newer dopamine agonists have largely replaced bromocriptine in the treatment of PD.

TABLE 20.1 Comparison of Drugs Used to Treat Parkinson Disease (PD)—cont'd

Drug	Purpose
Cabergoline	*Cabergoline* is a synthetic ergoline-derived dopamine agonist beneficial for motor fluctuations associated with PD. Its advantage over bromocriptine is once-daily dosing due to its longer half-life. It is used after other approved treatments have been unsuccessful due to risk of cardiac valvulopathy.
Pramipexole	*Pramipexole* differs from other dopamine drugs in that it is not an ergot alkaloid and is less likely to cause fibrotic and valvular complications.
Ropinirole	*Ropinirole* is an oral, nonergot, alkaloid dopamine agonist for the treatment of idiopathic PD in adults as early monotherapy and in combination with levodopa.
Rotigotine	*Rotigotine* is a transdermal nonergoline dopamine agonist used for the treatment of idiopathic PD and restless leg syndrome. Its effectiveness with and without concomitant levodopa treatment was established in patients with advanced and early-stage PD.
Monamine Oxidase B Inhibitors	
Safinamide	*Safinamide* is a selective and reversible inhibitor of monoamine oxidase (MAO) Type B. MAO exists as two catabolic isoenzymes, MAO-A and MAO-B. The neurotransmitters serotonin and norepinephrine are primarily catabolized by MAO-A, and dopamine is primarily catabolized by MAO-B. Due to its dopaminergic properties, safinamide is effective in the treatment of PD and is Food and Drug Administration approved as an adjunct to carbidopa-levodopa therapy to treat "off" episodes in adults with PD.
Selegiline	*Selegiline* is a selective MAO-B. It works by inhibiting the catabolic enzymes of dopamine and extends its action. It is available orally for treatment of PD as an adjunct to carbidopa-levodopa. Recommend decreasing dietary tyramine intake to decrease the risk of hypertensive crisis.
Rasagiline	*Rasagiline* is a potent, irreversible MAO-B that inhibits the breakdown of dopamine at synapses in the brain and allows neurons to reabsorb more dopamine for use later. It is 5 times more potent an inhibitor than selegiline. If dosing guidelines are followed, tyramine restrictions are not required; however, very high doses of tyramine (aged cheese) may result in hypertensive reaction.
Catechol-O-Methyltransferase Inhibitors	
Entacapone	*Entacapone* is a reversible inhibitor of the COMT enzyme that increases the concentration of levodopa and is used in combination with carbidopa-levodopa as an adjunct allowing the dosage of levodopa to be lowered.
Opicapone	*Opicapone* is an oral COMT inhibitor used once daily as adjunctive treatment to carbidopa-levodopa in adults with PD experiencing "off" episodes.
Tolcapone	*Tolcapone* is an oral peripherally and centrally acting COMT inhibitor used as an adjunct to carbidopa-levodopa therapy in the treatment of PD. By improving levodopa availability in the central nervous system, the patient's dose of levodopa can be lowered.
Dopamine Receptor Antagonist	
Amantadine	*Amantadine* decreases the symptoms of PD and drug-induced extrapyramidal reactions. Amantadine is a synthetic antiviral agent with dopamine agonist properties that cause symptomatic improvement in PD. It is a weak, uncompetitive antagonist of the NMDA receptor. It is used for early treatment of PD, which will delay the necessity of levodopa.
Istradefylline	*Istradefylline* is a xanthine derivative and an oral adenosine A2A receptor antagonist. It is used as an adjuvant with carbidopa-levodopa therapy in adults with PD who experience "off" episodes.
Atypical Antipsychotic	
Pimavanserin	*Pimavanserin* is an atypical antipsychotic, indicated for the treatment of hallucinations and delusions associated with PD psychosis.

COMT, Catechol-*O*-methyltransferase; *DA*, dopamine agonists; *DRA*, dopamine receptor antagonist; *MAO-B*, monoamine oxidase B; *NMDA*, *N*-methyl-D-aspartate; *PD*, Parkinson disease; *RLS*, restless leg syndrome.

CLINICAL JUDGMENT [NURSING PROCESS]
Antiparkinson Anticholinergic Agent

Concept: Mobility
- *Mobility* refers to the ability to move and refers to walking, exercise, and performing self-care. In nursing care, nurses assist the patient in the preservation and rehabilitation of mobility as well as the identification and avoidance of problems with immobility.

Recognize Cues [Assessment]
- Obtain a health history on the patient. Report any history of glaucoma, gastrointestinal (GI) dysfunction, urinary retention, angina, or myasthenia gravis. All anticholinergics are contraindicated if a patient has glaucoma.
- Obtain a drug history on the patient. Report any probable drug-drug interactions, such as with phenothiazines, tricyclic antidepressants (TCAs), and antihistamines, which increase the effect of trihexyphenidyl.
- Assess baseline vital signs for future comparisons. (The pulse rate may increase.)
- Assess the patient's knowledge regarding the medication regimen.
- Assess the patient's ability to ambulate and perform self-care interventions.
- Determine usual urinary output as a baseline for comparison. Urinary retention may occur with continuous use of anticholinergics.

Continued

CLINICAL JUDGMENT [NURSING PROCESS]—CONT'D
Antiparkinson Anticholinergic Agent

Analyze Cues and Prioritize Hypothesis [Patient Problems]
- Confusion
- Elimination
- Decreased mobility
- Potential for falls

Generate Solutions [Planning]
- The patient will have decreased involuntary symptoms caused by Parkinson disease (PD) or drug-induced parkinsonism.

Take Action [Nursing Interventions]
- Monitor vital signs, urine output, and bowel sounds. Increased pulse rate, urinary retention, and constipation are side effects of anticholinergic drugs.
- Observe and assess the patient for involuntary movements.
- Assess personal beliefs of patients and family, and modify communications to meet the patient's needs; use an interpreter and community nurse follow-up as needed.

Safety
- Discuss with the patient and family the need for "safety always." Depending on the progression of the disease, the patient may need assistance ambulating.
- Discuss bathroom changes such as a safety bar in the shower, an elevated toilet seat, and a shower chair.
- Discuss with the patient and family a home safety assessment: Remove all throw rugs, add extra lighting, and avoid anything that can block the patient's view when ambulating.

Patient Teaching
General
- Advise patients to avoid alcohol, cigarettes, caffeine, and aspirin to decrease gastric acidity.

Side Effects
- Encourage patients to relieve dry mouth with hard candy, ice chips, or sugarless chewing gum. Anticholinergics may decrease salivation.
- Suggest that patients use sunglasses in direct sunlight because of possible photophobia.
- Advise patients to void before taking the drug to minimize urinary retention.
- ⚡ Counsel patients who take an anticholinergic for control of symptoms of PD to have routine eye examinations because anticholinergics are contraindicated in patients with glaucoma.

Diet
- Encourage patients to ingest foods high in fiber and to increase fluid intake to prevent constipation.
- Instruct patients to avoid alcohol, cigarettes, and caffeine when taking anticholinergic drugs.

Evaluate Outcomes [Evaluation]
- Evaluate the patient's response to trihexyphenidyl or benztropine mesylate to determine whether PD symptoms are controlled and the patient can perform self-care.

TABLE 20.2 Antiparkinson Drugs: Anticholinergics

Drug	Route and Dosage	Uses and Considerations
Benztropine	A: PO/IM: Start 0.5–1 mg/d; increase as needed, 0.5 mg at 5- to 6-d intervals; *max*: 6 mg/d Drug-induced extrapyramidal symptoms: A: PO/IM/IV: 1–4 mg (once or twice daily per MD orders) *max*: IM/PO/IV: 8 mg/d	To decrease involuntary symptoms of Parkinson disease, tremor, and drug-induced parkinsonism May cause constipation, blurred vision, ocular hypertension, xerostomia (dry mouth), nausea, anhidrosis, and urinary retention Contraindications: Dementia, tachycardia, cardiac disease, autonomic neuropathy, prostatic hypertrophy, psychosis, glaucoma, myasthenia gravis, hyperthermia, alcoholism, toxic megacolon, confusion, depression, hallucinations; ❗ Contraindicated for use in older adults and children PB: 95%; t½: 36 h
Trihexyphenidyl	A: PO: Initially 1 mg, then increase by 2 mg every 3–5 d; *maint*: 6–10 mg/d, usually tid with meals and at bedtime; *max*: 15 mg/d Treatment of drug-induced extrapyramidal symptoms: A: PO: 1 mg daily, increase as needed/usual dose: 5–15 mg/d divided into 3–4 doses; *max*: 15 mg/d	Used for parkinsonism and drug-induced EPS; ⚡ Contraindicated for use in older adults and children May cause dizziness, anxiety, confusion, insomnia, nausea, restlessness, sinus tachycardia, NMS, toxic megacolon, ocular hypertension, and urinary retention Precautions: Abrupt discontinuation, alcoholism, cardiac disease, closed-angle glaucoma, hepatic disease May cause drug interaction: Tricyclic antidepressant, antihistamine PB: UK; t½: 5.6–10.2 h (some studies say t½: 33 h)

A, Adult; *bid*, two times a day; *d*, day; *h*, hour; *EPS*, extrapyramidal symptoms; *IM*, intramuscular; *IV*, intravenous; *maint*, maintenance; *max*, maximum; *mg*, milligram; *NMS*, neuroleptic malignant syndrome; *PB*, protein binding; *PO*, by mouth; *t½*, half-life; *tid*, three times day; *UK*, unknown.

Dopaminergics
Levodopa

The first dopaminergic drug was levodopa, which was introduced in 1961. When introduced, levodopa was effective in diminishing symptoms of PD and increasing mobility; this is because the blood-brain barrier admits levodopa but not DA. The enzyme *dopa decarboxylase* converts levodopa to DA in the brain, but this enzyme is also found in the peripheral nervous system and allows 99% of levodopa to be converted to DA *before* it reaches the brain. Therefore only about 1% of levodopa taken is available to be converted to DA once it reaches the brain, and large doses are needed to achieve a pharmacologic response. These high doses may cause many side effects, including nausea, vomiting, dyskinesia, orthostatic hypotension, cardiac dysrhythmias, and psychosis. Dopaminergic medications are contraindicated in glaucoma patients.

Levodopa was unavailable in the United States until December 21, 2018. The US Food and Drug Administration (FDA) approved the first and only inhaled levodopa used for intermittent treatment of "off episodes" in people with PD taking the regimen of carbidopalevodopa.

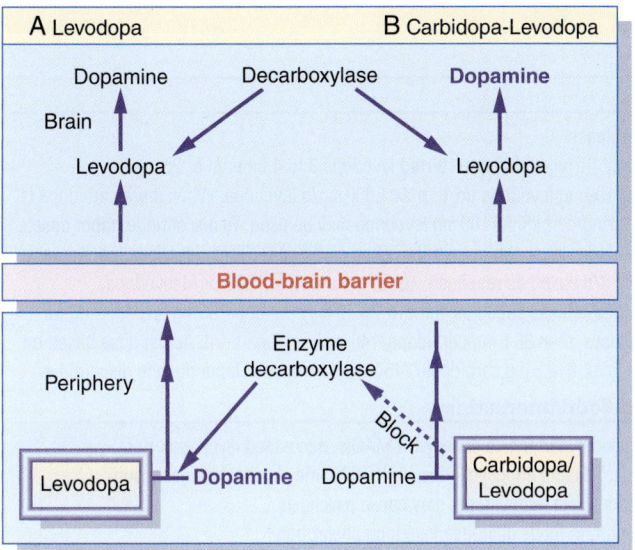

Fig. 20.1 (A) When levodopa is used alone, only 1% reaches the brain because 99% converts to dopamine while in the peripheral nervous system. (B) By combining carbidopa with levodopa, carbidopa can inhibit the enzyme decarboxylase in the periphery, thereby allowing more levodopa to reach the brain.

Off episodes, also known as *off periods*, are defined as the return of Parkinson symptoms that result from low levels of DA between doses of oral carbidopa/levodopa (http://www.FDA.gov) This inhalation therapy enters the blood stream directly via the lungs and does not depend upon absorption in the digestive tract.

Carbidopa-Levodopa

Due to the side effects of levodopa and the fact that so much levodopa is metabolized before it reaches the brain, an alternative drug, carbidopa, was developed to inhibit the enzyme *dopa decarboxylase*. By inhibiting the enzyme in the peripheral nervous system, more levodopa reaches the brain. The carbidopa is combined with levodopa in a ratio of 1 part carbidopa to 10 parts levodopa.

Fig. 20.1 illustrates the comparative action of levodopa and carbidopa-levodopa. By combining levodopa with carbidopa, more DA reaches the basal ganglia and smaller doses of levodopa are required to achieve the desired effect. The disadvantage of the carbidopa-levodopa combination is that with more available levodopa, more side effects may occur, which may include nausea, vomiting, **dystonic movement** (involuntary abnormal movement), and psychotic behavior. The peripheral side effects of levodopa are not as prevalent; however, angioedema, palpitations, and orthostatic hypotension may occur. Also, perspiration may be dark and can stain the patient's clothing.

Prototype Drug Chart: Carbidopa-Levodopa lists the pharmacologic behavior of carbidopa-levodopa.

Dopamine Agonists

DA agonists, also called *dopaminergics*, stimulate DA receptor activation and provide relief from PD symptoms such as tremor and rigidity. *Bromocriptine* acts directly on DA receptors in the CNS, cardiovascular system, and GI tract. Bromocriptine is an effective anticholinergic that works by blocking acetylcholine. It is not as effective as carbidopa-levodopa in alleviating PD symptoms. Patients who do not tolerate carbidopa-levodopa are frequently given bromocriptine. If bromocriptine is taken with carbidopa-levodopa, usually the drug dosages are reduced, and side effects and drug intolerance decrease.

Apomorphine is a DA agonist and a nonnarcotic derivative of the drug morphine. It contains DA receptor agonist properties and is used for acute, intermittent treatment of off episodes and with advanced PD. Apomorphine has a short duration of action and is inconvenient in the subcutaneous injection form (other forms of administration are being researched); however, the drug has several advantages. These advantages include a quick onset of action, a significant effect on parkinsonian hypomobility (off episodes) unresponsive to oral medications, safety in patients who have a history of psychosis from other DA agonists, and a therapeutic effect comparable to levodopa. Apomorphine is administered under close supervision of the health care provider (HCP) to observe the effect of the drug on the patient's blood pressure and heart rate.

Cabergoline carries a severe risk of cardiac valvulopathy. Prior assessment and close monitoring is necessary. This drug is rarely used in clinical practice due to this risk. *Pramipexole and Ropinirole* both include side effects causing hallucinations, psychotic like behavior, impulse control symptoms, and sleep attacks (falling asleep during ADL's) and is used with careful patient assessment.

Monoamine Oxidase B Inhibitors

The enzyme MAO-B causes catabolism (breakdown) of DA. *Selegiline* inhibits MAO-B and thus prolongs the action of levodopa. Selegiline increases the level of dopamine in the brain. It may be ordered for patients newly diagnosed with PD. The use of selegiline could delay carbidopa-levodopa therapy by 1 year. It decreases "on/off" fluctuations. Large doses of selegiline may inhibit MAO-A, an enzyme that promotes metabolism of tyramine in the GI tract. If not metabolized by MAO-A, ingestion of foods high in tyramine—such as aged cheese, red wine, and bananas—can cause a hypertensive crisis. Severe adverse drug interactions can occur between selegiline and various tricyclic antidepressants (TCAs) or selective serotonin reuptake inhibitors (SSRIs).

Catechol-*O*-Methyltransferase Inhibitors

The enzyme COMT inactivates DA. When taken with a levodopa preparation, COMT inhibitors increase the amount of levodopa concentration in the brain. *Tolcapone* was the first COMT inhibitor to be given with levodopa for advanced PD. This drug can affect liver cell function; therefore serum liver enzymes should be closely monitored.

Entacapone does not affect liver function. It is a combination drug of dopaminergics (carbidopa and levodopa) and a COMT inhibitor. With various dosage strengths available, this drug combination of carbidopa, levodopa, and entacapone provides greater dosing flexibility and individualization to the patient. It lessens the "wearing off" effects of levodopa that are sometimes experienced before the next dose.

Table 20.3 lists dopaminergics, dopamine agonists, MAO-B inhibitors, COMT inhibitors, DRAs, and atypical antipsychotics with their dosages, uses, and considerations.

Dopamine Receptor Antagonists
Amantadine

Amantadine, a synthetic antiviral agent, acts on DA receptors. It was introduced as an agent for prophylaxis of seasonal influenza and was later found to cause symptomatic improvement in PD. Although FDA approved for the prophylaxis and treatment of influenza, the Centers for Disease Control and Prevention (CDC) recommends against using amantadine due to the development of resistant viral strains. The exact mechanism of amantadine in the treatment of PD is unknown. Amantadine may be taken alone or in combination with carbidopa-levodopa or an anticholinergic drug. Initially, it produces improvement in symptoms of PD in approximately two-thirds of patients, but this improvement is usually not sustained because drug tolerance develops. Amantadine can also be used to treat drug-induced parkinsonism. It has few side effects, but the side effects may intensify when the drug is combined with other PD drugs. ⚡ Amantadine is contraindicated in patients with renal failure, patients undergoing dialysis, and patients with hypersensitivities to amantadine and rimantadine.

PROTOTYPE DRUG CHART

Carbidopa-Levodopa

Drug Class	Dosage
Dopaminergic Antiparkinson: Dopamine replacement	Immediate release: A: PO: Initially, 10 mg carbidopa/100 mg levodopa 3 to 4 times/d or 25 mg carbidopa/100 mg levodopa tid/d; *max:* 2000 mg/d levodopa. When more carbidopa is required 25 mg/carbidopa/100 mg levodopa may be used. To discontinue, taper dose. A: PO: Extended-release tablet: Initially 50 mg carbidopa/200 mg levodopa bid; Adjust dose every 3/d based on response. *Usual dose:* 400 to 1600 mg/d levodopa. A: PO Extended-release capsules: Initially 23.75 mg carbidopa/95 mg levodopa tid for the first 3 days, then 36.5 mg carbidopa/145 mg levodopa tid/d. Adjust dose based on response. *max:* 612.5 mg carbidopa/2450 mg/d levodopa. Taper dose to discontinue.
Contraindications	**Drug-Lab-Food Interactions**
Hypersensitivity to carbidopa-levodopa, closed–angle glaucoma, cardiovascular disease, hepatic disease, suspicious skin lesions (activates malignant melanoma), MAOI therapy, dyskinesia, pulmonary disease ⚡ *Caution:* Peptic ulcer, impulse control syndrome, orthostatic hypotension, myocardial infarction, psychosis, seizure disorder; avoid abrupt discontinuation. May cause suicidal ideation, glaucoma, and phenylketonuria.	Drug: Increased hypertensive crisis with MAOIs, decreased levodopa effect with anticholinergics and antipsychotics; with TCAs, may cause dyskinesia and hypertension; with methyldopa, may cause psychosis. Food: High-protein foods decrease levodopa absorption. Lab: LFT, Neurologic function testing, skin cancer screening.
Pharmacokinetics	**Pharmacodynamics**
Levodopa —10–30%; PB: Carbidopa: 36% Metabolism: t½: Levodopa is 50 min; in the presence of carbidopa, it is increased to 1.5 h; The half-life of carbidopa is about 2 h	Immediate release: Oral: Peak: 0.5 h Duration: 5 h Extended Release tablets: Peak: 2 h Duration: 4–6 h Extended Release capsule: Peak: 1 h Duration: 4–5 h
Therapeutic Effects/Uses	
To treat Parkinson disease and parkinsonism; relieves tremor and rigidity. Mechanism of Action: Transmission of levodopa to brain cells for conversion to dopamine; carbidopa blocks the conversion of levodopa to dopamine in the intestine and peripheral tissues. Carbidopa is added to levodopa to inhibit the peripheral destruction of levodopa; thus more levodopa is available for transport to the brain cells for conversion to dopamine.	
Side Effects	**Adverse Reactions**
Anorexia, nausea, vomiting, dysphagia, tardive dyskinesia, erythema, fatigue, dizziness, headache, dry mouth, constipation, bitter taste, twitching, blurred vision, insomnia, psychotic behavior, excess dark sweating, urine discoloration (red, brown, or black)	Involuntary movements, angioedema, palpitations, orthostatic hypotension, urinary retention, priapism, psychosis, depression with suicidal ideation, hallucinations, sudden sleep onset, impulse control symptoms ⚡ *Life-threatening:* Agranulocytosis, hemolytic anemia, leucopenia, thrombocytopenia, cardiac dysrhythmias; abrupt discontinuation may cause neuroleptic malignant syndrome

A, Adult; *ALP*, alkaline phosphatase; *ALT*, alanine aminotransferase; *AST*, aspartate aminotransferase; *bid*, two times a day; *BUN*, blood urea nitrogen; *d*, day; *h*, hour; *LDH*, lactic dehydrogenase; *LFT*, liver function test; *maint*, maintenance; *MAOI*, monoamine oxidase inhibitor; *max*, maximum; *min*, minute; *PB*, protein binding; *PO*, by mouth; *qid*, four times a day; *t½*, half-life; *TCA*, tricyclic antidepressant; *tid*, three times a day; *UK*, unknown.

Istradefylline

Istradefylline is an adenosine receptor antagonist used to treat PD. It reduces "off" periods resulting from long-term treatment with the antiparkinson drug levodopa. An "off" period is a time when a patient's medications are not working well, causing an increase in PD symptoms, such as tremors and difficulty walking. It is a selective antagonist.

Atypical Antipsychotic

Pimavanserin is a DA antagonist further classified as an atypical antipsychotic and is the first drug approved by the FDA to treat hallucinations and delusions associated with PD psychosis. Hallucinations or delusions may occur in as many as 50% of patients with PD at some time during their illness. People who experience them see or hear things that are not there (hallucinations) and/or have false beliefs (delusions). These are serious symptoms that can lead to thinking and emotions that are so impaired that people experiencing them may not relate to loved ones well or take appropriate care of themselves. ⚡ In January 2018 the nonprofit Institute for Safe Medication Practices (ISMP) requested that the FDA include stronger warnings on the label for pimavanserin, such as that it may lead to severe adverse effects, including death (https://www.ismp.org/best/practices).

CLINICAL JUDGMENT [NURSING PROCESS]
Antiparkinson Dopaminergic Agents: Carbidopa-Levodopa

Concept: Mobility
- *Mobility* refers to the ability to move and refers to walking, exercise, and performing self-care. In nursing care, nurses assist the patient in the preservation and rehabilitation of mobility as well as the identification and avoidance of problems with immobility.

Recognize Cues [Assessment]
- Obtain vital signs to use for future comparisons.
- Assess patients for signs and symptoms of PD, including stooped forward posture, shuffling gait, masked facies, and resting tremors.
- Obtain a patient history that includes glaucoma, heart disease, peptic ulcers, kidney or liver disease, and psychosis.
- Obtain a drug history. Report if drug-drug interaction is probable. Drugs that should be avoided or closely monitored are carbidopa-levodopa, bromocriptine, and anticholinergics.

Analyze Cues and Prioritize Hypothesis [Patient Problems]
- Reduced motor function
- Decreased functional ability
- Potential for falls
- Need for health teaching

Generate Solutions [Planning]
Patient's symptoms of PD will be decreased or absent after 1–4 weeks of drug therapy.

Take Action [Nursing Interventions]
- Monitor vital signs and electrocardiogram. Orthostatic hypotension may occur during early use of carbidopa-levodopa and bromocriptine. Instruct patients to rise slowly to avoid faintness.
- Observe for weakness, dizziness, or syncope, which are symptoms of orthostatic hypotension.
- Administer carbidopa-levodopa with low-protein foods. High-protein diets interfere with drug transport to the central nervous system (CNS).
- Observe for symptoms of PD.
- Recognize that elderly patients will need guidance in understanding the disease process of PD.
- Support the patient and their family members who may be dismayed about the diagnosis of PD and lack knowledge of the disease process.
- Secure an interpreter for patients who may have a language barrier.
- Instruct the patient in side effects to report to the health care provider.

Safety
- Ask the doctor for an occupational/physical therapist order to visit the patient's home after discharge. Depending on how the disease progresses, safety changes must be made in the patient's home.

Patient Teaching
General
- ⚡ Urge patients not to abruptly discontinue the medication. Rebound PD (increased symptoms of PD) can occur.
- Inform patients that urine may be discolored and will darken with exposure to air. Perspiration may also be dark. Explain that both are harmless, but clothes may be stained.
- Advise patients to avoid chewing or crushing extended-release tablets.

Side Effects
- Instruct the patient in side effects to report to the health care provider.
- Encourage patients to report symptoms of dyskinesia.
- Explain that it may take weeks or months before side effects are controlled.

Diet
- Suggest to patients that taking carbidopa-levodopa with food may decrease gastrointestinal (GI) upset, but food will slow the rate of drug absorption.
- Urge patients who take high doses of selegiline to avoid foods high in tyramine such as aged cheese, red wine, cream, yogurt, chocolate, bananas, and raisins to prevent hypertensive crisis.

Amantadine and Bromocriptine
- Urge patients taking amantadine to report any signs of skin lesions, seizures, or depression.
- A history of health problems should have been previously reported to a health care provider; however, it is important for the nurse to review health problems with the patient.
- Advise patients taking bromocriptine to report symptoms of lightheadedness when changing positions, a symptom of orthostatic hypotension.
- Warn patients to avoid alcohol when taking bromocriptine.
- Teach patients to check their heart rate and report rate changes or irregularity.
- Counsel patients not to abruptly stop the drug without first notifying the health care provider.

Evaluate Outcomes [Evaluation]
- Evaluate effectiveness of drug therapy in controlling symptoms of PD.
- Determine whether there is an absence of side effects.
- Determine whether the patient and family have increased knowledge of the drug regimen.

TABLE 20.3 Antiparkinson Medications

Drug	Route and Dosage	Uses and Considerations
Dopaminergics		
Levodopa	Respiratory oral inhalation: 84 mg, by mouth, up to 5 times a day; *max:* 8 mg/d/PO; 420 mg/d divided into equal doses via oral inhalation.	Uses: Oral inhalation: Treatment of "off" episodes of PD Absolute contraindications: Closed-angle glaucoma and MAOI therapy. May cause dyskinesia, chest pain, and skin laceration, agranulocytosis, akinesia, angioedema, broncho spasm, GI bleed, myocardial infarction, suicidal ideation; PB: unknown, t½: 2.3 h
Carbidopa-levodopa		See Prototype Drug Chart: Carbidopa-Levodopa

Continued

TABLE 20.3 Antiparkinson Medications—cont'd

Drug	Route and Dosage	Uses and Considerations
Dopamine Agonists (DA)		
Apomorphine	A: SQ: Initially 0.2 mL (2 mg) during "off" state. May increase dose by 0.1 mL (1 mg) dose every few days, based on response, may repeat dose up to 5 times daily as needed for "off" episodes. *max:* 5 doses/d and 0.6 mL (6 mg) dose. A: SL: Initially 10 mg for recurring "off" episodes. If tolerable, increase dose by 5 mg/dose, may repeat dose up to 5 times daily as needed for recurring "off" episodes. *max:* 5 doses/day 30 mg dose. If in effective do not administer any additional doses for "off" episodes as safety has not be studied.	⚡ Apomorphine is administered in a health care setting where the HCP can monitor the patient's BP and pulse. Used as acute, intermittent treatment of "off" episodes and advanced PD. Absolute contraindications: sulfite hypersensitivity. May cause angina, (unspecified) chest pain, dizziness, drowsiness, dyskinesia, ecchymosis, peripheral edema, hallucinations, hypotension, injection site reaction, nausea, orthostatic hypertension, peripheral edema, rhinorrhea, vomiting, and yawning. PB: 85%–90; SQ: t½: 30–60 min; SL: t½: 0.8–3 h
Bromocriptine	A: PO: Initially 1.25 mg bid, gradually increase the total daily dose by 2.5 mg every 14–28 days as needed. *max:* 30 mg/day PO	Used for or treatment of idiopathic or postencephalitic PD. May cause asthenia (weakness), rhinitis, sinusitis, headache, fatigue, nausea, constipation, GI bleeding, hypoglycemia, and hypotension. Avoid alcohol use. Contraindicated in uncontrolled HTN, use cautiously in patients with cardiac disease. PB: 90%–96%; t½: 4.8–6 h
Cabergoline	A: Oral: Initially 0.5 mg/d, titrate up as needed; doses range from 1–4 mg/d; *max:* 1 mg 2x/wk	Used for motor fluctuations (RLS) resulting from PD. May cause constipation, visual impairment, cardiac valvulopathy, heart failure, peripheral edema, palpitations, hypotension, pulmonary fibrosis. PB: 40%–42%; t½: 63–69 h ⚡ Caution: Only used if other treatments fail due to risk for cardiac valvulopathy. A full cardiac exam is required before use.
Pramipexole	PD: Immediate release: A: PO: Initially: 0.125 mg PO tid; *max:* 4.5 mg/d Extended release: A: PO: Initially 0.375 mg/d; after 5 to 7 days increase up to 0.75 mg/d based on response. Max: 4.5 mg/d	Used for PD and moderate to severe RLS. May cause visual impairment, headache, confusion, abnormal dreams, insomnia, asthenia (weakness), orthostatic hypotension, hallucinations, dyskinesia, nausea, impotence, sudden sleep onset, depression, chest pain, hypertonia, and constipation. (Taper off drug gradually.) PB: 15%; t½: 8–12 h ⚡ In patients with cardiac disease or hypotension, close monitoring is required; abrupt discontinuation of drug is prohibited; taper off drug gradually
Ropinirole	PD: Immediate release: A: PO: Initially: 0.25 mg tid; titrate up by 0.25 mg/dose on weekly basis; *max for PD:* 24 mg/d Extended release: A: PO: Initially 2 mg/d for 1–2 wk, titrate up weekly based on response; *max for RLS:* 4 mg/d	Used for PD and restless leg syndrome. May cause dizziness, drowsiness, dyskinesia, asthenia (weakness), dyspepsia, hypertension, hallucination, somnolence, bradycardia, angioedema, visual impairment, atrial fibrillation, confusion, dysphagia, impotence, sinus tachycardia, and orthostatic hypotension. PB: 40%; t½: roughly 6 h ⚡ Monitor for cardiac adverse effects: hypotension, hypertension, syncope, changes in heart rate; taper before d/c over 7-day period as gradual reduction of daily dose is recommended.
Rotigotine	Transdermal patch: Early-stage PD: A: 2 mg/24 h; titrate up 2 mg/24 h per week based on response. Taper before d/c; *max:* 6 mg/24 h Advanced PD: Transdermal: A: 4 mg/24 h once daily. Increase by 2 mg/24 h weekly based on response. Max: 8 mg/24 h. Taper off 2 g/24 h every other day.	Used for early stage and advanced-stage of PD and RLS. May cause arthralgia, asthenia, dizziness, drowsiness, dyskinesia, fatigue, headache, hyperhidrosis, hypoglycemia, insomnia, nausea, orthostatic hypotension, peripheral edema, pharyngitis, antecollis, sudden sleep onset, visual impairment, depression, hallucinations, impotence, hypertension, sinus tachycardia, and vomiting. PB: 89.5%; t½ 5–7 h
Monoamine Oxidase B (MAO-B) Inhibitors		
Safinamide	A: 50 mg/PO initially; after weeks may increase to 100 mg/d; *max:* 100 mg/d	Used for adjunctive treatment to carbidopa-levodopa therapy in patients with PD experiencing "off" episodes. May cause dyskinesia, elevated hepatic enzymes, retinopathy, sudden sleep onset, serotonin syndrome, cataracts, dyspnea, hallucinations, impulse control, NMS, psychosis, and orthostatic hypertension. PB: 76%; t½ 20–26 h

TABLE 20.3 Antiparkinson Medications—cont'd

Drug	Route and Dosage	Uses and Considerations
Selegiline	A: PO: (capsule or tablet) 5 mg bid; *max:* 10 mg/d A: PO: ODT tab: 1.25 mg/d for 6 wk, based on response, may increase to 2.5 mg/d; *max:* 2.5 mg/d	Used for PD and parkinsonism in combination with levodopa or carbidopa-levodopa. May cause AV block, Atrial flutter, Atrial fibrillation, dizziness, dyskinesia, dysphagia, dyspnea, headache, orthostatic hypotension, nausea, hallucinations, constipation, impotence, depression, confusion, hypertension, hypokalemia, and ataxia. PB: 85%–90%; t½: 1.3–2 h ⚡ Contraindicated with any other MAOI, SSRI, or SNRI; titrate off drug; never abruptly d/c; avoid foods high in tyramine, such as aged cheese, red wine, and bananas ❗ **Black-Box Warning:** Absolute contraindication for use in children; increased risk for suicidal ideation
Rasagiline	A: PO: 1 mg/d, start 0.5 mg daily if levodopa adjunct; taper dose gradually to d/c. *max:* 1 mg/d	Used for PD in early disease and as an adjunct to levodopa in later disease. May cause anuria, apnea, AV block, headache, orthostatic HTN, ataxia, dyskinesia, dyspnea, dystonic reaction, and GI bleed, myasthenia, hematuria, hallucinations, bundle-branch block, depression, heart failure, myocardial infarction. PB: 88%–94%; t½: 3 h
Catechol-*O*-Methyltransferase (COMT) Inhibitors		
Entacapone	A: PO: 200 mg with each dose of carbidopa-levodopa (up to 8 doses/d); *max:* 1600 mg/d	Used for PD. Used as an adjunct to levodopa and carbidopa to treat end-of-dose "wearing-off" in patients with PD. Levodopa dose should be decreased when taken with a COMT inhibitor. May cause constipation, confusion, colitis, dizziness, diarrhea, abdominal pain, dyskinesia, orthostatic HTN, hallucinations, impulse control, gastritis, NMS, psychosis, pulmonary fibrosis, rhabdomyolysis, sudden sleep onset, ventricular tachycardia, dyspnea. PB: 98%; t½: 1–2 h
Opicapone	A: PO: 50 mg/d at bedtime; *max:* 50 mg/d	Used as a treatment of "off" episodes of PD as an adjunct to carbidopa-levodopa. May cause dyskinesia, constipation, hallucinations, HTN, hypotension, NMS, impulse control symptoms, psycosis, sudden sleep onset, and withdrawal. PB: 99%, t½: 1–2 h ⚡ Contraindicated with MAOI therapy and pheochromocytoma
Tolcapone	A: PO: Initially 100 mg tid; *max:* 600 mg/d	Used for signs of idiopathic PD. May cause atrial fibrillation, apnea, bradycardia, bronchospasm, chestpain, depression, dysarthria, dyspnea, dyspnea, dizziness, drowsiness, headache, confusion, dystonic reaction, insomnia, elevated hepatic enzymes, anorexia, nausea, constipation, dyskinesia, muscle cramps, hallucinations, vomiting, constipation, palpations, euphoria, GI bleed, and orthostatic hypotension. PB: 99.9%; t½: 2–3 h ❗ **Black-Box Warning:** Dyskinesia and hepatotoxicity. ***Absolute Contraindications:*** hepatic disease, MAO1 Therapy, rhabdomyolysis.
Dopamine Receptor Antagonist (DRA)		
Amantadine	Immediate release: (capsules, oral solution or tablets) A: PO: 100 mg bid. Patients with drug induced EPS may require 300 mg/d in divided doses. Patients receiving more than 200 mg/d monitor closely. *max:* 400 mg/d in divided doses Extended release: A: PO: 129 mg/d in morning (increase at weekly intervals as needed); *max:* 322 mg/d	Used for treatment of PD and drug-induced extrapyramidal symptoms (EPS) reactions. May cause cataracts, dizziness, headache, anxiety, confusion, insomnia, nausea, blurred vision, ataxia, orthostatic hypotension, suicidal ideation, corneal opacification, heart failure, seizures, visual impairment, anaphylactoid reactions, arrhythmia exacerbation, coma, NMS, pulmonary edema, and peripheral edema. Do not abruptly stop taking (titrate off drug). PB: 67%; t½: 17 h
Istradefylline	A: Oral: 20 mg/d, may increase to 40 mg/d based on response. *max:* 40 mg/d	Used as "off" episodes in PD as an adjunct to carbidopa/levodopa. May cause dyskinesia, confusion, constipation, delirium, psychosis, hallucinations, mania, and difficulty with impulse control. Use with caution in hepatic disease. PB: 98%; t½: 83 h

Continued

TABLE 20.3 Antiparkinson Medications—cont'd

Drug	Route and Dosage	Uses and Considerations
Atypical Antipsychotic		
Pimavanserin	A: PO 34 mg/d *without titration; max:* 34 mg/d	Used for the treatment of hallucinations and delusions associated with PD psychosis. May cause confusion, constipation, hallucinations, infection, nausea, peripheral edema, QT prolongation, angioedema, and stroke. PB: 95%; TMAX: (Time to maximal concentration) 6 h (range: 4–24 h) **⚠ Black-Box Warning:** Not approved for dementia-related psychosis unrelated to hallucinations and delusions associated with PD psychosis; increases mortality risk in elderly patients on antipsychotic treatment for dementia-related psychosis.

A, Adult; *ADLs*, activities of daily living; *bid*, twice daily; *BP*, blood pressure; *COMT*, catechol-*O*-methyltransferase; *d*, day; *d/c*, discontinue; *h*, hour; *HCP*, health care provider; *HTN*, hypertension; *incr*, increase; *max*, maximum; *maint*, maintenance; *MAOI*, monoamine oxidase inhibitor; *mg*, milligrams; *min*, minutes; *mL*, milliliters; *NMS*, neuroleptic malignant syndrome; *ODT*, orally disintegrating; *PD*, Parkinson disease; *PB*, protein binding; *PO*, by mouth; *RLS*, restless leg syndrome; *SL*, sublingual; *SSRI*, serotonin reuptake inhibitor; *SNRI*, norepinephrine reuptake inhibitor; *SQ*, subcutaneous; *t½*, half-life; *tid*, three times a day; *tx*, treatment; *w*, with; *wk*, weeks.

Precautions for Drugs Used to Treat Parkinson Disease

Side Effects and Adverse Reactions

The common side effects of anticholinergics include dry mouth and dry secretions, urinary retention, constipation, blurred vision, and an increase in heart rate. Mental effects such as restlessness and confusion may occur in older adults.

The side effects of carbidopa-levodopa are numerous. GI disturbances are common because DA stimulates the chemoreceptor trigger zone (CTZ) in the medulla, which stimulates the vomiting center. Taking the drug with food can decrease nausea and vomiting, but food slows the absorption rate. Dyskinesia, impaired voluntary movement, may occur with high levodopa dosages. Cardiovascular side effects include orthostatic hypotension and increased heart rate during early use of levodopa. Nightmares, sudden sleep onset, impulse control symptoms, mental disturbances, and suicidal tendencies may occur.

Pramipexole and *ropinirole* can cause nausea, dizziness, somnolence, weakness, and constipation. These drugs intensify the dyskinesia and hallucinations caused by levodopa. Pramipexole is also FDA approved for treatment of restless legs syndrome.

Tolcapone may cause fatal hepatotoxicity. It is recommended that liver enzymes be drawn frequently. Abrupt discontinuation of tolcapone can cause pyrexia, confusion, and neuroleptic malignant syndrome (NMS). The side effects for tolcapone are GI related (e.g., nausea, anorexia, diarrhea, and vomiting).

Entacapone is not known to affect liver function. With entacapone, the urine can have a brownish orange discoloration. Abrupt discontinuation of entacapone may cause NMS. Both tolcapone and entacapone can intensify the adverse reactions of levodopa (e.g., hallucinations, orthostatic hypotension, constipation, dizziness) because these drugs prolong the effect of levodopa. Both tolcapone and entacapone may lead to intense, uncontrollable urges (sex, gambling, spending money) in addition to suddenly falling asleep. Patients should be warned to avoid driving and other potentially dangerous activities.

Contraindications

Anticholinergics or any drugs that have anticholinergic effects are contraindicated for patients with glaucoma. Those with severe cardiac, renal, or psychiatric health problems should avoid levodopa drugs because of adverse reactions. Patients with chronic obstructive lung diseases such as emphysema can have dry, thick mucus secretions caused by large doses of anticholinergic drugs.

Drug-Drug Interactions

Antipsychotic drugs block the receptors for DA. Carbidopa-levodopa taken with a monoamine oxidase inhibitor (MAOI) antidepressant can cause a hypertensive crisis.

ALZHEIMER DISEASE

AD is an irreversible neurodegenerative disorder characterized by a decline in a patient's activities of daily living (ADL) and cognitive abilities, as well as changes in behavior.

Pathophysiology

Many physiologic changes contribute to AD. Currently, theories related to the changes that cause AD include the following:
- Degeneration of the cholinergic neuron and deficiency in ACh
- Neuritic plaques that form mainly outside of the neurons and in the cerebral cortex
- Apolipoprotein E_4 (apoE_4), which promotes formation of neuritic plaques, which binds beta-amyloid in the plaques
- Beta-amyloid protein accumulation in high levels that may contribute to neuronal injury
- Presence of tau and neurofibrillary tangles that block the neurons and disrupt signals

Fig. 20.2 illustrates a normal healthy neuron and the neuron affected by AD. The etiology of AD is unknown, although factors thought to influence the occurrence of AD are genetic predisposition, virus, infection, or inflammation that attacks brain cells as well as nutritional, environmental, and immunologic factors.

The three phases of AD—(1) preclinical (initial stage), (2) mild cognitive impairment (MCI), and (3) Alzheimer dementia (final stage)—have been modified to assist the clinicians without access to neuropsychological testing, advanced imaging, and cerebrospinal fluid analysis. The modified criteria listed below are reliable for a probable AD diagnosis.

In addition, the patient's deficit must involve at least two of the following five areas:
1. Impaired ability to acquire and remember new information: repetitive questions or conversations, misplacing personal belongings, forgetting events or appointments, getting lost on a familiar route;
2. Impaired reasoning and handling of complex tasks, poor judgment: poor understanding of safety risks, an inability to manage finances,

Fig. 20.2 Histologic changes in Alzheimer disease. (A) Healthy neuron. (B) Neuron affected by Alzheimer disease shows characteristic neuritic plaques and cellular neurofibrillary tangles.

poor decision-making ability, and an inability to plan complex or sequential activities;
3. Impaired visuospatial abilities: an inability to recognize faces or common objects or to find objects in direct view despite good acuity, an inability to operate simple implements, and difficulty in orienting clothing to the body;
4. Impaired language functions (speaking, reading, writing): difficulty thinking of common words while speaking, hesitations, and errors in speech, spelling, and writing;
5. Changes in personality, behavior, or comportment: uncharacteristic mood fluctuations, such as agitation; impaired motivation and initiative; apathy; loss of drive; social withdrawal; decreased interest in previous activities; loss of empathy; compulsive or obsessive behaviors; and socially unacceptable behaviors.

When the diagnosis of AD is unclear, neuropsychological testing is conducted and includes advanced imaging, cerebrospinal fluid analysis, and positron emission tomography (PET).

Acetylcholinesterase/Cholinesterase Inhibitors

The cure for AD is unknown. FDA-approved medications to treat AD symptoms include *acetylcholinesterase (AChE) inhibitors* also called *Cholinesterase Inhibitors*. AChE is an enzyme responsible for breaking down acetylcholine (ACh). The AChE inhibitors are *donepezil*, *galantamine*, and *rivastigmine*, a drug that permits more ACh in the neuron receptors. Rivastigmine has effective penetration into the CNS; thus cholinergic transmission is increased. These AChE inhibitors increase cognitive function for patients with mild to moderate AD. A reversible AChE inhibitor used to treat mild to moderate AD is galantamine. These drugs do not delay progression of AD. *Memantine* is an N-methyl-D-aspartate (NMDA) receptor antagonist for the management of moderate to severe AD. It can be used alone or along with the AChE inhibitor donepezil.

Rivastigmine

Rivastigmine, an AChE inhibitor, is prescribed to improve cognitive function for patients with mild to moderate AD (see Prototype Drug Chart: Rivastigmine). This drug increases the amount of ACh at the cholinergic synapses. Rivastigmine tends to slow the disease process and has fewer drug interactions than donepezil.

Table 20.4 lists the AChE inhibitors and other drugs used to treat AD.

Pharmacokinetics of AChE

Rivastigmine is absorbed faster through the GI tract without food. It has a relatively short half-life and is given twice a day. The dose is gradually increased. The protein-binding power is average. It readily crosses the blood-brain barrier and is widely distributed.

Pharmacodynamics

Rivastigmine has been successful in improving memory in mild to moderate AD. When given orally the peak of action is 1 hour and with transdermal administration the peak of action is 8 to 16 hours. This drug is contraindicated for patients with liver disease because hepatotoxicity may occur. Cumulative drug effect is likely to occur in older adults and in patients with liver and renal dysfunction.

Many organizations are tackling AD research. Drug companies, the US government, and the Alzheimer Association are funding research to learn more about the disease and to find treatments that will reduce symptoms and prevent or cure the disease. Only through clinical research can we gain insights and answers about the safety and effectiveness of new drugs to treat AD. Drug companies are making huge strides in the development and research of Alzheimer medications. The process is long, tedious, and expensive to get drugs approved and ready for marketing. Currently there are several promising drugs in clinical trials.

N-methyl-D-Aspartate Receptor (NMDA), *memantine*, is a receptor antagonist indicated for moderate to severe Alzheimer disease. It is used as a monotherapy and in combination with donepezil, a cholinesterase inhibitor. Small improvements in cognition and activities of daily living are noted with this combination, however, the drugs do not prevent or delay progression of the disease.

Amyloid Monoclonal Antibody (IgG1)

Aducanumab is an IV-administered amyloid beta-directed antibody indicated for the treatment of adults with AD. It was approved under the FDA's accelerated approval program, which provides patients experiencing a serious disease earlier access to drugs when there is an expectation of clinical benefit as measured by a surrogate endpoint despite some uncertainty about the overall clinical benefit of the drug. The surrogate endpoint that allowed for accelerated approval in 2021 was a reduction of amyloid beta plaque in treated patients. Treatment with *aducanumab* should be initiated in patients with mild cognitive impairment or mild dementia state of disease. The presence of the amyloid beta plaque must be confirmed by magnetic resonance imaging (MRI) of the brain prior to starting the infusion of *aducanumab* (see Table 20.4).

Lecanemab was approved by the FDA in January 2023 under the accelerated process based on reduction in amyloid beta plaques with full FDA approval in July 2023. It is administered intravenously and is another monoclonal antibody that targets amyloid beta plaque in the brain.

It targets a different structure of beta-amyloid, called N3pG, which is believed to play a key role in the formation of amyloid plaque. The difference between *aducanumab* and *lecanemab* is their mechanism of action. *Aducanumab* works by removing beta-amyloid from the brain, while *lecanemab* works by blocking the formation of amyloid plaques in the brain. Before starting *lecanemab* treatment, obtain recent (within 1 year) brain magnetic resonance imaging (MRI) to establish the patient's baseline for the presence of amyloid beta pathology.

CLINICAL JUDGMENT [NURSING PROCESS]
Drug Treatment for Alzheimer Disease: Rivastigmine

Concept: Cognition
- *Cognition* is the mental action or process of acquiring knowledge and understanding through thought, experience, and the senses. Nurses care for patients with problems in cognition because they may face problems with their physical position or direction, attention span, memories, speaking, and thinking processes.

Recognize Cues [Assessment]
- Assess the patient's mental and physical abilities. Note limitation of cognitive function and self-care.
- Obtain a history that includes any liver or renal disease or dysfunction.
- Assess for memory and judgment losses. Elicit from family members a history of behavioral changes such as memory loss, declining interest in people or home, difficulty in following through with simple activities, and a tendency to wander from home.
- Observe for signs of behavioral disturbances such as hyperactivity, hostility, and wandering.
- Examine the patient for signs of aphasia or difficulty in speech.
- Note the patient's physical and motor functions.
- Determine family members' ability to cope with the patient's mental and physical changes.

Analyze Cues and Prioritize Hypothesis [Patient Problems]
- Weight loss
- Decreased self-concept
- Bowel incontinence/Gastrointestinal distress
- Confusion
- Decreased adherence
- Decreased coping
- Injury

Generate Solutions [Planning]
- Patient's memory will be improved.
- Patient will maintain self-care of body functions with assistance.
- Patient will be provided with assistance for self-care maintenance.

Take Action [Nursing Interventions]
- Maintain consistency in care.
- Assist the patient in ambulation and activity.
- Monitor for side effects related to continuous use of acetylcholinesterase (AChE) inhibitors.
- Record vital signs periodically. Note signs of bradycardia and hypotension.
- Observe any patient behavioral changes, and note any improvement or decline.
- Monitor and assist the patient closely to maintain the correct use of the drug dosing plan.
- Provide an interpreter during instruction for the patient and family if a language barrier exists.
- Assist family members in understanding about Alzheimer disease as a neurologic problem that may be part of the aging process. Explain how symptoms may become more progressive.

Safety
- ⚡ Instruct family in "home safety"; for example, remove area throw rugs, ensure pathways are clear, and keep electrical cords behind furniture to avoid injury when the patient wanders.

Patient Teaching
General
- Explain to the patient and family the purpose for the prescribed drug therapy.
- Clarify times for drug dosing and schedule to the family member responsible for the patient's medications.
- Inform family members of available support groups such as the Alzheimer's Association.

Side Effects
- Inform patients and family members that the patient should rise slowly to avoid dizziness and loss of balance.
- Monitor routine liver function tests because hepatotoxicity is an adverse effect.
- Monitor the patient for gastrointestinal distress a common side effect among patients.

Diet
- Inform family members about foods that may be prepared for the patient's consumption and tolerance.

Evaluate Outcomes [Evaluation]
- Evaluate the effectiveness of the drug regimen by determining whether the patient's mental and physical status shows improvement from drug therapy.

TABLE 20.4 Acetylcholinesterase Inhibitors and Other Drugs for Alzheimer Disease

Drug Acetylcholinesterase Inhibitors	Route and Dosage	Uses and Considerations
Donepezil	Oral: A: PO: Initially 5 mg/d, upward titration to 10 mg/d once daily should not occur until 4–6 wk; Max: 23 mg/d Transdermal dosages: A: 5 mg/d every 7/d. May increase the dose to 10 mg/d transdermal every 7 d after 4–6 wks. When converting from oral to transdermal dose: 5 mg/transdermal every 7/d for 5 mg/d PO and 10 mg/d transdermal every 7/d for 10 mg/d/PO. Max: 10 mg/d transdermal	Used for the treatment of mild to moderate Alzheimer disease. May cause: Diarrhea, erythema, hemolytic anemia, atopic dermatitis, bleeding, chest pain, confusion, hallucinations, AV block, bradycardia, cholecystic, NMS, pancreatitis, and seizures. ⚡ Use with caution in older adults. Taper off medication. PB: 96%; t½: (oral) 70 h; (transdermal) 9 h
Rivastigmine		See Prototype Drug Chart: Rivastigmi

TABLE 20.4 Acetylcholinesterase Inhibitors and Other Drugs for Alzheimer Disease—cont'd

Drug Acetylcholinesterase Inhibitors	Route and Dosage	Uses and Considerations
Galantamine	**Immediate release or oral solution:** A: PO Initially 4 mg bid; if well tolerated, after 4 wks may increase to 8 mg PO bid; if well tolerated, after 4 wks may increase to 12 mg bid, then after 4 more wks 16 mg/d. Usual dose of galantamine is 16–24 mg/d; *max.* 24 mg/d **Extended release capsules:** A: PO: 8 mg/d, initially. After 4 wks increase to 16 mg/d, if tolerated, and then to 24 mg/d after a minimum of 4 wks. *Max.* 24 mg/d/f treatment is interrupted for more than 3 days, restart initial titration schedule.	Used for treatment of mild to moderate Alzheimer disease. GI bleeding, anorexia, abdominal pain, nausea, vomiting, diarrhea, erythema, weight loss, Stevens-Johnson Syndrome, AV block, bradycardia, seizures, pancreatitis, NMS, peptic ulcer, and dyspepsia. ⚡ Use with caution in older adults. PB: 18%; t½: 7 h
N-methyl-d-aspartate (NMDA) Receptor		
Memantine	Immediate release: A:PO: 5 m/d once daily, initially. Increase the dose by 5 mg/d every wk, if tolerable. Usual dose: 10 mg PO twice daily; *max.* 20 mg/d Extended release: A: PO: Initially 7 mg/d, increase the dose weekly by 7 mg/d if tolerated; Maintenance dose: 28 mg/d; *max:* 28 mg/d Combination memantine and donepezil oral dose *(Converting from those stabilized on donepezil 10 mg/d)* A: PO 7 mg memantine/10 mg donepezil daily; Increase dose weekly by 7 mg memantine if tolerated; *max:* memantine 28 mg/d/ donepezil 10 mg/d (Converting from memantine 20 or 28 mg/d and donepezil 10 mg/d) A: PO 28 mg memantine /10 mg donepezil once daily for those stabilized on memantine 10 mg twice/d or 28 mg once/d and donepezil 10 mg/d; *max.* 28/d memantine extended release with 10 mg/d donepezil.	Used for moderate to severe Alzheimer disease. May cause serious rash, Stevens-Johnson syndrome, dizziness, headache, drowsiness, confusion, diarrhea, depression, hallucinations, hypertension, hypotension, urinary incontinence, AV block, bradycardia, GI bleeding, Heart Failure, NMS, renal failure, suicidal ideation, and constipation. ⚡ Avoid use in older adults who experience syncope due to bradycardia. PB: 45%; t½: 60–80 h
Monoclonal Antibody		
Aducanumab Lecanemab ⚡ Donanemab	A: IV 1 mg/kg infusion every 4 wks for 2 doses, then 3 mg/kg IV infusion every 4 wks for 2 doses. Then 6 mg/kg IV infusion every 4 wks for 2 doses. At the seventh infusion and beyond 10 mg/kg IV infusion every 4 wks. *Max:* 10 mg/kg/dose IV infusion for maintenance dose A: IV Dosage: 10 mg/kg infusion every 2 wks *max.* 10 mg/kg infusion once every 2 wks. A: IV: 700 mg IV infusion every 4 wks for 3 doses, then 1,400 mg IV infusion every 4 wks for maintenance therapy.	Mild cognitive impairment or mild dementia stage of Alzheimer disease. Aducanumab reduces amyloid beta plaques in the brain by binding to forms of beta-amyloid protein in Alzheimer disease. ⚡ Side effects include intracranial bleeding, hemosiderosis, seizures, hypersensitivity, headache, confusion, visual impairment, angioedema, and cerebral edema. ❗ **Black-Box Warning**: Amyloid-related imaging abnormalities t½: 24.8/d Treatment of mild cognitive or mild dementia stage of Alzheimer disease ⚡ May cause: Intracranial bleed, Infusion-related reactions, atrial fibrillation, lymphopenia, anaphylactic shock, visual impairment, angioedema, seizures, bronchospasm, cerebral edema, confusion, erythema, hypertension, and hypotension. ❗ **Black-Box Warning**: Amyloid-related imaging abnormalities; Serious hypersensitivity reactions or anaphylaxis. t½: 5–7 days Used for mild cognitive impairment or mild dementia in Alzheimer disease. ⚡ May cause: Intracranial bleeding, visual impairment, seizures, antibody formation, anaphylactic shock, angioedema, GI obstruction, GI perforation. ❗ **Black-Box Warning**: Amyloid-related imaging abnormalities. t½: 12.1/d

A, Adult; *AV*, atrial ventricular; *bid*, twice a day; *d*, day; *GI*, gastrointestinal; *h*, hour; *IV*, intravenous; *kg*, kilogram; *maint*, maintenance; *max*, maximum; *mg*, milligrams; *NMS*, neuroleptic malignant syndrome; *PB*, protein binding; *PO*, by mouth; *t½*, half-life; *wk*, week; *wks*, weeks.

PROTOTYPE DRUG CHART

Revastigmine

Drug Class	Dosag
Acetylcholinesterase inhibitor	A: PO: Initially: 1.5 mg bid with food; increase gradually after 2 wk to 3 mg bid Maintenance: 6–12 mg day; *max:* 12 mg/d Transdermal: (50 kg or more) Initially 4.6 mg/24 h; may increase after 4 wk to 9.5 mg/d; *max:* 13.3 mg/24 h
Caution	**Drug-Lab-Food Interactions**
Liver and renal diseases, urinary tract obstruction, orthostatic hypotension, bradycardia, asthma, COPD, seizures, peptic ulcer disease, abrupt discontinuation of drug, and carbamate hypersensitivity. ⚡ Caution in the elderly: High risk of bradycardia, CNS depression, and extrapyramidal effects.	Drug: Increased effect of theophylline, general anesthetics; TCAs decrease effect; increased effect with cimetidine; NSAIDs increase GI effects; alcohol and tobacco can increase clearance of rivastigmine Lab: Increased ALT, AST Monitor: LFT, neurologic function, and weight
Pharmacokinetics	**Pharmacodynamics**
Absorption: PO: Food decreases absorption rate Distribution: PB: 40% Metabolism: t½: 1.5 h Excretion: In urine	PO: Onset: UK Peak: 1 h Duration: UK Transdermal: Onset: 30 min–1 h Peak: 8–16 h Duration: 24 h
Therapeutic Effects/Uses	
Improves memory loss in mild to moderate Alzheimer disease Mechanism of Action: Elevates acetylcholine concentration; A selective inhibitor of brain AChE and BChE.	
Side Effects	**Adverse Reactions**
Anorexia, abdominal pain, GI distress, nausea, vomiting, diarrhea, constipation, weight loss, dizziness, headache, depression, confusion, peripheral edema, dry mouth, dehydration, nystagmus, photophobia	Seizures, bradycardia, orthostatic hypotension, cataracts, myocardial infarction, heart failure ⚡ *Life-threatening:* Hepatotoxicity, dysrhythmias, suicidal ideation, Stevens-Johnson syndrome

A, Adult; *ALT*, alanine aminotransferase; *AST*, aspartate aminotransferase; *AChE*, acetylcholinesterase; *BChE*, butylcholinesterase; *bid*, two times a day; *CNS*, central nervous system; *COPD*, chronic obstructive pulmonary disease; *d*, day; *GI*, gastrointestinal; *h*, hour; *LFT*, liver function test; *max*, maximum; *min*, minute; *mg*, milligram; *NSAID*, nonsteroidal anti-inflammatory drug; *PB*, protein binding; *PO*, by mouth; *t½*, half-life; *TCA*, tricyclic antidepressant; *UK*, unknown; *wk*, weeks.

In July of 2024 the FDA approved *donanemab* another monoclonal antibody which targets amyloid beta plaque in the brain. However, it works differently than *aducanumab* and *lecanemab*. Donanemab employs a distinct approach by binding to a specific truncated form of amyloid-beta plaque called N-truncated pyroglutamate amyloid beta. Prior to use, plaque in the brain must be confirmed by MRI. Treatment is recommended for persons with mild cognitive impairment or mild dementia stage of the disease.

CLINICAL JUDGMENT CASE STUDY

A 79-year-old male was diagnosed with Parkinson disease 10 years ago. During his early treatment, he took selegiline. The drug dosage was increased to alleviate symptoms.

1. How does selegiline alleviate symptoms of Parkinson disease?
2. Which dietary changes are most important to adhere to when a patient is prescribed selegiline?
3. The patient has developed nausea, depression, and ataxia to selegiline. The health care provider stops selegiline and orders carbidopa-levodopa. What are the similarities and differences between selegiline and carbidopa-levodopa?
4. What are the advantages of carbidopa-levodopa?
5. The family knows of a patient with Parkinson disease who takes the antiviral drug amantadine and does well. They ask whether amantadine is the same as carbidopa-levodopa and, if not, whether their family member can take amantadine instead of carbidopa-levodopa. What is the effect of amantadine on symptoms of Parkinson disease?
6. What would be an appropriate response to the family's question concerning the use of amantadine?
7. What are the uses for dopamine agonists and catechol-O-methyltransferase (COMT) inhibitors?
8. Certain anticholinergic drugs may be used to control Parkinson disease symptoms. What is the action of these drugs, and what are their side effects? These anticholinergic drugs are usually prescribed for parkinsonism symptoms resulting from what?

REVIEW QUESTIONS

1. Which of the following assessment findings would the nurse see in a patient with Parkinson disease? **Select all that apply.**
   a. Abrupt onset of symptoms
   b. Muscle rigidity
   c. Involuntary tremors
   d. Bradykinesia
   e. Bilateral muscle weakness
2. A patient is receiving carbidopa-levodopa for Parkinson disease. What is most important for the nurse know about this drug?
   a. Carbidopa-levodopa may lead to bronchitis.
   b. Carbidopa-levodopa may lead to increased salivation.
   c. Dopaminergics may lead to drowsiness.
   d. Dopaminergics are contraindicated in glaucoma.
3. The nurse has initiated teaching for a family member of a patient with Alzheimer disease. The nurse realizes more teaching is needed when the family member makes which of the following statements?
   a. As the disease progresses, the memory loss will get worse.
   b. There are several theories about the cause of the disease.
   c. Personality changes, wandering, and hostility may occur.
   d. It may take several medications over time to cure the disease.
4. A patient is taking rivastigmine. The nurse should teach the patient and family which information about rivastigmine?
   a. Hepatotoxicity and jaundice are side effects.
   b. The initial dose is 6 mg three times a day.
   c. Gastrointestinal distress is a common side effect.
   d. Increased appetite and weight gain is a side effect.
5. Which is a Take Action [Nursing Intervention] for a patient taking carbidopa-levodopa for Parkinson disease?
   a. Encourage the patient to adhere to a high-protein, high-sodium diet.
   b. Inform the patient that perspiration may be dark and may stain clothing.
   c. Advise the patient that glucose levels should be checked with urine testing.
   d. Warn the patient that it may take 4 to 5 days before symptoms are controlled.
6. What would the nurse teach a patient who is taking anticholinergic therapy for Parkinson disease? **Select all that apply.**
   a. Avoid alcohol and tobacco.
   b. Relieve dry mouth with hard candy or ice chips.
   c. Use sunglasses to reduce photophobia.
   d. Urinate 2 hours after taking the drug.
   e. Receive routine eye examinations.
7. A patient is taking rivastigmine to improve cognitive function. What should the nurse teach the patient/family member to do? **Select all that apply.**
   a. Rise slowly to avoid dizziness that may cause injury.
   b. Remove obstacles from pathways to avoid injury.
   c. Closely follow the medication dosing schedule.
   d. Have daily blood pressure checks for hypertension.
   e. Receive a monthly glucose panel.

21

Drugs for Neuromuscular Disorders and Muscle Spasms

http://evolve.elsevier.com/McCuistion/pharmacology

OBJECTIVES

- Interpret the occurrence, nursing care, and treatment of patients with myasthenia gravis.
- Interpret the occurrence, nursing care, and treatment of patients with multiple sclerosis.
- Explain the general use of muscle relaxants.

OUTLINE

Myasthenia Gravis, 244
    Pathophysiology, 244
    Acetylcholinesterase Inhibitors, 245
    Pharmacokinetics, 245
    Pharmacodynamics, 245
    Side Effects and Adverse Reactions, 246
Multiple Sclerosis, 248
    Classifications of Multiple Sclerosis, 248
    Immunomodulators, 248

Skeletal Muscle Relaxants, 253
    Centrally Acting Muscle Relaxants, 253
    Pharmacokinetics and Pharmacodynamics of Cyclobenzaprine, 256
Clinical Judgment Case Study, 257
Review Questions, 257

Neuromuscular disorders affect the neuromuscular system causing communication problems between the nerves and muscles. Some causes are unknown; others are caused by autoimmune issues and specific triggers to the immune response. This occurs when the immune system overreacts and attacks healthy cells, tissues, or organs.

Muscle spasms have various causes, including motor neuron disease, which can lead to damage of the nervous system, resulting in muscle weakness and wasting. There are many causes for these diseases. Some are genetic and run in families. Others are autoimmune, and the cause is unknown. Many have no cure. Spasticity of muscles can be reduced with the use of skeletal muscle relaxants. This chapter will discuss pharmacology for myasthenia gravis and multiple sclerosis.

MYASTHENIA GRAVIS

Myasthenia gravis (MG) is an acquired autoimmune disease that impairs the transmission of messages at the neuromuscular junction, resulting in varying degrees of skeletal muscle weakness that increases with muscle use. Although MG can affect any voluntary muscle, those that control eye and eyelid movement (ptosis), facial expression, chewing, and swallowing are most frequently affected due to cranial nerve involvement. MG also affects the muscles of the respiratory system. Respiratory arrest may result from respiratory muscle paralysis. The symptoms of MG are caused by autoimmune destruction of acetylcholine (ACh) sites and a resultant decrease in neuromuscular transmission.

MG is a chronic autoimmune neuromuscular disease that affects approximately 20 in 100,000 persons. It is estimated that 70,000 Americans are affected. MG can occur in people of any ethnicity and sex; however, more males are affected than females. MG peaks in females around the childbearing years (20–30 years of age), whereas the peak onset in males is after 50 years of age. MG can also occur in people outside of this age range. Although it is not a genetic disorder, a familial tendency may be apparent.

Pathophysiology

MG is an autoimmune process in which antibodies attack ACh receptors (AChRs). The result is a decreased amount of AChR sites at the neuromuscular junction, causing an error in the transmission of nerve impulses to the muscles. Neurotransmitters are chemicals that neurons, or brain cells, use to communicate information. This prevents ACh molecules from attaching to receptors and stimulating normal muscular contraction. The result is ineffective muscle contraction and muscle weakness. About 90% of patients with MG have antibodies (immune proteins produced by the body's immune system). Anti-AChR antibodies can be detected through serum testing. The other 10% have muscle weakness related to autoantibodies from other proteins such as MuSK (muscle specific kinase). These are proteins that can impair transmission at the neuromuscular junction.

Thymic hyperplasia and tumors are common in patients with MG. The thymus gland is involved in systemic immunity that is active during infancy and early childhood, but the gland normally shrinks during adulthood. Approximately 70% of patients with MG have thymic hyperplasia. A thymectomy (removal of the thymus gland) is most beneficial because it can cause a reduction of symptoms after the surgery.

MG is characterized primarily by weakness and fatigue of the skeletal muscles. In 90% of cases, eyelid or extraocular muscles are involved.

The patients experience ptosis (drooping eyelids) and diplopia (double vision). Other characteristics of MG include dysphagia (difficulty chewing and swallowing), dysarthria (slurred speech), and respiratory muscle weakness (SOB), a change in facial expressions, and weakness in arms, hands, fingers, legs, and neck.

The most favored classification of drugs used to control MG are the acetylcholinesterase (AChE) inhibitors. They inhibit the action of the enzyme AChE. As a result of this action, more ACh is available to activate the cholinergic receptors and promote muscle contraction. The AChE inhibitors are classified as parasympathomimetics.

When muscular weakness in the patient with MG becomes generalized, myasthenic crisis can occur. It is caused by a rapid unrecognized progression of the disease, inadequate amount of medication, infection, fatigue, or stress. This complication is a severe, generalized muscle weakness that involves the muscles of respiration, such as the diaphragm and intercostal muscles. Triggers of myasthenic crisis include inadequate dosing of AChE inhibitors, infection, emotional stress, menses, pregnancy, surgery, trauma, hypokalemia, temperature extremes, and alcohol intake. Myasthenic crisis can also occur 3 to 4 hours after taking certain medications (e.g., aminoglycoside and fluoroquinolone antibiotics, beta-blockers, phenytoin, and neuromuscular blocking agents; see Box 21.1). If muscle weakness remains untreated, death can result from paralysis of the respiratory muscles. Neostigmine, a fast-acting AChE inhibitor, can relieve myasthenic crisis.

Overdosing with AChE inhibitors may cause another complication of MG called cholinergic crisis, which is an acute exacerbation of symptoms. A cholinergic crisis usually occurs within 30 to 60 minutes after taking anticholinergic drugs. This complication is due to continuous depolarization of postsynaptic membranes that create a neuromuscular blockade. The patient with cholinergic crisis often has severe muscle weakness that can lead to respiratory paralysis and arrest. Accompanying symptoms include miosis (abnormal pupil constriction), pallor, sweating, vertigo, excessive salivation, nausea, vomiting, abdominal cramping, diarrhea, bradycardia, hypotension, and fasciculations (involuntary muscle twitching).

Acetylcholinesterase Inhibitors

Acetylcholinesterase inhibitors (AChE inhibitors) are also called cholinesterase inhibitors (CHEI). Doses of AChE inhibitors must be individualized to the patient's needs. Patients should always receive the correct dose, at the correct time, to avoid myasthenia crisis and cholinergic crisis. Drug treatments for MG are individualized according to the needs of the client.

The first drug used to manage MG is neostigmine methylsulfate, a parasympathomimetic agent (AChE inhibitor). All other AChE drugs should be discontinued 8 hours before administration of neostigmine. Parenteral doses of neostigmine should be accompanied by intravenous (IV) atropine about 30 minutes before administering to counteract the adverse muscarinic effects of neotigmine (Table 21.1).

Pyridostigmine is a reversible AChE inhibitor, preventing the destruction of acetylcholine by cholinesterase and thereby allowing free transmission of nerve impulses across the neuromuscular junction. It has an intermediate action and is given in divided doses. Pyridostigmine is presented in Prototype Drug Chart: Pyridostigmine. Additional uses of pyridostigmine include reversal of neuromuscular blockers after surgery and the immediate threat of exposure to the nerve gas Soman by the US military (see Chapter 16).

The US Food and Drug Administration (FDA) recently approved a drug classified as a monoclonal antibody neonatal Fc receptor blocker for the treatment of generalized myasthenia gravis called Rozanolixizumab (see Table 21.1). It is for adult patients who are anti-acetylcholine receptor (AChR) or anti-muscle-specific tyrosine kinase (MuSK) antibody positive.

BOX 21.1 Medications That May Exacerbate Myasthenia Gravis

- Aminoglycoside antibiotics (gentamicin, neomycin, and tobramycin)
- Beta-blockers
- Botulinum toxin
- D-Penicillamine
- [a]Fluoroquinolone antibiotics (moxifloxacin to ciprofloxacin and levofloxacin)
- Chloroquine, hydroxychloroquine
- Immune inhibitors (pembrolizumab, nivolumab, atezolizumab, avelumab, durvalumab, and ipilimumab)
- Iodine radiologic contrast agents
- Macrolides (erythromycin, azithromycin, and clarithromycin)
- Magnesium
- Neuromuscular blocking agents (tubocurarine chloride, pancuronium, succinylcholine)
- Phenytoin
- Quinine, quinidine, procainamide
- Corticosteroids
- Statins (atorvastatin, pravastatin, rosuvastatin, simvastatin)
- Zithromax

[a]See https://myasthenia.org/Living-with-MG/MG-Emergency-Preparedness/Cautionary-Drugs

---

Monoclonal antibodies target the process by which acetylcholine antibodies injure the neuromuscular junction. Another classification of drugs used for MG is parenteral immunosuppressive agents and thiopurine analogs for patients who have MG that is poorly controlled with cholinesterase inhibitor therapy. Immunosuppressive agents improve muscle strength by suppressing the production of abnormal antibodies. They can cause significant side effects and must be carefully monitored by a physician. (See Table 21.1 for information on the drugs within these classifications.)

Pharmacokinetics

Pyridostigmine is poorly absorbed from the gastrointestinal (GI) tract. The half-life of oral pyridostigmine is 3 hours, and the half-life of IV administration is up to 1.5 hours. Because of its short half-life, pyridostigmine should be administered several times a day to avoid muscle weakness and prevent myasthenic crisis. The drug is metabolized by the liver and is excreted in the urine.

Pharmacodynamics

Pyridostigmine increases muscle strength in patients with muscular weakness resulting from MG. Pyridostigmine works to promote transmission of neuromuscular impulses across the myoneural junctions by preventing destruction of ACh. Failure of patients to show clinical improvement may reflect underdosing or overdosing. Overdosing of pyridostigmine can result in cholinergic crisis. This crisis requires emergency medical intervention because of respiratory muscle weakness that can result in respiratory distress. Atropine sulfate injection is the antidote for pyridostigmine overdose to counter the muscarinic effects of ACh. Patients who do not respond to AChE inhibitors may require additional drug treatment such as prednisone, plasma exchange, IV immune globulin, or immunosuppressive drugs.

Prednisone is the drug of choice, but like other immunosuppressants, it reduces the presence of antibodies. Corticosteroids do not produce permanent remission, and the long-term side effects are significant. The immunosuppressive agent azathioprine can be used in conjunction with a lower dose of prednisone. With azathioprine, the complete blood count, including the platelet count, is monitored

TABLE 21.1 Medications for Myasthenia Gravis

Drug	Route and Dosage	Uses and Considerations
Acetylcholinesterase Inhibitors		
Neostigmine methylsulfate	Neostigmine bromide A: PO: 15 mg 3 times daily. Increase at 1 d or more intervals. Maintenance dose: 15 mg–3759 mg/d in divided doses; *max*/PO: 375 mg/d A: IM: SC: 0.5 mg; *max*: 0.07 mg/kg Diagnosing MG: IM: 1.5 mg (0.022 mg/kg) single dose (if cholinergic reaction occurs, discontinue test and administer additional IV atropine) Neuromuscular blockade reversal: A: IV: 0.5–2 mg slow IV injection. Repeat as required; *max*: 5 mg total dose	Used for treatment of myasthenia gravis (MG) and for neuromuscular blockade reversal and the diagnosis of MG. May cause dizziness, headache, nausea, vomiting, bradycardia, hypotension, tachycardia, muscle cramps, seizures, dyspnea, miosis, visual impairment, urinary retention, and digestive and GI adverse events. PB: 15%–25%; t½: IM: 51–90 min; t½: IV: 24–113 min ⚡ Safety Alert: Do not use it in older adults due to drug-disease or drug-syndrome interactions that may exacerbate the disease and cause bradycardia and syncope. Only trained clinicians should administer. Always have atropine and drugs to treat anaphylaxis available. Large doses IV should be administered with Atropine to counteract muscarinic effects.
Pyridostigmine		See Prototype Drug Chart: Pyridostigmine
Monoclonal Antibody Neonatal Fc Receptor Blocker		
Rozanolixizumab	Weighing 100 kg and above A: SQ Infusion: 840 mg once wkly for 6 wks. Use infusion pump 20 mL/h. Max dose: 840 mg once weekly for 6 wks Weighing 50 kg to less than 100 kg A: SQ infusion: 560 mg once wkly for 6 wks. Use infusion pump 20 mL/h. Max dose: 560 mg once weekly for 6 wks Weighing less than 50 kg A: SQ infusion: 420 mg once wkly for 6 wks. Use infusion pump 20 mL/h. Max dose: 420 mg once weekly for 6 wks	Used for the treatment of generalized gMG in adults who are AChR or MuSK antibody positive. May cause headache, diarrhea, fever, infection, nausea, photophobia, and severe angioedema and aseptic meningitis.
Immunosuppressant		
Azathioprine	A: PO: 50 mg daily × 1 wk; *gradually increase* to 2–3 mg/kg/d; *max*: 250 mg/d *Dosage is based on total body weight.*	Used for MG poorly controlled with AChE inhibitors. May cause infection, leukopenia, nausea, and vomiting. CBC and platelet required: weekly for the first month; twice monthly for 2–3 months; thereafter, monthly Onset: 6–8 wks (slow) Duration: UK PB: 30%; t½: UK ❗ **Black-Box Warning:** Risk for new primary malignancy ⚡ Safety Alert: Extreme risk of harm if used in error

A, Adult; *AChE*, acetylcholinesterase; *AChR*, anti-acetylcholine receptor; *CBC*, complete blood count; *d*, day; *GI*, gastrointestinal; *gMG*, generalized myasthenia gravis; *h*, hour; *IM*, intramuscular; *IV*, intravenous; *kg*, kilogram; *max*, maximum dosage; *MG*, myasthenia gravis; *min*, minutes; *MuSK*, anti-muscle-specific tyrosine kinase antibody positive; *PB*, protein binding; *PO*, by mouth; *q*, every; *s*, second; *SC*, subcutaneous; *t½*, half-life; *UK*, unknown; *wk*, weeks.

weekly during the first week of treatment, twice monthly for the second and third months, and monthly, including serum amylase, thereafter. These tests will monitor for leukopenia and hepatotoxicity.

Overdosing and underdosing of AChE inhibitors have similar symptoms: generalized muscle weakness, which can include the muscles of respiration, the diaphragm, and the intercostal muscles, resulting in dyspnea (difficulty breathing) and dysphagia. Additional symptoms that may be present with overdosing are increased salivation (drooling), sweating, and bronchial secretions, along with miosis, bradycardia, and abdominal pain. Underdosing can result in myasthenia crisis, and overdosing can result in cholinergic crisis. All doses of AChE inhibitors should be administered on time because late administration of the drug may result in muscle weakness.

Side Effects and Adverse Reactions

Side effects and adverse reactions of AChE inhibitors include GI disturbances (nausea, vomiting, diarrhea, abdominal cramps), increased salivation and tearing, miosis (constricted pupil of the eye), blurred vision, and

CHAPTER 21 Drugs for Neuromuscular Disorders and Muscle Spasms

PROTOTYPE DRUG CHART

Pyridostigmine

Drug Class	Dosage
Acetylcholinesterase (AChE) inhibitors	Myasthenia gravis: RR: A: PO: 600 mg/d in divided doses; Syrup: 60 mg/5 mL in divided doses; average dose is 600 mg/d; *max:* RR: PO 1500 mg 1 or 2 daily in divided doses ER: A: PO: 180–540 mg/d bid with at least 6 h between doses. Note: *ER is equal to that of a 60-mg regular-release tablet; however, its duration of effectiveness, although varying in individual patients, averages 2.5 times that of a 60-mg dose; max: ER: PO: 180 mg/d.* ER:A: IV: 1–2 mg/h (gradually titrate up in increments of 0.5–1 mg/h up to a max rate of 4 mg/h) One-thirtieth of the usual oral dose IV or IM dose.
Contraindications	**Drug Interactions**
GI and GU obstructions, ileus, bladder obstruction *Caution:* Asthma, bradycardia, peptic ulcer, cardiac arrhythmias, renal impairment, pregnancy, breastfeeding, COPD, hypertension	Corticosteroids, neuromuscular blockers, aminoglycosides, local anesthetics, magnesium salts; increased toxicity with acetylcholinesterase inhibitors, atropine, tetracyclines, polymyxin B, bacitracin, digoxin, quinidine; atropine decreases the effect of pyridostigmine, tricyclic antidepressants; Atropine sulfate injection is an antidote for pyridostigmine.
Pharmacokinetics	**Pharmacodynamics**
Absorption: PO: Poorly absorbed ER: 50% absorbed	PO: RR: Onset: 30–45 min PO: ER: Onset: 0.5–1 h IM: Onset: 15 min IV: Onset: Within minutes PB: UK; t½: Oral 3 h; IV up to 1.5 h
Therapeutic Effects/Uses	
Used to control and treat myasthenia gravis, for neuromuscular blockade reversal, and for nerve gas (Soman) exposure prophylaxis Mechanism of Action: Promotes transmission of neuromuscular impulses across the myoneural junctions by preventing destruction of acetylcholine	
Side Effects	**Adverse Reactions**
Abdominal pain, confusion, depression, diarrhea, blurred vision, hyperesthesia, fecal and urinary incontinence, seizures	Bradycardia, cardiac dysrhythmias, COPD, hypertension, and seizures

A, Adult; *bid*, twice a day; *C*, child; *COPD*, chronic obstructive pulmonary disease; *d*, day; *ER*, extended release; *GI*, gastrointestinal; *GU*, genitourinary; *h*, hour; *IM*, intramuscular; *IV*, intravenous; *max*, maximum; *mg*, milligram; *min*, minute; *mL*, milliliter; *PB*, protein binding; *PO*, by mouth; *q*, every; *RR*, regular release; *t½*, half-life; *UK*, unknown.

CLINICAL JUDGMENT [NURSING PROCESS]
Drug Treatment for Myasthenia Gravis: Pyridostigmine

Concept: Sensory Perception
- Sensory perception involves interpreting one's surroundings. A good sensory perception depends on normal sensory receptors, an intact reticular activating system, and a functioning nervous system. The nurse is responsible for thorough assessment of the patient to ensure a functioning sensory perception of their environment. The nurse is also responsible for implementing patient care or altering the patient's plan of care when malfunction is present.

Recognize Cues [Assessment]
- Obtain a drug history from the patient, which includes all current medications.
- Observe the patient's drug profile for possible drug interactions.
- Record baseline vital signs.
- Assess the patient's current laboratory results.
- Assess the patient for signs and symptoms of overdosing/underdosing, such as muscle weakness and difficulty breathing and swallowing.
- Instruct the patient in signs and symptoms to report to health care provider (HCP).

Analyze Cues and Prioritize Hypothesis [Patient Problems]
- Decreased gas exchange
- Acute respiratory distress
- Decreased functional ability
- Decreased mobility
- Decreased visual acuity
- Decreased ability to cope
- Need for patient teaching

Generate Solutions [Planning]
- Patient's muscle weakness will see improvements with timely administration of pyridostigmine in evenly divided doses as ordered by HCP.
- Patient will identify factors that increase potential for injury.
- Patient will optimize activities of daily living within sensorimotor limitations.

Take Action [Nursing Interventions]
- Monitor the effectiveness of drug therapy (AChE inhibitors). Muscle strength should be increased. Both depth and rate of respirations should be assessed and maintained within normal range.

Continued

CLINICAL JUDGMENT [NURSING PROCESS]—CONT'D
Drug Treatment for Myasthenia Gravis: Pyridostigmine

- Administer the prescribed AChE inhibitor after dosage recommendations and nursing guidelines.
- Observe the patient for signs and symptoms of cholinergic crisis and myasthenia crisis. In cholinergic crisis the client will experience severe muscle weakness leading to respiratory failure and arrest. In myasthenic crisis the client can experience severe to generalized muscle weakness involving the muscles of respiration, such as the diaphragm and intercostal muscles.
- Involve family members in teaching about prescriptive therapies and disease processes using simple and clear instructions.
- Communicate respect for the patient's cultural beliefs.
- Assess the patient's understanding of adherence to the drug regimen.
- Instruct the patient to notify the HCP before taking any medications other than what the HCP has ordered.
- Stress that medications need to be taken as prescribed.

Patient Teaching
- Teach patients to take drugs as ordered to avoid recurrence of symptoms.
- Encourage patients to wear a medical identification bracelet or necklace that indicates health problems.

Safety
- Instruct the patient and family in factors that may contribute to injury.

Side Effects
- Teach patients about the side effects of medication and when to notify the HCP.
- Advise patients to report recurrence of symptoms of myasthenia gravis to the HCP.

Diet
- Inform patients to take the drug before meals for best absorption. If gastric irritation occurs, take the drug with food.

Evaluate Outcomes [Evaluation]
- Evaluate the effectiveness of drug therapy to maintain muscle strength.
- Determine the absence of respiratory distress.
- Evaluate the correct use of the drug by the patient.
- Evaluate the patient's feelings of safety, comfort, and security.

---

bradycardia. Pyridostigmine is used to control the symptoms of MG. It is important to ensure the client is familiar with the drug. The client must take the drug to control the signs and symptoms of MG. Encourage the client to maintain therapeutic blood levels and see their physician regularly to prevent weakness, because weakness can impair the client's ability to breathe and swallow. Suggest for the client to wear a Medic Alert bracelet. Inform the client about the services available from the Myasthenia Gravis Foundation. (See Clinical Judgment for Pyridostigmine.)

MULTIPLE SCLEROSIS

Multiple sclerosis (MS) is a neuromuscular autoimmune disorder that attacks the myelin sheath of nerve fibers in the brain and spinal cord, causing lesions known as *plaques*. Although there are no definitive diagnostic tests, the sclerotic plaques are usually detected and measured by magnetic resonance imaging (MRI). Pharmacologic treatment is necessary to control the symptoms of this disorder.

In lesions called *plaques*. In the United States, MS affects approximately 1 million people. Most people with MS are diagnosed between 20 and 50 years of age, with at least two to three times more females than males being diagnosed with the disease. Although the cause of MS is unknown, it is thought that the disease develops in a genetically susceptible person because of environmental exposure, like an infection. The onset of MS is usually slow. It is a condition in which there are remissions and exacerbations of multiple symptoms. Common manifestations of MS are motor, sensory, neurologic, cerebellar, and emotional problems. Motor symptoms include weakness or paralysis of the limbs, muscle spasticity, and diplopia. Patients with MS experience sensory abnormalities, including numbness, tingling, blurred vision, vertigo, and tinnitus. Patients may experience neuropathic pain, particularly in the low thoracic and abdominal areas. Cerebellar signs include nystagmus, ataxia, dysarthria, and dysphagia. Many patients experience severe fatigue. If the sclerotic plaque is in the central nervous system (CNS), problems with bowel and bladder function, sexual function, and cognitive dysfunction can occur.

MS is difficult to diagnose. Most physicians use at least one other test besides the medical history and neurologic examination, such as MRI, evoked potential (EP) testing (a test that measures the electrical activity of the brain), or analysis of cerebrospinal fluid (CSF), to confirm the diagnosis (see http://www.nationalmssociety.org).

Classifications of Multiple Sclerosis

MS is classified into four primary patterns for treatment purposes:

- *Relapsing-remitting MS (RRMS):* This is the most common pattern. The patient experiences a sudden attack of symptoms and may recover completely until the next attack, or some residual deficits may remain permanently (affects 85%).
- *Primary progressive MS (PPMS):* Slowly worsening neurologic function is evident from the beginning with no relapses or remissions (affects 10%).
- *Secondary progressive MS (SPMS):* The initial course is relapsing-remitting, followed by progression with or without occasional relapses, minor remissions, and plateaus (about 50% of people with RRMS develop SPMS within 10 years).
- *Progressive relapsing MS (PRMS):* This form is progressive from the onset, with clear acute relapses with or without full recovery (affects 5%).
- *Clinically isolated syndrome (CIS):* This form occurs when a patient has only one flare-up of MS. CIS does not always develop into MS. The symptoms for CIS are the same as MS.

There is no known cure for MS.

Immunomodulators

Immunomodulators are disease-modifying drugs (DMDs), and they are the first line of treatment for patients with MS. DMDs modulate the course of MS as either an immunosuppressant or immunomodulator. Immunomodulators regulate or modulate the immune system activity. Immunosuppressants suppress the immune response. Immunomodulators regulate or modulate the immune system activity. Immunosuppressants suppress the immune response. DMDs can slow the progression of the disease and prevent relapses. Immunomodulators include interferon beta-1a, interferon beta-1b, and peginterferon beta-1a, which are popular drugs in the treatment of MS (Prototype Drug Chart: Beta-Interferon). Both interferon beta-1a and interferon beta-1b have been declared orphan status by the FDA. Multiple sclerosis affects fewer than 200,000 people in the United States, and the drugs are not expected to recover costs of development and marketing expenses. The FDA has authority to grant orphan drug designation to a drug or biological product to prevent, diagnose, or treat a rare disease or condition. Orphan drug status qualifies sponsors for tax-saving incentives including potential 7 years of market exclusivity after approval

PROTOTYPE DRUG CHART

Beta-Interferon

Drug Class	Dosage

Immunomodulators:
   Interferon beta-1a
   Interferon beta-1b
   Peginterferon beta-1a
	Beta-1a: Treatment of Relapsing Form s MS, CIS, RRMS, and active SPMS
	A: IM: 7.5 mcg once wk, initially; increase by 7.5 mcg/wk up to target dose 30 mm cg/wk; *max:* A: IM 30 mcg/wk
	A: SC: 44 mcg 3× wk; give 48 h ap art for 2 wks, then 11 mcg 3× wk for 2 wks, then 22 mcg 3× wk; *max:* 44 mcg every 48 h.
	Beta-1b: Treatment of MS, CIS, RRMS, and active SPMS
	A: SC: 62.5 mcg every other day for 2 wks, then 125 mcg every other day for 2 wks, then 187.5 mcg every other day for 2 wks, then 250 mcg every other day. *Max:* A: SC: 250 mcg every other day.
	Peginterferon beta-1a: Treatment of relapsing forms of MS, including CIS, RRMS, and active SPMS
	A: SC: Initially 63 mcg once on day 1; then 94 mcg on day 15, then 125 mcg every 14 days; starting on day 29.
	A:IM: Initially 63 mcg once on day 1 then, 94 mcg on day 125 mcg every 14 days starting on day 29. *Max:* A: SC: IM: 125 mcg once every 14 days. Switching between SC and IM r outes of administration has not been studied for Peginterferon beta-1a.

Contraindications	**Drug Interactions**
Beta-1a: Albumin hypersensitivity, hamster protein hypersensitivity, alcoholism, autoimmune disease, bone marrow suppression, cardiac disease, children, dyspnea, orolingual edema, skin rash, urticaria, anaphylaxis. ***Beta-1b:*** Albumin hypersensitivity, bone marrow suppression, children, depression, *Escherichia coli* protein hypersensitivity, heart failure, hepatitis, seizures, thyroid disease. ***Peginterferon beta-1a:*** Hypersensitivity to beta-interferon, hepatitis, alcoholism, hepatic disease, autoimmune disease, cardiac disease, bone marrow suppression, preexisting seizure disorder, thrombocytopenic purpura, pulmonary hypertension.	***Interferon beta-1a and beta-1b:*** Antiretroviral NNRTIs; antiretroviral NRTIs; antiretroviral protease inhibitors; ethanol ***Peginterferon beta-1a:*** Abacavir, dolutegravir, lamivudine, zidovudine
Pharmacokinetics	**Pharmacodynamics**
Interferon beta-1a IM: Peak 15 h SQ: Peak 16 h ***Interferon beta-1b*** Peak Serum Concentration: 1–8 h ***Peginterferon beta-1a:*** Metabolism: Not extensively metabolized in the liver Peak: 1–5 d Excretion: Urine	***Interferon beta-1a:*** A: IM: t½: 19 h A: SQ: t½: 69 h ***Interferon beta-1b:*** A: SQ: t½: between 8 min and 4.3 h ***Peginterferon beta-1a:*** A: SQ: t½: 78 h

Therapeutic Effects/Uses

Interferon beta-1a is designated as an orphan drug by the FDA for treatment of MS.
Interferon beta-1b is designated as an orphan drug by the FDA for treatment of MS.
Peginterferon beta-1a is used with caution in patient's with preexisting hepatic disease.
Mechanism of Action: Interferon beta-1a, beta-1b, and Peginterferon beta-1a are available through recombinant DNA technology. Immune-regulatory properties are produced by interacting with specific receptor sites on cell surfaces. Beta-interferon suppresses the inflammatory response. It controls the secretions of proinflammatory and antiinflammatory cytokines suppressing T-cell activation.

Side Effects	Adverse Reactions
Depression, dizziness, fatigue, suicidal ideation, vision problems, dyspnea, chest pain, edema, abdominal pain, autoimmune hepatitis, cystitis, neutropenia, injection site reaction, myalgia, arthralgia, muscle spasm, anaphylaxis, flulike symptoms	Increased myelosuppression may occur with other myelosuppressives including antineoplastics; concurrent use of hepatotoxic agents may increase risk of hepatotoxicity. Avoid concomitant use with immunomodulating natural products such as astragalus, echinacea, and melatonin.

A, Adult; *CIS*, clinically isolated syndrome; *d*, day; *FDA*, Food and Drug Administration; *h*, hours; *IM*, intramuscular; *IU*, International Unit; *MS*, multiple sclerosis; *mcg*, microgram; *mg*, milligram; *NNRTI*, nonnucleoside reverse transcriptase inhibitor; *NRTI*, nucleoside reverse transcriptase inhibitor; *q*, every; *RRMS*, remitting-relapsing MS; *SC*, subcutaneous; *SPMS*, secondary progressive MS; *t½*, half- life; *UK*, unknown; *wk*, week.

(https://www.fda.gov/industry/medicalproducts-rare-diseases-and-conditions/designating-orphan-product-drugs-and-biological-products).

Glatiramer acetate is an antineoplastic immunomodulator prescribed for relapsing forms of MS. It is available in prefilled syringes, 20 or 40 mg/mL, and administered subcutaneously either once daily or three times a week depending on the health care provider's (HCP) orders. It has a favorable safety profile and must be used cautiously in patients with preexisting immunosuppression. Glatiramer modifies the human immune response. Glatiramer is designated as an orphan drug by the FDA. Teriflunomide is a pyrimidine synthesis inhibitor immunomodulator antineoplastic used for RRMS, including CIS and active SPMS. It is in oral form and is administered daily. Alemtuzumab, ocrelizumab, and natalizumab are monoclonal antibodies. Ocrelizumab is the first B-cell targeted drug to treat primary progressive MS in adults. Ublituximab is administered IV, and the monoclonal antibody binds to CD20 on the surface of the immune cells called B cells and depletes them from the circulation. It is approved for relapsing-remitting forms of MS. Monoclonal antibodies affect the actions of the body's immune system. They target and destroy certain cells while protecting the body's healthy cells from damage. Many have Black-Box Warnings along with Institute for Safe Medication Practices (ISMP) safety alerts and are generally reserved for patients who have had an inadequate response to two or more drugs indicated for the treatment of MS. Dimethyl fumarate is a selective immunosuppressant that can lower the patient's immunity, causing an increased risk of infection. It is a central nervous system MS agent that has both neuroprotective and antiinflammatory properties that can help delay disability and disease progression. Mitoxantrone is a potent immunosuppressant antineoplastic topoisomerase II inhibitor used to reduce the relapse rate in patients with clinically worsening forms of remitting and secondary progressive MS.

Siponimod is a sphingosine-1-phosphate receptor modulator approved by the FDA for the treatment of MS. Before starting treatment with siponimod, an antineoplastic immunomodulator, the patient must have CYP2C9 genotype testing. Ponesimod and ozanimod are sphingosine-1-phosphate receptor modulator approved by the FDA to treat relapsing forms of MS, which include CIS, RRMS, and active SPMS. Cladribine is a purine antimetabolite. Its drug mechanism of action has not been made clear but is thought to involve lymphocyte depletion through cytotoxic effects on B and T lymphocytes through impairment of the DNA synthesis. Cladribine is a synthetic purine nucleoside antimetabolite with Black-Box Warnings and ISMP high safety alert status.

No two cases of MS are alike, so the drugs are tailored to the disease pattern and manifestations of the patient. Table 21.2 lists medications used in the treatment of MS. Corticosteroids are used to manage

TABLE 21.2 Drugs for Multiple Sclerosis

Drugs	Route and Dosage	Uses and Considerations
Immunomodulators		

Beta-Interferon
  Interferon beta-1a
  Interferon beta-1b
  Peginterferon beta-1a
		See Prototype Drug Chart: Beta-Interferon for beta-1a and beta-1b and peginterferon beta-1a

Glatiramer acetate	A: SC: 20 mg/mL once daily Max dose: 20 mg/mL daily A: SC: 40 mg/mL 3 × wk (administer at least 48 h apart) Max dose: 40 mg/mL 3 × wk	Used for treatment of RRMS, CIS, and active SPMS. May cause chest pain, dyspnea, erythema, and peripheral vasodilation. Distribution: Enters lymphatic and systemic circulation and modifies the immune response Onset/Peak/Duration: UK PB: UK; t½: UK ⚡ Glatiramer 20 mg/mL and 40 mg/mL solutions for injection are NOT interchangeable.
Teriflunomide	A: PO: 7 mg or 14 mg once daily; max: 14 mg daily	Used for treatment of RRMS, CIS, and active SPMS. May cause alopecia, back pain, cystitis, elevated hepatic enzymes, hyperreflexia, hypophosphatemia, lymphopenia, and myasthenia Monitor: ALT and CBC at least monthly for 6 months Absorption: Well absorbed Distribution: UK PB: >99%; t½: 18–19 d. ❗ **Black-Box Warning:** Pregnancy, hepatotoxicity, and reproduction risk. ⚡ Safety Alert: High risk of client harm when administered in error.
Dimethyl fumarate	A: PO: 120 mg bid for 7 days, then, 240 mg bid. Max: 480 mg/d	Used for treatment of RRMS, including CIS and active SPMS. May cause leukopenia, nausea, erythema, progressive multifocal leukoencephalopathy, flushing, anaphylactoid reactions, angioedema, GI bleeding, obstruction and perforation, pancreatitis and peptic ulcer disease. Absorption: Converted to active metabolite (MMF) by enzymes in the GI tract, blood, and tissue. Distribution: UK PB: 27%–45%; t½: 1 h
Fingolimod	A: PO: 0.5 mg once daily for the capsule and orally disintegrating tablet. Max dose: A: PO: 0.5 mg/d	Used for treatment of RRMS, CIS, and active SPMS. May cause elevated hepatic enzymes, diarrhea, headache, infection, AV block, bradycardia, stroke, macular edema, seizure, skin cancer, and hepatic failure. Monitor: (initially and periodically) CBC, ECG, LFTs, ophthalmologic examination, serum bilirubin, and skin cancer screening examination; cardiac patients should be monitored overnight in the hospital for the first dose, with careful monitoring thereafter. Absorption: 93% after oral administration. Distribution: 86% of drug into RBCs. PB: >99.7%; t½: 6–9 d

TABLE 21.2 Drugs for Multiple Sclerosis—cont'd

Drugs	Route and Dosage	Uses and Considerations
Ozanimod	A: PO: Days 1–4: 0.23 mg/d; days 5–7: 0.46 mg/d; day 8 and after: 0.92 mg/d. If a dose is missed during the first 2 wks, reinitiate titration. Max dose: A: PO: 0.92 mg/d	Used for treatment of CIS, RRMS, and active SPMS. Multiple requirements prior to administration: CBC, lymphocyte count, ECG, assess patient's medical profile for drugs that could slow heart rate or AV conduction, test patient's exposure to chickenpox; ALT, AST, and total bilirubin labs; opthalmologic evaluation. May cause elevated hepatic enzymes, infection, cystitis, HTN, orthostatic hypotension, AV block, encephalopathy, MS exacerbation, visual impairment, new primary malignancy, hypertension, peripheral edema, and bradycardia. PB: approx 98.2%/99.8%/99.3%; $t\frac{1}{2}$: 21 h, 11 d (active metabolites) Metabolism: Liver Excretion: 37% feces, 26% urine
Ponesimod	A: PO: 14-d titration: days 1 and 2: 2 mg/d; days 3 and 4: 3 mg/d; days 5 and 6: 4 mg/d; day 7: 5 mg/d; day 8: 6 mg/d; day 9: 7 mg/d; day 10: 8 mg/d; day 11: 9 mg/d; days 12, 13, and 14: 10 mg/d; on day 15 and after that, the maintenance dose is 20 mg/d. Max: 20 mg/d	Used for the treatment of relapsing forms of MS, to include CIS, RRMS, and active SPMS. Before initiation of therapy: CBC, ALT, AST, and lymphocyte counts; ECG; under care of cardiologist; and ophthalmologic exam. May cause anemia, bleeding, dyspnea, edema, elevated hepatic enzymes, GI bleeding, neutropenia, hypocalcemia, and hyperglycemia. Requires first dose monitoring in patients with cardiac conditions. ⚡ PB: >99%; $t\frac{1}{2}$: ~33 h
Siponimod	*Oral dosage in client's with *1/*1, *1/*2, or *2/*2 CYP2C9 genotypes* A: PO: Titration regimen: 0.25 mg on days 1 and 2; 0.5 mg on day 3; 0.75 mg on day 4; 1.25 mg on day 5; begin maintenance dose of 2 mg once daily starting on day 6; max: 2 mg/d *Oral dosage in clients with *1/*3 or *2/*3 CYP2C9 genotypes* A: PO: Titration regimen: 0.25 mg on days 1 and 2; 0.5 mg on day 3; 0.75 mg on day 4, begin maintenance dose of 1 mg once daily on day 5. Max: 2 mg/d ⚡ First dose monitoring is recommended in clients with bradycardia, first or second-degree AV block, hx of MI or heart failure for both 2 and 1 mg dose. (Must be determined before use.)	Used for treatment of RRMS, CIS, and active SPMS. May cause increased risk of infections (CBC, liver function, and macular eye exam required before beginning treatment). Can cause: Headache, hypertension, macular edema, myocardial infarction, peripheral edema, lymphopenia, AV block, bradycardia, pulmonary embolism, seizure, and skin cancer. Excretion: Biliary/fecal Peak: ~4 h (range 3–8 h) $t\frac{1}{2}$: ~30 h PB: 99.9%
Alemtuzumab	Regimen consists of 2 treatment courses: A: IV: 12 mg daily for 5 consecutive days follow 12 months later with 12 mg IV for 3 consecutive days. Max: IV: 12 mg/dose This drug is reserved for those who have had an inadequate response to 1 or more drugs indicated for MS.	Used for the treatment of RRMS and active SPMS. A monoclonal antibody targeting the CD52 antigen inhibitor. May cause abdominal pain, anemia, antibody formation, arthralgia, candidiasis, chills, diarrhea, dyspnea, fever, hypotension, infection, infusion-related reactions, lymphopenia, neutropenia, sinus tachycardia, and thrombocytopenia; may increase risk of thyroid cancer, melanoma, hyperthyroidism, hypotension, and lymphoproliferative disease. Monitor: CBC diff; CD4 and T-cell count; serum creatinine, skin cancer screening examination, TFTs, urinalysis, ECG, Hepatits B serology, pregnancy testing Onset: UK Peak: UK PB: UK; $t\frac{1}{2}$: 2 wks ❗ **Black-Box Warning:** Autoimmune disease, infection, bone marrow suppression, infusion-related reactions, stroke, new primary malignancy (administration requires a specialized care setting) ⚡ Safety Alert: Hightened risk if administered in error.
Natalizumab	A: IV: 300 mg every 4 wks Max: IV: 300 mg every 4 wks	Used for treatment to reduce frequency of exacerbations of RRMS, CIS, active SPMS. May cause antibody formation, anaphylactic shock, arthralgia, depression, diarrhea, GI obstruction, infusion-related reactions, constipation, and elevated hepatic enzymes. Monitor: Anti-JCV antibodies, LFTs, serum bilirubin Distribution: UK PB: UK; $t\frac{1}{2}$: 11 ± 4 d ❗ **Black-Box Warning:** Increased risk for progressive multifocal leukoencephalopathy (consider benefits and risk prior to use). ⚡ Safety Alert: High risk to client if given in error.

Continued

TABLE 21.2 Drugs for Multiple Sclerosis—cont'd

Drugs	Route and Dosage	Uses and Considerations
Ocrelizumab	A: IV: 300 mg as a single infusion *followed by a second* 300 mg IV infusion 2 wks and later *Subsequent infusions of 600 mg IV are administered every 6 months after initial dose.* *Max:* 600 mg/dose IV ⚡ Administration is required by a qualified clinician able to manage severe infusion reactions.	Used for treatment of RRMS, CIS, active SPMS, and PPMS. An immunomodulator targeting CD20 antigen inhibitors. May cause infection (upper respiratory and infusion-related reactions), laryngeal edema, new primary malignancy, and sinus tachycardia, depression, peripheral edema, and anaphylactic reactions. Patients are premedicated with IV methylprednisolone 100 mg and PO diphenhydramine 30 min before starting infusion. Onset/Peak/Duration: UK Monitor: Hepatitis B serology, neurologic functions, IgG serum concentrations PB: UK; $t\frac{1}{2}$: 26 d
Ublituximab	A: IV: 150 mg infusion as a single dose, initially. A second 450 mg IV infusion is administered 2 wks later. Then, 450 mg IV at 24 wks after initial dose. *Max:* A: 450 mg/dose IV	Used for relapsing for ms of MS, including CIS, RRMS, and active SPMS. An immunomodulator targeting CD20 antigen inhibitor. May cause antibody formation, infection, infusion-related reactions, anaphylactoid reactions, erythema, hepatitis B exacerbation, progressive multifocal leukoencephalopathy, sinus tachycardia. $t\frac{1}{2}$: 22 days; PB: UK ❗. The drug must be administered under the close supervision of an experienced. Drugs Route and Dosage Uses and Considerations 32/54 clinician with access to appropriate medical support to manage severe reactions. Client is premedicated with corticosteroids and antihistamine prior to administration.
IMMUNOSUPPRESSANTS MitoXANTRONE	A: IV: 12 mg/m² IV every 3 months. *Max:* Cumulative lifetime dose is 140 mg/m² IV. ❗ **Black-Box Warning**: Bone marrow suppression, cardiac toxicity, risk of extravasation, subcutaneous administration, intramuscular administration/injections, and new primary malignancy. ⚡ Requires experienced clinician for administration. Not indicated for treatment of PPMS or for LVEF that is less than 50%. ⚡ Safety Concern: Heightened risk if administered in error	Used for the treatment of chronic SPMS, or progressive relapsing, worsening RRMS to reduce neurologic disability and/or frequencies of clinical relapses. A parenteral synthetic antineoplastic immunomodulating agent. May cause anemia, bleeding, constipation, dyspnea, edema, elevated hepatic enzymes, GI bleeding, hematuria, hyperglycemia, hypocalcemia, leukopenia, lymphopenia, neutropenia, stomatitis, and thrombocytopenia. PB: 78% $t\frac{1}{2}$: (terminal/median) 75 h
Cladribine	A: PO: (first cycle) 100 mg PO divided once daily for 4–5 days. (*Max:* 20 mg/d), followed by 100 mg (second cycle) divided once daily for 4–5 days (*Max:* 20 mg/day) starting 23–27 days after the last dose of first cycle. Repeat course once at least 43 weeks after the last dose of second cycle. *Max:* 1.75 mg/kg/course and 3.5 mg/kg. After two treatment courses, do not administer additional cladribine during the next 2 years due to increased risk of malignancy. The safety and efficacy of more courses of treatment with cladribine have not been studied.	Used for RRMS and active SPMS; recommended for patients who cannot tolerate other MS drugs, not recommended for CIS clients because of safety profile. May cause anemia, fatigue, fever, lymphopenia, neutropenia, and thrombocytopenia. ❗ **Black-Box Warning**: Contraindicated in pregnancy; may cause bone marrow suppression, nephrotoxicity, neurotoxicity, new primary malignancy, and reproductive risk. ⚡ **Safety and High Alert Drug:** Causing client harm when given in error and clinician must avoid contact of drug on skin when administering. Must be administered by a trained clinical professional. Monitor CBC/diff, hepatitis B serology, LFTs, pregnancy testing, serum creatinine/BUN, TB skin tet, and skin cancer screening exam. PB: 20% $t\frac{1}{2}$: 24 h.

A, Adult; *approx*, approximately; *AV*, atrioventricular; *AV block*, atrioventricular block; *bid*, twice daily; *BUN*, blood urea nitrogen; *d*, day; *CBC*, complete blood count; *CIS*, clinically isolated syndrome; *diff*, differential; *ECG*, electrocardiogram; *fnx*, function; *GI*, gastrointestinal; *h*, hour; *htn*, hypertension; *JCV*, John Cunningham virus (enzyme-linked immunosorbent assay test for immune compromised); *ISMP*, Institute for Safe Medication Practices; *IV*, intravenous; *LFT*, liver function test; *LVEF*, Left Ventricular Ejection Fraction; *MI*, myocardial infarction; *MMF*, metabolite monomethyl fumarate; *mo*, months; *MS*, multiple sclerosis; *PB*, protein binding; *PML*, progressive multifocal leukoencephalopathy; *PO*, by mouth; *PPMS*, primary progressive MS; *PRMS*, progressive relapsing MS; *RRMS*, relapsing-remitting MS; *SPMS*, secondary progressive MS; *q*, every; *RBC*, red blood cell; *SC*, subcutaneous; *TB*, tuberculosis; *TFT*, thyroid function test; $t\frac{1}{2}$, half-life; *UK*, unknown; *wk*, weeks.

exacerbations of MS. They work by reducing edema and acute inflammation at the site of demyelination.

The study of MS has seen many advances. New pharmacologic methods in medications and treatments are being researched. The study on how immune B cells can activate the advancement of MS led to the development of ocrelizumab. Studies to slow brain atrophy in progressive MS are underway. In addition, advancement in stem cell and genetic research are gaining success in the study of MS.

SKELETAL MUSCLE RELAXANTS

Muscle relaxants relieve muscular spasms and pain associated with traumatic injuries and spasticity from chronic debilitating disorders (e.g., MS, stroke [CVA], cerebral palsy, head and spinal cord injuries). Spasticity results from increased muscle tone from hyper excitable neurons; motor neurons transmit nerve signals from your spinal cord to your muscles. Spasticity is a result of demyelination that occurs in nerves that regulate muscle tone. When these nerve signals are disrupted, muscle weakening occurs. The centrally acting muscle relaxants depress neuron activity in the spinal cord or brain and enhance neuronal inhibition of the skeletal muscles.

Centrally Acting Muscle Relaxants

The mechanism of action of centrally acting muscle relaxants is not fully known. Centrally acting muscle relaxants are used in cases of spasticity to suppress hyperactive reflex and for muscle spasms that do not respond to antiinflammatory agents, physical therapy, or other forms of therapy. The centrally acting muscle relaxants are described in Table 21.3.

Prototype Drug Chart: Cyclobenzaprine explains the drug data for the centrally acting muscle relaxant cyclobenzaprine.

Spasticity

Skeletal muscle spasticity is muscular hyperactivity that causes contraction of the muscles, resulting in pain and limited mobility. Centrally acting muscle relaxants act on the spinal cord. Examples of centrally acting muscle relaxants used to treat spasticity are baclofen, and tizanidine. Diazepam, a benzodiazepine, has also been effective for treating spasticity. Dantrolene is a peripherally acting muscle relaxant which is used to treat spasticity.

COMPLEMENTARY AND ALTERNATIVE THERAPIES

Diazepam

Kava, valerian, and St. John's wort may potentiate central nervous system depression. (It is imperative to consult the health care provider before starting supplements.)

PROTOTYPE DRUG CHART

Cyclobenzaprine

Drug Class	Dosage
Centrally acting muscle relaxant	IR: A: PO 5 mg tid; if needed, may be increased to 7.5–10 mg tid; *max:* 30 mg/d ER: A: PO: cap: 15 mg/d, may be increased to 30 mg daily if required; *max:* 30 mg/d Treatment for both forms is not recommended beyond 3 wk.
Contraindications	**Drug-Lab-Food Interactions**
AV block, acute myocardial infarction, bundle branch block, cardiac arrhythmias, heart failure, hyperthyroidism, MAOI therapy, and QT prolongation, extended interval between the heart contracting and relaxing. *Caution:* Seizure disorder, alcohol, prostatic hypertrophy, urinary retention, hepatic disease, breastfeeding, driving or operating machinery, morbidity in older adults, sunlight UV exposure. ⚡ Not recommended for use in older adults.	Drug: Increased CNS depression with alcohol, kava (*Piper methysticum*), valerian, barbiturates, promethazine, TCAs, and other CNS depressants. ⚡ Check drug guide for multiple interactions. ⚡ Take with food or milk to decrease GI upset.
Pharmacokinetics	**Pharmacodynamics**
Absorption: PO: Well absorbed Metabolism: Liver Excretion: primary urine	PO: Onset: 1 h Peak: IR: ~4 h; ER 7–8 h Duration: 12–24 h Distribution: PB: 93%; t½: 8–37 h
Therapeutic Effects/Uses	
For short-term treatment of muscle spasms Mechanism of Action: Cyclobenzaprine relieves muscle spasms through a central action, possibly at the brain stem level, with no direct action on the neuromuscular junction or the muscle involved.	
Side Effects	**Adverse Reactions**
Anticholinergic effects: Blurred vision, constipation, dry mouth, urinary retention, confusion, drowsiness, nausea, nervousness, sinus tachycardia; palpitations.	Allergic reactions, angioedema, myocardial infarction, seizure, ileus, stroke.

A, Adult; *AV*, atrioventricular; *cap*, capsule; *CNS*, central nervous system; *d*, day; *ER*, extended release; *GI*, gastrointestinal; *h*, hour; *IR*, immediate release; *MAOI*, monoamine oxidase inhibitor; *mg*, milligram; *max*, maximum; *MI*, myocardial infarction; *PB*, protein binding; *PO*, by mouth; *SCI*, spinal cord injury; *t½*, half-life; *TCA*, tricyclic antidepressant; *tid*, three times a day; *UV*, ultraviolet; *wk*, week.

TABLE 21.3 Muscle Relaxants and Related Drugs

Drugs	Route and Dosage	Uses and Considerations
Anxiolytic/Muscle Relaxant		
Cyclobenzaprine	See Prototype Drug Chart: Cyclobenzaprine	
DiazePAM	A: PO: 2–10 mg bid/qid A: IV/IM: 5–10 mg, q3–4 h. *Max:* 40 mg/d PO in divided doses; IV: 0.2 mg/kg/dose.	Diazepam has many uses, one of which is to relieve muscle spasms and spasticity associated with MS and other motor neuron diseases. Diazepam is a long acting benzodiazepine. May cause sedation, memory impairment, urinary incontinence, ataxia, confusion, euphoria, hypotension, peripheral vasodilation, and urinary retention. Contraindicated in MG, glaucoma, respiratory insufficiency, and hepatic disease; not recommended for use in older adults, sleep apnea, abrupt discontinuation, coadministration with other CNS depressants, substance abuse. A: PB: 98%; t½: 1–3 h Metabolized: Liver Excreted: Urine ⚠ **Black-Box Warning:** Contraindicated in coadministration with other CNS depressants, substance abuse, and abrupt discontinuation. ⚡ Safety Alert Drug: Hightened risk if given in error; inappropriate drug in older adults.
Muscle Relaxants		
Centrally Acting Muscle Relaxants		
Baclofen	A: PO: Initially 5 mg tid; increase gradually by 5 mg dose every 3 d. *Max:* 80 mg/d divided over 4 doses. *Titrate off baclofen over 2–3 wks to avoid withdrawal side effects.*	For muscle spasms caused by MS and spinal cord injury. Most common side effects involve CNS (confusion, coma) and GI tract, constipation, depression, dyspnea, hypotension, and impotence. PB: 30%; t½: 2.5–5.7 h Metabolized: 15% liver Excreted: kidneys 70%–85% ⚠ **Black-Box Warning:** Abrupt discontinuation.
TiZANidine	A: PO: Starting dose is 2 mg, may be repeated q6–8 h *Gradually* increase the dose by 2–4 mg, with 1–4 d in between dose increases until satisfactory reduction in muscle tone is achieved. *Max:* 36 mg/d	Used to reduce muscle tone associated with spasticity related to cerebral or spinal cord injury, MS, or other spastic disorders. May cause bradycardia, cystitis, hypotension, dizziness, drowsiness, and fatigue; abrupt discontinuation is not recommended. ⚡ Use of drug is not recommended in older adults. PB: 30%; t½: 2 h Due to short duration should be reserved for activities when spasticity control is most important.
Carisoprodol	A: PO: 18–65 y 250–350 mg/tid and at bedtime. A: 66 y and older: Efficacy and safety not established. ⚡ *To reduce abuse potential, the duration of therapy should not exceed 2–3 doses/wk.*	Used for relaxation of acute, painful musculoskeletal conditions May cause drowsiness, xerostomia, dizziness, headache, and nausea Use with caution in older adults and in patients with hepatic dysfunction, seizures, and substance abuse. This drug has addictive properties and can increase CNS depression. PB: UK; t½: 2.4 h
Chlorzoxazone	A: PO: 250–500 mg tid/qid; *max:* 3000 mg/d ⚡ Use cautiously in older adults; not recommended in older adults.	Used as a centrally acting skeletal muscle-relaxing agent with sedative properties. May cause CNS depression, urine discoloration, dizziness, drowsiness, and malaise; has a sedative effect, anaphylactoid reactions, angioedema, GI bleed, hepatic failure, hepatic necrosis. PB: UK; t½: 1 h
Methocarbamol	A: PO: Initially 1500 mg qid for 48–72 h, then reduce dose to 1500 mg tid, 1000 mg qid, or 750 mg q4h. Up to 8 g/d can be used for severe conditions. *Max:* PO: 8 g/d A: IV: IM: 1 g single dose, may repeat every 8 h up to 3 g/d for 3 d. *Max:* IV: IM: 3 g/d for no more than 3 consecutive days.	Used for relief of acute musculoskeletal pain. May cause drowsiness, dizziness, angioedema, bradycardia, and anaphylactoid reactions, amnesia, blurred vision, confusion, hypotension, jaundice, and seizure. ⚡ Patients should not drive or operate machinery when taking this medication; not recommended for use in older adults. PB: 46%–50%; t½: 1–2 h

TABLE 21.3 Muscle Relaxants and Related Drugs—cont'd

Drugs	Route and Dosage	Uses and Considerations
Metaxalone	A: PO: 800 mg tid/qid; *max:* 3200 mg/d	Used for the treatment of acute and painful musculoskeletal pain. May cause anaphylactoid reactions, leukopenia, hemolytic anemia, serotonin syndrome, jaundice, dizziness, and drowsiness; ⚡ not recommended for use in older adults. PB: UK; t½: 9 ± 4.8 h
Orphenadrine	A: PO: 100 mg bid *Max:* 200 mg/d A: IM/IV: 60 mg q12h; *Max:* 120 mg/d	Used for adjunctive therapy for the relief of musculoskeletal pain. May cause anaphylactoid reactions, aplastic anemia, ocular hypertension, confusion, dizziness, and drowsiness, sinus tachycardia, and urinary retention. ⚡ *Contraindication:* MG and older adults. PB: UK; t½: 14 h
Peripherally Acting Muscle Relaxants		
Dantrolene	A: PO: Initially 25 mg/d; then 25 mg tid for 7 d, then 50 mg tid for 7 d, then 100 mg tid daily. May increase to 100 mg qid if needed. *Maint:* 400 mg daily	Used for chronic neurologic disorders that cause spasms, MS, SCI, stroke, and CP. May cause drowsiness, dysphagia, dysphonia, flushing, AV block, blurred vision, sinus tachycardia, anaphylactic shock and reactions, cirrhosis, GI bleed, heart failure, and headache. PB: UK; t½: 8.7 h ❗ **Black-Box Warning:** Hepatotoxicity ⚡ Use cautiously in older adults. Not indicated for skeletal muscle spasms due to rheumatic disorders. Discontinue if no benefits evident within 45 days.
Succinylcholine	*Muscle relaxation during nonemergent endotracheal intubation:* A: IV: 0.6 mg/kg; *max:* 1.5 mg/kg/dose A: IM: 3–4 mg/kg; *max:* 150 mg/dose *Neuromuscular blockade during surgery:* A: IV: 0.3–1.1 mg/kg once; followed by 0.04–0.07 mg/kg/dose as needed; adjust dose interval to patient's twitch response.	A parenteral, short-acting, depolarizing neuromuscular blocking agent used during surgical procedures for muscular relaxation and used to allow endotracheal intubation. May cause acute quadriplegic myopathy syndrome, anaphylactoid reactions, angioedema, apnea, arrhythmia, asystole, bradycardia, bronchospasm, and cardiac arrest. PB: UK; t½: UK Monitor: HR, BP, oxygen saturation, and ECG continuously. ❗ **Black-Box Warning:** Contraindicated in children, infants, and neonates, hyperkalemia, and rhabdomyolysis. ⚡ High-Alert Drug: Can cause significant client harm if used in error. Only experienced clinicians should administer. Pretreatment with atropine can reduce bradyarrhythmias.
Nondepolarizing Neuromuscular Blocking Agent		
Pancuronium	*Neuromuscular blockade during mechanical ventalation* A: IV: 0.05–0.1 mg/kg *Continuous IV infusion dosage* IV: A: 0.06–0.1 mg/kg titrate as needed. *Nonemergent endotracheal intubation:* A: IV: 0.06–0.1 mg/kg/dose *Neuromuscular blockade during surgery:* A: IV: 0.04–0.1 mg/kg	Used for long-acting neuromuscular blockade and paralysis in surgery as an adjunct to general anesthesia. May cause bronchospasm, hypotension, edema, acute quadriplegic myopathy, anaphylactic reactions, angioedema, apnea, bronchospasm, malignant hyperthermia, muscle paralysis, thrombosis, and erythema. PB: 87%; t½: 89–161 min ❗ **Black-Box Warning:** Requires experienced clinician to administer. ⚡ High-Alert Drug: Can cause significant harm if administered in error.
Vecuronium	*Nonemergent endotrachial intubation:* A: IV: 0.08–0.1 mg/kg/dose *Neuromuscular blockade during surgery:* A: IV: 0.08–0.1 mg/kg once, followed by 0.01–0.015 mg/kg/dose every 12–15 min as needed to maintain blockade	An intermediate-acting nondepolarizing agent used for maintenance of neuromuscular blockade and paralysis as an adjunct to general anesthesia after general anesthesia has been started. May cause bronchospasm, acute quadriplegic myopathy, anaphylactoid reactions, angioedema, apnea, malignant hyperthermia, muscle paralysis, thrombosis, erythema, hypotension, and sinus tachycardia. PB: 60%–80%; t½: 65–75 min ❗ **Black-Box Warning:** Must be administered by qualified clinician. ⚡ Safety Alert Drug: Will cause significant harm if administered in error.

A, Adult; *bid*, twice a day; *BP*, blood pressure; *cardio*, cardiovascular; *CNS*, central nervous system; *CP*, cerebral palsy; *CSS*, Controlled Substances Schedule; *d*, day; *ECG*, electrocardiogram; *g*, grams; *GI*, gastrointestinal; *h*, hour; *HR*, heart rate; *IM*, intramuscular; *IV*, intravenous; *maint*, maintenance; *max*, maximum; *MG*, myasthenia gravis; *min*, minutes; *mo*, months; *MS*, multiple sclerosis; *PB*, protein binding; *PO*, by mouth; *PRN*, as needed; *q*, every; *qid*, four times a day; *sec*, seconds; *SCI*, spinal cord injury; *t½*, half-life; *tid*, three times a day; *UK*, unknown; *wk*, weeks; *y*, year.

Muscle Spasms

Various centrally acting muscle relaxants are used for muscle spasm to decrease pain and increase range of motion. They have a sedative effect and should *not* be taken concurrently with CNS depressants such as barbiturates, narcotics, and alcohol. These agents, except for cyclobenzaprine, can cause drug dependence. Most muscle relaxants are not recommended for use in older adults. In addition, dizziness and drowsiness are common side effects. Examples of this group of centrally acting muscle relaxants are carisoprodol, chlorzoxazone, cyclobenzaprine, metaxalone, methocarbamol, and orphenadrine citrate.

Pharmacokinetics and Pharmacodynamics of Cyclobenzaprine

Cyclobenzaprine is well absorbed from the GI tract, and its half-life is moderate. Cyclobenzaprine is metabolized in the liver and excreted in urine.

Pharmacodynamics

Cyclobenzaprine alleviates muscle spasm associated with acute painful musculoskeletal conditions. When cyclobenzaprine is taken with alcohol, kava, valerian, sedative-hypnotics, barbiturates, or tricyclic antidepressants (TCAs), increased CNS depression can occur.

Side Effects and Adverse Reactions

The side effects from centrally acting muscle relaxants include drowsiness, dizziness, lightheadedness, headaches, and occasional GI sensitivity (e.g., nausea, vomiting, abdominal distress). Cyclobenzaprine and orphenadrine have anticholinergic effects.

COMPLEMENTARY AND ALTERNATIVE THERAPIES

Orphenadrine

> Valerian, St. John's wort, and kava may potentiate sedation. (It is imperative to consult health care provider before starting supplements.)

CLINICAL JUDGMENT [NURSING PROCESS]

Muscle Relaxant: Cyclobenzaprine

Concept: Cognition
- *Cognition* is the useful storing and managing of information to focus, acquire, and solve problems. Nurses care for patients who have problems with remembering, attention span, and recall of information. Patients on muscle relaxants may experience cognition problems.

Recognize Cues [Assessment]
- Obtain a medical history. ⚡ Cyclobenzaprine is contraindicated if the patient has cardiovascular disorders, hyperthyroidism, or hepatic impairment or is taking concurrent monoamine oxidase inhibitors (MAOIs).
- Obtain baseline vital signs.
- Assess the patient's health history to identify the cause of muscle spasm and determine whether it is acute or chronic.
- Observe the patient's drug history for possible drug interactions.
- Assess whether the patient has a history of narrow-angle glaucoma or myasthenia gravis (MG). Cyclobenzaprine and orphenadrine are contraindicated with these health problems.

Analyze Cues and Prioritize Hypothesis [Patient Problems]
- Decreased level of consciousness
- Confusion
- Decreased functional ability

Generate Solutions [Planning]
- The patient will take the muscle relaxants as prescribed by their health care provider (HCP).
- The patient will not drive while taking muscle relaxants.
- The patient will not make any major decisions while taking muscle relaxants.

Take Action [Nursing Interventions]
- Monitor serum liver enzyme levels of patients taking dantrolene and carisoprodol. Report to the HCP elevated levels of liver enzymes such as alkaline phosphatase (ALP), aspartate aminotransferase (AST), alanine aminotransferase (ALT), and gamma-glutamyl transferase (GGT).
- Record vital signs. Report abnormal results.
- Observe for central nervous system (CNS) side effects (e.g., dizziness, fatigue, and confusion).
- Instruct the patient and family members about the importance of taking prescribed medications as directed by the HCP.
- Provide for an interpreter if the patient has a language barrier.

Patient Teaching

General
- ⚡ Teach patients that the muscle relaxant should not be abruptly stopped. The drug should be tapered over 1 week to avoid rebound spasms.
- ⚡ Advise patients not to drive, operate dangerous machinery, or make important life-changing decisions when taking muscle relaxants. These drugs have a sedative effect and can cause drowsiness.
- Inform patients that most of the centrally acting muscle relaxants for acute spasms are usually taken for no longer than 3 weeks.
- ⚡ Teach patients to avoid alcohol and CNS depressants. If muscle relaxants are taken with these drugs, CNS depression may be intensified.
- Advise female patients these drugs must be used cautiously when pregnant or nursing.
- Patients should always check with the HCP before stopping medications.

Side Effects
- Encourage patients to report side effects of the muscle relaxant to their HCP. Common side effects are nausea, vomiting, dizziness, fainting, headache, and diplopia. Dizziness and fainting are most likely caused by orthostatic (postural) hypotension.

Diet
- Advise patients to take muscle relaxants with food to decrease gastrointestinal (GI) upset.

Evaluate Outcomes [Evaluation]
- Evaluate the effectiveness of the muscle relaxant, and determine whether the patient's muscular pain or spasms have decreased or disappeared.

CLINICAL JUDGMENT CASE STUDY

A 29-year-old female was diagnosed with myasthenia gravis (MG) 2 years ago. She is receiving pyridostigmine 120 mg three times a day. Last evening, the patient was involved in an automobile accident. She was taken to the emergency department unconscious and missed two evening doses of pyridostigmine.

1. How does pyridostigmine alleviate the symptoms of MG?
2. What are the potential side effects and adverse effects of pyridostigmine?
3. What problems are likely to develop after delayed pyridostigmine dosing?
4. What medication is the antidote for pyridostigmine overdose?
5. What problems may develop from pyridostigmine overdosing?
6. What are the similarities between myasthenic crisis and cholinergic crisis?

REVIEW QUESTIONS

1. What is the nurse's best explanation of the pathophysiology of myasthenia gravis?
   a. Degeneration of cholinergic neurons and a deficit in acetylcholine lead to neuritic plaques and neurofibrillary tangles.
   b. A decreased amount of acetylcholine to cholinergic receptors produces weak muscles and reduced nerve impulses.
   c. Myelin sheaths of nerve fibers in the brain and spinal cord develop lesions or plaques affecting the nervous system.
   d. An imbalance of dopamine and acetylcholine leads to degeneration of neurons in midbrain and extrapyramidal motor tracts.
2. The nurse is teaching a patient recently diagnosed with multiple sclerosis about the disease. Which statement is *not* correct concerning multiple sclerosis?
   a. The disease has periods of exacerbations followed by periods of remissions.
   b. Goals of treatment are to decrease the inflammation in the nervous system.
   c. Patients experience muscle weakness, fatigue, and vision and emotional problems.
   d. Multiple sclerosis is an autoimmune disorder that causes plaque to develop.
3. A patient with multiple sclerosis is having muscle spasticity. The nurse anticipates which drug will be prescribed to treat the patient's spasticity?
   a. Neostigmine
   b. Ropinirole
   c. Cyclobenzaprine
   d. Pyridostigmine
4. The nurse anticipates that the health care provider will prescribe which medication to treat a patient with relapsing-remitting multiple sclerosis?
   a. Ambenonium
   b. Pyridostigmine
   c. Mitoxantrone
   d. Glatiramer acetate
5. The nurse is providing medication instructions to a patient with acute muscle spasms who has been prescribed cyclobenzaprine. Which statement indicates to the nurse that the patient understands the instructions?
   a. I plan to take this medication with a glass of milk.
   b. Cyclobenzaprine should be taken once daily at bedtime.
   c. I will only drink one glass of wine a day before taking.
   d. I will be able to take this drug with grapefruit juice.
6. Which instructions will the nurse include in the teaching plan for a patient who is taking pyridostigmine? **Select all that apply.**
   a. Pyridostigmine must always be taken on time.
   b. Take the prescribed dose every other week.
   c. Underdosing can result in myasthenic crisis.
   d. Overdosing can result in cholinergic crisis.
   e. Report the adverse effect of tachycardia to the health care provider (HCP).
7. A patient is beginning to take cyclobenzaprine for treatment of acute back spasms. Which interventions will the nurse include in the care of this patient? **Select all that apply.**
   a. Advise the patient to always take this drug on an empty stomach.
   b. Inform the patient not to abruptly stop taking the muscle relaxant.
   c. Tell the patient to report dizziness and double vision to the health care provider (HCP).
   d. Advise the patient to avoid consuming alcohol beverages.
   e. Taking narcotics at the same time can cause serious side effects.
8. The patient was just prescribed cycobenzaprine for back spasms. The nurse is reviewing the patient's drug profile and plans to contact the HCP about which drug on the patient's daily profile?
   a. Atorvastatin
   b. Conjugated estrogen
   c. Valerian
   d. Penicillin G procaine
9. A patient taking cyclobenzaprine might experience which of the following anticholinergic side effects? **Select all that apply.**
   a. Blurred vision
   b. Dry mouth
   c. Salivation
   d. Constipation
   e. Urinary retention

UNIT VI Mental and Behavioral Health Drugs

22

Antipsychotics and Anxiolytics

http://evolve.elsevier.com/McCuistion/pharmacology

OBJECTIVES

- Explain the neurotransmitter action involved in psychopathology.
- Differentiate the use of traditional and atypical antipsychotics.
- Describe the advantages and disadvantages of atypical antipsychotics.
- Explain the different types of anxiolytics.

OUTLINE

Psychopathology, 259
    Neurotransmitters and Neurons, 259
    Psychosis, 260
Antipsychotics, 260
    Pharmacophysiologic Mechanisms of Action, 260
    Antipsychotic Categories, 260
    Phenothiazines, 261
    Nonphenothiazines, 263
    Atypical Antipsychotics, 264

Anxiety, 268
    Anxiety Disorders, 268
    Nonpharmacologic Measures, 268
Anxiolytics, 268
    Benzodiazepines, 268
    Miscellaneous Anxiolytics, 271
Clinical Judgment Single-Episode Case Study, 272
Review Questions, 273

Central nervous system (CNS) depressants used to manage symptoms of psychosis and anxiety disorders include antipsychotics and anxiolytics, which may cause psychosis. Antipsychotics are also known as neuroleptics or psychotropics, but the preferred name for this group is either antipsychotics or neuroleptics. The term *neuroleptic* refers to any drug that modifies psychotic behavior and exerts an antipsychotic effect. Anxiolytics are also called *antianxiety drugs* or *sedative-hypnotics*. Certain anxiolytics are used to treat sleep disorders, seizures, and withdrawal symptoms from alcohol or other abuse substances. Some of these drugs are also used for conscious sedation and anesthesia supplementation. However, the anxiolytics described in this chapter are used specifically to treat anxiety and psychotic behaviors.

PSYCHOPATHOLOGY

From moods and emotions flow the various thoughts and actions of individuals, which are communicated throughout the CNS by chemical neurotransmitters. An impulse is communicated by traveling through the presynaptic neuron across the synaptic cleft and binding to a receptor on the postsynaptic neuron, as illustrated in Fig. 22.1. Neurotransmitters are synthesized in the cytoplasm in the presynaptic neuron and are stored in vesicles, which safeguard neurotransmitters from being destroyed by enzymes. When an impulse arrives by way of an action potential at a presynaptic neuron, vesicles are triggered to move to the cell membrane wall and release the transmitter into the synaptic cleft.

Neurotransmitters function with the help of receptors, which are embedded in the membrane of the postsynaptic neuron. Receptors are configured in size and shape to interlock with specific transmitters. Immediately upon connection of neurotransmitters to receptors, an action is exerted and the transmitter is removed. Once released, transmitters can be broken down into inactive substances by enzymes, diffused away from the synapse into intracellular fluid, or returned to the presynaptic neuron in a process called *reuptake*.

Neurotransmitters and Neurons
Neurotransmitters
The major neurotransmitters that affect psychopathology include gamma-aminobutyric acid (GABA), serotonin, dopamine, norepinephrine, and acetylcholine. The GABA neurotransmitter is associated with the regulation of anxiety. When the level of GABA neurotransmitters is reduced, anxiety disorders may result. Benzodiazepines (antianxiety drugs) act by binding to a GABA receptor site, making the postsynaptic receptor more sensitive to GABA and its neurotransmission. This connection decreases the signs and symptoms of anxiety.

Fig. 22.1 Chemical neurotransmitters.

Faulty release, reuptake, or elimination of neurotransmitters may lead to an imbalance of neurotransmission and subsequent pathology. Disorders can then develop that can affect an individual's thoughts, feelings, and behaviors.

Neurons

Dopamine-containing neurons are thought to be involved in the regulation of cognition, emotional responses, and motivation. When dopamine levels are low, an individual can have decreased motivation and become less excited about situations. This predisposes one to schizophrenia, depression, and other psychoses.

Psychosis

Psychosis, or loss of contact with reality, is manifested in a variety of mental or psychiatric disorders. Psychosis is usually characterized by more than one symptom, such as difficulty in processing information, disorganized thoughts, distortion of reality, delusions, hallucinations, incoherence, catatonia, and aggressive or violent behavior. Schizophrenia, a chronic psychotic disorder, is the major category of psychosis in which many of these symptoms are manifested.

The symptoms of schizophrenia usually develop in adolescence or early adulthood and are divided into three groups: (1) cognitive symptoms, (2) positive symptoms, and (3) negative symptoms. *Cognitive symptoms* are characterized by disorganized thinking, memory difficulty, and decreased ability to focus attention. *Positive symptoms* may be characterized by exaggeration of normal function (e.g., agitation), incoherent speech, hallucinations, delusions, and paranoia. *Negative symptoms* are characterized by a decrease or loss in function and motivation. A poverty or simplicity of speech, blunted affect, inertia, poor self-care, and social withdrawal are apparent. Negative symptoms tend to be more chronic and persistent.

ANTIPSYCHOTICS

The typical, conventional, or traditional group of antipsychotics (first-generation antipsychotics) is more helpful for managing positive symptoms. A group of antipsychotics called *atypical* (second-generation antipsychotics) has been found to be the newest treatment for both positive and negative symptoms of schizophrenia.

Pharmacophysiologic Mechanisms of Action

Antipsychotics compose the largest group of drugs used to treat mental illness. Specifically, these drugs improve the thought processes and behavior of patients with psychotic symptoms by blocking dopamine receptors in the postsynaptic neurons, especially those with schizophrenia and other psychotic disorders. They are not used as a primary treatment for anxiety or depression. The theory is that psychotic symptoms result from an imbalance in the neurotransmitter dopamine in the brain. Sometimes these antipsychotics are called *dopamine antagonists*. There are five subtypes of dopamine receptors numbered D1 through D5. All antipsychotics block the D2 (dopaminergic) receptors in the brain and thus reduce psychotic symptoms. Many antipsychotics block the chemoreceptor trigger zone and vomiting (emetic) center in the brain, producing an antiemetic (prevents or relieves nausea and vomiting) effect. However, when dopamine is blocked, symptoms of extrapyramidal syndrome (EPS) or drug-induced pseudoparkinsonism (a chronic neurologic disorder that affects the extrapyramidal motor tract) such as tremors, masklike facies, rigidity, and shuffling gait may develop in varying degrees. Atypical antipsychotics have a weak affinity to D2 receptors and a stronger affinity to D4 receptors, and they block the serotonin receptor. These agents cause fewer EPS than the typical (phenothiazine) antipsychotic agents, which have a strong affinity to D2 receptors. Many patients who take high-potency antipsychotic drugs may require long-term medication for symptoms of parkinsonism.

Antipsychotic Categories

Antipsychotics are divided into two major categories: *typical* and *atypical*. The typical antipsychotics, introduced in 1952, are subdivided into phenothiazines and nonphenothiazines. *Nonphenothiazines* include butyrophenones, dibenzoxazepines, dihydroindolones, and thioxanthenes. The butyrophenones block only the neurotransmitter dopamine. The *phenothiazines* and the thioxanthenes block norepinephrine, causing sedative and hypotensive effects early in treatment.

Atypical antipsychotics make up the second category of antipsychotics. Clozapine, discovered in the 1960s and made available in Europe in 1971, was the first atypical antipsychotic agent. It was not marketed in the United States until 1990 because of adverse hematologic reactions. Atypical antipsychotics are effective for treating schizophrenia and other psychotic disorders in patients who do not respond to or are intolerant of typical antipsychotics. Because of their decreased side effects, atypical antipsychotics are often used instead of traditional typical antipsychotics as first-line therapy.

Adverse Reactions

Pseudoparkinsonism, which resembles symptoms of parkinsonism, is a major side effect of typical antipsychotic drugs. Symptoms of pseudoparkinsonism or EPS include stooped posture, masklike facies, rigidity, tremors at rest, shuffling gait, pill-rolling motions of the hands, and bradykinesia. When patients take high-potency typical antipsychotic drugs for extended periods, EPS is more pronounced. Patients who take low-strength antipsychotics such as chlorpromazine are not as likely to have symptoms of pseudoparkinsonism as those who take fluphenazine.

During early treatment with typical antipsychotic agents for schizophrenia and other psychotic disorders, two adverse extrapyramidal reactions that may occur are acute dystonia and akathisia. Tardive dyskinesia is a later phase of extrapyramidal reaction to antipsychotics. The use of anticholinergic drugs helps decrease pseudoparkinsonism symptoms, acute dystonia, and akathisia but has little effect on alleviating tardive dyskinesia. Complementary and Alternative Therapies: Antipsychotic Agents details interactions with antipsychotic agents.

CHAPTER 22 Antipsychotics and Anxiolytics

COMPLEMENTARY AND ALTERNATIVE THERAPIES

Antipsychotic Agents

- Kava kava may increase the risk and severity of dystonic reactions when taken with phenothiazines.
- Kava kava may increase the risk and severity of dystonia when taken concurrently with fluphenazine.
- Ginkgo may potentiate drug effects in patients with schizophrenia who are taking antipsychotics such as haloperidol, olanzapine, and clozapine.
- St. Johns wort may decrease drug levels of clozapine.

The symptoms of acute dystonia usually occur in 5% of patients within days of taking typical antipsychotics. Characteristics of the reaction include muscle spasms of the face, tongue, neck, and back; facial grimacing; abnormal or involuntary upward eye movement; and laryngeal spasms that can impair respiration. This condition is treated with an anticholinergic antiparkinson drug such as benztropine. The benzodiazepine lorazepam may also be prescribed.

Akathisia occurs in approximately 20% of patients who take a typical antipsychotic drug. With this reaction, the patient has trouble standing still, is restless, paces the floor, and is in constant motion (e.g., rocks back and forth). Akathisia is best treated with a benzodiazepine such as lorazepam or a beta-blocker such as propranolol.

Tardive dyskinesia is a serious adverse reaction that occurs in approximately 20% to 30% of patients who have taken a typical antipsychotic drug for more than 1 year. The prevalence is higher in cigarette smokers. The likelihood of developing tardive dyskinesia depends on the dose and duration of the antipsychotic factor. Characteristics of tardive dyskinesia include protrusion and rolling of the tongue, sucking and smacking movements of the lips, chewing motion, and involuntary movement of the body and extremities. In older adults, these reactions are more frequent and severe. The antipsychotic drug should be stopped in all who experience tardive dyskinesia, and another antipsychotic agent should be substituted. Benzodiazepines, calcium channel blockers, and beta blockers are sometimes helpful in decreasing tardive dyskinesia, although no one agent is effective for all patients. High doses of vitamin E may be helpful, and its use to treat tardive dyskinesia is currently under investigation. Clozapine has also been effective for treating tardive dyskinesia. Tetrabenazine, used to improve symptoms of Huntington disease, seems to be effective in treating tardive dyskinesia. Tetrabenazine reduces dopamine, norepinephrine, and serotonin levels. Amantadine has also been helpful in reducing drug-induced involuntary movements. Fig. 22.2 shows the characteristics of pseudoparkinsonism, acute dystonia, akathisia, and tardive dyskinesia.

Neuroleptic malignant syndrome (NMS) is a rare but potentially fatal adverse reaction associated with antipsychotic drugs. Predisposing factors include excess agitation, exhaustion, and dehydration. NMS symptoms involve muscle rigidity, hyperthermia, altered mental status, profuse diaphoresis, blood pressure fluctuations, tachycardia, dysrhythmias, seizures, rhabdomyolysis, acute renal failure, respiratory failure, and coma. Treatment of NMS involves immediate withdrawal of antipsychotics, adequate hydration, hypothermic blankets, and administration of antipyretics, benzodiazepines, and muscle relaxants such as dantrolene.

Phenothiazines

Chlorpromazine hydrochloride was the first phenothiazine introduced for treating psychotic behavior in patients in psychiatric hospitals. The phenothiazines are subdivided into three groups: aliphatic, piperazine, and piperidine, which differ mostly in their side effects.

The *aliphatic phenothiazines* produce a strong sedative effect and decreased blood pressure and may cause moderate EPS (pseudoparkinsonism). Chlorpromazine hydrochloride is in the aliphatic group and may produce pronounced orthostatic hypotension, low blood pressure that occurs when an individual assumes an upright position from a supine position.

The *piperazine phenothiazines* produce more EPS than other phenothiazines. They also cause dry mouth, blurred vision, weight gain, and

Fig. 22.2 Characteristics of pseudoparkinsonism, acute dystonia, akathisia, and tardive dyskinesia.

TABLE 22.1 Effects of Phenothiazines (Varies Within Class)

Group	Sedation	Hypotension	EPS	Antiemetic
Aliphatic	+++	+++	++	++
Chlorpromazine and triflupromazine				+++
Piperazine	++	+	+++	+++
Piperidine	+++	+++	+	–
Nonphenothiazines				
Haloperidol	+	+	+++	+++
Loxapine	++	++	+++	–
Molindone	+/++	+	+++	–
Thiothixene	+	+	+++	–
Atypical Antipsychotics				
Risperidone	+	+	+/0	–

–, No effect; +, mild effect; ++, moderate effect; +++, severe effect; *EPS*, symptoms of extrapyramidal syndrome.

agranulocytosis. Examples of piperazine phenothiazines are fluphenazine and perphenazine.

The *piperidine phenothiazines* have a strong sedative effect, cause few EPS, have a low to moderate effect on blood pressure, and have no antiemetic effect. Thioridazine is an example of piperidine phenothiazines. Table 22.1 summarizes the effects of the phenothiazines.

Most antipsychotics can be given orally (tablet or liquid), intramuscularly (IM), or intravenously (IV). For oral use, the liquid form might be preferred because some patients may hide tablets in their cheek or under their tongue to avoid taking them. Mouth checks are necessary for noncompliant patients. In addition, the absorption rate is faster with the liquid form, and a peak serum drug level occurs in 2 to 3 hours. The antipsychotics are highly protein bound (>90%), and excretion of the drugs and their metabolites is slow. Phenothiazines are metabolized by liver enzymes into phenothiazine metabolites. Metabolites can be detected in the urine several months after the medication has been discontinued. Phenothiazine metabolites may cause a harmless pinkish to red-brown urine color. The *full* therapeutic effects of oral antipsychotics may not be evident for 3 to 6 weeks after initiation of therapy, but an observable therapeutic response may be apparent after 7 to 10 days.

Noncompliance with antipsychotics is common. Medication teaching in the following areas is of utmost importance: (1) encourage the patient to take the medication as prescribed, (2) explain and emphasize

PROTOTYPE DRUG CHART
Fluphenazine

Drug Class
Antipsychotic: Neuroleptic piperazine phenothiazine

Dosage
Schizophrenia:
A: PO: Initially 2.5–10 mg/d in 2–3 divided doses, increase gradually; *max:* 20 mg/d
Older A: PO: 1–2.5 mg/d in 2–3 divided doses; *max:* 20 mg/d
A: IM/subcut: 12.5–25 mg single dose; *max:* 10 mg/d IM of immediate-release injection, 100 mg/dose IM/subcut of decanoate depot injection

Contraindications
Hypersensitivity, CNS depression, coma, children
Caution: Dysrhythmias, GI obstruction, ileus, cardiovascular disease, bradycardia, orthostatic hypotension, urinary retention, BPH, blood dyscrasias, infection, hepatic and renal damage, glaucoma, parkinsonism, seizure disorder, older adults, suicidal ideation, tardive dyskinesia, chemotherapy, hyperthermia, dehydration, electrolyte imbalances, alcohol use disorder, tobacco smoking

Drug-Lab-Food Interactions
Drug: Increased depressive effects when taken with alcohol or other CNS depressants; lithium, and beta blockers increase effects; antacids and antiparkinson drugs decrease effects
Complementary and alternative therapies: Kava kava may increase dystonia

Pharmacokinetics
Absorption: Rapidly absorbed
Distribution: PB 99%
Metabolism: t½:
4.4–16.4 h for PO, 6–9 d for IM single dose, and 14–26 d for multiple doses
Excretion: In urine

Pharmacodynamics
PO: Onset: UK
Peak: 2.8 h
Duration: UK
IM decanoate: Onset: 24 h
Peak: 48–96 h
Duration: 4–6 wk

Therapeutic Effects/Uses
To manage symptoms of psychosis including schizophrenia
Mechanism of Action: Blocks dopamine receptors in the brain to control psychotic symptoms

Side Effects
Drowsiness, dizziness, headache, dry mouth, blurred vision, photosensitivity, akathisia, hyperhidrosis, impaired body temperature regulation, weight gain, constipation, erectile/ejaculatory dysfunction, urinary retention, peripheral edema, skin hyperpigmentation

Adverse Reactions
Hyper/hypotension, tachycardia, ileus, EPS, seizures, psychosis, hyper/hypoglycemia, hyponatremia, cerebral edema
Life threatening: Dysrhythmias, aplastic anemia, agranulocytosis, hemolytic anemia, leukopenia, eosinophilia, neutropenia, thrombocytopenia, angioedema, bronchospasm, NMS

A, Adult; *BPH*, benign prostatic hyperplasia; *CNS*, central nervous system; *d*, day; *EPS*, symptoms of extrapyramidal syndrome; *GI*, gastrointestinal; *h*, hours; *IM*, intramuscular; *max*, maximum; *NMS*, neuroleptic malignant syndrome; *PB*, protein binding; *PO*, by mouth; *q*, every; *subcut*, subcutaneous; *t½*, half-life; *UK*, unknown; *wk*, weeks.

> **BOX 22.1 Symptoms and Suggested Treatment for Overdose of Phenothiazines**
>
> **Symptoms**
> - Unable to arouse; blood pressure fluctuations; tachycardia; agitation; delirium; convulsions; dysrhythmias; neuroleptic malignant syndrome; extrapyramidal symptoms; and renal, cardiac, and respiratory failure
>
> **Treatment**
> - Maintain airway, gastric lavage, activated charcoal administration, adequate hydration, anticholinergics, and norepinephrine

essential information to compensate for the patient's knowledge deficit, and (3) provide an interpreter for patients whose first language is not English.

Prototype Drug Chart: Fluphenazine shows the drug characteristics of fluphenazine, a phenothiazine antipsychotic used to manage psychosis. Box 22.1 shows the symptoms and suggested treatment for overdose of phenothiazines.

Pharmacokinetics

Oral absorption of fluphenazine is rapid and unaffected by food. This drug is strongly protein bound and has a long half-life; therefore, the drug may accumulate in the body. Fluphenazine is metabolized by the liver, crosses the blood-brain barrier and placenta, and is excreted as metabolites primarily in the urine. With hepatic dysfunction, the phenothiazine dose may need to be decreased. Lack of drug metabolism in the liver will cause an elevation in serum drug level.

Pharmacodynamics

Fluphenazine blocks postsynaptic dopamine receptors increasing dopamine turnovers and is prescribed primarily for psychotic disorders. This drug has anticholinergic properties and should be cautiously administered to patients with glaucoma, especially narrow-angle glaucoma. Because hypotension is a side effect of these phenothiazines, any antihypertensives simultaneously administered can cause an additive hypotensive effect. Narcotics and sedative-hypnotics administered simultaneously with these phenothiazines can cause an additive CNS depression. Antacids decrease the absorption rate of both drugs and all phenothiazines, so they should be given 1 hour before or 2 hours after an oral phenothiazine.

The peak action of fluphenazine is 2.8 hours. Fluphenazine decanoate has delayed absorption, with an onset of action of 24 hours and a duration of 4 to 6 weeks.

Nonphenothiazines

The many groups of nonphenothiazine antipsychotics include butyrophenones, dibenzoxazepines, dihydroindolones, and thioxanthenes.

In the *butyrophenone* group, a frequently prescribed nonphenothiazine is haloperidol. Haloperidol's pharmacologic behavior is similar to that of the phenothiazines. It is a potent antipsychotic drug in which the equivalent prescribed dose is smaller than that of drugs of lower potency, such as chlorpromazine. The initial oral drug dose for haloperidol is 0.5 to 2 mg, whereas the drug dose for chlorpromazine is 10 to 25 mg. Long-acting preparations of haloperidol decanoate and fluphenazine decanoate are given for slow release via injection every 2 to 4 weeks. Administration precautions should be taken to prevent soreness and inflammation at the injection site. Because the medication is a viscous liquid, a large-gauge needle (e.g., 21 gauge) should be used with the Z-track method for administration in a deep muscle; Chapter 10 provides further explanation of the Z-track method of injection. The injection site should not be massaged, and sites should be rotated. These medications should not remain in a plastic syringe longer than 15 minutes. Prototype Drug Chart: Haloperidol and Haloperidol Decanoate provides the drug data related to haloperidol.

Pharmacokinetics

Haloperidol is absorbed well through the gastrointestinal (GI) mucosa. It has a long half-life and is highly protein bound, so the drug may accumulate. Haloperidol is metabolized in the liver and is excreted in urine and feces.

Pharmacodynamics

Haloperidol alters the effects of dopamine by blocking dopamine receptors; thus, sedation and EPS may occur. The drug is used to control psychosis and to decrease agitation in adults and children. Dosages need to be decreased in older adults because of decreased liver function and potential side effects. Haloperidol may be prescribed for children with hyperactive behavior. Because it has anticholinergic activity, care should be taken when administering it to patients with a history of glaucoma.

Haloperidol has a similar onset of action, peak time of concentration, and duration of action as the phenothiazines. It has strong EPS effects. Skin and sun protection is necessary for prolonged use because of the possible side effect of photosensitivity.

From the *dibenzoxazepine* group, loxapine is a moderately potent agent. It has moderate sedative and orthostatic hypotensive effects and strong EPS effects.

The typical antipsychotic molindone hydrochloride from the *dihydroindolone* group is a moderately potent agent. It has low sedative and orthostatic hypotensive effects and strong EPS effects.

In the nonphenothiazine group known as *thioxanthenes* is thiothixene, a highly potent typical antipsychotic drug. It has side effects similar to those of molindone with low sedative and orthostatic hypotensive effects and strong EPS effects.

Side Effects and Adverse Reactions

Several side effects are associated with antipsychotics. The most common side effect for all antipsychotics is drowsiness. Many of the antipsychotics have some anticholinergic effects: dry mouth, increased heart rate, urinary retention, and constipation can occur. Blood pressure decreases with the use of antipsychotics; aliphatics and piperidines cause a greater decrease in blood pressure than the others.

EPS can begin within 5 to 30 days after initiation of antipsychotic therapy and are most prevalent with the phenothiazines, butyrophenones, and thioxanthenes. These symptoms include pseudoparkinsonism, akathisia, **dystonia** (prolonged muscle contractions with twisting, repetitive movements), and tardive dyskinesia. Tardive dyskinesia may develop in 20% of patients taking antipsychotics for long-term therapy. Antiparkinson anticholinergic drugs may be given to control EPS, but they are not always effective in treating tardive dyskinesia.

High dosing or long-term use of some antipsychotics can cause **blood dyscrasias** (blood cell disorders) such as agranulocytosis. The white blood cell (WBC) count should be closely monitored and reported to the health care provider if an extreme decrease in leukocytes is observed.

Dermatologic side effects seen early in drug therapy are pruritus and marked photosensitivity. Patients are urged to use sunscreen, hats, and protective clothing, as well as to stay out of the sun.

Drug Interactions

Because phenothiazines lower the seizure threshold, dosage adjustment of an anticonvulsant may be necessary. If either aliphatic phenothiazine or the thioxanthene group is administered, a higher dose of anticonvulsant might be necessary to prevent seizures.

PROTOTYPE DRUG CHART
Haloperidol and Haloperidol Decanoate

Drug Class	Dosage
Antipsychotic: Neuroleptic (nonphenothiazine)	Schizophrenia: A: PO: Initially 0.5–2 mg bid/tid; *max:* 100 mg/d Decanoate: A: IM: Initially 10–15 times previous PO dose of haloperidol equivalents
Contraindications	**Drug-Lab-Food Interaction**
Parkinsonism, CNS depression, coma *Caution:* Alcohol use disorder, dementia, glaucoma, dehydration, liver damage, urinary retention, cerebrovascular disease, bradycardia, cardiovascular disease, RA, prostatic hypertrophy, neutropenia, leukopenia, agranulocytosis, seizures, hyperthermia, prostatic hypertrophy, electrolyte imbalances, older adults, tobacco smoking, pregnancy, breast-feeding	Effects of haloperidol may be increased by amiodarone, kava kava, magnesium sulfate, metoclopramide, promethazine, antidepressants, antidysrhythmics; haloperidol may increase effects of anticholinergics, CNS depressants, glucagon, opioid agonists, oxycodone, potassium chloride, thiazide diuretics; effects of haloperidol may be decreased by acetylcholinesterase inhibitors, glycopyrrolate; haloperidol may decrease the effects of amphetamines, systemic epinephrine, nitroglycerine
Pharmacokinetics	**Pharmacodynamics**
Absorption: PO: 60% absorbed Distribution: PB: 92% Metabolism: t½: 12–37 h PO, 3 weeks decanoate depot IM Excretion: In urine and feces	PO: Onset: 60–90 min Peak: 4–6 h Duration: 24–72 h IM: Onset: 15–30 min Peak: 20–40 min Duration: 4–8 h IM: Decanoate: Onset: UK Peak: 6 d Duration: 3 wk
Therapeutic Effects/Uses	
To treat acute psychoses, schizophrenia Mechanism of Action: Alters the effect of dopamine on the CNS; the mechanism for antipsychotic effects is unknown	
Side Effects	**Adverse Reactions**
Drowsiness, edema, headache, blurred vision, depression, confusion, euphoria, cataracts, photosensitivity, lethargy, tremor, dry mouth, constipation, weight gain/loss, restlessness, hyperhidrosis, erectile dysfunction, urinary retention, impaired body temperature regulation	Tachycardia, orthostatic hypotension, EPS, hyper/hypoglycemia, hyponatremia, seizures, retinopathy, osteopenia *Life threatening:* Laryngeal edema/spasm, bronchospasm, dysrhythmias, eosinophilia, aplastic anemia, hemolytic anemia, leukopenia, agranulocytosis, thrombocytopenia, neutropenia, pancytopenia, hepatic failure, NMS, rhabdomyolysis

A, Adult; *bid*, twice a day; *CNS*, central nervous system; *d*, day; *EPS*, symptoms of extrapyramidal syndrome; *h*, hour; *IM*, intramuscularly; *max*, maximum; *min*, minute; *NMS*, neuroleptic malignant syndrome; *PB*, protein binding; *PO*, by mouth; *RA*, rheumatoid arthritis; *t½*, half-life; *tid*, three times a day; *UK*, unknown; *wk*, week.

Antipsychotics interact with alcohol, hypnotics, sedatives, narcotics, and benzodiazepines to potentiate the sedative effects of antipsychotics. Atropine counteracts EPS and potentiates antipsychotic effects. Use of antihypertensives can cause an additive hypotensive effect.

Antipsychotics should *not* be given with other antipsychotic or antidepressant drugs except to control psychotic behavior for selected individuals who are refractory to drug therapy. Under ordinary circumstances, if one antipsychotic drug is ineffective, a different one is prescribed. Individuals should *not* take alcohol or other CNS depressants (e.g., narcotic analgesics, barbiturates) with antipsychotics because additive depression is likely to occur.

When discontinuing antipsychotics, the drug dosage should be reduced gradually to avoid sudden recurrence of psychotic symptoms and seizures. Table 22.2 lists common antipsychotic drugs—phenothiazines and nonphenothiazines—and their dosages, uses, and considerations, including common side effects and a few serious adverse effects.

Antipsychotic Dosage for Older Adults

Older adults usually require smaller doses of antipsychotics—from 25% to 50% less than young and middle-aged adults. Regular to high doses of antipsychotics increase the risk of severe side effects. Dosage amounts need to be individualized according to the patient's age and physical status. In addition, dosage changes may be necessary during antipsychotic therapy. Antipsychotics have a black-box warning that states mortality is increased in elderly patients with dementia-related psychosis.

Atypical Antipsychotics

Atypical antipsychotics differ from typical traditional antipsychotics in that the atypical agents are effective in treating both positive and negative symptoms of schizophrenia. The typical antipsychotics have not been effective in the treatment of negative symptoms. Two advantages of the atypical agents are that they are effective in

TABLE 22.2 Phenothiazines and Nonphenothiazines

Drug	Route and Dosage	Uses and Considerations
Chlorpromazine hydrochloride	Schizophrenia: A: PO: Initially 10–25 mg 2–4 times/d	For acute psychosis, schizophrenia, intractable hiccups, nausea, and vomiting. May cause drowsiness, dizziness, weight gain, dry mouth, nasal congestion, blurred vision, photosensitivity, orthostatic hypotension, jaundice, constipation, urinary retention, erectile/ejaculation dysfunction, and EPS. PB: 90%–99%; t½: 2–30 h
Fluphenazine hydrochloride	See Prototype Drug Chart: Fluphenazine	
Perphenazine	Schizophrenia: A: PO: Initially 4–16 mg bid/qid; after obtaining maximum response, gradually reduce dose; *max:* 24 mg/d (64 mg/d for short periods)	For schizophrenia, severe nausea, and vomiting. May cause blurred vision, photosensitivity, dry mouth, drowsiness, hypo/hypertension, constipation, akathisia, urinary retention, and EPS. PB: 91%–99%; t½: 9–12 h
Thioridazine hydrochloride	A: PO: Initially 50–100 mg tid; *maint:* 200–800 mg/d; *max:* 800 mg/d	For schizophrenia. May cause dizziness, drowsiness, photosensitivity, dry mouth, weight gain, appetite stimulation, nausea, vomiting, constipation, akathisia, hypotension, and EPS. PB: 96%–99%; t½: 21–24 h
Haloperidol and Haloperidol Decanoate	See Prototype Drug Chart: Haloperidol and Haloperidol Decanoate	
Loxapine	Schizophrenia: A: PO: Initially 10 mg bid (50 mg in severely disturbed patients); *maint:* 60–100 mg/d; *max:* 250 mg/d for severe symptoms, 100 mg/d for outpatients	For schizophrenia and bipolar disorder. May cause dizziness, drowsiness, dry mouth, throat irritation, insomnia, dysgeusia, constipation, hypotension, EPS, and bronchospasm. PB: 96.6%; t½: 5–19 h
Molindone hydrochloride	A: PO: Initially: 50–75 mg/d in 3–4 divided doses; *max:* 225 mg/d	For schizophrenia. May cause blurred vision, dry mouth, hypersalivation, drowsiness, amenorrhea, gynecomastia, urinary retention, nausea, constipation, and EPS. PB: UK; t½: 1.5 h
Thiothixene hydrochloride	A: PO: Initially 2 mg tid; *maint:* 20–30 mg/d; *max:* 60 mg/d	For schizophrenia. May cause blurred vision, drowsiness, appetite stimulation, dry mouth, hypersalivation, nausea, weight gain, akathisia, amenorrhea, gynecomastia, constipation, erectile/ejaculation dysfunction, hypotension, peripheral edema, and EPS. PB: 90%; t½: 3.4–34 h
Clozapine	A: PO: Initially: 12.5 mg/qd or bid; gradually increase to *maint:* 300–450 mg/d in 3 divided doses; *max:* 900 mg/d	For schizophrenia. May cause dizziness, drowsiness, insomnia, dyspepsia, hypersalivation, nausea, vomiting, constipation, hypo/hypertension, tachycardia, and EPS. PB: 97%; t½: 4–12 h
Olanzapine	*Schizophrenia:* A: PO: Initially 5–10 mg/d; *max:* 20 mg/d Older A: PO: Initially 5 mg/d; *max:* 20 mg/d	For schizophrenia, bipolar disorder, and depression. May cause headache, dizziness, drowsiness, insomnia, fatigue, weakness, dry mouth, weight gain, dyspepsia, constipation, akathisia, depression, hyperglycemia, elevated hepatic enzymes, hypercholesterolemia, hypertriglyceridemia, appetite stimulation, hyperprolactinemia, and EPS. PB: 93%; t½: 21–54 h
Quetiapine	Schizophrenia: Immediate release: A: PO: Initially 25 mg/bid; *maint:* 400–800 mg/d in divided doses; *max:* 800 mg/d Extended release: A: PO: Initially 300 mg at bedtime; *max:* 800 mg/d Older A: PO: Initially 50 mg/d; *max:* 800 mg/d	For schizophrenia, bipolar disorder, and depression. May cause dizziness, drowsiness, headache, agitation, dry mouth, hypercholesterolemia, appetite stimulation, weight gain, constipation, hypertriglyceridemia, fatigue, weakness, and hyper/hypotension, and EPS. PB: 83%; t½: 6–12 h
Asenapine	Schizophrenia: A: SL: Initially 5 mg bid; may increase after 1 wk; *max:* 20 mg/d A: Transdermal: Initially 3.8 mg patch/d; *max:* 7.6 mg patch/d	For schizophrenia and bipolar disorder. May cause dizziness, drowsiness, insomnia, headache, paresthesia, fatigue, hypertriglyceridemia, weight gain, hypercholesterolemia, appetite stimulation, erythema, hyperglycemia, and EPS. PB: 95%; t½: 24 h SL, 30 h patch
Risperidone	Schizophrenia: A: PO: Initially 2 mg/d; *maint:* 4–8 mg/d; *max:* 16 mg/d Older A: PO: Initially 0.5 mg bid; *maint:* 4–8 mg/d; *max:* 16 mg/d A: IM: 25 mg deep IM q2wks; max: 50 mg q2wks A: subcut Perseris: 90–120 mg/month; max: 120/month A: subcut Uzedy: 50–125 mg/month or 100–250 mg q2months	For management of schizophrenia and bipolar disorder. May cause dizziness, drowsiness, fever, headache, cough, weight gain, anxiety, dry mouth, rhinorrhea, hypo/hyperglycemia, insomnia, fatigue, appetite stimulation, abdominal pain, nausea, vomiting, constipation, and EPS. PB: 90%; t½: 3 h

Continued

TABLE 22.2 Phenothiazines and Nonphenothiazines—cont'd

Drug	Route and Dosage	Uses and Considerations
Ziprasidone	Schizophrenia: A: PO: 20 mg bid with food; may increase q2d; *max:* 80 mg bid	For schizophrenia and bipolar disorder. May cause dizziness, drowsiness, headache, insomnia, nausea, constipation, dyspepsia, weight gain, urinary retention, and EPS. PB: 99%; t½: 7 h
Iloperidone	A: PO: Initially 1 mg bid; *maint:* 6–12 mg bid; *max:* 24 mg/d	For schizophrenia and bipolar disorder. May cause dizziness, drowsiness, nasal congestion, diarrhea, hyperlipidemia, hyperprolactinemia, dry mouth, hypertriglyceridemia, weight gain, nausea, orthostatic hypotension, fatigue, and tachycardia. PB: 95%; t½: 18–33 h
Aripiprazole	See Prototype Drug Chart: Aripiprazole	
Cariprazine	Schizophrenia: A: PO: Initially 1.5 mg/d; *max:* 6 mg/d	For schizophrenia and bipolar disorder. May cause insomnia, drowsiness, dizziness, headache, restlessness, weight gain, dyspepsia, nausea, vomiting, constipation, and EPS. PB: 91%–97%; t½: 2–4 d
Brexpiprazole	Schizophrenia: A: PO: Initially 1 mg/d; *maint:* 2–4 mg/d; *max:* 4 mg/d	For schizophrenia and depression. May cause headache, drowsiness, dizziness, fatigue, dyspepsia, weight gain, pharyngitis, hypertriglyceridemia, tremor, and EPS. PB: 99%; t½: 91 h
Paliperidone	Extended-release tablet: A: PO: Initially 6 mg/d; may increase dose q5d; *max:* 12 mg/d A: IM: Initially 234 mg, then 1 wk later 156 mg; *maint:* 5 wk after first dose begin 117 mg/month; *max:* 234 mg q1month	For schizophrenia. May cause anxiety, drowsiness, headache, agitation, tachycardia, hypercholesterolemia, hypertriglyceridemia, hyperlipidemia, hyperglycemia, hyperprolactinemia, hyperkinesis, vomiting, weight gain, tremor, akathisia, and EPS. PB: 74%; t½: 23 h for PO, 25–49 for IM
Lumateperone	A: PO: 42 mg/d; *max:* 42 mg/d	For schizophrenia and bipolar disorder. May cause drowsiness, headache, dizziness, fatigue, dry mouth, nausea, vomiting, hypercholesterolemia, EPS, hypertriglyceridemia, and elevated hepatic enzymes. PB: 97.4%; t½: 18 h
Olanzapine and samidorphan	Schizophrenia: A: PO: Initially 5 mg olanzapine/10 mg samidorphan/d or 10 mg olanzapine/10 mg samidorphan/d; *max:* 20 olanzapine/10 mg samidorphan/d	For schizophrenia and bipolar disorder. May cause dizziness, drowsiness, headache, dry mouth, appetite stimulation, weight gain, constipation, hyperglycemia, hypertriglyceridemia, hyperprolactinemia, and orthostatic hypotension. PB: olanzapine 93%, samidorphan 23%–33%; t½: olanzapine 21–54 h, samidorphan 7–11 h
Dexmedetomidine	Mild/moderate agitation: A: SL/buccal: 120 mcg, if agitation persists give 2 more doses of 60 mcg/dose 2 h apart *max:* 240 mcg/d Severe Agitation: A: SL/buccal: 180 mcg, if agitation persists give 90 mcg *max:* 360 mcg/d	For agitation associated with bipolar disorders or schizophrenia. May cause drowsiness, brady/tachycardia, hypo/hypertension, nausea, constipation, and respiratory depression. Do not eat/drink for 15 min after SL dose or 1 h after buccal dose. PB: 94%; t½: 2.8 h

A, Adult; *bid*, twice a day; *d*, day; *EPS*, symptoms of extrapyramidal syndrome; *ER*, extended release; *h*, hour; *IM*, intramuscular; *maint*, maintenance; *max*, maximum; *NMS*, neuroleptic malignant syndrome; *PB*, protein binding; *PO*, by mouth; *q2d*, every 2 days; *subcut*, subcutaneous; *SL*, sublingual; *t½*, half-life; *tid*, three times a day; *UK*, unknown; *wk*, weeks; *y*, years.

---

treating negative symptoms and that they are unlikely to cause symptoms of EPS, including tardive dyskinesia. Atypical drugs (Serotonin/Dopamine Antagonists) available include clozapine, risperidone, olanzapine, ziprasidone, and aripiprazole. These agents have a greater affinity for blocking serotonin and dopaminergic D_4 receptors than primarily blocking the dopaminergic D_2 receptor responsible for mild and severe EPS. Weight gain, drowsiness, unsteady gait, headache, insomnia, depression, diabetes mellitus, and dyslipidemia are common side effects of atypical antipsychotics.

Clozapine was the first atypical antipsychotic agent used to treat schizophrenia and other psychoses. It is not as likely to cause symptoms of EPS, although they may occur. Tremors have been reported. Serious adverse reactions of clozapine are seizures and agranulocytosis, a decrease in the production of granulocytes that involves the body's immune defenses. Currently, clozapine is only indicated for the treatment of severely ill schizophrenic patients who have not responded to traditional antipsychotic drugs. The WBC (leukocyte) count needs to be closely monitored for leukopenia; if the level falls below 3000 mm^3, clozapine should be discontinued. Seizures have been reported in 3% of patients taking the drug. Dizziness, sedation, tachycardia, orthostatic hypotension, and constipation are common side effects.

Another atypical agent used to treat the positive and negative symptoms of schizophrenia is risperidone. Its action is similar to that of clozapine, and the occurrence of EPS and tardive dyskinesia is low. It does not cause agranulocytosis. Risperidone should be swallowed whole after being dissolved and not chewed, split, or crushed. The most common adverse effects include EPS, drowsiness, fatigue, appetite stimulation, insomnia, headache, and weight gain.

CLINICAL JUDGMENT [NURSING PROCESS]

Phenothiazines and Nonphenothiazines

Concept: Cognition
- Mental activities used to process and apply information

Recognize Cues [Assessment]
- Assess baseline vital signs for use in future comparisons.
- Obtain a patient health history that includes present drug therapy. If the patient is taking an anticonvulsant, the drug dose might need to be increased because antipsychotics tend to lower the seizure threshold.
- Assess mental status and cardiac, eye, and respiratory disorders before starting drug therapy, and continue daily assessment.

Analyze Cues and Prioritize Hypothesis [Patient Problems]
- Confusion
- Anxiety
- Decreased functional ability
- Decreased ability to cope

Generate Solutions [Planning]
- Patient will appear calmer.
- Patient will communicate coherently.
- Patient will carry out personal activities of daily living.
- Patient will demonstrate organized thoughts.
- Patient will communicate understanding of reality.

Take Action [Nursing Interventions]
- Monitor vital signs. Orthostatic hypotension is likely to occur.
- Remain with patients while medication is taken and swallowed; some patients hide antipsychotics in the mouth to avoid taking them.
- Avoid skin contact with liquid concentrates to prevent contact dermatitis. Liquid must be protected from light and should be diluted with fruit juice.
- Administer oral doses with food or milk to decrease gastric irritation.
- Dilute oral solution of fluphenazine in fruit juice, water, or milk. Avoid apple juice and caffeinated drinks.
- Administer deep into muscle because drug irritates fatty tissue. Do *not* administer intravenously.
- Check blood pressure for marked decrease or increase 30 minutes after drug is injected.
- Do *not* mix in same syringe with heparin, pentobarbital, cimetidine, or dimenhydrinate.
- Chill suppository in refrigerator for 30 minutes before removing foil wrapper.
- Observe for extrapyramidal syndrome (EPS) symptoms such as acute dystonia, akathisia, pseudoparkinsonism, and tardive dyskinesia (see Fig. 22.2) and report these promptly to the health care provider.
- ⚡ Assess for symptoms of neuroleptic malignant syndrome: increased fever, pulse, and blood pressure; muscle rigidity; increased creatine phosphokinase and white blood cell (WBC) count; altered mental status; acute renal failure; varying levels of consciousness; pallor; diaphoresis; tachycardia; and dysrhythmias.
- Record urine output; urinary retention may result.
- Monitor serum glucose level.
- Engage patient in interactions with staff, other patients, and attending therapies.

Patient Teaching
General
- Encourage patients to take the drug exactly as ordered. In schizophrenia and other psychotic disorders, antipsychotics do not cure the mental illness but do alleviate symptoms. Many patients on medication can function outside of an institutional setting. Adherence to a drug regimen is extremely important.
- Inform patients that medication may take 6 weeks or longer to achieve full clinical effect.
- ⚡ Caution patients not to consume alcohol or other central nervous system depressants such as narcotics; these drugs intensify the depressant effect on the body.
- Recommend that patients not abruptly discontinue the drug. Seek advice from a health care provider before making any changes in dosage.
- Encourage patients to read labels on over-the-counter preparations. Some are contraindicated when taking antipsychotics.
- Teach smoking cessation because smoking increases the metabolism of some antipsychotics.
- Guide patients to maintain good oral hygiene by frequently brushing and flossing teeth.
- Encourage patients to talk with a health care provider regarding family planning. The effect of antipsychotics on the fetus is not fully known; however, there may be teratogenic effects.
- Explain to the breast-feeding patient that phenothiazine passes into breast milk, possibly causing drowsiness and unusual muscle movement in the infant.
- Warn patients about the importance of routine follow-up examinations.
- ⚡ Encourage patients to obtain laboratory tests on schedule. WBCs are monitored for 3 months, especially during the start of drug therapy. Leukopenia, or decreased WBCs, may occur. Be alert to symptoms of malaise, fever, and sore throat, which may be an indication of agranulocytosis, a serious blood dyscrasia.
- Teach patients, especially those taking clozapine, to report symptoms of infection promptly to the health care provider.
- Advise patients to wear an identification bracelet indicating the medication taken.
- Inform patients that tolerance to the sedative effect develops over a period of days or weeks.

Side Effects
- ⚡ Direct patients to avoid potentially dangerous situations, such as driving, until drug dosing has been stabilized.
- Inform patients about EPS, and instruct them to promptly report symptoms to a health care provider.
- Encourage patients to wear sunglasses for photosensitivity, to limit exposure to direct sunlight, and to use sunscreen and protective clothing to prevent a skin rash.
- Warn patients about orthostatic hypotension and possible dizziness.
- Teach patients who are taking aliphatic phenothiazines such as chlorpromazine that the urine might be pink or red-brown; this discoloration is harmless.
- Inform patients that changes may occur related to sexual functioning and menstruation. Women could have irregular menstrual periods or amenorrhea, and men might experience impotence and gynecomastia (enlargement of breast tissue).
- Suggest lozenges or hard candy if mouth dryness occurs. Advise patients to consult a health care provider if dry mouth persists for more than 2 weeks.
- Encourage patients to avoid extremes in environmental temperatures and exercise.
- Advise patients to rise slowly from sitting or lying to standing to prevent a sudden decrease in blood pressure.

Evaluate Outcomes [Evaluation]
- Evaluate the effectiveness of the drug and whether the patient has acceptably reduced psychotic symptoms at the *lowest* dose possible.
- Ascertain whether the patient can cope with everyday living situations and attend to activities of daily living.
- Determine whether any side effects or adverse reactions to the drug have occurred.

Like clozapine and risperidone, the atypical antipsychotic olanzapine is effective for treating the positive and negative symptoms of schizophrenia.

Like all the other atypical antipsychotics, quetiapine is less likely to cause EPS. Severe tardive dyskinesia may occur, but it is rare.

For individuals with cardiac dysrhythmias, ziprasidone must be prescribed with caution because its use may lead to a prolonged QT interval; electrocardiograms (ECGs) should be monitored. Ziprasidone is contraindicated in patients with a history of prolonged QT interval or with other concurrent drugs known to prolong QT interval. Patients taking quetiapine, clozapine, risperidone, olanzapine, ziprasidone, and aripiprazole should be monitored for hyperglycemia and other symptoms of diabetes mellitus.

Prototype Drug Chart: Aripiprazole illustrates drug characteristics of aripiprazole, an atypical antipsychotic. When anxiety, hallucinations, agitation, mania, confusion, or depression and other symptoms are noted, the health care provider should check the medications that the patient is taking.

ANXIETY

A certain amount of anxiety may make a person more alert and energetic, but when anxiety is excessive, it can be disabling, and anxiolytics may be prescribed. The action of anxiolytics resembles that of the sedative-hypnotics but not that of the antipsychotics.

Anxiety Disorders

An estimated 264 million people have an anxiety disorder. Excessive anxiety may be characterized by sweating palms, pacing, palpitations, tachycardia, restlessness, irritability, difficulty concentrating, disturbed sleep, nausea, diarrhea, urinary frequency, and dyspnea. Common anxiety disorders include general anxiety disorder, social anxiety disorder, obsessive-compulsive disorder, panic disorder, and posttraumatic stress disorder. These agents treat the symptoms but do not cure them. Long-term use of anxiolytics is discouraged because tolerance develops within weeks or months, depending on the agent. Drug tolerance can occur in less than 2 to 3 months in patients who take phenobarbital.

Nonpharmacologic Measures

Some of the symptoms of a severe attack of anxiety, or panic attack, include dyspnea (difficulty in breathing), choking sensation, chest pain, heart palpitations, dizziness, faintness, sweating, trembling and shaking, and fear of losing control. Before giving anxiolytics, nonpharmacologic measures should be used for decreasing anxiety. A thorough assessment may avoid more anxiety caused by an alternative measure. These measures might include using a relaxation technique, psychotherapy, or support groups.

ANXIOLYTICS

Anxiolytics, or *antianxiety drugs*, are primarily used to treat excessive anxiety. The major anxiolytic group is benzodiazepines, a minor tranquilizer group. Long before benzodiazepines were prescribed for anxiety and insomnia, barbiturates were used. Benzodiazepines are considered more effective than barbiturates because they enhance the action of GABA, an inhibitory neurotransmitter within the CNS. Benzodiazepines have fewer side effects and may be less dangerous in overdosing. Long-term use of barbiturates causes drug tolerance and dependence and may cause respiratory distress. Currently, barbiturates are not drugs of choice for treating anxiety. Benzodiazepine-like drugs are used to treat insomnia. Selective serotonin reuptake inhibitors (SSRIs), serotonin-norepinephrine reuptake inhibitors (SNRIs), tricyclic antidepressants (TCAs), and monoamine oxidase inhibitors (MAOIs) are used to treat various anxiety disorders. These drugs are discussed in Chapter 23.

Table 22.3 lists approved uses for benzodiazepines. Drugs used to treat insomnia, including benzodiazepines, are discussed in Chapter 18.

Benzodiazepines

Benzodiazepines have multiple uses as anticonvulsants, sedative-hypnotics, preoperative drugs, substance abuse withdrawal agents, and anxiolytics. Most of the benzodiazepines are used mainly for severe or prolonged anxiety. Examples include chlordiazepoxide, diazepam, clorazepate dipotassium, lorazepam, and alprazolam. The most frequently prescribed benzodiazepine is lorazepam. Many of the benzodiazepines are used for more than one purpose.

Benzodiazepines are lipid soluble and are absorbed readily from the GI tract. They are highly protein bound (80%–98%). Benzodiazepines are primarily metabolized by the liver and are excreted in urine, so the drug dosage for patients with liver or renal disease should be lowered accordingly to avoid possible cumulative effects. Traces of benzodiazepine metabolites could be present in the urine for weeks or months after the person has stopped taking the drug. These are Controlled Substance Schedule IV (CSS IV) drugs.

The first benzodiazepine, chlordiazepoxide, became widely used for its sedative effect in 1962. Diazepam was the most frequently prescribed drug in the early 1970s. Lorazepam is the prototype drug of benzodiazepine and is described in Prototype Drug Chart: Lorazepam.

TABLE 22.3 Approved Uses for Benzodiazepines

Prescribed Uses	Drugs
Anxiety	Alprazolam Chlordiazepoxide Chlorazepate Diazepam Lorazepam
Anxiety associated with depression	Alprazolam Clonazepam Lorazepam
Insomnia, short-term use	Estazolam Flurazepam Quazepam Temazepam Triazolam
Seizures and status epilepticus	Clonazepam Clorazepate Diazepam Lorazepam
Alcohol withdrawal	Clorazepate Chlordiazepoxide Diazepam Lorazepam
Skeletal muscle spasms	Diazepam
Preoperative medications	Chlordiazepoxide Diazepam Lorazepam Midazolam

PROTOTYPE DRUG CHART
Aripiprazole

Drug Class	Dosage
Nonphenothiazine: Atypical antipsychotic	Schizophrenia: Immediate-release tablets: A: PO: Initially 10–15 mg/d, may increase q2wk; *maint:* 10–30 mg/d; *max:* 30 mg/d Extended release (Abilify Maintena): A: IM: Initially 400 mg/month; *max:* 400 mg/month
Contraindications	**Drug-Lab-Food Interactions**
Hypersensitivity *Caution:* Dysrhythmias, dehydration, CNS depression, dementia, hypovolemia, heart failure, hypotension, bradycardia, cerebro/cardiovascular disease, myocardial infarction, hyperglycemia, parkinsonism, RA, seizures, electrolyte imbalances, diabetes mellitus, hypercholesterolemia, hypertriglyceridemia, agranulocytosis, suicidal ideation, alcohol use disorder, older adult, children, pregnancy, breast-feeding	Drug: Antidiabetic agents decrease drug levels and increase risk of hyperglycemia; alpha blockers and antihypertensives increase risk of hypotension; other antipsychotics enhance risk of NMS, EPS, anticholinergic effects, hypotension, and seizures; CNS depressants may increase sedation and orthostatic hypotension; SSRIs may increase risk of serotonin syndrome; calcium channel blockers may increase blood levels Food: Grapefruit juice may increase blood levels Herbal: St. Johns wort may decrease blood levels Lab: Increased blood glucose
Pharmacokinetics	**Pharmacodynamics**
Absorption: Well absorbed, not affected by food Distribution: PB: 99% Metabolism: t½: 75 h; extended release 30–47 d Excretion: In urine and feces	PO: Onset: UK Peak: 3–5 h Duration: UK IM: Immediate release: Onset: UK Peak: 1–3 h Duration: UK IM: ER: Peak: 5–7 d Duration: UK
Therapeutic Effects/Uses	
To manage schizophrenia, bipolar disorder, autism, depression, Tourette syndrome Mechanism of Action: Interferes with the binding of dopamine to dopamine (D_2) and serotonin 5-hydroxytryptamine ($5-HT_2$) receptors	
Side Effects	**Adverse Reactions**
Drowsiness, dizziness, memory impairment, weight gain/loss, headache, fatigue, blurred vision, photosensitivity, peripheral edema, insomnia, anxiety, agitation, fever, dry mouth, pharyngitis, appetite stimulation, dyspepsia, nausea, vomiting, constipation, rash, tremor, urinary retention, impulse control symptoms, hyperhidrosis, erectile dysfunction	Hyper/hypotension, tachycardia, palpitations, bradycardia, hypokalemia, hyponatremia, rhabdomyolysis, hypertriglyceridemia, hypercholesterolemia, dysrhythmias, seizures, depression, EPS, hyper/hypoglycemia, diabetes mellitus *Life threatening:* Suicidal ideation, NMS, angioedema, agranulocytosis, neutropenia, leukopenia, laryngospasm, stroke

A, Adult; *CNS*, central nervous system; *d*, day; *EPS*, symptoms of extrapyramidal syndrome; *ER*, extended release; *h*, hour; *IM*, intramuscularly; *maint*, maintenance; *max*, maximum; *NMS*, neuroleptic malignant syndrome; *PB*, protein binding; *PO*, by mouth; *q2dwk*, every 2 weeks; *RA*, rheumatoid arthritis; *SSRI*, selective serotonin reuptake inhibitor; *t½*, half-life; *UK*, unknown; *wk*, week.

Pharmacokinetics
Lorazepam is highly lipid soluble, and the drug is rapidly absorbed from the GI tract. The drug is highly protein bound, and the half-life is 12 hours for immediate release and 13 to 27.2 for extended release. Lorazepam is excreted primarily in the urine.

COMPLEMENTARY AND ALTERNATIVE THERAPIES
Benzodiazepines
Kava kava should not be combined with benzodiazepines because it increases the sedative effect.

Pharmacodynamics
Lorazepam acts on the limbic, thalamic, and hypothalamic levels of the CNS. The onset of action is 20 to 30 minutes for IM administration and 2 to 3 minutes IV. The serum level of oral lorazepam peaks in 2 hours.

It is recommended that benzodiazepines be prescribed for no longer than 3 to 4 months. Beyond 4 months, the effectiveness of the drug lessens. Table 22.4 lists the anxiolytics and their dosages, uses, and considerations, including common side effects and a few serious adverse effects.

Side Effects and Adverse Reactions
The side effects associated with benzodiazepines are sedation, dizziness, headaches, dry mouth, blurred vision, rare urinary incontinence, and constipation. Adverse reactions include leukopenia (decreased WBC count) with symptoms of fever, malaise, and sore throat; tolerance

PROTOTYPE DRUG CHART

Lorazepam

Drug Class	Dosage
Anxiolytic: Benzodiazepine	Anxiety: A: PO: initially 2–3 mg/d in divided doses; increase gradually PRN; *maint:* 2–6 mg/d in divided doses; *max:* 10 mg/d Older A: PO: Initially 1–2 mg/d in divided doses; *maint:* 2–6 mg/d; *max:* 10 mg/d

Contraindications	Drug-Lab-Food Interactions
Hypersensitivity, glaucoma, sleep apnea *Caution:* Hepatic or renal dysfunction, COPD, alcohol and substance use disorder, depression, seizures, CNS depression, myasthenia gravis, psychosis, pregnancy, suicidal ideation, older adults, breast-feeding	Drug: Increases CNS depression when taken with alcohol, CNS depressants, and anticonvulsants; cimetidine increases lorazepam plasma levels, increases phenytoin levels, decreases levodopa effects; smoking and caffeine decrease antianxiety effects; oral contraceptives decrease effects

Pharmacokinetics	Pharmacodynamics
Absorption: Rapid from GI tract Distribution: PB: 85% Metabolism: t½: 12 h for immediate release, 13–27.4 h for extended release Excretion: In urine	PO: Onset: UK Peak: 2 h Duration: UK IM: Onset: 20–30 min Peak: 3 h Duration: 6–8 h IV: Onset: 2–3 min Peak: UK Duration: 6–8 h

Therapeutic Effects/Uses

To control anxiety, and to treat status epilepticus; for sedation induction; for insomnia
Mechanism of Action: Potentiates GABA effects by binding to specific benzodiazepine receptors and inhibiting GABA neurotransmission

Side Effects	Adverse Reactions
Drowsiness, dizziness, weakness, headache, confusion, depression, euphoria, amnesia, ataxia, blurred vision, restlessness, tremor, constipation, erectile dysfunction, injection site reaction	Hyper/hypotension, bradycardia, tachycardia, hearing loss, tolerance, dependence, seizures, hyponatremia, heart failure, psychosis *Life threatening:* Suicidal ideation, NMS, agranulocytosis, pancytopenia, thrombocytopenia, respiratory depression

A, Adult; *CNS*, central nervous system; *COPD*, chronic obstructive pulmonary disease; *d*, day; *GABA*, gamma-aminobutyric acid; *GI*, gastrointestinal; *h*, hour; *IM*, intramuscularly; *IV*, intravenously; *maint*, maintenance; *max*, maximum; *min*, minute; *PB*, protein binding; *PO*, by mouth; *PRN*, as needed; *t½*, half-life; *UK*, unknown.

TABLE 22.4 Anxiolytics

Drug	Route and Dosage	Uses and Considerations
Benzodiazepines		
Alprazolam CSS IV	Panic disorders: Immediate release: A: PO: Initially 0.5 mg tid, may increase q3–4d; *max:* 10 mg/d Older A: PO: Initially 0.25 bid/tid, may increase q3–4d; *max:* 10 mg/d Extended release: A: PO: Initially 0.5–1 mg/d in the morning, may increase q3–4d; *max:* 10 mg/d Older A: PO: Initially 0.5 mg/d, may increase q3–4d; *max:* 10 mg/d	For anxiety, panic disorders, and generalized anxiety disorder. May cause dizziness, drowsiness, ataxia, impaired memory/cognition, dry mouth, nasal congestion, irritability, dysarthria, fatigue, depression, weight gain/loss, constipation, withdrawal, and appetite stimulation. PB: 80%; t½: 6.3–26.9 h immediate release, 11–16 h extended release
Chlordiazepoxide hydrochloride CSS IV	Anxiety disorders: A: PO: 5–10 mg bid/qid; for severe anxiety: 20–25 mg tid/qid; *max:* 100 mg/d Older A: PO: 5 mg bid/qid	For anxiety, alcohol withdrawal syndrome (DTs). May cause nausea, drowsiness, confusion, ataxia, tolerance, dependence, and withdrawal. PB: 96%; t½: 5–30 h

TABLE 22.4 Anxiolytics—cont'd

Drug	Route and Dosage	Uses and Considerations
Clorazepate dipotassium CSS IV	Anxiety: A: PO: Initially 7.5–15 mg bid or 15 mg at bedtime; *maint:* 15–60 mg/d; *max:* 60 mg/d Older A: PO: 3.75–7.5 mg bid or 7.5 mg at bedtime; *maint:* 15–60 mg/d; *max:* 60 mg/d	For anxiety, alcohol withdrawal syndrome, and partial seizures. May cause drowsiness, dizziness, blurred vision, hypotension, ataxia, depression, memory impairment, suicidal ideation, tolerance, dependence, and withdrawal. PB: 97%–98%; t½: 40–50 h
Diazepam CSS IV	Anxiety: A: PO: 2–10 mg bid/qid; *max:* 40 mg/d Older A: PO: 2–2.5 mg qd/bid; *max:* 40 mg/d A: IM/IV: 2–10 mg; repeat in 3–4 h PRN	For anxiety, muscle spasms, alcohol withdrawal, seizures, status epilepticus, and sedation induction. May cause drowsiness, dizziness, headache, memory impairment, respiratory depression, rash, nasal irritation, ataxia, fatigue, diarrhea, and urinary retention/incontinence. PB: 95%–98%; t½: 48–100 h
Lorazepam CSS IV	See Prototype Drug Chart: Lorazepam	
Oxazepam CSS IV	Anxiety: A: PO: Initially 10–15 mg tid/qid; for severe symptoms, 15–30 mg tid/qid; *max:* A 120 mg/d Older A: PO: Initially 10 mg tid; *max:* 60 mg/d	For anxiety and acute alcohol withdrawal. May cause dizziness, rash, drowsiness, headache, memory impairment, hypotension, dependence, tolerance, and withdrawal. PB: 85%–95%; t½: 5–15 h
Azapirones Buspirone hydrochloride	A: PO: Initially: 7.5 mg bid; *maint:* 20–30 mg/d in divided doses; *max:* 60 mg/d	For anxiety and generalized anxiety disorder. May cause drowsiness, ataxia, dizziness, blurred vision, headache, confusion, excitability, hostility, nausea, diarrhea, edema, erectile/ejaculatory dysfunction, and EPS. PB: 86%; t½: 2–3 h
Benzodiazepine Antagonists Flumazenil	Benzodiazepine toxicity: A: IV: Initially 0.2 mg; may give 0.3 mg in 30 s, then may give 0.5 mg at 1-min intervals to a max of 3 mg	For sedation reversal and benzodiazepine toxicity. May cause dizziness, dyspnea, hyperventilation, blurred vision, headache, anxiety, ataxia, agitation, insomnia, hyperhidrosis, vomiting, dry mouth, palpitations, and tremor. PB: 50%; t½: 40–80 min

A, Adult; *bid*, twice a day; *CNS*, central nervous system; *CSS*, Controlled Substances Schedule; *d*, day; *DTs*, delirium tremens; *EPS*, symptoms of extrapyramidal symptoms; *h*, hour; *IM*, intramuscularly; *IV*, intravenously; *maint*, maintenance; *max*, maximum; *min*, minute; *PB*, protein binding; *PO*, by mouth; *PRN*, as needed; *q*, every; *q4–6h*, every 4 to 6 hours; *qd*, every day; *qid*, four times a day; *s*, seconds; *t½*, half-life; *tid*, three times a day; *y*, years.

BOX 22.2 Suggested Treatment for Overdose of Benzodiazepines

1. Administer an emetic, and follow with activated charcoal if the patient is conscious; use gastric lavage if the patient is unconscious.
2. Administer the benzodiazepine antagonist flumazenil intravenously if required.
3. Maintain an airway, give oxygen as needed for decreased respirations, and monitor vital signs.
4. Give intravenous vasopressors for severe hypotension.
5. Request a mental health consultation for the patient.

to the drug dosage with continuous use; and physical dependency. Box 22.2 lists guidelines for treating benzodiazepine overdose.

Benzodiazepines should not be abruptly discontinued because withdrawal symptoms are likely to occur. Withdrawal symptoms caused by short-term benzodiazepine use are similar to those from the sedative-hypnotics: agitation, nervousness, insomnia, tremor, anorexia, muscular cramps, and sweating; however, they are slow to develop, taking 2 to 10 days, and can last several weeks, depending on the benzodiazepine's half-life. When discontinuing a benzodiazepine, the drug dosage should be gradually decreased over a period of days, depending on the dose or length of time on the drug. Withdrawal symptoms from long-term, high-dose benzodiazepine therapy include paranoia, delirium, panic, hypertension, and status epilepticus. Convulsions during withdrawal may be prevented with simultaneous substitution of an anticonvulsant. Alcohol and other CNS depressants should *not* be taken with benzodiazepines because respiratory depression can result. Tobacco, caffeine, and sympathomimetics decrease the effectiveness of benzodiazepines. Benzodiazepines are contraindicated during pregnancy because of possible teratogenic effects.

Miscellaneous Anxiolytics

The anxiolytic buspirone hydrochloride binds to serotonin and dopamine receptors. It may not be effective until 1 to 2 weeks after continuous use. It has fewer of the side effects of sedation and physical and psychological dependency associated with many benzodiazepines. The most common side effects of buspirone include drowsiness, dizziness, headache, nausea, nervousness, and excitement. It is important to note that buspirone has an interaction with grapefruit juice that can lead to toxicity. To avoid this interaction, buspirone users should be advised to limit intake of grapefruit juice to 8 ounces daily or half of a grapefruit.

CLINICAL JUDGMENT [NURSING PROCESS]
Benzodiazepines

Concept: Anxiety
- More intense worry about everyday issues than situation demands

Recognize Cues [Assessment]
- Assess for suicidal ideation.
- Obtain a history of the patient's anxiety reaction.
- Determine the patient's support system (family, friends, groups).
- Obtain a drug history. Report possible drug–drug interactions.

Analyze Cues and Prioritize Hypothesis [Patient Problems]
- Anxiety
- Insomnia
- Decreased ability to cope
- Decreased functional ability

Generate Solutions [Planning]
- Patient will appear calmer after nonpharmacologic methods, anxiolytic drugs, or support/group therapy.
- Patient will sleep better.
- Patient will appear to cope better with everyday situations.
- Patient will carry out own activities of daily living.

Take Action [Nursing Interventions]
- Observe patient for side effects of anxiolytics. Recognize that drug tolerance and physical and psychological dependency can occur with most anxiolytics.
- Recognize that anxiolytic dosages should be lower for older adults, children, and debilitated persons than for middle-aged adults.
- Monitor vital signs, especially blood pressure and pulse; orthostatic hypotension may occur.
- Encourage family to be supportive of the patient.

Patient Teaching
General
- ⚠️ Advise patients not to drive a motor vehicle or operate dangerous equipment when taking anxiolytics because sedation is a common side effect.
- ⚠️ Warn patients not to consume alcohol or central nervous system (CNS) depressants such as narcotics while taking an anxiolytic.
- Teach patients ways to control excess stress and anxiety with relaxation techniques such as long walks.
- Inform patients that an effective response may take 1 to 2 weeks.
- Encourage patients to follow drug regimens and not to abruptly stop taking a drug after prolonged use because withdrawal symptoms can occur. The drug dose is usually tapered when a drug is discontinued.

Side Effects
- Encourage patients to rise slowly from sitting to standing positions to avoid dizziness from orthostatic hypotension.

Evaluate Outcomes [Evaluation]
- Evaluate the effectiveness of drug therapy by determining whether the patient is less anxious and more able to cope with stresses and anxieties.
- Determine whether the patient is taking the anxiolytic drug as prescribed and is adhering to patient teaching instructions.

CLINICAL JUDGMENT SINGLE-EPISODE CASE STUDY

Cognitive Skill: Enhanced Hot Spot
Objective: Knowledge of medication side effects.

A 35-year-old woman with a diagnosis of schizophrenia has stopped taking her medication. After experiencing agitation, delusions, and hallucinations, she was admitted to the hospital for evaluation. The physician prescribed risperidone 2 mg per day. After several days, the patient is stabilized and ready for discharge. The nurse teaches the patient about the side effects of risperidone.

Place a check mark next to the side effect of risperidone that is most important for the patient to report to the physician.
- ____ A. Dizziness
- ____ B. Weight loss
- ____ C. Drowsiness
- ____ D. Blurred vision
- ____ E. Appetite stimulation
- ____ F. Diarrhea
- ____ G. Akathisia

Answers
- ✓ A. Dizziness
- ____ B. Weight loss
- ✓ C. Drowsiness
- ____ D. Blurred vision
- ✓ E. Appetite stimulation
- ____ F. Diarrhea
- ✓ G. Akathisia

Rationale
Risperidone is an atypical antipsychotic drug and is the first line of treatment options for the management of schizophrenia. Risperidone exhibits strong antagonist activity at alpha-1 receptors, which likely contributes to adverse cardiovascular effects such as orthostatic hypotension, which may cause dizziness, syncope, drowsiness, and akathisia (muscle quivering and restlessness). It has a high affinity at H-1 histamine receptor sites and has been demonstrated to partially account for adverse effects such as sedation, drowsiness, appetite stimulation, and weight gain. It does not cause weight loss, blurred vision, or diarrhea.

Reference
Pharmacology: A patient centered pharmacology approach. 10th ed. McCuistion, L., et al (2021) Elsevier; www.clinicalkey.com/pharmacology; *Lehne's pharmacology for nursing care* (10th ed). Rosenack, J, etal (2019) Elsevier.

REVIEW QUESTIONS

1. The nurse suspects that a patient who is experiencing facial grimacing, involuntary upward eye movement, and muscle spasms of the tongue and face may have which condition?
   a. Akathisia
   b. Acute dystonia
   c. Tardive dyskinesia
   d. Pseudoparkinsonism
2. A patient asks the nurse to explain how antipsychotic drugs work to make him feel better. The nurse understands that antipsychotics act in which way?
   a. Blocking actions of dopamine
   b. Blocking actions of epinephrine
   c. Promoting prostaglandin synthesis
   d. Enhancing the action of gamma-aminobutyric acid
3. An antipsychotic agent, fluphenazine, is ordered for a patient with psychosis. The nurse understands that this agent can lead to symptoms of extrapyramidal syndrome (EPS). What are the symptoms of EPS?
   a. Hypertension
   b. Nausea and vomiting
   c. Hyperthermia and dysrhythmias
   d. Tremors, rigidity, and shuffling gait
4. An atypical antipsychotic is prescribed for a patient with psychosis. The nurse understands that this category of medications includes which drugs? **Select all that apply**.
   a. Clozapine
   b. Fluphenazine
   c. Haloperidol
   d. Olanzapine
   e. Aripiprazole
5. A patient is prescribed lorazepam. What does the nurse know to be true regarding lorazepam?
   a. It is used to treat anxiety, status epilepticus, insomnia, and sedation induction.
   b. It has a maximum adult dose of 25 mg/day.
   c. It causes plasma levels to be decreased when combined with cimetidine.
   d. It interferes with the binding of dopamine receptors.
6. A patient is receiving aripiprazole. Which nursing intervention(s) will the nurse include in the patient's care plan? **Select all that apply.**
   a. Administer before meals on an empty stomach to facilitate absorption.
   b. Remain with the patient until medication is swallowed.
   c. Monitor vital signs to detect orthostatic hypotension.
   d. Assess the patient for evidence of neuroleptic malignant syndrome.
   e. Observe the patient for acute dystonia, akathisia, and tardive dyskinesia.
7. A patient appears to have had an overdose of phenothiazines. The nurse anticipates that which intervention(s) may be used to treat phenothiazine overdose? **Select all that apply.**
   a. Gastric lavage
   b. Adequate hydration
   c. Maintaining an airway
   d. Fluphenazine
   e. Risperidone
   f. Activated charcoal administration

23

Antidepressants and Mood Stabilizers

http://evolve.elsevier.com/McCuistion/pharmacology

OBJECTIVES

- Explain the characteristics, contributing causes, and various types of depression.
- Contrast the five groups of antidepressants.
- Explain the use of mood stabilizers.

OUTLINE

Depression, 274
   Pathophysiology, 274
   Complementary and Alternative Therapy for Depression 275
Antidepressant Agents, 275
   Tricyclic Antidepressants, 275
   Selective Serotonin Reuptake Inhibitors, 275
   Serotonin-Norepinephrine Reuptake Inhibitors, 276
   Atypical Antidepressants, 277
   Monoamine Oxidase Inhibitors, 277
Mood Stabilizers, 277
   Lithium, 277
   Special Considerations for Lithium, 284
Clinical Judgment Case Study, 285
Review Questions, 285

Antidepressants are used for depressive episodes accompanied by feelings of hopelessness and helplessness. They can be prescribed for 1 month to 12 months or perhaps longer.

Mood-stabilizing agents such as lithium are effective for bipolar disorder. Drug therapy for treating bipolar disorder is discussed in this chapter.

DEPRESSION

Depression is the most common mental illness, affecting approximately 14.8 million Americans. Fewer than 50% of individuals with depression seek treatment despite the fact that about 70% of individuals with depression have a full remission with effective treatment. Females between the ages of 25 and 45 years are two to three times more likely than males to experience major depression. Depression is characterized primarily by mood changes and loss of interest in normal activities and is second only to hypertension as the most common chronic clinical condition.

Contributing causes of depression include genetic predisposition, social and environmental factors, and biologic conditions. Some signs of major depression include loss of interest in most activities, depressed mood, weight loss or gain, insomnia or hypersomnia, loss of energy, fatigue, feelings of despair, decreased ability to think or concentrate, and suicidal thoughts. Approximately 66% of all suicides are related to depression. Males with depression, especially older White males, are more likely to commit suicide successfully than females with depression. Antidepressants can mask suicidal ideation.

The three types of depression are (1) *reactive*, (2) *major*, and (3) *bipolar disorder*, previously referred to as *manic depression*. **Reactive depression** usually has a sudden onset after a precipitating event (e.g., depression resulting from a loss, such as death of a loved one). The patient knows why they are depressed and may call this "the blues." Usually, this type of depression lasts for months, and a benzodiazepine agent may be prescribed. *Major depression* is characterized by loss of interest in work and home, inability to concentrate and complete tasks, difficulty sleeping or excessive sleeping, feelings of fatigue and worthlessness, and deep depression, also known as **dysphoria**. Major depression can be either *primary* (unrelated to other health problems) or *secondary* to a health problem such as a physical or psychiatric disorder or drug use. Antidepressants have been effective in treating major depression. **Bipolar disorder** involves swings between two moods: manic (euphoric) and depressive (dysphoric). Lithium was originally the drug of choice for treating this type of disorder. Other mood stabilizers such as carbamazepine, valproic acid or divalproex, and lamotrigine are also currently first-line drugs of choice for bipolar disorder.

Pathophysiology

Many theories exist as to the cause of major depression. A common one suggests an insufficient amount of brain monoamine neurotransmitters (norepinephrine, serotonin, perhaps dopamine). It is thought that decreased levels of serotonin permit depression to occur, and decreased levels of norepinephrine cause depression. However, there can be other physiologic causes of depression, and social and environmental factors play a role.

Serotonin neurotransmission is associated with arousal and general activity levels of the central nervous system (CNS). Serotonin functions to regulate sleep, wakefulness, and mood as well as the delusions, hallucinations, and withdrawal of schizophrenia. Antidepressants block the reuptake of serotonin into the presynaptic neuron. A structurally specific drug is more likely to affect only the specific receptors for which it is intended and not the receptors specific for other neurochemicals, which would produce unintended effects. Selective serotonin reuptake inhibitor (SSRI) drugs are specific and generally produce fewer side effects in the treatment of depression than older antidepressants such as monoamine oxidase inhibitors (MAOIs).

Norepinephrine is associated with control of arousal, attention, vigilance, mood, affect, and anxiety. This neurotransmitter is involved with thinking, planning, and interpreting. Tricyclic antidepressants (TCAs) block the reuptake of norepinephrine into the presynaptic neuron and effectively treat depressive disorders. MAOIs inactivate norepinephrine, dopamine, and serotonin by inhibiting the MAO enzyme to relieve signs and symptoms of depression.

Faulty release, reuptake, or elimination of neurotransmitters may lead to an imbalance of neurotransmission and subsequent pathology. Disorders can then develop that can affect an individual's thoughts, feelings, and behaviors.

Complementary and Alternative Therapy for Depression

St. Johns wort and ginkgo biloba have been suggested for the management of mild depression, but these should not be taken along with prescription antidepression medications. St. Johns wort can decrease reuptake of the neurotransmitters serotonin, norepinephrine, and dopamine. The use of these and many complementary and alternative products should be discontinued 1 to 2 weeks before surgery. The patient should check with a health care provider regarding complementary and alternative therapies.

> **COMPLEMENTARY AND ALTERNATIVE THERAPIES**
>
> *Selective Serotonin Reuptake Inhibitors*
>
> - Feverfew may interfere with SSRI antidepressants such as fluoxetine.
> - St. Johns wort interacts with SSRIs, which may cause serotonin syndrome (dizziness, headache, sweating, and agitation).

ANTIDEPRESSANT AGENTS

Antidepressants are divided into five groups: (1) tricyclic antidepressants (TCAs), or tricyclics; (2) SSRIs; (3) serotonin-norepinephrine reuptake inhibitors (SNRIs); (4) atypical antidepressants that affect various neurotransmitters; and (5) MAOIs. TCAs and MAOIs were marketed in the late 1950s, and many of the SSRIs and atypical antidepressants were available in the 1980s. The SSRIs and SNRIs are popular antidepressants because they do not cause sedation, hypotension, anticholinergic effects, or cardiotoxicity as do many of the TCAs. However, users of SSRIs can experience sexual dysfunction, but this can be managed. With unpleasant side effects or lack of improvement, the patient is usually changed to another category of drug.

Tricyclic Antidepressants

Tricyclic antidepressants (TCAs) are used to treat major depression because they are effective and less expensive than SSRIs and other drugs. Imipramine was the first TCA marketed in the 1950s.

The action of TCAs is to block the uptake of the neurotransmitters norepinephrine and serotonin in the brain. The clinical response of TCAs occurs after 2 to 4 weeks of drug therapy. If there is no improvement after 2 to 4 weeks, the antidepressant is slowly withdrawn and another antidepressant is prescribed. *Polydrug therapy,* the practice of giving several antidepressants or antipsychotics together, should be avoided if possible because of potential serious side effects.

The effectiveness of TCAs in treating major depression is well documented. This group of drugs elevates mood, increases interest in daily living and activity, and decreases insomnia. For persons who are agitated and depressed, amitriptyline, doxepin, or trimipramine may be prescribed because of their highly sedative effect. TCAs are often given at night to minimize problems caused by their sedative action. When discontinuing TCAs, the drugs should be gradually decreased to avoid withdrawal symptoms such as nausea, vomiting, anxiety, and akathisia. Imipramine hydrochloride is used for the treatment of enuresis (involuntary discharge of urine during sleep in children).

The TCA drugs include amitriptyline, imipramine, trimipramine, doxepin, desipramine, mirtazapine, nortriptyline, and protriptyline. The TCA drugs desipramine and nortriptyline are major metabolites of imipramine and amitriptyline.

Pharmacokinetics

Amitriptyline is strongly protein bound. The half-life is 10 to 50 hours, and a cumulative drug effect may result. Amitriptyline is primarily excreted in urine.

Pharmacodynamics

Amitriptyline is well absorbed, but antidepressant effects develop slowly over several weeks. The onset of the antidepressant effect of amitriptyline is 1 to 3 weeks, and the peak concentration is 2 to 5 hours. Drug doses are decreased for older patients to reduce side effects.

Side Effects and Adverse Reactions

The TCAs have many side effects: orthostatic hypotension, sedation, anticholinergic effects, cardiotoxicity, and seizures. Rising from a sitting position too rapidly can cause dizziness and lightheadedness *(orthostatic hypotension)*, so the patient should be instructed to rise slowly to an upright position. The TCAs block the histamine receptors; thus sedation is likely to occur initially but decreases with continuous use of the drug. Because TCAs block the cholinergic receptors, they can cause anticholinergic effects such as tachycardia, urinary retention, constipation, dry mouth, and blurred vision. Other side effects of TCAs include allergic reactions (skin rash, pruritus, and weight gain), sexual dysfunction (erectile dysfunction, ejaculatory dysfunction), and suicidal ideation. Most TCAs can cause blood dyscrasias (leukopenia, neutropenia, thrombocytopenia, and agranulocytosis) that require close monitoring of blood cell counts. Amitriptyline may lead to symptoms of extrapyramidal syndrome (EPS) and neuroleptic malignant syndrome (NMS). Because the seizure threshold is decreased by TCAs, patients with seizure disorders may need TCA dose adjustment. The most serious adverse reaction to TCAs is cardiotoxicity, such as dysrhythmias that may result from high doses of the drug. The therapeutic serum range of TCAs should be monitored.

Drug Interactions

Alcohol, hypnotics, sedatives, and barbiturates potentiate CNS depression when taken with TCAs. Concurrent use of MAOIs with amitriptyline may lead to cardiovascular instability and toxic psychosis. Antithyroid medications taken with amitriptyline may increase the risk of dysrhythmias.

Selective Serotonin Reuptake Inhibitors

SSRIs block the reuptake of serotonin into the nerve terminal of the CNS, thereby enhancing its transmission at the serotonergic synapse. These drugs do *not* block the uptake of dopamine or norepinephrine, and they do *not* block cholinergic and alpha$_1$-adrenergic receptors. SSRIs are more commonly used to treat depression than TCAs, and they have fewer side effects than TCAs.

The primary use of SSRIs is for major depressive disorders. They are also effective for treating anxiety disorders such as obsessive-compulsive disorder (OCD), panic disorders, phobias, posttraumatic stress disorder, and other forms of anxiety. Fluvoxamine is useful for treating OCD in children and adults. SSRIs have also been used to treat eating disorders and selected drug abuses. Miscellaneous uses for SSRIs include decreasing premenstrual tension syndrome, preventing migraine headaches, and preventing or minimizing aggressive behavior in patients with borderline personality disorder.

The SSRIs include fluoxetine, sertraline, paroxetine, citalopram, and escitalopram. Fluoxetine has been effective in 50% to 60% of patients who fail to respond to TCA therapy (*TCA-refractory depression*). The US Food and Drug Administration approved a weekly delayed-release fluoxetine dose of 90 mg. However, before taking the weekly dose, the patient should respond to a daily maintenance dose of 20 mg/day without serious effects.

Many SSRIs have an interaction with grapefruit juice that can lead to possible toxicity. It is recommended that daily intake be limited to 8 ounces of grapefruit juice or one-half of a grapefruit.

Prototype Drug Chart: Fluoxetine describes the drug characteristics of the SSRI fluoxetine.

Pharmacokinetics

Fluoxetine is strongly protein bound, and the half-life is 4 to 6 days; therefore a cumulative drug effect may result from long-term use. Fluoxetine is metabolized and excreted by the kidneys.

Pharmacodynamics

Fluoxetine is well absorbed; however, its antidepressant effect develops slowly over several weeks. The onset of fluoxetine's initial antidepressant effect is between 3 and 4 weeks, and peak concentration with consistent therapy is at 6 to 8 hours after ingestion. The drug dose for older adults should be decreased to reduce side effects.

Side Effects and Adverse Reactions

Fluoxetine produces common side effects such as dry mouth, weakness, insomnia, headache, anorexia, nausea, diarrhea, and suicidal ideation. Fluoxetine has fewer side effects than amitriptyline.

Some patients may experience sexual dysfunction when taking SSRIs. Males have discontinued taking fluoxetine after experiencing a decrease in sexual arousal. Some females have become anorgasmic, whereas males reported erectile dysfunction and delayed ejaculation when taking paroxetine HCl. The side effects often decrease or cease over the 1- to 4-week period of waiting for the therapeutic effect to emerge.

Serotonin-Norepinephrine Reuptake Inhibitors

SNRIs inhibit the reuptake of serotonin and norepinephrine, increasing availability in the synapse. SNRIs are used for major depression. Other approved uses are for generalized anxiety disorder and social

PROTOTYPE DRUG CHART

Fluoxetine

Drug Class	Dosage
Antidepressant: Selective serotonin reuptake inhibitor	Depression: Immediate release: A: PO: Initially 20 mg/d in the morning; *max:* 80 mg/d Delayed release: A: PO: 90 once weekly; *max:* 90 mg/wk
Contraindications	**Drug-Lab-Food Interactions**
Hypersensitivity, MAOI therapy *Caution:* Dehydration, bipolar, stroke, cardiac disease, bradycardia, thyroid disease, dysrhythmias, hepatic disease, celiac disease, glaucoma, seizures, diabetes mellitus, anticoagulant therapy, anorexia nervosa, diarrhea, electrolyte imbalance, hyperparathyroidism, rheumatoid arthritis, osteoporosis, suicidal ideation, abrupt discontinuation, older adults, children, pregnancy, breast feeding	Drug: Increased effects of CNS and respiratory depression, hypotensive effect with alcohol and CNS depressants; increased bleeding potential with aspirin, NSAIDs, and anticoagulants; MAOIs and SSRIs increase risk of serotonin syndrome. Complementary and alternative therapy: St. Johns wort increases risk for serotonin syndrome; increased effect of hypoglycemics
Pharmacokinetics	**Pharmacodynamics**
Absorption: PO: well absorbed Distribution: PB: 94.5% Metabolism: Fluoxetine: t½: 4–6 d Excretion: Excreted primarily in urine	PO: Onset: 3–4 wk initially Peak: 6–8 h Duration: UK
Therapeutic Effects/Uses	
To treat depression, bipolar disorder, bulimia disorder, obsessive-compulsive disorder, panic disorder, and premenstrual dysphoric disorder Mechanism of Action: Serotonin action is enhanced in nerve cells because of selective serotonin reuptake blockade at neuronal membranes.	
Side Effects	**Adverse Reactions**
Headache, dizziness, drowsiness, yawning, insomnia, anxiety, weakness, abnormal dreams, tremors, hyperhidrosis, rash, urticaria, pharyngitis, dry mouth, anorexia, dyspepsia, nausea, diarrhea, constipation, peripheral edema, akathisia, urinary retention, erectile/ejaculatory dysfunction	Seizures, angioedema, hypo/hyperkalemia, hyponatremia, hypocalcemia, dehydration, gastrointestinal bleeding/obstruction, osteoporosis, bone fractures, tachycardia, orthostatic hypotension, hypertension, dysrhythmias, hearing loss, diabetes mellitus, hypo/hyperglycemia *Life-threatening:* Stevens-Johnson syndrome, hepatic/renal failure, thrombocytopenia, leukopenia, serotonin syndrome, stroke, suicidal ideation

A, Adult; *CNS*, central nervous system; *d*, day; *MAOI*, monoamine oxidase inhibitor; *max*, maximum; *NSAID*, nonsteroidal antiinflammatory drug; *PB*, protein binding; *PO*, by mouth; *SSRI*, selective serotonin reuptake inhibitor; *t½*, half-life; *UK*, unknown; *wk*, week.

anxiety disorder. Other SNRIs include duloxetine, levomilnacipran, and desvenlafaxine.

Side Effects and Adverse Effects
Side effects for this classification include drowsiness, dizziness, insomnia, headache, amnesia, blurred vision, hyperhidrosis, nausea, diarrhea, and erectile/ejaculation dysfunction. Adverse effects of this drug are hypertension, orthostatic hypotension, tachycardia, palpitations, seizures, serotonin syndrome, Stevens-Johnson syndrome, and suicidal ideation.

Atypical Antidepressants
Atypical antidepressants, or *second-generation antidepressants*, became available in the 1980s and have been used for major depression, reactive depression, and anxiety. They affect one or two of the three neurotransmitters: serotonin, norepinephrine, and dopamine. One of the first atypical antidepressants marketed was amoxapine; another atypical antidepressant drug is maprotiline.

Maprotiline is sometimes considered to be aTCA because of their pharmacologic similarities. Atypical antidepressants should *not* be taken with MAOIs and should not be used within 14 days after discontinuing MAOIs.

Side Effects and Adverse Effects
Side effects for atypical antidepressants include dizziness, drowsiness, dry mouth, constipation, orthostatic hypotension, tachycardia, palpitations, and erectile/ejaculatory dysfunction. Adverse effects include seizures.

Monoamine Oxidase Inhibitors
Another group of antidepressants is the *monoamine oxidase inhibitors (MAOIs)*. The enzyme MAO inactivates norepinephrine, dopamine, epinephrine, and serotonin. By inhibiting MAO, the levels of these neurotransmitters rise. Two forms of MAO enzyme exist in the body: MAO-A and MAO-B. These enzymes are found primarily in the liver and brain. MAO-A inactivates dopamine in the brain, whereas MAO-B inactivates norepinephrine and serotonin. The MAOIs are nonselective and inhibit both MAO-A and MAO-B. Inhibition of MAO by MAOIs is thought to relieve the symptoms of depression. Four MAOIs are currently prescribed: (1) tranylcypromine sulfate, (2) isocarboxazid, (3) selegiline HCl, and (4) phenelzine sulfate. These MAOIs are detailed in Table 23.1.

For the treatment of depression, MAOIs are as effective as TCAs; however, because of adverse reactions, such as the risk of hypertensive crisis resulting from food and drug interactions, only 1% of patients who take antidepressants take an MAOI. Currently, MAOIs are not the antidepressants of choice and are usually prescribed when the patient does not respond to TCAs or second-generation antidepressants. However, MAOIs are still used for mild, reactive, and atypical depression (chronic anxiety, hypersomnia, fear). MAOIs and TCAs should not be taken together when treating depression.

Drug and Food Interactions
Certain drug and food interactions with MAOIs can be fatal. Any drugs that are CNS stimulants or sympathomimetics, such as vasoconstrictors and cold medications that contain phenylephrine and pseudoephedrine, can cause a hypertensive crisis when taken with an MAOI. In addition, foods that contain tyramine—aged cheese (cheddar, Swiss, bleu), cream, yogurt, coffee, chocolate, bananas, raisins, Italian green beans, liver, pickled foods, sausage, soy sauce, yeast, beer, and red wines—have sympathomimetic-like effects and can cause a hypertensive crisis. MAOI users *must avoid* these types of food and drugs. Frequent blood pressure monitoring is essential, and patient teaching regarding foods and over-the-counter (OTC) drugs to avoid is an important nursing responsibility. Because of the danger associated with hypertensive crisis, many psychiatrists will not prescribe MAOIs for depression unless other drugs have failed to be effective for the patient. However, this group of drugs is effective for treating depression if taken properly.

> ### COMPLEMENTARY AND ALTERNATIVE THERAPIES
> #### Monoamine Oxidase Inhibitors
>
> - Ginseng, ephedra (ma-huang), and St. Johns wort may lead to palpitations, heart attack, and hypertensive crisis when taken with antidepressant MAOIs.
> - Ginseng may lead to manic episodes when taken in combination with MAOIs such as tranylcypromine sulfate.
> - An excessive dose of anise may interfere with MAOIs.
> - An increased use of brewer's yeast with MAOIs can increase blood pressure.

In teaching patients about the foods and drugs to avoid when taking MAOIs, some individuals respond better to verbal instructions and education with reinforcement from videos than to printed communications. Complementary and Alternative Therapies: Monoamine Oxidase Inhibitors details complementary and alternative therapy interactions with MAOIs.

Side Effects and Adverse Reactions
Side effects of MAOIs include dizziness, drowsiness, headache, insomnia, dry mouth, nausea, diarrhea, weight gain, erectile/ejaculation dysfunction, peripheral edema, orthostatic hypotension, hypertension, tachycardia, and palpitations. Adverse effects of MAOIs include serotonin syndrome, EPS, and suicidal ideation.

MOOD STABILIZERS
Mood stabilizers are used to treat bipolar affective disorder. These drugs can aid in the reduction of mood swings and relieve acute manic and depressive occurrences. Lithium, carbamazepine, valproic acid or divalproex, lamotrigine, cariprazine, and aripiprazole are currently first-line drugs for bipolar disorder.

Lithium
Lithium was the first drug used to manage this disorder. Some refer to lithium as an *antimania drug* effective in controlling manic behavior that arises from underlying bipolar disorder. Lithium has a calming effect but may cause some memory loss and confusion. It controls any evidence of flight of ideas and hyperactivity. If the person stops taking lithium, manic behavior may return.

Lithium is an inexpensive drug that must be closely monitored, and it has a narrow therapeutic serum range of 0.8 to 1.2 mEq/L. Serum lithium levels greater than 1.5 mEq/L may produce early signs of toxicity. The serum lithium level should be monitored biweekly until the therapeutic level has been obtained, and then it must be monitored at least every 1 to 2 months on the maintenance dose. Serum sodium levels also need to be monitored because lithium tends to deplete sodium.

◎ CLINICAL JUDGMENT [NURSING PROCESS]
Antidepressants

Concept: Mood and Affect
- A conscious state of mind or feeling

Recognize Cues [Assessment]
- Assess the patient's baseline vital signs and weight for future comparisons. Tricyclic antidepressants (TCAs) should be avoided in patients with cardiovascular disease and hypertension and should be used cautiously in patients with seizure disorders.
- Note the patient's hepatic and renal function by assessing urine output (>1500 mL/day), blood urea nitrogen (BUN), and serum creatinine and hepatic enzyme levels.
- Obtain a health history of episodes of depression; assess mental status, and assess for suicidal tendencies.
- Secure a drug history of the current drugs, alcohol, and herbs the patient is taking. CNS depressants can cause an additive effect. Antidepressants that cause anticholinergic-like symptoms are contraindicated if a patient has glaucoma.
- Assess for tardive dyskinesia and neuroleptic malignant syndrome (NMS), including hyperpyrexia, muscle rigidity, tachycardia, and cardiac dysrhythmias.

Analyze Cues and Prioritize Hypothesis [Patient Problems]
- Confusion
- Anxiety
- Hopelessness
- Decreased ability to cope
- Social isolation

Generate Solutions [Planning]
- Patient will display a calmer attitude.
- Patient will cope with at least one current issue.
- Patient will interact with others.

Take Action [Nursing Interventions]
- Observe patients for signs and symptoms of depression: mood changes, insomnia, apathy, or lack of interest in activities.
- Monitor vital signs. Orthostatic hypotension is common. Check for anticholinergic-like symptoms such as dry mouth, increased heart rate, urinary retention, and constipation. Check weight two to three times per week.
- ⚡ Monitor patients for suicidal tendencies when marked depression is present.
- Observe patients for seizures when anticonvulsants are taken; antidepressants lower the seizure threshold, and the anticonvulsant dose might need to be increased.
- ⚡ Monitor for drug-drug and drug-food interactions. Sympathomimetic-like drugs and foods that contain tyramine may cause a hypertensive crisis if taken with MAOIs.
- Check patients for extremely high blood pressure when taking MAOIs.
- Provide patients with a list of foods to avoid when taking MAOIs to avoid hypertensive crisis. These foods include cheese, red wine, beer, liver, bananas, yogurt, and sausage.

Patient Teaching
General
- Teach patients to take the medication as prescribed. Compliance is important.
- Inform patients that full effectiveness of a drug may not be evident until 1 to 2 weeks after the start of therapy.
- Encourage patients to keep medical appointments.
- Caution patients not to consume alcohol or any CNS depressants because of their addictive effect.
- ⚡ Inform patients that many complementary and alternative therapy products interact with antidepressants, especially MAOIs and SSRIs. Complementary and alternative therapies may need to be discontinued, or the antidepressant drug dosage may need to be modified (see Complementary and Alternative Therapies: Selective Serotonin Reuptake Inhibitors and Monoamine Oxidase Inhibitors).
- ⚡ Warn patients not to drive or be involved in potentially dangerous mechanical activity until stabilization of the drug dose has been established.
- Advise patients not to abruptly stop taking the drug. A health care provider should gradually decrease the drug dose.
- Encourage patients planning pregnancy to consult with a health care provider about possible teratogenic effects of the drug on the fetus.
- Advise patients to take the drug with food if gastrointestinal (GI) distress occurs.

Side Effects
- Advise patients that antidepressants may be taken at bedtime to decrease dangers from the sedative effect, and suggest they check with a health care provider. Transient side effects include nausea, drowsiness, headaches, and nervousness.

Evaluate Outcomes [Evaluation]
- Evaluate the effectiveness of the drug therapy regarding whether a patient's depression is controlled or has ceased.

TABLE 23.1 Antidepressants

Drug	Route and Dosage	Uses and Considerations
Tricyclic Antidepressants (TCAs)		
Amitriptyline hydrochloride	A: PO: Initially 75–100 mg/d for inpatients; 50–100 mg/d for outpatients; both in divided doses; *max:* 300 mg/d for inpatients, 150 mg/d for outpatients Older A: PO: 10 mg tid with 20 mg at hs; *max:* 150 mg/d for outpatients Therapeutic serum range: 120–150 ng/mL	For depression. May cause drowsiness, dizziness, orthostatic hypotension, blurred vision, memory impairment, insomnia, dry mouth, hyperhidrosis, constipation, nausea, weight gain, lethargy, tremor, weakness, and EPS. PB: 95%; t½: 10–50 h
Desipramine hydrochloride	A: PO: 100–200 mg/day or in divided doses; *max:* 300 mg/d for inpatients, 200 mg/d for outpatients Older A: PO: 25–100 mg/day; *max:* 150 mg/day Therapeutic serum range: 125–300 ng/mL	For depression. May cause dizziness, drowsiness, headache, blurred vision, tremor, dry mouth, dyspepsia, nausea, constipation, orthostatic hypotension, weight gain, erectile/ejaculation dysfunction, and withdrawal. PB: 90%; t½: 7–60 h
Doxepin hydrochloride	A: PO: Initially 75 mg/d at bedtime; or in 2–3 divided doses; *maint:* 75–150 mg/d; *max:* 300 mg/d Therapeutic serum range: 50–150 ng/mL	For insomnia, depression and anxiety. May cause dizziness, drowsiness, blurred vision, orthostatic hypotension, dyspepsia, dry mouth, constipation, lethargy, urinary retention, erectile/ejaculatory dysfunction, weight gain, withdrawal, and skin irritation. PB: 80%; t½: 6–8 h
Imipramine hydrochloride	A: PO: Initially 75 mg/d for outpatients and 100 mg/d in divided doses for inpatients; *maint:* 50–150 mg/d for outpatients; *max:* 200 mg/d for outpatients, 300 mg/d for inpatients Older A: Initially 30–40 mg/d at bedtime; *max:* 100 mg/d Therapeutic serum range: 125–250 ng/mL	For depression. May cause dizziness, drowsiness, headache, blurred vision, fatigue, dry mouth, dyspepsia, nausea, constipation, orthostatic hypotension, tremor, urinary retention, weight gain, withdrawal, and erectile/ejaculatory dysfunction. PB: 85–95%; t½: 8–16 h
Mirtazapine	A: PO: Initially 15 mg at bedtime; *maint:* 15–45 mg/d; *max:* 45 mg/d	For depression. May cause dizziness, drowsiness, weakness, abnormal dreams, appetite stimulation, dry mouth, constipation, hypercholesterolemia, weight gain, and hypertriglyceridemia. PB: 85%; t½: 20–40 h
Nortriptyline hydrochloride	A: PO: Initially 25 mg tid/qid; *max:* 150 mg/d Older A: PO: 30–50 mg/d or in divided doses; *max:* 50 mg/d Therapeutic serum range: 50–150 ng/mL	For depression. May cause dizziness, drowsiness, headache, fatigue, blurred vision, weight gain, dry mouth, dyspepsia, nausea, vomiting, constipation, appetite stimulation, erectile/ejaculatory dysfunction, withdrawal, and tremor. PB: 93%–95%; t½: 16–90 h
Protriptyline hydrochloride	A: PO: Initially 5–10 mg tid/qid; *max:* 60 mg/d Older A: PO: Initially 5 mg tid; *max:* 30 mg/d Therapeutic serum range: 70–250 ng/mL	For depression. May cause dizziness, drowsiness, headache, blurred vision, insomnia, tremor, dysarthria, dry mouth, erectile/ejaculatory dysfunction, dyspepsia, nausea, vomiting, constipation, and withdrawal. PB: 90%; t½: 54–92 h
Trimipramine maleate	A: Initially 75 mg/d in divided doses for outpatients, 100 mg for inpatients; *max:* 200 mg/d for outpatients, 300 mg/d for inpatients Older A: Initially 50 mg/d in divided doses; *max:* 100 mg/d Therapeutic serum range: 150–300 ng/mL	For depression. May cause dizziness, drowsiness, fatigue, tremor, headache, dry mouth, appetite stimulation, dyspepsia, nausea, constipation, weight gain, erectile/ejaculatory dysfunction, and withdrawal. PB: 95%; t½: 20–26 h
Selective Serotonin Reuptake Inhibitors (SSRIs)		
Citalopram	A: <60 y: PO: Initially 20 mg/day, may increase after 1 wk; *max:* 40 mg/day A >60 y: PO: 20 mg/d; *max:* 20 mg/d	For depression. May cause drowsiness, insomnia, dry mouth, hyperhidrosis, nausea, diarrhea, tremor, ejaculation dysfunction, and dyspepsia. PB: 80%; t½: 35 h
Fluoxetine hydrochloride	See Prototype Drug Chart: Fluoxetine	
Paroxetine hydrochloride	Depression: Immediate-release tablets: A: PO: Initially 20 mg/d in a.m.; *max:* 60 mg/d Older A: PO: Initially 10 mg/d; *max:* 40 mg/d Controlled-release tablets: A: PO: Initially 25 mg/d in a.m.; *max:* 75 mg/d Older A: PO: Initially 12.5 mg/d; *max:* 50 mg/d	For depression, general anxiety disorder, social anxiety disorder, panic disorder, PTSD, and OCD. May cause dizziness, drowsiness, insomnia, headache, asthenia, hyperhidrosis, dry mouth, nausea, constipation, diarrhea, tremors, and erectile/ejaculatory dysfunction. PB: 93%–95%; t½: 21 h for immediate release, 15–20 h for controlled release

Continued

TABLE 23.1 Antidepressants—cont'd

Drug	Route and Dosage	Uses and Considerations
Sertraline hydrochloride	Depression: A: PO: Initially 50 mg/d; max: 200 mg/d	For depression, OCD, PTSD, panic disorder, social anxiety disorder. May cause dizziness, drowsiness, agitation, insomnia, fatigue, hyperhidrosis, tremor, dry mouth, erectile/ejaculatory dysfunction, dyspepsia, nausea, constipation, and diarrhea. PB: 98%; t½: 26 h
Escitalopram	Depression: A: PO: Initially 10 mg/d, may increase to 20 mg/d after 1 wk; max: 20 mg/d Older A: PO: 10 mg/d; max: 10 mg/d	For depression and generalized anxiety disorder. May cause drowsiness, dizziness, fatigue, headache, insomnia, dry mouth, nausea, diarrhea, constipation, hyperhidrosis, and erectile/ejaculation dysfunction. PB: 56%; t½: 27–32 h
Atypical (Second-Generation) Antidepressants		
Amoxapine	A: PO: Initially 50 mg bid/tid; max: 400 mg/d for outpatients, 600 mg/d for inpatients Older A: PO: 25 mg bid/tid; max: 300 mg/d Therapeutic serum range is 200–400 ng/mL	For depression. May cause drowsiness, blurred vision, dry mouth, constipation, orthostatic hypo/hypertension, palpitations, tachycardia, edema, and erectile/ejaculatory dysfunction. PB: 90%; t½: 8 h
Maprotiline hydrochloride	A <60 y: PO: Initially 25–75 mg/d in divided doses for outpatients, 100–150 mg/d for inpatients; max: 225 mg/d Older A: Initially 25 mg/d; max: 150 mg/d	For depression. May cause dizziness, drowsiness, blurred vision, headache, confusion, dry mouth, constipation, tachycardia, palpitations, seizures, urinary retention, fatigue, ataxia, and erectile dysfunction. PB: 88%; t½: 51 h
Aminoketone Antidepressants		
Bupropion hydrochloride	Depression: Immediate release: A: PO: Initially 100 mg bid; max: 450 mg/d, 150 mg/dose Sustained release: A: PO: Initially 150 mg/d in the morning; maint: 200 mg bid; max: 400 mg/d, 200 mg single dose Extended release: A: PO: 150 mg/d in the morning; max: 450 mg/d	For depression, seasonal affective disorder, and tobacco cessation. May cause dizziness, blurred vision, insomnia, headache, dry mouth, anorexia, nausea, vomiting, constipation, hyperhidrosis, agitation, tachycardia, weight gain/loss, tremor, and erectile/ejaculatory dysfunction. PB: 84%; t½: 8–24 h immediate release, 21 h sustained and extended release
Miscellaneous Antidepressants		
Mirtazapine	Initially 15 mg at bedtime; max: 45 mg/d	For depression. May cause dizziness, drowsiness, weakness, abnormal dreams, appetite stimulation, dry mouth, constipation, hypercholesterolemia, weight gain, hypertriglyceridemia, and erectile/ejaculatory dysfunction. PB: 85%; t½: 20–40 h
Esketamine	A: Nasal spray: 56 mg Day 1; 56 or 84 mg 2 times/wk during wk 1–4; 56 or 84 mg/once a week during wk 5–8; thereafter 56 or 84 mg q1wk or q2wk; max: 84 mg 2 times/wk in induction phase, 84 mg/wk in maintenance phase	For treatment-resistant depression in addition to an oral antidepressant. May cause dizziness, drowsiness, dissociation, headache, anxiety, lethargy, hypoesthesia, hypertension, nausea, vomiting, dysgeusia, constipation. PB: insignificant; t½: 7–12 h
Vilazodone	A: PO: Initially 10 mg/d for 1 wk; maint: 20–40 mg/d with food; max: 40 mg/d	For depression. May cause drowsiness, dizziness, blurred vision, abnormal dreams, fatigue, insomnia, headache, dry mouth, dyspepsia, nausea, vomiting, diarrhea, and erectile/ejaculatory dysfunction. PB: 96%–99%; t½: 25 h
Nefazodone	A: PO: Initially 50–100 mg bid; maint: 300–600 mg/d in 2 divided doses; max: 600 mg/d Older A: Initially 50 mg bid; maint: 300–600 mg/d in 2 divided doses; max: 600 mg/d	For depression. May cause headache, drowsiness, dizziness, confusion, insomnia, blurred vision, scotomata, dry mouth, weakness, infection, nausea, diarrhea, and constipation. PB: 99%; t½: 2–4 h
Trazodone hydrochloride	Immediate release: A: PO: Initially 150 mg/d in divided doses; max: 400 mg/d for outpatients, 600 mg/d for inpatients Extended release: A: PO: Initially 150 mg/d at bedtime, max: 375 mg/d	For depression. May cause drowsiness, dizziness, blurred vision, headache, fatigue, insomnia, tachycardia, palpitations, dry mouth, nausea, vomiting, constipation, diarrhea, and hypo/hypertension. PB: 89%–95%; t½: 10 h

TABLE 23.1 Antidepressants—cont'd

Drug	Route and Dosage	Uses and Considerations
Vortioxetine	A: PO: Initially 5–10 mg/d; *maint:* 5–20 mg/d; *max:* 20 mg/d	For depression. May cause dizziness, dry mouth, nausea, vomiting, diarrhea, constipation, and orgasm/erectile/ejaculatory dysfunction. PB: 98%; t½: 66 h
Gepirone	A: PO: Initially 18.2 mg/d, on day 4 may increase to 36.3 mg/d, on day 7 may increase to 54.5 mg/d, on day 14 may increase to 72.6 mg/d; *max:* 72.6 mg/d	For major depression. May cause headache, dizziness, insomnia, fatigue, nausea, vomiting, diarrhea, abdominal pain dyspepsia, and dry mouth. Give with food. PB: 72%; t1/2: 5 h
Dextromethorphan, bupropion	A: PO: Initially 45 mg destromethorphan/105 mg bupropion daily, day 4 increase to bid; *max:* 90 mg/210 mg/d	For major depression. May cause headache, drowsiness, dizziness, anorexia, nausea, diarrhea, hyperhidrosis, and orgasm/erectile dysfunction. PB: dextromethorphan 60-70%, bupropion 84%; t1/2: dextromethorphan 22 h, bupropion 15 h
Serotonin-Norepinephrine Reuptake Inhibitors (SNRIs)		
Desvenlafaxine	A: PO: Initially 50 mg/d; *max:* 400 mg/d	For depression. May cause dizziness, drowsiness, fatigue, insomnia, hyperhidrosis, dry mouth, anorexia, nausea, vomiting, constipation, hypercholesterolemia, orthostatic hypotension, tremor, proteinuria, orgasm dysfunction, withdrawal, and erectile/ejaculatory dysfunction. PB: 30%; t½: 9–15 h
Duloxetine	Depression: A: PO: Initially 20–30 mg/bid or 60 mg daily; *max:* 120 mg/d	For major depression, diabetic neuropathy, fibromyalgia, generalized anxiety disorder, and chronic musculoskeletal pain. May cause dizziness, drowsiness, headache, insomnia, fatigue, weakness, dry mouth, anorexia, abdominal pain, nausea, constipation, weight loss, and erectile/ejaculatory dysfunction. PB: >90%; t½: 8–17 h
Levomilnacipran	A: PO: Initially 20 mg/d for 2 d, then 40 mg/d; *maint:* 40–120 mg/d; *max:* 120 mg/d	For depression. May cause orthostatic hypotension, hyperhidrosis, nausea, vomiting, constipation, tachycardia, erectile/ejaculatory dysfunction, urinary retention, and palpitations. PB: 22%; t½: 12 h
Monoamine Oxidase Inhibitors (MAOIs)		
Isocarboxazid	A: PO: Initially 10 mg bid; *max:* 60 mg/d	For depression. May cause dizziness, headache, insomnia, dry mouth, nausea, constipation, weight gain, withdrawal, elevated hepatic enzymes, and erectile/ejaculatory dysfunction. PB: UK; t½: 2.5 h
Phenelzine sulfate	A: PO: Initially 15 mg tid; *max:* 90 mg/d	For depression. May cause dizziness, drowsiness, headache, insomnia, blurred vision, hyperhidrosis, dry mouth, constipation, weight gain, elevated hepatic enzymes, withdrawal, peripheral edema, and erectile/ejaculation dysfunction. PB: UK; t½: 12 h
Tranylcypromine sulfate	A: PO: Initially 15 mg bid; *max:* 60 mg/d	For treatment-resistant depression. May cause dizziness, drowsiness, insomnia, constipation, orthostatic hypotension, peripheral edema, dry mouth, diarrhea, weight gain, erectile/ejaculatory dysfunction, and withdrawal. PB: UK; t½: 2.5 h
Selegiline hydrochloride	Depression: A: Transdermal: Initially 6 mg patch/d; *max:* 12 mg patch/d	For depression and parkinsonism. May cause dizziness, headache, confusion, insomnia, rhinitis, dry mouth, abdominal pain, nausea, diarrhea, orthostatic hypotension, dyskinesia, and hallucinations. PB: 85%–90%; t½: 1.3–2 h

Continued

TABLE 23.1 Antidepressants—cont'd

Drug	Route and Dosage	Uses and Considerations
Mood Stabilizers		
Lithium citrate	See Prototype Drug Chart: Lithium	
Carbamazepine	Bipolar disorder: Immediate release: A: PO: Initially 200 mg bid; *max:* 1600 mg/d in 3–4 divided doses Extended-release capsule: A: PO: Initially 200 mg bid; *max:* 1600 mg/d in 2 divided doses Therapeutic serum level: 4–12 mcg/mL	For bipolar disorder, seizures, and neuropathic pain. May cause dizziness, drowsiness, blurred vision, weakness, ataxia, oligospermia, rash, pruritus, dry mouth, nausea, vomiting, and constipation. PB: 76%; t½: 25–65 h
Valproic acid, divalproex	Bipolar disorder: Delayed release: A: PO: Initially 750 mg/d in 2–3 divided doses; *max:* 60 mg/kg/d Extended release: A: PO: Initially 25 mg/kg/d; *max:* 60 mg/kg/d Therapeutic range: 50–125 mcg/mL	For bipolar disorder, seizures, and migraine prophylaxis. May cause dizziness, drowsiness, insomnia, weakness, diplopia, abdominal pain, dyspepsia, anorexia, nausea, vomiting, diarrhea, weakness, thrombocytopenia, oligomenorrhea, and suicidal ideation. PB: 90%; t½: 9–16 h
Lamotrigine	Bipolar disorder: A: PO: Initially 25 mg/d for 2 wk, then 50 mg/d for 2 wk, then 100 mg/d for 1 wk; thereafter give 200 mg/d	For bipolar disorder, seizures, and Lennox-Gastaut syndrome. May cause dizziness, drowsiness, blurred vision, diplopia, fever, rash, pharyngitis, nausea, vomiting, diarrhea, abdominal/back pain, tremor, and ataxia. PB: 55%; t½: 14–59 h
Cariprazine	Bipolar depression: A: PO: Initially 1.5 mg/d; *max:* 3 mg/d	For bipolar disorder, major depression, and schizophrenia. May cause dizziness, drowsiness, fatigue, headache, insomnia, dyspepsia, vomiting, weight gain, nausea, constipation, restlessness, akathisia, and EPS. PB: 91%–97%; t½: 2–4 d
Aripiprazole	Bipolar disorder: Immediate release: A: PO: Initially 10–15 mg/d; *max:* 30 mg/d Extended-release maintenance: A: IM: 400 mg/month while continuing PO for 14 d, then may reduce to 300 mg/month Extended-release Asimtufii: A: IM: 960 mg q2months, then may reduce to 720 mg q2months	For bipolar disorder, schizophrenia, autism, depression, and Tourette syndrome. May cause drowsiness, dizziness, headache, anxiety, agitation, insomnia, nausea, vomiting, constipation, weight gain, fatigue, hyperglycemia, tremor, akathisia, skin irritation, and blurred vision. PB: 99%; t½: 75 h immediate release, 30–47 d extended release
Olanzapine and samidorphan	Bipolar disorder: A: PO: Initially 10 mg olanzapine/10 mg samidorphan/d or 15 mg olanzapine/10 mg samidorphan/d; *maint:* 5–20 mg olanzapine/10 mg samidorphan/d; *max:* 20 mg olanzapine/10 mg samidorphan/d	For bipolar disorder and schizophrenia. May cause hyperprolactinemia, weight gain, hyperglycemia, dizziness, drowsiness, hypertriglyceridemia, dry mouth, weakness, elevated hepatic enzymes, hypercholesterolemia, and appetite stimulation. PB: Olanzapine 93%, samidorphan 23%–33%; t½: olanzapine 35–52 h, samidorphan 7–11 h
Dexmedetomidine	Mild/moderate agitation: A: SL/buccal: 120 mcg, if agitation persists give 2 more doses of 60 mcg/dose 2 h apart; *max:* 240 mcg/d Severe agitation: A: SL/buccal: 180 mcg, if agitation persists give 2 more doses of 90 mcg/dose 2 h apart; *max:* 360 mcg/d	For agitation associated with bipolar disorders or schizophrenia. May cause drowsiness, agitation, brady/tachycardia, hypo/hypertension, nausea, constipation, and respiratory depression. Do not eat/drink for 15 min after SL dose or 1 h after buccal dose. PB: 94%; t½: 2.8 h

A, Adult; *bid*, twice a day; *CNS*, central nervous system; *d*, day; *EPS*, extrapyramidal syndrome symptoms; *FDA*, Food and Drug Administration; *GI*, gastrointestinal; *h*, hour; *maint*, maintenance; *MAOI*, monoamine oxidase inhibitor; *max*, maximum; *OCD*, obsessive-compulsive disorder; *PB*, protein binding; *PO*, by mouth; *PTSD*, posttraumatic stress disorder; *qid*, four times a day; *t½*, half-life; *tid*, three times a day; *TCA*, tricyclic antidepressant; *UK*, unknown; *wk*, week(s); *y*, year.

Lithium must be used with caution, if at all, by patients taking diuretics. Prototype Drug Chart: Lithium lists the pharmacologic behavior of lithium.

Pharmacokinetics

More than 95% of lithium is absorbed through the gastrointestinal (GI) tract. The protein-binding capacity of lithium is 15%. The half-life of lithium ranges from 18 to 36 hours. Because of its long half-life, cumulative drug action may result. The liver metabolizes lithium, and most of the drug is excreted unchanged in the urine.

Pharmacodynamics

Lithium is prescribed mostly for the stabilization of bipolar affective disorder. The onset of action is fast, but the patient may not achieve the desired effect for 5 to 6 days. Increased sodium intake increases renal excretion, so the sodium intake needs to be closely monitored. Increased urine output can result in body fluid loss and dehydration; therefore adequate fluid intake of 1 to 2 L should be maintained daily.

Antiseizure drugs such as carbamazepine, lamotrigine, and valproic acid/valproate/divalproex have been used in place of lithium for some patients. These antiseizure agents are further discussed in Chapter 19. The antipsychotic drugs olanzapine, ziprasidone, and aripiprazole are approved to treat acute mania and mixed episodes of bipolar disorder. Antipsychotic drugs are discussed in Chapter 22.

Side Effects and Adverse Reactions

The many side effects of lithium—dry mouth, thirst, polyuria (loss of water and sodium in increased urination), weight gain, metallic taste,

PROTOTYPE DRUG CHART
Lithium

Drug Class	Dosage
Mood stabilizer	Immediate release: A: PO: Initially 300 mg tid; *maint:* 300–600 mg/bid–tid Extended release: A: PO: Initially 900 mg bid; *maint:* 1800 mg/d Therapeutic drug range: 0.8–1.2 mEq/L
Contraindications	**Drug-Lab-Food Interactions**
Hypersensitivity *Caution:* Renal disease, pregnancy, breast-feeding, cardiac disease, bradycardia, stroke, dehydration, hyponatremia, hypo/hypercalcemia, hypokalemia, celiac disease, diarrhea, children, older adults, infection, parkinsonism, thyroid disease, hypoparathyroidism, seizures, suicidal ideation	Drug: May increase lithium level with thiazide diuretics, methyldopa, haloperidol, NSAIDs, antidepressants, carbamazepine, calcium channel blockers, spironolactone, ACE inhibitors, sodium bicarbonate, phenothiazines; may increase lithium excretion with theophylline, aminophylline; may increase risk of serotonin syndrome with SSRIs and SNRIs; may increase hyperglycemia with antidiabetics; caffeine may decrease lithium levels; CNS stimulants and direct renin inhibitors may increase risk of mania Lab: Increased urine and blood glucose, protein; decreased serum sodium level Food: Increase sodium intake; lithium may cause sodium depletion Complementary and alternative therapy: Use of St. Johns wort, kava kava, and valerian may lead to neurotoxicity
Pharmacokinetics	**Pharmacodynamics**
Absorption: PO: Well absorbed Distribution: PB: 15% Metabolism: t½: 18–36 h Excretion: 98% in urine, mostly unchanged	PO: Onset: UK Peak: 0.25–3 h Duration: 24 h Extended release: Onset: UK Peak: 4–6 h Duration: UK
Therapeutic Effects/Uses	
To treat bipolar disorder, manic episodes Mechanism of Action: Alteration of ion transport in muscle and nerve cells; increased receptor sensitivity to serotonin	
Side Effects	**Adverse Reactions**
Headache, memory impairment, blurred vision, metallic taste, thirst, dry mouth/skin, dental caries, drowsiness, dizziness, fatigue, ataxia, tremor, anorexia, nausea, vomiting, diarrhea, polyuria, dehydration, hypotension, abdominal pain, restlessness, erectile dysfunction, weight gain/loss, peripheral edema, rash	Urinary and fecal incontinence, thyroid disease, hyperglycemia, proteinuria, polyuria, leukocytosis, bradycardia *Life-threatening:* Dysrhythmias, seizures, angioedema, cardiac arrest, diabetes insipidus, serotonin syndrome, neuroleptic malignant syndrome, nephrotoxicity, coma

A, Adult; *ACE*, angiotensin-converting enzyme; *bid*, twice a day; *CNS*, central nervous system; *h*, hour; *maint*, maintenance; *NSAID*, nonsteroidal antiinflammatory drug; *PB*, protein binding; *PO*, by mouth; *SNRI*, serotonin-norepinephrine reuptake inhibitor; *SSRI*, selective serotonin reuptake inhibitor; *t½*, half-life; *tid*, three times a day; *UK*, unknown.

and peripheral edema of the hands and ankles—can be annoying to the patient. If taken during pregnancy, lithium may have teratogenic effects.

Special Considerations for Lithium

Lithium and NSAIDs should *not* be given together, because NSAIDs may increase lithium levels. Caffeine and loop diuretics may decrease lithium levels. Lithium should be prescribed with extreme caution for patients who have a cardiovascular disease due to an increased risk of lithium toxicity. Frequent monitoring of lithium levels is necessary. Caution must also be used in patients with thyroid disease, as hypothyroidism may occur.

CLINICAL JUDGMENT [NURSING PROCESS]

Mood Stabilizer: Lithium

Concept: Mood and Affect
- A conscious state of mind or feeling

Recognize Cues [Assessment]
- Assess for suicidal ideation.
- Assess baseline vital signs for future comparisons.
- Evaluate neurologic status, including gait, level of consciousness, reflexes, and tremors.
- Note hepatic and renal function by assessing urine output (>600 mL/day) and whether blood urea nitrogen (BUN) and serum creatinine and liver enzyme levels are within normal range. Assess for toxicity. Draw weekly blood levels initially and then every 1 to 2 months. Therapeutic serum levels for lithium are 0.8 to 1.2 mEq/L. Signs and symptoms of serum levels above 1.5 mEq/L are nausea and vomiting, diarrhea, ataxia, blurred vision, confusion, and tremors. Above 2.5 mEq/L, signs and symptoms of toxicity progress to include seizures, cardiac dysrhythmias, coma, and permanent neurologic impairment. At 3.5 mEq/L or higher, signs of toxicity are potentially lethal. Withhold medication and notify a health care provider immediately if any of these occur.
- Obtain a health history of episodes of depression or manic depressive behavior.
- Obtain a drug history. Diuretics, tetracyclines, methyldopa, probenecid, and nonsteroidal antiinflammatory drugs (NSAIDs) such as ibuprofen decrease renal clearance of lithium, causing drug accumulation.

Analyze Cues and Prioritize Hypothesis [Patient Problems]
- Diarrhea
- Confusion
- Anxiety
- Decreased visual acuity
- Hopelessness
- Decreased ability to cope
- Social isolation

Generate Solutions [Planning]
- Patient will display a calmer attitude.
- Patient will cope with at least one current issue.
- Patient will interact with others.

Take Action [Nursing Interventions]
- Observe patients for signs and symptoms of depression: mood changes, insomnia, apathy, or lack of interest in activities.
- Monitor vital signs. Hypotension is common.
- Draw blood samples for lithium levels immediately before the next dose (8 to 12 hours after the previous dose).
- ⚡ Monitor for signs of lithium toxicity. Report high (>1.5 mEq/L) serum lithium levels immediately to a health care provider.
- ⚡ Monitor patients for suicidal tendencies when marked depression is present.
- Evaluate urine output and body weight. Fluid volume deficit may occur as a result of polyuria.
- Observe patients for fine and gross motor tremors and presence of slurred speech, which are signs of adverse reaction.
- Assist patients in conserving energy when in a manic phase.
- Check cardiac monitor, blood pressure, and heart rate. Loss of fluids and electrolytes may cause electrolyte imbalance and cardiac dysrhythmias.
- Monitor serum electrolytes, and report abnormal findings.

Patient Teaching

General
- Teach patients to take lithium as prescribed. Emphasize the importance of adherence to the therapy, laboratory tests, and follow-up visits with a health care provider. If lithium is stopped, manic symptoms will reappear.
- Encourage patients to keep medical appointments. Have patients check with a health care provider before taking over-the-counter (OTC) preparations.
- Warn patients not to drive a motor vehicle or engage in potentially dangerous mechanical activity until a stable lithium level is established.
- Advise patients to maintain adequate fluid intake (2 to 3 L/day initially and 1 to 2 L/day maintenance). Fluid intake should increase in hot weather.
- Teach patients to take lithium with meals to decrease gastric irritation.
- Inform patients that effectiveness of the drug may not be evident until 1 to 2 weeks after the start of therapy. Compliance in taking the prescribed lithium doses on a daily basis is a major problem with patients with bipolar disorder. Sometimes, when a patient has a period of emotional stability, they do not believe that the drug is needed and may stop taking the lithium.
- Advise patients planning pregnancy to consult with a health care provider about possible teratogenic effects of the drug on the fetus, especially during the first 3 months.
- Encourage patients to wear or carry an identification tag or bracelet indicating the drug taken.

Diet
- Advise patients to avoid caffeine products (coffee, tea, cola) because they can aggravate the manic phase of bipolar disorder by decreasing lithium levels.
- Advise patients to maintain adequate sodium intake and to avoid crash diets that affect physical and mental health.

Side Effects
- Advise patients to contact a health care provider if they experience symptoms of toxicity. Early symptoms include diarrhea, drowsiness, loss of appetite, muscle weakness, nausea, vomiting, slurred speech, and trembling. Late symptoms include blurred vision, confusion, increased urination, convulsions, severe trembling, and unsteadiness.

Evaluate Outcomes [Evaluation]
- Evaluate the effectiveness of the drug therapy and determine if the patient is free of bipolar behavior.
- Allow patients to verbalize their understanding of symptoms of toxicity.
- Determine whether the patient demonstrates a subsiding or resolution of symptoms.

CLINICAL JUDGMENT CASE STUDY

A 37-year-old female is receiving fluoxetine 20 mg in the morning for depression. The patient complains of insomnia and gastrointestinal (GI) upset.

1. What could you suggest to help her avoid insomnia? Explain your answer.
2. How might the patient avoid GI upset when taking fluoxetine? What food should be avoided?

The patient states that she does not think the fluoxetine is helping. She states that she has heard about complementary and alternative therapies that may be taken for depression. She has also heard that fluoxetine can be taken weekly.

3. Is the patient's fluoxetine dose within the normal dosage range? Explain your answer.
4. How would you respond to the patient about the use of certain complementary and alternative therapies for depression?
5. What would your response be concerning the use of fluoxetine in a weekly dose?

REVIEW QUESTIONS

1. A patient is admitted with bipolar affective disorder. Which medication would the nurse acknowledge as one used to treat this disorder for some patients in place of lithium?
   a. Thiopental
   b. Ginkgo biloba
   c. Fluvoxamine
   d. Divalproex

2. The nurse realizes that some complementary and alternative therapies interact with selective serotonin reuptake inhibitors. Which complementary and alternative therapy interactions may cause serotonin syndrome? **Select all that apply.**
   a. Feverfew
   b. Ma-huang
   c. St. Johns wort
   d. Ginkgo biloba

3. A selective serotonin reuptake inhibitor is prescribed for a patient. The nurse knows that which drug is a selective serotonin reuptake inhibitor?
   a. Paroxetine
   b. Amitriptyline
   c. Divalproex sodium
   d. Bupropion hydrochloride

4. A patient is taking tranylcypromine sulfate for depression. What advice should the nurse include in the teaching plan for this medication?
   a. Warn the patient about weight loss.
   b. Instruct the patient to avoid beer and cheddar cheese.
   c. Encourage the patient to take ginseng and ephedra.
   d. Encourage the patient to eat fruit such as bananas.

5. Which statement is true concerning lithium?
   a. The maximum dose is 3.4 g/day.
   b. The therapeutic drug range is 2.5 to 3.5 mEq/L.
   c. Lithium increases receptor sensitivity to gamma-aminobutyric acid.
   d. Concurrent nonsteroidal antiinflammatory drugs (NSAIDs) may increase lithium levels.

6. When a patient is taking an antidepressant, what should the nurse do? **Select all that apply.**
   a. Monitor the patient for suicidal tendencies.
   b. Observe the patient for orthostatic hypotension.
   c. Teach the patient to take the drug with food if gastrointestinal distress occurs.
   d. Tell the patient that the drug may not have full effectiveness for 1 to 2 weeks.
   e. Advise the patient to maintain adequate fluid intake of 2 L/day.

7. A patient is taking lithium. The nurse should be aware of the importance of which nursing intervention(s)? **Select all that apply.**
   a. Observe the patient for motor tremors.
   b. Monitor the patient for hypotension.
   c. Draw lithium blood levels immediately after a dose.
   d. Advise the patient to drink 750 mL/day of fluid in hot weather.
   e. Advise the patient to avoid caffeinated foods and beverages.
   f. Teach the patient to take lithium with meals to decrease gastric irritation.

UNIT VII Pain and Inflammation Management Drugs

24

Antiinflammatories

http://evolve.elsevier.com/McCuistion/pharmacology

OBJECTIVES

- Explain tissue injury response in inflammation and how antiinflammatory agents affect it.
- Explain the action of nonsteroidal antiinflammatory drugs and corticosteroids.
- Discuss the drug groups included in disease-modifying antirheumatics.
- Describe characteristics of gout and its treatment.

OUTLINE

Inflammation and Antiinflammatory Agents, 287
    Pathophysiology, 287
    Antiinflammatory Agents, 288
Nonsteroidal Antiinflammatory Drugs and Corticosteroids, 288
    Salicylates, 289
    Para-Chlorobenzoic Acid, 292
    Propionic Acid Derivatives, 292
    Fenamates, 293
    Oxicams, 293
    Selective COX-2 Inhibitors, 294
    Use of NSAIDs in Older Adults, 294

    Corticosteroids, 295
Disease-Modifying Antirheumatic Drugs, 295
    Immunosuppressive Agents, 295
    Immunomodulators, 298
    Antimalarials, 298
Antigout Drugs, 298
    Antiinflammatory Gout Drug: Colchicine, 299
    Xanthine Oxidase Inhibitors, 299
    Uricosurics, 299
Clinical Judgment Case Study, 301
Review Questions, 302

INFLAMMATION AND ANTIINFLAMMATORY AGENTS

Inflammation is a response to tissue injury caused by the release of chemical mediators that trigger both a vascular response and the migration of fluid and cells—leukocytes, or white blood cells—to the injured site. The chemical mediators are histamines, kinins, and prostaglandins. The process of inflammation is a protective mechanism in which the body attempts to neutralize and destroy harmful agents at the site of injury and to establish conditions for tissue repair.

Although a relationship exists between inflammation and infection, these terms should *not* be used interchangeably. Infection is caused by microorganisms and *results* in inflammation, but not all inflammations are caused by infections. Only a small percentage of inflammations are caused by infection. Other causes of inflammation include trauma, surgical interventions, extreme heat or cold, and caustic chemical agents. Antiinflammatory drugs reduce fluid migration and pain, lessening loss of function and increasing the patient's mobility and comfort.

Pathophysiology

The five characteristics of inflammation, called *the cardinal signs of inflammation*, are (1) redness, (2) swelling (edema), (3) heat, (4) pain, and (5) loss of function. Table 24.1 gives the description and explanation of the cardinal signs of inflammation. Inflammation also has two phases: the *vascular phase*, which occurs 10 to 15 minutes after an injury; and the *delayed phase*. The vascular phase is associated with vasodilation and increased capillary permeability, during which blood substances and fluid leave the plasma and go to the injured site. The delayed phase occurs when leukocytes infiltrate the inflamed tissue.

Various chemical mediators are released during the inflammation process (Fig. 24.1). *Histamine*, the first mediator in the inflammatory process, causes dilation of the arterioles and increases capillary permeability, allowing fluid to leave the capillaries and flow into the injured area. *Kinins*, such as bradykinin, also increase capillary permeability and the sensation of pain.

Among these are *prostaglandins*, chemical mediators that have been isolated from the exudate at inflammatory sites. Prostaglandins have many effects, which include vasodilation, relaxation of smooth muscle, increased capillary permeability, and sensitization of nerve cells to pain.

TABLE 24.1	Cardinal Signs of Inflammation
Signs	**Description and Explanation**
Erythema (redness)	Redness occurs in the first phase of inflammation. Blood accumulates in the area of tissue injury because of the release of the body's chemical mediators (kinins, prostaglandins, and histamine). These chemical mediators dilate the arterioles.
Edema (swelling)	Swelling is the second phase of inflammation. Plasma leaks into the interstitial tissue at the injury site. Kinins and histamine increase capillary permeability.
Heat	Heat at the inflammatory site can be caused by increased blood accumulation and may result from pyrogens, substances that produce fever, which interfere with the temperature-regulating center in the hypothalamus.
Pain	Pain is caused by tissue swelling and release of chemical mediators.
Loss of function	Function is lost because of the accumulation of fluid at the tissue injury site and because of pain, which decreases mobility at the affected area.

Cyclooxygenase (COX) is the enzyme responsible for converting arachidonic acid into prostaglandins and their products. This synthesis of prostaglandins causes inflammation and pain at a tissue injury site. COX has two enzyme forms, COX-1 and COX-2. *COX-1* protects the stomach lining and regulates blood platelets, and *COX-2* triggers inflammation and pain.

Antiinflammatory Agents

Drugs such as aspirin inhibit the biosynthesis of prostaglandin and are therefore called *prostaglandin inhibitors*. Because prostaglandin inhibitors affect the inflammatory process, they are more commonly called *antiinflammatories or antiinflammatory drugs*.

Antiinflammatories also relieve pain (analgesic), reduce elevated body temperature (antipyretic), and inhibit platelet aggregation (anticoagulant). Aspirin is the oldest antiinflammatory drug, but it was first used for its analgesic and antipyretic properties. As a result of searching for a more effective drug with fewer side effects, many other antiinflammatories or prostaglandin inhibitors have been discovered. Although these drugs have potent antiinflammatory effects that mimic the effects of corticosteroids (cortisone), they are *not* chemically related to corticosteroids and therefore are called *nonsteroidal antiinflammatory drugs (NSAIDs)*. Most NSAIDs are used to decrease inflammation and pain for patients who have some type of musculoskeletal condition.

NONSTEROIDAL ANTIINFLAMMATORY DRUGS AND CORTICOSTEROIDS

NSAIDs include aspirin and aspirin-like drugs that inhibit the enzyme COX, which is needed for the biosynthesis of prostaglandins.

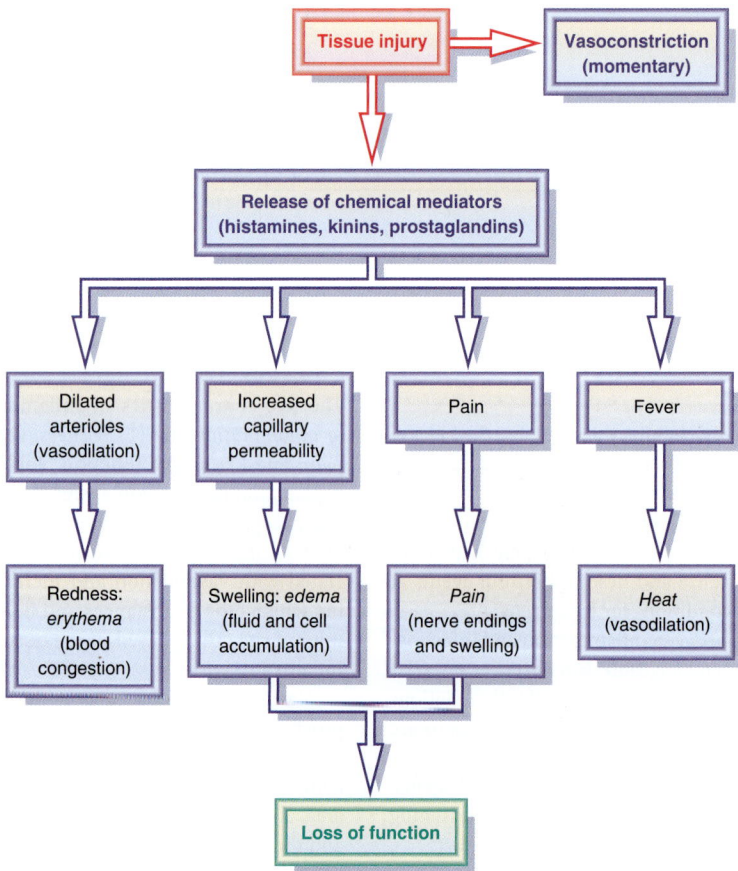

Fig. 24.1 Chemical mediator response to tissue injury.

Chapter 25 present expanded discussions of NSAIDs in their roles as analgesics and anticoagulants, respectively. These drugs may be called *prostaglandin inhibitors* with varying degrees of analgesic and antipyretic effects, but they are used primarily as antiinflammatories to relieve inflammation and pain. Their antipyretic effect is less than their antiinflammatory effect. With several exceptions, NSAID preparations are not suggested for use in alleviating mild headaches and mildly elevated temperature. Preferred drugs for headaches and fever are aspirin (adults only for fever), acetaminophen, and ibuprofen. NSAIDs are more appropriate for reducing swelling, pain, and stiffness in joints.

Most NSAIDs cost more than aspirin. Other than aspirin, the only NSAIDs that can be purchased over the counter (OTC) are ibuprofen and naproxen. All other NSAIDs require a prescription. Examples of prescription products on the market that contain NSAID contents alone or in combination include celecoxib, meloxicam, oxaprozin, nabumetone, sulindac, and ketorolac. If a patient can take aspirin for the inflammatory process without gastrointestinal (GI) upset, salicylate products are usually recommended.

There are six groups of NSAIDs:
1. Salicylates
2. *Para*-chlorobenzoic acid derivatives, or indoles
3. Propionic acid derivatives
4. Fenamates
5. Oxicams
6. Selective COX-2 inhibitors

The first five NSAID groups on the list are known as *first-generation NSAIDs*, and the COX-2 inhibitors are called *second-generation NSAIDs*.

Table 24.2 provides dosage information and considerations for use for the most commonly used NSAIDs. The half-lives of NSAIDs differ greatly; some have a short half-life of 1 hour, and others have a moderate to long half-life of 50 hours. Aspirin should not be taken with an NSAID because of the potentiation of side effects. In addition, combined therapy does not increase effectiveness.

Salicylates

Aspirin comes from the family of salicylates derived from salicylic acid. Aspirin is also called *acetylsalicylic acid (ASA)* after the acetyl group used in its composition.

Adolph Bayer developed aspirin in 1899, making it the oldest antiinflammatory agent. It was the most frequently used antiinflammatory agent before the introduction of ibuprofen. Aspirin is a prostaglandin inhibitor that decreases the inflammatory process. It is also considered an antiplatelet drug for patients with cardiac or cerebrovascular disorders; aspirin decreases platelet aggregation, and thus blood clotting is decreased. Because high doses of aspirin are usually needed to relieve inflammation, gastric distress—which includes anorexia, dyspepsia, nausea, vomiting, abdominal pain, and gastritis—is a common problem. In such cases, enteric-coated (EC) tablets may be used. Aspirin should *not* be taken with other NSAIDs because it decreases the blood level and effectiveness of NSAIDs.

TABLE 24.2 Antiinflammatory Agents: Nonsteroidal

Drug	Route and Dosage	Uses and Considerations
First-Generation NSAIDs		
Salicylates		
Aspirin	See Prototype Drug Chart: Aspirin	
Diflunisal	Osteoarthritis: A: PO: 250–500 mg bid; *max:* 1500 mg/d	For mild to moderate pain, osteoarthritis, and RA. Avoid if hypersensitive to aspirin. May cause headache, hearing loss, abdominal pain, dyspepsia, nausea, diarrhea, peptic ulcer, GI bleeding/perforation, elevated hepatic enzymes, and rash. PB: 99%; $t\frac{1}{2}$: 8–12 h
Salicylate Derivatives		
Olsalazine sodium	A: PO: 500 mg q12h; *max:* 1 g/d	For ulcerative colitis. May cause headache, abdominal pain, dyspepsia, nausea, and diarrhea. PB: 99%; $t\frac{1}{2}$: 1 h
Sulfasalazine	RA: A: PO: Initially 500 mg qd/bid for 1 wk, then may increase to 1 g bid or 3 g qd if needed; *max:* 3 g/d	For ulcerative colitis and RA. Avoid if allergic to sulfonamides or aspirin. May cause dizziness, headache, stomatitis, fever, abdominal pain, dyspepsia, anorexia, nausea, vomiting, oligospermia, elevated hepatic enzymes, and rash. PB: 99%; $t\frac{1}{2}$: 5–7 h
***Para*-Chlorobenzoic Acid (Indoles)**		
Indomethacin	RA: Regular release: A: PO: 25 mg bid/tid with food; *max:* 200 mg/d Sustained release: A: PO: 75 mg/d; *max:* 150 mg/d	For mild to severe pain, RA, acute gouty arthritis, and ankylosing spondylitis. May cause dizziness, headache, tinnitus, fluid retention, fatigue, weight gain, dyspepsia, anorexia, abdominal pain, nausea, vomiting, diarrhea, constipation, oliguria, peripheral edema, hypertension, hyperkalemia, and hyponatremia. Take with food. Avoid if allergic to aspirin. PB: 99%; $t\frac{1}{2}$: 2.6–11.2 h
Sulindac	RA: A: PO: 150–200 mg bid; *max:* 400 mg/d	For arthritis, bursitis, ankylosing spondylitis, and tendinitis. May cause dizziness, headache, abdominal pain, dyspepsia, nausea, vomiting, diarrhea, constipation, hypertension, rash, edema, and elevated hepatic enzymes. Take with food or milk. PB: 93%; $t\frac{1}{2}$: 8 h

Continued

TABLE 24.2 Antiinflammatory Agents: Nonsteroidal—cont'd

Drug	Route and Dosage	Uses and Considerations
Etodolac	Arthritis: Immediate release: A: PO: Initially 300 mg bid/tid; *maint:* 600 mg/d; *max:* 1200 mg/d Extended release: A: PO: 400–1000 mg/d; *max:* 1200 mg/d	For mild to moderate pain, RA, and osteoarthritis. May cause dizziness, weakness, abdominal pain, dyspepsia, nausea, diarrhea, flatulence, hypertension, and pyrosis. Take with food. PB: 99%; t½: 6–7 h
Propionic Acid		
Fenoprofen calcium	RA: A: PO: Initially 400–600 mg tid/qid; *max:* 3200 mg/d	For mild to moderate pain, osteoarthritis, and RA. May cause drowsiness, dizziness, headache, tinnitus, dyspepsia, nausea, constipation, rash, pruritus, palpitations, weakness, and peripheral edema. Take with food. PB: 99%; t½: 2.5–3 h
Flurbiprofen sodium	Arthritis: A: PO: 200–300 mg/d in 2–4 divided doses; *max:* 300 mg/d, 100 mg/dose	For mild to moderate pain, osteoarthritis, and RA. May cause dizziness, headache, blurred vision, insomnia, flatulence, abdominal pain, dyspepsia, nausea, diarrhea, constipation, and GI bleeding. Take with food. PB: 99%; t½: 3–9 h
Ibuprofen	See Prototype Drug Chart: Ibuprofen	
Ketoprofen	Arthritis: Immediate release: A: PO: Initially 50 mg qid or 75 mg tid (older A, initially 50 mg tid or 75 mg bid); *max:* 300 mg/d Extended release: A: PO: 200 mg/d; *max:* 200 mg/d Older A: PO: 100–150 mg/d; *max:* 200 mg/d	For mild to moderate pain, osteoarthritis, and RA. May cause headache, insomnia, abdominal pain, dyspepsia, nausea, diarrhea, flatulence, and constipation. PB: 99%; t½: immediate release, 0.9–3.3 h; extended release, 5.4 h
Naproxen	RA: A: PO: 250–500 mg bid; *max:* 1500 mg/d Delayed release: A: PO: 375–500 mg bid; *max:* 1500 mg/d Controlled release: A: PO: Initially 750–1000 mg/d; *max:* 1500 mg/d	For mild to moderate pain, osteoarthritis, RA, ankylosing spondylitis, and gout. May cause dizziness, drowsiness, headache, tinnitus, pharyngitis, rhinitis, sinusitis, dyspnea, dyspepsia, abdominal pain, nausea, vomiting, diarrhea, flatulence, constipation, GI bleeding/perforation/ulcer, back pain, edema, influenza, infection, and elevated hepatic enzymes. Take with food or with a full glass of water. PB: 99%; t½: 12–17 h
Oxaprozin	A: PO: 600–1200 mg/d based upon weight; *max:* 1200 mg/d	For osteoarthritis and RA. May cause edema, dizziness, drowsiness, weakness, confusion, headache, tinnitus, rash, pruritis, abdominal pain, dyspepsia, nausea, vomiting, diarrhea, constipation, and GI bleeding/perforation/ulcer. PB: 99%; t½: 41.4 h
Anthranilic Acids (Fenamates)		
Meclofenamate	Arthritis: A: PO: Initially 200 mg/d in 3–4 divided doses; *max:* 400 mg/d	For mild to moderate pain, dysmenorrhea, osteoarthritis, and RA. May cause dizziness, headache, rash, abdominal pain, nausea, vomiting, diarrhea, flatulence, and pyrosis. PB: 99%; t½: 2 h
Mefenamic acid	Pain: A: PO: Initially: 500 mg once, then 250 mg q6h PRN for 7 d; *max:* 1250 mg/d	For mild to moderate pain and dysmenorrhea. May cause dizziness, headache, tinnitus, abdominal pain, dyspepsia, nausea, vomiting, diarrhea, flatulence, constipation, and GI bleeding/perforation/ulcer, rash, pruritis, and edema. PB: 90%; t½: 2 h
Oxicams		
Piroxicam	A: PO: 20 mg/d; *max:* 20 mg/d	For osteoarthritis and RA. May cause dizziness, headache, tinnitus, edema, rash, pruritus, abdominal pain, anorexia, nausea, vomiting, diarrhea, flatulence, constipation, GI, and bleeding/perforation/ulcer. PB: 99%; t½: 50 h
Meloxicam	A: PO tablets: 7.5–15 mg/d; *max:* 15 mg/d	For moderate to severe pain, osteoarthritis and RA. May cause dizziness, headache, edema, pharyngitis, laryngitis, sinusitis, abdominal pain, dyspepsia, eructation, nausea, diarrhea, constipation, GI bleeding/perforation, and arthralgia. PB: 99.4%; t½: 15–20 h
Naphthylalkanones		
Nabumetone	A: PO: 1000 mg/d or 500 mg bid; *max:* 2000 mg/d	For osteoarthritis and RA. May cause dizziness, headache, tinnitus, abdominal pain, dyspepsia, nausea, vomiting, diarrhea, flatulence, constipation, rash, pruritus, and edema. PB: 99%; t½: 24 h
Second-Generation NSAIDs		
COX-2 inhibitors		
Celecoxib	See Prototype Drug Chart: Celecoxib	

TABLE 24.2 Antiinflammatory Agents: Nonsteroidal—cont'd

Drug	Route and Dosage	Uses and Considerations
Miscellaneous		
Tolmetin	A: PO: Initially: 400 mg tid; *maint*: 600–1800 mg/d in 3–4 divided doses; *max*: 1800 mg/d	For osteoarthritis and RA. May cause dizziness, headache, weakness, abdominal pain, dyspepsia, nausea, vomiting, diarrhea, flatulence, hypertension, edema and weight loss/gain. PB: 99%; $t½$: 1–5 h
Diclofenac sodium	Osteoarthritis: Immediate release Zorvolex: A: PO: 35 mg tid; *max*: 150 mg/d Extended release Voltaren XR: A: PO: 100 mg/d; *max*: 150 mg/d	For mild to severe pain, RA, osteoarthritis, migraine, and ankylosing spondylitis. May cause lacrimation, ocular hypertension/pain, xerophthalmia, blurred vision, keratitis, contact dermatitis, dyspepsia, GI bleeding/perforation, anemia, elevated hepatic enzymes, injection-site reaction, prolonged bleeding time, and edema. Take with food. PB: 99%; $t½$: 2 h
Ketorolac tromethamine	Short-term pain (continuation therapy from IV/IM only): A >50 kg: PO: Initially 20 mg dose, then 10 mg q4–6 h; *max*: 40 mg/d A <50 kg and Older A: PO: Initially 10 mg dose, then 10 mg q4–6 h; *max*: 40 mg/d A >50 kg: IM/IV: 30 mg q6h; *max*: 120 mg/d A <50 kg and Older A: IM/IV: 15 mg q6h; *max*: 60 mg/d Nasal spray: A >50 kg: Intranasal: 1 spray (15.75 mg/spray) q6–8h each nostril; *max*: 4 doses/d A <50 kg and Older A: Intranasal: 1 spray q6–8h 1 nostril; *max*: 4 doses/d	For short-term moderate to severe pain management of 5 days or less and for ocular inflammation. First injectable NSAID. May cause drowsiness, dizziness, ocular inflammation/irritation/infection and pain, corneal edema, iritis, keratitis, nasal irritation, rhinalgia, stomatitis, rash, pruritus, diaphoresis, injection-site reaction abdominal pain, dyspepsia, nausea, vomiting, diarrhea, flatulence, constipation, GI bleeding/perforation, peptic ulcer, and hypertension. PB: 99%; $t½$: PO, 2.4–9 h; IM, 3.5–9.2 h, intranasal 5.2 h

A, adult; *bid*, twice a day; *COX*, cyclooxygenase; *d*, day; *GI*, gastrointestinal; *h*, hour; *IM*, intramuscular; *IV*, intravenous; *maint*, maintenance; *max*, maximum; *NSAID*, nonsteroidal antiinflammatory drug; *PB*, protein binding; *PO*, by mouth; *PRN*, as needed; *q12h*, every 12 hours; *qd*, every day; *qid*, four times a day; *RA*, rheumatoid arthritis; *t½*, half-life; *tid*, three times a day; *wk*, week.

Aspirin and other NSAIDs relieve pain by inhibiting the COX enzyme, which is needed for the biosynthesis of prostaglandins. As mentioned earlier, the two enzyme forms of COX, COX-1 and COX-2 (Fig. 24.2), serve different purposes: COX-1 protects the stomach lining and regulates blood platelets, promoting blood clotting, whereas COX-2 triggers pain and inflammation at the injured site. NSAIDs usually inhibit or block *both* COX-1 and COX-2. Inhibition of COX-1 produces the desirable effect of decreasing platelet aggregation, but it has the undesirable effect of decreasing protection to the stomach lining; therefore stomach bleeding and ulcers may occur with aspirin and NSAID agents. When COX-2 is inhibited, pain and fever are reduced and inflammation is suppressed, but COX-2 inhibitors do *not* cause gastric ulceration, and they have no effect on platelet function.

Newer NSAIDs, called COX-2 inhibitors, block only COX-2 and not COX-1. These drugs leave protection for the stomach lining intact, so no gastric bleeding or ulcers result, but they still deliver relief for pain and inflammation.

A COX-2 inhibitor approved by the US Food and Drug Administration (FDA) is celecoxib. Drugs similar to COX-2 inhibitors include meloxicam and nabumetone, which allow some stomach protection. Patients at risk for stroke or heart attack who take aspirin to prevent blood clotting (decreased platelet aggregation) would not benefit from COX-2 inhibitors. If the COX-1 enzyme were not blocked, increased blood clotting would remain even though the stomach lining is protected.

Many researchers believe that COX-2 inhibitors may prevent some types of cancer, such as colon cancer. Fruits and vegetables block the COX-2 enzyme naturally, protecting the colon from malignant growths.

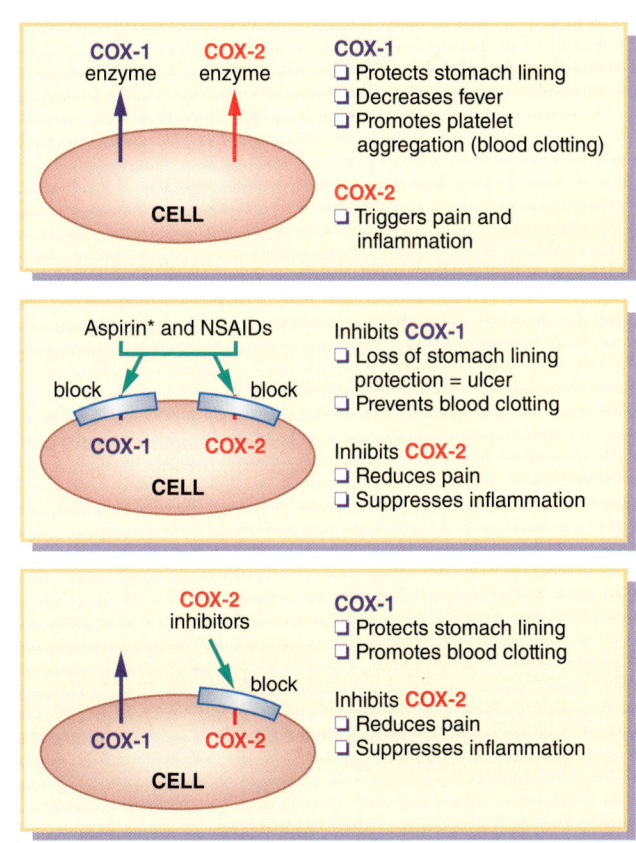

*Aspirin is only one of the NSAIDs.

Fig. 24.2 Uses of COX-1 and COX-2 inhibitors.

PROTOTYPE DRUG CHART
Aspirin

Drug Class	Dosage
Analgesic: Antiinflammatory drug	Mild pain: A: PO: 325 or 650 mg q4h PRN; *max:* 3900 mg/d A: R: 300–600 mg q4–6h PRN; *max:* 3600 mg/d Toxic serum salicylate level: >300 mcg/mL
Contraindications	**Drug-Lab-Food Interactions**
Hypersensitivity to salicylates or NSAIDs *Caution:* Renal or hepatic disorders, alcohol misuse, anticoagulant therapy, asthma, influenza, peptic ulcer disease, Reye syndrome, hemophilia, older adults, pregnancy, breast-feeding, children	Drug: Increased risk of bleeding with anticoagulants and other NSAIDs; increased risk of hypoglycemia with oral hypoglycemic drugs; increased ulcerogenic effect with glucocorticoids; decreased effects of ACE inhibitors, loop diuretics, and probenecid; effects are decreased by corticosteroids. Lab: Decreased cholesterol, potassium, T_3, and T_4 levels; increased uric acid, PT, and bleeding time
Pharmacokinetics	**Pharmacodynamics**
Absorption: PO: 80%–100% Distribution: PB: 90%–94%, crosses placenta Metabolism: t½: 15–20 min Excretion: 50% in urine	PO: Onset: 15–30 min Peak: 1–2 h Duration: 4–6 h
Therapeutic Effects/Uses	
To reduce pain and fever; use for prophylaxis for arterial thromboembolism, MI, TIA, and stroke Mechanism of Action: Inhibits prostaglandin synthesis, hypothalamic heat regulator center, and platelet aggregation	
Side Effects	**Adverse Reactions**
Dizziness, headache, confusion, agitation, lethargy, dyspepsia, anorexia, gastritis, abdominal pain, nausea, vomiting diaphoresis, pruritus, rash, and dehydration	Tinnitus, hearing loss, hypokalemia, hypernatremia, elevated hepatic enzymes, hypo/hyperglycemia, proteinuria, metabolic acidosis, cerebral edema, hyperuricemia, GI bleeding, peptic ulcer disease, intracranial bleeding *Life-threatening:* Reye syndrome, respiratory alkalosis, renal/hepatic failure

A, Adult; *ACE*, angiotensin-converting enzyme; *d*, day; *GI*, gastrointestinal; *h*, hour; *max*, maximum; *MI*, myocardio infarction; *min*, minute; *NSAID*, nonsteroidal antiinflammatory drug; *PB*, protein binding; *PO*, by mouth; *PRN*, as needed; *PT*, prothrombin time; *q*, every; *R*, rectal; *t ½*, half-life; T_3, triiodothyronine; T_4, thyroxine; *TIA*, transient ischemic attack.

Pharmacokinetics

Aspirin is well absorbed from the GI tract (Prototype Drug Chart: Aspirin). It can cause GI distress, which includes anorexia, nausea, vomiting, diarrhea, and abdominal pain, so it should be taken with water, milk, or food. The EC or buffered form can decrease gastric distress. EC tablets should not be crushed or broken.

Aspirin has a short half-life. It should not be taken during the last trimester of pregnancy because it could cause premature closure of the ductus arteriosus in the fetus. Children with flu symptoms should not take aspirin because it may cause the potentially fatal Reye syndrome.

Pharmacodynamics

Like other NSAIDs, aspirin inhibits prostaglandin synthesis by inhibiting COX-1 and COX-2; thus it decreases inflammation and pain. The onset of action for aspirin is within 30 minutes. It peaks in 1 to 2 hours, and the duration of action is an average of 4 to 6 hours. The action for the rectal preparation of aspirin can be erratic because of blood supply and fecal material in the rectum; it may take a week or longer for a therapeutic antiinflammatory effect.

Hypersensitivity to Salicylate Products

Patients may be hypersensitive to aspirin. Tinnitus (ringing in the ears), and vertigo (dizziness) are symptoms of aspirin overdose or hypersensitivity to aspirin.

Salicylates are present in numerous foods such as prunes, raisins, and licorice, as well as in spices such as curry and paprika.

Para-Chlorobenzoic Acid

One of the first NSAIDs introduced was indomethacin, a *para*-chlorobenzoic acid. It is used for rheumatoid arthritis (RA), gouty arthritis, and osteoarthritis, and it is a potent prostaglandin inhibitor. It is highly protein bound (99%) and displaces other protein-bound drugs, resulting in potential toxicity. It has a moderate half-life (2.6–11.2 hours). Indomethacin is very irritating to the stomach and should be taken with food.

Two other *para*-chlorobenzoic acid derivatives—sulindac and etodolac—produce less severe adverse reactions than indomethacin. These drugs are also highly protein bound at 93% to 99% and have a half-life of 6 to 8 hours. This group of NSAIDs may cause peripheral edema, weight gain, and increased blood pressure.

Propionic Acid Derivatives

The propionic acid group is a relatively new group of NSAIDs. These drugs are aspirin-like but have stronger effects and create less GI irritation. Drugs in this group are highly protein bound, so drug interactions might occur, especially when given with another highly protein-bound drug. Propionic acid derivatives are better tolerated than other NSAIDs. Gastric upset occurs, but it is not as severe as with aspirin

CLINICAL JUDGMENT [NURSING PROCESS]
Salicylate: Aspirin

Concept: Inflammation
- An immunologic response of the body to injury or infection involving redness, swelling, warmth, and pain

Recognize Cues [Assessment]
- Determine a medical history. Ask the patient about previous gastric distress, gastric bleeding, or liver disease. Aspirin can cause gastric irritation, and it prolongs bleeding time by inhibiting platelet aggregation.
- Obtain a drug history. Report if a drug–drug interaction is probable.

Analyze Cues and Prioritize Hypothesis [Patient Problems]
- Acute pain
- Injury
- Nausea
- Reduced functional ability

Generate Solutions [Planning]
- The patient will report a pain level has decreased within 1 hour of medication administration.
- The patient's swelling and redness will be reduced.

Take Action [Nursing Interventions]
- Monitor serum salicylate (aspirin) level when a patient takes high doses of aspirin for chronic conditions such as arthritis. The normal therapeutic range is 15–30 mg/dL. Mild toxicity occurs at a serum level greater than 30 mg/dL, and severe toxicity occurs above 50 mg/dL.
- Observe the patient for signs of bleeding such as dark, tarry stools; bleeding gums; petechiae (round red spots); ecchymosis (excessive bruising); and purpura (large red spots) when the patient takes high doses of aspirin.

Patient Teaching
General
- Advise patients not to take aspirin with alcohol or with drugs that are highly protein bound, such as the anticoagulant warfarin. Aspirin displaces drugs like warfarin from the protein-binding site, causing increased anticoagulant levels.
- Suggest that patients inform their dentist before a dental visit if they are taking high doses of aspirin.
- Instruct patients to discontinue aspirin approximately 7 days before surgery to reduce risk of bleeding (with the health care provider's approval).
- Advise patients to keep aspirin bottles out of reach of children.
- ⚡ Educate parents to call the poison control center immediately if a child has taken a large or unknown amount of aspirin or acetaminophen.
- Instruct patients not to cut or break an enteric-coated (EC) aspirin tablet.
- ⚡ Warn patients not to administer aspirin for virus or flu symptoms in children. Reye syndrome (vomiting, lethargy, delirium, and coma) has been linked with aspirin and viral infections. Acetaminophen is usually prescribed for cold and flu symptoms.
- Inform patients that aspirin tablets can cause gastrointestinal (GI) distress.
- Inform patients with dysmenorrhea to take acetaminophen instead of aspirin 2 days before and during the first 2 days of the menstrual period.

Side Effects
- Direct patients to report side effects such as drowsiness, tinnitus (ringing in the ears), headaches, flushing, dizziness, GI distress, GI bleeding, visual changes, and seizures.

Diet
- Instruct patients to take aspirin and ibuprofen with food, at mealtime, or with plenty of fluids. EC aspirin helps prevent GI distress.

Evaluate Outcomes [Evaluation]
- Evaluate the effectiveness of aspirin in relieving pain. If pain persists, another analgesic such as ibuprofen may be prescribed.
- Determine whether the patient shows any of the side effects of aspirin.

---

and indomethacin. Severe adverse reactions such as blood dyscrasias are not frequently seen. Ibuprofen is the most widely used propionic acid NSAID, and it may be purchased OTC in lower doses (200 mg). Prototype Drug Chart: Ibuprofen details the pharmacologic behavior of ibuprofen. Five other propionic acid agents are fenoprofen calcium, naproxen, ketoprofen, flurbiprofen, and oxaprozin.

Pharmacokinetics
Ibuprofens are well absorbed from the GI tract. Most of these drugs have a short half-life but are highly protein bound. If ibuprofen is taken with another highly protein-bound drug, severe side effects may occur. The drug is metabolized in the liver to inactive metabolites and is excreted as inactive metabolites in the urine.

Pharmacodynamics
Ibuprofen inhibits prostaglandin synthesis and is therefore effective in alleviating inflammation and pain. It has a short onset of action, peak concentration time, and duration of action. It may take several days for the antiinflammatory effect to be evident.

Many drug interactions are associated with ibuprofen. Because ibuprofen can increase the effects of warfarin and phenytoin, it should be avoided with these drugs. However, when taken with aspirin, its effect can be decreased. Hypoglycemia may result when ibuprofen is taken with insulin or an oral hypoglycemic drug. The risk of side effects are high when ibuprofen is taken concurrently with selective serotonin reuptake inhibitors, ACE inhibitors, beta-blockers, loop diuretics, and potassium sparing diuretics.

Fenamates
The fenamate group includes potent NSAIDs used for acute and chronic arthritic conditions. Fenamates decrease prostaglandin synthesis by inhibition of COX-1 and COX-2. As with most NSAIDs, gastric irritation is a common side effect; patients with a history of peptic ulcer should avoid taking fenamates. Other side effects include edema, dizziness, tinnitus, and headache. Two fenamates are meclofenamate sodium monohydrate and mefenamic acid.

Oxicams
Piroxicam and meloxicam, oxicams, are indicated for long-term arthritic conditions such as RA and osteoarthritis. Oxicams decrease prostaglandin synthesis by inhibition of COX-1 and COX-2. They too can cause gastric problems such as ulceration and epigastric distress, but the incidence is lower than for some other NSAIDs. Oxicams are well tolerated, and their major advantage over other

PROTOTYPE DRUG CHART

Ibuprofen

Drug Class	Dosage
NSAID: Propionic acid derivative	Rheumatoid arthritis: A: PO: 300 mg qid or 400–800 mg tid/qid; *max:* 3200 mg/d
Contraindications	**Drug-Lab-Food Interactions**
Hypersensitivity to salicylates and NSAIDs, coronary artery bypass graft surgery *Caution:* Bleeding disorders, anticoagulant therapy, cardiac disease, dysrhythmias, asthma, acute bronchospasm, cerebrovascular disease, chemotherapy, renal or hepatic disease, peptic ulcer, Crohn disease, GI bleeding/perforation, ulcerative colitis, systemic lupus erythematosus, bone marrow suppression, dehydration, alcohol use disorder, tobacco smoking, corticosteroid therapy, older adults, pregnancy, breast-feeding	Drug: Increased bleeding time with oral anticoagulants; increased effects of phenytoin, warfarin; decreased effect with aspirin; may increase severe side effects of lithium, SSRIs, ACE inhibitors, beta-blockers, loop diuretics, and potassium sparing diuretics
Pharmacokinetics	**Pharmacodynamics**
Absorption: PO: Well absorbed Distribution: PB: 99% Metabolism: t½: 1.7–2.5 h Excretion: In urine, mostly as inactive metabolites; some in bile	PO: Onset: 30 min–1 h Peak: 3–4 h Duration: 6–8 h
Therapeutic Effects/Uses	
To reduce inflammatory process; to relieve pain; antiinflammatory effect for arthritic conditions; to reduce fever, dysmenorrhea, headache Mechanism of Action: Inhibits COX-1 and COX-2 by blocking arachidonate binding, thus relieving pain and inflammation	
Side Effects	**Adverse Reactions**
Dizziness, drowsiness, headache, blurred vision, dyspepsia, pyrosis, abdominal pain, flatulence, nausea, vomiting, diarrhea, constipation, rash, pruritus, fluid retention, edema	Hearing loss, GI bleeding/perforation/ulcer, tinnitus, seizure, hypokalemia *Life-threatening:* Anemia, neutropenia, hemolytic anemia, aplastic anemia, agranulocytosis, thrombocytopenia, pancytopenia, renal failure, Stevens-Johnson syndrome

A, Adult; *ACE*, angiotensin-converting enzyme; *d*, day; *GI*, gastrointestinal; *h*, hour; *max*, maximum; *min*, minute; *NSAID*, nonsteroidal antiinflammatory drug; *PB*, protein binding; *PO*, by mouth; *qid*, four times a day; *SSRIs*, selective serotonin reuptake inhibitors; *t ½*, half-life; *tid*, three times a day.

NSAIDs is their long half-life, which allows them to be taken only once daily.

Full clinical response to piroxicam may take 1 to 2 weeks. This drug is also highly protein bound and may interact with another highly protein-bound drug when taken together. Piroxicam should *not* be taken with aspirin or other NSAIDs.

Side Effects and Adverse Reactions of First-Generation NSAIDs

Most NSAIDs tend to have fewer side effects than aspirin when taken at antiinflammatory doses, but gastric irritation is still a common problem when NSAIDs are taken without food. In addition, fluid retention, peripheral edema, weight gain, and hypertension may occur. Alcoholic beverages consumed with NSAIDs may increase gastric irritation and should be avoided.

COMPLEMENTARY AND ALTERNATIVE THERAPIES

Nonsteroidal Antiinflammatory Drugs

> Dong quai, feverfew, garlic, ginger, and ginkgo may cause bleeding when taken with nonsteroidal antiinflammatory drugs (NSAIDs).

Selective COX-2 Inhibitors

Cyclooxygenase-2 (COX-2) inhibitors, second-generation NSAIDs, became available in the past several years to decrease inflammation and pain. Most NSAIDs are nonselective inhibitors that inhibit COX-1 and COX-2. By inhibiting COX-1, protection of the stomach lining is decreased, and clotting time is also decreased, which may benefit the patient with cardiovascular or coronary artery disease (CAD). Selective COX-2 inhibitors are the drugs of choice for patients with severe arthritic conditions who need high doses of an antiinflammatory drug, because large doses of NSAIDs may cause peptic ulcer and gastric bleeding.

Currently, only one drug, celecoxib, is classified as a COX-2 inhibitor. Nabumetone and meloxicam are similar drugs that can be used; however, they are not considered true COX-2 inhibitors, although they do inhibit COX-2 more than COX-1. Celecoxib is described in Prototype Drug Chart: Celecoxib.

Use of NSAIDs in Older Adults

Older adults frequently use NSAIDs to treat pain associated with inflammation caused by osteoarthritis, RA, and neuromuscular-skeletal disorders. As older adults age, the number of drugs taken daily increases; therefore drug interactions are more common, especially when numerous drugs are taken with NSAIDs. With the use of NSAIDs, GI distress—including ulceration—is four times more common in older adults, and hospitalization is often necessary.

CLINICAL JUDGMENT [NURSING PROCESS]

Nonsteroidal Antiinflammatory Drug (NSAID): Ibuprofen

Concept: Inflammation
- An immunologic response of the body to injury or infection involving redness, swelling, warmth, and pain

Recognize Cues [Assessment]
- Check the patient's history for allergy to NSAIDs such as ibuprofen. If an allergy is present, notify the health care provider.
- Obtain a drug and herbal history, and report any possible drug–drug or drug–herb interactions. NSAIDs can increase the effects of phenytoin, sulfonamides, and warfarin. Most NSAIDs are highly protein bound and can displace other highly protein-bound drugs like warfarin.
- Determine the medical history. NSAIDs are contraindicated if a patient has severe renal or liver disease, peptic ulcer, or bleeding disorder.
- Assess for gastrointestinal (GI) distress and peripheral edema, which are common side effects of NSAIDs.

Analyze Cues and Prioritize Hypothesis [Patient Problems]
- Acute pain
- Injury
- Nausea
- Reduced functional ability
- Decreased mobility

Generate Solutions [Planning]
- The patient will report a pain level has decreased within 1 hour of medication administration.
- The patient's swelling and redness will be reduced within 1 week.

Take Action [Nursing Interventions]
- Observe the patient for bleeding gums, petechiae, ecchymoses, or black, tarry stools. Bleeding time can be prolonged when NSAIDs are taken, especially with a highly protein-bound drug such as warfarin (anticoagulant).
- Report if a patient has GI discomfort. Administer NSAIDs at mealtime or with food to prevent GI upset.
- Monitor vital signs, and check for peripheral edema, especially in the morning.
- Do not give directions such as "take one blue pill" at a specified time. Instead, provide the name and the dosage of medications.

Patient Teaching
General
- ⚡ Advise patients not to take aspirin and acetaminophen with NSAIDs. Taking an NSAID with aspirin could cause GI upset and possibly GI bleeding.
- Advise patients to avoid alcohol when taking NSAIDs. GI distress or gastric ulcer may result.
- Alert patients that many complementary and alternative therapy products may interact with NSAIDs and could cause bleeding. Doses of NSAIDs and/or herbs may need to be modified to avoid possible bleeding.
- Direct patients to inform the dentist or surgeon before a procedure if they are taking ibuprofen or other NSAIDs for a continuous period.
- Warn female patients not to take NSAIDs 1–2 days before menstruation to avoid heavy menstrual flow. If discomfort occurs, acetaminophen is usually prescribed.
- ⚡ Advise pregnant patients to avoid NSAIDs. Congenital abnormalities may occur when NSAIDS are taken during early pregnancy, and excess bleeding might occur during delivery.
- Inform patients that it may take several weeks to experience the desired drug effect of some NSAIDs and disease-modifying antirheumatic drugs (DMARDs).

Side Effects
- Educate patients about the common side effects of NSAIDs. GI distress, peripheral edema, purpura or petechiae, and dizziness can occur. Report occurrences of side effects.

Diet
- Advise patients to take NSAIDs with meals or snacks to reduce GI distress.

Evaluate Outcomes [Evaluation]
- Evaluate the effectiveness of the drug therapy, such as a decrease in pain and in swollen joints and an increase in mobility.

The introduction of COX-2 inhibitors (second-generation NSAIDs) has decreased the incidence of GI problems associated with NSAID use; however, edema is likely to occur. Renal function should be evaluated, and older adults should increase their fluid intake for adequate hydration. To decrease possible complications, the NSAID dose should be lowered.

Corticosteroids

Corticosteroids such as prednisone, prednisolone, and dexamethasone are frequently used as antiinflammatory agents. This group of drugs controls inflammation by suppressing or preventing many of the components of the inflammatory process at the injured site. Corticosteroids have been widely prescribed for arthritic conditions, and although they are not the drug of choice for arthritis because of their numerous side effects, they are frequently used to control arthritic flare-ups.

The half-life of a corticosteroid is long (>24 hours), and it is administered once a day in a large prescribed dose. When discontinuing long-term steroid therapy, the dosage should be tapered over a period of 5 to 10 days. Steroids are discussed in more detail in Chapter 46.

DISEASE-MODIFYING ANTIRHEUMATIC DRUGS

When NSAIDs do not control immune-mediated arthritic disease sufficiently, other drugs, although more toxic, can be prescribed to alter the disease process. The disease-modifying antirheumatic drugs (DMARDs) include immunosuppressive agents, immunomodulators, and antimalarials. DMARDs help alleviate the symptoms of RA for the 2 million persons in the United States affected by the disorder. DMARDs are described in Table 24.3. Other indications for use of DMARDs include osteoarthritis, psoriatic arthritis, severe psoriasis, ankylosing spondylitis, Crohn disease, and ulcerative colitis.

Immunosuppressive Agents

Immunosuppressives are used to treat refractory RA, arthritis that does not respond to antiinflammatory drugs. In low doses, selected immunosuppressive agents have been effective in the treatment of RA. Drugs such as azathioprine, cyclophosphamide, and methotrexate—primarily used to suppress cancer growth and proliferation—might be used to suppress the inflammatory process of RA when other

TABLE 24.3 Antiinflammatory Drugs: Disease-Modifying Antirheumatic Drugs

Drug	Route and Dosage	Uses and Considerations
Golimumab	RA: A: Subcut: 50 mg every month A: IV: 2 mg/kg/dose over 30 min, repeat after 4 wk, then q8wk	For RA, psoriatic arthritis, ankylosing spondylitis, and ulcerative colitis. May cause injection-site reaction, antibody formation, hypertension, elevated hepatic enzymes, influenza, and infection. PB: UK; t½: 10–18 days
Anakinra	RA: A: Subcut: 100 mg/d; max: 100 mg/d	For RA and investigational use for COVID-19. May cause headache, anxiety, fever, pharyngitis, sinusitis, nausea, vomiting, diarrhea, constipation, injection-site reaction, antibody formation, arthralgia, hyperkalemia, hypernatremia, and infection. PB: UK; t½: 4–6 h
Etanercept	RA: A: Subcut: 50 mg q wk max: 50 mg/wk	For RA, psoriatic arthritis, psoriasis, and ankylosing spondylitis. May cause pharyngitis, sinusitis, diarrhea, injection-site reaction, antibody formation, rash, influenza, and infection. PB: UK; t½: 72–132 h
Infliximab	See Prototype Drug Chart: Infliximab	
Rituximab	RA: A: IV: 1000 mg on day 1 and day 15, then repeat the 2-dose course q24wk	For RA, lymphocytic leukemia, and non-Hodgkin lymphoma. May cause headache, depression, weakness, fever, chills, pharyngitis, stomatitis, alopecia, abdominal pain, nausea, diarrhea, peripheral edema/neuropathy, antibody formation, infection, lymphopenia, elevated hepatic enzymes, hypo/hyperkalemia, and anemia. PB: UK; t½: 6–77 d
Adalimumab	RA: A: Subcut: 40 mg q2wk; max: 40 mg/wk or 80 mg q2wk	For RA, psoriatic arthritis, Crohn disease, ulcerative colitis, psoriasis, and ankylosing spondylitis. May cause headache, sinusitis, abdominal pain, nausea, influenza, infection, rash, injection-site reaction, hyperlipidemia, and antibody formation. PB: UK; t½: 10–20 d
Leflunomide	A: PO: Initially 100 mg/d for 3 d; maint: 10–20 mg/d	For RA. May cause dizziness, headache, weakness, alopecia, rash, pruritus, dyspepsia, abdominal pain, nausea, diarrhea, hypertension, back pain, elevated hepatic enzymes, and infection. PB: 99%; t½: 18–19 d
Abatacept	RA: A >100 kg: IV: 1 g over 30 min q2wk for 3 doses, then 1 g q4wk A 60–100 kg: IV: 750 mg over 30 min q2wk for 3 doses, then q4wk A <60 kg: IV: 500 mg over 30 min q2wk for 3 doses, then q4wk A: Subcut: 125 mg/wk	For RA and psoriatic arthritis. May cause headache, fever, epistaxis, pharyngitis, sinusitis, antibody formation, infection, hypo/hypertension, influenza, anemia, hypermagnesemia, lymphopenia, nephrotoxicity, and infusion-related reaction. PB: UK; t½: 14.3 d
Tofacitinib	RA: Immediate release: A: PO: 5 mg bid; max: 20 mg/d Extended release: A: PO: 11 mg/d; max: 22 mg/d	For RA, psoriatic arthritis, ankylosing spondylitis, and ulcerative colitis. May cause headache, pharyngitis, gastritis, nausea, diarrhea, infection, anemia, and rash. PB: 40%; t½: 3 h immediate release, 6–8 h extended release
Tocilizumab	RA: A: IV: Initially 4 mg/kg over 1 h q4wk A <100 kg: Subcut: 162 mg qowk A >100 kg: Subcut: 162 mg/wk	For RA, juvenile idiopathic arthritis and investigational use of COVID-19. May cause headache, pharyngitis, constipation, infusion/injection-related reaction, hyperlipidemia, elevated hepatic enzymes, neutropenia, infection, and hypertension. PB: UK; t½: subcut, every wk 18.3–18.9 d, qowk 4.2–7.9 d; IV, 11–13 d
Secukinumab	Psoriasis: A: Subcut: 300 mg wk 0–4, followed by 300 mg q4wk; max: 300 mg/dose	For psoriasis, psoriatic arthritis, and ankylosing spondylitis. May cause oral ulceration, pharyngitis, rhinorrhea, rhinitis, diarrhea, hives, neutropenia, infection, and antibody formation. PB: UK; t½: 22–31 d
Apremilast	Psoriatic arthritis: A: PO: Initially 10 mg in the morning on day 1; 10 mg bid on day 2, 10 mg in morning and 20 mg in evening on day 3; 20 mg bid on day 4; 20 mg in morning and 30 mg in evening on day 5; maint: 30 mg bid starting on day 6; max: 60 mg/d	For psoriatic arthritis and psoriasis. May cause headache, abdominal pain, nausea, vomiting, diarrhea, weight loss, arthralgia, back pain, and infection. PB: 68%; t½: 6–9 h
Canakinumab	A: Subcut: 4 mg/kg q4wk; max: 300 mg/dose	For systemic juvenile idiopathic arthritis. May cause dizziness, headache, rhinitis, pharyngitis, nausea, abdominal pain, diarrhea, weight gain, injection-site reaction, influenza, infection, neutropenia, thrombocytopenia and musculoskeletal pain. PB: UK; t½: 26 d
Sarilumab	RA: A: Subcut: 200 mg q2wk; max: 200 mg/dose	For moderate to severe RA and investigational use of COVID-19. May cause fatigue, pharyngitis, infection, constipation, myalgia, elevated hepatic enzymes, antibody formation, erythema, pruritus, leukopenia, neutropenia, injection-site reaction, hypertriglyceridemia, and hypercholesterolemia. PB: UK; t½: 8–43 d depending upon concentration
Ixekizumab	Psoriatic arthritis: A: Subcut: LD: 160 mg/wk, then 80 mg q4wk	For psoriatic arthritis, active ankylosing spondylitis, and plaque psoriasis. May cause conjunctivitis, ocular infection, nausea, antibody formation, infection, injection-site reaction, neutropenia, hives, and influenza. PB: UK; t½: 13 d

TABLE 24.3 Antiinflammatory Drugs: Disease-Modifying Antirheumatic Drugs—cont'd

Drug	Route and Dosage	Uses and Considerations
Certolizumab pegol	RA: A: Subcut: 400 mg qowk for 3 doses; then 200 mg qowk; *maint*: 400 mg q4wk; *max*: 400 mg/dose	For Crohn disease, RA, psoriatic arthritis, ankylosing spondylitis, and plaque psoriasis. May cause headache, pharyngitis, cough, fatigue, antibody formation, infection, arthralgia, back pain, hypertension, and rash. PB: UK; t½: 14 d
Baricitinib	RA: A: PO: 2 mg/d	For RA, alopecia areata, and investigational use of COVID-19. May cause headache, abdominal pain, nausea, infection, thrombocytosis, acne vulgaris, acneiform rash, and elevated hepatic enzymes. PB: 45%–50%; t½: 12 h
Upadacitinib	RA: A: PO: 15 mg/d	For RA, psoriatic arthritis, active ankylosing spondylitis, atopic dermatitis, moderate to severe ulcerative colitis, Crohn disease. May cause headache, fever, infection, acne vulgaris, anemia, neutropenia, and elevated hepatic enzymes. PB: 52%; t½: 8–14 h
Etrasimod	A: PO: 2 mg/d	For moderate to severe ulcerative colitis. May cause headache, migraine, dizziness, visual impairment, nausea, arthralgia, infection, and elevated hepatic enzymes. PB: 97.9%; t½: 30 h
Mirikizumab	Induction: A: IV: 300 mg infusion over at least 30 min at wk 0, 4, 8; Maintenance: A: Subcut: Begin 4 wks after last induction 200 mg at wk 12 then q4wk	For moderate to severe active ulcerative colitis. May cause headache, antibody formation, infection, arthralgia, rash, and injection-site reaction. PB: UK; t½: 9.3 d
Ustekinumab	Ulcerative colitis: A: IV: >85 kg: 520 mg as a single dose A: IV: 56–85 kg: 390 mg as a single dose A: 55 kg or <: 260 mg as a single dose A: Subcut: 8 wks after IV single dose, give 90 mg q8wks	For plaque psoriasis, psoriatic arthritis, Crohn's, and ulcerative colitis. May cause antibody formation, headache, infection, pharyngitis, abdominal pain, candidiasis, diarrhea, erythema, fever, influenza, and injection site reaction. PB: UK; t½: 19 d

A, Adult; *bid*, twice daily; *d*, day; *h*, hour; *IV*, intravenous; *maint*, maintenance; *max*, maximum; *min*, minute; *PB*, protein binding; *PO*, by mouth; *q2*, every two; *qowk*, every other week; *RA*, rheumatoid arthritis; *Subcut*, subcutaneous; *t ½*, half-life; *UK*, unknown; *wk*, week; *y*, year; *>*, greater than.

PROTOTYPE DRUG CHART

Celecoxib

Drug Class	Dosage
Nonsteroidal antiinflammatory: COX-2 inhibitor	Rheumatoid Arthritis: A: PO: 100–200 mg bid; *max*: 800 mg/d, older adult 400 mg/d

Contraindications	Drug-Lab-Food Interactions
Hypersensitivity, coronary artery bypass surgery *Caution*: Angina, hypertension, dysrhythmias, heart failure, cardiac disease, asthma, cerebrovascular disease, peripheral vascular disease, anticoagulant therapy, peptic ulcer disease, GI bleeding/perforation, renal or hepatic dysfunction, dehydration, alcohol misuse, tobacco smoking, older adults, breast-feeding, children	Drug: Decreased effect of ACE inhibitors; increased INR and GI bleeding with warfarin and SNRIs; may increase toxicity with lithium; fluoroquinolones may increase the risk of seizures; fluconazole increases celecoxib levels Complementary and alternative therapies: Ginkgo biloba may increase bleeding risk

Pharmacokinetics	Pharmacodynamics
Absorption: Well absorbed in GI tract Distribution: PB: 97% Metabolism: t½: 11.2 h Excretion: Primarily in feces	PO: Onset: UK Peak: 3 h Duration: UK

Therapeutic Effects/Uses

To treat osteoarthritis and rheumatoid arthritis; to relieve dysmenorrhea and moderate to severe pain; for ankylosing spondylitis, migraine
Mechanism of Action: Inhibits COX-2, which normally promotes prostaglandin synthesis and inflammatory response, but does not inhibit COX-1

Side Effects	Adverse Reactions
Dizziness, drowsiness, headache, sinusitis, pharyngitis, cough, anorexia, abdominal pain, nausea, dyspepsia, flatulence, vomiting, diarrhea, constipation, infection, arthralgia, peripheral edema, diaphoresis, rash	Hearing loss, tinnitus, dyspnea, angina, hypertension, GI bleeding/obstruction/ulcer/perforation, tendon rupture, hypo/hypernatremia, hypo/hyperkalemia, hypercholesterolemia, thromboembolism, hypo/hyperglycemia *Life-threatening*: Anaphylaxis, angioedema, bronchospasm, aplastic anemia, agranulocytosis, leukopenia, pancytopenia, thrombocytopenia, renal/hepatic failure, Stevens-Johnson syndrome

A, Adult; *ACE*, angiotensin-converting enzyme; *bid*, twice a day; *COX*, cyclooxygenase; *d*, day; *GI*, gastrointestinal; *h*, hour; *INR*, international normalized ratio; *max*, maximum; *PB*, protein binding; *PO*, by mouth; *qd*, every day; *SNRI*, serotonin norepinephrine reuptake inhibitor; *t ½*, half-life; *UK*, unknown.

PROTOTYPE DRUG CHART

Infliximab

Drug Class	Dosage
Immunomodulator: Tumor necrosis factor blocker	Crohn disease: A: IV: Initially 5 mg/kg over 2 h on wk 0, 2, and 6; *maint:* 5–10 mg/kg/dose q8wk; *max:* 10 mg/kg/dose
Contraindications	**Drug-Lab-Food Interactions**
Hypersensitivity *Caution:* Heart failure, COPD, diabetes mellitus, hepatic dysfunction, bone marrow suppression, immunosuppression, multiple sclerosis, seizures, corticosteroid therapy, infection, leukopenia, breast-feeding, children	Drug: May decrease effectiveness of vaccines; concurrent immunosuppressives may increase risk for infection or adverse effects
Pharmacokinetics	**Pharmacodynamics**
Absorption: UK Distribution: UK Metabolism: t½: 7.7–9.5 d Excretion: UK	IV: Onset: RA: 3–7 d; Crohn disease: 1–2 wk Peak: UK Duration: RA: 6–12 wk; Crohn disease 8–48 wk
Therapeutic Effects/Uses	
To treat psoriasis, RA, psoriatic arthritis, ankylosing spondylitis, ulcerative colitis, and Crohn disease Mechanism of Action: Binds to TNF and blocks it from attaching to TNF receptors on synovial cell surfaces; reduces infiltration of inflammatory cells and delays inflammatory process	
Side Effects	**Adverse Reactions**
Dizziness, headache, visual impairment, edema, phlebitis, fatigue, chills, flushing, fever, cough, sinusitis, pharyngitis, dyspepsia, abdominal pain, nausea, diarrhea, constipation, weight loss, hyperhidrosis, dehydration, rash, arthralgia, myalgia, candidiasis, infusion-related reaction	Hypo/hypertension, chest pain, bradycardia, dyspnea, pulmonary edema, GI obstruction, seizures, bone fractures, anemia, severe infection, antibody formation, elevated hepatic enzymes *Life-threatening:* Bronchospasm, anaphylaxis, agranulocytosis, leukopenia, neutropenia, pancytopenia, hemolytic anemia, thrombocytopenia, hepatotoxicity, Stevens-Johnson syndrome

A, Adult; *COPD*, chronic obstructive pulmonary disease; *d*, day; *GI*, gastrointestinal; *h*, hour; *IV*, intravenous; *maint*, maintenance; *max*, maximum; *PB*, protein binding; *RA*, rheumatoid arthritis; *q8*, every 8; *t ½*, half-life; *TNF*, tumor necrosis factor; *UK*, unknown; *wk*, week.

---

treatments fail. In one study of patients receiving cyclophosphamide, few new erosions of joint cartilage were present, suggesting that the disease process was not active.

Immunomodulators

Immunomodulators treat moderate to severe RA by disrupting the inflammatory process and delaying disease progression. Interleukin 1 (IL-1) receptor antagonists and tumor necrosis factor (TNF) blockers are two groups of drugs classified as immunomodulators.

Anakinra, an IL-1 receptor antagonist, blocks activity of IL-1 by inhibiting it from binding to interleukin receptors located in cartilage and bone. IL-1 is a proinflammatory cytokine that contributes to synovial inflammation and joint destruction. Anakinra is administered subcutaneously. The peak is 3 to 7 hours, and the half-life is 4 to 6 hours.

TNF blockers bind to TNF and block it from attaching to TNF receptors on synovial cell surfaces. By neutralizing TNF, a contributor to synovitis, the inflammatory disease process is delayed. Etanercept was the first TNF blocker developed. It is administered subcutaneously, and the half-life ranges from 72 to 132 hours. Signs and symptoms of RA are suppressed rapidly with etanercept therapy but reappear if the drug is discontinued. Other TNF blockers include infliximab, adalimumab, and certolizumab pegol. Infliximab is administered intravenously over at least 2 hours, adalimumab is administered subcutaneously, and leflunomide is administered orally. Infliximab is described in Prototype Drug Chart: Infliximab.

Both IL-1 receptor antagonists and TNF blockers predispose the patient to severe infections; they are contraindicated in active infection and should be discontinued when an infection occurs. Immunomodulators are usually very expensive.

Antimalarials

Antimalarial drugs may be used to treat RA when other methods of treatment fail. The mechanism of action of antimalarials in suppressing RA is unclear. The effect may take 4 to 12 weeks to become apparent. Antimalarials are usually used in combination with NSAIDs in patients whose arthritis is not under control.

ANTIGOUT DRUGS

Gout is an inflammatory condition that attacks joints, tendons, and other tissues. It may be called *gouty arthritis*. The most common site of acute gouty inflammation is at the joint of the hallux (big toe). Gout is characterized by a uric acid metabolism disorder and a defect in purine (products of certain proteins) metabolism, which results in an increase in urates (uric acid salts) and an accumulation of uric acid (hyperuricemia) or an ineffective clearance of uric acid by the kidneys. Uric acid solubility is poor in acid urine, and urate crystals may form, causing urate calculi. Gout may appear as bumps, or *tophi*, in the subcutaneous tissue of earlobes, elbows, hands, and at the base of the great toe. In addition to tophi, the complications of untreated or prolonged periods of gout include gouty arthritis, urinary calculi, and gouty nephropathy.

To promote uric acid excretion and to prevent renal calculi, fluid intake should be increased while taking antigout drugs. Foods high in

CLINICAL JUDGMENT [NURSING PROCESS]
Disease-Modifying Antirheumatic Drug: Infliximab

Concept: Inflammation
- An immunologic response of the body to injury or infection involving redness, swelling, warmth, and pain

Recognize Cues [Assessment]
- Determine a medical history. Ask the patient if there is any history of seizures, diabetes mellitus, multiple sclerosis, or kidney or liver disease. Infliximab may increase the risk of bleeding time.
- Obtain baseline complete blood count (CBC) and renal and liver function tests.

Analyze Cues and Prioritize Hypothesis [Patient Planning]
- Acute pain
- Injury
- Nausea
- Reduced functional ability
- Decreased mobility

Generate Solutions [Planning]
- The patient will report that pain level has decreased within 1 hour of medication administration.
- The patient's swelling and redness will be reduced within 1 week.

Take Action [Nursing Interventions]
- Obtain a negative tuberculosis skin test before initiating infliximab therapy.
- Monitor patients for signs and symptoms of infection. If a serious infection occurs while a patient is receiving infliximab therapy, antibiotic therapy should be initiated, and infliximab should be discontinued.
- Monitor laboratory tests for blood dyscrasias (CBC) and renal and liver function (blood urea nitrogen [BUN], serum creatinine, alkaline phosphatase [ALP], aspartate aminotransferase [AST], alanine aminotransferase [ALT]).
- Flush intravenous (IV) tubing with normal saline before and after administration. Deliver IV medication through a 1.2-micron or smaller filter.
- Administer each dose over a minimum of 2 hours.
- Discontinue IV dose of infliximab if the patient develops acute infusion reaction (e.g., chest pain, fever, chills, dyspnea, pruritus, urticaria, hypotension, or hypertension).
- Monitor patients up to 2 hours after infusion for acute infusion reaction.

Patient Teaching
General
- Encourage patients to keep medical appointments and to have regularly scheduled laboratory tests that include CBC and renal and liver function tests for early detection of blood dyscrasias and renal and liver damage.
- Advise patients to avoid live vaccines while taking infliximab.

Side Effects
- ⚡ Teach patients to report dizziness, chills, depression, dyspnea, severe infections, seizures, fatigue, or rash immediately.
- Teach patients to report severe infections immediately.

Evaluate Outcomes [Evaluation]
- Evaluate patient response to the disease-modifying antirheumatic drug (DMARD). If pain persists, the drug regimen may need modification.
- Determine the presence of adverse reactions. Drug therapy for pain may need to be changed.

---

purine—such as organ meats, sardines, salmon, gravy, herring, liver, and meat soups—and alcohol, especially beer, should be avoided. Alcohol causes both an overproduction and underexcretion of uric acid. To reduce acidity, acetaminophen should be taken for discomfort instead of aspirin (salicylic acid).

Antiinflammatory Gout Drug: Colchicine

The first drug used to treat gout was colchicine, introduced in 1936. This antiinflammatory gout drug reduces several proinflammatory pathways and increases levels of antiinflammatory mediators linked to gout. It prevents the activation of neutrophils in its interference of the inflammatory response. It is effective in alleviating acute symptoms of gout, but it is not effective for decreasing inflammation that occurs in other inflammatory disorders. Colchicine does not inhibit uric acid synthesis and does not promote uric acid excretion. It should not be used if the patient has a severe renal, cardiac, or GI problem. Gastric irritation is a common problem, so colchicine should be taken with food. With high doses, nausea, vomiting, diarrhea, or abdominal pain occurs in approximately 75% of patients taking the drug.

Colchicine is well absorbed in the GI tract, and its peak concentration time is within 3 hours. Most of the drug is excreted in the feces, but 10% to 20% is excreted in the urine.

Xanthine Oxidase Inhibitors

Allopurinol, first marketed in 1963, is *not* an antiinflammatory drug; instead, it increases uric acid excretion in the urine by inhibiting the xanthine oxidase enzyme, which blocks metabolism of xanthine to uric acid. It also reduces uric acid production, preventing the precipitation of an attack. This drug is frequently used as a prophylactic to prevent gout, and it is a drug of choice for patients with chronic tophaceous gout. Allopurinol is also indicated for gout patients with renal impairment. It is useful for patients who have renal obstructions caused by uric acid stones and for patients with blood disorders such as leukemia and polycythemia vera. It is also given to patients who do not respond well to uricosuric drugs such as probenecid. Increased fluid intake is recommended to promote diuresis and alkalinization of the urine.

Febuxostat was FDA approved in 2009 for the treatment of hyperuricemia associated with gout. This drug is more selective for xanthine oxidase than allopurinol. Febuxostat may cause gout exacerbations as allopurinol does. It has a greater risk of promoting cardiovascular adverse events. Febuxostat is eliminated by both hepatic and renal pathways.

Prototype Drug Chart: Febuxostat presents the pharmacologic behavior of febuxostat, another uric acid biosynthesis inhibitor.

Pharmacokinetics

The half-life of febuxostat is 5 to 8 hours. The protein-binding percentage is 99.2%. Approximately 49% is excreted in urine and 45% in feces.

Pharmacodynamics

Febuxostat inhibits the production of uric acid by inhibiting the enzyme xanthine oxidase, which is needed in the synthesis of uric acid. Its onset of action is unknown; its peak time averages 1 to 1.5 hours. The duration of action of febuxostat is unknown.

Uricosurics

Uricosurics increase the rate of uric acid excretion by inhibiting its reabsorption. These drugs are effective in alleviating chronic gout, but they should not be used during acute attacks. Probenecid is a uricosuric that has been available since 1945. It blocks the reabsorption of uric acid and promotes its excretion. Probenecid can be taken with colchicine. To begin initial therapy for relieving symptoms of gout and inhibiting uric acid reabsorption, small doses of colchicine should be given before adding probenecid. If gastric irritation occurs, probenecid should be taken with meals. It has an average half-life of 3 to 12 hours and is 75% to 95% protein bound. Table 24.4 gives dosages and considerations for the commonly used antigout drugs.

TABLE 24.4 Antigout Drugs

Drug	Route and Dosage	Uses and Considerations
Antiinflammatory Gout Drugs		
Colchicine	Acute gout attack: A: PO: Initially 1.2 mg; then 0.6 mg in 1 h; *max:* 1.8 mg over 1-h period Prophylaxis: A: PO: 0.6 mg qd/bid; *max:* 1.2 mg/d	For gout and familial Mediterranean fever. Not for patients with renal/hepatic disorders. May cause headache, fatigue, abdominal pain, nausea, vomiting, diarrhea, myalgia, and peripheral neuropathy. Take with food. PB: 34%–44%; $t\frac{1}{2}$: 1.7–31.9 h
Xanthine Oxidase Inhibitors		
Allopurinol	Gout: A: PO: Initially 50–100 mg/d; maint: 200–300 mg/d for mild gout, 400–600 mg/d for moderate to severe gout; *max:* 800 mg/d in divided dose	For gout, hyperuricemia, and renal calculi. May cause nausea, vomiting, diarrhea, rash, renal failure, and GI bleeding/obstruction. PB: UK; $t\frac{1}{2}$: 1–2 h
Febuxostat	See Prototype Drug Chart: Febuxostat	
Uricosurics		
Probenecid	A: PO: Initially 250 mg bid for 1 wk; *maint:* 500 mg bid; *max:* 2 g/d	For hyperuricemia and gout. May cause dizziness, headache, alopecia, fever, flushing, anorexia, nausea, vomiting, nephrolithiasis, and anemia. PB: 75%–95%; $t\frac{1}{2}$: 3–12 h

A, Adult; *bid*, twice a day; *d*, day; *GI*, gastrointestinal; *h*, hour; *maint*, maintenance; *max*, maximum; *PB*, protein binding; *PO*, by mouth; *qd*, every day; *t ½*, half-life; *UK*, unknown; *wk*, week; *y*, year; *>*, greater than.

PROTOTYPE DRUG CHART

Febuxostat

Drug Class	Dosage
Antigout: Xanthine oxidase inhibitor	A: PO: Initially 40 mg/d; *max:* 120 mg/d
Contraindications	**Drug-Lab-Food Interactions**
Hypersensitivity *Caution:* Cardiac disease, stroke, renal/hepatic disorder, chemotherapy, dialysis, pregnancy, breast-feeding	Drug: Increased effect of theophylline, azathioprine, mercaptopurine, pegloticase Lab: Increased AST, ALT, BUN
Pharmacokinetics	**Pharmacodynamics**
Absorption: PO: 49% absorbed Distribution: PB: 99.2% Metabolism: $t\frac{1}{2}$: 5–8 h Excretion: 49% in urine and 45% in feces	PO: Onset: UK Peak: 1–1.5 h Duration: UK
Therapeutic Effects/Uses	
To treat hyperuricemia in patients with gout Mechanism of Action: Blocks hypoxanthine and xanthine metabolism to reduce uric acid synthesis to decrease uric acid blood and urine concentrations	
Side Effects	**Adverse Reactions**
Dizziness, headache, flushing, fatigue, blurred vision, epistaxis, dry mouth, dysgeusia, anorexia, abdominal pain, nausea, dyspepsia, vomiting, diarrhea, constipation, flatulence, arthralgia, myalgia, weakness, edema, dehydration, rash, pruritus, erectile dysfunction	Bradycardia, tachycardia, chest pain, hypo/hypertension, stroke, dyspnea, diabetes mellitus, hyperglycemia, hypo/hyperkalemia, hyperlipidemia, hypertriglyceridemia, hypercholesterolemia, cholelithiasis, Guillain-Barre syndrome, anemia, elevated hepatic enzymes, cholecystitis, rhabdomyolysis *Life-threatening:* Thrombocytopenia, neutropenia, leukopenia, pancytopenia, angioedema, hepatic/renal impairment, dysrhythmias, Stevens-Johnson syndrome

A, Adult; *ALT*, alanine aminotransferase; *AST*, aspartate aminotransferase; *BUN*, blood urea nitrogen; *d*, day; *h*, hour; *max*, maximum; *PB*, protein binding; *PO*, by mouth; *t ½*, half-life; *UK*, unknown.

CLINICAL JUDGMENT [NURSING PROCESS]

Antigout Drug: Allopurinol

Concept: Inflammation
- An immunologic response of the body to injury or infection involving redness, swelling, warmth, and pain

Recognize Cues [Assessment]
- Obtain a medical history of any gastric, renal, cardiac, or liver disorders. Antigout drugs are excreted via the kidneys, so sufficient renal function is needed. Drug dosage and drug selection might need to be changed.
- Obtain a drug history. Report possible drug–drug interactions.
- Assess serum uric acid value for future comparisons.
- Record urine output. Use initial urine output for future comparisons.
- Check laboratory tests such as blood urea nitrogen (BUN), serum creatinine, alkaline phosphatase (ALP), aspartate aminotransferase (AST), alanine aminotransferase (ALT), and lactate dehydrogenase (LDH), and compare with future laboratory test results.

Analyze Cues and Prioritize Hypothesis [Patient Problems]
- Acute pain
- Injury
- Nausea
- Reduced functional ability
- Decreased mobility

Generate Solutions [Planning]
- The patient will report that pain level has decreased within 1 hour of medication administration.
- The patient's swelling and redness will be reduced within 1 week.

Take Action [Nursing Interventions]
- Report gastrointestinal (GI) symptoms, gastric pain, nausea, vomiting, or diarrhea for patients taking antigout drugs. Administer these drugs with food to alleviate gastric distress.
- Record urine output. Because the drugs and uric acid are excreted through the urine, kidney stones might occur, so both water intake and urine output should be increased.
- ⚡ Monitor laboratory tests for renal and liver function (BUN, serum creatinine, ALP, AST, ALT).

Patient Teaching
General
- ⚡ Encourage patients to keep medical appointments and to have regularly scheduled laboratory tests for renal and liver function and complete blood count (CBC). Some antigout drugs may cause blood dyscrasias, so blood tests should be monitored.
- Instruct patients to increase fluid intake; it will increase drug and uric acid excretion.

Side Effects
- Advise patients to report to a health care provider any side effects of antigout drugs such as anorexia, nausea, vomiting, diarrhea, stomatitis, dizziness, rash, pruritus, and metallic taste.
- Advise patients to have a yearly eye examination because visual changes can result from prolonged use of allopurinol.

Diet
- Warn patients to avoid alcohol and caffeine because they can increase uric acid levels.
- Suggest that patients not take large doses of vitamin C while taking allopurinol; kidney stones may occur.
- Tell patients not to ingest foods high in purine content such as organ meats, salmon, sardines, gravy, and legumes. Foods with purine increase uric acid levels.
- Direct patients to report any gastric distress. Encourage them to take antigout drugs with food or at mealtime.

Evaluate Outcomes [Evaluation]
- Evaluate the response to the antigout drug. If pain persists, the drug regimen may need modification.
- Determine the presence of adverse reactions. Drug therapy for gout pain may need to be changed.

Side Effects and Adverse Reactions

Side effects of uricosurics may include flushed skin, fever, dizziness, and headache. Kidney stones resulting from the uric acid could be prevented by increasing water intake and maintaining a urine pH above 6. Blood dyscrasias may occur. Aspirin use should be avoided with probenecid because it inhibits the action of probenecid.

CLINICAL JUDGMENT CASE STUDY

A 72-year-old female had taken 650 mg of aspirin four times a day for 8 months to alleviate her chronic symptoms of pain and inflammation associated with arthritis. Four weeks ago, a peptic ulcer developed.

1. Explain the process by which the patient could have a peptic ulcer. How could this have been prevented?
2. Compare the similarities and differences in the side effects of salicylates with those of acetic acid agents, propionic acid agents, COX-2 inhibitors, and phenylacetic acid.
3. What teaching points should the patient receive before and during the time she takes aspirin?
4. How would COX-2 inhibitors prevent the development of a peptic ulcer?

REVIEW QUESTIONS

1. A patient is taking ibuprofen. The nurse understands that COX-1 and COX-2 inhibitors are different in that ibuprofen is more likely than celecoxib to cause which adverse effect?
   a. Fever
   b. Constipation
   c. Peptic ulcer disease
   d. Metallic taste when eating

2. When teaching a patient who is receiving allopurinol, what should the nurse encourage the patient to do?
   a. Eat more meat.
   b. Increase vitamin C intake.
   c. Have annual eye examinations.
   d. Take medication 2 hours before meals.

3. A patient is admitted to the hospital with an acute gout attack. The nurse expects that which medication will be ordered to treat acute gout?
   a. Colchicine
   b. Allopurinol
   c. Probenecid
   d. Sulfinpyrazone

4. A patient is taking aspirin for arthritis. Which adverse reaction should the nurse teach the patient to report to the health care provider?
   a. Tinnitus
   b. Weight loss
   c. Sinusitis
   d. Palpitations

5. The nurse is teaching a patient about taking aspirin. Which are important points to include? **Select all that apply**.
   a. Advise the patient to avoid alcohol while taking aspirin.
   b. Instruct the patient to take aspirin before meals on an empty stomach.
   c. Instruct the patient to inform the dentist of the aspirin dosage before having dental work.
   d. Instruct the patient to inform the surgeon of the aspirin dosage before having surgery.
   e. Suggest that aspirin may be given to children for flu symptoms.
   f. Advise patient that urine may be a harmless pinkish-red or reddish-brown color.

6. A patient is taking infliximab and asks the nurse what side effects/adverse reactions to expect from this drug. The nurse lists which side effects? **Select all that apply**.
   a. Fatigue
   b. Headache
   c. Chest pain
   d. Renal damage
   e. Severe infections

25

Analgesics

http://evolve.elsevier.com/McCuistion/pharmacology

OBJECTIVES

- Explain the pathophysiology of pain as well as concepts that inform pain management approaches.
- Explain common uses and mechanisms of action of nonopioid analgesics.
- Explain usage considerations of opioid analgesics.
- Summarize considerations of medications administered with opioids.
- Contrast characteristics and treatments of migraine and cluster headaches.

OUTLINE

Pain, 303
    Pain Classification, 303
    Pathophysiology, 304
    Undertreatment of Pain, 304
Nonopioid Analgesics, 305
    Nonsteroidal Antiinflammatory Drugs, 305
    Acetaminophen, 305
    Side Effects and Adverse Reactions, 306
Opioid Analgesics, 306
    Morphine, 309
    Meperidine, 310
    Hydromorphone, 312
    Combination Drugs, 312

Patient-Controlled Analgesia, 312
Transdermal Opioid Analgesics, 312
Analgesic Titration, 312
Opioid Use in Special Populations, 312
Adjuvants, Agonists, and Antagonists, 313
    Adjuvant Therapy, 313
    Opioid Agonist-Antagonists, 313
    Opioid Antagonists, 314
Headaches: Migraine and Cluster, 314
    Pathophysiology, 316
    Treatment of Migraine Headaches, 316
Clinical Judgment Single-Episode Case Study, 318
Review Questions, 319

PAIN

Pain is an unpleasant sensory and emotional experience related to tissue injury. Due to the subjective nature of pain, the nurse must be knowledgeable and skillful in the assessment and measurement of pain to achieve optimal pain management.

Pain management is regarded as such a significant component of nursing care that pain has become known as the "fifth vital sign." The Joint Commission (TJC) has incorporated the assessment, documentation, and management of pain into its standards, which reflect the importance of this vital sign. The nurse's role is to assess the patient's pain level, alleviate the patient's pain through nonpharmacologic and pharmacologic treatments, thoroughly document the patient's response to treatment, and teach patients and their significant others to manage pain control when appropriate.

An individual's **pain threshold** reflects the level of stimulus needed to create a painful sensation, and individual genetic makeup contributes to the variations in pain threshold from person to person. The mu (μ) opioid receptor gene controls the number of μ-receptors present. When an individual has a large number of μ-receptors, the pain threshold is high, and pain sensitivity is reduced.

The amount of pain a person can endure without having it interfere with normal functioning is called **pain tolerance**. This psychological aspect of pain varies greatly in individuals because it is subjective and because pain tolerance is influenced by factors such as age, sex, culture, ethnicity, previous experience, anxiety level, and specific circumstances, such as a traumatic event.

Analgesics, both nonopioid and opioid, are prescribed for the relief of pain. The choice of analgesic depends on the severity of the pain. Mild to moderate pain is frequently relieved with the use of nonopioid, also known as *nonnarcotic*, analgesics. Moderate to severe pain usually requires an opioid, or *narcotic*, analgesic.

Drugs used for pain relief are presented in this chapter. Many of the same nonopioid analgesics that are taken for pain, such as the **nonsteroidal antiinflammatory drugs (NSAIDs)**, are also taken for antiinflammatory purposes. This application for these drugs is covered in Chapter 24.

Pain Classification

The most common classification of pain is by duration. Acute pain can be mild, moderate, or severe, and it is usually associated with a specific tissue injury. The onset of acute pain is usually sudden and of short duration, lasting less than 3 months. Chronic pain usually has a vague origin and gradual onset with a prolonged duration (more than 3 months) of long-lasting discomfort.

TABLE 25.1 Types of Pain

Type of Pain	Definition	Drug Treatment
Acute	Pain occurs suddenly, is of short duration (less than 3 months), and responds to treatment; it can result from trauma, tissue injury, inflammation, or surgery.	Mild pain: Nonopioid drugs, such as acetaminophen and NSAIDs Moderate pain: Combination of nonopioid and opioid drugs, such as oxycodone and acetaminophen Severe pain: Potent opioids, such as morphine or hydrocodone
Chronic	Pain persists for more than 3 months and is difficult to treat or control.	Nonopioid drugs are suggested. Opioids, if used, should meet these criteria: • Oral or transdermal • Long duration of action • Include adjunct therapy • Cause minimal respiratory depression
Cancer	Pain occurs from pressure on nerves and organs, blockage to blood supply, or metastasis to bone.	NSAIDs and opioid drugs administered PO, transdermally, via IM or IV routes, intrathecally, or with PCA
Somatic	Pain is in skeletal muscle, ligaments, and joints.	Nonopioids: NSAIDs; also act as antiinflammatories and muscle relaxants
Superficial	Pain is from surface areas such as skin and mucous membranes.	Mild pain: Nonopioid Moderate pain: Combination of opioid and nonopioid analgesic drugs
Vascular	Pain occurs from vascular or perivascular tissues contributing to headaches or migraines.	Nonopioid drugs
Visceral	Pain is from smooth muscle and organs.	Opioid drugs

IM, Intramuscular; *IV*, intravenous; *NSAIDs*, nonsteroidal antiinflammatory drugs; *PCA*, patient-controlled analgesia; *PO*, by mouth.

Pain may also be classified by its origin. Nociceptors, sensory receptors for pain, are activated by noxious stimuli—mechanical, thermal, and chemical—in peripheral tissues. When tissue damage occurs, injured cells release chemical mediators that affect the exposed nerve endings of the nociceptors. Pain that originates from tissue injury is nociceptor pain, which includes somatic pain—that is, pain from structural tissues such as bones and muscles—and visceral (organ) pain. Neuropathic pain is an unusual sensory disturbance that often involves neural supersensitivity. This pain is due to injury or disease of the peripheral nervous system (PNS) or central nervous system (CNS). The patient with neuropathic pain usually complains of burning, tingling, or electric shock sensations in the affected area, often triggered by light touch. Diabetic neuropathy associated with diabetes mellitus is an example of peripheral neuropathic pain. Severe, intractable pain from a herniated disk or spinal cord injury is evidence of neuropathic pain from the CNS.

Pathophysiology

The most common pain theory is called the *gate theory*, proposed by Melzack and Wall in 1965. According to this theory, tissue injury activates nociceptors and causes the release of chemical mediators, such as substance P, prostaglandins, bradykinin, histamine, serotonin, acetylcholine, glutamate, adenosine triphosphate, leukotrienes, and potassium. These substances initiate an action potential along a sensory nerve fiber and sensitize pain receptors. Nociceptive action potentials are transmitted via afferent nerve fibers. One type of pain fiber that primarily transmits impulses from the periphery is the A-delta (A-δ) fiber. Because A-δ pain fibers are wrapped in a myelin sheath, they transmit impulses rapidly in acute pain. The C-fiber is a type of pain fiber that is small and unmyelinated, and because C-fibers are unmyelinated, they transmit impulses slowly. C-fibers are more often associated with chronic, dull pain.

A pain signal begins at the nociceptors in the periphery and proceeds throughout the CNS. Knowing how and where pharmacologic agents work is essential to controlling pain. The body produces neurohormones called **endorphins** (peptides) that naturally suppress pain conduction, although the method is not completely understood. Opioids such as morphine activate the same receptors as endorphins to reduce pain. NSAIDs control pain at the peripheral level by blocking the action of cyclooxygenase, a pain-sensitizing chemical, and interfering with the production of prostaglandins. Cortisone decreases pain by blocking the action of phospholipase, reducing the production of both prostaglandins and leukotrienes. In neuropathic pain, anticonvulsant drugs inhibit the transmission of nerve impulses by stabilizing the neuronal membrane and inactivating peripheral sodium channels.

To ascertain severity of pain, the health care provider should ask the patient to rate the degree of pain on a scale of 0 to 10, with 10 being the worst or most severe pain. For example, a patient who indicates a pain level of 9 may verbalize a decrease in pain to a level of 7 within 30 to 45 minutes after receiving pain medication. Many scales and instruments are available to the nurse for assessment and measurement of the patient's pain level. Table 25.1 lists the types of pain and the drug groups that may be effective in relieving each type.

Undertreatment of Pain

Undertreatment of pain is a major issue in health care today. Postoperative pain is inadequately managed in 80% or more of patients in the United States. When acute postoperative pain is poorly controlled, associated factors include delayed recovery time, extended duration of opioid use, functional ability, impaired quality of life, higher health care costs, and increased morbidity. Some reasons for undertreatment are sociocultural variables that mediate a patient's willingness to acknowledge being in pain, the patient's inability to describe pain, the patient's fear of substance use disorder, the nurse's inability to measure pain, lack of regular pain assessment rounds, attitudes of the health care team, an unwillingness to believe the patient's report of pain, inaccurate knowledge on the part of the health care provider concerning substance use disorder and tolerance, and prescription of an inadequate analgesic dose.

Unrelieved pain leads to a multitude of harmful effects that involve almost all organs of the body. As a result of unrelieved pain, the patient may develop increased respiratory and heart rates, hypertension, increased stress response, urinary retention, fluid overload, electrolyte imbalance, glucose intolerance, hyperglycemia, pneumonia, atelectasis, anorexia, paralytic ileus, constipation, weakness, confusion, infection, or psychological and physical suffering.

Inadequate pain management leads to high health care costs. It is estimated that the cost of extended hospital stays, readmissions to the hospital, and outpatient visits due to inadequate pain management exceeds $200 billion per year.

NONOPIOID ANALGESICS

Nonopioid analgesics such as aspirin, acetaminophen, ibuprofen, and naproxen are less potent than opioid analgesics and are used to treat mild to moderate pain. Nonopioids are usually purchased over the counter, but cyclooxygenase 2 (COX-2) inhibitors require a prescription. Nonopioids are effective for the dull, throbbing pain of headaches; dysmenorrhea (menstrual pain); inflammation; minor abrasions; muscular aches and pain; and mild to moderate arthritis. Most analgesics also have an antipyretic effect and will lower an elevated body temperature. Some, such as aspirin, have antiinflammatory and antiplatelet effects as well.

Nonsteroidal Antiinflammatory Drugs

All NSAIDs have an analgesic effect as well as an antipyretic and antiinflammatory action. NSAIDs such as aspirin, ibuprofen, and naproxen can be purchased as over-the-counter (OTC) drugs. Aspirin, a salicylate NSAID, is the oldest nonopioid analgesic drug still in use. Adolf Bayer marketed the original formulation in 1899, and currently aspirin can be purchased under many names and with added ingredients.

The American Academy of Pediatrics, Centers for Disease Control and Prevention (CDC), US Food and Drug Administration (FDA), National Reye's Syndrome Foundation, US Surgeon General, and World Health Organization (WHO) recommend aspirin products not be given to children and adolescents younger than 19 years of age during episodes of fever or viral illnesses because of the danger of Reye syndrome. Reye syndrome is a rare but serious condition associated with viral infections treated with salicylates that cause swelling of the brain and liver. In these circumstances, acetaminophen is recommended instead of aspirin.

In addition to its analgesic, antipyretic, and antiinflammatory properties, aspirin decreases platelet aggregation (clotting). Some health care providers may therefore prescribe one 81-mg, 162-mg, or 325-mg aspirin tablet every day or one 325-mg tablet every other day as a preventive measure against transient ischemic attacks (TIAs, or ministrokes), heart attacks, or any thromboembolic episode. Aspirin is discussed in depth in Chapter 24 along with other NSAIDs.

Aspirin and other NSAIDs relieve pain by inhibiting biosynthesis of prostaglandin by different forms of the COX enzyme. As explained in Chapter 24, NSAIDs inhibit or block both COX-1 and COX-2 enzymes, whereas COX-2 inhibitors are selective and only inhibit COX-2 enzyme. Inhibition of COX-1 decreases protection of the stomach lining, whereas inhibition of COX-2 decreases inflammation and pain. As a result of an NSAID's inhibition of COX-1, gastric irritation and bleeding may occur. Aspirin is the drug of choice for alleviating pain and inflammation in arthritic conditions, but when given in high doses, severe gastrointestinal (GI) irritation and possible ulceration develop in approximately 20% of patients. Some pharmaceutical companies have developed antiinflammatory and analgesic drugs that inhibit only COX-2. The COX-2 inhibitors were developed to eliminate the GI side effects associated with aspirin and other NSAIDs. COX-2 inhibitors are discussed in depth in Chapter 24.

Side Effects and Adverse Reactions

A common side effect of NSAIDs is gastric distress, including anorexia, nausea, vomiting, and diarrhea. These drugs should be taken with food, at mealtime, or with a full glass of fluid to help reduce this problem. Excessive bleeding might occur as a side effect if an NSAID is taken for dysmenorrhea during the first 2 days of menstruation. Adverse effects of salicylate toxicity include tinnitus, vertigo, hyperventilation, pulmonary edema, and kidney failure.

Some patients are hypersensitive to aspirin. Dyspnea, bronchospasm, and urticaria are some of the symptoms that indicate anaphylaxis to salicylate products. Certain foods also contain salicylates: prunes, raisins, paprika, lentils, beans, cauliflower, strawberries, raspberries, plums, and licorice. Those with a hypersensitivity to aspirin and salicylate products may be sensitive to other NSAIDs. This hypersensitivity may be related to inhibition of the COX enzyme by the salicylate. It is recommended that aspirin not be given to children or adolescents unless specifically directed by a health care provider because of the danger of Reye syndrome.

Acetaminophen

The analgesic acetaminophen, a para-aminophenol derivative, was first marketed in the mid-1950s as an analgesic and antipyretic drug used for muscular aches and pains, and for fever caused by viral infections in infants, children, adults, and older adults. It is a popular nonprescription drug; it constitutes 25% of all OTC drugs sold. Acetaminophen is a nonopioid drug, but it is *not* an NSAID. Because acetaminophen does not have the antiinflammatory properties of aspirin, it is not the drug of choice for any inflammatory process. Acetaminophen is a safe, effective drug when used at therapeutic doses, causes little to no gastric distress, and does not interfere with platelet aggregation. Complementary and Alternative Therapies: Capsaicin describes the use of these products in pain relief. An intravenous (IV) formulation of acetaminophen was approved by the FDA for treating pain and fever. It should be administered undiluted over 15 minutes. There is no link between acetaminophen and Reye syndrome, and unlike aspirin and NSAIDs, it does not increase the potential for excessive bleeding if taken for dysmenorrhea (Prototype Drug Chart: Acetaminophen).

COMPLEMENTARY AND ALTERNATIVE THERAPIES

Capsaicin

Capsaicin, which is found naturally in cayenne pepper, is selective for C-fiber nociceptors and relieves some arthritis pain in topical cream or gel form.

Pharmacokinetics

Acetaminophen is well absorbed from the GI tract. Rectal absorption may be erratic because of the presence of fecal material or a decrease in blood flow to the colon. Because of acetaminophen's short half-life, it can be administered every 4 hours as needed with a maximum dose of 4 g/day for adults. However, it is suggested that a patient who frequently takes acetaminophen limit the dose to 2000 mg/day (2 g/day) to avoid the possibility of hepatic or renal dysfunction. More than 85% of acetaminophen is metabolized to drug metabolites by the liver.

Large doses or overdoses can be toxic to the hepatic cells, so when large doses are administered over a long period, the serum level of acetaminophen should be monitored. The therapeutic serum range is 10 to 20 mcg/mL. Hepatic enzyme levels (aspartate aminotransferase [AST], alanine aminotransferase [ALT], alkaline phosphatase [ALP]) and serum bilirubin should also be monitored. Ingesting alcohol concurrently with acetaminophen may lead to hepatic injury, hepatic failure, and death. When acetaminophen toxicity occurs, acetylcysteine is the antidote, which reduces liver injury by converting toxic metabolites to a nontoxic form.

PROTOTYPE DRUG CHART

Acetaminophen

Drug Class	Dosage
Analgesic	Mild pain: Immediate release: A: PO/PR: 325–650 mg q4–6h PRN; *max:* 4 g/d (1000 mg/dose) Extended release: A: PO: 650–1300 mg q8h PRN; *max:* 3900 mg/d (1300 mg/dose)
Contraindications	**Drug-Lab-Food Interactions**
Hypersensitivity *Caution:* Renal/hepatic disease, hypertension, diabetes mellitus, alcohol use disorder, tobacco smoking, infection, hypovolemia, malnutrition, neutropenia, phenylketonuria, pregnancy, breast-feeding, children	Increased effect with caffeine, diflunisal Decreased effect with oral contraceptives, antacids, anticholinergics, cholestyramine, charcoal, barbiturates, carbamazepine, and phenytoin
Pharmacokinetics	**Pharmacodynamics**
Absorption: Rapidly absorbed PO; rectal absorption is erratic. Distribution: PB: 10%–25%; crosses the placenta, excreted in breast milk Metabolism: t½: 2–3 h Excretion: In urine as metabolites	PO: Onset: 10–30 min Peak: 30–60 min Duration: 4–6 h Rectal: Onset: UK Peak: UK Duration: UK
Therapeutic Effects/Uses	
To decrease mild pain and fever Mechanism of Action: Inhibition (weak) of prostaglandin synthesis, inhibition of hypothalamic heat regulator center	
Side Effects	**Adverse Reactions**
Headache, insomnia, anxiety, fatigue, anorexia, nausea, vomiting, constipation, peripheral edema	Oliguria, hearing loss, hypomagnesemia, elevated hepatic enzymes *Life-threatening:* Hepatic/renal failure, hypokalemia, rhabdomyolysis, anemia, hemolytic anemia, agranulocytosis, neutropenia, thrombocytopenia, pancytopenia

A, Adult; *d,* day; *h,* hour; *max,* maximum; *min,* minute; *PO,* by mouth; *PR,* per rectum; *PRN,* as needed; *q,* every; *t½,* half-life; *UK,* unknown.

Pharmacodynamics

Acetaminophen weakly inhibits prostaglandin synthesis, which decreases pain sensation. It is effective in eliminating mild to moderate pain and headaches and is useful for its antipyretic effect. Acetaminophen does not possess antiinflammatory action. When given orally, its onset of action is within 10 to 30 minutes, and the peak concentration occurs within 30 to 60 minutes. Severe adverse reactions may occur with an overdose, so acetaminophen in liquid or chewable form should be kept out of children's reach.

Side Effects and Adverse Reactions

An overdose of acetaminophen can be extremely toxic to liver cells; death could occur in 1 to 4 days from hepatic necrosis. If a child or adult ingests excessive amounts of acetaminophen tablets or liquid, a poison control center should be contacted immediately, and the child or adult should be taken to the emergency department. Early symptoms of hepatic damage include nausea, vomiting, diarrhea, and abdominal pain.

Table 25.2 lists the commonly used nonopioid analgesics and their dosages, uses, and considerations.

OPIOID ANALGESICS

Opioid analgesics, called **opioid agonists**, are prescribed for moderate and severe pain. In the United States the Harrison Opioid Act of 1914 required that all forms of opium be sold with a prescription and that it no longer be used as a nonprescription drug. The Controlled Substances Act of 1970 classified drugs with high misuse potential, opioids among them, in five schedule categories according to their potential for drug misuse (see Chapter 8). **Addiction**, or substance use disorder, is defined as a psychological and physical dependence upon a substance beyond normal voluntary control, usually after prolonged use of a substance.

Morphine, a prototype opioid, is obtained from the sap of seedpods of the opium poppy plant. Codeine is another drug obtained from opium. In the past decades, many synthetic and semisynthetic opioids have been developed; for example, meperidine.

Although nonopioid analgesics act on the PNS at the pain receptor sites, opioid analgesics act mostly on the CNS. Opioids act primarily by activating the μ-receptors, but they also exert a weak activation of the kappa (κ) receptors. Analgesia, respiratory depression, euphoria, and sedation are effects of μ-receptor activation. Activation of κ-receptors leads to analgesia and sedation but has no effect on respiratory depression and euphoria.

Opioids not only suppress pain impulses but also suppress respiration and coughing by acting on the respiratory and cough centers in the medulla of the brain stem. One example of such an opioid is morphine, a potent analgesic that can readily depress respirations. Codeine is not as potent as morphine (1/15–1/20 as potent), but it also relieves mild to moderate pain and suppresses cough, which allows it also to be classified as an antitussive. Most opioids, with the exception of meperidine, have an antitussive (cough suppression) effect. The opioids have two isomers, levo and dextro. The levo-isomers of opioids produce

CLINICAL JUDGMENT [NURSING PROCESS]
Analgesic: Acetaminophen

Concept: Pain
- An unpleasant feeling of discomfort usually associated with tissue damage

Recognize Cues [Assessment]
- Obtain a medical history of liver dysfunction. Overdosing or extremely high doses of acetaminophen can cause hepatotoxicity, hepatic failure, and death.
- Ascertain the severity of pain. Nonopioid nonsteroidal antiinflammatory drugs (NSAIDs), such as ibuprofen, or an opioid may be necessary to relieve pain.

Analyze Cues and Prioritize Hypothesis [Patient Problems]
- Injury
- Acute pain
- Nausea
- Diarrhea
- Discomfort
- Decreased mobility

Generate Solutions [Planning]
- The patient will report pain has decreased within 1 hour after medication administration.

Take Action [Nursing Interventions]
- Check hepatic enzyme tests such as alanine aminotransferase (ALT), alkaline phosphatase (ALP), gamma-glutamyl transferase (GGT), 5′-nucleotidase, and bilirubin for elevations in patients who take high doses of acetaminophen or overdoses.

Patient Teaching
General
- Teach patients to keep acetaminophen out of children's reach. Acetaminophen for children is available in flavored tablets and liquid, and high doses can cause hepatotoxicity, hepatic failure, and death.
- Advise patients not to self-medicate with acetaminophen for more than 10 days. Teach adult caregivers not to medicate children for more than 5 days without a health care provider's approval.
- ⚡ Direct parents to call a poison control center immediately if a child has taken a large or unknown amount of acetaminophen.
- ⚡ Teach patients to check acetaminophen dosages on the label of over-the-counter (OTC) drugs. Do not exceed the recommended dosage. The suggested safe maximum adult acetaminophen dosage is 4 g/day to avoid hepatic damage (see Prototype Drug Chart: Acetaminophen).
- Teach patients to avoid alcohol ingestion while taking acetaminophen.

Side Effects
- Encourage patients to report side effects. Overdosing can cause severe hepatic damage, hepatic failure, and death.
- ⚡ Check the serum acetaminophen level if toxicity is suspected. The therapeutic serum level is 10–20 mcg/mL; the toxic level is greater than 200 mcg/mL 4 hours after ingestion and is usually associated with hepatotoxicity. The antidote for acetaminophen is acetylcysteine. Dosage is based on the serum acetaminophen level.

Evaluate Outcomes [Evaluation]
- Evaluate the effectiveness of acetaminophen in relieving pain using a consistent pain scale. If the pain persists, another analgesic may be needed.
- Determine whether the patient is taking the recommended dosage. Observe and report any side effects.

TABLE 25.2 Analgesics

Generic	Route and Dosage	Uses and Considerations
Para-Aminophenol		
Acetaminophen	See Prototype Drug Chart: Acetaminophen	
Nonsteroidal Antiinflammatory Drugs (NSAIDs)		
Aspirin	Mild pain: A: PO: 325–650 mg q4h PRN; *max:* 3900 mg/d	For relief of mild pain, fever, inflammation, or thromboembolism and stroke prevention or to treat angina and AMI. May cause dizziness, hearing loss, tinnitus, nausea, vomiting, anorexia, dyspepsia, abdominal pain, gastritis, elevated hepatic enzymes, and GI/intracranial bleeding. Aspirin should be taken with food. Avoid with alcohol. Avoid in children and teenagers younger than 19 years during episodes of fever or viral illnesses to prevent Reye's syndrome. PB: 20%–95%; t½: 15–20 min
Diflunisal	Pain: A: PO: Initial LD 500 mg–1 g; *maint:* 250–500 mg q8–12h PRN; *max:* 1500 mg/d	For mild to moderate pain, osteoarthritis, and RA. May cause headache, tinnitus, hearing loss, abdominal pain, dyspepsia, nausea, vomiting, diarrhea, GI ulcer/bleeding/perforation, rash, and elevated hepatic enzymes. PB: 99%, t½: 8–12 h
Ibuprofen	Mild to moderate pain: A: PO: 400 mg q4–6h PRN; *max:* 3200 mg/d Severe Pain: A: IV: 400–800 mg q6h PRN, infuse over at least 30 min; *max:* 3200 mg/d	For reducing fever, mild to severe pain, osteoarthritis, RA, and dysmenorrhea. May cause dizziness, headache, tinnitus, nausea, dyspepsia, vomiting, diarrhea, flatulence, abdominal pain, constipation, rash, hypokalemia, fluid retention, edema, prolonged bleeding time, thrombocytosis, neutropenia, and anemia. Should be taken with food, milk, or with plenty of fluids. PB: 99%; t½: 1.7–2.5 h

Continued

TABLE 25.2 Analgesics—cont'd

Generic	Route and Dosage	Uses and Considerations
Propionic Acids		
Naproxen	Osteoarthritis: A: PO: 250–500 mg bid; *max:* 1500 mg/d up to 6 months	For mild to moderate pain, fever, osteoarthritis, RA, bursitis, tendinitis, ankylosing spondylitis, acute gout, and dysmenorrhea. May cause dizziness, drowsiness, headache, tinnitus, rhinitis, sinusitis, pharyngitis, back pain, dyspnea, abdominal pain, dyspepsia, nausea, vomiting, flatulence, diarrhea, constipation, rash, pruritus, ecchymosis, infection, GI bleeding/ulcer/perforation, edema, influenza, and elevated hepatic enzymes. PB: 99%; *t½:* 12–17 h
Acetic Acids (Indoles)		
Indomethacin	Acute Gouty Arthritis: Immediate release capsules: A: PO: 50 mg tid until pain is tolerable, then rapidly reduce dose to discontinue	For mild to severe pain, gouty arthritis, tendinitis, osteoarthritis, RA, and ankylosing spondylitis. May cause dizziness, headache, nausea, vomiting, dyspepsia, constipation, hyperkalemia, and hyponatremia. Take with food. Avoid if allergic to aspirin. PB: 99%; *t½:* 2.6–11.2 h
Ketorolac	A ≥50 kg: Intranasal: 1 spray (15.75 mg spray) each nostril, q6–8 h; *max:* 4 doses/d, no more than 5 d Older A and A <50 kg: Intranasal: 1 spray 1 nostril q6–8 h; *max:* 4 doses/d (15.75 mg/spray), Total systemic therapy should not exceed 5 days	For short-term pain management (5 days or less). May cause ocular pain, nasal irritation, rhinalgia, dyspepsia, abdominal pain, nausea, vomiting, diarrhea, and GI bleeding/ulcer/perforation. PB: 99%; *t½:* 5–6 h
Nabumetone	A: PO: 1000 mg/d or 500 mg bid; *max:* 2000 mg/d	For pain from osteoarthritis and RA. May cause dizziness, headache, tinnitus, dyspepsia, abdominal pain, nausea, vomiting, flatulence, diarrhea, constipation, rash, pruritus, and edema. PB: 99%; *t½:* 24 h
Oxicams		
Meloxicam	A: PO: 7.5–15 mg/d; *max:* 15 mg/d	For pain from osteoarthritis and RA. May cause headache, pharyngitis, laryngitis, sinusitis, dyspepsia, eructation, abdominal pain, nausea, diarrhea, constipation, peripheral edema, arthralgia, cystitis, and influenza. PB: 99.4%; *t½:* 15–20 h
Cyclooxygenase 2 (COX-2) Inhibitors		
Celecoxib	Moderate to severe pain: A: PO: Initially 400 mg followed by additional 200 mg on day 1 if needed; *maint:* 200 mg bid; *max:* 800 mg/d, older A 400 mg/d	For moderate to severe pain, osteoarthritis, and RA. May cause headache, pharyngitis, sinusitis, dyspepsia, abdominal pain, nausea, vomiting, diarrhea, peripheral edema, hypertension, infection, elevated hepatic enzymes, and arthralgia. Use caution in patients with severe renal or liver disorders and contraindicated for those allergic to salicylates or sulfonamides. PB: 97%; *t½:* 11.2 h
Miscellaneous		
Baricitinib	A: PO: 2 mg/d	For severe RA in adults with inadequate response to 1 or more TNF inhibitors. Hgb must be 8 g/dL or more, ANC must be 1000 cells/mm^3 or more, and ALC must be 500 cells/mm^3 or more. May cause headache, nausea, abdominal pain, infection, elevated hepatic enzymes, acneiform rash, acne vulgaris, and thrombocytosis. PB: 45%; *t½:* 12–16 h
Norepinephrine and Serotonin Reuptake Inhibitors		
Tramadol	Severe pain: Immediate release: A: PO: Initially: 25 mg/d; *maint:* 50–100 mg q4–6 h PRN; *max:* 400 mg/d, 300 mg/d for A >75 y Extended release: A: PO: 100 mg/d; *max:* 300 mg/d	For severe pain. May cause drowsiness, dizziness, headache, anxiety, agitation, euphoria, flushing, weakness, fatigue, dry mouth, dysgeusia, anorexia, nausea, dyspepsia, vomiting, diarrhea, constipation, weight loss, and tremor. PB: 20%; *t½:* 6.3–7.4 h for immediate release, 7.9–8.8 h for extended release
Milnacipran	A: PO: Initially 12.5 mg on day 1, 12.5 bid on days 2–3, 25 mg bid days 4–7, then 50 mg bid; *max:* 200 mg/d	For management of fibromyalgia. May cause dizziness, headache, hot flashes, insomnia, nausea, and constipation. Withdraw gradually upon discontinuation. PB: 13%; *t½:* 4–10 h

<, Less than; >, greater than; *A*, adult; *alc*, absolute lymphocyte count; *anc*, absolute neutrophil count; *AMI*, acute myocardial infarction; *bid*, twice a day; *d*, day; *GI*, gastrointestinal; *hgb*, hemoglobin; *h*, hour; *IV*, intravenous; *maint*, maintenance; *max*, maximum; *min*, minute; *PB*, protein binding; *PO*, by mouth; *PRN*, as needed; *q*, every; *RA*, rheumatoid arthritis; *t ½*, half-life.

an analgesic effect only; however, both levo- and dextro-isomers possess an antitussive response. The dextro-isomers do not cause physical dependence, but the levo-isomers do. Synthetic cough suppressants are discussed in Chapter 35.

In addition to pain relief and antitussive effects, many opioids possess antidiarrheal effects. Common side effects with high doses of most opioids include nausea and vomiting, particularly in ambulatory patients; constipation; a moderate decrease in blood pressure; and orthostatic hypotension. High doses of opioids may also cause respiratory depression; urinary retention, usually in older adults; and antitussive effects. See Complementary and Alternative Therapies: Sedatives for interactions with opioids.

COMPLEMENTARY AND ALTERNATIVE THERAPIES

Sedatives

Opioids taken with kava, valerian, and St. John's wort may increase sedation.

Morphine

Morphine, an extraction from opium, is a potent opioid analgesic (Prototype Drug Chart: Morphine Sulfate). Morphine is effective against acute pain resulting from acute myocardial infarction (AMI) and cancer, relieves dyspnea resulting from pulmonary edema, and

PROTOTYPE DRUG CHART

Morphine Sulfate

Drug Class	Dosage
Opioid CSS II	Immediate release: A: PO: Initially 15–30 mg q4h PRN Extended release: A: PO: Initially 15 mg q8–12h PRN or 30 mg/d A: IM/subcut: 5–20 mg q4h PRN A: IV: 2–10 mg q4h PRN

Contraindications	Drug-Lab-Food Interactions
Hypersensitivity, CNS or respiratory depression, status asthmaticus, alcohol use disorder, ileus, shock, GI obstruction, status epilepticus, children *Caution:* Respiratory insufficiency, COPD, asthma, arteriosclerosis, coagulopathy, pancreatitis, seizures, increased intracranial pressure, hypovolemia, shock, renal or hepatic disorders, biliary tract disease, diarrhea, bladder obstruction, urinary retention, obesity, sleep apnea, older adults, pregnancy, breast-feeding	Drug: Increased effects of alcohol, sedative-hypnotics, antipsychotic drugs, muscle relaxants; concurrent use with MAOIs can lead to severe respiratory depression, hypotension, coma Complementary and Alternative Therapies: St. John's wort may decrease drug effect (see Complementary and Alternative Therapies: Sedatives). Lab: Increased AST, ALT

Pharmacokinetics	Pharmacodynamics
Absorption: PO, varies; IV, rapid Distribution: PB: 20%–35%; crosses placenta, excreted in breast milk Metabolism: t½: 2–4 h Excretion: 90% in urine	PO: Onset: 30 min Peak: IR 1 h, ER 3–4 h Duration: IR 3–5 h; ER 8–24 h Subcut: Onset: 15–30 min Peak: 50–90 min Duration: 3–6 h IM: Onset: 15–30 min Peak: 30–60 min Duration: 3–6 h IV: Onset: 5–10 min Peak: 20 min Duration: 3–6 h

Therapeutic Effects/Uses
To relieve severe pain
Mechanism of Action: Depression of the CNS; depression of pain impulses by binding with opiate receptors in the CNS

Side Effects	Adverse Reactions
Anorexia, dry mouth, dyspepsia, dysphagia, nausea, abdominal pain, vomiting, diarrhea, constipation, flatulence, fever, drowsiness, dizziness, amnesia, delirium, agitation, anxiety, dysgeusia, hiccups, confusion, depression, bladder spasms, oliguria, urinary retention, rash, dry skin, blurred vision, diplopia, miosis, ocular pain, weakness, ataxia, tremor, flushing, euphoria, peripheral edema, paresthesia, diaphoresis, pruritus, infection, back pain, insomnia, weight loss, hypoesthesia, erectile dysfunction	Orthostatic hypo/hypertension, bradycardia, tachycardia, palpitations, seizures, ileus, psychological dependence, withdrawal, dyspnea, hypoxia, biliary obstruction *Life-threatening:* Respiratory depression, anemia, leukopenia, thrombocytopenia, pulmonary edema, GI obstruction, dysrhythmias, coma

A, Adult; *ALT*, alanine aminotransferase; *AST*, aspartate aminotransferase; *CNS*, central nervous system; *COPD*, chronic obstructive pulmonary disorder; *CSS*, Controlled Substances Schedule; *ER*, extended release; *GI*, gastrointestinal; *h*, hour; *IM*, intramuscular; *IR*, immediate release; *IV*, intravenous; *MAOI*, monoamine oxidase inhibitor; *min*, minute; *PB*, protein binding; *PO*, by mouth; *PRN*, as necessary; *q*, every; *subcut*, subcutaneous; *t½*, half-life.

may be used as a preoperative medication to relieve anxiety. Although it is effective in relieving severe pain, it can cause respiratory depression, orthostatic hypotension, miosis, urinary retention, constipation resulting from reduced bowel motility, and cough suppression. An antidote for morphine excess or overdose is the opioid antagonist naloxone.

Pharmacokinetics

Morphine may be taken orally, although GI absorption can be somewhat erratic. For quick relief of severe pain, such as with AMI, or for fast relief of anxiety and to reduce hypertension, it is given intravenously. Morphine is 20% to 35% protein bound and may also be administered rectally and epidurally. Oral morphine undergoes first-pass hepatic metabolism, meaning the liver metabolizes the drug before morphine is available to the rest of the body. Only a small amount of morphine crosses the blood-brain barrier to produce an analgesic effect. It has a short half-life of 2 to 4 hours, and 90% is excreted in the urine. Morphine crosses the placenta and is excreted in breast milk.

Pharmacodynamics

Morphine binds with the opiate receptor in the CNS. Parenterally, the onset of action is rapid, especially when administered intravenously. The onset of action is 15 to 30 minutes for subcutaneous (subcut) and intramuscular (IM) injections. The duration of action with most types of drug administration is 3 to 6 hours; with controlled-release morphine sulfate tablets, the duration is 8 to 24 hours.

COMPLEMENTARY AND ALTERNATIVE THERAPIES

St. John's Wort

St. John's wort may potentiate the drug effects of oral morphine and decrease drug levels of oxycodone.

Meperidine

One of the first synthetic opioids, meperidine became available in the mid-1950s. It is classified as a Schedule II drug according to the Controlled Substances Act. Meperidine has a shorter duration of action than morphine, and its potency varies according to the dosage. Meperidine can be given orally or via IM and IV routes, and it is primarily effective in GI procedures. It does not have the antitussive property of opium preparations.

CLINICAL JUDGMENT [NURSING PROCESS]

Opioid Analgesic: Morphine Sulfate

Concept: Pain
- An unpleasant feeling of discomfort usually associated with tissue damage

Recognize Cues [Assessment]
- Obtain a medical history. Contraindications for morphine include severe respiratory disorders, increased intracranial pressure, and severe renal disease. Morphine may cause seizures.
- Determine a drug history, and check for drug allergies. Report if a drug–drug interaction is probable. Morphine increases the effects of alcohol, sedatives and hypnotics, antipsychotic drugs, and muscle relaxants, and it can cause respiratory depression.
- Assess vital signs, noting the rate and depth of respirations, as well as pupil size for future comparisons; opioids commonly decrease respirations and systolic blood pressure and may cause miosis.
- Monitor urinary output; morphine can cause urinary retention.
- Assess the type of pain, location, and duration before giving opioids.

Analyze Cues and Prioritize Hypothesis [Patient Problems]
- Decreased gas exchange
- Injury
- Acute pain
- Hypotension
- Falls
- Urinary retention
- Constipation
- Discomfort

Generate Solutions [Planning]
- The patient will report pain is decreased within 1 hour after medication administration.

Take Action [Nursing Interventions]
- Administer morphine before pain reaches its peak to maximize effectiveness of the drug.
- Monitor vital signs at frequent intervals to detect respiratory changes and hypotension. Fewer than 10 respirations per minute can indicate respiratory distress.
- Record the patient's urine output because urinary retention is a side effect of morphine. Urine output should be at least 600 mL/day.
- Check bowel sounds for decreased peristalsis; constipation is a side effect of morphine. A dietary change or mild laxative might be needed.
- ⚡ Check for pupil changes and reaction. Pinpoint pupils can indicate morphine overdose.
- ⚡ Have naloxone available as an antidote to reverse respiratory depression if morphine overdose occurs.
- Validate the dose of morphine before administration. Check older adults for alertness and orientation because confusion is a side effect of morphine. Use side rails, and take other safety precautions as necessary.

Patient Teaching

General
- Encourage patients not to use alcohol or central nervous system (CNS) depressants with any opioid analgesics such as morphine. Respiratory depression can result, as well as dizziness and the potential fall risk.
- Suggest nonpharmacologic measures to relieve pain as the patient recuperates from surgery. As recovery progresses, a nonopioid analgesic may be prescribed.

Side Effects
- Alert patients that with continuous use, opioids such as morphine can become a substance use disorder. If this occurs, inform patients about methadone treatment programs and other resources in the area.
- Encourage patients to report dizziness while taking morphine. Dizziness could be due to orthostatic hypotension. Advise patients to ambulate with caution or only with assistance.
- ⚡ Teach patients to report difficulty in breathing, blurred vision, and headaches.

Evaluate Outcomes [Evaluation]
- Evaluate the effectiveness of morphine in lessening or alleviating pain using a consistent pain scale. If the pain persists after several days, the dose should be increased or the opioid should be changed.
- Determine the stability of vital signs. Any decrease in respiration or blood pressure should be reported.

TABLE 25.3 Opioids: Opium and Synthetics

Generic	Route and Dosage	Uses and Considerations
Codeine sulfate, codeine phosphate CSS II	A: PO: 15–60 mg q4h PRN; *max:* 360 mg/d	For mild to moderate pain. May cause drowsiness, dizziness, euphoria, miosis, weakness, fatigue, orthostatic hypotension, diarrhea, constipation, and dependence. PB: 7%–25%, $t\frac{1}{2}$: 3 h
Hydrocodone bitartrate CSS II	Pain: A: PO: Initially 10 mg q12h, may increase 10 mg q3–7d PRN	For severe pain. May cause headache, flushing, anxiety, dyspnea, dyspepsia, abdominal pain, nausea, vomiting, constipation, arthralgia, back pain, dehydration, peripheral edema, and infection. Taper off upon discontinuation. PB: 36%; $t\frac{1}{2}$: 7–12 h
Hydromorphone hydrochloride CSS II	A: PO: Initially 2–4 mg q4–6h PRN A: IM/subcut: 1–2 mg q2–3 h PRN A: IV: 0.2–1 mg over 2–3 min q2–3 h PRN Rectal: 3 mg suppository q6–8h PRN	For severe pain. May cause dizziness, drowsiness, headache, fatigue, weakness, insomnia, hyperhidrosis, anorexia, abdominal pain, nausea, vomiting, diarrhea, constipation, pruritus, peripheral edema, and arthralgia. PB: 8%–19%; $t\frac{1}{2}$: 2–3 h
Meperidine CSS II	Severe Pain: A: PO/subcut/IM/IV: 50–150 mg q3–4 h PRN, give IV slowly; *max:* 150 mg/dose	For severe pain and sedation induction and anesthesia maintenance. May cause dizziness, drowsiness, visual impairment, confusion, euphoria, flushing, weakness, dry mouth, nausea, vomiting, constipation, orthostatic hypotension, bradycardia, urinary retention, dependence, and respiratory depression. PB: 65%–75%; $t\frac{1}{2}$: 2–5 h
Morphine sulfate CSS II	See Prototype Drug Chart: Morphine Sulfate	
Oxycodone hydrochloride CSS II	Severe pain: Immediate release: A: PO: 5–15 mg q4–6 h PRN Extended release: A: PO: 10 mg q12h PRN	For severe pain. Avoid taking drug over an extended period of time. May cause drowsiness, blurred vision, miosis, weakness, euphoria, dry mouth, nausea, vomiting, diarrhea, constipation, edema, and urinary retention. Take with food to avoid GI distress. PB: 45%; $t\frac{1}{2}$: Immediate release: 3.2 h, Extended release: 3.8–4.5 h
Oxycodone with acetaminophen and oxycodone with aspirin CSS II	Immediate release: A: PO: 1–2 tabs (2.5–10 mg oxycodone/325 mg acetaminophen) q6h PRN Extended release: A: PO: 2 tabs q12h With aspirin: A: PO: 1 tab (4.8355 mg oxycodone/325 mg aspirin) q6h PRN; *max:* 12 tabs/d	For moderate to severe pain. May cause dizziness, drowsiness, headache, rhinitis, confusion, nausea, vomiting, constipation, and urticaria. Take with food or milk. PB: oxycodone 45%, acetaminophen 10%–25%, ASA 20%–95%; $t\frac{1}{2}$: oxycodone 3.2 h, acetaminophen 4 h, ASA 15–20 min
Fentanyl CSS II	Pain: A: IM/IV: 50–100 mcg 30–60 min before surgery (slow IV over 1–3 min); may repeat in 1–2 h for postoperative pain	For severe pain. May cause dizziness, drowsiness, headache, euphoria, confusion, fatigue, weakness, hypokalemia, nausea, vomiting, constipation, rash, and tolerance. PB: 80%–85%; $t\frac{1}{2}$: IV, 2–4 h
Methadone CSS II	Pain: A: PO: Initially 2.5 mg q8–12 h PRN A: IV/subcut/IM: 2.5–10 mg q8–12 h	For moderate to severe pain, opiate agonist dependence and withdrawal. May cause dizziness, drowsiness, blurred vision, confusion, euphoria, orthostatic hypotension, edema, constipation, urinary retention, dependence, and respiratory depression. PB: 85%–90%; $t\frac{1}{2}$: 2–3 h

A, Adult; *ASA*, aspirin; *CSS*, Controlled Substances Schedule; *d*, day; *GI*, gastrointestinal; *h*, hour; *IM*, intramuscular; *IV*, intravenous; *max*, maximum; *min*, minute; *PB*, protein binding; *PO*, by mouth; *PRN*, as necessary; *q*, every; *subcut*, subcutaneous; *t ½*, half-life; *tab*, tablet.

During pregnancy, meperidine is preferred to morphine because it does not diminish uterine contractions and causes less neonatal respiratory depression. Meperidine causes less constipation and urinary retention than morphine. Meperidine is not indicated for patients with chronic pain, severe liver dysfunction, sickle cell disease, a history of seizures, severe coronary artery disease (CAD), or cardiac dysrhythmias. When older adults and patients with advanced cancer receive large doses of meperidine, neurotoxicity (e.g., nervousness, tremors, agitation, irritability, seizures) is reported. Meperidine should *not* be prescribed for long-term use; the dosage is frequently limited to 150 mg/dose for a period no longer than 48.

Meperidine is metabolized in the liver to an active metabolite; therefore the dose should be decreased for patients with hepatic or renal insufficiency. It is excreted in the urine in a metabolite form called *normeperidine*. Meperidine should not be taken with alcohol or sedative-hypnotics because the combination of these drugs causes an additive CNS depression. A major side effect of meperidine is a decrease in blood pressure, which should be monitored, especially if the patient is an older adult.

Table 25.3 lists opioids and their dosages, uses, and considerations.

> ⚡ **PATIENT SAFETY**
>
> **Do Not Confuse...**
> - **Meperidine** (opioid analgesic) with **morphine** (opioid analgesic), **meprobamate** (antianxiety), or **hydromorphone** (opioid analgesic).
> - **Demerol** (opioid analgesic) with **Desyrel** (antidepressant) or **Dilaudid** (opioid analgesic).

Hydromorphone

Hydromorphone is a semisynthetic opioid similar to morphine. The analgesic effect is approximately six times more potent than that of morphine with fewer hypnotic effects and less GI distress. This opioid has a faster onset and shorter duration of action than morphine. Hydromorphone is classified as a Schedule II drug according to the Controlled Substances Act. Tolerance to hydromorphone increases gradually.

This drug is given orally, rectally, or via subcut, IM, and IV routes for the relief of moderate to severe pain. When given intravenously, dilute with sterile water or normal saline. Direct IV administration should be given slowly over 2 to 3 minutes. Hydromorphone is readily absorbed in the body and is excreted in the urine. Respirations should be monitored closely, and adequate hydration should be provided.

Side Effects and Adverse Reactions

Many side effects are known to accompany the use of opioids. Of particular importance are signs of respiratory depression (respiration <10 breaths/min). Other side effects include *orthostatic hypotension* (decrease in blood pressure when rising from a sitting or lying position), drowsiness, dizziness, weakness, confusion, constipation, and urinary retention. In addition, pupillary constriction (a sign of toxicity), tolerance, and psychological and physical dependence may occur with prolonged use.

Increased metabolism of opioids contributes to tolerance, which causes an increased need for higher doses of the opioid. If chronic use of the opioid is discontinued, symptoms of withdrawal that result from cessation of drug administration usually occur within 24 to 48 hours after the last opioid dose. *Withdrawal syndrome* is caused by physical dependence. Symptoms of opioid withdrawal syndrome include pupillary dilation, rhinorrhea, diaphoresis (sweating), hyperactivity, myalgia, tachycardia, and increased blood pressure. Withdrawal symptoms from opioids are unpleasant but not as severe or life-threatening as those that accompany withdrawal from sedative-hypnotics, a process that may lead to seizures.

Contraindications

The use of opioid analgesics is contraindicated for patients with head injuries. Opioids decrease respiration, which promotes carbon dioxide (CO_2) retention, leading to increased intracranial pressure.

Opioid analgesics given to a patient with a respiratory disorder only intensify the respiratory distress. In a patient with asthma, opiates decrease respiratory drive while simultaneously increasing airway resistance.

Opioids may cause hypotension and are not indicated for patients in shock or for those who have very low blood pressure. If an opioid is necessary, the dosage needs to be adjusted accordingly; otherwise, the hypotensive state may worsen. For an older adult or a person who is debilitated, the opioid dose usually needs to be decreased.

Morphine is the opioid analgesic prototype; all other opioids are measured in comparison to morphine.

Combination Drugs

To treat moderate to severe pain, combination drugs that comprise an NSAID and an opioid analgesic may be used. Examples are ibuprofen and hydrocodone, a combination of an NSAID and an opioid. Another combination for the treatment of mild to moderate pain is acetaminophen and codeine. When using a combination of drugs, smaller doses of each drug are required, thereby decreasing side effects. Also, using a combination of drugs for pain helps to decrease drug dependency that may result from possible long-term use of an opioid agent.

Patient-Controlled Analgesia

Patient-controlled analgesia (PCA) is an alternative route for opioid administration for self-administered pain relief as needed. Usually a loading dose (e.g., 2–10 mg of morphine) is given initially to achieve pain relief. Within predetermined safety limits, the patient controls administration of the opioid analgesic based on the amount of pain. To receive the opioid, the patient pushes a button on the PCA device, which releases a specific dose of analgesic (e.g., 1 mg morphine) into the IV line. The nurse sets the PCA pump with the opioid analgesic dose prescribed by the health care provider by regulating the time intervals (every several minutes) at which the drug can be received. A lockout mechanism on the electronically controlled infusion pump prevents the patient from constantly pushing the button and causing a drug overdose. The PCA device maintains a near-constant analgesic level, avoiding episodes of severe pain or oversedation. It is imperative that the patient, not the family or the nurse, control the PCA device to avoid overdosing. Morphine is used most often for PCA, but fentanyl and hydromorphone may also be given.

Transdermal Opioid Analgesics

Transdermal opioid analgesics provide continuous, around-the-clock pain control that is helpful to patients who experience chronic pain. The transdermal method is not useful for acute or postoperative pain. An example of a transdermal opioid analgesic is fentanyl, which is administered via a transdermal patch. This patch comes in various strengths—12.5, 25, 50, 75, and 100 mcg/h. Maximum serum fentanyl levels occur within 24 hours of when the patch is first applied. Fentanyl is also available for IM and IV use. Fentanyl is more potent than morphine. For older adults, the use of a lower fentanyl transdermal dose is usually suggested. The health care provider must exercise caution when prescribing fentanyl for patients who weigh less than 110 pounds.

Analgesic Titration

Analgesics may be titrated to increase or decrease the dosage. Usually, postoperative pain will decrease over time, and analgesics will be titrated downward. However, the patient with cancer-related pain usually has a continual increase in pain and will require an upward titration. Titration can be accomplished by changing the dose, the interval between doses, the route of administration, or the drug. When titrating analgesics, the dosage is decided after assessing the patient's respiratory rate and pain level.

Opioid Use in Special Populations
Children

Pain management in children is complex because it is more difficult to assess their pain. Some children will not verbalize discomfort when they are in severe pain, and some are fearful of treatments like injections that relieve pain. Nurses should use age-appropriate communication skills to ascertain a child's need for pain relief. The "ouch scale" illustrated in Fig. 25.1 can be helpful in determining a child's level of pain. Also, the parent may help identify the presence and degree of the

0	2	4	6	8	10
No Hurt	Hurts Little Bit	Hurts Little More	Hurts Even More	Hurts Whole Lot	Hurts Worst

Fig. 25.1 Wong-Baker FACES Pain Rating Scale. (From Wong-Baker FACES Foundation: *Wong-Baker FACES Pain Rating Scale*, 2019. Published with permission from http://www.WongBakerFACES.org. Originally published in *Whaley & Wong's nursing care of infants and children*, Elsevier Inc.)

child's pain. Crying and whining may be indicators of a need for pain relief or may represent other needs.

A child, like an adult, should be given medication before the pain becomes severe. The use of oral liquid medication for pain relief, if appropriate, is generally more acceptable to the child. The nurse may alleviate the child's fear and help with drug compliance by using drawings and pictures related to areas of pain in the body and pain relief with smiling faces.

Older Adults
Usually, adults who are 65 years of age or older require adjustment to drug doses to avoid severe side effects. Merely decreasing the usual adult dosage of opioid analgesic is not always the answer for older adults. Many take an array of medications for their health problems, increasing the possibility of drug interactions and drug side effects. In older adults, side effects from the use of opioids are more pronounced; therefore the nurse must closely monitor for adverse reactions in older adults who take opioid analgesics. As a person ages, liver and renal functions decrease, causing the rate of metabolism and excretion of the drug to decrease. As a result, drug accumulation may occur.

Older adults tend to have different beliefs and fears than younger generations regarding opioids. They may believe that pain is inevitable due to aging, or they may fear addiction. Older adults may not want to report pain because they do not want to be a burden. The nurse must perform pain assessment with a supportive approach in an unhurried manner and should give the patient accurate drug information.

Pain assessment may be more difficult with older adults due to the decrease in cognitive and sensory perceptual abilities. Dementia or hearing and visual deficits may interfere with communication. The nurse may need to rely on a more thorough physical assessment to discover the presence of pain, because self-reporting may not be reliable.

In the presence of decreased renal and hepatic function, drugs that tend to be more toxic in older adults include meperidine and pentazocine. Analgesics are usually metabolized in the liver and are excreted in the urine. Usual doses of analgesics in older adults may result in excessive sedation and prolonged duration of action. Chronologic age is one of several factors that influence medication use and dosage. Comorbidity must also be considered.

Patients With Cognitive Impairment
Any individual with cognitive impairment may be unable to report pain adequately. The nurse should use a measurement scale that is appropriate for the patient. Some physical signs of pain include moans, grimacing, clenched teeth, noisy respirations, and restlessness.

Patients With Cancer
Cancer pain is managed according to three levels of analgesia based on the WHO "ladder" as follows:

Step 1—Mild Pain: Nonopioids with or without an adjuvant medication

Step 2—Moderate Pain: Nonopioids and mild opioids with or without an adjuvant medication

Step 3—Severe Pain: Stronger opioids at higher dosage levels with or without an adjuvant medication

Opioids are titrated for oncology patients until pain relief is achieved or the side effects become tolerable. For effective pain management in patients with cancer, extremely high doses may be required. There are no set dosage limits for oncology patients.

Patients Who Have a History of Substance Use Disorder
Often patients with a history of substance use disorder require pain medication. A thorough pain assessment is necessary to find out the cause of pain. The nurse needs to know that opioids are effective and safe in this population, even though larger doses in greater frequency may be required. Studies have shown that withholding opioids in this population has not increased recovery from addiction. However, opioid agonist-antagonists such as pentazocine should be avoided in chemically dependent patients because these drugs may precipitate withdrawal syndrome.

ADJUVANTS, AGONISTS, AND ANTAGONISTS

Adjuvant Therapy
Medications used as **adjuvant analgesics** have been developed for other purposes and were later found to be effective for pain relief in neuropathy. Adjuvant therapy is usually used along with a nonopioid and opioid analgesic. Examples of adjuvant analgesics include anticonvulsants, antidepressants, corticosteroids, antidysrhythmics, and local anesthetics.

Antiseizure medications such as gabapentin act on the peripheral nerves and CNS by inhibiting spontaneous neuronal firing. They are used for neuropathic pain and for prevention of migraine headaches. Tricyclic antidepressants (TCAs) such as amitriptyline prevent the reuptake of serotonin and norepinephrine in the cells. Lower doses of TCAs than those usually prescribed for depression are effective in treating peripheral neuropathy. Corticosteroids serve as effective analgesics by reducing nociceptive stimuli. Antidysrhythmics such as mexiletine block sodium channels to reduce pain. Local anesthetics—for example, a lidocaine patch—can provide effective analgesia by interrupting the transmission of pain signals to the brain.

Adjuvant medications potentiate opioid analgesia for severe persistent pain in diabetic neuropathy, cancer, migraine headaches, and rheumatoid arthritis. When any of the adjuvant medications are used in conjunction with an NSAID and an opioid, dosages may be kept lower to reduce adverse effects.

Opioid Agonist-Antagonists
Opioid agonist-antagonists, medications in which an opioid antagonist is added to an opioid agonist, may be used to decrease substance

use disorder. Pentazocine, an opioid agonist-antagonist analgesic, can be given by injection (subcut, IM, and IV). Pentazocine is classified as a Schedule IV drug. Butorphanol tartrate, buprenorphine, and nalbuphine hydrochloride are examples of other opioid agonist-antagonist analgesics. This drug classification can cause dependence. Opioid agonist-antagonist drugs are not given for cancer pain because of the risk of potential CNS toxicity from the high doses required. These analgesics are considered safe for use during labor, but their safety during early pregnancy has not been established.

Prototype Drug Chart: Nalbuphine details the pharmacologic behavior of nalbuphine, and Table 25.4 lists the various opioid agonist-antagonists.

Pharmacokinetics

Nalbuphine can be administered IM, subcut, or IV routes. It is rapidly absorbed parenterally. Nalbuphine has a short half-life of 3 to 6 hours. It is metabolized in the liver and excreted in the urine.

Pharmacodynamics

Nalbuphine is effective in alleviating severe pain. The onset of action is rapid, and peak time occurs within 30 minutes with IV administration. The duration of action is 3 to 4 hours for IV administration and 3 to 6 hours for intramuscular/subcutaneous administration.

Opioid Antagonists

Opioid antagonists are antidotes for drug toxicity of natural and synthetic opioid analgesics. The opioid antagonists have a higher affinity to the opiate receptor site than the opioid being taken. An **opioid antagonist** blocks the receptor and displaces any opioid that would normally be at the receptor, which inhibits the opioid action. Indications for opioid antagonists include reversal of postoperative opioid depression and opioid overdose.

Naloxone is administered via an IM or IV route, and naltrexone hydrochloride is administered orally by tablet or liquid. These drugs are perfect examples of pharmacologic antagonists because they reverse the respiratory and CNS depression (sedation and hypotension) caused by opioids. Table 25.5 lists the opioid antagonists.

When receiving opioid antagonists, the patient should be monitored continuously. The opioid action may exceed that of opioid antagonists, and further analgesia may be needed. For example, fentanyl and a combination of drugs given during surgery may lead to excessive respiratory depression. Naloxone may be given as an opioid antidote. The patient's respiratory and CNS status should be monitored closely for indications of analgesic reversal (tachycardia, nausea, vomiting, and sweating) and the possible need for further analgesia.

HEADACHES: MIGRAINE AND CLUSTER

Migraine headaches are characterized by a unilateral throbbing head pain accompanied by nausea, vomiting, and photophobia. These symptoms frequently persist for 4 to 24 hours and for several days in some cases. Two-thirds of migraine headaches are experienced by females in their 20s and 30s. Symptoms usually decrease or are absent during pregnancy and menopause. The intensity of migraine pain can disrupt daily activities.

> ⚡ **PATIENT SAFETY**
>
> **Do Not Confuse...**
> - **Nubain**, a narcotic agonist-antagonist analgesic for moderate to severe pain, with **Nebcin**, an aminoglycoside antibiotic, or **Nuprin**, an over-the-counter analgesic, antipyretic nonsteroidal antiinflammatory drug.

PROTOTYPE DRUG CHART

Nalbuphine

Drug Class	Dosage
Opioid agonist-antagonist	Pain: A: IV/IM/subcut: 10 mg q3–6 h PRN; *max:* 20 mg/dose, 160 mg/d

Contraindications	Drug-Lab-Food Interactions
Hypersensitivity, respiratory depression, GI obstruction, ileus *Caution:* Alcohol or drug use disorder, asthma, respiratory insufficiency, COPD, hypoxemia, head injury, increased ICP, brain tumor, pancreatitis, biliary tract disease, hypovolemia, renal or hepatic dysfunction, coma, sleep apnea, seizures, older adults, pregnancy, breast-feeding	Drug: CNS depression is potentiated with alcohol or other CNS depressants.

Pharmacokinetics	Pharmacodynamics
Absorption: Readily occurs parenterally Distribution: PB: 50%; crosses placenta, excreted in breast milk Metabolism: $t\frac{1}{2}$: 5 h Excretion: In urine	Onset: 2–3 min IV; <15 min IM/subcut Peak: 30 min IV; 30 min IM Duration: 3–4 h IV; 3–6 h IM/subcut

Therapeutic Effects/Uses	
To relieve severe pain and for anesthesia induction and maintenance Mechanism of Action: Inhibits pain impulses transmitted in the CNS by binding with opiate receptors and increasing pain threshold	

Side Effects	Adverse Reactions
Dizziness, drowsiness, headache, confusion, euphoria, depression, restlessness, weakness, blurred vision, flushing, dry mouth, nausea, vomiting, diaphoresis, tremor, rash, erectile dysfunction	Bradycardia, tachycardia, withdrawal, hypo/hypertension, dyspnea *Life-threatening:* Respiratory depression, laryngeal edema, seizures, dependence

<, Less than; *A*, adult; *CNS*, central nervous system; *COPD*, chronic obstructive pulmonary disorder; *d*, day; *GI*, gastrointestinal; *h*, hour; *ICP*, increased intracranial pressure; *IM*, intramuscular; *IV*, intravenous; *max*, maximum; *min*, minute; *PB*, protein binding; *PRN*, as needed; *q*, every; *subcut*, subcutaneous; *t ½*, half-life.

TABLE 25.4 Opioid Agonist-Antagonists and Opioid Agonist

Generic	Route and Dosage	Uses and Considerations
Buprenorphine hydrochloride CSS V	Pain: A: IM/IV: Initially, 0.3 mg; may repeat in 30–60 min, then q6–8 h PRN; *max:* 0.6 mg/dose IM, 0.3 mg/dose IV A: Transdermal: 5 mcg/h patch q7d; *max:* 20 mcg/h A: Transmucosal: 75 mcg/d or q12h; *max:* 900 mcg q12h	For moderate to severe pain, opiate dependence. May cause dizziness, drowsiness, headache, anxiety, weakness, insomnia, depression, pruritus, diaphoresis, back/abdominal pain, nausea, constipation, infection, and withdrawal. PB: 96%; $t\frac{1}{2}$: IV 1.2–7.2 h, transdermal 26 h
Butorphanol tartrate CSS IV	Severe pain: A: IM: 1–4 mg q3–4h PRN A: IV: 0.5–2 mg q3–4h PRN A: Nasal spray: 1 mg (1 spray into 1 nostril), may repeat in 60–90 min, then may repeat sequence q3–4h PRN	For severe pain, migraine, and anesthesia induction and maintenance. May cause dizziness, drowsiness, insomnia, nasal congestion, nausea, vomiting, withdrawal, and tolerance. PB: 80%; $t\frac{1}{2}$: 2–9 h
Nalbuphine hydrochloride CSS IV	See Prototype Drug Chart: Nalbuphine	
Pentazocine lactate, Naloxone CSS IV	A: PO: 1 tablet (50 mg pentazocine/0.5 mg naloxone) q3–4 h PRN; *max:* 600 mg/6 mg/d	For severe pain. May cause dizziness, drowsiness, confusion, nausea, vomiting, and tolerance. PB: UK; $t\frac{1}{2}$: UK
Sufentanil	A: SL: 30 mcg q1h PRN up to 72 h; *max:* 360 mcg/d	For acute severe pain when alternative treatment options are inadequate, and anesthesia induction/maintenance. May cause dizziness, headache, nausea, vomiting, chest wall rigidity, and hypo/hypertension. PB: 93%; $t\frac{1}{2}$: 13.4 h
Oliceridine	A: IV: 1.5 mg, then 0.75 mg q1h PRN; *max:* 3 mg/dose, 27 mg/d for 48 h	For acute severe pain. May cause dizziness, drowsiness, headache, nausea, vomiting, constipation, back pain, pruritus, and hypoxia. PB: 77%; $t\frac{1}{2}$: 1.3-3 h
Celecoxib, tramadol	A: PO: 112 mg celecoxib/88 mg tramadol (2 tablets) q12h PRN; *max:* 224 mg celecoxib/176 mg tramadol/d	For acute severe pain. May cause headache, dizziness, drowsiness, anorexia, nausea, and vomiting. PB: celecoxib 97%, tramadol 20%; $t\frac{1}{2}$: celecoxib 11 h, tramadol 6.5–9 h

A, adult; *CSS,* Controlled Substances Schedule; *d,* day; *h,* hour; *IM,* intramuscular; *IV,* intravenous; *max,* maximum; *min,* minutes; *PB,* protein binding; *PRN,* as needed; *q,* every; *SL,* sublingual; *t ½,* half-life; *UK,* unknown.

TABLE 25.5 Opioid Antagonists

Generic	Route and Dosage	Uses and Considerations
Naloxone hydrochloride	Opiate agonist overdose: A: IV/IM/Subcut: 0.4–2 mg q2–3min PRN up to total dose of 10 mg A: Intranasal: 1 spray (2 or 4 mg) may repeat dose in alternate nostrils q2–3min PRN	For opioid overdose and opioid agonist–induced respiratory depression. May cause dizziness, headache, weakness, confusion, agitation, dyspnea, flushing, paresthesia, bradycardia, tachycardia, hyperhidrosis, nausea, vomiting, diarrhea, constipation, and hypo/hypertension. PB: UK; $t\frac{1}{2}$: 0.5–2 h
Naltrexone hydrochloride	A: PO: Initially 25 mg/d, may increase to 50 mg/d if no withdrawal signs occur; *max:* 150 mg/d A: IM: 380 mg/dose q4wk; *max:* 380 mg/dose	For opioid agonist and alcohol dependence. May cause dizziness, chills, headache, anxiety, insomnia, weakness, anorexia, abdominal pain, nausea, vomiting, diarrhea, constipation, elevated hepatic enzymes, arthralgia, and injection-site reaction. PB: 21%–28%; $t\frac{1}{2}$: PO 4 h, IM 5–10 d
Lofexidine	A: PO: Initially 0.54 mg qid during peak withdrawal symptoms, generally for 5–7 d after last opioid; *max:* 2.88 mg/d or 0.72 mg/dose	For opioid-agonist withdrawal. May cause dizziness, drowsiness, insomnia, tinnitus, dry mouth, bradycardia, orthostatic hypotension, and withdrawal. PB: 55%; $t\frac{1}{2}$: 17–22 h
Nalmefene	Non–opioid dependent A: IV: 0.5/70 kg, if needed 2-5 min later give 1 mg/70 kg Opioid dependent A: IV: Initially 0.1 mg/70 kg, if needed in 2 min give 0.5 mg/70 kg, if needed in 2-5 min give 1 mg/70 kg A: IM/Subcut: 1 mg as single dose A: Intranasal: 1 spray (2.7 mg) q2-5 min in alternating nostrils as needed	For opioid overdose and opioid agonist–induced respiratory depression. May cause dizziness, headache, flushing, chills, rhinalgia, nasal irritation/congestion, nausea, hypertension, and tachycardia. PB: 45%; $t1/2$: 5.6–16 h

<, Less than; >, greater than; *A,* adult; *d,* day; *IM,* intramuscular; *IV,* intravenous; *max,* maximum; *min,* minute; *PB,* protein binding; *PO,* by mouth; *q,* every; *subcut,* subcutaneous; *t ½,* half-life; *UK,* unknown; *wk,* weeks.

CLINICAL JUDGMENT [NURSING PROCESS]
Opioid Agonist-Antagonist Analgesic: Nalbuphine

Concept: Pain
- An unpleasant feeling of discomfort associated usually with tissue damage

Recognize Cues [Assessment]
- Obtain a drug history from the patient. Report if a drug–drug interaction is probable. When taken with nalbuphine, central nervous system (CNS) depressants can cause respiratory depression.
- Note baseline vital signs for future comparisons.
- Assess the type of pain, duration, and location before giving the drug.

Analyze Cues and Prioritize Hypothesis [Patient Problems]
- Decreased gas exchange
- Acute pain
- Discomfort
- Constipation

Generate Solutions [Planning]
- The patient will report that pain has decreased within 1 hour after medication administration.

Take Action [Nursing Interventions]
- Monitor vital signs. Note any changes in respirations.
- Check bowel sounds and the date of the last bowel movement to identify constipation. Decreased peristalsis may result in constipation. A mild laxative may be necessary.
- Determine urine output. Report if urine output is less than 30 mL/h or less than 600 mL/day.
- Administer intravenous (IV) nalbuphine undiluted. Do not mix with barbiturates.

Patient Teaching
General
- ⚡ Warn patients not to use alcohol or CNS depressants while taking nalbuphine. Respiratory depression can occur.
- Suggest nonpharmacologic methods for lessening pain, such as changing position or ambulation.

Side Effects
- Advise patients to report side effects of nalbuphine: dizziness, headaches, constipation, dysuria, rash, or blurred vision. Hallucinations, tachycardia, and respiratory depression are adverse reactions that might occur.

Evaluate Outcomes [Evaluation]
- Evaluate the effectiveness of nalbuphine in relieving pain. If ineffective, another opioid analgesic may need to be ordered.
- Determine stability of vital signs. Note whether a change in respirations, pulse rate, or blood pressure occurs. Report abnormal findings.

Pathophysiology

The exact etiology of migraine headaches is unknown, although many theories exist. A common theory suggests a series of neurovascular events initiates a migraine headache. Neuronal hyperexcitability occurs in the cerebral cortex, especially in the occipital cortex. Specific factors that trigger a migraine headache include foods, monosodium glutamate, aspartame, fatigue, stress, too much or too little sleep, missed meals, odors, light, hormone changes, drugs, and weather. Foods such as cheese, chocolate, and red wine can trigger an attack.

The two types of migraine are *migraines associated with an aura*, which occurs minutes to 1 hour before onset, and *migraines without aura*.

Cluster headaches are characterized by a severe, unilateral, nonthrobbing pain usually located around the eye. They occur in a series of cluster attacks in which one or more attacks occur every day for several weeks. Cluster headaches are not associated with an aura and do not cause nausea and vomiting. Males are more commonly affected by cluster headaches than females.

Treatment of Migraine Headaches

Preventive treatment for migraines includes (1) beta-adrenergic blockers, such as propranolol and atenolol; (2) anticonvulsants, such as valproic acid and gabapentin; and (3) TCAs, such as amitriptyline and imipramine.

Treatment of a migraine attack depends on the intensity of pain. Drugs used to treat migraines include analgesics, opioid analgesics, ergot alkaloids, and selective serotonin (5-HT) receptor agonists, also known as *triptans*. For mild migraine attacks, aspirin, acetaminophen, or NSAIDs such as ibuprofen or naproxen may be prescribed. Aspirin may be used in combination with caffeine. Meperidine and butorphanol nasal spray are opioid analgesics that are occasionally used.

Antimigraine medication should be taken early during a migraine attack. Nausea and vomiting might occur, and antiemetics decrease these symptoms. Dihydroergotamine, an ergot alkaloid, can be administered subcutaneously, intramuscularly, intravenously, and by means of a nasal spray.

The triptans, 5-HT receptor agonists, are the most recently developed group of drugs for the treatment of migraine headaches. Sumatriptan, a selective serotonin receptor agonist with a short duration of action, was the first triptan drug. It is considered more effective than ergot alkaloids in treating acute migraine attacks. Table 25.6 lists the ergot alkaloids and the 5-HT receptor agonists and their dosages, uses, and considerations.

> ⚡ **PATIENT SAFETY**
> **Do Not Confuse...**
> - **Sumatriptan** with **zolmitriptan**. Both drugs are triptans but have different dosages.
> - **Amerge**, a triptan used for migraines, with **Amaryl**, a sulfonylurea used for diabetes mellitus, or **Altace**, an angiotensin-converting enzyme (ACE) inhibitor used for hypertension and heart failure.

Prototype Drug Chart: Sumatriptan provides further information on the pharmacology of sumatriptan.

TABLE 25.6 Drugs Used to Treat Severe Migraine Headaches

Drug	Route and Dosage	Uses and Considerations
Ergot Alkaloids		
Dihydroergotamine mesylate	A: Intranasal: 1 spray (0.5 mg) in each nostril; may repeat in 15 min; *max*: 3 mg/d, 4 mg/wk A: IM/subcut/IV: initially 1 mg; may repeat q1h until resolved; *max*: Subcut/IM 3 mg/d (6 mg/wk), IV 2 mg/d (6 mg/wk)	For migraine and cluster headaches. May cause dizziness, drowsiness, rhinitis, sinusitis, epistaxis, pharyngitis, dysgeusia, nausea, vomiting, diarrhea, and paresthesia. PB: 93%; t½: 9–12 h
Selective Serotonin Receptor Agonists (Triptans)		
Sumatriptan	See Prototype Drug Chart: Sumatriptan	
Naratriptan	A: PO: 1–2.5 mg as a single dose; may repeat in 4 h; *max*: 5 mg/d	For migraines. May cause dizziness, drowsiness, photophobia, fatigue, malaise, nausea, vomiting, chest pain, and paresthesia. PB: 28%–31%; t½: 6 h
Rizatriptan benzoate	A: PO: 5–10 mg as a single dose; may repeat in 2 h; *max*: 30 mg/d	For migraines. May cause dizziness, drowsiness, fatigue, weakness, dry mouth, nausea, chest pain, and paresthesia. PB: 14%; t½: 2–3 h
Zolmitriptan	A: PO tabs: 1.25–2.5 mg as a single dose; may repeat in 2 h; *max*: 5 mg/dose; 10 mg/d A: Oral disintegrating tab: 2.5 mg as a single dose, may repeat in 2 h; *max*: 5 mg/dose, 10 mg/d Nasal inhalation: A: 2.5 mg in 1 nostril as a single dose; may repeat in 2 h; *max*: 5 mg/dose, 10 mg/d	For migraines. May cause dizziness, drowsiness, weakness, dry mouth, dysgeusia, nausea, myasthenia, hyperhidrosis, paresthesia, and hyperesthesia. PB: 25%; t½: 3 h
Almotriptan	A: PO: 6.25–12.5 mg as a single dose; may repeat in 2 h; *max*: 25 mg/d	For migraines. May cause dizziness, drowsiness, headache, nausea, vomiting, and paresthesia. PB: 35%; t½: 3–4 h
Frovatriptan	A: PO: 2.5 mg as a single dose; may repeat in 2 h; *max*: 7.5 mg/d	For migraines. May cause dizziness, headache, fatigue, flushing, dry mouth, dyspepsia, nausea, vomiting, diarrhea, muscular skeletal pain, and paresthesia. PB: 15%; t½: 26 h
Eletriptan	A: PO: 20–40 mg as a single dose; may repeat in 2 h; *max*: 80 mg/d	For migraines. May cause dizziness, drowsiness, headache, weakness, flushing, dry mouth, and nausea. PB: 85%; t½: 13 h
Lasmiditan	A: PO: 50, 100, or 200 mg as a single dose; *max*: 1 dose/24 h or 200 mg/d	For migraines. May cause dizziness, drowsiness, fatigue, malaise, weakness, nausea, vomiting, hypoesthesia, and paresthesias. PB: 55%–60%; t½: 5.7 h
Gene-Related Peptide Antagonist		
Erenumab	A: Subcut: 70–140 mg/mo; *max*: 140 mg/mo	For migraine prophylaxis. May cause antibody formation, injection-site reaction, constipation, alopecia, muscle cramps, erythema, and pruritus. PB: UK; t½: 28 d
Fremanezumab	A: Subcut: 225 mg/mo or 675 mg q3mo	For migraine prophylaxis. May cause antibody formation, injection-site reaction, constipation, erythema, rash, urticaria, and pruritus. PB: UK; t½: 31 d
Galcanezumab	A: Subcut: LD 240 mg, then 120 mg q1mo; *max*: 300 mg/mo	For migraine prophylaxis and cluster headaches. May cause antibody formation, injection-site reaction, constipation, erythema, rash, hives, and pruritus. PB: UK; t½: 27 d
Rimegepant	A: PO: 75 mg as single dose; *max*: 75 mg/d	For migraines. May cause dyspnea, dyspepsia, abdominal pain, nausea, and rash. PB: 96%; t½: 11 h
Ubrogepant	A: PO: 50 or 100 mg as single dose, may repeat in 2 h PRN; *max*: 200 mg/d	For migraines. May cause fatigue, dry mouth, rash, hives, pruritus, and nausea. PB: 87%; t½: 5–7 h
Eptinezumab	A: IV: 100 mg q3mo over 30 min infusion; *max*: 300 mg q3mo	For migraine prophylaxis. May cause flushing, pharyngitis, rash, urticaria, angioedema, and antibody formation. PB: UK; t½: 27 d
Atogepant	A: PO: 10, 30, or 60 mg/d; *max*: 60 mg/d	For episodic migraine prophylaxis. May cause drowsiness, fatigue, anorexia, nausea, constipation, and weight loss. PB: 98%; t½: 11 h
Zavepepant	A: Intranasal: 10 mg in 1 nostril as a single dose; *max*: 10 mg/d	For acute treatment of migraine. May cause nasal irritation, dysgeusia, nausea, vomiting, and urticaria. PB: 90%; t½: 6.55 h
Miscellaneous Drugs for Migraines		
Topiramate	Immediate release: 25 mg q evening for 1 wk, then 25 mg bid for 1 wk, then 25 mg qam & 50 mg qpm for 1 wk, then 50 mg bid Extended release: A: PO: 25 mg/d for 1 wk, then 50 mg/d for 1 wk, then 75 mg/d for 1 wk, then 100 mg/d; *max*: 100 mg/d	For migraine prophylaxis Lennox-Gastaut syndrome, and seizures. May cause drowsiness, dizziness, confusion, ataxia, diplopia, dysgeusia, anorexia, abdominal pain, fatigue, hyperammonemia, metabolic acidosis, infection, paresthesias, and weight loss. PB: 15%–41%; t½: Immediate release 21 h, Extended release 31–56 h

>, Greater than; *A*, adult; *bid*, two times a day; *CAD*, coronary artery disease; *d*, day; *GI*, gastrointestinal; *h*, hour; *IHD*, ischemic heart disease; *IM*, intramuscular; *IV*, intravenous; *LD*, loading dose; *max*, maximum; *MI*, myocardial infarction; *min*, minute; *mo*, month; *PB*, protein binding; *PO*, by mouth; *q*, every; *subcut*, subcutaneous; *t½*, half-life; *tab*, tablet; *wk*, week; *y*, years.

PROTOTYPE DRUG CHART

Sumatriptan

Drug Class	Dosage
Selective serotonin receptor agonist: Antimigraine	Migraine: A: PO: Initially 25, 50, or 100 mg as a single dose, may repeat in 2 h; *max:* 200 mg/d or 100 mg/dose A: Subcut: 3–6 mg as a single dose, may repeat after 1 h; *max:* 12 mg/d A: Intranasal: 5, 10, or 20 mg in 1 nostril as a single dose, may repeat after 2 h; *max:* 40 mg/d

Contraindications	Drug-Lab-Food Interactions
Hypersensitivity, CAD, AMI, peripheral vascular disease, hypertension, cardiac/cerebrovascular disease, stroke *Caution:* Renal or hepatic dysfunction, dysrhythmias, intracranial bleeding, visual disturbance, colitis, hypercholesterolemia, obesity, DM, smoking, seizures, Raynaud's phenomenon, older adults, pregnancy, breast-feeding	Drug: Risk of vasospasm and blood pressure elevation with dihydroergotamine and other ergot alkaloids; increased levels and toxicity within 2 wk of MAOIs; increased risk of serotonin syndrome or neuroleptic malignant syndrome with SSRIs

Pharmacokinetics	Pharmacodynamics
Absorption: Rapidly absorbed after subcut injection Distribution: PB: 14%–21% Metabolism: t½: 2 h Excretion: Urine and feces	PO: Onset: 60 min Peak: 2–4 h; duration: 24–48 h Subcut: Onset: 10 min Peak: 5–20 min; duration: 24–48 h Intranasal: Onset: 15 min Peak: 1–1.75 h; duration: 24–48 h

Therapeutic Effects/Uses
To treat migraine and cluster headaches
Mechanism of Action: Causes vasoconstriction of cranial arteries to relieve migraine attacks

Side Effects	Adverse Reactions
Dizziness, headache, blurred vision, rhinorrhea, rhinalgia, malaise, paresthesia, fatigue, flushing, drowsiness, dysgeusia, myalgia, hyperhidrosis, nausea, vomiting, injection-site reaction, contact dermatitis, pruritus, skin/ocular irritation	Hypotension, hypertensive crisis, angina, dysrhythmias, bradycardia, tachycardia, thrombosis, seizures, hearing loss, tinnitus, ocular hemorrhage, GI bleeding/obstruction, myasthenia *Life-threatening:* Coronary artery vasospasm, renal failure, angioedema, hemolytic anemia, pancytopenia, thrombocytopenia, intracranial hemorrhage, stroke, MI, cardiac arrest, suicidal ideation

A, adult; *AMI*, acute myocardial infarction; *CAD*, coronary artery disease; *d*, day; *DM*, diabetes mellitus; *GI*, gastrointestinal; *h*, hour; *MAOI*, monoamine oxidase inhibitor; *max*, maximum; *MI*, myocardial infarction; *min*, minute; *PB*, protein binding; *PO*, by mouth; *SSRI*, selective serotonin reuptake inhibitor; *subcut*, subcutaneous; *t½*: half-life.

CLINICAL JUDGMENT SINGLE-EPISODE CASE STUDY

Cognitive Skill: Prioritize Hypotheses
Objective: Prioritize nursing care for a postoperative patient receiving a prescribed analgesic.

A 79-year-old male client on the medical surgical unit is reporting abdominal pain. This patient has a history of ulcerative colitis and 24 hours prior received emergent resection of the colon. During the morning assessment the nurse notes his last dose of 2 mg IV morphine was administered on the previous shift 6 hours prior. It is ordered every 4 hours. The nurse administers the patient's prescribed dose of 2 mg IV morphine after the morning assessment and vital signs check.

Which nursing actions are required related to the client's condition and prescribed pain medication? Choose the most likely options for the information missing from the statements below by selecting from the lists of options provided.

The nurse will continue to monitor the patient's _____(A)_____ and assess the depth and rate of the patient's _____(A)_____. Instruct the patient to report signs and symptoms of _____(A)_____, _____(A)_____, and _____(A)_____. Monitor and observe for changes in the patient's _____(B)_____. The nurse will withhold pain medication for any difficulty in the patient's _____(B)_____ and respirations below _____(B)_____. Instruct the patient to notify the nurse immediately upon return or increase of the patient's _____(B)_____.

OPTION A	OPTION B
tinnitus	dry skin
dizziness	breathing
vital signs	pedal edema
sore throat	mental status
respirations	abdominal pain
constipation	episodes of sneezing
hypotension	12 breaths per minute
feeling of fullness	20 breaths per minute

CLINICAL JUDGMENT SINGLE-EPISODE CASE STUDY—CONT'D

Answers
The nurse will continue to monitor the patient's **vital signs** and asses the depth and rate of the patient's **respirations**. Instruct the patient to report signs and symptoms of **dizziness, constipation**, and **hypotension**. Monitor and observe for changes in the patient's **mental status**. The nurse will withhold pain medication for any difficulty in the patient's **breathing** and respirations below **12 breaths per minute**. Instruct the patient to notify the nurse immediately upon return or increase of the patient's **abdominal pain**.

Rationale
Morphine binds with the opiate receptors in the central nervous system, producing analgesia and sedation. The onset of action when administered parenterally is 15–20 min. Morphine injection has high risk for low respiratory rate, which can result in respiratory depression. If the patient is experiencing breathing difficulty and their respirations are below 12 breaths per minute, the nurse should withhold the medication and notify the provider because the patient may be developing respiratory distress. Also, it is known to cause sedation, hypotension, constipation, and changes in mental status. It is important to administer the morphine before pain reaches its peak to maximize the effectiveness of the drug, so instruct the patient to report any periods of increased abdominal pain.

Reference
McCuistion, et al.: Pharmacology, Chapter 25 (see Prototype Drug Chart), In Burchum J, Rosenthal L, editors: *Lehne's Pharmacology for Nursing Care*, 10th ed, 2019,.

REVIEW QUESTIONS

1. A patient requires a nonopioid medication. The nurse knows that which medication will cause the least gastrointestinal distress?
    a. Aspirin
    b. Ketorolac
    c. Celecoxib
    d. Ibuprofen

2. A patient states during a medical history that he takes several acetaminophen tablets throughout the day for acute pain. The nurse teaches the patient that the dosage should not exceed which amount?
    a. 1 g/day
    b. 3 g/day
    c. 4 g/day
    d. 6 g/day

3. For the patient receiving periodic morphine via intravenous push, which of the following findings would be of utmost concern to the nurse?
    a. Increased temperature
    b. Decreased bowel sounds
    c. Decreased respirations
    d. Increased red blood cell count

4. A patient is admitted to the emergency department with signs of respiratory depression after self-injection with hydromorphone. The admitting nurse knows that which drug will reverse respiratory depression caused by opioid overdose?
    a. Fentanyl
    b. Naloxone
    c. Butorphanol
    d. Sufenta

5. Assessing a patient after intravenous morphine administration, the nurse notes cold, clammy skin; a pulse of 40 beats/min; respirations of 10 breaths/min; and constricted pupils. Which medication will the patient likely need next?
    a. Naloxone
    b. Meloxicam
    c. Pentazocine
    d. Propoxyphene

6. For the patient taking acetaminophen, what should the nurse do? **Select all that apply**.
    a. Monitor routine liver enzyme tests.
    b. Encourage the patient to check package labels of over-the-counter drugs to avoid overdosing.
    c. Report side effects immediately, as toxicity can cause severe hepatic damage.
    d. Teach the female patient that oral contraceptives can increase the effect of acetaminophen.
    e. Teach the patient that caffeine decreases the effects of acetaminophen.

7. For the patient who is taking nalbuphine, what should the nurse do? **Select all that apply**.
    a. Monitor any changes in respirations.
    b. Instruct the patient to report hypohidrosis.
    c. Administer intravenous nalbuphine undiluted.
    d. Explain to the patient to expect an excessive amount of urine output.
    e. Instruct the patient to avoid alcohol when taking nalbuphine to avoid respiratory depression.

8. A patient is having a migraine attack. The nurse should know that which drugs are used to treat migraine attacks?
    a. Triptans
    b. Anticonvulsants
    c. Tricyclic antidepressants
    d. Beta-adrenergic blockers

UNIT VIII Antimicrobial Drugs

26

Penicillins, Other Beta-Lactams, and Cephalosporins

http://evolve.elsevier.com/McCuistion/pharmacology

OBJECTIVES

- Recall the pathophysiology of disease-producing microorganisms.
- Describe components involved in destroying bacteria.
- Explain the mechanism of action of penicillins and other beta-lactam antibacterials.
- Discuss the use and mechanism of action of cephalosporins.

OUTLINE

Pathophysiology, 321
    Gram Staining, 321
    Cell Lysis, 321
Antibacterials/Antibiotics, 322
    Mechanisms of Antibacterial Action, 322
    Body Defenses, 323
    Resistance to Antibacterials, 323
    Use of Antibiotic Combinations, 324
    Narrow-Spectrum and Broad-Spectrum Antibiotics, 324
Penicillins and Other Beta-Lactam Antibacterials, 324
    Broad-Spectrum Penicillins (Aminopenicillins), 325
    Penicillinase-Resistant Penicillins (Antistaphylococcal Penicillins), 325

Extended-Spectrum Penicillins (Antipseudomonal Penicillins), 325
    Beta-Lactamase Inhibitors, 325
    Side Effects and Adverse Reactions, 327
    Other Beta-Lactam Antibacterials, 328
Cephalosporins, 328
    First-, Second-, Third-, Fourth-, and Fifth-Generation Cephalosporins, 328
    Side Effects and Adverse Reactions, 332
    Drug Interactions, 332
Clinical Judgment Case Study, 332
Review Questions, 332

This chapter discusses penicillins, other beta-lactam antibacterials, and cephalosporins and their effects. It includes mechanisms of antibacterial action, body defenses, resistance to antibacterials, use of antibacterial combinations, general adverse reactions to antibacterials, and narrow- and broad-spectrum antibiotics.

PATHOPHYSIOLOGY

Disease-producing microorganisms may be gram-positive or gram-negative bacteria, viruses, protozoans, or fungi. The degree to which they are pathogenic depends on the microorganism and its virulence.

    Bacteria, known as *prokaryotes*, are single-celled organisms that lack a true nucleus and nuclear membrane. Most bacteria have a rigid cell wall, and the structure of the cell wall determines the shape of the bacteria. One classification of bacteria involves the appearance or shape under a microscope. A *bacillus* is a rod-shaped organism, and *cocci* are spherical. When cocci appear in clusters, they are called *staphylococci*; when they are arranged in chains, they are called *streptococci*. Bacteria reproduce by cell division about every 20 minutes.

Gram Staining

Another classification of bacteria involves staining properties of the cell. The Gram staining method was devised in 1882 by Hans Christian Gram, a Danish bacteriologist. Gram staining determines the ability of the bacterial cell wall to retain a purple stain by a basic dye. Crystal violet is normally used in the staining process but may be substituted with methylene blue. If bacteria retain a purple stain, they are classified as gram-positive microorganisms. Those bacteria that are not stained are known as gram-negative microorganisms. Examples of gram-positive bacteria include *Staphylococcus aureus, Streptococcus pneumoniae*, group B *Streptococcus* (GBS), and *Clostridium perfringens*. Examples of gram-negative bacteria include *Neisseria meningitides, Escherichia coli*, and *Haemophilus influenzae*.

Cell Lysis

Bacteria produce toxins that cause cell lysis (cell breakdown). Many bacteria produce the enzyme beta-lactamase, which destroys beta-lactam antibiotics such as penicillins and cephalosporins.

ANTIBACTERIALS/ANTIBIOTICS

Although the terms *antibacterial*, *antimicrobial*, and *antibiotic* are frequently used interchangeably, there are some subtle differences in meaning. Antibacterials and antimicrobials are substances that inhibit bacterial growth or kill bacteria and other microorganisms—microscopic organisms that include viruses, fungi, protozoa, and rickettsiae. Technically, the term *antibiotic* refers to chemicals produced by one kind of microorganism that inhibit the growth of or kill another. For practical purposes, however, these terms may be used interchangeably. Several drugs, including antiinfective and chemotherapeutic agents, have actions similar to those of antibacterial and antimicrobial agents. Antibacterial drugs do not act alone in destroying bacteria. Natural body defenses, surgical procedures to excise infected tissues, and dressing changes may be needed along with antibacterial drugs to eliminate the infecting bacteria.

Antibacterial drugs are either obtained from natural sources or manufactured. The use of moldy bread on wounds to fight infection dates back 3500 years. In 1928 British bacteriologist Alexander Fleming noted that a mold that had contaminated his bacterial cultures was inhibiting bacterial growth. The mold was *Penicillium notatum*; thus Fleming called the substance *penicillin*. In 1939 Howard Florey expanded on Fleming's findings and purified penicillin so it could be used commercially. Penicillin was used during World War II and was marketed in 1945.

Mechanisms of Antibacterial Action

Five mechanisms of antibacterial action are responsible for the inhibition of growth or destruction of microorganisms: (1) inhibition of bacterial cell wall synthesis, (2) alteration of membrane permeability, (3) inhibition of protein synthesis, (4) inhibition of the synthesis of bacterial ribonucleic acid (RNA) and deoxyribonucleic acid (DNA), and (5) interference with metabolism within the cell (Table 26.1).

Pharmacokinetics

Antibacterial drugs must not only penetrate the bacterial cell wall in sufficient concentrations but also have an affinity for (attraction to) the binding sites on the bacterial cell. The length of time the drug remains at the binding sites increases the effect of the antibacterial action. This time factor is controlled by the pharmacokinetics—the distribution, half-life, and elimination—of the drug.

Antibacterials that have a longer half-life usually maintain a greater concentration at the binding site; therefore frequent dosing is not required. Most antibacterials are not highly protein bound, with a few exceptions (e.g., oxacillin, ceftriaxone, cefotetan, dicloxacillin, nafcillin, clindamycin). Protein binding does not have a major influence on the effectiveness of most antibacterial drugs. The steady state of the antibacterial drug occurs after the fourth to fifth half-lives, and after the seventh half-life, the drug is eliminated from the body, mainly through urine.

Pharmacodynamics

The drug concentration at the site and the exposure time for the drug play important roles in bacterial eradication. Antibacterial drugs are used to achieve the minimum effective concentration (MEC) necessary to halt the growth of a microorganism. Many antibacterials have a bactericidal effect against the pathogen when the drug concentration remains constantly above the MEC during the dosing interval. Duration of use of the antibacterial varies according to the type of pathogen, site of infection, and immunocompetence of the host. With some severe infections, a continuous infusion regimen is more effective than intermittent dosing because of constant drug concentration and time exposure. Once-daily antibacterial dosing—such as with aminoglycosides, macrolides, and fluoroquinolones—has been effective in eradicating pathogens and has not caused severe adverse reactions (ototoxicity, nephrotoxicity) in most cases. The ease of compliance with once- or twice-daily drug dosing also increases the patient's adherence to the drug regimen.

TABLE 26.1 Mechanisms of Action of Antibacterial Drugs

Action	Effect	Drugs
Inhibition of cell wall synthesis	Bactericidal effect Enzyme breakdown of cell wall Inhibition of enzyme in synthesis of cell wall	Penicillin Cephalosporins Bacitracin Vancomycin
Alteration of membrane permeability	Bacteriostatic or bactericidal effect Increases membrane permeability Cell lysis caused by loss of cellular substances	Amphotericin B Nystatin Polymyxin Colistin
Inhibition of protein synthesis	Bacteriostatic or bactericidal effect Interferes with protein synthesis without affecting normal cell Inhibits steps of protein synthesis	Aminoglycosides Tetracyclines Erythromycin Lincomycin
Inhibition of synthesis of bacterial RNA and DNA	Inhibits synthesis of RNA and DNA in bacteria Binds to nucleic acid and enzymes needed for nucleic acid synthesis	Fluoroquinolones
Interference with cellular metabolism	Bacteriostatic effect Interferes with steps of metabolism within cells	Sulfonamides Trimethoprim Isoniazid Nalidixic acid Rifampin

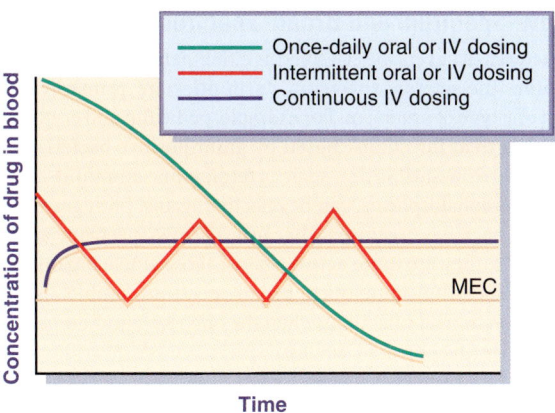

Fig. 26.1 Effects of concentrated drug dosing. *MEC,* Minimum effective concentration.

Fig. 26.1 illustrates the effect of three methods of drug dosing. The drug dose is effective when it remains above the MEC.

Body Defenses

Body defenses and antibacterial drugs work together to stop the infectious process. The effect that antibacterial drugs have on an infection depends not only on the drug but also on the host's defense mechanisms. Factors such as age, nutrition, immunoglobulins, white blood cells (WBCs), organ function, and circulation influence the body's ability to fight infection. Older adults and individuals who are undernourished have less resistance to infection than younger, well-nourished populations. If the host's natural body defense mechanisms are inadequate, drug therapy might not be as effective. As a result, drug therapy may need to be closely monitored or revised. When circulation is impeded, an antibacterial drug may not be distributed properly to the infected area. In addition, immunoglobulins—antibody proteins such as IgG and IgM—and other elements of the immune response system, such as WBCs needed to combat infections, may be depleted in individuals with poor nutritional status.

Resistance to Antibacterials

Bacteria can be either sensitive or resistant to certain antibacterials. When bacteria are *sensitive* to a drug, the pathogen is inhibited or destroyed; however, if bacteria are *resistant*, the pathogen continues to grow despite administration of that antibacterial drug.

Bacterial resistance can result naturally, called inherent resistance, or it may be acquired. A natural, or inherent, resistance occurs without previous exposure to the antibacterial drug. For example, the gram-negative bacterium *Pseudomonas aeruginosa* is inherently resistant to penicillin G. An acquired resistance is caused by prior exposure to the antibacterial. Although *S. aureus* was once sensitive to penicillin G, repeated exposures have caused this organism to evolve and become resistant to that drug. Penicillinase, an enzyme produced by the microorganism, is responsible for causing its penicillin resistance. Penicillinase metabolizes penicillin G, causing the drug to be ineffective; however, penicillinase-resistant penicillins that are effective against *S. aureus* are now available.

Antibiotic resistance is a major problem. In the early 1980s pharmaceutical companies thought that enough antibiotics were on the market, so they concentrated on developing antiviral and antifungal drugs. As a result, fewer new antibiotics were developed during the 1980s. Now pharmaceutical companies have developed many new antibiotics, but antibiotic resistance continues to develop, especially when antibiotics are used frequently. As bacteria reproduce, some mutation occurs, and eventually the mutant bacteria survive the effects of the drug. One explanation is that the mutant bacterial strain may have grown a thicker cell wall.

In large health care institutions, there is a tendency toward drug resistance in bacteria. Mutant strains of organisms have developed, thus increasing their resistance to antibiotics that were once effective against them. Infections acquired while patients are hospitalized are called health care-acquired infections (previously known as nosocomial infections). Many of these infections are caused by drug-resistant bacteria, and this can prolong hospitalization, which is costly to both the patient and third-party health care insurers.

Another problem related to antibiotic resistance is that bacteria can transfer their genetic instructions to another bacterial species, and the other bacterial species then becomes resistant to that antibiotic as well. Bacteria can also pass along high resistance to a more virulent and aggressive bacterium (e.g., *S. aureus*, enterococci).

Methicillin was the first penicillinase-resistant penicillin; it was developed in 1959 in response to the resistance of *S. aureus*. In 1968 strains of *S. aureus* were beginning to become resistant to methicillin. Highly resistant bacteria, so-called methicillin-resistant *S. aureus* (MRSA), became resistant not only to methicillin but to all penicillins and cephalosporins as well. Resistance that was once found only in hospitals began to emerge in 1981 in the community. Methicillin is now off the market, and the treatment of choice for MRSA is vancomycin. Other effective drugs used to treat MRSA include linezolid, tedizolid, daptomycin, TMP-SMZ, doxycycline, clindamycin, and telavancin, a glycopeptide antiinfective.

Many enterococcal strains are resistant to penicillin, ampicillin, gentamicin, streptomycin, and vancomycin. Another big resistance problem is vancomycin-resistant *Enterococcus faecium* (VREF), which can cause death in persons with weakened immune systems. The incidence of VREF in hospitals has increased, and a strain of MRSA has also been reported to be resistant to vancomycin (vancomycin-resistant *S. aureus*, or VRSA). One antibiotic after another is ineffective against new resistant strains of bacteria, and major medical problems result. As new drugs are developed, drug resistance will probably also develop.

Pharmaceutical companies and biotech firms are working on new classes of drugs to overcome the problem of bacterial resistance to antibiotics. A class of antibiotics known as *oxazolidinones* was discovered by a pharmaceutical company in 1988, but the company could not overcome the toxicity problems with this class of drug; however, another pharmaceutical company has taken the compound and made it less toxic. This antibiotic, linezolid, is effective against MRSA, VREF, and penicillin-resistant streptococci. Quinupristin-dalfopristin, which consists of two streptogramin antibacterials, is marketed in a 30:70 combination for intravenous (IV) use against life-threatening infection caused by VREF and for treatment of bacteremia, *S. aureus*, and *Streptococcus pyogenes*.

Another way to attack antimicrobial resistance is to develop drugs that disable the antibiotic-resistant mechanism in the bacteria. Patients would take the antibiotic-resistance disabler along with the antibiotic already on the market, making the drug effective again. Developing a bacterial vaccine is another way to combat bacteria and lessen the need for antibiotics. The bacterial vaccine against pneumococcus has been effective in decreasing the occurrence of pneumonia and meningitis among various age groups.

Antibiotic misuse, a major problem today, increases antibiotic resistance. Studies reveal that 23% to 37.8% of patients in hospitals receive antibiotics, and 50% of this population is receiving antibiotics inappropriately. When antibiotics are taken unnecessarily—such as for viral infections when no bacterial infection is present—or incorrectly (e.g., skipping doses, not taking the full antibiotic regimen), resistance to antibacterials may develop. Consumer education is important because many patients demand antibiotics for viral conditions, even though antibiotics are ineffective against viruses; however, viral infections that persist could compromise the body's immune system and thus promote a secondary bacterial infection. The nurse should teach patients about the proper use of antibiotics to prevent situations that promote drug resistance to bacteria.

Cross-resistance can also occur among antibacterial drugs that have similar actions, such as the penicillins and cephalosporins. To ascertain the effect antibacterial drugs have on a specific microorganism, culture and sensitivity (C&S) or antibiotic susceptibility laboratory testing is performed. C&S can detect the infective microorganism present in a sample (e.g., blood, sputum, swab) and the best drug to kill it. The organism causing the infection is determined by culture, and antibiotics the organism is sensitive to are determined by sensitivity. The susceptibility or resistance of one microorganism to several antibacterials can be determined by the C&S test. Multiantibiotic therapy, or daily use of several antibacterials, delays the development of microorganism resistance.

Use of Antibiotic Combinations

Combination antibiotics should not be routinely prescribed or administered except for specific uncontrollable infections. Usually a single antibiotic will successfully treat a bacterial infection; however, when severe infection persists and is of an unknown origin or has been unsuccessfully treated with several single antibiotics, a combination of two or three antibiotics may be suggested. Before beginning antibiotic therapy, a culture or cultures should be taken to identify the bacteria.

When two antibiotics are combined, the result may be additive, potentiative, or antagonistic. The *additive* effect is equal to the sum of the effects of two antibiotics. The *potentiative* effect occurs when one antibiotic potentiates the effect of the second antibiotic, *increasing* its effectiveness. The *antagonistic* result is achieved with combination of a drug that is bactericidal, such as penicillin, and a drug that is bacteriostatic, such as tetracycline; when these two drugs are used together, the desired effect may be greatly *reduced*.

General Adverse Reactions to Antibacterials

Three major adverse reactions associated with the administration of antibacterial drugs are (1) allergic (hypersensitivity, anaphylaxis) reactions, (2) superinfection, and (3) organ toxicity. Table 26.2 describes these adverse reactions, all of which require close monitoring of the patient.

Narrow-Spectrum and Broad-Spectrum Antibiotics

Antibacterial drugs can be classified as either narrow spectrum or broad spectrum. The narrow-spectrum antibiotics are primarily effective against one type of organism. For example, penicillin and erythromycin are used to treat infections caused by gram-positive bacteria. Certain broad-spectrum antibiotics, such as tetracycline and third- and fifth-generation cephalosporins, can be effective against both gram-positive and gram-negative organisms. Because narrow-spectrum antibiotics are selective, they are more active against those single organisms than the broad-spectrum antibiotics. Broad-spectrum antibiotics are frequently used to treat infections when the offending microorganism has not been identified by the C&S test.

PENICILLINS AND OTHER BETA-LACTAM ANTIBACTERIALS

Penicillin, a natural antibacterial agent obtained from the mold genus *Penicillium*, was introduced to the military during World War II and is considered to have saved many soldiers' lives. It became widely used in 1945 and was considered a "miracle drug." With the advent of penicillin, many patients survived who would have normally died from wound and severe respiratory infections.

Penicillin's beta-lactam ring structure interferes with bacterial cell wall synthesis by inhibiting the bacterial enzyme necessary for cell division and cellular synthesis. The bacteria die of cell lysis (cell breakdown). The penicillins can be both bacteriostatic (inhibit growth) and bactericidal (kill bacteria), depending on the drug, dosage, serum level, and pathogen (disease-producing microorganism). Penicillin G is primarily bactericidal.

Penicillins are mainly referred to as *beta-lactam antibiotics*. Bacteria can produce a variety of enzymes, such as beta-lactamases, that can inactivate penicillin and other beta-lactam antibiotics such as the cephalosporins. The beta-lactamases, which attack penicillins, are called *penicillinases*.

Penicillin G was the first penicillin administered orally and by injection. With oral administration, only about one-third of the dose is absorbed. Because of its poor absorption, penicillin G given by injection (IV and intramuscular [IM]) is more effective in achieving a therapeutic serum penicillin level. Because it is an aqueous drug solution, aqueous penicillin G has a short duration of action, and the IM injection is very painful. As a result, a longer-acting form of penicillin, procaine penicillin (milky color), was produced to extend the activity of

TABLE 26.2	General Adverse Reactions to Antibacterial Drugs
Type	**Considerations**
Allergy or hypersensitivity	Allergic reactions to drugs may be mild or severe. Examples of mild reactions are rash, pruritus, and hives. An example of a severe response is anaphylactic shock, which results in vascular collapse, laryngeal edema, bronchospasm, and cardiac arrest. Severe allergic reaction generally occurs within 20 minutes, and shortness of breath is often the first symptom of anaphylaxis. Mild allergic reaction is treated with an antihistamine, whereas anaphylaxis requires treatment with epinephrine, bronchodilators, and antihistamines.
Superinfection	Superinfection is a secondary infection that occurs when the normal microbial flora of the body are disturbed during antibiotic therapy. Superinfections can occur in the mouth, respiratory tract, intestine, genitourinary tract, and skin. Fungal infections frequently result in superinfections, although bacterial organisms (e.g., *Proteus, Pseudomonas, Staphylococcus*) may be the offending microorganisms. Superinfections rarely develop when the drug is administered for less than 1 week, and they occur more commonly with the use of broad-spectrum antibiotics. For fungal infection of the mouth, nystatin is frequently used.
Organ toxicity	The liver and kidneys are involved in drug metabolism and excretion, and antibacterials may result in damage to these organs. For example, aminoglycosides can be nephrotoxic and ototoxic.

the drug. Procaine (an anesthetic) in the penicillin decreases the pain related to injection.

Penicillin V was the next type of penicillin produced. Although two-thirds of the oral dose is absorbed by the gastrointestinal (GI) tract, it is a less potent antibacterial drug than penicillin G. Penicillin V is effective against mild to moderate infections, including anthrax as a weapon of bioterrorism.

Initially, penicillin was overused. It was first introduced for the treatment of staphylococcal infections, but after a few years, mutant strains of *Staphylococcus* developed that were resistant to penicillins G and V because of the bacterial enzyme penicillinase, which destroys penicillin. This led to the development of new broad-spectrum antibiotics with structures similar to penicillin to combat infections resistant to penicillins G and V.

Food in the stomach does not significantly alter absorption of penicillin V, so it should be taken after meals. Amoxicillins are penicillins that are unaffected by food.

Broad-Spectrum Penicillins (Aminopenicillins)

Broad-spectrum penicillins are used to treat both gram-positive and gram-negative bacteria. They are not, however, as broadly effective against all microorganisms as they were once considered to be. This group of drugs is costlier than penicillin and therefore should not be used when ordinary penicillins, such as penicillin G, are effective. The broad-spectrum penicillins are effective against some gram-negative organisms such as *E. coli*, *H. influenzae*, *Shigella dysenteriae*, *Proteus mirabilis*, and *Salmonella* species. However, these drugs are not penicillinase resistant; because they are readily inactivated by beta-lactamases, they are ineffective against *S. aureus*. Examples of this group are ampicillin and amoxicillin (Table 26.3). Amoxicillin is the most prescribed penicillin derivative for adults and children.

Penicillinase-Resistant Penicillins (Antistaphylococcal Penicillins)

Penicillinase-resistant penicillins (antistaphylococcal penicillins) are used to treat penicillinase-producing *S. aureus*. Dicloxacillin is an oral preparation of these antibiotics, whereas nafcillin and oxacillin are IM and IV preparations. This group of drugs is *not* effective against gram-negative organisms and is less effective than penicillin G against gram-positive organisms. See Prototype Drug Chart: Amoxicillin and Table 26.3 to compare the similarities and differences in the broad-spectrum penicillin amoxicillin and the penicillinase-resistant penicillin dicloxacillin.

Extended-Spectrum Penicillins (Antipseudomonal Penicillins)

The antipseudomonal penicillins are a group of broad-spectrum antibiotics effective against *P. aeruginosa*, a gram-negative bacillus that is difficult to eradicate. These drugs are also useful against many gram-negative organisms such as *Proteus*, *Serratia*, *Enterobacter*, and *Acinetobacter* species, and also *Klebsiella pneumoniae*. The antipseudomonal penicillins are *not* penicillinase resistant. Their pharmacologic action is similar to that of aminoglycosides, but they are less toxic.

Table 26.3 lists the drugs in the four categories of penicillin-type antibacterials. The administration routes (oral, IM, or IV) of various types of penicillins, along with the cephalosporins, are available on the Evolve website.

Beta-Lactamase Inhibitors

When a broad-spectrum antibiotic such as amoxicillin is combined with a beta-lactamase enzyme inhibitor such as clavulanic acid, the resulting antibiotic combination inhibits the bacterial beta-lactamases, making the antibiotic effective and extending its antimicrobial effect. There are three beta-lactamase inhibitors: (1) clavulanic acid, (2) sulbactam, and (3) tazobactam. These inhibitors are not given alone but are combined with a penicillinase-sensitive penicillin such as amoxicillin, ampicillin, or piperacillin. The combination drugs currently marketed include amoxicillin-clavulanic acid (for oral use), and ampicillin-sulbactam and piperacillin tazobactam (for use parenterally).

PROTOTYPE DRUG CHART
Amoxicillin

Drug Class	Dosage
Amoxicillin: Broad-spectrum penicillin	Lower respiratory infections: Immediate release: A: PO: 875 mg q12h or 500 mg q8h; max: 1750 mg/d

Contraindications	Drug-Lab-Food Interactions
Penicillin hypersensitivity *Caution:* Cephalosporin hypersensitivity, renal impairment, diarrhea, CDAD, pseudomembranous colitis, mononucleosis, dialysis, pregnancy, breast-feeding	Drug: Increased effect with aspirin, probenecid, acetaminophen; increased bleeding with oral anticoagulants; increased effect of methotrexate; decreased effect with tetracycline Lab: Increased serum AST, ALT, BUN, and creatinine; increased PT, INR Food: Decreased effect with acidic fruits and juices

Pharmacokinetics	Pharmacodynamics
Absorption: PO: >80% in the GI tract Distribution: PB: 20% Metabolism: t½: 1–1.5 h Excretion: 70% in urine	PO: Onset, duration: UK Peak: 1–2 h

Therapeutic Effects/Uses
For treating otitis media, pharyngitis, tonsillitis, sinusitis, and skin, respiratory, and urinary tract infections. Amoxicillin is effective against *Helicobacter pylori* and *Escherichia coli* and species of *Haemophilus*, *Enterococcus*, *Proteus*, *Staphylococcus*, and *Streptococcus*.
Mechanism of Action: Amoxicillin inhibits the enzyme in cell wall synthesis and has a bactericidal effect.

Side Effects	Adverse Reactions
Dizziness, headache, anxiety, confusion, insomnia, dermatitis, rash, pruritus, hives, tongue/tooth discoloration, esophagitis, dysgeusia, dysphagia, abdominal pain, nausea, vomiting, diarrhea, candidiasis, crystalluria	Superinfection, prolonged bleeding time, seizures *Life threatening:* Anaphylaxis, angioedema, eosinophilia, leukopenia, thrombocytopenia, agranulocytosis, hemolytic anemia, elevated hepatic enzymes, pseudomembranous colitis, CDAD, Stevens-Johnson syndrome

A, adult; *ALT*, alanine aminotransferase; *AST*, aspartate aminotransferase; *BUN*, blood urea nitrogen; *CDAD*, *Clostridium difficile*–associated diarrhea; *d*, day; *GI*, gastrointestinal; *h*, hour; *INR*, international normalized ratio; *max*, maximum dosage; *PB*, protein binding; *PO*, by mouth; *PT*, prothrombin time; *q*, every; *t½*, half-life; *UK*, unknown.

TABLE 26.3 Antibacterials: Penicillins

Generic	Route and Dosage	Uses and Considerations
Basic Penicillins		
Penicillin G procaine	Pneumococcal pneumonia: A: IM: 600,000–1.2 million units/d for at least 10 d; max: 2.4 million units/d	For treating diphtheria, skin infections, staphylococcal/streptococcal, syphilis, bacterial endocarditis, scarlet fever, and respiratory infections. May cause rash, dermatitis, hives, chills, fever, edema, injection site reaction, tongue discoloration, nausea, vomiting, diarrhea, anaphylaxis, CDAD, pseudomembranous colitis, superinfection and arthralgia. PB: 60%; t½: UK
Penicillin G benzathine	Upper respiratory infection: A: IM: 1.2 million units as a single dose; max: 2.4 million units/d	For streptococcal, syphilis, and respiratory infections and for rheumatic fever prophylaxis. May cause rash, hives, fever, fatigue, weakness, injection site reaction, tongue discoloration, edema, nausea, vomiting, diarrhea, anaphylaxis, arthralgia, CDAD, pseudomembranous colitis, and superinfection. PB: 60%; t½: UK
Penicillin G potassium	Endocarditis: A: IM/IV: 12–24 million units/d divided q4–6 h; max: 24 million units/d	For anthrax, bacteremia, diphtheria, skin, respiratory, and clostridial infections, gonorrhea, syphilis, pericarditis, and endocarditis. May cause fever, malaise, tongue discoloration, rash, hives, injection site reaction, arthralgia, myalgia, nausea, vomiting, diarrhea, hyperkalemia, anaphylaxis, CDAD, pseudomembranous colitis, and superinfection. PB: 45%–68%; t½: 20–30 min
Penicillin V potassium	Skin infection: A: PO: 250–500 mg q6–8h for at least 5–14 d; max: 2 g/d	For streptococcal infections, ulcerative gingivitis, otitis media, skin infections, and endocarditis prophylaxis. May cause tongue discoloration, contact dermatitis, rash, hives, fever, nausea, vomiting, diarrhea, anaphylaxis, peripheral neuropathy, pseudomembranous colitis, CDAD, and superinfection. PB: 75%–89%; t½: UK
Broad-Spectrum Penicillins		
Amoxicillin	See Prototype Drug Chart: Amoxicillin	
Amoxicillin-clavulanate	Lower respiratory infection: Immediate release: A: PO: 875 mg amoxicillin and 125 mg clavulanate q12h or 500 mg amoxicillin/125 mg clavulanate q8h Extended release: A: PO: 2000 mg amoxicillin and 125 mg clavulanate q12h for at least 5 d	For treating otitis media, sinusitis, and respiratory, skin, and urinary tract infections. May cause tooth/tongue discoloration, pruritus, dermatitis, rash, hives, nausea, vomiting, diarrhea, anaphylaxis, CDAD, pseudomembranous colitis, superinfection, and candidiasis. PB: amoxicillin 18%, clavulanate 25%; t½: amoxicillin 1–1.3 h, clavulanate 1 h
Ampicillin	Respiratory infection: A: PO: 250 mg qid; max: 2 g/dput max	For endocarditis, bacteremia, gonorrhea, and gastrointestinal, skin, respiratory, and urinary tract infections. May cause tongue discoloration, stomatitis, rash, hives, dermatitis, pruritus, glossitis, erythema multiform, serum sickness, dysphagia, nausea, vomiting, diarrhea, anaphylaxis, CDAD, pseudomembranous colitis, and superinfection. PB: 20%; t½: 1–1.5 h
Ampicillin-sulbactam	Skin infections: A: IM/IV: 1 g ampicillin/0.5 g sulbactam q6h or 2 g ampicillin 1 g sulbactam q6h; max: 8 g ampicillin 4 g sulbactam	For skin, intraabdominal, and gynecologic infections. May cause headache, chills, fatigue, tongue discoloration, hives, rash, dermatitis, pruritus, glossitis, stomatitis, phlebitis, edema, injection site reaction, nausea, vomiting, diarrhea, anaphylaxis, CDAD, pseudomembranous colitis, candidiasis, and superinfection. PB: sulbactam 38%, ampicillin 15%–25%; t½: both 1–1.5 h
Penicillinase-Resistant Penicillins		
Dicloxacillin sodium	Skin infections: A: PO: 250 mg qid for 5–7 d; max: 1 g/d	For mastitis and skin infections. May cause fever, malaise, serum sickness, tongue, discoloration, rash, pruritus, stomatitis, arthralgia, myalgia, abdominal pain, nausea, vomiting, diarrhea, anaphylaxis, CDAD, and superinfection. PB: 95%–99%; t½: 30–42 min
Nafcillin	Endocarditis: A: IV: 2 g q4h or 3 g q6h for 6 wk	For treating endocarditis, meningitis, bacteremia, mastitis, and skin, respiratory, and bone/joint infections. May cause fever, serum sickness, malaise, tongue discoloration, stomatitis, rash, pruritus, hives, arthralgia, myalgia, phlebitis, injection site reaction, abdominal pain, nausea, vomiting, diarrhea, anaphylaxis, CDAD, and superinfection. PB: 70%–90%; t½: 30–90 min
Oxacillin sodium	Meningitis: A: IV: 2 g q4h	For endocarditis, meningitis, bacteremia, mastitis, and skin, and bone/joint infections. May cause malaise, fever, tongue discoloration, serum sickness, rash, pruritus, stomatitis, injection site reaction, arthralgia, myalgia, abdominal pain, nausea, vomiting, diarrhea, elevated hepatic enzymes, hepatitis, anaphylaxis, CDAD, and superinfection. PB: 89%–94%; t½: 30 min
Extended-Spectrum Penicillins		
Piperacillin tazobactam	Community-acquired pneumonia: A: IV: 4 g piperacillin/0.5 g tazobactam over 30 min q6h at least 7 d; max: 16 g piperacillin/2 g tazobactam/d	For intraabdominal, skin, urinary tract, and respiratory infections. May cause headache, fever, insomnia, rash, pruritus, hives, dyspepsia, abdominal pain, nausea, vomiting, diarrhea, constipation, CDAD, pseudomembranous colitis, candidiasis, anaphylaxis, and superinfection. PB: 30%; t½: 0.7–1.5 h

A, adult; *CDAD*, *Clostridium difficile*–associated diarrhea; *d*, day; *h*, hour; *IM*, intramuscular; *IV*, intravenous; *max*, maximum; *min*, minutes; *PB*, protein binding; *PO*, by mouth; *q*, every; *t½*, half-life; *UK*, unknown; *wk*, weeks.

Pharmacokinetics

Amoxicillin is well absorbed from the GI tract, whereas dicloxacillin is only partially absorbed. Protein-binding power differs between the two drugs—amoxicillin is 20% protein bound, but dicloxacillin is highly protein bound (95%–99%). Drug toxicity may result when other highly protein-bound drugs are used with dicloxacillin. Both drugs have short half-lives. Sixty percent of amoxicillin is excreted in the urine; dicloxacillin is excreted in bile and urine.

Pharmacodynamics

Both amoxicillin and dicloxacillin are penicillin derivatives and are bactericidal. These drugs interfere with bacterial cell wall synthesis, causing cell lysis. Amoxicillin may be produced with or without clavulanic acid, an agent that prevents the breakdown of amoxicillin by decreasing resistance to the antibacterial drug. The addition of clavulanic acid intensifies the effect of amoxicillin. The amoxicillin-clavulanic acid preparation and amoxicillin trihydrate have similar pharmacokinetics and pharmacodynamics as well as similar side effects and adverse reactions. When probenecid is taken with amoxicillin or dicloxacillin, the serum antibacterial levels may be increased. The effects of amoxicillin are decreased when taken with erythromycin and tetracycline. The onset of action, serum peak concentration time, and duration of action for amoxicillin and dicloxacillin are very similar.

Older Adults

Most beta-lactam antibiotics are excreted via the kidneys. For older adults, assessment of renal function is most important. Serum blood urea nitrogen (BUN) and serum creatinine should be monitored. With a decrease in renal function, the antibiotic dose should be decreased.

Side Effects and Adverse Reactions

Common adverse reactions to penicillin administration are hypersensitivity and superinfection, the occurrence of a secondary infection when the flora of the body are disturbed (see Table 26.2). Anorexia, nausea, vomiting, and diarrhea are common GI disturbances, often referred to as *GI distress*. This may be alleviated some by taking penicillin with food. Rash is an indicator of a mild to moderate allergic reaction; severe allergic reaction leads to anaphylactic shock. Clinical manifestations of a severe allergic reaction include laryngeal edema, severe bronchoconstriction with stridor, and hypotension. Allergic effects occur in 5% to 10% of persons receiving penicillin compounds; therefore close monitoring during the first and subsequent doses of penicillin is essential.

Drug Interactions

The broad-spectrum penicillins, amoxicillin and ampicillin, may decrease the effectiveness of oral contraceptives. Potassium supplements can increase serum potassium levels when taken with potassium penicillin G or V. When penicillin is mixed with an aminoglycoside in IV solution, the actions of both drugs are inactivated.

CLINICAL JUDGMENT [NURSING PROCESS]
Antibacterials: Penicillins

Concept: Infection
- A condition in which microorganisms enter the body and release toxins

Recognize Cues [Assessment]
- Assess for allergy to penicillin or cephalosporins. The patient who is hypersensitive to amoxicillin should not take *any* type of penicillin products because severe allergic reaction could occur. A small percentage of patients who are allergic to penicillin could also be allergic to a cephalosporin product.
- Evaluate laboratory results, especially liver enzymes. Report elevated alkaline phosphatase (ALP), alanine aminotransferase (ALT), and aspartate aminotransferase (AST).
- Record urine output. If the amount is inadequate (<30 mL/h or <600 mL/d), the drug or drug dosage may need to be changed.

Analyze Cues and Prioritize Hypothesis [Patient Problems]
- Tissue injury
- Vomiting
- Nausea

Generate Solutions [Planning]
- The patient's white blood cells (WBCs) will be within normal limits.

Take Action [Nursing Interventions]
- Obtain a sample (e.g., swab, blood, sputum) for laboratory culture and antibiotic sensitivity testing (C&S test) to discern the infective organism before antibiotic therapy is started.
- Monitor for signs and symptoms of superinfection, especially in patients taking high doses of an antibiotic for a prolonged time. Signs and symptoms include stomatitis (mouth ulcers), genital discharge (vaginitis), and anal or genital itching.
- ⚡ Examine the patient for allergic reaction to the penicillin product, especially after the first and second doses. This may be a mild reaction, such as a rash, or a severe reaction, such as respiratory distress or anaphylaxis.
- ⚡ Have epinephrine available to counteract a severe allergic reaction.
- Do not mix aminoglycosides with a high-dose or extended-spectrum penicillin G because this combination may inactivate the aminoglycoside.
- Assess the patient for bleeding if high doses of penicillin are being given; a decrease in platelet aggregation (clotting) may result.
- Monitor body temperature and the infected area.
- Dilute antibiotic for IV use in an appropriate amount of solution as indicated in the package insert.

Patient Teaching
General
- Teach patients to always take the *entire* prescribed penicillin product, such as amoxicillin, until the bottle is empty. If only a portion of the penicillin is taken, drug resistance to that antibacterial agent may develop in the future.
- Advise patients allergic to penicillin to wear a medical alert bracelet or necklace and to carry a card that indicates the allergy. Patients should notify their health care providers of any allergy to penicillin when reporting their health history.
- Keep drugs out of reach of small children. Request childproof containers.
- Tell patients to report any side effects or adverse reactions that may occur while taking the drug.
- Encourage patients to increase fluid intake; fluids can aid in regulating body temperature and in excreting the drug.
- Warn patients or the parents of children taking antibiotics that chewable tablets must be chewed or crushed before swallowing.
- Advise female patients of childbearing years to use an additional form of birth control while taking penicillins.

Diet
- Advise patients to take medication with food to avoid gastric irritation.

Evaluate Outcomes [Evaluation]
- Evaluate the effectiveness of antibacterial agents by determining whether the infection has resolved and whether any side effects, including superinfection, have occurred.

TABLE 26.4 Other Beta-Lactam Antibiotics

Generic	Route and Dosage	Uses and Considerations
Aztreonam	Skin infections: A: IV: 1–2 g q8–12 h; *max:* 8 g/d A: IM: 1 g q8–12 h; *max:* 8 g/d	For bacteremia and intraabdominal, skin, respiratory, gynecologic, and urinary tract infections. May cause fever, rash, nasal congestion, cough, wheezing, injection site reaction, abdominal pain, vomiting, neutropenia, elevated hepatic enzymes, eosinophilia, thrombocytosis, CDAD, and superinfection. PB: 56%–65%; $t\frac{1}{2}$: 1.7 h
Ertapenem	Skin infections: A: IM/IV: 1 g/d for 7–14 d; *max:* 1 g/d	For bacteremia, community-acquired pneumonia, and complicated urinary tract, skin, pelvic, and intraabdominal infections. May cause drowsiness, headache, confusion, agitation, injection site reaction, abdominal pain, nausea, vomiting, diarrhea, anemia, infection, CDAD, superinfection, and elevated hepatic enzymes. PB: 95%; $t\frac{1}{2}$: 4 h
Imipenem and cilastatin	UTI: A: IV: 500 mg q6h or 1 g q8h; *max:* 4 g/d	For sepsis, endocarditis, and gynecologic, intraabdominal, respiratory, urinary tract, skin, and bone/joint infections. May cause rash, phlebitis, injection site reaction, nausea, vomiting, diarrhea, urine discoloration, oliguria, anuria, seizures, CDAD, and superinfection. PB: imipenem 20%, cilastatin 40%; $t\frac{1}{2}$: both 1 h
Meropenem	Skin infections: A: IV: 500 mg–1 g q8h for 5–14 d; *max:* 3 g/d	For treating meningitis and intraabdominal and skin infections. May cause headache, rash, injection site reaction, nausea, vomiting, diarrhea, constipation, hyperbilirubinemia, anemia, CDAD, and superinfection. PB: 2%; $t\frac{1}{2}$: 1 h
Meropenem, vaborbactam	A: IV: 2 g meropenem and 2 g vaborbactam q8h for 7–14 d; administer over 3 h; *max:* 6 g meropenem and 6 g vaborbactam/d	For complicated UTIs. May cause headache, fever, phlebitis, injection site reaction, nausea, diarrhea, CDAD, superinfection, hypokalemia, and elevated hepatic enzymes. PB: meropenem 2%, vaborbactam 33%; $t\frac{1}{2}$: meropenem 1.22 h, vaborbactam 1.68 h
Imipenem, cilastatin, relebactam	Intraabdominal infections: A: IV: 500 mg imipenem, 500 mg cilastatin, 250 mg rebebactam q6h for 4–14 d; *max:* 2 g imipenem, 2 g cilastatin, 1 g relebactam/d	For UTIs, nosocomial pneumonia, and complicated intraabdominal infections. May cause headache, fever, erythema, rash, phlebitis, injection site reaction, nausea, vomiting, diarrhea, constipation, anemia, elevated hepatic enzymes, hypokalemia, hyponatremia, thrombocytopenia, and hypertension. PB: imipenem 20%, cilastatin 40%, relebactam 22%; $t\frac{1}{2}$: imipenem 1 h, cilastatin 1 h, relebactam 1.2 h
Sulbactam, durlobactam	A: IV: Sulbactam 1 g & durlobactam 1 g over 3 h q6h for 7–14 d; *max:* 4 g sulbactam & 4 g durlobactam/d	For nosocomial pneumonia. May cause dysrhythmias, anaphylaxis, hypokalemia, anemia, thrombocytopenia, elevated hepatic enzymes, constipation, diarrhea, CDAD, pseudomembranous colitis, superinfection, and renal failure. PB: Sulbactam 38%, durlobactam 10%; $t\frac{1}{2}$: Sulbactam 0.99–3.31 h, durlobactam 1.75–3.29 h

A, Adult; *CDAD*, *Clostridium difficile*–associated diarrhea; *d*, day; *h*, hour; *IM*, intramuscular; *IV*, intravenous; *max*, maximum; *PB*, protein binding; *q*, every; *t½*, half-life; *UTI*, urinary tract infection.

Other Beta-Lactam Antibacterials

Like penicillins, these beta-lactam antibacterials preferentially bind to specific penicillin-binding proteins located inside the bacterial cell wall and are bactericidal. This group includes aztrenam, imipenem/cilastatin, meropenem, ertapenem, meropenem/vaborbactam, imipenem/cilastin/relebactam, and sulbactam/durlobactam. Aztreonam's effectiveness is limited to aerobic gram-positive infections. Imipenem/cilastatin and meropenem are effective against a broader spectrum of activity than many other beta-lactam antibacterials. These three antibacterials are less nephrotoxic than many other antibacterials. Table 26.4 describes these other beta-lactam antibacterials and their dosages, uses, and considerations.

Side Effects and Adverse Reactions

Side effects and adverse reactions to aztrenam, imipenem/cilastatin, and meropenem include headache, nausea, vomiting, diarrhea, anemia, eosinophilia, and neutropenia. Rash may also occur. Severe adverse reactions include anaphylaxis, angioedema, seizures, and *Clostridium difficile*–associated diarrhea.

CEPHALOSPORINS

In 1948 a fungus called *Emericellopsis minimum* (*Cephalosporium acremonium*) was discovered in seawater at a sewer outlet off the coast of Sardinia. This fungus was found to be active against gram-positive and gram-negative bacteria and resistant to beta-lactamase, an enzyme that acts against the beta-lactam structure of penicillin. In the early 1960s cephalosporins were used with clinical effectiveness. For cephalosporins to be effective against numerous organisms, their molecules were chemically altered, and semisynthetic cephalosporins were produced. Like penicillin, the cephalosporins have a beta-lactam structure and act by inhibiting the bacterial enzyme necessary for cell wall synthesis. Cephalosporins are bactericidal as lysis to the cell occurs, and the bacterial cell dies.

First-, Second-, Third-, Fourth-, and Fifth-Generation Cephalosporins

Cephalosporins are a major antibiotic group used in hospitals and in health care offices. These drugs are bactericidal with actions similar to those of penicillin. For antibacterial activity, the beta-lactam ring of cephalosporins is necessary.

Five groups of cephalosporins have been developed, identified as *generations*. Each generation is effective against a broader spectrum of bacteria, an increased resistance to destruction by beta-lactamases, and an increased ability to reach cerebrospinal fluid (Table 26.5).

Not all cephalosporins are affected by the beta-lactamases. First-generation cephalosporins are effective against most gram-positive bacteria and are destroyed by beta-lactamases, but not all

TABLE 26.5 Activity of the Five Generations of Cephalosporins

Generation	Activity
First	Effective mostly against gram-positive bacteria (streptococci and most staphylococci) and some gram-negative bacteria (*Escherichia coli* and species of *Klebsiella, Proteus, Salmonella,* and *Shigella*)
Second	Same effectiveness as first generation but with a broader spectrum against other gram-negative bacteria such as *Haemophilus influenzae, Neisseria gonorrhoeae* and *N. meningitidis, Enterobacter* species, and several anaerobic organisms
Third	Same effectiveness as first and second generations and also effective against gram-negative bacteria (*Pseudomonas aeruginosa* and *Serratia* and *Acinetobacter* species) but with increased resistance to destruction by beta-lactamases
Fourth	Similar to third-generation drugs and highly resistant to most beta-lactamase bacteria with broad-spectrum antibacterial activity and good penetration to cerebrospinal fluid; effective against *E. coli; P. aeruginosa; Klebsiella, Proteus,* and *Streptococcus* species; and certain staphylococci
Fifth	Similar characteristics of third and fourth generations, also broad spectrum, and the only cephalosporins effective against methicillin-resistant *Staphylococcus aureus* (MRSA)

PROTOTYPE DRUG CHART

Ceftriaxone

Drug Class	Dosage
Ceftriaxone: Third-generation cephalosporin	Bacteremia and sepsis: A: IV: 1–2 g q12–24 h; *max:* 4 g/d

Contraindications	Drug-Lab-Food Interactions
Cephalosporin hypersensitivity, jaundice, premature neonates *Caution:* Penicillin hypersensitivity, calcium IV coadministration, vitamin K deficiency, malnutrition, hepatic/renal dysfunction, diarrhea, CDAD, pseudomembranous colitis, pregnancy, breast-feeding	Drug: Increased nephrotoxicity with loop diuretics; increased bleeding with anticoagulants; decreased effect of oral contraceptives Lab: May increase AST, ALT, ALP, LDH, PT, and INR

Pharmacokinetics	Pharmacodynamics
Absorption: IM, IV Distribution: PB: 85%–95% Metabolism: $t\frac{1}{2}$: 6–9 h Excretion: In urine	IM: Onset, duration: UK Peak: 1.5–4 h IV: Onset: Immediate; duration: UK Peak: 30 min

Therapeutic Effects/Uses

For treating otitis media, bacteremia, sepsis, surgical infection prophylaxis, and skin, respiratory, and urinary tract infections.
Ceftriaxone is effective against *Klebsiella, Haemophilus, Clostridium, Citrobacter, Bacteroides, Acinetobacter, Neisseria, Proteus, Salmonella, Serratia, Shigella, Staphylococcus, Streptococcus,* and *Escherichia coli.*
Mechanism of Action: Inhibits bacterial cell wall synthesis causing cell lysis; bactericidal effect

Side Effects	Adverse Reactions
Dizziness, drowsiness, headache, confusion, chills, fever, flushing, diaphoresis, rash, pruritus, epistaxis, stomatitis, glossitis, dysgeusia, dyspepsia, abdominal cramps, nausea, vomiting, diarrhea, flatulence, edema, phlebitis, injection site reaction, vaginitis, azotemia, candidiasis, elevated hepatic enzymes	Superinfection, bleeding, palpitations, cholelithiasis, nephrolithiasis, jaundice, hyperbilirubinemia, anemia, hematuria, hypoprothrombinemia, pancreatitis, biliary obstruction, coagulopathy *Life threatening:* Seizures, anaphylaxis, angioedema, bronchospasm, agranulocytosis, aplastic anemia, hemolytic anemia, leukopenia, thrombocytopenia, neutropenia, eosinophilia, renal failure, CDAD, Stevens-Johnson syndrome, thrombocytosis

A, Adult; *ALP,* alkaline phosphatase; *ALT,* alanine aminotransferase; *AST,* aspartate aminotransferase; *CDAD, Clostridium difficile*–associated diarrhea; *d,* day; *h,* hour; *IM,* intramuscular; *INR,* international normalized ratio; *IV,* intravenous; *LDH,* lactic dehydrogenase; *max,* maximum; *min,* minute; *PB,* protein binding; *PT,* prothrombin time; *q,* every; *t½,* half-life; *UK,* unknown.

second-generation cephalosporins are affected by beta-lactamases. Second-generation cephalosporins are effective against gram-positive and some gram-negative bacteria. Third-generation cephalosporins are resistant to beta-lactamases. They have broad-spectrum antibacterial activity and are effective against *P. aeruginosa*. The fourth-generation cephalosporin, cefepime, has broad-spectrum activity, is highly resistant to beta-lactamases, and has good penetration to cerebrospinal fluid. The fifth-generation cephalosporins are broad-spectrum drugs effective against MRSA.

Approximately 10% of persons allergic to penicillin are also allergic to cephalosporins because both groups of antibacterials have similar molecular structures. If a patient is allergic to penicillin and taking a cephalosporin, the nurse should watch for a possible allergic reaction to the cephalosporin, although the likelihood of a reaction is small.

TABLE 26.6 Antibacterials: Cephalosporins

Generic	Route and Dosage	Uses and Considerations
First Generation		
Cefadroxil	UTI: A: PO: 1–2 g/d in 1–2 divided doses; *max:* 2 g/d	For treating pharyngitis, tonsillitis, and urinary tract and skin infections. May cause rash, pruritus, nausea, vomiting, diarrhea, angioedema, elevated hepatic enzymes, CDAD, and superinfection. PB: UK; t½: 1–2 h
Cefazolin sodium	Respiratory infection: A: IV/IM: 250–500 q8h	For endocarditis, bacteremia, mastitis, prostatitis, epididymitis, and skin, bone/joint, biliary, respiratory, and urinary tract infections. May cause headache, rash, pruritus, hives, injection site reaction, anorexia, nausea, vomiting, diarrhea, CDAD, superinfection, candidiasis, elevated hepatic enzymes, eosinophilia, and thrombocytopenia. PB: 80%; t½: 2 h
Cephalexin	URI: A: PO: 250 mg q6h or 500 mg q12h for 7–14 d; *max:* 4 g/d	For treating mastitis, otitis media and skin, bone/joint, respiratory, and genitourinary infections. May cause headache, rash, hives, nausea, vomiting, diarrhea, elevated hepatic enzymes, eosinophilia, thrombocytopenia, CDAD, and superinfection. PB: 10%–15%; t½: 1 h
Second Generation		
Cefaclor	Lower respiratory infection: Immediate release: A: PO: 250–500 mg q8h; *max:* 1.5 g/d Extended release: A: PO: 500 mg q12h for 5–7 d; *max:* 1 g/d	For pharyngitis, tonsillitis, otitis media, and skin, respiratory, and urinary tract infections. May cause headache, cough, pharyngitis, rhinitis, rash, pruritus, nausea, abdominal pain, diarrhea, CDAD, pseudomembranous colitis, candidiasis, vaginitis, eosinophilia, elevated hepatic enzymes, and superinfection. PB: 25%; t½: 1 h
Cefotetan	UTI: A: IM/IV: 500 mg q12h or 1–2 g q24h; *max:* 6 g/d IV, 4 g/d IM	For intraabdominal, respiratory, urinary tract, skin, and bone/joint infections. May cause rash, pruritus, phlebitis, nausea, diarrhea, CDAD, elevated hepatic enzymes, eosinophilia, and superinfection. PB: 78%–91%; t½: 3–4.6 h
Cefoxitin sodium	Intraabdominal infection: A: IV: 1–2 g q6h for 3–7 d; *max:* 12 g/d	For bacteremia, intraabdominal, gynecologic, skin, respiratory, bone/joint, and urinary tract infections. May cause rash, pruritus, hives, diarrhea, CDAD, thrombocytopenia, elevated hepatic enzymes, and superinfection. PB: 73%; t½: 40–60 min
Cefprozil	Skin infection: A: PO: 250–500 mg q12h for 10 d or 500 mg/d for 10 d; *max:* 1 g/d	For treating sinusitis, tonsillitis, pharyngitis, otitis media, and respiratory and skin infections. May cause rash, pruritus, nausea, diarrhea, CDAD, elevated hepatic enzymes, vaginitis, eosinophilia, and superinfection. PB: 36%; t½: 1.3 h
Cefuroxime	Chronic bronchitis: A: PO: 250–500 mg q12h for 5–7 d; *max:* 1 g/d	For meningitis, otitis media, gonorrhea, bacteremia, pharyngitis, tonsillitis, sinusitis, and skin, respiratory, urinary tract, and bone/joint infections. May cause dermatitis, rash, phlebitis, nausea, vomiting, diarrhea, CDAD, vaginitis, elevated hepatic enzymes, anemia, eosinophilia, and superinfection. PB: 50%; t½: 1–2 h
Third Generation		
Cefdinir	Skin infection: A: PO: 300 mg q12h for 10 d; *max:* 600 mg/d	For treating otitis media, acute sinusitis, tonsillitis, and respiratory, and skin infections. May cause headache, rash, nausea, diarrhea, CDAD, elevated hepatic enzymes, proteinuria, candidiasis, and superinfection. PB: 60%–70%; t½: 1.7 h
Cefixime	Bronchitis: A: PO: 400 mg/d in divided doses q12–24h for at least 5–7 d; *max:* 400 mg/d	For treating otitis media, tonsillitis, gonorrhea, pharyngitis, bronchitis, and UTIs. May cause dizziness, headache, rash, dyspepsia, abdominal pain, nausea, vomiting, flatulence, diarrhea, CDAD, and superinfection. PB: 65%–70%; t½: 3–4 h
Cefotaxime	Skin infection: A: IV/IM: 1 g q8–12h; *max:* 12 g/d	For treating bacteremia, sepsis, meningitis, and gynecologic, skin, bone/joint, intraabdominal, respiratory, and urinary tract infections. May cause rash, pruritus, fever, injection site reaction, nausea, vomiting, diarrhea, CDAD, colitis, eosinophilia, and superinfection. PB: 13%–38%; t½: 1–1.5 h
Cefpodoxime	Community-acquired pneumonia: A: PO: 200 mg q12h for at least 5 d; *max:* 800 mg/d	For treating otitis media, tonsillitis, sinusitis, gonorrhea, pharyngitis, and skin, community-acquired pneumonia, and urinary tract infections. May cause headache, abdominal pain, nausea, vomiting, diarrhea, pseudomembranous colitis, CDAD, and superinfection. Food enhances drug absorption. PB: 22%–33%; t½: 3 h
Ceftazidime	Sepsis: A: IV: 2 g q8h; *max:* 6 g/d	For treating bacteremia, sepsis, meningitis, gynecologic, intraabdominal, skin, respiratory, bone/joint, and urinary tract infections. May cause dizziness, headache, fever, paresthesias, rash pruritis, phlebitis, injection site reaction, abdominal pain, nausea, vomiting, diarrhea, CDAD, eosinophilia, thrombocytosis, and superinfection. PB: 10%; t½: 1.4–2 h
Ceftriaxone	See Prototype Drug Chart: Ceftriaxone	
Ceftazidime and avibactam	UTI: A: IV: 2 g ceftazidime/0.5 g avibactam over 2 h q8h for 3–7 d; *max:* 6 g ceftazidime/1.5 g avibactam/d	For treating intraabdominal, respiratory, and urinary tract infections. May cause dizziness, headache, pruritus, nausea, vomiting, diarrhea, constipation, CDAD, and superinfection. PB: 5%–8% avibactam, 10% ceftazidime; t½: 2 h avibactam, 1.5–2 h ceftazidime
Fourth Generation		
Cefepime	Pneumonia: A: IV: 1–2 g q8–12h for 10 d; *max:* 6 g/d	For treating febrile neutropenia, bacteremia, and respiratory, intraabdominal, and urinary tract infections. May cause headache, injection site reaction, rash, nausea, vomiting, diarrhea, CDAD, hypoprothrombinemia, eosinophilia, hypophosphatemia, elevated hepatic enzymes, and superinfection. PB: 20%; t½: 2 h

TABLE 26.6 Antibacterials: Cephalosporins—cont'd

Generic	Route and Dosage	Uses and Considerations
Fifth Generation		
Ceftaroline fosamil	Skin infections: A: IV: 600 mg q12h for 5–14 d; *max:* 1200 mg/d	For treating skin and respiratory infections. May cause headache, fever, rash, pruritus, nausea, vomiting, diarrhea, CDAD, elevated hepatic enzymes, and superinfection. PB: 20%; t½: 1.6 h
Ceftolozane and tazobactam	Intraabdominal infection: A: IV: 1 g ceftolozane/0.5 g tazobactam q8h for 4–14 d; *max:* 6 g ceftolozane, 3 g tazobactam/d	For treating intraabdominal, respiratory, and urinary tract infections. May cause headache, fever, phlebitis, abdominal pain, nausea, vomiting, diarrhea, CDAD, elevated hepatic enzymes, neutropenia, thrombocytosis, anemia, and renal failure. PB: ceftolozane 16%–21%, tazobactam 30%; t½: ceftolozane 3–4 h, tazobactam 2–3 h
Ceftobiprole	Skin infection: A: IV: 667 mg q8h for 5–14 d	For treating pneumonia, bacteremia, skin, and MRSA. May cause headache, anemia, hypokalemia, hypertension, nausea, vomiting, diarrhea, rash, insomnia, and elevated hepatic enzymes. PB: 16%; t½: 3.3 h

A, adult; *CDAD*, Clostridium difficile–associated diarrhea; *d*, day; *h*, hour; *IM*, intramuscularly; *IV*, intravenously; *max*, maximum; *min*, minutes; *MRSA*, methicillin-resistant *Staphylococcus aureus*; *PB*, protein binding; *PID*, pelvic inflammatory disease; *PO*, by mouth; *q*, every; *t½*, half-life; *UK*, unknown; *URI*, upper respiratory infection; *UTI*, urinary tract infection.

CLINICAL JUDGMENT [NURSING PROCESS]
Antibacterials: Cephalosporins

Concept: Infection
- A condition in which microorganisms enter the body and release toxins

Recognize Cues [Assessment]
- Assess for allergy to cephalosporins or penicillins. If a patient is allergic to one type or class of cephalosporin, that patient should not receive any other type of cephalosporin or penicillin.
- Record vital signs and urine output. Report abnormal findings, which may include elevated temperature or decreased urine output.
- Evaluate laboratory results, especially those that indicate renal and liver function (blood urea nitrogen [BUN], serum creatinine, aspartate aminotransferase [AST], alanine aminotransferase [ALT], alkaline phosphatase [ALP], and bilirubin). Use these laboratory results for baseline values, and report any abnormal findings.

Analyze Cues and Prioritize Hypothesis [Patient Problems]
- Tissue injury
- Vomiting
- Nausea

Generate Solutions [Planning]
- The patient's white blood cells (WBCs) will be within normal limits.

Take Action [Nursing Interventions]
- Culture the infected area before cephalosporin therapy is started. The organism causing the infection can be determined by culture, and the antibiotics the organism is sensitive to are determined by sensitivity. If antibiotic therapy is started before culture result is reported, the antibiotic may need to be changed after culture and sensitivity (C&S) test results are received.

Patient Teaching
General
- Keep drugs out of reach of children. Request childproof containers.
- Tell patients to report signs of superinfection, such as mouth ulcers or discharge from the anal or genital area.
- Advise patients to ingest buttermilk, yogurt, or an acidophilus supplement to prevent superinfection of the intestinal flora.
- Instruct patients to take the complete course of medication, even when symptoms of infection have ceased.
- Infuse all IV cephalosporins over 30 minutes or as ordered to prevent pain and irritation.
- Observe for hypersensitivity reactions.

Side Effects
- Warn patients to report any side effects from use of oral cephalosporin drugs; these may include anorexia, nausea, vomiting, headache, dizziness, itching, and rash.

Diet
- Advise patients to take medication with food if gastric irritation occurs.
- Encourage patients to take an adequate amount of fluids to avoid dehydration from diarrhea.

Evaluate Outcomes [Evaluation]
- Evaluate the effectiveness of the cephalosporin by determining whether the infection has ceased and that no side effects, including superinfection, have occurred.

Only a few cephalosporins are administered orally. These include cephalexin, cefadroxil, cefaclor, cefuroxime, cefdinir, cefprozil, cefixime, cefpodoxime, cefditoren, and ceftibuten. The rest of the cephalosporins are administered IM and IV. Prototype Drug Chart: Ceftriaxone describes the drug data related to ceftriaxone.

Pharmacokinetics
Cefazolin is administered IM and IV, and cefaclor is given orally. The protein-binding power of cefazolin is greater than that of cefaclor. The half-life of each drug is short, and the drugs are excreted 60% to 80% unchanged in the urine.

Pharmacodynamics
Cefazolin and cefaclor inhibit bacterial cell wall synthesis and produce a bactericidal action. For IM and IV use of cefazolin, the onset of action is almost immediate, and peak concentration time is 5 to 15 minutes with IV use. The peak concentration time for an oral dose of cefaclor is 30 to 60 minutes.

When probenecid is administered with either of these drugs, urine excretion of cefazolin and cefaclor is decreased, which increases the action of the drug. The effects of cefazolin and cefaclor can be decreased if the drug is given with tetracyclines or erythromycin. These drugs can cause false-positive laboratory results for proteinuria and glucosuria, especially when they are taken in large doses.

Table 26.6 lists the cephalosporins by their designated generation and also gives dosages, uses, and considerations.

Side Effects and Adverse Reactions

The side effects and adverse reactions to cephalosporins include GI disturbances (nausea, vomiting, diarrhea), alteration in blood clotting time (increased bleeding) with administration of large doses, and nephrotoxicity (toxicity to the kidney) in individuals with a preexisting renal disorder.

Drug Interactions

Drug interactions can occur with certain cephalosporins and alcohol. For example, alcohol consumption may cause a disulfiram-like reaction (flushing, dizziness, headache, nausea, vomiting, and muscular cramps) while taking cefotetan. Alcohol should be avoided while taking cefotetan and for 2 to 3 days after discontinuation. Cefotetan may increase the effects of warfarin, salicylates, and aminoglycosides.

CLINICAL JUDGMENT CASE STUDY

A child 6 years of age has otitis media. The health care provider ordered amoxicillin 250 mg every 8 hours. The nurse asks the child's parent if he is allergic to any drugs, and the parent says that he is allergic to penicillin.

1. What are the similarities and differences in penicillin and amoxicillin? Explain your answer.
2. What nursing action should the nurse take? Why? The health care provider changed the amoxicillin order to cefaclor 250 mg every 8 hours. The therapeutic dosage for children is 20–40 mg/kg/d in three divided doses. The child weighs 40 pounds.
3. What are the similarities and differences in amoxicillin and cefaclor? Explain your answer.
4. Is the prescribed cefaclor dosage for the child within safe parameters? Explain your answer.
5. What should the nurse include in patient teaching for the child and his parent?

REVIEW QUESTIONS

1. Amoxicillin is prescribed for a patient who has a respiratory infection. The nurse is teaching the patient about this medication and realizes that more teaching is needed when the patient makes which statement?
    a. This medication should not be taken with food.
    b. I will take my entire prescription of medication.
    c. I should report to the physician any genital itching.
    d. If I experience any excess bleeding, I will contact the health care provider.
2. A patient is taking a cephalosporin. The nurse anticipates which appropriate nursing intervention(s) for this medication? **Select all that apply.**
    a. Monitoring renal function studies
    b. Monitoring liver function studies
    c. Infusing intravenous medication over 30 minutes
    d. Monitoring the patient for mouth ulcers
    e. Advising the patient to stop the medication when they feel better
3. Penicillin G has been prescribed for a patient. Which nursing intervention(s) should the nurse perform for this patient? **Select all that apply.**
    a. Collect culture and sensitivity before the first dose.
    b. Monitor the patient for mouth ulcers.
    c. Instruct the patient to limit fluid intake to 1000 mL/day.
    d. Have epinephrine on hand for a potential severe allergic reaction.
    e. No particular interventions are required for this patient.
4. A patient is receiving amoxicillin. The nurse understands that the action of this drug is by which process?
    a. Inhibition of protein synthesis
    b. Alteration of membrane permeability
    c. Inhibition of bacterial cell wall synthesis
    d. Alteration of bacterial ribonucleic acid synthesis
5. A patient is prescribed dicloxacillin. For which adverse effect should the nurse monitor the patient?
    a. Constipation
    b. Tongue discoloration
    c. Hypertension
    d. Hemolytic anemia
6. A patient has been prescribed amoxicillin. What does the nurse know is true about this medication?
    a. It has a normal adult dose of 2 g q6h.
    b. It has a common side effect of hypotension.
    c. It has an intramuscular administration route.
    d. It is used to treat respiratory infections.

27

Macrolides, Oxazolidinones, Lincosamides, Glycopeptides, and Lipopeptides

http://evolve.elsevier.com/McCuistion/pharmacology

OBJECTIVES

- Explain the use and administration route of macrolides.
- Describe the mechanism of action and uses of oxazolidinones.
- Differentiate between the use of clindamycin and lincomycin.
- Contrast the use of vancomycin and telavancin.
- Discuss the mechanism of action and use of daptomycin.

OUTLINE

Macrolides, 333
    Pharmacology, 335
    Side Effects and Adverse Reactions, 335
    Drug Interactions, 335
    Extended Macrolide Group, 335
Oxazolidinones, 336
    Side Effects and Adverse Reactions, 336
    Drug Interactions, 336
Lincosamides, 336
    Side Effects and Adverse Reactions, 336
    Drug Interactions, 337

Glycopeptides, 337
    Pharmacology, 337
    Side Effects and Adverse Reactions, 337
    Drug Interactions, 337
Lipopeptides, 337
    Pharmacology, 337
    Side Effects and Adverse Reactions, 337
    Drug Interactions, 337
Clinical Judgment Case Study, 338
Review Questions, 338

Disease-producing microorganisms may be gram-positive or gram-negative bacteria, viruses, protozoans, or fungi. The degree to which they are pathogenic depends on the microorganism and its virulence. This chapter discusses drugs prescribed to combat disease-producing microorganisms.

The groups of antibacterials discussed in this chapter include macrolides (erythromycin, clarithromycin, and azithromycin), lincosamides, glycopeptides, lipopeptides, and oxazolidinones.

The macrolides, oxazolidinones, and lincosamides, are primarily **bacteriostatic** drugs, those that inhibit bacterial growth, but they may also be bactericidal (bacteria killing), depending on the drug dose, serum level, and **pathogen** (the disease-producing microorganism). Glycopeptides and lipopeptides are bactericidal drugs.

Macrolides, oxazolidinones, lincosamides, and glycopeptides are discussed together because they have spectrums of antibiotic effectiveness similar to that of penicillin, although they differ in structure. Drugs from these groups are used as penicillin substitutes, especially in individuals who are allergic to penicillin. Erythromycin is the drug frequently prescribed if the patient has a hypersensitivity to penicillin.

MACROLIDES

Macrolide antibiotics—which include azithromycin, clarithromycin, and erythromycin—are called *broad-spectrum antibiotics*. Erythromycin, the first macrolide, was derived from the fungus-like bacteria *Streptomyces erythreus* and was first introduced in the early 1950s. Macrolides bind to the 50 S ribosomal subunits and inhibit protein synthesis. At low to moderate drug doses, macrolides have a bacteriostatic effect, and with high drug doses, their effect is bactericidal. Macrolides can be administered orally or by IV but not intramuscularly because it is too painful. IV macrolides should be infused slowly to avoid unnecessary pain (phlebitis).

Gastric acid destroys erythromycin in the stomach; therefore acid-resistant salts are added (e.g., ethylsuccinate, stearate, estolate) to decrease breakdown into small particles (dissolution) in the stomach. This allows the drug to be absorbed in the intestine. Normally, food does not hamper the absorption of acid-resistant macrolides. Table 27.1 lists the dosages, uses, and considerations of macrolides.

Macrolides are active against most gram-positive bacteria and are moderately active against some gram-negative bacteria, although resistant organisms may emerge during treatment. Macrolides are used to treat mild to moderate infections of the respiratory tract, sinuses, GI tract, and skin and soft tissue in addition to treating diphtheria, impetigo contagiosa, and sexually transmitted infections (STIs).

Erythromycin is the drug of choice for the treatment of mycoplasmal pneumonia and Legionnaires disease. Clarithromycin is also available in a once-a-day extended-release tablet to be taken for 7 days. Azithromycin is frequently prescribed for upper and lower respiratory infections, STIs, and uncomplicated skin infections. Table 27.1 lists the drugs developed from the derivatives of erythromycin, and Prototype Drug Chart: Azithromycin details the pharmacologic behavior of azithromycin.

TABLE 27.1 Antibacterials: Macrolides, Oxazolidinones, Lincosamides, Glycopeptides, and Lipopeptides

Generic	Route and Dosage	Uses and Considerations
Macrolides		
Azithromycin	See Prototype Drug Chart: Azithromycin	
Clarithromycin	Skin infections: Immediate release: A: PO: 250 mg q12h for 7–14 d; *max:* 1.5 g/d	For treating otitis media, tonsillitis, sinusitis, pharyngitis, and *Helicobacter pylori*, skin, and respiratory infections. May cause headache, rash, dysgeusia, dyspepsia, nausea, vomiting, diarrhea, flatulence, CDAD, abdominal pain, elevated hepatic enzymes, and superinfection. PB: 42%–70%; t½: 3–7 h
Erythromycin base	Respiratory infections: A: PO: 250 mg q6h or 500 mg q12h; *max:* 4 g/d A: IV: 15–20 mg/kg/d in divided doses q6h; *max:* 4 g/d	For treating acne, impetigo, tonsillitis, urethritis, STIs, Legionnaires disease, PID, diphtheria, listeriosis, pertussis, and respiratory, GI, and skin infections. May cause dry, irritated skin; superinfection; CDAD; anorexia; pruritus; erythema; phlebitis; jaundice; elevated hepatic enzymes; nausea; vomiting; diarrhea; and abdominal pain. PB: 75%–90%; t½: 1.5 h
Fidaxomicin	A: PO: 200 mg bid for 10 d; *max:* 400 mg/d	For treating CDAD. May cause nausea, vomiting, diarrhea, abdominal pain, GI bleeding, constipation, fever, rash, pruritus, and elevated hepatic enzymes. PB: UK; t½: 6.9–16.5 h
Oxazolidinones		
Linezolid	Nosocomial pneumonia: A: PO/IV: 600 mg q12h for at least 7 d; *max:* 1200 mg/d	For treating bacteremia, sepsis, MRSA, VREF, tuberculosis, respiratory and skin infections. May cause headache, pruritus, tongue/tooth discoloration, nausea, vomiting, diarrhea, abdominal pain, dizziness, anemia, thrombocytopenia, serotonin syndrome, CDAD, and superinfection. PB: 31%; t½: 4.26–5.4 h
Tedizolid	A: PO/IV: 200 mg/d for 6 d; *max:* 200 mg/d	For treating skin infections. May cause headache, nausea, vomiting, diarrhea, infusion-related/injection site reactions, phlebitis, erythema, serotonin syndrome, CDAD, and superinfection. PB: 70%–90%; t½: 12 h
Lincosamides		
Clindamycin	Lower respiratory infection: A: PO: Initially 150–450 mg q6h; *max:* 1800 mg/d A: IM/IV: 300–600 mg q6–12 h; *max:* 2700 mg/d IV, 2400 mg/d IM	For treating PID, acne, bacteremia, sepsis, mastitis, MRSA, and respiratory, intraabdominal, skin, gynecologic, and bone/joint infections. May cause dry skin, nausea, vomiting, diarrhea, CDAD, erythema, pruritus, superinfection, headache, candidiasis, vaginitis, and back pain. Should be taken with full glass of water. PB: 80%–95%; t½: 2–3 h
Lincomycin	A: IM: 600 mg q12–24h; *max:* 1.2 g/d A: IV: 600 mg–1 g q8–12h; *max:* 8 g/d	For treating severe infections. May cause glossitis, stomatitis, headache, candidiasis, dizziness, nausea, vomiting, diarrhea, CDAD, superinfection, injection site reaction, and rash. PB: 77%–82%; t½: 4.4–6.4 h
Glycopeptides		
Vancomycin hydrochloride	Clostridium difficile infection: A: PO: 125 mg qid for 10 d, *max:* 2 g/d	For treating bacteremia, mastitis, endocarditis, enterocolitis, *Staphylococcus aureus*, MRSA, CDAD, and respiratory, skin, and bone/joint infections. May cause fever, headache, fatigue, back pain, peripheral edema, nausea, vomiting, flatulence, diarrhea, abdominal pain, hypokalemia, tinnitus, CDAD, vancomycin flushing syndrome (red man syndrome), infection, neutropenia, ototoxicity, nephrotoxicity, and superinfection. PB: 55%; t½: 4–6 h
Oritavancin	Skin infection: A: IV: 1200 mg as a single dose over 3 h; *max:* 1200 mg	For treating skin infections. May cause erythema, nausea, vomiting, diarrhea, dizziness, headache, peripheral edema, infusion-related reaction, elevated hepatic enzymes, phlebitis, tachycardia, infection, vancomycin infusion reaction (red man syndrome), superinfection, and CDAD. PB: 85%; t½: 245 h
Telavancin	Respiratory infections: A: IV: 10 mg/kg/dose over 60 min q24h for 7–21 d; *max:* 10 mg/kg/dose	For treating MRSA and respiratory and skin infections. May cause erythema, chills, dizziness, pruritus, rash, renal failure, metallic taste, nausea, vomiting, diarrhea, infusion site reaction, CDAD, and superinfection. PB: 93%; t½: 8–9 h
Lipopeptides		
Daptomycin	Skin infection: A: IV: 4 mg/kg/dose for 7–14 d; *max:* 6 mg/kg/dose	For treating endocarditis, bacteremia, and skin infections. May cause rash, pruritus, insomnia, edema, dizziness, hypo/hypertension, chest pain, headache, hyperhidrosis, nausea, vomiting, diarrhea, abdominal pain, CDAD, and superinfection. PB: 90%–93%; t½: 8–9 h

A, Adult; *bid*, twice daily; *CDAD*, *Clostridium difficile*–associated diarrhea; *d*, day; *GI*, gastrointestinal; *h*, hour; *IM*, intramuscular; *IV*, intravenous; *max*, maximum; *MRSA*, methicillin-resistant *Staphylococcus aureus*; *PB*, protein binding; *PID*, pelvic inflammatory disease; *PO*, by mouth; *q*, every; *qid*, 4 times a day; *STI*, sexually transmitted infection; *t½*, half-life; *UK*, unknown; *VREF*, vancomycin-resistant *Enterococcus faecium*.

Pharmacology

Pharmacokinetics
Clarithromycin and erythromycin are readily absorbed from the GI tract, mainly by the duodenum. Azithromycin is incompletely absorbed from the GI tract, and only 37% reaches systemic circulation. Azithromycin and erythromycin can be administered intravenously, but intermittent infusions should be diluted in normal saline (NS) or in 5% dextrose in water (D_5W) to prevent phlebitis or burning sensations at the injection site. Azithromycin 500 mg should be diluted in 250 to 500 mL of fluid, and erythromycin lactobionate 1 g should be diluted in 200 to 1000 mL. Macrolides are excreted in bile, feces, and urine. Because only a small amount is excreted in urine, renal insufficiency is not a contraindication for macrolide use.

Pharmacodynamics
Macrolides suppress bacterial protein synthesis. The onset of action of oral preparations of erythromycin is 1 hour, peak concentration time is 4 hours, and duration of action is 6 hours. Newer macrolides have a longer half-life and are administered less frequently. Clarithromycin is administered twice a day for immediate release, and the extended-release formulation is administered once a day. Azithromycin has a 68-hour half-life.

Side Effects and Adverse Reactions
Side effects and adverse reactions to macrolides include GI disturbances such as nausea, vomiting, diarrhea, and abdominal cramping. Severe diarrhea occurs when antibacterials kill normal flora, allowing an overgrowth of *Clostridium difficile*. This superinfection is called *Clostridium difficile*-associated diarrhea (CDAD), also known as pseudomembranous colitis. A release of bacterial toxins causes injury, inflammation, and bleeding in the colon lining. This condition causes abdominal cramping, 5 to 10 watery diarrheal stools per day, and bloody stools. Frequency of stools may increase to 20 per day in severe cases. Conjunctivitis may develop as a side effect of azithromycin, and the patient should avoid wearing contact lenses if this occurs. Allergic reactions to erythromycin are rare. Hepatotoxicity (liver toxicity) can occur when erythromycin and azithromycin are taken in high doses with other hepatotoxic drugs, such as acetaminophen (high doses), phenothiazines, and sulfonamides. Liver damage is usually reversible when the drug is discontinued. Erythromycin should not be taken with clindamycin or lincomycin because they compete for receptor sites.

Drug Interactions
Macrolides can increase serum levels of theophylline (a bronchodilator), carbamazepine (an anticonvulsant), and warfarin (an anticoagulant). If these drugs are given with macrolides, their drug serum levels should be closely monitored. To avoid severe toxic effects, erythromycin should not be used with other macrolides. Antacids may reduce azithromycin peak levels when taken at the same time.

Extended Macrolide Group
Derivatives of erythromycin have been effective in the treatment of numerous organisms. Like erythromycin, they also inhibit protein synthesis. Many of these macrolides have a longer half-life and are administered once a day. After the introduction of erythromycin, the first extended macrolide drug developed was clarithromycin, which has been effective against many bacterial infections. Clarithromycin is administered twice a day for immediate-release form, and the extended-release formulation is given once a day. Another extended macrolide is azithromycin. This drug has a long half-life of up to 68 hours.

PROTOTYPE DRUG CHART
Azithromycin

Drug Class	Dosage
Antibacterial macrolide	Chronic bronchitis exacerbation: Immediate release: A: PO: 500 mg for 1 d, or 500 mg/d for 3 d, then follow with 250 mg/d for 4 d; *max*: 500 mg/d

Contraindications	Drug-Lab-Food Interactions
Hypersensitivity to macrolides, jaundice *Caution:* Bradycardia, hypokalemia, hypomagnesemia, dysrhythmias, renal dysfunction, diarrhea, CDAD, hypocalcemia, rheumatoid arthritis, cardiac disease, MI, CVA, myasthenia gravis, thyroid disorder, breast-feeding, older adults, contact lens, pregnancy	Drug: Increases effects of digoxin, cyclosporine, and warfarin; increases risk of QT prolongation with alfuzosin and adagrasib; decreases effects of penicillins and clindamycin

Pharmacokinetics	Pharmacodynamics
Absorption: PO: 38% absorbed Distribution: PB: 51% Metabolism: t½: 40–68 h Excretion: In bile, a small amount in urine	PO: Onset, duration: UK Peak: 2–3 h Extended release: Peak: 3–5 h IV: Onset, duration, peak: UK

Therapeutic Effects/Uses
For treating bacterial conjunctivitis, otitis media, tonsillitis, pharyngitis, sinusitis, PID, STIs, and skin and respiratory infections. For patients who are allergic to penicillin. Azithromycin is effective against species of *Clostridium*, *Haemophilus*, *Chlamydia*, *Mycobacterium*, *Neisseria*, *Staphylococcus*, and *Streptococcus*.

Mechanism of Action: Inhibits the steps of protein synthesis; bacteriostatic or bactericidal effect

Side Effects	Adverse Reactions
Blurred vision, ocular irritation/pain, photosensitivity, headache, tinnitus, edema, drowsiness, dizziness, fever, erythema, fatigue, tongue discoloration, dysgeusia, anorexia, nausea, vomiting, diarrhea, flatulence, abdominal cramps, pruritus, rash, injection site reaction, weakness, agitation, vaginitis, constipation	Superinfection, hearing loss, seizures, hyperbilirubinemia, hypotension, azotemia, cholestasis, myasthenia gravis exacerbation, hypo/hyperkalemia, dyspnea, hyponatremia, hypo/hyperglycemia *Life-threatening:* Hepatotoxicity, anemia, eosinophilia, anaphylaxis, bronchospasm, angioedema, CDAD, leukopenia, thrombocytopenia, Stevens-Johnson syndrome, renal failure

A, Adult; *CDAD*, *Clostridium difficile*–associated diarrhea; *CVA*, cerebral vascular accident; *d*, day; *h*, hour; *IV*, intravenous; *max*, maximum; *MI*, myocardial infarction; *PB*, protein binding; *PID*, pelvic inflammatory disease; *PO*, by mouth; *STI*, sexually transmitted infection; *t½*, half-life; *UK*, unknown.

CLINICAL JUDGMENT [NURSING PROCESS]
Antibacterials: Macrolides

Concept: Infection
- A condition in which microorganisms enter the body and release toxins

Recognize Cues [Assessment]
- Assess vital signs and urine output. Report abnormal findings.
- Check laboratory tests (liver enzyme values) to determine liver function. Order liver enzyme tests periodically for patients taking large doses of azithromycin for a continuous period.
- Obtain a history of drugs the patient currently takes. The peak level of azithromycin may be decreased by antacids.

Analyze Cues and Prioritize Hypothesis [Patient Problems]
- Tissue injury
- Nausea
- Vomiting

Generate Solutions [Planning]
- The patient's white blood cells (WBCs) will be within normal limits.

Take Action [Nursing Interventions]
- Obtain a sample from the infected area, and send it to the laboratory for culture and sensitivity (C&S) testing before starting azithromycin therapy. Antibiotic therapy can be initiated after obtaining the culture sample.
- Monitor vital signs, urine output, and laboratory values, especially liver enzymes (alkaline phosphatase [ALP], alanine aminotransferase [ALT], aspartate aminotransferase [AST], and bilirubin).
- Monitor the patient for liver damage resulting from prolonged use and high dosage of macrolides such as azithromycin. Signs of liver dysfunction include elevated liver enzyme levels and jaundice.
- Administer oral azithromycin 1 hour before or 2 hours after meals. Give with a full glass of water, *not* fruit juice. Give the drug with food if gastrointestinal (GI) upset occurs. Chewable tablets should be chewed, *not* swallowed whole.
- Dilute in an appropriate amount of solution as indicated in the drug circular for intravenous (IV) azithromycin.
- Administer antacids either 2 hours before or 2 hours after azithromycin.

Patient Teaching
General
- Instruct patients to take the full course of the antibacterial agent as prescribed. Drug compliance is most important for all antibacterials (antibiotics).

Side Effects
- Encourage patients to report side effects, including adverse reactions (nausea, vomiting, diarrhea, abdominal cramps, itching).
- Teach patients to report any evidence of superinfection, secondary infection resulting from drug therapy; for some patients, stomatitis or vaginitis may occur.
- ⚡ Tell patients to report the onset of loose stools or diarrhea. *Clostridium difficile*-associated diarrhea (CDAD) should be ruled out.

Evaluate Outcomes [Evaluation]
- Evaluate the effectiveness of azithromycin by determining whether the infection has been controlled or has ceased and that no side effects, including superinfection, have occurred.

Elimination of these drugs is via bile and feces. Azithromycin is frequently prescribed for upper and lower respiratory tract infections, STIs, and uncomplicated skin infections.

When erythromycin is given concurrently with verapamil, diltiazem, clarithromycin, fluconazole, ketoconazole, and itraconazole, erythromycin blood concentration and the risk of sudden cardiac death increase. Table 27.1 lists the drugs developed from the derivatives of erythromycin.

Common side effects of clarithromycin are nausea, diarrhea, and abdominal discomfort. With azithromycin, the side effects of nausea, diarrhea, and abdominal pain are common.

OXAZOLIDINONES

Like macrolides, oxazolidinones inhibit protein synthesis on the 50S ribosomal subunit of bacteria. This action prevents the formation of 70S initiation complex, which is necessary for bacterial reproduction. Linezolid and tedizolid are examples of oxazolidinones. Drugs in this antibacterial classification are bacteriostatic or bactericidal and are effective against gram-positive infections. Table 27.1 lists the oxazolidinones.

Side Effects and Adverse Reactions

Side effects and adverse reactions to linezolid and tedizolid include headache, nausea, vomiting, diarrhea, anemia, and thrombocytopenia. Severe adverse reactions include CDAD and serotonin syndrome.

Drug Interactions

Linezolid can cause hypertensive crisis when given with a monoamine oxidase (MAO) inhibitor. When Linezolid is given with a selective serotonin reuptake inhibitor (SSRI), serotonin syndrome may result. The serotonin content of CNS neurons is increased when MAO is inhibited. Deaths have occurred. Tramadol, tricyclic antidepressants, and trazodone may elevate serotonin to dangerous levels.

LINCOSAMIDES

Like erythromycin, lincosamides inhibit bacterial protein synthesis and have both bacteriostatic and bactericidal actions, depending on drug dosage. Clindamycin and lincomycin are examples of lincosamides. Clindamycin is more widely prescribed than lincomycin because it is active against most gram-positive organisms, including *S. aureus* and anaerobic organisms. It is not effective against gram-negative bacteria (e.g., *E. coli* and *Proteus* and *Pseudomonas* species). Clindamycin is absorbed better than lincomycin through the GI tract and maintains a higher serum drug concentration. Clindamycin is considered more effective than lincomycin and has fewer toxic effects. Table 27.1 lists the lincosamides.

Side Effects and Adverse Reactions

Side effects and adverse reactions to clindamycin and lincomycin include GI irritation, which may manifest as nausea, vomiting, and stomatitis. Rash may also occur. Severe adverse reactions include colitis and anaphylactic shock.

Drug Interactions

Clindamycin and lincomycin are incompatible with aminophylline, phenytoin, barbiturates, and ampicillin.

GLYCOPEPTIDES

Vancomycin, a glycopeptide bactericidal antibiotic, was widely used in the 1950s to treat staphylococcal infections. Vancomycin is used against drug-resistant *S. aureus* and in cardiac surgical prophylaxis for individuals with penicillin allergies. Serum vancomycin levels should be monitored.

Vancomycin has become ineffective for treating enterococci. Antibiotic-resistant enterococci can cause staphylococcal endocarditis.

Telavancin, a glycopeptide, treats selected gram-positive bacteria and skin infections. This drug is a semisynthetic derivative of vancomycin with bactericidal action against MRSA. Telavancin has an advantage of once-daily dosing. Oritavancin has the further advantage of being administered in a single dose.

Pharmacology
Pharmacokinetics

Vancomycin is given orally for treatment of staphylococcal enterocolitis and antibiotic-associated pseudomembranous colitis due to *C. difficile*. When vancomycin is given orally, it is not absorbed systemically and is excreted in the feces. Vancomycin is also given intravenously for septicemia; for severe infections due to MRSA; and for bone, skin, and lower respiratory tract infections that do not respond or are resistant to other antibiotics. Intermittent vancomycin doses should be diluted in 100 mL for 500 mg and 200 mL for 1 g of D_5W, NS, or lactated Ringer's (LR), and should be administered over 60 to 90 minutes. Vancomycin is excreted in the urine when given by IV route. It is 55% protein bound, and the half-life is 4 to 6 hours.

Pharmacodynamics

Vancomycin inhibits bacterial cell wall synthesis and is active against several gram-positive microorganisms. The peak action is 30 minutes after the end of the infusion.

Side Effects and Adverse Reactions

Vancomycin may cause nephrotoxicity and ototoxicity. Ototoxicity results in damage to the auditory or vestibular branch of cranial nerve VIII. Such damage can result in permanent hearing loss (auditory branch) or temporary or permanent loss of balance (vestibular branch). Side effects may include headache, dizziness, fatigue, fever, nausea, vomiting, flatulence, abdominal pain, diarrhea, back pain, infusion site reaction, and peripheral edema. Adverse effects include angioedema, eosinophilia, neutropenia, phlebitis, CDAD, hypokalemia, renal failure, ototoxicity, and Stevens-Johnson syndrome.

Too-rapid infusion of IV vancomycin can cause a condition known as vancomycin flushing syndrome, previously known as *red man syndrome* or *red neck syndrome*. Characterized by red flushing of the face, neck, arms, upper body, and back, this is a toxic effect rather than an allergic reaction. Other effects include weakness, hypotension, tachycardia, chest pain, wheezing, dyspnea, muscle spasms of the back, paresthesias, erythema, pruritus, and urticaria, and may lead to cardiac arrest. Slowing (10 mg/min or less) or stopping the infusion rate may reduce the incidence or severity of reaction. Signs and symptoms usually resolve within 20 minutes but may last several hours.

Drug Interactions

Dimenhydrinate can mask ototoxicity when taken with vancomycin. The risk of nephrotoxicity and ototoxicity may be potentiated when vancomycin is taken with furosemide, aminoglycosides, amphotericin B, colistin, cisplatin, and cyclosporine. Vancomycin may inhibit methotrexate excretion and can increase methotrexate toxicity. The absorption of oral vancomycin may be decreased when given with cholestyramine and colestipol.

LIPOPEPTIDES

Daptomycin is a US Food and Drug Administration (FDA)-approved antibiotic in the category of *lipopeptides*. Daptomycin acts by binding to the bacterial membrane and causing rapid depolarization of its membrane potential, inhibiting protein, DNA, and RNA synthesis. This action results in bacterial cell death.

Indications for daptomycin include complicated skin infections due to gram-positive microorganisms, septicemia due to *S. aureus* infection, and infective endocarditis due to MRSA infection.

Pharmacology
Pharmacokinetics

Daptomycin is administered by IV at a dose of 4 mg/kg daily. Each 500-mg vial of the medication is diluted in 10 mL of NS 0.9% and allowed to stand for 10 minutes. After gentle rotation of the vial to ensure dilution, further dilute in 50 to 100 mL of NS and administer over 30 minutes. Drug should *not* be mixed with dextrose-containing diluents. The protein-binding capacity is 90% to 93%, and half-life averages 8 to 9 hours. Daptomycin is primarily excreted by the kidneys.

Pharmacodynamics

Daptomycin binds to the bacterial membrane and causes cell death. An effective trough concentration of 5.9 mcg/mL is usually achieved by the third dose.

Side Effects and Adverse Reactions

Side effects that may occur when taking daptomycin include hypertension, hypotension, dizziness, insomnia, nausea, vomiting, and diarrhea. More serious adverse reactions that have occurred with daptomycin are chest pain, anemia, peripheral neuropathy, anaphylaxis, rhabdomyolysis, angioedema, *Clostridium difficile*-associated diarrhea, Stevens-Johnson syndrome, and renal failure.

Drug Interactions

When daptomycin is given with 3-hydroxy-3-methylglutaryl coenzyme A (HMG-CoA) reductase inhibitors (statins, e.g., simvastatin or atorvastatin), the risk of rhabdomyolysis and elevated levels of creatine phosphokinase (CPK) is increased. Daptomycin toxicity may be increased when given concurrently with tobramycin, and warfarin may lead to increased bleeding when taken with daptomycin.

CLINICAL JUDGMENT CASE STUDY

A 54-year-old male is ordered clarithromycin 250 mg every 12 hours for his newly developed chronic bronchitis.

1. Is the dose within normal dosage range? Explain your answer.
2. What side effects should the nurse teach the patient about?
3. What are some adverse effects that the patient should report to the health care provider?

REVIEW QUESTIONS

1. A patient is prescribed daptomycin. Which action(s) should the nurse implement? **Select all that apply.**
   a. Monitor blood values for toxicity.
   b. Dilute in 50 to 100 mL of normal saline and administer intravenously over 30 minutes.
   c. Monitor the patient for allergic reactions such as rhabdomyolysis.
   d. Advise the patient to take the medication on an empty stomach, even if gastrointestinal distress occurs.
   e. Culture the infected area before administering the first dose.

2. A patient is taking azithromycin. Which nursing intervention(s) would the nurse plan to implement for this patient? **Select all that apply.**
   a. Monitor periodic liver function tests.
   b. Dilute with 50 mL of 5% dextrose in water for intravenous administration.
   c. Instruct the patient to report any loose stools or diarrhea.
   d. Instruct the patient to report evidence of superinfection.
   e. Teach the patient to take oral drug 1 hour before or 2 hours after meals.
   f. Advise the patient to avoid antacids from 2 hours before or 2 hours after administration.

3. For which serious adverse effect should the nurse closely monitor a patient who is taking lincosamides?
   a. Seizures
   b. Ototoxicity
   c. Hepatotoxicity
   d. *Clostridium difficile*-associated diarrhea

4. The nurse enters a patient's room to find that his heart rate is 120 beats per minute, his blood pressure is 70/50 mm Hg, and he has red blotching of his face and neck. Vancomycin is running intravenous piggyback. The nurse believes that this patient is experiencing a severe adverse effect called *red man syndrome*. What action will the nurse take?
   a. Stop the infusion, and call the health care provider.
   b. Reduce the infusion to 10 mg/min.
   c. Encourage the patient to drink more fluids, up to 2 L/d.
   d. Report onset of Stevens-Johnson syndrome to the health care provider.

28

Tetracyclines, Glycylcyclines, Aminoglycosides, and Fluoroquinolones

http://evolve.elsevier.com/McCuistion/pharmacology

OBJECTIVES

- Explain the use of tetracyclines.
- Discuss the mechanism of action and use of glycylcyclines.
- Explain the mechanism of action and use of aminoglycosides.
- Describe the mechanism of action and use of fluoroquinolones.

OUTLINE

Tetracyclines, 339
　Side Effects and Adverse Reactions, 339
　Drug Interactions, 340
Glycylcyclines, 340
　Pharmacology, 340
　Side Effects, Adverse Reactions, and Drug Interactions, 343
Aminoglycosides, 343
　Pharmacology, 343
　Side Effects and Adverse Reactions, 344
　Drug Interactions, 344
Fluoroquinolones, 346
　Pharmacology, 346
　Side Effects, Adverse Reactions, and Drug Interactions, 347
Clinical Judgment Case Study, 347
Review Questions, 347

The groups of antibacterials discussed in this chapter include tetracyclines, glycylcyclines, aminoglycosides, and fluoroquinolones (quinolones).

TETRACYCLINES

Tetracyclines, isolated from *Streptomyces aureofaciens* in 1948, were the first broad-spectrum antibiotics effective against gram-positive and gram-negative bacteria and many other organisms such as rickettsiae, *Escherichia coli*, *Klebsiella*, *Neisseria*, *Staphylococcus*, *Streptococcus*, and chlamydia. Tetracyclines act by inhibiting bacterial protein synthesis and have a bacteriostatic effect.

Tetracyclines are not effective against *Staphylococcus aureus* (except for the newer tetracyclines) or *Pseudomonas* or *Proteus* species, but they can be used against *Mycoplasma pneumoniae*. Tetracycline in combination with metronidazole and bismuth subsalicylate is useful in treating *Helicobacter pylori*, a bacterium in the stomach that can cause peptic ulcers. For years, oral and topical tetracyclines have been used to treat severe acne vulgaris, and low doses are usually prescribed to minimize the toxic effect of the drug.

Tetracyclines are frequently prescribed for oral use although they are also available for intravenous (IV) use to treat severe infections (see Prototype Drug Chart: Doxycycline). The newer oral preparations of tetracyclines (i.e., doxycycline, minocycline) are more rapidly and completely absorbed. Tetracyclines should not be taken with magnesium and aluminum antacid preparations, milk products containing calcium, or iron-containing drugs because these substances bind with tetracycline and prevent absorption of the drug. It is suggested that tetracyclines, except for doxycycline and minocycline, be taken on an empty stomach 1 hour before or 2 hours after mealtime; the absorption of doxycycline and minocycline is improved with food ingestion. Table 28.1 describes the tetracycline preparations and their dosages, uses, and considerations. The tetracyclines are listed according to whether they are short- or intermediate acting drugs, as well as miscellaneous.

Continuous use of tetracyclines has resulted in bacterial resistance to the drugs. Tetracycline resistance has increased in the treatment of pneumococcal and gonococcal infections; therefore tetracyclines are not as useful in treating these infections. Although tetracyclines are widely used, they have numerous side effects, adverse reactions, toxicities, and drug interactions.

Side Effects and Adverse Reactions

GI disturbances such as nausea, vomiting, and diarrhea are side effects of tetracyclines. **Photosensitivity** (sunburn reaction) may occur in persons taking tetracyclines, especially demeclocycline. Pregnant patients should *not* take tetracycline during the first trimester of pregnancy because of possible teratogenic effects. Women in the last trimester of pregnancy and children younger than 8 years of age should also *not* take tetracycline because it irreversibly discolors the permanent teeth. Minocycline can cause damage to the vestibular part of the inner ear, which may result in difficulty maintaining balance. Outdated tetracyclines should always be discarded because the drug breaks down into a toxic by-product. Renal failure results with some tetracyclines, especially when given in high doses with other nephrotoxic drugs. Because tetracycline can disrupt the microbial flora of the body, superinfection (secondary infection resulting from drug therapy) is another adverse reaction that might result. Blood dyscrasias may occur with tetracyclines.

PROTOTYPE DRUG CHART
Doxycycline

Drug Class	Dosage
Antibacterial: Tetracycline	Urinary tract infection: Delayed release: A: PO: 100 mg q12h on day 1, then 100 mg/d or 50 mg q12h A: IV: 200 mg q12–24h on day 1, then 100 mg/d or 200 mg/d q12–24h
Contraindications	**Drug-Lab-Food Interactions**
Hypersensitivity *Caution:* Radiation therapy, chemotherapy, periodontal disease, asthma, diabetes mellitus, obesity, sulfite hypersensitivity, HIV, diarrhea, CDAD, immunosuppression, sunlight exposure, breastfeeding, pregnancy, children	Drug: May increase effects of digoxin and warfarin; doxycycline absorption decreases with sucralfate, antacids, iron, calcium, magnesium/aluminum hydroxide, zinc, bismuth, vitamin C, barbiturates, phenytoin, quinapril, and rifampin; decreases effects of oral contraceptives, neuromuscular blockers, amoxicillin, and penicillin Lab: Decreases serum potassium level Food: Dairy products decrease the effect
Pharmacokinetics	**Pharmacodynamics**
Absorption: PO: 100% absorbed Distribution: PB: 80%–90% Metabolism: t½: 12–25 h Excretion: Urine and feces	PO: Onset: 2–3 h Duration: 16–24 h Peak: 3 h IV: Onset: Rapid Peak: 2 h Duration: 16–24 h
Therapeutic Effects/Uses	
For treating acne, anthrax, amebiasis, brucellosis, psittacosis, epididymitis, tularemia, plague, STIs, rickettsia, malaria prophylaxis, and respiratory, urinary tract, and skin infections. Doxycycline is effective against *Escherichia coli* and MRSA, and species of *Clostridium, Haemophilus, Enterococcus, Chlamydia, Neisseria, Klebsiella, Staphylococcus, Streptococcus,* and *Shigella* Mechanism of action: Inhibits the steps of protein synthesis; bacteriostatic or bactericidal	
Side Effects	**Adverse Reactions**
Headache, anxiety, photosensitivity, blurred vision, diplopia, throat irritation, sinusitis, cough, pharyngitis, nasal congestion, glossitis, dry mouth, tooth/nail discoloration, dyspepsia, dysphagia, abdominal pain, nausea, vomiting, diarrhea, rash, injection site reaction, skin hyperpigmentation, musculoskeletal/back pain, influenza, elevated hepatic enzymes, candidiasis, Jarisch-Herxheimer reaction	Superinfection, hypertension, hyperglycemia, enterocolitis, pancreatitis, esophageal ulceration *Life-threatening:* Anaphylaxis, angioedema, eosinophilia, thrombocytopenia, hemolytic anemia, neutropenia, hepatotoxicity, CDAD, increased intracranial pressure, Stevens-Johnson syndrome

A, Adult; *CDAD, Clostridium difficile*–associated diarrhea; *d*, day; *h*, hour; *HIV,* human immunodeficiency virus infection; *IV,* intravenous; *MRSA,* methicillin-resistant *Staphylococcus aureus; PB,* protein binding; *PO,* by mouth; *q,* every; *STI,* sexually transmitted infection; *t½,* half-life; *UK,* unknown.

Drug Interactions

Antacids and iron-containing drugs can prevent the absorption of tetracycline from the GI tract. Milk and foods high in calcium can inhibit tetracycline absorption. To avoid drug interaction, these should be taken at least 2 hours apart from tetracycline. Be aware that lipid-soluble tetracyclines, such as doxycycline and minocycline, are actually better absorbed from the GI tract when taken *with* milk products and food.

The desired action of oral contraceptives can be lessened when taken with tetracyclines. The activity of penicillins given with a tetracycline can be decreased because the tetracyclines could cause bacterial resistance to the action of penicillin.

GLYCYLCYCLINES

Tigecycline is an antibiotic in a category called *glycylcyclines*, synthetic analogues of the tetracyclines (see Table 28.1). It acts by blocking protein synthesis in bacterial cells, resulting in a bacteriostatic action. Indications for use are community-acquired pneumonia, complicated skin infections, and intraabdominal infections, including *S. aureus, E. coli, Streptococcus pyogenes, Klebsiella pneumoniae,* and *Clostridium perfringens.*

Pharmacology
Pharmacokinetics

Tigecycline is administered IV at an initial loading dose of 100 mg over 30 to 60 minutes, followed by 50 mg every 12 hours. The protein-binding capacity of tigecycline ranges from 71% to 89%, and the half-life is 27 to 42 hours. The drug is eliminated from the body in bile, feces, and urine, but biliary excretion is the primary route.

Pharmacodynamics

Tigecycline binds to the 30S ribosomal subunit and causes cell death. It has broad-spectrum activity against Gram-positive and Gram-negative bacterial pathogens.

TABLE 28.1 Antibacterials: Tetracyclines and Glycylcyclines

Generic	Route and Dosage	Uses and Considerations
Short-Acting Tetracycline		
Tetracycline	Mild to moderate URI: A: PO: 500 mg bid or 250 mg q6h; *max:* 2 g/d	For treating acne, tularemia, shigellosis, intestinal amebiasis, psittacosis, anthrax, plague, gingivitis, cholera, MRSA, STIs, Rocky Mountain Spotted fever, and *Helicobacter pylori*, skin, urinary tract, and respiratory infections. May cause headache, dermatitis, glossitis, tooth/tongue/nail discoloration, nausea, vomiting, diarrhea, CDAD, blood dyscrasias, and superinfection. PB: 65%; t½: 6–12 h
Intermediate-Acting Tetracycline		
Demeclocycline hydrochloride	Respiratory infection: A: PO: 150 mg q6h or 300 mg q12h; *max:* 1.2 g/d	For treating acne, gingivitis, anthrax, amebiasis, cholera, plague, STIs, and skin, rickettsial, respiratory, and urinary tract infections. May cause headache, tooth discoloration, glossitis, nausea, vomiting, diarrhea, CDAD, blood dyscrasias, renal failure, myasthenia, elevated hepatic enzymes, and superinfection. PB: 65%–90%; t½: 10–17 h
Miscellaneous Tetracyclines		
Doxycycline hyclate	See Prototype Drug Chart: Doxycycline	
Minocycline hydrochloride	Respiratory infection: Immediate release: A: PO/IV: Initially 200 mg/d, then 100 mg q12h; *max:* 200 mg/d PO; 400 mg/d IV	For treating anthrax, cholera, plague, meningitis, MRSA, STIs, acne, and respiratory, rickettsial, urinary tract, and skin infections. May cause headache, fatigue, dizziness, tinnitus, flushing, erythema, pruritus, xerosis, stomatitis, dental caries/pain, gingivitis, tooth/tongue discoloration, oral ulceration, dry mouth, anorexia, nausea, vomiting, CDAD, telangiectasia, blood dyscrasias, renal failure, and superinfection. PB: 76%; t½: 11–24 h
Omadacycline	Pneumonia: A: IV: LD 200 mg once or 100 mg bid on day 1, then 100 mg/d for 7–14 d; *max:* 200 mg/d A: PO: After IV LD, 300 mg bid on day 1, then 300 mg/d for 7–14 d; *max:* PO 600 mg/d. IV 200 mg/d	For community-acquired pneumonia and skin infections. May cause headache, insomnia, tooth discoloration, nausea, vomiting, diarrhea, constipation, injection site reaction, hypertension, elevated hepatic enzymes, superinfection, and CDAD. PB: 20%; t½: 15.5–16.83 h
Eravacycline	A: IV: 1 mg/kg q12h for 4–14 d; *max:* 2 mg/kg/d	For complicated intraabdominal infections. May cause tooth discoloration, nausea, vomiting, diarrhea, injection site reaction, hypotension, CDAD, and wound dehiscence. PB: 79%–90%; t½: 20 h
Glycylcyclines		
Tigecycline	Skin infections: A: IV: Initially: 100 mg over 30–60 min; *maint:* 50 mg q12h for 7–14 d; *max:* 100 mg/d	For treating MRSA, community-acquired pneumonia, and skin/intraabdominal infections. May cause dizziness, tooth discoloration, headache, photosensitivity, weakness, abdominal pain, nausea, vomiting, diarrhea, rash, superinfection, anemia, azotemia, elevated hepatic enzymes, anaphylaxis, and CDAD. PB: 71%–89%; t½: 27–42 h

A, Adult; *CDAD*, *Clostridium difficile*–associated diarrhea; *d*, day; *h*, hour; *IV*, intravenous; *LD*, loading dose; *maint*, maintenance; *max*, maximum; *min*, minutes; *MRSA*, methicillin-resistant *Staphylococcus aureus*; *PB*, protein binding; *PO*, by mouth; *q*, every; *STI*, sexually transmitted infection; *t½*, half-life.

CLINICAL JUDGMENT [NURSING PROCESS]

Antibacterials: Tetracyclines

Concept: Infection
- A condition in which microorganisms enter the body and release toxins

Recognize Cues [Assessment]
- Assess vital signs and urine output. Report abnormal findings.
- Check laboratory results, especially those that indicate renal and liver function (blood urea nitrogen [BUN], serum creatinine, aspartate aminotransferase [AST], alanine aminotransferase [ALT], bilirubin).
- Obtain a history of dietary intake and drugs the patient currently takes. Dairy products, antacids, iron, calcium, and magnesium decrease drug absorption. Digoxin absorption is increased, which may lead to digitalis toxicity.

Analyze Cues and Prioritize Hypothesis [Patient Problems]
- Tissue injury
- Vomiting
- Nausea

Generate Solutions [Planning]
- The patient's white blood cells will be within normal limits.

Take Action [Nursing Interventions]
- Obtain a sample for culture from the infected area, and send it to the laboratory for culture and sensitivity (C&S). Antibiotic therapy can be started after the culture sample has been taken.
- Administer tetracycline 1 hour before or 2 hours after meals for optimum absorption.
- Monitor laboratory values to assess liver and kidney function (in particular, liver enzymes, BUN, and serum creatinine).
- Record vital signs and urine output.

Continued

CLINICAL JUDGMENT [NURSING PROCESS]—CONT'D
Antibacterials: Tetracyclines

Patient Teaching

General
- Instruct patients to store tetracycline away from light and extreme heat. Tetracycline decomposes in light and heat and causes the drug to become toxic.
- Advise patients to check expiration dates on bottles of tetracycline; out-of-date tetracycline can be toxic.
- ⚡ Inform female patients who are contemplating pregnancy to avoid taking tetracycline because of possible teratogenic effects.
- Warn parents that children younger than 8 years should not take tetracycline because it can cause discoloration of permanent teeth.
- Encourage patients to take the complete course of tetracycline as prescribed.

Side Effects
- Advise patients to use a sunblock and protective clothing during sun exposure. Photosensitivity is associated with tetracycline.
- Encourage patients to report signs of a superinfection (mouth ulcers, anal or genital discharge).
- Advise patients to use additional contraceptive techniques and *not* to rely on oral contraceptives when taking the drug because contraceptive effectiveness may decrease.
- Teach patients to use effective oral hygiene several times a day to prevent or alleviate mouth ulcers (stomatitis).

Diet
- Educate patients to avoid milk products, iron, and antacids. Tetracycline should be taken 1 hour before or 2 hours after meals with a full glass of water. If gastrointestinal (GI) upset occurs, the drug can be taken with nondairy foods.

Evaluate Outcomes [Evaluation]
- Evaluate the effectiveness of tetracycline by determining whether the infection has been controlled or has ceased and that there are no side effects.

PROTOTYPE DRUG CHART
Gentamicin Sulfate

Drug Class	Dosage
Antibacterial: Aminoglycoside	Respiratory infection: A: IM/IV: 3–5 mg/kg/d in q6–8h Extended-interval dosing: A: IM/IV: 5–7 mg/kg/dose q24h TDM: Peak: 5–8 mcg/mL Trough: <1–2 mcg/mL
Contraindications	**Drug-Lab-Food Interactions**
Hypersensitivity *Caution:* Renal disease, neuromuscular disorders (myasthenia gravis, parkinsonism), neurotoxicity, electrolyte imbalance, dehydration, corneal abrasion, hearing impairment, diarrhea, CDAD, ototoxicity, tinnitus, respiratory depression, older adults, pregnancy, breastfeeding	Drug: Increases risk of ototoxicity with loop diuretics; increases risk of nephrotoxicity with NSAIDs, amphotericin B, cephalosporins, cisplatin, furosemide, and vancomycin Lab: Increases BUN, serum AST, ALT, LDH, bilirubin, and creatinine; decreases serum potassium and magnesium
Pharmacokinetics	**Pharmacodynamics**
Absorption: IM, IV Distribution: PB: 0%–30% Metabolism: $t\frac{1}{2}$: 2 h Excretion: Unchanged in urine	IM/IV: Onset: rapid Peak: IM 30–60 min, IV 30 min Duration: UK
Therapeutic Effects/Uses	
For treating blepharitis, conjunctivitis, endocarditis, bacteremia, sepsis, and respiratory, intraabdominal, bone/joint, skin, and urinary tract infections. Aminoglycosides are effective against *Pseudomonas aeruginosa*, *Escherichia coli*, and species of *Proteus*, *Enterococcus*, *Haemophilus*, *Klebsiella*, *Salmonella*, *Serratia*, *Staphylococcus*, and *Streptococcus* Mechanism of action: Inhibits bacterial protein synthesis; bactericidal effect	
Side Effects	**Adverse Reactions**
Headache, dizziness, confusion, depression, hallucinations, conjunctivitis, photosensitivity, ocular/skin irritation, fever, erythema, rash, pruritus, alopecia, tinnitus, hypersalivation, stomatitis, nausea, vomiting, weakness, arthralgia, phlebitis, injection site reaction, paresthesias, vitamin B_6 and B_{12} deficiency, impaired wound healing, oliguria, elevated hepatic enzymes	Peripheral neuropathy, neurotoxicity, laryngeal edema, hearing loss, ototoxicity, myasthenia, hypokalemia, hypomagnesemia, hyponatremia, hypocalcemia, hyperbilirubinemia, azotemia, superinfection, hypo/hypertension, CDAD *Life-threatening:* Anaphylaxis, agranulocytosis, thrombocytopenia, anemia, eosinophilia, leukopenia, nephrotoxicity, hepatomegaly, increased intracranial pressure

<, Less than; *A*, adult; *ALT*, alanine aminotransferase; *AST*, aspartate aminotransferase; *BUN*, blood urea nitrogen; *CDAD*, *Clostridium difficile*-associated diarrhea; *d*, day; *h*, hour; *IM*, intramuscular; *IV*, intravenous; *LDH*, lactic dehydrogenase; *min*, minutes; *NSAID*, nonsteroidal antiinflammatory drug; *PB*, protein binding; *q*, every; $t\frac{1}{2}$, half-life; *TDM*, therapeutic drug monitoring; *UK*, unknown.

Side Effects, Adverse Reactions, and Drug Interactions

Because of their related structural formulas, many side effects of tigecycline are similar to those of tetracycline. The most common side effects of tigecycline involve the GI tract and include nausea, vomiting, abdominal pain, and diarrhea. *Clostridium difficile*–associated diarrhea (CDAD) may occur but is rare. Other side effects are photosensitivity, tooth discoloration, weakness, headache, dizziness, anemia, and thrombocythemia. Elevated hepatic enzymes, hepatic failure, and Stevens-Johnson syndrome may also occur.

Drug Interactions

Oral contraceptives may be less effective when given concurrently with tigecycline. Warfarin levels may be increased and may lead to bleeding when taken with tigecycline.

AMINOGLYCOSIDES

Aminoglycosides act by inhibiting bacterial protein synthesis. The aminoglycoside antibiotics are used against Gram-negative bacteria such as *E. coli* and *Proteus* and *Pseudomonas* species. Some Gram-positive cocci are resistant to aminoglycosides, so penicillins or cephalosporins may be used.

Streptomycin sulfate, derived from the bacterium *Streptomyces griseus* in 1944, was the first aminoglycoside available for clinical use and was used to treat tuberculosis. Because of its ototoxicity and the bacterial resistance that can develop, it is infrequently used today. Despite its toxicity, streptomycin is the drug of choice to treat tularemia and plague.

Aminoglycosides are used for serious infections, and they cannot be absorbed from the GI tract or cross into the cerebrospinal fluid; they cross the blood-brain barrier in children but not in adults. These agents are primarily administered intramuscularly (IM) and IV, except for a few aminoglycosides (e.g., neomycin) that may be given orally to decrease bacteria and other organisms in the bowel. Neomycin is frequently used as a preoperative bowel antiseptic.

The aminoglycosides currently used to treat *Pseudomonas aeruginosa* infection include gentamicin, tobramycin, and amikacin. *P. aeruginosa* is sensitive to gentamicin. Amikacin may be used when there is bacterial resistance to gentamicin and tobramycin. Prototype Drug Chart: Gentamicin Sulfate lists the drug data related to the aminoglycoside gentamicin.

Pharmacology

Pharmacokinetics

Gentamicin is administered IM and IV. This drug has a short half-life, and the drug dose can be given three to four times a day. Excretion of this drug is primarily unchanged in the urine.

Pharmacodynamics

Gentamicin inhibits bacterial protein synthesis and has a bactericidal effect. The onset of action is rapid or immediate, and the peak action for gentamicin is 30 minutes to 1 hour for IM and 30 minutes for IV administration.

To ensure a desired blood level, aminoglycosides are usually administered IV. The patient's blood levels are drawn periodically to determine the drug's peak (highest concentration) and trough (lowest

---

CLINICAL JUDGMENT [NURSING PROCESS]
Antibacterials: Aminoglycosides

Concept: Infection
- A condition in which microorganisms enter the body and release toxins

Recognize Cues [Assessment]
- Record vital signs and urine output. Compare these results with future vital signs and urine output. Nephrotoxicity is an adverse reaction to most aminoglycosides.
- Assess laboratory results to determine renal and liver function, including blood urea nitrogen (BUN), serum creatinine, alkaline phosphatase (ALP), alanine aminotransferase (ALT), aspartate aminotransferase (AST), and bilirubin. Serum electrolytes should also be checked. Aminoglycosides may decrease serum potassium and magnesium levels.
- Obtain a medical history related to renal or hearing disorders. Large doses of aminoglycosides could cause nephrotoxicity or ototoxicity.

Analyze Cues and Prioritize Hypothesis [Patient Problems]
- Tissue injury
- Vomiting
- Nausea

Generate Solutions [Planning]
- The patient's white blood cells will be within normal limits.

Take Action [Nursing Interventions]
- Send a sample from the infected area to the laboratory for culture to determine the organism and its antibiotic sensitivity before the aminoglycoside is started.
- Monitor intake and output. Urine output should be at least 600 mL/day. Immediately report any decrease in urine output. Urinalysis may be ordered daily, and results should be checked for proteinuria, casts, blood cells, and appearance.
- ⚡ Check for hearing loss. Aminoglycosides can cause ototoxicity.
- Evaluate laboratory results, and compare with baseline values. Report abnormal results.
- Monitor vital signs. Note whether body temperature has decreased.
- Dilute gentamicin in 50 to 200 mL of normal saline or 5% dextrose in water (D_5W) solution, and administer IV over 30 to 60 minutes.
- ⚡ Check that therapeutic drug monitoring (TDM) has been ordered for peak and trough drug levels. Blood should be drawn 45 to 60 minutes after the drug has been administered for peak levels and minutes before next drug dosing for trough levels. Gentamicin peak values should be 5 to 8 mcg/mL, and trough values should be less than 1 to 2 mcg/mL.
- Monitor for signs and symptoms of superinfection; these include stomatitis (mouth ulcers), genital discharge (vaginitis), and anal or genital itching.

Patient Teaching
General
- Encourage patients to increase fluid intake unless fluids are restricted.

Side Effects
- Advise patients to report aminoglycoside side effects, which include nausea, vomiting, tremors, tinnitus, pruritus, and muscle cramps.
- Direct patients to use a sunblock and protective clothing during sun exposure because aminoglycosides can cause photosensitivity.

Evaluate Outcomes [Evaluation]
- Evaluate the effectiveness of the aminoglycoside by determining whether the infection has ceased and whether any side effects have occurred.

PROTOTYPE DRUG CHART

Ciprofloxacin

Drug Class	Dosage
Antibacterials: Quinolone, fluoroquinolone	UTI: Immediate release: A: PO: 250 mg q12h for 3 d; *max:* 1.5 g/d Extended release: A: PO: 500 mg/d for 3 d; *max:* 1 g/d
Contraindications	**Drug-Lab-Food Interactions**
Hypersensitivity to other quinolones *Caution:* Renal/hepatic dysfunction, stroke, peripheral neuropathy, fever, dehydration, electrolyte imbalance, contact lenses, corticosteroid therapy, dialysis, hyperparathyroidism, hypothyroidism, rheumatoid arthritis, seizures, dysrhythmias, bradycardia, hypertension, myasthenia gravis, tendon rupture, diarrhea, diabetes mellitus, cardiovascular, HIV, CDAD, tendinitis, neurotoxicity, older adults, females, pregnancy, breastfeeding, children	Drug: Increases effects of theophylline, and caffeine; increases levels of ciprofloxacin with NSAIDs, and probenecid; decreases drug absorption with iron, and calcium; may increase warfarin effects Lab: Increased AST, ALT; prolonged bleeding time
Pharmacokinetics	**Pharmacodynamics**
Absorption: PO: rapidly absorbed Distribution: PB: 20%–40% Metabolism: t½: 4 h Excretion: 35%–50% excreted in urine, 20%–35% excreted in feces	Immediate Release: PO: Onset: 0.5–1 h Peak: 1–2 h Duration: UK Extended Release: PO: Onset: UK Peak: 1–4 h Duration: UK
Therapeutic Effects/Uses	
For treating sinusitis, plague, anthrax, typhoid fever, febrile neutropenia, STIs, prostatitis, and respiratory, intraabdominal, bone/joint, urinary tract, and skin infections, as well as corneal ulcers, bacterial conjunctivitis, and otitis media/externa. Ciprofloxacin is effective against *Escherichia coli* and species of *Enterobacter, Haemophilus, Klebsiella, Neisseria, Proteus, Pseudomonas, Serratia, Chlamydia, Enterococcus, Staphylococcus,* and *Streptococcus* Mechanism of action: Inhibits the enzyme DNA gyrase, which is needed for bacterial DNA synthesis; bactericidal effect	
Side Effects	**Adverse Reactions**
Headache, dizziness, drowsiness, syncope, confusion, anxiety, irritability, nightmares, hallucinations, depression, psychosis, insomnia, fever, flushing, restlessness, weakness, ataxia, conjunctival hyperemia, blurred vision, diplopia, corneal deposits, photosensitivity, nystagmus, ocular irritation/pain/ulceration/pruritus, rhinorrhea, tinnitus, pharyngitis, dry mouth, dysgeusia, dyspepsia, anorexia, abdominal pain, nausea, vomiting, diarrhea, constipation, increased urinary frequency, myalgia, arthralgia, tremor, injection site reaction, rash, peripheral neuropathy, paresthesia, phlebitis, candidiasis	Neurotoxicity, crystalluria, myasthenia, ileus, GI bleeding, hypercholesterolemia, cholestasis, tendon rupture, tendinitis, superinfection, hearing loss, bradycardia, tachycardia, hypo/hyperglycemia, hypertriglyceridemia, hypo/hypertension, angina, myocardial infarction, pancreatitis, hematuria *Life-threatening:* Anaphylaxis, angioedema, bronchospasm, anemia, aplastic anemia, leukopenia, agranulocytosis, thrombocytopenia, eosinophilia, hemolytic anemia, pancytopenia, increased intracranial pressure, Stevens-Johnson syndrome, seizures, CDAD, hepatic/renal failure, dysrhythmias, cardiac/respiratory arrest, suicidal ideation

A, Adult; *ALT,* alanine aminotransferase; *AST,* aspartate aminotransferase; *CDAD, Clostridium difficile*–associated diarrhea; *d,* day; *DNA,* deoxyribonucleic acid; *h,* hour; *HIV,* human immunodeficiency virus infection; *NSAID,* nonsteroidal antiinflammatory drug; *PB,* protein binding; *PO,* by mouth; *STIs,* sexually transmitted infections; *t½,* half-life; *UK,* unknown, *UTI,* urinary tract infection.

concentration) blood levels. A therapeutic drug level can be maintained by monitoring the trough level, and peak levels are useful to monitor for toxicity. Many other antibiotics should be monitored as well to maintain adequate blood levels.

IV aminoglycosides can be given concurrently with penicillins and cephalosporins but should not be mixed together in the same container. When combinations of antibiotics are given by IV, the IV line is flushed after each antibiotic has been administered to ensure that the antibiotic was completely delivered.

Side Effects and Adverse Reactions

Serious adverse reactions to aminoglycosides include ototoxicity and nephrotoxicity. Renal function, drug dose, and age are all factors that determine whether a patient will develop nephrotoxicity from aminoglycoside therapy. Careful drug dosing is especially important with younger and older patients. The nurse must assess changes in a patient's hearing, balance, and urinary output. Prolonged use of aminoglycosides could result in a superinfection, and specific serum aminoglycoside levels should be closely monitored to avoid adverse reactions. Table 28.2 lists the aminoglycosides and their dosages, uses, and considerations.

Drug Interactions

When aminoglycosides are administered concurrently with penicillins, the desired effects of the aminoglycosides are greatly decreased; preferably these drugs should be given several hours apart. The drug action of oral anticoagulants such as warfarin can increase when taken

TABLE 28.2 Antibacterials: Aminoglycosides

Generic	Route and Dosage	Uses and Considerations
Amikacin sulfate	Respiratory infections: Conventional dosing: A: IM/IV: 15 mg/kg/d in divided doses q8–12 h; *max:* 1.5 g/d Extended interval dosing: A: IM/IV: 15–20 mg/kg/dose q24h; *max:* 1.5 g/d TDM: Peak: 25–40 mcg/mL; *trough:* <5 mg/mL	For treating bacteremia, sepsis, respiratory, urinary, bone/joint, skin, and intraabdominal infections. May cause cough, throat irritation, laryngitis, wheezing, bronchospasm, dyspnea, hemoptysis, ototoxicity, dysphonia, aphonia, nausea, diarrhea, myalgia, arthralgia, fatigue, weakness, back pain, CDAD, and nephrotoxicity. PB: 0%–11%; $t\frac{1}{2}$: 2 h
Gentamicin sulfate	See Prototype Drug Chart: Gentamicin Sulfate	
Streptomycin sulfate	Respiratory infection: A: IM: 1–2 g/d in divided doses q6–12 h; *max:* 2 g/d TDM: Peak: 40–50 mcg/mL; *trough:* <5 mcg/mL	For treating meningitis, endocarditis, bacteremia, tuberculosis, tularemia, plague, and respiratory and urinary tract infections. May cause tinnitus, hearing loss, fever, weakness, injection site reaction, rash, paresthesia, vitamin B_6/B_{12} deficiency, superinfection, CDAD, ototoxicity, neurotoxicity, and nephrotoxicity. PB: negligible; $t\frac{1}{2}$: 2–3 h
Tobramycin sulfate	Bone/joint infection: Conventional dosing: A: IV: 3–5 mg/kg/d in 3–4 divided doses for 4–6 wks; give IV over 30–60 min; *max:* 10 mg/kg/d; older A 7.5 mg/kg/d Extended interval dosing: A: IV/IM: 5–7 mg/kg/dose q24h for 4–6 weeks TDM: Peak: 5–8 mcg/mL, *trough:* 1–2 mcg/mL	For treating bacteremia, sepsis, respiratory, urinary tract, intraabdominal, skin, external eye, and bone/joint infections. May cause fever, headache, pharyngitis, rhinitis, cough, hemoptysis, dyspnea, dysphonia, ototoxicity, anorexia, abdominal pain, nausea, vomiting, weakness, chest pain, nephrotoxicity, superinfection, weight loss, and CDAD. PB: negligible; $t\frac{1}{2}$: 2–3 h

<, Less than; *A,* adult; *CDAD, Clostridium difficile*–associated diarrhea; *d,* day; *h,* hour; *IM,* intramuscular; *IV,* intravenous; *max,* maximum; *PB,* protein binding; *q,* every; *t½,* half-life; *TDM,* therapeutic drug monitoring.

CLINICAL JUDGMENT [NURSING PROCESS]
Antibacterials: Fluoroquinolones

Concept: Infection
- A condition in which microorganisms enter the body and release toxins

Recognize Cues [Assessment]
- Record vital signs along with intake and urine output. Compare these results with future vital signs and urine output. Fluid intake should be at least 2000 mL/day.
- Assess laboratory results (blood urea nitrogen [BUN] and serum creatinine) to determine renal function.
- Obtain a drug and diet history. Antacids and iron preparations decrease the absorption of fluoroquinolones such as levofloxacin, and levofloxacin can increase the effects of theophylline and caffeine. It can also increase the effects of oral hypoglycemics. When levofloxacin is taken with nonsteroidal antiinflammatory drugs, CNS reactions may occur, including seizures.

Analyze Cues and Prioritize Hypothesis [Patient Problems]
- Tissue injury
- Vomiting
- Nausea

Generate Solutions [Planning]
- The patient's white blood cells will be within normal limits.

Take Action [Nursing Interventions]
- Obtain a specimen from the infected site, and send it to the laboratory for culture and sensitivity (C&S) before initiating antibacterial drug therapy.
- Monitor intake and output. Urine output should be at least 750 mL/day. The patient should be well hydrated, and fluid intake should be greater than 2000 mL daily to prevent crystalluria (crystals in the urine). Urine pH should be below 6.7.
- Record vital signs and report any abnormal findings.
- Check laboratory results, especially BUN and serum creatinine. Elevated values may indicate renal dysfunction.
- Administer levofloxacin 2 hours before or after antacids and iron products for best absorption. Give with a full glass of water. If GI distress occurs, the drug may be taken with food.
- Dilute IV levofloxacin in the recommended amount of solution (NS, D_5W, D_5NS). Infuse over 60 to 90 minutes.
- Check for signs and symptoms of superinfection: stomatitis (mouth ulcers), furry black tongue, and anal or genital discharge or itching.
- ⚡ Monitor serum theophylline levels when taken concurrently with levofloxacin, which can increase theophylline levels. Check for symptoms of CNS stimulation such as nervousness, insomnia, anxiety, and tachycardia.
- ⚡ Monitor blood glucose. Levofloxacin can increase the effects of oral hypoglycemics.

Patient Teaching
General
- Teach patients to drink at least 6 to 8 glasses (8 oz) of fluid daily.
- Encourage patients to avoid caffeinated products.

Side Effects
- Direct patients to avoid operating motor vehicles or hazardous machinery while taking the drug, at least until drug stability has occurred, because of possible drug-related dizziness.
- Inform patients that photosensitivity is a side effect of most fluoroquinolones. Patients should wear sunglasses, sunblock, and protective clothing when in the sun.
- Encourage patients to report side effects such as dizziness, nausea, vomiting, diarrhea, flatulence, abdominal cramps, tinnitus, rash, and tendon rupture (very rare). Older adults are more likely to develop side effects.

Evaluate Outcomes [Evaluation]
- Evaluate the effectiveness of the fluoroquinolone by determining whether the infection has resolved and the body temperature has returned within normal range.

simultaneously with aminoglycoside administration, and the risk of ototoxicity increases when ethacrynic acid and an aminoglycoside are given.

FLUOROQUINOLONES

The mechanism of action of fluoroquinolones (quinolones) is to interfere with the enzyme DNA gyrase, which is needed to synthesize bacterial DNA. Their antibacterial spectrum includes bactericidal action on both gram-positive and gram-negative organisms. The fluoroquinolones are effective against some gram-positive organisms, such as *Streptococcus pneumoniae*, and also against *Haemophilus influenzae*, *P. aeruginosa*, and *Salmonella* and *Shigella* species. This group of antibiotics is useful in the treatment of urinary tract, bone, and joint infections; bronchitis; pneumonia; gastroenteritis; and gonorrhea. Table 28.3 lists the various fluoroquinolones.

Ciprofloxacin is a synthetic antibacterial. This fluoroquinolone has a broad spectrum of action on gram-positive and gram-negative organisms, including *P. aeruginosa*. Ciprofloxacin is approved for use in urinary tract and lower respiratory tract infections and in skin, soft tissue, bone, and joint infections.

The use of fluoroquinolones as urinary antibiotics is discussed in Chapter 51. Prototype Drug Chart: Ciprofloxacin illustrates pharmacological data of ciprofloxacin. Other fluoroquinolones include levofloxacin, moxifloxacin, Ofloxacin, and delafloxacin. Levofloxacin is used primarily to treat respiratory problems, such as, community-acquired pneumonia, chronic bronchitis, acute sinusitis, uncomplicated skin infections, and urinary tract infections.

Moxifloxacin is available for once-a-day oral and parenteral dosing. This drug is prescribed to treat the same infections other fluoroquinolones are effective against. Moxifloxacin is more active than levofloxacin against *S. pneumoniae*. It is also effective against some strains of *S. aureus* and enterococci but not against vancomycin-resistant *Enterococcus faecium*. The fluoroquinolones are included in Table 28.3.

> ### ⚡ PATIENT SAFETY
>
> Fluoroquinolones, especially levofloxacin, should be reserved for patients who have no other treatment options for uncomplicated urinary tract infection, acute bacterial exacerbation of chronic bronchitis, or acute bacterial sinusitis due to disabling and potentially irreversible serious adverse reactions. These adverse reactions include tendon rupture, tendinitis, peripheral neuropathy, central nervous system (CNS) effects, and exacerbation of myasthenia gravis. (Black Box Warning.)

Pharmacology
Pharmacokinetics

Ciprofloxacin is rapidly absorbed from the GI tract. It has a low protein-binding effect of 20% to 40% and a moderately short half-life of 4 hours. Ciprofloxacin is excreted in the urine and feces.

TABLE 28.3 Antibacterials: Fluoroquinolones (Quinolones)

Generic	Route and Dosage	Uses and Considerations
Fluoroquinolones		
Ciprofloxacin hydrochloride	See Prototype Drug Chart: Ciprofloxacin	
Levofloxacin	Chronic bronchitis: A: PO/IV: 500 mg/d for 5–7 d; *max:* 750 mg/d	For acute bacterial sinusitis, UTI, exacerbation of chronic bronchitis, community-acquired pneumonia, skin infections, tuberculosis, conjunctivitis, plaque, and anthrax. May cause headache, dizziness, visual impairment, ocular irritation/pain, photophobia, pharyngitis, insomnia, dysgeusia, abdominal pain, nausea, vomiting, diarrhea, constipation, CDAD, superinfection, tendon rupture, and Stevens-Johnson syndrome. PB: 24%–38%; $t\frac{1}{2}$: 6–8 h
Moxifloxacin	Sinusitis: A: PO/IV: 400 mg/d for 5–10 d; *max:* 400 mg/d	For treating sinusitis, conjunctivitis, plague, respiratory, intraabdominal, and skin infections. May cause headache, dizziness, cough, pharyngitis, rhinitis, ocular irritation/bleeding/pain/lacrimation, fever, rash, pruritus, nausea, diarrhea, CDAD, tendon rupture, and superinfection. PB: 30%–50%; $t\frac{1}{2}$: 12 h
Ofloxacin	UTI: A: PO: 200 mg q12h for 3–7 d; *max:* 800 mg/d	For treating otitis media/externa, PID, STIs, prostatitis, chronic bronchitis, and, urinary tract, ophthalmic, and skin infections. May cause headache, dizziness, insomnia, dysgeusia, dry mouth, abdominal pain, nausea, vomiting, diarrhea, rash, pruritus, CDAD, superinfection, candidiasis, vaginitis, polyuria, and tendon rupture. PB: 20%–32%; $t\frac{1}{2}$: 4–8 h
Delafloxacin	Skin infection: A: PO: 450 mg q12h for 5–14 d; *max:* 900 mg/d A: IV: 300 mg q12h for 5–14 d; *max:* 600 mg/d	For community-acquired pneumonia, and skin infections. May cause headache, dizziness, anxiety, dysgeusia, nausea, diarrhea, abdominal pain, hyperglycemia, tendon rupture, CDAD, elevated hepatic enzymes, and superinfection. PB: 84%; $t\frac{1}{2}$: 4.2–8.5 h PO, 3.7 h IV

A, Adult; *CDAD*, *Clostridium difficile*–associated diarrhea; *d*, day; *h*, hour; *IV*, intravenous; *max*, maximum; *PB*, protein binding; *PID*, pelvic inflammatory disease; *PO*, by mouth; *q*, every; *STI*, sexually transmitted infection; $t\frac{1}{2}$, half-life; *UTI*, urinary tract infection.

Pharmacodynamics

Ciprofloxacin inhibits bacterial DNA synthesis by inhibiting the enzyme DNA gyrase. The drug has a high tissue distribution. If possible, it should be taken before meals because food slows the absorption rate; antacids also decrease the absorption rate. Ciprofloxacin increases the effect of theophylline and caffeine.

Ciprofloxacin has an average onset of action of 30 minutes to 1 hour, and the peak concentration time is 1 to 2 hours. The duration of action is unknown.

Side Effects, Adverse Reactions, and Drug Interactions

Adverse reactions to ciprofloxacin include GI effects such as dysgeusia, nausea, vomiting, abdominal pain, and diarrhea. CNS reactions include headache, restlessness, dizziness, and confusion. Patients taking fluoroquinolones may experience *Candida* infections of the pharynx and vagina, as well as *Clostridium difficile* infection in the bowel. Side effects may include photosensitivity, corneal deposits, conjunctival hyperemia, and ocular ulceration and irritation. Tendon rupture, usually involving the Achilles tendon, may develop. Individuals age 60 years or older are at the highest risk. Also, those who have received a heart, lung, or kidney transplant are at risk.

Drug Interactions

Antacids containing aluminum or magnesium, iron salts, zinc salts, calcium supplements, sucralfate, and dairy products (milk) can reduce ciprofloxacin absorption. These items should be given at least 2 hours before ciprofloxacin or 6 hours after administration. Ciprofloxacin can elevate the plasma level of theophylline and warfarin, leading to toxicity.

CLINICAL JUDGMENT CASE STUDY

A 46-year-old female patient has a wound infection. The culture report states that the infection is due to *P. aeruginosa*, and the patient's temperature has risen to 104°F (40°C). Amikacin sulfate is to be administered IV in 100 mL of 5% dextrose in water (D$_5$W solution) over 45 minutes every 8 hours. The dosage is 15 mg/kg/day in three divided doses. The patient weighs 165 pounds.

1. What is the drug classification of amikacin? How many milligrams of amikacin should the patient receive every 8 hours?
2. What type of IV infusion should be used? What would be the IV flow rate?
3. When would a wound culture be obtained to determine the appropriate antibacterial agent? Explain your answer.
4. What are the similarities of amikacin to other aminoglycosides such as gentamicin? Would one aminoglycoside be preferred over another? Explain your answer.
5. The nurse assesses the patient for hearing and urinary function before and during amikacin therapy. Why should a hearing assessment be included?
6. The patient's urine output in the last 8 hours was 125 mL. Explain the possible cause for the amount of urine output. What nursing action should be taken?
7. What laboratory tests monitor renal function?
8. The health care provider requests peak and trough serum amikacin levels. When should the nurse draw the blood samples to determine peak and trough serum levels?

REVIEW QUESTIONS

1. A patient is receiving tetracycline. Which advice should the nurse include when teaching this patient about tetracycline?
   a. Take sunscreen precautions when at the beach.
   b. Take an antacid with the drug to prevent severe gastrointestinal distress.
   c. Obtain frequent hearing tests for early detection of hearing loss.
   d. Obtain frequent eye checkups for early detection of retinal damage.
2. A patient is taking levofloxacin. What does the nurse know to be true regarding this drug?
   a. It is administered intravenous only.
   b. Levofloxacin may cause hypertension.
   c. This drug is classified as an aminoglycoside.
   d. An adverse effect is tendon rupture.
3. Which instruction(s) will the nurse include when teaching patients about gentamicin? **Select all that apply.**
   a. Patients should report any hearing loss.
   b. Patients should use sunscreen when taking gentamicin.
   c. Intravenous gentamicin will be given over 20 minutes.
   d. Patients are monitored for mouth ulcers and vaginitis.
   e. Peak levels will be drawn 30 minutes before the intravenous dose.
   f. Patients should increase fluid intake.
4. Which nursing intervention(s) should the nurse consider for the patient taking ciprofloxacin? **Select all that apply.**
   a. Obtain a culture before drug administration.
   b. Tell the patient to avoid taking ciprofloxacin with antacids.
   c. Monitor the patient for tinnitus.
   d. Encourage fluids to prevent crystalluria.
   e. Infuse intravenous ciprofloxacin over 60 minutes.
   f. Monitor blood glucose because ciprofloxacin can decrease effects of oral hypoglycemics.

29

Sulfonamides and Nitroimidazoles Antibiotics

http://evolve.elsevier.com/McCuistion/pharmacology

OBJECTIVES

- Explain the action and use of sulfonamides.
- Describe the action of trimethoprim-sulfamethoxazole (TMP-SMZ).
- Explain the use of sulfacetamide sodium, nitromidazoles, and miscellaneous antibaterials.

OUTLINE

Sulfonamides, 348
    Pharmacology, 348
    Side Effects and Adverse Reactions, 348
Trimethoprim-Sulfamethoxazole, 349
    Pharmacology, 349
    Side Effects and Adverse Reactions, 349

Sulfonamides, Nitromidazoles, Miscellaneous Antibacterials, 349
    Topical and Ophthalmic Sulfonamides, 349
    Nitroimidazoles, 350
Miscellaneous Antibacterial Drugs, 352
Clinical Judgment Case Study, 353
Review Questions, 353

SULFONAMIDES

Sulfonamide, a synthetic antibacterial, was introduced in 1935. Sulfonamides are one of the oldest antibacterial agents used to combat infection. When penicillin was initially marketed, the sulfonamide drugs were not widely prescribed because penicillin was considered a "miracle drug." However, the use of sulfonamides has increased as a result of newer sulfonamides and drugs that combine a sulfonamide with an antibacterial agent in preparations such as trimethoprim-sulfamethoxazole (TMP-SMZ). This chapter discusses sulfonamides and nitroimidazoles.

Sulfonamides were first isolated from a coal tar derivative compound in the early 1900s and were produced for clinical use against coccal infections in 1935. Sulfonamides were the first group of drugs used against bacteria, although they are not classified as antibiotics because they were not obtained from biological substances. The sulfonamides are bacteriostatic because they inhibit bacterial synthesis of folic acid, which is essential for bacterial growth. Humans do not synthesize folic acid; rather, they acquire it through their diet. Therefore sulfonamides selectively inhibit bacterial growth without affecting normal cells. Folic acid (folate) is required by cells for biosynthesis of RNA, DNA, and proteins.

The clinical usefulness of sulfonamides alone, not in combination, has decreased for several reasons. The availability and effectiveness of penicillin and other antibiotics have increased, and bacterial resistance to some sulfonamides can develop. Sulfonamides may be used as an alternative drug for patients who are allergic to penicillin. They are still used to treat urinary tract and ear infections and may be used for newborn eye prophylaxis. Sulfonamides are approximately 90% effective against *E. coli*; therefore they are frequently a preferred treatment for urinary tract infections, which are often caused by *E. coli*. They are also useful in the treatment of meningococcal meningitis and against *Chlamydia* species and *Toxoplasma gondii*. Sulfonamides are *not* effective against viruses and fungi.

Pharmacology
Pharmacokinetics
Sulfonamide drugs are well absorbed by the gastrointestinal (GI) tract, and they are well distributed to body tissues and the brain. The liver metabolizes the sulfonamide drug, and the kidneys excrete it.

Pharmacodynamics
Many sulfonamides are for oral administration because they are absorbed readily by the GI tract. They are also available in solution and as ointments for ophthalmic use and in cream form (silver sulfadiazine and mafenide acetate) for burns. Most of the early sulfonamides were highly protein-bound and displaced other drugs by competing for protein sites. The two categories of sulfonamides, classified according to their duration of action, are *short-acting sulfonamides* that have a rapid absorption and excretion rate and *intermediate-acting sulfonamides* with moderate to slow absorption and a slow excretion rate.

Sulfadiazine is useful in prophylactic treatment of streptococcal infections in patients with rheumatic fever who are hypersensitive to penicillin. Older sulfonamides such as sulfadiazine are poorly soluble in urine and can cause crystallization, which could damage the kidneys if fluid and water intake are insufficient; however, newer sulfonamides have greater water solubility. Therefore crystal formations in the urine and renal damage are unlikely. Table 29.1 describes the sulfonamides.

Side Effects and Adverse Reactions
Side effects of sulfonamides may include an allergic response such as skin rash and itching. Anaphylaxis is uncommon. Blood disorders

TABLE 29.1 Antibacterials: Sulfonamides

Generic	Route and Dosage	Uses and Considerations
Sulfadiazine	UTI: A: PO: LD 2–4 g, then 2–4 g/d in 3–6 divided doses; *max:* 4 g/d	For treating otitis media, meningitis, malaria, nocardiosis, toxoplasmosis, chancroid, chlamydial conjunctivitis, and UTIs and for rheumatic fever prophylaxis. May cause headache, insomnia, crystalluria, stomatitis, abdominal pain, arthralgia, hypoglycemia, anorexia, nausea, vomiting, and diarrhea. Increase fluid intake to maintain urine output at 1200–1500 ml/d. PB: 38%–48%; t½: 17 h
Sulfasalazine	Ulcerative colitis: Uncoated tablets: A: PO: Initially 1 g q6–8 h; *maint:* 500 mg q6–12 h; *max:* 4 g/d Enteric-coated tablets: A: PO: Initially 1 g q6–8 h; *maint:* 500 mg q6–12 h; *max:* 4 g/d	For treating ulcerative colitis and rheumatoid arthritis. May cause headache, dizziness, stomatitis, fever, dyspepsia, abdominal pain, anorexia, nausea, vomiting, oligospermia, elevated hepatic enzymes, rash, and pruritus. Take drug after eating. PB: 99%; t½: 5.7–7.6 h
Trimethoprim-sulfamethoxazole	See Prototype Drug Chart: Trimethoprim-Sulfamethoxazole	

A, adult; *d*, day; *h*, hour; *LD*, loading dose; *maint*, maintenance; *max*, maximum; *PB*, protein binding; *PO*, by mouth; *q*, every; *t½*, half-life; *UTI*, urinarytract infection.

such as hemolytic anemia, aplastic anemia, and low white blood cell (WBC) and platelet counts could result from prolonged use and high dosages. GI disturbances such as anorexia, nausea, and vomiting may also occur. The early sulfonamides were insoluble in acid urine, and **crystalluria** (crystals in the urine) and hematuria (blood in the urine) were common problems. Increasing fluid intake dilutes the drug, which helps prevent crystalluria. Photosensitivity, an excessive reaction to direct sunlight or ultraviolet (UV) light that leads to redness and burning of the skin, can also occur; therefore the patient should avoid sunbathing and excess ultraviolet light. **Cross-sensitivity**, a sensitivity or allergy to one sulfonamide that leads to sensitivity to another sulfonamide, might occur with the different sulfonamides but does not occur with other antibacterial drugs. Sulfonamides should be avoided during pregnancy to avoid congenital malformations, neural tube defects, and kernicterus.

TRIMETHOPRIM-SULFAMETHOXAZOLE

TMP-SMZ contains one part trimethoprim and five parts sulfamethoxazole to produce a **synergistic effect** that increases the desired drug response. Trimethoprim is an antibacterial agent that interferes with bacterial folic acid synthesis just as sulfonamides do; it is classified as a urinary tract antiinfective that may be used alone for uncomplicated urinary tract infections, and it is also effective against the gram-negative bacteria *E. coli* and also *Proteus* and *Klebsiella* species. In the 1970s trimethoprim was combined with sulfamethoxazole, an intermediate-acting sulfonamide, to prevent bacterial resistance to sulfonamide drugs and to obtain a better response against many organisms. Giving both drugs together in one compounded form causes bacterial resistance to develop much more slowly than if only one of the drugs were to be used alone.

TMP-SMZ is effective in treating urinary, intestinal, lower respiratory tract, and middle ear (otitis media) infections; prostatitis; and gonorrhea. It is also used to prevent *Pneumocystis carinii* in patients with acquired immunodeficiency syndrome (AIDS). Increased fluid intake is strongly recommended to avoid complications such as crystalluria. Prototype Drug Chart: Trimethoprim-Sulfamethoxazole describes the pharmacologic behavior of TMP-SMZ.

Pharmacology
Pharmacokinetics
TMP-SMZ is well absorbed from the GI tract and is moderately protein-bound. Sulfamethoxazole's half-life ranges from 6 to 12 hours, and trimethoprim's half-life ranges from 8 to 10 hours; thus it is administered twice a day. It is excreted as unchanged metabolites in the urine.

Pharmacodynamics
Trimethoprim, a nonsulfonamide antibiotic, enhances the activity of the drug combination. TMP-SMZ blocks steps in the bacterial synthesis of protein and nucleic acid, producing a bactericidal effect.

TMP-SMZ can be administered orally or intravenously (IV). Orally the drug has a moderately rapid onset of action; drug action is immediate via the IV route. Serum peak concentration time for oral use is 1 to 4 hours and 30 minutes to 1 hour for IV use. TMP-SMZ increases the hypoglycemic response when taken with sulfonylureas (oral hypoglycemic agents). It can also increase the activity of oral anticoagulants.

Side Effects and Adverse Reactions
Side effects of TMP-SMZ may include mild to moderate rashes, anorexia, nausea, vomiting, diarrhea, stomatitis, crystalluria, and photosensitivity. Serious adverse reactions are rare; however, agranulocytosis, aplastic anemia, and myocarditis have been reported as possible life-threatening conditions.

SULFONAMIDES, NITROIMIDAZOLES, MISCELLANEOUS ANTIBACTERIALS

Topical and Ophthalmic Sulfonamides
Sulfonamides can be administered for topical and ophthalmic uses, but because topical use of sulfonamides can cause hypersensitivity reactions, they are used infrequently. Mafenide acetate is a sulfonamide derivative prescribed to prevent sepsis in cases of second- and third-degree burns. Silver sulfadiazine is another topical sulfonamide used to treat burns. Both of these drugs are discussed in more detail in Chapter 45.

Sulfacetamide sodium is a sulfonamide for ophthalmic and topical uses. In ophthalmic preparations (liquid drops and ointments), sulfacetamide sodium is used to treat ocular infections. It is often used as prophylactic treatment after an eye injury or after the removal of a foreign body. Do *not* use ointment for the eye unless it has *ophthalmic* printed on the drug label. Sulfacetamide sodium is discussed in more detail in Chapter 47.

Topical sulfacetamide sodium *for the skin* is a cream, gel, lotion, or cleanser and is used to treat seborrheic dermatitis and acne. This dermatologic form is *not* used for the eye.

Nitroimidazoles

Nitroimidazoles act by disrupting DNA and protein synthesis in susceptible bacteria and protozoa. The nitroimidazoles are effective against *Helicobacter pylori* and bacterial species (e.g., *Bacteroides, Clostridium, Gardnerella, Prevotella, Peptococcus, Giardia*), and protozoa (e.g., *Trichomonas vaginalis*). Nitroimidazoles are used for prophylaxis for surgical infections and to treat *Clostridium difficile*–associated diarrhea (CDAD), anaerobic infections, amebiasis, giardiasis, trichomoniasis, bacterial vaginosis, and acne rosacea. Metronidazole and tinidazole are two of the most effective drugs available to treat anaerobic bacterial infections. Both nitroimidazoles are used with other agents to treat *H. pylori* infections associated with peptic and duodenal ulcers. Metronidazole was FDA approved in 1963, and tinidazole was approved in 2004.

Nitroimidazoles are primarily administered orally, parenterally, and topically. When metronidazole is given IV intermittently, it should be administered slowly over 30 to 60 minutes. Avoid contact with the eyes when using topical product. Table 29.2 lists nitroimidazoles and their dosages, uses, and considerations.

⚡ PATIENT SAFETY
Preventing Medication Errors

Do Not Confuse...
- **Septra**, an antibacterial sulfonamide, with **Sectral**, a beta-adrenergic antagonist used to manage dysrhythmias.
- **Sulfadiazine**, a short-acting antibacterial sulfonamide, with **sulfasalazine**, an intermediate-acting antibacterial sulfonamide.

🌿 COMPLEMENTARY AND ALTERNATIVE THERAPIES
Milk thistle may decrease absorption of metronidazole.

📋 PROTOTYPE DRUG CHART
Trimethoprim-Sulfamethoxazole (TMP-SMZ)

Drug Class	Dosage
Antibacterial: Sulfonamide	Acute exacerbation of chronic bronchitis: A: PO: TMP 160 mg, SMZ 800 mg q12h for 10–14 d; *max:* 1600 mg/d
Contraindications	**Drug-Lab-Food Interactions**
Severe renal/hepatic disease, hypersensitivity to sulfonamides, thrombocytopenia, infants *Caution:* Thyroid disorder, electrolyte imbalance, hypoglycemia, folate deficiency, bradycardia, dysrhythmias, CDAD, celiac disease, diarrhea, cardiac disease, older adults, pregnancy, breastfeeding	Drug: Increased anticoagulant effect with warfarin; increased hypoglycemic effect with oral hypoglycemic drugs, increased potassium levels with ACE inhibitors and spironolactone, increased digoxin and sulfonylurea levels, increased phenytoin and methotrexate toxicity Lab: May increase BUN, serum creatinine, AST, ALT, and ALP
Pharmacokinetics	**Pharmacodynamics**
Absorption: PO: Well absorbed Distribution: PB: 44% for TMP; 70% for SMZ; crosses placenta Metabolism: t½: 8–10 h for TMP, 6–12 h for SMZ Excretion: In urine as metabolites	PO: Onset: 2 h Peak: 1–4 h Duration: 12 h
Therapeutic Effects/Uses	
For treating otitis media, MRSA, respiratory, and urinary tract infections. TMP-SMZ is effective against *Salmonella* and species of *Haemophilus, Staphylococcus, Streptococcus, Proteus, Escherichia coli, Shigella flexneri,* and *Klebsiella*. Mechanism of action: Inhibits folic acid synthesis and protein synthesis of nucleic acids; bactericidal effect	
Side Effects	**Adverse Reactions**
Anorexia, stomatitis, glossitis, fever, nausea, vomiting, diarrhea, abdominal pain, weakness, ataxia, rash, depression, headache, insomnia, photosensitivity, tinnitus, arthralgia, myalgia	Rhabdomyolysis, lupus-like symptoms, crystalluria, hypotension, hypo/hyperthyroidism *Life-threatening:* Anaphylaxis, angioedema, seizures, myocarditis, leukopenia, thrombocytopenia, hemolytic anemia, aplastic anemia, agranulocytosis, eosinophilia, neutropenia, hyperkalemia, hyponatremia, hypoglycemia, CDAD, Stevens-Johnson syndrome, renal/hepatic impairment

A, Adult; *ACE,* angiotensin-converting enzyme; *ALP,* alkaline phosphatase; *ALT,* alanine aminotransferase; *AST,* aspartate aminotransferase; *BUN,* blood urea nitrogen; *CDAD, Clostridium difficile*–associated diarrhea; *d,* day; *h,* hour; *MRSA,* methicillin-resistant *Staphylococcus aureus; PB,* protein binding; *PO,* by mouth; *q,* every; *SMZ,* sulfamethoxazole; *TMP,* trimethoprim; *t½,* half-life.

TABLE 29.2 Antibacterials: Nitroimidazoles

Generic	Route and Dosage	Uses and Considerations
Metronidazole	Amebiasis: A: PO: 500 or 750 mg q8h for 5–10 d; *max:* 4 g/d A: IV: 750 mg q8h for 5–10 d; *max:* 4 g/d	For treating acne, amebiasis, bacterial vaginosis, endocarditis, meningitis, trichomoniasis, and bone/joint, gynecologic, skin, intraabdominal, and respiratory infections and for surgical infection prophylaxis. May cause headache, rash, dizziness, weakness, dry mouth, metallic taste, candidiasis, nausea, vomiting, diarrhea, abdominal pain, rhinitis, pruritus, influenza, vaginitis/irritation, vaginal discharge, and superinfection. PB: <20%; t½: 8 h
Tinidazole	Intestinal amebiasis: A: PO: 2 g/d with food for 3 d; *max:* 2 g/d	For treating amebiasis, giardiasis, trichomoniasis, and bacterial vaginosis. May cause candidiasis, metallic taste, nausea, vomiting, anorexia, vaginitis, weakness, tongue/urine discoloration, and superinfection. PB: 12%; t½: 12–14 h
Secnidazole	Bacterial vaginosis: A: PO: 2 g single dose; *max:* 2 g	For trichomoniasis and bacterial vaginosis. May cause headache, candidiasis, abdominal pain, dysgeusia, nausea, vomiting, diarrhea, and vaginitis. PB: <5%; t½: 17 h

>, Greater than; *A*, adult; *d*, day; *h*, hour; *IV*, intravenous; *max*, maximum; *PB*, protein binding; *PO*, by mouth; *q*, every; *t½*, half-life; *y*, year.

CLINICAL JUDGMENT [NURSING PROCESS]
Antibacterials: Sulfonamides

Concept: Infection
- A condition in which microorganisms enter the body and release toxins

Recognize Cues [Assessment]
- Assess the patient's renal function by checking urinary output (>600 mL/day), blood urea nitrogen (BUN; normal, 8–25 mg/dL), and serum creatinine (normal, 0.5–1.5 mg/dL).
- Obtain a medical history from the patient. Sulfonamides such as trimethoprim-sulfamethoxazole (TMP-SMZ) are contraindicated for patients with severe renal or liver disease.
- Determine whether the patient is hypersensitive to sulfonamides. An allergic reaction can include rash, skin eruptions, and itching. A severe hypersensitivity reaction includes erythema multiforme—an erythematous macular, papular, or vesicular eruption that can cover the entire body—or exfoliative dermatitis, characterized by desquamation, scaling, and itching of the skin.
- Obtain a history of drugs the patient currently takes. Oral antidiabetic drugs (sulfonylureas) given with sulfonamides increase the hypoglycemic effect; use of warfarin with sulfonamides increases the anticoagulant effect.
- Assess baseline laboratory results, especially complete blood count (CBC). Blood dyscrasias may occur as a result of high doses of sulfonamides over a continuous period, causing life-threatening conditions.

Analyze Cues and Prioritize Hypothesis [Patient Problems]
- Tissue injury
- Vomiting
- Nausea

Generate Solutions [Planning]
- The patient's white blood cells (WBCs) will be within normal limits.

Take Action [Nursing Interventions]
- Administer sulfonamides with a full glass of water. Extra fluid intake can prevent crystalluria and kidney stone formation.
- Record intake and output. To decrease the risk of crystalluria, fluid intake should be at least 2000 mL/day, and urine output should be at least 1200 mL/day. Sulfonamide sulfadiazine is more likely to cause crystalluria than combination drugs.
- Monitor vital signs. Note whether the patient's temperature has gone down.
- Observe the patient for hematologic reactions that may lead to life-threatening anemias. Early signs are sore throat, purpura, and decreasing WBC and platelet counts. Check CBC, and compare values with baseline findings.
- Check for signs and symptoms of superinfection. Symptoms include stomatitis (mouth ulcers), furry black tongue, anal or genital discharge, and itching.

Patient Teaching
General
- Encourage patients to drink several quarts of fluid daily while taking sulfonamides to avoid crystalluria.
- Advise pregnant patients to avoid sulfonamides during the last 3 months of pregnancy.
- Counsel patients not to take antacids with sulfonamides because antacids decrease the absorption rate of sulfonamide drugs.
- ⚡ Warn patients with an allergy to one sulfonamide that all sulfonamide preparations should be avoided, with health care provider's approval, because of the possibility of cross-sensitivity. Observe the patient for rash or any skin eruptions.

Self-Administration
- Teach patients to take sulfonamides 1 hour before or 2 hours after meals with a full glass of water.

Side Effects
- ⚡ Direct patients to report bruising or bleeding that could be a result of a drug-induced blood disorder. Advise patients to have their blood cell count monitored on a regular basis.
- Warn patients to wear sunglasses, avoid direct sunlight, and use sun block and protective clothing to decrease the risk of photosensitive reactions.

Evaluate Outcomes [Evaluation]
- Evaluate the effectiveness of sulfonamide therapy by determining whether the infection has been alleviated and the blood cell count is within normal range.

TABLE 29.3 Miscellaneous Antibacterial Drugs

Generic	Route and Dosage	Uses and Considerations
Chloramphenicol; Unclassified	Salmonella: A: IV: 50–100 mg/kg/d in 4 divided doses, reduce dose to 50 mg/kg/d as quickly as possible; *max:* 100 mg/kg/d TDM: Peak: 10–20 mcg/mL Trough: 5–10 mcg/mL	Due to the risk of potentially fatal toxicities, this drug is only used for treating only serious infections, such as bacteremia, salmonella, rickettsial infection, and typhoid fever. This drug is only used when other drugs are ineffective or contraindicated. When handling, use double chemotherapy gloves and protective gown, as well as, eye/face and respiratory protection. May cause headache, glossitis, confusion, depression, rash, nausea, vomiting, diarrhea, peripheral neuropathy, blood dyscrasias, bone marrow toxicity, CDAD, angioedema, and anaphylaxis. PB: 60%; t½: 4.1 h
Quinupristin-dalfopristin; Streptogramins classification	Skin infections: A: IV: 7.5 mg/kg/dose given over 1 h, q12 h for at least 7 d; *max:* 15 mg/kg/d	For treating skin infections. May cause infusion site reaction, rash, arthralgia, myalgia, CDAD, nausea, vomiting, diarrhea, hyperbilirubinemia, edema, and superinfection. PB: 11%–19%; t½: Dalfopristin 0.7 h, Quinupristin 0.85 h
Obiltoxaximab; Unclassified	A >40 kg: IV: 16 mg/kg as single dose A: <40 kg: IV: 24 mg/kg as single dose	For prophylaxis and treatment of anthrax. May cause hypersensitivity, headache, cough, nasal congestion, vomiting, hematoma, rash, pruritus, and injection site reaction. PB: UK; t½: UK
Lefamulin; Pleuromutilin classification	A: PO: 600 mg q12h for 5 d; *max:* 1200 mg/d A: IV: 150 mg q12h for 5–7 d; *max:* 300 mg/d	For community-acquired pneumonia. May cause headache, injection site reaction, nausea, vomiting, diarrhea, hypokalemia, CDAD, superinfection, and elevated hepatic enzymes. PB: 94.8%–97.1%; t½: 3–20 h

>, Greater than; <, less than; *A*, adult; *CDAD*, Clostridium difficile–associated diarrhea; *d*, day; *h*, hour; *IV*, intravenous; *max*, maximum; *PB*, protein binding; *PO*, by mouth; *q*, every; *t½*, half-life; *TDM*, therapeutic drug monitoring; *UK*, unknown; *UTI*, urinary tract infection; *y*, year.

Pharmacokinetics

Both metronidazole and tinidazole are well absorbed from the GI tract and are usually not given parenterally unless the patient cannot tolerate oral medications. The protein-binding capacity of nitroimidazoles ranges from 5% to 20%, and the half-life is 8 to 17 hours. These drugs are eliminated from the body via urine and feces.

Pharmacodynamics

Nitroimidazoles disrupt DNA and protein synthesis becoming bactericidal, amebicidal, and trichomonacidal. It is recommended that tinidazole be taken with food, but metronidazole can be given without regard to food. When metronidazole is used in the extended-release form, it should be taken on an empty stomach. The topical form is only minimally absorbed. The peak action for both agents is 1 to 3 hours.

Side Effects and Adverse Reactions

Common side effects that may occur when taking nitroimidazoles include headache, dizziness, insomnia, weakness, dry mouth, dysgeusia, anorexia, nausea, vomiting, diarrhea, tongue/urine discoloration, and superinfection. More serious adverse reactions that have occurred with metronidazole and tinidazole are leukopenia, peripheral neuropathy, seizures, and Stevens-Johnson syndrome. A disulfiram-like reaction may occur when metronidazole is taken with excessive amounts of alcohol. Symptoms of disulfiram-like reaction include flushing, throbbing headache, visual disturbance, confusion, dyspnea, nausea, vomiting, tachycardia, syncope, and circulatory collapse.

MISCELLANEOUS ANTIBACTERIAL DRUGS

Chloramphenicol does not belong to any major drug group. Table 29.3 discusses miscellaneous antibacterial drugs. Chloramphenicol was discovered in 1947 and exerts its bacteriostatic action by inhibiting bacterial protein synthesis. Because of the toxic effects of chloramphenicol, including blood dyscrasias related to bone marrow suppression, it is used only to treat serious infections. It is effective against gram-negative and gram-positive bacteria, and many other microorganisms, such as rickettsiae, *Mycoplasma*, and *Haemophilus influenzae*.

Quinupristin-dalfopristin is in a class of drugs called streptogramin antibiotics. It is effective for treating vancomycin-resistant *Enterococcus faecium* bacteremia and skin infected by *S. aureus* and *S. pyogenes*. It acts by disrupting the protein synthesis of the organism. When administering the drug through a peripheral IV line, pain, edema, and phlebitis may occur.

Obiltoxaximab is a monoclonal antibody and was FDA approved in 2016 for prophylaxis and treatment of anthrax. It prevents the lethal factor of anthrax from intracellular entry by inhibiting the binding of the protective antigen of *Bacillus anthracis* toxin to cellular receptors. This drug is administered IV as a single dose over 90 minutes.

Lefamulin is first in its class of pleuromutilin antibiotics, which is used for the treatment of community-acquired pneumonia. It can be bacteriostatic or bactericidal. Lefamulin inhibits bacterial protein synthesis. The most common side effects are diarrhea, injection site reaction, nausea, and vomiting.

CHAPTER 29 Sulfonamides and Nitroimidazoles Antibiotics

CLINICAL JUDGMENT CASE STUDY

A 46-year-old female has a severe urinary tract infection. She takes trimethoprim-sulfamethoxazole 160 mg/800 mg every 6 hours.
1. What are the similarities and differences between trimethoprim-sulfamethoxazole and sulfadiazine?
2. Is the dose within the recommended drug dose and dosing interval?
3. Patient teaching is an important part of nursing interventions. Explain the nurse's role regarding patient teaching concerning the following:
   a. What is the required amount of daily fluid intake?
   b. What time of day should sulfonamides be taken?
   c. Why should bruising and bleeding be reported?
   d. What effect does trimethoprim-sulfamethoxazole have on warfarin?

REVIEW QUESTIONS

1. A patient is taking sulfasalazine. What should the nurse teach the patient to do?
   a. Drink at least 10 glasses of fluid per day.
   b. Monitor blood glucose carefully to avoid hyperglycemia.
   c. Avoid operating a motor vehicle because this drug may cause drowsiness.
   d. Take this drug with an antacid to decrease the risk of gastrointestinal distress.
2. The nurse is teaching a patient about sulfadiazine. Which instructions will the nurse include in the teaching?
   a. Avoid caffeine during sulfonamide treatment.
   b. Administer in 50 mL of fluid over 30 minutes.
   c. Avoid sulfonamides during the third trimester of pregnancy.
   d. Use an ultraviolet light to enhance drug effectiveness.
3. A patient is ordered to take trimethoprim-sulfamethoxazole. The nurse knows to be aware of which adverse effect?
   a. Bronchospasm
   b. Tendon rupture
   c. Red man syndrome
   d. *Clostridium difficile*–associated diarrhea
4. The nurse is teaching a patient about trimethoprim-sulfamethoxazole. Which instructions will the nurse plan to include? **Select all that apply.**
   a. Report any bruising or bleeding.
   b. Report any diarrhea or bloody stools.
   c. Report any fever, rash, or sore throat.
   d. Avoid unprotected exposure to sunlight.
   e. Report thirst and polyuria.
5. A patient is taking a sulfonamide for an acute urinary tract infection. Which medication does the nurse realize is a short-acting sulfonamide?
   a. Sulfadiazine
   b. Sulfasalazine
   c. Seconidazole
   d. Trimethoprim-sulfamethoxazole

30

Antituberculars, Antifungals, and Antivirals

http://evolve.elsevier.com/McCuistion/pharmacology

OBJECTIVES

- Summarize the pathophysiology and clinical manifestations of tuberculosis.
- Outline drug therapy for tuberculosis.
- Summarize the pathophysiology and treatment for fungal infection.
- Summarize the pharmacological profile of antivirals and the viruses they treat.

OUTLINE

Tuberulosis, 354
    Pathophysiology, 354
    Clinical Manifestations, 354
Antitubercular Drugs, 354
    First-line Drugs, 355
    Drug-Resistant Tuberculosis, 355
    Prophylactic Antituberculars, 356
    Treatment Plan, 356
    Tuberculosis Treatment in Special Populations, 357
Fungus: Pathophysiology, 358
    Antifungals: Polyenes–Amphotericin B and Nytstatin, 359

    Antifungals: Azole, 361
    Antifungals: Antimetabolites and Echinocandins, 361
Viruses: Pathophysiology, 361
    Herpesviruses, 362
    Non-HIV Antivirals: Influenza, 363
    Non-HIV Antivirals: Herpes Antivirals, 366
    Non-HIV Antivirals: Cytomegalovirus Antivirals, 366
    Non-HIV Antivirals: Hepatitis Antivirals, 366
Clinical Judgment Case Study, 368
Review Questions, 368

TUBERCULOSIS

Tuberculosis (TB) is caused by the acid-fast bacillus *Mycobacterium tuberculosis*. The number of TB cases had declined until the mid-1980s when the number of cases started to increase. The increase in cases of TB was attributed to multiple factors, such as human immunodeficiency virus (HIV), increased immigration, and the spread of multidrug-resistant TB (MDR TB). According to the World Health Organization (WHO), TB is the 13th leading cause of death. After COVID-19, it is the world's leading cause of death due to infectious diseases. In 2022 the Centers for Disease Control and Prevention (CDC) reported a total of 8300 active TB cases. Another 13 million people in the United States are reported to have latent TB. Treatment for TB consists of a multidrug regimen. MDR TB occurs because the medications are mismanaged or they are misused. Patients started on therapy for TB who do not finish the prescribed therapy can develop and spread resistant strains of *M. tuberculosis*.

Pathophysiology

TB is transmitted from one person to another by droplets dispersed in the air through coughing, sneezing, and speaking. TB microorganisms can be inhaled into the lungs; therefore persons in close contact with the infected patient are at the highest risk of becoming infected. Others at high risk for contracting the disease include the immunocompromised (e.g., patients with HIV, diabetes, and renal failure, and those taking certain medications, such as cortisol), people living or working in high-risk residential settings (e.g., nursing homes, shelters, correctional facilities), those who inject illegal drugs, and health care workers who serve high-risk patients.

Nurses should be aware that persons coming to the United States from high-risk countries where TB disease is common may have been vaccinated with bacille Calmette-Guérin (BCG) as a child. This vaccine is seldom used in the United States. Previous vaccination with BCG may cause a positive reaction to skin testing; however, interferon-gamma release assay (IGRA) is not affected and false-positive results are not expected for IGRA.

Clinical Manifestations

Not everyone infected with TB will develop clinical manifestations; rather, some will harbor the microorganisms and will have what is called latent tuberculosis infection; these persons are at risk of developing TB disease later, and only those with active TB disease can infect others. Symptoms of active TB include anorexia, cough with blood-tinged sputum, chest pain, fever, night sweats, weight loss, and positive acid-fast bacilli in the sputum. Isolating infectious persons and initiating treatment for TB disease as soon as possible is the best way to decrease transmission.

ANTITUBERCULAR DRUGS

Antitubercular drugs (Table 30.1), which include antimycobacterials, are prescribed to people with active TB and those exposed to TB. Streptomycin was the first drug used in the treatment of TB disease in 1943. However, it was noted that patients began to deteriorate after 3 months of therapy due to drug resistance. In 1952 isoniazid (INH) began to see widespread use in the treatment of TB disease and was felt to be a "wonder drug."

First-Line Drugs

Antitubercular drugs are divided into two categories: first-line drugs that form the core of treatment regimens and drugs used in the treatment of drug-resistant TB. **First-line drugs**—those drugs chosen first, such as INH, rifampin, pyrazinamide, and ethambutol—are considered more effective and less toxic than drugs used in the treatment of drug-resistant TB. To this day, INH remains the first-line treatment for TB disease. INH is a bactericidal drug that inhibits tubercle cell wall synthesis and interferes with the metabolism of pyridoxine (vitamin B_6). When INH is prescribed, pyridoxine may be prescribed to avoid vitamin B deficiency and to minimize peripheral neuropathy. INH is administered orally. Prototype Drug Chart: Isoniazid lists the data for INH.

However, single-drug therapy is ineffective in the treatment of TB disease due to drug resistance. Using a combination of antitubercular drugs has been shown to decrease bacterial resistance. In addition, using combination therapy has decreased the duration of treatment from 2 years to 6 to 9 months. Different combinations of drugs can be used with INH, rifampin, ethambutol, and pyrazinamide.

Drug-Resistant Tuberculosis

Drugs used in the treatment of drug-resistant TB, in which *M. tuberculosis* is resistant to at least one first-line drug, or MDR TB, in which *M. tuberculosis* is resistant to INH and rifampin plus one other first-line drug, are used in combination with first-line drugs to treat drug-resistant *M. tuberculosis*. See Table 30.1 for drugs used in the treatment of drug-resistant TB. Combination therapy against active TB is more effective in eradicating infection than any single drug. Combination therapy for drug-resistant TB disease consists of a minimum of three drugs, but preferably four to five drugs, administered as part of directly observed therapy to ensure adherence. Drug therapy should be managed by an expert in the disease, and susceptibility testing to determine drug resistance should be performed before drug therapy; however, treatment with first-line therapy should not be delayed if active TB is suspected.

TABLE 30.1 Antitubercular Drugs

Generic	Route and Dosage	Uses and Considerations
Treatment for Tuberculosis Disease		
Ethambuto (First-line drug)	Dependent upon body weight	For drug-susceptible/resistant tuberculosis as combination therapy. May cause headache, dizziness, confusion, visual impairment, anorexia, nausea, vomiting, gout, peripheral neuropathy, leukopenia, thrombocytopenia, and anaphylaxis. Give with food to decrease GI disturbance. Monitor LFTs. PB: 20%–30%; t½: 3–4 h
Isoniazid (INH) (First-line drug)	See Prototype Drug Chart: Isoniazid	
Pyrazinamide (First-line drug)	Dependent upon body weight	For drug-susceptible/resistant tuberculosis as combination therapy. May cause photosensitivity, anorexia, nausea, vomiting, arthralgia, myalgia, gout, elevated hepatic enzymes, hepatitis, hepatotoxicity, and thrombocytopenia. Monitor LFTs and serum uric acid. PB: 50%; t½: 9–10 h
Rifabutin	A: PO: 5 mg/kg/d; *max:* 300 mg/d or	For drug-susceptible/resistant tuberculosis infections as combination therapy. May cause contact lens/urine discoloration, nausea, rash, leukopenia, neutropenia, anemia, thrombocytopenia, and elevated hepatic enzymes. Monitor LFTs. PB: 85%; t½: 45 h
Rifampin (First-line drug)	A: PO/IV: 10 mg/kg/d or 5 d/wk; *max:* 600 mg/d	For drug-susceptible/resistant tuberculosis as combination therapy. Take 1 h before or 2 h after eating. Aminosalicylate blocks absorption of rifampin so do not take at same time. Contents of capsules may be mixed with applesauce or jelly. May cause headache, dizziness, confusion, fatigue, visual impairment, tooth/urine discoloration, anorexia, nausea, vomiting, blood dyscrasias, and hepatotoxicity. PB: 80%; t½: 3–5 h
Rifapentine	A: PO: 600 mg twice weekly for 2 months, then 600 mg once weekly for 4 months	For drug-susceptible tuberculosis in combination therapy. May cause headache, cough, hemoptysis, diaphoresis, anorexia, anemia, neutropenia, lymphopenia, and elevated hepatic enzymes. PB: 98%; t½: 13 h
Drugs for Multidrug-Resistant Tuberculosis **(Used in combination with first-line drugs based on sensitivity)**		
Aminosalicylate	Drug-susceptible TB: A: PO: 8–12 g/d or 5 d/wk in divided doses Drug-resistant TB: A: PO: 6–12 g/d in divided doses	For drug-susceptible/resistant TB as combination therapy. May cause optic neuritis, abdominal pain, nausea, vomiting, diarrhea, vitamin B_{12} deficiency, thrombocytopenia, and leukopenia. Aminosalicylate blocks absorption of rifampin so do not take at same time. PB: 50%–60%; t½: 26 min
Capreomycin	A: IV/IM: 1 g/d or 5 d/wk for 60–120 d, then 1 g/d 2–3 times/wk for 12–24 months	For drug-susceptible TB. May cause tinnitus, hearing loss, vertigo, injection site reaction, hypomagnesemia, hypokalemia, blood dyscrasias, and nephrotoxicity. Inject deep into a large muscle mass. PB: UK; t½: 5.2–6.8 h

Continued

TABLE 30.1 Antitubercular Drugs—cont'd

Generic	Route and Dosage	Uses and Considerations
Cycloserine	Tuberculosis: A: PO: 10–15 mg/kg/d in divided doses; max: 1000 mg/d TDM: Target peak 20–35 mcg/mL to avoid CNS toxicity	For drug-susceptible/resistant tuberculosis and UTI. May cause drowsiness, memory impairment, folate/vitamin B_6 deficiency, seizures, psychosis, and suicidal ideation. Contraindicated in patients with a history of ETOH abuse, anxiety, depression, psychosis, renal impairment, and seizure disorders. PB: 0%; t½: 10 h
Ethionamide	A: PO: 15–20 mg/kg/d as a single dose or twice daily; max: 1 g/d	For drug-susceptible/resistant tuberculosis as combination therapy. Contraindicated in hepatic disease. May cause visual impairment, metallic taste, hypersalivation, stomatitis, anorexia, abdominal pain, nausea, vomiting, diarrhea, peripheral neuropathy, and weight loss. May be taken with meals or at hs. PB: 30%; t½: 2 h
Streptomycin	A: IM/IV: 15 mg/kg/d or 5 d/wk; TDM: Peak >40–50 mcg/mL; trough >5 mcg/mL	For drug-susceptible/resistant tuberculosis, gram neg bacillary bacteremia, endocarditis, UTI, plague, and tularemia. Inject into a large muscle mass. Contraindicated in aminoglycoside hypersensitivity. May cause weakness, hearing loss, injection site reaction, vitamin B_{12}/B_6 deficiency, anaphylaxis, blood dyscrasias, ototoxicity, nephrotoxicity, and neurotoxicity. PB: Negligible; t½: 2–3 h

A, Adult; *CNS*, central nervous system; *d*, day; *ETOH*, ethanol (alcohol); *GI*, gastrointestinal; *h*, hour; *hs*, hour of sleep; *HIV*, human immunodeficiency virus; *IM*, intramuscular; *IV*, intravenous; *LFT*, liver function test; *max*, maximum; *min*, minutes; *PB*, protein binding; *PO*, by mouth; *t½*, half-life; *TB*, tuberculosis; *TDM*, therapeutic drug monitoring; *UK*, unknown; *UTI*, urinary tract infection; *wk*, week; *y*, year; >, greater than; ≥, greater than or equal to; ≤, less than or equal to.
a Rifampin is the preferred agent from the class of rifamycins (rifabutin, rifampin, and rifapentine).

Prophylactic Antituberculars

Prophylactic antituberculars are drugs to prevent TB disease in individuals with latent TB infection. Prophylaxis is recommended for those who have a clinically significant result on tuberculin skin testing (≥5 mm for immunocompromised individuals or ≥10 mm for high-risk groups; Box 30.1) or a positive IGRA result. Patients who have converted from a negative to a positive TB skin test (TST) or from a negative to positive IGRA should be considered candidates for prophylactic therapy as well. Prototype Drug Chart: Isoniazid shows guidelines for latent TB infection treatment with INH.

Prophylactic therapy is contraindicated for persons with liver disease because INH is the primary antitubercular drug used, and it may cause INH-induced liver damage. Other antitubercular drugs may also cause liver damage if given in high doses over an extended period.

Treatment Plan

The treatment regimen is divided into two phases: the initial phase lasts 2 months, and the continuation phase consists of the next 4 or 7 months. The total treatment plan can be up to 9 months or longer, depending on response to drug therapy. If drug resistance develops, other antibacterial drugs such as aminoglycosides (streptomycin, kanamycin, amikacin) or fluoroquinolones (levofloxacin, ciprofloxacin, or ofloxacin) may be given as part of combination therapy. Aminoglycoside antibiotics should not be taken if kidney dysfunction is present. When antibacterial agents are used continuously or at high doses, serum drug levels should be closely monitored to avoid drug toxicity.

Many drug-drug interactions and side effects occur with antituberculars. To increase adherence to drug therapy, direct observation therapy (DOT) is recommended.

BOX 30.1 Determining When to Treat Latent Tuberculosis Infection

People with a positive tuberculin skin test (TST) reaction of ≥5 mm if they are:
HIV positive
Recent contacts of someone with active tuberculosis (TB disease)
Persons with fibrotic changes on chest radiography consistent with old TB
Organ transplant recipients
Persons who are immunosuppressed for other reasons (e.g., those taking the equivalent of >15 mg/day of prednisone for 1 month or longer, those taking tumor necrosis factor–alpha [TNF-α] antagonists)
People with a positive TST reaction of ≥10 mm if they are:
Recent immigrants (<5 years) from high-prevalence countries
Injection drug users
Residents and employees of high-risk congregate settings (e.g., correctional facilities, nursing homes, homeless shelters, hospitals, and other health care facilities)
Mycobacteriology laboratory personnel
Children under 4 years of age or children or adolescents exposed to adults in high-risk categories

From http://www.cdc.gov/tb/topic/treatment/decideltbi.htm.

Side Effects and Adverse Reactions

Side effects and adverse reactions to antituberculars differ according to the drug prescribed. For INH, peripheral neuropathy can be a problem, especially for those who are malnourished, have diabetes mellitus, or are alcoholics. This condition can be prevented if pyridoxine (vitamin B_6) is administered. Hepatotoxicity (liver toxicity) is an adverse reaction to many antituberculars. Patients with moderate to severe liver dysfunction should *not* take these drugs. Patients with liver disease should have hepatic transaminases monitored closely. Patients may also develop headaches, blood dyscrasias, paresthesias, gastrointestinal (GI) distress (e.g., nausea, vomiting), and ocular toxicity. An ophthalmic examination before and during treatment is warranted. INH may cause memory impairment, hyperglycemia, seizures, hypotension, and neuropathy. Rifampin turns body fluids orange, and soft contact lenses/teeth may be permanently discolored. It may also cause thrombocytopenia and GI intolerance. The patient taking ethambutol may develop dizziness, confusion, visual impairment, and joint pain. Streptomycin may lead to many adverse effects such as ototoxicity, encephalopathy, angioedema, neurotoxicity, and nephrotoxicity.

⚡ PATIENT SAFETY

Do Not Confuse...
- **Rifampin** with other antituberculars such as **rifabutin** and **rifapentine**.

Tuberculosis Treatment in Special Populations

Pregnancy
The benefits of treating a pregnant female with TB disease outweigh the risks of treatment. Females with untreated TB disease are at risk for passing the infection to the fetus and delivering a newborn with low birthweight. The drugs used in initial treatment of TB do cross the placenta but do not appear to harm the fetus.

Treatment of latent TB infection in the pregnant female includes INH daily or twice weekly for 9 months with pyridoxine supplementation. Three-month combination therapy of INH with rifapentinem, referred to as 3HP, is not recommended for pregnant females or those planning to become pregnant within 3 months.

The pregnant female with active TB should be treated with INH, rifampin, and ethambutol daily for 2 months followed by INH and rifampin daily or twice weekly for 7 months for a total of 9 months. Streptomycin should *not* be used due to potential harmful effects on the fetus.

HIV Coinfection
HIV is a risk factor for the development of TB, and TB disease is one of the leading causes of death for people coinfected with HIV. Left untreated, latent TB infection can quickly develop into TB disease. The recommended treatment for an adult with latent TB infection and HIV is INH and rifapentine weekly for 12 weeks.

Adults with HIV and TB disease should be treated for 2 months with INH, rifampin, pyrazinamide, and ethambutol during the initial phase. The 4-month continuation phase should consist of INH and rifamycin. A pregnant female with HIV and TB disease should be treated the same as a nonpregnant female but with concern for the fetus when choosing drug therapy.

Pediatrics
Children are more likely than adults to become sick more quickly by TB. Because of this, children with latent TB infection should be treated to prevent development of TB disease. The recommended treatment is INH for 6 to 9 months or INH in combination with rifampin for 4 months. Treatment of TB disease should be managed by a pediatric TB expert in conjunction with drug susceptibility studies. It is very important for the nurse to make sure parents understand that if a child stops taking the drugs before therapy is finished, the child can become sick again. In addition, nurses should stress to parents that if drugs are not taken correctly, the bacteria may become resistant to the drug. Drug-resistant TB is harder and more expensive to treat.

📋 PROTOTYPE DRUG CHART
Isoniazid

Drug Class	Dosage
Antimycobacterial (first-line antitubercular)	Latent TB infection: A: PO/IM: 5 mg/kg/d up to 300 mg/d or 15 mg/kg 2–3 d/wk; max: 900 mg 2–3 × wk. Do not give with food.

Contraindications	Drug-Lab-Food Interactions
Hepatic disease, hepatitis, jaundice Caution: Alcohol use disorder, HIV, AIDS, diabetes mellitus, malnutrition, peripheral neuropathy, gout, renal impairment, Hispanics, African Americans, females, older adults, pregnancy, breastfeeding	Drug: Potent inhibitor of CYP450 enzyme system; many drug-drug interactions can occur (see the package insert for a complete list). Increased effect with alcohol, rifampin, and cycloserine; decreased GI absorption while taking aluminum antacids; inhibits the metabolism of benzodiazepines, phenytoin, fosphenytoin, SSRIs, SNRIs, and valproic acid. MAOIs could potentiate the effects of INH. Food: Avoid tyramine-containing foods. Herb: Green tea, guarana, and ginseng could potentiate the effects of INH. Lab: Increases LFTs, bilirubin, and glucose; decreases platelets and granulocytes

Pharmacokinetics	Pharmacodynamics
Absorption: Rapidly absorbed in the GI tract when given PO; absorption slowed with food Distribution: PB: Insignificant Metabolism: t½: 1–4 h Excretion: 75% in urine; remainder in feces, saliva, and sputum	PO/IM: Onset: Rapid Peak: 1–2 h Duration: 6–8 h

Therapeutic Effects/Uses
To treat active tuberculosis and as a prophylactic measure against tuberculosis
Mechanism of Action: Bactericidal; inhibits bacterial cell wall synthesis by interfering with lipid and DNA synthesis. No cross-resistance with other antitubercular drugs occurs except with ethionamide. Pyridoxine supplementation reduces neurotoxic side effects.

Side Effects	Adverse Reactions
Syncope, chills, fever, cough, psychosis, memory impairment, abdominal pain, nausea, vomiting, injection site reaction, rash, dermatitis, paresthesias, peripheral neuropathy, myalgia,	Vitamin B6/D deficiency, neuropathy, optic neuritis/atrophy, hypotension, elevated hepatic enzymes, hyperglycemia, nephritis, seizures *Life-threatening:* Agranulocytosis, hemolytic anemia, aplastic anemia, thrombocytopenia, eosinophilia, hepatitis, encephalopathy, and Steven's-Johnson syndrome

A, Adult; *CYP450*, cytochrome P450; *d*, day; *GI*, gastrointestinal; *h*, hour; *IM*, intramuscular; *INH*, isoniazid; *LFT*, liver function test; *MAOI*, monoamine oxidase inhibitor; *max*, maximum; *PB*, protein binding; *PO*, by mouth; *SNRI*, serotonin-norepinephrine reuptake inhibitor; *SSRI*, selective serotonin reuptake inhibitor; *t½*, half-life; *TB*, tuberculosis; *UK*, unknown; *wk*, week; *y*, year.

Other Special Populations

Consideration of other special populations for TB includes the homeless and foreign-born, including Hispanics/Latinos and Asians. According to the CDC, 1% of the US population experiences homelessness in a given year. Of the foreign-born people with TB, 32% were Hispanics/Latinos. Lack of resources and reduced public health capacity increase the challenges faced in treating people with TB. There are many barriers in properly treating these vulnerable populations in eradicating TB. Socioeconomic, cultural, and language barriers are just a few that increase the risk for latent TB infection.

FUNGUS: PATHOPHYSIOLOGY

An infection caused by a fungus may also be called *mycosis, tinea,* or *candidiasis*. A fungal infection may be local or systemic. Local fungal infections can be acquired by contact with an infected person. Fungi known as *dermatophytes* can cause local fungal infections involving the integumentary system, which includes mucous membranes, hair, nails, and moist skin areas. When *Candida albicans* affects the mouth, it is called *oral candidiasis* or *thrush*. Vaginal candidiasis is common in females who are pregnant, diabetic, immunocompromised, or taking certain medications (e.g., antibiotics, oral contraceptives, and dapagliflozin). Systemic fungal infections may involve the lungs, CNS, or abdomen and are usually transmitted to an individual through inhalation into the lungs. Fungal infections may be mild, such as tinea pedis (athlete's foot), or severe, such as fungal disease of the lungs or fungal meningitis.

Fungal infections are also classified as *opportunistic* or *primary*. Opportunistic infections usually occur in the immunocompromised or debilitated population (e.g., patients who have cancer or AIDS) or in those taking antibiotics, corticosteroids, chemotherapy, or other immunosuppressive drugs. Fungi such as *Candida* species (yeast) are part of the normal flora of the mouth, skin, intestine, and vagina. An opportunistic infection, such as systemic candidiasis, may occur when the body's defense mechanisms are impaired such that they allow overgrowth of the fungus. Other opportunistic infections are aspergillosis, mucormycosis, *Pneumocystis* pneumonia, and fusariosis. Primary infections typically occur in immunocompetent persons and result from inhaled spores. Primary infections include coccidioidomycosis, blastomycosis, paracoccidioidomycosis, cryptococcosis, and histoplasmosis, including progressive disseminated histoplasmosis.

CLINICAL JUDGMENT [NURSING PROCESS]
Antitubercular Drugs

Concept: Drug Adherence
- The ability or lack of the ability to take drugs as prescribed

Concept: Safety
- Protection of the patient from potential or actual harm; a basic human need

Recognize Cues [Assessment]
- Assess for financial means to obtain drugs for tuberculosis (TB).
- Assess the means to follow up with the appropriate person.
- Determine any past instances of TB in the patient's health history—including the last purified protein derivative tuberculin test and the reaction or the serum interferon-gamma release assay result, the last chest radiograph and result, and the last ophthalmic examination—along with any allergies.
- Obtain a general medical history from the patient. Most antitubercular drugs are contraindicated if the patient has severe hepatic disease.
- Check laboratory results for liver function studies, bilirubin, blood urea nitrogen, and serum creatinine. These baseline values can be compared with future laboratory test results.
- Evaluate the patient for signs and symptoms of paresthesia (tingling, numbness, or burning).
- Assess for hearing changes if the antitubercular drug regimen includes streptomycin. Drug-induced ototoxicity is the major irreversible toxicity of aminoglycosides.

Analyze Cues and Prioritize Hypothesis [Patient Problems]
- Pulmonary infection

Generate Solutions [Planning]
- Patient will verbalize understanding for strict adherence to drug treatments.
- Patient will be free of symptoms of new infections.
- Patient will have a negative sputum test for acid-fast bacilli 2 to 3 months postantitubercular treatment.

Take Action [Nursing Interventions]
- Consult case management for financial help with drug treatment.
- Obtain initial follow-up appointment before discharge.
- If isoniazid (INH) is ordered, administer the drug 1 hour before or 2 hours after meals because food decreases the absorption rate. Other antitubercular drugs are given without regard to meals.
- Give pyridoxine (vitamin B_6) as prescribed with INH to prevent peripheral neuropathy.
- Monitor serum liver enzyme levels. Elevated levels may indicate liver toxicity.
- Collect sputum specimens for acid-fast bacilli early in the morning. Usually three consecutive morning sputum specimens are sent to the laboratory.
- Encourage eye examinations for patients taking INH and ethambutol because these antitubercular drugs may cause visual disturbances.
- Emphasize the importance of complying with the drug regimen.
- Tell patients who take INH to take the drug 1 hour before meals or 2 hours after meals for better absorption.
- ⚡ Direct patients to take antitubercular drugs as prescribed. Ineffective treatment and development of drug resistance might occur if drugs are taken intermittently or discontinued when symptoms are decreased or when the patient is feeling better. *Adherence to the drug regimen is essential to prevent the spread of drug-resistant* M. tuberculosis.
- Advise patients to keep medical appointments and to participate in sputum testing, which is important in evaluating the effectiveness of drug regimens.
- Warn patients contemplating pregnancy to first check with their health care provider about taking the antitubercular drugs ethambutol and rifampin.
- Increase access to health care. Community involvement and culturally sensitive patient education are important. Explain to patients who have active TB that family members should get a TB skin test and may receive a prophylactic drug for 6 months to 1 year. Emphasize the importance of family members seeking medical care.
- Provide a written sheet for drug and treatment regimens in the language the patient speaks or reads most easily. Explain the importance of good hygiene (e.g., discarding tissues that contain sputum, separating dishes, using a dishwasher to clean dishes if possible).
- Understand the significance of community if multiple individuals in the same community are treated for latent TB infection. Make all attempts to place

CLINICAL JUDGMENT [NURSING PROCESS]—CONT'D

Antitubercular Drugs

- community members on a treatment plan to increase compliance through social support.
- Instruct patients not to take antacids while taking antitubercular drugs because they decrease drug absorption. Patients should also avoid alcohol because it increases the risk of hepatotoxicity.
- Alert patients receiving ethambutol to take daily single doses to avoid visual problems. Divided doses of ethambutol may cause visual disturbances.
- Inform patients taking rifampin that urine, feces, saliva, sputum, sweat, and tears may turn a harmless red-orange color. Soft contact lenses may be permanently stained.
- Guide patients to report any numbness, tingling, or burning of hands and feet. Peripheral neuropathy is a common side effect of INH. Vitamin B_6 prevents peripheral neuropathy.
- Encourage patients to avoid direct sunlight to decrease the risk of photosensitivity. Patients should use a sunscreen with a minimum sun protection factor of 30 and ultraviolet A and B protection while in the sun.

Evaluate Outcomes [Evaluation]
- Evaluate the effectiveness of the antitubercular drugs. Sputum specimens for acid-fast bacilli should be negative after taking antitubercular drugs for several weeks or months.

Antifungals: Polyenes—Amphotericin B and Nystatin

Antifungals, also called antimycotics, are used to treat fungal infections. The antifungal drugs are classified into the following groups (Table 30.2). Typically, antifungals are fungistatic or fungicidal depending on the susceptibility of the fungus and the dosage.

Amphotericin B is a polyene antifungal and is used for severe, life-threatening systemic fungal infection is amphotericin B, which is effective against numerous fungal diseases that include histoplasmosis, cryptococcosis, coccidioidomycosis, aspergillosis, blastomycosis, zygomycosis, including mucormycosis, and systemic candidiasis. Polyene antifungals act by binding to the fungal cell membrane to form open channels that increase cell permeability and leakage of intracellular components, especially potassium. Because of its toxicity, amphotericin B is administered with close supervision. It must be given intravenously since the drug is not absorbed from the GI tract.

TABLE 30.2 Antifungal Drugs

Generic	Route and Dosage	Uses and Considerations
Polyenes		
Amphotericin B	CNS infections: A: IV: 0.25–0.3 mg/kg/d, may increase to 0.5–0.7 mg/kg/d, give slowly over 2–6 h using in-line filter and protected from light	For patients with potentially life-threatening fungal infections. Premedicate with an analgesic, antihistamine, antipyretic, antiemetic, and corticosteroid for infusion-related reactions. Hydrate prior to protect from nephrotoxicity. May cause headache, fever, chills, visual impairment, hearing loss, abdominal pain, nausea, vomiting, diarrhea, hypotension, injection site reaction, electrolyte imbalances, and elevated hepatic enzymes. PB: 90%–95%; t½: 24 h
Nystatin	See Prototype Drug Chart: Nystatin	
Azole Antifungals		
Fluconazole	See Prototype Drug Chart: Fluconazole	
Itraconazole	Fluconazole refractory oropharyngeal candidiasis: A: PO: 200 mg/d for up to 28 d TDM: Trough 1–2 mg/L Peak >4 mg/L	For a variety of fungal infections. Targets CYP450 enzymatic pathway. Contraindicated in coadministration with other drugs and in pregnancy. May cause headache, rhinitis, sinusitis, fever, rash, abdominal pain, nausea, vomiting, diarrhea, infection, and hypokalemia. Take with full meal. PB: 99%; t½: 16–28 h single dose, 34–42 h repeated dosing
Ketoconazole	Systemic: A: PO: 200–400 mg/d Tinea corporis/cruris: A: Topical: Apply a sufficient amount to affected and surrounding areas once daily for 2 wk	For a variety of fungal infections. May cause dizziness, drowsiness, headache, chills, fever, nausea, vomiting, diarrhea, nail/hair discoloration, vitamin D deficiency, hepatotoxicity, and QT prolongation. PB: 84–99%; t½: 2–8 h
Posaconazole	Oral candidiasis: Immediate-release suspension: A: PO: 100 mg bid for 1 d, then 100 mg/d for 13 d TDM: Trough: Prophylaxis >0.7 mcg/mL Treatment >1 mcg/mL	For prophylaxis and treatment of *Aspergillus* and *Candida* infections. May cause headache, cough, fever, abdominal pain, nausea, vomiting, diarrhea, anemia, rash, hypokalemia, and blood dyscrasias. Do not chew, divide, or crush. PB: >98%; t½: 20–66 h for immediate-release suspension

Continued

TABLE 30.2 Antifungal Drugs—cont'd

Generic	Route and Dosage	Uses and Considerations
Voriconazole	Candidiasis: A: PO: Weight-based dosing: 100–400 mg q12h A: IV: 6 mg/kg q12h on day 1, then 3–4 mg/kg q12h TDM: Trough 1–5.5 mg/L	For fungal infections including aspergillosis, candidiasis, fusariosis, cryptococcus, and scedosporiosis. Take PO 1 h before or after meals. May cause headache, fever, epistaxis, visual impairment, rash, hypokalemia, elevated hepatic enzymes, and hyperbilirubinemia. PB: 58%; t½: 6 h, after prolonged use 6 d
Isavuconazole	A: PO/IV: Initially 372 (isavuconazole 200 mg) q8h times 6, then 372 (isavuconazole 200 mg) daily for 6–12 wk	For aspergillosis. Do not chew, crush, dissolve, or open. May cause headache, anxiety, fatigue, abdominal pain, nausea, vomiting, diarrhea, constipation, pruritus, rash, hypomagnesemia, hypokalemia, peripheral edema, hepatotoxicity, elevated hepatic enzymes, and renal failure. Monitor electrolytes, LFTs, and BUN. PB: >99%; t½: 130 h
Antimetabolites		
Flucytosine	A: PO: 50–150 mg/kg/d in divided doses q6h; *max:* 150 mg/kg/d TDM: Peak <100 mcg/mL	Usually given in conjunction with amphotericin B for treatment of systemic candidiasis and cryptococcosis, to decrease the development of resistance to flucytosine. May cause headache, dry mouth, confusion, hearing loss, fatigue, anorexia, abdominal pain, nausea, vomiting, diarrhea, GI bleeding, and renal/hepatotoxicity. Monitor renal/LFTs. PB: 2%–4%; t½: 2.5–4 h
Echinocandins		
Anidulafungin	Esophageal candidiasis: A: IV: 100 mg loading dose on day 1, then 50 mg/d for 14–21 d Give 100 mg dose over 90 min	For *Candida* and *Aspergillus* infections. Infusion time is dose dependent. Monitor liver function tests. May cause insomnia, dyspnea, fever, nausea, vomiting, diarrhea, hypo/hypertension, peripheral edema, hypomagnesemia, and hypokalemia. PB: 99%; t½: 30–60 min
Caspofungin	A: IV: 70 mg on day 1, then 50 mg/d, give infusion over 1 h	For *Aspergillus* and *Candida* infections. Monitor CBC and LFTs. May cause headache, fever, chills, diarrhea, hypotension, rash, phlebitis, and injection site reaction. PB: 97%; t½: 9–50 h
Micafungin	Esophageal candidiasis: A: IV: 100–150 mg/d for 14-21 d, infuse over 1 h	For *Candida* infection. May cause headache, insomnia, abdominal pain, nausea, vomiting, diarrhea, hypokalemia, pruritus, rash, tachycardia, and thrombocytopenia. To minimize excessive foaming, do not vigorously shake the vial. PB: 99%; t½: 13–17.2 h
Rezafungin	A: IV: 400 mg one time, then 200 mg/wk	For candidiasis and candidemia. May cause headache, dizziness, fever, photosensitivity, abdominal pain, nausea, vomiting, diarrhea, constipation, infusion-related reactions, electrolyte imbalances, hypervolemia, and elevated hepatic enzymes. PB: UK; t½: 152 h
Miscellaneous Antifungals		
Griseofulvin	Tinea cruris/tinea barbae: Microsize: A: PO: 500 mg/d in divided doses Ultramicrosize A: PO: 375 mg/d in divided doses Give both until organism completely eradicated	For tinea infection. May cause headache, dizziness, confusion, fatigue, abdominal pain, nausea, vomiting, diarrhea, and GI bleeding. Give with a fatty meal to increase absorption. Tablets can be crushed and mixed with food; can be swallowed whole. Avoid during pregnancy and caution is advised while breastfeeding. PB: UK; t½: 9–24 h
Ibrexafungerp	A: PO: 300 mg q12h for 1 d	For vulvovaginal candidiasis. May cause headache, dizziness, fatigue, abdominal pain, nausea, vomiting, and diarrhea. PB: 99%; t½: 20 h

A, Adult; *bid,* twice daily; *CBC,* complete blood count; *CNS,* central nervous system; *CYP450,* cytochrome P450; *d,* day; *GI,* gastrointestinal; *h,* hour; *HIV,* human immunodeficiency virus; *IV,* intravenous; *max,* maximum; *min,* minute; *mo,* month; *PB,* protein binding; *PO,* by mouth; *PPI,* proton pump inhibitor; *q,* every; *t½,* half-life; *TDM,* therapeutic drug monitoring; *tid,* three times daily; *UK,* unknown; *wk,* weeks; *y,* year; >, greater than; ≥, greater than or equal to.

Nystatin is another polyene antifungal drug that is administered orally or topically to treat *Candida* infection. It is available in suspension, cream, and ointment forms. Nystatin is poorly absorbed by the GI tract. The more common use of nystatin is as an oral suspension for *Candida* infection of the mouth (oral thrush). The suspension is swished in the mouth for several minutes to ensure contact with the mucous membranes and then is either disposed of or swallowed. If the throat area is involved, the patient should also gargle with nystatin before swishing and swallowing or spitting. Prototype Drug Chart: Nystatin lists the data for nystatin.

Side Effects and Adverse Reactions

Side effects and adverse reactions for amphotericin B include fever, chills, flushing, loss of appetite, dizziness, nausea, vomiting, headache, shortness of breath, and tachypnea. These symptoms may occur 1 to 3 hours after the infusion has started. Pretreatment with acetaminophen, diphenhydramine, or hydrocortisone administered 30 to 60 minutes before infusion may alleviate these symptoms. In addition, patients may experience hypotension, paresthesia, and phlebitis. Amphotericin B is *highly toxic* and can cause nephrotoxicity and electrolyte imbalance, especially hypokalemia and hypomagnesemia (low serum potassium and magnesium levels). Urinary output, BUN, and serum creatinine levels must be closely monitored. Amphotericin B is also toxic to bone marrow; therefore complete blood counts (CBCs) should be monitored periodically.

Antifungals: Azole

The azole group is effective against candidiasis (local and systemic), coccidioidomycosis, cryptococcosis, histoplasmosis, and paracoccidioidomycosis. Ketoconazole was the first effective antifungal drug that was orally absorbed. Fluconazole, itraconazole, posaconazole, and voriconazole are other azole drugs used to treat systemic fungal infections. These antifungals can be taken orally, unlike amphotericin B and caspofungin, which are administered by the IV route only. Fluconazole, a systemic azole antifungal agent, is described in Prototype Drug Chart: Fluconazole.

Azoles inhibit cytochrome P450 (CYP450) in fungal cells, interfering with the formation of ergosterol. Because ergosterol is a major sterol in the fungal cell membrane, cell permeability and leakage are increased. Numerous azoles are used in topical preparations (e.g., creams, ointments, powders, shampoos, sprays, and solutions) to treat candidiasis and tinea infections. Azoles and other topical antifungal agents are presented in Table 30.2.

Antifungals: Antimetabolites and Echinocandins

The antimetabolite flucytosine acts by selectively penetrating the fungal cell, which converts the drug into fluorouracil, an antimetabolite that disrupts fungal DNA and RNA synthesis. Flucytosine is well absorbed from the GI tract, and it is used in combination with other antifungal drugs, such as amphotericin B. Antimetabolites are discussed further in Chapter 35.

Echinocandins are the newest class of antifungals. Three echinocandins are available in the United States: anidulafungin, caspofungin, and micafungin. The action of echinocandins is to inhibit biosynthesis of essential components of the fungal cell wall, which interferes with growth and reproduction of *Candida* and *Aspergillus* species. Echinocandins are administered intravenously because they are not absorbed in the GI tract. Phlebitis at the IV site and increased aspartate aminotransferase (AST) and alanine aminotransferase (ALT) are common adverse effects. Rapid infusion can cause histamine-mediated reactions.

> ### ⚡ PATIENT SAFETY
>
> **Amphotericin B**
> The two formulations of amphotericin B are amphotericin B deoxycholate and liposomal amphotericin B. Dosing for each formulation is different; therefore, caution is advised.

VIRUSES: PATHOPHYSIOLOGY

A **virus** is an obligate intracellular organism that must reside within a living host cell to survive and reproduce. Viruses enter healthy cells, live and reproduce within living cells, and use their DNA and RNA to generate more viruses. The growth cycle of viruses depends on host cell enzymes and cell substrates for viral replication. With the exception of HIV and certain kinds of viral hepatitis, viruses are self-limiting

📋 PROTOTYPE DRUG CHART
Nystatin

Drug Class	Dosage
Polyene antifungal	Candidiasis: A: PO susp: 400,000–600,000 units swished in the mouth then swallowed qid for 7–14 d A: Top: Apply to affected area bid until healed. A: PO tablets: 500,000–1 million units tid for at least 48 h
Contraindications	**Drug-Lab-Food Interactions**
Caution: Pregnancy, breastfeeding.	Drug: Avoid azole antifungals
Pharmacokinetics	**Pharmacodynamics**
Absorption: Poorly absorbed in the GI tract when given PO Absorption: Susp/top: Not absorbed from intact skin or mucous membranes Distribution: PB: Not subject to plasma PB Metabolism: t½: Not metabolized Excretion: PO: In feces, unchanged	PO: Onset symptom relief: 24–72 h; peak and duration: UK Susp/top: Onset, peak, and duration: UK
Therapeutic Effects/Uses	
To treat cutaneous and mucocutaneous mycotic infections including *Candida* and *Trichophyton* Mechanism of Action: Binds to sterols (ergosterol), causing the loss of intracellular potassium and other cellular contents	
Side Effects	**Adverse Reactions**
PO: Diarrhea, dyspepsia, nausea, vomiting, abdominal pain, rash, pruritus, skin irritation, urticaria, myalgia	Top/susp: Hypersensitivity reaction, tachycardia *Life-threatening:* Bronchospasm, Stevens-Johnson syndrome

A, Adult; *bid*, twice daily; *cap*, capsule; *d*, day; *GI*, gastrointestinal; *h*, hour; *PB*, protein binding; *PO*, by mouth; *qid*, four times a day; *susp*, suspension; *t½*, half-life; *tid*, three times daily; *top*, topical; *UK*, unknown.

illnesses that usually do *not* require treatment with a specific antiviral. Current antivirals target influenza, herpes, and hepatitis.

Influenza, commonly called *the flu*, is a highly contagious viral infection that causes mild to severe illness that can result in hospitalization or even death. Influenza is usually seasonal and is more prevalent from fall to spring. There are three main types of influenza: A, B, and C. *Influenza A* causes a moderate to severe infection. There are two subtypes of A found in humans, designated by the hemagglutinin (H) and neuraminidase (N) proteins. These subtypes (H1N1 and H3N2), found on the viral surface. *Influenza B* usually causes mild illness in children. Two strains are currently found in humans: B/Yamagata and B/Victoria. *Influenza C* infection is a mild respiratory illness not thought to cause epidemics. Influenza is transmitted easily via contaminated droplets during coughing, sneezing, or talking. Droplets enter into the respiratory tract of the unaffected person and begin replication 24 hours before the appearance of symptoms. Usually influenza has an abrupt onset, with the first symptoms being high fever, headache, fatigue, and myalgia (muscle aches). Chills; sore throat; nonproductive cough; watery nasal discharge; weakness; red, watery eyes; and photophobia can also occur.

Herpesviruses

Herpesviruses are large viruses that cause infections. Among the most familiar are herpes simplex virus type 1 (HSV-1) and type 2 (HSV-2); varicella-zoster viruses (HSV-3, or VZV), more commonly known as *chickenpox* and *shingles*; Epstein-Barr virus (EBV, or human herpesvirus 4 [HHV-4]); and cytomegalovirus (CMV, or human herpesvirus 5 [HHV-5]).

Herpes Simplex Virus Types 1 and 2

HSV-1 is usually associated with cold sores (vesicular lesions) and is capable of latency, the establishment and maintenance of latent infection in nerve cell ganglia proximal to the site of infection.

HSV-2 is usually associated with vesicular lesions and small ulcerations on the genitalia (genital herpes). The HSV-2 virus remains dormant by traveling through the peripheral nerves to the sacral dorsal nerve root ganglia. The reactivation and replication of latent HSV always occur in the area supplied by the ganglia in which latency was established. Reactivation can be induced by various factors that include fever, trauma, emotional stress, sunlight, and menstruation. Both HSV-1 and HSV-2 are capable of causing recurrent infections, and both can replicate in the mucous membranes and skin of the oropharynx or genitalia. Virus is transmitted by contact with infectious lesions or secretions. Signs and symptoms usually include eruption of small pustules and vesicles, fever, headache, malaise, myalgia, and tingling, itching, and pain in the affected area.

Varicella-Zoster Virus

VZV causes chickenpox and shingles. Chickenpox is a highly contagious viral infection that causes generalized pruritic vesicles and fever. Serious illness, hospitalizations, and deaths from VZV have decreased by 90% since vaccination began in 1995; however, some outbreaks still occur. When a person who has previously been infected with chickenpox becomes older or develops a weakened immune system, VZV that has lain dormant in nerve root ganglia can reactivate. The reactivation, called shingles, is a painful vesicular rash along the region of skin innervated by the nerve root ganglia, or dermatome, where the virus had lain dormant. In addition to the rash, the patient may also develop fever, malaise, myalgia, and pain along the involved dermatome.

PROTOTYPE DRUG CHART
Fluconazole

Drug Class	Dosage
Azole antifungal	Systemic candidiasis (candidemia): A: PO/IV: 800 mg on day 1, then 400 mg daily until 2 wks after symptoms resolved and is cleared from bloodstream Candidiasis, oropharyngeal: A: PO/IV: 200 mg on day 1, then 100 mg/d for at least 14 d
Contraindications	**Drug-Lab-Food Interactions**
Caution: Hypersensitivity, fever, QT prolongation, renal or hepatic disease, celiac disease, HF, cardiomyopathy, bradycardia, MI, CVA, HIV, hypokalemia, hypomagnesemia, hypocalcemia, hypothyroidism, hypothermia, fever, sleep deprivation, sickle cell disease, RA, SLE, females, older adults, neonates, pregnancy, breastfeeding	Drug: Because this drug inhibits the CYP450 isoenzyme, many drug-drug interactions are possible. Increases PT in patients taking warfarin; increases hypoglycemia when taken with oral sulfonylureas; increases phenytoin, cyclosporine, and haloperidol levels; decreases fluconazole level with cimetidine and rifampin; decreases the effect of clopidogrel; increases incidences of QT prolongation with cisapride, thioridazine, ondansetron, and other CYP3A4 substrates Food: May be administered without regard to food Herb: None significant
Pharmacokinetics	**Pharmacodynamics**
Absorption: PO: Oral administration with 90% bioavailability Distribution: PB: 11%–12% Metabolism: t½: 20–50 h; does not undergo first-pass metabolism Excretion: 80% in urine unchanged, 11% as metabolites	Lab: May increase LFTs PO: Onset: Rapid Peak: 1–2 h Duration: UK IV: Onset, peak, and duration: UK
Therapeutic Effects/Uses	
To treat *Candida* infections and cryptococcal meningitis; as prophylaxis for patients undergoing BMT or chemo/radiation therapy Mechanism of Action: Increases permeability of the fungal cell membrane by inhibiting ergosterol synthesis	
Side Effects	**Adverse Reactions**
PO: Dizziness, drowsiness, headache, insomnia, weakness, fatigue, fever, dry mouth, dysgeusia, dyspepsia, nausea, vomiting, diarrhea, abdominal pain, dyspepsia, rash, pruritus, jaundice, alopecia, myalgia, paresthesias, tremor	Seizures, anemia, adrenocortical insufficiency, elevated hepatic enzymes, hypokalemia, hypercholesterolemia, hypertriglyceridemia, *Life-threatening:* Anaphylaxis, angioedema, hepatotoxicity, leukopenia, neutropenia, agranulocytosis, thrombocytopenia, Stevens-Johnson syndrome, QT prolongation, torsade de pointes, renal failure, fatal cardiac arrhythmias, toxic epidermal necrolysis

A, Adult; *BMT*, bone marrow transplant; *CVA*, cerebralvascular accident; *CYP*, cytochrome P; *d*, day; *GI*, gastrointestinal; *HF*, heart failure; *h*, hour; *IV*, intravenous; *LFT*, liver function test; *MI*, myocardial infarction; *PB*, protein binding; *PO*, by mouth; *PT*, prothrombin time; *RA*, rheumatoid arthritis; *SLE*, systemic lupus erythematosus; *t½*, half-life; *UK*, unknown.

Epstein-Barr Virus

EBV most commonly causes infectious mononucleosis, a condition manifested by fever, fatigue, tonsillitis, and enlarged lymph nodes in the neck. EBV resides in lymphocytes, epithelial cells, and muscle cells and has a latency period.

Cytomegalovirus

CMV is a common viral infection that affects people of all ages. Most people infected with CMV do not exhibit symptoms and are unaware they have the virus. However, people with weakened immune systems (e.g., those with HIV, transplant recipients, and those taking immunosuppressant drugs), along with pregnant females, unborn babies, and neonates, are at risk for developing signs and symptoms (e.g., lymphadenopathy and splenomegaly). In susceptible individuals, CMV infection can lead to blindness (CMV retinitis) or fatal pneumonia.

Viral Hepatitis

Most viral hepatitis infections are caused by hepatitis B and C viruses (HBV and HCV, respectively). Many people with HBV and HCV are unaware they have the virus. These viruses can persist undetected for years, increasing the likelihood of transmitting the disease to others. HBV and HCV are blood-borne pathogens spread through blood and body fluids. They are the leading causes of hepatic cancer and the most common reason for hepatic failure and subsequent liver transplant. Signs and symptoms of viral hepatitis include fatigue, jaundice, abdominal pain, malaise, and nausea.

Non-HIV Antivirals: Influenza

Antiviral drugs are used to prevent or delay the spread of viral infections. They inhibit viral replication by interfering with viral nucleic acid synthesis in the cell. The non-HIV antiviral drugs are listed in Table 30.3. Some groups of antiviral drugs are effective against various viruses, such as influenzas A and B, herpesviruses, HBV and HCV, and HIV. Interferon alfa-2a and -2b used to treat HBV and HCV are discussed in Chapter 37. Drugs for HIV are discussed in Chapter 32.

Current recommendations for the treatment of influenza type A and B are oseltamivir or zanamivir. These are neuraminidase inhibitors, a group of drugs that decrease the release of the virus from infected cells by inhibiting the activity of neuraminidase, a viral glycoprotein, thus decreasing viral spread and shortening the duration of flu symptoms. Zanamivir and oseltamivir should be taken within 48 hours of flu symptoms, but they are *not* substitutes for the influenza vaccines. Due to high resistance among H3N2 and H1N1 strains, the CDC recommends that amantadine and rimantadine not be used for prophylaxis or treatment of currently circulating influenza A viruses.

CLINICAL JUDGMENT [NURSING PROCESS]
Antifungals

Concept: Drug Adherence
- The ability or lack of the ability to take drugs as prescribed

Concept: Safety
- Protection of the patient from potential or actual harm; is a basic human need

Recognize Cues [Assessment]
- Obtain a medical history that includes any serious renal or hepatic disorders. Antifungal agents such as amphotericin B, fluconazole, flucytosine, and ketoconazole are contraindicated if the patient has a serious renal or liver disease.
- Assess the ability to swallow. Oral candidiasis can impede swallowing, which can decrease appropriate nutritional intake.
- Check laboratory tests for liver function (alkaline phosphatase [ALP], alanine aminotransferase [ALT], aspartate aminotransferase [AST], gamma-glutamyl transferase), blood urea nitrogen (BUN), bilirubin, and serum creatinine because elevated levels can indicate liver or renal dysfunction. Use these test results for future comparisons.
- Assess any prior use of antifungals.

Analyze Cues and Prioritize Hypothesis [Patient Problems]
- Potential for nonadherence
- Potential for decreased tissue integrity
- Potential for decreased nutrition

Generate Solutions [Planning]
- Patient will list potential complications and when to call the medical provider.
- Patient will verbalize appropriate means to protect self from further injury.
- Patient will identify proper nutrition while on antifungals to prevent further injury and improve healing.

Take Action [Nursing Interventions]
- Obtain a culture to determine the fungus type (e.g., *Candida*).
- Monitor the patient's urinary output; many antifungal drugs can cause nephrotoxicity.
- Check laboratory results for BUN, serum creatinine, ALP, ALT, AST, bilirubin, and electrolytes and compare these with baseline findings. Certain antifungals can cause hepatotoxicity and nephrotoxicity when high doses are taken for an extended period.
- Record vital signs and compare these with baseline findings.
- Observe for side effects and adverse reactions to antifungal drugs, which may include nausea, vomiting, headache, phlebitis, and signs and symptoms of electrolyte imbalance.
- Advise patients to take drugs as prescribed. Compliance is of the utmost importance because discontinuing a drug too soon may result in relapse.
- Instruct patients to keep appointments to monitor laboratory testing of serum liver enzymes, BUN, creatinine, and electrolytes.
- Advise patients not to consume alcohol.
- Educate patients on proper administration of topical preparations.
- Respect the patient's apprehension and fear concerning the use of topical antifungal drugs and the desire to use alternative methods. Evaluate the patient's method of topical administration in regard to safe practice. If the method is considered unsafe, explain why and suggest modifications. If appropriate, involve other persons for clarification.
- Teach patients to avoid operating hazardous equipment or motor vehicles when taking antifungals that may cause visual changes, sleepiness, dizziness, or lethargy (e.g., amphotericin B, ketoconazole, or flucytosine).
- Encourage patients to report side effects such as nausea, vomiting, diarrhea, dermatitis, rash, dizziness, tinnitus, edema, and flatulence. These symptoms may occur when taking certain antifungal drugs.

Evaluate Outcomes [Evaluation]
- Evaluate the effectiveness of the antifungal drug by noting the diminishing or absence of the fungal infection.

TABLE 30.3 Non-HIV Antivirals

Generic	Route and Dosage	Uses and Considerations
Antivirals: Influenza		
Cidofovir	A: IV: 5 mg/kg/wk for 2 wks, give over 1 h with concurrent probenecid and hydration to minimize renal toxicity	For CMV, herpesvirus, and adenovirus infections. May cause headache, fever, weakness, nausea, vomiting, diarrhea, rash, infection, neutropenia, proteinuria, and nephrotoxicity. Use hazardous drug precautions. PB: <6%; t½: 2.6 h
Foscarnet	Acyclovir-resistant herpesvirus: A: IV: 40 mg/kg q8–12h for 2–3 wks or until lesions are healed, give infusion over 1 h	For CMV retinitis and acyclovir-resistant mucocutaneous HSV. May cause headache, fever, nausea, vomiting, diarrhea, blood dyscrasias, electrolyte imbalance, and nephrotoxicity. Patient must be hydrated with 750 to 1000 mL 0.9% NS prior and during treatment to minimize renal toxicity. Monitor renal function. PB: 14%–17%; t½: 3.3–6.8 h
Oseltamivir	Influenza A & B treatment: A: PO: 75 mg bid for 5 d Prophylaxis: A: PO: 75 mg daily for at least 10 d up to wks, start within 48 h of exposure or symptom onset	For prevention and treatment of acute uncomplicated seasonal influenza A and B virus infections. May cause headache, nausea, vomiting, diarrhea, and dermatitis. Monitor renal function. PB: 3%, t½: 1–3 h
Zanamivir	Treatment: Inhaler: A: 2 oral inhalations (5 mg/inhalation) bid for 5 d Prophylaxis: A: 2 oral inhalations (5 mg/inhalation) once daily for 10 d	For treatment of uncomplicated influenzas A and B, as well as prophylaxis. Treatment should begin within 36 h of exposure or 48 h of onset of symptoms. Take bronchodilators before zanamivir when taking drugs concurrently. May cause headache, cough, chills, fatigue, malaise, and infection. PB: <10%; t½: 2.5–5 h
Peramivir	A: IV: 600 mg as single dose within 48 h symptom onset, give over 15–30 min	For treatment of uncomplicated influenzas A and B. May cause insomnia, vomiting, diarrhea, constipation, hypertension, hyperglycemia, neutropenia, elevated hepatic enzymes, and proteinuria. PB: <30%; t½: 20 h
Baloxavir marboxil	A >80 kg: PO: 80 mg as single dose A <80 kg: PO: 40 mg as single dose Both within 48 h of symptom onset	For treatment and prophylaxis of uncomplicated influenzas A and B. May cause headache, sinusitis, nausea, vomiting, and diarrhea. Gently swirl suspension, do not shake. Avoid coadministration with dairy products, calcium fortified beverages, laxatives, antacids, oral supplements of calcium, iron, magnesium, zinc, and selenium. PB: 92.9%; t½: 79.1 h
Antivirals: Herpes Species		
Acyclovir	See Prototype Drug Chart: Acyclovir	Also available as a topical
Famciclovir	Herpes zoster: A: PO: 500 mg q8h for 7 d, give within 48 h of rash onset	For herpes zoster and herpes simplex virus. May cause headache, fatigue, abdominal pain, nausea, vomiting, diarrhea, flatulence, and dysmenorrhea. Monitor renal function. PB: <20%; t½: 2–3 h
Ganciclovir	CMV retinitis: A: IV: 5 mg/kg/dose q 12 h for 14–21 d	For treatment and prophylaxis of CMV infection in immunocompromised patients, herpes simplex, varicella zoster, and human herpesvirus. May cause blurred vision, fever, anorexia, diarrhea, infection, and blood dyscrasias. Monitor renal/liver function, CBC, and ophthalmic exam. PB: 1%–2%; t½: 3.5 h
Penciclovir	A: Topical: Apply q2h while awake for 4 d	For recurrent herpes labialis (cold sores). May cause headache, dysgeusia, rash pruritus, erythema, skin discoloration, and paresthesias. Start at onset of symptoms. Do not administer on or near eyes or to mucous membranes. PB: UK; t½: UK
Trifluridine	A: Ophthal: 1 gtt q2h to each affected eye while awake until corneal ulcer completely re-epithelialized, then 1 gtt in affected eye q4h while awake (minimum 5 gtts/d) for 7 d; max: 9 gtts/d, not to exceed 21 d treatment	For HSV including keratoconjunctivitis. May cause ocular irritation/hypertension, corneal edema, and blepharedema. Remove contact lenses before use. If more than one ophthalmic drug is used, separate instillations by at least 5–10 min. Store under refrigeration. PB: UK; t½: 12 min
Valacyclovir	Herpes simplex labialis A: PO: 2 g q12h for 1 d at first sign of cold sore Herpes zoster (shingles): A: PO: 1 g tid for 7 d, give within 1 h rash onset	For varicella zoster and HSV. May cause headache, pharyngitis, abdominal pain, nausea, neutropenia, and elevated hepatic enzymes. Monitor renal function. PB: 14%–18%; t½: 2.5–3.3 h

TABLE 30.3 Non-HIV Antivirals—cont'd

Generic	Route and Dosage	Uses and Considerations
Valganciclovir	CMV retinitis: A: PO: 900 mg q12h for 14–21 d CMV prophylaxis: A: PO: 900 mg once daily, start within 10 d after transplant	For CMV disease prophylaxis in transplant recipients and CMV retinitis in AIDS patients. May cause headache, fever, insomnia, nausea, vomiting, diarrhea, tremor, and blood dyscrasias. Monitor kidney function. Monitor CBC. Do not crush or break tablets. Oral solution is not recommended for adults and should not be mixed with other liquids. PB: 1%–2% as ganciclovir; t½: 2.8–6 h
Letermovir	A: PO/IV: 480 mg/d Start between day 0–28 posttransplant until day 100, may continue to day 200 for late CMV infection	For CMV prophylaxis. May cause headache, nausea, vomiting, diarrhea, anemia, peripheral edema, neutropenia, and thrombocytopenia. PB: 99%; t½: 12 h
Maribavir	A: PO: 400 mg bid	For CMV refractory to treatment with ganciciovit, valganciclovir, cidofovir, or foscarnet. May cause dysgeusia, fatigue, nausea, vomiting, diarrhea, decreased hemoglobin/platelets, infection, and increased creatinine. PB: UK; t½: 4.3 h
Antivirals: Hepatitis		
Adefovir	A: PO: 10 mg/d	For chronic HBV, used in combination with lamivudine. May cause headache, weakness, abdominal pain, dyspepsia, nausea, diarrhea, flatulence, and hepatitis B exacerbation. Monitor renal/liver function and HBV serology. PB: <4%; t½: 7.5 h
Entecavir	A: PO: 0.5–1 mg/d	For chronic HBV. Take 2 h before or after a meal. May cause fever, peripheral edema, ascites, infection, elevated hepatic enzymes, and hepatic encephalopathy. Follow hazardous drug precautions. Monitor liver function and HBV DNA viral load. PB: 13%; t½: 128–149 h
Lamivudine	HBV without HIV: A: PO: 100 mg/d HBV with HIV: A: PO: 150 mg bid or 300 mg/d	For HBV and HIV combination treatment. May cause headache, fever, malaise, fatigue, nausea, infection, and elevated hepatic enzymes. Monitor glucose, CBC, LFTs, and cholesterol. PB: 36%; t½: 13–19 h
Ledipasvir/sofosbuvir	A: PO: ledipasvir 90 mg/sofosbuvir 400 mg fixed dose tab; 1 tab daily for 8–12 wks	For chronic HCV. May cause headache, cough, dyspnea, weakness, fatigue, irritability, nausea, diarrhea, and myalgia. Monitor liver function, HCV RNA concentration, and renal function. Must be taken with food. PB: ledipasvir 99.8%, sofosbuvir 61%–65% t½: ledipasvir 47 h, sofosbuvir 0.4 h
Peginterferon alfa-2a	HBV: A: Subcut: 180 mcg/wk for 48 wks HCV: A: Subcut: 180 mcg/wk for 12 wks	For HBV and HCV. May cause fever, weakness, fatigue, nausea, vomiting, myalgia, injection site reaction, elevated hepatic enzymes, hypertriglyceridemia, and lymphopenia. PB: UK; t½: 50–140 h
Ribavirin	HBV: Dependent upon weight Other dosing regimens are available	For HCV and RSV. Contraindicated during pregnancy. May cause headache, weakness, fatigue, fever, anxiety, irritability, nausea, vomiting, injection site reaction, myalgia, and anemia. Do not open, crush, or chew capsules; give with food. Use hazardous drug precautions. PB: 0%; t½: capsule single dose 44 h; tablet single dose 120–170 h
Sofosbuvir	A: PO: 400 mg once daily for 12–24 wks	For chronic HCV as combination therapy, monotherapy is not recommended. May cause headache, weakness, fatigue, insomnia, nausea, pruritus, and anemia. Monitor HCV RNA and renal/liver function. PB: 61%–65%; t½: 0.4 h
Tenofovir disoproxil	HBV: A: PO: 300 mg once daily	For chronic HBV and HIV. Monotherapy not recommended. May cause headache, dizziness, weakness, insomnia, abdominal pain, nausea, vomiting, diarrhea, and hypercholesterolemia. Monitor CBC, renal/liver function, cholesterol, and pregnancy. PB: Minimal; t½: 17 h

A, Adult; *AIDS*, acquired immunodeficiency syndrome; *bid*, twice daily; *CBC*, complete blood count; *CMV*, cytomegalovirus; *gtt*, drops; *h*, hour; *HBV*, hepatitis B virus; *HCV*, hepatitis C virus; *HIV*, human immunodeficiency virus; *HSV*, herpes simplex virus; *IM*, intramuscular; *IV*, intravenous; *LFT*, liver function test; *max*, maximum; *min*, minutes; *mo*, month; *NA*, not applicable; *NS*, normal saline; *Ophthal*, ophthalmic solution; *PB*, protein binding; *PO*, by mouth; *q*, every; *RSV*, respiratory syncytial virus; *subcut*, subcutaneous; *t½*, half-life; *tab*, tablet; *tid*, three times daily; *UK*, unknown; *wk*, weeks; *y*, year; >, greater than; ≥, greater than or equal to; <, less than.

Side Effects and Adverse Reactions

The side effects and adverse reactions of these two neuraminidase inhibitors include dizziness, headache, fatigue, and GI disturbances such as nausea, vomiting, and diarrhea. ⚡ Nurses must be aware of a US Food and Drug Administration (FDA) advisory that persons receiving oral oseltamivir should be monitored closely for abnormal behavior. Incidence of self-injury and delirium have been reported in postmarketing surveillance.

PROTOTYPE DRUG CHART
Acyclovir

Drug Class	Dosage
Nucleotide analog antiviral	Herpes genitalis: Initial infection A: PO: 200 mg q4h for 7–10 days. A: IV: 5 mg/kg/dose over 1 h q8h for 5 d Herpes zoster (shingles): A: PO: 800 mg 5 times/d for 7–10 d Varicella (chickenpox): A: PO: 800 mg q4h for 5 d at first sign of symptoms

Contraindications	Drug-Lab-Food Interactions
Known hypersensitivity to acyclovir, valacyclovir, and milk protein *Caution:* Renal/hepatic impairment, electrolyte imbalance, dehydration, neurological disorder, seizure disorder, immunosuppression, obesity, older adults, children, breastfeeding	Drug: Increased nephrotoxicity with aminoglycosides, probenecid, and ibuprofen; decreases effect of phenytoin; increases serum concentrations of other antivirals (e.g., tenofovir, entecavir) Lab: May increase AST, ALT, serum creatinine, BUN Food: Food does not affect absorption. Herb: None significant

Pharmacokinetics	Pharmacodynamics
Absorption: PO: Poorly absorbed, 10%–30% Distribution: PB: 9%–33% Metabolism: t½: PO: 2.5–3.3 h Excretion: Unchanged in urine (90%–92%)	PO: Onset: UK; peak: 1.5–2.5 h; duration: UK IV: Onset: UK; peak: 1 h; duration: UK

Therapeutic Effects/Uses
To treat herpes simplex type 1 and 2 and varicella-zoster viruses
Mechanism of Action: Inhibits viral DNA synthesis and inhibits viral DNA polymerase and viral DNA chain; inactivates viral DNA polymerase

Side Effects	Adverse Reactions
Stomatitis, anorexia, nausea, vomiting, diarrhea, headache, lethargy, rash, skin irritation, pruritus, phlebitis, injection site reaction, malaise	Leukopenia, hepatitis, elevated hepatic enzymes, kidney dysfunction, agitation, hemolytic uremic syndrome, and TTP *Life-threatening:* Coma, seizures, Steven-Johnsons syndrome, toxic epidermal necrolysis, and erythema

A, Adult; *ALT*, alanine aminotransferase; *AST*, aspartate aminotransferase; *BUN*, blood urea nitrogen; *d*, day; *h*, hour; *HSV*, herpes simplex virus; *IV*, intravenous; *mo*, months; *PB*, protein binding; *PO*, by mouth; *q*, every; *t½*, half-life; *TTP*, thrombotic thrombocytopenic purpura; *UK*, unknown.

Non-HIV Antivirals: Herpes Antivirals

The synthetic purine nucleoside antiviral group is effective in interfering with the steps of viral nucleic acid (DNA) synthesis. Drugs in this group of nucleoside analogues include ribavirin, acyclovir, famciclovir, ganciclovir sodium, valacyclovir, and valganciclovir. These drugs are effective in managing herpes simplex viruses (HSV-1, HSV-2) and VZV (chickenpox and shingles).

Acyclovir, famciclovir, and valacyclovir appear equally effective in the treatment of initial episodes and recurrent episodes of genital herpes, but famciclovir appears somewhat less effective for suppression of viral shedding. Topical antivirals for herpes simplex viruses include acyclovir, penciclovir, and trifluridine.

Non-HIV Antivirals: Cytomegalovirus Antivirals

Four antivirals are effective in treating CMV retinitis in persons with acquired immunodeficiency syndrome (AIDS): ganciclovir, valganciclovir, cidofovir, and foscarnet. Ganciclovir and valganciclovir are synthetic purine nucleoside analogues. Ganciclovir was the first drug approved for treatment of CMV retinitis. Cidofovir is a nucleotide analogue that suppresses viral replication by inhibiting DNA polymerase. Foscarnet selectively inhibits viral-specific DNA polymerases and reverse transcriptases. Due to the emergence of drug resistance, many times it is necessary to use a combination of agents to effectively manage CMV retinitis (Prototype Drug Chart: Acyclovir).

Side Effects and Adverse Reactions

A limiting factor in all antiviral therapy for CMV and herpes is hematologic toxicity. All patients should be closely monitored for signs of bone marrow suppression and toxicity, including thrombocytopenia, granulocytopenia, and leukopenia. In addition, all antivirals should be dose adjusted in the setting of kidney dysfunction. Kidney function should be closely monitored during drug therapy because acute kidney failure can occur.

Side effects and adverse reactions to antiviral drugs include nausea, vomiting, and diarrhea; headache; dizziness; rash and pruritus; and hematuria. In addition, when antiviral drugs are administered IV, extravasation may lead to sloughing of the skin. Topical preparations can cause local irritations, and contact lenses should be removed before instilling ophthalmic antivirals.

Non-HIV Antivirals: Hepatitis Antivirals

Viral hepatitis can be caused by at least five distinct viruses that affect the liver: hepatitis A virus (HAV), HBV, HCV, hepatitis D (delta hepatitis, HDV), and hepatitis E. Hepatitis A and E are self-limiting illnesses and do not usually require antiviral therapy. HBV and HCV can develop into chronic hepatitis; individuals with HBV can be coinfected with HDV. The CDC and the World Health Organization have developed guidelines for screening, treatment, and surveillance of persons with HBV and HCV. Currently, HAV and HBV are vaccine preventable. Vaccines are discussed in Chapter 34.

No specific therapy exists for people with acute HBV. Instead, treatment is mostly supportive. Antivirals are given for people with chronic HBV and signs of liver disease progression to attempt to suppress viral replication and potentially halt liver disease and liver-related deaths. Treatment with antivirals is recommended for all people with chronic HBV who are at high risk of disease progression regardless of age. Currently, five antiviral drugs are approved for this indication: lamivudine, adefovir, entecavir, tenofovir, and peginterferon alfa-2a. Except for peginterferon alfa-2a, all of these are nucleoside analogues, and all have been shown to delay the progression of liver disease (e.g., cirrhosis, hepatic carcinoma). Adefovir inhibits

CLINICAL JUDGMENT [NURSING PROCESS]
Antiviral: Acyclovir

Concept: Infection
- The introduction of pathogen eliciting an immune response

Concept: Safety
- Protection of the patient from potential or actual harm; is a basic human need

Recognize Cues [Assessment]
- Obtain a medical history from the patient that includes any serious renal or hepatic diseases.
- Determine baseline vital signs and obtain a complete blood count (CBC). Use these findings for comparisons with future results.
- Assess baseline laboratory results, particularly blood urea nitrogen (BUN), serum creatinine, liver function studies, bilirubin, and electrolytes. Use these results for future comparisons.
- Evaluate baseline vital signs and urine output. Report abnormal findings.

Analyze Cues and Prioritize Hypothesis [Patient Problems]
- Decreased immunity

Generate Solutions [Planning]
- Patient will exhibit decreased symptoms of viral infections.

Take Action [Nursing Interventions]
- Check the patient's CBC. Report abnormal results (leukopenia, thrombocytopenia, low hemoglobin, and hematocrit).
- Monitor other laboratory tests (BUN, serum creatinine, liver function studies); compare with baseline values.
- Record the patient's urinary output. An antiviral drug such as acyclovir can affect renal function.
- Monitor vital signs, especially blood pressure. Acyclovir may cause hypotension.
- Observe for signs and symptoms of side effects. Most antiviral drugs have many side effects.
- Check for superimposed infection (superinfection) caused by high doses and prolonged use of an antiviral drug such as acyclovir.
- Administer oral acyclovir as prescribed. Oral doses can be taken at mealtime.
- Dilute the antiviral drug in an appropriate amount of solution as indicated in the drug circular when giving intravenously. Administer intravenous (IV) drug over 60 minutes. Never give acyclovir as a bolus (IV push).
- Advise patients to maintain adequate fluid intake to ensure sufficient hydration for drug therapy and to increase urine output.
- Instruct patients with genital herpes to avoid spreading infection by practicing sexual abstinence or by using condoms correctly and consistently. Patients must be aware that although condoms reduce the transmission of disease, they may not eliminate it. Advise females with genital herpes to have a Pap test done as indicated by their health care provider. Cervical cancer is more prevalent in females with genital herpes simplex.
- Teach non-English-speaking patients and family members how to properly use antivirals by providing materials in the patient's first language. Pictures may be helpful.
- Guide patients to report adverse reactions, including a decrease in urine output and central nervous system changes such as dizziness, anxiety, or confusion.
- Warn patients with dizziness resulting from orthostatic hypotension to arise slowly from a sitting to a standing position.
- Tell patients to report any side effects associated with the antiviral drug; this may include nausea and vomiting, diarrhea, increased bleeding time, rash, and urticaria.

Evaluate Outcomes [Evaluation]
- Evaluate the effectiveness of the antiviral drug in eliminating the virus or in decreasing symptoms.
- Determine whether any side effects are present.

---

reverse transcription, entecavir inhibits several major stages of viral replication, and lamivudine and tenofovir inhibit the synthesis of viral DNA; however, no antiviral therapy cures HBV. Lamivudine and adefovir are no longer the preferred agents in the treatment of HBV.

Hepatitis C is more prevalent among people who inject drugs. HCV is an RNA virus, whereas HBV is a DNA virus. As with HBV, HCV can cause chronic infection that leads to liver cirrhosis, liver failure, and hepatic carcinoma. No vaccine against HCV is currently available. In addition to peginterferon alfa-2a, NS5A inhibitors (e.g., ledipasvir) and polymerase inhibitors (e.g., sofosbuvir) can treat HCV. Many of these antivirals are prepackaged as combination therapy.

Persons with HCV should have genotype testing; HCV has 6 genotypes and more than 50 subtypes, and genotyping can help predict treatment response and duration of treatment. For example, genotypes 2 and 3 respond better to peginterferon alfa-2a or a combination of peginterferon alfa-2a and ribavirin than does genotype 1. Genotypes 2 and 3 only need 24 months of treatment, whereas genotype 1 requires 48 months. Genotype 1 is the most common genotype in the United States. The Infectious Diseases Society of America (IDSA) and the American Association for the Study of Liver Diseases (AASLD) have published treatment guidelines based on genotype (see https://www.hcvguidelines.org).

Table 30.3 lists the antivirals, uses, and considerations for viral hepatitis. Chapter 32 further illustrates nucleoside analogues.

Side Effects and Adverse Effects

Side effects range from mild to life-threatening. Transient exacerbations of viral hepatitis can occur if antivirals are suddenly stopped. HBV and HCV can become resistant to antivirals; therefore routine monitoring of renal and hepatic functions is warranted in addition to monitoring viral load. Nucleoside analogues can cause hepatotoxicity or lactic acidosis, and dose adjustments are recommended in patients with renal impairment. Side effects for peginterferon include depression, fatigue, flulike symptoms, pancytopenia, alopecia, arthralgia, myalgia, anorexia, dysgeusia, thyroid dysfunction, and infection. Ophthalmic dysfunction can also occur (e.g., papilledema, vasculature obstruction). Ribavirin is teratogenic and can also cause hemolytic anemia, and protease inhibitors can cause skin reactions and dysgeusia.

CLINICAL JUDGMENT CASE STUDY

A 41-year-old homeless male has had a constant cough and night sweats for several months. He consumes about a fifth of liquor over 2 days. Acid-fast bacilli (AFB) smear on the sputum is positive. The health care provider orders a 6- to 9-month antitubercular drug regimen, with the time of therapy to be determined according to sputum and radiograph test results. For 2 months, the patient takes isoniazid (INH), rifampin, and pyrazinamide daily. For the next 4 to 7 months, he takes INH and rifampin biweekly.

1. What are some of the patient's risk factors for contracting tuberculosis (TB)? Give other risk factors for contracting TB.
2. The patient received first-line antitubercular drugs for treatment of TB. How can the health professional determine whether the drugs are effective in eradicating the bacillus *Mycobacterium tuberculosis*? Explain your answer.
3. What is the nurse's role in patient teaching concerning the drug regimen?
4. Name at least two serious adverse reactions that can occur when antitubercular drugs are given over an extended period.
5. What laboratory tests should the nurse monitor while the patient takes isoniazid and rifampin? Why?
6. The health care provider orders pyridoxine to be given daily. Give the rationale for the use of pyridoxine.

REVIEW QUESTIONS

1. A patient is beginning isoniazid and rifampin treatment for tuberculosis. The nurse gives the patient which instruction?
   a. Do not skip doses.
   b. Take both drugs three times daily.
   c. Take an antacid with the drugs.
   d. Take rifampin initially.
2. A patient taking isoniazid is worried about the negative effects of the drug. The nurse provides information knowing that which is an adverse effect of the drug?
   a. Ototoxicity
   b. Hepatotoxicity
   c. Nephrotoxicity
   d. Optic nerve toxicity
3. The nurse teaches a patient taking amphotericin B to report which signs and symptoms to the health care provider?
   a. Change in sight
   b. Decrease in hearing
   c. Decrease in urine
   d. Painful red rash and blisters
4. A patient has been diagnosed with tuberculosis and will begin antitubercular therapy with isoniazid, rifampin, and ethambutol. Which actions are appropriate for the nurse to do? (**Select all that apply.**)
   a. Encourage periodic eye examinations.
   b. Instruct the patient to take medications with meals.
   c. Suggest that the patient take antacids with medications to prevent gastrointestinal distress.
   d. Advise the patient to report numbness and tingling of the hands or feet.
   e. Alert the patient that body fluids may develop a red-orange color.
   f. Teach the patient to avoid direct sunlight and to use sunblock.
5. Zanamivir is ordered for a patient with which disorder?
   a. Herpes simplex virus type 2
   b. Herpes simplex virus type 1
   c. Varicella-zoster virus
   d. Influenza
6. Acyclovir has been ordered for a patient with genital herpes. Which nursing interventions are appropriate for this patient? (**Select all that apply.**)
   a. Monitor the patient's blood urea nitrogen and creatinine.
   b. Monitor the patient's blood pressure for hypertension.
   c. Administer intravenous acyclovir over 30 minutes.
   d. Advise maintenance of adequate fluid intake.
   e. Monitor complete blood count for blood dyscrasias.
7. A mother of two children was just diagnosed with hepatitis C virus. Which of the following is *incorrect* about hepatitis C virus?
   a. A vaccine has been available for 5 years.
   b. Hepatitis C virus can be transmitted by blood and body fluids.
   c. Hepatitis C virus can cause hepatic carcinoma.
   d. Persons with hepatitis C virus can become chronic carriers.

31

Antimalarials, Anthelmintics, and Peptides

http://evolve.elsevier.com/McCuistion/pharmacology

OBJECTIVES

- Relate the various aspects of the usage of antimalarial drugs.
- Interpret the various aspects of the usage of anthelmintic drugs.
- Relate principles of nursing care to the use of peptides.

OUTLINE

Antimalarial Drugs, 369
    Malarial Drug Treatment, 369
    Side Effects and Adverse Reactions, 370
Anthelmintic Drugs, 372
    Anthelmintics Drug Treatment, 372
    Side Effects and Adverse Reactions, 374
Peptides, 374

Colistimethate, 375
Polymyxins, 376
Bacitracin, 377
Metronidazole, 377
Clinical Judgment Case Study, 379
Review Questions, 379

ANTIMALARIAL DRUGS

Malaria is a life-threatening disease that was eliminated from the United States in the early 1950s. Since that time, about 2000 to 2500 cases of malaria have been diagnosed each year in the United States. An estimated 247 million cases of malaria occurred worldwide, and 619,000 people died, mostly children in the sub-Saharan African region (https://www.WHO.int/malaria). Malaria is caused by multiple species of protozoan parasites of the genus *Plasmodium* that are carried by infected *Anopheles* mosquitoes, and it remains one of the most prevalent protozoan diseases. After the mosquito infects humans, the protozoan parasite passes through two phases: the tissue phase and the erythrocytic phase. The tissue phase (invasion of body tissue) produces no clinical symptoms in humans, but the erythrocytic phase (invasion of the red blood cells) causes symptoms of chills, fever, and sweating. The incubation period is 10 to 35 days, followed by flu-like symptoms. Preventing transmission of malaria can be done by controlling the mosquito first through insecticide-treated mosquito nets and second with spraying.

There are approximately 50 species of *Plasmodium*, 5 of which cause malaria: *P. malariae, P. ovale, P. vivax,* and *P. falciparum. Plasmodium vivax* is the most prevalent, whereas *P. falciparum* is the most severe. Despite having more than 200 million cases of malaria globally, in the United States malaria is confined mainly to persons who enter the country after having traveled abroad, primarily because of travel to regions in the world where malaria is endemic and drug-resistant malaria parasites have evolved (www.WHO.int).

Malarial Drug Treatment

Treatment of malaria depends on the type of *Plasmodium* and the organism's life cycle. Quinine was the only antimalarial drug available from 1820 until the early 1940s. Antimalarial drugs provide treatment and prophylaxis, and synthetic antimalarial drugs have since been developed that are as effective as quinine and cause fewer toxic effects (www.CDC.gov/malaria). When drug-resistant malaria occurs, combinations of antimalarials are used to facilitate effective treatment. Chloroquine is a commonly prescribed drug for malaria. Antimicrobial resistance to chloroquine therapy is widespread, so it is critical to determine whether chloroquine is appropriate for use. If drug resistance occurs to chloroquine, other antimalarials or combinations of antimalarials with or without antibiotics (e.g., tetracycline, aminoglycosides, fluoroquinolones) (see Chapter 28) may be prescribed.

Three methods used to eradicate malaria are prophylaxis (prevention), treatment for the acute attack, and prevention of relapse. Many synthetic antimalarials, including chloroquine and primaquine, are used prophylactically. Chloroquine and mefloquine are frequently used to treat an acute malarial attack.

(Table 31.1) lists commonly ordered antimalarial drugs and their dosage, uses, and considerations.

Pharmacokinetics

Chloroquine is well absorbed from the gastrointestinal (GI) tract. It is moderately protein binding, and the drug has a long half-life. Chloroquine is metabolized in the liver to active metabolites and is largely excreted in the urine, with small amounts in the feces. The elimination half-life is 108 to 291 hours. This drug has two absolute contraindications: chloroquine hypersensitivity and ocular disease. Antimalarial drugs concentrate first in the liver; if the patient drinks large amounts of alcohol or has a liver disorder, the liver enzymes will require closer monitoring. Renal impairment may also occur as an adverse effect of antimalarials.

PROTOTYPE DRUG CHART

Antimalarial

Drug Class Antimalarial Drugs	Dosage
Chloroquine (4-aminoquinoline antiprotozoal agent)	Malaria treatment (uncomplicated): A: PO: 16.6 mg (10 mg base) kg/dose. Max: 1,000 mg/dose (600 mg base/dose) in 6-8 h, then 8.3 (5 mg base) kg/dose. Max: 500 mg/dose (300 mg base/dose) once daily for 2 days. Malaria prophylaxis: A: PO: 500 mg weekly (300 mg/base), beginning 1–2 wks before entry and continuing for 4 wks after visiting endemic area. Max: A: PO: 1,000 mg/d (600 mg base/d)

Contraindications	Drug-Lab-Food Interactions
Chloroquine hypersensitivity and ocular disease (retinal and visual field changes) *Caution:* Cardiomyopathy, heart failure, renal disease, psoriasis, alcoholism, G6PD deficiency, hepatic disease, GI disease, neurologic disorders (seizures), increased sensitivity to the sun, hearing impairment, hypokalemia, and hypoglycemia	Use appropriately to avoid chloroquine antimicrobial resistance. Multiple drug-drug interactions; please refer to drug reference. Drug: Increases effects of digoxin, neuromuscular blockers; decreased absorption with antacids and laxatives. Monitor Labs: Blood glucose, CBC, ophthalmic exam, and ECG Food: Take with food to avoid GI upset.

Pharmacokinetics	Pharmacodynamics
Absorption: Well absorbed from GI tract Distribution: Widely distributed into body tissue PB: 55% Metabolism: in the liver Excretion: Excreted slowly in urine, feces, breast milk; crosses placenta	Onset: Rapid Peak: 1–2 h Duration: Days to weeks t½: 108–291 h

Therapeutic Effects/Uses

Treatment and prophylaxis of uncomplicated malaria due to susceptible strains of *Plasmodium: P. falciparum, P. knowlesi, P. ovale, P. malariae,* and *P. vivax.*
Mechanism of action: Chloroquine, a 4-aminoquinoline, is an antiprotozoal agent. The precise mechanism is unknown. Chloroquine may exert its effect against *Plasmodium* species by concentrating in the acid vesicles of the parasite and by inhibiting polymerization of heme. It can also inhibit certain enzymes by its interaction with DNA.

Side Effects	Adverse Reactions
Anorexia, nausea, vomiting, diarrhea, abdominal cramps, fatigue, pruritus, headache, nervousness, visual impairment, insomnia, photosensitivity, hair discoloration, skin and eyes may appear yellowish	Extrapyramidal reaction, Stevens-Johnson syndrome, toxic epidermal necrolysis, DRESS syndrome, heart block, cardiac arrhythmia, ECG changes, hypotension, psychosis, dermatologic reactions (pruritus, urticaria), seizures; may cause dizziness, so use caution driving a vehicle; avoid sun exposure. *Life-threatening:* Loss of consciousness, agranulocytosis, aplastic anemia, corneal opacity, macular degeneration, thrombocytopenia, ototoxicity, cardiovascular collapse, anaphylactic shock

CBC, Complete blood count; *d,* day; *ECG,* electrocardiogram; *GI,* gastrointestinal; *h,* hour; *max,* maximum; *PO,* by mouth; *t½,* half-life; *wk,* week.

Pharmacodynamics

Chloroquine, an antiprotozoal agent, inhibits the malaria parasite's growth by interfering with protein synthesis. The onset of action for chloroquine is rapid. The duration of effect of the drug is very long, from days to weeks.

Side Effects and Adverse Reactions

General side effects and adverse reactions to antimalarials include GI upset, retinal damage, cranial nerve VIII involvement, renal impairment, and cardiovascular effects. The manufacturer of malarial drugs indicates these drugs have been shown to be active against most strains of microorganisms either in vitro or in clinical infections. However, the safety and effectiveness in treating clinical infections due to organisms in vitro data have not been established in adequate and well-controlled clinical trials.

Caution is advised when using quinidine. Both quinine and quinidine are easily confused drugs. Quinine is an antimalarial drug; Quinidine is an antidysrhythmic drug. If confused can be fatal quinidine is an antidysrhythmic drug. The black-box warning prescribed by the Food and Drug Administration (FDA) on quinine is muscle weakness. The adverse reactions of artesunate include anemia, elevated hepatic enzymes, renal failure, acute respiratory distress syndrome, and disseminated intravascular coagulation.

The FDA has added a black-box warning to mefloquine due to reports of neurological side effects (dizziness, loss of balance, and ringing in the ear), which remain permanent. Adverse effects of mefloquine include severe anxiety, restlessness, disorientation, depression, hallucinations, paranoia, and suicidal thoughts, which may continue after the drug is discontinued. Primaquine is reported to cause methemoglobinemia in clients with nicotinamide adenine dinucleotide (NADH), a coenzyme central to metabolism, causing bluish fingernails, lips, or skin; dizziness; breathing difficulty; tiredness; and weakness during therapy with primaquine.

⚡ PATIENT SAFETY

Do Not Confuse...
- **quiNINE** (antimalarial) with **quiNIDine** (antidysrhythmic).
- **Hydroxychloroquine** (antimalarial drug) and **hydroxyurea** (chemotherapy drug).

TABLE 31.1 Antimalarials

Generic	Route and Dosage	Uses and Considerations
Artesunate (artemisinin derivative)	A: IV: PO: 2.4 mg/kg/dose IV, initially at 0h, 12h, 24h. Then switch to oral therapy starting 4h–24h following final IV dose. For patients who cannot tolerate oral therapy, 2.4 mg/kg/dose IV administered at 0, 12, and 24h, then 2.4mg/kg/dose IV once daily for up to 6 days. After 7 total days of IV therapy, proceed with full treatment course with oral regimen. max: A: IV: 2.4 mg/kg/dose IV.	Used to treat severe malaria and active against microorganism strains of *Plasmodium (P.)* such as *P. falciparum, P. malariae, P. ovale, P. sp,* and *P. vivax.* *Contraindicated:* Not recommended for client's breastfeeding and pregnant contraindicated in hypersensitivity to drug. Monitor: Hemoglobin, hematocrit, and LDH PB: 93%; t½: 1.3 h
Chloroquine	See Prototype Drug Chart: Chloroquine	
Hydroxychloroquine (disease-modifying antirheumatic)	*Uncomplicated Malaria* A: PO: 800 mg (620 mg/base) then 400 mg (310 mg/base) at 6, 24, 48 h for a total dose of 2000 mg (1550 mg/base). *Max:* A: PO: 800 mg/dose (620 mg base/dose) up to a total of 2000 mg (1515 mg/base) within 48 hrs. Malaria prophylaxis: A: PO: 400 mg (310 mg/base) 1–2 wks before entering endemic area and 4 wks after leaving. Max: A: PO: 400 mg (310 mg/dose) wk.	Used to treat and prevent malaria due to susceptible strains of *P. falciparum, P. vivax, P. malariae, P. ovale,* and *P. knowlesi*; also an alternative to chloroquine sensitivity. Give with meals or milk to reduce GI distress. *Contraindicated:* Irreversible retinal damage, life-threatening and fatal cardiomyopathy including life-threatening and fatal cardiomyopathy, ventricular arrhythmias, torsade de pointes. *Adverse reactions:* Not recommended in pregnancy, or patients with psoriasis, renal impairment, ocular disturbances, history of alcoholism or hepatic impairment. Can cause sensorimotor disorder including neuropathy, GI upset, cardiomyopathy, hypoglycemia, and suicidal ideation. Consider monitoring complete blood count (CBC), electrocardiogram (ECG), and ophthalmologic examination. PB: 50%; t½: 40–50 d
Mefloquine (antiparasitic/ antiprotozoal/ antiinfective)	Treatment of uncomplicated and severe malaria A: PO: 750 mg as initial dose, then 500 mg 6–12 h after initial dose. Max: 1250 mg single dose for treatment Malaria prophylaxis: A: PO: 250 mg PO weekly, starting at least 2 wks prior to entering the endemic area and continuing for 4 wks after leaving the area. Max: A: PO: 250 mg once a week for prophylaxis.	Used for treatment of malaria prophylaxis or for treatment of susceptible strains of malaria like *P. falciparum, P. vivax, P. ovale, P. malariae,* and *P. knowlesi.* *Adverse reactions:* Agranulocytosis, aplastic anemia, AV block, bradycardia, hepatic failure, Stevens Johnsons, visual impairment *Absolute contraindications:* Anxiety, depression, hypersensitivities with mefloquine, quinidine, or quinine, psychosis, schizophrenia, hepatic disease, cardiac conditions, and seizures. ⚡ **Black-Box Warning:** psychiatric events Safety/Monitoring: Ophthalmic exam; and CBC. PB: 98–99%; t½: 13–33 d
Primaquine (antiparasitic/ antiprotozoal/ antiinfective)	*Prevention of relapse of malaria:* Adults weighing 70 kg or more: A: PO: 52.6 mg (30 mg base) once daily until cumulative dose of 10.52 mg/kg (6 mg/kg/base). Adults weighing 69 kg or less: A: PO: 52.6 mg (30 mg base) PO × 14 days. *Malaria prophylaxis:* A: PO: 52.6 mg (30 mg base) 30 mg before entering malaria-risk area continue 7 d after leaving the endemic area. Max: A: PO: 15 mg daily; however, higher doses of 30 mg daily have been used.	Used to treat malaria caused by *P. vivax, P. ovale,* and *P. falciparum, P. malariae, Pneumocystis jirovecii.* Also, for Malaria Prevention of Relapse. *Adverse reactions:* GI distress, rash, cardiac arrhythmias, acute hemolytic anemia in clients with G6PD deficiency, leukopenia, nausea, QT prolongation, nausea, and vomiting. Pregnancy test at baseline, CBC, ECG if risk of prolonged QT interval, Glucose-6-phosphate dehydrogenase. *Contraindications:* Cardiac disease, rheumatoid arthritis, pregnancy, systemic lupus erythematosus (SLE). ❗ **High Alert Drug:** Heightened risk of harm when used in error. PB: UK; t½: 6 h
quiNINE (antiparasitic/ antiprotozoal/ antiinfective)	Uncomplicated/Severe malaria: A: PO: 648 mg every 8 h for 3–7 d. Max: A: PO 1944 mg/d.	Used to treat malaria caused by *P. falciparum, P. vivax, P. ovale, P. malariae, P. knowlesi* including chloroquine-resistant strains and chloroquine-resistant strains of *P. vivax.* ⚡ **Black-Box Warning:** Muscular cramps (severe) *Adverse Reactions:* Abdominal pain, blurred vision, hearing loss, peripheral vasodilation, aphasia, bradycardia, cardiac arrest. *Absolute Contraindications:* Blackwater fever, hemolytic-uremic syndrome, long QT syndrome, myasthenia gravis, optic neuritis, QT prolongation, thrombocytopenia, and thrombotic thrombocytopenic purpura. PB: 70%; t½: 8–21 h.

Continued

TABLE 31.1 Antimalarials—cont'd

Generic	Route and Dosage	Uses and Considerations
Combination Antimalarial Drugs		
Atovaquone; Proguanil (oral antimalarial combination/ antiinfective/ antiparasitic/ antiprotozoal)	Malaria both acute and uncomplicated and prophylaxis A: PO: 1,000 mg Atovaquone, 400 mg proguanil PO once daily for 3 consecutive days. Malaria prophylaxis: A: PO: 250 mg atovaquone; 100 mg proguanil per tab for a day. Begin 1–2 d before entering the endemic area. Continue daily during the stay and for 7 d after leaving the area. Max: A: PO: Total of atovaquone 250 mg/100 mg (1 tablet) proguanil per day PO for prophylaxis; total of atovaquone 1 g/400 mg proguanil (4 tablets) per day PO for treatment (3 d only).	Treatment of malaria due to *P. falciparum* or *P. vivax, P. ovale, P. malariae, P. knowlesi*; effective for chloroquine-resistant strains. *Adverse reactions*: GI distress, elevated hepatic enzymes, headache, insomnia, visual disturbances. Take with food or milk at same time each day. *Contraindication*: Renal and hepatic impairment, GI disease, pulmonary edema, vomiting, sunlight (UV) exposure, precaution in Asian, African clients, children, and geriatric clients. Atovaquone: PB: 99% t½: 2–3 d. Proguanil: PB: 75% t½: 12–21 h.
Artemether; Lumefantrine (artemisimin-based combination/ antiinfective/ antiparasitic/ antiprotozoal)	Acute, uncomplicated malaria: A:PO: 80 mg artemether, 480 mg lumefantrine as initial dose and 8h after initial dose; then, twice daily for 2 days for a total course of 6 doses. Max: A: PO: 35 kg or more: 8 tabs/d A: PO: 25kg to 34 kg: 6 tabs/day	Used to treat malaria in patients with infections due to *P. vivax, P. ovale, P. malariae*, and *P. knowlesi*. *Adverse Effects*: Abdominal pain, arthralgia, chills, fever, peptic ulcer disease, proteinuria, ataxia, wheezing, anorexia, palpitations, and hepatomegaly. *Contraindications*: AV block, bradycardia, cardiomyopathy, fever, hepatic disease, human immunodeficiency, rheumatoid arthritis, sickle cell disease, stroke. Caution in breastfeeding Artemether: PB: 95% t½: 2–3 h Lumefantrine: PB: 99.7% t½: 3–6 d

<, Less than; >, greater than; *A*, adult; *Adol*, adolescent; *CBC*, complete blood count; *d*, day; *d/c*, discharge; *G-6-PD*, glucose-6-phosphate dehydrogenase; *GI*, gastrointestinal; *h*, hour; *IV*, intravenous; *LDH*, lactate dehydrogenase; *LFT*, Liver function test; *max*, maximum; *P*, plasmodium; *PB*, protein binding; *PO*, by mouth; *q*, every; *t½*, half-life; *tabs*, tablets; *UK*, unknown; *WBC*, white blood cell; *wk*, week; *y*, year.

ANTHELMINTIC DRUGS

Helminths are parasitic worms that cause disease worldwide. Transmission occurs in areas of poor sanitation and hygiene from infected soil to the person, whereupon the helminth then feeds on host tissue (https://www.cdc.gov/sth/about/). Helminth infection affects the host's immunity resulting in disability in the host and, if left untreated, causes developmental delays in children. The most common site for **helminthiasis** (worm infection) is the intestine. Other sites for parasitic infection are the lymphatic system, blood vessels, and liver.

The classification of helminths includes (1) cestodes (tapeworms), (2) trematodes (flukes), (3) intestinal nematodes (roundworms), and (4) extraintestinal tissue-invading nematodes (trichinosis, onchocerciasis, and filariae). They enter the human host via contaminated food, bites of carrier insects, or direct penetration of the skin.

The cestodes (tapeworms) enter the intestine via contaminated food and attach to the intestinal wall. There are four types of cestodes: *Taenia solium* (pork tapeworm), *T. saginata* (beef tapeworm), *Diphyllobothrium latum* (fish tapeworm), and *Hymenolepis nana* (dwarf tapeworm). Cestodes have heads and hooks or suckers that attach to the tissue.

The trematodes (flukes) are flat parasites that feed on the host and include *Fasciola hepatica* (liver fluke), which inhabits the biliary track; *Fasciolopsis buski* (intestinal fluke) common in Southeast Asia; *Paragonimus westermani* (lung fluke); and *Schistosoma* species (blood flukes), which are acquired outside the United States.

Intestinal nematodes infect and feed on intestinal tissue: *Ascaris lumbricoides* (a giant roundworm) is prevalent worldwide, *Necator americanus* (a hookworm) is common in rural areas, *Enterobius vermicularis* (a pinworm) is most common in the United States, *Strongyloides stercoralis* (a threadworm) is common in the southern United States, and *Trichuris trichiura* (a whipworm) is common worldwide.

Extraintestinal nematodes are tissue-invading: *Trichinella spiralis* (pork roundworm) can cause **trichinosis**, a disease caused by ingestion of raw or inadequately cooked pork that contains larvae of the *T. spiralis* parasite, which can be diagnosed by muscle biopsy. By thoroughly cooking pork, the roundworm is destroyed. *Onchocerciasis volvulus* (river blindness) is transmitted by an infected fly causing worm-filled skin lesions and ocular lesions, leading to blindness.

Anthelmintics Drug Treatment

Ivermectin is a broad-spectrum antiparasitic agent of the *Avermectin Class*. Ivermectin has structural similarities to the macrolide antibiotics but lacks antibacterial activity.

Ivermectin lotion is used topically to treat *Pediculosis capitis* (head lice). Ivermectin cream is used topically for the treatment of inflammatory lesions of rosacea. Oral ivermectin is used to treat infections caused by *Onchocerca volvulus, Sarcoptes scabiei, Wuchereria bancroft*, or *S. stercoralis*. Ivermectin is recommended by the World Health Organization (WHO) for treating onchocerciasis (river blindness) and lymphatic filariasis (Bancroft's filariasis). Resistance to ivermectin has not been reported. Ivermectin oral tables were approved by the FDA in November 1996. Ivermectin lotion was approved in February 2012. Ivermectin cream was approved in December 2014. Prototype Drug Chart: Ivermectin lists dosages and drug data for ivermectin. Ivermectin is not an antiviral drug and is not FDA approved for treating or preventing COVID-19. Off-label use of any drug can cause serious harm. Ivermectin is intended for veterinary use in animals.

Animal products are often highly concentrated, and such high doses can be toxic to humans. Do not use veterinary ivermectin products as substitutes for FDA-approved human ivermectin products prescribed by a health care provider for appropriate indications. Praziquantel treats liver flukes, Pyrantel pamoate is used for pinworms, and Triclabendazole treats fascioliasis. These medications are listed in Table 31.2.

TABLE 31.2 Anthelmintics

Generic	Route and Dosage	Uses and Considerations
Ivermectin	See Prototype Drug Chart: Ivermectin	
Praziquantel (antiparasitic)	*Liver flukes (clonorchiasis and opisthorchiasis):* A: PO: 25 mg/kg/dose tid for 1 d, separate doses for 4–6 h *Schistosomiasis:* A: PO 20 mg/kg/dose tid (q4–6/h) × 1 d *Cysticercosis (tapeworms):* A: PO: 50 mg/kg/d given in 3 divided doses for 2–4 wk *Taeniasis (tapeworms):* A: PO: 5–10 mg/kg as a single dose *Neurocysticercosis (pork tapeworm infection):* 50 mg/kg/d given in 3 divided doses for 10–14 d, usually in combination with other medications. Max: A: PO: 75 mg/kg/d	Used for schistosomiasis, clonorchiasis, and opisthorchiasis; also effective for certain cestode (tapeworm) infections. *Absolute Contraindication:* Retinal cysticercosis. *Contraindicated:* In hypersensitivity to drug class; hepatic impairment, AV block, bradycardia, cardiac arrhythmias, driving or operating machinery, and seizures. *Adverse reactions:* Urticaria, drowsiness, abdominal pain and distension, vertigo, anorexia, asthenia, pruritus, vomiting, diarrhea, myalgia, fatigue, dizziness, nausea, weakness, headache, rash, fever, arrhythmia, AV block, bradycardia, and malaise. In neurocysticercosis, anticonvulsive therapy is recommended for those with seizure disorders. PB: 80%–85%; t½: 0.8–1.5 h Metabolized: Liver Excreted: Kidney
Pyrantel (antiparasitic)	*Enterobiasis and trichostrongylosis (pinworms):* A: PO: 11 mg/kg base (*max.* 1 g) as single dose repeat in 2 wk *Uncinariasis (hookworm):* A: PO: 11 mg/kg base (max. 1 g) daily × 3 d *Ascariasis (intestinal roundworm):* A: PO: 11 mg/kg base (*max.* 1 g) daily × 3 d as an alternative to other treatments; *Max.* A: PO: 11 mg/kg/dose, not to exceed 1 g/dose	Antihelminthic for treating pinworm infections. *Contraindicated:* hypersensitivity to drug class; use with caution in hepatic impairment, breastfeeding, and pregnancy. *Adverse reactions:* abdominal cramps, nausea, vomiting, diarrhea, and dizziness. Metabolized: Liver Excreted: 7% or < in urine 50% in feces Peak: 1–3 h PB: UK; t½: UK
Triclabendazole (antiparasitic)	*Fascioliasis:* A: PO: 10 mg/kg/dose for 2 doses given 12 h apart *Max:* 20 mg/kg/d	Antiparasitic used to treat infections of worms. *Contraindicated* in hypersensitivity to triclabendazole, irregular heartbeat, heart failure, bradycardia, celiac disease, geriatric, hepatic disease, pregnancy, and breastfeeding. *Adverse reactions:* Chest pain, changes in heart rate, constipation, dizziness, palpitations, breathing problems, hyperbilirubinemia, elevated hepatic enzymes. PB: 96.7%, 98.4%, 98.8%, respectively t½: 8, 14, 11 h, respectively
Albendazole (antiparasitic)	*Neurocysticercosis:* A: PO: 15 mg/kg/d (max 1200 mg/d) in 2 divided doses 10–14 d Max: 800 mg/d for 8–30 d *Ascariasis (roundworm)* A: PO: 400 mg single dose *Capillariasis:* A: PO: 200 mg twice daily for 10 d Max: A: PO: 15 mg/kg/d or 800 mg/d for most indications, up to 3200 mg/d PO in HIV pts with microsporidosis	Used for Cestodes, Nematodes, and Trematodes worms. *Adverse reactions:* Headache, dizziness, nausea, vertigo, elevated haptic enzymes, headache, increased intracranial pressure, agranulocytosis, aplastic anemia, hepatic failure, Steven-Johnson syndrome. *Contraindications:* Anemia, biliary obstruction, bone marrow suppression, chemotherapy, driving or operating machinery, children, pregnancy, seizures. PB: 70% t½: 8–12 h Metabolized: Liver Excreted: Bile

<, Less than; >, greater than; *A*, adult; *d*, day; *h*, hour; *HIV*, human immunodeficiency virus; *max*, maximum; *PB*, protein binding; *PO*, by mouth; *t½*, half-life; *tid*, three times a day; *UK*, unknown; *wk*, week; *y*, year.

Side Effects and Adverse Reactions

The common side effects of anthelmintics (agents that destroy worms) include various manifestations of GI distress, such as anorexia, nausea, vomiting, and occasionally diarrhea and stomach cramps. The neurologic problems associated with anthelmintics are dizziness, weakness, headache, and drowsiness. Adverse reactions do not occur frequently because the drugs are usually given for a short period (1–3 days).

PEPTIDES

Antimicrobial peptides (AMPs) are broad-spectrum, powerful defenses that kill parasites, fungi, and viruses. The Center for Communicable Disease, a governmental health agency that prevents and reduces communicable diseases in the United States and globally, has launched an initiative for health care providers and patients to prevent drug-resistant infection. There is ongoing research in combining antibiotics as multidrug regimens, which can reduce antibiotic resistance. Mismanagement of antibiotics has created an increased antibiotic resistance whereby a drug is no longer able to treat a disease. Examples include methicillin-resistant *Staphylococcus aureus* (MRSA) and carbapenem-resistant *Enterobacteriaceae* (CRE), *Clostridium difficile*, and vancomycin resistant enterococcus.

Im clueless this must be a message among your team. The missing paragraph is listed directly under Peptides and perhaps you want to add it here because it is split by the tables.

Peptides are generally considered to be short chains of two or more amino acids. Meanwhile, longer molecule proteins comprising multiple peptide subunits are known as polypeptides.

Peptide classifications include antiviral, antimicrobial, antifungal, and antiparasitic. The two groups of peptides used as antibiotics are polymyxins and bacitracin. Peptides are derived from cultures of *Bacillus subtilis*, and this group appears to weaken the bacterial cell membrane function, causing cell death.

CLINICAL JUDGMENT [NURSING PROCESS]
Antimalarials

Concept: Infection
- Invasion and growth of malaria parasitic microorganisms in body tissues resulting in cellular infection and destruction

Concept: Nutrition
- Optimal cellular metabolism during antimalarial prophylaxis and treatment

Concept: Immunity
- Protective physiologic response to the malarial protozoa

Recognize Cues [Assessment]
- Assess the patient's hearing by establishing an auditory baseline and hearing tests at scheduled intervals. Drugs such as quinine or chloroquine may affect cranial nerve VIII.
- Assess the patient for visual changes including establishing a baseline and checking vision at scheduled intervals.
- Note the patient's level of consciousness.
- Secure a history of whether the patient has traveled out of the country to a malaria-endemic area.
- Obtain a patient history of malaria and whether antimalarial drugs were taken.
- Note renal function by assessing urinary color, output (>600 mL/day), and blood urea nitrogen (BUN).
- Assess the patient for the presence of allergies including skin rash, tissue swelling, and altered ventilation.
- Monitor electrocardiogram (ECG).

Analyze Cues and Prioritize Hypothesis [Patient Problems]
- Decreased visual acuity
- Decreased level of consciousness
- Decreased immunity
- Need for health teaching
- Skin rash with pruritus
- Diarrhea
- Nausea and vomiting

Generate Solutions [Planning]
- The patient will exhibit vital signs at baseline level showing the absence of malarial symptoms.
- The patient will take antimalarial drugs at the times and dosages prescribed.
- The Patient will use preventive measures when in the outside environment.

Take Action [Nursing Interventions]
- ⚡ Monitor renal and liver function by checking urine output (>600 mL/d) and liver enzymes.
- ⚡ Report if the patient's serum liver enzymes are elevated and if renal function tests are abnormal.
- ⚡ Observe the patient for side effects and adverse reactions from antimalarial drugs such as chloroquine and quinine; impaired consciousness, headache, or seizures; ventricular fibrillation monitored by ECG; skin and eyes that appear yellowish, and skeletal muscle weakness.
- Identify home-based safety measures to avoid injuries during periods of weakness, decreased vision, and difficulty hearing.

Patient Teaching
- ⚡ Advise patients traveling to malaria-endemic countries to receive prophylactic doses of an antimalarial drug before leaving, during the visit, and upon their return.
- Teach patients to take oral antimalarial drugs with food or at mealtime if gastrointestinal (GI) upset occurs.
- ⚡ Monitor patients returning from malaria-endemic areas for malarial symptoms of nausea, vomiting, diarrhea, abdominal cramps, pruritus, visual changes, and dizziness.
- ⚡ Inform patients who take chloroquine or hydroxychloroquine to report vision changes immediately, such as blurred and low vision, redness, and irritation.
- Provide patients with information on herbal supplements that may be harmful when taking prescribed medications.

Side Effects
- ⚡ Direct patients to report signs and symptoms of anorexia, nausea, vomiting, diarrhea, abdominal cramps, pruritus, visual disturbances, hearing loss, skin and eyes that appear yellowish, and dizziness.

Evaluate Outcomes [Evaluation]
- ⚡ Evaluate the effectiveness of the antimalarial drug by determining that the patient is free of symptoms.
- Evaluate the patients' self-management in prophylaxis and medication regimen.

PROTOTYPE DRUG CHART
Ivermectin

Drug Class Anthelmintic Drug	Dosage
Ivermectin (broad-spectrum anthelmintic/antiparasitic)	Administered both topically and orally: *Onchocerca volvulus infection:* A (>=15 kg): PO: Doses are prescribed to provide approximately 150 mcg/kg as a single dose. Repeated doses may be necessary. Dosage based on weight. *Strongyloidiasis/Scabies:* A (80kg or more): PO: 200 mcg/kg dose daily for 1–2 d. Doses are based on weight; Follow-up treatment is required. *Pediculosis capitis:* A: Topical: 1 tube; Follow instructions on tube A: PO: 200–400 mg/kg/dose for 2 doses; administer 7 days apart. *Pediculosis corporis:* A: PO: 200–400 mcg/kg/dose for 2 doses, administer 7 d apart. *Ascariases/Roundworms:* A: PO: 150–200 mcg, single dose *Enterobiasis/Pinworms:* A: PO: 200 mcg/dose single dose repeat in 2 w. Max Dose: A:PO: 150-200 mcg/kg single dose for most indications Max: A:PO 150-200 mcg/kg single dose Topical application: 4 oz.

Contraindications	Drug-Lab-Food Interactions
Contraindicated: For those who are hypersensitive to the drug's components; asthma, hepatic impairment, pregnancy, and immunosuppression; not recommended with breastfeeding.	*Drug Interactions:* Use with caution with aprepitant or fosaprepitant. Do not use with idelalisib and mirabegron. Mitotane decreases effectiveness; posaconazole increases the risk of toxicity; may increase INR when used concurrently with warfarin. Food: Take on an empty stomach with water. Lab: Monitor ophthalmic examinations; obtain and monitor stool examinations, LFTs, and pregnancy testing.

Pharmacokinetics	Pharmacodynamics
Absorption: Oral: Well absorbed Distribution: Widely distributed within the body; does not cross blood-brain barrier. Metabolism: Liver; PB: 93%; $t\frac{1}{2}$: Oral: 16–28 h Lotion: $t\frac{1}{2}$: 6.5 d Excretion: In feces (over 12 d) and urine (<1%)	Peak: 4 h Onset: UK Duration: UK

Therapeutic Effects/Uses
An antiparasitic agent, drug of choice for strongyloidiasis and onchocerciasis. Used topically for pediculosis capitis.
Mechanism of action: Binds with chloride ions, increases cell permeability to kill parasites.

Side Effects	Adverse Reactions
Pruritus, urticaria, fever, arthralgia, dizziness, diarrhea, nausea, skin irritation, xerosis, ocular irritation, back pain, lethargy, lymphadenopathy, rash, asthenia, fatigue, vomiting, anorexia, abdominal pain, vertigo, tremor, drowsiness	Angioedema, Stevens-Johnson syndrome, toxic epidermal necrolysis, seizures, ocular hemorrhage, coma, keratitis, uveitis, visual impairment

<, Less than; *A*, adult; *ALT*, alanine aminotransferase; *AST*, aspartate aminotransferase; *d*, day; *h*, hour; *INR*, international normalized ratio; *LFT*, Liver Function Test; *PB*, protein binding; *PO*, by mouth; *UK*, unknown.

Colistimethate

Colistimethate/Colistin is a polypeptide antibiotic that targets aerobic gram-negative bacteria. It is used to treat *Pseudomonas aeruginosa*, *Klebsiella* and *Shigella* species. This antibiotic has the capacity to penetrate and disrupt the bacterial cell. Colistimethate is available in forms administrated IM, intravenously (IV), and by inhalation. Common reactions include dyspepsia, tingling, slurred speech, dizziness, paresthesia, pruritus, rash, and fever. Serious reactions include nephrotoxicity, neurotoxicity, neuromuscular blockade, respiratory distress, apnea, superinfection, and *C. difficile*–associated diarrhea. Acute respiratory distress syndrome can occur when the antibiotic is administered by inhalation.

CLINICAL JUDGMENT [NURSING PROCESS]
Anthelmintics

Concept: Nutrition
- Deficient nutrients needed for cellular metabolism resulting from intestinal parasites leading to nutritional deficiencies

Concept: Infection
- The presence of tissue inflammation from invading helminths causing gastrointestinal (GI) distress and neurologic effects

Recognize Cues [Assessment]
- ⚡ Note whether the patient has traveled to countries outside the United States or has been in areas that are overcrowded with poor sanitation.
- ⚡ Identify the close contacts with the patient infected by helminths.
- Assess the patient's health behavior when at home; also assess handwashing facilities, disposal of waste, access to safe drinking water, and whether the patient walks barefoot in soil.
- Secure a history of foods (especially beef and pork) the patient has eaten and how the food was prepared to determine if it was raw, undercooked, or contaminated.
- Document whether any other person in the household has been checked for helminths.
- ⚡ Determine the presence and intensity of anal itching, diarrhea, and abdominal discomfort in the patient before and during treatment and medication management.
- Assess the patient's baseline vital signs and then monitor changes at prescribed intervals while the patient is responding to anthelmintic medications.
- Note the type of helminthiasis to ensure the anthelmintic drug is specific to the organisms.

Analyze Cues and Prioritize Hypothesis [Patient Problems]
- Coping
- Decreased adherence to medication regimen
- Decreased functional ability when performing self-care management
- Decreased immunity
- Need for health teaching
- Reduced sensory perception (vision)
- Diarrhea, nausea, and vomiting

Generate Solutions [Planning]
- The patient will demonstrate handwashing before eating.
- The patient will explain how to prepare foods properly to avoid recurrence.
- The patient will identify changes needed at home to ensure sanitation in food preparation.
- The patient will describe methods of infection control within the home.

Take Action [Nursing Interventions]
- Discuss the benefits of handwashing before eating and after working in the soil or with animals.
- Monitor the patient's fluid and urinary output during anthelmintic medication use, checking for fluid loss from vomiting, diarrhea, and inadequate fluid intake.
- Collect the stool specimen in a clean container. Avoid having stool come in contact with water, urine, or chemicals, which could destroy parasitic worms.
- Administer the prescribed anthelmintic after meals to prevent or minimize the occurrence of GI distress.
- Monitor adverse reactions, including wheezing, abdominal pain, abdominal distention, and high fever.
- Check laboratory values of iron, iodine, and vitamin A to monitor nutritional status.
- Obtain an interpreter when necessary. Avoid relying on family members who may not fully disclose or understand medical terminology.
- Provide community-based resources for patients discharged to areas at high risk for poor sanitation.

Patient Teaching
- ⚡ Explain to the patient the importance of handwashing before meals and after going to the toilet. The parasite can be transferred within the family if proper hygiene is not used.
- Advise the patient to take daily showers and not baths.
- Encourage the patient to change sheets, bedclothes, towels, and underwear daily.
- Advise the patient that a second course of anthelmintic may be necessary if helminthiasis persists after therapy.
- Emphasize the importance of taking the prescribed drug at the designated times and keeping health care appointments.
- Teach the patient to read all directions regarding over-the-counter (OTC) drugs before use and avoid self-medication.
- ⚡ Warn the patient that drowsiness may occur and that operating a car or machinery should be avoided if this should happen.
- Encourage collaboration between family, patient, and health care provider when reporting side effects or adverse reactions.

Evaluate Outcomes [Evaluation]
- Evaluate the effectiveness of anthelmintic therapy and the absence of side effects.
- Determine the patient's self-management ability in proper hygiene, handwashing, and cleaning bed linen to avoid the spread of parasitic worms.
- Evaluate the patient's knowledge of maintaining adequate food and fluid intake to provide strength and healing.

Colistimethate/Colistin is used for severe bacterial infections due to multi-drug resistant gram-negative bacteria. To avoid errors in dosing and administration, colistimethate sodium should only be prescribed as colistin in terms of colistin base activity. Approximately 33 mg colistin base activity corresponds to approximate 80 mg of colistimethate sodium and 1 million IU of colistimethate sodium.

Polymyxins

Polymyxins were one of the early groups of antimicrobials, but many of the early drugs were discontinued because of severe toxic reactions such as neurotoxicity and nephrotoxicity. Polymyxins are polypeptide antibiotics that consist of five different chemical compounds, polymyxins A through E. Currently, polymyxin B and polymyxin E (also known as *colistin*) are used in clinical practice. Polymyxins produce a bactericidal effect by interfering with the cell membrane of the bacterium, thereby causing cell death. They affect most gram-negative bacteria, such as *P. aeruginosa*, *Escherichia coli*, and *Klebsiella* and *Shigella* species.

The polymyxins are not absorbed through the oral route except for colistin, which exerts action on the colon and is excreted in the feces. Intramuscular injection of polymyxins produces intense pain at the injection site. Consequently, parenteral polymyxins are administered at a slow IV infusion rate.

Table 31.3 lists antiinfective peptides with dosage and uses.

TABLE 31.3 Antiinfectives

Generic	Route and Dosage	Uses and Considerations
Peptides		
Bacitracin/Polymyxin B (polypeptide/antiinfective)	A: Topical: Apply a thin layer to affected area 1–3 times daily. Continue for full course of treatment; therapy should be limited to 7 days. A: Ophthalmic ointment: Apply a thin flim (0.5 inch ribbon) to the affected eye every 3–4 h for 7–10 d. *Max:* Ophthalmic Ointment: 8 applications/d up to 10 days *Max:* Topical: 3 applications/for up to 7 d	Available topical ointment for skin infections; ophthalmic ointment for eye infections involving the conjunctiva and cornea. *Adverse reactions:* Hypersensitivity and anaphylactoid reactions: puritus and failure to heal. *Contraindications:* In patients with viral, fungal and myobacterial infections. Monitor: BUN/Creatinine in patients with renal dysfunction; Ophtalmologic exam. PB: <20%; t½: UK for Bacitracin/Polymyxin B
Metronidazole	See Prototype Drug Chart: Metronidazole	
Colistimethate/Colistin (polypeptide/antiinfective/polymyxin E)	A: IV: IM: 300 mg colistin base activity loading dose; then, 150–180 mg/d of colistin base activity divided q12h *Note: Approximately 33 mg colistin base is approximately 80 mg of colistimethate. Max: 5 mg/kg/day colistin base activity IV/IM is FDA-approved with 360 mg/day colistin base activity IV used off-label.	Used for gram-negative infections like bacteremia, including infections related to resistant gram-negative organisms. *Adverse reactions:* Anaphylactoid reactions, anuria, apnea, bronchospasm, confusion, hearing loss, renal failure, seizures *Absolute Contraindication:* Polymyxin hypersensitivity *Contraindications:* Renal disease and impairment, neuromuscular disease, asthma, breastfeeding, *C. difficile*, COPD, myasthenia Gravis, pregnancy. Monitor BUN/Creatinine at baseline, then frequently PB: UK; t½: 2–3 h

<, Less than; *A*, adult; *bid*, twice daily; *BUN*, blood urea nitrogen; *COPD*, chronic obstructive pulmonary disease; *Cr*, creatinine; *d*, day; *GI*, gastro-intestinal; *h*, hour; *IM*, intramuscular; *IV*, intravenous; *kg*, kilogram; *max*, maximum; *PB*, protein binding; *PO*, by mouth; *q*, every; *t½*, half-life; *UK*, unknown; *UTI*, urinary tract infection.

Severe Adverse Effects

High serum levels of polymyxins can cause nephrotoxicity and neurotoxicity. In nephrotoxicity, the blood urea nitrogen (BUN) and serum creatinine levels are elevated, but when the serum drug level decreases, renal toxicity is usually reversed. Signs and symptoms of neurotoxicity (toxicity of the nerves) include paresthesias—abnormal sensations such as numbness, tingling, burning, and prickling—and dizziness. Neurotoxicity is usually reversible when the drug is discontinued.

Bacitracin

Bacitracin has a polypeptide structure and acts by inhibiting bacterial cell wall synthesis and damaging the cell wall membrane, which results in cell death. The drug action can be bacteriostatic or bactericidal. Bacitracin is not absorbed by the GI tract; if given orally, it is excreted in the feces. Bacitracin is effective against most gram-positive bacteria and some gram-negative bacteria. Over-the-counter (OTC) bacitracin ointment is available for application to the skin. The side effects of bacitracin include skin redness and rash, nausea, and vomiting. Severe adverse reactions are renal damage and ototoxicity, and mild to severe allergic reactions that range from hives to anaphylaxis may occur. Intramuscular (IM) bacitracin is not recommended in adults or children. Oral bacitracin was NOT proven efficacious in reducing carriage of vancomycin-resistant enterococcus (VRE) beyond the 2-week treatment period in studies. Bacitracin and polymyxin B products are approved for the treatment and prevention of infections caused by susceptible bacteria and should not be used in patients with viral infection, fungal infection, or mycobacterial infection.

Metronidazole

Metronidazole is a synthetic antibiotic and antiprotozoal (nitroimidazole class) that works by disrupting the bacterial DNA and inhibiting cell synthesis, which causes cell death. Metronidazole is lethal to anerobic organisms. It is a protozoal that treats *Trichomonas vaginalis including both initial and resistant forms and* bacterial vaginosis; as an antibiotic, it is used for anaerobic bacteria, including *Helicobacter pylori*, a pathogen in GI infections. In addition, this drug has immunosuppressive and antiinfective properties that treat rosacea. This drug can be added to multidrug regimens to reduce antibiotic resistance, which occurs when the bacteria are not sensitive to the antibiotic. Metronidazole can be administered orally, parenterally, topically, and intravaginally. Toxic reactions include neurologic disturbances such as seizures and peripheral neuropathies. The Prototype Drug Chart: Metronidazole provides information on metronidazole.

⚡ PATIENT SAFETY

To avoid antibiotic resistance, use health care provider-patient/family collaboration to counsel patients in antibiotic management by:
- Checking if the patient can be treated without antibiotics.
- Completing antibiotics as prescribed.
- Teaching the patient the correct use of the antibiotic, including not skipping doses or self-medicating with someone else's medication.
- Reinforcing self-management skills in personal hygiene.

PROTOTYPE DRUG CHART
Metronidazole (metroNIDAZOLE)

Drug Class (Antibacterial Peptide/Antiprotozoal Agent/Nitroimidazole Class)	Dosage
Reduces the development of drug-resistant organisms and maintains the effectiveness of antimicrobial drugs	*Initial trichomoniasis*: A: PO: Immediate Release: Female: 500 mg bid for 7 d or 2 g PO as a single dose A: PO: Male: 2 g single dose times 7 d *Resistant trichomoniasis* A: Females: PO: 500 mg bid daily for 7 d if failure occurs with reexposure, treat with 2 g once daily for 7 d. A: Male: PO: 2 g as a single dose. If failure occurs with reexposure, treat with 500 mg bid /d for 7 d *Bacterial Vaginosis*: A: PO: Immediate release: 500 mg bid daily for 7 d. A: PO: Extended release: 750 mg once daily for 7 d *Helicobacter pylori (H pylori) eradication*: A: PO: Immediate release 500 mg 3 times a day in combination with clarithromycin and proton pump inhibitor for 14 days. Max: A: IV/PO is usual maximum, however FDA has approved up to 4 g/d IV/PO.

Contraindications	Drug-Lab-Food Interactions
Absolute contraindication: AV block, corticosteroid therapy, Crohn's disease, dialysis, hepatic disease, HIV positive, pregnancy, breastfeeding, alcoholism (drinking alcohol is not recommended will cause gastrointestinal upset), sickle cell disease, lupus disease, cardiac and neoplastic disease. **Black-Box Warning:** New primary malignancy	Drug: Alcohol may cause disulfiram-type reaction. Disulfiram may increase the risk of toxicity. May increase the effects of oral anticoagulants. Herbal: None significant Food: None known Lab: May increase serum LDH, ALT, AST; Monitor: CBC w/diff

Pharmacokinetics	Pharmacodynamics
Absorption: Well absorbed orally Distribution: Widely distributed; crosses blood-brain barrier Metabolized in liver; PB: <20%; t½: 8 h Excretion: In urine (60%–80%) and feces (6%–15%)	Administered IV, intravaginally, topically IV: Onset immediate, peak end of infusion PO: Peak 1–2 h

Therapeutic Effects/Uses
Produces bactericidal, antiprotozoal, amebicidal, trichomonacidal effects. Produces antiinflammatory, immunosuppressive effects when applied topically.
Mechanism of action: Diffuses into an organism, interacting with DNA and causing a loss of helical DNA structure and strand breakage, inhibiting protein synthesis.

Side Effects	Adverse Reactions
Anorexia, metallic taste, headache, dizziness, vomiting, diarrhea, abdominal cramps, candidiasis, vaginitis, hypertension, constipation, depression.	Seizures, aseptic meningitis, pseudomembranous colitis, pancreatitis leukopenia, bone marrow suppression, aplasia, thrombocytopenia, Stevens-Johnson syndrome, toxic epidermal necrolysis

<, Less than; *A*, adult; *ALT*, alanine aminotransferase; *AST*, aspartate aminotransferase; *bid*, twice daily; *CBC*, complete blood count; *d*, day; *diff*, differential; *DNA*, deoxyribonucleic acid; *h*, hour; *HIV*, human immunodeficiency virus; *IV*, intravenous; *LDH*, lactate dehydrogenase; *PB*, protein binding; *PO*, by mouth; *q*, every; *t½*, half-life; *wk*, week.

CLINICAL JUDGMENT [NURSING PROCESS]
Antiinfectives: Peptides

Concept: Immunity
- Protective immunologic response of microbial peptides in patients with bacterial diseases

Concept: Infection
- The presence of drug-resistant bacteria causing infectious disease

Recognize Cues [Assessment]
- ⚡ Obtain a health history listing all prescribed and over-the-counter (OTC) medications and medication allergies.
- ⚡ Assess the patient's prior use of antibiotics, use of a multidrug regimen, and presence of untreated infections.
- Assess the patient's level of consciousness.
- Assess renal function and urinary output.
- Assess skin integrity, and evaluate for skin rash and pruritus.

Analyze Cues and Prioritize Hypothesis [Patient Problems]
- Sensory-perceptual impairment: decreased hearing, decreased vision
- Disrupted fluid and electrolyte balance: nephrotoxicity
- Decreased functional ability: dizziness
- Allergic skin rash
- Need for health teaching
- Nausea and vomiting

CLINICAL JUDGMENT [NURSING PROCESS]—CONT'D
Antiinfectives: Peptides

Generate Solutions [Planning]
- The laboratory values at baseline level by assessing urine output, blood urea nitrogen (BUN), and hepatic enzymes.
- The patient's skin will be intact without pruritus, swelling, or rash.
- The patient will be able to identify the dose and explain how to properly take the prescribed drug.
- The patient will describe the side effects and adverse reactions that require notification of a health care provider.

Take Action [Nursing Interventions]
- ⚡ Monitor laboratory values, including liver function tests (aspartate aminotransferase [AST], alanine aminotransferase [ALT]) and evaluation of renal function (BUN, creatinine clearance [CrCl]) and blood serum (platelet count, hemoglobin, hematocrit).
- Check urinary function by monitoring intake and output.
- Monitor the patient for an altered level of consciousness.

Patient Teaching
- Teach patients to read all instructions before taking medications.
- Inform patients to take all prescribed medication.
- Discuss possible side effects that can occur as a reaction to the drug.
- ⚡ Instruct patients to check for signs of superinfection, such as white patches on the tongue.
- ⚡ Advise patients to report all adverse reactions to a health care provider, including fever, diarrhea, trouble breathing, and decreased urination.
- Describe urinary signs that indicate impairment, such as decreased urinary flow.
- Caution patients not to replace a prescribed medication with an herbal supplement.
- ⚡ Use safety measures during activities of mobility.
- Encourage self-management skills, reporting all side effects and adverse reactions.

Evaluate Outcomes [Evaluation]
- Evaluate the effectiveness of treatment by the absence of manifestations.
- Evaluate the patient's understanding of the medication regimen by encouraging patient feedback and questions.

CLINICAL JUDGMENT CASE STUDY

A 40-year-old male has returned to the United States after working in a missionary health clinic in a malaria-endemic area. He was admitted to the hospital with fever, chills, and severe unrelieved headache. A diagnosis of acute malaria was made.

Chloroquine was ordered, and the patient was discharged. One week later, he returned to the emergency department with worsening symptoms and signs of confusion. The patient states he took his pills every other day and then stopped because they made him sick. He decided to take over-the-counter (OTC) antinausea medication. The patient was readmitted to the hospital. A care coordination meeting was scheduled with the patient, family, health care provider, and pharmacist to determine ways to improve medication adherence.

1. Which key factors should be assessed in this patient's history?
2. What is the significance of monitoring liver function tests, blood urea nitrogen (BUN)/creatinine (Cr), and complete blood count (CBC)?
3. Describe the correct method of preventive prophylaxis when taking antimalarial drugs.

REVIEW QUESTIONS

1. An international traveler diagnosed with malaria is admitted to the emergency department and is prescribed mefloquine. The nurse anticipates which laboratory test will be ordered.
    a. Liver function test (LFT)
    b. Blood glucose
    c. Sputum culture and sensitivity
    d. White blood cell count
2. A patient is admitted to the hospital with a multidrug-resistant urinary tract infection. Laboratory tests show *Pseudomonas aeruginosa*. Colistimethate sodium is ordered in powder form and must be diluted for intramuscular injection. The nurse understands which of the following is the purpose of this drug.
    a. This drug prevents toxic adverse reactions.
    b. This drug treats gram-negative bacteria.
    c. This drug is safe for patients with renal impairments.
    d. This drug prevents antibiotic resistance.
3. Which of the following is a priority to evaluate in a patient being treated for *Taeniasis* tapeworm)?
    a. Increased appetite
    b. Abdominal distension
    c. Fatigue
    d. Constipation
4. A patient with a history of malaria who is being treated with chloroquine is in the clinic for a follow-up visit. What should the nurse advise the patient to do?
    a. Avoid eating pork.
    b. Take antimalarials before meals.
    c. Get frequent testing of stool specimens.
    d. Avoid sun exposure.
5. A 50-year-old female is being discharged from the hospital after treatment for malaria. Which teaching topic would best inform the patient about adverse reactions?
    a. The occurrence of headaches
    b. Experiencing dizziness
    c. Developing mild pruritus
    d. Skin and eyes that appear yellowish
6. A 30-year-old female presents with a recurrence of *Trichomonas vaginalis* infection, and metronidazole is ordered. Which of the following contraindications does the patient's history reveal?
    a. A recent pregnancy test is negative.
    b. She previously took metronidazole and had no side effects.
    c. She drinks a glass of wine before bedtime.
    d. She takes an oral contraceptive.

UNIT IX Immunologic Drugs

32

HIV- and AIDS-Related Drugs

http://evolve.elsevier.com/McCuistion/pharmacology

OBJECTIVES

- Discuss the strides made toward HIV and AIDS.
- Summarize a treatment plan with ART.
- Discuss the role of the nurse for patients receiving antiretroviral therapy.

OUTLINE

Overview of HIV and AIDS, 381
   HIV Pathophysiology, 381
   HIV Transmission, 382
   Laboratory Testing, 382
   Classification, 382
   Indications for Antiretroviral Therapy, 382
Antiretroviral Drugs, 383
   Nucleoside/Nucleotide Reverse Transcriptase Inhibitors, 383
   Nonnucleoside Reverse Transcriptase Inhibitors, 383
   Protease Inhibitors, 388
   Fusion (Entry) Inhibitors, 389

   Chemokine (CCR5) Coreceptor Antagonists, 390
   Integrase Strand Transfer Inhibitors, 390
The Nurse's Role in Antiretroviral Therapy, 391
   Adherence, Assessment, and Education, 391
   Immune Reconstitution Inflammatory Syndrome, 392
   Opportunistic Infections, 392
   Antiretroviral Therapy in Pregnancy, 392
   Occupational HIV Exposure and Postexposure Prophylaxis, 393
Clinical Judgment Case Study, 394
Review Questions, 394

OVERVIEW OF HIV AND AIDS

Since the acquired immunodeficiency syndrome (AIDS) epidemic began in the United States in the early 1980s, the advancement of antiretroviral therapy (ART) has dramatically improved human immunodeficiency virus (HIV)-related morbidity and mortality, and has reduced perinatal and behaviorally associated HIV transmission. The Centers for Disease Control and Prevention (CDC) reports that more than 1 million people in the United States are infected with HIV; 87% knew they had the virus upon diagnosis. In 2021 over 36,000 people were newly diagnosed with HIV; however, this number may be skewed due to the recent COVID-19 pandemic. Improvement of health, prolonging lives, reducing transmission risk, and suppression of HIV necessitate the use of combination treatments with antiretroviral (ARV) drugs. Current clinical guidelines recommend ART for all persons infected with HIV-1, regardless of their viral load (CD4+ cell count). Prophylactic treatment of HIV-negative partners minimizes their risk of contracting HIV. It is critical that nurses educate patients regarding ART and, in partnership with the patient, develop strategies to optimize adherence.

Although strides have been made in the treatment of HIV/AIDS, challenges remain. One important aspect is increased drug resistance to current therapies. The makeup of the HIV DNA strands allows the virus to mutate from a drug-sensitive to a drug-resistant form. To minimize resistant strains, clinical and nonclinical providers and health departments need to strive for the highest possible adherence to ART. At each health care visit, persons with HIV and their partners should receive ongoing counseling to reinforce HIV prevention measures, screening for high-risk behaviors, diagnosis and treatment of sexually transmitted infections (STIs), and reinforcement of the importance of medication adherence. Open communication between the health care provider and patient should be fostered.

The goals for initiating ART are to (1) reduce HIV-associated morbidity and mortality, (2) prolong the duration and quality of life, (3) restore and preserve immunologic function, (4) maximally and durably suppress plasma HIV viral load, and (5) prevent HIV transmission.

HIV Pathophysiology

HIV is an RNA retrovirus. It is unable to survive and replicate unless it is inside a living human cell. HIV destroys CD4+ T cells, also called *helper T cells* or *CD4+ T lymphocytes*; these cells play a critical role in the human immune response through recognition of infectious and neoplastic processes. The destruction of CD4+ cells by HIV results in immune deficiency, so the CD4+ cell count is an indicator for immune function in those with HIV.

Normal CD4+ counts range from 500 to 1500 cells/mm^3. After initial infection, rapid viral replication occurs, resulting in a high level of HIV in circulation (high viral load); the virus then attacks and destroys CD4+ cells. There is a corresponding drop in CD4+ cells, which triggers an immune response that results in CD4+ cell replacement and HIV antibody production. HIV uses the CD4+ cell's apparatus to replicate itself and spread throughout the body. The CD4+ cells continue to drop as HIV viral load increases, which further weakens the person's natural immune system such that it cannot fight off infection and disease (e.g., cancer). Symptoms of HIV infection range from mild to severe and include fever, fatigue, pharyngitis, myalgia or arthralgia, lymphadenopathy, headache, and night sweats in those recently infected; these symptoms can be experienced 2 to 12 weeks after HIV exposure. This period is called *acute retroviral syndrome, acute seroconversion syndrome*, or *primary HIV infection*. At this stage, people are highly infectious, and symptoms can often be mistaken, by both the patient and the health care provider, for a transient flu-like illness. Consequently, few people are diagnosed during this time. In addition, the time delay from infection to a positive HIV test result—the **window period**—averages 10 to 14 days, but some do not seroconvert for 3 to 4 weeks. Almost all patients seroconvert within 6 months. For this reason, patients who are at risk for HIV infection and test negative should be counseled to have the test repeated in 3 months (the close of the window period). If HIV is strongly suspected, an HIV RNA quantitative test can be done. A viral load of 10,000 copies/mL usually indicates the virus is adequately suppressed.

HIV Transmission

HIV is spread via intimate contact with blood, semen, vaginal fluids, and breast milk. Transmission of the virus occurs primarily by (1) sexual contact, which includes oral, vaginal, and anal sex; (2) direct blood contact, including intravenous (IV) drug use with shared needles or shared drug works, shared contaminated personal care items such as razors, and blood transfusions (now extremely rare in the United States); and (3) mother-to-child contact through shared maternal-fetal blood circulation, direct blood contact during delivery, or breast milk. Included in these modes are accidental needle injury, artificial insemination with donated semen, and organ transplant. Those at highest risk include persons who engage in unprotected sex, those with multiple sexual partners (either the patient or partner[s] of the patient), IV drug users who share needles or drug works, and infants born to females with HIV. The risk of mother-to-child transmission (MTCT) is 25% without ART; the risk decreases to 1% to 2% with successful use of ART. Other factors that increase the risk of MTCT are a mother with a viral load greater than 1000 copies/mL at delivery, premature rupture of the membranes, hepatitis C virus coinfection, preterm gestation, and vaginal delivery. HIV is not spread by air or water, mosquitoes or ticks, shaking hands, hugging, sharing toilets, sharing dishes or drinking glasses, or drinking fountains.

Laboratory Testing

Several laboratory tests are important for initial patient evaluation upon entry to care, during follow-up evaluation for those not on ART, and before and after initiation or modification of ART to assess for immunologic and virologic efficacy of treatment.

The laboratory tests used to determine when to initiate medication therapy and to monitor efficacy of therapy and indications for changing therapy are CD4+ T-cell count, plasma HIV RNA quantitative assay (or **viral load** test), and HIV resistance testing.

The count reflects the number of CD4+ cells circulating in the blood. The CD4+ percentage is a more stable reflection of the immune system and is used in conjunction with the absolute count to monitor health status and response to medication therapy. The patient should be encouraged to use the same laboratory at approximately the same time of day to promote consistency of results. The nurse should monitor the laboratory used because laboratory value references vary from laboratory to laboratory. The HIV viral load is indicative of the level of virus circulating in the blood and is the best determinant of treatment efficacy. Effective treatment is evidenced by less than 200 copies/mL, which indicates the HIV is suppressed. A key goal of therapy is to achieve and maintain a viral load below the limits of detection (<40–75 copies/mL, depending on the assay used). This goal should be achieved in 16 to 24 weeks of therapy. A person with undetectable viral load is not transmittable. Resistance to ART is possible and leads to treatment failure, which increases the risk of transmitting drug-resistant virus. Determination of the presence of a drug-resistant strain of HIV is important to prevent ineffective treatment. Individuals who experience failure of ART should have drug resistance testing, assessment of drug adherence, and a review of possible drug-drug and drug-food interactions. Other assessments include drug intolerability, treatment history, and HIV RNA and CD4+ cell counts.

Classification

HIV disease staging and classification systems are important tools for tracking and monitoring the HIV epidemic and for providing the clinician and patient with information about HIV disease stage and clinical management. Treatment for HIV slows or prevents disease progression to stage 3. Major classification system by the CDC includes the following:

- Stage 1—Acute HIV infection: The viral load is high, and persons in stage 1 typically exhibit flu-like symptoms.
- Stage 2—Chronic HIV infection: The viral load is lower, but the virus is still being produced in the body. Persons in this stage may not exhibit symptoms of HIV but can still transmit HIV to others.
- Stage 3—AIDS: This stage is the severest. Persons in this stage have very high viral load, and their immune systems are damaged. They are prone to opportunistic infections. Survival rate without treatment is about 3 years.

Indications for Antiretroviral Therapy

ART has dramatically reduced HIV-associated morbidity and mortality. However, the CDC reported that, in the United States, 66% of adults and adolescents with HIV have adequate viral suppression. Many individuals with HIV infection are undiagnosed or they are not retained within the health care system for routine monitoring.

A set of guidelines was developed by the US Department of Health and Human Services Expert Panel on Antiretroviral Guidelines for Adults and Adolescents (the Panel). The Panel last updated the guidelines in 2019 and recommends ART for all HIV-infected individuals regardless of CD4+ count to reduce HIV-related morbidity and mortality and to prevent HIV transmission. The Panel also seeks to educate patients on the benefits and considerations for ART, especially the importance of adherence. The current guidelines for treatment-naïve persons with HIV include initial therapy with two nucleoside reverse transcriptase inhibitors (NRTIs) in combination with a third-active ARV drug from one of three drug classes: an integrase strand transfer inhibitor (INSTI), a nonnucleoside reverse transcriptase inhibitor

(NNRTI), or a protease inhibitor (PI) with a pharmacokinetic (PK) enhancer (booster) (cobicistat or ritonavir). All HIV-infected persons diagnosed with active tuberculosis (TB) should be started on ARV and TB therapy. Rifamycin (rifabutin, rifampin) should be included in the TB regimen despite drug interactions. Chapter 29 further discusses antituberculars.

Suppression of HIV with ART may decrease inflammation and immune activation thought to contribute to higher rates of cardiovascular, kidney, and liver disease; neurologic complications; and malignancy in HIV-infected cohorts. If therapy is to be initiated, medications are selected based on results of genotypic resistance testing where applicable, comorbidities (e.g., liver disease, renal dysfunction, depression), potential drug-drug interactions, pregnancy status, and assessment of the patient's willingness and readiness to start therapy. Evaluation of medication readiness should include dosage regimen, pill burden, dosing frequency, food restrictions, side effects, and the patient's daily routine. Tools for promoting medication adherence (e.g., alarms, pill planners) and plans for management of potential medication side effects should be reviewed before medication initiation. The patient should be instructed in the need for 100% medication adherence, the potential for development of medication resistance with less than optimal adherence, and the clinical implications of resistance.

ANTIRETROVIRAL DRUGS

NRTIs, NNRTIs, PIs, fusion (entry) inhibitors, CCR5 antagonists, and INSTIs make up the drugs used as ART. Table 32.1 lists dosages, uses, and considerations for several ARVs. More than 25 different ARVs have received US Food and Drug Administration (FDA) approval, and various combination of drugs are available in fixed-dose combinations that contain two or more HIV medications from one or more drug classes. In addition to the previously mentioned classes of ARVs, PK enhancers are approved to be taken with some ARVs (e.g., PIs and certain INSTIs).

Since the 1980s, when zidovudine monotherapy showed survival benefits in advanced HIV patients, much progress has been made. Newer drugs have improved adherence (e.g., fewer pills for more convenient dosing, formulation changes that reduce dosing frequency or pill burden, combination dosage forms with two or three drugs in one pill). Other improvements include increased potency, improved side effect profile (e.g., decreased gastrointestinal [GI] effects), and PI enhancers.

ART is the standard of care in the treatment of HIV infection. Currently, there are six recommended regimens for treatment-naïve patients, five of which are INSTI based and one that is ritonavir-boosted-PI based. For treatment-naïve patients, ART generally consists of two NRTIs plus an INSTI, NNRTI, or PK-enhanced PI. Treatment-experienced patients who encounter drug resistance should begin a new regimen that includes two to three fully active drugs. Adding a single ARV is not recommended because of the increased risk of drug resistance to all ARVs. Furthermore, drug interruption is not recommended due to a risk of rapid increase of HIV RNA viral load and a decrease in CD4+ cell count.

The Panel reports that nevirapine (NVP) should not be given to ARV-naïve women whose CD4+ count is greater than 250 cells/mm^3 or to males with CD4+ greater than 400 cells/mm^3 due to a high incidence of hepatotoxicity; however, if no other ARV option is available, NVP can be administered, but patients should be closely monitored. On the other hand, the Panel reports no exceptions to stavudine plus zidovudine (antagonistic effect) and unboosted darunavir, saquinavir, or tipranavir (inadequate bioavailability).

Nucleoside/Nucleotide Reverse Transcriptase Inhibitors

Of the ARV drugs, NRTIs were the first type of drug to treat HIV. NRTIs act by interfering with HIV viral RNA-dependent DNA polymerase, resulting in inhibition of viral replication. Seven NRTIs, also known as "nukes," are approved for use in the United States: zidovudine, didanosine, stavudine, lamivudine, abacavir, tenofovir, and emtricitabine. All but didanosine and stavudine are available in a fixed-dose combination with other classes of ARV drugs.

All NRTIs except didanosine can be taken without regard to food. Didanosine should be taken 30 minutes before or 2 hours after meals for optimal absorption. Fifty percent or more of NRTIs are excreted by the kidneys; therefore NRTIs require dosage adjustment in persons with renal insufficiency. With abacavir, dosage adjustment is recommended in individuals with hepatic insufficiency.

Side and Adverse Drug Effects

As a class, NRTIs are associated with changes in the body's metabolism secondary to mitochondrial toxicity. GI side effects such as nausea, diarrhea, and abdominal pain are transient and improve within the first 2 weeks of therapy. Rash is a common hypersensitivity reaction. Complications include peripheral neuropathy, myopathy, pancreatitis, and lipoatrophy. Lipoatrophy—or wasting of fat on the extremities, face, and buttocks—is associated with chronic NRTI administration. Rare fatalities have occurred due to lactic acidosis and hepatic steatosis associated with NRTIs. Persons coinfected with hepatitis B virus (HBV) are at risk for severe acute exacerbation of their HBV upon discontinuation of emtricitabine, lamivudine, or tenofovir disoproxil fumarate.

Drug Interactions

Drug interactions are minimal with NRTIs because these drugs are not metabolized by the cytochrome P450 (CYP450) isoenzymes. However, drug interactions can still occur: for example, ribavirin inhibiting phosphorylation of zidovudine can cause hematologic toxicities, and coadministration of ribavirin with didanosine is contraindicated because fatal hepatic failure can occur; didanosine coadministered with stavudine can worsen lactic acidosis and pancreatitis; allopurinol is contraindicated in individuals taking didanosine; and PIs can increase serum concentration of tenofovir disoproxil fumarate.

Prototype Drug Chart: Zidovudine gives pharmacologic data for zidovudine, and Prototype Drug Chart: Tenofovir Disoproxil Fumarate shows the data for tenofovir.

Nonnucleoside Reverse Transcriptase Inhibitors

Five NNRTIs are used in the United States: delavirdine, efavirenz (EFV), etravirine, nevirapine (NVP), and rilpivirine. NNRTIs ("non-nukes") do not require intracellular metabolism; they directly bind to the reverse transcriptase (RT) enzymes and block DNA polymerization. The primary advantage of using NNRTIs is to reserve a PI-based therapy for future use. In general, an NNRTI regimen has a lower pill burden compared with most PI-based regimens. Major disadvantages are the prevalence of NNRTI-resistant viral strains and the low genetic barrier of NNRTIs for development of resistance. (Resistance testing is recommended for treatment-naïve patients before starting therapy.)

EFV and rilpivirine are available as components of fixed-dose regimens. EFV should be taken on an empty stomach; delavirdine and NVP can be taken without regard to food; all other NNRTIs should to be taken with food to enhance absorption. Except for NVP, all NNRTIs are metabolized by the liver and excreted in feces, whereas NVP is mostly excreted in urine.

TABLE 32.1 Antiretroviral Age Integrase Strand Transfer Inhibitors (INSTIs)

Generic	Route and Dosage	Uses and Considerations
Nucleoside/NRTIs		
ABC Also available as a component of fixed-dose combinations	Tablets and solution: A: PO: 300 mg bid or 600 mg once daily	Used in combination with other ARVs. Screen for HLA-B*5701 before initiation. Hypersensitivity reactions are highest in patients who test positive for HLA-B*5701. Avoid in persons with cardiovascular risk factors. A black-box warning exists for hepatotoxicity or lactic acidosis. May be administered without regard to meals. Metabolized by alcohol dehydrogenase and glucuronyl transferase; ethanol decreases elimination of ABC. A reduced dose is recommended in persons with hepatic impairment.
DDI	Extended-release capsule and powder for oral solution: A: ≥60 kg: PO: 400 mg once daily A: <60 kg: PO: 250 mg once daily *Dosages are decreased if administered with TDF.*	DDI is not recommended for initial therapy due to inferior virologic efficacy. Used in combination with other ARVs. Metabolized by the liver. A black-box warning exists for hepatotoxicity or lactic acidosis and pancreatitis. Take on an empty stomach. ER capsules must be swallowed whole. Reduce the dose in persons with renal impairment.
FTC Also available as a component of fixed-dose combinations	Capsule: A: PO: 200 mg once daily Solution: A: PO: 240 mg once daily	Used in combination with other ARVs. Metabolized by oxidation. A black-box warning exists for acute severe exacerbation of hepatitis B upon discontinuation of FTC and hepatitis or lactic acidosis. Otherwise, minimal toxicity is noted with FTC. Take without regard to meals. Reduce dose in patients with renal impairment.
Lamivudine (3TC) Also available as a component of fixed-dose combinations	Tablet and solution: A: PO: 300 mg once daily or 150 mg bid	Used in combination with other ARVs for treating HIV. Minimal toxicity with 3TC; a black-box warning exists for acute severe exacerbation of hepatitis B upon discontinuation of 3TC and hepatitis or lactic acidosis. Take without regard to meals. Adjust dosage in patients with renal insufficiency.
Stavudine (d4T)	A: ≥60 kg: PO: 40 mg q12h A: <60 kg: PO: 30 mg q12h	Used in combination with other ARVs for treating HIV. Crosses the blood-brain barrier. A black-box warning exists for hepatotoxicity or lactic acidosis and pancreatitis. Take without regard to meals. Adjust dosage in patients with renal insufficiency.
TDF	See Prototype Drug Chart: Tenofovir disoproxil fumarate	
ZDV Also available as a component of fixed-dose combinations	See Prototype Drug Chart: Zidovudine	
NNRTIs		
DLV	A: PO: 400 mg tid	Used in combination with NRTIs. Take without regard to meals. Acidic food improves absorption, and 100-mg tablets may be dispersed in liquid before administration. DLV is metabolized extensively by the CYP450 isoenzymes.
EFV Also available as a component of fixed-dose combinations	See Prototype Drug Chart: Efavirenz	
ETR	A: PO: 200 mg bid	Used in combination with NRTIs. However, patients with virologic failure on NNRTIs should not receive ETR solely with NRTIs. Administer after meals to enhance absorption. Tablets may be dispensed in water. Do not use grapefruit juice, carbonated beverages, or warm liquids. Do not add ETR to juice or milk without first adding it to water. Add more fluids to the glass to ensure the full dose is consumed. Metabolized by CYP450 enzymes; numerous drug-drug interactions exist. No dosage adjustment is needed in patients with renal insufficiency. Hypersensitivity reactions include rash, including Stevens-Johnson syndrome and hepatitis that includes hepatic necrosis.

TABLE 32.1 Antiretroviral Age Integrase Strand Transfer Inhibitors (INSTIs)—cont'd

Generic	Route and Dosage	Uses and Considerations
NVP	Immediate release: A: PO: 200 mg/d for 14 d, then 200 mg bid. Extended release: A: PO: Initial dosing with IR as previously discussed for 14 d, then 400 mg ER once daily	NVP should not be used as an initial treatment option for treatment-naïve patients because fatal toxicities can occur. Used in combination with other ARVs (NRTIs, NNRTIs, PIs). A black-box warning exists for females whose CD4+ counts are >250/mm^3 because risk of hepatotoxicity is increased. Take without regard to meals. Do not crush or chew ER tablets. Metabolized by CYP450. NVP is contraindicated in persons with hepatic impairment because of increased risk for hepatotoxicity. Numerous drug-drug interactions exist. Discontinue with hepatotoxicity or rash, including Stevens-Johnson syndrome.
RPL Also available as a component of fixed-dose combinations	A: ≥35 kg: PO: 25 mg once daily	Must be administered in combination with other ARVs. Take with a meal. Primarily metabolized by the liver. Numerous drug-drug interactions exist, and hepatotoxicity can occur. Monitor for depression, insomnia, cephalgia.
PIs ATV Also available as a component of fixed-dose combinations	See Prototype Drug Chart: Atazanavir	
DRV Also available as a component of fixed-dose combinations	A: PO: 600–800 mg bid	Used in combination with other ARVs. Must be administered with PK enhancer (cobicistat or low-dose ritonavir). Administer with food. DRV is metabolized by CYP450 isoenzymes. Adjust dosage in patients with hepatic insufficiency. Caution in patients with sulfa hypersensitivity. Monitor closely for rash, including Stevens-Johnson syndrome, toxic epidermal necrolysis, acute generalized exanthematous pustulosis, and erythema multiforme. Hepatotoxicity, DKA, and pancreatitis can occur. Other adverse effects include lipodystrophy, elevated transaminases, nausea, and diarrhea.
FPV	A: PO: 700 mg bid with ritonavir 100 mg PO bid	Used in combination with other ARVs. A PK enhancer with low-dose ritonavir and twice-daily dosing are recommended. Monitor in patients with sulfa hypersensitivity; cross-reaction can occur. Metabolized by CYP450 isoenzymes and drug transporters. Dose adjustment is required in patients with hepatic impairment. Tablets can be taken without regard to meals. Oral suspension is taken on an empty stomach in adults and with food in children. Can readminister dose if emesis occurs within 30 min of administration. Adverse effects include rash, diarrhea, nausea, vomiting, headache, hyperlipidemia, elevated transaminase levels, hyperglycemia, fat maldistribution, and possible increased bleeding in patients with hemophilia.
IDV	A: PO: 800 mg q12h	Used in combination with other ARVs and PK enhancers (e.g., ritonavir). CYP450 3A4 inhibitor and substrate. Adjust dosage in patients with hepatic insufficiency. For optimal absorption, take on an empty stomach. Hydrate with at least 1.5 L of fluid during a 24-h period. Adverse effects include nephrolithiasis, GI intolerance, nausea, indirect hyperbilirubinemia, headache, asthenia, blurred vision, dizziness, rash, metallic taste, thrombocytopenia, alopecia, hemolytic anemia, hyperlipidemia, elevated transaminase levels, hyperglycemia, fat maldistribution, and risk of increased bleeding in patients with hemophilia.
Lopinavir-ritonavir (LPV/r)	A: PO: 400/100 mg bid *or* 800/200 mg once daily	Used in combination with other ARVs. CYP450 3A4 inhibitor and substrate. May take tablet with or without food; take oral solution with food. Adverse effects include GI intolerance, asthenia, PR interval prolongation, pancreatitis, hyperlipidemia, elevated transaminase levels, hyperglycemia, fat maldistribution, and risk of increased bleeding in patients with hemophilia.

Continued

TABLE 32.1 Antiretroviral Age Integrase Strand Transfer Inhibitors (INSTIs)—cont'd

Generic	Route and Dosage	Uses and Considerations
NFV	A: PO: 1250 mg bid or 750 mg tid	Used in combination with other ARVs. Not recommended in treatment-naïve patients as initial therapy. CYP450 3A4 inhibitor and substrate. Take with food; do not mix with acidic food or juice. Tablets can be dispersed in a small amount of water before mixing with food or juice. Nelfinavir oral powder may be added to water, milk, formula, soymilk, or dietary supplements. Do not mix nelfinavir oral powder with acidic food or juice (orange juice, apple juice, or applesauce). Do not mix nelfinavir with water in the original container. Adverse effects include diarrhea, hyperlipidemia, elevated transaminase levels, hyperglycemia, fat maldistribution, and risk of increased bleeding in patients with hemophilia. ⚡ Persons with phenylketonuria should not take nelfinavir powder as it contains phenylalanine.
RTV	Other ARVs: A: PO: 600 mg bid Booster: A: PO: 100–400 mg in 1–2 divided doses	Used in combination with other ARVs and as a PK enhancer (booster) of other PIs. Dosage depends on use of RTV. CYP450 3A4 potent inhibitor; use extreme caution when administering other drugs, especially antihistamines, sedative hypnotics, antiarrhythmics, and ergot alkaloids. If coadministering with didanosine, separate drugs by 2 h. Take with food. Swallow tablets and capsules whole. Refrigerate capsules; RTV oral solution should not be refrigerated but left at room temperature for up to 30 d. Adverse effects include GI intolerance, paresthesia, hepatitis, asthenia, hyperlipidemia, hyperglycemia, fat maldistribution, and risk of increased bleeding in patients with hemophilia. Titrating the dosage may help reduce side effects. ⚡ RTV oral solution contains significant amounts of ethanol (43.2%) and propylene glycol (26.57%). Accidental ingestion by small children may lead to deadly ethanol or propylene glycol toxicity.
SQV	A: PO: 1000 mg bid	*Must* be dosed concurrently with low-dose ritonavir. SQV is not recommended for treatment-naïve adults due to its serious adverse effects. CYP450 3A4 inhibitor and substrate. Take with food. Adverse effects include nausea, diarrhea, headache, hyperlipidemia, elevated transaminase levels, hyperglycemia, PR and QT interval prolongation, fat maldistribution, and risk of increased bleeding in patients with hemophilia. Contraindicated in patients with PR or QT prolongation, hypokalemia, or hypomagnesemia.
TPV	A: PO: 500 mg bid	Used in combination with other ARVs; *must* be coadministered with ritonavir. TPV has a black-box warning for hepatotoxicity and intracranial bleeding. CYP450 3A4 inducer and substrate. Take with food if coadministered with RTV tablets; if administered with RTV capsules or solutions, TPV can be taken regardless of food. Adverse effects include hepatotoxicity, rash hyperlipidemia, hyperglycemia, fat maldistribution, and risk of increased bleeding in patients with hemophilia. Use with caution in patients with sulfa hypersensitivity.
FIs Enfuvirtide (T20)	A: subcut: 90 mg bid	Used in treatment-experienced patients in combination with other ARVs. Administer via subcut, and rotate site. Store vial at room temperature; once reconstituted, refrigerate and use within 24 h. Adverse effects include local injection site reaction (pain, erythema, induration, nodules, cysts, pruritus, ecchymosis), increased rate of bacterial pneumonia, hypersensitivity reaction (rash, fever, nausea, vomiting, chills, rigors, hypotension, elevated transaminases), fatigue. To minimize local reactions, apply ice or heat after injection or gently massage the site to better disperse the drug.

TABLE 32.1 Antiretroviral Age Integrase Strand Transfer Inhibitors (INSTIs)—cont'd

Generic	Route and Dosage	Uses and Considerations
Ibalizumab	A: IV: 2000 mg ×1, then 2 wk later, 800 mg every 2 wk	Used in treatment-experienced patients with multidrug-resistant virus. Before administering, must be further diluted. May store the diluted drug at room temperature for 4 h; refrigerated for up to 24 h. Do not administer via IVP or as bolus. Infuse first dose over 30 min. Succeeding doses can be infused over 15–30 min. Observe patient for 1 h after infusion. Common adverse reactions include diarrhea, dizziness, nausea, and rash.
CCR5 Antagonists		
MRV	A: PO: 150–600 mg bid	Used in combination with other ARVs. MRV is administered *only* to patients with CCR5-tropic HIV infection. Dosing depends on other drugs taken concomitantly. CYP3A substrate; drugs that inhibit or induce the enzymes will alter the pharmacokinetics of MRV. May take without regard to food. Concentration may increase in kidney dysfunction (CrCl <30); therefore caution is advised when used in renal-compromised patients; it is contraindicated in patients with CrCl <30 who are taking strong inhibitors and/or inducers of CYP3A. May need to adjust dose with concomitant CYP3A inhibitors or inducers (because of interactions) or with postural hypotension. Adverse effects include fever, upper respiratory tract infection, flatulence, orthostatic hypotension, hepatotoxicity, rash, cough, abdominal pain, and dizziness.
INSTIs		
DTG Also available as a component of fixed-dose combinations	A: ≥40 kg: PO: 50 mg once daily	Used in treatment-naïve or -experienced patients in combination with other ARVs. Metabolized by CYP3A4 enzyme. Can be taken without regard to meals. Take polyvalent cation products (e.g., Mg^{++}, Fe, and Ca^{++} salts); ASA on an empty stomach can reduce bioavailability of DTG. Adverse effects include headache, insomnia, rash, and liver injury.
EVG Also available as a component of fixed-dose combinations	A: PO: 85–150 mg once daily depending on ritonavir and other ARVs taken concurrently	Used in treatment-naïve or -experienced patients in combination with other ARVs; unboosted EVG is not recommended. EVG is metabolized by CYP3A. Take with food. Adverse effects are rare, but nausea and vomiting can occur; suicidal ideation, albeit rare, can also occur, especially in those with a history of psychiatric illness.
RTG	A: PO: 400 mg bid	Used in treatment-naïve or -experienced patients in combination with other ARVs. Does not affect the CYP450 isoenzymes, nor is it a substrate of CYP450 enzymes. Can be taken without regard to meals. Coated tablets are not bioequivalent with chewable tablets or powder for oral suspension; swallow coated tablets whole. Adverse effects include GI symptoms, headache, pyrexia, increased total cholesterol, fatigue, rhabdomyolysis, insomnia, and rash that includes Stevens-Johnson syndrome and epidermal necrolysis.

<, Less than; >, greater than; ≤, less than or equal to; ≥, greater than or equal to; *A*, adult; *ABC*, abacavir; *ARV*, antiretroviral; *ASA*, acetylsalicylic acid (aspirin); *ATV*, atazanavir; *bid*, twice a day; Ca^{++}, calcium; *CrCl*, creatinine clearance; *CYP450*, cytochrome P450; *d*, day; *DDI*, didanosine; *DKA*, diabetic ketoacidosis; *DLV*, delavirdine; *DRV*, darunavir; *DTG*, dolutegravir; *EFV*, efavirenz; *ER*, extended release; *ETR*, etravirine; *EVG*, elvitegravir; *Fe*, iron; *FIs*, fusion (entry) inhibitors; *FPV*, fosamprenavir; *FTC*, emtricitabine; *GI*, gastrointestinal; *h*, hour; *HIV*, human immunodeficiency virus; *HLA*, human leukocyte antigen; *IDV*, indinavir; *IR*, immediate release; *IV*, intravenous; *IVP*, intravenous push; *LPV/r*, lopinavir-ritonavir; Mg^{++}, magnesium; *min*, minute; *mo*, months; *MRV*, maraviroc; *NFV*, nelfinavir; *NNRTIs*, nonnucleoside reverse transcriptase inhibitors; *NVP*, nevirapine; *PI*, protease inhibitor; *PIs*, protease inhibitors; *PK*, pharmacokinetic; *PO*, by mouth; *q*, every; *RPL*, rilpivirine; *RTG*, raltegravir; *RTV*, ritonavir; *SQV*, saquinavir; *subcut*, subcutaneous; *TDF*, tenofovir; *tid*, three times a day; *TPV*, tipranavir; *wk*, week; *y*, years; *ZDV*, zidovudine.

PROTOTYPE DRUG CHART
Zidovudine (ZDV)

Drug Class	Dosage
Nucleoside/nucleotide reverse transcriptase inhibitor (NRTI) Also available as a component of fixed-dose combinations	Treatment in combination with other antiretrovirals: A: PO: 200 mg q8h or 300 mg q12h A: IV: 1 mg/kg over 1 h q4h (total daily dose: 6 mg/kg/day). Initiate oral therapy as soon as possible.

Contraindications	Drug-Lab-Food Interactions
Life-threatening allergies to ZDV or components of the preparation *Black-Box Warning:* Hepatotoxicity, lactic acidosis, myopathy, bone marrow suppression *Caution:* Severe anemia (interruption of therapy or reduction in daily dose should be considered); renal impairment/failure; viral hepatitis	*Drug:* Ganciclovir, probenecid, valproic acid may increase concentration/adverse effects. Rifampin, interferon, and ritonavir may decrease concentration/effects. May potentiate hematologic toxicity with other drugs (e.g., interferon alfa, ganciclovir, primaquine), causing myelosuppression; interferon beta can increase ZDV levels, leading to drug toxicity. Can be taken without regard to food. *Lab:* May increase ALT, AST

Pharmacokinetics	Pharmacodynamics
Absorption: PO: 66%–70% Distribution: PB: <38%, crosses blood-brain barrier, crosses placenta, excreted in breast milk Metabolism: t½: 0.5–3 h; extensive first-pass effect in liver to GZDV (metabolite) Excretion: 63%–95% in urine as GZDV (metabolite)	Route: PO/IV Onset: UK Peak: 30–90 min; can be taken without regard to meals Duration: UK

Therapeutic Effects/Uses
Management of patients with HIV infection, prevention of maternal-fetal HIV transmission
Mechanism of action: Inhibits viral enzyme reverse transcriptase and thymidine kinase, enzymes necessary for viral HIV replication.

Side Effects	Adverse Reactions
Headache, malaise, nausea, anorexia, vomiting, asthenia (abnormal weakness and loss of energy), constipation, abdominal cramps/pain, arthralgia, rigors, dyspepsia, fatigue, insomnia, musculoskeletal pain, myalgia, neuropathy, elevated liver enzymes, anemia, fever, cough, hepatomegaly, rash, diarrhea, lipodystrophy, and stomatitis	Severe anemia, lactic acidosis, pancreatitis, neutropenia, pancytopenia, seizures, congestive heart failure, myelosuppression, rhabdomyolysis, anaphylaxis, hyperlipidemia, insulin resistance, Stevens-Johnson syndrome, and toxic epidermal necrolysis

Side and Adverse Drug Effects
EFV is the first-choice drug within the NNRTI class, and it is the only NNRTI that penetrates the cerebrospinal fluid (CSF). It should be used with caution in pregnancy because neural tube defects have been reported after early human gestational exposure. Because of CSF involvement, neuropsychiatric symptoms such as dizziness, sedation, nightmares, euphoria, or loss of concentration can occur. Common complications among all the NNRTIs are rashes, which includes Stevens-Johnson syndrome. Elevated liver transaminases and hepatotoxicity, including hepatic failure, can also occur.

Drug Interactions
Drug-drug interactions are many because of the extensive metabolizing effects by cytochrome P3A4 (CYP3A4). Acid reducers (e.g., antacids, H_2-receptor antagonists, proton pump inhibitors [PPIs]) can decrease the bioavailability of rilpivirine, so coadministration of rilpivirine with PPIs is contraindicated; all other acid reducers can be taken at least 2 hours before or 4 hours after rilpivirine. Coadministration with drugs that induce or inhibit any of the CYP isoenzymes can alter the therapeutic effects of other drugs (e.g., anticonvulsants, antidepressants, anticoagulants, antiplatelets, antifungals, antimycobacterials, statins, and calcium channel blockers [CCBs]). Other drugs used concomitantly can alter NNRTI serum levels (e.g., corticosteroids, hepatitis antivirals, and St. John's wort). NNRTIs can decrease the efficacy of hormonal contraceptives, so individuals should use alternative means of contraception or additional contraceptive methods.

Prototype Drug Chart: Efavirenz presents the pharmacologic data for EFV.

Protease Inhibitors
PI-based regimens (one or two PIs plus two NRTIs) have revolutionized the treatment of HIV infection, especially with PK enhancement (boosters such as cobicistat and ritonavir); this has led to sustained viral suppression, improved immunologic function, and prolonged patient survival. PIs that have been approved by the FDA include atazanavir (ATV), atazanavir/cobicistat (ATV/c), darunavir (DRV), darunavir/cobicistat (DRV/c), fosamprenavir (FPV), indinavir (IDV), lopinavir/ritonavir (LPV/r), nelfinavir (NFV), saquinavir (SQV), ritonavir (RTV), and tipranavir (TPV). RTV as the sole PI is not recommended; instead, it should be used as a boosting agent with other PIs. TPV is only approved for ARV-experienced patients. Unlike NRTIs and NNRTIs, PIs act at the end of the HIV life cycle to target viral assembly by inhibiting the activity of protease, an enzyme used to cleave nascent proteins for final assembly of new virions, resulting in formation and release of immature, defective, and noninfectious virus particles. Each PI has unique characteristics based on clinical efficacy, side effect profile, and PK properties. PIs are highly protein bound, metabolized by the liver, and primarily eliminated in feces.

PROTOTYPE DRUG CHART
Tenofovir Disoproxil Fumarate (TDF)

Drug Class	Dosage
Nucleoside/nucleotide reverse transcriptase inhibitor (NRTI) Also available as a component of fixed-dose combinations	HIV treatment: A: ≥35 kg: PO: 300 mg once daily
Contraindications	**Drug-Lab-Food Interactions**
Black-Box Warning: Hepatitis B exacerbation, hepatotoxicity, lactic acidosis *Caution:* Renal and hepatic dysfunction	*Drug:* Concomitant use with streptozocin is contraindicated because it can increase risk of nephrotoxicity and ototoxicity. Tenofovir can decrease levels of some drugs (e.g., dabigatran, edoxaban) and increase levels of other drugs (e.g., adefovir, bacitracin, diltiazem, metformin); acyclovir, amikacin, cisplatin, ganciclovir, and gentamicin may increase levels and adverse effects of TDF. *Lab:* May increase triglycerides, AST, ALT, ALP
Pharmacokinetics	**Pharmacodynamics**
Absorption: PO: 25%–40% Distribution: PB: 7.2% Metabolism: $t\frac{1}{2}$: 17 h; is not metabolized by CYP450 isoenzymes; converted intracellularly by hydrolysis and phosphorylated to active tenofovir diphosphate Excretion: 70%–80% primarily in urine as unchanged drug	Route: PO Onset: UK Peak: 1 h (fasting), 2 h (food) Duration: UK
Therapeutic Effects/Uses	
Management of patients with HIV infection, treatment of chronic hepatitis B Mechanism of action: Inhibits viral enzyme reverse transcriptase, an enzyme necessary for viral HIV replication, by competing with AMP as substrate	
Side Effects	**Adverse Reactions**
Diarrhea, nausea, vomiting, flatulence, insomnia, dizziness, depression, fever, hyperlipidemia, elevated transaminases, chest pain	Lactic acidosis, hepatomegaly, bone fractures, renal insufficiency, Fanconi syndrome

The Panel's recommended PI regimen is DRV/r plus two NRTIs (tenofovir disoproxil fumarate/emtricitabine [TDF/FTC]). RTV boosting is a relatively new concept and one of the mainstays of PI therapy. The potent inhibitory effect of RTV on the cytochrome P450 3A4 isoenzyme (CYP3A4) allows the addition of 100 to 400 mg of RTV to other PIs as a PK booster. This helps reduce dietary restrictions, increase drug exposure, inhibit metabolism, and maximize blood levels of the coadministered PI, thus reducing dosing frequency and pill burden and overcoming viral resistance. Because "boosted" regimens may be less complex, patients may be able to follow and tolerate them better.

Side and Adverse Drug Effects
Selection of a PI-based regimen should consider dosing frequency, food and fluid requirements, pill burden, drug interaction potential, and side effect profile. PIs result in numerous metabolic abnormalities that include dyslipidemia and insulin resistance; PK enhancers can alter these adverse effects. Some PIs come with a risk factor for causing myocardial infarction (MI). When initiating therapy with PIs, GI side effects (nausea, vomiting, and diarrhea) can be bothersome and may negatively affect adherence. Skin reactions such as rash, which includes Stevens-Johnson syndrome, can occur with PIs. Other adverse effects include hemolytic anemia, electrocardiogram changes, and MI.

Drug Interactions
In patients with hepatic impairment, dosing adjustment may be necessary. All PIs inhibit the CYP450 system, which can lead to many drug-drug interactions. Drugs such as H_2-receptor antagonists (e.g., cimetidine, famotidine, or ranitidine) should be given 10 or more hours before PIs. PPIs are not recommended in PI-experienced patients, and concomitant use with anticoagulants/antiplatelets should also be avoided. Ritonavir-boosted PIs can decrease warfarin levels. Anticonvulsants (e.g., carbamazepine, phenobarbital, phenytoin) are contraindicated with certain PIs, whereas some antidepressants (e.g., bupropion, selective serotonin reuptake inhibitors [SSRIs]) may need dose adjustments. Trazodone is contraindicated with saquinavir/ritonavir, and antimycobacterials and cardiac drugs can worsen cardiac toxicities. Many PIs without the ritonavir boost can increase drug levels of hormonal contraceptives, whereas boosted PIs can decrease the levels. It is important that nurses instruct patients to use an alternative contraceptive method when taking boosted PIs. Rifoampin and rifapentine are contraindicated with PIs, as are many other classes of drugs (e.g., antiarrhythmics, antivirals for viral hepatitis, St. John's wort, hydroxymethylglutaryl coenzyme A [HMG-CoA] reductase inhibitors, and some hypnotics) due to a decrease in PI drug levels and toxic drug levels in the other classes of drugs. Benefits of corticosteroid use should outweigh the risks with concomitant administration with corticosteroids.

Prototype Drug Chart: Atazanavir presents the pharmacologic data for ATV.

Fusion (Entry) Inhibitors
Enfuvirtide (T20) was the first approved in this class. T20 acts by a mechanism that inhibits the fusion of the virus to healthy cell membranes, thus preventing HIV entry into healthy cells. T20 is indicated only in combination with other ARVs for patients with limited treatment options who require salvage therapy. It is not indicated for HIV-2. Before initiating a fusion (entry) inhibitor, immunoassay and subsequent testing for HIV-1/HIV-2 are recommended.

PROTOTYPE DRUG CHART
Efavirenz (EFV)

Drug Class	Dosage
Nonnucleoside reverse transcriptase inhibitor (NNRTI) Also available as a component of fixed-dose combination.	Note: Take dose at bedtime to minimize CNS adverse effects; take on an empty stomach to reduce adverse reactions. A: PO: 600 mg at bedtime Do not crush tablets. Capsules may be opened and sprinkled into a small amount of age-appropriate soft food or formula; administer within 30 min of mixing; no additional food for 2 h after dosing.
Contraindications	**Drug-Lab-Food Interactions**
Life-threatening allergies to EFV or components of the preparation; concurrent use with rifapentine, St. John's wort, dasabuvir, ombitasvir, paritaprevir, simeprevir, triazolam *Caution:* Patients with history of mental illness or drug abuse; liver impairment; seizure disorder	*Drug:* EFV can increase or decrease levels of warfarin, carbamazepine, nevirapine, phenobarbital, bupropion, sertraline, phenytoin, rifampin, CCBs, hormonal contraceptives, HMG-CoA reductase inhibitors; EFV can increase the levels of triazolam. Drugs that can increase or decrease EFV include dexamethasone, boceprevir, St. John's wort. *Food:* Avoid alcohol because of liver/CNS adverse effects; high-fat meals increase absorption. *Lab:* May cause a false-positive result for cannabinoid and benzodiazepine screening assays.
Pharmacokinetics	**Pharmacodynamics**
Absorption: PO: Increased after high-fat meal Distribution: PB: >99%, widely distributed (found in CSF) Metabolism: t½: 40–76 h; metabolized in liver; CYP3A4 inducer/inhibitor Excretion: 16%–61% in feces, primarily as unchanged drug; 14%–34% in urine, primarily as metabolite	Route: PO Onset: UK Peak: 3–5 h Duration: UK
Therapeutic Effects/Uses	
Treatment of HIV-1 infections Mechanism of action: Binds directly to reverse transcriptase, blocking RNA- and DNA-dependent DNA polymerase activities, including HIV-1 replication	
Side Effects	**Adverse Reactions**
Rash, nausea, diarrhea, CNS effects (dizziness, insomnia, abnormal dreams/thinking, impaired concentration, amnesia, agitation, hallucinations, euphoria, anxiety)	Aggressive reaction, allergic reaction, convulsion, liver failure, neuropathy, suicide, abnormal vision, hyperlipidemia

Enfuvirtide T20 does not require dosage adjustment in patients with renal failure or hepatic impairment. It is not metabolized by the CYP enzymes and is not associated with any CYP-mediated drug-drug interactions. Injection site reactions (e.g., subcutaneous nodules, redness) occur in up to 98% of patients. Other side effects reported include rash and diarrhea. Serious allergic reactions—including anaphylaxis, fever, and hypotension—have occurred in less than 1% of patients.

Ibalizumab is newly approved fusion inhibitors to treat HIV-1. Similar to T20, ibalizumab is indicated for patients with multiple drug-resistant infection. It is also used in combination with other ART drugs. Dose modification is not required. Reported side effects include diarrhea, dizziness, nausea, and rash.

Chemokine (CCR5) Coreceptor Antagonists

Maraviroc (MVC), the only drug in this class, blocks the CCR5 coreceptor needed for CCR5-tropic HIV entry into immune cells, thus preventing viral replication. MVC is indicated in combination with other ARVs for treatment-experienced adult patients with evidence of viral replication and HIV-1 strains resistant to multiple ART.

Side and Adverse Drug Effects
The most common side effects are cough, pyrexia, upper respiratory tract infection, rash, abdominal pain, and dizziness. Because MVC is metabolized by the liver, drug-drug interactions exist.

Drug Interactions
MVC is metabolized by the CYP3A substrate. Coadministration with St. John's wort or rifampin or other CYP3A inducers is not recommended due to reduced effectiveness of MVC. Rifapentine and some NRTI fixed-drug combinations are contraindicated with CCR5 coreceptor antagonists. Possible drug-induced hepatotoxicity with allergy-type features has been reported. Use caution in patients with liver or heart disease or a history of orthostatic hypotension and in those on medication that lowers blood pressure. Other adverse reactions include rash, musculoskeletal symptoms, upper respiratory infections, and pyrexia.

Integrase Strand Transfer Inhibitors
INSTIs such as dolutegravir (DTG), elvitegravir (EVG), and raltegravir (RTG) exert their action by interfering with integrase, the enzyme that HIV needs to multiply and divide, thus limiting the ability of the virus

PROTOTYPE DRUG CHART
Atazanavir (ATV)

Drug Class	Dosage
Protease inhibitor Also available as a component of fixed-dose combinations.	Note: HIV guidelines recommend administering concurrently with a PK enhancer (cobicistat or RTV). Capsules and powder packets are not interchangeable. Capsules: A: PO: 300 mg plus RTV 100 mg once daily Capsules must be swallowed whole. Powder may be mixed with food; use oral dosing syringe in persons unable to drink from a cup.

Contraindications	Drug-Lab-Food Interactions
Hypersensitivity to ATV or any component, concurrent use with alfuzosin, ergot derivatives, lovastatin, midazolam (oral), rifampin, simvastatin, St. John's wort *Caution:* Patients with preexisting conduction abnormalities (may prolong PR interval), hepatitis B or C, hepatic impairment, hemophilia A or B	*Drug:* Drug-drug interactions are numerous. Some known interactions include drugs that can decrease or decrease ATV; acid reducers, including H_2-receptor antagonists and PPIs; carbamazepine, phenytoin, phenobarbital, itraconazole, rifampin, boceprevir, and St. John's wort. ATV can increase or decrease levels of dabigatran, warfarin, buspirone, rifabutin, amiodarone, BBs, CCBs, digoxin, corticosteroids, hormonal contraceptives, lovastatin, and simvastatin *Lab:* May increase liver function tests, cholesterol, triglycerides, glucose *Food:* Bioavailability increases when taken with food

Pharmacokinetics	Pharmacodynamics
Absorption: PO: Rapidly, increased with food Distribution: PB: 86% Metabolism: $t\frac{1}{2}$: 7–8 h (9–18 h when boosted with RTV). Metabolized in the liver; inhibitor of CYP450 isoenzymes Excretion: Primarily in feces (79%) but also in urine (13%)	Route: PO Onset: UK Peak: 2–3 h Duration: UK

Therapeutic Effects/Uses
Treatment of HIV-1 infection
Mechanism of action: Inhibits HIV protease, rendering enzyme incapable of processing polyprotease precursors, thus rendering immature HIV particles noninfectious

Side Effects	Adverse Reactions
Rash, nausea, vomiting, diarrhea, cough, fever	Atrioventricular block, hyperglycemia, diabetes mellitus, jaundice, hyperlipidemia, lipodystrophy, cholelithiasis, nephrolithiasis, elevated liver transaminases

to replicate and infect new cells. INSTIs are used for the treatment of HIV-1 infections with at least two or three other ARVs in both treatment-naïve (recommended initial agent) and treatment-experienced patients. DTG and EVG are also available in fixed-dose combinations. INSTIs distribute into the CSF. DTG and RTG are metabolized by the UDP-glucuronosyltransferases (UGTs) 1A1-mediated glucuronidation pathway; EVG is metabolized by the CYP450 enzymes. Strong inducers (e.g., EFV, rifampin, rifabutin) or inhibitors (e.g., tenofovir, atazanavir) of UGT1A1 can significantly alter the concentration of RTG. DTG distributes into the CSF. Common side effects include rash, nausea, headache, insomnia, diarrhea, and pyrexia; liver injury can also occur. Caution is advised in patients at increased risk for muscle problems (e.g., myopathy, rhabdomyolysis), which includes patients who take medications that can cause these adverse effects, such as statins.

THE NURSE'S ROLE IN ANTIRETROVIRAL THERAPY
Adherence, Assessment, and Education

Adherence challenges are common with any drug therapy, but ART presents a greater challenge because patients are asked to achieve an adherence of 100%. Nonadherence can result in HIV viral replication and can potentiate drug resistance. Multiple strategies for adherence are available and should be discussed with patients. Drug organizers, alarms on cell phones or mobile devices, medication "maps" with pictures, and drug diaries are available tools to improve adherence. Friends, family members, and personal support systems can also assist patients with adherence. Nurses can facilitate adherence by allowing sufficient time to educate patients about drugs, developing a trusting relationship, and building a partnership with the patient.

Assessment
Thorough assessment of the patient's physiological and psychosocial health needs and literacy levels is required initially and for the duration of care. Follow-up assessment after ART initiation should include drug side effects, adherence to the therapy regimen, and issues that affect medication adherence. Patients may confuse drug side effects with new onset of symptoms. Careful follow-up assessment can detect the need for additional medical care or drug management.

Nursing assessment for adherence should include asking the reasons for missing drug dosages. Reasons commonly include stigma, forgetting, feeling ill, side effects, not having the medicine when doses are due, pill fatigue (nonadherence due to the stress and monotony of constant pill swallowing), drug costs, loss of health insurance, and lack of transportation to the pharmacy. If barriers to adherence are identified, individualized plans should be addressed with the patient and the prescriber.

Nurses should identify problems that require additional investigation and research. Because of individual needs, research on strategies to promote adherence is needed. Whenever drug regimens change, nurses should contribute to the ongoing evaluation of the drug regimen, any side effects, and adverse event reporting.

Education

Patient education should include the purpose of each drug, the dosage schedule, food and fluid restrictions, recommended food choices, and storage of drugs. Additional suggestions include taking drugs during a daily routine, such as brushing teeth, or using a drug calendar to track drugs taken. The nurse should assess whether scheduled appointments to assist the patient with filling a drug organizer would be helpful until the patient is comfortable with completing this task. Discussion of anticipated drug side effects and management of drug side effects is necessary. See Box 32.1 for HIV resources.

Immune Reconstitution Inflammatory Syndrome

Immune reconstitution inflammatory syndrome (IRIS) is related to a disease- or pathogen-specific inflammatory response in patients with ART being initiated or changed. IRIS comprises two distinct entities: *paradoxical IRIS* is an exacerbation of treated (successful or partial) opportunistic infection (OI), whereas *unmasking IRIS* is a response to undiagnosed or subclinical OI. Diagnosis is a challenge because there are no laboratory markers; it is a condition of exclusion. For example, new OI or concurrent illness must be excluded before IRIS can be diagnosed. CD4+ cells usually increase in patients with IRIS because of the acute inflammatory response. IRIS may occur in response to many diseases and pathogens, such as Kaposi sarcoma or infection with mycobacteria, viruses, bacteria, or fungi.

Risk factors for developing IRIS include a low CD4+ cell count when ART is initiated and a high baseline HIV RNA. Starting ART soon after initiation of treatment for recognized OI also increases risk for IRIS. Severity of IRIS ranges from mild to life-threatening. Treatment varies according to the specific pathogen and clinical situation but typically includes continuing ART if possible, treating the OI as indicated, and adding antiinflammatory therapy (including corticosteroids) as needed.

Opportunistic Infections

As HIV advances, patients are more vulnerable to malignancies and opportunistic infections (OIs). Since the introduction of ART, there has been a dramatic reduction in the incidence of OIs among HIV-positive patients receiving ARVs. Although hospitalizations and deaths have decreased, OIs continue to be a leading cause of morbidity and mortality among patients with HIV. Prevention and treatment of OIs remain essential. The most common HIV-related OIs include pulmonary TB, pneumococcal pneumonia, *Cryptosporidium*, fungal infections, Kaposi sarcoma, toxoplasmosis, histoplasmosis, and cytomegalovirus, among others.

> **BOX 32.1 HIV Resources**
>
> **Acquired Immunodeficiency Syndrome Info**
> The website https://hivinfo.nih.gov/home-page provides information on HIV/AIDS clinical research, treatment, and prevention.
>
> **National HIV/AIDS Clinicians' Consultation Center**
> The website www.nccc.ucsf.edu provides up-to-date HIV/AIDS information to pharmacists, physicians, and nurses and is staffed by pharmacists, physicians, and nurse practitioners.

Tuberculosis infection predominantly affects the lungs but can affect other organs, such as the bowel, brain, and lining of the heart, lungs, central nervous system (CNS), or integument. The CD4+ cell count is not a reliable predictor of increased risk for TB disease. Treatment for TB is discussed in Chapter 30.

Kaposi sarcoma causes dark blue lesions that can occur in a variety of locations, including the skin, mucous membranes, GI tract, lungs, or lymph nodes; they usually appear early in the course of HIV infection. Treatment depends on the symptoms and location, but chemotherapy is the preferred treatment for severe widespread disease.

Pneumocystis jiroveci pneumonia (PJP) is caused by a fungus that shares biologic characteristics with protozoa that infect the lungs. Symptoms include fever, dry cough, chest pain, and dyspnea. Even though PJP is classified as a fungal infection, it does not respond to antifungals. Trimethoprim-sulfamethoxazole, dapsone plus trimethoprim, pentamidine, or atovaquone is recommended treatment for persons with HIV and PJP.

Toxoplasmosis encephalitis caused by a protozoan can be found in uncooked meat and cat feces. Infection in the brain can cause headache, confusion, motor weakness, and fever. If left untreated, the disease progression results in seizures, stupor, and coma. Treatment includes pyrimethamine, sulfadiazine, and clindamycin. Leucovorin is added to decrease hematologic toxicities associated with pyrimethamine therapy.

Cryptosporidiosis is an infection caused by the protozoan parasite *Cryptosporidium*, usually in the bowel mucosa; in persons with low CD4+ counts, *Cryptosporidium* may involve the biliary tract or respiratory tract. GI symptoms include profuse, watery diarrhea, often with nausea, vomiting, and lower abdominal cramping. In addition to symptomatic therapy, treatment includes nitazoxanide or paromomycin combined with azithromycin. Treatment may be only partially effective in the setting of a low CD4+ count.

Mycobacterium avium complex (MAC) is a blood infection caused by bacteria related to *Mycobacterium tuberculosis*, the pathogen in TB. MAC generally affects multiple organs with symptoms that include fever, night sweats, weight loss, fatigue, diarrhea, and abdominal pain. Localized syndromes include pneumonitis, osteomyelitis, skin or soft tissue abscesses, or CNS infections. Treatment includes clarithromycin, azithromycin, ethambutol, amikacin, moxifloxacin, rifabutin, or rifampin.

Cytomegalovirus (CMV) infection is caused by a virus that infects the entire body, but it most commonly appears as retinitis, causing blurred vision that can lead to blindness. CMV can also affect other organs and can cause fever, diarrhea, nausea, pneumonia-like symptoms, and dementia. Treatment includes ganciclovir, valganciclovir, foscarnet, or cidofovir.

Antiretroviral Therapy in Pregnancy

Optimal drug therapy should be used for women of reproductive age and for those who are pregnant. When initiating ART for women of reproductive age, the criteria for starting therapy and the goals of treatment are identical to those for other adults and adolescents. Because of considerations related to the prevention of HIV transmission to the fetus during pregnancy, the timing of initiation of treatment and the selection of regimens for pregnant patients may differ from those for nonpregnant adults or adolescents. Women of childbearing potential should undergo a pregnancy test before initiation of EFV. If the patient expresses interest in becoming pregnant, and EFV is considered as part of the ARV regimen, a risk-benefit discussion must take place regarding the risk of neural tube defects related to EFV use in the first 5 to 6 weeks of pregnancy. EFV can be continued in pregnant patients receiving an EFV-based regimen who present for antenatal care in the first trimester, provided the regimen produces virologic suppression.

CLINICAL JUDGMENT [NURSING PROCESS]
Antiretroviral Therapy

Concept: Drug Adherence
- The ability or lack of the ability to take drugs as prescribed

Recognize Cues [Assessment]
- Obtain an in-depth patient history, and assess physiologic and psychosocial needs.
- Assess for signs and symptoms related to clinical progression of human immunodeficiency virus (HIV), and refer to medical care and psychological support as indicated.
- Perform a drug reconciliation that includes all prescription, over-the-counter (OTC), and herbal products. Assess for use of illegal and other nonprescription drugs. Report potential drug-drug or drug-herb interactions.
- Obtain a nutritional history to assess for nutritional deficits and for potential drug-food interactions. Assess for the potential need for therapeutic lifestyle change.
- Assess readiness to learn and discern the preferred method of instruction (written, verbal, pictorial).
- With each patient visit, conduct a pill count to determine treatment adherence.

Analyze Cues and Prioritize Hypothesis [Patient Problems]
- Risk for nonadherence
- Need for health teaching
- Coping
- Decreased immunity

Generate Solutions [Planning]
- The patient will adhere to the drug regimen and will report any difficulties related to adherence.
- The patient will participate in medical treatment and in the spiritual and psychological support that best fits the patient's needs and belief system; the patient will verbalize fears.
- The patient will verbalize ways of maintaining self-health management such as a daily calendar and reminders.
- The patient will verbalize ways to cope with side effects of the drug regimen.
- The patient will verbalize signs and symptoms of potential infection and can reiterate when to notify the health care provider.
- The patient will have undetectable viral load at end of therapy.
- The patient will not experience secondary or opportunistic infections.

Take Action [Nursing Interventions]
- Provide information on the necessity of adhering to the drug regimen and regular health care. Inconsistent dosing can promote drug resistance. Effectiveness and side effects of antiretroviral therapy (ART) need to be monitored and/or treated.
- Provide information on various methods of remembering to take drugs. Inconsistent dosing can increase the risk of drug resistance.
- Refer the patient for health care maintenance and appropriate health screening examinations, including Pap tests, ophthalmologic and dental examinations, and age- or risk-related colonoscopies. Side effects and adverse reactions are common in patients receiving ART.
- Refer the patient for spiritual support and for mental health or substance use counseling as needed.
- Provide opportunities for the patient and/or support persons to verbalize feelings.
- Encourage strategies to cope with the side effects of medications.
- Monitor laboratory reports for indications of decreasing CD4+ counts and/or rising viral load; inform the HIV health care provider.
- Refer the patient for nutritional counseling as needed.

Patient Teaching
General
- Educate patients about adherence to the therapeutic regimen by providing information on drugs and a timetable of dosing in patients' preferred method of learning.
- Explain common emotional responses.
- For patients of childbearing age, explain how HIV transmission to the unborn baby can occur.
- Teach about safe sex practices and other ways to prevent transmission of HIV.
- Inform patients that certain drugs—including OTC medications—and foods and herbal products may interact with antiretrovirals.
- Assist patients in developing a system for taking the correct dose of the correct drugs at the correct time.
- Counsel patients about the importance of having an adequate supply of drugs to avoid interruption in the dosing schedule. Omission of drugs may result in deterioration of the patient's condition.

Side Effects
- Explain how HIV can damage the immune system and promote infection.
- To decrease risk for exposure to infection, emphasize protective precautions as necessary, such as frequent handwashing, avoiding crowds, and receiving influenza vaccines.
- Inform the patient to report unmanageable side effects, such as nausea and diarrhea.

Evaluate Outcomes [Evaluation]
- The patient will maintain a 100% drug adherence. The patient will maintain a pill calendar or reminder to maintain drug adherence.
- Viral load will decrease or become undetectable.
- The patient and/or the significant other will openly discuss any fears or concerns related to HIV and ART.
- The patient will verbalize safe sex practices and methods to reduce HIV transmission.

A pregnant patient infected with HIV can transmit the virus during pregnancy, labor, and delivery and through breast-feeding. To prevent MTCT of HIV, ART is recommended in all pregnant patients who test positive for HIV infection, regardless of virologic, immunologic, or clinical parameters. Combination drug therapy is considered the standard of care for both treatment of maternal HIV infection and prophylaxis to reduce the risk for perinatal HIV transmission. The goal of ART is to achieve maximal and sustained viral suppression during pregnancy to prevent perinatal transmission of HIV. If viral load is greater than or equal to 400 copies/mL, IV zidovudine is recommended regardless of current ART. Prototype Drug Chart: Zidovudine presents the pharmacologic data for zidovudine.

Occupational HIV Exposure and Postexposure Prophylaxis

Treatment regimens after percutaneous exposure to HIV are called **postexposure prophylaxis (PEP)** regimens. Many PEP regimens are available, with varying degrees of tolerability and probability of patients completing 4 weeks of treatment. PEP management of potential HIV exposure should be initiated within 72 hours of the event and should be continued for 4 weeks. Health care workers who take PEP have reported adverse reactions, with the most common being nausea, malaise, and fatigue. More information from the Panel on the treatment of HIV/AIDS can be found at https://clinicalinfo.hiv.gov/en/guidelines.

CLINICAL JUDGMENT CASE STUDY

A 35-year-old female patient was recently diagnosed with HIV. Other than a recent "case of the flu" approximately 1 month ago, the patient reported being healthy. She has been divorced for 2 years and has a 3-year-old child from her previous marriage. The patient tested negative for HIV in the first trimester of her pregnancy and was not retested during the third trimester. She reports that the relationship with her partner was monogamous and that they did not use "protections." She began a relationship with a new partner 1 year after her divorce, who denied having HIV, and they did not use protective barriers (the patient takes oral contraceptives for pregnancy prevention). The patient denies a history of IV drug use and other high-risk behaviors. Her baseline labs include a CD4+ count of 450 cells/mm^3 and a viral load of 75,000 copies/mL. Her genotypic resistance assay shows no baseline resistance. Her preference is for a once-a-day regimen. She may want to have another child but is not certain.

1. The patient asks the nurse when she may have become infected with HIV. What are some of the responses that the nurse should include in a discussion with the patient? What else should the nurse discuss with the patient about HIV transmission?
2. Considering the patient's preference for a daily antiretroviral regimen and in view of her history, which medication regimens could be considered? What, if any, risk-benefit discussion should occur with regard to choices?
3. The patient is told she will begin therapy with a fixed-dose combination regimen containing three different antiretrovirals. The patient asks why she needs to be on more than one drug. How would the nurse explain the reason for the multidrug regimen?
4. At her next routine visit, the patient says that she missed two doses of her medications because she had an unplanned overnight stay during a trip. What counseling and interventions would the nurse include in discussion with the patient?

REVIEW QUESTIONS

1. During routine prenatal testing, a patient is diagnosed with human immunodeficiency virus (HIV) infection. To help prevent perinatal transmission of HIV to the fetus, which nursing action is best?
    a. Provide the patient with contact information for an acquired immunodeficiency syndrome support group.
    b. Educate the patient about the risks of human immunodeficiency virus disease to the fetus.
    c. Notify the Centers for Disease Control and Prevention of the patient's diagnosis.
    d. Provide written and oral education about the use of antiretroviral therapy during pregnancy.
2. A recent laboratory result indicated an "undetectable" viral load. Which response by the nurse is best?
    a. Inform the patient that they must be seen immediately because the undetectable viral load indicates that the medication stopped working.
    b. Have the patient reschedule the clinic visit.
    c. Congratulate the patient on the treatment success.
    d. Educate the patient about the continued need for medications and ongoing laboratory monitoring.
3. The nurse advises human immunodeficiency virus (HIV)-positive patients about blood draws to obtain a CD4+ count. Which information would be correct?
    a. Laboratory tests should be done at the same laboratory at approximately the same time of day.
    b. A 10-hour fast is required for laboratory tests.
    c. Laboratory tests will need to be obtained approximately 1 hour after taking antiretroviral medications.
    d. It does not matter where the labs are conducted as long as they are done.
4. In collaboration with a patient on antiretroviral therapy, the nurse formulates a plan of care. Which items are appropriate to include in planning? **Select all that apply.**
    a. Viral load will become and remain undetectable.
    b. The patient will not experience secondary infection.
    c. New onset of symptoms and side effects will be promptly reported.
    d. Laboratory blood work will be within normal limits.
    e. The patient will adhere to the medication regimen and will report any difficulties related to adherence.
5. A patient is to start on efavirenz. Which points are important for the nurse to include in health teaching for this patient? **Select all that apply.**
    a. The dose is given at bedtime to minimize central nervous system adverse effects.
    b. Alcohol should be avoided because of adverse effects to the liver.
    c. The dose should be taken after breakfast to minimize central nervous system adverse effects.
    d. High-fat meals can increase absorption of the medication.
    e. Hyperglycemia, jaundice, and diabetes mellitus are side effects.

33

Transplant Drugs

http://evolve.elsevier.com/McCuistion/pharmacology

OBJECTIVES

- Explain the principles of immunosuppression and the therapies used to address it.
- Summarize the use of drugs to treat transplant rejection.
- Summarize the use of drugs for bacterial, fungal, and viral infections associated with organ transplantation.
- Describe the issues and considerations in the promotion of adherence to a posttransplant regimen.

OUTLINE

Principles of Immunosuppression and Immunosuppressant Drugs, 395
   Immunosuppression, 395
   Induction Therapy, 395
   Maintenance Therapy, 397
Drugs for Transplant Rejection, 402
   Antithymocyte Globulin, 402
Drugs for Infection, 403
   Bacterial, 403

   Fungal, 403
   Viral, 403
Promoting Adherence, 403
   Importance of Adherence, 403
   Nurse's Role in Adherence, 403
Clinical Judgment Unfolding Case Study, 404
Review Questions, 406

Organ transplantation is a life-saving procedure. In **cadaveric transplantation**, a healthy organ donated at the time of a person's death is transplanted into the body of a patient with end-stage organ failure. In **living-donor transplantation**, a kidney or a portion of a liver donated by a living person is transplanted into the body of a patient with end-stage kidney or liver disease. Organ transplant is an acceptable treatment option when organs fail (e.g., kidney, heart, liver, and lung). More than 100,000 people are currently waiting for an organ transplant. Every 10 minutes, another person is added to the wait list, and more than 8000 people die each year while waiting for a donor organ. The average wait time is 3 to 5 years.

PRINCIPLES OF IMMUNOSUPPRESSION AND IMMUNOSUPPRESSANT DRUGS

Immunosuppression

The immune system remains the biggest barrier to transplantation as a routine medical treatment because it has effective mechanisms to fight off foreign organisms. These same mechanisms are involved in the rejection of transplanted organs, which are recognized as foreign by the recipient's immune system. The underlying premise of **immunosuppression** is to use multiple drugs that alter different aspects of the immune system (Fig. 33.1), thereby reducing the chances of transplant rejection and enabling the use of lower doses of individual drugs, which reduces the likelihood of drug toxicity. Transplantation has revolutionized care for patients with end-stage organ failure, yet significant problems remain with treatments designed to promote transplant survival and prevent rejection. When patients are immunosuppressed, they have a diminished capacity to fight infection and other diseases. Immunosuppressant drugs are not always effective; in addition, they are expensive, must be taken daily, and are associated with toxic effects. Prolonged immunosuppression presents a malignancy risk.

Induction Therapy

Induction therapy is immunosuppressive therapy administered pretransplantation and early posttransplantation to provide intense immunosuppression with drugs designed to diminish antigen presentation and T-cell response, thus reducing the risk for acute rejection during the initial transplant period.

Basiliximab

Basiliximab is a monoclonal antibody that inhibits the activation of lymphocytes, a critical component of the cellular immune response involved in transplant rejection. By inhibiting the activation of lymphocytes, it prevents the body from mounting an immune response against the transplanted organ. Basiliximab has been approved for induction therapy in kidney transplants.

   Pharmacokinetics. Basiliximab is readily adsorbed. The protein binding capacity is unknown. The half-life is 4 to 10.7 days.

   Pharmacodynamics. The duration of action is 22 to 50 days.

   Basiliximab is administered intravenously (IV), 20 mg within 2 hours before transplant surgery, followed by a second 20-mg dose 4 days after transplantation. The second dose should be withheld if complications occur (including severe hypersensitivity reactions or loss of the transplanted organ). Children under 35 kg should receive

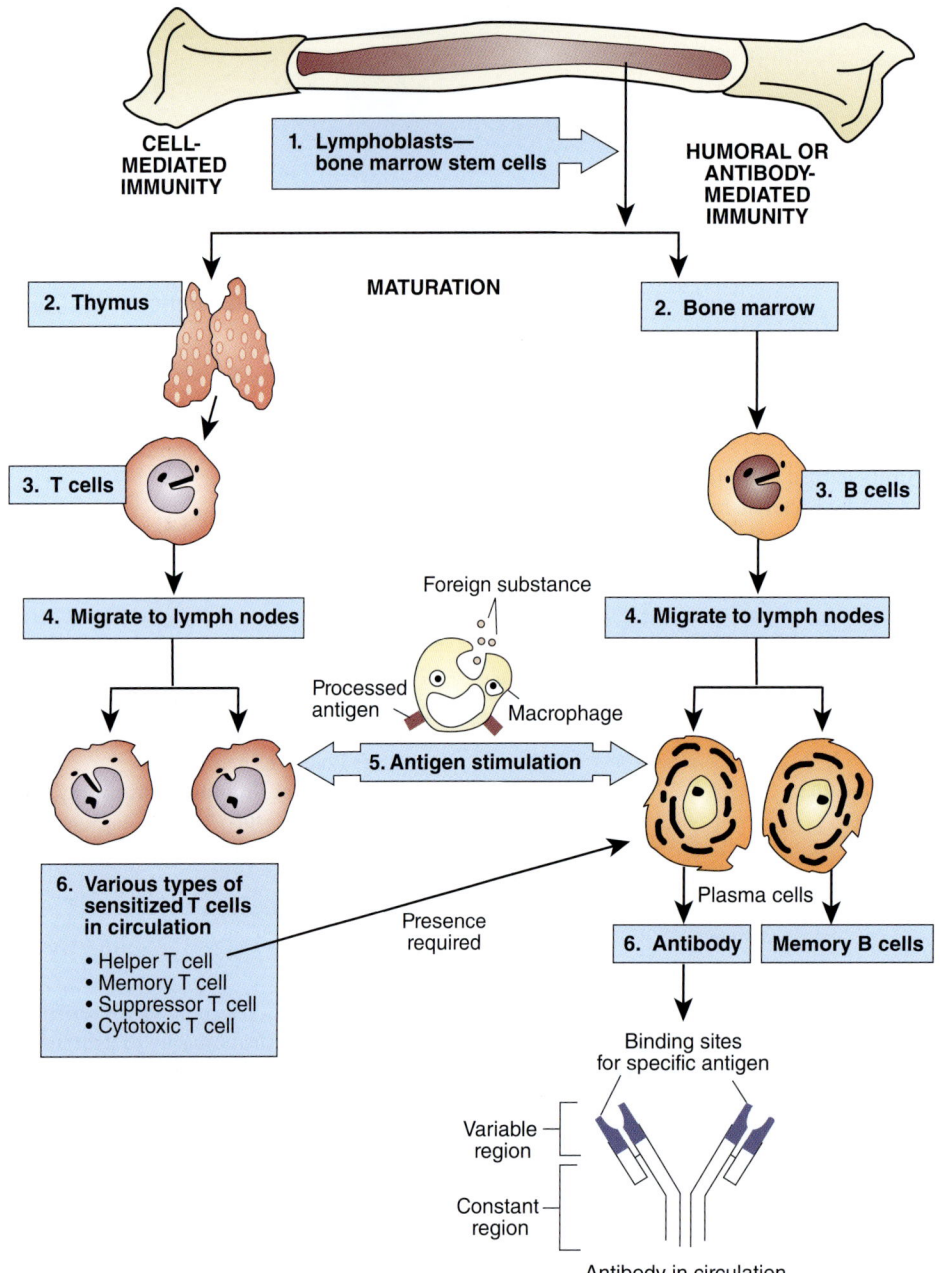

Fig. 33.1 The immune response. (From Gould B, Dyer R: *Pathophysiology for the health professions*, ed 4, St Louis, 2011, Saunders.)

10 mg IV within 2 hours before transplant surgery, followed by a second 10-mg dose 4 days after transplantation; the second dose should be withheld if complications occur (including severe hypersensitivity reactions or loss of the transplanted organ); children over 35 kg should receive the adult dose.

Side Effects and Adverse Reactions. Side effects of basiliximab include abdominal and back pain, cough, dizziness, fever or chills, fatigue, weakness, dysuria, dyspnea, pharyngitis, edema, tremor, nausea and vomiting, and anemia. Serious reactions include sepsis, opportunistic infections, malignancy, lymphoproliferative disorders, thrombocytopenia, leukopenia, diabetes mellitus, anaphylaxis, capillary leak syndrome, and cytokine release syndrome (Box 33.1).

Transplant recipients who receive basiliximab should not receive live vaccines because they may produce an inadequate immune response and are at risk for disseminated infection resulting from the live virus. Caution is advised when basiliximab is administered with other drugs that lower the immune response because of the increased risk of serious infection.

No adequate and well-controlled studies have been done on basiliximab's use in pregnant patients; however, since it is known to cross the placenta, it is not recommended during pregnancy as it may cause birth defects. Females of childbearing potential should use effective contraceptive measures before beginning treatment, during treatment, and for 4 months after completion of therapy. It is not known whether basiliximab is excreted in breast milk. Because of the potential for adverse drug reactions, a decision should be made whether to discontinue nursing or to discontinue the drug, taking into account the importance of the drug to the mother.

BOX 33.1 Cytokine Release Syndrome

Cytokine release syndrome is a symptom complex associated with the use of anti-T-cell antibody infusions, such as antithymocyte globulin (rabbit) and muromonab-CD3. Commonly referred to as an *infusion reaction*, cytokine release syndrome results from the release of cytokines from cells targeted by the antibody. When cytokines are released into the circulation, systemic symptoms such as fever, nausea, chills, hypotension, tachycardia, asthenia, headache, rash, scratchy throat, and dyspnea can result. In most patients, the symptoms are mild to moderate in severity and are managed easily. Premedication with corticosteroids or acetaminophen plus an antihistamine has been reported to be effective in reducing the severity of symptoms caused by cytokine release. Other management measures include a reduction of the infusion rate. However, some patients may experience life-threatening reactions; therefore nurses must closely monitor patients receiving anti-T-cell antibody infusions. Patients with asthma, autoimmune disease, history of drug allergies, and previous exposure to the drug are at increased risk of developing cytokine release syndrome. During infusions, nurses must assess the patient frequently, monitoring vital signs and watching for any signs or symptoms of a reaction. Reactions are most likely to occur in the first hour, but a reaction could occur at any time. Any delay in recognition of the signs of anaphylaxis can compromise the patient's outcome.

From Vogel WH: Infusion reactions: diagnosis, assessment and management, *Clin J Oncol Nursing* 14(2):E10–E21, 2010.

Maintenance Therapy

Calcineurin Inhibitors

Maintenance therapy is used throughout life to prevent rejection. The calcineurin inhibitors (CNIs) suppress the immune system by binding to cytoplasmic proteins that inhibit calcineurin phosphatase, ultimately resulting in the inhibition of T-lymphocyte proliferation. There are two CNIs, cyclosporine and tacrolimus; the prototype CNI is cyclosporine (see Prototype Drug Chart: Cyclosporine [Modified]). The drug became available in 1983 and was modified to improve bioavailability in 1994. Cyclosporine carries a boxed warning for malignancies and serious infections.

Grapefruit and grapefruit juice affect drug metabolism, increasing the concentration of cyclosporine in the blood; for this reason, grapefruit should be avoided. To make the cyclosporine oral solution USP modified more palatable, it should be diluted with room-temperature orange juice or apple juice; patients should avoid switching diluents frequently. Cyclosporine is also available as immediate-release capsules (25 and 100 mg) and as an IV solution (250 mg/5 mL).

Transplant recipients taking cyclosporine should not receive live vaccines because they may have inadequate immune responses and are at risk for disseminated infection resulting from the live virus.

In addition to therapeutic drug monitoring (TDM; drug levels should be drawn just before the dose), patients taking cyclosporine should have frequent monitoring of blood urea nitrogen (BUN), creatinine, potassium, and magnesium levels in addition to liver function tests (LFTs) and lipid profiles.

Cyclosporine does not appear to be a major human teratogen; however, it may be associated with increased rates of prematurity. Cyclosporine is present in breast milk. Because of the potential for serious adverse drug reactions in nursing infants, a decision should be made whether to discontinue nursing or discontinue the drug, taking into account the importance of the drug to the mother.

Tacrolimus

Approved by the US Food and Drug Administration (FDA) in 1994, tacrolimus is the second CNI approved for prophylaxis of rejection in heart, liver, lung, and kidney transplants. It carries a boxed warning for malignancies and serious infections. Patients taking this drug are at increased risk for developing lymphoma and other malignancies. In addition, patients taking tacrolimus are at risk for developing bacterial, viral, fungal, and protozoal infections.

Dosing for heart transplant recipients begins no sooner than 6 hours posttransplant with a continuous infusion at 0.01 mg/kg per day IV. When oral dosing begins, it should be at a dose of immediate-release 0.075 mg/kg per day orally in two divided doses every 12 hours. For patients with a liver transplant, tacrolimus is administered with a continuous infusion at 0.03 to 0.05 mg/kg per day IV. When oral dosing begins, it should be dosed with immediate-release capsules of 0.1 to 0.15 mg/kg per day orally in two divided doses every 12 hours. Dosing after lung transplantation begins 6 hours after surgery with immediate-release oral capsules of 0.075 mg/kg per day in two divided doses, every 12 hours or by continuous infusion of 0.01 to 0.03 mg/kg per day. Kidney transplant recipients should begin tacrolimus within 24 hours of receiving the transplanted organ. Dosing ranges from 0.1 to 0.2 mg/kg per day orally in two divided doses every 12 hours or if the patient is unable to tolerate oral, 0.03 to 0.05 mg/kg per day IV as a continuous infusion and may vary based on other drugs used for induction.

For all transplant recipients, dosing is adjusted based on serum drug levels, with trough levels ranging between 5 and 20 ng/mL, depending on organ transplanted and length of time since transplant.

Tacrolimus is highly nephrotoxic and should be administered at the lowest recommended dose for those with renal impairment. For those with postoperative oliguria, the use of tacrolimus may be delayed until kidney function is adequate. All patients on tacrolimus should have their kidney function monitored periodically during therapy.

Tacrolimus may prolong the QT/QTc interval and may cause torsades de pointes. Avoid tacrolimus in patients with congenital long QT syndrome. In patients with congestive heart failure, bradycardia, those taking certain antiarrhythmic medications or other medicinal products that lead to QT prolongation, and those with electrolyte disturbances such as hypokalemia, hypocalcemia, hyponatremia, or hypomagnesemia, consider obtaining electrocardiograms and monitoring electrolytes (magnesium, potassium, calcium) periodically during treatment.

Pharmacokinetics. Tacrolimus is slowly absorbed in the gastrointestinal (GI) tract, making absorption variable. Food, especially food high in fat, slows absorption and reduces bioavailability. Tacrolimus is highly bound (>99%) to plasma proteins. The half-life ranges from approximately 22.9 to 41.3 hours. It is metabolized extensively in the liver and is over 90% excreted in the feces, with the remaining excreted in the urine.

Pharmacodynamics. Bioavailability is incomplete and variable averaging 25%. Peak serum concentration is reached in 0.5 to 6 hours.

Side Effects and Adverse Reactions. Tacrolimus has multiple common side effects in addition to those mentioned in Table 33.1 anemia, anorexia, arthralgia, cough, constipation, infection, rash, pruritus, and paresthesias may occur. Adverse reactions that are associated with tacrolimus include hyperglycemia, diabetes mellitus, elevated lipid levels, electrolyte imbalances, nephrotoxicity, neurotoxicity, blood dyscrasias, and hepatic failure.

Costimulation Blockers

Belatacept is a first-in-class selective T-cell costimulation blocking agent indicated for use in combination with basiliximab induction, mycophenolate mofetil, and corticosteroids to prevent kidney transplant rejection. It inhibits T-cell activation and proliferation, thereby inhibiting T-lymphocyte proliferation and the production of inflammatory mediators.

PROTOTYPE DRUG CHART
Cyclosporine (Modified)

Drug Class	Dosage
Calcineurin inhibitors	Kidney transplant 4–12 h before transplant for induction therapy: A: PO: 15 mg/kg single dose A: IV: 5–6 mg/kg single dose over 2–6 h Kidney transplant 4–12 h after transplant for maintenance therapy: A: PO: 15 mg/kg/d divided into two immunosuppressives can lead to infection doses A: IV: 5–6 mg/kg/d may be continuous infusion until able to tolerate and switch to PO TDM: Trough 150–400 ng/mL
Contraindications/Cautions	**Drug-Lab-Food Interactions**
Hypersensitivity, HTN, renal impairment, radiation therapy Caution: Concurrent immunosuppressants, alcohol abuse, electrolyte imbalance, gout, hepatic disease, vaccination, sunlight (UV) exposure, infection, contact lenses, biliary tract disease, malignancy, older adult, children, pregnancy, breastfeeding	Live vaccines and immunosuppressives can lead to infection; abrocitinib and P-glycoprotein drugs (e.g., diltiazem, erythromycin, ketoconazole) may increase adverse effects; grapefruit and grapefruit juice can increase the levels of cyclosporine Lab: Monitor CBC, LFTs, creatinine, BUN
Pharmacokinetics	**Pharmacodynamics**
Absorption: Variable Distribution: Distributed widely throughout the body, crosses placenta, and found in breast milk. PB: 90%–98% Metabolism: Extensive Elimination: Bile, feces, urine	Onset: UK Peak: 1.5–6 h Duration: UK Half-life: 10–40 h
Therapeutic Effects/Uses	
For kidney, heart, and liver organ transplant rejection prophylaxis; RA, psoriasis, and dry eye syndrome.	
Side Effects	**Adverse Reactions**
Headache, dizziness, drowsiness, insomnia, weakness, anxiety, depression, hearing loss, tinnitus, glossitis, dysgeusia, gingival overgrowth, gingivitis, rhinitis, dysphagia, cough, dyspnea, ocular irritation, blurred vision, dyspepsia, anorexia, abdominal pain, nausea, vomiting, diarrhea, constipation, flatulence, alopecia, acne, hypertrichosis, infection, influenza, tremor, edema, myalgia, arthralgia, paresthesias, peripheral neuropathy, bone fractures, rash, pruritus, dry mouth/skin, weight loss/gain, urine urgency/incontinence	Hypertension, hypo/hyperglycemia, anemia, electrolyte imbalances, chest pain, MI, HF, seizures, diabetes mellitus, hyperuricemia, hyperbilirubinemia, hypercholesterolemia, peptic ulcer, GI bleeding, *Life-threatening:* Angioedema, malignancy, thrombocytopenia, hemolytic anemia, neurotoxicity, nephrotoxicity, hepatotoxicity

<, Less than; >, greater than; *bid*, twice a day; *BP*, blood pressure; *BUN*, blood urea nitrogen; *CBC*, complete blood count; *Cr*, creatinine; *d*, day; *GI*, gastrointestinal; *h*, hour; *HF*, heart failure; *HTN*, hypertension; *K*, potassium; *LFT*, liver function test; *Mg*, magnesium; *MI*, myocardial infarction; *min*, minute; *mo*, month; *PO*, by mouth; *q*, every; *RA*, rheumatoid arthritis; *TDM*, therapeutic drug monitoring; *UK*, unknown; *wk*, weeks.

Initial dosing is 10 mg/kg to the nearest 12.5 increment IV before surgery on the day of transplant; the dose is repeated on day 5 and at the end of weeks 2, 4, 8, and 12 after transplantation. Maintenance dosing is 5 mg/kg IV at the end of week 16 after transplantation and then every 4 weeks thereafter. Belatacept is not approved for pediatric use.

⚡ This drug carries a black-box warning for increased risk of developing posttransplant lymphoproliferative disorder (PTLD), predominantly involving the central nervous system (CNS). In addition, recipients without immunity to Epstein-Barr virus (EBV) are at a particularly increased risk; therefore, belatacept is for use in patients who are EBV-seropositive only.

Pharmacokinetics. Proteolytic enzymes degrade belatacept into smaller peptides and amino acids. The route of excretion is unknown. The half-life is 10 days.

Pharmacodynamics. Drug half-life is 8.2 to 9.8 days.

Side Effects and Adverse Reactions. Common side effects of belatacept in addition to those in Table 33.1 include anemia, constipation, cough, leukopenia, hypophosphatemia, arthralgia, and proteinuria. Serious reactions include malignancy, neutropenia, renal failure, atrial fibrillation, and diabetes mellitus.

Transplant recipients receiving belatacept should not receive live vaccines because their immune response may be inadequate, and they are at risk for disseminated infection resulting from the live virus. Caution is advised when belatacept is administered with other drugs that lower the immune response because of the increased risk of serious infection.

Adverse events have been observed in animal studies with belatacept. According to the manufacturer, belatacept should not be used in pregnancy unless the potential benefit to the mother outweighs the potential risk to the fetus. ⚡ A pregnancy registry has been established to monitor outcomes of the females exposed to belatacept during pregnancy (1-877-955-6877). Safety during breastfeeding is unknown; therefore a decision should be made whether to discontinue nursing

TABLE 33.1 Immunosuppressant Drugs Used in Organ Transplantation

Drug Name and Type	Route and Dosage	Uses and Considerations
Monoclonal Antibodies (Induction Therapy)		
Basiliximab	A: PO: 20 mg within 2 h before transplant, then 20 mg 4 d after transplant, withhold second dose if complications occur	For kidney transplant rejection prophylaxis. May cause headache, dizziness, weakness, chills, fever, dyspnea, hypertension, insomnia, abdominal pain, nausea, vomiting, infection, peripheral edema, tremor, hypo/hyperkalemia, and blood dyscrasias. PB: UK; $t\frac{1}{2}$: 7.2 d
Calcineurin Inhibitors (Maintenance Therapy)		
Tacrolimus	Liver transplant: A: PO: 0.1–0.15 mg/kg/d in 2 divided doses q12h, initial dose should be at least 6 h after transplantation A: IV: 0.03–0.05 mg/kg/d at least 6 h after transplant	For prophylaxis of liver, kidney, heart, and lung transplant rejection. Use hazardous drug precautions. Do not give with grapefruit or grapefruit juice. Give at the same time qd consistently with or without food. Do not crush, chew, or divide capsules. May cause headache, weakness, fever, insomnia, infection, abdominal pain, nausea, vomiting, diarrhea, tremor, and hypertension. PB: 99%; $t\frac{1}{2}$: 16–32 h
Cyclosporine	Kidney transplant: A: PO: 15 mg/kg as single dose A: IV: 5–6 mg/kg over 2–6 h as single dose Both PO and IV are given 4–12 h before transplantation TDM: Trough 150–400 ng/mL	For prophylaxis of kidney and heart transplant rejection in combination therapy. Also, it is effective in autoimmune conditions, such as RA, inflammatory disease. Use hazardous drug precautions. Give at a consistent time of day. Do not crush, chew, or swallow whole. Do not take with grapefruit juice. Remove contact lens before administration; may reinsert 15 min after administration. May cause headache, gingival overgrowth, hypertension, infection, hyperkalemia, weight gain/loss, abdominal pain, nausea, and tremor. PB: 90%–98%; $t\frac{1}{2}$: 16–27 h
Costimulation Blockers		
Belatacept	A: IV: 10 mg/kg over 30 min on day 1 before transplantation, on d 5 and at end of wk 2, 4, 8, 12, then 5 mg/kg over 30 min at end of wk 16 and q4wk thereafter Base patients' weight on day of transplantation Infusion must be completed within 24 h of drug reconstitution	For prophylaxis of kidney transplant rejection. Used in combination with basilixiab induction, mycophenolate mofetil, and corticosteroids. Only indicated for use in Epstein-Barr virus seropositive patients. Contraindicated if seronegative. May cause headache, fever, insomnia, abdominal pain, nausea, vomiting, diarrhea, hypertension, infection, and peripheral edema. PB: UK; $t\frac{1}{2}$: 10 d
mTOR Inhibitors Sirolimus Everolimus	See Prototype Drug Chart: Sirolimus Kidney transplant (Zortress): A: PO: Initially 0.75 mg q12h ASAP transplant, before 48 h postop Liver transplant: Initially 1 mg q12h, begin at least 30 postop TDM: Trough 3–8 ng/mL	For kidney and liver transplant rejection prophylaxis. The most common side effects and adverse reactions. include anemia, rash, fatigue, peripheral edema, infection, stomatitis, prolonged bleeding time, elevated hepatic enzymes, thrombocytopenia, hypercholesterolemia, hypertriglyceridemia, and hyperglycemia. PB: 74%; $t\frac{1}{2}$: 30 h
Purine Antimetabolites		
Azathioprine	A: PO: 3–5 mg/kg/d start on day of transplant or 1–3 d before, then 1–3 mg/kg/d A: IV: Same dose only if unable to tolerate PO	For prophylaxis of kidney transplant rejection and treat symptoms of RA. Use hazardous drug precautions. May cause fever, nausea, vomiting, diarrhea, infection, hypotension, arthralgia, and myalgia. PB: 30%; $t\frac{1}{2}$: 2 h
Inosine Monophosphate Dehydrogenase Inhibitors		
Mycophenolate mofetil	Kidney transplant: A: PO/IV: 1 g bid over at least 2 h IV, begin within 24 h of transplant, may continue for 14 d, max: 2 g/d	For prophylaxis of kidney, heart, liver transplant rejection in combination therapy. Hazardous drug precautions. Do not crush or open capsules. May cause headache, dizziness weakness, fever, cough, insomnia, abdominal pain, nausea, vomiting, diarrhea, hyper/hypoglycemia, and hypertension. PB: 82%–97%; $t\frac{1}{2}$: PO 11.4–24.4 h, IV 10.8–22.4 h
Corticosteroids		
Prednisone	A: PO: 5–30 g/d	For prophylaxis of kidney transplant rejection in combination therapy with tacrolimus and mycophenolate. Also used for inflammatory conditions such as RA, autoimmune conditions. Give with food. May cause headache, euphoria, fever, insomnia, fluid retention, nausea vomiting, diarrhea, infection, hyperglycemia, and visual impairment. PB: <50%; $t\frac{1}{2}$: 2–3 h
Polyclonal Antibody		
Antithymocyte globulin (ATG) (rabbit)	A: IV (Atgam): 10–15 mg/kg/d for 14 d A: IV (Thymoglobulin): 1.5 mg/kg/d for 7–14 d	For treatment of kidney organ transplant rejection in combination therapy. This drug is derived from rabbits. May cause headache, fever, dyspnea, chills, abdominal pain, nausea, vomiting, diarrhea, constipation, rash, infection, and antibody formation. PB: UK; $t\frac{1}{2}$: 2–3 d

<, Less than; *ASAP*, as soon as possible; *bid*, twice a day; *d*, day; *h*, hour; *PB*, protein binding; *PO*, by mouth; *q*, every; *RA*, rheumatoid arthritis; *t½*, half-life; *TDM*, therapeutic drug monitoring; *UK*, unknown; *wk*, weeks.

PROTOTYPE DRUG CHART

Sirolimus

Drug Class	Dosage
mTOR inhibitors	A >40 kg: PO: 6 mg loading dose ASAP after transplant, then 2 mg/d A <40 kg: PO: 3 mg/m² loading dose ASAP after transplant, then 1 mg/m²/d TDM: Trough 5–15 ng/mL
Contraindications/Cautions	**Drug-Lab-Food Interactions**
Hypersensitivity Caution: Dialysis, vaccination, angioedema, anaphylaxis, immunosuppression, infection, diabetes mellitus, renal/hepatic impairment, hypercholesterolemia, hypertriglyceridemia, hyperlipidemia, UV sunlight exposure, dehiscence, malignancy, African American individuals, children, pregnancy, breastfeeding	Drug: Live vaccinations and concurrent immunosuppressives can lead to infection; CYP3A and P-glycoprotein drugs may increase adverse effects Labs: CBC, cholesterol, lipid profile, potassium, creatinine/BUN, trough
Pharmacokinetics	**Pharmacodynamics**
Absorption: Rapid Distribution: PB: 92% Metabolism: Extensive Excretion: feces 91%, urine 2.2%	Onset: UK Peak: 1–3 h solution; 1–6 h tablets Duration: UK Half-life: 46–78 h
Therapeutic Effects/Uses	
For the prophylaxis of organ transplant rejection	
Side Effects	**Adverse Reactions**
Headache, dizziness, fever, pharyngitis, gingivitis, stomatitis, cough, dyspnea, oral irritation/ulceration, photosensitivity, epistaxis, acne, rash, pruritus, alopecia, folliculitis, dry skin, hypertrichosis, abdominal pain, nausea, diarrhea, constipation, arthralgia, myalgia, edema, impaired wound healing/dehiscence, infection, peripheral edema, osteonecrosis	Anemia, hypertension, tachycardia, chest pain, hypokalemia, hypercholesterolemia, hypertriglyceridemia, hyperlipidemia, hypophosphatemia, diabetes mellitus, hyperglycemia, proteinuria, pancreatitis, immunosuppression, pancreatitis, malignancy *Life-threatening:* Anaphylaxis, angioedema, leukopenia, neutropenia, thrombocytopenia, pancytopenia thrombo/pulmonary embolism, pericardial/pleural effusion, nephrotoxicity, hepatic necrosis

<, Less than; >, greater than; *ASAP*, as soon as possible; *BUN*, blood urea nitrogen; *CBC*, complete blood count; *d*, day; *h*, hour; *PB*, protein binding; *PO*, by mouth; *q*, every; *TDM*, therapeutic drug monitoring; *UK*, unknown; *UV*, ultraviolet.

mTOR Inhibitors

There are two mammalian target of rapamycin (mTOR) inhibitors approved for the prevention of organ rejection in kidney transplant recipients aged 13 years and older: sirolimus and everolimus. Sirolimus is the prototype drug (see Prototype Drug Chart: Sirolimus); it inhibits T-lymphocyte activation and proliferation and inhibits antibody production.

⚡ There are two black-box warnings for sirolimus: use of sirolimus increases susceptibility to infection and the possible development of lymphoma and other malignancies, and the safety and efficacy have not been established in liver or lung transplant recipients; therefore, use is not advised in liver or lung transplant recipients due to increased morbidity and mortality.

It is recommended that the maintenance dose of sirolimus tablets be reduced by approximately one-third in patients with mild or moderate hepatic impairment and by half in patients with severe hepatic impairment. Dosing should not exceed 40 mg/day.

When taking sirolimus, hazardous drug precautions must be used. This drug should not be taken with grapefruit juice. It should be taken consistently regarding food and time of day.

Some side effects of sirolimus include headache, dizziness, fever, pharyngitis, stomatitis, epistaxis, abdominal pain, nausea, diarrhea, constipation, infection, peripheral edema, acne, rash, and dry skin. More serious adverse effects include anemia, arthralgia, myalgia, hypertension, hypertriglyceridemia, thrombocytopenia, hepatic necrosis, diabetes mellitus, nephrotoxicity, and thromboembolism.

Transplant recipients taking sirolimus should not receive live vaccines because their immune response may be inadequate, and they are at risk for disseminated infection resulting from the live virus. Caution is advised when sirolimus is administered with other drugs that lower the immune response because of the increased risk of serious infection.

No adequate and well-controlled studies of sirolimus have been done in pregnant patients; therefore effective contraception must be initiated before sirolimus therapy, and it should continue during sirolimus therapy and for 12 weeks after therapy has been stopped. Sirolimus should be used during pregnancy only if the potential benefit outweighs the potential risk. Whether sirolimus is excreted in breast milk is unknown; therefore a decision should be made whether to discontinue nursing or to discontinue the drug, taking into account the importance of the drug to the mother.

The second mTOR inhibitor is everolimus. This drug is FDA approved for preventing kidney and liver transplant rejection. It is approved for use with cyclosporine, a modified formulation only. Safety and effectiveness have not been established for patients with a high immunologic risk.

Pharmacokinetics. Everolimus is rapidly absorbed. The metabolism is extensive. It is excreted in the feces and urine. The protein binding is 74%, and the half-life is approximately 30 hours.

Pharmacodynamics. The peak for everolimus is 1 to 2 hours.

Side Effects and Adverse Reactions. Some of the most common side effects are those in Table 33.1. Others are headache, acne, dizziness, agitation, anxiety, weakness, blurred vision, cough, back pain, arthralgia, myalgia, fluid retention, abdominal pain, dysgeusia, nausea, vomiting, diarrhea, and constipation. More serious reactions include electrolyte imbalance, blood dyscrasias, proteinuria, impaired wound healing, nephrotoxicity, and malignancy.

Precautions for everolimus administration include using hazardous drug precautions. When taking everolimus, the tablets should not be broken or crushed. One should follow a set schedule, taking it always at the same time of day. It should be taken consistently with or without food. The laboratory tests to be monitored include glucose, complete blood count (CBC), liver function tests, lipids, electrolytes, and creatinine.

Purine Antimetabolites

Azathioprine, a purine antimetabolite, blocks purine metabolism and DNA and RNA synthesis, thereby suppressing T- and B-lymphocyte proliferation. It is indicated for the prevention of kidney transplant rejection.

Pharmacokinetics. Azathioprine is well absorbed after oral administration. Azathioprine and its metabolite are moderately bound to serum proteins (30%) and undergo extensive metabolism in the liver. It is rapidly eliminated from blood and excreted in the urine. The half-life of azathioprine is 2 hours.

Pharmacodynamics. The onset of action is unknown; the drug reaches a peak in 1 to 2 hours; the duration of action is unknown.

⚡ Azathioprine has a black-box warning that chronic immunosuppression with azathioprine increases the risk of malignancy in humans.

Dosing ranges from 1 to 2 mg/kg per day orally (an IV form is not currently available in the United States). In the setting of kidney dysfunction, the dose should be reduced by 25% for a creatinine clearance (CrCl) between 10 and 50 mL/min; if CrCl is less than 10 mL/min, the dose should be reduced by 50%.

Side Effects and Adverse Reactions. Common side effects in addition to those listed in Table 33.1 include leukopenia, thrombocytopenia, anemia, pancytopenia, anorexia, elevated LFTs, malaise, arthralgia, myalgia, and rash. Serious side effects include pancreatitis, hepatotoxicity, lymphomas, leukoencephalopathy, and other malignancies.

Transplant recipients taking azathioprine should not receive live vaccines because their immune response may be inadequate, and they are at risk for disseminated infection resulting from the live virus. Caution is advised when azathioprine is administered with other drugs that lower the immune response because of an increased risk of serious infection. Combining azathioprine with antihypertensive drugs increases the risk of leukopenia.

Patients who receive azathioprine should have a CBC. LFTs and bilirubin should be monitored.

Azathioprine can cause fetal harm when given to pregnant patients and should be avoided; however, maternal benefit may outweigh fetal risk in serious or life-threatening situations. Azathioprine is found in breast milk and is possibly unsafe during breastfeeding; therefore a decision should be made whether to discontinue nursing or to discontinue the drug, taking into account the importance of the drug to the mother.

Inosine Monophosphate Dehydrogenase Inhibitors

Mycophenolate mofetil blocks synthesis of purine nucleotides, thereby preventing the proliferation of T cells and lymphocytes and preventing the formation of antibodies from B cells; it also may inhibit recruitment of leukocytes to inflammatory sites.

Recommended dosing for kidney transplant recipients is 1 g orally twice daily; for heart and liver transplant recipients, the dosage is 1.5 g orally twice daily. The maximum dosage for kidney transplantation is 1 g twice daily. In pediatric transplant recipients, the recommended dose of mycophenolate mofetil oral suspension is $600\,mg/m^2$ twice daily, up to a maximum of $1800\,mg/m^2$ per day.

Pharmacokinetics. Mycophenolate mofetil is rapidly absorbed after oral administration with 94% bioavailability, and it is protein bound (82%–97%). It is a prodrug that is metabolized in the liver to mycophenolic acid; it is excreted in the urine (93%) and in feces (6%). The drug half-life for the oral formulation is 18 hours; the half-life for the IV formulation is 17 hours.

Pharmacodynamics. Oral mycophenolate mofetil reaches a peak in 2 hours.

Side Effects and Adverse Reactions. Common side effects of mycophenolate mofetil in addition to those in Table 33.1 include infection, edema, anemia, constipation, dyspnea, hypercholesterolemia, tremor, hypokalemia, and acne. Serious reactions include thrombocytopenia, leukopenia, neutropenia, infection, nephropathy, lymphoma, lymphoproliferative disorders, malignancy, GI bleeding, and renal failure (Box 33.2).

Transplant recipients taking mycophenolate mofetil should not receive live vaccines because their immune response may be inadequate, and they are at risk for disseminated infection resulting from the live virus. Caution is advised when mycophenolate mofetil is administered with other drugs that lower the immune response because of the increased risk of serious infection. Combining mycophenolate mofetil with nonsteroidal antiinflammatory drugs increases the risk of GI bleeding.

Mycophenolate mofetil is associated with an increased risk of first-trimester pregnancy loss and an increased risk of congenital malformations. ⚡ Females of reproductive potential must be made aware of the increased risk of first-trimester pregnancy loss and congenital malformations and must be counseled regarding pregnancy prevention and planning. It is unknown whether mycophenolate mofetil is found in breast milk; therefore a decision should be made whether to discontinue breastfeeding or to discontinue the drug, taking into account the importance of the drug to the mother.

Corticosteroids

Prednisone, a corticosteroid, is a glucocorticoid receptor agonist. It decreases inflammation by suppression of leukocytes and reversal of increased capillary permeability. It suppresses the immune system by reducing the activity and volume of the lymphatic system.

Pharmacokinetics. Prednisone is readily absorbed from the GI tract (up to 90%). Plasma protein binding is less than 50% but is concentration dependent. Prednisone is metabolized by the liver to its active metabolite, prednisolone. It is excreted in the urine.

Pharmacodynamics. Prednisone reaches peak plasma concentration in 1 to 2 hours for the immediate-release formulation and 6 to 6.5 hours for the delayed-release formulation. Prednisone has a plasma half-life of 2 to 3 hours and should be administered after meals or with food or milk to decrease GI upset.

Side Effects and Adverse Reactions. Common side effects of corticosteroid use in addition to those in Table 33.1 include edema, hypokalemia, hypo/hypertension, diaphoresis, petechiae and ecchymosis, facial erythema, acne, rash, dizziness and vertigo, emotional lability, depression, anxiety, hyperglycemia, menstrual irregularities, hirsutism, appetite stimulation, and weight gain. Serious reactions include anaphylaxis, adrenal insufficiency, psychosis, diabetes mellitus, seizures,

BOX 33.2 Neutropenic Precautions

In addition to receiving treatment from your doctor, the following suggestions can help prevent infections:
- Clean your hands frequently.
- Try to avoid crowded places and contact with people who are sick.
- Do not share food, drink cups, utensils, or other personal items, such as toothbrushes.
- Shower or bathe daily, and use an unscented lotion to prevent your skin from becoming dry and cracked.
- Cook meat and eggs all the way through to kill any germs.
- Carefully wash raw fruits and vegetables.
- Protect your skin from direct contact with pet bodily waste (urine or feces) by wearing vinyl or household cleaning gloves when cleaning up after your pet. Wash your hands immediately afterward.
- Use gloves for gardening.
- Clean your teeth and gums with a soft toothbrush, and if your doctor or nurse recommends one, use a mouthwash to prevent mouth sores.
- Try and keep all your household surfaces clean.
- Get the seasonal flu shot as soon as it is available.
- If you go to the emergency department, you should not sit in the waiting room for a long time; when you check in, tell them right away you are receiving immunosuppressant drugs.
- Know the signs and symptoms of an infection:
  - Fever that is 100.4°F (38°C) or higher for more than 1 hour, or a one-time temperature of 101°F or higher
  - Chills and sweats
  - Change in cough or new cough
  - Sore throat or new mouth sore
  - Shortness of breath
  - Nasal congestion
  - Stiff neck
  - Burning or pain with urination
  - Unusual vaginal discharge or irritation
  - Increased urination
  - Redness, soreness, or swelling in any area, including surgical wounds
  - Diarrhea
  - Vomiting
  - Pain in the abdomen or rectum
  - New onset of pain
  - Changes in skin, urination, or mental status

Center for Disease Control and Prevention: *Neutropenia and risk for infection*, Author, n.d. https://www.cdc.gov/cancer/preventinfections/pdf/neutropenia.pdf.

---

heart failure, peptic ulcer disease and GI bleeding/perforation, and tendon rupture. Long-term use may lead to impaired wound healing, skin atrophy, Cushing syndrome, cataracts, and growth suppression in children. Cessation of corticosteroids may lead to withdrawal symptoms with high doses or long-term use.

Transplant recipients taking corticosteroids should not receive live vaccines because their immune response may be inadequate, and they are at risk for disseminated infection resulting from the live virus. Caution is advised when corticosteroids are administered with other drugs that lower the immune response because of the increased risk of serious infection. Combining corticosteroids with certain antibiotics increases the risk of dysrhythmias; combining corticosteroids with diuretics increases the risk of hypokalemia.

Transplant recipients taking corticosteroids should have periodic monitoring of their electrolytes, blood pressure, weight, and glucose levels. Pediatric patients should have their height monitored. Chest x-rays and ophthalmic examinations are indicated with long-term use.

Caution is advised during pregnancy, especially in the first trimester or with long-term use, because of the possible risk of low birthweight and premature birth. Hypoadrenalism can cause fetal harm. Caution is also advised during breastfeeding.

DRUGS FOR TRANSPLANT REJECTION

> **TYPES OF REJECTION:** Organ rejection happens due to a normal immune response to foreign tissue. The use of immunosuppression therapy lowers the risk of rejection. Rejection may be hyperacute, acute, or chronic. Hyperacute rejection occurs within a few minutes to hours after transplant due to rapid destruction of blood vessels and preexisting antibodies that attack the transplanted organ, resulting in irreversible damage. This type of rejection is extremely rare. As there is no treatment for hyperacute rejection, the organ must be removed.
>
> Acute rejection occurs in the first weeks to 3 months after transplant. It is a cell-mediated response. Symptoms include an increase in serum creatinine, hypertension, decreased urine output, flu-like symptoms, fever, and tenderness over the graft site. Acute rejection is confirmed with a biopsy. Early detection and treatment can reverse rejection.
>
> Chronic rejection develops after months or years and is irreversible. The body's immune system slowly damages the transplanted organ and results in a slow but progressive decline in organ function. Indications of chronic rejection include hypertension and proteinuria. Controlling glucose, cholesterol, and blood pressure levels can possibly prevent chronic rejection. Chronic rejection can last for months or years, and the patient may receive a second transplant.

Antithymocyte Globulin

Antithymocyte globulin, or *ATG*, is a drug composed of antibodies obtained from either a rabbit, ATG (Thymoglobulin) or a horse, ATG (Atgam). It is thought that Thymoglobulin is more effective in treating graft rejection and patient survival. It is a polyclonal (depleting) antibody that blocks T-cell membrane proteins; this causes altered T-cell function and lysis, and prolonged T-cell depletion, which begins within 24 hours, but the drug half-life is 2 to 3 days.

Dosing should be on a set schedule. The first dose should be infused over 6 hours and subsequent doses over 4 hours. Dosage should be decreased by 50% if the white blood cell (WBC) count decreases to 2000 to 3000 or the platelet count is 50,000 to 75,000. Treatments should be discontinued if the WBC count falls to less than 2000 or the platelet count falls to less than 50,000.

Common side effects of ATG in addition to those in Table 33.1 include weakness, anxiety, arthralgia, myalgia, paresthesias, anemia, hypo/hyperkalemia, hypo/hypertension, hyperglycemia, hyperlipidemia, peripheral edema, and increased risk for infection. Serious side effects include anaphylaxis, severe infusion reaction, cytokine release syndrome, serum sickness, leukopenia, neutropenia, hemolytic anemia, thrombocytopenia, pancytopenia, GI bleed/perforation, seizures, renal failure, and malignancy. Premedication with corticosteroids, acetaminophen, and allergy medications given at least 1 hour prior to each dose is recommended to help prevent an infusion reaction. ⚡ Close supervision of the patient is required during and after IV infusion, to include frequent vital signs and assessment of the site for signs of extravasation.

Transplant recipients receiving ATG should not receive live vaccines because their immune response may be inadequate, and they are at risk for disseminated infection resulting from the live virus. Caution is advised when ATG is administered with other drugs that lower the immune response because of the increased risk of serious infection.

Patients should have WBC and platelets monitored frequently during treatment. There are no adequate and well-controlled studies of ATG in pregnant patients. Inadequate information is available to assess the risk of ATG when breastfeeding; therefore a decision should be made whether to discontinue nursing or to discontinue the drug, taking into account the importance of the drug to the mother.

DRUGS FOR INFECTION

Bacterial

Pneumocystis jiroveci pneumonia (PJP) is a life-threatening illness in patients who are immunocompromised. Routine prophylaxis with trimethoprim-sulfamethoxazole (TMP-SMZ) has significantly reduced the morbidity and mortality of PJP after transplantation. TMP-SMZ is dosed once every morning or one tablet three times a week (Monday, Wednesday, and Friday). TMP-SMZ can make the skin more sensitive to sunlight; therefore patients should be instructed to use a lotion with a minimum sun protection factor of 25 when in the sun. See Chapter 29 for further information regarding sulfonamides.

Fungal

Transplant recipients use nystatin to prevent or treat thrush in the mouth and esophagus. This is usually given when the patient is on a high-dose immunosuppression regimen. Nurses must instruct the transplant recipient in the proper administration of nystatin liquid:
- Shake the preparation well before measuring the dose.
- Swish the dose around in the mouth before swallowing.
- Allow the nystatin to coat the mouth for as long as possible.
- Do not eat or drink anything for 5 to 10 minutes after taking the medication.

See Chapter 30 for further information regarding antifungal drugs.

Viral

One common virus that patients develop after transplantation is cytomegalovirus (CMV). It may present as a viral syndrome or as an invasive disease, and it plays a role in organ rejection. Transplant recipients receive antiviral prophylaxis with oral ganciclovir or valganciclovir for 3 to 6 months after surgery. If untreated, CMV can cause serious complications, particularly in the liver, intestine, pancreas, kidneys, heart, lungs, blood, and eyes. See Chapter 30 for further information regarding antiviral drugs.

PROMOTING ADHERENCE

Importance of Adherence

Upon discharge from the hospital, transplant recipients begin a lifelong journey of close medical supervision that includes frequent visits to their health care provider, monitoring of blood work, and maintenance of a complex drug regimen. The 1-year survival rates are over 80% for liver and lung transplants and over 90% for kidney and heart transplants; most recipients experience an improved quality of life. However, long-term adherence is a problem, with reports of nonadherence being approximately 50%. Nonadherence to the posttransplant regimen (e.g., drug regimen, exercise, and health promotion) is one of the top three reasons for transplant failure. Typically, 80% or more adherence is needed for optimal therapeutic efficacy.

Nurse's Role in Adherence

Factors that affect adherence include episodes of rejection, comorbid illness and disease, side effects of drugs, and health care costs. Nurses play a key role in promoting adherence by incorporating education, motivational strategies, and coping skills into an individually tailored posttransplant plan of care.

CLINICAL JUDGMENT [NURSING PROCESS]

Organ Transplants: Immunosuppression

Concept: Safety
- Protecting the patient from potential or actual harm, a basic human need

Concept: Immunity
- The body's protective response to infection and disease

Recognize Cues [Assessment]
- Assess for clinical signs of rejection including malaise, fever, edema, pain over the transplant site, and increased weight.
- Assess for the presence of risk factors for infection, including drugs, travel, and exposure to individuals with active infections.
- Assess for signs and symptoms of infection, including redness, swelling, pain, and elevated temperature.
- Assess immunization status.
- Assess nutritional status, including weight and history of weight loss.

Analyze Cues and Prioritize Hypothesis [Patient Problems]
- Decreased immunity
- Self-concept
- Need for health teaching

Generate Solutions [Planning]
- Infection is recognized early to allow prompt treatment.
- The transplant recipient and family members will verbalize understanding of early signs and symptoms of rejection.
- The transplant recipient will remain free of infection.

Take Action [Nursing Interventions]
- Instruct the transplant recipient on the benefits of a balanced and healthy diet accompanied by exercise.
- Instruct the transplant recipient on proper adherence to the drug regimen. Teach the transplant recipient the purpose of each drug and how to administer each drug, then reinforce that each drug should be taken exactly as prescribed. Also, teach the most common side effects associated with each drug and what to do if they occur.
- Patients should be instructed to avoid anyone with an active infection and to be careful not to injure themselves, which may increase the chance of acquiring a wound infection. They should stay away from anyone who has a cold, mumps, measles, chickenpox, or other communicable diseases.
- Promote health education with patients and families to recognize and minimize the risk of complications and rejection and to facilitate optimum quality of life.
- Teach the transplant recipient the signs and symptoms of rejection and infection, then instruct them on when to call their health care provider.
- Teach the transplant recipient to self-monitor vital signs, daily weights, and blood glucose (if appropriate); ensure the recipient knows when to call the health care provider.
- Transplant recipients and their families should be taught to wash hands properly, especially after toileting, before meals, and before administering drugs.

Evaluate Outcomes [Evaluation]
- Evaluate the effectiveness of the plan, including adherence to the immunosuppressive drug regimen and freedom from infection and transplant rejection.

CLINICAL JUDGMENT UNFOLDING CASE STUDY

Phase I: Induction Therapy
NGN Item Type: Enhanced hot spot
Cognitive Skills: Recognize cues

A 42-year-old African American female with a 6-year history of chronic kidney disease requiring hemodialysis (HD), secondary to polycystic kidney disease, is admitted for a cadaveric kidney transplant. She lives alone and has been on disability for the past 4 years. She had become too fatigued with HD to continue her job as an elementary school teacher. She denies a history of substance use. On admission, her blood pressure (BP) is 145/90 mm Hg, temperature (T) is 98.4 °F, respiratory rate (RR) is 18 breaths per minute, and heart rate (HR) is 100 beats per minute; height is 68 inches and weight is 185 pounds. While receiving basiliximab 20 mg intravenously 2 hours prior to surgery, the patient tells the nurse that she is both excited and scared; she has a lot of questions about her induction therapy. Three days after surgery, the patient reports fatigue, headache (pain rated a 5 on a scale of 0–10), and dizziness. On assessment, her T is 101.6 °F, HR is 115 beats per minute, RR is 16 breaths per minute, and BP is 100/62 mm Hg. In addition, she did not eat breakfast due to nausea and abdominal discomfort. Intake and output from the previous shift are 1000 mL/250 mL.

1. **Use an "X" to indicate the potential issues listed in the left column that may place this patient at risk while in the hospital.**

Potential Issues	Risk to Patient
Acute pain	
Decreased immunity	
Cognitive decline	
Social isolation	
Need for health teaching	

Answers

1. **Highlight the assessment findings that require immediate follow-up.**

A 42-year-old African American female with a 6-year history of chronic kidney disease requiring hemodialysis (HD), secondary to polycystic kidney disease, is admitted for a cadaveric kidney transplant. She lives alone and has been on disability for the past 4 years. She had become too fatigued with HD to continue her job as an elementary school teacher. She denies a history of substance use. On admission, her blood pressure (BP) is 145/90 mm Hg, temperature (T) is 98.4 °F, respiratory rate (RR) is 18 breaths per minute, and heart rate (HR) is 100 beats per minute; height is 68 inches and weight is 185 pounds. While receiving basiliximab 20 mg intravenously 2 hours prior to surgery, the patient tells the nurse that she is both excited and scared; she has a lot of questions about her induction therapy. Three days after surgery, the patient reports **fatigue, headache (pain rated a 5 on a scale of 0–10)**, and dizziness. On assessment, her **T is 101.6 °F, HR is 115 beats per minute, RR is 16 breaths per minute**, and **BP is 100/62 mm Hg**. In addition, she did not eat breakfast due to **nausea** and **abdominal discomfort**. Intake and output from the previous shift are **1000 mL/250 mL**.

2. **Use an "X" to indicate the potential issues listed in the left column that may place this patient at risk while in the hospital**

Potential Issues	Risk to Patient
Acute pain	X
Decreased immunity	X
Cognitive decline	
Social isolation	
Need for health teaching	X

Rationale
Signs and symptoms of cytokine release syndrome resulting from basiliximab include fever, nausea, chills, hypotension, tachycardia, asthenia, headache, rash, scratchy throat, and dyspnea. Signs and symptoms of acute rejection include flu-like symptoms, fever, tenderness over the kidney, decreased urine output, and hypertension.

Phase II: Discharge
NGN Type Item: Matrix
Cognitive Skills: Analyze Cues

The nurse is completing final preparations for the patient's discharge home, 9 days following cadaveric kidney transplant. Her discharge drugs include cyclosporine (modified), mycophenolate mofetil, and prednisone, as well as nifedipine, furosemide, sulfamethoxazole/trimethoprim, nystatin, and valganciclovir. The patient is voicing concerns about taking so many drugs and their side effects; she is worried about how she is going to pay for all of them. Her BP on discharge is 145/88 mm Hg, T is 99.5 °F, RR is 16 breaths per minute, and HR is 90 beats per minute. This morning her creatinine is 2.0 mg/dL (was 1.7 mg/dL yesterday) and her blood urea nitrogen (BUN) is 30 mg/dL; her K is 5.3 mEq/L, Na is 136 mEq/L, and glucose is 110 mg/dL. Her cyclosporin trough concentration is 325 ng/mL. Her adult daughter has flown in from across the country and will stay with her for a couple of weeks after discharge.

1. **Based on the patient's condition at discharge, which information MUST be included in the patient education prior to discharge home? Select all that apply.**
   a. When to call the provider about drug side effects
   b. Systems to promote adherence to drug regimen
   c. A balanced diet accompanied by exercise
   d. Support groups for transplant recipients
   e. Drug assistance programs
   f. Catch-up immunization schedule and pretravel vaccines
   g. Glucose monitoring

2. Place a checkmark to indicate which assessment data listed in the left column may place this patient at risk during the discharge phase of treatment.

Assessment Data	Risk to Patient
Lives alone	
BP 145/88 mm Hg	
Creatinine 2.0 mg/dL	
K 5.3 mEq/L	
Glucose 110 mg/dL	
Cyclosporin trough concentration 325 ng/mL	
T 99.5 °F	

Answers

1. Based on the patient's condition at discharge, which information MUST be included in the patient educaon prior to discharge home? **Select all that apply.**
   a. When to call the provider about drug side effects
   b. Systems to promote adherence to drug regimen
   c. A balanced diet accompanied by exercise
   d. Drug assistance programs

Rationale
The patient is voicing concerns about taking so many drugs (b) and their side effects (a); she is worried about how she is going to pay for all of them (e). Her BP and glucose are borderline; her prescribed drugs have side effects related to

CLINICAL JUDGMENT UNFOLDING CASE STUDY—CONT'D

weight gain, hypertension, electrolyte imbalance, and elevated lipids. Diet and exercise are an important part of discharge planning (c). While the other options may be important, they are not a priority for the discharge of this patient.

2. Place a checkmark to indicate which assessment data listed in the left column may place this patient at risk during the discharge phase of treatment.

Assessment Data	Risk to Patient
Lives alone	
BP 145/88 mm Hg	
Creatinine 2.0 mg/dL	✓
K 5.3 mEq/L	✓
Glucose 110 mg/dL	
Cyclosporin trough concentration 325 ng/mL	
T 99.5	✓

Rationale
Living alone does not put the patient at risk during the discharge phase. Although an isolated BP of 145/88 mm Hg is borderline, it can be managed as an outpatient, as can glucose of 110 mg/dL; therefore they do not put the patient at risk during the discharge phase. The cyclosporine trough concentration is within range for a patient immediately posttransplant. The rise in creatinine level accompanied by an elevated potassium level and low-grade fever are indicators of acute rejection and put the patient at risk during the discharge phase.

Phase III: Acute Rejection
NGN Type Item: Extended multiple response; Matrix
Cognitive Skills: Take Action; Evaluate Outcomes

Six months after kidney transplant surgery, the patient experiences another episode of acute rejection. In addition to cyclosporine (modified), mycophenolate mofetil, and prednisone, this morning she is starting antithymocyte globulin (rabbit), having failed high-dose steroid treatment over the last 3 days as the initial treatment for her acute rejection. The patient tearfully admits to being scared about losing her transplant, going back on HD, and never being able to teach again. Her weight this morning is 215 pounds. She had a complete blood count (CBC) with differential drawn; her white blood cell (WBC) count is $3.0 \times 10^3/\mu L$, segmented neutrophils are 14.8%, and the segmented bands are 5% (absolute neutrophil count of 594 cells/μL); platelets are 100,000/μL. Her cyclosporin trough concentration is 150 ng/mL, creatinine is 2.5 mg/dL, and BUN is 38 mg/dL; her K is 4.4 mEq/L, and glucose is 150 mg/dL. Her BP is 148/90 mm Hg, T is 99.5 °F, RR is 20 breaths per minute, and HR is 106 beats per minute. Urine output for the last 12 hours was 336 cc.

1. Which nursing actions are appropriate for the patient at this time? **Select all that apply.**
   a. Refer to counseling and psychology
   b. Social work referral
   c. Administer acetaminophen and diphenhydramine
   d. Refer for dietary counseling
   e. Administer insulin per sliding scale
   f. Instruct on using a soft toothbrush
   g. Remove flowers from the patient's room
   h. Instruct on the side effects of antithymocyte globulin
2. The nurse administers the diphenhydramine/acetaminophen premedication; then, 1 hour later the nurse administers ATG and teaches the patient the drug side effects and when to call the health care provider. The nurse also instructs the patient regarding neutropenic precautions.
   Use an "X" to indicate whether assessment findings in the left column indicate effectiveness, ineffectiveness, or being unrelated to the nursing interventions.

Assessment Finding	Effective	Ineffective	Unrelated
The patient requests assistance to the bathroom			
The patient reports pain 1 on a scale of 0–10			
The patient reports shakes and chills			
T 98.4°F			
The patient reports bleeding gums after oral care			

Answers
1. Which nursing actions are appropriate for the patient at this time? **Select all that apply.**
   a. Administer acetaminophen and diphenhydramine
   b. Instruct on using a soft toothbrush
   c. Instruct on the side effects of antithymocyte globulin

Rationale
Side effects of antithymocyte globulin include high fever and chills; premedication with corticosteroids or acetaminophen and antihistamines will decrease the severity. The patient is neutropenic. Neutropenic precautions include using a soft toothbrush. Safe and effective nursing care includes educating patients on the side effects of the drugs they are receiving.

2. The nurse administers the diphenhydramine/acetaminophen premedication; then, 1 hour later the nurse administers ATG and teaches the patient the drug side effects and when to call the health care provider. The nurse also instructs the patient regarding neutropenic precautions.
   Use an X to indicate whether assessment findings in the left column indicate effectiveness, ineffectiveness, or being unrelated to the nursing interventions.

Assessment Finding	Effective	Ineffective	Unrelated
The patient requests assistance to the bathroom			X
The patient reports pain 1 on a scale of 0–10	X		
The patient reports shakes and chills		X	
T 98.4°F	X		
The patient reports bleeding gums after oral care		X	

Rationale
Requesting assistance to the bathroom does not reflect nursing actions taken immediately prior to drug administration. A report of pain as a 1 on a scale of 0–10 reflects the administration of premedication. A potential side effect of antithymocyte globulin is headache. Experiencing shakes and chills would indicate high fever; premedication is administered to reduce the severity of adverse reactions. However, a high fever indicates that the administration of the premedication was not effective. A temperature of 98.4°F would indicate that the administration of the premedication was effective. The patient reporting bleeding gums after oral care indicates instructions regarding neutropenic precautions did not prevent bleeding, creating an access point for infection.

REVIEW QUESTIONS

1. All transplant drugs have the same advisory: to use caution when administering them with another immunosuppressant drug because of the increased risk for what?
   a. Nausea and vomiting
   b. Edema
   c. Anemia
   d. Infection
2. Which virus has been associated with posttransplant lymphoproliferative disorder?
   a. Cytomegalovirus
   b. Herpes simplex virus
   c. Epstein-Barr virus
   d. Human immunodeficiency virus
3. Nurses are key to promoting adherence in transplant recipients. What factors influence whether a recipient adheres to a drug regimen? **Select all that apply.**
   a. Drug side effects
   b. Episodes of rejection
   c. Cost
   d. Infection
   e. Marital status
4. Your patient is receiving basiliximab and develops cytokine release syndrome. You would expect to see what symptom?
   a. Coughing
   b. Chills
   c. Tremors
   d. Weakness
5. Your patient taking belatacept becomes pregnant. After a discussion with her partner, her health care provider, and you, she decides the best thing to do is continue taking the drug while pregnant. In addition to making this informed decision, what else should she do?
   a. Discontinue all other drugs
   b. Contact the pregnancy registry
   c. Ensure her blood level stays between 16 and 24 ng/mL
   d. Decrease her dose by 50%

34

Vaccines

http://evolve.elsevier.com/McCuistion/pharmacology

OBJECTIVES

- Differentiate active, passive, and community immunity.
- Describe the different types of vaccines and their composition
- Differentiate vaccine-preventable diseases and vaccine recommendations for various populations and international travel.
- Discuss issues and considerations regarding vaccine safety.
- Describe the development and use of the varicella vaccine.
- Discuss the history and plans for future developments of various vaccines.

OUTLINE

Immunity, 408
  Active Immunity, 408
  Passive Immunity, 408
  Community Immunity, 408
Vaccines, 408
  Attenuated Viruses, Toxoids, and Conjugate Vaccines, 408
  Recombinant Subunit Vaccines, Messenger RNA Vaccines, and Adjuvants, 409
Vaccine-Preventable Diseases and Vaccine Recommendations, 409
  Vaccine-Preventable Diseases, 409
  Vaccination Recommendations, 413
  Immunization Before International Travel, 414
Vaccine Safety: Reporting Diseases and Adverse Reactions, 414
  Contraindications, 414
  Reporting, 414
Varicella Vaccine, 415
  Pharmacokinetics and Pharmacodynamics, 415
  Contraindications, 415
  Drug Interactions, 415
Future Developments in Vaccines, 416
  Anthrax, Smallpox, and Pertussis, 416
  Zoster, Rotavirus, and HPV, 416
  Pneumococcal Disease and Bacterial Meningitis, 416
  Respiratory Syncytial Virus, 417
Clinical Judgment Case Study, 418
Review Questions, 418

November 17, 2019, marked the first case of what was to become known as the COVID-19 (novel coronavirus, or 2019-nCoV, or SARS-CoV-2; Fig. 34.1) pandemic, the worst pandemic since the 1918 Spanish flu killed 50 million people worldwide. By January 9, 2020, there were 59 cases of pneumonia from this virus in Wuhan, China, where it began. It spread to the United States by January 21; by January 31 the World Health Organization (WHO) issued a Global Health Emergency. By March 11, 2020, the WHO declared COVID-19 a pandemic. Phase I vaccine trials began in March. On December 11, 2020, the Food and Drug Administration (FDA) granted emergency use authorization (EUA) for Pfizer-BioNTech's vaccine. On December 14, 2020, the first vaccine was administered in Queens, with shipments heading to all 50 states. On this date, there were 16.9 million cases of COVID-19 in the United States, with 307,803 deaths. The COVID-19 public health emergency ended on May 11, 2023, by which time there were more than 1.1 million deaths in the United States. The virus is by no means eradicated. In the last week of January 2024, there were 26,607 hospitalizations in the United States due to COVID-19. The virus mutates constantly, with the JN.1 variant accounting for 93.1% of current infections.

Over the years, immunizations have prevented global epidemics, such as smallpox in 1977 and the eradication of polio in the United States in 1979. The US National Immunization Survey (NIS; https://www.cdc.gov/vaccines/imz-managers/nis/index.html) tracks vaccination coverage of children 19 to 35 months and teens 13 to 17 years. In 2017 overall vaccination rates for children between 19 and 35 months was at 70.4%. Specific vaccination rates were 83.2% for diphtheria, tetanus, and pertussis; 92.7% for polio; 91.5% for measles, mumps, and rubella; 80.7% for *Haemophilus influenzae* type b; 91.4% for hepatitis B; 91% for chickenpox; and 82.4% for pneumococcal conjugate vaccine. Children below the federal poverty level have lower coverage for all vaccinations compared with children at or above the poverty level, and those with insurance or Medicaid.

The NIS estimated that in 2019, among teens aged 13 to 17 years, vaccination rates continued to increase. For tetanus, diphtheria, and acellular pertussis (Tdap) coverage rates were 90.2% and 88.9% for ≥1 dose of meningococcus 4-valent conjugate (MenACWY). Vaccination coverage for human papillomavirus (HPV) continues to improve. In 2019, 71.5% of teens had received their first dose, and 54.2% had completed the series. Coverage exceeded 90% for ≥2 doses of measles, mumps, and rubella vaccine (MMR), ≥3 doses of hepatitis B vaccine, and ≥1 and ≥2 doses of varicella vaccine among adolescents without a history of varicella disease. These results indicate an increase in all vaccinations for teens, with a continued need to improve HPV coverage.

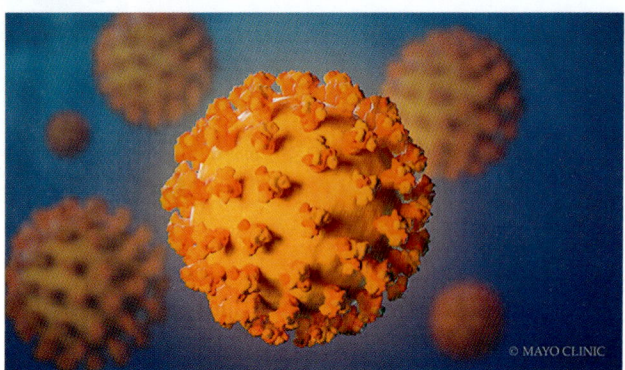

Fig. 34.1 Microphotograph of the novel coronavirus.

IMMUNITY

Active Immunity

The body can obtain immunity in different ways. **Active immunity** occurs when the body's **immune response** is stimulated by an **antigen** or when a **pathogen** enters the body. The body recognizes this pathogen as a foreign substance and produces **antibodies**, also called *immunoglobulins*, which defend the body against pathogens. The immune response is slow, taking several days or weeks to develop immunity. Yet the immunity is often long-lasting. During this process, the immune system retains memory of the pathogen then produces antibodies to defend against the disease. **Natural acquired active immunity** occurs from exposure to a pathogen or disease. **Active acquired artificial immunity** occurs when a weakened antigen or immunoglobulin (Ig) is injected into an individual as a vaccination, which then stimulates an immune response.

Passive Immunity

When an individual is unable to make antibodies and memory cells, antibodies are given from another source to provide passive immunity. These antibodies may be produced using recombinant deoxyribonucleic acid (DNA) technology or pooled antigens from several human or animal sources that have been exposed to disease-causing pathogens.

Passive immunity can be natural, in which case the body produces its own antibodies, or it can be acquired—that is, the body receives antibodies from an outside source. Either way the immunity is immediate and short-lived, lasting no more than several weeks to a few months; the recipient does not induce their own immune response. One example of natural immunity passively acquired is in infants, who are unable to protect against disease because of immature immune systems but instead require antibodies from an outside source, such as the mother's placenta and breast milk. Another example is receiving an Ig to provide antibodies against a specific disease. Passive acquired immunity is essential when (1) time does not permit active vaccination alone, (2) the exposed individual is at high risk for complications of the disease, or (3) the individual experiences an immune system deficiency that renders that person unable to produce an effective immune response.

Community Immunity

Community immunity, also known as *herd immunity*, occurs when most of the community is immunized against contagious diseases, allowing protection of those not immunized. In contrast, when most of the community is *not* immunized, there is an increased risk for the spread of contagious disease within the community (Fig. 34.2). For more information, see https://www.vaccines.gov/basics/work/protection/index.html.

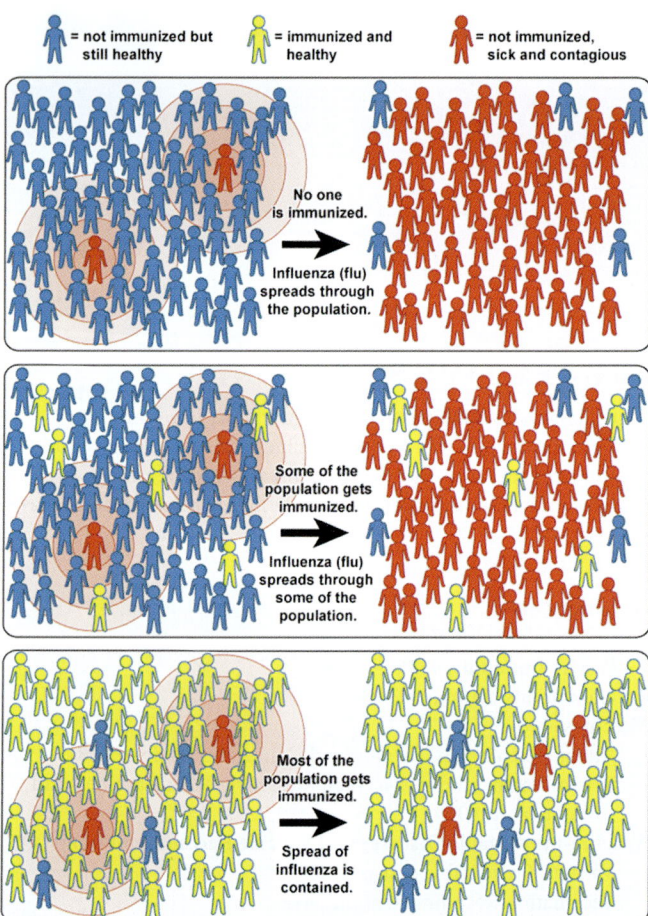

Fig. 34.2 Community immunity. (Courtesy National Institute of Allergy and Infectious Diseases.)

VACCINES

Vaccination involves administering a small amount of antigen that, although capable of stimulating an immune response, does not typically produce the disease. Different types of vaccines are available, but the type used in vaccinations depends on the person's immune response. The antigen in vaccines may be produced in several ways. Traditional vaccines contain the whole or components of an inactivated (killed) microorganism.

Attenuated Viruses, Toxoids, and Conjugate Vaccines
Attenuated Viruses

Other vaccines are **attenuated viruses** composed of live, attenuated (weakened) microorganisms. Individuals who are immunocompromised because of illness or take medication that causes immunosuppression should avoid live vaccines.

Toxoids

Toxoids are inactivated toxins that can no longer produce harmful diseases but do stimulate the formation of antitoxins, which produce active immunity (e.g., tetanus toxoid).

Conjugate Vaccines

Newer vaccines, called **conjugate vaccines**, require a protein or toxoid from an unrelated organism to link to the outer coating of the disease-causing microorganism. This linkage creates a substance that the immature immune system of young infants can recognize. Examples include the *H. influenzae* type B vaccine, and the newest COVID-19 vaccine, Novavax COVID-19 vaccine.

Recombinant Subunit Vaccines, Messenger RNA Vaccines, and Adjuvants

Recombinant Subunit Vaccines

Recombinant subunit vaccines involve inserting some of the genetic material (e.g., DNA) of a pathogen into another cell or organism, where the antigen is produced in massive quantities. These antigens are then used as a vaccine instead of the whole pathogen. The HepB vaccine is an example of this type of vaccine.

Adenovector vaccines have been in development for the past 20 years. In these vaccines, a modified adenovirus is injected into an individual, triggering an immune response. After administration, the vaccine enters the cells and teaches the immune cells to make the desired protein. The first such adenovector vaccine approved for general use is a vaccine for Ebola. Trials of adenovector vaccines are underway for HIV and Zika.

Messenger RNA Vaccines

One of the newest vaccines in the arsenal against infectious diseases is the severe acute respiratory syndrome coronavirus 2 (SARS-CoV-2) vaccine, a **messenger RNA (mRNA)** vaccine. Messenger RNA vaccines have been 30 years in the making, with mRNA vaccines in development for Ebola, cytomegalovirus, Zika virus, and influenza. With an mRNA vaccine, scientists synthesize an mRNA strand with an altered code so the body does not identify it as foreign. The synthetic mRNA tells the body to create the spike protein found on the SARS-CoV-2 virus, which in turn triggers the immune system to produce cells designed to fight the spike protein, protecting the body against SARS-CoV-2 (Fig. 34.3). The Centers for Disease Control and Prevention (CDC) has launched v-safe, the after-vaccination health checker, to monitor side effects experienced by persons receiving the COVID-19 vaccine (see https://www.cdc.gov/vaccinesafety/ensuringsafety/monitoring/v-safe/index.html for further information).

Adjuvants

An **adjuvant**—often an aluminum salt such as aluminum hydroxide, aluminum phosphate, or aluminum potassium sulfate—is a substance added to a vaccine to increase the body's immune response to the vaccine. One value of adding an adjuvant to a vaccine is to reduce the amount of antigen needed to produce a dose of vaccine. Vaccines with adjuvants are rigorously tested for safety before being licensed. In the United States, vaccines against measles, mumps, rubella, chickenpox, rotavirus, polio, and seasonal influenza do *not* contain adjuvants.

Regardless of the composition of the vaccine, each vaccine is designed to stimulate an immune response against a specific pathogen. Some vaccines require booster doses to maintain sufficient immunity. The immune system's memory responds rapidly to prevent disease when exposed to a booster, which provides an active, albeit artificially acquired, immunity.

VACCINE-PREVENTABLE DISEASES AND VACCINE RECOMMENDATIONS

Vaccine-Preventable Diseases

Vaccinations maintain health by preventing disease. In the United States, more than 20 infectious diseases may be prevented by active vaccination. Many of these vaccines are routinely administered to healthy children and adults. Others are reserved for special populations such as health care providers, military personnel, immigrants, adults with special health needs, individuals with chronic illness, and travelers to certain foreign countries. Table 34.1 provides an overview of the disease manifestations and vaccine information, including route of administration and storage temperature. Vaccine-preventable

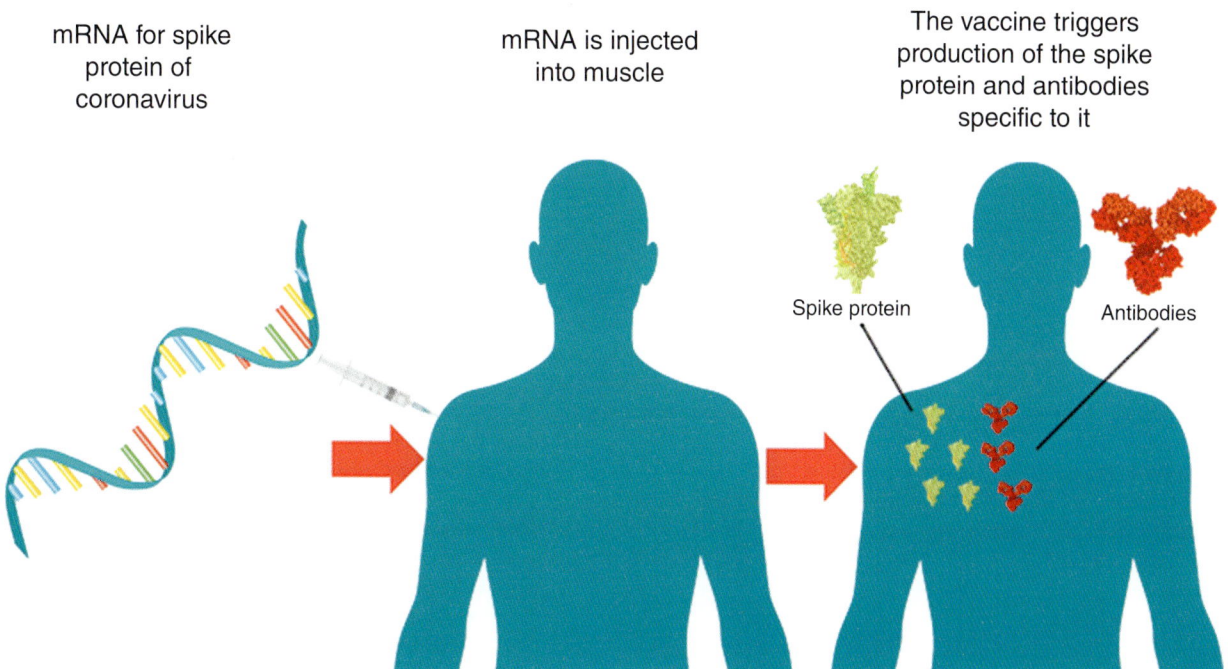

Fig. 34.3 COVID-19 mRNA vaccines give instructions for our cells to make **a harmless piece** of what is called the *spike protein*.

TABLE 34.1 Vaccine-Preventable Diseases

Disease, Route of Administration, Storage	Manifestations	Vaccine
Anthrax, subcut 2°C–8°C Do not freeze.	*Cutaneous:* An itchy sore that may blister and form a black ulcer (eschar). The sore is usually painless but may have surrounding edema. *Gastrointestinal:* Abdominal pain, vomiting, mouth sores, bloody diarrhea, toxemia, shock, and possibly death *Inhaled:* Wool sorter's disease or associated with the use of biologic warfare: Fever, malaise, headache, cough, shortness of breath, and chest pain (due to bleeding and swelling in chest cavity) are often followed by shock within 36 h of symptom onset due to bacteremia.	Routine vaccinations are not recommended but are administered to specific groups: laboratory workers who work with anthrax; people who handle animals or animal products, such as some veterinarians; some members of the US military. These persons should receive five shots over 18 mo with annual boosters. When used as postexposure prophylaxis, the vaccine is given as a three-dose series, administered at 0, 2, and 4 wk after exposure, along with 60 d of antibiotic therapy (ciprofloxacin and doxycycline).
Diphtheria, IM (diphtheria toxoids) 35°F–46°F (2°C–8°C) Do not freeze.	Respiratory infection, blocked airway, myocardial damage, nerve damage, sore throat, weakness, swollen glands	Toxoid A single-antigen toxoid is not available. Currently combined as DTaP, Tdap, DT, and Td. DTaP is used for active immunity in those 6 wk–6 y. Tdap (active booster) is given as a single dose for those 10 y and older.
Haemophilus influenzae type B (Hib), IM 35°F–46°F (2°C–8°C) Do not freeze.	Sepsis, arthritis, skin and throat infections, meningitis, intellectual disability, epiglottitis, pneumonia, and death Increased severity is seen in those younger than 5 y and older than 65 y.	Bacterial conjugate is contained in Hib vaccine. There are different types of influenza; Hib is specific to influenza B. Not all influenza bacteria have vaccines.
Hepatitis A virus (HAV), IM 36°F–46°F (2°C–8°C) Do not freeze.	Fever; can cause liver damage or failure, malaise, jaundice, anorexia, nausea, arthralgia, kidney, pancreatic, and blood disorders This acute, self-limited illness is highly contagious.	Inactivated viral antigen is available as HepA vaccine and in HepA/HepB. Routinely administered to children 12–23 mo, high-risk populations, close contacts to persons with HAV, and persons traveling to certain countries. Because it is inactivated, the vaccine can be given to persons who are immunocompromised.
Hepatitis B virus (HBV), IM 35°F–46°F (2°C–8°C) Do not freeze.	Fever, headache, malaise, anorexia, arthralgia, arthritis, jaundice Chronic infection can occur, leading to liver cirrhosis, liver cancer, and death.	Recombinant viral antigen is available as HepB and HepA/HepB vaccines. Vaccines are recommended for at-risk infants, health care personnel, those who share injectable/IV drug needles and equipment, males who have sex with males, those whose sex partners are HBV positive, and those not in a monogamous relationship. HepB vaccine is available as a single dose and as a combined vaccine. Administer monovalent HepB to all infants at birth. Combination HepA-HepB is recommended only for those 18 y and older and for at-risk infants.
Human papillomavirus (HPV; various disease strains), IM 35°F–46°F (2°C–8°C) Protect from light, and shake well before administering. Pregnancy: Administer only if needed.	Sexually transmitted and seen as cervical, vaginal, anal, and oropharyngeal cancers and genital warts	The HPV vaccine is recommended for preteens 11 or 12 y so they are protected before ever being exposed to the virus. Adults can receive the HPV vaccine through age 26 y.
Influenza, IM/ID/IN Inactivated influenza vaccine (IIV) 35°F–46°F (2°C–8°C): Administer IM/ID Live attenuated influenza vaccine (LAIV) ≤5°F (−15°C): Administer IN.	Fever, chills, headaches, malaise, myalgias, nasal congestion, and cough Can cause pneumonia	*Trivalent flu vaccine* (influenza A [H1N1 and an H3N2] and influenza B). *Quadrivalent flu vaccine* (2 influenza A and 2 influenza B). Everyone 6 mo and older should have the flu vaccine annually, particularly those at high risk. Those who should NOT receive the flu shot include infants <6 mo old, those with allergies to the flu vaccine or any of its components, those with allergies to eggs, and those with or who have recovered from Guillain-Barré syndrome. The IN flu vaccine should not be administered to children <2 y or adults >50 y, or children >2 y or <17 y receiving aspirin-containing therapy or with asthma.

TABLE 34.1 Vaccine-Preventable Diseases—cont'd

Disease, Route of Administration, Storage	Manifestations	Vaccine
Measles, subcut (rubeola) 35°F–46°F (2°C–8°C) or colder; may be frozen. Protect from light, and discard after 8 hours.	Rash, fever, cough, nasal congestion, conjunctivitis, pneumonia Occasionally results in encephalitis	Live virus is contained in measles, MMR, and MMRV vaccines. ⚠ Contraindicated in pregnancy.
Meningococcal disease, subcut/IM 35°F–46°F (2°C–8°C) Groups A, C, W, Y Meningococcal *H. influenzae* type b conjugate vaccine	Fever, sepsis, rash, meningitis	Meningococcal conjugate vaccines MenACWY: quadrivalent (protects against serogroups A, C, W, and Y). Recommended for children 2 mo–10 y who are at increased risk and children/adolescents 11–18 years. First dose is recommended between 11y and 12y with booster at 16 y. Also for adults after splenectomy, persons working with the pathogen, college freshmen, and military recruits. Meningococcal polysaccharide vaccine (MPSV4): quadrivalent (protects against serogroups A, C, W, and Y) meningococcal vaccine. For adults after splenectomy, persons working with the pathogen, college freshmen, and military recruits. Serogroup B meningococcal vaccine (MenB): monovalent (protects against serogroup B) meningococcal vaccine. Recommended for children/adolescents 10–18 y who are at increased risk.
Mumps, subcut 35°F–46°F (2°C–8°C), but may be frozen	Swelling of salivary glands, fever, headache, fatigue, and myalgia Can cause meningitis, encephalitis, inflammation of testicles or ovaries, deafness	Live attenuated virus is contained in MMR and MMRV. ⚠ Contraindicated in pregnancy
Pertussis ("whooping cough"), IM 35°F–46°F (2°C–8°C)	Highly contagious Severe coughing spasms; can cause pneumonia, seizures, encephalitis, and death. Symptoms are more severe in infants and young children.	Antigenic components of inactivated bacteria (acellular) are contained in the two vaccines that are available, DTap and Tdap.
Pneumococcal disease, IM/subcut 35°F–46°F (2°C–8°C)	Ear infections, sinus infections, pneumonia; can cause sepsis, meningitis, and death	Pneumococcal polysaccharide vaccine (PPSV23) protects against 23 types of pneumococcal bacteria (IM/subcut). PPSV23 is recommended for all adults ≥ 65 y. Patients who are immunocompromised ≥ 2 but ≤ 64 y should also receive PPSV23. Pneumococcal conjugate vaccine (PCV13) protects against 13 types of pneumococcal bacteria (IM). PCV13 is recommended for all children <5 y as a series of 4 injections starting at 2 mo, then 4 mo, 6 mo, and between 12 and 15 mo; adults ≥ 65 y, and people ≥ 6 y with certain chronic illnesses should also receive the vaccine.
Poliomyelitis, subcut/IM 35°F–46°F (2°C–8°C)	Invades brain and spinal cord; the milder form causes fever, sore throat, nausea, and headaches; the severe form causes paralysis and death.	Children should receive a series of 4 inactive polio vaccine (IPV) injections starting at 2 mo, then at 4 mo, 6–18 mo, and a booster at 4–6 y.
Rabies, IM 35°F–46°F (2°C–8°C)	Anxiety, difficulty swallowing, seizures; life threatening; almost always progresses to death	Administer killed virus to high-risk groups (e.g., veterinarians, animal handlers) and to persons traveling to areas where rabies is common. The preexposure schedule for rabies vaccination is three doses, given on the following schedule: 1st dose: before potential exposure 2nd dose: 7 d after the first dose 3rd dose: 21 d or 28 d after the second dose

Continued

TABLE 34.1 Vaccine-Preventable Diseases—cont'd

Disease, Route of Administration, Storage	Manifestations	Vaccine
Two respiratory syncytial virus (RSV) vaccines are approved for people ages 60 y and older. • Arexvy (GSK adjuvanted RSV vaccine) • Abrysvo (Pfizer RSV vaccine) Administer IM in the deltoid with a 1- to 1.5-in needle. Arexvy adjuvant suspension component vial and lyophilized antigen component vials must be refrigerated in the original package at temperature of 36°F–46°F (2°C–8°C). Protect vials from light. Do not freeze. Abrysvo kit (vial of lyophilized antigen component [a sterile white powder] and prefilled syringe containing sterile water and diluent component) must be refrigerated at 36°F–46°F (2°C–8°C) in the original carton. Do not freeze.	Causes mild, cold-like symptoms. Most people recover in 1–2 wk, but RSV can be serious. Infants and older adults are more likely to develop severe RSV and need hospitalization.	Vaccination should occur before the onset of the fall and winter RSV season. RSV vaccines appear to provide some protection for at least two RSV seasons. Additional surveillance and evaluation activities are planned to assess how long the vaccines protect against RSV and whether additional doses will be needed. Adults 60 y and older, a single dose is recommended. 1 dose of maternal RSV vaccine during weeks 32–36 of pregnancy, administered September through January. Abrysvo is the only RSV vaccine recommended during pregnancy.
Rotavirus, PO 35°F–46°F (2°C–8°C)	Acute gastroenteritis; contagious and may be particularly severe in infants and young children but mild in adults	Two vaccines are available: RV5 is given in 3 doses at ages 2 mo, 4 mo, and 6 mo. RV1 is given in 2 doses at ages 2–4 mo. ⚠ Due to the small increase in cases of intussusception from rotavirus vaccination, health care providers should weigh the potential risks and benefits of administering rotavirus vaccine to infants with a previous history of intussusception.
Rubella ("German measles"), subcut 35°F–46°F (2°C–8°C) May be frozen.	Rash, fever, swollen lymph nodes Congenital disorders occur if rubella is acquired by a pregnant patient.	The rubella vaccine is a live attenuated virus. Recommended vaccination schedule: 1st dose: 12–15 mo 2nd dose: 4–6 y ⚠ Contraindicated in pregnancy
SARS-Cov-2 (COVID-19), IM into the deltoid muscle See https://www.cdc.gov/vaccines/hcp/admin/storage/toolkit/index.html for storage and handling information.	The virus spreads by airborne particles and droplets, close person-to-person contact, mainly via airborne particles and droplets 2–14 d after exposure. Fever/chills, cough, dyspnea, fatigue, myalgia, headache, new-onset loss of taste or smell, sore throat, rhinorrhea, nausea, vomiting, or diarrhea. May progress to acute respiratory distress syndrome and death. Serious complications include arrhythmias, cardiomyopathy and acute cardiac injury, coagulation disorders, sepsis, shock, and multiorgan failure. Children may develop multisystem inflammatory syndrome. Some individuals develop COVID-19 syndrome, or "long COVID," and experience persistent symptoms including cognitive impairment, fatigue, anxiety, depression, PTSD, headaches, dizziness, persistent shortness of breath, and permanent lung damage.	The 2023–24 updated COVID-19 vaccines more closely target the XBB lineage of the Omicron variant and could restore protection against severe COVID-19 that may have decreased over time. CDC recommends the 2023–2024 updated COVID-19 vaccines: Pfizer-BioNTech, Moderna, or Novavax, to protect against serious illness from COVID-19. Everyone aged 5 y and older should get 1 dose of an updated COVID-19 vaccine to protect against serious illness from COVID-19. Children aged 6 mo–4 y need multiple doses of COVID-19 vaccines to be up to date, including at least 1 dose of updated COVID-19 vaccine. People who are moderately or severely immunocompromised may get additional doses of updated COVID-19 vaccine.

TABLE 34.1 Vaccine-Preventable Diseases—cont'd

Disease, Route of Administration, Storage	Manifestations	Vaccine
Smallpox, percutaneous skin prick of 15 jabs using a steel bifurcated needle 35°F–46°F (2°C–8°C) Protect from light and use within 6–8 h after reconstitution, then discard.	High fever, severe headache, backache, abdominal pain, and lethargy that lasts 2–5 d; then an extensive rash develops that begins as macules and progresses to papules; then firm vesicles form; and finally, deep-seated, hard pustules form that cause significant scarring.	Smallpox vaccine (live vaccinia virus) is stockpiled in case of an outbreak and emergency. Immunization program for at-risk laboratory personnel and health care providers, emergency personnel, and military personnel Vaccinate only if exposed to smallpox. ⚠ Contraindicated in pregnancy; can cause stillbirth. Can cause myocarditis and pericarditis.
Tetanus ("lockjaw"), IM 35°F–46°F (2°C–8°C)	Stiffness in neck and abdominal muscles, difficulty swallowing, muscle spasms, fever; can cause broken bones, breathing difficulty, and death	Toxoid conjugate contained in tetanus, DTaP, DT, Tdap, and Td vaccines. Children should receive a series of 5 doses of DTaP vaccine, beginning at 2 mo; then at 4 and 6 mo; then between 15 and 18 mo; and between 4 and 6 y. The Td booster should be given every 10 y.
Tuberculosis (TB), ID (preferred)/subcut 35°F–46°F (2°C–8°C)	Highly contagious respiratory infection Symptoms include cough lasting 3 wk or longer, pleuritic chest pain, coughing up blood or sputum, weakness or fatigue, weight loss, anorexia, fever and night sweats. May also cause meningitis and bone, joint, and skin infections	Live attenuated bacteria Called *bacille Calmette-Guérin (BCG)* Not routinely administered in the United States, it prevents severe disease but does not prevent infection with the bacterium. Should only be considered for children who have a negative tuberculin skin test and who are continually exposed, or for select health care workers.
Typhoid, subcut/PO 35°F–46°F (2°C–8°C)	Sustained high fever, headache, anorexia, abdominal pain, enlarged liver and spleen, constipation, and, later, diarrhea	Vaccine given in exposure to *Salmonella paratyphi* and *S. typhi* B is available as live attenuated bacteria (Ty21a; PO) or inactivated components of the typhoid bacterial capsule (Vi; subcut). Routine vaccinations are not required in the United States but are recommended for travelers to certain foreign countries.
Varicella (chickenpox), subcut ≤5°F (−15°C) Contraindicated in pregnancy	Fever and rash, consisting of a few to hundreds of itchy, blisterlike lesions; symptoms are more severe in older children and adults. Complications may include encephalitis, bacterial skin infections, pneumonia, Reye syndrome, and death.	Varicella vaccine, live, is recommended as a two-dose series, first at 12–15 mo, then again between 4 and 6 y. ⚠ Contraindicated in pregnancy
Yellow fever, subcut 35°F–46°F (2°C–8°C)	Fever, jaundice, and gastrointestinal hemorrhage	Yellow fever vaccine, live A single primary dose is recommended for persons ≥9 mo traveling to, or living in, areas at risk for yellow fever virus transmission (e.g., South America and Africa). The vaccine is required by international regulations for travel to and from certain countries.
Herpes zoster (shingles), subcut ≤5°F (−15°C) Contraindicated in pregnancy	A painful, blisterlike rash in a dermatomal distribution occurs due to reactivation of varicella virus. After resolution of the rash, prolonged severe pain (postherpetic neuralgia) may occur.	Herpes zoster vaccine approved by the FDA for people ≥50 y.

<, Less than; >, greater than; ≤, less than or equal to; ≥, greater than or equal to; *DT*, diphtheria-tetanus; *DTaP*, diphtheria-tetanus–acellular pertussis; *FDA*, US Food and Drug Administration; *HepA*, hepatitis A; *HepB*, hepatitis B; *ID*, intradermal; *IM*, intramuscular; *IN*, intranasal; *IV*, intravenous; *MMR*, measles-mumps-rubella; *MMRV*, measles-mumps-rubella-varicella; *mo*, months; *PO*, by mouth; *PTSD*, posttraumatic stress disorder; *subcut*, subcutaneous; *Td*, tetanus-diphtheria; *Tdap*, tetanus-diphtheria–acellular pertussis; *wk*, weeks; *y*, years.

diseases for children, adolescents, and adults include—but are not limited to—anthrax, diphtheria, *H. influenzae* type B, hepatitis A and B, HPV, influenza (flu), measles, meningococcal disease, mumps, pertussis, pneumococcal disease, poliomyelitis, rabies, respiratory syncytial virus, rotavirus, rubella, smallpox, tetanus, tuberculosis (TB), typhoid, varicella, yellow fever, SARS-CoV-2, and herpes zoster.

Vaccination Recommendations

Immunization schedules are approved by the Advisory Committee on Immunizations (ACIP). Each schedule identifies recommended vaccinations, ages to vaccinate, dosage, and route for children, adolescents, and adults. For the most current information on childhood immunizations, consult the CDC website at www.cdc.gov/vaccines. A vaccine information statement (VIS) is also produced by the CDC for each vaccine and provides information on the (1) route of administration, (2) schedule for routine vaccine administration, (3) minimum dosing intervals, (4) contraindications, and (5) standing orders for administering vaccines.

The childhood immunization schedule from birth to 6 years recommends HepB, RV, DTaP, Hib, PCV, inactivated polio virus (IPV),

MMR, varicella, and HepA. Before immunizations are administered, screen for medical conditions that put the child at risk, use of prescription and over-the-counter (OTC) drugs to include herbal preparations, and any food or drug allergies.

The adolescent immunization schedule from ages 7 to 18 years recommends Tdap, influenza, HPV, and meningococcal vaccinations. Adolescents may also need to catch up on any vaccines missed, such as MMR, HepA, HepB, IPV, and varicella (chickenpox).

A catch-up immunization schedule is available for those up to 18 years of age who fall behind or start late with immunizations. Childhood and adolescent immunization schedules are also available as a combined schedule (birth to 18 years).

Adult (19 years and older) vaccination rates remain low, which indicates a need to improve. One way is to increase awareness that routine vaccines for adults are important for well-being, to provide information on how vaccines protect from diseases, and to assess routine vaccinations for adults are important for well-being, to provide information on how vaccines protect from diseases, and to assess immunization status during clinical visits. Adult vaccines are based on factors such as age and health status and include Tdap, tetanus-diphtheria (Td) booster, influenza, pneumococcal polysaccharide vaccine (PPSV23), HPV, MMR, varicella vaccine (chickenpox), and zoster vaccine (shingles). Adults may also be immunized with certain additional vaccines, including HepA, HepB, smallpox (routine for laboratory personnel handling vaccine cultures), and meningococcal vaccine. Current recommendations for adult immunization can be found at www.cdc.gov/vaccines/schedules/.

> ### ⚡ PATIENT SAFETY
>
> **Do Not Confuse...**
> - Hepatitis A, inactivated/hepatitis B (recombinant) vaccine provides active immunity against both hepatitis A virus (HAV) and hepatitis B virus (HBV) for adults >18 years of age who are at high risk for HAV and HBV.
> - There are different types of **meningococcal vaccine:** MCV4 or MenACWY (conjugate; administered to preteens 11–12 years old), MenB (serogroup B; administered to teens and young adults ages 16–23), and MPSV4 (polysaccharide; for adults ≥56 who require a single dose [traveling or at risk due to community outbreak]).
> - **HepA** and **HepB** vaccines are *dosed differently* for children, adolescents, and adults.
> - Do not confuse **HepB** *vaccine* and **HepB** *immunoglobulin*.
> - **Zoster vaccine**, a vaccine administered to adults to prevent shingles, and **varicella vaccine**, which prevents chickenpox and is approved for use in susceptible children and adults.
> - ⚠ **DTaP**, for active immunization in children 6 weeks to 6 years, and **Tdap**, the active booster for those aged 10 years and older; antigens in both are the same, but the amount of antigen component varies.

Immunization Before International Travel

International travel warrants the updating of routine vaccines based on age and immunization history, and travelers to some areas should consider additional vaccines (https://wwwnc.cdc.gov/travel/page/travel-vaccines). For example, the CDC currently recommends US travelers 6 months and older to have an updated MMR vaccine based on the travel destination.

Travelers may need to consider vaccination against typhoid and yellow fever. Typhoid fever is caused by a bacterium, *Salmonella typhi*, which is generally spread via contaminated food and water (see Table 34.1). Risk of contracting this infection is greatest for travelers to India, Pakistan, Mexico, Bangladesh, the Philippines, and Haiti. Even stays of less than 2 weeks pose significant risk. Two forms of typhoid vaccine are available for use in the United States. Typhoid vaccine live oral contains the Ty21a strain of *S. typhi* and is a live attenuated vaccine, which can be administered to persons 6 years of age and older and consists of four capsules, one taken every 48 hours, with the series completed 1 week before potential exposure. A booster dose consisting of the same four-capsule regimen is recommended every 5 years. The other vaccine, parenteral typhoid Vi polysaccharide vaccine, is an inactivated vaccine that contains purified cell surface polysaccharide antigens extracted from *S. typhi* of the Ty2 strain and may be administered to travelers 2 years of age and older. It is administered at least 2 weeks before expected exposure as a single, intramuscular (IM) injection. A booster dose is recommended every 2 years for those who remain at risk.

Yellow fever is a mosquito-borne viral illness endemic to sub-Saharan Africa and tropical South America. The vaccine is administered as a single injection for persons older than 9 months. In the United States, the vaccine is administered only at authorized vaccine centers nationwide. Other vaccines needed for travel may include those for cholera, meningococcus, rabies, hepatitis A and B, and polio.

VACCINE SAFETY: REPORTING DISEASES AND ADVERSE REACTIONS

Contraindications

Vaccines are generally safe, although mild reactions include swelling at the injection site and low-grade fever. Awareness of the contraindications for use of vaccines decreases the incidence of serious adverse reactions. Contraindications include moderate or severe illness or anaphylaxis, a serious, life-threatening allergic reaction to a specific vaccine or vaccine component. Therefore it is important to review vaccine-specific contraindications before administering any vaccine. Vaccines may be given in cases of mild acute illness or the convalescent phase of illness, antimicrobial therapy, exposure to infectious disease, or premature birth.

Reporting

Health care providers are responsible for reporting cases of vaccine-preventable diseases and adverse reactions after immunizations. These data identify whether an outbreak is occurring and assess the effect of immunization policies and procedures. Providers must report adverse reactions to the Vaccine Adverse Events Reporting System (VAERS). Information and forms are available at http://vaers.hhs.gov/index. VAERS is a surveillance system that receives and acts on reports of adverse events. The National Childhood Vaccine Injury Act of 1986 initiated the National Vaccine Injury Compensation Program (NVICP), which provides compensation for injury or death caused by a vaccination. More information is available at www.hrsa.gov/vaccinecompensation. To provide safety through communication, the NVICP requires providers to distribute a VIS before vaccines are administered. Federal law requires health care providers to provide information to those receiving vaccines. These information statements include indications, age recommendations, schedule of doses, side effects, special circumstances, and resources to notify if an adverse reaction occurs. For more information, visit www.cdc.gov/vaccines/hcp/vis.

PROTOTYPE DRUG CHART
Varicella Vaccine

Drug Class	Dosage
Vaccine	0.5 mL subcut × 2 doses First dose: 12–15 mo; second dose: 4–6 y Catch-up initiated any time after 12–15 mo <13 y, space doses at least 3 mo apart ≥13 y, space doses 4–8 wk apart *For varicella prophylaxis; for outbreak control of local epidemics of wild-type varicella virus in susceptible persons after varicella exposure,* consult the current recommendations of the CDC (https://www.cdc.gov/chickenpox/php/outbreak-control/).
Contraindications	**Drug-Lab-Food Interactions**
Previous anaphylaxis to this vaccine or to any of its components; pregnancy or possibility of pregnancy within 1 mo; vaccine recipient who is immunocompromised; presence of moderate to severe acute illness; active untreated tuberculosis	Drug: Separate from other live virus vaccines (e.g., MMR, intranasal flu) by 4 wk if not given on the same day; delay VV for up to 11 mo after blood transfusion or Ig; delay Ig for 2 mo after VV, high-dose immunosuppressant medications; avoid salicylates for 6 wk after VV.
Pharmacokinetics	**Pharmacodynamics**
Not applicable	Seroconversion rates: 12 mo–12 y: >98% at 4–6 wk after vaccination ≥13 y: ~75% 4 wk after first dose and 99% 4 wk after second dose
Therapeutic Effects/Uses	
For prevention of chickenpox, when administered to susceptible individuals, the vaccine results in complete protection from chickenpox for most persons. For the minority in whom breakthrough chickenpox develops after vaccination, the disease is typically very mild. The vaccine may also provide prophylaxis protection if administered within 3–5 d of exposure to chickenpox. Mechanism of Action: Stimulates active immunity against natural disease	
Side Effects	**Adverse Reactions**
Pain and redness at the injection site, fever, chickenpox-like rash (generalized or confined to the area surrounding injection site)	Anaphylaxis, thrombocytopenia, encephalitis, Stevens-Johnson syndrome

VARICELLA VACCINE

Before the development of the varicella vaccine in 1995, about 4 million people came down with varicella zoster virus (VZV), resulting in 10,600 hospitalizations and close to 150 deaths per year. Since implementation of the varicella vaccine, cases of VZV have declined more than 75%, hospitalizations have declined more than 90%, and deaths from VZV have been reduced by 85% or more.

Prototype Drug Chart: Varicella Vaccine provides the pharmacologic data for varicella vaccine.

Pharmacokinetics and Pharmacodynamics
Pharmacokinetics
Biologic products such as vaccines do not undergo the pharmacokinetic processes associated with other drug therapy.

Pharmacodynamics
Seroconversion is the acquisition of detectable levels of antibodies in the bloodstream. In the case of varicella vaccine, seroconversion occurs in more than 98% of 12-month-old to 12-year-old recipients approximately 6 weeks after receiving a single dose of vaccine. Susceptible persons 13 years and older who receive two doses of varicella vaccine 4 to 8 weeks apart show a seroconversion rate of approximately 75% 4 weeks after the first dose and 99% 4 weeks after the second dose. Despite the high rate of initial seroconversion among children 12 months to 12 years of age, clinical trials have shown that, over 10 years, the vaccine's effectiveness in preventing disease was 94% for children who received one dose of vaccine and 98% for those who received two doses. Therefore, beginning in 2007, a second varicella vaccine dose was recommended for all susceptible individuals, including children.

Contraindications
Varicella vaccine should be avoided in patients with a history of previous anaphylaxis to this vaccine or to any of its components, including gelatin and neomycin. It is also contraindicated in the presence of moderate to severe acute illness or active untreated TB.

Although varicella infection can cause fetal harm, the possible effects of the vaccine on fetal development are currently unknown. Therefore, varicella vaccine is contraindicated during pregnancy. Pregnancy should also be avoided for at least 1 month after each dose of the vaccine. It is important to note that this recommendation differs from the product package insert, which suggests a 3-month delay in pregnancy.

Patients who are immunocompromised because of malignancies, high-dose systemic steroids, or other immunosuppressive therapy should avoid varicella vaccine. Likewise, the vaccine is generally contraindicated in the presence of primary or acquired immunodeficiencies. However, vaccination may be considered in children with certain classes of human immunodeficiency virus (HIV) infection.

Drug Interactions
Frequently a patient is eligible for several immunizations at a visit. A patient receiving varicella vaccine may receive all other vaccines concurrently if each is administered at a separate site. If the MMR

or other live virus vaccine is not given the same day as the varicella vaccine, administration of the two vaccines should be separated by at least 4 weeks.

If a patient has received a transfusion of blood or blood products, including Ig, administering the varicella vaccine will need to be deferred for as long as 11 months. Likewise, such blood products should be avoided for at least 2 months after vaccination if possible. Blood products and Ig interfere with the body's production of antibodies specific to chickenpox, thereby decreasing the likelihood that active immunity will develop.

Reye syndrome has occasionally occurred in children after natural chickenpox infection. Most of these children also received salicylate medications (e.g., aspirin). Therefore patients should avoid salicylates for 6 weeks after vaccination.

FUTURE DEVELOPMENTS IN VACCINES

Anthrax, Smallpox, and Pertussis

A small outbreak of anthrax cases in the United States in 2001 increased the level of awareness of the anthrax vaccine. Anthrax is caused by the bacteria *Bacillus anthracis*. A serious disease, cutaneous anthrax is the most common form (95% of cases). Anthrax can also occur in the gastrointestinal (GI) tract and lungs. As a biologic weapon, anthrax is highly lethal. It is easily produced, stored, and spread over large areas. Proper vaccination is an essential part of protection against this disease. Approved by the US Food and Drug Administration (FDA) in 1970, anthrax vaccine adsorbed (AVA) has been routinely and safely administered to laboratory and military personnel, livestock farmers, and veterinarians. The vaccine requires five injections over 18 months with annual boosters. No serious side effects have been reported, but the vaccination is contraindicated during pregnancy. In the event of a bioterrorism attack, persons exposed to anthrax should receive three doses of vaccine over 4 weeks and be given ciprofloxacin and doxycycline for 60 days to prevent anthrax. Additional information is available at https://www.cdc.gov/anthrax/prevention/.

Smallpox, caused by the variola virus, is transmitted through human body fluids or contaminated materials. Smallpox was eradicated in the United States by 1972 and worldwide by 1977; therefore the United States discontinued routine childhood immunization against smallpox in 1972. The vaccine is no longer in use except in persons who have a high risk of exposure. When the vaccine is administered, most people usually have a mild reaction, such as a sore arm, fever, and body aches. However, persons with a weakened immune system may experience more serious side effects, including death. Since the events of September 2001, concern has arisen that smallpox could be used as a bioterrorist weapon. A smallpox immunization response plan is available for outbreaks or emergencies (https://www.cdc.gov/smallpox/bioterrorism/public/index.html).

It has long been known that immunity to pertussis, or "whooping cough," weakens over time and that adolescents and adults are often responsible for transmitting this infection to vulnerable, incompletely immunized infants and young children. In 2018 there were more than 15,500 cases of pertussis in the United States. Pertussis in infants is associated with significant morbidity and mortality; a quarter of infants with pertussis develop pneumonia, and 1 in 100 infants die. Tdap contains tetanus and diphtheria toxoids along with acellular pertussis; these are licensed for use in older children and adults. Tdap may be used as an active booster for people 11 to 64 years of age, and DTaP is approved for use in children 6 weeks to 6 years. Each vaccine contains the same antigens, but the quantities of diphtheria and acellular pertussis vary. It is recommended that, for booster immunization, adolescents and adults receive a one-time dose of Tdap in lieu of the Td vaccine.

Research is underway to update the current vaccine, as the causative bacterium, *Bordetella pertussis*, has undergone genetic changes.

Zoster, Rotavirus, and HPV

Herpes zoster, commonly known as *shingles* or *zoster*, occurs due to reactivation of the varicella virus. The virus persists after a primary varicella infection (chickenpox) but becomes dormant in the body, usually settling in a dorsal root ganglion. Zoster often occurs decades after the primary varicella infection. The development of zoster may be related to a decline in immunity to the VZV. Zoster is characterized by a painful rash that presents in a dermatomal distribution. Especially in older adults, the resolution of the rash may be followed by a chronic, severe, sometimes debilitating pain, referred to as *postherpetic neuralgia*. A live attenuated vaccine (zoster vaccine, live) is licensed for use as a one-time injection in adults 50 and older. The vaccine has been shown to boost VZV immunity among vaccine recipients. In clinical trials, zoster vaccine prevented zoster in about 50% of people who received the vaccine. Effectiveness appears to decrease with increasing age of the vaccine recipient. In those who received the vaccine yet went on to develop zoster, the duration of pain was reduced.

Rotavirus is a leading cause of severe acute gastroenteritis in infants and young children. Rotavirus vaccine, live oral, containing five strains of rotavirus, is effective in protecting against severe gastroenteritis and significantly reduces the need for hospitalization among infected children. The vaccine is administered as a three-dose series at 2, 4, and 6 months of age. It is recommended that the third dose be administered before 8 months.

HPV is a sexually transmitted virus that causes cancer of the cervix, vagina, vulva, and penis and can cause genital warts. It also causes anal and oropharyngeal cancers in both males and females. There are more than 100 different types of this disease. Two vaccines are approved as routine prophylaxis to prevent HPV disease: HPV quadrivalent vaccine (recombinant) and HPV 9-valent vaccine (recombinant).

Both HPV vaccines are administered as a three-dose series to 9- to 26-year-old males and females. The HPV vaccine is contraindicated in pregnancy. The FDA denied Merck's request for expanded use in females 27 to 45 years of age. Because HPV is sexually transmitted, the vaccine is most effective if administered before initiation of sexual intercourse.

Pneumococcal Disease and Bacterial Meningitis

The pneumococcal vaccine provides protection against multiple strains of *Streptococcus pneumoniae* (pneumococcus). Pneumococcal disease includes serious infections of the blood, brain, and lungs. Each year in the United States, around 22,000 persons (both children and adults) die of this vaccine-preventable disease. Two forms of the vaccine are available: pneumococcal 23-valent polysaccharide vaccine (PPV) targeting 23 of the most common serotypes, and pneumococcal 13-valent conjugate vaccine (PCV13) targeting 13 serotypes. PPV is indicated in high-risk persons between the ages of 2 and 65 years (e.g., those undergoing splenectomy, cochlear implant, or immunosuppression) and in all persons older than 65 years. PPV should be repeated after 5 years. PCV13 is recommended for all high-risk persons and for all persons older than 65 years. Since initiation of pneumococcal vaccination, the incidence of antibiotic-resistant disease has dropped significantly.

Bacterial meningitis is a potentially life-threatening infection. Annually more than 1000 cases occur in the United States; 10% to 15% of patients die and one out of five who live have permanent disability, including brain damage, hearing loss, amputations, or loss of kidney function. ACIP recommends routine vaccination to prevent meningococcal infection for those aged 2 to 55 years. The quadrivalent meningococcal conjugate vaccine (MCV4) and meningococcal polysaccharide vaccine (MPSV4) are approved in the United States. MCV4 is preferred for those between the ages of 2 and 55 years; MPSV4 should be used for those older than 55 years of age. For those receiving MCV4, the first dose should be given at 11 or 12 years, with a booster at 16 years. For those who receive the first dose between 13 and 15 years, a one-time booster should be given between 16 and 18 years. If the first dose of MCV4 is given after 16 years, a booster is not needed unless the individual remains at high risk (e.g., microbiologists exposed to *Neisseria meningitidis*, military recruits, those traveling outside the United States, or those with asplenia).

Respiratory Syncytial Virus

The respiratory syncytial virus (RSV) vaccine can prevent lower respiratory tract infections caused by the RSV. This virus is highly contagious and causes cold-like symptoms (runny nose, decreased appetite, cough, sneezing, fever, and wheezing), which can be serious for infants, older adults, those with chronic cardiac and pulmonary disease, those with a weakened immune system, and individuals residing in the long-term care environment. RSV spreads through direct contact with the virus from droplets coming into contact with the eyes, nose, and mouth, and through contact with contaminated surfaces. Each year, as many as 120,000 older adults are hospitalized with RSV and nearly 10,000 older adults die from RSV each year; up to 80,000 children are hospitalized each year and up to 300 deaths occur each year. It is the second largest cause of death in children younger than 1 year of age.

Both RSV vaccines that are available are recombinant protein vaccines that cause the immune system to produce antibodies to RSV. Vaccination is recommended for pregnant individuals during weeks 32 to 36 (Abrysvo), to provide the baby maternal antibodies to RSV from birth to 6 months. The vaccine is also recommended to those 60 and older (Arexvy). The vaccines appear to provide protection for at least two RSV seasons. It is not yet known if additional vaccine doses will be needed.

Common reactions to the IM injection include pain, redness at injection site, and fatigue. Some may also experience diarrhea, and muscle pain. During vaccine trials, very rarely, patients experienced Guillain-Barre syndrome; however, it is unknown if it was due to chance or if the vaccination increases the risk of inflammatory neurologic events.

CLINICAL JUDGMENT [NURSING PROCESS]
Vaccines

Concept: Safety
- Protection of the patient from potential or actual harm; a basic human need

Concept: Health, Wellness, and Illness
- Health, wellness, and illness are dynamic responses to a continuum of biopsychosocial states experienced through all stages of life.

Recognize Cues [Assessment]
- Identify benefits and barriers to timely and complete immunization (e.g., beliefs that vaccine-preventable diseases no longer exist, misunderstanding of true contraindications to immunization, concerns regarding vaccine safety and efficacy, fear of multiple injections, cost).
- Obtain a medical history, including history of malignancy or other immune deficiency.
- Determine history of pregnancy or possible pregnancy within the next month. Many vaccines are contraindicated during pregnancy.
- Obtain a drug history that includes high-dose immunosuppressants, blood transfusions, and Ig.
- Obtain a list of complementary and alternative therapies used, and in the case of a breastfed infant, include herbal products used by the mother.
- Determine a complete allergy history that includes drugs, vaccines, food, and environmental allergies.
- Assess for adverse reactions (other than allergic) to previous doses of vaccine or any vaccine component.
- Assess for symptoms of moderate to severe acute illness with or without fever.
- Screen for household contacts who are unvaccinated or immunocompromised at every visit.
- Obtain an immunization history and a history of vaccine-preventable diseases to determine current vaccine needs. For example, a person with a reliable history of chickenpox or herpes zoster (shingles) does not need the varicella vaccine; natural immunity is assumed.

Analyze Cues and Prioritize Hypothesis [Patient Problems]
- Need for health teaching
- Potential for decreased adherence

Generate Solutions [Planning]
- The patient or the patient's parent or guardian will possess knowledge of vaccine-preventable diseases and risks and benefits of vaccination.
- The patient or the patient's parent or guardian will adhere to the recommended immunization schedule for vaccine-preventable diseases unless contraindications exist.
- The patient will be free of adverse reactions.

Take Action [Nursing Interventions]
- Strictly adhere to individual vaccine storage requirements to ensure potency of the product.
- Upon preparation, including reconstitution of a given vaccine, administer within the time limits stated in the package insert to ensure potency.
- ⚡ Administer at separate sites all vaccines for which a patient is eligible at the time of the visit. Do *not* mix vaccines in the same syringe.
- ⚡ Document in a patient's record the vaccination date, route, and site of administration; the vaccine type, manufacturer, lot number, and expiration date; and the name, business address, and title of the person administering the vaccine.
- ⚡ Observe the patient for signs and symptoms of adverse reactions to vaccines.
- Keep epinephrine readily available for immediate use in case of an anaphylactic reaction.
- Provide the patient with a record of immunizations administered.
- Modify communications to meet the cultural needs of the patient and the patient's family.
- Use a professional interpreter when necessary.
- Provide the patient and the patient's family with a VIS in the patient's preferred language (available at www.immunize.org).
- Discuss vaccine-preventable diseases with the patient and/or the patient's family, including manifestations and risk of contracting the disease.
- Answer all questions regarding vaccine safety, effectiveness, and risk factors in clear, understandable language.
- Advise female patients of childbearing age to avoid pregnancy for 1 month, depending on the vaccines administered.

Continued

CLINICAL JUDGMENT [NURSING PROCESS]—CONT'D

Vaccines

- Advise patients to avoid contact with persons who are immunocompromised, depending on the vaccines to be administered.
- Provide the patient or the patient's family with a current vaccine information statement (VIS), available from the Centers for Disease Control and Prevention (CDC), for each vaccine before its administration as required by federal law.
- Remind the patient or the patient's family to maintain a vaccine immunization record and to bring it to all visits.
- Provide the patient or the patient's family with a return date for the next vaccination(s) based on assessment of the immunization history.
- Discuss common side effects of vaccines, such as injection site soreness, fever, and side effects specific to individual vaccines.
- Offer suggestions for management of common side effects (e.g., cold compresses for injection site soreness, acetaminophen for soreness or fever).
- Advise the patient or the patient's family to contact the health care provider if signs of a serious reaction are noted.

Evaluate Outcomes [Evaluation]
- Evaluate patient and family understanding of the rationale for immunizations.
- Evaluate patient adherence to the recommended immunization schedule.
- Evaluate whether the patient is free from adverse reactions.

PATIENT SAFETY

Don't Wait! Vaccinate!
Use the SHARE method (see https://www.cdc.gov/vaccines/hcp/adults/downloads/standards-immz-practice-recommendation.pdf):

Share reasons why the vaccine is right for the patient.
Highlight positive experiences.
Address the patient's questions about the vaccine.
Remind the patient that vaccines protect against diseases.
Explain the costs and consequences of getting the disease.

CLINICAL JUDGMENT CASE STUDY

A 22-year-old college student is in the wellness clinic with their 3-month-old baby and their 13-year-old sister. They live with their grandmother, who is 68 years old. The student requests immunizations for the baby and asks if there are any immunizations the student and their sibling need.

1. The patient says the baby needs the "regular shots." The baby received their first hepatitis B vaccine while in the newborn nursery but has not had any shots since coming home. What is the hepatitis B vaccine catch-up schedule for the baby? What is the routine schedule for hepatitis B vaccine in infants and children?
2. The patient is worried that they will need to start their immunizations over because "my baby is so far behind." How should the nurse respond to the concern?
3. Which vaccines are due for the baby today? When would the baby be due for another series of immunizations?
4. The nurse asks the patient about their vaccine history. The student says they had their "baby shots" a long time ago but did not keep a personal vaccine record; however, the student remembers receiving a flu shot 2 years ago. What immunizations will the student need at this point? How can they best keep track of their immunizations?
5. After the nurse administers the patient's meningitis vaccine, the 13-year-old sister mentions that they heard that high school students should get a vaccination for human papillomavirus (HPV). They want to know if they should get one or if it is too late. Who is eligible to receive the HPV vaccine, and what assessment questions would the nurse ask? What type and dosage of vaccine would the nurse administer?
6. After the visit, how does the nurse ensure that the vaccines were safely administered?

REVIEW QUESTIONS

1. The parent of a 4-month-old infant calls in to the clinic reporting that their baby is having a reaction to immunizations. Which piece of information is **most** important for the nurse to elicit?
   a. The time the immunization was received
   b. Whether the parent has given the infant any acetaminophen
   c. The signs and symptoms the infant is experiencing
   d. The sites used to administer the immunizations
2. The nurse is preparing to administer varicella vaccine to a young adult. Which finding has the **greatest** implication for this young adult's care?
   a. The patient tells the nurse they are "deathly afraid of needles."
   b. The medical record indicates that the patient is allergic to eggs.
   c. Medical history indicates that the patient had leukemia as a young child.
   d. The patient appears to be pregnant.
3. A 38-year-old migrant farm worker is seen in the clinic with a cut to their arm from an old metal drum. The patient has sutures placed, and a tetanus, diphtheria, and acellular pertussis vaccine is given. Which action is **most** important for the nurse to take after the vaccine has been administered?
   a. The nurse provides the patient with a vaccine information statement about the tetanus, diphtheria, and acellular pertussis vaccine in the patient's primary language.
   b. The nurse determines the exact date of the patient's last tetanus booster.
   c. The nurse documents that the patient did not experience any side effects immediately after immunization.
   d. The nurse provides the patient with a record of the immunization administered at the visit.

4. The nurse is preparing to administer routine, recommended immunizations to an immunocompromised 1-year-old child. Which information is the **most** important to know before administering a vaccination?
   a. The type of vaccine to be administered to the child
   b. The child presents with a temperature of 99.8°F.
   c. The child's vaccine report shows immunizations were received on time.
   d. The child did not experience adverse reactions to prior immunizations.

5. A 14-year-old requests a vaccination for human papillomavirus. After the nurse administers the first dose, which information is important to include in the patient's teaching?
   a. Human papillomavirus prevents all sexually transmitted diseases.
   b. Pap smears are no longer needed after the human papillomavirus vaccination.
   c. The patient needs to notify the health care provider about pain at the injection site.
   d. The date the patient needs to return to the clinic for the next human papillomavirus dose.

6. Which patient would be eligible to receive the influenza vaccine?
   a. One taking care of a sibling with AIDS
   b. A pregnant patient
   c. Someone with an egg allergy
   d. An 18-month-old child

7. With the help of an interpreter, the nurse has just immunized a young adult with the tetanus, diphtheria, and acellular pertussis vaccine and the vaccine against measles, mumps, and rubella. Which action is essential for the nurse to take? **Select all that apply**.
   a. Provide a vaccine information statement in the patient's preferred language for each vaccine received.
   b. Document in the patient's record the date; site and route of administration; vaccine type, manufacturer, lot number, and expiration date; and the name, business address, and title of the person administering the vaccine.
   c. Administer a dose of ibuprofen to prevent postimmunization fever.
   d. Instruct the patient to call about any injection site soreness.
   e. Administer a dose of acetaminophen to prevent postimmunization fever.

8. It would be **priority** to notify the health care provider if a live vaccine was prescribed for a person in which situation?
   a. Child whose parent is receiving chemotherapy
   b. A child with an active viral infection
   c. A patient undergoing chemotherapy
   d. An HIV-positive patient with no active infections

UNIT X Antineoplastics and Biologic Response Modifiers

35

Anticancer Drugs

http://evolve.elsevier.com/McCuistion/pharmacology

OBJECTIVES

- Summarize the development of cancer cells.
- Summarize anticancer drug treatment for cancer.
- Discuss how alkylating drugs affect cancer cells.
- Discuss the general effects of antimetabolites to cancer cells.
- Discuss the general effects of antitumor antibiotics on cancer cells.
- Discuss the general effects of plant alkaloids.
- Explain the actions of immunomodulators, targeted therapies, hormones, hormonal agonists, and antagonists on cancer cells.

OUTLINE

Overview of Cancer, 421
    Genetic, Inflammatory, Infective, Environmental, and Dietary Influences, 421
    Cell Cycle-Nonspecific and Cell Cycle-Specific Anticancer Drugs, 423
Cancer Chemotherapy, 423
    Combination Chemotherapy, 425
    Liposomal Chemotherapy, 425
    General Side Effects and Adverse Reactions, 426
Alkylating Drugs, 427
    Cyclophosphamide, 427
Antimetabolites, 429
    Methotrexate, 429
    Fluorouracil, 429
Antitumor Antibiotics, 433
    Anthracyclines: Doxorubicin, 434
Plant Alkaloids, 436
    Vincristine, 439
Other Drugs to Treat Cancer, 440
    Immunomodulators, 440
    Targeted Therapies, 440
    Hormones and Hormonal Agonists and Antagonists, 442
Clinical Judgment Single-Episode Case Study, 444
Review Questions, 445

OVERVIEW OF CANCER

Cancer-related deaths rank second only to deaths by heart disease in the United States. Even though cancer-related mortality has decreased since the early 1990s, 39.5% of the population is projected to develop cancer over their lifetime. Excluding basal and squamous cell skin cancers, the highest incidences of cancer in males are prostate, lung, and colorectal cancer. In females, the highest frequency includes breast, lung, and colorectal cancers. Cancer mortality continues to be higher among males than females. Lung cancer remains the leading cause of cancer-related death regardless of gender.

The incidences and mortality rates of cancer differ by ethnicity. Non-Hispanic Blacks (henceforth "African Americans") have higher incidences (except breast cancer) and higher death rates from cancer (except breast and lung) than any racial or ethnic group. African American females have lower incidences of breast cancer but higher mortality rates than Caucasian females do. Hispanics have the lowest incidences and mortality rates of lung cancer. Incidences and mortality rates for liver and stomach cancers due to hepatitis B virus (HBV) and *Helicobacter pylori* are the highest among Asians and Pacific Islanders. Incidences of cancer increase among all immigrants as they adopt a more Westernized lifestyle.

Cancer is a group of diseases in which abnormal cells grow out of control and can spread to other areas of the body. DNA is the genetic substance in the body cells that transfers information necessary for the production of enzymes and protein synthesis. In most cases cancer is caused by damage to the DNA within the cell. Although some cancers are inherited, most develop when genes in a normal cell become damaged or lost. More than one mutation is required before a malignancy can develop; therefore, the development of cancer is a multistep process that may take years to complete.

Genetic, Inflammatory, Infective, Environmental, and Dietary Influences

Cancer can be influenced by genetic mutations, inflammation, infectious organisms, environment, and an unhealthy diet. Box 35.1 gives examples of environmental substances, viruses, and foods that have a carcinogenic effect in humans. Genes provide the instructions for

> **BOX 35.1 Environmental, Infective, and Dietary Influences on Cancer Development**
>
> **Environmental**
>
> *Tobacco*
> Gastric cancers and cancer of the bladder, cervix, colon, esophagus, head and neck, kidney and ureter, liver, lung, pancreas, trachea and bronchus, and acute myeloid leukemia
>
> *Asbestos*
> Lung cancer
>
> *Benzene*
> Acute myelogenous leukemia
>
> *Formaldehyde*
> Cancer of the nose, throat, and trachea
>
> *Vinyl Chloride*
> Sarcoma, leukemia
>
> *Arsenic*
> Cancer of the lung and skin, sarcoma
>
> *Ionizing Radiation*
> Leukemia; cancer of the thyroid, breast
>
> *Ultraviolet Rays*
> Skin cancer
>
> *Aflatoxin*
> Liver cancer
>
> **Infective**
>
> *Herpes Simplex 2 Virus (Genital Herpes)*
> Cervical and penile cancer
>
> *Hepatitis B and C Viruses*
> Cancer of the liver
>
> *Epstein-Barr Virus*
> Non-Hodgkin lymphoma, Hodgkin disease, nasopharyngeal cancers
>
> *Human Papillomavirus*
> Cancer of the cervix, vulva, vagina, anus, penis, head and neck
>
> *Human Immunodeficiency Virus*
> Kaposi sarcoma, non-Hodgkin lymphoma, cervical cancer
>
> *Human T-Cell Lymphotropic Virus*
> T-cell leukemia
>
> *Helicobacter pylori*
> Cancer of the stomach, gastric mucosa-associated lymphoid tissue lymphoma
>
> **Dietary**
>
> *Animal Fat*
> Cancer of the colon, rectum, breast, uterus, prostate, ovary
>
> *Heterocyclic Amines (Found in Some Smoked Meats)*
> Cancer of the stomach, colon, rectum, pancreas, breast
>
> *Alcohol*
> Cancer of the mouth, throat, esophagus, liver, breast

the production and function of cellular proteins essential for normal cellular activities. Genetic defects may occur in a variety of ways, including deletion, translocation, duplication, inversion, or insertion of genetic material. When defects cannot be effectively repaired, cells exhibit abnormal characteristics and unregulated growth. More than 2000 genes have been causally implicated in the formation of cancer. Cancers with a proven genetic influence include breast, ovarian, prostate, endometrial, colon, pancreatic, and lung cancers; retinoblastoma; and malignant melanoma, to name a few. Many more genetic influences are expected to be found as cancer research continues.

Genes can cause cells to become cancerous in several ways. **Proto-oncogenes** are normal genes involved in cell differentiation and division, and they regulate cell death, also known as **apoptosis**. These processes are necessary for healthy tissues and organs. An **oncogene** is a mutation in a proto-oncogene that affects cellular growth-control proteins and triggers unregulated cell division. Some genes, called **antioncogenes**, protect others. One such gene is the tumor-suppressor (TS) genes that signal a cell to cease multiplying and stop the action of oncogenes. Uncontrollable cell growth can occur if TS genes become lost or dysfunctional. Other genes repair damage to DNA. If these DNA-repair genes are damaged, mutations are not corrected and are subsequently passed on to the next generation of daughter cells. These and other gene mutations can take place over a long time before cancer develops. As a result, cancers more commonly occur in older individuals.

Inflammation

Inflammation is a normal physiologic process to heal injured tissues. Chronic inflammation, such as chronic inflammatory bowel disease (IBD), is an ongoing inflammatory process. The continued inflammation can lead to DNA damage and can result in cancer.

Viruses

A number of viruses are associated with the development of cancer. The human papillomavirus (HPV) has been found in most females with invasive cervical cancer. Individuals with human immunodeficiency virus (HIV) may develop lymphomas and rectal or genital cancers. The Epstein-Barr virus is found in almost all people with Burkitt lymphoma in central Africa and has been implicated in the development of nasopharyngeal cancer. Hepatocellular carcinoma (liver cancer) is linked to hepatitis B and C viruses. Other viruses linked to cancer include human T-cell lymphotropic virus and Kaposi sarcoma-associated herpesvirus.

Bacteria

Bacteria can play a role in the development of cancer. The presence of *H. pylori* in the stomach is associated with an increased risk of gastric cancer. Some reports have indicated a link between certain bacteria and cancer of the gallbladder, colon, and lung. However, no clear evidence supports a link between bacterial infection and other cancers.

Environmental Factors

Environmental factors associated with the development of cancer include tobacco use, poor diet, decreased physical activity, chemicals, and excessive sun and radiation exposures. According to the Centers for Disease Control and Prevention (CDC), 80% to 90% of lung cancers occur due to smoking. In 2019 a sharp increase in the use of electronic cigarettes (e-cigs) increased smoking-associated lung injury and death from these injuries. The CDC continues to research the long-term health effects from e-cigs. Other cancer-causing environmental agents include alcohol consumption on a regular basis, which

CHAPTER 35 Anticancer Drugs

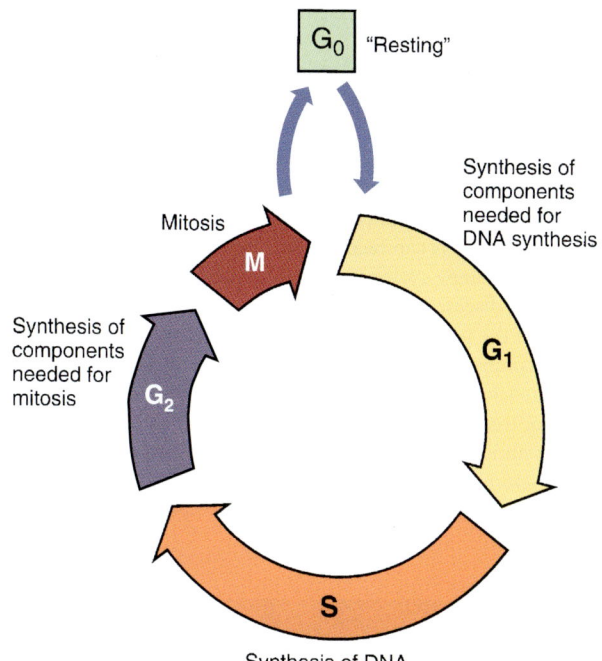

Fig. 35.1 Cell cycle G₁ phase (postmitotic gap): Production of RNA, protein, and enzymes for DNA synthesis; the G₁ phase lasts 15–18 h. S phase (synthesis): All the components of DNA are synthesized, and the cells have doubled; the S phase lasts 10–20 h. G₂ phase (premitotic gap): The cell continues to grow and ensures it is not defective; the G₂ phase lasts approximately 3 hours. M phase (mitosis): Cell growth has stopped, and the cell divides into two identical (daughter) cells; the M phase lasts approximately 1 h. G₀ phase (resting): cells remain in this phase and leave the cell cycle or return to the cell cycle for cell replication. Cells in this phase are not as sensitive to many antineoplastic drugs. The cells must pass through a series of checkpoints to continue through the cycle. Defective cells undergo apoptosis (self-destruction). (From Burcham J, Rosenthal L. *Lehne's Pharmacology for Nursing Care*. 9th ed. Elsevier; 2016.)

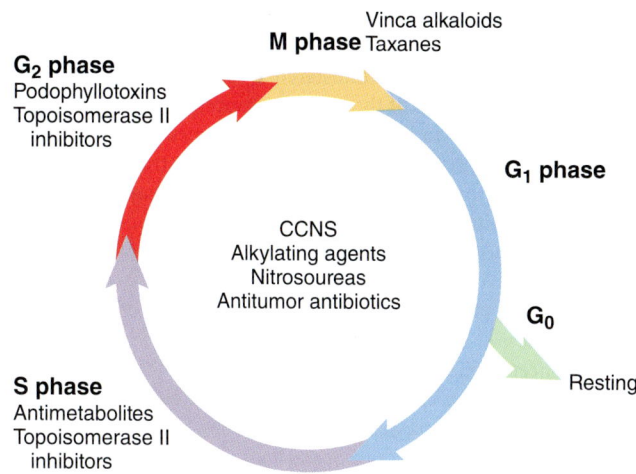

Fig. 35.2 Selected anticancer drugs and the phases of the cell cycle in which they are most effective. *CCNS*, cell cycle nonspecific.

raises the risk of mouth, larynx, and throat cancers; being overweight or obese, which increases the risk of uterine, breast, prostate, and colorectal cancers; and excessive exposure to sun and other forms of ultraviolet (UV) rays, which promotes skin cancers. Many of these cancers can be prevented. According to the American Cancer Society, about 606,520 people were expected to succumb to cancer during the year 2020.

Cell Cycle-Nonspecific and Cell Cycle-Specific Anticancer Drugs

The cell cycle progress through five distinct phases or cycles, four of which are directed toward cell replication and a fifth phase in which the cell stops dividing. The five phases include *gap 1* (G_1), *synthesis* (S), *gap 2* (G_2), *mitosis* (M), and *gap 0* (G_0). G_0 is a dormant phase, and most cells in the human body are in the G_0 phase. Fig. 35.1 illustrates the cell cycle.

Anticancer drugs stop or slow the growth of cancer cells by interfering with cell replication and are classified according to their action. **Cell cycle-nonspecific (CCNS)** drugs act during any phase of the cell cycle, including the G_0 phase. CCNS drugs include most alkylating drugs, antitumor antibiotics, and hormones. **Cell cycle-specific (CCS)** drugs exert their influence during a specific phase of the cell cycle and are most effective against rapidly growing cancer cells. The CCS drugs include antimetabolites, some alkylating agents, and vinca alkaloids.

Fig. 35.2 shows selected categories of anticancer drugs and the phase of the cell cycle in which they are most effective.

Growth fraction and doubling time are two factors that play a major role in how the cancer cells respond to anticancer drugs. **Growth fraction**, the percent of actively dividing cells, decreases as the tumor enlarges, and doubling time increases. **Doubling time** is defined as the time it takes for a tumor to double in size. Anticancer drugs are more effective against neoplastic cells that have a high growth fraction. Leukemia and some lymphomas have high growth fractions and thus respond well to anticancer drug therapy.

Solid tumors have a large percentage of their cell mass in the G_0 phase; thus they generally have a low growth fraction and are less sensitive to anticancer drugs. As the tumor grows, the blood supply decreases, thereby slowing the growth rate. High-dose chemotherapy results in better tumor-killing (tumoricidal) effects. Depending on the type of cancer, malignant cell growth is usually faster in the earlier stages of tumor development. Adequate vascularization is needed for the anticancer drugs to be effective. Anticancer drugs are more effective against small, fast-growing tumors with sufficient blood supply. The vascularization in solid tumors can be inconsistent. Some areas of tumor may have an adequate blood supply, whereas other areas are poorly perfused. This characteristic may make some large tumors resistant to anticancer drugs and therefore difficult to treat.

CANCER CHEMOTHERAPY

Pharmaceuticals are often used to destroy cancer cells and are called by different names, including *anticancer drugs, cancer chemotherapeutic agents*, **antineoplastic drugs**, or **cytotoxic therapy**. In the 1970s **combination chemotherapy**—the use of two or more chemotherapy agents to treat cancer—was adopted and led to improved response rates and increased survival times. Chemotherapy may be used as the only treatment of cancer, or it may be used in conjunction with other modalities such as radiation, surgery, and biologic response modifiers. **Chemotherapy** is the use of chemicals to kill cancer cells. Combination chemotherapy increases the chance for months to years of cancer remission. If cancer can no longer be controlled, palliative treatment with chemotherapy may be used to relieve disease-related symptoms and improve quality of life.

Anticancer drugs do not affect just cancer cells; instead, the drugs affect both cancer and healthy cells. The side effects of chemotherapy are largely related to the toxic effects on these healthy cells.

Healthy cells are able to repair themselves and continue to grow; thus, the side effects of chemotherapeutic agents are often temporary. Chemotherapy is usually administered systemically for cancer that has spread to other parts of the body, for cancers in multiple sites, or for cancers too large to be removed by other means (e.g., surgery). The most common route of chemotherapy administration is through intravenous (IV) infusion, although other routes may be used and include oral, intramuscular, subcutaneous, intraperitoneal, intraventricular (intrathecal), intrapleural, intravesicular, intraarterial, and topical routes.

Some types of cancer can be cured with chemotherapy (e.g., Hodgkin disease, Burkitt lymphoma, and testicular cancer). Other types of cancer (e.g., breast and colon cancer) may be treated with surgery first, followed by chemotherapy to eliminate any residual cancer cells (microscopic metastases) that may remain in the body. This is referred to as **adjuvant therapy**. Sometimes **neoadjuvant chemotherapy** may be given first to help shrink a large tumor so that it can be surgically removed. **Palliative chemotherapy**, used to relieve symptoms associated with advanced disease (e.g., pain and shortness of breath), can improve quality of life.

Chemotherapy administration is guided by specific **protocols** based on the results of controlled research studies. The length of treatment is determined by the type and extent of the malignancy, the type of chemotherapy given, expected side effects of the drugs, and the amount of time that normal cells need to recover. Chemotherapy is usually given in cycles to improve the likelihood that cancer cells will be destroyed and that normal cells can recover. The duration, frequency, and number of chemotherapy cycles are based on the cancer type and size, the spread of the disease to other areas of the body (**metastasis**), and the condition of the patient. Chemotherapy treatment may consist of one drug or a combination of drugs. Combination chemotherapy may be administered in 1 day or may be spread out over several days. The duration of treatment is based on the protocol being followed; it can vary from minutes to days and may be repeated weekly, biweekly, or monthly. Selected anticancer drugs are listed in Box 35.2 according to classification.

BOX 35.2 Anticancer Drugs by Classification[a]

High-Alert Medications
All chemotherapeutic agents are categorized as high-alert medications for all routes of drug delivery.

Alkylating Agents
Nitrogen Mustard Gas Derivatives
Bendamustine
Chlorambucil
Cyclophosphamide
Estramustine
Ifosfamide
Mechlorethamine hydrochloride
Melphalan

Nitrosoureas
Carmustine (*bis*-chloroethylnitrosourea [BCNU])
Lomustine (1-[2-chloroethyl]-3-cyclohexyl-1-nitrosourea [CCNU])
Streptozocin

Alkyl Sulfonates
Busulfan

Alkylating-Like Agents
Altretamine
Carboplatin
Cisplatin
Dacarbazine
Oxaliplatin

Antimetabolites
Folic Acid Antagonists
Methotrexate
Pemetrexed disodium

Pyrimidine Analogues
Azacitidine
Capecitabine
Cytarabine
Floxuridine
Fluorouracil injection (5-Fluorouracil [5-FU])
Gemcitabine hydrochloride

Purine Analogues
Cladribine
Clofarabine
Fludarabine
Mercaptopurine (6-MP)
Nelarabine
Pentostatin
Thioguanine (6-TG)

Ribonucleotide Reductase Inhibitors (Enzyme Inhibitors)
Hydroxyurea

Antitumorals
Anthracyclines
Daunorubicin hydrochloride
Daunorubicin liposomal
Doxorubicin
Epirubicin
Idarubicin
Mitoxantrone
Valrubicin

Other Antitumor Antibiotics
Bleomycin sulfate
Dactinomycin
Doxorubicin liposomal
Mitomycin

Plant Alkaloids
Antimicrotubules and Taxanes
Docetaxel
Paclitaxel

Camptothecin Analogues
Irinotecan
Topotecan

Epipodophyllotoxins
Etoposide
Teniposide

BOX 35.2 Anticancer Drugs by Classification[a]—cont'd

Immunomodulators
Alemtuzumab
Interleukin 2 (IL-2)
Rituximab
Thalidomide

Retinoids
Bexarotene

Vinca Alkaloids
Vinblastine sulfate
Vincristine sulfate
Vincristine, liposomal
Vinorelbine

Sex Hormones, Hormonal Agonists and Antagonists, Selective Estrogen Receptor Modulators, Luteinizing Hormone-Releasing Hormone Agonists, Aromatase Inhibitors, Enzymes, and Vaccines
Androgens
Fluoxymesterone

Hormonal Agonists and Antagonists
Abiraterone
Anastrozole
Bicalutamide
Enzalutamide
Exemestane
Flutamide
Fulvestrant
Goserelin acetate
Histrelin acetate implant
Letrozole
Leuprolide acetate
Medroxyprogesterone
Megestrol acetate
Mitotane
Nilutamide
Raloxifene
Tamoxifen citrate
Toremifene citrate

Enzymes
Asparaginase *Erwinia chrysanthemi*
Pegaspargase

Vaccines
Hepatitis B
Quadrivalent human papillomavirus subtypes 6, 11, 16, and 18
Human papillomavirus bivalent vaccine

[a]See Chapter 36 for monoclonal antibodies and targeted therapies and Chapter 37 for biologic therapies.

TABLE 35.1 Selected Combinations of Anticancer Drugs

Generic	Acronym[a]	Selected Uses
Cytarabine, daunorubicin, etoposide	ADE	Acute myelogenous leukemia
Fluorouracil, doxorubicin, cyclophosphamide	FAC	Breast cancer
Leucovorin, fluorouracil, irinotecan, oxaliplatin	FOLFIRIFOLFOX	Colorectal cancer
Capecitabine, irinotecan	XELIRI	Esophageal cancer, gastric cancer
Bortezomib (PS-341), doxorubicin, dexamethasone	PAD	Multiple myeloma
Carboplatin, paclitaxel	CARBOPLATIN-TAXOL	Non-small cell lung cancer
Cyclophosphamide, doxorubicin, vincristine, prednisone	CHOP	Non-Hodgkin lymphoma
Rituximab, cyclophosphamide, doxorubicin, vincristine, prednisone	R-CHOP	
Gemcitabine, cisplatin	(None)	Pancreatic cancer
Gemcitabine, fluorouracil, leucovorin	OFF	
Bleomycin, etoposide, cisplatin	BEP	Testicular cancer
Vinblastine, ifosfamide, cisplatin	VIP	

[a]Acronyms are based on the generic or trade name of the chemotherapy drugs used in a specific protocol (e.g., ABVD [Adriamycin, bleomycin, vinblastine, dacarbazine], FAC [fluorouracil, Adriamycin, cyclophosphamide]). Not all acronyms for combination chemotherapy treatments are listed.

Combination Chemotherapy

Single-agent drug therapy is not usually used to treat cancer because combination therapy with two or more anticancer drugs has demonstrated more effective tumoricidal activity. Combination therapy increases the likelihood of affecting cancer cells in all phases of the cell cycle.

To maximize cell death, CCNS and CCS drugs are often combined to increase synergistic effects. Each individual drug used in combination therapy should have a proven tumoricidal activity, a different mechanism of action, and different dose-limiting toxicities. A combination of antineoplastic drugs has the advantage of decreasing drug resistance while increasing cancer cell destruction. Table 35.1 presents some of the combined anticancer drugs.

Liposomal Chemotherapy

A more recent change in the delivery of chemotherapy involves the use of anticancer drugs packaged inside synthetic fat globules called **liposomes**. The fatty coating helps the chemotherapy drug remain in the system longer and increases the duration of therapeutic effects;

it also decreases side effects such as hair loss, nausea, and cardiotoxicity. Encapsulated forms of liposomal doxorubicin, daunorubicin, vincristine, and cytarabine are examples of liposomal chemotherapy.

General Side Effects and Adverse Reactions

Anticancer drugs exert adverse effects on rapidly growing normal cells, such as skin and hair. These drugs can also affect cells in the gastrointestinal (GI) tract, mucous membranes, bone marrow, and reproductive system. Myelosuppression can occur when there is a significant decrease in the bone marrow activity that results in decreased white blood cells, platelets, and red blood cells. After chemotherapy administration, the nadir—the time at which the blood count is at the lowest—typically occurs 7 to 10 days after treatment. Table 35.2 lists the general adverse effects anticancer drugs exert on the fast-growing cells of the body. Patients receiving highly potent drugs will need to be closely monitored for severe adverse effects. Selected nursing measures and considerations are included. Because of the toxic effects of chemotherapy, care in handling of such drugs must be considered, and protective gear that includes gloves specific for handling chemotherapy drugs must be used. When a chemotherapy drug is given, a health care provider qualified to administer anticancer drugs follows the policies provided by the oncologist and the health care agency. By following strict protocols, the nurse reduces exposure to hazardous chemotherapy drugs during administration.

TABLE 35.2 General Adverse Reactions to Anticancer Drugs[a]

Adverse Reactions	Nursing Measures and Considerations
Bone Marrow Suppression, Myelosuppression	
Low RBC count (anemia)	Assess for fatigue, shortness of breath, low blood pressure, increased heart rate, increased respiratory rate, and oliguria. Assess for cyanosis. Plan rest periods. Administer oxygen as prescribed. Elevate the head of the bed to facilitate breathing. Provide pain mediation if pain is increasing oxygen consumption. Provide assistance with activities. Monitor for mental status changes. Anemia may be treated with ferrous sulfate or infusions of RBCs. EPO may be administered to stimulate RBC production. Monitor RBCs, hemoglobin, and hematocrit.
Low WBC count (leukopenia)	Susceptibility to infection increases as WBCs decrease. Patients should avoid people with infections and report fever, chills, URIs, or sore throat to their HCP. Hand hygiene before and after contact with the patient is important. Monitor for changes in body temperature; elevated temperature is considered a sign of infection. Avoid medications that may mask fever. Immediately report temperatures of 101°F (38.3°C) or above to the HCP. Appropriate cultures (e.g., blood, urine, sputum) are collected before antibiotics are started if applicable, and an antibiotic regimen is initiated. Assess for localized infections. Auscultate breath sounds. Colony-stimulating factors (e.g., filgrastim) may be administered to stimulate WBC production. Monitor WBCs, especially ANCs.
Low platelet count (thrombocytopenia)	Petechiae, bruising, bleeding of gums, and nosebleeds are signs of a low platelet count; report these signs to an HCP. Assess for bleeding, petechiae, and ecchymosis. Assess for occult bleeding in urine, feces, and emesis. Apply pressure to injection sites until bleeding has stopped. Platelet transfusions may be needed. Avoid medications that may promote bleeding (aspirin, heparin). Avoid invasive procedures (injections, indwelling urinary catheters, rectal temperature, and suppositories). Monitor platelet counts and bleeding time.
Gastrointestinal Disturbances	
Anorexia	Loss of appetite may be related to anemia, pain, fatigue, or altered taste caused by chemotherapy drugs. Provide small, frequent meals that are high in calories and protein. Plan rest periods. Address issues of pain control. Hard candy or ice chips may help relieve bitter taste.
Nausea and vomiting	Antineoplastic drugs often stimulate the CTZ, leading to nausea and vomiting, which can be caused by irritation of the GI tract; effects of radiation to chest, abdomen, or brain; anxiety; constipation; pain; electrolyte imbalances; or other medications. Grading scales are useful to assess severity. Provide antiemetics before, during, and after chemotherapy. Assess for GI upset, and medicate appropriately. Minimize noise, stimulation, and odors. Frequent mouth care is recommended. Monitor fluid balance and serum electrolytes.
Diarrhea	Diarrhea may be one of three types: *osmotic* (absorption defects), *secretory* (bacterial infection or neoplasm), or *exudative* (secondary to chemotherapy). Chemotherapeutic drugs most commonly associated with diarrhea are alkylating agents, antitumor antibiotics, and antimetabolites. Treatment (e.g., medications, diet changes) will depend on cause and severity. Diarrhea may be caused by other medications, such as antibiotics, comorbid conditions (e.g., Crohn's disease), or enteral (tube) feedings. Assess normal bowel habits, and monitor for electrolyte imbalances and dehydration. Administer appropriate antidiarrheal medications (antibiotics, anticholinergics, antispasmodics, psyllium, kaolin and pectin, or octreotide acetate). Teach patients to eat small, frequent meals; follow a low-residue diet; limit spicy, fatty foods; limit intake of salty foods, whole grains, fresh fruits and vegetables, and caffeinated and carbonated drinks; and avoid very hot or very cold foods (may stimulate peristalsis). Monitor intake and output.
Mucositis (stomatitis)	Many antineoplastic drugs cause changes in oral mucosa that generally occur 2–14 days after initiation of therapy. Assess for taste changes, tissue swelling, redness, pain, dry mouth, white patches, or a white coating on the oral mucosa. Mucositis ranges from mild to severe. Symptomatic treatment may include frequent mouth rinses, topical anesthetics, antibiotics, antifungal medication, saliva substitutes, and pain medication. Patients should avoid commercial mouthwashes that contain alcohol. A soft toothbrush is recommended. Offer ice chips or ice pops to help relieve pain. Assess intake and output. Evaluate caloric needs. A grading scale may be useful to assess severity.

TABLE 35.2 General Adverse Reactions to Anticancer Drugs—cont'd

Adverse Reactions	Nursing Measures and Considerations
Other	
Alopecia	Not all chemotherapeutic drugs cause hair loss. Hair thinning, patchy baldness, or complete alopecia may occur, depending on the drug. Hair on all areas of the body is affected. Hair loss may be gradual, progressing with each cycle of chemotherapy, or rapid. Hair regrowth usually occurs once chemotherapy is completed, although the texture may be changed. Before therapy, discuss potential hair loss and ways to address the discomforts (e.g., baldness and scalp hypothermia) due to hair loss (wigs, scarves, hats, or turbans). Assess for body image changes and concerns.
Fatigue	Fatigue may be caused by chemotherapy, sleep disturbances, emotional distress, depression, bone marrow suppression, infection, pain, or electrolyte imbalances. Assess fatigue using a visual analogue grading scale (0 = no fatigue; 10 = worst fatigue). Address conditions that might be contributing to fatigue (lack of sleep, pain, depression). Plan ways to help patients conserve energy. Plan a well-balanced diet, and encourage participation in regular (but not strenuous) exercise and stress reduction measures, such as relaxation and guided imagery.
Infertility	If infertility occurs, it may be permanent. Pretreatment counseling is advised.

ANC, Absolute neutrophil count; *CTZ*, chemoreceptor trigger zone; *EPO*, erythropoietin; *GI*, gastrointestinal; *HCP*, health care provider; *RBC*, red blood cell; *URI*, upper respiratory infection; *WBC*, white blood cell.
^aThe list in the table is not all-inclusive. Some more serious reactions are discussed in the Prototype Drug Charts.

ALKYLATING DRUGS

One of the largest groups of anticancer drugs is the alkylating compounds. **Alkylating drugs** damage the cell's DNA by cross-linkage of DNA strands, abnormal base pairing, or DNA strand breaks, thus preventing the reproduction of cancer cells. Drugs in this group belong to the CCNS category and kill cells in all phases of the cell cycle. They are used to treat many different types of cancer, including leukemia, lymphoma, multiple myeloma, sarcoma, and solid tumors such as those of the breast, ovary, uterus, lung, bladder, and stomach. Even though alkylating drugs are effective in all phases of the cell cycle, they are most effective in the G_0 phase. Alkylating drugs are divided into five different classes: (1) nitrogen mustards, (2) nitrosoureas, (3) alkyl sulfonates, (4) triazines, and (5) ethylenimines. Table 35.3 lists some of the alkylating drugs, their uses, and considerations. Of the alkylating drugs, nitrosoureas cross the blood-brain barrier, making them useful in the treatment of brain cancer. General adverse effects to anticancer drugs are discussed in Table 35.2. In addition, alkylating drugs given in high doses can cause long-term damage to the bone marrow, resulting in acute leukemia. The platinum (alkylating-like) drugs—cisplatin, carboplatin, and oxaliplatin—kill cells in a similar fashion but are less likely to cause leukemia later.

Cyclophosphamide

Cyclophosphamide, an alkylating drug, is an analogue of nitrogen mustard and has activity against many neoplastic diseases, including Hodgkin and non-Hodgkin lymphoma (NHL), acute and chronic lymphocytic leukemia (CLL), multiple myeloma, breast and ovarian carcinoma, lung cancer, and retinoblastoma. The drug is also used for immunologic disorders such as lupus nephritis and has been shown to prevent progressive renal scarring, preserve renal function, induce renal remission, and decrease end-stage renal failure. This drug is a severe **vesicant** that causes tissue necrosis if it infiltrates into the tissues. Cyclophosphamide can be administered orally or intravenously. The patient should be well hydrated while taking cyclophosphamide to prevent hemorrhagic cystitis (bleeding due to severe bladder inflammation). Sodium 2-mercaptoethanesulfonate is a **chemoprotectant** drug often given with high-dose cyclophosphamide to inactivate urotoxic metabolites to reduce the incidence of hemorrhagic cystitis.

> ⚡ **PATIENT SAFETY**
>
> Patients should be well hydrated before and during therapy.
> **Do Not Confuse...**
> - **Myleran** with **Alkeran**
> - **Cisplatin** with **Carboplatin**
> - **Paraplatin** with **Platinol**
> - **Cyclophosphamide** with **Cyclosporine**

Pharmacokinetics

Oral cyclophosphamide is well absorbed in the GI system. Cyclophosphamide is a prodrug that is activated and extensively metabolized by the liver. About 5% to 25% of the drug is eliminated by the kidney as unchanged, and its elimination half-life is 3 to 12 hours. Approximately 20% is bound to plasma protein, and this is not dose dependent. Some cyclophosphamide metabolites are greater than 60% protein bound. Less than 10%, mostly in the form of metabolites, is excreted in feces.

Pharmacodynamics

Cyclophosphamide is an early antineoplastic drug used alone or with other drugs to treat a variety of cancers. Average time to peak plasma concentration (T_{max}) is 1 hour. Several drug interactions can occur with cyclophosphamide. Patients should report all medications they are taking, including over-the-counter (OTC) medicines, vitamins, minerals, and herbal supplements. Anthracycline (e.g., doxorubicin) has been reported to induce cardiotoxicity when taken with cyclophosphamide, and it exacerbates hemorrhagic cystitis. Other serious drug interactions can occur when taking cyclophosphamide concomitantly with aspirin, allopurinol, phenobarbital, warfarin, thiazide diuretics, and some psychiatric medications. The Complementary and Alternative Therapies box lists herbal supplements that may also interact with cyclophosphamide.

TABLE 35.3 Antineoplastics: Alkylating Drugs

- Visually inspect parenteral products for particulate matter and discoloration before use.
- Observe and exercise precautions when handling, preparing, and administering cytotoxic drugs.
- The correct dose of chemotherapeutic drugs will vary from protocol to protocol. Consult appropriate references to verify doses.

Drug	Route and Dosage	Uses and Considerations
Nitrogen Mustards		
Bendamustine	CLL: A: IV: 100 mg/m² on days 1 and 2, repeated q28d for up to 6 cycles NHL: A: IV: 120 mg/m² on days 1 and 2, repeated q21d for up to 8 cycles	For CLL and NHL. Monitor for bone marrow depression. Assess for tumor-lysis syndrome and skin reactions PB: 94%–96%; t½: 40 min
Chlorambucil	Palliative CLL, Hodgkin disease, and NHL: A: PO: 0.1–0.2 mg/kg/d (4–10 mg/d) for 3–6 wk	For CLL, Hodgkin disease, and NHL. Monitor for bone marrow suppression or pancytopenia PB: 99%; t½: 1.5 h
Estramustine	A: PO: 14 mg/kg/d or 600 mg/m²/d in 3–4 divided doses	For palliative treatment of prostate cancer. Gynecomastia and impotence may occur PB: UK; t½: 20–24 h
Ifosfamide	A: IV: 1.2–2 g/m²/d for 5 d in combination with mesna; repeat every 3 wk after recovery from hematologic toxicity. Mesna is usually given concomitantly to prevent hemorrhagic cystitis	For testicular cancer. Monitor for hemorrhagic cystitis PB: negligible; t½: 7–15 h
Mechlorethamine hydrochloride	Hodgkin disease: A: IV: 0.2 mg/kg or 6 mg/m² as single dose CLL: A: IV: 6 mg/m² q4wk CML: A: IV: 0.4 mg/kg or 6 mg/m² monthly Other dosing regimen and routes are available	For Hodgkin disease, leukemias, solid tumors, and effusions caused by cancer. This drug is contraindicated in patients with active infections PB: UK; t½: Minutes
Melphalan	Multiple myeloma: A: PO: 6 mg daily for 2–3 wk; *maint:* 2 mg/d; adjust 1–3 mg/d based on hematologic response A: IV: 16 mg/m² q2wk for 4 doses; *maint:* 16 mg/m² q4wk Ovarian cancer: A: PO: 200 mcg/kg/d for 5 d; repeat q4–5wk based on hematologic response	For multiple myeloma and ovarian cancer. *Do not confuse Alkeran with Leukeran or Myleran* PB: 20%–30%; t½: 1.25–1.5 h
Nitrosoureas		
Carmustine (BCNU)	A: IV: 150–200 mg/m² single dose q6wk or 75–100 mg/m²/d for 2 days q6wk	For Hodgkin disease, NHL, multiple myeloma, and brain tumors. Monitor for bone marrow suppression and pulmonary symptoms PB: UK; t½: 5–30 min
Lomustine (CCNU)	Hodgkin disease and malignant glioma: A: PO: 100–130 mg/m² q6wk	For Hodgkin disease and malignant gliomas. Monitor for bone marrow suppression and liver function PB: UK; t½: 16 h–2 d
Streptozocin	A: IV: 500 mg/m²/d for 5 d q4–6wk; doses above 500 mg/m² are not recommended	*Do not confuse with streptomycin.* For pancreatic cancer PB: UK; t½: 30–45 min
Alkyl Sulfonates		
Busulfan	A: PO: 4–8 mg/d	For myelocytic leukemia. Monitor for seizures and cerebral hemorrhage PB: 32%; t½: 2.5 h
Alkylating-Like Drugs		
Altretamine	A: PO: 260 mg/m²/d in 4 divided doses after meals and at bedtime for 14 or 21 d in a 28-d cycle; drug holiday for ≥14 d then restart at 200 mg/m²/d	For ovarian cancer PB: Weakly; t½: 4.7–10.2 h
Carboplatin	New cancer: A: IV: 300 mg/m² in combination with cyclophosphamide q4wk for 6 cycles Recurrent cancer: A: IV: 360 mg/m² q4wk	For advanced ovarian cancer. Usually given as combination therapy PB: UK; t½: 1.5–2.5 h

TABLE 35.3 Antineoplastics: Alkylating Drugs—cont'd

Drug	Route and Dosage	Uses and Considerations
Cisplatin	Bladder cancer: A: IV: 50–70 mg/m² q3–4wk Ovarian cancer: A: IV: 50–75 mg/m² q21d Testicular cancer: A: IV: 20 mg/m² for 5 d; repeat q3wk for 2 more cycles	For bladder, ovarian, testicular, and NSCLC. Monitor for CNS function; reversible posterior leukoencephalopathy may occur PB: 90%; t½: 30–100 h, dose related
Dacarbazine	Melanoma: A: IV: 250 mg/m²/d for 5 d repeated q3wk Hodgkin disease: A: IV: 375 mg/m² days 1 and 15 q28d	For Hodgkin disease and malignant melanoma. Monitor hepatic function PB: Minimal; t½: 5 h
Oxaliplatin	A: IV: 85 mg/m² on day 1 q2wk for 12 cycles	For metastatic colorectal cancer. Used with 5-FU and leucovorin (FOLFOX4). Assess for pulmonary complications PB: >90%; t½: 391 h

Note: Chemotherapeutic doses and schedules will vary depending on protocol, body surface area (m²), age, functional status, and comorbid conditions. For a full discussion of body surface area in dosage calculation, see Chapter 11.
5-FU, 5-Fluorouracil; *A*, adult; *CLL*, chronic lymphocytic leukemia; *CML*, chronic myelogenous leukemia; *CNS*, central nervous system; *d*, day; *h*, hour; *IV*, intravenous; *maint*, maintenance; *min*, minute; *NHL*, non-Hodgkin lymphoma; *NSCLC*, non–small cell lung cancer; *PB*, protein binding; *PO*, by mouth; *q*, every; *t½*, half-life; *UK*, unknown; *wk*, week; >, greater than; ≥, greater than or equal to.

COMPLEMENTARY AND ALTERNATIVE THERAPIES

Cyclophosphamide

- Use cautiously with garlic (antiplatelet activity), ginkgo (increased antiplatelet effect), echinacea (decreased effects of immunosuppressive drugs), ginseng (altered bleeding time), St. John's wort (may interfere with chemotherapy), and kava kava (increased risk for bleeding). Toxicity and actions of both cyclophosphamide and vitamin A are altered if given together. *Do not use with mistletoe because it may promote cancer growth.*
- Astragalus (Huang-qi; milk vetch root) stimulates the immune system and may help speed recovery from immunosuppressive chemotherapy. Astragalus has blood clot-fighting properties and may increase risk of bleeding when given with cyclophosphamide.

Side Effects and Adverse Reactions

The side effects of cyclophosphamide reflect those seen in the general class of antineoplastic drugs. (For the general side effects, see Table 35.2.) Hemorrhagic cystitis is a serious problem that can arise when high doses of cyclophosphamide are given. Patients who receive a high dose should be assessed for cardiomyopathy and syndrome of inappropriate antidiuretic hormone (SIADH) during treatment. In addition, cyclophosphamide may increase pigmentation of the skin or nail beds. Prototype Drug Chart: Cyclophosphamide details the pharmacologic behavior of cyclophosphamide.

ANTIMETABOLITES

Molecularly, antimetabolites resemble natural substances, building blocks that not only synthesize but also recycle and break down organic compounds used by the body. However, antimetabolites interfere with substances needed for normal cell function. Most antimetabolites are classified as CCS, and they exert their effects during the S phase (DNA synthesis and metabolism) of the cell cycle. Few antimetabolites (e.g., 5-fluorouracil [5-FU], floxuridine) have cytotoxic effects in multiple phases of the cell cycle. Antimetabolites are classified according to the substances with which they interfere. Substances can include folate, pyrimidine, purine analogues, and ribonucleotide reductase inhibitors. Table 35.4 lists the antimetabolite drugs, uses, and considerations.

Methotrexate

Methotrexate, a folate antimetabolite, is used to treat malignant and nonmalignant conditions (e.g., rheumatoid arthritis, psoriasis). Methotrexate affects cells that have high metabolic rates, such as neoplasms, hair follicles, endothelium, cells of the GI tract, fetal cells, and bone marrow; it is used to treat leukemias and cancers of the GI tract, head and neck, breast, and ovaries. Because methotrexate causes apoptosis to fetal cells, it can be used for ectopic pregnancies. Methotrexate inhibits the biosynthesis of a purine nucleotide, 5-aminoimidazole-4-carboxamide ribonucleotide (AICAR) transformylase, which provides antiinflammatory properties that result in metabolites; AICARs are immunotoxic. Leucovorin can be given 12 to 24 hours after methotrexate administration (not simultaneously) to reduce AICAR concentrations, thereby diminishing the adverse effects of methotrexate. Leucovorin should not be referred to as *folinic acid* because it can be confused with *folic acid*, which can lead to severe methotrexate toxicity. Other interactions are seen with methotrexate. Nonsteroidal antiinflammatory drugs (NSAIDs) given just before, concomitantly with, or after intermediate or high doses of methotrexate have resulted in severe hematologic and GI toxicity. Furthermore, NSAIDs may mask fever, swelling, and other signs and symptoms of infection. Several corticosteroids can reduce the cytotoxicity of methotrexate. Protein-bound drugs such as salicylates (aspirin), sulfonylureas (glyburide), hydantoin (phenytoin) anticonvulsants, and sulfonamides can induce methotrexate toxicity. Penicillins, proton pump inhibitors, and probenecid, among other drugs, can cause methotrexate toxicity. Acidic food and drink can also cause elevated methotrexate concentrations.

Fluorouracil

Fluorouracil (5-FU), an antimetabolite agent similar to uracil with an addition of fluoride, is a component of chemotherapy for many cancers, including breast, colorectal, GI, and head and neck. 5-FU is administered intravenously to treat solid tumors and is applied topically for superficial basal cell carcinoma and actinic keratosis. A microsponge delivery system for a cream-based 5-FU was approved in 2000 to provide a sustained-release formulation administered once daily. It is not administered orally because of the inconsistent bioavailability.

TABLE 35.4 Antineoplastics: Antimetabolites

- Visually inspect parenteral products for particulate matter and discoloration before use.
- Observe and exercise precautions when handling, preparing, and administering cytotoxic drugs.
- Chemotherapeutic drug dosages will vary from protocol to protocol. Consult appropriate references to verify doses.

Drug	Route and Dosage	Uses and Considerations
Folic Acid Antagonists		
Methotrexate	ALL: A: PO/IM/IV: 3.3 mg/m^2/d for 4–6 wk followed by maintenance dosing NHL: A: IV: 200 mg/m^2 days 8 and 15 q21d in a combination regimen Head/Neck: A: IV: 40 mg/m^2 days 1 and 15 q21d A: PO: 25–50 mg/m^2 q7d Osteogenic sarcoma: A: IV: 12 g/m^2 q2wk	For ALL, NHL, sarcomas, solid tumors, head and neck cancers, choriocarcinomas, lymphomas, and some autoimmune disorders. Older adults may be more sensitive to toxicity and adverse events. PB: 50%–60%; t½: 10–12 h Leucovorin is used with high doses of methotrexate as rescue therapy to prevent fatal toxicity.
Pemetrexed	A: IV: 500 mg/m^2 day 1 of a 21-d cycle	For mesothelioma and non–small cell lung cancer. Folic acid and vitamin B$_{12}$ IM injections are recommended to prevent hematologic and GI adverse reactions. PB: 81%; t½: 3.5 h
Pyrimidine Analogues		
Azacitidine	A: IV/Subcut: 75 mg/m^2/d for 7 d q4wk	For myelomonocytic syndrome (MDS). Absolutely contraindicated in those with mannitol hypersensitivity. PB: UK; t½: 4 h
Capecitabine	Breast cancer and colorectal cancer: A: PO: 1250 mg/m^2 twice daily for 2 wk, repeated q3wk for a total of 8 cycles	For breast and colorectal cancer. Usually reserved for patients resistant to anthracyclines. Converted in tissue to 5-FU. Monitor for GI symptoms. PB: <60%; t½: 0.75 h
Cytarabine	AML: A: IV: 100–200 mg/m^2/d continuous infusion for 7 d A: Subcut (maint): 100 mg/m^2/d for 5 d q28d ALL: A: IV: 1–3 g/m^2 every 12 h for 8–12 doses CML: A: IV: 200 mg/m^2/d continuous infusion for 9 d, but other doses have been used Carcinomatous meningitis: A/C: Intrathecal: 5–70 mg/m^2	For ALL, AML, CML, carcinomatous meningitis. Use preservative-free diluent. PB: 15%; t½: 3–6 h in plasma; 2–11 h in CSF
Floxuridine	A: Intraarterial: 0.1–0.6 mg/kg/d continuous infusion	For colorectal cancer with liver metastasis. Given as an intraarterial infusion into the hepatic artery; catabolized to 5-FU. PB: UK; t½: UK, but CSF concentrations can be sustained for several hours.
5-Fluorouracil (fluorouracil, 5-FU)	See Prototype Drug Chart: 5-Fluorouracil (5-FU)	
Gemcitabine hydrochloride	NSCLC and breast cancer: A: IV: 1250 mg/m^2 on days 1 and 8 of a 21-d cycle (usually given with another chemotherapeutic drug) Pancreatic cancer: A: IV: 1000 mg/m^2 weekly for up to 7 wk followed by 1 wk of rest Ovarian cancer: A: IV: 1000 mg/m^2 days 1 and 8 of a 21-d cycle	For breast, ovarian, pancreatic, and NSCLC. Pulmonary and cardiac toxicity may occur. PB: 10%; t½: 32–94 min (birth gender and dose dependent)
Purine Analogues		
Cladribine	A: IV: 0.09 mg/kg/d continuous infusion for 7 d	For hairy cell leukemia. Chemical conversion to the active form takes place intracellularly. PB: 20%; t½: 7 h

TABLE 35.4 Antineoplastics: Antimetabolites—cont'd

Drug	Route and Dosage	Uses and Considerations
Fludarabine	A: IV: 25 mg/m²/d for 5 d q28d	For CLL. Absolutely contraindicated in those with hemolytic anemia and renal disease. PB: UK; t½: 7–12 h
Mercaptopurine (6-MP)	A: PO: 1.5–2.5 mg/kg/d followed by maintenance dosage	For ALL. Significant first-pass metabolism occurs after oral administration; significant metabolic variability. PB: UK; t½: 1–2 h
Nelarabine	A: IV: 1500 mg/m² on days 1, 3, and 5 repeated q21d	For T-cell leukemia/lymphoma. Assess for neurologic symptoms. PB: <25%; t½: 0.5–1 h
Pentostatin	A: IV: 4 mg/m² every other wk	*Do not confuse with pentosan.* For hairy cell leukemia. Monitor pulmonary, hepatic, and renal function; assess for seizures. Concomitant use with fludarabine is not recommended. PB: 4%; t½: 2.6–15 h
Thioguanine (6-TG)	A: PO: 100 mg/m² q12h for 5–10 d	For AML. Not recommended for maintenance therapy or long-term continuous treatments due to liver toxicity. PB: UK; t½: Variable
Ribonucleotide Reductase Inhibitors (Enzyme Inhibitors)		
Hydroxyurea	CML: A: PO: 20–30 mg/kg/d Head and neck: A: PO: 80 mg/kg q3d	For CML and head and neck cancer. Monitor for infection and bone marrow suppression. PB: UK; t½: 3.5–4.5 h

Note: Chemotherapeutic doses and schedules will vary depending on protocol, body surface area (m²), age, functional status, and comorbid conditions. For a full discussion of body surface area in dosage calculation, see Chapter 11.
5-FU, 5-Fluorouracil; *A*, adult; *ALL*, acute lymphocytic leukemia; *AML*, acute myelogenous leukemia; *CLL*, chronic lymphocytic leukemia; *CSF*, cerebrospinal fluid; *CML*, chronic myelogenous leukemia; *d*, day; *GI*, gastrointestinal; *h*, hour; *IM*, intramuscular; *IV*, intravenous; *maint*, maintenance dose; *min*, minute; *NHL*, non-Hodgkin lymphoma; *NSCLC*, non–small cell lung cancer; *PB*, protein binding; *PO*, by mouth; *q*, every; *subcut*, subcutaneous; *t½*, half-life; *UK*, unknown; *WBC*, white blood cell; *wk*, weeks; >, greater than; <, less than; ≤, less than or equal to.

PROTOTYPE DRUG CHART
Cyclophosphamide

Drug Class	Dosage
Alkylating drug: Nitrogen mustard Generic Name: Cyclophosphamide	Acute lymphocytic leukemia (ALL): A: IV: 40–50 mg/kg/d A: PO: 1–5 mg/kg/d Breast cancer: A: IV: 500–1000 mg/m² q15d Various protocols exist, including combination therapy. Dosage varies based on indicated use and response. Adjust dose if bone marrow suppression (myelosuppression) occurs.
Contraindications	**Drug-Lab-Food Interactions**
Absolute contraindications: Hypersensitivity, severe urinary outflow obstruction, bladder obstruction *Caution:* Myelosuppression, tumor-lysis syndrome, liver or kidney disease, hemorrhagic cystitis, or heart failure. Many other precautions are necessary when administering cyclophosphamide.	Drug: Doxorubicin may potentiate cardiac toxicity, and busulfan may potentiate lung toxicity. Other antineoplastic and immunosuppressive drugs may have an additive effect on immunosuppressive activity. Drugs metabolized by the cytochrome P450 can increase toxic effects of cyclophosphamide. Doxorubicin decreases digoxin level and increases drug action of barbiturates, chloramphenicol half-life, and effects of anticoagulant drugs. Duration of leukopenia may be prolonged if given with thiazide diuretics. Actions and toxicities of allopurinol, probenecid, colchicine, phenothiazines, potassium iodide, imipramine, warfarin, and succinylcholine are altered if given with cyclophosphamide. Toxicity is increased if given with corticosteroids, phenytoin, or sulfonamides. Many other possible drug-drug interactions are not listed here. Lab: Suppresses positive reaction to uric acid, purified protein derivative, mumps, *Candida*. Cyclophosphamide may cause Papanicolaou test (Pap smear) to be falsely positive.

Continued

PROTOTYPE DRUG CHART—CONT'D
Cyclophosphamide

Pharmacokinetics	Pharmacodynamics
Absorption: PO: Well absorbed Distribution: PB: 20%, not dose dependent Metabolism: t½: 3–12 h Excretion: 5%–25% in urine unchanged; 4% in feces mostly as metabolites	PO/IV: Onset: 7 d PO/IV: Peak: 7–15 d PO/IV: Duration: 21 d

Therapeutic Effects/Uses

Leukemias, breast and ovarian cancer, lymphomas, multiple myeloma, lung cancer, and retinoblastoma
Mechanism of action: Cell cycle–nonspecific alkylating drugs inhibit the protein synthesis by interfering with DNA replication by alkylation of DNA.

Side Effects	Adverse Reactions
Nausea, vomiting, diarrhea, anorexia, leukopenia, febrile neutropenia, fever, weight loss, alopecia, amenorrhea, gonadal suppression, impaired wound healing, stomatitis, pain	Anaphylaxis, hematologic toxicity, pulmonary toxicity (pneumonitis, pulmonary fibrosis, pulmonary thrombosis), hemorrhagic cystitis, urotoxicity, nephrotoxicity, secondary neoplasm, cardiotoxicity, hepatotoxicity, tumor-lysis syndrome

Note: Chemotherapy drug doses are based on body weight and are prescribed either as milligrams per kilogram (mg/kg) or milligrams per meter squared (mg/m²). Doses will also vary based on drug protocol, type and stage of cancer, age, functional status, and comorbid conditions (e.g., heart disease).
A, Adult; *d*, day; *DNA*, deoxyribonucleic acid; *h*, hour; *IV*, intravenous; *q*, every; *PB*, protein binding; *PO*, by mouth; *t½*, half-life.

PATIENT SAFETY

Obtain a complete medication list that includes over-the-counter, herbal preparations, and other alternative therapies.
Do Not Confuse…
- **Hydroxyurea** with **Hydroxychloroquine**
- **Xeloda** with **Xenical**

COMPLEMENTARY AND ALTERNATIVE THERAPIES
Fluorouracil

- Use cautiously with ginseng and St. John's wort (may interfere with chemotherapy). *Do not use with mistletoe because it may promote cancer growth.*
- Astragalus stimulates the immune system and may help speed recovery from immunosuppressive chemotherapy. Astragalus has blood clot–fighting properties and may increase risk of bleeding when given with 5-fluorouracil (5-FU).

Pharmacokinetics

5-FU crosses the blood-brain barrier and is distributed widely throughout the body tissues. The concentration of 5-FU can be sustained for several hours in the cerebrospinal fluid. It is also effective for ascites and pleural effusions. The bioavailability and elimination half-life of IV 5-FU is nonlinear with high dosages, most likely due to saturation of metabolic processes. Approximately 15% is protein bound, and the rest (85%) is distributed throughout the body, including in the liver, GI mucosa, and peripheral WBCs. The major catabolizer is the liver; however, with continuous IV infusion, significant extrahepatic metabolism occurs. After IV administration, the mean elimination half-life is 16 minutes, with a range of 8 to 20 minutes, and it is dose dependent. A small amount of unchanged 5-FU is eliminated by the biliary and renal systems. After topical administration, approximately 6% is absorbed systemically. Also, 5-FU can be administered to patients with hepatic impairment with serum bilirubin less than 5 mg/dL without reducing the dose. No dose adjustments are needed for patients with renal impairment.

Pharmacodynamics

5-FU converts into multiple active metabolites, inhibiting normal cell growth by interfering with the cell's RNA and DNA. Cytotoxicity involving the DNA is noted during the S phase of the cell cycle during the first 24 hours after drug exposure. The cell's RNA is affected after 24 hours during the G_1 phase. 5-FU is used alone or with other anticancer drugs and has a low therapeutic index. Dosing of 5-FU can vary from protocol to protocol. High IV boluses of 5-FU can result in severe hemorrhagic colitis or bone marrow suppression. Administering high doses as continuous therapy has reduced the incidences of hematologic toxicity. The Complementary and Alternative Therapies box lists herbal supplements that may interact with 5-FU.

Side Effects and Adverse Reactions

See Table 35.2 for general side effects. GI bleeding and bone marrow suppression can occur with high bolus doses of 5-FU, and patients who previously received myelosuppressive therapy and/or radiation treatment have increased risk for bone marrow suppression. 5-FU can potentiate the effects of radiation therapy and should be discontinued at the first visible sign of WBCs less than 3500/mm³, a rapidly falling WBC count, or a platelet count below 100,000/mm³. Prototype Drug Chart: Fluorouracil, 5-Fluorouracil (5-FU) details the pharmacologic behavior of 5-FU.

CLINICAL JUDGMENT [NURSING PROCESS]
Alkylating Drug: Cyclophosphamide

Concept: Immunity
- The protective response of the body toward inflammation and infection

Recognize Cues [Assessment]
- To avoid drug-drug interactions, obtain a detailed medication history that includes prescriptions, over-the-counter medicines, antacids, dietary supplements, vitamins, and herbal supplements.
- Obtain a list of the patient's drug and food allergies.
- Obtain baseline information about the patient's physical status. Include height, weight, vital signs, cardiopulmonary assessment, intake and output, skin assessment, nutritional status, and information on any underlying disease.
- Assess baseline laboratory values (complete blood count [CBC], uric acid, chemistry panel) for future comparisons.
- Assess baseline results of pulmonary function tests, chest radiographs, electrocardiography (ECG), and renal and liver function studies.
- Assess the patient's current level of comprehension.

Analyze Cues and Prioritize Hypotheses [Patient Problems]
- Decreased immunity
- Need for patient teaching

Generate Solutions [Planning]
- The patient will verbalize understanding of the signs and symptoms of infection.
- The patient will maintain adequate white blood cell (WBC), red blood cell (RBC), and platelet counts.
- The patient will remain free from infection and hemorrhagic cystitis.
- The patient will demonstrate understanding of protection from sun exposure.
- The patient/family/caregiver will demonstrate understanding of chemotherapeutic protocol (e.g., dose administration).

Take Action [Nursing Interventions]
- Monitor labs (CBC, blood urea nitrogen [BUN], creatinine, liver panel, and electrolytes) before and during treatment.
- Monitor the IV site frequently for irritation and phlebitis.
- Maintain strict medical asepsis during dressing changes and invasive procedures.
- Encourage small, frequent meals high in calories and protein.
- Monitor fluid intake and output and nutritional intake during therapy.
- Encourage patients to drink at least 2 L of fluid per day to promote excretion of cellular breakdown products and to reduce the risk of hemorrhagic cystitis.
- Assess the need for IV hydration.
- Maintain hydration before and during chemotherapy.
- Assess for signs and symptoms of hematuria, urinary frequency, or dysuria.
- Administer premedications as ordered 30 to 60 minutes before administering cyclophosphamide.
- Provide drug information verbally and in print to the patient/family/caregiver.
- Encourage patients to use sunblock with a sun protection factor (SPF) of 50 or greater and to use other means to protect skin from sun exposure.

Patient Teaching
General
- Teach patients to take cyclophosphamide early in the day to prevent accumulation of drug in the bladder during the night.
- Remind patients to consult with a health care provider before administration of any vaccines.
- Advise patients to promptly report signs of infection (e.g., elevated temperature, fever, chills, sore throat, frequent urination or burning on urination, and redness/swelling/pain near a wound), bleeding (e.g., bleeding gums, petechiae, bruises, hematuria, blood in the stool), and anemia (e.g., increased fatigue, dyspnea, and orthostatic hypotension).
- Advise patients not to visit anyone who has a respiratory infection. A decreased WBC count puts patient at high risk for infections.
- Emphasize protective precautions as necessary (e.g., hand washing and personal hygiene).
- Teach patients to empty their bladder every 2 to 3 hours.
- Teach methods of sun protection (e.g., sunblock with SPF 50 or greater, brimmed hats, and lightweight, long-sleeved shirts).

Side Effects
- Advise patients about good oral hygiene with a soft toothbrush for stomatitis; have patients use a soft toothbrush when the platelet count is less than 50,000/mm^3.
- Assess for use of alternative and complementary therapies that may interact with chemotherapy drugs.
- Advise patients to report any signs of bleeding.

Diet
- Advise patients to follow a diet low in purines—such as low fat dairy products, beans, peas, and eggs—to alkalize urine.
- Advise patients to avoid citric acid.
- Offer patients food and fluids that may decrease nausea (e.g., cola, crackers, and ginger ale).
- Plan small, frequent meals.

Evaluate Outcomes [Evaluation]
- The patient is free from infection.
- The patient does not develop hemorrhagic cystitis.
- The patient/family/caregiver education needs are met.

ANTITUMOR ANTIBIOTICS

Antitumor antibiotics are similar to natural antibiotics; however, they do *not* treat infections; instead, they interfere with DNA replication and RNA transcription of cancer cells. All antitumor antibiotics except for bleomycin have their major effects in all phases of the cell cycle (cell cycle nonspecific). Bleomycins affect cells during the G_2 phase. Types of antitumor antibiotics are anthracyclines (daunorubicin, doxorubicin, epirubicin, and idarubicin) and other antitumor antibiotics (actinomycin D, bleomycin, mitomycin C, and mitoxantrone). Antitumor antibiotics are used to treat leukemias and many solid tumors. Table 35.5 lists the antitumor antibiotics, and their uses and considerations.

Adverse reactions to the antitumor antibiotics are similar to those of other antineoplastics and include alopecia, nausea, vomiting, stomatitis, and myelosuppression. Antitumor antibiotics are capable of causing vesication (blistering of tissue); exceptions to this are bleomycin and plicamycin. General adverse reactions to chemotherapeutic drugs are listed in Table 35.2.

TABLE 35.5 Antineoplastics: Antitumorals

- Visually inspect parenteral products for particulate matter and discoloration before use.
- Observe and exercise precautions when handling, preparing, and administering cytotoxic drugs.
- Dosages of chemotherapeutic drugs vary from protocol to protocol. Consult appropriate references to verify dosages.

Drug	Route and Dosage	Uses and Considerations
Anthracyclines		
Daunorubicin	AML: A $\leq$60 y: IV: 45 mg/m²/d for 3 d for first course, then 2 d for subsequent courses A $\geq$60 y: IV: 30 mg/m²/d for 3 d for first course, then 2 d for subsequent courses ALL: A: IV: 45 mg/m²/d on days 1–3.	*Do not confuse with doxorubicin.* For ALL and AML. Given with other antineoplastic drugs. Monitor for cardiotoxicity PB: 80%; t½: 45–55 h
Doxorubicin	See Prototype Drug Chart: Doxorubicin	*Do not confuse with daunorubicin*
Epirubicin	A: IV: 75 mg/m² q21d for 4 cycles	Adjuvant treatment for breast cancer. Assess for signs of infection PB: 77%; t½: 30 h
Idarubicin	AML and APL: A: IV: 12 mg/m²/d for 3 d	For AML and APL. May cause red or orange urine discoloration PB: 97%; t½: 22 h
Mitoxantrone	AML: A: IV: 12 mg/m²/d; duration of treatment is different for induction and consolidation therapy Prostate cancer: A: IV: 12–14 mg/m² q21d	*Do not confuse with mitomycin.* For AML and prostate cancer PB: 78%; t½: 23–215 h
Valrubicin	Intravesicular: A: 800 mg q1wk for 6 wk; *max:* 800 mg intravesically	For bladder cancer. Systemic exposure is dependent on the integrity of the bladder wall PB: UK; t½: UK
Other Antitumor Antibiotics		
Bleomycin	Hodgkin disease and cervical, head and neck, and vulvar cancers: A: IV/IM/subcut: 5–20 units/m² 1 or 2 times/wk; other dosing is available NHL and testicular cancer: A: IV/IM/subcut: 10–20 units/m² once a wk 1 or 2 times/wk	For head and neck cancer; Hodgkin disease; NHL; cervical, penile, testicular, and vulvar cancer; and malignant effusion. Monitor for pulmonary complications PB: 10%; t½: 2–4 h
Dactinomycin, actinomycin D	Testicular cancer: A: IV: 1000 mcg/m² q3wk for 12 wk Malignant melanoma: A: IA: 50 mcg/kg for legs; 35 mcg/kg for arms Other dosing regimen available	For testicular cancer, Ewing sarcoma, Wilms tumor, malignant melanoma, and rhabdomyosarcoma. Nausea and vomiting may occur during first 24 h. Absolutely contraindicated with herpes infection or varicella PB: UK; t½: 36 h
Mitomycin	A: IV: 20 mg/m² q6–8wk	For gastric and pancreatic cancer. Monitor for pulmonary complications PB: UK; t½: 0.25–1.5 h

Note: Chemotherapeutic doses and schedules vary depending on protocol, body surface area (m²), age, functional status, and comorbid conditions. For a full discussion of body surface area in dosage calculation, see Chapter 11.

A, Adult; *ALL*, acute lymphocytic leukemia; *AML*, acute myelocytic leukemia; *APL*, acute promyelocytic leukemia; *d*, day; *h*, hour; *IA:* intraarterial; *IM*, intramuscular; *IV*, intravenous; *max*, maximum dosage; *NHL*, non-Hodgkin lymphoma; *PB*, protein binding; *q*, every; *subcut*, subcutaneous; *t½*, half-life; *UK*, unknown; *wk*, week; $\geq$, greater than or equal to; $\leq$, less than or equal to.

Anthracyclines: Doxorubicin

Doxorubicin is an anthracycline antitumor antibiotic antineoplastic agent used to treat many solid and hematogenous tumors except for acute myelogenous leukemias (AMLs), due to the increased incidences of stomatitis and cardiotoxicity compared with other anthracyclines. Doxorubicin is a component of many combination chemotherapy treatments because of its broad antitumor activity and flexible dosing schedule. However, patients receiving IV doxorubicin must be monitored for cardiotoxicity. Doxorubicin has a maximum dose of 550 mg/m² due to cardiotoxicity. Patients taking other cardiotoxic drugs, who are older, who have preexisting cardiac problems, or who have had radiation therapy to the chest are at increased risk for cardiotoxicity. Dexrazoxane, a chemoprotectant, is administered before anthracyclines to prevent cardiotoxicity. Cardiac function should be assessed before administering doxorubicin or other anthracyclines. Liposomal doxorubicin was developed to be carried by a liposomal carrier, which decreases the incidence of severe toxicity; however, the dosages vary greatly from conventional doxorubicin, and the indications for use are different.

PROTOTYPE DRUG CHART
Fluorouracil, 5-Fluorouracil (5-FU)

Drug Class	Dosage
Antimetabolite	A: IV: 300–1000 mg/m^2/d for 4–5 d continuous infusion q4wk Topical: 1%–5% cream once or twice daily for 3–12 wk Various protocols exist, including topical; IV drugs are often used with other chemotherapeutic drugs.

Contraindications	Drug-Lab-Food Interactions
Bone marrow suppression, dihydropyrimidine dehydrogenase deficiency, infection, malnutrition, pregnancy *Caution:* GI bleeding, liver and renal impairment, biliary tract disease, coronary artery disease Many other precautions are present when administering fluorouracil.	Drug: Bone marrow depressants increase chances of toxicity. Avoid live virus vaccines, which may potentiate infection. Leucovorin may potentiate adverse effects of 5-FU. Drugs that can increase the systemic cytotoxicity of 5-FU include cimetidine, dipyridamole, interferon-alfa, and levamisole. Metronidazole may cause blood dyscrasias. Synergistic reaction can occur with cisplatin and 5-FU. Lab: May decrease albumin; may increase excretion of 5-HIAA in urine

Pharmacokinetics	Pharmacodynamics
Absorption: IV and topical: 5%–10% Distribution: PB: 15%; readily crosses the blood-brain barrier Metabolism (IV): t½: 8–20 min, dose dependent Excretion: 7%–20% via urine unchanged within 6 h; inactive metabolites via respiratory system as CO_2 and the urinary system as urea	IV onset: 1–9 d Topical onset: 2–3 d IV peak: 9–21 d Topical peak: 2–6 wk IV duration: 30 d Topical duration: 1–2 mo This information provides two examples of pharmacodynamics. Clinical pharmacology is complex and is dependent on route of administration and patient condition.

Therapeutic Effects/Uses
Basal cell carcinoma; breast, colorectal, pancreas, and gastric cancers; given in combination with levamisole after surgical resection in patients with Duke stage C colon cancer
Mechanism of action: Some cell cycle–specific effects during the S and G_1 phases; prevention of thymidine synthase production interferes with RNA synthesis and function and has some effects to DNA

Side Effects	Adverse Reactions
Nausea, vomiting, anorexia, leukopenia, febrile neutropenia, fever, weight loss, alopecia, amenorrhea, gonadal suppression, impaired wound healing, stomatitis, pain, dry/cracked skin	Bone marrow suppression, bleeding, stomatitis, esophagopharyngitis, intractable vomiting, diarrhea, palmar-plantar erythrodysesthesia (hand and foot syndrome), cardiac toxicity, thrombocytopenia, myelosuppression, renal failure

5-FU, Fluorouracil; *5-HIAA*, 5-hydroxyindoleacetic acid; *A*, adult; CO_2, carbon dioxide; *d*, day; *GI*, gastrointestinal; *h*, hour; *IV*, intravenous; *min*, minute; *mo*, months; *PB*, protein binding; *q*, every; *RNA*, ribonucleic acid; *t½*, half-life; *UK*, unknown; *wk*, week.

Pharmacokinetics
Doxorubicin is administered intravenously and is distributed throughout the body tissues but does not cross the blood-brain barrier. It is extensively bound to DNA, 75% bound to plasma proteins, and not dose dependent up to 1.1 mcg/mL. Doxorubicin does not cross the placenta but appears to pass into breast milk. It is extensively metabolized by the liver into active (doxorubicinol) and inactive (hydroxylated conjugates or glucuronide) metabolites. Clearance of doxorubicinol from the blood decreases as the dose of conventional doxorubicin increases. The metabolites are excreted in the bile (50%), feces, and urine (<10%).

Pharmacodynamics
Doxorubicin is a part of standard regimens for breast, lung, gastric, and ovarian cancers; Hodgkin and non-Hodgkin lymphomas; sarcoma and myeloma; and acute lymphocytic leukemia (ALL). The terminal half-life for doxorubicin is 30 to 50 hours. The clearance of doxorubicin was found to be reduced in patients with elevated serum bilirubin levels; therefore, a dose reduction is recommended in patients with a bilirubin level greater than 1.2 mg/dL. Drug clearance was also reduced in patients whose weight was greater than 130% of ideal body weight. Administration of doxorubicin is not recommended to patients who received the maximum allowable dose of other anthracyclines. Cardiotoxicity is a major concern with doxorubicin. Mitochondrial damage to cardiac cells can be extensive and can cause cardiomyopathy, dysrhythmias, congestive heart failure (CHF), and cardiogenic shock. Mitochondrial damage occurs because superoxide radicals cannot be converted back to oxygen; the heart is nearly devoid of glutathione peroxidase, an enzyme necessary for the conversion. Dexrazoxane is a parenteral chemoprotectant agent used to decrease anthracycline-associated cardiomyopathies; it is administered 30 minutes before the doxorubicin infusion. It is also used to treat anthracycline extravasation and is administered intravenously close to the affected area. The Complementary and Alternative Therapies box lists herbal supplements that may also interact with doxorubicin.

CLINICAL JUDGMENT [NURSING PROCESS]
Antimetabolite: Fluorouracil

Concept: Immunity
- The protective response of the body toward inflammation and infection

Recognize Cues [Assessment]
- To avoid drug-drug and drug-supplement interactions, conduct a detailed current medication history that includes prescriptions, over-the-counter medicines, antacids, dietary supplements, vitamins, and herbal supplements.
- Obtain a list of drug and food allergies.
- Obtain baseline information about the patient's physical status. Include height, weight, vital signs, cardiopulmonary assessment, intake and output, skin assessment, daily activities status, nutritional status, and any underlying disease.
- Obtain baseline laboratory values (complete blood count [CBC], uric acid, and chemistry panel) to compare with future laboratory results.
- Assess baseline results of pulmonary function tests, chest radiographs, electrocardiograms, and renal and hepatic studies.
- Assess the ability for comprehension.

Analyze Cues and Prioritize Hypotheses [Patient Problems]
- Decreased immunity
- Need for patient teaching

Generate Solutions [Planning]
- The patient will be free of infection.
- The patient will remain free from signs and symptoms of bleeding.
- The patient/family/caregiver will demonstrate understanding of chemotherapeutic protocol (dose, administration, side effects, and adverse reactions).

Take Action [Nursing Intervention]
- Monitor the intravenous (IV) site frequently. Extravasation produces severe pain and can promote infection.
- Maintain strict medical asepsis during dressing changes and invasive procedures.
- Monitor blood counts and laboratory values.
- Administer an antiemetic 30 to 60 minutes before the drug to prevent nausea and emesis.
- Monitor fluid intake and output and nutritional intake.
- Offer the patient food and fluids that may decrease nausea (e.g., crackers, cola, and ginger ale).
- Assist with the planning of small, frequent meals.
- Record the number and consistency of stools; monitor perineal skin condition.

Patient Teaching
General
- Advise patients to promptly report signs of infection (fever, sore throat, chills, urinary frequency or burning on urination; redness, swelling, or pain near a wound), bleeding (bleeding gums, petechiae, bruises, hematuria, or blood in the stool), or signs of anemia (increased fatigue, dyspnea, or orthostatic hypotension).
- Teach patients to examine their mouth daily and report signs of stomatitis (soreness, ulcerations, or white patches in the mouth).
- Advise patient not to visit anyone who has a respiratory infection.
- Emphasize protective precautions such as hand washing and personal hygiene.
- Emphasize the importance of maintaining sound nutrition, and assist in the development of small, frequent meals high in calories and protein.

Side Effects
- Advise patients about good oral hygiene with a soft toothbrush for mucositis/stomatitis; have patients use a soft toothbrush when the platelet count is 50,000/mm^3 or less. Instruct patients to rinse their mouth every 2 hours with saline solution of 1/4 teaspoon of salt in 1 cup of water and to avoid use of commercial mouthwashes that contain alcohol.
- Assess for use of alternative or complementary therapies that may interact with chemotherapy.

Diet
- Encourage small, frequent meals to decrease incidences of nausea and emesis.
- Encourage use of cool, bland foods when the patient is nauseated.
- Offer ice chips or ice pops to help relieve mouth pain.
- Encourage foods high in calories and protein.

Evaluate Outcomes [Evaluation]
- The patient is free from infection.
- Oral mucosa is free from erythema and swelling.
- Skin integrity remains intact.
- Patient/family/caregiver education needs are met.
- The patient's weight is maintained at the desired level.

COMPLEMENTARY AND ALTERNATIVE THERAPIES
Doxorubicin

- St. John's wort is a potent cytochrome P450 inducer and moderate P-glycoprotein inducer that may decrease the concentration of doxorubicin.
- Grapefruit is a potent cytochrome P3A4 inhibitor that may increase the concentration and effect of doxorubicin.
- Black cohosh and Dong-quai should be avoided in estrogen-dependent tumors.
- Many complementary therapies—such as acupuncture, art therapy, and music therapy—have been used to improve patients' sense of well-being.

PATIENT SAFETY

Monitor for cardiac toxicity and infection.
Do Not Confuse...
- **Doxorubicin** with **daunorubicin, doxorubicin liposomal,** or **idarubicin**

Side Effects and Adverse Reactions

Doxorubicin has adverse drug effects similar to those of other chemotherapeutic agents. Table 35.2 lists the common side effects and adverse reactions. One common side effect of doxorubicin includes a change of the urine color to pink or light red. Life-threatening effects include cardiotoxicity, CHF, severe myelosuppression, and ECG abnormalities. The amount of myelosuppression tends to be dose dependent, dose limiting, and reversible. Prototype Drug Chart: Doxorubicin presents the pharmacologic data for doxorubicin.

PLANT ALKALOIDS

Plant alkaloids are derived from plants and are cell cycle specific; they block cell division at the M phase of the cell cycle. The **vinca alkaloids** (vinblastine, vincristine, and vinorelbine) and the **taxanes** (docetaxel and paclitaxel) are considered antimicrotubule compounds that cause disruption and interference with vital cell functions when cells are dividing (mitosis), which leads to cell apoptosis.

Microtubules also involve many nonmitotic functions and thereby affect malignant and nonmalignant cells.

The vinca alkaloids are derived from the periwinkle plant, and taxanes are derived from the yew tree. When the natural resources became scarce, a semisynthetic form of taxanes was developed. Epipodophyllotoxins (etoposide, teniposide) come from apple trees and interfere with topoisomerases, enzymes that separate strands of DNA during the S phase of the cell cycle. Another group of plant alkaloids, camptothecin analogues (irinotecan, topotecan) isolated from a Chinese tree, are water soluble and have a broad range of antitumor properties. Retinoids (bexarotene), a natural derivative of vitamin A, are an important regulator for cell reproduction, proliferation, and differentiation. However, retinoids do not convert into the rhodopsin needed for night vision. Retinoids are given orally or topically. Table 35.6 lists the plant alkaloids and their uses and considerations.

Adverse reactions to plant alkaloids include leukopenia, hypersensitivity reactions, partial to complete alopecia, constipation, and nausea.

Vomiting, diarrhea, and phlebitis. The plant alkaloids damage peripheral nerve fibers and may cause reversible or irreversible neurotoxicity. Signs and symptoms of neurotoxicity include a decrease in muscular strength numbness and tingling of fingers and toes (stocking-glove syndrome), constipation, and motor instability. Other adverse effects of these drugs include loss of deep tendon reflexes, muscle weakness, joint pain, and bone marrow suppression. Docetaxel may cause fluid retention. General adverse effects to chemotherapeutic drugs are listed in Table 35.2.

TABLE 35.6 Antineoplastics: Plant Alkaloids

- Visually inspect parenteral products for particulate matter and discoloration before use.
- Observe and exercise precautions when handling, preparing, and administering cytotoxic drugs.
- Antineoplastic drug dosages vary from protocol to protocol. Consult appropriate references to verify doses.

Drug	Route and Dosage	Uses and Considerations
Antimicrotubules/Taxanes		
Docetaxel	Breast cancer: A: IV: 60–100 mg/m^2 day 1, repeat q3wk All other cancers: A: IV: 75 mg/m^2 q3wk	For breast, gastric, prostate, and head and neck cancers and NSCLC. Monitor for pulmonary and cardiac complications. PB: 94%; t½: 11 h
Paclitaxel	Breast cancer: A: IV: 175 mg/m^2 q3wk Ovarian, NSCLC, and Kaposi sarcoma: A: IV: 135 mg/m^2 q3wk	*Do not confuse Taxol with Taxotere.* For breast and ovarian cancers, NSCLC, and Kaposi sarcoma. PB: 95%–98%; t½: 19 h
Camptothecin Analogues		
Irinotecan	A: IV: 125 mg/m^2 once a week for 4 wk Other dosing regimen is available	For colorectal cancer. Consider lower doses in older adults. PB: 30%–68%; t½: 6–12 h
Topotecan	Ovarian cancer and SCLC: A: IV: 1.5 mg/m^2/d for 5 d q21d Cervical cancer: A: IV: 0.75 mg/m^2 for 3 d q3wk	For cervical and ovarian cancers and SCLC. Do not give for severe renal impairment (creatinine >1.5 mg/dL). PB: >35%; t½: 2–6 h (route dependent)
Epipodophyllotoxins		
Etoposide	SCLC: A: IV: 35–50 mg/m^2/d for 4–5d q21d for 4 cycles Testicular cancer: A: IV: 100 mg/m^2/d for 5 d, repeat q3–4wk Other dosing regimen is available	For testicular cancer and SCLC. Contraindicated in known benzyl alcohol intolerance. PB: 95%; t½: 5–10 h
Teniposide	A: IV: 165 mg/m^2 on days 1, 4, 8, and 11.	For ALL. Contraindicated with polyoxyethylated castor oil hypersensitivity. PB: 99%; t½: 5 h
Immunomodulators		
Thalidomide	ENL: A: PO: 100–300 mg/d at bedtime Multiple myeloma: A: PO: 200 mg/d at bedtime	For multiple myeloma and ENL. Do not administer to pregnant patients; severe birth defects have occurred. PB: 55%–66%; t½: 5.5–7.3 h
Retinoids		
Bexarotene	A: PO: 300 mg/m^2/d (round to nearest 75 mg)	For cutaneous T-cell lymphoma. Do *not* administer to pregnant patients. PB: >99%; t½: 7 h

Continued

TABLE 35.6 Antineoplastics: Plant Alkaloids—cont'd

Drug	Route and Dosage	Uses and Considerations
Vinca Alkaloids		
Vinblastine	Breast cancer: A: IV: 4.5 mg/m²/d every 21 d NHL: A: IV: 4 mg/m² days 1 and 2, repeated q28d for 3 cycles Hodgkin disease: A: IV: 6 mg/m² days 1 and 15, repeated q28d Other dosing regimen is available	For solid organ cancers, choriocarcinoma, cutaneous T-cell lymphoma, Hodgkin disease, and NHL. Usually given with combination therapy. Monitor for any pulmonary complications. PB: 50%; t½: 23–85 h
Vincristine	See Prototype Drug Chart: Vincristine	
Vinorelbine	A: IV: 30 mg/m²/wk	For NSCLC. Dose must be adjusted with hepatic impairment. PB: 79.6%–91.2%; t½: 27.7–43.6 h

Note: Chemotherapeutic doses and schedules vary depending on protocol, body surface area (m²), age, functional status, and comorbid conditions. For a full discussion of body surface area in dosage calculation, see Chapter 11.
A, Adult; *ALL*, acute lymphocytic leukemia; *d*, day; *ENL*, erythema nodosum leprosum; *h*, hour; *IV*, intravenous; *NHL*, non-Hodgkin lymphoma; *NSCLC*, non–small cell lung cancer; *PB*, protein binding; *PO*, by mouth; *q*, every; *SCLC*, small cell lung cancer; *t½*, half-life; *UK*, unknown; *wk*, week: >, greater than; ≥, greater than or equal to.

PROTOTYPE DRUG CHART

Doxorubicin

Drug Class	Dosage
Antitumor antibiotic: Anthracycline	A: IV: 60–75 mg/m² once q21d as a single agent, 20–75 mg/m² q21–28d if used in combination with other drugs Various protocols exist, including combination therapy. Dose varies based on indicated use and response. Adjust dose with hepatic impairment.

Contraindications	Drug-Lab-Food Interactions
Anthracycline hypersensitivity, hepatic disease, myocardial infarction or severe myocardial insufficiency, neutropenia, those who received the maximum dose of doxorubicin or daunorubicin. *Caution:* Bone marrow suppression, extravasation, heart failure, impaired hepatic or renal function	Drug: Other cytotoxic drugs combined with doxorubicin may increase hematologic and GI toxicities. Cardiotoxicity may result with concomitant use with paclitaxel and verapamil. Hematologic toxicity can occur when used with cyclosporine and cyclophosphamide. Secondary malignancies have been noted with use of progesterone. Cytarabine has been known to cause necrotizing colitis. Lab: Abnormal hepatic function tests; may induce tumor-lysis syndrome and hyperuricemia, ECG changes; increases uric acid and may reduce neutrophil and RBC counts.

Pharmacokinetics	Pharmacodynamics
Absorption: IV Distribution: PB: 70% Metabolism: t½: 20–48 h Excretion: 40% in bile and 5%–12% in urine	IV: Onset: 10 d Peak: 14 d Duration: 21–24 d

Therapeutic Effects/Uses
Breast, gastric, lung, and ovarian cancers; hematogenous tumors; soft tissue and bone sarcomas; leukemias; lymphomas
Mechanism of action: Inhibits DNA and RNA synthesis; has immunosuppressant activity; it is cell cycle specific for the S phase.

Side Effects	Adverse Reactions
Complete alopecia, stomatitis, anorexia, nausea, vomiting, diarrhea, rash, reddish-colored urine, hyperpigmentation of nail beds, dermal creases, fever, chills Dexrazoxane, a cytoprotectant drug, is used to treat extravasation and reduce the incidence and/or severity of cardiotoxicity due to anthracycline toxicity.	Cardiotoxicity (cardiomyopathy, dysrhythmias, CHF, and cardiogenic shock); myelosuppression (hematologic toxicity [leukopenia, anemia, and thrombocytopenia])

A, Adult *CHF*, congestive heart failure; *d*, day; *DNA*, deoxyribonucleic acid; *ECG*, electrocardiogram; *GI*, gastrointestinal; *h*, hour; *IV*, intravenous; *PB*, protein binding; *q*, every; *RBC*, red blood cell; *RNA*, ribonucleic acid; *t½*, half-life.

Vincristine

Vincristine was developed from the periwinkle plant and has an increased cellular retention compared with vinblastine. Neurotoxicity is a dose-limiting adverse effect of vincristine, whereas other vinca alkaloids have a dose-limiting myelosuppression. Vincristine is used for leukemias, breast carcinoma, NHL, multiple myeloma, soft tissue and osteogenic sarcomas, and brain tumors.

Pharmacokinetics

Vincristine is given parenterally. It is distributed widely throughout many tissues and binds to RBCs and platelets. Approximately 50% is metabolized by the liver and is excreted as metabolites or as the parent drug in the bile and feces. Approximately three-fourths of the drug is eliminated through the biliary tree within 72 hours. The final elimination half-life is between 23 and 85 hours. Patients with significant biliary obstruction may need dose adjustment.

Pharmacodynamics

Vincristine exerts cytotoxic effects by interfering with microtubules in the M phase in addition to having other effects, such as inhibition of RNA, DNA, and protein synthesis; inhibition of glycolysis; and disruption of cell membrane integrity. It has a high-volume distribution and rapid distribution half-life of less than 5 minutes due to extensive tissue binding. Vincristine does not cross the blood-brain barrier. The Complementary and Alternative Therapies box lists herbal supplements that may also interact with vincristine.

COMPLEMENTARY AND ALTERNATIVE THERAPIES

Vincristine

> St. John's wort and echinacea are cytochrome P450 inducers, which cause decreased levels of vincristine. Many complementary therapies—such as acupuncture, art therapy, and music therapy—have been used to improve patients' sense of well-being.

Side Effects and Adverse Reactions

Vincristine is associated with neurotoxicity with an intracellular concentration above a certain critical threshold. Continuous infusion is associated with longer tissue exposure above the critical cytotoxic

---

CLINICAL JUDGMENT [NURSING PROCESS]
Antitumor Antibiotic: Doxorubicin

Concept: Perfusion
- The ability for the cardiopulmonary and vascular systems to deliver oxygen and nutrients to body tissues

Recognize Cues [Assessment]
- Conduct a detailed medication history that lists all concurrent medications and includes prescriptions, over-the-counter medicines, antacids, dietary supplements, vitamins, and herbal supplements to avoid drug-drug and drug-supplement interactions.
- Obtain baseline information about the patient's physical status. This should include height, weight, vital signs, cardiopulmonary assessment, intake and output, skin assessment, daily activities status (e.g., sleep-wake cycle, ability to perform activities of daily living), nutritional status, presence or absence of any underlying disease, and past or current use of medications and treatment.
- Assess laboratory values (complete blood count with differentials, uric acid, electrolytes, serum bilirubin, and hepatic and renal studies) and electrocardiogram (ECG) for comparison with future labs.
- Assess patient and family knowledge related to the therapeutic regimen.

Analyze Cues and Prioritize Hypothesis [Patient Problems]
- Decreased tissue perfusion, general
- Risk for dysrhythmias
- Need for patient teaching

Generate Solutions [Planning]
- The patient will remain free from infection.
- The patient will be free from cardiac abnormalities.
- The patient will have intact skin.
- The patient/family/caregiver will demonstrate understanding of the chemotherapy regimen, including side effects.
- The patient/family/caregiver will exhibit behavior appropriate for the chemotherapeutic protocol.

Take Action [Nursing Interventions]
- Maintain strict medical asepsis during dressing changes and invasive procedures.
- Assess cardiac status, and check for any ECG abnormalities before and during treatment. Prepare to administer dexrazoxane.
- Monitor the intravenous (IV) site frequently, and stop the infusion immediately if signs of extravasation are apparent.
- Give the drug through a large-bore, quickly running IV infusion. Monitor blood counts and laboratory values.
- Handle the drug with care during preparation, and avoid direct skin contact with the drug.

Patient Teaching
General
- Teach patients/family/caregivers when to call the health care provider.
- Explain to patients that the anticancer drug can decrease immune response and blood count.
- Emphasize protective precautions such as hand washing, personal hygiene, and avoiding people with respiratory infection.

Side Effects
- Teach patients about changes in urine color (pink or red) caused by this drug.
- Advise patients when to call a health care provider about cardiac abnormalities (chest pain, shortness of breath, or palpitations).
- Advise patients to promptly report signs of infection (fever, sore throat), bleeding (bleeding gums, petechiae, bruises, hematuria, or blood in stool), and anemia (increased fatigue, dyspnea, or orthostatic hypotension).
- Stress to patients the importance of notifying their health care provider immediately if burning or pain is experienced at the IV site.

Diet
- Encourage small, frequent, bland meals high in calories and protein.

Evaluate Outcomes [Evaluation]
- The patient is free from infection.
- Cardiac function is maintained.
- The patient and family educational needs are met.
- Side effects of therapy are controlled.

level. Neurotoxicity is a dose-limiting adverse effect, and neuropathy may occur with single weekly vincristine doses but usually resolves within a week. If the total calculated dose is administered in divided doses, more severe neuritic pain occurs. Sensory loss, paresthesias, difficulty walking, hyporeflexia, and muscle wasting may occur and may become progressively worse as therapy continues. Neurologic symptoms usually resolve within 6 months; however, residual effects have been prolonged in some patients. Other adverse effects from vincristine include bronchospasm, hepatic venoocclusive disease, transient cortical blindness and optic atrophy with blindness, and bladder atony. Glutamic acid given with vincristine has been known to decrease the adverse effects. Nonneurologic symptoms are similar to those of other anticancer drugs.

Vincristine is a substrate for the cytochrome P450 system. Several drug interactions may occur with vincristine, so the patient should report all medications being taken, including OTC medicines, vitamins, minerals, and herbal supplements. Other CYP3A4 inhibitors—including L-asparaginase, calcium channel blockers, amiodarone, statin drugs, proton pump inhibitors, and grapefruit juice—can decrease metabolism of vincristine, thereby increasing tissue exposure. CYP3A4 inducers such as phenytoin, barbiturates, and nafcillin decrease vincristine efficacy. Prototype Drug Chart: Vincristine details the pharmacologic behavior of vincristine.

OTHER DRUGS TO TREAT CANCER

Immunomodulators

Chapter 24 provides information on other immunomodulators used as antiinflammatories. Thalidomide has antiangiogenic, immunomodulatory, and antitumor properties. The exact mechanism of action is unknown; however, thalidomide selectively reduces levels of tumor necrosis factor alpha (TNF-α), inhibits interleukin 12 (IL-12), increases IL-2, and increases interferon (IFN) gamma. Thalidomide is used to treat moderate to severe erythema nodosum leprosum (ENL; leprosy), and it is used with dexamethasone to treat patients with multiple myeloma. Thalidomide is well known for its teratogenicity; hence availability is limited. Other immunomodulators designed to strengthen the immune system to attack cancer cells include monoclonal antibody therapy (i.e., rituximab and alemtuzumab), nonspecific immunotherapies, and vaccines.

> ⚡ **PATIENT SAFETY**
>
> Serious drug interactions can occur. Obtain a complete medication list that includes over-the-counter preparations and herbal supplements.
> **Do Not Confuse...**
> - **Taxol** with **Taxotere** or **Paxil**
> - **Vincristine** with **vinblastine**

Vaccines

Recombinant vaccines include hepatitis B to prevent infection with HBV, which can cause liver cancer, and HPV quadrivalent, HPV-9 valent, and HPV bivalent, given to males and females aged 9 to 26 years to prevent HPV infections that can cause cervical cancer in females and genital warts in males. Sipuleucel-T is composed of autologous blood mononuclear cells and antigen-presenting cells (APCs) fused in protein, and it is given to stimulate T-cell immunity against the prostate cancer antigen prostatic acid phosphatase. Sipuleucel-T is the first immunotherapy to treat prostate cancer.

Biologic Response Modifiers

Biologic response modifiers (i.e., IL-2 and interferon-alfa) are also immunomodulators in that they stimulate or suppress the immune system. These are further discussed in Chapter 37. Adverse effects from immunomodulators include suppressed immune system, fatigue, nausea, and vomiting. Table 35.2 provides more information for general adverse effects from anticancer drugs.

Targeted Therapies

Targeted therapy is a relatively new approach to treating cancers. Some monoclonal antibodies are also considered targeted therapy. Targeted therapy attacks specific cells (proteins) interfering with tumor growth without harming healthy cells. Chapter 36 provides in-depth information on this treatment modality.

> ⚡ **PATIENT SAFETY**
>
> Thalidomide is a known human teratogen.
> **Do Not Confuse...**
> - **Thalomide** and **thalidomide** with **thiamine**

📋 PROTOTYPE DRUG CHART

Vincristine

Drug Class	Dosage
Plant alkaloid/vinca alkaloid	A: IV: 1.4 mg/m² q7d for 4 wk Various protocols exist, including combination therapy. Dosage varies based on indicated use and response. Adjust dose if hepatic impairment.
Contraindications	**Drug-Lab-Food Interactions**
Demyelinating form of Charcot-Marie-Tooth syndrome, hypersensitivity to vincristine, pregnancy *Caution:* Liver impairment, history of viral infections, neurotoxicity, electrolyte imbalances, patients receiving radiation through ports (including liver), elderly *Hyaluronidase* may be given for extravasation.	Drug: Many drug-drug interactions exist. Vincristine can increase serum concentrations of methotrexate and bleomycin. Neurotoxicity can result if asparaginase or pegaspargase is coadministered with vincristine. Many drugs increase the concentration of vincristine; some include amiodarone, statin drugs, proton pump inhibitors, and testosterone. All these drugs inhibit the P-glycoprotein system. Lab: May increase serum uric acid, may cause leukopenia, may cause hyponatremia

PROTOTYPE DRUG CHART—CONT'D

Vincristine

Pharmacokinetics	Pharmacodynamics
Absorption: IV	Onset: UK
Distribution: PB: 44%	Peak: 4 d
Metabolism: Liver; t½: triphasic 19–155 h	Duration: 7 d
Excretion: 80% in feces; 10%–20% in urine	

Therapeutic Effects/Uses
Hodgkin disease, non-Hodgkin lymphoma, neuroblastoma, rhabdomyosarcoma, Wilms tumor, acute lymphocytic leukemia
Mechanism of action: Affects cells in the M and S phase of the cell cycle by inhibiting microtubule formation; inhibits cell division and RNA, DNA, and protein synthesis

Side Effects	Adverse Reactions
Peripheral neuropathy, loss of deep tendon reflexes, phlebitis, constipation, cramps, nausea, vomiting, muscle weakness, reversible alopecia *Glutamic acid* may decrease adverse effects. *Leucovorin* may be given as a cytoprotectant from the toxic effects of vincristine.	Hepatic venoocclusive disease, neurotoxicity (dose dependent), sensory loss, hypotension, visual disturbances, ptosis, ileus, SIADH, hyponatremia, hyperuricemia, severe local reaction with extravasation, fever *Life-threatening:* Intestinal necrosis, seizures, coma, acute bronchospasm, bone marrow suppression

A, Adult; *d*, day; *DNA*, deoxyribonucleic acid; *h*, hour; *IV*, intravenous; *PB*, protein binding; *q*, every; *RNA*, ribonucleic acid; *SIADH*, syndrome of inappropriate antidiuretic hormone; *t½*, half-life; *UK*, unknown; *wk*, weeks; <, less than; ≥, greater than or equal to.

CLINICAL JUDGMENT [NURSING PROCESS]
Plant Alkaloid: Vincristine

Concept: Sensory Perception
- Receiving and interpreting various stimuli for functional nervous system pathways to the brain

Recognize Cues [Assessment]
- Conduct a detailed medication history that lists all concurrent medications and includes prescriptions, over-the-counter medicines, antacids, dietary supplements, vitamins, and herbal supplements to avoid drug interactions.
- Obtain baseline information about the patient's physical status. This should include height, weight, vital signs, cardiopulmonary assessment, intake and output, skin assessment, daily activities status (i.e., ability to perform activities of daily living), sleep-wake cycle, nutritional status, presence or absence of underlying symptoms of disease, and the use of current or past medications and treatments. Be especially aware of evidence of neurotoxicity such as peripheral neuropathy (numbness or tingling in fingers or toes), loss of deep tendon reflexes, foot drop, slapping gait, and difficulty walking.
- Assess baseline laboratory values (complete blood count, liver and renal function tests, serum sodium, and serum bilirubin) for comparison with future values.
- Monitor for acute bronchospasm.
- Monitor bowel and urinary function. Autonomic neuropathy may lead to constipation, paralytic ileus, and bladder atony.
- Obtain baseline data regarding psychosocial status that include the patient's educational level, ability and desire to learn, support systems, past coping strategies, presence or absence of emotional difficulties, and self-care abilities.

Analyze Cues and Prioritize Hypothesis [Patient Problems]
- Risk for reduced sensory perception
- Risk for constipation
- Risk for urinary elimination
- Need for teaching

Generate Solutions [Planning]
- The patient will be free from neuropathic dysfunction.
- The patient will be free from respiratory complications (bronchospasm).
- The patient will maintain adequate bowel function.
- The patient will maintain adequate urinary function.
- The patient/family/caregiver will demonstrate understanding of the chemotherapy regimen, including side effects.

Take Action [Nursing Interventions]
- Assess for signs of respiratory distress during and after drug administration.
- Monitor for signs of peripheral neuropathy (numbness or tingling in hands or feet, sensory loss, loss of deep tendon reflexes, paresthesia, foot drop or wrist drop, ataxia).
- Assess the intravenous (IV) site carefully. Give the drug through a large-bore, quickly running IV infusion.
- Monitor the IV site for extravasation, and if it occurs, stop the infusion immediately and follow the drug protocol for extravasation.
- Monitor blood counts and laboratory values.
- Maintain strict medical asepsis during dressing changes and invasive procedures.
- Administer stool softener or laxative as prescribed.
- Monitor fluid intake and output and nutritional intake.

Patient Teaching
General
- Teach patients the signs and symptoms of neurotoxicity: numbness or tingling in hands or feet, sensory loss, loss of deep tendon reflexes, paresthesia, foot or wrist drop, and ataxia.
- Emphasize the importance of notifying the health care provider of any breathing difficulties such as wheezing, shortness of breath, and anxiety.
- Advise patients to promptly report signs of infection (fever, sore throat), bleeding (bleeding gums, petechiae, bruises, hematuria, blood in the stool), and anemia (increased fatigue, dyspnea, orthostatic hypotension).
- Emphasize protective precautions such as hand washing and personal hygiene.

Side Effects
- Teach patients the signs of peripheral neuropathy.
- Teach patients the signs of respiratory compromise.

Continued

CLINICAL JUDGMENT [NURSING PROCESS]—CONT'D
Plant Alkaloid: Vincristine

- Teach patients to report constipation, abdominal pain, and difficulty with urination.
- Teach patients the signs of drug extravasation into tissue, which can occur 3 to 4 weeks after administration of the drug.

Diet
- Encourage bulky high-fiber foods and moderate exercise to reduce the risk of constipation.

- Encourage adequate hydration to prevent electrolyte imbalances and renal toxicity.

Evaluate Outcomes [Evaluation]
- Bowel function is maintained.
- Electrolytes and renal function are maintained.
- Peripheral neuropathy did not occur.
- Patient/family/caregiver educational needs are met.

Hormones and Hormonal Agonists and Antagonists

Although hormones are not considered true chemotherapeutic agents, several classes of hormonal agents are used in the treatment of cancer. These hormones do not work in the same ways as standard chemotherapy drugs. Instead, the hormones mask the cancer cells and prevent them from using or producing hormones. These include corticosteroids, estrogens, antiestrogens, aromatase inhibitors, gonadotropin-releasing hormone, progestins, and antiandrogens.

Corticosteroids

Corticosteroids are natural hormones and hormone-like drugs used to treat many types of cancer and noncancerous disorders. They are divided into glucocorticoids and mineralocorticoids. These steroids should not be confused with anabolic steroids (i.e., growth hormone). *Glucocorticoids* assist with protein metabolism; examples of such steroids are prednisone, methylprednisolone, hydrocortisone, and dexamethasone. Steroids suppress the inflammatory process associated with tumor growth. In addition, they are also considered immunosuppressives, which depress the patient's immune system. Steroids are used to treat leukemias, multiple myeloma, IBD, and transplant rejection, among other disorders. Because steroids suppress both the immune and the inflammatory systems, they can mask infection. Other common adverse effects include delirium, elevated serum glucose, insomnia, irritability, and other psychological problems. Because of its deleterious effects, it is recommended to avoid the use of prednisone among older adults who are at high risk for delirium. Prednisone is the most common steroid prescribed and is four times as potent as a glucocorticoid. Prednisone has little mineralocorticoid activity. Other adverse effects of prednisone include fluid retention, muscle weakness, irregular menstrual bleeding, atherosclerosis, and thrombosis, among others. It is metabolized in the liver to its active metabolite prednisolone, and the drug is excreted in the urine.

Sex Hormones

The sex hormones (estrogen, androgen) and hormone-like drugs are used to slow the growth of hormone-dependent tumors (e.g., prostate cancer and breast cancer). Exogenous estrogens maintain all the properties of endogenous estrogens, and estrogen therapy is a palliative treatment used to slow the progression of prostatic cancer by decreasing testosterone production. Estrogen has also been used for the improvement of bone metastasis. An example of this group of drugs is conjugated estrogens. Synthetic progestin (e.g., hydroxyprogesterone caproate, megestrol, and medroxyprogesterone acetate) is used for renal and endometrial cancers. Both estrogen and progesterone are mainly metabolized by the liver, excreted through the biliary system, and eliminated by the kidneys. Adverse effects of estrogens and progestins include fluid retention, thrombosis, menstrual irregularities, and osteoporosis, among others. Testosterone is the primary androgen synthesized by the cells in the testes, ovaries, and adrenal cortex. Exogenous androgen opposes the activity of estrogen and is most effective for palliative treatment of breast cancer among postmenopausal females.

Table 35.7 lists sex hormones, hormonal agonists and antagonists, selective estrogen receptor modulators, luteinizing hormone–releasing hormone agonists, aromatase inhibitors, miscellaneous enzymes, and vaccines, as well as their uses and considerations.

Antiandrogens

Antiandrogens, such as bicalutamide and flutamide, and antiestrogens such as fulvestrant block the effects of testosterone and estrogen, respectively, thereby slowing or shrinking cancers.

Selective Estrogen Receptor Modulators

Selective estrogen receptor modulators such as tamoxifen and raloxifene have both estrogenic and antiestrogenic effects on various tissues. Tamoxifen is primarily used for breast cancer in both males and females. Raloxifene produces estrogenic effects in bone and lipids and has an antiestrogenic property in mammary tissues. It is used as a prophylactic against breast cancer in high-risk postmenopausal females with osteoporosis.

Luteinizing Hormone–Releasing Hormone Agonists

Luteinizing hormone–releasing hormone (LHRH), also known as *gonadotropin-releasing hormone* (GnRH) analogues or agonists (leuprolide, goserelin), suppresses the secretion of follicle-stimulating hormone and luteinizing hormone from the pituitary gland. In males, the continued suppression of the male hormone decreases the size of the prostate gland and produces an improvement in symptoms. In females, continued suppression of LHRH decreases serum estradiol and reduces the size and function of the ovaries, uterus, and mammary glands.

Aromatase Inhibitors

Aromatases are enzymes that convert other hormones into estrogen, and aromatase inhibitors are drugs that stop the enzyme from converting other hormones into estrogen. For example, in postmenopausal females, the ovaries no longer produce estrogen, but aromatase converts androgen to estrogen in this group of females. The aromatase inhibitors block the peripheral conversion of androgens to estrogens, thus suppressing the postmenopausal synthesis of estrogen and slowing tumor growth. Aromatase inhibitors are used in the treatment of hormonally sensitive breast cancer in postmenopausal females and premenopausal females who have had their ovaries removed. Anastrozole, letrozole, and exemestane are examples of aromatase inhibitors currently in use. Increasingly these agents are being used before tamoxifen in postmenopausal females with hormonally responsive metastatic breast cancer. Table 35.7 lists hormonal agents and their uses and considerations.

TABLE 35.7 Antineoplastics: Sex Hormones, Hormonal Agonists and Antagonists, Selective Estrogen Receptor Modulators, Luteinizing Hormone–Releasing Hormone Agonists, Aromatase Inhibitors, Enzymes, and Vaccines

- Visually inspect parenteral products for particulate matter and discoloration before use.
- Observe and exercise precautions when handling, preparing, and administering cytotoxic drugs.
- Antineoplastic drug dosages will vary from protocol to protocol. Consult appropriate references to verify doses.

Drug	Route and Dosage	Uses and Considerations
Sex Hormones		
Androgens		
Fluoxymesterone	Females: PO: 10–40 mg/d in divided doses	For breast cancer. Do *not* give to pregnant patients. PB: UK; t½: 9.2 h
Hormonal Agonists and Antagonists		
Abiraterone	Males: PO: 1 g/d	For prostate cancer. Assess liver function. PB: 99%; t½: 7–17 h
Anastrozole	PO: 1 mg/d	For advanced breast cancer. Monitor for cardiac toxicity and angioedema. PB: 40%; t½: 50 h
Bicalutamide	Males: PO: 50 mg/d	For prostate cancer. Monitor for hepatotoxicity. PB: 99%; t½: 6–10 d
Enzalutamide	PO: 160 mg/d	For prostate cancer. Given after docetaxel failure. PB: 97%; t½: 2.8–10.2 d
Exemestane	Postmenopausal females: PO: 25 mg/d	For breast cancer. Adjuvant treatment for those who have estrogen receptor–positive early disease and have received tamoxifen. PB: 90%; t½: 24 h
Flutamide	PO: 250 mg q8h; max daily dose: 750 mg	For prostate cancer. Assess for any suicidal thoughts or tendencies. Do not use with MAOIs. PB: 95%; t½: UK
Fulvestrant	IM: 500 mg on days 1, 15, and 29 and once monthly thereafter	For breast cancer. Avoid IV administration. PB: 99%; t½: UK
Goserelin acetate	Subcut: 3.6 mg q28d Implants available for prostate cancer	For breast and prostate cancers. Slow absorption for first 8 days of therapy. PB: <30%; t½: 4.2 h
Histrelin acetate implant	Males: Subcut implant: 50 mg q12mo	For prostate cancer. Contraindicated in children, females, and pregnancy. Proper surgical technique is critical to minimize adverse events. PB: UK; t½: 3.92 h
Letrozole	Postmenopausal females: PO: 2.5 mg/d	For breast cancer. Dose adjustment is needed for severe hepatic impairment. PB: UK; t½: 2 d
Leuprolide	Leuprolide acetate lyophilisate: Subcut: 1 mg/d Leuprolide acetate suspension: IM: Depot 7.5 mg q1mo	For prostate cancer. Cardiac, pulmonary, and hepatic toxicity can occur. PB: 43%–49%; t½: 3 h
Medroxyprogesterone	IM: Depot 400–1000 mg/wk; attempt to decrease to 400 mg/mo	For endometrial and renal cell cancers. Monitor hepatic and renal function. PB: >90%; t½: 30–50 d (dose dependent)
Megestrol acetate	Breast: PO: 40 mg qid Endometrial: PO: 40–320 mg/d divided doses	For breast and endometrial cancers. Risk for thromboembolism increases. PB: >90%; t½: 15–105 h
Mitotane	PO: 2–6 g/d in 3–4 divided doses, then 9–10 g/d	For adrenocortical cancer. Monitoring parameters include neurologic function and serum cortisol and potassium. PB: UK; t½: 18–159 d
Nilutamide	PO: 300 mg/d for 30 d, then 150 mg/d maintenance dose	For prostate cancer. Absolutely contraindicated in hepatic and respiratory disease. Use with caution in Asians. PB: UK; t½: 38–59 h
Raloxifene	Postmenopausal females: PO: 60 mg/d	For breast cancer prophylaxis. Increases risk of embolism and thromboembolism with estrogen products. PB: UK; t½: 25.8–86.6 h
Tamoxifen citrate	PO: 20–40 mg bid	For breast cancer. May cause abnormal Papanicolaou and vaginal smears; regular gynecologic examinations should be performed; uterine malignancy can occur. PB: UK; t½: 5–7 d
Toremifene citrate	Females: PO: 60 mg/d	For breast cancer. Absolutely contraindicated in those with hypokalemia, hypomagnesemia, and prolonged QT intervals. PB: >99%; t½: 5 d

Continued

TABLE 35.7 Antineoplastics: Sex Hormones, Hormonal Agonists and Antagonists, Selective Estrogen Receptor Modulators, Luteinizing Hormone–Releasing Hormone Agonists, Aromatase Inhibitors, Enzymes, and Vaccines—cont'd

Drug	Route and Dosage	Uses and Considerations
Miscellaneous Enzymes		
Asparaginase *Erwinia chrysanthemi*	To substitute pegaspargase: A: IV: 25,000 u/m² 3/wk for 6 doses To substitute L-asparaginase *Escherichia coli*: A: IV: 25,000 u/m² for each scheduled dose of L-asparaginase	For ALL. Used as part of combination treatment. Assess for any pancreatic complications. PB: UK; t½: 8–30 h
Pegaspargase	IV/IM: 2500 units/m² q14d	For ALL. Assess for any pancreatic complications or seizures. PB: UK; t½: 3.24–5.07 d
Vaccines		
Hepatitis B virus (HBV)	IM: Given in a series of 3 doses at 0, 1, and 3 mo	As prophylaxis against HBV. Contraindicated with known yeast hypersensitivity. PB: UK; t½: UK
Quadrivalent human papillomavirus (HPV; types 6, 11, 16, and 18) recombinant vaccine	IM: 0.5 mL given in a series of 3 doses (0, 2, and 6 mo)	As prophylaxis against HPV types 6, 11, 16, and 18 for prevention of cervical cancer. Contraindicated with known yeast hypersensitivity. PB: UK; t½: UK
HPV bivalent vaccine	IM: 0.5 mL given in a series of 3 shots (0, 1, and 6 mo) in deltoid region of upper arm	As prophylaxis against HPV for prevention of cervical cancer and precancerous lesions associated with the most common cancer-causing HPV types. PB: UK; t½: UK

Note: Chemotherapeutic doses and schedules vary depending on protocol, body surface area (m²), age, functional status, and comorbid conditions. For a full discussion of body surface area in dosage calculation, see Chapter 11.

ALL, acute lymphocytic leukemia; *bid*, twice daily; *d*, day; *h*, hour; *IM*, intramuscular; *IV*, intravenous; *MAOI*, monoamine oxidase inhibitor; *max*, maximum; *mo*, month; *PB*, protein binding; *PO*, by mouth; *q*, every; *qid*, four times daily; *subcut*, subcutaneous; *t½*, half-life; *UK*, unknown; *wk*, week; >, greater than; <, less than.

CLINICAL JUDGMENT SINGLE-EPISODE CASE STUDY

SLO: Apply knowledge of drug pharmacodynamics to determine which medication effects require a follow-up by the nurse.
NGN Item Type: Extended multiple response
Cognitive Skills: Recognize cues

A 43-year-old female with metastatic colorectal cancer has been receiving Bolus-IFL, which consists of irinotecan, fluorouracil (5-FU), and leucovorin 5 mg/kg IV every 2 weeks. The patient weighs 140 pounds. The patient presents to the oncology unit for the third round of treatment. Before starting treatment, the nurse documents the assessment findings.

Place a check mark next to the assessment data that requires a follow-up by the nurse.

Assessment
Temperature of 99.3°F
Blood pressure of 118/60 mm Hg
Heart rate at 94 beats per minute with occasional irregularities
Respiratory rate of 19 breaths per minute
Reports right upper quadrant abdominal pain
Reports being able to walk down the driveway to retrieve mail
States nausea but is able to tolerate oral intake
Weight gain of 2 pounds in 1 week
Electrocardiogram with premature ventricular contractions
States hands and feet have felt hot since last treatment

Answers

	Assessment
X	Temperature of 99.3°F for 5 days
	Blood pressure of 118/60 mm Hg
X	Heart rate at 94 beats per minute with occasional irregularities
	Respiratory rate of 19 breaths per minute
X	Reports right upper quadrant abdominal pain
	Reports being able to walk down the driveway to retrieve mail
	States nausea but is able to tolerate oral intake
	Weight gain of 2 pounds in 1 week
X	Electrocardiogram with premature ventricular contractions
X	States hands and feet have felt hot since last treatment

CLINICAL JUDGMENT SINGLE-EPISODE CASE STUDY—CONT'D

Rationale
Fluorouracil (5-FU) is an antimetabolite used to treat colorectal cancer. The mechanism of action of 5-FU affects cells during the S and G_1 phases of the cell cycle and interferes with healthy and cancer cell RNA synthesis. Anticancer drugs such as 5-FU can result in many side effects and adverse drug reactions because of their effect on healthy cells. Some of 5-FU negative effects include leukopenia, including neutropenia, increasing the patient's risk for infection. Fever is usually the first hallmark sign of an infection. Therefore, the nurse would follow up for any elevated temperature. A temperature of 99.3°F is slightly elevated. Anticancer drugs can also cause serious adverse drug reactions, such as hematologic toxicity, cardiotoxicity, and hepatotoxicity. Cardiac rhythm irregularities, such as skipped beats on palpation and premature ventricular contractions on electrocardiogram, would need further investigation. If these cardiac abnormalities are new, the dose of 5-FU may need to be adjusted. 5-FU is metabolized by the liver, and a report of right upper quadrant abdominal pain can indicate hepatic involvement. Reports of hands and feet feeling hot can indicate palmar-plantar erythrodysesthesia, an adverse hand-foot syndrome that includes erythema, swelling, and intense pain to the palms of the hands and soles of the feet. If the hand-foot syndrome is severe, the dose of 5-FU may need to be adjusted.

Reference
Chidharia A, Kanderi T, Kasi A. Chemotherapy acral erythema. *StatPearls [Internet]*. 2020. https://www.ncbi.nlm.nih.gov/books/NBK459375/.

REVIEW QUESTIONS

1. A patient is to receive a chemotherapy protocol that includes an alkylating agent, an antimetabolite, and an antitumor antibiotic. Which response by the nurse would be best when the patient asks the nurse why so much chemotherapy is needed?
   a. Combination of chemotherapeutic drugs works in the S phase to kill cells.
   b. Combination chemotherapy increases the extent of tumor cell killing.
   c. Combination chemotherapy uses drugs that work the same way.
   d. Combination chemotherapy has no dose-limiting toxicities.

2. A patient is scheduled to receive chemotherapy drugs that will cause myelosuppression. Which action by the nurse would be most important?
   a. Monitor for a change in temperature.
   b. Evaluate gastrointestinal function.
   c. Assess for evidence of cardiac compromise.
   d. Question the patient about changes in sense of taste.

3. The nurse is caring for a patient with colorectal cancer who is to receive fluorouracil. Which symptom would be most important for the nurse to report to the health care provider?
   a. Nausea
   b. Decreased appetite
   c. Bleeding gums
   d. Constipation

4. A patient in the outpatient oncology clinic reports fatigue after receiving chemotherapy. Which initial nursing action would be most appropriate?
   a. Assess for other factors contributing to their fatigue, such as trouble sleeping.
   b. Encourage a high-protein, high-calorie diet, and design it with the patient.
   c. Refer the patient to a physical therapist to develop a strenuous exercise program.
   d. Encourage the patient to sleep as much as possible during the day to ease fatigue.

5. A patient in the outpatient oncology clinic has developed mucositis after receiving fluorouracil. Which statement made by the patient indicates the need for additional teaching about mucositis?
   a. I will frequently rinse out my mouth with normal saline.
   b. To relieve my mouth pain, I will use ice pops or ice chips.
   c. I will use mouthwash with alcohol to clean my mouth.
   d. Using a soft toothbrush will clean my teeth and freshen my breath.

6. A patient is scheduled to receive high-dose cyclophosphamide via an intravenous infusion as treatment for cancer. Which patient teaching would be most important for the nurse to include on cyclophosphamide?
   a. An indwelling urinary catheter will be placed.
   b. Drink at least 2 liters of fluid per day.
   c. Empty the bladder every 4 to 6 hours.
   d. Limit fluid intake during chemotherapy.

7. A nurse is administering doxorubicin to a patient in the outpatient oncology clinic. Which information would be most important for the nurse to include in patient teaching?
   a. Blood counts will most likely remain normal.
   b. Complete alopecia rarely occurs with this drug.
   c. Report any shortness of breath, palpitations, or edema to the health care provider.
   d. Tissue necrosis usually occurs 2 to 3 days after administration.

8. A patient diagnosed with cancer is scheduled to receive vincristine. Which assessment would have the highest priority when providing care for this patient?
   a. Degree of alopecia
   b. Increased digoxin levels
   c. Decreased phenytoin effects
   d. Peripheral neuropathy

9. A patient is experiencing mucositis (stomatitis) after receiving chemotherapy. Which symptomatic treatment will be appropriate? **Select all that apply.**
   a. Frequent mouth rinses
   b. Antiemetics
   c. Topical anesthetics
   d. Stress reduction
   e. Antibiotics

10. A nurse is teaching a patient who will receive chemotherapy that can cause thrombocytopenia. Which instructions would the nurse include in the patient's teaching plan? **Select all that apply.**
    a. Use an electric razor when shaving.
    b. Use a soft-bristled toothbrush.
    c. Use aspirin for pain or headache.
    d. Monitor oral temperature daily.
    e. Report any bleeding (gums, petechiae, bruises, hematuria, melena) to the health care provider.

36

Targeted Therapies to Treat Cancer

http://evolve.elsevier.com/McCuistion/pharmacology

OBJECTIVES

- Summarize how targeted therapy treats cancer.
- Describe how angiogenesis inhibitors prevent tumor growth.
- Discuss how epidermal growth factor receptor inhibitors prevent tumor growth.
- Explain how tyrosine kinase and multikinase inhibitors prevent tumor growth.
- Describe how mTOR kinase inhibitors and proteasome inhibitors prevent tumor growth.
- Discuss the general actions of monoclonal antibodies in the treatment of cancer.

OUTLINE

Overview of Targeted Therapy, 446
    Approaches to Targeted Therapy, 446
    General Mechanisms of Action of Targeted Therapy, 447
    Limitations of Targeted Therapy, 447
Angiogenesis Inhibitors/Vascular Endothelial Growth Factor Receptor Inhibitors, 447
    Angiogenesis Inhibitors Mechanisms, 447
    Ziv-Aflibercept, 447
Epidermal Growth Factor Receptor Inhibitors, 448
    Gefitinib, 448
    Osimertinib, 451
Tyrosine Kinase Inhibitors and Multikinase Inhibitors, 452
    Alectinib, 453
    Nilotinib, 454
    Dasatinib, 454
    Sorafenib, 455
    Sunitinib, 455
mTOR Kinase Inhibitors and Proteasome Inhibitors, 455
    Temsirolimus, 456
    Carfilzomib, 457
    Ixazomib, 457
Monoclonal Antibodies, 459
    Alemtuzumab, 459
    Cetuximab, 460
    Ibritumomab Tiuxetan, 461
    Panitumumab, 461
    Tositumomab, 461
    Trastuzumab, 464
Clinical Judgment Case Study, 464
Review Questions, 464

OVERVIEW OF TARGETED THERAPY

As discussed in Chapter 35, traditional chemotherapy is systemic, and its chemical makeup is cytotoxic such that it directly damages or kills normal, healthy cells, and cancer cells. Chemotherapeutic drugs inhibit *mitosis*, which can damage the RNA and DNA and thus prevent cell division, eventually causing apoptosis, or programmed cell death. Even though traditional chemotherapy treatments improve cancer control and increase long-term survival, adverse effects of traditional chemotherapy can be life-threatening. Furthermore, traditional chemotherapy's cancer cell–killing effect is limited by the dosages and scheduling regimens needed to reduce toxic side effects on normal cells. Drugs that molecularly target cells associated with cancer are currently the focus of much research.

In 1998 *targeted therapy* was first recognized as a potential cancer therapy against certain cell receptors. Targeted therapy for cancer treatment differs from traditional cancer chemotherapy in that targeted therapies are specific, deliberate, and cytostatic, whereas most standard chemotherapies are not specific but rather are cytotoxic to normal and abnormal cells. Targeted therapy is the cornerstone of precision medicine because it directs the treatment according to the person's genes and proteins. The National Cancer Institute defines *targeted therapy* as drugs or other substances that block the growth and spread of cancer by interfering with specific molecules involved in tumor growth, progression, and spread.

The rapid identification of specific cancer cell targets in recent years has led to an increased development of targeted therapies. Management of patient issues related to targeted therapies is an evolving area of study. With many targeted therapies being new to the market, costs can be prohibitive.

Approaches to Targeted Therapy

The ability to treat cancers with targeted therapy continues to expand. Currently, there are three approaches to targeted therapy. One approach compares individual proteins in cancer cells with those of normal cells. An example of a differentially expressed target is the human epidermal growth factor receptor 2 protein (*ERBB2*), which is expressed at high levels in breast and gastric cancers. Targeted therapy directed at *ERBB2* includes trastuzumab, which has been approved by the US Food and Drug Administration (FDA) to treat certain breast and gastric cancers. A second approach identifies mutant proteins that can cause cancer progression. An example of a mutant cell is the *BRAF* gene in its altered form, *BRAF V600E*, in melanomas. Vemurafenib targets this altered form of *BRAF* and has been approved to treat metastatic or inoperable melanomas. A third approach looks for abnormal chromosomes present in cancer cells but not in normal cells. Chromosomal abnormalities can result in gene fusion, wherein parts of two different genes are incorporated as one gene. These fusion proteins can increase cancer development. Imatinib mesylate is one example of a therapy that targets the *BCR-ABL1* fusion protein responsible for the growth of some leukemic cells.

General Mechanisms of Action of Targeted Therapy

According to the American Cancer Society, targeted therapies have five ways to attack cancer cells. One way is for the drug to block or turn off chemical signals. In cancer cells, the cells are stimulated to divide continuously without being prompted by external growth factors. Signal transduction inhibitors (STIs) block signals to cancerous cells by blocking signals passed from one molecule to another; this prevents cancer cells from growing and dividing. Second, targeted drugs can change proteins within the cancer cells causing cell lysis. Third, targeted drugs can prevent cancer cells from angiogenesis, the formation of new vessels. Fourth, targeted therapies can trigger the immune system to kill cancer cells. Lastly, targeted therapy is toxic to cancer cells but not to noncancerous cells.

Targeted cancer therapies are STIs that block signal transduction among specific molecules, which block the growth and spread of cancerous cells. Drugs that target specific cells inhibit cancer cell division by blocking cancer membrane receptors and tyrosine kinase (TK) activities, interfering with signal transduction, stimulating immune system attacks on cancer cells, or inducing cells to undergo apoptosis.

Targeted therapies are more selective for specific molecular targets than cytotoxic anticancer drugs; thus, they are able to kill cancer cells with less damage to normal cells compared with chemotherapy. They are the cornerstone of precision medicine that uses a person's genes and proteins to prevent, diagnose, and treat cancer. Targeted therapies are sometimes known as *molecular targeted drugs* and *precision medicines*. Most targeted therapies consist of either small molecules or large molecules. Small molecular drugs enter cancer cells, whereas large molecules affect the surfaces of cancer cells. Drug classes used for targeted therapies include angiogenesis inhibitors, epidermal growth factor receptor (EGFR)-TK inhibitors, BCR-ABL1 TK inhibitors, proteasome inhibitors, and monoclonal antibodies (mAbs). All but the mAbs are small-molecule drugs, and they are *not* antibodies. Most generic small-molecule drugs have *-nib* or *-mib* suffixes, such as imatinib and bortezomib. Large-molecule drugs are mAbs and generally have *-mab* suffixes, such as rituxi*mab*. Table 36.1 identifies other suffixes common to small- and large-molecule drugs. Small-molecule drugs are usually administered orally, whereas mAbs are given intravenously. All targeted therapies are categorized as high-alert medications. Targeted drugs may be used as monotherapy (a single agent), in combination with traditional chemotherapy, and with radiotherapy. Side effects and risks associated with targeted therapy include diarrhea, hepatitis, thrombus formation, poor wound healing, hypertension, fatigue, stomatitis, and skin changes, among others.

Limitations of Targeted Therapy

Targeted therapies do have limitations. One limitation is that cancers that do not have enough of the specific molecular targets will not respond to targeted therapy. Another limitation involves cancer cells mutating and becoming drug resistant. Finally, yet another limitation of targeted therapy is the difficulty of developing drugs for some identified targets.

TABLE 36.1 Suffixes of Targeted Cancer Therapies

Suffix	Meaning
-mab	A monoclonal antibody
-momab	A monoclonal antibody composed of only murine (mouse) proteins
-imab	A monoclonal antibody composed of more human proteins (>60%) than murine proteins (~30%)
-zumab	A monoclonal antibody composed of mostly human proteins (95% or more) and only a few murine proteins (<5%)
-umab	A monoclonal antibody composed of only human proteins and no murine proteins
-nib	A tyrosine kinase inhibitor
-mib	A proteasome inhibitor

⚡ PATIENT SAFETY

Do Not Confuse…
- **Trastuzumab**, a chemotherapy drug, with **tositumomab**, a murine monoclonal antibody
- **Bortezomib**, a chemotherapy drug for multiple myeloma and mantle cell lymphoma, with **bevacizumab**, a chemotherapy drug for colorectal, lung, ovary, and kidney cancers and glioblastoma

ANGIOGENESIS INHIBITORS/VASCULAR ENDOTHELIAL GROWTH FACTOR RECEPTOR INHIBITORS

Angiogenesis Inhibitors Mechanisms

Most angiogenesis inhibitors are small-molecule drugs that prevent new blood vessels from forming; blood vessels are required for tumors to spread and grow. Some angiogenesis inhibitors interfere with the action of vascular endothelial growth factor (*VEGF*), a substance that stimulates new blood vessel formation. Others prevent the formation of platelet-derived growth factor (*PDGF*) that is intricate in the formation of new blood vessels and in the growth of preexisting blood vessels. Some angiogenesis inhibitors are large-molecule drug (mAbs), such as bevacizu*mab*. Prototype Drug Chart: Bevacizumab lists specific drug information for bevacizumab.

Ziv-Aflibercept

Ziv-aflibercept is a fully humanized recombinant fusion protein that inhibits angiogenesis. It is indicated in combination with 5-fluorouracil (5-FU), leucovorin, and irinotecan (FOLFIRI) for the treatment of metastatic colorectal cancer that is resistant to or has progressed after receiving an oxaliplatin-containing regimen.

Pharmacokinetics

Ziv-aflibercept is administered by intravenous (IV) infusion. Its elimination half-life is approximately 6 days, which appears to be dose dependent. The steady state is also dose dependent, with the average steady state reached by the second dose in a 2-week regimen. The metabolic and elimination pathways are unknown. However, free ziv-aflibercept does not seem to be affected by mild to moderate hepatic or renal impairment.

Pharmacodynamics

Ziv-aflibercept is an angiogenesis inhibitor that acts as a soluble receptor to bind VEGFs A and B and placental growth factors 1 and 2, which prevents other native receptors from binding. This action can result in decreased neovascularization and decreased vascular permeability.

Side Effects and Adverse Reactions

Ziv-aflibercept can cause severe bleeding, including gastrointestinal (GI) bleeding, intractable bleeding, and pulmonary hemorrhage. GI perforations, some fatal, have also been reported. Other adverse events include compromised wound healing and/or wound dehiscence, reversible posterior leukoencephalopathy syndrome, hypertensive crisis, nephrotic syndrome, or thrombotic microangiopathy. Common side effects include diarrhea, dizziness, asthenia, weight loss, and dehydration.

Drug Interactions

No interactions have been reported.

EPIDERMAL GROWTH FACTOR RECEPTOR INHIBITORS

The largest class of targeted therapy that attacks a particular molecular target is EGFR inhibitors. These receptors are overexpressed, dysregulated, or mutated in many epithelial cancers. EGFR expression has been associated with poor prognosis, metastasis, chemotherapy resistance, hormonal therapy, and radiation therapy. The activation of *EGFRs* is important in cancer cell growth and proliferation. Most EGFR inhibitors also inhibit TK indirectly. However, two other classes of EGFR inhibitors target *EGFR* extracellularly (mAbs) and also target the receptor catalytic domain of *EGFR* (TK inhibitors). These two classes are further discussed under the headings *Monoclonal Antibodies* and *Tyrosine Kinase Inhibitors and Multikinase Inhibitors*. The EGFR inhibitors that inhibit TK indirectly include erlotinib, gefitinib, and osimertinib. The growth factor receptors on the cell membrane can activate TKs, which then turn on signal transduction pathways that promote cell division. The EGFR inhibitors bind to different areas of the *EGFR*, blocking its activity so that it cannot activate TK. As a result, the downstream signal transduction pathway for promotion of cell division is inhibited, and cell proliferation is severely limited. Table 36.2 lists the EGFR inhibitors and their dosages, routes, uses, and considerations. Prototype Drug Chart: Erlotinib lists the specific drug information for erlotinib.

Gefitinib

Gefitinib is a synthetic anilinoquinazoline that selectively inhibits the epidermal growth factor receptor tyrosine kinase (EGFR-TK). It is most commonly used in the management of locally or advanced metastatic non–small cell lung cancer (NSCLC).

TABLE 36.2 Small-Molecule Inhibitors

Drug Name and Type	Route and Dosage	Uses and Considerations
Angiogenesis Inhibitors/Vascular Endothelial Growth Factor Receptor Inhibitors		
Bevacizumab (VEGFR/mAb; prototype)	See Prototype Drug Chart: Bevacizumab	
Ziv-aflibercept (VEGFR)	A: IV: 4 mg/kg over 1 h, followed by FOLFIRI. Steady state is reached by the second dose.	For metastatic colorectal cancer. Fully humanized angiogenesis inhibitor. Monitor ANC and UA. Discontinue for severe bleeding, GI perforation, fistula formation, wound dehiscence, hypertensive crisis/hypertensive encephalopathy, arterial thromboembolic events, and reversible posterior leukoencephalopathy syndrome. PB: UK; t½: 6 d
Epidermal Growth Factor Receptor Inhibitors		
Erlotinib (prototype)	See Prototype Drug Chart: Erlotinib	
Gefitinib	A: PO: 250 mg once daily. Steady state is achieved in 10 d.	For NSCLC. Monitor LFTs, and increase the dose if used concomitantly with strong CYP3A4 inducers. Drug may be held for up to 14 d if patient develops poorly managed diarrhea, worsening ocular or pulmonary disorders, or worsening rash. Discontinue if GI perforation or interstitial lung disease is present. PB: 90%; t½: 48 h
Osimertinib	A: PO: 80 mg/d	For NSCLC. Dose adjustment is required for treatment-related toxicities. Contraindicated in patients with interstitial lung disease/pneumonitis and symptomatic heart failure. Monitor ECG, ejection fraction, and serum electrolytes. PB: Likely high based on physiochemical properties; t½: 48 h
Tyrosine Kinase Inhibitors/Multikinase Inhibitors		
Alectinib (TKI)	A: PO: 600 mg bid with food until disease progression or unacceptable toxicity occurs	For *ALK*-positive metastatic NSCLC in a patient who has progressed or is intolerant to crizotinib. Monitor LFTs, worsening respiratory symptoms, heart rate and blood pressure, and CPK levels. PB: >99%; t½: 31–33 h

TABLE 36.2 Small-Molecule Inhibitors—cont'd

Drug Name and Type	Route and Dosage	Uses and Considerations
Dasatinib (MKI)	A: PO: Advanced CML, resistance or intolerance to prior therapy: 100–140 mg/d; can be increased to 180 mg/d if response is inadequate with the initial dose. Newly diagnosed CML: 100 mg/d; may be increased to 140 mg/d if response is inadequate.	For Ph+ CML and ALL. Adjust dose with concomitant use of a strong CYP3A4 inhibitor/inducer. Avoid grapefruit juice and concomitant use with H_2-receptor antagonists or proton pump inhibitors. Monitor CBC, serum electrolytes, and uric acid. PB: 96%; t½: 3–5 h
Imatinib mesylate, STI-571 (TKI) prototype	See Prototype Drug Chart: Imatinib Mesylate, STI-571	
Nilotinib (TKI)	A: PO: Resistance or intolerance to imatinib: 400 mg bid on an empty stomach. Newly diagnosed Ph+ CML: 300 mg bid on an empty stomach	For Ph+ CML. No food should be given 1 hour after or 2 hours before dose is taken. Capsule may be opened and dispersed in 1 teaspoon of applesauce. Monitor ECG, CBC, electrolytes, LFTs, pancreatic functions, uric acid, and weight. *Absolute contraindications:* Hypokalemia, hypomagnesemia, long QT syndrome, and QT prolongation. PB: 98%; t½: 17 h
Sorafenib (MKI)	A: PO: 400 mg bid; administer without food, at least 1 h before or 2 h after meal.	For hepatocellular, renal cell, and thyroid cancers. Adjust the dose if use is concomitant with a strong CYP3A4 inhibitor/inducer. Monitor CBC and LFTs. PB: 99.5%; t½: 25–48 h
Sunitinib (MKI)	GIST and RCC: A: PO: 50 mg/d on a schedule of 4 wk on treatment followed by 2 wk off treatment. PNET: A: PO: 37.5 mg/d; administer with or without food.	For GIST, PNET, and advanced RCC. Avoid concomitant use with a strong CYP3A4 inhibitor/inducer. Monitor UA and cardiac function. PB: sunitinib 95%; metabolite 90%; t½: sunitinib 40–60 h, major metabolite 80–110 h
mTOR Kinase Inhibitors (mTOR)/Proteasome Inhibitors (PIs)		
Bortezomib (prototype)	See Prototype Drug Chart: Bortezomib	
Carfilzomib (PI)	A: IV: Progressive disease on or within 60 d after completing therapy: Cycle 1: 20 mg/m² on days 1 and 2; if tolerated, increase to 27 mg/m² on days 8, 9, 15, and 16. Treatment cycles are repeated q28d. Cycles 2–12: 27 mg/m² on days 1, 2, 8, 9, 15, and 16. Cycles 13 and beyond: 27 mg/m² on days 1, 2, 15, and 16. Relapsed multiple myeloma: Give carfilzomib as discussed earlier with lenalidomide daily for 21 d of each cycle and dexamethasone on days 1, 8, 15, and 22 of each cycle. Treatment cycles are repeated q28d.	For relapsed multiple myeloma refractory to previous one to three lines of therapy, in combination with lenalidomide and dexamethasone. Premedicate with dexamethasone 30 min to 4 h before carfilzomib. Prehydrate and maintain hydration with oral and IV fluids. Monitor CBC, liver and renal function, and uric acid. PB: 97%; t½: ≤1 h
Ixazomib (PI)	A: PO: 4 mg on days 1, 8, and 15 in combination with lenalidomide on days 1 through 21 and dexamethasone on days 1, 8, 15, and 22. Repeat treatment cycles q28d.	For relapsed multiple myeloma refractory to one previous therapy. Give with lenalidomide and dexamethasone; and adjust dose for hepatic or renal impairment. Adjust or hold dose for hematologic toxicity, moderate-grade rash, peripheral neuropathy, and other nonhematologic toxicity. PB: 99%; t½: 9.5 d
Temsirolimus (mTOR)	A: IV: 25 mg given over 30–60 min once per wk	For advanced RCC. Premedicate with antihistamine intravenously approximately 30 min before the start of infusion. Two dilutions are required before IV infusion; use only the supplied diluent for initial dilution. Avoid strong CYP3A4 inducers/inhibitors. Dose reduction is required in patients with mild hepatic impairment. *Contraindication:* Moderate to severe hepatic impairment. PB: UK; t½: 17 h

A, Adult; *ALL*, acute lymphoblastic leukemia; *ANC*, absolute neutrophil count; *bid*, twice daily; *CBC*, complete blood count; *CML*, chronic myelogenous leukemia; *CPK*, creatine phosphokinase; *CYP3A4*, cytochrome P3A4; *d*, day; *ECG*, electrocardiograph; *FOLFIRI*, folinic acid, fluorouracil, and irinotecan; *GI*, gastrointestinal; *GIST*, gastrointestinal stromal tumor; *h*, hour; *IV*, intravenous; *LFT*, liver function test; *mAb*, monoclonal antibody; *min*, minutes; *MKI*, multikinase inhibitor; *mTOR*, mechanistic target of rapamycin; *NSCLC*, non–small cell lung cancer; *PB*, protein bound; *Ph+*, Philadelphia chromosome positive; *PI*, proteasome inhibitor; *PNET*, pancreatic neuroendocrine tumor; *PO*, oral; *q*, every; *RCC*, renal cell carcinoma; *t½*, half-life; *TKI*, tyrosine kinase inhibitor; *UA*, urinalysis; *UK*, unknown; *VEGFR*, vascular endothelial growth factor receptor; *wk*, week; >, greater than; ≤, less than or equal to.

Pharmacokinetics

Gefitinib is taken orally and is absorbed slowly in the GI tract, with 60% reaching systemic circulation. Peak plasma level occurs 3 to 7 hours after dosing. No significant alteration in its bioavailability was noted when gefitinib was taken with food. It is metabolized mainly by the hepatic system primarily through the CYP3A4 enzyme. Gefitinib is primarily excreted in the feces, mostly in the form of its metabolites. The elimination half-life is approximately 48 hours.

Pharmacodynamics

Gefitinib reversibly binds to the adenosine triphosphate (ATP) binding site and completely inhibits autophosphorylation by EGFR-TK; EGFR-TK functions as a mediator of cell growth, differentiation, and death. This action results in blockage of downstream EGFR-TK–mediated signal transduction pathways, cell cycle arrest, and inhibition of angiogenesis.

Side Effects and Adverse Reactions

Common side effects include skin reactions, diarrhea, anorexia, vomiting, and elevated transaminases. Gefitinib can cause conjunctivitis and abnormal eyelash growth, and rash occurs in about 47% of patients. Patients can also experience acne, pruritus, and nail disorders. Interstitial lung disease and GI perforation were also reported.

PROTOTYPE DRUG CHART

Bevacizumab

Drug Class	Dosage
Monoclonal antibody/angiogenesis inhibitor (VEGF inhibitor)	A: IV: *Colorectal cancer:* 5 or 10 mg/kg q2wk in combination with 5-FU; or 5 or 7.5 mg/kg q2–3wk with fluoropyrimidine and irinotecan or fluoropyrimidine and oxaliplatin. *NSCLC:* 15 mg/kg q3wk with carboplatin and paclitaxel. *Metastatic RCC:* 10 mg/kg q2wk in combination with interferon-alfa. *Progressive glioblastoma:* 10 mg/kg q2wk on a 28-d cycle. *Ovarian cancer:* 10 mg/kg q2wk in combination with paclitaxel, topotecan, or pegylated liposomal doxorubicin. *Cervical cancer:* 15 mg/kg with cisplatin on day 2 in combination with paclitaxel q3wk. Other treatment protocols exist (see full prescriber's information).
Contraindications	**Drug-Lab-Food Interactions**
No absolute contraindications. Warnings and precautions during treatment include serious bleeding (e.g., GI, intracranial), GI obstruction/perforation, wound dehiscence, and nephrotic syndrome. *Caution:* Known murine protein hypersensitivity, hamster protein hypersensitivity, or sensitivity to any other component of the drug; preexisting hypertension, cardiovascular disease, renal disease, history of glaucoma (see full prescriber's information for a complete list).	Drug: When used as combination therapy with irinotecan, incidence of grade 3–4 diarrhea and neutropenia increased and serum concentration of irinotecan active metabolites increased. Concomitant use with sunitinib increased incidences of microangiopathic hemolytic anemia. Concomitant use with daunorubicin, doxorubicin, and epirubicin, among others, has an increased risk of cardiotoxicity. Lab: None known Food: None known
Pharmacokinetics	**Pharmacodynamics**
Absorption: IV, bioavailability UK Distribution: PB: UK; steady-state levels achieved at approximately 100 d Metabolism: UK; t½: 11–50 d, dose dependent Excretion: Clearance of drug varies by weight, sex, and tumor burden	Onset: UK Peak: UK Duration: UK
Therapeutic Effects/Uses	
For cervical, colorectal, and ovarian cancers; metastatic RCC; NSCLC; and relapsed glioblastoma multiforme Mechanism of Action: Recombinant humanized monoclonal antibody binds to VEGF and prevents the binding of VEGF with its receptors, which are found on the surface of endothelial cells. The role of VEGF is critical in angiogenesis, the formation of new blood vessels. In human cancers, increased VEGF expression is associated with increased microvascular density, tumor growth, metastasis, and poor prognosis. The result of bevacizumab therapy is the reduction of microvascular growth and inhibition of metastatic disease progression.	
Side Effects	**Adverse Reactions**
Hypertension, proteinuria, cephalgia, rhinitis, taste alteration, dry skin, rectal hemorrhage, lacrimation disorder, back pain, and exfoliative dermatitis	Perforation or fistula, thromboembolic events, hypertensive crisis/encephalopathy, nephrotic syndrome, infusion reactions, embryonic/fetal toxicity, ovarian failure, PRES, exogenous endophthalmitis, gallbladder perforation, and congestive heart failure have been associated with bevacizumab (see full prescriber's information for a complete list)

5-FU, 5-Fluorouracil; *A*, adult; *d*, day; *GI*, gastrointestinal; *IV*, intravenous; *NSCLC*, non–small cell lung cancer; *PB*, protein bound; *PRES*, posterior reversible encephalopathy syndrome; *q*, every; *RCC*, renal cell cancer; *t½*, half-life; *UK*, unknown; *VEGF*, vascular endothelial growth factor; *wk*, week.

Drug Interactions

Gefitinib is extensively metabolized by CYP3A4. Other drugs metabolized by the hepatic system can affect the concentrations of gefitinib and other drugs. Drugs that inhibit CYP3A4, increasing the gefitinib level, include thioridazine, amiodarone, bupropion, diphenhydramine, promethazine, and metoclopramide. Other CYP3A4 inhibitors, such as venlafaxine, may decrease the levels of gefitinib. Gefitinib can increase the concentration of other drugs that have a narrow therapeutic index, such as amitriptyline, warfarin, and eliglustat. Patients taking warfarin concomitantly with gefitinib had an elevated international normalized ratio (INR) and/or hemorrhage. CYP3A4 inducers—such as acetaminophen, butalbital, caffeine, and aspirin—can increase gefitinib metabolism, thereby decreasing concentrations of the drug. When given concomitantly with gefitinib, drugs that decrease gastric pH (e.g., omeprazole and lansoprazole) can lower plasma concentrations of gefitinib.

Osimertinib

Osimertinib is one of the newest FDA-approved EGFR-TK inhibitors for *T790M* mutation–positive NSCLC. It is currently being studied in the treatment of other types of cancer.

Pharmacokinetics

Osimertinib is taken orally, and absorption is dose dependent. High-fat, high-calorie meals increase the absorption rate by 14%. It is metabolized primarily by the hepatic system through the CYP3A isoenzyme and by oxidation and dealkylation. Osimertinib is primarily excreted in the feces and to a lesser extent in the urine. The elimination half-life is approximately 48 hours.

Pharmacodynamics

Osimertinib is a CYP3A4 and CYP1A2 inducer that irreversibly binds to certain mutant forms of *EGFR* (*T790M*, *L858R*, and *exon 19* deletion). In vitro, it exhibits inhibition of *ERBB2*, *ERBB3*, *ERBB4*, *ACK1*, and *BLK* receptors.

Side Effects and Adverse Reactions

Common side effects include pancytopenia, rash, dry skin, anorexia, constipation, hyponatremia, nausea, pruritus, fatigue, cough, back pain, and stomatitis. Other side effects include eye disorders and cephalgia. Adverse reactions include venous thromboembolism, interstitial lung disease, pneumonitis, increased QTc, and cardiomyopathy.

PROTOTYPE DRUG CHART
Erlotinib

Drug Class	Dosage
Epidermal growth factor receptor inhibitor	*NSCLC:* 150 mg PO once daily *Pancreatic cancer:* 100 mg PO once daily as combination therapy. Take without food, 1 h before or 2 h after meal.
Contraindications	**Drug-Lab-Food Interactions**
No absolute contraindications. Precautions are warranted in patients who may become pregnant, are pregnant, or are breast-feeding; who have preexisting respiratory problems (pulmonary fibrosis may occur); or who are dehydrated or have liver impairment. Use cautiously in patients with history of peptic ulcer disease or diverticulitis (increases risk for GI perforation). Advise smokers to stop smoking while taking erlotinib; tobacco decreases the effectiveness of the drug.	Drug: Concomitant use with drugs that alter the pH of the upper GI tract is contraindicated (e.g., esomeprazole, lansoprazole, omeprazole, or pantoprazole). CYP3A4 inhibitors such as ketoconazole, atazanavir, clarithromycin, indinavir, itraconazole, nefazodone, nelfinavir, ritonavir, saquinavir, telithromycin, and voriconazole increase blood levels of erlotinib and may lead to increased adverse reactions or toxicities. Concomitant use with competitive inhibitors of CYP3A4, such as midazolam and statin drugs, can increase the competitor's concentration. CYP3A4 inducers such as rifampicin, dexamethasone, phenytoin, carbamazepine, phenobarbital, St. John's wort, H_2-receptor blockers, and proton pump inhibitors reduce the effectiveness of erlotinib. Lab: Erlotinib may increase INR and can lead to increased risk for bleeding. Food: Drug must be given on an empty stomach; administering with food increases the risk of side effects.
Pharmacokinetics	**Pharmacodynamics**
Absorption: Bioavailability is 60%. Distribution: 93% PB. Steady-state levels are achieved in 7–8 d. Metabolism: Liver (CYP3A4 and CYP1A2 enzymes); t½: 36 h. Excretion: Mainly in feces, some renal elimination; 24% higher among smokers	Give drug on an empty stomach, either 1 h before or 2 h after meals (administering with food increases risk for side effects). Administer at the same time each day between meals. Increase dose if used concomitantly with strong CYP3A4 inducers. Onset: Slowly absorbed with oral dosage with 60% bioavailability. Peak: 4 h; duration: UK
Therapeutic Effects/Uses	
Approved for treatment of NSCLC and pancreatic cancer. Mechanism of Action: Erlotinib selectively inhibits activation of *EGFR* tyrosine kinase, possibly blocking angiogenesis and cellular proliferation.	
Side Effects	**Adverse Reactions**
Diarrhea, skin changes (acne vulgaris, acneiform rash), alopecia, anorexia, anxiety, bone pain, cough, constipation, anorexia, diarrhea, fatigue, vomiting, pruritus	Ocular changes (inflammation, corneal perforation), GI perforation, skin desquamation, renal failure, hepatic failure, interstitial pulmonary disease

CYP, Cytochrome P; *d*, day; *GI*, gastrointestinal; *h*, hour; H_2, histamine 2; *INR*, international normalized ratio; *NSCLC*, non–small cell lung cancer; *PB*, protein bound; *PO*, by mouth; *t½*, half-life; *UK*, unknown.

Drug Interactions

Osimertinib is a CYP3A inducer. Drugs metabolized by the liver can affect their concentrations and the osimertinib plasma level. Osimertinib can cause a prolonged QT interval. Other drugs that can prolong QT intervals, causing torsade de pointes, should be avoided or monitored closely when used concomitantly with osimertinib (e.g., thioridazine, beta agonists, chlorpromazine, ofloxacin, desipramine, moxifloxacin, metronidazole, promethazine, and trimethoprim or sulfamethoxazole-trimethoprim). CYP3A inhibitors such as aldesleukin, alfentanil, and ethanol can alter osimertinib concentration. Osimertinib can alter plasma concentration of other drugs, which can worsen adverse reactions and can alter the efficacy of drugs such as acetaminophen, amlodipine, amitriptyline, and alprazolam.

TYROSINE KINASE INHIBITORS AND MULTIKINASE INHIBITORS

Several types of targeted therapies inhibit TKs. Specific drugs that cause this action as their main mechanism are referred to as TK inhibitors (TKIs). TKIs primarily exert their effects on an enzyme known as *BCR-ABL TK*. The *BCR-ABL* gene is an important pathogenesis for chronic myelogenous leukemia (CML). CML cells make abnormal active *BCR-ABL TK* enzyme. *BCR-ABL TK* enzymes are present in cancer cells that have a specific gene mutation known as the *Philadelphia chromosome*.

When activated and expressed, *BCR-ABL TK* turns on a strong pro-cell-division signal transduction pathway that leads to the proliferation of cancer cells. TKIs prevent activation of TKs, which then inhibits further activation of the signal transduction pathway and stops the

🎯 CLINICAL JUDGMENT [NURSING PROCESS]

Angiogenesis Inhibitors, Vascular Endothelial Growth Factor Receptor Inhibitors, and Epidermal Growth Factor Receptor Inhibitors

Concept: Cellular Regulation
- The ability for cells to maintain homeostasis, including its responses to extracellular signals

Recognize Cues [Assessment]
- Obtain a detailed medication history that includes current prescriptions, over-the-counter medicines, antacids, dietary supplements, vitamins, and herbal supplements and compare them to the targeted therapy for possible drug reactions.
- Obtain a list of all drug and food allergies.
- Obtain baseline information about the patient's physical status that includes height, weight, vital signs, cardiopulmonary assessment, intake and output, skin assessment, nutritional status, and any underlying diseases.
- Obtain baseline laboratory values (complete blood count [CBC], uric acid, chemistry panel) before and during treatment.
- Assess baseline results of pulmonary function tests, chest radiographs, electrocardiographs (ECGs), and renal and liver function studies.
- Assess patient's and caregiver's current level of comprehension related to the therapeutic regimen.

Analyze Cues and Prioritize Hypothesis [Patient Problems]
- Altered potential for inflammation
- Potential for altered clotting
- Potential for decreased immunity
- Need for teaching

Generate Solutions [Planning]
- The patient will remain free of skin breakdown.
- The patient will remain free from infection.
- The patient and family will verbalize understanding of targeted therapy as part of an anticancer treatment regimen.
- The patient and family will verbalize strategies to minimize risks related to targeted therapy–related side effects.
- The patient and family will demonstrate understanding of the importance of reporting targeted therapy–related side effects and adverse reactions.
- The patient will have tolerable side effects.

Take Action [Nursing Interventions]
- Examine the patient's skin closely at each visit for the presence of erythema, rash, peeling, or blister formation; rate the severity of dermatologic reactions.
- Monitor for any evidence of infection, such as fever, chills, leukocytosis or leukopenia, and neutropenia.
- Assess for evidence of thromboembolic events.
- Monitor for any signs of perforation, such as abdominal pain/distension, absent bowel sounds, and changes in blood pressure and heart rate.
- Monitor laboratory values, such as renal function, hepatic function, CBC, chemistry, and urinalysis.
- Administer prescribed premedications according to established protocols for specific targeted therapies.
- Assess for any cardiac events, such as new chest pain and ECG changes.
- Assess for any pulmonary complications, such as dyspnea or cough.

Patient Teaching

General
- Advise patients to notify the health care provider if foamy urine occurs (an indication of protein in the urine).
- Teach patients to avoid taking nonsteroidal antiinflammatory drugs such as aspirin, celecoxib, ibuprofen, and naproxen to decrease the risk of bleeding.
- Teach patients ways to promote venous return and avoid deep venous thrombosis, such as avoiding dehydration, constrictive clothing, and smoking cigarettes.

Side Effects
- Advise patients to immediately report worsening of skin rash; severe or persistent diarrhea, nausea, anorexia, or vomiting; onset or worsening of unexplained shortness of breath or cough; or eye irritation.
- Teach patients to avoid direct sunlight and tanning beds to prevent worsening of skin side effects.
- Advise patients to seek medical help immediately if chest pain, severe abdominal pain, or swelling associated with redness or pain in one leg occurs.
- Report symptoms of adverse effects or severe side effects promptly, especially fever, chills, persistent sore throat, swelling, weight gain, or increasing shortness of breath.
- Report symptoms of bleeding immediately, including black stools, coffee ground emesis, and easy bleeding or bruising.

Evaluate Outcomes [Evaluation]
- Patient, family, and caregiver education needs are met.
- The patient, family, and caregivers understand therapy-related side effects and adverse reactions.
- The patient, family, and caregivers understand strategies to minimize side effects and adverse reactions.
- Side effects are managed effectively.
- The patient is free from infection.
- The patient is free from injury, perforation, or internal fistula.

proliferation of cancer cells. This action can control the disease but cannot eradicate it alone. Receptors on the cell membrane can activate TKs, which then turn on signal transduction pathways that promote cell division. Table 36.2 lists some of the TKI drugs and their uses and considerations. Of the TKIs, alectinib and nilotinib are further discussed under those headings in text. Prototype Drug Chart: Imatinib Mesylate, STI-571 lists specific drug information about the TKI imatinib.

The multikinase inhibitors (MKIs) are chemicals that directly inhibit the activity of multiple kinase enzymes in cancer cells. (Recall that kinases are enzymes that activate other proteins, including those that activate signal transduction pathways that promote cancer cell division.) Table 36.2 lists some of the MKIs and their dosages, routes, uses, and considerations. Of the MKIs, dasatinib, sorafenib, and sunitinib are discussed.

Alectinib

Alectinib is a TKI that targets anaplastic lymphoma kinase (*ALK*) and the RET proto-oncogene (*RET*). It is indicated for the treatment of patients with *ALK*-positive metastatic NSCLC whose disease has progressed or who are intolerant to crizotinib.

PROTOTYPE DRUG CHART
Imatinib Mesylate, STI-571

Drug Class	Dosage
Signal transduction inhibitor/tyrosine kinase inhibitor	A: PO: For Ph+ leukemias, myelodysplastic syndrome, myeloproliferative disease, GI stromal tumors (GISTs), hypereosinophilic syndrome (HES) or chronic eosinophilic leukemia (CEL), aggressive systemic mastocytosis, metastatic dermatofibrosarcoma protuberans. Dose depends on disease; starting dose is 400 mg/d; may increase if no serious adverse reactions occur. Other protocols exist, including twice-daily dosing.
Contraindications	**Drug-Lab-Food Interactions**
Contraindicated among patients who may be or could become pregnant or who are breast-feeding. *Caution:* Patients with renal impairment, cardiac disease, hepatic impairment, bone marrow suppression, or infection, and in children. Avoid concomitant strong CYP3A4 inducers. See full prescriber's information for a complete list of contraindications.	Drug: Any drug that *inhibits* CYP450 or CYP3A4 (e.g., nefazodone, itraconazole, fluvoxamine, fluconazole, erythromycin) can decrease the metabolism of imatinib and increase the concentration, leading to an increased incidence of adverse reactions. Any drug that *induces* CYP450 (e.g., St. John's wort, phenytoin, fosphenytoin, rifampin, barbiturates, dexamethasone, phenobarbital) can increase the metabolism of imatinib and decrease imatinib concentrations and clinical effects. Imatinib is a CYP450 inhibitor and serum concentrations of any drug that is metabolized by CYP450 (e.g., ergot alkaloids, carbamazepine, cyclosporine, quinidine, clonazepam, fentanyl, calcium channel blockers, sertraline, acetaminophen) can increase. Taking imatinib with thrombolytic agents, NSAIDs, platelet inhibitors, aspirin, and other anticoagulants/antiplatelets may increase risk of bleeding. Concomitant use of flibanserin and moderate CYP3A4 inhibitors, such as imatinib, is contraindicated due to severe hypotension and syncope. Lab: May affect serum levels of liver enzymes, CBC, electrolytes, renal function, and uric acid. Food: Grapefruit juice increases imatinib plasma concentrations.
Pharmacokinetics	**Pharmacodynamics**
Absorption: Bioavailability is 98%. Distribution: 95% PB with extensive distribution. Metabolism: Mainly by CYP3A4; inhibits CYP2D6 and CYP3A4; t½: imatinib is 18 h, major metabolite is 40 h. Clearance is 8–14 L/h. Excretion: Mainly in the feces as metabolites.	Well absorbed after oral administration with Cmax achieved within 2–4 h. Imatinib should be taken with food and a large glass of water to decrease the risk of GI irritation. Drug may be dispersed in water or apple juice for patients who cannot swallow tablets. Suspension should be administered immediately after complete disintegration of the tablets. Onset: UK Peak: 2–4 h Duration: UK
Therapeutic Effects/Uses	
Approved for ALL, CEL, CML, dermatofibrosarcoma protuberans, GIST, HES, myelodysplastic syndrome, and systemic mastocytosis. Mechanism of Action: Imatinib competitively inhibits the ATP-binding site on *BCR-ABL* tyrosine kinase (TK) that results in inhibition of proliferation and induces apoptosis in *BCR-ABL*–positive cell lines and in fresh leukemic cells of Philadelphia chromosome–positive CML. Receptors for TKs include various growth factors (e.g., *EGF, PDGF, SGF, VEGF, NGF*). Imatinib also acts as a mediator for many nonreceptor TKs (e.g., G-protein–coupled receptors, B- and T-cell receptors, and interferon gamma receptors). Imatinib also interacts with lipids, proteins, and DNA. Imatinib inhibits proliferation in vitro and induces apoptosis in GIST cells, which express an activating *KIT* mutation. Imatinib inhibits CYP2C9, CYP2D6, and CYP3A4.	
Side Effects	**Adverse Reactions**
Edema, fluid retention, GI irritation, nausea, vomiting, hematologic dyscrasias, hepatotoxicity, electrolyte abnormalities	The most common adverse reactions include cerebral edema, cardiac tamponade, increased ICP and papilledema, pleural effusions, heart failure, renal failure, GI perforation and bleeding, avascular necrosis, cardiac events, and tumor lysis syndrome.

A, Adult; *ALL*, acute lymphoblastic leukemia; *ATP*, adenosine triphosphate; *CBC*, complete blood count; *CEL*, chronic eosinophilic leukemia; *Cmax*, maximum serum concentration; *CML*, chronic myelogenous leukemia; *CYP3A4*, cytochrome P3A4; *CYP450*, cytochrome P450; *d*, day; *EGF*, epidermal growth factor; *h*, hour; *GI*, gastrointestinal; *GIST*, gastrointestinal stromal tumor; *HES*, hypereosinophilic syndrome; *ICP*, intracranial pressure; *NGF*, nerve growth factor; *NSAID*, nonsteroidal antiinflammatory drug; *PDGF*, platelet-derived growth factor; *PB*, protein bound; *Ph+*, Philadelphia chromosome positive; *PO*, oral; *SGF*, sarcoma growth factor; *t½*, half-life; *UK*, unknown; *VEGF*, vascular endothelial growth factor; *y*, year; >, greater than; ≤, less than or equal to.

Pharmacokinetics
Alectinib is administered orally. Alectinib and its major metabolite, M4, are more than 99% bound to plasma proteins. Steady state is reached by day 7 of administration. Alectinib is metabolized by CYP3A4 to its major active metabolite, M4. The elimination half-lives for alectinib and M4 are 33 and 31 hours, respectively. Alectinib and its metabolite are excreted in the feces (84% and 6%, respectively). No significant effect was noted in patients with mild to moderate hepatic and renal impairment.

Pharmacodynamics
Alectinib is a TKI that targets *ALK* and *RET*. Alectinib is a central nervous system (CNS)-active and highly selective ALK inhibitor that inhibits *ALK* phosphorylation and *ALK*-mediated activation of the downstream signaling proteins.

Side Effects and Adverse Reactions
Common side effects include anemia, elevated transaminases, fatigue, constipation, bradycardia, edema, hypocalcemia, hypokalemia, and myalgia. Serious adverse events include hepatotoxicity, pneumonitis, bradycardia, and elevated creatine phosphokinase (CPK).

Drug Interactions
No interactions with alectinib that require dose adjustment have been identified.

Nilotinib
Nilotinib is a TKI that has a high affinity for the ATP-binding site of *BCR-ABL* kinase, inhibiting cell proliferation in cell lines and in primary Philadelphia chromosome–positive (Ph+) CML cells. It is indicated for the treatment of Ph+ CML that is resistant or intolerant to imatinib in the chronic or accelerated phase.

Pharmacokinetics
Nilotinib is administered orally, and approximately 98% is protein bound in plasma. The elimination half-life is approximately 17 hours. Peak serum concentration occurs 3 hours after oral administration, and steady state is achieved on day 8. The bioavailability of the drug is significantly increased with food. Nilotinib is metabolized in the liver by CYP3A4; no active metabolites have been identified. The primary metabolic pathways are oxidation and hydroxylation. The majority of the drug is eliminated mainly in the feces within 7 days. Caution is advised in administering nilotinib to patients with hepatic impairment.

Pharmacodynamics
Nilotinib is an oral TK that selectively inhibits *BCR-ABL* kinase. It is a competitor inhibitor at the ATP-binding site of *BCR-ABL* and prevents tyrosine phosphorylation of downstream intracellular signal transduction proteins. Blocking the TK prevents proliferation of cancer cells and induces cell death.

Side Effects and Adverse Reactions
The most common adverse effects are pancytopenia, rash, pruritus, nausea, fatigue, cephalgia, and constipation. Severe adverse events include dysrhythmias due to prolonged QT interval, which can cause sudden cardiac death. Pulmonary toxicity has been reported in patients with CML.

Drug Interactions
Concomitant administration of strong CYP3A4 inhibitors or inducers may significantly alter nilotinib concentrations. If CYP3A4 inhibitor drugs (e.g., ketoconazole, clarithromycin, ritonavir, fluoroquinolones, ibutilide, lithium) are unavoidable, dose reduction should be considered, and the QT interval should be monitored on a frequent basis. Electrolyte imbalances should be corrected before administering nilotinib.

Dasatinib
Dasatinib is an MKI approved for newly diagnosed Ph+ CML and acute lymphocytic leukemia (ALL); Ph+ CML in chronic, accelerated, or myeloid or lymphoid blast phases resistant or intolerant to prior therapy, including imatinib; and Ph+ ALL with resistance or intolerance to prior therapy.

Pharmacokinetics
Dasatinib is an oral drug that is readily absorbed from the GI tract, and it can be taken with or without food. Dasatinib and its active metabolite are highly protein bound (96% and 93%, respectively). The drug is extensively metabolized in the liver by the CYP3A4 isoenzyme. Dasatinib is also a weak time-dependent inhibitor of CYP3A4. Unlike other tyrosine inhibitors, dasatinib does not have the multidrug-resistant protein P-glycoprotein. Dasatinib is eliminated primarily through feces, with only minimal amounts recovered in the urine. Antacids slow the absorption.

Pharmacodynamics
Dasatinib specifically targets *BCR-ABL TK*, *SRC* family kinases, and imatinib-resistant mutations mostly found in CML and ALL, possibly blocking angiogenesis and cell proliferation. Inhibiting the activity of these enzymes further inhibits activation of the signal transduction pathway, thereby stopping the proliferation of cancer cells. The drug has the greatest effects on Ph+-expressing cancer cells.

Side Effects and Adverse Reactions
Dasatinib often causes electrolyte imbalances, especially hypokalemia, hypocalcemia, and hypophosphatemia. Other common side effects include diarrhea, cephalgia, fatigue, skin rash, nausea, vomiting, anorexia, arthralgia, pyrexia, and dyspnea, among others. Hemorrhage, vascular disorders, and severe dermatologic reactions have been associated with dasatinib. Another adverse reaction includes ECG abnormalities, especially prolonged QT intervals, and development of arrhythmias. Hematologic side effects of myelosuppression with anemia, thrombocytopenia, and neutropenia are relatively common and are usually reversible. Bleeding, including GI and intracranial bleeding, was reported that required treatment interruptions and transfusions.

Drug Interactions
CYP3A4 enzyme inhibitors decrease dasatinib metabolism, resulting in an increased serum concentration and increased risk for toxicity. Other drugs that strongly increase the serum concentration of dasatinib include atazanavir, clarithromycin, indinavir, itraconazole, ketoconazole, nefazodone, nelfinavir, telithromycin, triazolobenzodiazepines, and voriconazole.

Drugs that enhance the activity of the CYP3A4 enzyme decrease dasatinib serum levels and reduce its effectiveness. Such drugs include aminoglutethimide, barbiturates, carbamazepine, dexamethasone, griseofulvin, nafcillin, phenytoin, primidone, and rifampin. Other drugs that appear to reduce the effectiveness of dasatinib include antacids, histamine 2 (H_2) receptor blockers, and proton pump inhibitors. Dasatinib may interfere with the metabolism of other drugs that use the CYP3A4 enzyme system, such as alfentanil, terfenadine, cisapride, cyclosporine, fentanyl, quinidine, tacrolimus, and ergot alkaloids.

Sorafenib

Sorafenib is an MKI that specifically targets serine/threonine and receptor TKs, which are activated because of gene mutations. Gene mutations are most commonly found in pancreatic cancer, colon cancer, and NSCLC. In addition, the drug may be used in hepatocellular carcinomas and renal cell carcinomas (RCCs) that overexpress the target.

Pharmacokinetics

Sorafenib is an oral drug whose absorption and bioavailability are inhibited when taken with a high-fat meal. The drug is metabolized in the liver, mainly by the CYP3A4 enzyme system. It is 99.5% protein bound and reaches steady state within 7 days. The peak plasma level is about 3 hours; the mean half-life is 25 to 48 hours. Eight metabolites have been identified, with pyridine N-oxide being the major circulating active metabolite. The drug is eliminated in the feces unchanged and in the urine as glucuronidated metabolites (77% and 19%, respectively).

Pharmacodynamics

Sorafenib inhibits multiple kinase receptors to inhibit cell proliferation and angiogenesis. Some of the targeted kinases include *RAF* kinase, *VEGF* receptors, *PDGFR*, and *RET*. When cytokines or growth factors activate these TK receptors, a protein kinase–mediated cascade starts that leads to uncontrolled cellular proliferation. The inhibition of these signaling pathways decreases cancer cellular proliferation. In addition, sorafenib specifically inhibits two *VEGF* receptors, thereby inhibiting angiogenesis.

Side Effects and Adverse Reactions

Sorafenib has many common adverse effects, such as hypertension, cephalgia, alopecia, pruritus, xerosis, exfoliative dermatitis, acne, flush, anorexia, nausea/vomiting, diarrhea, constipation, abdominal pain, dyspepsia, dysphagia, hand and foot syndrome, and mild neutropenia. More severe adverse events include QT prolongation, especially in patients with heart failure or electrolyte abnormalities and in those taking other drugs that prolong QT interval. Other severe adverse events were hemorrhage, especially in patients taking anticoagulants or antiplatelets; cardiac ischemia/infarction; GI perforation; and pulmonary toxicity.

Drug Interactions

Sorafenib levels are not increased by the presence of other drugs, even those that inhibit the enzyme that metabolizes sorafenib. However, drugs that induce metabolizing enzyme activity can reduce the blood levels and the effectiveness of sorafenib. These include primidone, phenobarbital, rifampicin, phenytoin, carbamazepine, and dexamethasone. If drugs that prolong QT intervals—such as methadone, daunorubicin, epirubicin, and doxorubicin—are coadministered with sorafenib, close ECG monitoring is warranted. Sorafenib can increase the blood levels of repaglinide, amiodarone, ibuprofen, loperamide, irinotecan, propofol, and warfarin.

Sunitinib

Sunitinib is an MKI with antiangiogenic and antitumor activities. It selectively inhibits several receptor TKs (RTKs). This inhibition results in regression of tumor growth, especially in advanced RCC; gastrointestinal stromal tumors (GISTs); and progressive, well-differentiated pancreatic neuroendocrine tumors in patients with unresectable or metastatic disease.

Pharmacokinetics

Sunitinib is an oral MKI that is well absorbed with or without food. Sunitinib and its active metabolites are highly protein bound (95% and 90%, respectively). Sunitinib reaches peak plasma level in 6 to 12 hours. The drug and its metabolite are metabolized in the liver, mainly by the CYP3A4 enzyme system; elimination half-life is 40 to 60 hours, and the drug is eliminated primarily in the feces. No dose adjustment is warranted in patients with renal impairment or in patients with mild to moderate hepatic impairment.

Pharmacodynamics

Sunitinib inhibits more than 80 RTKs, including PDGFR, vascular endothelial growth factor receptor (*VEGFR*), stem cell factor receptor, and glial cell line–derived neurotrophic factor receptor. In addition, it inhibits the phosphorylation of RTKs, and it has demonstrated inhibition of tumor growth, tumor regression, and tumor angiogenesis. Several adverse effects of sunitinib, including hair and skin discoloration, are associated with the inhibition of the multiple signaling pathways.

Side Effects and Adverse Reactions

Side effects and adverse reactions are more widespread as a result of the number of different types of kinases sunitinib inhibits. Cardiovascular effects include hypertension, peripheral edema, left ventricular dysfunction, prolonged QT interval, and venous thromboembolism. GI effects include nausea, vomiting, diarrhea, stomatitis, and dyspepsia. Neuromuscular effects include fatigue, asthenia, headache, dizziness, peripheral neuropathy, mild arthralgia, limb pain, myalgia, and back pain. Liver impairment may occur with elevated liver enzymes and jaundice of the skin and sclera. Common integumentary changes include depigmentation of the skin, skin discoloration, rash, dry skin, and palmar-plantar erythrodysesthesia. Endocrine changes may include hypothyroidism and adrenal insufficiency, hematologic changes may include myelosuppression, and respiratory effects may include mild dyspnea and cough.

Drug Interactions

Plasma concentration and the activity of sunitinib are increased by drugs that inhibit CYP3A4 enzyme levels, including atazanavir, clarithromycin, ketoconazole, itraconazole, nefazodone, nelfinavir, telithromycin, diltiazem, and verapamil. When these drugs are used during sunitinib therapy, side effects of sunitinib are more common and more severe. Drugs that increase sunitinib elimination and reduce its effectiveness include rifampin, phenytoin, phenobarbital, carbamazepine, dexamethasone, rifabutin, and rifapentine.

mTOR KINASE INHIBITORS AND PROTEASOME INHIBITORS

Mechanistic target of rapamycin (mTOR) is an atypical serine/threonine protein kinase that helps regulate cell growth, proliferation, and survival. Inhibitors of mTOR lead to G_1 arrest and apoptosis. They are not without adverse effects, which are common and include weakness, rash, mucositis, nausea, edema, anorexia, and fever. Effects on laboratory values include pancytopenia, hyperglycemia, hypercholesterolemia, hypertriglyceridemia, and hypophosphatemia. Severe adverse events include hepatic necrosis, pericardial effusion, cardiac tamponade, nephrotic syndrome, hemolytic uremic syndrome, and exfoliative dermatitis. Like other targeted drugs, adverse effects of mTOR and other CYP3A4 inhibitor drugs are increased when mTOR is administered concomitantly. CYP3A4 inducers can cause drug levels to decrease.

Proteasomes are multienzyme complexes that degrade proteins intracellularly. The degraded proteins can accumulate and can disrupt a cell's physiologic properties, such as regulating transcription, cell adhesion, apoptosis, and progression of mitosis. In cancer cells, proteasome inhibitors promote the accumulation of proteins that promote programmed cell death. It has limited action on normal, healthy cells. Table 36.2 lists the mTOR kinase inhibitors and the proteasome inhibitors. Prototype Drug Chart: Bortezomib lists specific drug information on bortezomib.

Temsirolimus

Temsirolimus is an inhibitor of mTOR. When temsirolimus or sirolimus binds to the intracellular protein *FKBP-12*, a protein-drug complex forms that directly inhibits the activity of mTOR. Inhibition of mTOR greatly reduces the concentration of VEGF. In addition, by its inhibition of mTOR, a variety of downstream pro-cell-division signal transduction pathways are disrupted, especially in RCC cells. This drug is most commonly used to treat advanced RCC.

Pharmacokinetics

Temsirolimus is administered by IV infusion. It is extensively metabolized in the liver by CYP3A4 into five active metabolites, including sirolimus. The half-life of temsirolimus is 17 hours, and the half-life of sirolimus is 54 hours. Temsirolimus and its metabolites are primarily excreted in the feces. Approximately 82% of total radioactivity is eliminated within 14 days. Serum concentration of the metabolite, sirolimus, peaks at 0.5 to 2 hours. Caution is advised in patients with mild hepatic impairment. In patients with moderate to severe hepatic impairment, the drug is contraindicated.

Pharmacodynamics

Temsirolimus and its metabolites bind to an intracellular protein to form a drug-protein complex that inhibits the activity of mTOR, and mTOR regulates messenger RNA (mRNA) translation through phosphorylation. Inhibition of mTOR activity results in G_1 growth arrest in treated RCC cells.

Side Effects and Adverse Reactions

Hypersensitivity reactions to temsirolimus are common, and premedication with an IV antihistamine (e.g., diphenhydramine) is recommended. Adverse effects are common and include weakness, rash, mucositis, nausea, edema, anorexia, dyspnea, pain, elevated transaminases, pancytopenia, hyperlipidemia, diarrhea, hypophosphatemia, hypercholesterolemia, and hypertriglyceridemia. Hyperglycemia is also common in patients receiving temsirolimus; patients may require treatment with oral antidiabetic agents or with insulin. Respiratory adverse effects of interstitial pneumonitis or other interstitial lung disease are possible. Liver impairment and renal impairment have been reported. Cardiovascular effects of edema formation, chest pain, hypertension, venous thromboembolism, and thrombophlebitis are possible.

Drug Interactions

Drugs that inhibit the CYP3A4 enzyme can lead to increased serum levels of temsirolimus, which increases the risk for severe side effects. These drugs include ketoconazole, clarithromycin, indinavir, itraconazole, nefazodone, telithromycin, voriconazole, diltiazem, fluconazole, verapamil, and cimetidine.

Drugs that induce CYP3A4 enzyme activity may lower temsirolimus blood serum levels and can reduce its effectiveness. These drugs include rifampin, carbamazepine, and phenytoin.

CLINICAL JUDGMENT [NURSING PROCESS]
Tyrosine Kinase Inhibitors and Multikinase Inhibitors for Cancer Treatment

Concept: Cellular Regulation
- The ability for cells to maintain homeostasis, including responses to extracellular signals

Recognize Cues [Assessment]
- Obtain a detailed current medication history that includes prescriptions, over-the-counter medicines, antacids, dietary supplements, vitamins, and herbal supplements and compare with the targeted therapy drug for possible drug-drug interactions.
- Obtain a list of drug and food allergies.
- Obtain baseline information about the patient's physical status that includes height, weight, vital signs, cardiopulmonary assessment, intake and output, skin assessment, nutritional status, and any underlying diseases.
- Assess baseline laboratory values (complete blood count [CBC], uric acid, chemistry panel) to compare with future ones.
- Assess baseline results of pulmonary function tests, chest radiographs, electrocardiograms, and renal and liver function studies.
- Assess the patient's and caregiver's current level of comprehension ability related to the therapeutic regimen.

Analyze Cues and Prioritize Hypothesis [Patient Problems]
- Potential for altered clotting
- Potential for decreased immunity
- Need for teaching

Generate Solutions [Planning]
- The patient/family member/caregiver will verbalize understanding of the signs and symptoms of infection.
- The patient will maintain white blood cell, red blood cell, and platelet counts in the desired range.
- The patient will remain free from infection and from pulmonary, cardiac, and gastrointestinal (GI) complications.
- The patient will verbalize ways to decrease GI disturbances to improve nutrition intake.
- The patient/family/caregiver will demonstrate understanding of the chemotherapeutic protocol (e.g., dose administration).

Take Action [Nursing Interventions]
- Monitor labs (CBC, blood urea nitrogen [BUN], creatinine, liver panel, and electrolytes) before administration and during treatment.
- Monitor for any signs of bleeding.
- Monitor for any dysrhythmias, decreased cardiac output, heart rate, and blood pressure.
- Monitor intravenous (IV) site frequently for irritation and phlebitis.
- Maintain strict medical asepsis during dressing changes and invasive procedures.
- Encourage small, frequent meals that are high in calories and protein.
- Monitor fluid intake and output, weight, and nutritional intake during therapy.
- Assess the need for IV hydration.

CLINICAL JUDGMENT [NURSING PROCESS]—CONT'D
Tyrosine Kinase Inhibitors and Multikinase Inhibitors for Cancer Treatment

- Administer premedications as ordered 30 to 60 minutes before giving the drug.
- Provide drug information—such as therapeutic effects, side effects, and drug-drug/drug-food interactions—verbally and in print to the patient/family/caregiver.
- Monitor for any vision changes.

Patient Teaching
General
- Teach patients when to take medications as it relates to food intake.
- Teach patient to weigh daily and report a weight gain of more than 2 pounds in 1 day or 4 pounds in 1 week to the health care provider.
- Remind women with childbearing potential to avoid pregnancy throughout treatment and for up to 12 months after treatment is complete.
- Advise breast-feeding patients to stop breast-feeding during and for 60 days after therapy.
- Teach patients to avoid using St. John's wort while on treatment.

Side Effects
- Avoid alcohol and nonessential drugs that are metabolized by the liver or that have hepatotoxic effects (e.g., acetaminophen).
- Report symptoms of adverse effects or severe side effects promptly, especially fever, chills, persistent sore throat, swelling, weight gain, or increasing shortness of breath.
- Report symptoms of bleeding immediately, including black stools, coffee ground emesis, or easy bleeding or bruising.
- Report symptoms of stomach or abdominal pain, yellowing of eyes or skin, dark urine, or unusual fatigue.
- Teach patients to avoid grapefruit juice, which can increase blood levels of drug to a dangerous level, leading to worsening side effects or adverse events.

Evaluate Outcomes [Evaluation]
- Patient, family, and caregiver education needs are met.
- The patient, family, and caregivers understand therapy-related side effects and adverse reactions.
- The patient, family, and caregivers understand strategies to minimize side effects and adverse reactions.
- Side effects are managed effectively.
- The patient is free from infection.
- The patient's fluid balance and electrolytes are maintained at expected normal ranges.

Patients taking antihypertensive drugs such as angiotensin-converting enzyme (ACE) inhibitors or angiotensin II–receptor antagonists during temsirolimus therapy are at increased risk for angioedema of the face and upper airways. The combination of temsirolimus and sunitinib may result in dose-limiting integumentary toxicities of erythematous maculopapular rash and gout/cellulitis that require hospitalization. The use of live vaccines such as intranasal influenza; measles, mumps, rubella; oral polio; bacille Calmette-Guérin; yellow fever; varicella; and typhoid vaccines should be avoided during treatment with temsirolimus.

Carfilzomib
Carfilzomib is a proteasome inhibitor that prevents the proliferation of cancerous cells and promotes apoptotic activity in solid and hematologic tumor cells. Carfilzomib is indicated in the treatment of multiple myeloma.

Pharmacokinetics
Carfilzomib is administered intravenously, and in vitro, 97% of the drug is protein bound. Its metabolites have no known biologic activity. The elimination half-life is 1 hour or less. Carfilzomib is extensively metabolized in the plasma rather than in the liver. The drug clearance exceeds hepatic blood flow, suggesting a large extrahepatic clearance. About 25% of the drug's metabolite is excreted in the feces.

Pharmacodynamics
Carfilzomib irreversibly binds to the N-terminal threonine-containing active sites of the 20 S proteasome, unlike bortezomib. Carfilzomib may be more selective for the chymotrypsin protease, leading to more sustained and selective proteasome activity. It has minimal cross-reactivity with other protease classes.

Side Effects and Adverse Reactions
Adverse effects include fatigue, pancytopenia, dyspnea, diarrhea, pyrexia, cephalgia, cough, peripheral edema, nausea, vomiting, arthralgia, hypertension, asthenia, insomnia, and back pain. Cardiac toxicity (e.g., congestive heart failure, cardiac arrest, myocardial ischemia/infarction) has been reported. Pulmonary arterial hypertension and pulmonary edema were noted in some patients. Renal and hepatic toxicity was also noted; therefore, close monitoring of renal and hepatic functions is warranted.

Drug Interactions
Specific drug interactions have not been reported with this drug. Because carfilzomib is not metabolized by the liver, it is unlikely to be affected by concomitant administration of cytochrome P450 (CYP450) inhibitors and inducers.

Ixazomib
Ixazomib is a reversible proteasome inhibitor that binds and inhibits 20 S proteasome. It is indicated for the treatment of multiple myeloma in patients who have received at least one prior therapy.

Pharmacokinetics
Ixazomib is administered orally and is highly bound to plasma proteins (99%) with distribution into erythrocytes. Terminal half-life is 9.5 days. The drug is metabolized by CYP450 isoenzymes and non-CYP proteins. Approximately 62% of the dose radioactivity is recovered in the urine and 22% in the feces. The concentration of the drug is decreased with food; therefore, the drug should be given at least 1 hour before or at least 2 hours after food consumption.

Pharmacodynamics
Ixazomib is a reversible proteasome inhibitor that preferentially binds to the beta-5 subunit of the 20 S proteasome, and it inhibits its chymotrypsin-like activity. It induces apoptosis of multiple myeloma cells and has a cytotoxic effect on myeloma cells in patients who relapse after receiving prior therapies with other drugs.

PROTOTYPE DRUG CHART

Bortezomib

Drug Class
Proteasome inhibitor

Dosage
A: IV or Subcut:

Mantle cell lymphoma: 1.3 mg/m² on days 1, 4, 8, and 11 followed by a 10-d rest period (days 12–21) for six 3-wk cycles in combination with rituximab, cyclophosphamide, doxorubicin, and prednisone.

Multiple myeloma (FDA-designated orphan drug for multiple myeloma): Treatment is administered for nine 6-wk cycles.

Cycles 1–4: Admin 1.3 mg/m²/dose on days 1, 4, 8, and 11 followed by a 10-d rest period (days 12–21); then 1.3 mg/m²/dose on days 22, 25, 29, and 32 followed by another 10-d rest period (days 33–42) in combination with melphalan and prednisone.

Cycles 5–9: Admin 1.3 mg/m²/dose on days 1, 8, 22, and 29 in combination with melphalan and prednisone.

Other protocols exist. See full prescribing information.

At least 72 h should elapse between consecutive doses of bortezomib. IV doses should be given as a bolus over 3–5 s.

Subcut injections should be administered in the thigh or abdomen; rotate sites and *do not* admin to areas that are tender, bruised, erythematous, or indurated.

Dose adjustment is needed for moderate to severe hepatic impairment; no adjustments are needed with renal impairment. Admin bortezomib after dialysis procedure; dialysis may reduce bortezomib blood levels.

Contraindications
Absolute contraindications: Intrathecal administration, patients with mannitol, bortezomib, or boron hypersensitivity

Avoid during pregnancy; breast-feeding should be discontinued.

Caution: Cardiac, pulmonary, and liver disorders; bleeding dyscrasias; pancytopenia; dehydration; diabetes mellitus; herpes infection; bleeding; history of tumor lysis syndrome; and in neonates and children.

Drug-Lab-Food Interactions
Drug: Dialysis may reduce bortezomib drug level; bortezomib may increase serum levels of eliglustat, amobarbital, axitinib, and tamsulosin by inducing CYP2D6 metabolism.

CYP3A4 inhibitor drugs (e.g., idelalisib, mefloquine, cimetidine, clarithromycin, cyclosporine, erythromycin, fluconazole, nifedipine) can increase the serum level of bortezomib if given concomitantly.

CYP2C19 inhibitor drugs can decrease the effects of clopidogrel and diazepam.

Drugs metabolized by CYP3A4 (e.g., dexamethasone, diazepam, St. John's wort, phenobarbital) can decrease the level or effect of bortezomib. Bortezomib may increase the level or effect of omeprazole and pantoprazole through CYP2C19 metabolism.

See full prescriber's information for a complete list of drug interactions.

Lab: Bortezomib may alter other drug levels if given concomitantly (e.g., phenytoin and phenobarbital).

Food: Green tea decreases bortezomib's effects; grapefruit juice may increase the level of bortezomib.

Pharmacokinetics
Absorption: Bioavailability is unknown.
Distribution: Range, 498–1884 L/m² distributed widely into peripheral tissues; >83% PB.
Metabolism: CYP3A4, CYP2C19, and CYP1A2; t½: 40–193 h; dose dependent.
Excretion: UK

Pharmacodynamics
Onset: UK
Peak: 509 ng/mL
Duration: UK

Therapeutic Effects/Uses
Mantle cell lymphoma (MCL) and multiple myeloma.

Mechanism of Action: Bortezomib is a signal transduction inhibitor and a reversible inhibitor of the 26 S proteasome in mechanistic cells. Proteasome is a large multiprotein particle present in the cytosol and cell nucleus that regulates protein expression and degradation of damaged or obsolete proteins within the cell; it regulates the expression of proteins that mediate cell cycle progression, oncogenes, and apoptosis. Proteasome inhibition affects malignant cells more so than normal cells.

Side Effects
See full prescriber's information for a complete list.

Nausea, vomiting, diarrhea, constipation, anorexia, abdominal pain, dyspepsia, dysgeusia, hypotension, neuropathy, pancytopenia, rash, urticaria, vasculitis, pruritus, injection site reaction (e.g., pain, erythema, hematoma, skin irritation, and phlebitis), arthralgia, myalgia, back pain, bone pain, bone fractures, hyperglycemia, hypoglycemia, fatigue, fever, insomnia

Adverse Reactions
See full prescriber's information for a complete list.

Severe sensory and peripheral neuropathy, cardiotoxicity, heart failure, QT prolongation, arrhythmias, pulmonary hypertension, acute respiratory distress syndrome, pneumonitis, interstitial pneumonia, GI perforation, GI toxicity, hepatotoxicity, toxic epidermal necrolysis, acute febrile neutrophilic dermatosis (Sweet syndrome)

A, Adult; *admin*, administer; *CYP*, cytochrome P; *d*, day; *FDA*, US Food and Drug Administration; *GI*, gastrointestinal; *h*, hour; *IV*, intravenous; *PB*, protein bound; *s*, second; *Subcut*, subcutaneous; *t½*, half-life; *UK*, unknown; *wk*, week; *>*, greater than.

Side Effects and Adverse Reactions
Ixazomib causes multiple adverse effects that include pancytopenia, diarrhea, peripheral neuropathies, peripheral edema, back pain, upper respiratory tract infection, nausea, vomiting, dry eye, and grade 3 rash. Severe adverse effects include drug-induced hepatotoxicity, Stevens-Johnson syndrome, and grade 3 or 4 GI toxicity.

Drug Interactions
Ixazomib is metabolized by CYP3A4; levels of ixazomib can be altered by drugs that induce or inhibit CYP3A4. Such drugs include carbamazepine, fosphenytoin, primidone, rifabutin, rifampin, and St. John's wort.

MONOCLONAL ANTIBODIES

Monoclonal antibodies (mAbs) are larger molecules that exert their effects mostly on specific cell membrane surface proteins. Some mAbs act more like immunotherapy drugs because of their effects in improving the person's immune system to find and attack cancer cells. Chapter 37 provides more information on immunotherapies. All FDA-approved mAbs currently used in cancer treatment are given intravenously because the GI tract could alter the drug's structure and render it inactive. Ideal target antigens for cancer treatment should (1) be specific to tumor cells, (2) be located on the surface of the tumor cell and not shed into the bloodstream, (3) occur in high numbers, and (4) play a role in tumor cell survival.

mAb therapy is aimed specifically at tumor cells that express the target antigen. The side effects of mAbs are related to activation of the immune system, location of the target antigen, and the type of mAb. Binding of a mAb to its specific target antigen on the cancer cell inactivates or destroys the cell by one or more of the following mechanisms:

- Causing neutralization of tumor cell growth by direct interference with normal biologic activities of the antigen, such as signal transduction of cell growth messages. This cytostatic process can slow growth of the tumor cells.
- Promoting antibody-dependent cell-mediated cytotoxicity (ADCC) that recruits effector cells such as phagocytes, T cells, and natural killer cells of the immune system to release cytokines that destroy the target cell.
- Initiating complement-dependent cytotoxicity (CDC) that activates the complement system, a cascade of naturally circulating blood proteins, thus enhancing immune system destruction of antibody-bound cells.
- Directly inducing apoptosis, or programmed cell death.

Fully human antibodies are engineered to contain only human antibody protein sequences. Murine mAbs are derived from mice. Mouse antibodies have a very short half-life in the human body, are not as effective as human antibodies in eliciting a response from the CDC and ADCC systems, and can cause development of human anti-mouse antibodies (HAMAs) that neutralize the mouse antibodies and render them ineffective against the tumor. Chimeric mAbs contain both human and mouse protein sequences (typically 70% human and 30% mouse). Humanized mAbs also contain human and gene mouse sequences; however, they are not considered chimeric because they contain more human sequences than do chimeric mAbs, usually 90% to 95% human and 5% to 10% mouse.

mAbs can also be transporters for other anticancer agents (e.g., chemotherapy agents, toxins, or radioisotopes). Although agents attached to conjugated antibodies specifically target tumor cells, nearby healthy cells can still be negatively affected, especially if radioisotopes are used. If the specific target antigen is found on normal cells, these antibodies also cause damage to these cells.

Table 36.3 lists some of the mAbs currently in use. Bevacizumab has angiogenesis-inhibiting properties. Prototype Drug Chart: Bevacizumab lists specific information on bevacizumab. Prototype Drug Chart: Rituximab lists specific drug information on rituximab.

Alemtuzumab
Alemtuzumab is an unconjugated, humanized mAb against the cell surface antigen CD52 that promotes antigen-dependent cell lysis of leukemic cells. CD52 is found on most B and T lymphocytes; on the majority of monocytes, macrophages, and natural killer (NK) cells; and on some granulocytes, stem cells, and mature spermatozoa. Although normal cells may express this antigen, malignant cells are much more sensitive to the destructive activity of this antibody. This drug is most commonly used for management of chronic lymphocytic leukemia (CLL) and multiple sclerosis (MS). However, alemtuzumab should be

TABLE 36.3 Monoclonal Antibodies

Drug Name and Type	Route and Dosage	Uses and Considerations
Alemtuzumab	Chronic lymphocytic leukemia: A: IV: Initially, 3 mg over 2 h once daily. When tolerated, escalate dose to 10 mg/d until infusion reactions are grade 2 or less, then start maintenance dose: 30 mg 3 × weekly on alternate days (e.g., Monday, Wednesday, Friday). Total therapy duration including dose escalation is 12 wk. MS with inadequate response to two or more previous treatments: A: IV: First treatment: 12 mg daily for 5 d Second treatment: 12 months later, 12 mg daily for 3 d (Not FDA approved for subcut use).	For CLL and MS. Premedicate 30 min before infusion with diphenhydramine and acetaminophen and an antiinfective prophylaxis to reduce risk of opportunistic infection. Monitor for infusion-related reaction. *Absolute contraindication:* HIV PB: UK; t½: 12 d
Bevacizumab (*VEGFR*/mAb; prototype)	See Prototype Drug Chart: Bevacizumab	
Cetuximab	A: IV: Initial infusion dose is 400 mg/m² over 2 h, then continue weekly infusions of 250 mg/m² over 60 min.	For colorectal and head and neck cancers. Monitor for infusion-related reactions and worsening symptoms of cardiac or respiratory problems. PB: UK; t½: 41–213 h

Continued

TABLE 36.3 Monoclonal Antibodies—cont'd

Drug Name and Type	Route and Dosage	Uses and Considerations
Ibritumomab tiuxetan	A: IV: Given in two steps: Step 1: Day 1, admin rituximab 250 mg/m² with initial rate at 50 mg/h; increase as tolerated to a max of 400 mg/h. Step 2: Day 7, 8, or 9 repeat rituximab; within 4 h of second rituximab infusion, give ibritumomab 0.4 mCi/kg over 10 min; *max:* 32 mCi. Adjust dose for thrombocytopenia.	For untreated or relapsed/refractory follicular B-cell NHL. Premedicate with diphenhydramine and acetaminophen 30 min before each rituximab dose. Use actual body weight to calculate dose, not to exceed 32 mCi. *Do not* exceed 10% of the prescribed dose. *Do not* give Y-90 ibritumomab tiuxetan if platelets are <100,000 cells/mm³. Monitor CBC and platelet count. PB: UK; t½: 30 h
Panitumumab	A: IV: 6 mg/kg admin over 60 min given once q2wk.	Fully human Ab against EGFR colorectal cancer. Not indicated for *RAS* mutation–positive or *RAS* mutation–unknown cancers. Monitor for acute or worsening dermatologic changes; monitor serum electrolytes. PB: nonlinear, dose dependent; t½: 7.5 d
Trastuzumab	A: IV: Breast cancer: Week 1: 4 mg/kg over 90 min Week 2: If patient tolerates initial infusion, admin 2 mg/kg over 30 min once weekly. Other treatment protocols exist (see full prescriber's information). Gastric/GEJ adenocarcinoma given in combination with other chemotherapeutic drugs: Day 1: 8 mg/kg over 90 min. Day 22: 6 mg/kg over 30–90 min every 21 d.	*ERBB2*-positive metastatic breast cancer and not previously treated *ERBB2*-metastatic gastric or GEJ adenocarcinoma. *Do not* substitute trastuzumab for or with ado-trastuzumab emtansine. Monitor CBC and cardiac function; hold or adjust dose for LVEF ≥16% absolute decrease from baseline; may need to permanently discontinue. Monitor for infusion-related reactions such as fever, chills, and dyspnea. PB: UK; t½: dose dependent, 6–16 d

A, Adult; *Ab*, antibody; *admin*, administer; *CBC*, complete blood count; *CLL*, chronic lymphocytic leukemia; *d*, day; *EGFR*, epidermal growth factor receptor; *FDA*, US Food and Drug Administration; *GEJ*, gastroesophageal junction; *h*, hour; *HIV*, human immunodeficiency virus; *IV*, intravenous; *LVEF*, left ventricular ejection fraction; *mAb*, monoclonal antibody; *max*, maximum dosage; *mCi*, millicurie; *min*, minutes; *MS*, multiple sclerosis; *NHL*, non-Hodgkin lymphoma; *PB*, protein bound; *q*, every; *subcut*, subcutaneous, *t½*, half-life; *UK*, unknown; *VEGFR*, vascular endothelial growth factor receptor; *wk*, week; *Y-90*, yttrium-90; <, less than; ≥, greater than or equal to.

reserved for patients who have had an inadequate response to two or more drugs for the treatment of MS.

Pharmacokinetics
Alemtuzumab is administered as an IV infusion. Its average half-life is 12 days, and steady-state levels are reached by about 6 weeks. Alemtuzumab is largely confined to blood and interstitial spaces. mAbs bind to target cell surfaces and are destroyed along with the target cell; they are then cleared as debris from the blood and are eliminated in the feces.

Pharmacodynamics
Alemtuzumab binds to leukemic cells that express the CD52 cell surface antigen and induces antibody-dependent lysis. Alemtuzumab seems to have preferential effects in the blood and bone marrow, as opposed to the spleen or lymph nodes, which indicates that alemtuzumab is most effective in hematologic disease. As an unconjugated mAb, this drug relies on inducing apoptotic signals and activation of mechanisms such as complement or T cells to attack and kill the target cells. Alemtuzumab is also associated with the release of tumor necrosis factor, interleukin 6, and interferon gamma.

Side Effects and Adverse Reactions
The most common side effect of alemtuzumab that is not related to infusion reactions or pancytopenia is fatigue. Another common side effect is flulike symptoms. Subcutaneous injections, compared with IV infusion, have been shown to decrease the incidence of flulike symptoms. Additional reactions include nausea, blood pressure changes, hyperglycemia, and hypoxia; these are common and often require premedication with antihistamines and acetaminophen. Alemtuzumab can cause severe lymphopenia and a rapid, sustained lymphocyte count decrease in addition to fatal autoimmune pancytopenia and prolonged myelosuppression. Because of severe lymphopenia, patients are at increased risk for infections. Other adverse events include nonlethal arrhythmias, heart failure, cardiomyopathy, and decreased ejection fraction along with infusion reactions and rash. Some patients have reduced reactions with subsequent infusions.

Drug Interactions
Specific drug interactions have not been reported with this drug; however, concomitant administration of drugs with similar pharmacologic effects may cause additive side effects, including toxicity.

Cetuximab
Cetuximab is a recombinant human/mouse chimeric mAb that binds specifically to the extracellular domain of the human *EGFR*. However, cetuximab differs in mechanism of action from small-molecule TK inhibitors (e.g., imatinib) that inhibit the TK activity of *EGFR* by interfering with ATP binding; cetuximab blocks the *EGFR* receptor. It is most commonly used for the management of colorectal and head and neck cancers.

Pharmacokinetics
Cetuximab is administered as an IV infusion, and it exhibits nonlinear pharmacokinetics. The mean half-life ranges from 41 to 213 hours. Steady-state half-life ranges from 75 to 188 hours. The pharmacokinetics do not seem to have any effect on patients with renal or hepatic impairments.

Pharmacodynamics
Cetuximab still contains about 30% mouse protein. It binds specifically to *EGFR* on both normal and tumor cells and prevents formation of a ligand that usually attaches epidermal growth factor (*EGF*) to the receptor. This action prevents the receptor from binding to agonists that activate it. As a result, *EGFR*-TKs are not activated, and the signals are not conducted downstream. Other effects of this drug include inhibition of cell growth, induction of apoptosis, decreased proinflammatory cytokine and vascular growth factor production, and internalization of the *EGFR*. Cetuximab may make cancer cells more vulnerable to other cancer chemotherapy agents and radiation therapy. The drug is most effective in causing regression in tumors that have the wild-type *KRAS* oncogene and overexpress *EGFR*.

Side Effects and Adverse Reactions
Cetuximab carries a black-box warning for infusion reactions, usually with the initial dosing, although severe reactions also have been reported during later infusions. Manifestations include rapid onset of airway obstruction, including bronchospasm, stridor, hoarseness, urticaria, and hypotension. Cetuximab is associated with dermatologic changes that typically involve the face, upper chest, and back. An acneiform rash occurred in 90% of patients, usually within the first 2 weeks of therapy. Most patients continued to have the rash for at least 28 days after therapy was discontinued.

Drug Interactions
Minimal information is available on drug interactions, although cisplatin and radiation therapy increased the incidence of adverse events.

Ibritumomab Tiuxetan
Ibritumomab tiuxetan is a conjugated murine mAb. Yttrium-90 (Y-90), a pure beta-radionuclide ibritumomab, binds specifically to the human B lymphocytes that express the CD20 cell surface antigen. This drug is most commonly used for management of B-cell types of non-Hodgkin lymphoma (NHL).

Pharmacokinetics
Ibritumomab tiuxetan is administered as an IV infusion. Its physical half-life is 64 hours, and its biologic half-life (determined by radioactivity detection) is 30 hours. The drug is excreted to a slight degree by the kidneys (7.2%) but is mostly eliminated in the feces. Y-90 decays by emission of beta particles with a half-life of 64.1 hours.

Pharmacodynamics
Ibritumomab tiuxetan binds to the CD20 antigen on B lymphocytes and lymphoma cells. After binding with the CD20 antigen, beta-wave radioactive emissions from the attached radionuclide, Y-90, induce cellular damage by the formation of free radicals in the target and neighboring cells. This cellular damage prevents cells from dividing.

Side Effects and Adverse Reactions
Ibritumomab tiuxetan carries a black-box warning for infusion reactions, bone marrow suppression, and exfoliative dermatitis. Severe infusion reactions warrant discontinuing the drug. Less severe infusion reactions may be managed using premedication with antihistamines and acetaminophen. Some patients experienced reduced reactions with the second and subsequent infusions. Common adverse effects include pancytopenia, asthenia, fever, chills, nausea, vomiting, cephalgia, abdominal pain, and infections.

Drug Interactions
Ibritumomab tiuxetan increases the risk for bleeding or hemorrhage when used along with anticoagulant or antiplatelet drugs, including nonsteroidal antiinflammatory drugs, aspirin, salicylate derivatives, thrombolytic therapy, and anticoagulants. Immunization with live viruses is not recommended for 12 months after therapy because of the patient's immunosuppressed state. No other formal studies have been conducted with other drugs to determine specific drug interactions.

Panitumumab
Panitumumab is a fully human mAb with a high affinity for the *EGFR* extracellularly. It is most commonly used in the management of advanced metastatic colorectal carcinomas that express or overexpress *EGFR*.

Pharmacokinetics
Panitumumab is administered as an IV infusion. It is a small immunoglobulin that appears to be eliminated in the feces. The half-life ranges from 3.6 to 10.9 days, and the steady state is reached by the third infusion. Mild to moderate hepatic and renal impairment do not affect the drug's action.

Pharmacodynamics
Panitumumab binds strongly to the *EGFR* when it is overexpressed on malignant cells. It binds specifically to the *EGFR* on both normal and tumor cells. As a result, *EGFR*-TKs are not activated, and the signals are not conducted downstream. Other effects of this drug include inhibition of cell growth, induction of apoptosis, and decreased proinflammatory cytokine and vascular growth factor production. Tumors must express *EGFR* for patients to be candidates for panitumumab.

Side Effects and Adverse Reactions
Panitumumab carries a black-box warning for dermatologic toxicity. Manifestations usually occur within the first 2 weeks of therapy and include dry skin, skin fissures, erythema, acneiform rash, pruritus, exfoliation, and nail disorders, such as paronychia. Electrolyte imbalances, specifically hypomagnesemia and hypocalcemia, may occur and require replacement. Severe diarrhea can occur when panitumumab is given along with irinotecan. Severe infusion reactions, including angioedema and anaphylaxis, have occurred with hypotension and bronchospasm. Although this reaction is rare, patients should be monitored closely throughout the infusion. Full resuscitative equipment should be available during infusion, including epinephrine, corticosteroids, IV antihistamines, bronchodilators, and oxygen.

Drug Interactions
Panitumumab is not recommended for use in combination with other antineoplastic drug regimens because of the increased toxic reactions. No other information on drug interactions is available.

Tositumomab
Tositumomab is a murine mAb conjugated with the radioactive isotope Iodine I-131. Like rituximab and ibritumomab tiuxetan, the antibody portion of this drug binds specifically to the human B lymphocytes that express the CD20 cell surface antigen. This drug is most commonly used to manage B-cell NHL that does not respond to rituximab.

Pharmacokinetics

Tositumomab is administered as four IV infusions in two distinct steps. It has a median blood clearance of 68.2 mg/h (with a 485-mg dosage). The mean total-body effective half-life is 67 hours. The Iodine I-131 decays with beta and gamma emissions with a half-life of 8.04 days. The elimination of Iodine I-131 occurs by decay and is excreted in the urine. Whole-body clearance was 67% of the injected dose, with elimination occurring mostly in the urine. Patients with high tumor burden, splenomegaly, or bone marrow involvement had faster clearance, shorter terminal half-life, and larger volume distribution.

Pharmacodynamics

A tositumomab therapeutic regimen is administered as a two-step process. Each step consists of unlabeled tositumomab administered intravenously followed by Iodine I-131 tositumomab. The unlabeled tositumomab is given to decrease splenic targeting and to increase the terminal half-life of the Iodine I-131 tositumomab. The regimen induces cytotoxicity by combining the immunologic effects of antibody binding to nonmalignant B lymphocytes in the circulation, liver, and spleen. Actions of the antibody include the induction of complement-mediated cytolysis, antibody-dependent cellular cytotoxicity, and apoptosis. Radiation activity is cytotoxic not only to the cells bound by the radiolabeled antibody but also to adjacent normal cells, a process called the *cross-fire effect*. Together, these actions result in sustained depletion of circulating CD20-positive lymphocytes and lymphoma cells.

Side Effects and Adverse Reactions

Tositumomab carries a black-box warning for fetal damage when used during pregnancy, for severe hypersensitivity reactions (anaphylaxis), severe bone marrow suppression, and radiation exposure.

PROTOTYPE DRUG CHART

Rituximab

Drug Class	Dosage
Humanized monoclonal antibody	*Relapsed/refractory low-grade or follicular CD20-positive B-cell NHL:* A: IV: 375 mg/m^2 once weekly for 4 doses; may be retreated for an additional 4 doses Combination chemotherapy treatment: A: IV: Day 1 of each cycle, 375 mg/m^2 for up to 8 infusions Maintenance therapy with Y-90 ibritumomab: Day 1, admin 250 mg/m^2; day 7, 8, or 9, admin second rituximab dose within 4 h after Y-90 ibritumomab. *CD20-positive CLL in combination with fludarabine and cyclophosphamide:* Cycle 1: 375 mg/m^2 1 d before fludarabine and cyclophosphamide Cycles 2–6: 500 mg/m^2 plus fludarabine 25 mg/m^2/d on days 1–3 and cyclophosphamide 250 mg/m^2/d on days 1–3, repeated every 28 d for 6 cycles *RA, in combination with methotrexate:* 1000 mg on days 1 and 15. Admin subsequent courses every 16–24 wk based on clinical evaluation. Admin methylprednisolone 30 min before each infusion for RA. Premedicate 30 min before rituximab with diphenhydramine and acetaminophen.
Contraindications	**Drug-Lab-Food Interactions**
Patients who are or may become pregnant and those who are breast-feeding; those who have previously had hepatitis B; have active bacterial or viral infection; those who have moderate to severe renal, liver, and/or cardiac disease; and those with preexisting pulmonary fibrosis.	Drug: Hypotension is potentiated when drug is coadministered with antihypertensive drugs. Bone marrow suppression is potentiated when drug is coadministered with drugs that also cause bone marrow suppression, increasing risk for infection and bleeding. Rituximab reduces effectiveness of vaccinations. Lab: None known Food: None known
Pharmacokinetics	**Pharmacodynamics**
Absorption: Bioavailability is 100% after IV infusion. Distribution: Throughout extracellular fluid, bone marrow, and secondary lymphoid tissues (primarily the spleen); t½: first infusion, 76.3 h; fourth infusion, 205.8 h. Metabolism: Degraded by circulating and liver-based phagocytic cells. Excretion: As cellular debris in feces	Antibody binding specifically to the CD20 cell surface antigen on B lymphocytes
Therapeutic Effects/Uses	
Relapsed or refractory, low-grade, or follicular CD20-positive B-cell NHL, CLL, RA, Wegener granulomatosis. Mechanism of Action: Binds to CD20-positive B lymphocytes and lymphoma cells, leading to complement-dependent cytotoxicity, antibody-dependent cellular cytotoxicity, and apoptosis.	
Side Effects	**Adverse Reactions**
Bone marrow suppression with pancytopenia, tumor lysis syndrome, hypotension, night sweats, joint and muscle aches, headaches, soreness at injection site	Infusion reactions, pulmonary fibrosis, cardiac dysrhythmias, heart failure, reactivation of dormant viruses

A, Adult; *admin*, administer; *CLL*, chronic lymphocytic leukemia; *d*, day; *h*, hour; *IV*, intravenous; *min*, minute; *NHL*, non-Hodgkin lymphoma; *RA*, rheumatoid arthritis; *t½*, half-life; *wk*, week; *Y-90*, yttrium-90.

Specific tositumomab side effects and adverse effects include asthenia, headache, hypotension, nausea, vomiting, abdominal pain, diarrhea, hypothyroidism, cough, dyspnea, pleural effusion, and pneumonia. Toxicities associated with radioimmunotherapy can be acute, delayed, or long term. The most common acute toxicities are fever, rigors, fatigue, headache, and nausea, whereas hypotension and allergic reactions are less common. Delayed toxicities include shortness of breath, fever, signs of infection, inflammation, pain with urination, rash, sore joints, and bone marrow suppression. Long-term toxicities are myelodysplasia or acute leukemia, secondary malignancies, and hypothyroidism. Just as with other mAbs, this drug causes profound bone marrow suppression that may require dose interruptions or reductions, based on severity, and is more profound in patients who are also receiving standard cytotoxic chemotherapy. In addition, infusion reactions with fever, nausea, chills, blood pressure changes, hyperglycemia, and hypoxia are common and often require premedication with antihistamines and acetaminophen. Some patients have reduced reactions with subsequent infusions.

CLINICAL JUDGMENT [NURSING PROCESS]
mTOR Inhibitors, Proteasome Inhibitors, and Monoclonal Antibodies

Concept: Cellular Regulation
- The ability for cells to maintain homeostasis, including responses to extracellular signals

Recognize Cues [Assessment]
- Obtain a detailed current medication history that includes prescription drugs, over-the-counter medicines, antacids, dietary supplements, vitamins, and herbal supplements and check for possible drug-drug interactions with targeted therapy drugs.
- Obtain a list of the patient's drug and food allergies.
- Obtain baseline information about the patient's physical status. Include height, weight, vital signs, cardiopulmonary assessment, intake and output, skin assessment, nutritional status, and any underlying diseases.
- Assess baseline laboratory values (complete blood count [CBC], uric acid, chemistry panel) to compare with future ones.
- Assess baseline results of pulmonary function tests, chest radiographs, electrocardiograms (ECGs), and renal and liver function studies.
- Assess patient, family, and caregiver knowledge related to the therapeutic regimen.

Analyze Cues and Prioritize Hypothesis [Patient Problems]
- Disrupted fluid and electrolyte balance
- Potential for altered clotting
- Potential for decreased immunity
- Need for teaching

Generate Solutions [Planning]
- The patient will remain free from infection.
- The patient and family will verbalize understanding of targeted therapy as part of an anticancer treatment regimen.
- The patient and family will verbalize strategies to minimize risks related to targeted therapy–related side effects.
- The patient and family will demonstrate understanding of the importance of reporting targeted therapy–related side effects and adverse reactions.
- The patient's side effects will be managed to a tolerable level and are not life-threatening.

Take Action [Nursing Interventions]
- Assess for any cardiac events, such as new chest pain and ECG changes.
- Monitor appropriate labs according to established protocol for specific targeted therapy (e.g., CBC with differential, electrolytes, renal and hepatic function, glucose, phosphate).
- Assess for any bleeding, especially if the patient is taking anticoagulants, antiplatelets, or nonsteroidal antiinflammatory drugs.
- Monitor liver function tests and renal function tests at baseline and at least once monthly during therapy.
- Examine the patient's skin closely at each visit for the presence of erythema, rash, peeling, or blister formation; rate the severity of dermatologic reactions, and determine whether infection is present in any nonintact skin.
- Administer prescribed premedications according to established protocols for specific targeted therapies (e.g., allopurinol, antiinfectives, antivirals, antihistamines).
- Have resuscitative equipment on standby as per protocol.
- Ensure appropriate supervising personnel are present according to protocols for specific targeted therapy.

Patient Teaching
General
- Ensure patient understands to avoid alcohol and nonessential drugs that are cleared by the liver or that have hepatotoxic effects (e.g., acetaminophen).
- Remind women with childbearing potential to avoid pregnancy throughout treatment and for up to 12 months after treatment is completed.
- Advise breast-feeding patients to stop breast-feeding during and for 60 days after therapy.
- Teach diabetic patients to monitor their glucose more frequently, and advise them when to seek medical help.
- Teach proper waste disposal to patients receiving monoclonal antibodies conjugated to radioisotopes (ibritumomab tiuxetan and tositumomab) to prevent unnecessary radiation exposure.

Side Effects
- Report symptoms of bleeding immediately, including black stools, vomit that looks like coffee grounds, and easy bleeding or bruising.
- Report symptoms of adverse effects or severe side effects promptly, especially fever, chills, persistent sore throat, swelling, weight gain, or increasing shortness of breath.
- Report symptoms of liver impairment immediately, including stomach/abdominal pain, yellowing eyes or skin, dark urine, or unusual fatigue.
- Advise the patient or a family member to immediately report convulsions, persistent headache, reduced eyesight, increased blood pressure, or blurred vision.

Evaluate Outcomes [Evaluation]
- Patient, family, and caregiver education needs are met.
- The patient, family, and caregiver understand therapy-related side effects and adverse reactions.
- The patient, family, and caregiver understand strategies to minimize side effects and adverse reactions.
- Side effects are managed effectively.
- The patient is free from infection.
- The patient's fluid balance and electrolytes are maintained at expected normal ranges.

Drug Interactions

Tositumomab increases the risk for bleeding or hemorrhage when used along with anticoagulant or antiplatelet therapy. When patients are immunosuppressed, immune response to vaccines and toxoids is decreased, and higher doses or more frequent boosters may be required. Other specific drug interactions have not been reported with this drug; however, concomitant administration of drugs with similar pharmacologic effects may cause additive side effects, including toxicity.

Trastuzumab

Trastuzumab is an mAb that binds to the *ERBB2* protein on the surface of cancer cells. The *ERBB2* receptor is structurally related to *VEGFR*. The *ERBB2* receptor is overexpressed in some breast, ovarian, and colon cancers. Proliferation and angiogenesis of cancer cells are increased with the overexpression of *ERBB2* receptors. When the VEGF pathway is inhibited, tumor growth is suppressed. Trastuzumab is most commonly used in combination with chemotherapy agents to manage breast and gastric cancers that have demonstrated overexpression of the *ERBB2* receptor. Trastuzumab and ado-trastuzumab emtansine are not interchangeable.

Pharmacokinetics

Trastuzumab is administered as a weekly IV infusion. Its half-life is 6 days. The steady state is reached within 9 weeks in patients with gastric cancer and 12 weeks in breast cancer patients. Elimination is unknown.

Pharmacodynamics

Trastuzumab is a mostly humanized mAb that binds to the *ERBB2* protein on the surface of breast, ovarian, and colon cancer cells that overexpress this receptor. This drug specifically inhibits the proliferation of cancer cells that overexpress *ERBB2* receptors. In addition, binding of trastuzumab to the cancer cell receptor increases killing of these cells through attack by immune system cells, especially NK cells and monocytes.

> ⚡ **PATIENT SAFETY**
>
> **Do Not Confuse…**
> **Trastuzumab** with **ado-trastuzumab emtansine**

Side Effects and Adverse Reactions

Trastuzumab carries a black-box warning for cardiomyopathy manifesting as congestive heart failure when the drug is used as a monotherapy. This risk is increased when the drug is given in combination with other drugs that cause cardiotoxicity, such as the anthracyclines and cyclophosphamide. Another black-box warning includes infusion-related reactions (anaphylaxis) and pulmonary toxicity. Hypersensitivity reactions, including anaphylaxis, may occur but are not common. Trastuzumab is associated with headache, dizziness, hypotension, fever, chills, and nausea during the initial infusion. After the initial infusion, these symptoms typically do not recur. Other common side effects include headache, muscle aches, and loss of appetite.

Drug Interactions

Trastuzumab can increase the incidence and severity of cardiac dysfunction in patients who receive trastuzumab in combination with anthracyclines and cyclophosphamide. Elevated INR can occur in patients taking warfarin concomitantly with trastuzumab. This drug may increase the myelosuppressive effects of other antineoplastic agents.

CLINICAL JUDGMENT CASE STUDY

A 64-year-old is diagnosed with stage III B-cell non-Hodgkin lymphoma (NHL). The patient is scheduled to receive rituximab and a traditional chemotherapy regimen of cyclophosphamide, doxorubicin, vincristine, and prednisolone, a combination known as "CHOP." The dosage and schedule of rituximab for the patient is 375 mg/m^2 IV on day 1 before the first CHOP chemotherapy cycle, which will be administered on day 8. The next two doses will be administered 2 days before the third and fifth cycles, and the remaining two cycles of rituximab will be administered after the sixth cycle of CHOP on days 134 and 141. The patient has a friend who is taking imatinib daily as an oral drug for CML and asks why rituximab must be taken intravenously through the implanted port. The patient also asks if a family member, who is a licensed practical nurse, could administer it at home rather than having to travel to the clinic for the chemotherapy.

1. What is the nurse's best response about why rituximab must be administered intravenously?
2. How are rituximab and imatinib different?
3. Why can the patient's family member *not* administer rituximab at home?
4. What side effects are specific for rituximab?
5. What are the most common adverse effects of rituximab?
6. What would the nurse teach the patient specifically in relation to rituximab therapy?

REVIEW QUESTIONS

1. A patient undergoing chemotherapy for breast cancer asks why she is not receiving trastuzumab like her sister. Which response by the nurse is correct?
   a. Your breast cancer cells are estrogen receptor positive, and targeted therapy is not needed.
   b. You are much older than your sister and would not tolerate the treatment well.
   c. The drug is expensive, and your insurance does not cover it.
   d. Your cancer cells do not have the target for trastuzumab.

2. Which instruction is important for the nurse to include when teaching a patient about imatinib therapy?
   a. Do not drink grapefruit juice while taking this drug.
   b. Go immediately to the emergency department if you develop a headache.
   c. This drug will only work for about 2 months.
   d. Be sure to take this drug on an empty stomach.

3. Which patient problem is a priority for patients receiving epidermal growth factor receptor inhibitors?
   a. Potential for decreased clotting related to bone marrow suppression and neutropenia
   b. Potential for tissue injury related to skin side effects
   c. Potential for injury related to reduced platelet activity
   d. Disturbed self-concept related to alopecia
4. Which class of targeted therapy would cause the nurse the most concern in regard to a possible infusion reaction?
   a. Tyrosine kinase inhibitors
   b. Multikinase inhibitors
   c. Monoclonal antibodies
   d. Proteasome inhibitors
5. A patient taking sunitinib reports that the skin on the hands and feet is red and painful, and has some blisters. Which action is appropriate for the nurse to take?
   a. The only action needed is to document the finding because this is a mild side effect.
   b. Advise the patient to wear gloves and mittens when going outdoors in cold weather.
   c. Advise the patient to avoid getting hands wet and touching food.
   d. Notify the oncologist to determine whether a dosage reduction is needed.
6. Which action is most important for the nurse to teach a patient who is taking tositumomab?
   a. Avoid drinking alcohol for 1 week after receiving this drug.
   b. Avoid smoking cigarettes for the entire treatment period.
   c. Use a separate bathroom and sit while urinating for 1 week after receiving this drug.
   d. Be sure to take this drug on an empty stomach, either 1 hour before or 2 hours after eating.
7. Which activity has a higher priority for the nurse to advise the patient to do while taking ixazomib?
   a. Drinking alcoholic beverages
   b. Taking aspirin or aspirin-containing drugs
   c. Socializing in crowds or with persons who are ill
   d. Taking the drug 1 hour before or 2 hours after food
8. A patient receiving a targeted therapy asks the nurse why St. John's wort must be avoided. Which response by the nurse is most appropriate?
   a. This herbal drug increases blood levels of most targeted therapies and increases the risk for severe side effects or adverse reactions.
   b. This herbal drug decreases blood levels of most targeted therapies and reduces their effectiveness.
   c. Targeted therapies increase blood levels of St. John's wort, increasing the risk of an overdose of this herbal agent.
   d. Targeted therapies bind with St. John's wort in the intestinal tract, preventing absorption of both the drug and the herbal agent.
9. A patient taking imatinib voices concern about gaining 5 pounds in the past week. Which statement is correct about imatinib and weight gain?
   a. Weight gain is an expected side effect of this drug because it increases the appetite.
   b. Weight gain is an indication of slow metabolism and possible hypothyroidism.
   c. Weight gain is an indication of water retention and possible renal impairment.
   d. Weight gain is an indication of a drug interaction between imatinib and loop diuretics.

37

Biologic Response Modifiers

http://evolve.elsevier.com/McCuistion/pharmacology

OBJECTIVES

- Discuss how biologic response modifiers affect the immune system.
- Describe the general actions of interferons to deter cancer cell growth.
- Summarize the benefits of colony-stimulating factors when used with chemotherapy drugs.
- Explain the effects interleukin-2 has on the immune system.

OUTLINE

Overview of Biologic Response Modifiers, 466
　Biologic Response Modifier Mechanisms, 466
　Chimeric Antigen Receptor T Cells, 467
Interferons, 467
　Interferon Alfa, 467
　Interferon Beta, 470
　Interferon Gamma, 470
Colony-Stimulating Factors, 470
　Erythropoietin-Stimulating Agents, 471
　Granulocyte Colony-Stimulating Factor, 473
　Granulocyte-Macrophage Colony–Stimulating Factor, 473
Interleukin-2, 473
　Interleukins, 473
　Aldesleukin, 474
Clinical Judgment Case Study, 476
Review Questions, 476

OVERVIEW OF BIOLOGIC RESPONSE MODIFIERS

Biologic Response Modifier Mechanisms

The immune system recognizes and protects the body from foreign invaders, such as bacteria or viruses; it also destroys damaged, diseased, or abnormal cells, including cancer cells. When the body detects an invader, an immune response is triggered, and substances such as white blood cells (WBCs), cytokines, and natural killer cells (NKCs) provide a certain level of protection. Biologic response modifiers (BRMs), also called *immunomodulators*, are a class of pharmacologic drugs used to enhance, direct, or restore the body's immune system. BRMs are made naturally in the body and are also developed in a laboratory. They can be targeted directly or indirectly toward cancer cells and toward disease-causing mechanisms that cause some autoimmune disorders. BRMs that directly target cancer cells are also called *targeted therapy*, and these are discussed in Chapter 36. Indirect therapies stimulate the body's immune system and do not directly target cancer cells. Biologic therapies are used to treat the cancer or the side effects caused by other cancer treatments. Recombinant DNA, the genetic engineering process that combines two human DNA strands artificially, and hybridoma technology, the process that genetically makes monoclonal antibodies, are two advances that have led to commercial mass production of BRMs (Fig. 37.1). Interferons (IFNs; alfa, beta, and gamma), tumor necrosis factor (TNF) inhibitors, erythropoietin (EPO), vaccines, colony-stimulating factors (CSFs), interleukins, and monoclonal antibodies (mAbs) are some currently known BRMs. With the exception of monoclonal antibodies, BRMs are a complex set of proteins produced by the immune system (Fig. 37.2). Monoclonal antibodies are considered for targeted therapies and are further discussed in Chapter 36. Like chemotherapy, BRMs suppress the immune system; people in an immunocompromised state are at risk for complications such as infection. BRMs should not be taken by those with active infections, immunodeficiency syndromes, and demyelinating disease (e.g., multiple sclerosis). BRMs assist the immune system in several ways:

- They enhance the immune system's ability to kill abnormal cells (immunomodulation).
- They change cancer cells to make them behave more like healthy cells.
- They inhibit normal cells from changing into cancer cells.
- They enhance the body's ability to repair or replace damaged cells caused by other cancer treatments.
- They prevent cancer cells from metastasizing (spreading to other parts of the body).

New BRMs are always under development and investigation for clinical effectiveness. One newly emerged method of immunotherapy is chimeric antigen receptor T cell (CAR T cell). A patient's T cells are removed and genetically modified to eradicate cancer cells. In 2017, the US Food and Drug Administration (FDA) approved two CAR T-cell therapies (tisagenlecleucel and axicabtagene ciloleucel) to treat children and young adults with acute lymphoblastic leukemia and diffuse large B-cell lymphoma in adults. Four other CAR T-cell therapies have been approved since then to target other lymphomas, leukemias, and multiple myelomas. Other categories of BRMs have been approved by the FDA. Of the BRMs, IFNs, CSFs, and interleukin-2 (IL-2) are further discussed later in this chapter.

Chimeric Antigen Receptor T Cells

A patient's T cells are removed and sent to a lab to genetically modify and grow proteins on the cell called chimeric antigen receptors (CARs). The cells are allowed to multiply and once enough CAR T cells are made, they are infused into the patient (Fig. 37.3). These CARs are able to recognize and bind to cancer cells and eliminate them. In addition, these cells are able to multiply in the patient's body for continued activity. CAR T-cell therapy is individualized to each patient; therefore each CAR is created to specific cancer's antigen. Currently, there are six therapies approved. Table 37.1 provides information on CAR T-cell therapies with their dosages, uses, and considerations. CAR T-cell therapy is generally used after other conventional treatments failed because of its serious or even life-threatening adverse effects. CAR T cells release large amounts of cytokines that can cause cytokine release syndrome (CRS). Signs and symptoms of CRS include high fever, dyspnea, severe GI disturbances, tachycardia, fatigue, and muscle and joint pains. Other adverse effects include changes in level of consciousness, seizures, dysphasia, and confusion. Table 37.3 provides information on the adverse effects, and Table 37.4 lists the black-box warnings for CAR T cells.

INTERFERONS

Interferons (IFNs) are a family of cytokines that occur naturally in the body. They are also produced in the laboratory. Various subtypes of IFNs have different mechanisms of action, with some overlapping actions. IFNs work directly on cancer cells to slow their growth or cause cancer cells to behave more like normal cells. Some IFNs also stimulate certain types of WBCs to fight cancer, which includes NKCs, T cells, and macrophages. Other IFNs have antiviral activity. The two main types of IFNs are type I and type II. *Type I interferons* include IFN-α (leukocyte IFN) and IFN-β (fibroblast and epithelial cell IFN). *Type II interferon* includes IFN-γ produced by $CD4^+$, $CD8^+$, NKCs, and lymphokine-activated killer (LAK) cells. Table 37.2 provides information on IFNs with their dosages, uses, and considerations.

Interferon Alfa

B-lymphocyte cells; non–B- and non–T-lymphocyte cells; and macrophages (mature monocytes) produce interferon alfa-2b (IFN-α-2b) endogenously in response to viral infection and other various exogenous inducers. Exogenous α-2b IFNs used as BRMs are considered second-generation IFNs. IFN-α-2a, a first-generation IFN, is currently not being marketed; however, both subtypes have similar actions. IFNs bind to cell receptors for biologic activities followed by activation of the tyrosine kinases (TKs). IFNs have been shown to have antiviral,

Fig. 37.1 Recombinant DNA.

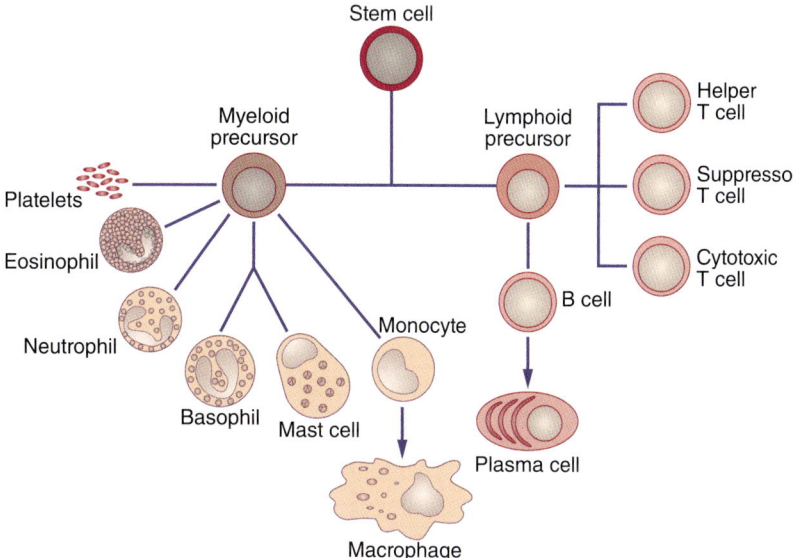

Fig. 37.2 Cells of the immune system.

Fig. 37.3 CAR T-cell therapy. Artificial leukocyte receptors. (From iStock.com/ttsz.)

TABLE 37.1 Biologic Response Modifiers: CAR T-Cell

Generic Drug Name	Route and Dosage	Uses and Considerations
Tisagenlecleucel	IV: Dosing varies: $0.2–6 \times 10^8$ CAR-positive viable T cells $\times 1$ after lymphodepleting regimen	For B-cell precursor acute lymphoblastic leukemia, large B-cell lymphoma, follicular lymphoma. Distribution is restricted due to cytokine release syndrome and neurological toxicity, which can be fatal. Screen for HBV, HCV, HIV, pregnancy, and infection. PB: UK; $t\frac{1}{2}$: 2.5–45.3 days
Axicabtagene ciloleucel	A: IV: Dosing varies: 2×10^6 CAR-positive viable T cells/kg/dose $\times 1$. Start 2 days after lymphodepleting regimen.	For follicular lymphoma and large B-cell lymphoma. Distribution limited due to cytokine release syndrome and neurological toxicity, which can be fatal. Screen for HBV, HCV, HIV, pregnancy, and infection. Metabolized by the liver. PB: UK; $t\frac{1}{2}$: UK
Brexucabtagene autoleucel	A: IV: Dosing varies: 2×10^6 CAR-T positive viable T cells/kg/dose $\times 1$. Start 2 days after lymphodepleting regimen.	For mantle cell lymphoma and B-cell precursor acute lymphoblastic leukemia. Distribution limited due to cytokine release syndrome and neurological toxicity which can be fatal. Screen for HBV, HCV, HIV, pregnancy, and infection. PB: UK; $t\frac{1}{2}$: UK
Lisocabtagene maraleucel	A: IV: Dosing varies: $90–110 \times 10^6$ CAR-T positive viable T cells $\times 1$. Start 2–7 days after lymphodepleting regimen.	For large B-cell lymphoma. Distribution limited due to cytokine release syndrome and neurological toxicity which can be fatal. Screen for HBV, HCV, HIV, pregnancy, and infection. PB: UK; $t\frac{1}{2}$: UK
Idecabtagene vicleucel	A: IV: Dosing varies: $300–460 \times 10^6$ CAR-T positive viable T cells $\times 1$. Start 2–7 days after lymphodepleting regimen.	For multiple myeloma. Distribution limited due to cytokine release syndrome and neurological toxicity which can be fatal. Screen for CMV, HBV, HCV, HIV, pregnancy, and infection. PB: UK; $t\frac{1}{2}$: UK
Ciltacabtagene autoleucel	A: IV: Dosing varies: $0.5–1 \times 10^6$ CAR-T positive viable T cells/kg/day $\times 1$. Start 2–4 days after lymphodepleting regimen.	Distribution limited due to cytokine release syndrome and neurological toxicity, which can be fatal. Screen for CMV, HBV, HCV, HIV, pregnancy, and infection. PB: UK; $t\frac{1}{2}$: 3–395 days

A, Adult; *CAR-T*, chimeric antigen receptor T cell; *CMV*, cytomegalovirus; *HBV*, hepatitis B virus; *HCV*, hepatitis C virus; *HIV*, human immunodeficiency virus; *IV*, intravenous; *kg*, kilogram; *PB*, protein binding; $t\frac{1}{2}$, half-life; *UK*, unknown.

TABLE 37.2 Biologic Response Modifiers: Interferons

Generic Drug Name	Route and Dosage	Uses and Considerations
Interferon alfa-2b	Hairy cell leukemia: A: IM/Subcut: 2 million units/m^2 3 times/wk for up to 6 mo Kaposi sarcoma: A: IM/Subcut: Initially: 30 million units/m^2 3 times/wk until severe intolerance or maximal response after 16 wk Malignant melanoma as adjuvant treatment: A: IV: Induction: 20 million units/m^2 for 5 consecutive d/wk for 4 wk Subcut: *Maint:* 10 million units/m^2 3 times/wk for 48 wk Non-Hodgkin's lymphoma (NHL): A: Subcut: 5 million units 3 times/wk for up to 18 mo	For hairy cell leukemia, adjuvant to surgical resection of malignant melanoma, follicular NHL, condyloma acuminata, AIDS-related Kaposi sarcoma, and chronic hepatitis B and non-A hepatitis. Monitor CBC, AST, ALT, ALP, LDH. PB: UK; t½: 2–3 h
Interferon gamma	Body surface area: >0.5 m^2: A: Subcut: 50 mcg/m^2 3 times/wk Body surface area: <0.5 m^2: A: Subcut: 1.5 mcg/kg per dose 3 times/wk	For chronic granulomatous disease and malignant osteopetrosis. PB: UK; t½: 0.5–6 h
Interferon beta-1b	Relapsing-remitting forms of MS: A: Subcut 250 mcg every other day. Incremental titration q2wk is recommended at 62.5 mcg every other day during wk 1 and 2, 125 mcg every other day during wk 3 and 4, and 187.5 mcg every other day during wk 5 and 6.	For MS. PB: UK; t½: 8 min–4.3 h

<, Less than; >, greater than; *A*, adult; *AIDS*, acquired immunodeficiency syndrome; *ALP*, alkaline phosphatase; *ALT*, alanine aminotransferase; *AST*, aspartate aminotransferase; *CBC*, complete blood count; *d*, day; *h*, hour; *IM*, intramuscular; *IV*, intravenous; *LDH*, lactate dehydrogenase; *maint*, maintenance; *min*, minute; *mo*, month; *MS*, multiple sclerosis; *NHL*, non-Hodgkin lymphoma; *PB*, protein binding; *q*, every; *subcut*, subcutaneous; *t½*, half-life; *UK*, unknown; *wk*, week; *y*, year.

antiproliferative, and immunomodulatory effects, and they affect cellular differentiation, regulation of cell surface major histocompatibility complex (MHC) antigen expression, and cytokine induction.

IFN-α-2b is approved for hairy cell leukemia, AIDS-related Kaposi sarcoma, malignant melanoma, and non-Hodgkin lymphoma (NHL); hepatitis B and C viruses; and human papillomavirus (HPV) infection. In addition, it has been used in combination with antiviral or anticancer drugs in patients with Philadelphia chromosome–positive (Ph$^+$) chronic myelogenous leukemia (CML), renal cell cancer (RCC), and T-cell leukemia/lymphoma.

Pharmacokinetics

IFN-α-2b is administered parenterally via intravenous (IV), intramuscular (IM), or subcutaneous routes. Mean serum concentrations after IM and subcutaneous administration were similar. IFN is catabolized by the renal system. Maximum concentration occurs in 3 to 12 hours, and elimination half-life is 2 to 3 hours. After the IV route, the half-life is reached in about 2 hours and is undetectable in the serum in about 4 hours. IFN-α-2b is not cleared by hemodialysis.

Pharmacodynamics

IFN-α-2b has similar actions to native IFN-α. Endogenous IFNs are secreted by leukocytes in response to viral infection or various synthetic and biologic inducers. Once the IFN binds to cell surface receptors, TKs are activated, which produce several IFN-stimulated enzymes that cause antiviral, antiproliferative, and immunomodulatory effects; cellular differentiation; regulation of cell surface MHC antigen expression; and cytokine induction. Antiviral effects include inhibiting viral replication by inhibiting translation of viral proteins; inhibition of viral penetration and uncoating and/or viral assembly and release; and enhancement of the lytic (killing) effects of cytotoxic T lymphocytes. Viruses affected include hepatitis B, C, and D; herpes simplex virus types 1 and 2; human immunodeficiency virus (HIV); HPV; and rhinovirus, among others.

Antineoplastic effects may result from IFN's ability to induce a host response to the tumor (e.g., immunomodulatory effects), cause a cytostatic effect on tumor cells, and slow the rate of cell proliferation by enhancing or inhibiting the synthesis of specific proteins, modifying cell surface antigen expression, and/or modulating the immune system. IFNs prolong all phases of the cell cycle and promote cells to enter the G$_0$ (resting) phase, which is thought to be important in treating hairy cell leukemia.

Side Effects and Adverse Reactions

Side effects are not usually severe but, when present, persons may report flulike symptoms, fatigue, and loss of appetite. Table 37.3 lists the common adverse effects for BRMs, including IFNs, and any dosage adjustments or discontinuation of the drug for toxicity. The black-box warning includes the risk of fatal or life-threatening neuropsychiatric, autoimmune, ischemic, and infectious disorders. Patients must be closely monitored with periodic clinical and laboratory evaluations. Table 37.4 compares the black-box warnings for IFN, IL-2, and EPO. While taking IFN-α, close monitoring of complete blood count (CBC), chest radiography (CXR), electrocardiography (ECG), liver function tests (LFTs), triglycerides, and thyroid function tests (TFTs) should be conducted.

Drug Interactions

It is unknown whether IFN-α-2b is metabolized by the liver; therefore caution is advised when IFN-α-2b is taken with other drugs metabolized through the hepatic cytochrome P450 enzyme system. The effect of IFN on the CYP450 system might increase enzyme degradation or inhibit CYP450 system. IFN-α-2b with concomitant use of theophylline may result in a 100% increase in theophylline concentrations. Caution is also warranted when taking drugs (e.g., antiretroviral nonnucleoside reverse transcriptase inhibitors [NNRTIs] and antiretroviral protease inhibitors) that can cause liver toxicity because IFNs also can cause liver damage. Hearing loss has been associated with IV eflornithine in

TABLE 37.3 Adverse Effects and Dosage Modifications for Biologic Response Modifiers

Drug Class	Side Effects/Adverse Effects	Dose Adjustment or Discontinuation
Colony-stimulating factors: Erythropoietin (EPO)	Hypertension, flulike symptoms, rash, anaphylactoid reactions, antibody formation, arthralgia, myalgia, cephalgia, edema, red cell aplasia, thromboembolism, injection site reaction, urticaria, bronchospasm, cough, encephalopathy	Stop treatment: Anaphylactoid reactions, red cell aplasia secondary to antibody formation Adjust dosage: Hgb rise >1 g/dL in 2 wk, CKD
Colony-stimulating factors: Granulocyte colony-stimulating factor (G-CSF), granulocyte-macrophage colony-stimulating factor (GM-CSF)	Peripheral edema, flulike symptoms, chest pain, splenomegaly, anaphylactoid reactions, elevated hepatic enzymes, rash, cardiac arrhythmia, cephalgia, arthralgia, leukocytosis, asthenia, antibody formation, pulmonary disorders, capillary leak syndrome	Stop treatment: Anaphylactoid reaction, capillary leak syndrome, ANC >10,000/mm^3; ARDS, splenic involvement, sickle cell crisis, alveolar hemorrhage Adjust dosage: Vasculitis, renal disorders
Erythropoietin-stimulating drugs (ESAs; interferons)	Flulike symptoms (fever, chills, tachycardia, malaise, myalgia, cephalgia), chest pain, fatigue, depression, drowsiness, dizziness, irritability, paresthesia, insomnia, alopecia, skin rash, amenorrhea, nausea, diarrhea, vomiting, xerostomia, abdominal pain, pancytopenia, dyspnea, cough, pharyngitis, infection	Stop treatment: Severe depression, hypersensitivity reactions, hematologic toxicity (ANC <500/mm^3 or platelets <25,000/mm^3); severe hepatic decompensation Adjust dosages for other hematologic toxicity.
Interleukin (IL-2)	Hypotension, peripheral edema, tachycardia, SVT, flulike symptoms, rash, pruritus, electrolyte imbalances, diarrhea, vomiting, nausea, weight gain, anorexia, abdominal pain, pancytopenia, elevated liver function tests, weakness, renal impairment, respiratory disorders, antibody formation, infection	See Table 37.5.

<, Less than; >, greater than; ANC, absolute neutrophil count; ARDS, acute respiratory distress syndrome; CKD, chronic kidney disease; Hgb, hemoglobin; SVT, supraventricular tachycardia; wk, week.

TABLE 37.4 US Food and Drug Administration Black-Box Warnings for CAR T cell, Interferon, Interleukin-2, and Erythropoietin

CAR T Cell	Interferon	Aldesleukin (IL-2)	Erythropoietin
Cytokine release syndrome	Autoimmune disorders	Cardiac disease	Hgb concentration >11 g/dL
Neurological toxicity	Infectious disorders	Coma	Myocardial infarction
Do not administer if active infection.	Ischemic disorders	Capillary leak syndrome	Neoplastic disease
	Neuropsychiatric disorders	Infection	Surgery
		Pulmonary disease	Thromboembolic disease
		Treatment requires a specialized setting and experienced clinician.	

>, Greater than; CAR T cell, chimeric antigen receptor T cell; Hgb, hemoglobin; IL, interleukin.

combination with IFN-α-2b. Other drugs that may interact with IFN include barbiturates, colchicine, chemotherapy, and hydroxyurea. No information is available on drug-food or drug-herbal interactions.

Interferon Beta

Interferon beta (IFN-β) is a type I IFN produced by fibroblasts, macrophages, and epithelial cells. It has both antiviral and immune regulatory activities, especially against herpesvirus, HPV, hepatitis B and C, and HIV. IFN-β-1a is indicated for the treatment of multiple sclerosis (MS); IFN-β-1a inhibits the proinflammatory cytokines responsible for triggering the autoimmune reaction that leads to MS. IFN-β-1a also reduces T-cell migration across the blood-brain barrier and increases the production of nerve growth factor, which promotes axonal recovery; this may result in remyelination.

Interferon Gamma

Interferon gamma (IFN-γ) is a type II IFN produced endogenously by targeting macrophages, T lymphocytes, and NKCs, and it is genetically produced from *Escherichia coli*. IFN-γ regulates the immune system and interacts with other interleukins, and it has direct and indirect antiviral activities by affecting attachment, penetration, uncoating, transcription, assembly, and maturation of viruses. It is also the primary factor for macrophage activation to kill parasites and cancer cells. IFN-γ enhances antigen processing and presentation by increasing the expression of MHC. It also increases humoral immunity and the expression of tumor suppressor genes, and it enhances recruitment of leukocytes to the sites of inflammation. IFN-γ is used for the treatment of chronic granulomatous disease and osteopetrosis.

COLONY-STIMULATING FACTORS

Hematopoietic colony-stimulating factors (CSFs) are proteins that stimulate or regulate the growth, maturation, and differentiation of bone marrow stem cells. Like IFNs, CSFs are a subgroup of cytokines. Although CSFs are not directly tumoricidal, they are useful in cancer treatment. Chemotherapy depletes normal stem cells and the blood cells that they produce; CSFs promote the growth of these blood cells, which increases the opportunity to continue with chemotherapy. More specifically, CSFs have other functions:

- CSFs decrease the length of posttreatment neutropenia—the length of time neutrophils, a type of WBC, are decreased secondary to chemotherapy—thereby reducing the risk, incidence, and duration of infection.
- CSFs permit the delivery of higher doses of chemotherapy drugs. Myelosuppression, suppression of bone marrow activity, is often a dose-limiting toxicity of chemotherapy. Higher, possibly tumoricidal doses of these drugs cannot be administered because of potentially life-threatening side effects. CSFs can minimize the myelosuppressive toxicity, thus allowing the delivery of the higher doses.
- CSFs reduce bone marrow recovery time after bone marrow transplantation.
- CSFs enhance macrophage or granulocyte tumor-, virus-, and fungus-destroying abilities.
- CSFs prevent severe thrombocytopenia after myelosuppressive chemotherapy.

CSFs have been used to treat patients with neutropenia secondary to disease or treatment and can be administered both intravenously and subcutaneously. The CSFs that are FDA approved for clinical use are erythropoietin-stimulating agents (ESAs), granulocyte colony-stimulating factors (G-CSFs), and granulocyte-macrophage colony-stimulating factors (GM-CSFs).

Erythropoietin-Stimulating Agents

Erythropoietin (EPO) is a glycoprotein produced by the kidney; it stimulates red blood cell (RBC) production in the bone marrow. Specifically, EPO stimulates the division and differentiation of committed RBC progenitors (parent cells destined to become circulating RBCs) in the bone marrow. RBCs contain hemoglobin, which is necessary to transport oxygen in the body.

Erythropoietin-stimulating agents (ESAs) include epoetin alfa and darbepoetin alfa. ESAs are administered as an injection to stimulate RBC production in the bone marrow to increase oxygen-carrying capacity. They must be used cautiously and only as indicated because of the potential for serious complications (e.g., myocardial infarction, stroke, venous thromboembolism, thrombosis of vascular access, and tumor progression or recurrence) and even death. Table 37.3 lists the common adverse effects for BRMs, including ESAs, dosage adjustments, and whether discontinuation of the drug is warranted. Prototype Drug Chart: Epoetin Alfa (Erythropoietin) provides specific drug information for epoetin alfa.

Pharmacokinetics

EPO can be administered either subcutaneously or intravenously. The IV route for either drug results in a more rapid peak, whereas the subcutaneous route, with its delayed systemic absorption, gives a more sustained response. Serum half-life for darbepoetin alfa after IV administration is 22.1 hours in patients without chronic renal failure (CRF). With subcutaneous injections, peak plasma concentrations occur at 71 to 123 hours (in CRF, peak is 24–72 hours), and the half-life of darbepoetin alfa in patients with CRF ranges from 27 to 89 hours. The pharmacokinetics in children suggests darbepoetin is absorbed more rapidly after subcutaneous injection compared with adults.

Pharmacodynamics

EPO stimulates erythropoiesis as endogenous EPO. Exogenous EPO stimulates the bone marrow in the production of RBCs to transport oxygen.

Side Effects and Adverse Reactions

Absolute contraindications for EPO include hypertension or hypersensitivity to albumin, hamster protein, or polysorbate 80. Black-box warnings include patients with a hemoglobin (Hgb) concentration greater than 11 g/dL, those who have had myocardial infarction (MI) or stroke, and patients with neoplastic or thromboembolic disease, because of the increased risk of death. Other side effects and adverse reactions are similar to those of epoetin alfa. Table 37.4 compares the black-box warnings for IFNs, IL-2, and EPO.

Drug Interactions

Darbepoetin alfa and epoetin alfa should not be used concomitantly because of the danger of adverse reactions. Concurrent administration of androgens can increase the patient's response to EPO. In addition, the patient's iron stores should be repleted because inadequate iron interferes with EPO's therapeutic response.

PROTOTYPE DRUG CHART
Epoetin Alfa (Erythropoietin)

Drug Class	Dosage
Biologic response modifier	*Black Box Warning:* ESAs increase the risk for death when given to target Hgb >11 g/dL in cancer patients. A: Modify dose to keep target Hgb <11 g/dL. CKD: A/Adol ≥17 y: IV/Subcut: 50–100 units/kg 3 times/wk Dialysis patients: Initiate IV treatment when Hgb <10 g/dL Anemia as a result of myelosuppression: A: Subcut: 150 units/kg 3 times/wk or 40,000 units once/wk
Contraindications	**Drug-Lab-Food Interactions**
Absolute contraindications: Benzyl alcohol hypersensitivity *Black Box Warning:* Hgb concentration >11 g/dL; myocardial infarction; stroke; neoplastic disease; surgery; thromboembolic disease *Precautions:* Hypertension, anticoagulant therapy, cardiac disease, coagulopathy, dialysis, folate deficiency, heart failure, electrolyte imbalance, hyperparathyroidism, iron-deficiency hematologic disease, renal disease, seizure disorders, vitamin B$_{12}$ deficiency	Drug: Use with darbepoetin alfa has additive effects that increase adverse reactions. Androgens have an additive effect to epoetin alfa. Probenecid and amphotericin B may inhibit the response of epoetin. Lab: Inadequate iron stores interfere with the therapeutic response to epoetin alfa. Monitor transferrin saturation and serum ferritin before and during treatment. Administer iron therapy when serum ferritin is <100 mcg/L or when transferrin saturation is <20%. Food: None known

Continued

PROTOTYPE DRUG CHART—cont'd
Epoetin Alfa (Erythropoietin)

Pharmacokinetics	Pharmacodynamics
Absorption: Subcut, IV Distribution: PB: UK Metabolism: t½: Affected by renal function; 4–13 h in patients with CKD (IV); 20% less in those with normal renal function Excretion: Majority in feces, 10% in urine; dialysis does not remove EPO	Onset: Several days Peak: 5–24 h (subcut); IV with more rapid peak Duration: UK

Therapeutic Effects/Uses
Approved for use in the treatment of anemia to increase the Hgb concentration to the lowest level sufficient to avoid the need for RBC transfusions
Mechanism of Action: Regulates the production of RBCs by stimulating the committed erythroid progenitor cells to divide and differentiate in the bone marrow to maintain optimal red cell mass for oxygen transport

Side Effects	Adverse Reactions
Injection site reaction, myalgia, arthralgia, cephalgia, nausea, emesis, pruritus, cough, urticaria, dizziness, insomnia, anemia, fever, hypokalemia	Anaphylactoid reactions, angioedema, bronchospasm, MI, seizures, stroke, thromboembolism, red cell aplasia, hypertension, antibody formation, heart failure, encephalopathy

<, Less than; >, greater than; ≥, greater than or equal to; *A*, adult; *Adol*, adolescent; *CKD*, chronic kidney disease; *EPO*, erythropoietin; *ESA*, erythropoietin-stimulating agent; *h*, hour; *Hgb*, hemoglobin; *IV*, intravenous; *MI*, myocardial infarction; *PB*, protein binding; *RBC*, red blood cell; *subcut*, subcutaneous; *t½*, half-life; *UK*, unknown; *wk*, week; *y*, year.

PROTOTYPE DRUG CHART
Filgrastim

Drug Class	Dosage
Granulocyte colony-stimulating factor	Chronic neutropenia, chemotherapy-induced neutropenia prophylaxis, after induction or consolidation therapy for AML; prophylaxis in nonmyeloid cancer A: IV/subcut: 5 mcg/kg per d HIV or drug therapy-induced neutropenia: A: Subcut: 5–10 mcg/kg per day 1–3 times weekly to maintain ANC of 2000–10,000/mm³ Refer to specific protocols.

Contraindications	Drug-Lab-Food Interactions
Absolute: Hypersensitivity to *Escherichia coli*–derived proteins or 24 h before or after cytotoxic chemotherapy *Precautions:* Pregnancy, lactation, latex hypersensitivity, leukemia, leukocytosis, obstetric delivery, pulmonary bleeding, radiation therapy, respiratory distress syndrome, sickle cell disease, vasculitis, thrombocytopenia	Drug: No clinically important drug interactions have been noted, but drugs that can increase the release of neutrophils (e.g., lithium) should be used with caution. Lab: Leukocytosis, thrombocytopenia, proteinuria, elevated LDH, and increased ALP Food: None known

Pharmacokinetics	Pharmacodynamics
Absolute bioavailability with subcut route is 60%–70%. Absorption: Subcut: Well absorbed Distribution: PB: UK Metabolism: t½: 1.8–3.5 h Excretion: Mainly by the kidneys; clearance is nonlinear and dependent on drug concentration and neutrophil count	Onset: UK Peak: 2–8 h Duration: ANC decreases to baseline in approximately 4 d.

Therapeutic Effects/Uses
To decrease incidence of infection in patients with MDS; in those receiving myelosuppressive chemotherapeutic drugs, including patients with AML undergoing induction or consolidation therapy; in aplastic anemia; and for mobilization of progenitor stem cells used in autologous transplant; also for treatment of patients with severe chronic neutropenia
Mechanism of Action: Increases production, maturation, and activation of neutrophils and enhances their migration and cytotoxicity

Side Effects	Adverse Reactions
Most common side effects include nausea, vomiting, arthralgia, alopecia, diarrhea, fever, fatigue, skin rash, anorexia, cephalgia, cough, chest pain, sore throat, constipation, dizziness, and dyspnea.	Splenomegaly, thrombocytopenia, MI, ARDS, splenic rupture, capillary leak syndrome, anaphylactoid reactions, glomerulonephritis, pulmonary bleeding/alveolar hemorrhage, and cutaneous vasculitis

A, Adult; *ALP*, alkaline phosphatase; *AML*, acute myelogenous leukemia; *ANC*, absolute neutrophil count; *ARDS*, acute respiratory distress syndrome; *d*, day; *h*, hour; *IV*, intravenous; *LDH*, lactate dehydrogenase; *MDS*, myelodysplastic syndrome; *MI*, myocardial infarction; *PB*, protein binding; *subcut*, subcutaneous; *t½*, half-life; *UK*, unknown.

Granulocyte Colony-Stimulating Factor

Endogenous **granulocyte colony-stimulating factor (G-CSF)** is produced by macrophages, endothelium, and other immune cells, and stimulates the synthesis of neutrophils. Neutrophils are the most abundant WBCs that take part in the inflammatory response system, and their main function is to detect and destroy harmful bacteria. Recombinant DNA technology can produce CSFs for human granulocytes to be used for myelodysplastic syndrome (MDS) and for patients receiving myelosuppressive cancer chemotherapy, induction or consolidation chemotherapy for acute myeloid leukemia (AML), and bone marrow transplantation for cancer; for severe, chronic neutropenia; and to increase the hematopoietic stem cells in stem cell donors before leukapheresis. Two commercially available forms are filgrastim and pegfilgrastim. Unlike filgrastim, pegfilgrastim is administered once per chemotherapy cycle. Prototype Drug Chart: Filgrastim provides specific drug information for filgrastim.

Granulocyte-Macrophage Colony–Stimulating Factor

Granulocyte-macrophage colony–stimulating factor (GM-CSF), or *sargramostim*, belongs to a group of growth factors that support survival, proliferation, and differentiation (maturation) of hematopoietic **progenitor cells**. It induces partially committed progenitor (parent) cells to divide and differentiate in the granulocyte-macrophage pathway. GM-CSF, unlike G-CSF, is a multilineage factor that promotes proliferation of myelomonocytic, megakaryocytic, and erythroid progenitors. It is primarily produced by the bone marrow, B and T lymphocytes, and monocytes (immature macrophages). Commercially prepared GM-CSF came about through recombinant DNA technology and is FDA approved for use to reduce neutropenia and promote myeloid recovery in patients receiving myelosuppressive chemotherapy or bone marrow transplant (BMT), for mobilization of autologous peripheral blood progenitor cells, and in BMT failure or delayed engraftment. Prototype Drug Chart: Sargramostim provides specific drug information for sargramostim.

INTERLEUKIN-2

Interleukins

Interleukins are a group of signaling molecule proteins produced by leukocytes, more specifically by T lymphocytes. Because interleukins are hormone-like glycoproteins manufactured by T lymphocytes, they are sometimes called **lymphokines**. Interleukins also increase the growth and activity of other T cells and B cells, which affects the immune response system. One of the most widely studied interleukins

PROTOTYPE DRUG CHART
Sargramostim

Drug Class	Dosage
Granulocyte-macrophage colony-stimulating factor	After reinfusion of BMT: A: 250 mcg/m² per day subcut or IV over 2 h After failed or delayed engraftment from BMT: A: 250 mcg/m² per day subcut or IV over 2 h for 14 d; may repeat after having 7 d off therapy. If a third dose is warranted, give 500 mcg/m² per day for 14 d after 7 d off therapy. Other dosing protocols are available.
Contraindications	**Drug-Lab-Food Interactions**
Absolute: Concomitant use with chemotherapy and/or radiation therapy or within 24 h of chemotherapy administration or within 12 h after last dose of radiation therapy; yeast hypersensitivity; excessive leukemic blasts (≥10%) in the bone marrow or peripheral blood *Caution:* Pregnancy, lactation, cardiac arrhythmias, heart failure, leukemia, mannitol hypersensitivity, neonates, pulmonary disorders, leukocytosis	Drug: Drugs having synergistic effects may increase leukocytosis (e.g., lithium and corticosteroids); however, formal drug interaction data are currently not available. Sargramostim may increase the activity of zidovudine. Lab: Leukocytosis including neutrophilia, hyperbilirubinemia, elevated transaminases and serum creatinine Food: None known
Pharmacokinetics	**Pharmacodynamics**
Absorption: IV: Essentially complete Distribution: PB: UK Metabolism: t½: 1 h (IV); 2.7 h (subcut) Excretion: Mostly in urine as inactive protein fragments	Onset: 7–14 d Peak: 1–3 h (subcut) Duration: Baseline WBCs within 1 wk of stopping therapy
Therapeutic Effects/Uses	
To accelerate growth and development of myeloid cell lines to shorten neutropenic state, to mobilize peripheral blood progenitor cells for collection, and for bone marrow graft failure or engraftment delay Mechanism of Action: Stimulates the proliferation and differentiation of myeloid cell lines to enhance immune defense mechanism; enhances the function of mature granulocytes and monocytes; enhances bacteriocidal activity of neutrophils	
Side Effects	**Adverse Reactions**
Generally well tolerated, but SEs may occur. Common SEs include arthralgia, myalgia, diarrhea, fatigue, chills, weakness, asthenia, cephalgia, malaise, unspecified chest pain, local irritation at injection site, peripheral edema, rash, and fever.	Pleural/pericardial effusion, capillary leak syndrome, anaphylactoid reactions, rigors, GI hemorrhage, dyspnea, hypotension

≥, Greater than or equal to; *A*, Adult; *BMT*, bone marrow transplant; *d*, day; *GI*, gastrointestinal; *h*, hour; *IV*, intravenous; *PB*, protein binding; *SEs*, side effects; *subcut*, subcutaneous; *t½*, half-life; *UK*, unknown; *WBC*, white blood cell; *wk*, week.

TABLE 37.5 Interleukin-2[a]

Generic	Route and Dosage	Uses and Considerations
Aldesleukin	Two 5-d treatment periods are separated by a rest period. A: IV: 600,000 units/kg (0.037 mg/kg) over 15 min q8h; *max:* 14 doses. After 9 d of rest, repeat the schedule for another 14 doses; *max:* 28 doses per course	For metastatic renal cancer and metastatic melanoma *Do not* give dexamethasone during treatment unless absolutely necessary; it may negate the effects of IL-2.

A, Adult; *d*, day; *h*, hour; *IL*, interleukin; *IV*, intravenous; *max*, maximum; *min*, minute; *q*, every.
[a]Patients receiving IL-2 by any route, in any dose, and in any setting—inpatient or outpatient—should be monitored closely for signs of toxicity.

is IL-2. Table 37.5 provides information on IL-2 and includes dosages, uses, and considerations.

Aldesleukin

IL-2 is produced commercially through recombinant DNA technology as aldesleukin. It is FDA approved for treatment of metastatic renal cell carcinoma and metastatic melanoma by inducing proliferation and differentiation of B and T cells along with other cells involved in the immune system. Table 37.3 lists common adverse effects with IL-2 therapy.

Pharmacokinetics

Aldesleukin is administered intravenously or subcutaneously and is rapidly distributed to the extravascular and extracellular spaces and to the liver, spleen, kidneys, and lungs. After IV administration, the serum distribution and elimination half-life is 13 and 85 minutes, respectively. After subcutaneous injection, the serum levels were slightly prolonged. Aldesleukin is cleared from the systemic circulation by the kidneys and is then metabolized into amino acids by the renal cells; the drug is also affected by the cytochrome P450 isoenzymes.

Pharmacodynamics

Aldesleukin has essentially identical effects to those of endogenous IL-2. The interaction of the drug with the IL-2 receptors stimulates the cytokine cascade and involves various IFNs, interleukins, and TNFs. Along with these other cytokines, aldesleukin induces proliferation and differentiation of B and T lymphocytes, monocytes, macrophages, and NKCs, among others.

Side Effects and Adverse Reactions

The black-box warning includes patients with cardiac disease, coma, capillary leak syndrome, infection, and pulmonary disease, and warns that the drug must be administered in a specialized care setting by an experienced clinician. Table 37.4 compares the black-box warnings for IFNs, IL-2, and EPO. Box 37.1 lists absolute contraindications for aldesleukin.

⚠ Conventional high-dose IV bolus aldesleukin is associated with significant adverse reactions that affect almost every organ system. Many of the adverse effects may be due to capillary leak syndrome, which results from extravasation of plasma proteins and fluid into the extravascular space, which leads to vascular atony. Vascular tone is lost within 2 to 12 hours of starting aldesleukin and causes decreased arterial pressure and decreased organ perfusion, resulting in multiorgan dysfunction that leads to death. Once the drug is discontinued, the capillary leak syndrome resolves within a few hours. Other side effects and adverse reactions include hyperglycemia, diabetes, metabolic and respiratory acidosis, and electrolyte imbalance (e.g., hypomagnesemia and hypocalcemia). Because of the many potential adverse effects, patients must be selected with care, and those with significant cardiac, pulmonary, renal, hepatic, or central nervous system impairments must be excluded. Table 37.6 provides information on aldesleukin for dose interruption or discontinuation for drug toxicity.

Drug Interactions

Because of the number of serious adverse effects associated with aldesleukin therapy, almost any other drug represents a potential interaction. Aldesleukin is associated with kidney and liver toxicity, and other drugs known to cause such toxicity can exacerbate the impairment caused by aldesleukin (e.g., vancomycin, cyclosporine, nonsteroidal antiinflammatory drugs [NSAIDs], methotrexate, isoniazid [INH], and ethanol). Antihypertensives (e.g., beta blockers and calcium channel blockers) can worsen hypotension. The immune response from vaccines may be decreased if given to those who are immunocompromised and receiving aldesleukin.

⚡ PATIENT SAFETY

Do Not Confuse…
- **Interferon alfa-2a** with **interferon alfa-2b**
- **Interferon alfa** with **interferon beta** or **interferon gamma**
- **Interleukin-2** with **interferon 2**
- **Darbepoetin alfa** with **epoetin alfa**

⚡ BOX 37.1 Absolute Contraindications for Aldesleukin

Angina	Organ transplant
Cardiac arrhythmias	Psychosis
Cardiac disease	Pulmonary disease
Cardiac tamponade	Renal failure
Coma	Respiratory insufficiency
Gastrointestinal bleeding	Seizures
Gastrointestinal perforation	Ventricular tachycardia
Myocardial infarction	

TABLE 37.6 Aldesleukin[a] Dose Interruption or Discontinuation

Body System	Interruption[b]	Discontinue Permanently
Mental health	Any changes to mental status, including confusion or agitation	Coma or toxic psychosis lasting more than 48 h, poorly managed seizures
Skin, hair, and nails	New bullous dermatitis or worsening of preexisting skin condition; may treat with antihistamines; *do not* treat with topical steroids.	
⚠ Cardiovascular	Atrial fibrillation, SVT, or bradycardia that is persistent, recurrent, or needs treatment SBP <90 mm Hg if it requires vasopressors ECG changes consistent with MI, ischemia, or myocarditis	Sustained ventricular tachycardia ≥5 beats Uncontrolled cardiac rhythm disturbances ECG changes that show MI or cardiac tamponade
Pulmonary	O_2 saturation <90%	Requiring intubation >72 h
Endocrine	Hypoglycemia	
Hematology	Sepsis	
GI/GU	Stool guaiac repeatedly >3–4+; serum creatinine >4.5 mg/dL or ≥4 mg/dL with severe volume overload, acidosis, or hyperkalemia; persistent oliguria, UO <10 mL/h for 16–24 h with increasing serum creatinine	Renal failure that requires dialysis >72 h; bowel ischemia or perforation or GI bleeding that requires surgery
Hepatobiliary	Hepatic failure, including encephalopathy, ascites, liver pain, hypoglycemia	

<, Less than; >, greater than; ≥, greater than or equal to; *ECG*, Electrocardiograph; *GI/GU*, gastrointestinal/genitourinary; *h*, hours; *MI*, myocardial infarction; O_2, oxygen; *SBP*, systolic blood pressure; *SVT*, supraventricular tachycardia; *UO*, urine output.

[a] ⚠ Aldesleukin must be withheld or interrupt a dose due to drug toxicity; *do not reduce dose*.
[b] May be resumed with dose adjustment once toxicity has resolved.

CLINICAL JUDGMENT [NURSING PROCESS]
Biologic Response Modifiers

Concept: Immunity
- The protective response of the body toward inflammation and infection

Recognize Cues [Assessment]
- Conduct a detailed current medication history that includes prescriptions, over-the-counter (OTC) medicines, antacids, dietary supplements, vitamins, and herbal supplements.
- Obtain a list of the patient's drug and food allergies.
- Obtain baseline information about physical status that includes height, weight, vital signs, cardiopulmonary assessment, intake and output, skin assessment, nutritional status, and any underlying diseases.
- Obtain baseline laboratory values (complete blood count [CBC] with differentials and platelet count, uric acid, chemistry panel, lipid panel, and thyroid panel) before and during treatment.
- ⚡ With erythropoietin-stimulating agents, assess serum ferritin and serum iron–transferrin saturation. Most patients will need supplemental iron.
- Assess baseline results of pulmonary function tests, chest radiographs, electrocardiogram (ECG), and kidney and liver function studies.
- Assess patient's and caregiver's level of comprehension and physical ability related to the therapeutic regimen.

Analyze Cues and Prioritize Hypothesis [Patient Problems]
- Decreased immunity
- Need for teaching

Generate Solutions [Planning]
- The patient and caregivers will verbalize signs and symptoms of significant reactions (e.g., wheezing; chest pain; swelling of face, neck, lips, throat, or tongue; emotional instability; altered speaking or thinking; and excessive weight gain or loss).
- The patient and caregivers will verbalize when to notify the health care provider or seek emergency treatment.
- The patient will remain free from infection.
- The patient and caregivers will verbalize understanding of immunotherapy as part of an anticancer treatment regimen.

Take Action [Nursing Interventions]
- Assess for any cardiac events, such as new chest pain and ECG changes.
- ⚡ Monitor appropriate labs according to established protocol for the specific immunotherapy (e.g., CBC with differential, electrolytes, renal and hepatic function, and glucose).
- Assess for bleeding, especially in patients taking anticoagulants, antiplatelets, or nonsteroidal antiinflammatory drugs (NSAIDs).
- Monitor renal and hepatic function at baseline and per treatment protocol.
- Examine the patient's skin closely at each visit for the presence of erythema, rash, peeling, or blister formation, and rate the severity of any dermatologic reactions.
- ⚡ During treatment, monitor patients for any indications of adverse effects such as fever, chills, hypoxia, wheezing, bradycardia or tachycardia, hypotension or hypertension, arrhythmia, or seizures.
- Premedicate patients with acetaminophen to reduce chills and fever, and with diphenhydramine to reduce histamine effects.
- Have resuscitative equipment on standby as per protocol.
- Actively listen to patient and caregiver concerns, and explain in laymen's terms the immunotherapy being used as part of the patient's cancer treatment regimen.

Patient Teaching
General
- Report flulike symptoms, such as chills, fever, myalgia, and weakness.
- Report unmanageable nausea and vomiting.
- Instruct the patient to not receive vaccines with live viruses.
- Inform the patient of the need for frequent laboratory tests.
- Teach the patient to avoid crowds and people with infection.

Continued

CLINICAL JUDGMENT [NURSING PROCESS]—CONT'D

Biologic Response Modifiers

Side Effects
- Report symptoms of bleeding immediately; these include black stools, vomit that looks like coffee grounds, easy bleeding/bruising, or hematuria.
- Report symptoms of adverse effects or severe side effects promptly, especially chest pain; swelling of the face, neck, tongue, or lips; weight gain or loss; increasing shortness of breath; fever or chills; convulsions; or difficulty speaking.
- Advise patients and caregivers to immediately report convulsions, persistent headache, reduced eyesight, increased blood pressure, decreased urine output, or blurred vision.

Evaluate Outcomes [Evaluation]
- The patient is free of further injury related to immunotherapy.
- Side effects are managed effectively.
- The patient is free from infection.
- Patient, family, and caregiver education needs are met.
- The patient, family, and caregivers understand therapy-related side effects and adverse reactions.
- The patient, family, and caregivers understand strategies to minimize side effects and adverse reactions.

CLINICAL JUDGMENT CASE STUDY

A 75-year-old patient has metastatic non–small-cell cancer of the lung. The patient's past treatment regimen included external-beam chest irradiation and combination chemotherapy. Two weeks before hospitalization, the patient received a course of carboplatin and paclitaxel as an outpatient, with subsequent admission to the hospital with neutropenia, thrombocytopenia, and anemia. Upon assessment, the patient was cachectic and weak but was able to perform activities of daily living with only minimal assistance. Admitting laboratory data were hemoglobin (Hgb) 6.9 g/dL, hematocrit (Hct) 20.6%, platelets $16 \times 10^3/\mu L$, a white blood cell (WBC) count of $6 \times 10^3/\mu L$ with absolute neutrophil count (ANC) of $0.096 \times 10^3/\mu L$. The patient was prescribed units subcutaneously once a week and filgrastim, G-CSF 5 mcg/kg per day given subcutaneously. Parenteral antibiotic therapy was also initiated.

1. Why were filgrastim and erythropoietin (EPO) indicated?
2. What must be monitored closely in patients receiving EPO and why?
3. List three patient problems for this patient.
4. Identify three nursing actions for each of the patient problems identified in Question 3.

REVIEW QUESTIONS

1. Which action is primary for interferon alfa?
   a. Enhancing immune function and producing antigen/antibody reaction
   b. Causing allergic reactions, producing red blood cells, and producing interferon
   c. Immunomodulation, causing cytotoxic/cytostatic effects, and differentiating stem cells
   d. Producing cytokines, producing interleukin, and fighting infection
2. A patient diagnosed with malignant melanoma, a skin cancer, is treated with interferon alfa-2a. The nurse teaches this patient about which side effect?
   a. Increase in white blood cells
   b. Increase in red blood cells
   c. Flulike syndrome
   d. Gastrointestinal symptoms
3. The nurse reviews the list of medications and is aware that red blood cell production can be stimulated with which drug for anemia?
   a. Epoetin alfa
   b. Filgrastim
   c. Interleukin-2
   d. Sargramostim
4. Which drug must be administered intravenously?
   a. Epoetin alfa
   b. Interleukin-2
   c. Granulocyte colony-stimulating factor
   d. Granulocyte-macrophage colony-stimulating factor
5. In developing a plan of care for the patient, the nurse understands that the order for pegfilgrastim was prescribed for which reason?
   a. Pegfilgrastim is eliminated via the kidneys.
   b. Pegfilgrastim is a pegylated filgrastim.
   c. Pegfilgrastim is not easily eliminated from the body.
   d. Pegfilgrastim requires injection once per chemotherapy cycle.
6. A patient receiving erythropoietin-stimulating drug has the following laboratory values: hemoglobin, 12.8 mg/dL; platelet count, 148,000/mm²; white blood cell count, 4800/mm². Which action is most appropriate for the nurse to implement?
   a. Discuss with the health care provider the potential need for a colony-stimulating factor such as granulocyte colony-stimulating factor based on the laboratory results.
   b. Contact the health care provider to discuss the laboratory results and a possible discontinuation of the ordered erythropoietin-stimulating agent.
   c. Discuss the laboratory values with the health care provider to determine whether a colony-stimulating factor such as interleukin-2 should be given.
   d. Discuss with the health care provider the potential need for more laboratory tests before administration of the erythropoietin-stimulating agent.

UNIT XI Respiratory Drugs

38

Upper Respiratory Disorders

http://evolve.elsevier.com/McCuistion/pharmacology

OBJECTIVES

- Summarize the concepts of ventilation and respiration.
- Differentiate treatments for acute rhinitis and allergic rhinitis.
- Identify the treatment of sinusitis and acute pharyngitis.

OUTLINE

Respiratory System, 477
   Physiology, 477
   Upper Respiratory Infections, 477
Common Cold, Acute Rhinitis, and Allergic Rhinitis, 477
   Antihistamines, 478
   Nasal and Systemic Decongestants, 479
   Intranasal Glucocorticoids, 482

   Antitussives, 482
   Expectorants, 484
Other Upper Respiratory Disorders, 484
   Sinusitis, 484
   Acute Pharyngitis, 484
Clinical Judgment Case Study, 485
Review Questions, 485

RESPIRATORY SYSTEM

Physiology

The respiratory tract is divided into two major parts: the *upper respiratory tract*, which consists of the nares, nasal cavity, pharynx, and larynx, and the *lower respiratory tract*, which consists of the trachea, bronchi, bronchioles, alveoli, and alveolar-capillary membrane. Air enters through the upper respiratory tract and travels to the lower respiratory tract, where gas exchanges occur. Fig. 38.1 illustrates these components.

Ventilation and *respiration* are distinct terms and should not be used interchangeably. Ventilation is the movement of air from the atmosphere through the upper and lower airways to the alveoli. *Respiration* is the process whereby gas exchange occurs at the alveolar-capillary membrane. Respiration has three phases:

- *Ventilation* is the phase in which oxygen passes through the airways. With every inspiration, air is moved into the lungs, and with every expiration, air is transported out of the lungs.
- *Perfusion* involves blood flow at the alveolar-capillary bed. Perfusion is influenced by alveolar pressure. For gas exchange to occur, the perfusion of each alveolus must be matched by adequate ventilation. Factors such as mucosal edema, secretions, and bronchospasm increase resistance to air flow and decrease ventilation and diffusion of gases.
- *Diffusion*, the movement of molecules from higher to lower concentrations, takes place when oxygen passes into the capillary bed to be circulated and carbon dioxide leaves the capillary bed and diffuses into the alveoli for ventilatory excretion.

Upper Respiratory Infections

Upper respiratory infections (URIs) include the common cold, acute rhinitis, sinusitis, and acute pharyngitis. The common cold is the most prevalent type of URI. Adults have an average of 2 to 4 colds per year, and children have an average of 4 to 12 colds per year. Incidence is seasonally variable: approximately 50% of the population experiences a winter cold, and 25% experience a summer cold. A cold is not considered a life-threatening illness, but it does cause physical and mental discomfort and lost time at work and school. The common cold is an expensive illness in the United States—more than $60 billion is spent each year on over-the-counter (OTC) cold and cough preparations in addition to missed time at work and school.

COMMON COLD, ACUTE RHINITIS, AND ALLERGIC RHINITIS

The common cold is caused by the rhinovirus and affects primarily the nasopharyngeal tract. Acute rhinitis, acute inflammation of the mucous membranes of the nose, usually accompanies the common cold. Acute rhinitis is not the same as allergic rhinitis, often called *hay fever*, which is caused by pollen or a foreign substance such as animal dander. Nasal secretions increase in both acute and allergic rhinitis.

A cold is most contagious 1 to 4 days before the onset of symptoms (the incubation period) and during the first 3 days of the cold. Transmission occurs more frequently from touching contaminated surfaces and then touching the nose or mouth than it does from contact with viral droplets released by sneezing.

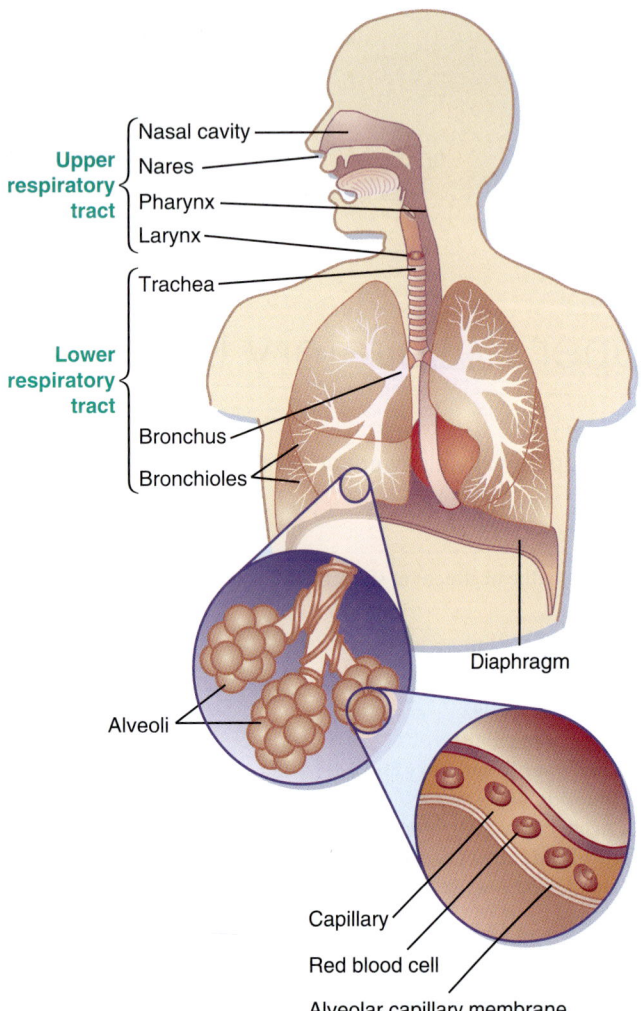

Fig. 38.1 Basic structures of the respiratory tract.

The groups of drugs used to manage cold symptoms include antihistamines (H_1 blockers), decongestants (sympathomimetic amines), antitussives, and expectorants. These drugs can be used singly or in combination preparations.

Symptoms of the common cold include **rhinorrhea** (watery nasal discharge), nasal congestion, cough, and increased mucosal secretions. If a bacterial infection secondary to the cold occurs, infectious rhinitis may result, and nasal discharge becomes tenacious, mucoid, and yellow or yellow green. The nasal secretions are discolored by white blood cells and cellular debris that are byproducts of the fight against the bacterial infection. Antibiotics used to treat bacterial respiratory infections are discussed in Chapter 26.

Antihistamines

Antihistamines, H_1 blockers or H_1 antagonists, compete with histamine for receptor sites and prevent a histamine response. The two types of histamine receptors, H_1 and H_2, cause different responses. When the H_1 receptor is stimulated, the extravascular smooth muscles—including those lining the nasal cavity—are constricted. With stimulation of the H_2 receptor, an increase in gastric secretions occurs, which is a cause of peptic ulcer (see Chapter 46). These two types of histamine receptors should not be confused. Antihistamines decrease nasopharyngeal secretions by blocking the H_1 receptor.

Although antihistamines are commonly used as cold remedies, these agents can also treat seasonal allergies that cause allergic rhinitis. However, antihistamines are not useful in an emergency situation such as anaphylaxis. Most antihistamines are rapidly absorbed in 15 minutes, but they are not potent enough to combat anaphylaxis.

First-Generation Antihistamines

The antihistamine group can be divided into first and second generations. Most *first-generation antihistamines* cause drowsiness, dizziness, dry mouth, and other anticholinergic symptoms, whereas *second-generation antihistamines* have fewer anticholinergic effects and a lower incidence of drowsiness. Many OTC cold remedies contain a first-generation antihistamine, which can cause drowsiness; therefore patients should be alerted not to drive or operate dangerous machinery when taking such medications. The anticholinergic properties of most antihistamines cause dryness of the mouth and decreased secretions, making them useful in treating rhinitis caused by the common cold. Antihistamines also decrease the nasal itching and tickling that cause sneezing.

The first-generation antihistamine diphenhydramine has been available for years and is frequently combined with other ingredients in cold remedy preparations. Its primary use is to treat rhinitis. Prototype Drug Chart: Diphenhydramine lists the pharmacologic behavior of diphenhydramine.

Pharmacokinetics

Diphenhydramine can be administered orally, intramuscularly (IM), or intravenously (IV). It is well absorbed from the gastrointestinal (GI) tract, but systemic absorption from topical use is minimal. It is highly protein-bound (98%) and has an average half-life of 2 to 8 hours. Diphenhydramine is metabolized by the liver and is excreted as metabolites in the urine.

Pharmacodynamics

Diphenhydramine blocks the effects of histamine by competing for and occupying H_1 receptor sites. It has anticholinergic effects and should be used with caution by patients with closed-angle glaucoma. Drowsiness is a major side effect of the drug; in fact, it is sometimes used in sleep aid products. Diphenhydramine is also used as an antitussive to alleviate cough. Its onset of action can occur in as few as 15 minutes when taken orally and IM. IV administration results in an immediate onset of action. The duration of action for oral use is 3 to 6 hours.

Diphenhydramine can cause central nervous system (CNS) depression if taken with alcohol, narcotics, hypnotics, or barbiturates.

> ⚡ **PATIENT SAFETY**
>
> **Do Not Confuse ...**
> - **Benadryl**, an antihistamine, with **benazepril**, an angiotensin-converting enzyme (ACE) inhibitor

Side Effects of Most First-Generation Antihistamines

The most common side effects of first-generation antihistamines are drowsiness, dizziness, fatigue, and disturbed coordination. Anticholinergic symptoms such as dry mouth, urine retention, blurred vision, and wheezing may also occur.

PROTOTYPE DRUG CHART
Diphenhydramine

Drug Class	Dosage
Antihistamine	Allergic reaction: A: PO: 25–50 mg tid/qid PRN; *max:* 300 mg/d A: IM/IV: 10–50 mg IV or IM q4–6h; *max:* 400 mg/d

Contraindications	Drug-Lab-Food Interactions
Breast-feeding *Caution:* Asthma, hepatic disease, COPD, closed-angle glaucoma, cardiac disease, hypertension, prostatic hypertrophy, urinary retention, GI obstruction, ileus, increased intraocular pressure, contact lens, older adults, pregnancy, children	Drug: Increased CNS depression with alcohol, opioids, and barbiturates; avoid use with MAOIs

Pharmacokinetics	Pharmacodynamics
Absorption: PO: Well absorbed Distribution: PB: 98% Metabolism: t½: 2–8 h Excretion: In urine as metabolites	PO: Onset: 15–30 min Peak: 2–4 h Duration: 4–6 h IM: Onset: 15–30 min Peak: 1–4 h Duration: 4–7 h IV: Onset: Immediate Peak: 0.5–1 h Duration: 4–7 h

Therapeutic Effects/Uses
To treat insomnia and allergic reactions including allergic rhinitis, the common cold, cough, sneezing, pruritus, and urticaria and to prevent motion sickness
Mechanism of Action: Competes with histamine for binding at H_1-receptor sites and antagonizes histamine effects

Side Effects	Adverse Reactions
Drowsiness, dizziness, headache, irritability, weakness, insomnia, fatigue, blurred vision, photosensitivity, dermatitis, rash, paresthesia, dry mouth, dry mucous, membranes, restlessness, confusion, anorexia, nausea, vomiting, diarrhea, constipation, urinary retention, tremor	Seizures, hypotension, tachycardia, palpitations *Life-threatening:* Agranulocytosis, hemolytic anemia, thrombocytopenia

A, Adult; *CNS*, central nervous system; *COPD*, chronic obstructive pulmonary disease; *d*, day; *GI*, gastrointestinal; *h*, hour; *IM*, intramuscular; *IV*, intravenous; *MAOI*, monoamine oxidase inhibitor; *max*, maximum; *min*, minute; *PB*, protein binding; *PO*, by mouth; *PRN*, as needed; *q4–6h*, every 4 to 6 hours; *qid*, four times a day; *t½*, half-life; *tid*, three times as day; *y*, years.

Second-Generation Antihistamines
The second-generation antihistamines cause fewer anticholinergic symptoms. Although a moderate amount of alcohol and other CNS depressants may be taken with second-generation antihistamines, many clinicians advise against such use.

The second-generation antihistamines cetirizine, fexofenadine, azelastine, desloratadine, and loratadine have half-lives between 3 and 30 hours. Some are administered by nasal spray. Table 38.1 lists the first- and second-generation antihistamines used to treat allergic rhinitis.

Nasal and Systemic Decongestants
Nasal congestion results from dilation of nasal blood vessels caused by infection, inflammation, or allergy. With this dilation, a transudation of fluid into the tissue spaces occurs that results in swelling of the nasal cavity. Nasal **decongestants** (sympathomimetic amines) stimulate the alpha-adrenergic receptors, producing vascular constriction (vasoconstriction) of the capillaries within the nasal mucosa. The result is shrinking of the nasal mucous membranes and a reduction in fluid secretion (runny nose).

Nasal decongestants are administered by nasal spray or drops or in tablet, capsule, or liquid form. Frequent use of decongestants, especially nasal spray or drops, can result in tolerance and **rebound nasal congestion**, rebound vasodilation instead of vasoconstriction. Rebound nasal congestion is caused by irritation of the nasal mucosa.

Systemic decongestants (alpha-adrenergic agonists) are available in tablet, capsule, and liquid form, and are used primarily for allergic rhinitis, including hay fever and acute coryza (profuse nasal discharge). Examples of systemic decongestants are tetrahydrozoline, phenylephrine, oxymetazoline, and pseudoephedrine. In the past, phenylpropanolamine was used in many cold remedies; however, the US Food and Drug Administration (FDA) ordered its removal from OTC cold remedies and weight loss aids because reports suggest that the drug might cause stroke, hypertension, and cardiac dysrhythmias. Pseudoephedrine is frequently combined with an antihistamine, analgesic, or antitussive in oral cold remedies. The advantage of systemic decongestants is that they relieve nasal congestion for a longer period than nasal decongestants; however, long-acting nasal decongestants are now available. Nasal decongestants usually act promptly and cause fewer side effects than systemic decongestants.

National regulatory measures control pseudoephedrine drug sales with individual limits of 3.6 g/day and 9 g within 30 days. Identifications are scanned with each purchase. The database is linked nationally and keeps a 2-year tally. Table 38.2 lists systemic and nasal decongestants and their dosages, uses, and considerations.

TABLE 38.1 Antihistamines for Treatment of Allergic Rhinitis

Drug	Route and Dosage	Uses and Considerations
First-Generation Antihistamines		
Alkylamine Derivatives		
Brompheniramine tannate	Extended release: A: PO: 6–12 mg q12h; *max:* 24 mg/d	For allergic rhinitis, rhinorrhea, and conjunctivitis. May cause drowsiness, dizziness, restlessness, euphoria, irritability, blurred vision, dry mouth, constipation, urinary retention, palpitations, and tachycardia. PB: 39%–49%; t½: 11.8–34.7 h
Chlorpheniramine	Immediate release: A: PO: 4 mg q4–6h; *max:* 24 mg/d Extended release: A: 8–12 mg bid; *max:* 24 mg/d	For allergic conjunctivitis, allergic rhinitis, seasonal allergies, symptoms of the common cold, rhinorrhea, sneezing, pruritus, and hives. May cause drowsiness, dizziness, headache, blurred vision, confusion, ataxia, dry mouth, nausea, constipation, restlessness, tachycardia, palpitations, and urinary retention. PB: 70%; t½: 21–24 h
Ethanolamine Derivatives		
Clemastine fumarate	A: PO: 1 tab (1.34 mg) q12h; *max:* 2 tabs/d	For common cold, allergic rhinitis, pruritus, and urticaria. May cause drowsiness, dizziness, blurred vision, restlessness, euphoria, headache, confusion, irritability, dry mouth, nausea, constipation, urinary retention, palpitations, and tachycardia. PB: UK; t½: 4–6 h
Diphenhydramine	See Prototype Drug Chart: Diphenhydramine	
Piperidine Derivatives		
Cyproheptadine	A: Initially 4 mg tid; *maint:* 4–20 mg/d in divided doses; *max:* 32 mg/d or 0.5 mg/kg/d whichever is less	For allergies rhinitis, conjunctivitis, pruritus, and urticaria. May cause drowsiness, dizziness, irritability, excitability, euphoria, blurred vision, restlessness, wheezing, anorexia, dry mouth, nausea, diarrhea, constipation, urinary retention, hypotension, and tachycardia. PB: UK; t½: 1–4 h
Piperazine Derivatives		
Levocetirizine	A: PO: 2.5–5 mg/d in the evening; *max:* 5 mg/d	For chronic urticaria and symptoms of seasonal allergies including allergic rhinitis. May cause drowsiness, dizziness, blurred vision, fever, fatigue, pharyngitis, epistaxis, cough, dry mouth, nausea, diarrhea, constipation, urinary retention, hypotension, palpitations, and tachycardia. PB: 91%–92%; t½: 8–9 h
Chlorcyclizine	A: PO: 25 mg q6–8h PRN; *max:* 75 mg/d	For allergic rhinitis and hay fever. May cause dizziness, drowsiness, headache, blurred vision, euphoria, weakness, restlessness, confusion, dry mouth, nausea, diarrhea, constipation, urinary retention, and tachycardia. PB: 85%–90%; t½: 12 h
Combination Antihistamines		
Azelastine and fluticasone	A: Nasal spray: 1 spray per nostril bid; *max:* 2 sprays/nostril/d	For symptoms of seasonal allergies including allergic rhinitis. May cause drowsiness, dizziness, blurred vision, headache, dysphonia, dysgeusia, rhinitis, nasal irritation, hoarseness, epistaxis, nausea, diarrhea, tachycardia, and palpitations. PB: 88% azelastine, 91% fluticasone; t½: 25 h azelastine, 7.8 h fluticasone
Second-Generation Antihistamines		
Azelastine	Nasal spray: A: 1–2 sprays in each nostril q12h; *max:* 4 sprays/nostril/d	For seasonal allergies including allergic rhinitis. May cause drowsiness, headache, confusion, fatigue, blurred vision, dyspnea, rhinitis, pharyngitis, cough, ocular irritation/pain, conjunctivitis, dry mouth, and pruritus. PB: 88%; t½: 22 h
Cetirizine	Seasonal allergies: A: PO: 5–10 mg/d; *max:* 10 mg/d Older A>77 y: PO: 5 mg/d; *max:* 5 mg/d	For ocular pruritus, urticaria, and seasonal allergies including allergic rhinitis. May cause drowsiness, dizziness, headache, blurred vision, conjunctival hyperemia, insomnia, fatigue, euphoria, ataxia, hearing loss, pharyngitis, cough, epistaxis, dry mouth, abdominal pain, nausea, vomiting, diarrhea, and urinary retention. PB: 93%; t½: 6.5–10 h
Fexofenadine	A: PO: 60 mg q12h or 180 mg qd; *max:* 120 mg/d if 2 divided doses or 180 mg/d if given qd	For chronic urticaria and seasonal allergies including allergic rhinitis. May cause dizziness, headache, fever, fatigue, restlessness, cough, dyspepsia, vomiting, and diarrhea. PB: 60%–70%; t½: 14.4 h
Loratadine	A: PO: 10 mg/d; *max:* 10 mg/d	For chronic urticaria and seasonal allergies including allergic rhinitis. May cause drowsiness, blurred vision, headache, confusion, fatigue, wheezing, pharyngitis, stomatitis, dry mouth, and vomiting. PB: 97%; t½: 3–20 h
Desloratadine	A: PO: 5 mg/d; *max:* 5 mg/d	For chronic urticaria, and seasonal allergies including allergic rhinitis. May cause drowsiness, dizziness, fatigue, headache, fever, infection, irritability, restlessness, insomnia, rhinorrhea, pharyngitis, cough, dry mouth, anorexia, nausea, vomiting, and diarrhea. PB: 82%–87%; t½: 20–30 h

A, Adult; *bid*, twice a day; *d*, day; *GI*, gastrointestinal; *h*, hour; *max*, maximum; *PB*, protein binding; *PO*, by mouth; *q*, every; *qd*, every day; *t½*, half-life; *tid*, three times a day; *UK*, unknown; *y*, years.

TABLE 38.2 Systemic and Nasal Decongestants (Sympathomimetic Amines)

Drug	Route and Dosage	Uses and Considerations
Oxymetazoline hydrochloride	Nasal congestion: A: gtt or spray; 2–3 sprays in each nostril q10–12h PRN; max: 2 doses/d for no more than 3 d	For nasal congestion, ocular pruritus, and facial erythema due to acne. May cause headache, blurred vision, dry eyes, ocular pain/irritation, keratitis, and conjunctival hyperemia. Limit use to less than 3 days to avoid rebound congestion. PB: 57%; t½: 5.6–13.9 h
Phenylephrine hydrochloride	A: Intranasal: 2–3 sprays/gtt in each nostril q4h PRN for 3 d A: PO: 10–20 mg q4–6h; max: 60 mg/d	For nasal congestion. May cause blurred vision, headache, excitability, nasal irritation, dyspnea, nausea, and hypertension. PB: UK; t½: 2.1–3.4 h
Pseudoephedrine	Regular release: A: PO: 60 mg q4–6h; max: 240 mg/d 12-h extended release: A: PO: 120 mg q12h for 12 h; max: 240 mg/d 24-h extended release: A: PO: 240 mg/d; max: 240 mg/d	For rhinitis, nasal congestion, and the common cold. May cause dizziness, headache, restlessness, insomnia, nausea, diarrhea, palpitations, dysrhythmia, hypertension, and tachycardia. PB: UK; t½: 9–16 h
Tetrahydrozoline (0.1% sol)	Nasal congestion: A: Nasal: 2–4 drops (3–4 sprays) each nostril q3h PRN	For nasal congestion and eye redness. May cause drowsiness, headache, blurred vision, insomnia, nasal irritation, and dryness. PB: UK; t½: UK

A, Adult; *bid*, twice a day; *d*, day; *GI*, gastrointestinal; *gtt*, drops; *h*, hour; *max*, maximum; *PB*, protein binding; *PO*, by mouth; *PRN*, as necessary; *q4h*, every 4 hours; *sol*, solution; *t½*, half-life; *UK*, unknown; *y*, year.

Side Effects and Adverse Reactions

The incidence of side effects is low with topical preparations such as nose drops. However, decongestants can lead to nasal and ocular irritation, dry eyes, blurred vision, insomnia, restlessness, and dysrhythmias.

Use of nasal decongestants for as little as 3 days could result in rebound nasal congestion. Instead of the nasal membranes constricting, vasodilation occurs, causing increased stuffy nose and nasal congestion. The nurse should emphasize the importance of limiting the use of nasal sprays and drops.

As with any alpha-adrenergic drug such as decongestants, blood pressure levels can increase. These drugs are contraindicated or used with extreme caution in patients with hypertension, cardiac disease, hyperthyroidism, and diabetes mellitus.

CLINICAL JUDGMENT [NURSING PROCESS]
Antihistamine: Diphenhydramine

Concept: Gas Exchange
- The lungs deliver oxygen to the pulmonary capillaries, carried by hemoglobin to body cells, and carbon dioxide is carried away from body cells to the lungs and exhaled from the body.

Recognize Cues [Assessment]
- Determine baseline vital signs.
- Obtain a drug history, and report if a drug-drug interaction is probable.
- Assess for signs and symptoms of urinary dysfunction, including retention, dysuria, and altered frequency.
- Note complete blood count (CBC) during drug therapy.
- Assess cardiac and respiratory status.
- Obtain a history of environmental exposures that includes drugs, recent foods eaten, and stress.

Analyze Cues and Prioritize Hypothesis [Patient Problems]
- Airway obstruction
- Decreased gas exchange
- Hypoxemia
- Discomfort

Generate Solutions [Planning]
- Patient will have decreased nasal congestion, mucosal secretions, and cough.
- Patient will sleep 6–8 hours per night.

Take Action [Nursing Interventions]
- Give the oral form of the drug with food to decrease gastric distress.
- Administer the intramuscular form in a large muscle. *Avoid subcutaneous injection.*

Patient Teaching
General
- ⚡ Warn patients to avoid driving a motor vehicle and performing other dangerous activities if drowsiness occurs or until stabilized on the drug.
- ⚡ Advise patients to avoid alcohol and other central nervous system (CNS) depressants.
- Encourage patients to take drugs as prescribed. Notify a health care provider if confusion or hypotension occurs.
- Teach patients on prophylaxis for motion sickness to take the drug at least 30 minutes before the offending event, and also before meals and at bedtime during the event.
- Inform breast-feeding mothers that small amounts of drug pass into breast milk. Because children are more susceptible to the side effects of antihistamines (e.g., unusual excitement or irritability), breast-feeding is not recommended while using these drugs.

Side Effects
- Advise family members or parents that children are more sensitive to the effects of antihistamines. Nightmares, nervousness, and irritability are more likely to occur in children.
- Inform older adults that they are more sensitive to the effects of antihistamines and more likely to experience confusion, difficult or painful urination, dizziness, drowsiness, feeling faint, and dryness of the mouth, nose, or throat.
- Suggest using sugarless candy or gum, ice chips, or a saliva substitute for temporary relief of mouth dryness.

Evaluate Outcomes [Evaluation]
- Evaluate effectiveness of the drug in relieving allergic symptoms or as a sleep aid.

Drug Interactions

When using decongestants with other drugs, drug interactions can occur. Pseudoephedrine may decrease the effect of beta blockers. Taken together with monoamine oxidase inhibitors (MAOIs), decongestants may increase the possibility of hypertension or cardiac dysrhythmias. The patient should also avoid large amounts of caffeine (coffee, tea) because it can increase restlessness and palpitations caused by decongestants.

Intranasal Glucocorticoids

Intranasal glucocorticoids and steroids are effective for treating allergic rhinitis because they have an antiinflammatory action, thus decreasing the allergic rhinitis symptoms of rhinorrhea, sneezing, and congestion. The following are examples of intranasal steroids:

- Beclomethasone
- Budesonide
- Flunisolide
- Fluticasone
- Mometasone
- Triamcinolone

These drugs may be used alone or in combination with an H_1 antihistamine. The spray should be directed away from the nasal septum, and the patient should sniff gently. With continuous use, dryness of the nasal mucosa may occur. Common side effects include headache, nasal irritation, pharyngitis, fatigue, and candidiasis.

Intranasal glucocorticoids undergo rapid deactivation after absorption. Most allergic rhinitis is seasonal; therefore the drugs are for short-term use unless otherwise indicated by the health care provider. Table 38.3 lists the intranasal glucocorticoids and their dosages, uses, and considerations.

Antitussives

Antitussives act on the cough control center in the medulla to suppress the cough reflex. The cough is a naturally protective way to clear the airway of secretions or any collected material. A sore throat may cause coughing that increases throat irritation. If the cough is nonproductive and irritating, an antitussive may be taken. Hard candy may decrease the constant, irritating cough. Dextromethorphan, a nonnarcotic antitussive, is widely used in OTC cold remedies. Prototype Drug Chart: Dextromethorphan Hydrobromide lists the drug data related to dextromethorphan.

The three types of antitussives are nonopioid, opioid, or combination preparations. Antitussives are usually used in combination with other agents (Table 38.4).

PROTOTYPE DRUG CHART
Dextromethorphan Hydrobromide

Drug Class	Dosage
Antitussive	Immediate release: A: PO: 10–20 mg q4h PRN or 30 mg q6–8h PRN; *max:* 120 mg/d Extended release: A: PO: 60 mg q12h; *max:* 120 mg/d

Contraindications	Drug-Lab-Food Interactions
Hypersensitivity, MAOI therapy *Caution:* Asthma, emphysema, hepatic disease, tobacco smoking, pregnancy, breast-feeding, children	Drugs: Avoid use with codeine and MAOIs. Hallucinations and seizures may occur when taken with grapefruit/grapefruit juice as drug actions are increased.

Pharmacokinetics	Pharmacodynamics
Absorption: PO: Rapidly absorbed Distribution: PB: 60%–70% Metabolism: t½: 2–24 h Excretion: In urine	PO: Onset: 15–30 min Peak: 2–3 h Duration: 3–6 h

Therapeutic Effects/Uses

For temporary cough relief, especially a nonproductive cough due to sore throat, irritation, the common cold, inhaled irritants, or chronic bronchitis
Mechanism of Action: Decreases excitability of cough center in the medulla

Side Effects	Adverse Reactions
Dizziness, drowsiness, confusion, fatigue, ataxia, nausea, vomiting, restlessness, rash urticaria	Psychosis, tachycardia *Life-threatening:* Respiratory depression, serotonin syndrome, anaphylaxis

A, Adult; *d*, day; *GI*, gastrointestinal; *h*, hour; *MAOI*, monoamine oxidase inhibitor; *max*, maximum; *min*, minute; *PB*, protein binding; *PO*, by mouth; *PRN*, as necessary; *q*, every; *t½*, half-life.

TABLE 38.3 Intranasal Glucocorticoids

Drug	Route and Dosage	Uses and Considerations
Beclomethasone	Rhinitis: A: 1–2 sprays (42 mcg/spray) each nostril bid	For asthma, nasal polyps, and seasonal allergies including allergic rhinitis. May cause headache, nasal irritation, nasopharyngitis, rhinitis, epistaxis, dysphonia, infection, candidiasis, nausea, and hoarseness. PB: 87%; t½: 2.8–15 h
Budesonide	Rhinitis: A: 1–2 sprays/d each nostril qd	For asthma, seasonal allergies including allergic rhinitis. May cause dizziness, headache, emotional lability, fatigue, epistaxis, rhinitis, cough, acne vulgaris, muscle cramps, ecchymosis, peripheral edema, hypertension, Cushing syndrome, abdominal pain, nausea, vomiting, flatulence, and diarrhea. PB: 85–90%; t½: 2–3.6 h

TABLE 38.3 Intranasal Glucocorticoids—cont'd

Drug	Route and Dosage	Uses and Considerations
Flunisolide	A: 2 sprays each nostril bid; max: 8 sprays/d each nostril	For seasonal allergies including allergic rhinitis. May cause headache, nasal irritation/congestion, pharyngitis, sneezing, epistaxis, dysgeusia, and candidiasis. PB: UK; t½: 1.8–2 h
Fluticasone	A: 2 sprays/d each nostril week 1, then 1–2 sprays each nostril qd PRN	For asthma and seasonal allergies including allergic rhinitis. May cause headache, fatigue, malaise, epistaxis, nasal congestion, pharyngitis, rhinitis, sinusitis, candidiasis, throat irritation, dysphonia, nausea, and vomiting. PB: 91%; t½: 7.8 h
Mometasone furoate	Allergic rhinitis prophylaxis: A: 2 sprays/d each nostril	For asthma, nasal polyps, and seasonal allergies with allergic rhinitis. May cause headache, fatigue, arthralgia, candidiasis, earache, rhinitis, nasopharyngitis, cough, sinusitis, wheezing, and epistaxis. PB: 98%–99%; t½: 5–6 h
Triamcinolone	A: 2 sprays/d each nostril	For seasonal allergies with allergic rhinitis, ocular inflammation, and asthma. Common side effects are ocular hypertension/pain, skin irritation/dryness, rash, pruritus, hyperglycemia, arthralgia, and erythema. PB: UK; t½: 88 min

A, Adult; *bid*, twice a day; *d*, day; *GI*, gastrointestinal; *h*, hour; *IOP*, intraocular pressure; *max*, maximum; *PB*, protein binding; *t½*, half-life; *UK*, unknown; *y*, year.

TABLE 38.4 Antitussives and Expectorants

Drug	Route and Dosage	Uses and Considerations
Opioid Antitussives		
Codeine CSS II	Cough: A: PO: 10–20 mg q4–6h PRN; max: 360 mg/d	For cough and pain. May cause drowsiness, dizziness, headache, euphoria, fatigue, miosis, orthostatic hypotension, weakness, dry mouth, anorexia, nausea, vomiting, diarrhea, constipation, and respiratory depression. PB: 7%–25%; t½: 3 h
Dextromethorphan	See Prototype Drug Chart: Dextromethorphan Hydrobromide	
Guaifenesin 200 mg and codeine 9 mg CSS V	A: PO: 2 capsules q4h PRN; max: Codeine 12 capsules qd (120 mg/d and guaifenesin 2400 mg/d)	For nonproductive cough. May cause drowsiness, dizziness, headache, euphoria, confusion, miosis, hypotension, dependence, nausea, vomiting, constipation, abdominal pain, urinary retention, and respiratory depression. PB: Guaifenesin UK, codeine 7%–25%; t½: guaifenesin 1 h, codeine 3 h
Homatropine 1.5 mg and hydrocodone 5 mg CSS III	A: PO: Hydrocodone 5 mg and homatropine 1.5 mg q4–6h PRN; max: hydrocodone 30 mg and homatropine 9 mg/d	For cough. May cause drowsiness, dizziness, headache, lethargy, blurred vision, euphoria, confusion, dry mouth, nausea, vomiting, constipation, urinary retention, respiratory depression, and dependence. PB: UK; t½: 4 h; hydrocodone, UK homatropine
Nonopioid Antitussives		
Benzonatate	A: PO: 100–200 mg tid; max: 600 mg/d	For cough. May cause drowsiness, dizziness, headache, confusion, pruritus, ocular irritation, dyspepsia, nausea, and constipation. PB: UK; t½: UK
Expectorants		
Guaifenesin	Immediate release: A: PO: 200–400 q4h PRN; max: 2400 mg/d Extended release: A: PO: 600–1200 mg q12h PRN; max: 2.4 g/d	For cough associated with URI and the common cold. May cause drowsiness, dizziness, headache, nausea, vomiting, and diarrhea. PB: UK; t½: 1 h

A, Adult; *CSS*, Controlled Substances Schedule; *d*, day; *GI*, gastrointestinal; *h*, hour; *max*, maximum; *PB*, protein binding; *PO*, by mouth; *PRN*, as necessary; *q*, every; *t½*, half-life; *tid*, three times a day; *UK*, unknown; *URI*, upper respiratory infection.

Pharmacokinetics

Dextromethorphan is available in numerous cold and cough remedy preparations in syrup or liquid form, chewable capsules, and lozenges. The drug is rapidly absorbed and exerts its effects 15 to 30 minutes after oral administration. Its protein-binding percentage is 60% to 70%, and the half-life is 2 to 24 hours. Dextromethorphan is metabolized by the liver and is excreted in the urine.

Pharmacodynamics

Dextromethorphan, an antitussive, provides temporary cough relief, especially for nonproductive cough due to sore throat, irritation, or the common cold. This drug acts by decreasing the excitability of the cough center in the medulla.

Dextromethorphan has a duration of 3 to 6 hours. Usually preparations that contain dextromethorphan can be used several times a day.

Expectorants

Expectorants loosen bronchial secretions so that they can be eliminated by coughing. They can be used with or without other pharmacologic agents. Expectorants are found in many OTC cold remedies along with analgesics, antihistamines, decongestants, and antitussives. The most common expectorant in such preparations is guaifenesin. Hydration is the best natural expectorant. When taking an expectorant, patients should increase fluid intake to at least 8 glasses per day to help loosen mucus. Table 38.4 lists the dosages, uses, and considerations for antitussives and expectorants.

OTHER UPPER RESPIRATORY DISORDERS

Sinusitis

Sinusitis is an inflammation of the mucous membranes of one or more of the maxillary, frontal, ethmoid, or sphenoid sinuses. A systemic or nasal decongestant may be indicated. Acetaminophen, fluids, and rest may also be helpful. For acute or severe sinusitis, an antibiotic may be prescribed.

Acute Pharyngitis

Acute pharyngitis, inflammation of the throat or "sore throat," can be caused by a virus, beta-hemolytic streptococci ("strep throat"), or other bacteria. It can occur alone or with the common cold and rhinitis or acute sinusitis. Symptoms include elevated temperature and cough. A throat culture should be obtained to rule out beta-hemolytic streptococcal infection. If the culture is positive for beta-hemolytic streptococci, a 10-day course of antibiotics is often prescribed. Saline gargles, lozenges, and increased fluid intake are usually indicated. Acetaminophen may be taken to decrease elevated temperature. Antibiotics are *not* effective for viral pharyngitis.

CLINICAL JUDGMENT [NURSING PROCESS]
Nasal Decongestant: Oxymetazoline

Concept: Gas Exchange
- The lungs deliver oxygen to the pulmonary capillaries, carried by hemoglobin to the body cells, and carbon dioxide is carried away from body cells to the lungs and exhaled from the body.

Recognize Cues [Assessment]
- Determine whether the patient has a history of hypertension, especially if a decongestant is an ingredient in the cold remedy being taken.
- Note baseline vital signs. An elevated temperature of 99°F–101°F (37.2°C–38.3°C) may indicate a viral infection caused by a cold.
- Obtain a drug history, and report if a drug-drug interaction is probable. Dextromethorphan hydrochloride (HCl) given with monoamine oxidase inhibitors (MAOIs), narcotics, sedative-hypnotics, barbiturates, antidepressants, and alcohol may increase toxicity.
- Assess cardiac and respiratory status.

Analyze Cues and Prioritize Hypothesis [Patient Problems]
- Airway obstruction
- Decreased gas exchange
- Hypoxemia
- Discomfort
- Fatigue

Generate Solutions [Planning]
- Patient's cough will be eliminated or diminished.
- Patient will be free from a secondary bacterial infection.

Take Action [Nursing Interventions]
- Monitor vital signs. Blood pressure can become elevated when a decongestant is taken, and dysrhythmias can also occur.
- Observe the color of bronchial secretions. Yellow or green mucus is indicative of a bronchial infection. Antibiotics may be needed.
- Warn patients that codeine preparations for cough suppression can lead to tolerance and physical dependence.

Patient Teaching
General
- Tell patients that hypotension and hyperpyrexia may occur when dextromethorphan is taken with MAOIs.
- Teach patients about proper use of nasal sprays and proper use of "puff" or squeeze products.
- Caution patients not to use more than 3 days, because rebound congestion can occur with overuse.
- ⚡ Advise patients to read labels on over-the-counter (OTC) drugs and to check with a health care provider before taking cold remedies. This is especially important when taking other drugs or when a patient has a major health problem such as hypertension or hyperthyroidism. Also, acetaminophen may be in many products, promoting an overdose.
- Inform patients that antibiotics are *not* helpful in treating common cold viruses. However, they may be prescribed if a secondary infection occurs.
- Encourage older patients with heart disease, asthma, emphysema, diabetes mellitus, or hypertension to contact a health care provider concerning the selection of drug, including OTC drugs.
- Direct patients not to drive during initial use of a cold remedy containing an antihistamine because drowsiness is common.
- Tell patients to maintain adequate fluid intake. Fluids liquefy bronchial secretions to ease elimination with coughing.
- Teach patients not to take a cold remedy before or at bedtime. Insomnia may occur if it contains a decongestant.
- Encourage patients to get adequate rest.
- Inform patients that common cold and flu viruses are transmitted frequently by hand-to-hand contact or by touching a contaminated surface. Cold viruses can live on the skin for several hours and on hard surfaces for several days.
- Advise patients to avoid environmental pollutants, fumes, smoking, and dust to lessen irritating cough.
- Teach patients to perform three effective coughs before bedtime to promote uninterrupted sleep.
- Direct patients and parents to store drugs out of reach of children; request childproof caps.
- Advise patients to contact a health care provider if cough persists for more than 1 week or is accompanied by chest pain, fever, or headache.

Self-Administration
- Teach patients to self-administer medications such as nose drops and inhalants.
- Encourage patients to cough effectively, to take deep breaths before coughing, and to be in an upright position.

Evaluate Outcomes [Evaluation]
- Evaluate effectiveness of drug therapy. Determine that the patient is free from nonproductive cough, has adequate fluid intake and rest, and is afebrile.

CLINICAL JUDGMENT CASE STUDY

A 35-year-old patient has allergic rhinitis. Her prescriptions include loratadine 5 mg/day and fluticasone, two nasal inhalations per day. Previously, she had taken over-the-counter (OTC) drugs and asked if she should continue to take the OTC drug with her prescriptions. She has never used a nasal inhaler before.

1. What additional information is needed from the patient concerning her health problem?
2. What is your response to the patient concerning the use of OTC drugs with her prescription drugs?
3. How would you instruct the patient to use a nasal inhaler? Explain your answer.
4. What are the similarities and differences between loratadine and diphenhydramine? Could one of these antihistamines be more effective than the other? Explain your answer.
5. What could you suggest to decrease allergens such as dust mites in the home?

REVIEW QUESTIONS

1. A patient tells the nurse that he has started to take an over-the-counter antihistamine, diphenhydramine. In teaching about side effects, what is most important for the nurse to tell the patient?
   a. To avoid insomnia, do not take this drug at bedtime.
   b. Avoid driving a motor vehicle until stabilized on the drug.
   c. Nightmares and nervousness are more likely in an adult.
   d. Medication may cause excessive secretions.
2. A patient reports a sore throat and has been told it is due to beta-hemolytic streptococcal infection. The nurse anticipates that the patient has which acute condition?
   a. Rhinitis
   b. Sinusitis
   c. Pharyngitis
   d. Rhinorrhea
3. A patient is prescribed a decongestant nasal spray that contains oxymetazoline. What will the nurse teach the patient?
   a. Take this drug at bedtime because it may cause drowsiness.
   b. Directly spray the medication away from the nasal septum and gently sniff.
   c. This drug may be used in maintenance treatment for asthma.
   d. Limit use of the drug to 3 days to prevent rebound nasal congestion.
4. A patient has been prescribed guaifenesin. The nurse understands that the purpose of the drug is to accomplish what?
   a. Treat allergic rhinitis and prevent motion sickness
   b. Loosen bronchial secretions so coughing can eliminate them
   c. Compete with histamine for receptor sites, thus preventing a histamine response
   d. Stimulate alpha-adrenergic receptors, thus producing vascular constriction of capillaries in nasal mucosa
5. Beclomethasone has been prescribed for a patient with allergic rhinitis. What should the nurse teach the patient regarding this medication?
   a. This medication may be used for an acute attack.
   b. An oral form is available if the patient prefers to use it.
   c. Avoid large amounts of caffeine intake because an increased heart rate may occur.
   d. With continuous use, dryness of the nasal mucosa/lining may occur.
6. The nurse is teaching a patient about diphenhydramine. Which instructions should the nurse include in the patient's teaching plan? **Select all that apply.**
   a. Take medication on an empty stomach to facilitate absorption.
   b. Avoid alcohol and other central nervous system depressants.
   c. Notify a health care provider if confusion or hypotension occurs.
   d. Use sugarless candy, gum, or ice chips for temporary relief of dry mouth.
   e. Avoid handling dangerous equipment or performing dangerous activities until stabilized on the medication.

39

Lower Respiratory Disorders

http://evolve.elsevier.com/McCuistion/pharmacology

OBJECTIVES

- Describe components of the lower respiratory system.
- Summarize the lower respiratory system disorders.
- Discuss the drug categories used to treat lower respiratory disorders.
- Contrast asthma drug therapy for special populations.

OUTLINE

Lower Respiratory System, 486
    Lung Compliance, 486
    Control of Respiration, 486
    Bronchial Smooth Muscle, 486
Lower Respiratory System Disorders, 487
    Asthma, 487
    Bronchitis and Bronchiectasis, 488
    Emphysema, 488
    Chronic Obstructive Pulmonary Disease, 488
    Restrictive Lung Disease, 489
Major Drug Categories That Treat Lower Respiratory Disorders, 489

    Sympathomimetics: Alpha- and Beta$_2$-Adrenergic Agonists, 489
    Anticholinergics, 490
    Methylxanthine (Xanthine) Derivatives, 492
    Leukotriene Receptor Antagonists and Synthesis Inhibitors, 493
    Glucocorticoids (Steroids), 495
    Cromolyn, 496
    Phosphodiesterese-3 and Phosphodiesterase-4 Inhibitors, 497
Asthma Drug Therapy for Special Populations, 498
    Drug Therapy for Asthma According to Severity, 498
    Drug Therapy for Asthma According to Age, 498
Clinical Judgment Single-Episode Case Study, 498
Review Questions, 498

LOWER RESPIRATORY SYSTEM

The chest cavity is a closed compartment bounded by 12 ribs, the diaphragm, thoracic vertebrae, the sternum, neck muscles, and intercostal muscles between the ribs. The pleurae are membranes that encase the lungs. The lungs are divided into lobes; the right lung has three lobes, and the left lung has two lobes. The heart, which is not attached to the lungs, lies on the mid-left side in the chest cavity.

Lung Compliance

Lung compliance is the lung volume based on the pressure in the alveoli. This volume determines the lung's ability to stretch. Factors that influence lung compliance include (1) connective tissue (collagen and elastin) and (2) surface tension in the alveoli, which is controlled by surfactant. Surfactant lowers the surface tension in the alveoli and prevents interstitial fluid from entering. Increased lung compliance is present with chronic obstructive pulmonary disease (COPD), and decreased lung compliance occurs with restrictive pulmonary disease. With low compliance, there is decreased lung volume resulting from increased connective tissue or increased surface tension. The lungs become "stiff," and it takes greater-than-normal pressure to expand lung tissue.

Control of Respiration

Oxygen (O_2), carbon dioxide (CO_2), and hydrogen (H^+) ion concentrations in the blood influence respiration. *Chemoreceptors* are sensors that are stimulated by changes in these gases and ions. The central chemoreceptors, located in the medulla near the respiratory center and cerebrospinal fluid, respond to an increase in CO_2 and a decrease in pH by increasing ventilation. However, if the CO_2 level remains elevated, the stimulus to increase ventilation is lost.

Peripheral chemoreceptors, located in the carotid and aortic bodies, respond to changes in oxygen (P_{O_2}) levels. A low blood oxygen level (P_{O_2} <60 mm Hg) stimulates the peripheral chemoreceptors, which in turn stimulate the respiratory center in the medulla, and ventilation is increased. If oxygen therapy increases the oxygen level in the blood, the P_{O_2} may be too high to stimulate the peripheral chemoreceptors, and ventilation will be depressed.

Bronchial Smooth Muscle

The tracheobronchial tube is composed of smooth muscle whose fibers spiral around the tracheobronchial tube, becoming more closely spaced as they near the terminal bronchioles (Fig. 39.1). Contraction of these muscles constricts the airway. The sympathetic and parasympathetic nervous systems affect the bronchial smooth muscle in opposite ways. The vagus nerve (parasympathetic nervous system) releases acetylcholine, which causes bronchoconstriction. The sympathetic nervous system releases epinephrine, which stimulates the beta$_2$ receptor in the bronchial smooth muscle, resulting in bronchodilation. These two nervous systems counterbalance each other to maintain homeostasis.

Cyclic adenosine monophosphate (cAMP) in the cytoplasm of bronchial cells increases bronchodilation by relaxing the bronchial smooth muscles. The pulmonary enzyme phosphodiesterase can

Fig. 39.1 Bronchial smooth muscle fibers become more closely spaced as they near the alveoli.

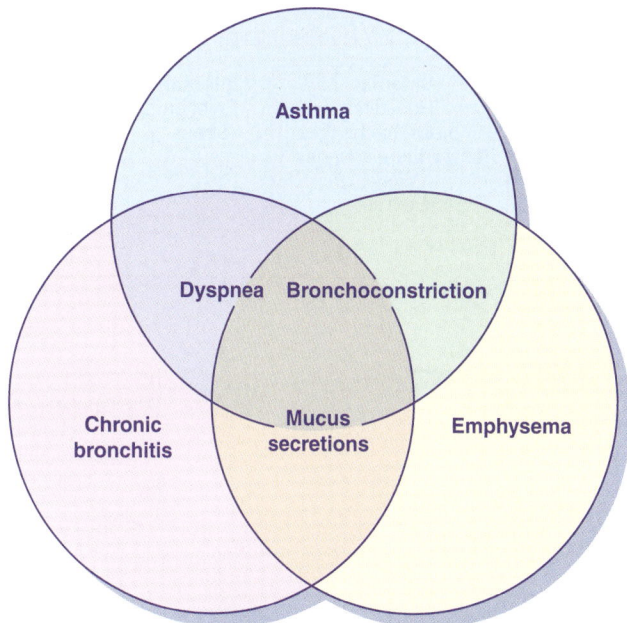

Fig. 39.2 Overlapping signs and symptoms of chronic obstructive pulmonary disease conditions.

inactivate cAMP. Drugs of the methylxanthine group (theophylline) inactivate phosphodiesterase, thus permitting cAMP to function.

This chapter discusses drugs used to alleviate and control airway obstruction. These include the sympathomimetics (adrenergics), particularly the beta$_2$ adrenergics; methylxanthines such as theophylline; leukotriene receptor antagonists; glucocorticoids; cromolyn; and mucolytics.

LOWER RESPIRATORY SYSTEM DISORDERS

Asthma

Asthma is an inflammatory disease in which airway walls are associated with a varying amount of airway obstruction. This disorder is triggered by stimuli such as stress, allergens, and pollutants. When activated by stimuli, the bronchial airways become inflamed and edematous, leading to constriction of air passages. Inflammation aggravates airway hyperresponsiveness to stimuli, causing bronchial cells to produce more mucus, which obstructs air passages. This obstruction contributes to wheezing, coughing, dyspnea (breathlessness), chest tightness, and bronchospasm, particularly at night or in the early morning.

Bronchial asthma is a COPD characterized by periods of bronchospasm (constricted bronchioles) resulting is wheezing, mucous secretions, and dyspnea. There is resistance to airflow caused by obstruction of the airway. Bronchospasm, or bronchoconstrictive, results when the lung tissue is exposed to extrinsic or intrinsic factors that stimulate a bronchoconstrictive response. Factors that can trigger an asthmatic attack (bronchospasm) include humidity, air pressure changes, temperature changes, smoke, fumes (exhaust, perfume), stress, emotional upset, exercise, and allergies to animal dander, dust mites, food, and drugs (e.g., aspirin, ibuprofen, beta-adrenergic blockers). Reactive airway disease is a cause of asthma that results from sensitivity stimulation from allergens, dust, temperature changes, and cigarette smoking. In acute and chronic asthma, minimal to no changes are seen in the structure and function of lung tissues when the disease process is in remission. In chronic bronchitis, emphysema, and bronchiectasis, irreversible damage is done to the physical structure of lung tissue.

Symptoms are similar to those of asthma in these three pulmonary disorders, except wheezing does not occur. Fig. 39.2 shows the overlapping symptoms of COPD conditions. Frequently, a steady deterioration occurs over a period of years.

Pathophysiology

Mast cells found in connective tissue throughout the body are directly involved in the asthmatic response, particularly to extrinsic factors. Allergens attach themselves to mast cells and basophils, resulting in an antigen-antibody reaction on the mast cells in the lung; thus the mast cells stimulate the release of chemical mediators such as histamines, cytokines, serotonin, eosinophil chemotactic factor of anaphylaxis (ECF-A), and leukotrienes. Eosinophil counts are usually elevated during an allergic reaction, which indicates that an inflammatory process is occurring. These chemical mediators stimulate bronchial constriction, mucus secretions, inflammation, and pulmonary congestion. Histamine and ECF-A are strong bronchoconstrictors. Bronchial smooth muscles are wrapped spirally around the bronchioles and contract as they are stimulated by these mediators. Exposure to an allergen results in bronchial hyperresponsiveness, epithelial shedding of the bronchial wall, mucous gland hyperplasia and hypersecretion, leakage of plasma that leads to swelling, and bronchoconstriction.

Fig. 39.3 shows factors that contribute to bronchoconstriction. Cyclic AMP, or cAMP, a cellular signaling molecule, is involved in many cellular activities and is responsible for maintaining bronchodilation. When histamine, ECF-A, and leukotrienes inhibit the action of cAMP, bronchoconstriction results. The sympathomimetic (adrenergic) bronchodilators and methylxanthines increase the amount of cAMP in bronchial tissue cells.

In an acute asthmatic attack, short-acting sympathomimetics (beta$_2$-adrenergic agonists) are the first line of defense. They promote cAMP production and enhance bronchodilation. Long-acting sympathomimetics are used for maintenance. Sympathomimetics (adrenergics) are also discussed in Chapter 15.

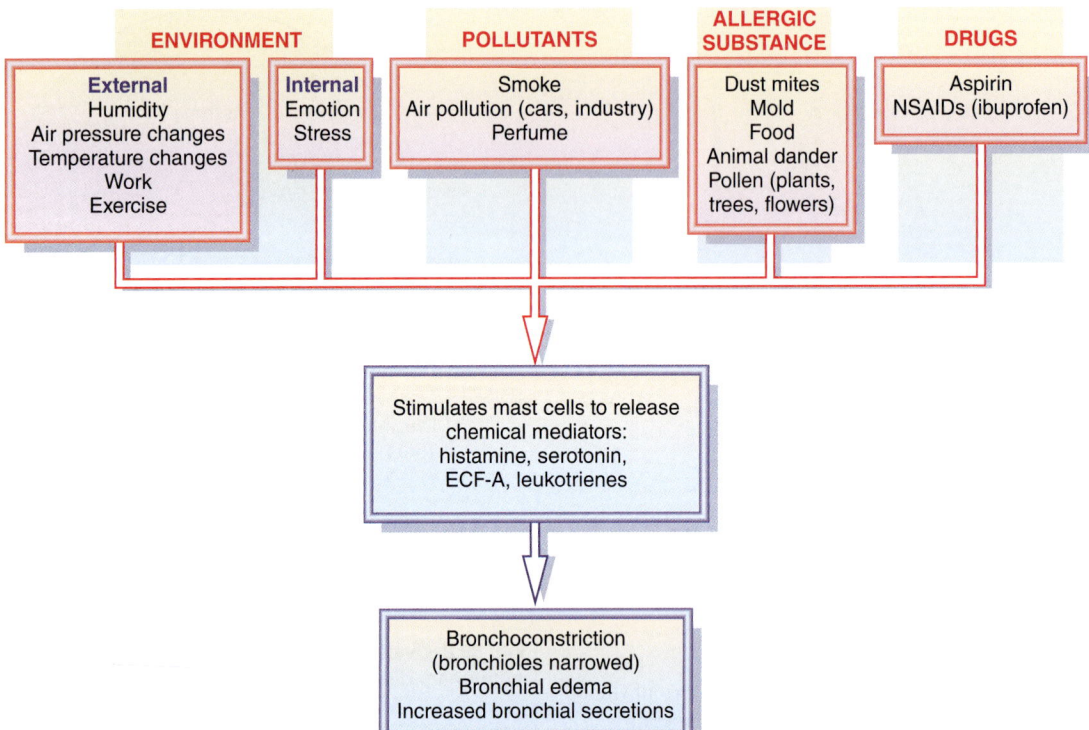

Fig. 39.3 Factors that contribute to bronchoconstriction. *ECF-A*, Eosinophil chemotactic factor of anaphylaxis; *NSAIDs*, nonsteroidal antiinflammatory drugs.

Bronchitis and Bronchiectasis

Chronic bronchitis is a progressive lung disease caused by smoking or chronic lung infections. Bronchial inflammation and excessive mucous secretion result in airway obstruction. Productive coughing is a response to excess mucus production and chronic bronchial irritation. Inspiratory and expiratory rhonchi may be heard on auscultation. Hypercapnia (increased carbon dioxide retention) and hypoxemia (decreased blood oxygen) lead to respiratory acidosis.

In bronchiectasis, dilation of the bronchi and bronchioles is abnormal secondary to frequent infection and inflammation. The bronchioles become obstructed by the breakdown of the epithelium of the bronchial mucosa, and tissue fibrosis may result.

Emphysema

Emphysema is a progressive lung disease caused by cigarette smoking, atmospheric contaminants, or lack of the alpha-1 antitrypsin protein that inhibits proteolytic enzymes that destroy alveoli (air sacs). Proteolytic enzymes are released in the lung by bacteria or phagocytic cells. The terminal bronchioles become plugged with mucus, causing a loss in the fiber and elastin network in the alveoli. Alveoli enlarge as many of the alveolar walls are destroyed. Air becomes trapped in the overexpanded alveoli, leading to inadequate gas exchange (oxygen and carbon dioxide).

In chronic bronchitis, emphysema, and bronchiectasis, irreversible damage is done to the physical structure of lung tissue. Symptoms are similar to those of asthma in these three pulmonary disorders, except wheezing does not occur. Fig. 39.2 shows the overlapping symptoms of COPD conditions. Frequently, a steady deterioration occurs over a period of years.

Chronic Obstructive Pulmonary Disease

Chronic obstructive pulmonary disease (COPD) and restrictive pulmonary disease are the two major categories of lower respiratory tract disorders. COPD is caused by airway obstruction with increased airway resistance of airflow to lung tissues. Four major pulmonary disorders cause COPD: (1) chronic bronchitis, (2) bronchiectasis, (3) emphysema, and (4) asthma. Chronic bronchitis, bronchiectasis, and emphysema frequently result in irreversible lung tissue damage. The lung tissue changes that result from an acute asthmatic attack are normally reversible; however, if the attacks are frequent and asthma becomes chronic, irreversible changes in the lung tissue may result. Patients with COPD usually have a decrease in forced expiratory volume in 1 second (FEV_1) as measured by pulmonary function tests.

Cigarette smoking is the most common risk factor for COPD, especially with chronic bronchitis and emphysema. There is no currently known cure for COPD; however, it remains preventable in most cases. Because cigarette smoking is the most directly related cause, not smoking significantly prevents COPD from developing. Quitting smoking will slow the disease process.

Medications frequently prescribed for COPD include the following:
- Bronchodilators such as sympathomimetics (adrenergics), parasympatholytics (anticholinergic drugs, ipratropium bromide), and methylxanthines (caffeine, theophylline) are used to assist in opening narrowed airways.
- Glucocorticoids (steroids) are used to decrease inflammation.
- Leukotriene modifiers reduce inflammation in the lung tissue, and cromolyn acts as an antiinflammatory agent by suppressing the release of histamine and other mediators from the mast cells.

- Expectorants are used to assist in loosening mucus from the airways.
- Antibiotics may be prescribed to prevent serious complications from bacterial infections.

Restrictive Lung Disease

Restrictive lung disease is a decrease in total lung capacity as a result of fluid accumulation or loss of elasticity of the lung. Pulmonary edema, pulmonary fibrosis, pneumonitis, lung tumors, thoracic deformities (scoliosis), and disorders that affect the thoracic muscular wall, such as myasthenia gravis, are among the types and causes of restrictive pulmonary disease.

Drugs discussed in this chapter are primarily used to treat COPD, particularly asthma. These drugs include bronchodilators (sympathomimetics [primarily beta$_2$-adrenergic agonists], methylxanthines [xanthines]), leukotriene antagonists, glucocorticoids, cromolyn, and anticholinergics. Some of these drugs may also be used to treat restrictive pulmonary diseases.

MAJOR DRUG CATEGORIES THAT TREAT LOWER RESPIRATORY DISORDERS

Sympathomimetics: Alpha- and Beta$_2$-Adrenergic Agonists

Sympathomimetics increase cAMP, causing dilation of the bronchioles. In an acute bronchospasm caused by anaphylaxis from an allergic reaction, the nonselective sympathomimetic epinephrine—an alpha$_1$, beta$_1$, and beta$_2$ agonist—is given subcutaneously to promote bronchodilation and elevate blood pressure. Epinephrine is administered in emergency situations to restore circulation and increase airway patency (see Chapter 58).

For bronchospasm associated with chronic asthma or COPD, selective beta$_2$-adrenergic agonists are given by aerosol or as a tablet. These drugs act primarily on the beta$_2$ receptors; therefore side effects are less severe than those of epinephrine, which acts on alpha$_1$, beta$_1$, and beta$_2$ receptors.

Albuterol

The newer beta-adrenergic drugs for asthma are more selective for beta$_2$ receptors. High doses or overuse of the beta$_2$-adrenergic agents for asthma may cause some degree of beta$_1$ response, such as nervousness, tremor, and increased pulse rate. The ideal beta$_2$ agonist is one that has a rapid onset of action, longer duration of action, and few side effects. Albuterol is a selective beta$_2$ drug that is effective for the treatment and control of asthma by causing bronchodilation with a long duration of action. (See Prototype Drug Chart: Albuterol for drug data related to albuterol.)

⚡ PATIENT SAFETY

Do Not Confuse...
- **Albuterol**, a beta$_2$-adrenergic, with **Accupril**, a cardiovascular agent

PROTOTYPE DRUG CHART

Albuterol

Drug Class	Dosage
Beta$_2$-adrenergic agonist	Exercise-induced bronchospasm: A: MDI: 2 actuations 15–30 min before exercise: *max:* 12 actuations/d

Contraindications	Drug-Lab-Food Interactions
Hypersensitivity *Caution:* Cardiac dysrhythmia, coronary artery disease, hypertension, hyperthyroidism, diabetes mellitus, diabetic ketoacidosis, thyrotoxicosis, hypokalemia, seizures, MAOI therapy, pregnancy, breast-feeding	Drug: Increased effect with other sympathomimetics; may increase effect with MAOIs, Antagonized effect with beta blockers Lab: May increase glucose level slightly; may decrease serum potassium level with thiazide and loop diuretics and carbonic anhydrase inhibitors

Pharmacokinetics	Pharmacodynamics
Absorption: Well absorbed from the GI tract after oral administration; well absorbed from respiratory tract after inhalation Distribution: PB: 10% Metabolism: *t½:* Oral inhal: 3.8–5 h, 100% excreted in the urine	Inhal: Onset: 5–15 min Peak: 0.5–2 h Duration: 2–6 h

Therapeutic Effects/Uses

To treat asthma exacerbation and for prophylaxis and treatment of bronchospasm
Mechanism of action: Stimulates beta$_2$-adrenergic receptors in the lungs, which relaxes the bronchial smooth muscle, thus causing bronchodilation

Side Effects	Adverse Reactions
Dizziness, drowsiness, headache, rhinitis, nasopharyngitis, dry mouth, throat irritation, cough, tooth discoloration, hyperhidrosis, fever, edema, agitation, anxiety, excitability, hyperkinesis, restlessness, insomnia, weakness, ataxia, tremor, muscle cramps, musculoskeletal pain, dyspepsia, nausea, vomiting, diarrhea, urinary retention	Palpitations, tachycardia, hypo/hypertension, chest pain, dyspnea, infection, hyperglycemia, hypokalemia *Life threatening:* Dysrhythmia, angioedema, bronchospasm, Stevens-Johnson syndrome

A, Adult; *d*, day; *GI*, gastrointestinal; *h*, hour; *inhal*, inhalation; *MAOI*, monoamine oxidase inhibitor; *max*, maximum; *MDI*, metered-dose inhaler; *min*, minute; *PB*, protein binding; *PO*, by mouth; *t½*, half-life; *UK*, unknown.

Metaproterenol

The beta-adrenergic agent metaproterenol has some beta$_1$ effect but is primarily used as a beta$_2$ agent. It can be administered orally or by inhalation with a metered-dose inhaler (MDI) or a nebulizer.

For long-term asthma treatment, beta$_2$-adrenergic agonists are frequently administered by inhalation. This route of administration usually delivers more of the drug directly to the constricted bronchial site. The effective inhalation drug dose is less than it would be by the oral route, and there are also fewer side effects using this route. The onset of action is 1 minute by oral inhalation, 5 to 30 minutes by nebulization, and 15 to 30 minutes when taken orally. The peak for inhalation and oral administration is 1 hour with a duration of 4 hours.

Use of an Aerosol Inhaler

If the beta$_2$ agonist is given by MDI or dry-powder inhaler (DPI), correct use of the inhaler and dosage intervals need to be explained to the patient. If the patient does not receive effective relief from the inhaler, either the technique is faulty or the canister is empty. A spacer device may be attached to the inhaler to improve drug delivery to the lung with less deposition in the mouth. If the patient does not use the inhaler properly to deliver the drug dose, the medication may be trapped in the upper airways. Because of drug inhalation, mouth dryness and throat irritation could result.

Excessive use of the aerosol drug can lead to tolerance and loss of drug effectiveness. Occasionally, severe paradoxic airway resistance (bronchoconstriction) develops with repeated excessive use of sympathomimetic oral inhalation. Frequent dosing can cause tremors, nervousness, and increased heart rate. Table 39.1 lists the sympathomimetics used as bronchodilators.

Side Effects and Adverse Reactions

The side effects and adverse reactions of epinephrine include throat irritation, rhinorrhea, sneezing, tremors, dizziness, hypertension, tachycardia, palpitations, dysrhythmias, and angina. The patient needs to be closely monitored when epinephrine is administered.

The side effects associated with beta$_2$-adrenergic drugs, such as albuterol, include tremors, headaches, restlessness, increased pulse rate, and palpitations (high doses). The beta$_2$ agonists may increase blood glucose levels, so patients with diabetes should be taught to closely monitor their serum glucose levels. Side effects of beta$_2$ agonists may diminish after 1 week or longer. The bronchodilating effects may decrease with continued use. It is believed that tolerance to these drugs can develop; if this occurs, the dose may need to be increased. Failure to respond to a previously effective dose may indicate worsening asthma that requires reevaluation before increasing the dose.

Anticholinergics

Tiotropium is an anticholinergic drug used for maintenance treatment of bronchospasms associated with COPD. This drug is administered by inhalation only with the HandiHaler device (DPI). Patients should discard any capsules that are opened and not used immediately. HandiHalers should be washed with warm water and dried. The most common adverse effects of tiotropium include pharyngitis, rhinitis, dry mouth, constipation, vomiting, dyspepsia, abdominal pain, depression, insomnia, headache, joint pain, and peripheral edema. Chest pain has been reported after tiotropium administration. Prototype Drug Chart: Tiotropium lists the drug data related to tiotropium.

PROTOTYPE DRUG CHART

Tiotropium

Drug Class	Dosage
Anticholinergic	COPD: A: Oral inhalation: 2 inhal/d (2.5 mcg/actuation) at the same time qd; *max*: 2 inhal/d

Contraindications	Drug-Lab-Food Interactions
Hypersensitivity *Caution:* Lactose hypersensitivity, cardiac dysrhythmias, closed-angle glaucoma, bladder obstruction, renal impairment, prostatic hypertrophy, contact lens, older adults, pregnancy, breast-feeding, children	Drug: Increased anticholinergic effects with aclidinium, atropine, flavoxate, opium, glycopyrrolate, neostigmine, oxybutynin, phenobarbital, scopolamine

Pharmacokinetics	Pharmacodynamics
Absorption: Minimally absorbed PO Distribution: 72% PB Metabolism: t½: 5–6 d Excretion: In urine as metabolites	Inhalation: PO: Onset: 30 min Peak: 1–4 h Duration: 24 h

Therapeutic Effects/Uses

For maintenance treatment of asthma and COPD
Mechanism of action: Blocks muscarinic cholinergic receptors and antagonizes acetylcholine action by inhibiting M3 receptor response to acetylcholine, thereby relaxing smooth muscle of bronchi; dilates bronchi

Side Effects	Adverse Reactions
Dizziness, headache, blurred vision, cough, oral ulceration, stomatitis, pharyngitis, laryngitis, dysphonia, sinusitis, rhinitis, epistaxis, fever, rash, pruritus, insomnia, depression, peripheral edema, arthralgia, myalgia, musculoskeletal pain, paresthesias, dry mouth, dyspepsia, GERD, abdominal pain, vomiting, diarrhea, constipation, urinary retention, candidiasis, infection	Tachycardia, palpitations, hypertension, chest pain, cataracts, dehydration, hyperglycemia, ileus, GI obstruction, hypercholesterolemia, elevated hepatic enzymes *Life threatening:* Dysrhythmias, anaphylaxis, angioedema

A, Adult; *COPD*, chronic obstructive pulmonary disease; *d*, day; *GERD*, gastroesophogeal reflux disease; *GI*, gastrointestinal; *inhal*, inhalation; *max*, maximum; *min*, minute; *PB*, protein binding; *PO*, by mouth; *qd*, every day; *UK*, unknown.

TABLE 39.1 Adrenergic Bronchodilators and Anticholinergics

Drug	Route and Dosage	Uses and Considerations
Alpha- and Beta-Adrenergics		
Epinephrine Alpha$_1$, beta$_1$, beta$_2$	Intermittent asthma: A: Oral inhal: 1 inhal (0.125 mg), may repeat after 1 min if needed, then wait 4 h between doses	For bronchospasm, anaphylaxis, angioedema, nasal congestion, asthma, and cardiac arrest. May cause headache, weakness, fatigue, rhinorrhea, sneezing, throat irritation, diaphoresis, nausea, vomiting, hypo/hyperglycemia, hypokalemia, angina, palpitations, tachycardia, hypertension, and dysrhythmias. PB: UK; t½: <5 min
Beta-Adrenergics		
Albuterol Beta$_2$	See Prototype Drug Chart: Albuterol	
Formoterol Beta$_2$	A: Inhalation: Inhale 20 mcg (one 2 mL unit) via nebulizer q12h; *max:* 40 mcg/d	For COPD. May cause dizziness, pharyngitis, sinusitis, infection, insomnia, nausea, diarrhea, hyperglycemia, hypokalemia, chest pain, tachycardia, and palpitations. PB: 61%–64%; t½: 10 h
Levalbuterol Beta$_2$	Bronchospasm: A: Inhalation: 0.63–1.25 mg q6–8 h PRN; *max:* 3.75 mg/d	For bronchospasm, asthma exacerbation, and COPD. May cause dizziness, headache, fever, rash, pharyngitis, cough, weakness, nausea, vomiting, diarrhea, hyperglycemia, hypokalemia, chest pain, tachycardia, candidiasis, and tremors. PB: UK; t½: 3.3–4 h
Metaproterenol sulfate Beta$_1$ (some) and beta$_2$	A: PO: 20 mg tid/qid; *max:* 80 mg/d A: Nebulizer: 1 vial (0.4%) tid/qid PRN	For bronchospasm and asthma exacerbation. May cause dizziness, drowsiness, headache, blurred vision, insomnia, fatigue, dysgeusia, nausea, diarrhea, hypokalemia, tremor, chest pain, tachycardia, and palpitations. PB: UK; t½: UK
Salmeterol Beta$_2$	COPD: A: Inhal: 1 puff (50 mcg) q12h; *max:* 2 doses/d Prevention of exercise-induced bronchospasm: A: Inhal MDI: 1 puff at least 30 min before exercise	For asthma, COPD, and exercise-induced bronchospasm prophylaxis. May cause dizziness, headache, pharyngitis, nasal congestion, rhinitis, tracheitis, influenza, rash, hypokalemia, hyperglycemia, musculoskeletal pain, palpitations, tachycardia, and hypo/hypertension. PB: 94%–98%; t½: 5 h
Terbutaline sulfate Beta$_2$	Asthma: A: PO: 5 mg tid; *max:* 15 mg/d	For asthma and bronchospasm. May cause dizziness, drowsiness, headache, dyspnea, weakness, tremors, hyperhidrosis, nausea, vomiting, chest pain, palpitations, and tachycardia. PB: 25%; t½: 2.9–14 h
Arformoterol tartrate Beta$_2$	A: Inhal nebulizer: 15 mcg q12h; *max:* 30 mcg/d	For COPD. May cause headache, sinusitis, dyspnea, rash, diarrhea, tremor, hyperglycemia, back pain, muscle cramps, peripheral edema, chest pain, and tachycardia. PB: 52%–65%; t½: 26 h
Olodaterol Beta$_2$	A: Oral inhal: 2 inhal/d of (2.5 mcg each) at the same time every day	For COPD. May cause dizziness, fever, cough, pharyngitis, rash, diarrhea, constipation, infection, hyperglycemia, hypokalemia, back pain, and arthralgia. PB: 60%; t½: 7.5 h
Anticholinergics		
Ipratropium bromide	Bronchospasm: A: Inhal MDI: 2 puffs tid/qid, *max:* 12 inhal/d	For rhinorrhea and bronchospasm. May cause dizziness, headache, blurred vision, pharyngitis, rhinitis, nasal dryness, infection, epistaxis, dyspnea, dry mouth, dysgeusia, dyspepsia, nausea, urinary retention, tachycardia, back pain, and palpitations. PB: UK; t½: 2 h
Aclidinium	A: Oral MDI inhal: 1 inhal (400 mcg aclidinium) bid; *max:* 2 inhal/d	For COPD. May cause headache, cough, pharyngitis, rhinitis, sinusitis, blurred vision, ocular hypertension, and diarrhea. PB: Minimal; t½: 5–8 h
Tiotropium	See Prototype Drug Chart: Tiotropium	
Umeclidinium	A: Inhal: 1 inhal (62.5 mcg)/d at the same time every day; *max:* 1 dose/d	For COPD. May cause dizziness, pharyngitis, cough, arthralgia, infection, urinary retention, and tachycardia. PB: 89%; t½: 11 h
Revefenacin	A: Inhal: 175 mcg/d by nebulizer: *max:* 1 dose/d	For treatment of COPD. May cause dizziness, headache, pharyngitis, cough, back pain, infection, and hypertension. PB: 71%; t½: 22–70 h
Monoclonal Antibody		
Omalizumab	Asthma: A 91–150 kg: Subcut: 300 mg q4wk; dose and frequency based on body weight and total IgE serum levels	For asthma and chronic urticaria. May cause dizziness, headache, pharyngitis, sinusitis, fatigue, abdominal pain, nausea, arthralgia, bone fractures, peripheral edema, injection-site reaction, and infection. Do not give more than 150 mg/injection site. PB: UK; t½: 26 d

Continued

TABLE 39.1 Adrenergic Bronchodilators and Anticholinergics—cont'd

Drug	Route and Dosage	Uses and Considerations
Reslizumab	A: IV: 3 mg/kg/dose infusion q4wk	For asthma. May cause pharyngitis, dyspnea, musculoskeletal pain, antibody formation, serious hypersensitivity reaction, myalgia, hypotension, and new primary malignancy. PB: UK; t½: 24 d
Dupilumab	A: Subcut: Initially 400 mg/single dose, then 200 mg as a single dose q2wk, or initially 600 mg as a single dose, then 300 mg q2wk	For moderate to severe asthma. May cause dizziness, ocular pruritus, conjunctivitis, blepharitis, keratitis, xerophthalmia, pharyngitis, diarrhea, injection-site reaction, eosinophilia, arthralgia, myalgia, infection, and antibody formation. PB: UK; t½: UK
Tezepelumab	A: Subcut: 210 mg q4wk	For severe asthma. May cause pharyngitis, conjunctivitis, injection-site reaction, back pain, arthralgia, and antibody formation. PB: UK; t½: 26 d
Combination Beta-Adrenergics and Anticholinergics		
Ipratropium and albuterol	A: Inhaled spray: 1 inhal (120 mcg albuterol, 20 mcg ipratropium) q6h; *max:* 6 inhal/d	For COPD. May cause headache, blurred vision, pharyngitis, cough, dyspnea, sinusitis, hyperglycemia, hypokalemia, infection, and angina. PB: 9% ipratropium, 10% albuterol; t½: 2 h ipratropium, 4 h albuterol
Indacaterol and glycopyrrolate	A: Inhal: 1 capsule (27.5 mcg indacaterol and 15.6 mcg glycopyrrolate) bid; *max:* 2 capsules/d	For COPD. May cause headache, blurred vision, pharyngitis, hyperglycemia, hypokalemia, diarrhea, infection, edema, chest pain, back pain, tachycardia, palpitation, and hypertension. PB: 38%–41% glycopyrrolate, 94%–96% indacaterol; t½: 33–53 h glycopyrrolate, 40–56 h indacaterol
Olodaterol and tiotropium	A: Inhal: 2 inhal/d (2.5 mcg olodaterol and 2.5 mcg tiotropium) at same time every day; *max:* 2 inhal/d	For COPD. May cause headache, blurred vision, ocular hypertension, pharyngitis, rhinitis, cough, insomnia, abdominal pain, vomiting, constipation, myalgia, back pain, peripheral edema, hyperglycemia, hypokalemia, chest pain, hypertension, tachycardia, and palpitations. PB: 60% olodaterol, 72% tiotropium; t½: olodaterol 45 h, tiotropium 5–6 d
Umeclidinium and vilanterol	A: Inhal: 1 inhal/d (62.5 mcg umeclidinium and 25 mcg vilanterol) at same time every day; *max:* 1 inhal/d	For COPD. May cause blurred vision, pharyngitis, diarrhea, constipation, hypokalemia, hyperglycemia, urinary retention, chest pain, and palpitations. PB: 89% umeclidinium, 94% vilanterol; t½: 11 h umeclidinium, 21.3 h vilanterol
Glycopyrrolate and formoterol	A: Inhal: 2 inhal (9 mcg glycopyrrolate and 4.8 mcg formoterol) bid in the morning and evening; *max:* 2 inhal/d	For COPD. May cause dizziness, blurred vision, ocular hypertension, cough, infection, hyperglycemia, hypokalemia, urinary retention, chest pain, and palpitations. PB: 38%–41% glycopyrrolate, 46%–58% formoterol; t½: 33–53 h glycopyrrolate, 11 h formoterol
Aclidinium bromide and formoterol fumarate	A: Inhalation: 1 oral inhal (400 mcg aclidinium and 12 mcg formoterol) morning and evening	For COPD. May cause dizziness, headache, blurred vision, insomnia, hyperglycemia, hypokalemia, muscle cramps, back pain, and infection. PB: UK aclidinium, 46%–58% formoterol; t½: 12 h aclidinium, 10 h formoterol

A, Adult; *bid*, two times a day; *COPD*, chronic obstructive pulmonary disease; *d*, day; *h*, hour; *IgE*, immunoglobulin E; *inhal*, inhalation; *max*, maximum; *MDI*, metered-dose inhaler; *min*, minute; *PB*, protein binding; *PO*, by mouth; *PRN*, as needed; *q*, every; *qid*, four times a day; *subcut*, subcutaneous; *t½*, half-life; *tid*, three times a day; *UK*, unknown; *wk*, week.

The anticholinergic drug ipratropium bromide is used to treat asthmatic conditions by dilating the bronchioles. Unlike other anticholinergics, ipratropium bromide has few systemic effects. It is administered by MDI.

The combination of ipratropium bromide with albuterol sulfate is used to treat COPD. The combination is more effective and has a longer duration of action than either agent used alone. These two agents combined increase the FEV_1, the index used to evaluate asthma and obstructive lung disease and the patient's response to bronchodilator therapy.

Methylxanthine (Xanthine) Derivatives

The second major group of bronchodilators used to treat asthma is the methylxanthine (xanthine) derivatives, which include theophylline and caffeine. Xanthines also stimulate the central nervous system (CNS) and respiration, dilate coronary and pulmonary vessels, and cause diuresis. Because of their effect on respiration and pulmonary vessels, xanthines are used in the treatment of asthma.

Theophylline

Theophylline relaxes the smooth muscles of the bronchi, bronchioles, and pulmonary blood vessels by inhibiting the enzyme phosphodiesterase, resulting in an increase in cAMP, which promotes bronchodilation.

Theophylline has a low therapeutic index and a narrow desired therapeutic range (5–15 mcg/mL). The serum or plasma theophylline concentration level should be monitored frequently to avoid severe adverse effects. Toxicity is likely to occur when the serum level is greater than 20 mcg/mL. Certain theophylline preparations can be given with sympathomimetic (adrenergic) agents, but the dose may need to be adjusted.

Theophylline was once used as the first-line drug for treating patients with chronic asthma and other COPDs. However, theophylline use has declined sharply because of a potential danger of serious adverse effects—including dysrhythmias, seizures, and cardiac arrest—and efficacy has not been found to be greater than that of beta agonists or glucocorticoids. Because of its numerous adverse reactions, drug-drug interactions, and narrow therapeutic drug range, theophylline is prescribed mostly for maintenance therapy in patients with chronic stable asthma and other COPDs when other drugs have failed to show improvement. Theophylline drugs are given with caution for patients with seizure disorders or cardiac, renal, or liver disease. Patients who receive theophylline preparations need to be closely monitored for serious side effects and drug interactions.

Table 39.2 lists theophylline and its dosages, uses, and considerations.

Pharmacokinetics

Theophylline is usually well absorbed after oral administration, but absorption may vary according to the specific dosage form. Theophylline is also well absorbed from oral liquids and uncoated plain tablets. Sustained-release dosage forms are slowly absorbed. Food and antacids may decrease the rate but not the extent of absorption; large volumes of fluid and high-protein meals may increase the rate of absorption. The protein binding capacity of aminophylline is 40%. The dose size can also affect the rate of absorption: larger doses are absorbed more slowly. Theophylline can also be administered in intravenous (IV) fluids.

Theophylline drugs are metabolized by liver enzymes, and 90% of the drug is excreted by the kidneys. Tobacco smoking increases metabolism of theophylline drugs, thereby decreasing the half-life. The half-life is also shorter in children. With a short half-life, theophylline is readily excreted by the kidneys, so the dose may need to be increased to maintain a therapeutic serum/plasma range. In nonsmokers and older adults, the average half-life of theophylline is 6.5 to 10.5 hours, and the dose requirements may be decreased. However, in smokers and children, the half-life is 4 to 5 hours, and the dose requirement may be increased. In premature infants, the half-life is 9.4 to 43 hours. In patients with heart failure (HF), cor pulmonale, COPD, or liver disease, the half-life is 24 hours. Kidney function may be decreased in older adults, so caution should be used regarding the theophylline dosage to avoid drug toxicity.

Pharmacodynamics

Theophylline increases the level of cAMP, resulting in bronchodilation. The average onset of action is 30 minutes for oral preparations and 1 to 2 hours for sustained-release (SR) capsules. The peak action is 30 minutes for IV administration and 1 to 2 hours when taken orally.

Side Effects and Adverse Reactions

Side effects and adverse reactions to theophylline include anorexia, nausea, vomiting, and diarrhea caused by increased gastric acid secretion, dysrhythmias, tachycardia, palpitations, and marked hypotension. Adverse CNS reactions—headaches, irritability, restlessness, insomnia, dizziness, and seizures—are often more severe in children than in adults. To decrease the potential for side effects, patients should not take other xanthines while taking theophylline.

Theophylline toxicity is most likely to occur when serum concentrations exceed 20 mcg/mL. Theophylline can cause hyperglycemia. Because of the diuretic effect of xanthines, including theophylline, patients should avoid caffeinated products such as coffee, tea, cola, and chocolate, and they should increase fluid intake.

Rapid IV administration of aminophylline, a theophylline product, can cause dizziness, hypotension, and palpitations. To avoid severe adverse effects, IV theophylline preparations *must be administered slowly* via an infusion pump.

Drug Interactions

Beta blockers, cimetidine, propranolol, and erythromycin decrease the liver metabolism rate and increase the half-life and effects of theophylline; barbiturates and carbamazepine decrease its effects. In both situations, the theophylline dosage would need adjustment. Theophylline decreases the effects of lithium. Phenytoin decreases theophylline levels. If theophylline and a beta-adrenergic agonist are given together, a synergistic effect can occur that can result in cardiac dysrhythmias.

Leukotriene Receptor Antagonists and Synthesis Inhibitors

Leukotriene is a chemical mediator that can cause inflammatory changes in the lung. The *cysteinyl leukotrienes* promote an increase in eosinophil migration, mucous production, and airway wall edema

TABLE 39.2 Theophylline Preparations

Drug	Route and Dosage	Uses and Considerations
Theophylline	A: 18–59 y: IV: 0.4 mg/kg per hour infusion; *max*: 900 mg/d for healthy nonsmokers, or 0.2 mg/kg per hour infusion to others, *max*: 400 mg/d Older adults >60 y: IV: Initially 0.3 mg/kg per hour infusion or 0.2 mg/kg per hour infusion to those with lung/liver dysfunction, sepsis, congestive heart failure, or shock; *max*: 400 mg/d Therapeutic range: 5–15 mcg/L.	For asthma exacerbation/maintenance and COPD. May cause dizziness, headache, restlessness, irritability, insomnia, hematemesis, abdominal pain, GERD, anorexia, nausea, vomiting, diarrhea, hypokalemia, hypercalcemia, seizures, palpitations, tachycardia, and dysrhythmias. Give on empty stomach, 30–60 min before meals or 2 h after meals. PB: 40%; t½: 6.5–10.5 h

A, Adult; *COPD*, chronic obstructive pulmonary disease; *d*, day; *GERD*, gastroesophageal reflux disease; *h*, hour; *IV*, intravenous; *max*, maximum; *min*, minute; *PB*, protein binding; *t½*, half-life; *y*, year.

TABLE 39.3 Antiinflammatory Drugs for Chronic Obstructive Pulmonary Disease and Asthma

Drug	Route and Dosage	Uses and Considerations
Leukotriene Modifiers (Do Not Administer for Acute Asthmatic Attack)		
Leukotriene Receptor Antagonists Zafirlukast	A: PO: 20 mg bid 1 h before or 2 h after meals; *max:* 40 mg/d	For asthma maintenance. May cause dizziness, headache, restlessness, nausea, vomiting, diarrhea, myalgia, hyperbilirubinemia, infection, and peripheral neuropathy. PB: 99%; t½: 10 h
Montelukast	See Prototype Drug Chart: Montelukast	
Leukotriene Synthesis Inhibitors Zileuton	Immediate release: A: PO: 600 mg qid with meals and at bedtime Extended release: A: PO: 1200 mg bid within 1 h after morning and evening meal; *max:* 2400 mg/d	For asthma maintenance. May cause headache, chills, sinusitis, weakness, fatigue, insomnia, myalgia, abdominal pain, dyspepsia, nausea, diarrhea, constipation, and elevated hepatic enzymes. PB: 93%; t½: 1–2.3 h
Phosphodiesterase-4 Inhibitor Roflumilast	A: PO: Initially 250 mcg/d for 4 wk; *maint:* 500 mcg/d; *max:* 500 mcg/d	For COPD. May cause dizziness, depression, headache, insomnia, anorexia, nausea, diarrhea, influenza, infection, weight loss, and back pain. PB: 99%; t½: 17 h
Glucocorticoids (Corticosteroids) (See Chapter 49)		
Combination Drugs: Glucocorticoid and Beta₂ Agonist Fluticasone and salmeterol	COPD: A: Inhal DPI diskus: 1 inhal (250 mcg fluticasone and 50 mcg salmeterol) bid in morning and evening; *max:* 2 inhal/d	For asthma and COPD. May cause headache, fever, throat irritation, cough, pharyngitis, sinusitis, oral candidiasis, nausea, vomiting, diarrhea, infection, and musculoskeletal pain. PB: 99% fluticasone, 94%–98% salmeterol; t½: 7.8 h fluticasone, 12.6 h salmeterol
Fluticasone furoate and vilanterol	COPD: A: Inhal: 1 inhal/d (100 mcg fluticasone and 25 mcg vilanterol) at same time every day	For asthma and COPD. May cause headache, fever, pharyngitis, cough, candidiasis, infection, peripheral edema, and arthralgia. PB: 99.6% fluticasone, 93.9% vilanterol; t½: 24 h fluticasone, 21.3 h vilanterol
Mast Cell Stabilizer Cromolyn sodium Phosphodiesterase-3 and Phosphodiesterase-4 inhibitors Ensifentrine	Asthma maintenance: A: Inhal: 20 mg nebulizer q6h A: Oral inhal nebulizer: 3mg (1 unit-dose ampule) bid, in morning and evening; *max:* 6 mg/d	For seasonal allergies, conjunctivitis, asthma, and exercise-induced bronchospasm prophylaxis. May cause headache, cough, hoarseness, nausea, diarrhea, rash, pruritus, and myalgia. Do not use for acute asthma attack. PB: UK; t½: 80–90 min For COPD. May cause anxiety, insomnia, diarrhea, back pain, depression, hypertension, paradoxical bronchospasm, and suicidal ideation. PB: 90%; t½: 10.6–12.6 h

A, Adult; *bid*, twice a day; *COPD*, chronic obstructive pulmonary disorder; *d*, day; *DPI*, dry-powder inhaler; *GI*, gastrointestinal; *h*, hour; *inhal*, inhalation; *maint*, maintenance; *max*, maximum; *MDI*, metered-dose inhaler; *min*, minute; *PB*, protein binding; *PO*, by mouth; *q*, every; *qd*, every day; *t½*, half-life; *UK*, unknown; *wk*, week; *y*, years.

that results in bronchoconstriction. Leukotriene receptor antagonists and leukotriene synthesis inhibitors, called *leukotriene modifiers*, are effective in reducing the inflammatory symptoms of asthma triggered by allergic and environmental stimuli. These drug groups are *not* recommended for treatment of acute asthmatic attacks; rather, they are used for asthma maintenance or exercise-induced asthma. Three leukotriene modifiers—zafirlukast, zileuton, and montelukast—are available in the United States. These drugs are listed in Table 39.3.

Zafirlukast was the first drug in the class of leukotriene modifiers. It acts as a leukotriene receptor antagonist, reducing the inflammatory process and decreasing bronchoconstriction. It is administered orally, is absorbed rapidly, and has a moderate to moderately long half-life; it is given twice a day. Zileuton is a leukotriene synthesis inhibitor. It decreases the inflammatory process and decreases bronchoconstriction. Zileuton has a short half-life of 1 to 2.3 hours. Montelukast has a short half-life of 2.7 to 5.5 hours and is considered safe for use in children 2 years of age and older (see Prototype Drug Chart: Montelukast).

PROTOTYPE DRUG CHART

Montelukast

Drug Class	Dosage
Bronchodilator: Leukotriene receptor antagonist	Asthma maintenance: A: PO: 10 mg/d in the evening or at least 2 h before exercise; *max:* 10 mg/d
Contraindications	**Drug-Lab-Food Interactions**
Hypersensitivity *Caution:* Bronchospasm, status asthmaticus, depression, behavioral changes, psychiatric event, suicidal ideation, corticosteroid withdrawal, alcohol abuse, hepatic disease, older adults, pregnancy, breast-feeding	Decreased drug effects with carbamazepine, hydantoins, isoniazid, phenobarbital, rifampin, St. John's wort; Gemfibrozil, increases drug levels Lab: Abnormal liver function tests (ALT, AST)
Pharmacokinetics	**Pharmacodynamics**
Absorption: Well absorbed Distribution: 99% PB Metabolism: t½: 2.7–5.5 h Elimination: In feces and urine	PO: Onset: UK Peak: 3–4 h Duration: 24 h
Therapeutic Effects/Uses	
For treatment of allergic rhinitis and asthma maintenance, for exercise-induced bronchospasm prophylaxis Mechanism of action: Binds with leukotriene receptors to inhibit smooth muscle contraction and bronchoconstriction	
Side Effects	**Adverse Reactions**
Dizziness, drowsiness, headache, cough, nasal congestion, rhinitis, sinusitis, pharyngitis, laryngitis, fatigue, agitation, restlessness, insomnia, confusion, depression, gastritis, nausea, vomiting, diarrhea, edema, palpitations, muscle cramps	Bleeding, seizures *Life threatening:* Anaphylaxis, angioedema, suicidal ideation, thrombocytopenia, Stevens-Johnson syndrome

A, Adult; *ALT*, alanine transaminase; *AST*, aspartate transaminase; *h*, hour; *max*, maximum; *PB*, protein binding; *PO*, by mouth; *t½*, half-life; *UK*, unknown.

Leukotriene receptor antagonists and synthesis inhibitors should not be used during an acute asthmatic attack. They are only for prophylactic and maintenance drug therapy for chronic asthma.

COMPLEMENTARY AND ALTERNATIVE THERAPIES

Lower Respiratory Disorders
- Ephedra may increase the effect of the theophylline group and may cause theophylline toxicity.
- St. John's wort may decrease montelukast concentration.

Glucocorticoids (Steroids)

Glucocorticoids, members of the corticosteroid family, are used to treat respiratory disorders, particularly asthma. These drugs have an antiinflammatory action and are indicated if asthma is unresponsive to bronchodilator therapy or if the patient has an asthmatic attack while on maximum doses of theophylline or an adrenergic drug. It is thought that glucocorticoids have a synergistic effect when given with a beta$_2$ agonist.

Glucocorticoids can be given using the following methods:
- *MDI inhaler:* Beclomethasone
- *Tablet:* Dexamethasone, prednisone
- *Intravenous:* Dexamethasone

Inhaled glucocorticoids are not helpful in treating a severe asthmatic attack because it may take 1 to 4 weeks for an inhaled steroid to reach its full effect. When maintained on inhaled glucocorticoids, asthmatic patients demonstrate an improvement in symptoms and a decrease in asthmatic attacks. Inhaled glucocorticoids are more effective for controlling symptoms of asthma than are beta$_2$ agonists, particularly in the reduction of bronchial hyperresponsiveness. The use of an oral inhaler minimizes the risk for adrenal suppression associated with oral systemic glucocorticoid therapy. Inhaled glucocorticoids are preferred over oral preparations unless they fail to control the asthma.

The National Asthma Education and Prevention Program guidelines recommend systemic glucocorticoids—prednisone, prednisolone, dexamethasone, or methylprednisolone—for management of moderate to severe asthma exacerbations. Oral or IV administration of methylprednisolone 40 to 80 mg/day in 1 to 2 divided doses may be given for 5 to 10 days. With a single dose or short-term use, glucocorticoids may be discontinued abruptly after symptoms are controlled. Suppression of adrenal function does not usually occur within 1 to 2 weeks.

When severe asthma requires prolonged glucocorticoid therapy, weaning or tapering of the dose may be necessary to prevent an exacerbation of asthma symptoms and suppression of adrenal function. Previously, alternate-day therapy with oral prednisone was used in some asthmatic patients. Currently, inhaled glucocorticoids are thought to be preferable in the treatment of most patients with asthma. Glucocorticoid preparations are discussed in detail in Chapter 49.

Glucocorticoids can irritate the gastric mucosa and should be taken with food to avoid ulceration. A combination inhalation drug containing the glucocorticoid fluticasone propionate and salmeterol is effective in controlling asthma symptoms by alleviating airway constriction and inflammation. This combination is used every day but requires only one inhalation in the morning and one at night. This drug does not replace fast-acting inhalers for sudden symptoms.

Side Effects and Adverse Reactions

Side effects associated with orally inhaled glucocorticoids are generally local (e.g., throat irritation, hoarseness, dry mouth, coughing) rather

CLINICAL JUDGMENT [NURSING PROCESS]
Bronchodilators

Concept: Oxygenation
- The addition of oxygen to the body

Recognize Cues [Assessment]
- Obtain a medical and drug history; report probable drug-drug interactions.
- Note baseline vital signs and pulse oximetry for abnormalities and future comparisons.
- Assess for wheezing, decreased breath sounds, cough, and sputum production.
- Assess sensorium for confusion and restlessness caused by hypoxia and hypercapnia.
- Determine hydration; diuresis may result in dehydration in children and older adults.
- Assess serum theophylline levels. Toxicity occurs at a higher frequency with levels greater than 20 mcg/mL.

Analyze Cues and Prioritize Hypothesis [Patient Problems]
- Airway obstruction
- Decreased gas exchange
- Dyspnea
- Fatigue

Generate Solutions [Planning]
- The patient will be free from wheezing, and lung fields will be clear within 2 to 5 days.
- The patient will self-administer oral drugs and will use an inhaler as prescribed.

Take Action [Nursing Interventions]
- Monitor vital signs. Blood pressure and heart rate can increase greatly. Check for cardiac dysrhythmias.
- Provide adequate hydration. Fluids help loosen secretions.
- Monitor drug therapy.
- Observe for side effects.
- Administer medication after meals to decrease gastrointestinal (GI) distress.
- Administer medication at regular intervals around the clock to have a sustained therapeutic level.
- Do *not* crush enteric-coated (EC) or sustained-released (SR) tablets or capsules.
- ⚡ Check serum theophylline levels (normal level is 5–15 mcg/mL).

Patient Teaching
General
- Teach patients to monitor their pulse rate.
- Encourage patients to monitor the amount of medication remaining in the canister.
- Advise patients not to take over-the-counter (OTC) preparations without first checking with a health care provider. Some OTC products may have an additive effect.
- Encourage patients contemplating pregnancy to seek medical advice before taking a theophylline preparation.
- Advise patients to avoid smoking. Avoid marked sudden changes in smoking amounts, which could affect theophylline blood levels. Smoking increases drug elimination, which may require an increased drug dose.
- Discuss ways to alleviate anxiety, such as relaxation techniques and music.
- ⚡ Advise patients having asthmatic attacks to wear an identification bracelet or MedicAlert tag.
- Inform patients that certain complementary and alternative therapies may interact with theophylline.
- ⚡ Advise patients to notify a health care provider of aggressive or altered behavior and suicidal thoughts.

Self-Administration
- Teach patients to correctly use the inhaler or nebulizer. Caution against overuse because side effects and tolerance may result.
- Teach patients to monitor pulse rate and report to a health care provider any irregularities in comparison with baseline values.

Diet
- Advise patients that a high-protein, low-carbohydrate diet increases theophylline elimination. Conversely, a low-protein, high-carbohydrate diet prolongs half-life; dosage may need adjustment.

Correct Use of a Metered-Dose Inhaler to Deliver Beta$_2$ Agonist
- Insert the medication canister into the plastic mouthpiece.
- Shake the inhaler well before use.
- Remove the cap from the mouthpiece.
- Hold the mouthpiece 1 to 2 inches from the mouth or place the inhaler mouthpiece in the mouth. A spacer may be used; discuss technique with a health care provider.
- Breathe out through the mouth, then take a *slow deep* breath in through the mouth; at the same time, push the top of the medication canister once.
- Hold the breath for a few seconds; exhale slowly through pursed lips.
- Wait 2 minutes if a second dose is required, and then repeat the procedure by first shaking the inhaler with the mouthpiece cap in place.
- Do a test spray into the air before administering the metered dose of a new inhaler or when the inhaler has not been used recently.

Evaluate Outcomes [Evaluation]
- Evaluate the effectiveness of the bronchodilator. The patient should be breathing without wheezing and should be unharmed from the side effects of the drug.
- Determine serum theophylline levels to ensure a therapeutic range.

---

than systemic. Oral, laryngeal, and pharyngeal fungal infections have occurred but can be reversed with discontinuation and antifungal treatment. *Candida albicans* oropharyngeal infections may be prevented by using a spacer with the inhaler to reduce drug deposits in the oral cavity, rinsing the mouth and throat with water after each dose, and washing the apparatus (cap and plastic nose or mouthpiece) daily with warm water.

Oral and injectable glucocorticoids have many side effects when used long term, but short-term use usually causes no significant side effects. Most adverse reactions are seen within 2 weeks of glucocorticoid therapy and are usually reversible. Side effects that may occur include headache, euphoria, mood changes, diaphoresis, insomnia, nausea, vomiting, weakness, and menstrual irregularities. Adverse effects include depression, peptic ulcer, loss of bone density and development of osteoporosis, and psychosis.

When oral and IV steroids are used for prolonged periods, electrolyte imbalance, fluid retention (puffy eyelids, edema in the lower extremities, moon face, weight gain), hypertension, thinning of the skin, purpura, abnormal subcutaneous fat distribution, hyperglycemia, and impaired immune response are likely to occur.

Cromolyn

Cromolyn sodium is used for prophylactic treatment of bronchial asthma, and it must be taken daily. It is not used for acute asthmatic attacks. Cromolyn does not have bronchodilator properties but instead acts by

CLINICAL JUDGMENT [NURSING PROCESS]
Leukotriene Receptor Antagonists

Concept: Oxygenation
- The addition of oxygen to the body

Recognize Cues [Assessment]
- Obtain a medical, drug, and herbal history; report probable drug-drug or drug-herb interactions.
- Note baseline vital signs for identifying abnormalities and for future comparisons.
- Assess for wheezing, decreased breath sounds, cough, and sputum production.
- Assess sensorium for confusion and restlessness caused by hypoxia and hypercapnia.
- Assess for a history of phenylketonuria when montelukast is prescribed because children's chewable tablets contain phenylalanine.
- Determine hydration; diuresis may result in dehydration in children and older adults.

Analyze Cues and Prioritize Hypothesis [Patient Problems]
- Airway obstruction
- Decreased gas exchange
- Dyspnea
- Fatigue

Generate Solutions [Planning]
- The patient will be free from wheezing, or wheezing will have significantly improved.
- The patient's lung fields will be clear within 2 to 5 days.
- The patient will take medications as prescribed.

Take Action [Nursing Interventions]
- Monitor respirations for rate, depth, rhythm, and type.
- Monitor lung sounds for rhonchi, wheezing, or rales.
- Observe lips and fingernails for cyanosis.
- Monitor drug therapy for effectiveness.
- Observe for side effects.
- Provide adequate hydration; fluids help loosen secretions.
- Monitor liver function tests; aspartate transaminase (AST) and alanine transaminase (ALT) may be elevated with zafirlukast and montelukast.
- Provide pulmonary therapy by chest clapping and postural drainage as appropriate.

Patient Teaching
General
- Advise patients that if an allergic reaction occurs (i.e., rash, urticaria), the drug should be discontinued, and a health care provider should be notified.
- Monitor hepatic function tests periodically.
- Direct patients not to take St. John's wort without first checking with a health care provider because this product may decrease montelukast concentration.
- Warn patients that black or green tea and guarana taken with montelukast and zafirlukast may cause increased stimulation.
- Encourage patients to stop smoking.
- Discuss ways to alleviate anxiety (relaxation techniques, music).
- ⚡ Advise patients who have frequent or severe asthmatic attacks to wear an identification bracelet or a MedicAlert tag.
- Encourage patients contemplating pregnancy to seek medical advice before taking montelukast.
- Caution patients and their significant others not to open oral granule packets until they are ready to use them. After opening a packet, the dose must be administered within 15 minutes. If mixed with baby formula or an approved food (applesauce, carrots, rice, or ice cream), do *not* store for future use.
- Advise patients with known aspirin sensitivity to avoid a bronchoconstrictor response by avoiding aspirin and nonsteroidal antiinflammatory drugs (NSAIDs) while taking montelukast.

Self-Administration
- Teach patients not to use montelukast for reversal of an acute asthmatic attack because it is only recommended for prevention of acute attacks and for treatment of chronic asthma.
- Advise patients to continue to use the usual regimen of inhaled prophylaxis and short-acting rescue medication for exercise-induced bronchospasm.
- ⚡ Encourage patients to inform a health care provider if short-acting inhaled bronchodilators are needed more often than usual with montelukast.
- Tell patients to comply with the medication regimen even during symptom-free periods.
- Advise patients, especially children, that chewable tablets are to be chewed thoroughly because swallowing whole may alter absorption.

Diet
- Tell patients to take leukotriene receptor antagonists in the evening for maximum effectiveness.

Evaluate Outcomes [Evaluation]
- Evaluate the effectiveness of the bronchodilators. The patient should be breathing without wheezing and without side effects of the drug.
- Evaluate tolerance to activity.

---

inhibiting release of histamine and other inflammatory mediators from mast cells to prevent an asthma attack. Its most common side effects include postnasal drip, irritation of the nose and throat, and a cough. These effects can be decreased by drinking water before and after using the drug.

Cromolyn is administered by oral inhalation via MDI or nebulizer and nasal inhalation via metered spray. It can be used with beta-adrenergics and xanthine derivatives. Rebound bronchospasm and laryngeal edema are serious side effects of cromolyn. The drug should not be discontinued abruptly because a rebound asthmatic attack can result.

Cromolyn has a low incidence of side effects but the drug is only moderately effective, and many newer drugs have replaced cromolyn use. Table 39.3 lists antiinflammatory drugs for COPD, including leukotriene receptor antagonists, leukotriene synthesis inhibitors, phosphodiesterase-4 inhibitors, glucocorticoids, combination drugs (glucocorticoid and beta$_2$ agonist), and cromolyn.

Phosphodiesterase-3 and Phosphodiesterase-4 Inhibitors

Ensifentrine is a new FDA approved drug in June 2024 to treat COPD, which inhibits phosphodiesterase-3 (PDE3) and Phosphodiesterase-4 (PDE4) enzymes. When PDE3 and PDE4 enzymes are inhibited, the degradation or breaking down of cyclic adenosine monophosphate (cAMP) and cyclic guanosine monophosphate (cGMP) is prevented. This action increases bronchial muscle relaxation and decreases inflammatory mediators.

Some side effects of ensifentrine include anxiety, insomnia, depression, diarrhea, and back pain. Adverse reactions are hypertension, paradoxical bronchospasm, and suicidal ideation. Patients and their families or caregivers should be advised to be on the alert for suicidal thoughts or mood changes and to contact their healthcare provider.

ASTHMA DRUG THERAPY FOR SPECIAL POPULATIONS

Drug Therapy for Asthma According to Severity
Chronic asthma may be controlled through a long-term medical treatment program and by a quick-relief program during an acute phase. The long-term program may vary according to the symptoms of the asthma and its severity, whereas the quick-relief therapy is the same for all classes of asthma.

Drug Therapy for Asthma According to Age
Young Children
Cromolyn is used to treat the inflammatory effects of asthma in children. Oral glucocorticoids may be prescribed for the young child to control a moderate to severe asthmatic state. An inhalation dose of a glucocorticoid should be about 1 to 2 inhalations 4 times a day. If the condition is severe, selected young children may be ordered an oral beta$_2$-adrenergic agonist.

Older Adults
Drug selection and dosage need to be considered for the older adult with an asthmatic condition. Beta$_2$-adrenergic agonists and methylxanthines such as theophylline can cause tachycardia, nervousness, and tremors in older adults, especially those with cardiac conditions. Frequent use of glucocorticoids can increase the risk of the patient developing cataracts, osteoporosis, and diabetes mellitus. If a theophylline drug is ordered, dosages of glucocorticoids are normally decreased.

CLINICAL JUDGMENT SINGLE-EPISODE CASE STUDY

Cognitive Skill: Prioritize hypothesis.

A 45-year-old female patient with a diagnosis of asthma was feeling short of breath. Earlier in the morning she performed outside gardening work. She used the rescue inhaler prescribed by her doctor. After not receiving any relief the symptoms worsened, so she went to the emergency department. Her oxygen saturation was 91% on room air. They immediately placed her on oxygen and called for the respiratory therapist, who started her on albuterol breathing treatment. After about 1 hour she started to improve. On discharge she received an order for the anticholinergic drug tiotropium bromide, two inhalations once a day, with instructions to continue her prescribed medications and to follow-up with her respiratory doctor.

During the discharge teaching, the nurse reviewed the new drug tiotropium inhaler, its therapeutic effectiveness, and its side effects.

Tiotropium is used to treat _____ (1). The therapeutic response of tiotropium is to _____ (1) and _____ (1). The side effects include _____ (2), _____ (2), _____ (2), and _____ (2).

Options for 1	Options for 2
Increase wheezing	Insomnia
Relax smooth muscle	Muscle cramping
Asthma	Tremor
Increase shortness of breath	Sinusitis

Options for 1	Options for 2
Dilate the bronchi	Coughing
Promote drowsiness	Headache
Sore throat	Increased appetite
Hypokalemia	Blurred vision

Answers
Tiotropium is used to treat asthma (1). The therapeutic response of tiotropium is to relax smooth muscle (1) and dilate the bronchi (1). The side effects include insomnia (2), sinusitis (2), headache (2), and blurred vision (2).

Rationale
Asthma is an inflammatory disorder of the airway walls associated with varying amount of airway obstruction. The patient's asthma was triggered by stimuli such as stress, allergens, and pollutants. When activated by stimuli, the bronchial airways become inflamed and edematous, leading to constriction of air passages. Inflammation aggravates airway hyperresponsiveness to stimuli, causing bronchial cells to produce more mucus, which obstructs air passages. Tiotropium blocks muscarinic cholinergic receptors and antagonizes acetylcholine action by inhibiting M3 receptor response to acetylcholine, thereby relaxing smooth muscle of bronchi and dilating the bronchi.

References
Pharmacology, McCuistion, et al. Pharmacology, Chapter 39 (Tiotropium Prototype Drug Chart) J. R. Burchum, et al: *Lehne's pharmacology for nursing care*, ed 9, p 930. Chapter 76.

REVIEW QUESTIONS

1. Fluticasone propionate and salmeterol combination inhalation is ordered for a patient with chronic obstructive pulmonary disease. What does the nurse know about this medication? **Select all that apply.**
   a. It can be used to treat an acute attack.
   b. It is delivered as a dry-powder inhaler.
   c. It contains a beta$_1$ agonist and cromolyn.
   d. It is taken as one puff two times a day.
   e. It promotes bronchodilation.

2. A patient with chronic obstructive pulmonary disease has an acute bronchospasm. The nurse anticipates that the health care provider will prescribe which medication?
   a. Zafirlukast
   b. Epinephrine
   c. Dexamethasone
   d. Beclomethasone

3. A patient is prescribed aminophylline-theophylline. For what adverse effect should the nurse monitor the patient?
   a. Drowsiness
   b. Hypoglycemia
   c. Increased heart rate
   d. Decreased white blood cell count
4. A patient is receiving intravenous aminophylline. The nurse checks the patient's laboratory values and sees the serum theophylline level is 32 mcg/mL. What action should the nurse take?
   a. Assess the patient's breath sounds for improvement.
   b. Increase the dosage per sliding scale directions.
   c. Notify the health care provider of the level.
   d. Have the laboratory collect another sample to verify the results.
5. A patient with chronic obstructive pulmonary disease is taking the leukotriene antagonist montelukast. The nurse is aware that this medication is given for which purpose?
   a. Maintenance treatment of asthma
   b. Treatment of acute asthmatic attack
   c. Reversing bronchospasm associated with chronic obstructive pulmonary disease
   d. Treatment of inflammation in chronic bronchitis

UNIT XII Cardiovascular Drugs

40

Cardiac Glycosides, Antianginals, and Antidysrhythmics

http://evolve.elsevier.com/McCuistion/pharmacology

OBJECTIVES

- Describe the components of the cardiovascular system.
- Describe laboratory tests to diagnose heart failure.
- Contrast the different treatments of heart failure.
- Describe angina pectoris.
- Differentiate the three types of antianginals.
- Explain cardiac dysrhythmias.
- Describe the four classes of antidysrhythmic drugs.

OUTLINE

Introduction, 501
Cardiovascular System, 501
   Heart, 501
   Conduction of Electrical Impulses, 502
   Regulation of Heart Rate and Blood Flow, 502
   Circulation, 503
   Blood, 503
Laboratory Tests to Diagnose Heart Failure, 503
   Atrial Natriuretic Hormone or Peptide, 503
   Brain Natriuretic Peptide, 503
Agents Used to Treat Heart Failure, 503
   Cardiac Glycosides, 503
   Digoxin, 504
   Phosphodiesterase Inhibitors, 505
   Other Agents Used to Treat Heart Failure (PDE), 506
   Nonpharmacologic Measures to Treat Heart Failure, 507
Angina Pectoris, 507

Types of Angina Pectoris, 507
Nonpharmacologic Measures to Control Angina, 507
Types of Antianginal Drugs, 507
   Nitrates, 508
   Beta-Blockers, 509
   Calcium Channel Blockers, 512
Cardiac Dysrhythmias, 512
   Cardiac Action Potentials, 513
   Antidysrhythmic Drugs, 514
Types of Antidysrythmic Drugs, 514
   Class I: Sodium Channel Blockers, 514
   Class II: Beta-Blockers, 514
   Class III: Drugs That Prolong Repolarization, 519
   Class IV: Calcium Channel Blockers, 519
   Side Effects and Adverse Reactions of Antidysrhythmic Drugs, 519
Clinical Judgment Unfolding Case Study, 520
Review Questions, 523

INTRODUCTION

The cardiovascular system includes the heart, blood vessels (arteries and veins), and blood flow. Blood that is abundant in oxygen (O_2), nutrients, and hormones move through vessels called *arteries*, which narrow to arterioles and then to capillaries. Capillaries transport nourished blood to body cells and absorb waste products, such as carbon dioxide (CO_2), urea, creatinine, and ammonia. The deoxygenated blood returns to circulation through small venules and larger veins to be eliminated by the lungs and kidneys with other waste products (Fig. 40.1).

The heart's pumping action serves as the energy source that circulates blood to the cells of the body. Blockage of vessels can inhibit blood flow.

CARDIOVASCULAR SYSTEM

Heart

The heart is composed of four chambers, including the right and left atria and the right and left ventricles (Fig. 40.2). The right atrium receives deoxygenated blood from the circulation, and the right ventricle pumps blood through the pulmonary artery to the lungs for gas exchange (carbon dioxide for oxygen). The left atrium receives oxygenated blood, and the left ventricle pumps the blood into the aorta for systemic circulation.

The heart muscle, called the *myocardium*, surrounds the ventricles and atria. The ventricles have thick walls, especially the left ventricle, to produce the muscular force needed to pump blood to the pulmonary and systemic circulations. The atria have thin walls, have less pumping action, and receive blood from the circulation and lungs.

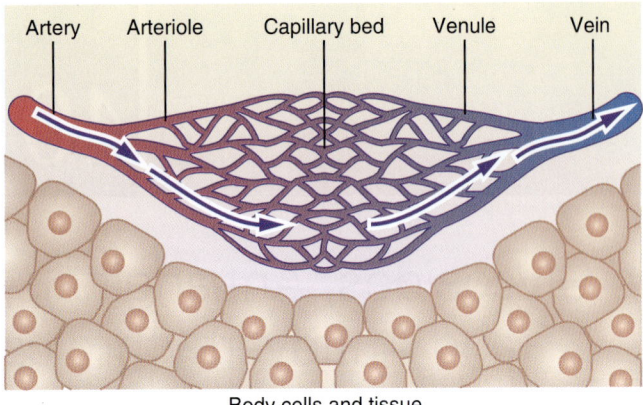

Fig. 40.1 Basic structures of the vascular system.

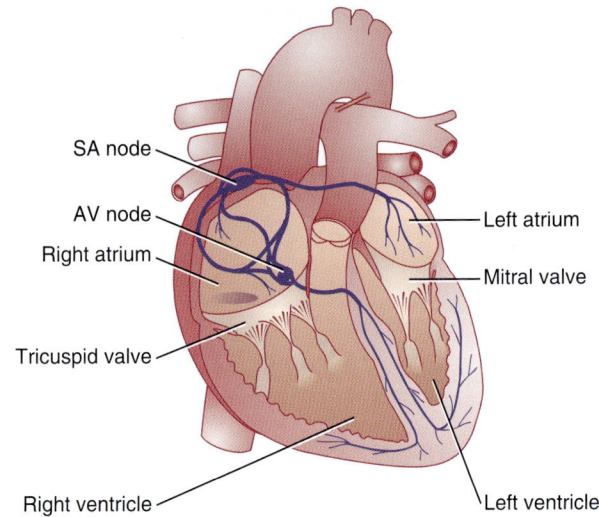

Fig. 40.2 Anatomy of the heart. *AV node*, Atrioventricular node; *SA node*, sinoatrial node.

The heart has a fibrous covering called the *pericardium*, which protects it from injury and infection. The *endocardium* is a three-layered membrane that lines the inner part of the heart chambers. Four valves—two atrioventricular (tricuspid and mitral) and two semilunar (pulmonic and aortic)—control blood flow between the atria and ventricles, and between the ventricles and the pulmonary artery and the aorta. There are two main coronary arteries: the right coronary artery divides into branches that supply blood to the right atrium and both ventricles of the heart, and the left coronary artery divides near its origin to form the left circumflex artery and the anterior descending artery, which supply blood to the left atrium and both ventricles of the heart. Blockage to one of these arteries can result in a myocardial infarction (MI), or heart attack.

Conduction of Electrical Impulses

The myocardium can generate and conduct its own electrical impulses. The cardiac impulse normally originates in the *sinoatrial (SA) node* located in the posterior wall of the right atrium. The SA node is frequently called the *pacemaker* because it regulates the heartbeat (firing of cardiac impulses), which is approximately 60 to 80 beats/min in the normal adult. The *atrioventricular (AV) node*, located in the posterior right side of the interatrial septum, has a continuous tract of fibers called the *bundle of His*, or the AV bundle. The AV node has an adult rate of 40 to 60 beats/min. If the SA node fails, the AV node takes over as the pacemaker, thus causing a slower heart rate; the AV node sends impulses to the ventricles. These two conducting systems, the SA and AV nodes, can act independently of each other. The ventricle can contract independently 30 to 40 times per minute.

Drugs that affect cardiac contraction include calcium, digitalis preparations, and quinidine and its related preparations. The autonomic nervous system (ANS) and drugs that stimulate or inhibit it influence heart contractions. The sympathetic nervous system and drugs that stimulate it *increase* heart rate; the parasympathetic nervous system and drugs that stimulate it *decrease* heart rate.

Regulation of Heart Rate and Blood Flow

The heart beats approximately 60 to 80 times per minute in an adult, pumping blood into the systemic circulation. As blood travels, resistance to blood flow develops, and arterial pressure increases. The average systemic arterial pressure, known as *blood pressure*, is 120/80 mm Hg. Arterial blood pressure is determined by peripheral resistance and *cardiac output*, which is the volume of blood expelled from the heart in 1 minute, calculated by multiplying the heart rate by the stroke volume.

Fig. 40.3 Cardiac output and stroke volume. Three groups of drugs—cardiac glycosides, antianginals, and antidysrhythmics—are discussed in this chapter. Drugs in these groups regulate heart contraction, heart rate and rhythm, and blood flow to the myocardium (heart muscle).

The average cardiac output is 4 to 8 L/min. *Stroke volume*, the amount of blood ejected from the left ventricle with each heartbeat, is approximately 70 mL/beat.

Three factors—preload, contractility, and afterload—determine the stroke volume (Fig. 40.3). *Preload* refers to the blood flow force that stretches the ventricle at the end of diastole. However, an increase in preload can increase stroke volume, and a decrease in preload can decrease stroke volume. *Contractility* is the force of ventricular contraction, and afterload is the resistance to ventricular ejection of blood, which is caused by opposing pressures in the aorta and systemic circulation. If afterload *increases*, stroke volume will *decrease*, and if afterload *decreases*, stroke volume will *increase*.

Specific drugs can increase or decrease preload and afterload, affecting both stroke volume and cardiac output. Most vasodilators decrease preload and afterload, thus decreasing arterial pressure and cardiac output.

Circulation

There are two types of circulation, pulmonary and systemic. With *pulmonary circulation*, the heart pumps deoxygenated blood from the right ventricle through the pulmonary artery to the lungs. The pulmonary artery carries blood that has a high concentration of carbon dioxide. Oxygenated blood returns to the left atrium by the pulmonary vein.

With *systemic circulation*, also called *peripheral circulation*, the heart pumps blood from the left ventricle to the aorta and into the general circulation. Arteries and arterioles carry the blood to capillary beds. Nutrients in the capillary blood are transferred to cells in exchange for waste products. Blood returns to the heart through venules and veins.

Blood

Blood is composed of plasma, red blood cells (RBCs; erythrocytes), white blood cells (WBCs; leukocytes), and platelets. Plasma, made up of 90% water and 10% solutes, constitutes 55% of the total blood volume. The solutes in plasma include glucose, protein, lipids, amino acids, electrolytes, minerals, lactic and pyruvic acids, hormones, enzymes, oxygen, and carbon dioxide.

The major function of blood is to provide nutrients, including oxygen, to body cells. Most of the oxygen is carried on the hemoglobin of RBCs. WBCs are the major defense mechanism of the body and act by engulfing microorganisms. They also produce antibodies. The platelets are large cells that cause blood to coagulate. RBCs have a life span of approximately 120 days, whereas the life span of a WBC is only 2 to 24 hours.

Three groups of drugs (cardiac glycosides, antianginals, and antidysrhythmics) are discussed in this chapter. Drugs in these groups regulate heart contraction, heart rate, heart rhythm, and blood flow to the myocardium.

LABORATORY TESTS TO DIAGNOSE HEART FAILURE

Atrial Natriuretic Hormone or Peptide

Reference values: 20 to 77 pg/mL; 20 to 77 ng/L (SI units). An elevated atrial natriuretic hormone (ANH) or atrial natriuretic peptide (ANP) may confirm heart failure (HF). ANH is secreted from the atria of the heart and acts as an antagonist to renin and aldosterone. Released during expansion of the atrium, it produces vasodilation and increases glomerular filtration rate (GFR). Results of ANH secretion include a large volume of urine that decreases blood volume and blood pressure.

Brain Natriuretic Peptide

Reference values: Desired value is less than 100 pg/mL; positive value is greater than 100 pg/mL. The brain natriuretic peptide (BNP) is primarily secreted from atrial cardiac cells and, when tested, aids in the diagnosis of HF. Diagnosing HF is difficult in persons with lung disease who are experiencing dyspnea and in those who are obese or older. An elevated BNP helps differentiate that dyspnea is due to HF rather than to lung dysfunction. Frequently the BNP is higher than 100 pg/mL in females who are 65 years of age or older. An 80-year-old female may have a BNP of 160 pg/mL; however, the BNP is markedly higher (i.e., 400 pg/mL) in HF. BNP is considered a more sensitive test than ANP for diagnosing HF. Today, a bedside/emergency department machine can be used to measure BNP.

AGENTS USED TO TREAT HEART FAILURE

Cardiac Glycosides

Digitalis use began as early as CE 1200, making it one of the oldest drugs. It is still used in a purified form. Digitalis is obtained from the purple and white foxglove plant, and it can be poisonous. Digitalis preparations have come to be known for their effectiveness in treating HF, also known as *cardiac failure* (CF), and previously referred to as congestive heart failure (CHF). When the heart muscle (*myocardium*) weakens and enlarges, it loses its ability to pump blood through the heart and into the systemic circulation. This is called heart failure, *pump failure*, or *chronic heart failure*. When compensatory mechanisms fail and the peripheral and lung tissues are congested, the condition is called *acute heart failure*. The causes of HF include chronic hypertension, MI, coronary artery disease (CAD), valvular heart disease, congenital heart disease, and arteriosclerosis.

HF can be left sided or right sided. The patient has *left-sided HF* when the left ventricle does not contract sufficiently to pump the blood returned from the lungs and left atrium out through the aorta into the peripheral circulation; this causes excessive amounts of blood to back up into the lung tissue. Usually the patient has shortness of breath (SOB) and dyspnea. *Right-sided HF* occurs when the heart does not sufficiently pump the blood returned into the right atrium from the systemic circulation. As a result, the blood and its constituents are backed up into peripheral tissues, causing peripheral edema. Left-sided HF may lead to right-sided HF and vice versa. Myocardial hypertrophy resulting in *cardiomegaly*, increased heart size, can be a major problem associated with chronic HF.

In the cardiac physiology of HF, an increase in *preload* and *afterload* occurs. The increased preload results from an excess of blood volume in the ventricle at the end of diastole. This occurs because of a pathologic increase in the stretching and thickening of the ventricular walls, which allows a greater filling pressure associated with a weakened heart. Increased afterload is an additional pressure or force in the ventricular wall caused by excess resistance in the aorta. This resistance must be overcome to open the aortic valve so blood can be ejected into the circulation. The American College of Cardiology Foundation (ACCF) and the American Heart Association (AHA) have classified HF in stages according to its severity. Table 40.1 lists the stages of HF according to the ACCF/AHA. In the early

TABLE 40.1 The American College of Cardiology Foundation/American Heart Association Stages of Heart Failure

Stage	Characteristics According to Stage
A	At high risk for heart failure but without structural heart disease or symptoms of heart failure
B	Structural heart disease but without signs or symptoms of heart failure
C	Structural heart disease with prior or current symptoms of heart failure
D	Refractory heart failure requiring specialized interventions

Source: Maddox, T, Januzzi, J, Allen, L. et al. 2021 Update to the 2017 ACC Expert Consensus Decision Pathway for Optimization of Heart Failure Treatment: Answers to 10 Pivotal Issues About Heart Failure With Reduced Ejection Fraction: A Report of the American College of Cardiology Solution Set Oversight Committee. *JACC.* 2021 Feb, 77 (6) 772–810. https://doi.org/10.1016/j.jacc.2020.11.022.

stage of HF, there are no symptoms, and no structural heart damage occurs. Detailed informaton related to the staging process of HF and the New York Heart Associations Functional classifications may be found at: https://www.heart.org/en/health-topics/heartfailure/whatisheartfailure/classesofheartfailure.

Naturally occurring cardiac glycosides are found in several plants, including *Digitalis*. Also called *digitalis glycosides*, this group of drugs inhibits the sodium-potassium pump, which results in an increase in intracellular sodium. This increase leads to an influx of calcium, which causes the cardiac muscle fibers to contract more efficiently. Digitalis preparations have three effects on heart muscle: (1) a positive inotropic action *increases* myocardial contraction stroke volume, (2) a negative chronotropic action *decreases* heart rate, and (3) a negative dromotropic action *decreases* conduction of heart cells. The increase in myocardial contractility strengthens cardiac, peripheral, and kidney function by enhancing cardiac output, decreasing preload, improving blood flow to the periphery and kidneys, decreasing edema, and promoting fluid excretion. As a result, fluid retention in the lungs and extremities is decreased. Digoxin does not prolong life; rather, it acts by increasing the force and velocity of myocardial systolic contraction.

Digoxin is a secondary drug for HF. First-line drugs used to treat acute HF include intravenous (IV) inotropic agents (dopamine and dobutamine) and phosphodiesterase (PDE) inhibitors, such as milrinone. Other drugs prescribed for HF include oral diuretics, beta-blockers, angiotensin-converting enzyme (ACE) inhibitors, angiotensin-receptor blockers (ARBs), calcium channel blockers (CCBs), and vasodilators, all of which are more convenient to self-administer. Oral administration allows the patient to go home on these medications.

Cardiac glycosides are also used to correct atrial fibrillation, cardiac dysrhythmia with rapid uncoordinated contractions of atrial myocardium, and atrial flutter, cardiac dysrhythmia with rapid contractions of 200 to 300 beats/min. This is accomplished by the negative chronotropic effects (decreased heart rate) and negative dromotropic effects (decreased conduction through the atrioventricular [AV] node).

When digoxin cannot convert atrial fibrillation to normal heart rhythm, the goal is to slow the heart rate by decreasing electrical impulses through the AV node. For management of atrial fibrillation, a CCB such as verapamil may be prescribed. To prevent thromboemboli resulting from atrial fibrillation, warfarin is prescribed concurrently with other drug therapy. Warfarin is discussed in Chapter 43.

Digoxin

Prototype Drug Chart: Digoxin gives the pharmacologic data for digoxin, a cardiac glycoside.

Pharmacokinetics

The absorption rate of digoxin in oral tablet form is 60% to 80%. The rate is 70% to 85% in liquid form. The protein-binding power for digoxin is 25%. The half-life is 36 to 48 hours. Because of its long half-life, drug accumulation can occur. Digoxin comes with a warning as a drug with a Narrow Therapeutic Index (NTI). This means a small change in the dose can lead to serious events. There is a <2-fold difference between the median lethal dose and effective dose or between minimum toxic and minimum effective concentrations. Digoxin requires careful titration and monitoring. In all populations, dosage is based on patient's weight and clinical response, renal function, clinical goals, and when needed, lab for serum digoxin concentration level.

Side effects should be closely monitored to detect digitalis toxicity. Patients should be made aware of side effects that need to be reported to the health care provider. Serum digoxin levels are most commonly drawn when actual digitoxicity is suspected. This allows the health care provider to ascertain the extent of such toxicity and to confirm elimination of the drug after it is stopped or decreased in dosage (see the Digitalis [Digoxin] Toxicity section).

Thirteen to sixteen percent of digoxin is metabolized by the liver, and 70% is excreted by the kidneys mostly unchanged. Kidney dysfunction can affect the excretion of digoxin. Thyroid dysfunction can alter the metabolism of cardiac glycosides. For patients with hypothyroidism, the dose of digoxin should be decreased; in hyperthyroidism, the dose may need to be increased.

PROTOTYPE DRUG CHART

Digoxin

Drug Class	Dosage
Cardiac glycoside	Atrial fibrillation and Heart failure: A: PO: 3.4–5.1 mcg/kg/dose once/d. A: IV/IM: 2.4–3.6 mcg/kg/dose once/d.

Contraindications	Drug-Lab-Food Interactions
Absolute Contraindication: Ventricular fibrillation hypersensitivity *Caution*: AMI, AV block, ventricular tachycardia, hypertension, thyroid disorder, renal/hepatic dysfunction, bradycardia, electrolyte imbalance, cardiomyopathy, breastfeeding Not recommended for use in older adults. **High-Alert Drug**: Significant client harm when used in error. NTI Drug	Drug: Increased digoxin serum level with quinidine, flecainide, verapamil, indomethacin; decreased digoxin absorption with antacids, ketoprofen, penicillins, potassium chloride, psyllium, acarbose, colestipol; increased risk for digoxin toxicity with thiazide diuretics, loop diuretics, proton pump inhibitors Labs: ECG, serum: calcium, creatinine/BUN, magnesium, potassium, digoxin serum plasma labwork. Hypokalemia, hypomagnesemia, hypercalcemia can increase digitalis (digoxin) toxicity

Pharmacokinetics	Pharmacodynamics
Absorption: PO tablet: 60%–80%; PO liquid: 70%–85% Distribution: PB: 25% Metabolism: t½: 36–48 h; 13%–16% metabolized in liver Excretion: 50%–70% in urine	PO: Onset: 30 min–2 h Peak: 1–3 h Duration: 3–4 d IV: Onset: 5–30 min Peak: 1–4 h Duration: UK

Therapeutic Effects/Uses

To treat heart failure, atrial fibrillation
Mechanism of Action: Inhibits sodium-potassium ATPase, promoting increased force of cardiac contraction, cardiac output, and tissue perfusion; decreases ventricular rate

Side Effects	Adverse Reactions
Anorexia, nausea, vomiting, diarrhea, abdominal pain, bowel ischemia, bradycardia, headache, blurred or yellow vision, dizziness, weakness, confusion, visual impairment, anxiety, hyperkalemia	Bradycardia, hallucinations, bowel necrosis, palpitations, cardiac arrest, atrial fibrillation, sinus tachycardia *Life-threatening*: Dysrhythmias, thrombocytopenia

A, Adult; *AMI*, acute myocardial infarction; *AV*, atrial ventricular; *BUN*, blood urea nitrogen; *d*, day; *ECG*, electrocardiogram; *h*, hour; *IM*, intramuscular; *IV*, intravenous; *maint*, maintenance; *min*, minute; *PB*, protein binding; *PO*, by mouth; *t½*, half-life; *UK*, unknown. *NTI*, Narrow Therapeutic Index

Pharmacodynamics

In patients with a failing heart, cardiac glycosides increase myocardial contraction, which increases cardiac output and improves circulation and tissue perfusion. Because these drugs decrease conduction through the AV node, the heart rate decreases. The onset and peak actions of oral and IV digoxin vary. The digoxin therapeutic serum level for dysrhythmias is 0.8 to 2.0 ng/mL. The target therapeutic serum level for HF is 0.5 to 1.0 ng/mL.

Digoxin can be administered orally or by the IV route. Table 40.2 lists the digitalis preparations and their dosages, uses, and considerations.

Digitalis (Digoxin) Toxicity

Overdose or accumulation of digoxin causes digitalis toxicity. Signs and symptoms include anorexia, diarrhea, nausea and vomiting, bradycardia (pulse rate below 60 beats/min), premature ventricular contractions, cardiac dysrhythmias, headaches, malaise, blurred vision, visual illusions (white, green, or yellow halos around objects), confusion, and delirium. Older adults are more prone to toxicity.

Cardiotoxicity is a serious adverse reaction to digoxin, and ventricular dysrhythmias result. Three cardiac-altered functions can contribute to digoxin-induced ventricular dysrhythmias: (1) suppression of AV conduction, (2) increased automaticity, and (3) a decreased refractory period in ventricular muscle. The antidysrhythmics phenytoin and lidocaine are effective in treating digoxin-induced ventricular dysrhythmias. Lidocaine should be limited to short-term treatment.

Antidote for Cardiac/Digitalis Glycosides

Digoxin-immune Fab may be given to treat severe digitalis toxicity. This agent binds with digoxin to form complex molecules that can be excreted in the urine; thus digoxin is unable to bind at the cellular site of action. Serum digoxin levels should be closely monitored, and signs and symptoms of digoxin toxicity should be reported promptly to the health care provider. Digitalis toxicity may result in first-degree, second-degree, or complete heart block. Failure to respond to Digoxin-immune Fab can alert the clinician to the possibility that the problem may not be caused by Digoxin.

Drug Interactions

Drug interaction with digitalis preparations can cause digitalis toxicity. Many of the potent diuretics, such as furosemide and hydrochlorothiazide, promote the loss of potassium from the body. The resultant hypokalemia, low serum potassium level, increases the effect of digoxin at its myocardial cell site of action, resulting in digitalis toxicity. Cortisone preparations taken systemically promote sodium retention and potassium excretion or loss and can also cause hypokalemia. Patients who take digoxin along with a potassium-wasting diuretic or a cortisone drug should consume foods rich in potassium or take potassium supplements to avoid hypokalemia and digitalis toxicity. Antacids can decrease digitalis absorption if taken at the same time to prevent this problem, doses should be staggered.

Phosphodiesterase Inhibitors

PDE inhibitors are another positive inotropic group of drugs given to treat acute HF. This drug group inhibits the enzyme PDE, which

TABLE 40.2 Cardiac Glycosides and Inotropic Agents

Drug	Route and Dosage	Uses and Considerations
Rapid-Acting Digitalis		
Digoxin	See Prototype Drug Chart: Digoxin	
Phosphodiesterase Inhibitors (Positive Inotropic Bipyridines)		
Milrinone lactate	A: IV: 50 mcg/kg infusion over 10 min; *maint:* 0.125–0.75 mcg/kg/min infusion; *max:* 0.75 mcg/kg/min infusion	For acute decompensated heart failure. May cause headache, hypotension, ventricular tachycardia, dysrhythmias, injection site reaction, tremor, nausea, vomiting, hypokalemia, thrombocytopenia, atrial fibrillation, atrial flutter, anaphylactic shock, bronchospasm, and angina. PB: 70%; t½: 2.4 h
Antidote for Digitalis Toxicity		
Digoxin-immune Fab	A: IV: 800 mg (20 vials) IV as a single dose or give 400 mg (10 vials) IV with careful monitoring of the patient, followed by 400 mg (10 vials) if necessary. Please Note: Administering 800 mg (20 vials) in a single dose may enhance the risk of a febrile reaction. *Max:* depends on age, amount of digoxin, and client's response	For digoxin overdose and toxicity and cardiac glycoside–induced dysrhythmias. May cause anaphylaxis, orthostatic hypotension, atrial fibrillation, heart failure exacerbation, angioedema, wheezing, infusion-site reactions, phlebitis, and hypokalemia. PB: UK; t½: 15–20 h
Guanylate Cyclase Stimulant		
Vericiguat	A: PO: 2.5 mg/d with food; double dose every 2 wks till target dose of 10 mg/d. *maint:* 10 mg/d is reached; *max:* 10 mg/d	For heart failure and ejection fraction less than 45%. May cause hypotension, anemia, syncope, and birth defects. ⚡ **Black-Box Warning:** Pregnancy ❗ **High Alert Drug:** Heightened risk of harm if administered in error. PB: 98%; t½: 30 h

A, Adult; *CV*, cardiovascular; *h*, hours; *HF*, heart failure; *IV*, intravenous; *maint*, maintenance; *max*, maximum; *min*, minute; *PB*, protein binding; *t½*, half-life; *UK*, unknown; *wk*, week.

COMPLEMENTARY AND ALTERNATIVE THERAPIES

Cardiac Glycosides, Antihypertensives, and Antidysrhythmics

Complementary and alternative therapies require extreme caution and can cause toxicity or drug interactions when taking cardiac medications.

- Ginseng may falsely elevate digoxin levels.
- St. John's wort decreases absorption of digoxin and thus decreases serum digoxin level.
- Psyllium may decrease digoxin absorption.
- Hawthorn may increase the effect of digoxin and hypotensive drugs.
- Licorice can potentiate the effect of digoxin; it promotes potassium loss (hypokalemia), which increases the effect of digoxin, and it may cause digitalis toxicity. Licorice also decreases the effectiveness of antihypertensives.
- Aloe may increase the risk of digitalis toxicity. It increases potassium loss, which increases the effect of digoxin.
- Ma-huang, or ephedra, increases the risk of digitalis toxicity.
- Goldenseal may decrease the effects of cardiac glycosides and may increase the effects of antidysrhythmics.
- Coleus may potentiate effects of antihypertensives.
- Ginger may cause a synergistic antiplatelet effect with nifedipine.
- Ginkgo may increase drug levels or side effects of nifedipine.
- Korean ginseng may decrease the effectiveness of antihypertensives.
- Laxative (anthraquinone-containing) herbs may potentiate cardiac glycosides and antidysrhythmics.
- Milk thistle may delay the absorption rate of nifedipine.
- https://www.heart.org/en/healthtopics/heartfailure/treatment

promotes a positive inotropic response and vasodilation. A drug in this group is milrinone lactate. This drug increases stroke volume and cardiac output and promotes vasodilation. It is administered intravenously for no longer than 48 to 72 hours. Severe cardiac dysrhythmias might result from the use of PDE inhibitors, so the patient's electrocardiogram (ECG) and cardiac status should be closely monitored.

! Milrinone is a high-alert medication that may cause significant harm to a patient when given inappropriately.

Other Agents Used to Treat Heart Failure (PDE)

Vasodilators, ACE inhibitors, angiotensin II–receptor antagonists (blockers), diuretics (thiazides, furosemide), spironolactone, nesiritide, and some beta-blockers are other drug groups prescribed to treat HF.

Vasodilators can be used to treat HF. The vasodilators decrease venous blood return to the heart and result in a decrease in cardiac filling, ventricular stretching (preload), and oxygen demand on the heart. Arteriolar dilators act in three ways: they (1) reduce cardiac afterload, which increases cardiac output; (2) dilate the arterioles of the kidneys, which improves renal perfusion and increases fluid loss; and (3) improve circulation to the skeletal muscles.

ACE inhibitors are usually prescribed for HF. ACE inhibitors dilate venules and arterioles, which improves renal blood flow and decreases blood fluid volume. ACE inhibitors also moderately decrease the release of aldosterone, which in turn reduces sodium and fluid retention.

ACE inhibitors can increase potassium levels, so serum potassium levels should be monitored, especially if potassium-sparing diuretics such as spironolactone are being taken concurrently. Angiotensin II–receptor blockers (ARBs) such as valsartan and candesartan have been approved for HF in patients who cannot tolerate ACE inhibitors.

CLINICAL JUDGMENT [NURSING PROCESS]

Cardiac Glycosides: Digoxin

Concept: Perfusion
- The passage of blood flow through the arteries and capillaries that deliver oxygen and nutrients to body cells

Recognize Cues [Assessment]
- Obtain a drug and herbal history. Report if a drug-drug or drug-herb interaction is probable. If a patient is taking digoxin and a potassium-wasting diuretic or cortisone drug, hypokalemia can result, causing digitalis toxicity. A low serum potassium level enhances the action of digoxin. Patients taking a thiazide and/or cortisone with digoxin should take a potassium supplement.
- Obtain a baseline pulse rate for future comparisons. Apical pulse should be taken for a full minute and should be greater than 60 beats/min.
- Assess for signs and symptoms of digitalis toxicity. Common symptoms include anorexia, nausea, vomiting, bradycardia, cardiac dysrhythmias, and visual disturbances. Report symptoms immediately to the health care provider.

Analyze Cues and Prioritize Hypothesis [Patient Problems]
- Decreased gas exchange
- Decreased tissue perfusion
- Hypoxemia
- Ischemia

Generate Solutions [Planning]
- The patient will demonstrate checking their pulse rate before taking digoxin.
- The patient will state that it is important to report the pulse rate when it is less than 60 beats/min or when a marked decline in pulse rate occurs.
- The patient will list six foods high in potassium to maintain a desired serum potassium level (see Patient Teaching and Diet sections).

Take Action [Nursing Interventions]
- Ascertain apical pulse rate before administering digoxin. Do *not* administer if pulse rate is below 60 beats/min.

- Determine signs of peripheral and pulmonary edema, which indicate heart failure is present.
- Monitor serum digoxin level (normal therapeutic drug range is 0.8–2 ng/mL). A serum digoxin level greater than 2 ng/mL is indicative of digitalis toxicity.
- Monitor serum potassium level (normal range is 3.5–5.0 mEq/L), and report if hypokalemia (<3.5 mEq/L) is present.

Patient Teaching
General
- Explain to patients the importance of adherence to drug therapy. A visiting nurse may ensure that medications are taken properly.
- Advise patients to avoid adverse drug interactions by not taking over-the-counter (OTC) drugs without first consulting a health care provider.
- Keep drugs out of reach of small children, and request childproof bottles.
- Teach patients and caregivers to check the pulse rate before administering drugs.
- Inform patients of possible drug-herb interactions.

Self-Administration
- Teach patients how to check the pulse rate before taking digoxin and to notify a health care provider if the pulse rate is irregular or less than 60 beats/min.

Side Effects
- Instruct patients to report side effects: pulse rate less than 60 beats/min, nausea and vomiting, headache, diarrhea, and visual disturbances, including diplopia.

Diet
- Advise patients to eat foods high in potassium, such as fresh and dried fruits, fruit juices, and vegetables, including potatoes.

Evaluate Outcomes [Evaluation]
- Evaluate the effectiveness of digoxin by noting the patient's response to a drug (decreased heart rate, decreased rales) and absence of side effects. Continue monitoring the pulse rate.

Refer to Chapter 39 for a complete discussion of ACE inhibitors and ARBs.

Diuretics are the first-line drug treatment for reducing fluid volume. They are frequently prescribed with digoxin or other agents.

Spironolactone, a potassium-sparing diuretic, is used in treating moderate to severe HF. Aldosterone secretions are increased in HF. This promotes body loss of potassium and magnesium needed by the heart and increases sodium and water retention. Spironolactone blocks the production of aldosterone. This drug improves heart rate variability and decreases myocardial fibrosis by its cardioprotective effect of blocking aldosterone in the heart and blood vessels to promote cardiac remodeling. The recommended dose for HF is initially 25 mg/d. Occurrence of hyperkalemia (excess serum potassium) is rare unless the patient is receiving 50 mg/day and has renal insufficiency. However, the serum potassium level should be closely monitored.

In the past, all beta-blockers were contraindicated for patients with HF because this drug class reduces cardiac contractility. With dosage control, beta-blockers (carvedilol, metoprolol, and bisoprolol) have been shown to improve cardiac performance. Doses should be low initially and gradually increased. It may take 1 to 3 months for a beneficial effect to develop. Refer to Chapters 15 and 39 for more information on beta-blockers.

A combination of hydralazine (for blood pressure) and isosorbide dinitrate (a dilator to relieve heart pain) has received US Food and Drug Administration (FDA) approval for treating HF, especially in African American individuals, who have more than twice the rate of HF as White individuals; a research study has shown this drug to be effective in treating HF in the African American population.

Vericiguat, a guanylate cyclase stimulant, treats HF. It helps regulate vascular tone, cardiac contractility, and cardiac remodeling. It is used for the reduction of cardiovascular mortality and reduction of HF hospitalizations and an ejection fraction less than 45%. This drug is contraindicated in pregnancy due to serious birth defects. A female of childbearing age must have a negative pregnancy test before treatment and use effective contraception. Vericiguat is not recommended with coadministration of phosphodiesterase type 5 inhibitors due to potentiated hypotension. Some side effects of vericiguat include hypotension, anemia, syncope, and serious birth defects.

Oral sodium-glucose co-transporter inhibitors (SGLT1 and SGLT2) were FDA approved for adult patients with type 2 diabetes mellitus. Many of the patients also had heart failure (HF). It was discovered those with heart failure showed significant success in reducing cardiovascular deaths and HF hospitalizations. Further studies showed a reduction in the risk of atherosclerotic cardiovascular disease (ADCVD). The SGLT1 inhibitor accounts for most of the dietary glucose uptake in the intestines. The SGLT2 inhibitor is responsible for the majority of glucose uptake in the tubular system of the kidneys. Empagliflozin, is a a sodium glucose co-transporter (SGLT2) Inhibitor. The adult oral dose is 10 mg once daily. The protein binding is 86.2% and half-life is 12.4 hours. Sotagliflozin, is both a (SGLT1) and (SGLT2) inhibitor. The recommended oral dose is 200 mg a day, if tolerated, it may be increased to 400 mg a day. The protein binding is 93% and the half life is 21–35 hours. Dapagliflozin is an SGLT2 inhibitor that works in the same way. The adult dosage is 5 mg PO once daily, initially. May increase the dose to 10 mg PO once daily if needed. It is 91% protein bound with a half of 12.9 hours. A common side effect of sodium-glucose co-transporter inhibitors is hypoglycemia.

Nonpharmacologic Measures to Treat Heart Failure

Nondrug therapy is an integral part of the regimen for controlling HF. The nondrug component of the regimen should be tailored to meet the needs of each patient, but the following are some general recommendations. The patient should limit salt intake to 2 g/day, approximately 1 teaspoon. Alcohol intake should be either decreased to 1 drink per day or completely avoided because excessive alcohol use can lead to cardiomyopathy. Fluid intake may be restricted. Smoking should be avoided because it deprives the heart of oxygen (O2). Obesity may increase cardiovascular problems if it is associated with unhealthy behaviors; thus patients with obesity should modify their behaviors as needed. Saturated fat intake should be decreased. Mild exercise, such as walking or bicycling, is recommended.

ANGINA PECTORIS

A condition of acute cardiac pain caused by inadequate blood flow to the myocardium due to either plaque occlusions within or spasms of the coronary arteries. With decreased blood flow, there is a decrease in oxygen to the myocardium, which results in pain. Anginal pain is frequently described by the patient as tightness, pressure in the center of the chest, and pain radiating down the left arm. Referred pain felt in the neck and left arm commonly occurs with severe angina pectoris. Anginal attacks may lead to MI (heart attack). Anginal pain usually lasts for only a few minutes. Stress tests, echocardiogram, cardiac profile laboratory tests, and cardiac catheterization may be needed to determine the degree of blockage in the coronary arteries and then also to treat the condition.

Types of Angina Pectoris

The frequency of anginal pain depends on many factors, including the type of angina. There are three types of angina:
- *Classic (stable) angina* occurs with predictable stress or exertion.
- *Unstable (preinfarction) angina* occurs frequently with progressive severity unrelated to activity and is unpredictable regarding stress/exertion and intensity.
- *Variant (Prinzmetal, vasospastic) angina* occurs during rest.

The first two types are caused by a narrowing or partial occlusion of the coronary arteries; variant angina is caused by vessel spasm (vasospasm). It is common for a patient to have both classic and variant angina. Unstable angina often indicates an impending MI; it is an emergency that needs immediate medical intervention.

Nonpharmacologic Measures to Control Angina

A combination of pharmacologic and nonpharmacologic measures is usually necessary to control and prevent anginal attacks. Nonpharmacologic methods of decreasing anginal attacks are to avoid heavy meals, smoking, extreme weather changes, strenuous exercise, and emotional upset. Proper nutrition, moderate exercise (only after consulting with a health care provider), adequate rest, and relaxation techniques are used as preventive measures.

TYPES OF ANTIANGINAL DRUGS

Antianginal drugs increase blood flow either by increasing oxygen supply or by decreasing oxygen demand by the myocardium. Three types of antianginals are (1) nitrates, (2) beta-blockers, and (3) Calcium Channel Blocker (CCB). The major systemic effect of nitrates is a reduction of venous tone, which decreases the workload of the heart and promotes vasodilation. Beta-blockers and CCBs decrease the workload of the heart and decrease oxygen demands.

Nitrates and CCBs are effective in treating variant (vasospastic) angina pectoris; beta-blockers are not effective for this type of angina and may aggravate it. With stable angina, beta-blockers can effectively be used to prevent angina attacks. Table 40.3 lists the effects of antianginal drug groups on angina.

With unstable angina, immediate medical care is necessary. Nitrates are usually given sublingually and intravenously as needed. If the cardiac pain continues, a beta-blocker is given intravenously, and if the patient is unable to tolerate beta-blockers, a CCB may be substituted.

Nitrates

Nitrates were the first agents used to relieve angina. They affect coronary arteries and blood vessels in the venous circulation. Nitrates cause generalized vascular and coronary vasodilation, which increases blood flow through the coronary arteries to the myocardial cells. This group of drugs reduces myocardial ischemia but can cause hypotension.

⚡ PATIENT SAFETY

Do Not Confuse...
- **Nitrostat**, a nitroglycerin drug that promotes coronary vasodilation and thus increases blood flow to the coronary arteries, with **Nystatin**, an antifungal antibiotic that has fungistatic and fungicidal activity against yeasts and fungi

TABLE 40.3 Effects of Antianginal Drug Groups on Angina

Drug Groups	Variant (Vasospastic) Anginas	Classic (Stable) Anginas
Nitrates	Relaxation of coronary arteries, which decreases vasospasms and increases oxygen supply	Dilation of veins, which decreases preload and decreases oxygen demand
Beta-blockers	Not effective	Decrease heart rate and contractility, which decreases oxygen demand
Calcium channel blockers (CCB)	Relaxation of coronary arteries, which decreases vasospasms and increases oxygen supply	Dilation of arterioles decreases afterload and decreases oxygen demand. Verapamil and diltiazem decrease heart rate and contractility.

The sublingual (SL) nitroglycerin tablet, which is absorbed under the tongue, comes in various dosages, but the average prescribed dose is no more than 3 tablets (300 to 600 mcg) within 15 minutes. If pain has not subsided, then 911 should be called. The effects of SL nitroglycerin last for 30 to 60 minutes. The SL tablets decompose when exposed to heat and light, so they must be kept in their original, airtight glass containers. The tablets themselves are normally dispensed in these original glass containers, which have screw-cap tops that are *not* childproof to facilitate emergency use by older adults who may have reduced manual dexterity and are experiencing an anginal attack. After a dose of nitroglycerin, the patient may experience dizziness, faintness, or headache as a result of the peripheral vasodilation. If pain persists, the patient should immediately call for medical assistance.

SL nitroglycerin is the most commonly used nitrate. It is not swallowed, because it undergoes first-pass metabolism by the liver, which decreases its effectiveness. Instead, it is readily absorbed into the circulation through the SL vessels. Nitroglycerin is also available in other forms: topical (ointment, transdermal patch), translingual, oral extended-release capsule and tablet, aerosol spray (inhalation), and IV. Prototype Drug Chart: Nitroglycerin summarizes the action of nitroglycerin (nitrates).

Among the various types of organic nitrates is *isosorbide dinitrate*, which can be administered in an SL tablet form and is also available as immediate-release tablet, and extended-release tablet or capsule. *Isosorbide mononitrate* can be given orally in immediate- and extended-release tablets.

Pharmacokinetics
When taken sublingually, nitroglycerin is absorbed rapidly and directly into the internal jugular vein and the right atrium. Nitrates absorbed through the gastrointestinal (GI) tract are inactivated by first-pass metabolism in the liver. The nitroglycerin in the ointment and in the patch is absorbed slowly through the skin and is excreted primarily in the urine. The protein binding is 60%, and the half-life is 1 to 4 minutes.

Pharmacodynamics
Nitroglycerin acts directly on the smooth muscle of blood vessels, causing relaxation and dilation. It decreases cardiac **preload** (amount of blood in the ventricle at the end of diastole) and **afterload** (peripheral vascular resistance) and reduces myocardial O_2 demand. With dilation of the veins, there is less blood return to the heart, and with dilation of the arteries, there is less vasoconstriction and resistance.

📋 PROTOTYPE DRUG CHART

Nitroglycerin

Drug Class	Dosage
Antianginal	Angina: A: SL: 300–600 mcg SL no more than 3 tabs in a 15-min period. ⚡ Seek medical help if pain is unrelieved after 3 tabs. Extended release: A: PO: 2.5–6.5 mg, 3–4 times/d, up to 26 mg PO 4 times a day has been used. Topical ointment 2%: 7.5 mg (0.5″) twice/d q6h, dose can be doubled. *Max.* 30 mg/dose Transdermal patch: 0.2–0.4 mg/h for 12–14 h/d with 10–12 h daily, then patch-off period, dose range 0.1 to 0.8 mg/hr. Translingual spray: 400–800 mcg on or under tongue 5–10 min; repeat 400 mcg q5min as needed: Recommended dose: 1200 mcg in 15-min period. Notify MD if chest pain persists Hypertensive emergency: IV: Initially: 5 mcg/min infusion, titrate up by 5 mcg/min q3–5min up to 20 mcg/min until control is achieved. *Max Titration:* 20 mcg/min q3–5min Max dose: IV: 200 mcg/min
Contraindications	**Drug-Lab-Food Interactions**
Increased intracranial pressure, AMI, cardiomyopathy, cardiac tamponade, shock, constrictive pericarditis, nitrate hypersensitivity *Caution:* Hepatic disease, hypotension, hypovolemia, anemia, diabetes mellitus, head trauma, pregnancy, breastfeeding, older adults	Drug: Increased effect with alcohol, beta-blockers, calcium channel blockers, antihypertensives, aspirin, benzodiazepines, vasodilators; decreased effects of heparin Herbs: Hawthorn increases nitroglycerin levels.

PROTOTYPE DRUG CHART—CONT'D
Nitroglycerin

Pharmacokinetics	Pharmacodynamics
Absorption: Oral/SL: Greater than 75% absorbed; ointment and patch: slow absorption Distribution: PB: 60% Metabolism: $t\frac{1}{2}$: 1–4 min Excretion: Liver and urine	Oral/SL: Onset: 1–3 min Duration: 30–60 min ER cap: Onset: 20–45 min Duration: 8–12 h Topical ointment: Onset: 20–60 min Duration: 4–8 h Transdermal patch: Onset: 40–60 min Duration: 18–24 h IV: Onset: Immediate Duration: several minutes (dose dependant)

Therapeutic Effects/Uses

To control angina, AMI, hypertensive emergency, pulmonary edema, and heart failure Mechanism of Action: Decreases myocardial demand for oxygen; decreases preload by dilating veins, indirectly decreasing afterload

Side Effects	Adverse Reactions
Headache, hypotension, blurred vision, dizziness, syncope, weakness, diaphoresis, flushing, nausea, faintness, vomiting, dry mouth, paresthesia, peripheral edema, rash, pharyngitis, tolerance	Orthostatic hypotension, chest pain, dyspnea, tachycardia, bradycardia, palpitations, methemoglobinemia *Life-threatening:* MI, pulmonary edema

A, Adult; *AMI*, acute myocardial infarction; *d*, day; *h*, hour; *IV*, intravenous; *MD*, medical doctor; *MI*, myocardial infarction; *min*, minute; *PB*, protein binding; *q*, every; *SL*, sublingual; $t\frac{1}{2}$, half-life.

The onset of action of nitroglycerin depends on the method of administration. With Oral/SL use, the onset of action is rapid (1–3 minutes); it is slower with the transdermal method (40–60 minutes). The duration of action of the transdermal nitroglycerin patch is approximately 18 to 24 hours. Because nitroglycerin ointment is effective for only 4 to 8 hours, it must be reapplied three to four times a day. The use of nitroglycerin ointment has declined since the advent of the transdermal nitroglycerin patch, which is applied only once a day. It is important to note that the patch should be removed nightly to allow for an 8- to 12-hour nitrate-free interval. This is also true for most other forms of nitroglycerin. This is necessary to avoid tolerance associated with uninterrupted use or continued dosage increases of nitrate preparations. Table 40.4 lists the nitrates and their dosages, uses, and considerations.

Side Effects and Adverse Reactions
Headaches are one of the most common side effects of nitroglycerin, but they may become less frequent with continued use. Otherwise, acetaminophen may provide some relief. Other side effects include hypotension, dizziness, flushing, weakness, and faintness. When nitroglycerin ointment or transdermal patches are discontinued, the dose should be tapered over several weeks to prevent the rebound effect of severe pain caused by *myocardial ischemia*, lack of blood supply to the heart muscle. In addition, *reflex tachycardia* may occur if the nitrate is given too rapidly. The heart rate increases greatly because of overcompensation of the cardiovascular system.

Drug Interactions
Beta-blockers, CCBs, vasodilators, and alcohol can enhance the hypotensive effect of nitrates. IV nitroglycerin may antagonize the effects of heparin.

Beta-Blockers
Beta-adrenergic blockers block the beta$_1$- and beta$_2$-receptor sites. Beta-blockers decrease the effects of the sympathetic nervous system by blocking the action of the catecholamines, epinephrine and norepinephrine, thereby decreasing the heart rate and blood pressure. Beta-blockers are used as antianginal, antidysrhythmic, and antihypertensive drugs. Beta-blockers are effective as antianginals because by decreasing the heart rate and myocardial contractility they reduce the need for oxygen consumption and consequently reduce anginal pain. These drugs are most useful for classic (stable) angina.

Beta-blockers should *not* be abruptly discontinued. The dose should be tapered over a specified number of days to avoid reflex tachycardia and recurrence of anginal pain. Patients who have decreased heart rate and blood pressure usually cannot take beta-blockers. Patients who have second- or third-degree AV block should not take beta-blockers.

Beta-blockers, discussed in detail in Chapters 15 and 39, are subdivided into *nonselective* beta-blockers that block beta$_1$ and beta$_2$ and *selective* (cardiac) beta-blockers that only block beta$_1$. Examples of nonselective beta-blockers are propranolol, nadolol, and pindolol. These drugs decrease the heart rate and can cause bronchoconstriction. The cardioselective beta-blockers act more strongly on the beta$_1$ receptor, which decreases heart rate but avoids bronchoconstriction because of their lack of activity at the beta$_2$-receptor. Examples of selective beta-blockers are atenolol and metoprolol. Selective beta-blockers are the group of choice for controlling angina pectoris. Table 40.4 lists the beta-blockers most frequently used for angina and their dosages, uses, and considerations.

Pharmacokinetics
Beta-blockers are well absorbed orally. Absorption of sustained-release capsules is slow. The half-life of propranolol is 2 to 6 hours. Of the selective beta-blockers, atenolol has a half-life of 6 to 7 hours, and metoprolol has a half-life of 3 to 7 hours. Propranolol and metoprolol are metabolized and excreted by the liver. Half an *oral* dose of atenolol is absorbed from the GI tract, with the remainder excreted unchanged in feces. Intravenous beta-blockers are reserved for high-risk patients.

Pharmacodynamics
Because beta-blockers decrease the force of myocardial contraction, oxygen demand by the myocardium is reduced. Therefore the patient can tolerate increased exercise with less oxygen requirement. Beta-blockers are effective for classic (stable) angina.

After oral administration of immediate release propranolol, a nonselective beta-blocker, the dose is almost completely absorbed, however, due to high first pass metabolism, bioavailability is only about 25%. Peak concentrations of immediate release tablets and long acting capsules are reached in 1 to 4 hours, and about 6 hours, respectively.

TABLE 40.4 Antianginals

Drug	Route and Dosages	Uses and Considerations
Nitrates		
Short Acting		
Nitroglycerin	See Prototype Drug Chart: Nitroglycerin	
Long Acting		
Isosorbide dinitrate	Immediate release: A: PO: Initially 5–20 mg bid/tid; *maint:* 10–40 mg bid/tid; *max:* 480 mg/d Extended release: A: PO: Initially 40 mg/d; increase dose as needed. *max:* 160 mg/d A: Sublingual: 5 mg 10–15 min before meals *max:* SL is unavailable	To prevent and treat angina. May cause headaches, dizziness, dry mouth, orthostatic hypotension, tachycardia, bradycardia, nausea, vomiting, methemoglobinemia, syncope, and flushing. PB: 28%; t½: 1 h
Isosorbide mononitrate	Immediate release: A: PO: 20 mg bid; initially given 7h apart. Increase dose to 10 mg bid daily by day 2 or 3. *max:* 40 mg/d Extended release: A: PO: 30–60 mg/d initially; Increase dose to 1220 mg/d after several days. *max:* 240 mg/d	To prevent angina. May cause headache, dizziness, flushing, fatigue, cough, anxiety, hypotension, dry mouth, abdominal pain, nausea, vomiting, rash, pruritus, chest pain. PB: <4%; t½: 5 h
Beta-Adrenergic Blockers		
Atenolol (beta₁)	Stable Angina: A: PO: Initially 50 mg/d; in 7 d increase to 100 mg/d *max:* 200 mg/d Unstable Angina: A: PO: 50 mg 10 to 60 min after final IV dose of IV beta blocker is administered then give 50 mg PO 12 h later. Continue PO 50 to 100 mg/d given in 1 to 2 doses. *max:* 200 mg/d	To treat both stable and unstable angina, hypertension, and AMI. May cause hypotension, bradycardia, fatigue, dizziness, nausea, diarrhea, depression, peripheral vasoconstriction, tachycardia, edema, and heart failure. PB: 10%; t½: 6–7 h **! High-Alert Drug:** Heightened risk if given in error **⚡ Black-Box Warning:** Abrupt discontinuation
Metoprolol tartrate (beta₁)	Chronic Stable Angina: Immediate release: A: PO: 50 mg bid; *maint:* 100–400 mg/d in divided doses. *max:* 450 mg/d Extended release: A: PO: 100 mg/d; increase dose weekly till desired response. *max:* 400 mg/d Unstable Angina: A: IV: 5 mg IV every 5 min for a total dose of 15 mg, then begin oral metoprolol 1–2.5 mg/d. (IV is reserved for high risk patients) Immediate release: A: PO: 25–50 mg every 6 h. May start with 12.5 mg PO every 6h, initially. *max:* 450 mg/d	To treat angina, AMI, hypertension, and heart failure. May cause dizziness, fatigue, drowsiness, blurred vision, depression, rash, pruritus, diarrhea, peripheral edema, erectile dysfunction, bradycardia, hypotension, heart failure, and palpitations. PB: 10%–12%; t½: 3–7 h **! High-Alert Drug:** Heightened risk if given in error **⚡ Black-Box Warning:** Abrupt discontinuation
Nadolol (beta₁ and beta₂)	Angina: A: PO: Initially 40 mg/d; *maint:* 40–80 mg/d; *max:* 240 mg/d	For long term management of angina and hypertension. May cause dizziness, drowsiness, headache, bradycardia, hypotension, palpitations, peripheral vasoconstriction, erectile dysfunction, and fatigue. PB: 30%; t½: 10–24 h **! High-Alert Drug:** Heightened risk if given in error **⚡ Black-Box Warning:** Abrupt discontinuation
Propranolol (beta₁ and beta₂)	Angina: Immediate release: A: PO: Initially 10–20 mg 2–4 times day; then increase 3 to 7 day intervals up to 160–320 mg/d in 2–4 divided doses; *max:* 320 mg/d Extended release capsules: A: PO: Initially 80 mg/d; then increase 3–7 day intervals up to 160–320 mg/d; *max:* 320 mg/d	For angina, hypertension, AMI, HF, dysrhythmias, and migraine prophylaxis. May cause dizziness, headache, visual impairment, bradycardia, depression, weakness, hyperkalemia, agitation, fatigue, erectile dysfunction, and bronchospasm. PB: 90%; t½: 2–6 h **! High-Alert Drug:** Heightened risk if administered in error **⚡ Black-Box Warning:** Abrupt discontinuation

TABLE 40.4 Antianginals—cont'd

Drug	Route and Dosages	Uses and Considerations
Calcium Channel Blockers		
AmLODIPine	Chronic Stable Angina: A: PO: 5–10 mg/d; usual dose 10 mg/d; *max:* 10 mg/d	For angina, CAD, and hypertension. May cause peripheral edema, dizziness, palpitations, flushing, bradycardia, orthostatic hypotension, constipation, nausea, hyperglycemia, peripheral neuropathy, visual impairment, edema, weakness, drowsiness, erectile dysfunction, and fatigue. PB: 93%; t½: 30–50 h
dilTIAZem	Angina: Immediate release: A: PO: 30 mg qid; gradually increase dose every 1–2 days until desired response, usual dose 180–360 mg/d in 3–4 divided doses; *max:* 360 mg/d Extended release capsules: A: PO: 120–180 mg/d, increase dose every 7–14 days until response is achieved; *max:* 540 mg/d Extended release tablets: A: PO: 180 mg/d. Increase dose every 7–14 days until response achieved; *max:* 360 mg/d	For angina, PSVT, atrial flutter or fibrillation, and hypertension. May cause headache, peripheral edema, dizziness, weakness, bradycardia, hypotension, dyspnea, fatigue, rhinitis, pharyngitis, infection, constipation, and dyspepsia PB: 70%–80%; t½: 3.5–9 h ⚠ **High-Alert Drug:** Heightened risk if given in error ⚡ Inappropriate drug for use in older adults
Felodipine	Angina: A: PO: Initially 5–10 mg/twice daily regimens have been used; *max:* 10 mg/d due to dose related adverse effects.	To treat angina and hypertension. May cause peripheral edema, palpitations, dizziness, weakness, infection, hypotension, erectile dysfunction, cough, rash, and headache. PB: 99%; t½: 11–16 h
Isradipine	Chronic Stable Angina: Regular release: A: PO: Initially 2.5 mg tid; *max:* 20 mg/d	To treat chronic stable angina and hypertension. May cause headache, palpitations, peripheral edema, fatigue, flushing, hypotension, tachycardia, angina, abdominal pain, erectile dysfunction, and dizziness. PB: 95%; t½: 8 h
NiCARdipine	Angina: Immediate release: A: PO: Initially 20 mg tid, titrate dosage as needed allow at least 3 days between dosage increases. Usual dose 20–40 mg tid; *max:* 120 mg/d	For chronic stable angina and hypertension. May cause peripheral edema, headache, dizziness, hypotension, palpitations, weakness, tachycardia, flushing, angina, nausea, and vomiting. PB: 95%; t½: 8.6 h
NIFEdipine	Angina: Immediate release: A: PO: Initially 10 mg tid; Increase the dose every 7 to 14 days until desired response is achieved. Usual dose: 10–20 mg/tid. Usual Max: 30 mg/dose and 120 mg/day. *max:* 180 mg/d Extended release: A: PO: 30–60 mg/d, initially. Increase dose every 7–14 days until desired response is achieved. Usual max: 90 mg/d *max:* 120 mg/d	For variant and chronic angina and hypertension. May cause dizziness, flushing, headache, peripheral edema, nausea, constipation, hypotension, pyrosis, tremor, muscle cramps, cough, fatigue, dyspnea, heart failure, erectile dysfunction, nasal congestion, and weakness. PB: 92%–98%; t½: 2–5 h ⚡ Inappropriate drug for use in older adults
Nisoldipine	Angina: Extended release: A: PO: Initially 17 mg/d; *maint:* –8.5–34 mg/d; *max:* 34 mg/d Older A: PO: Initially 8.5 mg/d; *max:* 34 mg/d	For variant angina (Prinzmetal angina), stable angina, and hypertension. May cause headache, dizziness, flushing, sinusitis, pharyngitis, orthostatic hypotension, palpitations, tachycardia, hypokalemia, visual impairment, and peripheral edema. PB: >99%; t½: 7–12 h
Verapamil	Angina: Immediate release: A: PO: 40–120 mg tid; *maint:* 80–120 mg/tid, adjust dose daily or weekly until desired response is achieved; *max:* 480 mg/d in 3–4 divided doses	For variant (Prinzmetal angina) and chronic angina, cardiac dysrhythmias, and hypertension. May cause dizziness, weakness, peripheral edema, nausea, constipation, tachycardia, headache, confusion, bradycardia, fatigue, blurred vision, erectile dysfunction, and orthostatic hypotension. PB: 90%; t½: 2–5 h ⚠ **High-Alert Drug:** Heightened risk if given in error ⚡ Inappropriate drug for use in older adults

>, Greater than; *A*, adult; *a.m.*, in the morning; *AMI*, acute myocardial infarction; *bid*, twice a day; *CAD*, coronary artery disease; *d*, day; *GI*, gastrointestinal; *h*, hour; *maint*, maintenance; *max*, maximum; *min*, minute; *PB*, protein binding; *PO*, by mouth; *PSVT*, paroxysmal supraventricular tachycardia; *q8h*, every 8 hours; *qid*, four times a day; *SL*, sublingual; *SR*, sustained release; *t½*, half-life; *tid*, three times a day.

The duration of action for metoprolol, a nonselective beta-blocker is 6–12 hours for the immediate release and approximately 24 hours for the extended release. In the elderly, begin the beta blocker with a conservative dose and titrate upward carefully. The elderly have an unpredictable response to beta-blockers.

Side Effects and Adverse Reactions

Both nonselective and selective beta-blockers cause a decrease in heart rate and blood pressure. For the nonselective beta-blockers, bronchospasm, agitation, dizziness, drowsiness, confusion, cool extremities, and erectile dysfunction (with use of propranolol) are potential adverse reactions.

Vital signs need to be closely monitored in the early stages of beta-blocker therapy. When discontinuing use, the dosage should be tapered for 1 or 2 weeks to prevent a rebound effect such as reflex tachycardia or life-threatening cardiac dysrhythmias.

Calcium Channel Blockers

Calcium channel blockers (CCBs), or *calcium blockers*, were introduced in 1982 for the treatment of stable and variant angina pectoris, certain dysrhythmias, and hypertension. Calcium activates myocardial contraction, increasing the workload of the heart and the need for more oxygen. CCBs relax coronary artery spasm (variant angina) and relax peripheral arterioles (stable angina), decreasing cardiac oxygen demand. They also decrease cardiac contractility (negative inotropic effect that relaxes smooth muscle), afterload, and peripheral resistance, and they reduce the workload of the heart, which decreases the need for oxygen. CCBs achieve their effect in controlling variant (vasospastic) angina by relaxing coronary arteries and in controlling classic (stable) angina by decreasing oxygen demand. Based on the findings of the CAMELOT trial, amlodipine is indicated for use in patients with recently documented CAD to reduce the risk of hospitalization due to angina and to reduce the risk of a coronary revascularization procedure. Fig. 40.4 shows the suggested steps for treating classic and variant angina pectoris. Table 40.4 presents the drug data for the CCBs used to treat angina and their dosages, uses, and considerations.

Pharmacokinetics

Three CCBs—verapamil, nifedipine, and diltiazem—have been effectively used for the long-term treatment of angina. Eighty to ninety percent of CCBs are absorbed through the GI mucosa. However, first-pass metabolism by the liver decreases the availability of free circulating drug, and only 20% of verapamil, 45% to 65% of diltiazem, and 35% to 40% of nifedipine are bioavailable. All three drugs are highly protein bound (70%–98%), and their half-lives are usually 2 to 5 hours.

Several other CCBs are available, such as nicardipine hydrochloride (HCl), amlodipine, felodipine, and nisoldipine. All are highly protein bound (greater than 93%).

Pharmacodynamics

Bradycardia is a common problem with the use of verapamil, the first calcium blocker. Nifedipine, the most potent of the calcium blockers, promotes vasodilation of the coronary and peripheral vessels, and hypotension can result. The onset of action is 1 to 2 hours for immediate release, oral, verapamil and 20 minutes for nifedipine immediate release and 30 to 60 minutes for diltiazem immediate release. Verapamil's duration of action is 6 to 8 hours when given orally and 0.5 to 6 hours when given intravenously.

Side Effects and Adverse Reactions

The side effects of calcium blockers include headache, hypotension (more common with nifedipine and less common with diltiazem), dizziness, and flushing of the skin. Reflex tachycardia can occur as a result of hypotension. Peripheral edema may occur with several CCBs, including nicardipine, nifedipine, and verapamil. CCBs can cause changes in liver and kidney function, and serum liver enzymes should be checked periodically. CCBs are frequently given with other antianginal drugs such as nitrates to prevent angina.

In its immediate-release form (10- and 20-mg capsules), nifedipine has been associated with an increased incidence of sudden cardiac death, especially when prescribed in high doses for outpatients. This is not true of the sustained-release preparations. For this reason, immediate-release nifedipine is usually prescribed only as needed in the hospital setting for acute increases in blood pressure.

CARDIAC DYSRHYTHMIAS

A cardiac dysrhythmia (arrhythmia) is defined as any deviation from the normal rate or pattern of the heartbeat. This includes heart rates that are too slow (bradycardia), too fast (tachycardia), or irregular. The

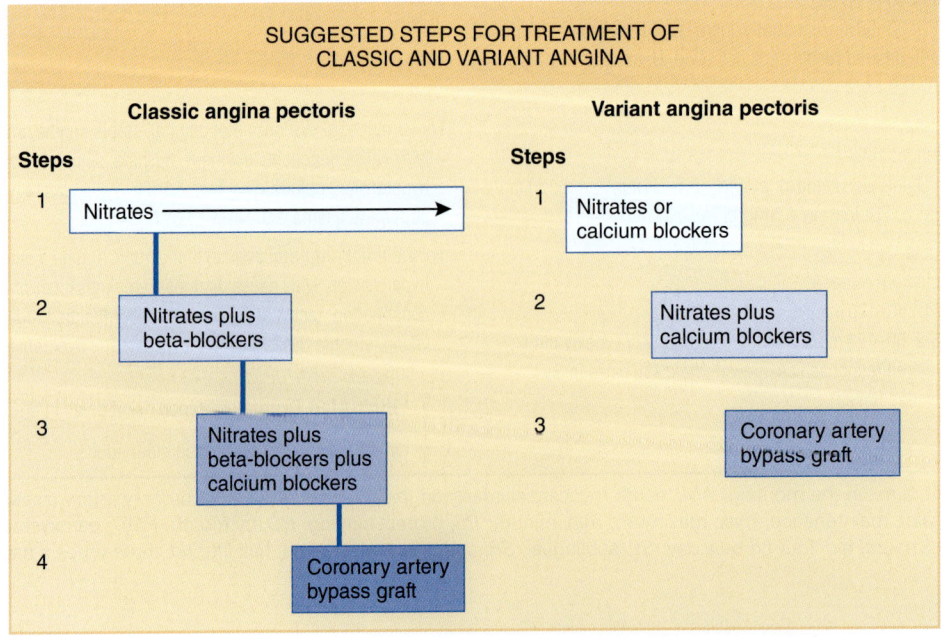

Fig. 40.4 Suggested steps for treating classic and variant angina pectoris.

CLINICAL JUDGMENT [NURSING PROCESS]
Antianginals

Concept: Perfusion
- The passage of blood flow through the arteries and capillaries that deliver oxygen and nutrients to body cells

Recognize Cues [Assessment]
- Obtain baseline vital signs for future comparisons.
- Obtain health and drug histories. Nitroglycerin is contraindicated for marked hypotension or acute myocardial infarction (AMI).

Analyze Cues and Prioritize Hypothesis [Patient Problems]
- Dyspnea
- Myocardial tissue injury
- Pain
- Decreased tissue perfusion
- Hypoxemia
- Anxiety
- Reduced functional ability

Generate Solutions [Planning]
- The patient will report that angina pain is controlled by nitroglycerin or other antianginals.

Take Action [Nursing Interventions]
- Monitor vital signs. Hypotension is associated with most antianginal drugs.
- Position the patient sitting or lying down when administering a nitrate for the first time. After administration, check vital signs while the patient is lying down and then sitting up. Have the patient rise slowly to a standing position.
- Offer sips of water before giving sublingual (SL) nitrates; dryness may inhibit drug absorption.
- ⚡ Monitor effects of intravenous (IV) nitroglycerin. Report angina that persists.
- ⚡ Apply nitroglycerin ointment to a designated mark on paper. Do not use fingers because drug can be absorbed; use tongue blade or gloves. When using a nitroglycerin patch, do not touch the medication portion.
- ⚡ Do *not* apply nitroglycerin ointment or a nitroglycerin patch in any area on the chest in the vicinity of defibrillator-cardioverter paddle placement. Explosion and skin burns may result.

Patient Teaching
General
- ⚡ Administer SL nitroglycerin tablet if chest pain occurs. If pain has not subsided or has worsened in 5 minutes, call 911.
- ⚡ Advise patients not to ingest alcohol while taking nitroglycerin to avoid hypotension, weakness, and faintness.
- ⚡ Advise patients to notify a health care provider if chest pain is not completely alleviated. Tolerance to nitroglycerin can occur.
- ⚡ Inform patients not to discontinue beta-blockers and calcium blockers without a health care provider's approval. Withdrawal symptoms (reflex tachycardia and pain) may be severe.

Self-Administration
- Demonstrate how SL nitroglycerin tablets are taken. The tablet is placed under the tongue for quick absorption. A stinging or biting sensation indicates that the tablet is fresh; however, with newer SL nitroglycerin tablets, the biting sensation may not be present.
- Teach patients to store medication bottles away from light in a dry place and to keep the drug in its original screw-cap, amber glass bottle. The amber color provides light protection, and the screw-cap closure protects from moisture in the air, which can easily reduce tablet potency.
- Teach patients about nitroglycerin patches, applied once a day, usually in the morning. Rotate skin sites. The patch is usually applied to the chest wall, but the thighs and arms may also be used. Avoid hairy areas.
- Advise patients to seek medical attention if nitroglycerin does not relieve pain.

Side Effects
- Suggest acetaminophen to patients for relief of headache, which commonly occurs when first taking nitroglycerin products and lasts about 30 minutes.
- ⚡ Place patients in a supine position with legs elevated if hypotension results from SL nitroglycerin.
- Instruct patients how to check their pulse rate.
- Advise patients taking beta-blockers and calcium blockers to notify a health care provider if dizziness or faintness occurs because it may indicate hypotension.

Evaluate Outcomes [Evaluation]
- Evaluate the patient's response to nitrate products for relieving anginal pain. Note headache, dizziness, or faintness.

---

terms *dysrhythmia* (disturbed heart rhythm) and *arrhythmia* (absence of heart rhythm) are used interchangeably despite the slight difference in meaning.

The ECG identifies the type of dysrhythmia. The *P wave* of the ECG reflects atrial activation, the *QRS complex* indicates ventricular depolarization, and the *T wave* reflects ventricular **repolarization** (return of cell membrane potential to resting after depolarization). The *PR interval* indicates AV conduction time, and the *QT interval* reflects ventricular action potential duration. Atrial dysrhythmias prevent proper filling of the ventricles and decrease cardiac output by 33%. Ventricular dysrhythmias are life-threatening because ineffective filling of the ventricle and ineffective pumping result in decreased or absent cardiac output. With ventricular tachycardia, ventricular fibrillation is likely to occur, followed by death. Cardiopulmonary resuscitation (CPR) is necessary to treat these patients.

Cardiac dysrhythmias frequently follow an MI (heart attack) or can result from **hypoxia** (lack of oxygen to body tissues), **hypercapnia** (increased carbon dioxide in the blood), thyroid disease, CAD, cardiac surgery, excess catecholamines, or electrolyte imbalance.

Cardiac Action Potentials

Electrolyte transfer occurs through the cardiac muscle cell membrane. When sodium and calcium enter the cardiac cell, **depolarization** (myocardial contraction) occurs. Sodium enters rapidly to start the depolarization, and calcium enters later to maintain it. Calcium influx leads to an increased release of intracellular calcium from the sarcoplasmic reticulum, resulting in cardiac contraction. In the presence of myocardial ischemia, the contraction can be irregular.

Cardiac action potentials are transient depolarizations followed by repolarizations of myocardial cells. Fig. 40.5 illustrates the action potential of a ventricular cardiac cell (myocyte) during a heartbeat. There are five phases: phase 0 is the rapid depolarization caused by an influx of sodium ions; phase 1 is initial repolarization, which coincides with termination of sodium ion influx; phase 2 is the plateau and is characterized by the influx of calcium ions, which prolong the action potential and promote atrial and ventricular muscle contraction; phase 3 is rapid repolarization caused by influx of potassium ions; and phase 4 is the resting membrane potential between heartbeats and is normally flat in ventricular muscle, but it begins to rise in the cells of the SA node as they slowly depolarize toward the threshold potential just before depolarization occurs, initiating the next heartbeat.

Antidysrhythmic Drugs

The desired action of antidysrhythmic (antiarrhythmic) drugs is to restore the cardiac rhythm to normal. Box 40.1 describes the various mechanisms by which this is accomplished. Antidysrhythmics are high-alert drugs that may cause significant harm to the patient when given inappropriately.

The antidysrhythmics are grouped into four classes: (1) sodium (fast) channel blockers IA, IB, and IC; (2) beta-blockers; (3) drugs that prolong repolarization; and (4) calcium (slow) channel blockers. Table 40.5 lists the classes, actions, and indications for cardiac antidysrhythmic drugs. Table 40.6 lists the commonly administered antidysrhythmics and their dosages, uses, and considerations.

TYPES OF ANTIDYSRHYTHMIC DRUGS

Class I: Sodium Channel Blockers

A sodium channel blocker decreases sodium influx into cardiac cells. Responses to the drug are decreased conduction velocity in cardiac tissues; suppression of automaticity, which decreases the likelihood of ectopic foci; and increased recovery time (repolarization or refractory period). There are three subgroups of sodium channel blockers: those in *class IA* slow conduction and prolong repolarization (quinidine, procainamide, disopyramide); those in *class IB* slow conduction and shorten repolarization (lidocaine, mexiletine HCl); and *class IC* drugs prolong conduction with little to no effect on repolarization (flecainide).

Lidocaine, a class IB sodium channel blocker, was used in the 1940s as a local anesthetic and is still used for this purpose. It was later discovered to have antidysrhythmic properties as well. Lidocaine is still used by some cardiologists to treat acute ventricular dysrhythmias. It slows conduction velocity and decreases action potential amplitude. Onset of action (IV) is rapid. About one-third of lidocaine reaches the general circulation, and a bolus of lidocaine is short lived. Another class IB sodium channel blocker is mexiletine.

Class II: Beta-Blockers

The drugs in the second class, beta-blockers, decrease conduction velocity, automaticity, and recovery time (refractory period). Examples are propranolol, acebutolol, esmolol, and sotalol. Beta-blockers are more frequently prescribed for dysrhythmias than are sodium channel blockers. This drug class should be gradually reduced in dose upon discontinuation. Propranolol is a drug that has a narrow therapeutic Index. A small change in the dose can lead to serious adverse events. This drug requires careful titration and monitoring. Prototype Drug Chart: Acebutolol Hydrochloride

Fig. 40.5 Action potential of a ventricular myocyte during the course of a heartbeat.

BOX 40.1 Pharmacodynamics of Antidysrhythmics

Mechanisms of Action
- Blocks adrenergic stimulation of the heart
- Depresses myocardial excitability and contractility
- Decreases conduction velocity in cardiac tissue
- Increases recovery time (repolarization) of the myocardium
- Suppresses automaticity (spontaneous depolarization to initiate beats)

TABLE 40.5 Classes, Actions, and Indications of Antidysrhythmic Drugs

Classes	Actions	Indications
Class I		
Sodium Channel Blockers		
IA	Slow conduction and prolong repolarization	Atrial and ventricular dysrhythmias, paroxysmal atrial tachycardia, supraventricular dysrhythmias
IB	Slow conduction and shorten repolarization	Acute ventricular dysrhythmias
IC	Prolong conduction with little to no effect on repolarization	Life-threatening ventricular dysrhythmias
Class II Beta-blockers	Reduce calcium entry. Decrease conduction velocity, automaticity, and recovery time (refractory period)	Atrial flutter and fibrillation, tachydysrhythmias, ventricular and supraventricular dysrhythmias
Class III Drugs that prolong repolarization	Prolong repolarization during ventricular dysrhythmias. Prolong action potential duration	Life-threatening atrial and ventricular dysrhythmias resistant to other drugs
Class IV Calcium channel blockers	Block calcium influx. Slow conduction velocity. Decrease myocardial contractility (negative inotropic). Increase refraction in atrioventricular node	Supraventricular tachydysrhythmias; prevention of paroxysmal supraventricular tachycardia

TABLE 40.6 Antidysrhythmics

Drug	Route and Dosage	Uses and Considerations
Class I		
Sodium Channel Blockers IA		
Disopyramide (antiarrhythmic class 1-A)	Immediate release: A: >18 y >50 kg: PO: 150–200 mg q6h; *max*: 800 mg/d A: >18 y <50 kg: PO: 100 mg q6h; *max*: 800 mg/d Extended release: A: >50 kg: PO: 300 mg q12h; *max*: 800 mg/d A: <50 kg: PO: 200 mg q12h; *max*: 800 mg/d	For life-threatening dysrhythmias, such as ventricular tachycardia. May cause dizziness, headache, fatigue, blurred vision, dry mouth, urinary urgency/frequency/retention, nausea, flatulence, abdominal pain, constipation, and inappropriate to use in older adults. PB: 90%; t½: 4–10 h ⚡ *Absolute contraindications*: AV block 2nd or 3rd degree; cardiogenic shock, Congenital long QT Syndrome. ⚡ **Black-Box Warning**: Mortality ❗ **High-Alert Drug**: Heightened risk if used in error
Procainamide (antiarrhythmic class 1-A)	Ventricular tachycardia: A: IV: 20–50 mg/min infusion or 100 mg IV every 5 minutes until arrythmia is suppressed. *maint*: 1–4 mg/min infusion if needed	For ventricular tachycardia and cardiopulmonary resuscitation. May cause anorexia, nausea, dyspepsia, vomiting, abdominal pain, and diarrhea. ⚡ *Absolute Contraindications*: SLE, torsade de pointes. ⚡ **Black Box**: Bone marrow suppression positive antinuclear antibodies, mortality ❗ **High-Alert Drug**: Heightened risk if used in error. NTI: Narrow Therapeutic Index drug PB: 15%; t½: 2.5–5.2 h ⚡ NTI Warning
Quinidine (antiarrhythmic class 1-A)	Immediate release: Quinidine sulfate: A: PO: Initially 200–300 mg q6–8 h Extended release: A: PO: 300–600 mg q8–12h TDM: Serum concentrations should be monitored, a range of 2–6 mcg/mL are recommended.	For atrial, ventricular, and supraventricular dysrhythmias and A-Fib, A-flutter. May cause headache, dizziness, fatigue, weakness, palpitations, fever, nausea, vomiting, esophagitis, pyrosis, diarrhea, and rash. ⚡ *Absolute contraindications*: AV block, bundle-branch block, MG, quinidine hypersensitivity ⚡ **Black-Box Warning**: Mortality ❗ **High-Alert Drug**: Heightened risk if used in error NTI: Narrow Therapeutic Index drug PB: 80%–90%; t½: 6–8 h
Sodium Channel Blockers IB		
Lidocaine (antiarrhythmic class 1-B)	Dysrhythmias: A: IV: LD: 1–1.5 mg/kg/loading dose (LD), follow with 1–4 mg/min infusion for an average 70K adult. *Max*: 100 mg IV loading dose, repeat max dose 300 mg over 1 hr period.	For ventricular dysrhythmias. May cause erythema, pruritus, edema, injection site reaction, petechiae, dizziness, nausea, and vomiting. ⚡ *Absolute contraindications*: Adams-Stokes syndrome, sepsis, Wolfe-Parkinson-White Syndrome, amideloccal anesthetic hypersensitivity. ⚡ **Black-Box Warning**: Teething Pain ❗ **High-Alert Drug**: Heightened risk if used in error PB: 60%–80%; t½: 1.5–2 h
Mexiletine (antiarrhythmic class 1-B)	A: PO: Initially 200 mg q8h; *maint*: 200–300 mg q8h; *max*: 1200 mg/d	For ventricular dysrhythmias. May cause weakness, nausea, pyrosis, vomiting, diarrhea, tremor, dizziness, headache, blurred vision, palpitations, chest pain, and ataxia. ⚡ *Absolute contraindications*: 2nd or 3rd AV block, cariogenic shock ⚡ **Black-Box Warning**: Hepatotoxicity, mortality ❗ **High-Alert Drug**: Heightened risk if used in error PB: 50%–60%; t½: 10–12 h
Sodium Channel Blockers IC		
Flecainide (antiarrhythmic class 1-C)	A: PO: Initially 100 mg q12h, usual dose 150 mg every 12 h; *max*: 400 mg/d	For prevention of life threatening ventricular arrythmias. May cause dizziness, palpitations, headache, fatigue, visual impairment, tremor, dyspnea, dysrhythmia exacerbation, weakness, chest pain, HF, nausea, and constipation. ⚡ *Absolute contraindications*: Cardiogenic shock ⚡ **Black-Box Warning**: A-fibrillation, mortality. Ventricular arrhythmias ❗ **High-Alert Drug**: Heightened risk if given in error PB: 40%–50%; t½: 12–30 h

Continued

TABLE 40.6 Antidysrhythmics—cont'd

Drug	Route and Dosage	Uses and Considerations
Propafenone (antiarrhythmics class 1-C)	Immediate release: *(Treatment initiated in hospital setting)* A: PO: Initially 150 mg q8h; *max:* 900 mg/d	For the treatment of life threatening arrhytimias such as sustained ventricular tachycardia. May cause dizziness, fatigue, headache, weakness, chest pain, anxiety, dyspnea, dysgeusia, nausea, vomiting, constipation, edema, infection, influenza, and blurred vision. ⚡ *Absolute contraindication:* Acute bronchospasm, asthma, AV block, cardiogenic shock, heart failure, hypotension, sick sinus syndrome ⚡ **Black-Box Warning**: Mortality ❗ **High-Alert Drug**: Heightened risk if given in error PB: 85%–97%; $t\frac{1}{2}$: 2–10 h
Class II		
Beta-Adrenergic Blockers		
Acebutolol (beta₁ blocker)	See Prototype Drug Chart: Acebutolol	
Esmolol (beta₁ blocker) selective adrenergic blocker and antiarrhythmic class-II)	Supraventricular tachycardia: A: IV: LD: 50 mcg/kg/min continuous infusion; *maint:* 25–200 mcg/kg/min; *max:* 300 mcg/kg/min (continuous infusion) Ventricular tachycardia: 500 mcg/kg, then 50 mcg/kg/min (continuous infusion) *max:* 500 mcg/kg/ loading dose.	To treat atrial flutter and fibrillation, PSVT, and HTN. May cause bradycardia, hypotension, dizziness, drowsiness, wheezing, infusion-site reaction, headache, confusion, agitation, and nausea. ❗ **High-Alert Drug**: Heightened risk if used in error PB: 55%; $t\frac{1}{2}$: 9 min
Propranolol (beta₁ and beta₂ blocker, class II antiarrhythmics)	A: IV: 1 mg every 2 min for up to 2 doses *main:* 1–3 mg IV every 2 min for up to 2 doses, further doses given after 4 h	For atrial fibrillation and flutter, and supraventricular dysrhythmias. May cause dizziness, agitation, headache, weakness, depression, fatigue, visual impairment, bradycardia, hyperkalemia, bronchospasm, and erectile dysfunction. ⚡ *Absolute contraindications:* Acute heart failure, asthma, AV block, bradycardia, cariogenic shock, neonates, sick sinus syndrome ⚡ **Black-Box Warning:** Abrupt discontinuation ❗ **High-Alert Drug:** Heightened risk if given in error PB: 90%; $t\frac{1}{2}$: 2–6 h
Sotalol (beta₁ and beta₂ blocker; and class II and class III antiarrhythmic activity)	Atrial flutter/fibrillation: A: PO: Initially 80 mg bid; *max:* 320 mg/d Life threatening VT: A: IV: Initially 75 mg bid; The IV loading dose depends on the target oral dose; *max:* IV: 600 mg/d	For atrial flutter and fibrillation and life-threatening ventricular tachycardia. May cause bradycardia, chest pain, hyperhidrosis, diarrhea, musculoskeletal pain, fatigue, dizziness, headache, palpitations, weakness, abdominal pain, nausea, vomiting, and dyspnea. ⚡ *Absolute contraindications*: Acute bronchospasm, asthma, AV block, heart failure, hypokalemia, renal failure, sick sinus syndrome ⚡ **Black-Box Warning**: QT prolongation, requires specialized care setting, ventricular arrythmias ❗ **High-Alert Drug**: Heightened risk if given in error PB: 0%; $t\frac{1}{2}$: 12 h
Class III		
Drugs That Prolong Repolarization		
Adenosine (antiarrhythmic)	A: IV: 6 mg as a single dose, if conversion does not occur in 1–2 min, administer 12 mg IV as a single dose. May repeat 12 mg dose once; *max:* 12 mg/dose, with total max dose 30 mg	For life-threatening ventricular tachycardia and fibrillation. May cause headache, dizziness, flushing, dyspnea, hypotension, nausea, and paresthesia. PB: UK; $t\frac{1}{2}$: <10 seconds ❗ **High-Alert Drug:** Heightened risk if administered in error

TABLE 40.6 Antidysrhythmics—cont'd

Drug	Route and Dosage	Uses and Considerations
Amiodarone (class III antiarrhythmic)	A: PO: Initially 800–1600 mg/d for 1–3 wk, in a monitored setting until an initial therapeutic response is achieved, followed by 600–800 mg/day for 1 month; then reduce to lowest effective dose (usually 400 mg/d) Patients in an Emergency setting receiving ACLS: A: IV: 150 mg over first 10 min, then 1 mg/min infusion for 6 h; then 0.5 mg/min for 18 h; after first 24 h *maint:* 0.5 mg/min *max:* A:PO: Up to 1600 mg/d. A: IV: 300 mg/dose IV, 1 mg/min continuous infusion.	For life-threatening ventricular tachycardia and fibrillation. May cause corneal deposits, anorexia, nausea, vomiting, constipation, hypo/hyperthyroidism, injection site reaction, bradycardia, hypotension, and photosensitivity. ⚡ *Absolute contraindication:* Cardiogenic shock, iodine hypersensitivity, sick sinus syndrome ⚡ **Black-Box Warning:** Amiodarone-induced liver toxicity and Amiodarone-induced lung toxicity, arrhythmia exacerbation ⚡ Inappropriate drug for use in older adults ❗ **High-Alert Drug:** Heightened risk if given in error PB: >99%; t½: 26–107 d
Dofetilide (Class III antiarrhythmic)	A: PO: 500 mg twice daily, initially, monitor QT interval at 2–3 h after each dose for 3 d or every 12 h until conversion occurs; *max:* 1000 mcg/d	For atrial flutter and fibrillation. May cause headache, dizziness, insomnia, chest pain, infection, dyspnea, influenza, tachycardia, and nausea. Monitor renal function. ⚡ *Absolute contraindication:* Long QT syndrome, QT prolongation, renal failure torsade de pointes ⚡ **Black-Box Warning:** Requires a specialized care setting ❗ **High-Alert Drug:** Heightened risk if given in error ⚡ Inappropriate drug for older adults PB: 60%–70%; t½: 10 h
Ibutilide (Class III antiarrhythmic)	A: >60 kg: IV: 1 mg as a single dose; may repeat with 1 mg in 10 min; *max:* 2 mg over 20 min A: <60 kg: IV: 0.01 mg/kg given as a single dose; may repeat after 10 min if no response; *max:* 2 mg in 20 min	For conversion of atrial flutter and fibrillation. May cause headache, palpitations, nausea, tachycardia, bradycardia, orthostatic hypotension, and dysrhythmia exacerbation. ⚡ **Black-Box Warning:** Requires a specialized care setting ❗ **High-Alert Drug:** Heightened risk if given in error PB: 40%; t½: 2–12 h
Sotalol (Class III antiarrhythmic, and Class II nonselective beta-block)	A: PO: Initially 80 mg bid; *maint:* 160–320 mg/d in 2–3 divided doses; *max:* 640 mg/d Substituting oral therapy for IV sotalol: A: IV: Initially 75 mg for 80 mg PO, 112.5 mg IV for 120 mg PO, or 150 mg IV for 160 mg PO at same oral dose frequency. *max:* 600 mg/d	For life threatening ventricular arrhythmia such as SVT. May cause bradycardia, hyperhidrosis, musculoskeletal pain, diarrhea, chest pain, abdominal pain, fatigue, dizziness, headache, palpitations, weakness, nausea, vomiting, and dyspnea. ⚡ *Absolute contraindications:* Heart failure, hypokalemia, long QT syndrome, QT prolongation, renal failure, sick sinus syndrome ⚡ **Black-Box Warning:** Requires specialized care setting, ventricular arrhythmias ❗ **High-Alert Drug:** Heightened risk if given in error PB: 0%; t½: 12 h
Class IV		
Calcium Channel Blockers		
Verapamil (Antiarrhythmic Class IV)	Conversion of PSVT: A: IV: 2.5–5 mg IV bolus followed by 5–10 mg IV bolus every 15–30 min as needed; *max:* 30 mg	For narrow complex PSVT including Wolf Parkinson White or Lown Ganong Levine, for rapid conversion. May cause peripheral edema, constipation, dizziness, fatigue, weakness, nausea, confusion, headache, blurred vision, erectile dysfunction, bradycardia, and orthostatic hypotension. ❗ **High-Alert Drug:** Heightened risk if given in error ⚡ Inappropriate drug for use in older adults PB: 90%; t½: 2–10 h
dilTIAZem (Antiarrhythmic, Class IV)	A: IV: 0.25 mg/kg (usual dose: 15 to 20 mg) IV bolus, followed by 5 to 10 mg/hr continuous IV infusion. Titrate by 5 mg/hr as needed. *max:* 15 mg/h. Extended release: A: PO: 120 to 360 mg daily. *max:* 360 mg/d	For short term control of ventricular rate in atrial arrhythmias and long term control of atrial flutter or atrial fibrillation. May cause headache, peripheral edema, dizziness, weakness, bradycardia, hypotension, fatigue, infection, dyspnea, pharyngitis, rhinitis, constipation, and dyspepsia. ❗ **High-Alert Drug:** Heightened risk if given in error ⚡ Inappropriate drug for use in older adults PB: 70%–80%; t½: 3.5–9 h

Continued

TABLE 40.6 Antidysrhythmics—cont'd

Drug	Route and Dosage	Uses and Considerations
Others		
Digoxin	See Prototype Drug Chart: Digoxin	
Dronedarone (antiarrhythmic/ miscellaneous)	A: PO: 400 mg bid with morning and evening meals; *max.* 800 mg/d. Dronedarone is contraindicated in patients with permanent a-fib who cannot be cardioverted to normal sinus rhythm.	For reduction in the risk of hospitalization for A-Fib in patients in sinus rhythm with a history of paroxysmal A-Fib or persistent A-Fib. Discontinue class 1 or III antiarrhythmic drugs before dronedarone. May cause rash, pruritus, nausea, diarrhea, vomiting, abdominal pain, and weakness. Avoid grapefruit and grapefruit juice. ⚡ *Absolute contraindications*: Amiodarone-induced liver toxicity, amiodarone-induced lung toxicity, AV block, QT prolongation, heart failure, bradycardia, sick sinus syndrome ⚡ **Black-Box Warning**: Heart failure, atrial fibrillation ❗ **High-Alert Drug**: Heightened risk if given in error PB: 98%; t½: 13–19 h

<, Less than; >, greater than; *A*, adult; *ACLS*, advanced cardiac life support; *A-Fib*, atrial fibrillation; *A-flutter*, atrial flutter; *AMI*, acute myocardial infarction; *AV block*, atrial ventricular block; *bid*, two times a day; *d*, day; *h*, hour; *HF*, heart failure; *HTN*, hypertension; *inf*, infusion; *IV*, intravenous; *LD*, loading dose; *maint*, maintenance; *max*, maximum; *MG*, myasthenia gravis; *min*, minute; *NSR*, normal sinus rhythm; *NTI*, narrow therapeutic index; *PB*, protein binding; *PO*, by mouth; *PSVT*, paroxysmal supraventricular tachycardia; *q*, every; *qd*, every day; *qid*, four times a day; *s*, second; *SLE*, systemic lupus erythematosus; *t½*, half-life; *TDM*, therapeutic drug monitoring; *tid*, three times a day; *UK*, unknown; *VT*, ventricular tachycardia; *wk*, week; *y*, year; *NTi*, Narrow Therapeutic Index.

lists the drug data related to the beta-blocker acebutolol hydrochloride, which can be prescribed to treat recurrent stable ventricular dysrhythmias.

Sotalol is a very unique beta-blocker as it is classified as both class II and III antiarrhythmic properties. As a Class II nonselective beta-blocker, it has no intrinsic sympathomimetic activity or membrane stabilizing activity.

As a Class III antiarrhythmic effects, like amiodarone, prolong the action potential duration and increase cardiac tissue refractoriness. Sotalol is used in the treatment of symptomatic atrial arrthythmias or

📋 PROTOTYPE DRUG CHART
Acebutolol

Drug Class	Dosage
Beta₁ blocker: Cardioselective beta-adrenergic antagonist (antiarrhythmic class II)	Premature ventricular arrhythmias (PVCS) and hypertension. A: PO: Initially 200 mg q12h; *maint:* 600–1200 mg/d in 2 divided doses; *max:* 1200 mg/d
Contraindications	**Drug-Lab-Food Interactions**
Second or third degree AV block, bradycardia, acute heart failure, cardiogenic shock *Caution:* Surgery, renal/hepatic impairment, diabetes mellitus, thyroid disorder, asthma, bronchitis, COPD, pulmonary edema, PVD, myasthenia gravis, acute bronchospasm, cerebrovascular disorder, depression, older adults, pregnancy, breastfeeding	Drug: Increased effects with diuretics, adenosine, amiodarone, class IC antidysrhythmics, cardiac glycosides, disopyramide; prolongs hypoglycemic effects of insulin and oral antidiabetics; antagonist effect with albuterol, metaproterenol, terbutaline Lab: May increase ALT, AST, ALP, ANA titer, BUN, lipoproteins, and potassium. Monitoring parameters: Blood pressure, heart rate, serum creatinine/BUN.
Pharmacokinetics	**Pharmacodynamics**
Absorption: Well absorbed Distribution: PB: 26% Metabolism: t½: 3–4 h	When discontinued reduce dose gradually over 2 wks. ❗ **High-Alert Drug**: Heightened risk if given in error
Therapeutic Effects/Uses	
To aid in treatment of premature ventricular contractions and hypertension Mechanism of Action: Blocks beta₁-adrenergic receptors in cariac tissues, anti-arrhythmics, Class II	
Side Effects	**Adverse Reactions**
Dizziness, headache, fatigue, insomnia, nightmares, anxiety, visual impairment, depression, arthralgia, myalgia, weakness, abdominal pain, flatulence, anorexia, nausea, vomiting, dyspepsia, constipation, diarrhea, edema, diaphoresis, erectile dysfunction	Palpitations, bradycardia, hypo/hypertension, tachycardia, chest pain, hyper/hypoglycemia, diabetes mellitus, lupus-like symptoms, hyperbilirubinemia, dyspnea ⚡ *Life-threatening:* Agranulocytosis, thrombocytopenia, HF

A, Adult; *ALP*, alkaline phosphatase; *ALT*, alanine aminotransferase; *ANA*, antinuclear antibody; *AST*, aspartate aminotransferase; *AV*, atrioventricular; *BUN*, blood urea nitrogen; *COPD*, chronic obstructive pulmonary disease; *d*, day; *h*, hour; *HF*, heart failure; *maint*, maintenance; *max*, maximum; *PB*, protein binding; *PO*, by mouth; *PVC*, premature ventricular contractions; *PVD*, peripheral vascular disease; *q12h*, every 12 hours; *t½*, half-life.

life-threatening ventriculr arrhythmias, including sustained ventricular tachycardia. It is not recommnded for mild arrhythmias. When used in emergency treatment of ventricular dysrhythmias requires hospitalization and cardiac monitoring.

Pharmacokinetics
The cardioselective beta drug acebutolol is well absorbed in the GI tract. It is metabolized in the liver to active metabolites; Excretion in the feces is (50%–60%) and in the urine (30%–40%). The half-life for the drug is 3 to 4 hours.

Pharmacodynamics
Acebutolol is prescribed for ventricular dysrhythmias and hypertension. As an antidysrhythmic drug, the bioavailability of acebutolol is 40%; peak time is 2.5 to 3.5 hours. Administration with food slightly affects rate of absorption and peak concentrations. When discontinued reduce dose gradually over 2 weeks.

Class III: Drugs That Prolong Repolarization
Drugs in the third class prolong repolarization and are used in emergency treatment of ventricular dysrhythmias when other antidysrhythmics are ineffective. Amiodarone increases the refractory period (recovery time) and prolongs the action potential duration (cardiac cell activity).

Class IV: Calcium Channel Blockers
The fourth class consists of the calcium channel blockers verapamil and diltiazem. Verapamil is a slow (calcium) channel blocker that blocks calcium influx, thereby decreasing the excitability and (negative inotropic) contractility of the myocardium. It increases the refractory period of the AV node, which decreases ventricular response. Verapamil is contraindicated for patients with AV block or HF.

Side Effects and Adverse Reactions of Antidysrhythmic Drugs
Quinidine, the first drug used to treat cardiac dysrhythmias, has many side effects, which include nausea, vomiting, diarrhea, confusion, and hypotension. It can also cause heart block and neurologic and psychiatric symptoms. Procainamide causes less cardiac depression than quinidine.

High doses of lidocaine can cause cardiovascular depression, bradycardia, hypotension, seizures, blurred vision, and double vision. Less serious side effects may include dizziness and confusion. The use of lidocaine is contraindicated in patients with advanced AV block, and it should be used with caution in patients with hepatic disorders or HF. Mexiletine has side effects similar to lidocaine, and both drugs are contraindicated for use in patients with cardiogenic shock or in those with second- or third-degree heart block.

The side effects of beta-blockers are bradycardia and hypotension. Amiodarone can cause nausea, vomiting, hypotension, and neurologic problems. The side effects of calcium blockers include nausea, vomiting, hypotension, and bradycardia.

It should be noted that *all* antidysrhythmic drugs are potentially prodysrhythmic. This is because of both the pharmacologic activity of the drug on the heart and the inherently unpredictable activity of a diseased heart, with or without the use of drugs. In some cases, life-threatening ventricular dysrhythmias can result from appropriate and skillful attempts at drug therapy to treat patients with heart disease. For these reasons, antidysrhythmic drug therapy is often initiated during continuous cardiac monitoring of the patient's heart rhythm in a hospital setting.

CLINICAL JUDGMENT [NURSING PROCESS]
Antidysrhythmics

Concept: Perfusion
- The passage of blood flow through the arteries and capillaries that deliver oxygen and nutrients to body cells

Recognize Cues [Assessment]
- Obtain health and drug histories. The history may include shortness of breath, heart palpitations, coughing, chest pain (type, duration, and severity), previous angina or cardiac dysrhythmias, and drugs the patient currently takes.
- Obtain baseline vital signs and electrocardiogram (ECG) for future comparisons.
- Monitor early cardiac enzyme results (aspartate aminotransferase [AST], lactate dehydrogenase [LDH], creatine phosphokinase) and cardiac-specific troponins for future comparisons.

Analyze Cues and Prioritize Hypothesis [Patient Problems]
- Decreased gas exchange
- Dysrhythmia
- Decreased tissue perfusion
- Hypoxemia
- Anxiety

Generate Solutions [Planning]
- The patient will be in normal sinus rhythm.
- The patient will comply with the antidysrhythmic drug regimen.

Take Action [Nursing Interventions]
- ⚡ Monitor vital signs because hypotension can occur.
- ⚡ Administer drug by IV push or bolus over a period of 2 to 3 minutes or as prescribed.
- ⚡ Monitor ECG for abnormal patterns, and report findings such as premature ventricular contractions (PVCs), increased PR and QT intervals, and/or widening of the QRS complex. Increased QT interval is a risk factor for *torsades de pointes*.

Patient Teaching
General
- Teach patients to take prescribed drugs as ordered because drug compliance is essential.
- Provide specific instructions for each drug (e.g., photosensitivity for amiodarone).

Side Effects
- ⚡ Tell patients to report side effects and adverse reactions to a health care provider, including dizziness, faintness, nausea, and vomiting.
- ⚡ Advise patients to avoid alcohol, caffeine, and tobacco. Alcohol can intensify a hypotensive reaction, caffeine increases catecholamine levels, and tobacco promotes vasoconstriction.

Evaluate Outcomes [Evaluation]
- Evaluate effectiveness of prescribed antidysrhythmics by comparing heart rates with baseline rates and assessing the patient's response to the drug.
- Report side effects and adverse reactions. Drug regimens may need to be adjusted, and drug-induced dysrhythmias may occur that can require discontinuation of a drug.

CLINICAL JUDGMENT UNFOLDING CASE STUDY

Question 1
Cognitive Skill: Recognize cues (enhanced hot spot). A 64-year-old female patient with a diagnosis of heart failure has been admitted to the emergency department. Her medication profile includes furosemide 20 mg/d, digoxin 0.25 mg/d, and potassium chloride (KCl) 20 mEq/d. The patient has experienced 3 days of flulike symptoms, including anorexia, nausea, vomiting, and diarrhea. Her fluid and food intake are diminished, and she refused to take the KCl, stating, "This drug makes me sick." The nurse's assessment includes:

- Normal skin turgor
- Complaints of stress
- Muscle weakness
- Pulse rate 90 beats per minute (bpm), irregular
- Hypoactive bowel sounds
- Complaints of feeling lightheaded
- Pedal pulses strong and palpable
- Patient alert and oriented

Highlight or place a check mark next to the patient's assessment data that needs an immediate response by the nurse.

Answers
- Normal skin turgor
- Complaints of stress
- **Muscle weakness**
- **Pulse rate 90 beats per minute (bpm), irregular**
- **Hypoactive bowel sounds**
- **Complaints of feeling lightheaded**
- Pedal pulses strong and palpable
- Patient alert and oriented

Rationale
The patient has refused to take her ordered dose of potassium chloride. Signs and symptoms of hypokalemia are flulike symptoms: anorexia, nausea, vomiting, and diarrhea.

References
Lewis's, et al (2020) *Medical sugical nursing*, 11th ed, Ch 16, Elsevier: MO.
McCuistion, et al (2023) *Pharmacology: A patient-centered nursing process approach*, 11th ed, Ch 40, Elsevier: MO.

Question 2
Cognitive Skill: Analyze cues (extended multiple response). A 64-year-old patient with a diagnosis of heart failure has been admitted to the emergency department. Her medication profile includes furosemide 20 mg/d, digoxin 0.25 mg/d, and potassium chloride (KCl) 20 mEq/d. The patient has experienced 3 days of flulike symptoms, including anorexia, nausea, vomiting, and diarrhea. Her fluid and food intake are diminished, and she refused to take the KCl, stating, "This drug makes me sick." The nurse's assessment includes:

- Normal skin turgor
- Complaints of stress
- Muscle weakness
- Pulse rate 90 beats per minute (bpm), irregular
- Hypoactive bowel sounds
- Complaints of feeling lightheaded
- Pedal pulses strong and palpable
- Patient alert and oriented

The nurse draws blood for STAT samples. Indicate which labs require priority intervention by placing an "X" next to the correct answers.

- Potassium (K) 3.0 mEq/L
- Sodium (Na) 135 mEq/L
- Creatinine 1.0 mg/dL
- Chloride (Cl) 90 mEq/L
- Blood urea nitrogen (BUN) 10 mg/dL
- Digoxin 3 ng/mL
- Hematocrit 38%
- B-type natriuretic peptide (BNP) 1000 pg/mL

Answers
- **X** a. Potassium (K) 3.0 mEq/L
- ____ b. Sodium (Na) 135 mEq/L
- ____ c. Creatinine 1.0 mg/dL
- **X** d. Chloride (Cl) 90 mEq/L
- ____ e. Blood urea nitrogen (BUN) 10 mg/dL
- **X** f. Digoxin 3 ng/mL
- ____ g. Hematocrit 38%
- **X** h. B-type natriuretic peptide (BNP) 1000 pg/mL

Rationale
The abnormal labs are potassium 3.0 mEq/L (normal 3.5–5.0 mEq/L; a low potassium level will exacerbate digoxin toxicity), chloride 90 mEq/L (normal 96–106 mEq/L; a low chloride level can cause vomiting), digoxin 3 ng/mL (normal 0.8–2.0 ng/mL; a high digoxin level indicates digoxin toxicity); BNP 1000 pg/mL (normal <100 pg/mL; a BNP >900 indicates heart failure).

References
Lewis's, et al (2020) *Medical surgical nursing*, 11th ed, Laboratory reference intervals/appendix c; Elsevier: MO.
McCuistion, et al (2023) *Pharmacology: A patient-centered nursing process approach*, 11th ed, Laboratory reference intervals; appendix C; Elsevier: MO.

Question 3
Cognitive Skill: Prioritize hypotheses (Cloze)
The 64-year-old female patient is admitted to the Telemetry Unit of the hospital for further care. She will receive cardiac monitoring, nausea medication, and sodium chloride 0.9% IV.

Based on the options below, which problems should the nurse consider priority?
The patient has a diagnosis of heart failure and is experiencing _____(1)_____.
The patient's history indicates a problem with _____(2)_____. The nurse recognizes the patient's lab indicates _____(3)_____.

Option 1	Option 2	Option 3
hyperkalemia	bowel incontinence	hyponatremia
hypokalemia	osteoarthritis	digoxin toxicity
hypotension	peptic ulcer disease	increased calcium levels
myocardial infarction	medication compliance	hypernatremia
tachycardia	high-protein diet	high blood sugar levels

Answers
The patient has a diagnosis of heart failure and is experiencing **hypokalemia** (1). The patient's history indicates a problem with **medication compliance** (2). The nurse recognizes the patient's digoxin lab indicates **digoxin toxicity** (3).

Rationale
In the state of hypokalemia, or low potassium, digitalis toxicity is worsened because digoxin normally binds to the ATPase pump on the same site as potassium. When potassium levels are low, digoxin can more easily bind to the ATPase pump, exerting the inhibitory effects.

CLINICAL JUDGMENT UNFOLDING CASE STUDY—CONT'D

References
Cummings E, Swoboda H: *Digoxin toxicity*, Treasure Island, 2021, StatPearls Publishing. www.ncbi.nlm.nih.gov/books/NBK470568

McCuistion, et al (2023) *Pharmacology: A patient centered nursing process approach*. 11th ed, Ch 40, Elsevier: MO.

Question 4
Cognitive Skill: Generate solutions (matrix). The provider orders much needed medications to be administered STAT. Use an X for the medication indicated for this patient that is most effective; if the medication is not recommended for this patient and could be harmful, place an X in the ineffective box. If the medication does not apply to this patient, place an X in the unrelated box.

Nursing Intervention	Effective	Ineffective
20 mEq (IV) potassium chloride over 4 h STAT		
400 mg single dose digoxin-immune fab IV STAT		
1 g ceftriaxone IV over 3 h STAT		
5 mcg/kg/min dopamine IV STAT		

Answers

Nursing Intervention	Effective	Ineffective
20 mEq (IV) potassium chloride over 4 h STAT	X	
400 mg single dose digoxin-immune fab IV STAT	X	
1 g ceftriaxone IV over 3 h STAT		X
5 mcg/kg/min dopamine IV STAT		X

Rationale
The antidote for digitalis toxicity is digoxin-immune fab. This agent binds with digoxin to form complex molecules that can be excreted in the urine, so digoxin is unable to bind at the cellular site of action. The patient has a low potassium level, which can add to the toxicity, so more potassium is being ordered. Ceftriaxone and dopamine are not indicated for this patient and are considered ineffective.

Reference
McCustion, et al (2023) *Pharmacology: A patient centered nursing process approach*. 11th ed, Ch 40, Elsevier: MO.

Question 5
Cognitive Skill: Generate solutions (extended multiple response). The patient is taking digoxin for heart failure and is experiencing digoxin toxicity and hypokalemia.

The nurse is instructing the patient about hypokalemia. Which of the following information is most important to prevent hypokalemia? (Select all that apply.)

Never skip your daily dose of potassium.
You do not need to report dizziness to your doctor.
Bananas and strawberries are high in potassium.
Weigh yourself daily.
Leg cramping is a sign of low potassium.
Drink 4 L of water each day.
Muscle weakness is a sign of low potassium..
It's OK to skip your potassium; just double the next dose.
Antacids can lower the amount of potassium in your blood if taken at the same time.

Answers
__X__ a. Never skip your daily dose of potassium.
____ b. You do not need to report dizziness to your doctor.
__X__ c. Bananas and strawberries are high in potassium.
__X__ d. Weigh yourself daily.
__X__ e. Leg cramping is a sign of low potassium.
____ f. Drink 4 L of water each day.
__X__ g. Muscle weakness is a sign of low potassium.
____ h. It's okay to skip your potassium; just double the next dose.
__X__ i. Antacids can lower the dose of potassium in your blood if taken at the same time.

Rationale
Hypokalemia can alter the resting membrane potential, which will cause a negative pressure within the cells and impaired muscle contraction. This change can affect the cardiac muscle. Hypokalemia also increases the risk for digoxin toxicity. It is important for the nurse to instruct the patient in how to avoid the risk of hypokalemia.

References
Lewis's, et al (2020) *Medical surgical nursing*, 11th ed, Ch 16, Elsevier: MO.
McCuistion, et al (2023) *Pharmacology: A patient centered nursing process approach*. 11th ed, Ch 40, Elsevier: MO.

Question 6
Cognitive Skills: Evaluate outcomes (extended drag and drop). In anticipation of discharge, the nurse is preparing to instruct the patient concerning furosemide, digoxin, and signs and symptoms of digoxin toxicity.

Indicate which nursing response listed in the far-left column is appropriate for the patient's questions by placing the number of the question under the appropriate nurse's response.

Nurse's Responses	Patient Questions	Appropriate Nurse's Response for Each Patient Question
1. Your digoxin dose will remain as 0.25 mg/d.	Why is the doctor putting me back on digoxin after experiencing toxicity?	
2. Can you explain how digoxin works on your heart to improve the heart failure?	I do not know but would like to learn.	
3. Name a side effect of digoxin toxicity.	The only side effects I know are nausea, vomiting, and diarrhea.	
4. You must follow your provider's orders for bloodwork.	Why must I have my blood drawn?	
5. You will have to take your pulse rate before taking digoxin. I will be happy to show you how it is done.	Why must I count my pulse rate before taking digoxin?	
6. It may affect your vision and can cause blurred or yellow vision.		

Continued

CLINICAL JUDGMENT UNFOLDING CASE STUDY—CONT'D

Nurse's Responses	Patient Questions	Appropriate Nurse's Response for Each Patient Question	Nurse's Responses	Patient Questions	Appropriate Nurse's Response for each patient question
7. Digoxin increases the force of your heart's contraction and decreases the heart rate. It increases your cardiac output.			2. Can you explain how digoxin works on your heart to improve heart failure?	I do not know but would like to learn.	7. Digoxin increases the force of your heart's contraction and decreases the heart rate. It increases your cardiac output.
8. The provider will request periodic lab draws to ensure your digoxin level and potassium level are within normal limits to prevent digoxin toxicity and hypokalemia.			3. Name a side effect of digoxin toxicity.	The only side effects I know are nausea, vomiting, and diarrhea.	6. It may affect your vision and can cause blurred or yellow vision.
9. You received digoxin-immune fab IV, which lowers the toxic level of digoxin in the blood. Your digoxin level this morning is in the normal range (1.8 ng/mL).			4. You must follow your provider's orders for bloodwork.	Why must I have my blood drawn?	8. The provider will request periodic lab draws to ensure your digoxin level and potassium level are within normal limits to prevent digoxin toxicity and hypokalemia.
10. If your pulse rate is less than 60 beats per minute, you must hold digoxin and notify your health provider.			5. You will have to take your pulse rate before taking digoxin. I will be happy to show you how it is done.	Why must I count my pulse rate before taking digoxin?	10. If your pulse is less than 60 beats per minute, you must hold digoxin and notify your health provider.

Answers

Nurse's Responses	Patient Questions	Appropriate Nurse's Response for each patient question
1. Your digoxin dose will remain as 0.25 mg/d.	Why is the doctor putting me back on digoxin after experiencing toxicity?	9. You received digoxin-immune fab IV, which lowers the toxic level of digoxin in the blood. Your digoxin level this morning is in the normal range (1.8 ng/mL).

Rationale
The nurse is instructing the client in medication compliance. Digoxin affects the heart by increasing the force of the contraction and decreasing the heart rate. The nurse explains the severity of digoxin toxicity. This is why she received digoxin-immune fab IV. It is most important for the patient to be compliant with all of her health care provider–prescribed medications. Also, the patient must know the signs and symptoms of digoxin toxicity to report to the provider. It is important for the patient to be taught how to count the pulse and, if it is under 60 bpm, not to take the digoxin and to notify the provider.

References
McCuistion, et al (2023) *Pharmacology: A patient centered nursing process approach*, 11th ed, Ch 40; Elsevier: MO.
Lewis's, et al (2020) *Medical surgical nursing*, 11th ed, Ch 34, Elsevier: MO.

REVIEW QUESTIONS

1. The patient is receiving digoxin for treatment of heart failure. Which finding would suggest to the nurse that the heart failure is improving?
   a. Pale and cool extremities
   b. Absence of peripheral edema
   c. Urine output of 60 mL every 4 hours
   d. Complaints of increasing dyspnea

2. The patient's serum digoxin level is 3.0 ng/mL. What does the nurse know about this serum digoxin level?
   a. It is in the high (elevated) range.
   b. It is in the low (decreased) range.
   c. It is within the normal range.
   d. It is in the low-average range.

3. The nurse is assessing a patient for possible evidence of digitalis toxicity. Which of these is included in the signs and symptoms for digitalis toxicity?
   a. Apical pulse rate of 100 beats/min
   b. Apical pulse of 72 beats/min with an irregular rate
   c. Apical pulse of 90 beats/min with an irregular rate
   d. Apical pulse of 48 beats/min with an irregular rate

4. A patient is taking a potassium-depleting diuretic and digoxin. The nurse expects that a low potassium level (hypokalemia) could have what effect on digoxin?
   a. Increases serum digoxin sensitivity level
   b. Decreases serum digoxin sensitivity level
   c. No effect on serum digoxin sensitivity level
   d. Causes a low-average serum digoxin sensitivity level

5. A patient takes an initial dose of a nitrate. Which symptom(s) will the nurse expect to occur?
   a. Nausea and vomiting
   b. Headaches
   c. Stomach cramps
   d. Irregular pulse rate

6. A patient is prescribed a beta-blocker. Beta-blockers are as effective as antianginals because they do what?
   a. Increase oxygen to the systemic circulation
   b. Maintain heart rate and blood pressure
   c. Decrease heart rate and decrease myocardial contractility
   d. Decrease heart rate and increase myocardial contractility

7. The health care provider is planning to discontinue a patient's beta-blocker. Which instruction will the nurse give the patient regarding the beta-blocker?
   a. The beta-blocker should be abruptly stopped when another cardiac drug is prescribed.
   b. The beta-blocker should not be abruptly stopped; the dose should be tapered down.
   c. The beta-blocker dose should be maintained while taking another antianginal drug.
   d. Half the beta-blocker dose should be taken for the next several weeks.

8. The beta-blocker acebutolol is prescribed for dysrhythmias. What is the primary purpose of the drug?
   a. Increase $beta_1$ and $beta_2$ receptors in cardiac tissues
   b. Increase the flow of oxygen to cardiac tissues
   c. Block $beta_1$-adrenergic receptors in cardiac tissues
   d. Block $beta_2$-adrenergic receptors in cardiac tissues

9. A patient who has angina is prescribed nitroglycerin. Which are appropriate nursing interventions for nitroglycerin? **Select all that apply**.
   a. Have the patient sit or lie down when taking a nitroglycerin sublingual tablet.
   b. Teach the patient who has taken nitroglycerin to call 911 if chest pain persists.
   c. Apply the nitroglycerin patch to a hairy area to protect skin from burning.
   d. Call the health care provider after taking five tablets if chest pain persists.
   e. Warn the patient against ingesting alcohol while taking nitroglycerin.
   f. Advise the patient not to drink water before taking nitroglycerin.

41

Diuretics

http://evolve.elsevier.com/McCuistion/pharmacology

OBJECTIVES

- Explain the use of diuretics.
- Describe the use and drug interactions of thiazides.
- Discuss the use and drug interactions of loop diuretics.
- Summarize usage considerations of osmotic diuretics and carbonic anhydrase inhibitors.
- Summarize usage considerations of potassium-sparing diuretics.

OUTLINE

Diuretics, 524
    Physiology, 524
    Antihypertensive Effect, 524
    Diuretic Categories, 524
Thiazides and Thiazide-Like Diuretics, 525
    Overview, 525
    Pharmacology, 527
Loop Diuretics, 528
    Overview, 528

    Pharmacology, 529
Osmotic Diuretics and Carbonic Anhydrase Inhibitors, 532
    Osmotic Diuretics, 532
    Carbonic Anhydrase Inhibitors, 532
Potassium-Sparing Diuretics, 532
    Overview, 532
    Side Effects and Adverse Reactions, 532
Clinical Judgment Case Study, 534
Review Questions, 535

DIURETICS

Diuretics are used for two main purposes: to decrease hypertension (lower blood pressure) and to decrease edema, typically peripheral and pulmonary, in heart failure (HF) and renal or liver disorders. Hypertension is an elevated blood pressure greater than 120/80 mm Hg. Diuretics discussed in this chapter are used either alone or in combination to decrease blood pressure and edema.

Diuretics produce increased urine flow, or diuresis, by inhibiting sodium and water reabsorption from the kidney tubules. Most sodium and water reabsorption occurs throughout the renal tubular segments (proximal, loop of Henle [descending loop and ascending loop], and collecting tubule). Diuretics can affect one or more segments of the renal tubules. Fig. 41.1 illustrates the renal tubule along with the normal process of water and electrolyte reabsorption and diuretic effects on the tubules.

Physiology

Every 1.5 hours, the total volume of the body's extracellular fluid (ECF) goes through the kidneys (glomeruli) for cleansing; this is the first process for urine formation. Small particles such as electrolytes, drugs, glucose, and waste products from protein metabolism are filtered in the glomeruli. Larger products such as protein and blood cells are not filtered with normal renal function, and they remain in the circulation. Sodium and water are the largest filtrate substances.

Normally, 99% of the filtered sodium that passes through the glomeruli is reabsorbed; 50% to 55% of sodium reabsorption occurs in the proximal tubules, 35% to 40% occurs in the loop of Henle, 5% to 10% occurs in the distal tubules, and less than 3% occurs in the collecting tubules. Diuretics that act on the tubules closest to the glomeruli have the greatest effect in causing natriuresis, sodium loss in the urine. A classic example is the osmotic diuretic mannitol. The diuretic effect depends on the drug reaching the kidneys and its concentration in the renal tubules.

Antihypertensive Effect

Diuretics have an antihypertensive effect because they promote sodium and water loss by blocking sodium and chloride reabsorption. This causes a decrease in fluid volume, which lowers blood pressure. With fluid loss, edema—fluid retention in body tissues—should decrease, but if sodium is retained, water is also retained, and blood pressure increases.

Many diuretics cause the loss of other electrolytes, including potassium, magnesium, chloride, and bicarbonate. The diuretics that promote potassium excretion are classified as potassium-wasting diuretics, and those that promote potassium retention are called potassium-sparing diuretics.

Diuretic Categories

The following five categories of diuretics are effective in removing water and sodium:
- Thiazide and thiazide-like diuretics
- Loop diuretics
- Osmotic diuretics
- Carbonic anhydrase inhibitors
- Potassium-sparing diuretics

Thiazide, loop, and potassium-sparing diuretics are most frequently prescribed for hypertension and for edema associated with HF. Except for those in the potassium-sparing group, all diuretics are potassium-wasting.

Fig. 41.1 **Diuretics act on different segments of the renal tubule.** Osmotic, mercurial, and carbonic anhydrase inhibitor diuretics affect the proximal tubule; loop diuretics affect the loop of Henle; thiazides affect the distal tubule; and potassium-sparing diuretics act primarily on the collecting tubules. *ADH*, Antidiuretic hormone; H_2O, water; K^+, potassium; Na^+, sodium.

Combination diuretics that contain both potassium-wasting and potassium-sparing drugs have been marketed primarily for the treatment of hypertension. Combinations have an additive effect in reducing blood pressure and are discussed in more detail in the Potassium-Sparing Diuretics section later in this chapter. Chapter 39 takes a closer look at the combinations of antihypertensive agents with hydrochlorothiazide.

THIAZIDES AND THIAZIDE-LIKE DIURETICS

Overview

Chlorothiazide was the first thiazide marketed, and hydrochlorothiazide was the second. There are numerous thiazide and thiazide-like preparations. Thiazides act on the distal convoluted renal tubule, beyond the loop of Henle, to promote sodium, chloride, and water excretion. Thiazides are used to treat hypertension and peripheral edema. They are not effective for immediate diuresis and should not be used to promote fluid loss in patients with severe renal dysfunction. Table 41.1 lists thiazide and thiazide-like diuretics and their dosages, uses, and considerations. Drug dosages for hypertension and edema are similar.

Thiazide diuretics are used primarily for patients with normal renal function. If the patient has a renal disorder and creatinine clearance is less than 30 mL/min, the effectiveness of the thiazide diuretic is greatly decreased. Thiazides cause a loss of sodium, potassium, and magnesium, but they promote calcium reabsorption. Hypercalcemia (calcium excess) may result, and the condition can be hazardous to the patient who is digitalized or has cancer that causes hypercalcemia. Thiazides affect glucose tolerance, so hyperglycemia can also occur. Thiazides should be used cautiously in patients with diabetes mellitus. Laboratory test results, such as electrolytes and glucose, need to be monitored.

Hydrochlorothiazide has been combined with selected angiotensin-converting enzyme (ACE) inhibitors, beta-blockers, alpha-blockers, angiotensin II blockers, and centrally acting sympatholytics to control hypertension. Prototype Drug Chart: Hydrochlorothiazide outlines the pharmacologic data for hydrochlorothiazide.

TABLE 41.1 Diuretics

Drug	Route and Dosage	Uses and Considerations
Thiazides		
Chlorothiazide	Edema: A: PO: 500–1000 mg/d in 1–2 divided doses; max: 1 g/d A: IV: 500–1000 mg qd/bid in 1–2 divided doses given slowly or as an infusion; max: 2 g/d	For hypertension and edema. May cause headache, dizziness, blurred vision, orthostatic hypotension, anorexia, nausea, vomiting, diarrhea, constipation, hypokalemia, hypomagnesemia, hyponatremia, hypochloremia, hypercholesterolemia, hypercalcemia, hyperglycemia, hyperuricemia, weakness, paresthesia, muscle cramps, and erectile dysfunction. PB: UK; t½: 45–120 min
Hydrochlorothiazide	See Prototype Drug Chart: Hydrochlorothiazide	
Thiazide-Like Diuretics		
Chlorthalidone	Edema: A: PO: Initially 50–100 mg/d or 100 qod; maint: 50–200 mg/d; max: 200 mg/d	For hypertension and edema. May cause dizziness, headache, orthostatic hypotension, anorexia, nausea, vomiting, diarrhea, constipation, hypomagnesemia, hyponatremia, hypokalemia, hypochloremia, hypercalcemia, hyperglycemia, hyperuricemia, and hypercholesterolemia. PB: 75%; t½: 40–60 h
Indapamide	HF: A: PO: Initially 2.5 mg/d; max: 5 mg/d	For hypertension and HF. May cause dizziness, headache, orthostatic hypotension, dry mouth, abdominal pain, nausea, vomiting, diarrhea, constipation, hypercholesterolemia, hypokalemia, hyperglycemia, hypochloremia, hyponatremia, hypercalcemia, hyperuricemia, and erectile dysfunction. PB: 71%–79%; t½: 14–18 h
Metolazone	Edema: A: PO: 5–20 mg/d; max: 20 mg/d	For hypertension and edema. May cause blurred vision, orthostatic hypotension, anorexia, nausea, vomiting, diarrhea, constipation, hypomagnesemia, hypochloremia, hypokalemia, hypophosphatemia, hyponatremia, hypercalcemia, hyperuricemia, hypovolemia, weakness, and hyperglycemia. PB: 33%; t½: 14 h

A, Adult; *bid*, twice a day; *d*, day; *HF*, heart failure; *h*, hour; *IV*, intravenous; *maint*, maintenance; *max*, maximum; *min*, minute; *PB*, protein binding; *PO*, by mouth; *qd*, every day; *qod*, every other day; *t½*, half-life; *UK*, unknown.

PROTOTYPE DRUG CHART
Hydrochlorothiazide

Drug Class	Dosage
Thiazide diuretic	Peripheral edema: A: PO: 12.5–100 mg/d in single or divided doses; max: 100 mg/d

Contraindications	Drug-Lab-Food Interactions
Anuria, hypersensitivity *Caution:* Hepatic/renal dysfunction, diabetes mellitus, gout, asthma, hypotension, electrolyte imbalance, hypovolemia, hypokalemia, hyponatremia, hypomagnesemia, hypercalcemia, hypochloremia, hyperuricemia, hyperglycemia, metabolic alkalosis, older adults, breast-feeding, pregnancy	Drug: Increased digitalis toxicity with digitalis if hypokalemia is present; increased renal toxicity with aspirin; increased potassium loss with steroids; decreased effect of antidiabetics; decreased thiazide absorption and effects with NSAIDs, cholestyramine, and colestipol Lab: Increased serum calcium, glucose, uric acid; decreased serum potassium, sodium, magnesium

Pharmacokinetics	Pharmacodynamics
Absorption: Readily absorbed from GI tract Distribution: PB: 40%–68% Metabolism: t½: 5.6–14.8 h Excretion: In urine	PO: Onset: 2 h Peak: 4 h Duration: 6–12 h

PROTOTYPE DRUG CHART—CONT'D
Hydrochlorothiazide

Therapeutic Effects/Uses

To increase urine output and to treat hypertension and peripheral edema due to HF, nephrotic syndrome, and ascites

Mechanism of Action: Action is on the renal distal tubules, promoting sodium, potassium, and water excretion and decreasing preload and cardiac output; also decreases edema; acts on arterioles and causes vasodilation, thus decreasing blood pressure

Side Effects	Adverse Reactions
Dizziness, headache, weakness, blurred vision, photosensitivity, restlessness, anorexia, nausea, abdominal cramps, vomiting, diarrhea, constipation, rash, muscle cramps, paresthesias, polyuria, erectile dysfunction	Ocular hypertension, orthostatic hypotension, hyponatremia, hypomagnesemia, hypochloremia, hyperglycemia, hypercalcemia, hyperuricemia, hypercholesterolemia, hypertriglyceridemia, metabolic alkalosis, pulmonary edema, gout *Life threatening*: Hypokalemia, aplastic anemia, leukopenia, hemolytic anemia, thrombocytopenia, agranulocytosis, renal failure, Stevens-Johnson syndrome

A, Adult; *h*, hour; *HF*, heart failure; *max*, maximum; *NSAID*, nonsteroidal antiinflammatory drug; *PB*, protein binding; *PO*, by mouth; *t½*, half-life.

TABLE 41.2 Serum Chemistry Abnormalities Associated With Thiazides

Serum Chemistry Parameter	Abnormal Results
Electrolytes, Normal Levels	
Potassium, 3.5–5.0 mEq/L	Hypokalemia (low serum potassium); potassium is excreted from the distal renal tubule.
Magnesium, 1.5–2.5 mEq/L	Hypomagnesemia (low serum magnesium); potassium and sodium loss prompt magnesium loss.
Calcium, 8.6–10.2 mg/dL	Hypercalcemia (elevated serum calcium); thiazides may block calcium excretion.
Chloride, 96–106 mEq/L	Hypochloremia (low serum chloride); sodium and potassium losses produce chloride loss.
Bicarbonate, 24–28 mEq/L	Minimal bicarbonate loss occurs from the proximal tubule.
Uric acid, 2.8–8.0 mg/dL	Hyperuricemia (elevated uric acid); thiazides can block uric acid excretion.
Blood glucose, 70–99 mg/dL	Hyperglycemia (increased blood glucose); thiazides increase fasting blood glucose levels and those of the prediabetic state.
Blood Lipids Cholesterol: <200 mg/dL LDL: <100 mg/dL Triglyceride: <150 mg/dL	Elevated cholesterol, LDL, and triglycerides

LDL, Low-density lipoprotein.

Pharmacology

Pharmacokinetics

Thiazides are well absorbed from the gastrointestinal (GI) tract. Hydrochlorothiazide has moderate protein-binding power. The half-life of the thiazide drugs is longer than that of the loop diuretics. For this reason, thiazides should be administered in the morning to avoid nocturia (nighttime urination) and sleep interruption.

Pharmacodynamics

Thiazides act directly on arterioles to cause vasodilation, which can lower blood pressure. Other action includes the promotion of sodium chloride and water excretion, resulting in a decrease in vascular fluid volume and a concomitant decrease in cardiac output and blood pressure. The onset of action of hydrochlorothiazide occurs within 2 hours. Peak concentration times are long (4 hours).

Side Effects and Adverse Reactions

Side effects and adverse reactions of thiazides include electrolyte imbalances (hypokalemia, hypercalcemia and hypomagnesemia), hyperglycemia (elevated blood glucose), hyperuricemia (elevated serum uric acid level), and hypercholesterolemia (elevated blood cholesterol level). Signs and symptoms of hypokalemia should be assessed, and serum potassium levels must be closely monitored. Potassium supplements are frequently needed. Serum calcium and uric acid levels should be checked because thiazides block calcium and uric acid excretion. Thiazides affect the metabolism of carbohydrates, and hyperglycemia can result, especially in patients with high to high-normal blood glucose levels. Thiazides can increase serum cholesterol, low-density lipoprotein, and triglyceride levels. A drug may be ordered to lower blood lipids. Other side effects include dizziness, headache, nausea, vomiting, constipation, and blood dyscrasias (rare). Table 41.2 summarizes the serum chemistry abnormalities that can occur with thiazide use.

Contraindications

Thiazides are contraindicated for use in renal failure. Symptoms of severe kidney impairment or shutdown include oliguria, a marked decrease in urine output; elevated blood urea nitrogen (BUN); and elevated serum creatinine.

Drug Interactions

Of the numerous thiazide drug interactions, the most serious occurs with digoxin. Thiazides can cause hypokalemia, which enhances the action of digoxin, and digitalis toxicity can occur. Potassium supplements are frequently prescribed, and serum potassium levels are monitored. Thiazides also induce hypercalcemia, which enhances the action of digoxin, resulting in possible digitalis toxicity. Signs and symptoms of digitalis toxicity—bradycardia, nausea, vomiting, and visual changes—should be reported. Thiazides enhance the action of lithium, and lithium toxicity can occur. Thiazides potentiate the action of other antihypertensive drugs, which may be used to advantage in combination drug therapy for hypertension.

LOOP DIURETICS

Overview

The loop diuretics act on the thick ascending loop of Henle to inhibit chloride transport of sodium into the circulation and inhibit passive reabsorption of sodium. Sodium and water are lost, together with potassium, calcium, and magnesium. Loop diuretics can affect blood glucose and can increase uric acid levels. Drugs in this group are extremely potent and cause marked depletion of water and electrolytes. The effects of loop diuretics are dose-related; that is, increasing the dose increases the effect and response of the drug. More potent than thiazides for promoting diuresis, inhibiting reabsorption of sodium two to three times more effectively, loop diuretics are less effective as antihypertensive agents.

COMPLEMENTARY AND ALTERNATIVE THERAPIES

Diuretics

- When taken with a potassium-wasting diuretic such as a thiazide, aloe can decrease the serum potassium level, thereby causing hypokalemia.
- Ginkgo may increase blood pressure when taken with a thiazide diuretic.
- Licorice can increase potassium loss, leading to hypokalemia.
- Hawthorn may potentiate hypotension.

CLINICAL JUDGMENT [NURSING PROCESS]

Diuretics: Thiazides

Concept: Elimination
- Excretion of body waste products through the urinary system

Recognize Cues [Assessment]
- Assess vital signs, weight, urine output, and serum chemistry values (electrolytes, glucose, uric acid) for baseline levels.
- Check peripheral extremities for the presence of edema. Note pitting edema.
- Obtain a history of drugs and herbal supplements taken daily. Review for drugs and herbs that may cause a drug interaction (digoxin, corticosteroids, antidiabetics, ginkgo, licorice).

Analyze Cues and Prioritize Hypothesis [Patient Problems]
- Disrupted fluid and electrolyte imbalance
- Fluid overload
- Hypokalemia
- Hypernatremia
- Elimination

Generate Solutions [Planning]
- The patient's blood pressure will be decreased or will return to a normal value.
- The patient's edema will be decreased.
- The patient's serum chemistry levels will remain within normal ranges.

Take Action [Nursing Interventions]
- ⚡ Monitor vital signs and serum electrolytes, especially potassium, glucose, uric acid, and cholesterol levels. Report changes. If a patient is taking digoxin and hypokalemia occurs, digitalis toxicity frequently results.
- Observe for signs and symptoms of hypokalemia such as muscle weakness, leg cramps, and cardiac dysrhythmias.
- Monitor the patient's weight at the same time every day with the same type of clothing. A weight gain of 2.2 lb is equivalent to 1 L of body fluids.
- Note urine output to determine fluid loss or retention.
- Observe for signs and symptoms of hyperglycemia.

Patient Teaching
General
- Emphasize the need for adherence to the therapy plan. The patient may not feel better for some time or may not feel worse if treatment is missed or discontinued.
- Suggest that the patient take the drug early in the morning to avoid sleep disturbance resulting from nocturia.
- Instruct patients to keep drugs out of reach of small children. Request a childproof bottle.
- Inform patients that certain herbal products may interact with thiazide diuretics.

Self-Administration
- Instruct patients or family members on how to take blood pressure and record daily results.

Side Effects
- ⚡ Instruct patients to slowly change positions from lying to standing because dizziness may occur as a result of orthostatic (postural) hypotension.
- Advise patients who may be prediabetic to have blood glucose checked periodically because large doses of hydrochlorothiazide increase blood glucose levels.
- Suggest that patients use sunblock when in direct sunlight to prevent photosensitivity.

Diet
- Teach patients to eat foods rich in potassium (fruits, fruit juices, and vegetables). Potassium supplements may be ordered.
- Instruct patients to take drugs with food to avoid gastrointestinal (GI) upset (anorexia, nausea, vomiting, diarrhea).

Evaluate Outcomes [Evaluation]
- Evaluate the effectiveness of drug therapy. The patient's blood pressure and edema will be reduced, and blood chemistry will remain within normal range.
- Determine an absence of side effects and adverse reactions to therapy.

Loop diuretics should not be prescribed if a thiazide could alleviate body fluid excess. If furosemide alone is not effective in removing body fluid, a thiazide may be added. Furosemide is usually administered as an oral dose in the morning or intravenously when the patient's condition warrants immediate removal of body fluid; for example, in cases of acute HF or pulmonary edema.

Loop diuretics can increase renal blood flow by up to 40%. Furosemide is a frequently prescribed diuretic for patients whose creatinine clearance is less than 30 mL/min and for those with end-stage renal disease. This group of diuretics causes excretion of calcium, unlike thiazides, which inhibit calcium loss.

The first loop diuretic marketed was ethacrynic acid, followed by furosemide and then bumetanide, which is more potent than furosemide on a milligram-for-milligram basis. Furosemide and bumetanide are derivatives of sulfonamides. Ethacrynic acid, a phenoxyacetic acid derivative, is a seldom-chosen loop diuretic. It is usually reserved for patients who are allergic to sulfa drugs. Prototype Drug Chart: Furosemide lists the drug data for the loop diuretic furosemide.

Pharmacology
Pharmacokinetics
Loop diuretics are rapidly absorbed by the GI tract. These drugs are highly protein bound with half-lives that vary from 0.5 to 2 hours. Loop diuretics compete for protein-binding sites with other highly protein-bound drugs.

Pharmacodynamics
Loop diuretics have a great saluretic (sodium chloride–losing) or natriuretic (sodium-losing) effect and can cause rapid diuresis, decreasing vascular fluid volume and causing a decrease in cardiac output and blood pressure. Because furosemide is more potent than thiazide diuretics, it causes a vasodilatory effect; thus renal blood flow increases before diuresis. Furosemide is used when other conservative measures, such as sodium restriction and use of less potent diuretics, fail. The oral dose of furosemide is usually twice that of an intravenous (IV) dose.

The onset of action of loop diuretics occurs within 30 to 60 minutes. The onset of action for IV furosemide is 5 minutes. The duration of action is shorter than that of the thiazides.

PROTOTYPE DRUG CHART
Furosemide

Drug Class	Dosage
Loop diuretic	Peripheral edema: A: PO: Initially 20–80 mg single dose/d; may repeat or increase by 20–40 mg/dose q6–8 h PRN; *maint:* 40–240 mg/d; *max:* 600 mg/d A: IM/IV: Initially 20–40 mg; May repeat or increase by 20 mg q2h PRN; *maint:* 40–240 mg/d; *max:* 6 g/d IV

Contraindications	Drug-Lab-Food Interactions
Hypersensitivity, hepatic disease, ascites, anuria *Caution:* HF, electrolyte imbalance, diabetes mellitus, hyperglycemia, diarrhea, orthostatic hypotension, acute myocardial infarction, gout, hearing impairment, hypovolemia, dehydration, hyperuricemia, oliguria, renal/hepatic disease, acid-base imbalance, metabolic alkalosis, thyroid disease, older adults, pregnancy, breastfeeding, children	Drug: Increased orthostatic hypotension with alcohol; increased ototoxicity and nephrotoxicity with aminoglycosides; increased bleeding with anticoagulants; increased potassium loss with steroids, amphotericin B; increased digitalis toxicity and cardiac dysrhythmias with digoxin and hypokalemia; increased lithium toxicity; increased amphotericin B nephrotoxicity Food: Licorice may increase potassium loss. Lab: Increased BUN, blood-urine glucose, serum uric acid, ammonia; decreased potassium, sodium, calcium, magnesium, chloride serum levels Complementary and Alternative Therapies: Hawthorn may potentiate hypotension, and ginseng may decrease the action of loop diuretics.

Pharmacokinetics	Pharmacodynamics
Absorption: PO: Absorbed erratically from oral dose Distribution: PB: 91%–99% Metabolism: t½: 0.5–2 h Excretion: In urine, some in feces; crosses the placenta	PO: Onset: 30–60 min Peak: 1–2 h Duration: 6–8 h IV: Onset: 5 min Peak: 20–30 min Duration: 2 h

Therapeutic Effects/Uses
To treat edema due to HF, renal dysfunction, hepatic cirrhosis, and nephrotic syndrome, and to treat hypertension
Mechanism of Action: Inhibition of sodium and water reabsorption from loop of Henle and distal renal tubules; increases excretion of potassium, chloride, magnesium, ammonium, phosphate, and calcium

Side Effects	Adverse Reactions
Dizziness, headache, weakness, blurred vision, photosensitivity, tinnitus, anorexia, abdominal cramps, nausea, vomiting, diarrhea, constipation, rash, muscle cramps, paresthesias, restlessness, polyuria, dehydration, injection-site reaction	Orthostatic hypotension, hearing loss, hypokalemia, hyponatremia, hypocalcemia, hypomagnesemia, hypochloremia, metabolic alkalosis, hypovolemia, hyperglycemia, hyperuricemia, hypertriglyceridemia, hypercholesterolemia, diabetes mellitus, thromboembolism, renal/hepatic impairment, gout *Life threatening:* Aplastic anemia, hemolytic anemia, eosinophilia, leukopenia, anemia, thrombocytopenia, agranulocytosis, Stevens-Johnson syndrome

A, Adult; *d*, day; *h*, hour; *HF*, heart failure; *IM*, intramuscular; *IV*, intravenous; *maint*, maintenance; *max*, maximum; *min*, minutes; *PB*, protein binding; *PO*, by mouth; *t½*, half-life.

Side Effects and Adverse Reactions

The most common side effects of loop diuretics are fluid and electrolyte imbalances such as hypokalemia, hyponatremia, hypocalcemia, hypomagnesemia, and hypochloremia. Hypochloremic metabolic alkalosis may result, which can worsen hypokalemia, and orthostatic hypotension can occur. Thrombocytopenia, skin disturbances, and transient hearing loss are rarely seen. Table 41.3 lists the physiologic and laboratory changes associated with loop diuretics.

Drug Interactions

The major drug interaction is with digitalis preparations. If the patient takes digoxin with a loop diuretic, digitalis toxicity can result. Hypokalemia enhances the action of digoxin and increases the risk for digitalis toxicity. The patient needs potassium replacement with food or supplements. Serum potassium levels should be closely monitored, especially when the patient is taking high dosages of loop diuretics. Table 41.4 lists the data for the four loop diuretics.

TABLE 41.3 Physiologic and Laboratory Changes Associated With Loop Diuretics

Physiologic/Laboratory Changes	Possible Effects of Loop (High-Ceiling) Diuretics
Physiologic Changes	
Hypotension	Postural (orthostatic) hypotension can result because of ECFV deficit.
Ototoxicity	Hearing impairment, although rare, may occur. It is more common with use of ethacrynic acid. Diuretics in other categories are not considered ototoxic. *Caution:* Avoid taking a loop diuretic with a drug that can be ototoxic, such as an aminoglycoside.
Skin disturbances	Pruritus, urticaria, exfoliative dermatitis, and purpura may occur in some persons allergic to the drug or when taking a loop diuretic in high doses over a long period.
Photosensitivity	When exposed to sun or a sunlamp for a prolonged time, severe sunburn could result. Patient should use sunblock and avoid long sun exposures.
Hypovolemia	Excess extracellular fluid is lost through increased urine excretion.
Laboratory Changes	
Hypokalemia, hypomagnesemia, hyponatremia, hypocalcemia, hypochloremia	Potassium, magnesium, sodium, calcium, and chloride are lost from the body from increased urine excretion. Chloride, an anion, is attached to the cations potassium and sodium; thus chloride is lost along with potassium and sodium.
Hyperglycemia	Increased glycogenolysis may contribute to elevated blood glucose level. Patients with diabetes should closely monitor blood glucose levels when taking a loop diuretic.
Hyperuricemia	Elevated uric acid levels are common in patients susceptible to gout.
Elevated BUN and creatinine	These elevations may result from ECFV loss. Hemoconcentration can cause elevated BUN and creatinine levels, which are reversible when fluid volume returns to normal levels.
Thrombocytopenia, leukopenia	Decreases in platelet and white blood cell counts are rare, but they should be closely monitored.
Elevated lipids	Loop diuretics can decrease HDL and increase LDL. Patients with elevated cholesterol levels should have their HDL and LDL levels checked. Regardless of the lipid effects, loop diuretics are useful for patients with serious fluid retention caused by a cardiac condition such as HF.

BUN, Blood urea nitrogen; *ECFV,* extracellular fluid volume; *HDL,* high-density lipoprotein; *HF,* heart failure; *LDL,* low-density lipoprotein.

TABLE 41.4 Diuretics: Loop, Osmotics, and Carbonic Anhydrase Inhibitors

Drug	Route and Dosage	Uses and Considerations
Loop		
Bumetanide	Edema: A: PO: Initially 0.5–1 mg/d; *maint:* 0.5–2 mg/d; *max:* 10 mg/d A: IM/IV: Initially 0.5–1 mg/dose slowly over 1–2 min when IVP; may give a second and third dose q2–3h PRN; *max:* 10 mg/d	For edema. May cause dizziness, headache, weakness, muscle cramps, abdominal pain, nausea, vomiting, diarrhea, orthostatic hypotension, hypokalemia, hyponatremia, hypochloremia, hypocalcemia, hypovolemia, hyperglycemia, hyperuricemia, polyuria, dehydration, metabolic alkalosis, and azotemia. PB: 96%; *t½:* 1–1.5 h
Ethacrynic acid	Pulmonary edema: A: IV: Initially 50 mg or 0.5–1 mg/kg slowly over several min, may repeat after 1 h at new injection site; *max:* 100 mg/dose	For pulmonary and peripheral edema. May cause headache, blurred vision, hearing loss, tinnitus, anorexia, nausea, vomiting, diarrhea, fatigue, orthostatic hypotension, hyperglycemia, hyperuricemia, hypochloremia, hypokalemia, hypomagnesemia, hyponatremia, hypocalcemia, metabolic alkalosis, and injection-site reaction. PB: 95%; *t½:* 2–4 h
Furosemide	See Prototype Drug Chart: Furosemide	

TABLE 41.4 Diuretics: Loop, Osmotics, and Carbonic Anhydrase Inhibitors—cont'd

Drug	Route and Dosage	Uses and Considerations
Torsemide	Hypertension: A: PO: Initially: 5 mg/d; *max*: 10 mg/d	For hypertension, edema, and ascites. May cause photosensitivity, tinnitus, hearing loss, abdominal pain, anorexia, orthostatic hypotension, hypokalemia, hypochloremia, hypocalcemia, hyponatremia, hypomagnesemia, frequency, polyuria, hypovolemia, dehydration, metabolic alkalosis, paresthesia, hyperglycemia, and hyperuricemia. PB: 99%; *t½*: 3.5 h
Osmotics		
Mannitol	Cerebral edema/ICP: A: IV: 0.25–2 g/kg/dose over 30–60 min; may repeat q6–8h PRN	For edema, cerebral edema, IOP, increased ICP, acute renal failure, and excretion of toxic substances. May cause dizziness, headache, blurred vision, cough, hemoptysis, nausea, vomiting, tachycardia, hypo/hypertension, weakness, arthralgia, hypo/hypernatremia, hypo/hyperkalemia, hypovolemia, polyuria, dehydration, metabolic acidosis/alkalosis, and injection-site reaction. PB: UK; *t½*: 30–150 min
Carbonic Anhydrase Inhibitors		
Acetazolamide	Edema: A: PO/IV: 250–375 mg/d or 5 mg/kg/dose; *max*: 1000 mg/d	For edema, seizures, altitude sickness, and glaucoma. May cause headache, dizziness, drowsiness, tinnitus, fatigue, anorexia, nausea, vomiting, diarrhea, photosensitivity, hyper/hypoglycemia, hypokalemia, hyponatremia, hyperchloremia, polyuria, crystalluria, hyperuricemia, and metabolic acidosis, and injection-site reaction. PB: 90%; *t½*: 10–15 h

A, Adult; *d*, day; *h*, hour; *ICP*, intracranial pressure; *IM*, intramuscular; *IVP*, intravenous push; *IOP*, intraocular pressure; *IV*, intravenous; *maint*, maintenance dose; *max*, maximum; *min*, minute; *PB*, protein binding; *PO*, by mouth; *PRN*, as needed; *q2–3h*, every 2–3 hours; *q6–8h*, every 6–8 hours; *t½*, half-life; *UK*, unknown.

CLINICAL JUDGMENT [NURSING PROCESS]
Diuretics: Loop

Concept: Elimination
- Excretion of body waste products through the urinary system

Recognize Cues [Assessment]
- Obtain a history of drugs taken daily. Note if the patient is taking a drug that may interact with a loop diuretic, such as alcohol, aminoglycosides, anticoagulants, corticosteroids, lithium, amphotericin B, or digitalis. Recognize that furosemide is highly protein bound and can displace other protein-bound drugs such as warfarin.
- Assess vital signs, serum electrolytes, weight, and urine output for baseline levels.
- Compare the patient's drug dose with the recommended dose, and report any discrepancy.
- Note whether the patient is hypersensitive to sulfonamides.

Analyze Cues and Prioritize Hypothesis [Patient Problems]
- Disrupted fluid and electrolyte imbalance
- Fluid overload
- Hypokalemia
- Hypernatremia

Generate Solutions [Planning]
- The patient's edema will be reduced.
- The patient's blood pressure will be decreased.
- The patient's serum chemistry levels will remain within normal ranges.

Take Action [Nursing Interventions]
- Monitor urinary output to determine body fluid gain or loss. Urinary output should be at least 30 mL/h or 600 mL/24 h.
- Notify a health care provider if urine output does not increase; a severe renal disorder may be present.
- Weigh the patient at the same time every day with the same type of clothing to determine fluid loss or gain. A loss of 2.2 lb is equivalent to a fluid loss of 1 L.
- Monitor vital signs, and be alert for marked decreases in blood pressure.
- Administer IV furosemide slowly; hearing loss may occur if it is rapidly injected.
- ⚡ Observe for signs and symptoms of hypokalemia (<3.5 mEq/L), such as muscle weakness, abdominal distension, leg cramps, and/or cardiac dysrhythmias.
- Monitor serum potassium levels, especially when a patient is taking digoxin. Hypokalemia enhances the action of digitalis, causing digitalis toxicity.

Patient Teaching
General
- Advise patients to take furosemide in the morning and *not* in the evening to prevent sleep disturbance and nocturia. Advise patients to request a child-proof medication bottle if children are around.

Side Effects
- Teach patients to rise slowly from lying or sitting to standing to prevent dizziness resulting from fluid loss.

Diet
- Suggest taking furosemide with food to avoid nausea.

Evaluate Outcomes [Evaluation]
- Evaluate effectiveness of the drug action, such as decreased fluid retention or fluid overload, decreased respiratory distress, and increased cardiac output.
- Check for side effects and increased urine output.

OSMOTIC DIURETICS AND CARBONIC ANHYDRASE INHIBITORS

Osmotic Diuretics

Osmotic diuretics increase the osmolality (concentration) and sodium reabsorption in the proximal tubule and loop of Henle. Sodium, chloride, potassium (to a lesser degree), and water are excreted. This group of drugs is used to decrease intracranial pressure (ICP, such as in cerebral edema) and decrease intraocular pressure (IOP, such as in glaucoma), and to promote excretion of toxic substances. Mannitol is a potent osmotic potassium-wasting diuretic frequently used in emergency situations such as ICP and IOP. In addition, mannitol can be used with cisplatin and carboplatin in cancer chemotherapy to induce a frank diuresis and decrease side effects of treatment.

Mannitol is the most frequently prescribed osmotic diuretic, followed by urea. Diuresis occurs within 1 to 3 hours after IV administration. Table 41.4 describes mannitol.

Side Effects and Adverse Reactions

The side effects and adverse reactions of mannitol include fluid and electrolyte imbalance, pulmonary edema from rapid shift of fluids, nausea and vomiting, tachycardia from rapid fluid loss, and acidosis. Crystallization of mannitol in the vial may occur when the drug is exposed to a low temperature; the vial should be warmed to dissolve the crystals. The mannitol solution should not be used for IV infusion if crystals are present and have not been dissolved.

Contraindications

Mannitol must be given with extreme caution to patients who have electrolyte imbalances and HF. It should be immediately discontinued if the patient develops hypovolemia or hypertension.

Carbonic Anhydrase Inhibitors

The carbonic anhydrase inhibitor acetazolamide blocks the action of the enzyme carbonic anhydrase, which is needed to maintain the body's acid-base balance (hydrogen and bicarbonate ion balance). Inhibition of this enzyme causes increased sodium, potassium, and bicarbonate excretion. With prolonged use, metabolic acidosis can occur.

This group of drugs is used primarily to decrease IOP in patients with open-angle (chronic) glaucoma. Other uses include management of epilepsy, and treatment of high-altitude sickness. Table 41.4 presents the drug data for carbonic anhydrase inhibitor diuretics.

Side Effects and Adverse Reactions

Acetazolamide can cause fluid and electrolyte imbalance, metabolic acidosis, nausea, vomiting, anorexia, and crystalluria. Hemolytic anemia and hepatic failure can also occur. These drugs are contraindicated in hypokalemia, hyponatremia, metabolic acidosis, and renal/hepatic disease.

POTASSIUM-SPARING DIURETICS

Overview

Potassium-sparing diuretics, which are weaker than thiazides and loop diuretics, are used as mild diuretics or in combination with another diuretic such as hydrochlorothiazide or an antihypertensive drug. Potassium supplements are *not* used when the patient takes a potassium-sparing diuretic; in fact, serum potassium excess, called hyperkalemia, typically results when a potassium supplement is taken with a potassium-sparing diuretic. The serum potassium should be periodically monitored when the patient continuously takes a potassium-sparing diuretic. If the serum potassium level is greater than 5.0 mEq/L, the patient should discontinue the potassium-sparing diuretic and restrict foods high in potassium.

Potassium-sparing diuretics act primarily in the collecting duct renal tubules and late distal tubule to promote sodium and water excretion and potassium retention. The drugs interfere with the sodium-potassium pump controlled by the mineralocorticoid hormone aldosterone (sodium retained and potassium excreted).

Spironolactone, an aldosterone antagonist, was the first potassium-sparing diuretic. Aldosterone is a mineralocorticoid hormone that promotes sodium retention and potassium excretion. Spironolactone blocks the action of aldosterone and inhibits the sodium-potassium pump (i.e., potassium is retained, and sodium is excreted). Spironolactone has been prescribed by cardiologists for patients with cardiac disorders because of its potassium-retaining effect. As a result of the action of spironolactone, the heart rate is more regular, and the possibility of myocardial fibrosis is decreased. The effects of spironolactone may take 48 hours.

Amiloride, triamterene, and eplerenone are additional commonly prescribed potassium-sparing diuretics. Amiloride and eplerenone are effective as antihypertensive agents. Triamterene is useful in the treatment of edema caused by HF or cirrhosis of the liver. Low doses of spironolactone and eplerenone are effective for chronic HF. Spironolactone, amiloride, triamterene, and eplerenone should not be taken with ACE inhibitors and angiotensin II receptor blockers (ARBs) because they can also increase serum potassium levels. Prototype Drug Chart: Spironolactone provides the pharmacologic data for spironolactone.

When potassium-sparing diuretics are used alone, they are less effective than when used in combination to reduce body fluid and sodium. These drugs are usually combined with a potassium-wasting diuretic, primarily hydrochlorothiazide or a loop diuretic. The combination of potassium-sparing and potassium-wasting diuretics intensifies the diuretic effect and prevents potassium loss. The common combination diuretics contain spironolactone and hydrochlorothiazide, amiloride and hydrochlorothiazide, and triamterene and hydrochlorothiazide. Table 41.5 lists the potassium-sparing diuretics and the combination potassium-wasting and potassium-sparing diuretics.

Side Effects and Adverse Reactions

The main side effect of potassium-sparing diuretics is hyperkalemia. Caution must be used when giving potassium-sparing diuretics to patients with poor renal function because the kidneys excrete 80% to 90% of potassium. Urine output should be at least 600 mL/day. Patients should *not* use potassium supplements while taking potassium-sparing diuretics, unless the serum potassium level is low. If a potassium-sparing diuretic is given with antihypertensive ACE inhibitors, hyperkalemia could become severe or life threatening because both drugs retain potassium. Monitoring serum potassium levels is essential to safe drug therapy. Headache, dizziness, asthenia (weakness), GI disturbances (nausea, vomiting, diarrhea) hyperuricemia, muscle cramps, and paresthesia (numbness and tingling of the hands and feet) can occur.

TABLE 41.5 Diuretics: Potassium-Sparing

Drug	Route and Dosage	Uses and Considerations
Single Agents		
Amiloride hydrochloride	A: PO: 5–10 mg/d; *max:* 20 mg/d	For hypokalemia, hypertension, HF, and edema. May cause dizziness, headache, cough, weakness, orthostatic hypotension, abdominal pain, anorexia, nausea, vomiting, diarrhea, constipation, hyperkalemia, hyponatremia metabolic acidosis, and erectile dysfunction. PB: 40%; t½: 6–9 h
Eplerenone	HF: A: PO: 25–50 mg/d; *max:* 50 mg/d	For hypertension and HF. May cause dizziness, headache, weakness, fatigue, cough, diarrhea, hyperkalemia, hyponatremia, hyperuricemia, hypertriglyceridemia, hypercholesterolemia, and vaginal bleeding. PB: 50%; t½: 4–6 h
Spironolactone	See Prototype Drug Chart: Spironolactone	
Triamterene	A: PO: Initially 100 mg bid; *max:* 300 mg/d	For peripheral edema. May cause dizziness, headache, weakness, nausea, vomiting, diarrhea, bradycardia, hypo/hyperkalemia, hyponatremia, hyperuricemia, and metabolic acidosis. PB: 67%; t½: 1–2 h
Combinations		
Amiloride hydrochloride and hydrochlorothiazide	A: PO: 1–2 tab/d (amiloride 5 mg/HCTZ 50 mg); *max:* 10 mg amiloride, 100 mg HCTZ	For hypertension and peripheral edema. May cause dizziness, headache, weakness, orthostatic hypotension, abdominal pain, anorexia, nausea, diarrhea, rash, pruritus, hypomagnesemia, hyponatremia, hypochloremia, hypovolemia, hypo/hyperkalemia, hypercalcemia, hyperglycemia, metabolic acidosis, and hyperuricemia. PB: 40% amiloride, 40%–68% HCTZ; t½: 6–9 h amiloride, 5.6–14.8 h HCTZ
Spironolactone and hydrochlorothiazide	Hypertension: A: PO: Initially 1 tab/d (25 mg spironolactone/25 mg HCTZ); *max:* 200 mg/d of each	For edema and hypertension. May cause dizziness, headache, abdominal pain, anorexia, nausea, vomiting, diarrhea, weakness, hyperkalemia, hypercalcemia, hyperuricemia, hyperglycemia, hypercholesterolemia, hypomagnesemia, hyponatremia, hypovolemia, and muscle cramps. PB: 90% spironolactone, 40%–68% HCTZ; t½: 1.3–2 h spironolactone, 5.6–14.8 h HCTZ
Triamterene and hydrochlorothiazide	A: PO: Initially 1 cap/d pc (37.5 mg triamterene, 25 mg HCTZ); maint: 1–2 cap/d pc; *max:* 75 mg triamterene, 50 mg HCTZ	For edema and HTN. May cause dizziness, headache, blurred vision, photosensitivity, rash, abdominal pain, anorexia, nausea, vomiting, diarrhea, constipation, weakness, muscle cramps, orthostatic hypotension, hyperglycemia, hypo/hyperkalemia, hypercalcemia, hypochloremia, hypomagnesemia, hyponatremia, hypovolemia, hyperuricemia, and erectile dysfunction. PB: 67% triamterene, 40%–68% HCTZ; t½: 1–2 h triamterene, 5.6–14.8 h HCTZ

A, Adult; *bid*, twice a day; *cap*, capsule; *d*, day; *h*, hour; *HCTZ*, hydrochlorothiazide; *HF*, heart failure; *HTN*, hypertension; *maint*, maintenance dose; *max*, maximum; *PB*, protein binding; *pc*, after meals; *PO*, by mouth; *t½*, half-life; *tab*, tablet.

PROTOTYPE DRUG CHART
Spironolactone

Drug Class	Dosage
Potassium-sparing diuretic	Edema: A: PO: Initially 100 mg/d in single or divided doses, *maint:* 25–200 mg/d in divided doses; *max:* 400 mg/d Hypertension: A: PO: 25–100 mg/d in single or divided doses; *max:* 400 mg/d
Contraindications	**Drug-Lab-Food Interactions**
Renal failure, anuria, hyperkalemia, adrenal insufficiency *Caution:* Renal/hepatic dysfunction, diabetes mellitus, ascites, acid-base imbalance, acidosis/alkalosis, older adults, pregnancy, breast-feeding, children	Drug: Increased serum potassium level with potassium supplements; increased effects of antihypertensives and lithium *Life threatening:* Hyperkalemia if given with an ACE inhibitor Lab: Increased serum potassium level; may increase BUN, AST, alkaline phosphatase levels; decreased serum sodium, chloride
Pharmacokinetics	**Pharmacodynamics**
Absorption: PO: Rapidly absorbed from GI tract Distribution: PB: 90% Metabolism: t½: 1–2 h Excretion: In urine, mostly as metabolites and bile	PO: Onset: UK Peak: 0.5–1.5 h Duration: 2–3 d or longer

Continued

PROTOTYPE DRUG CHART—CONT'D
Spironolactone

Therapeutic Effects/Uses
For edema, hypertension, HF, and hyperaldosteronism

Mechanism of Action: Inhibits aldosterone effects on distal renal tubules to promote sodium and water excretion and potassium retention

Side Effects	Adverse Reactions
Dizziness, drowsiness, headache, confusion, weakness, ataxia, nausea, abdominal cramps, vomiting, diarrhea, muscle cramps, gout, gynecomastia, menstrual irregularity, dehydration, erectile dysfunction	Orthostatic hypotension, bradycardia, hyperkalemia, hypomagnesemia, hyponatremia, hypocalcemia, hypovolemia, hyperglycemia, hyperuricemia, metabolic acidosis/alkalosis *Life threatening*: Agranulocytosis, leukopenia, thrombocytopenia, renal/hepatic failure, Stevens-Johnson syndrome

A, Adult; *ACE*, angiotensin-converting enzyme; *AST*, aspartate transaminase; *BUN*, blood urea nitrogen; *d*, day; *GI*, gastrointestinal; *h*, hour; *HF*, heart failure; *maint*, maintenance; *max*, maximum; *PB*, protein binding; *PO*, by mouth; *t½*, half-life; *UK*, unknown.

CLINICAL JUDGMENT [NURSING PROCESS]
Diuretics: Potassium Sparing

Concepts: Elimination
- Excretion of body waste products through the urinary system

Recognize Cues [Assessment]
- Obtain a history of drugs taken daily. Note whether the patient is taking a potassium supplement or using a salt substitute.
- Assess vital signs, serum electrolytes, weight, and urinary output for baseline levels.
- Compare the patient's drug dose with the recommended dose, and report any discrepancy.

Analyze Cues and Prioritize Hypothesis [Patient Problems]
- Fluid overload
- Hyperkalemia
- Diarrhea
- Nausea

Generate Solutions [Planning]
- The patient blood pressure will be decreased.
- The patient's serum electrolytes will remain within normal ranges.

Take Action [Nursing Interventions]
- Note the half-life of spironolactone. With a long half-life, the drug is usually administered once a day, sometimes twice a day.
- Monitor urinary output; it should increase. Report if urine output is less than 30 mL/h or less than 600 mL/day.
- Weigh the patient at the same time every day with the same type of clothing to determine fluid loss or gain. A loss of 2.2 lb is equivalent to a fluid loss of 1 L.
- Record vital signs, and report any abnormal changes.
- ⚡ Observe for signs and symptoms of hyperkalemia (serum potassium >5.0 mEq/L). Nausea, diarrhea, abdominal cramps, numbness and tingling of the hands and feet, leg cramps, tachycardia and later bradycardia, peaked narrow T wave on electrocardiogram, or oliguria may signal hyperkalemia.
- Administer spironolactone in the morning and not in the evening to avoid nocturia.

Patient Teaching
General
- Teach patients to take spironolactone with or after meals to avoid nausea.
- Encourage patients not to discontinue the drug without consulting a health care provider.

Side Effects
- Caution patients to avoid exposure to direct sunlight because spironolactone can cause photosensitivity.
- Advise patients to report possible side effects such as rash, dizziness, weakness, and gastrointestinal (GI) upset.

Diet
- Advise patients with high serum potassium levels to avoid foods rich in potassium when taking potassium-sparing diuretics.

Evaluate Outcomes [Evaluation]
- Evaluate the effectiveness of potassium-sparing diuretics (e.g., triamterene). Fluid retention (edema) should be decreased or absent.
- Determine whether urine output has increased and whether serum potassium level is within the normal range.

CLINICAL JUDGMENT CASE STUDY

A 58-year-old patient has been recently diagnosed with hypertension. His resting blood pressure is 158/92 mm Hg. He is prescribed hydrochlorothiazide 50 mg/day and is told to eat foods rich in potassium.

1. How does hydrochlorothiazide differ from furosemide? What are their similarities and differences?
2. Why is it necessary for the patient to eat foods rich in potassium when taking hydrochlorothiazide? Explain your answer.
3. What nursing interventions should be considered while the patient takes hydrochlorothiazide?
4. After 1 month on hydrochlorothiazide therapy, the patient becomes weak and reports nausea and vomiting. His muscles are "soft," and his serum potassium level is 3.3 mEq/L. The patient's diuretic is changed to triamterene and hydrochlorothiazide. Again, he is advised to eat foods rich in potassium. Explain the rationale for changing the patient's diuretic.
5. Should the patient receive a potassium supplement? Explain your answer.
6. What nursing interventions should the nurse follow for the patient?
7. What care plan should the nurse develop for the patient in relation to patient teaching?
8. What medical follow-up care is needed for the patient?

REVIEW QUESTIONS

1. A patient is taking hydrochlorothiazide 50 mg/day and digoxin 0.25 mg/day. The nurse plans to monitor the patient for which potential electrolyte imbalance?
   a. Hypocalcemia
   b. Hypokalemia
   c. Hyperkalemia
   d. Hypermagnesemia

2. The nurse knows that which statement is correct regarding nursing care of a patient receiving hydrochlorothiazide? **Select all that apply.**
   a. Monitor patients for signs of hypoglycemia.
   b. Administer ordered potassium supplements.
   c. Monitor serum potassium and uric acid levels.
   d. Assess blood pressure before administration.
   e. Notify the health care provider if a patient has had oliguria for 24 hours.
   f. Assess for decreased cholesterol and triglyceride levels.

3. A patient has heart failure, and a high dose of furosemide is ordered. What suggests a favorable response to furosemide?
   a. A decrease in level of consciousness occurs, and the patient sleeps more.
   b. Respiratory rate decreases from 28/min to 20/min, and the depth increases.
   c. Breath sounds reveal increased congestion, and the patient reports shortness of breath.
   d. Urine output is 50 mL/4 hours, and intake is 200 mL.

4. What does the nurse know to be correct concerning the use of mannitol in patients?
   a. It decreases intracranial pressure.
   b. It increases intraocular pressure.
   c. It causes sodium and potassium retention.
   d. It causes diuresis in several days.

5. What should the nurse do when a patient is taking furosemide?
   a. Instruct the patient to change positions quickly when getting out of bed.
   b. Assess blood pressure before administration.
   c. Administer the drug at bedtime for maximum effectiveness.
   d. Teach the patient to avoid fruits to prevent hyperkalemia.

6. For the patient taking a diuretic, a combination such as triamterene and hydrochlorothiazide may be prescribed. The nurse realizes that this combination is ordered for which purpose?
   a. To decrease serum potassium level
   b. To maintain serum potassium level
   c. To decrease glucose level
   d. To increase glucose level

7. The patient has been receiving spironolactone 50 mg/day for heart failure. The nurse should closely monitor the patient for which condition?
   a. Hypokalemia
   b. Hyperkalemia
   c. Hypoglycemia
   d. Hypermagnesemia

42

Antihypertensives

http://evolve.elsevier.com/McCuistion/pharmacology

OBJECTIVES

- Explain contributing factors leading to essential hypertension and guidelines for its treatment.
- Summarize the mechanism of action and uses of the seven categories of antihypertensive drugs.

OUTLINE

Hypertension, 536
    Guidelines for Hypertension, 536
    Selected Regulators of Blood Pressure, 536
    Physiologic Risk Factors, 537
    Variable Responses to Antihypertensive Agents, 537
    Hypertension in Older Adults, 537
    Nonpharmacologic Control of Hypertension, 537
Phamacologic Control of Hypertension, 537
    Diuretics, 538

    Sympatholytics, 538
    Direct-Acting Arteriolar Vasodilators, 543
    Angiotensin-Converting Enzyme Inhibitors, 544
    Angiotensin II Receptor Blockers, 547
    Direct Renin Inhibitors, 548
    Calcium Channel Blockers, 548
Clinical Judgment Case Study, 550
Review Questions, 550

HYPERTENSION

Hypertension is the most common condition leading to myocardial infarction (MI), stroke, renal failure, and death. **Essential hypertension** is the most common type of hypertension and affects 90% to 95% of persons with high blood pressure (BP). The exact origin of essential hypertension is unknown; however, contributing factors may include hyperlipidemia, a diet high in saturated fats and salt, being physically inactive, African American race, coexisting diabetes or kidney disease, aging, stress, excessive alcohol ingestion, smoking, obesity, and a family history of hypertension. Approximately 65% of female and 78% of male hypertension cases can be attributable to obesity. Five to ten percent of hypertension cases are related to renal and endocrine disorders and are classified as **secondary hypertension**.

Guidelines for Hypertension

BP data collected should be based on an average of more than two readings on more than two occasions. BP guidelines for determining hypertension have been revised and are contained in the Eighth Report of the Joint National Committee on Prevention, Detection, Evaluation, and Treatment of High Blood Pressure, or JNC 8, from 2017. The purpose of these guidelines is to decrease the risk of cardiovascular disease (CVD) in the American population. The guideline for normal BP is less than 120/80 mm Hg. *Elevated blood pressure* is defined as systolic blood pressure (SBP) of 120 to 129 and diastolic blood pressure (DBP) of less than 80. *Stage 1 hypertension* falls between 130/80 and 139/89, and *stage 2 hypertension* is 140/90 or greater.

Two out of three patients with hypertension have uncontrolled BP or are not optimally treated. SBP is more important than DBP as a CVD risk. According to the JNC 8, a BP of 140/90 is the goal for the population younger than 60 years, with a target of 150/90 for those older than 60.

Selected Regulators of Blood Pressure

The kidneys and blood vessels strive to regulate and maintain a "normal" BP. The kidneys regulate BP by control of fluid volume and via the renin-angiotensin-aldosterone system (RAAS; Fig. 42.1). Kidneys control sodium and water elimination and retention, which affects cardiac output and systemic arterial BP. Renin from the renal cells stimulates production of angiotensin II, a potent vasoconstrictor that causes the release of aldosterone, an adrenal hormone that promotes sodium retention and therefore water retention. Retention of sodium and water causes fluid volume to increase, elevating BP.

The baroreceptors in the aorta and carotid sinus and the vasomotor center in the medulla also assist in the regulation of BP. Catecholamines such as norepinephrine, released from the sympathetic nerve terminals, and epinephrine, released from the adrenal medulla, increase BP through vasoconstrictive activity.

Other hormones that contribute to BP regulation are antidiuretic hormone (ADH), atrial natriuretic peptide (ANP) hormone, and brain natriuretic peptide hormone. ADH is produced by the hypothalamus and is stored and released by the posterior pituitary gland (neurohypophysis). This hormone stimulates the kidneys to conserve and retain water when there is a fluid volume deficit. When there is fluid overload, ADH secretion is inhibited, and the kidneys then excrete more water.

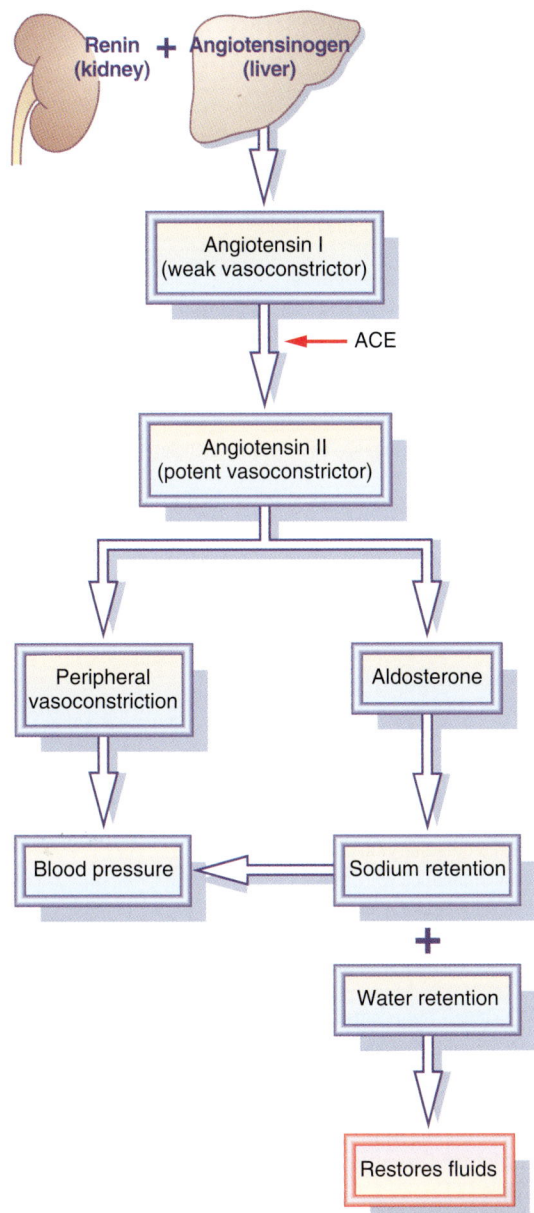

Fig. 42.1 The renin-angiotensin-aldosterone system (RAAS). Renin, an enzyme located in the juxtaglomerular cells of the kidney, is released when blood pressure decreases. This diagram shows how the RAAS restores fluid balance and stabilizes blood pressure. *ACE*, Angiotensin-converting enzyme.

Physiologic Risk Factors

Certain physiologic risk factors contribute to hypertension. A diet high in saturated fat and simple carbohydrates can increase BP. Carbohydrate intake can affect sympathetic nervous activity. Alcohol increases renin secretions, causing the production of angiotensin II. Obesity affects the sympathetic and cardiovascular systems by increasing cardiac output, stroke volume, and left ventricular filling. Two-thirds of hypertensive persons are obese. Normally weight loss can decrease hypertension, as can mild to moderate sodium restriction.

Variable Responses to Antihypertensive Agents

African American patients are more likely to develop hypertension at an earlier age than White patients. African American patients also have a higher mortality rate from hypertension than the White population. The use of beta-adrenergic blockers (beta blockers) and angiotensin-converting enzyme (ACE) inhibitors is less effective for the control of hypertension in African American patients unless the drug is combined or given with a diuretic. This group is susceptible to low-renin hypertension; therefore they do not respond well to beta blockers and ACE inhibitors. The antihypertensive drugs that are effective for African American patients are alpha$_1$ blockers and calcium channel blockers (calcium blockers). African American patients do respond to diuretics as the initial monotherapy for controlling hypertension. White patients usually have high-renin hypertension and respond well to all antihypertensive agents.

Asian American patients are twice as sensitive as White patients to beta blockers and other antihypertensives. A reduction in antihypertensive dosing is frequently needed. Native American patients have a reduced or lower response to beta blockers compared with White patients. Monitoring BP and drug dosing should be an ongoing assessment for patients in these cultural groups.

Hypertension in Older Adults

Approximately 70% of American adults have hypertension, which is 46% of the adult population. Of individuals older than 55 years of age, 65% have developed hypertension or two in three people. Only approximately 48% of hypertensive individuals have this condition under control. Typically, in the age range of 18 to 49, males have more prevalence of hypertension than females. Both systolic and diastolic hypertension are associated with increased cardiovascular morbidity and mortality. With antihypertensive therapy, the greatest decrease in cardiovascular disorders is 34% for stroke and 19% for coronary heart disease.

One of the troublesome side effects of the use of antihypertensive agents in older adults, especially frail individuals or persons living in institutions, is orthostatic (postural) hypotension. This episode of sudden low BP presents as dizziness due to blood pooling in the lower extremities when an individual repositions to an upright position. In older adults, the sympathetic nervous system does not respond as quickly to correct the situation, especially when potentiated by antihypertensive drug administration. If orthostatic hypotension occurs, the antihypertensive drug dose may need to be decreased or another antihypertensive drug may need to be used. Older adults with hypertension should be instructed to modify their lifestyle and activities. This includes restricting dietary sodium to 2400 mg daily, avoiding tobacco, modifying diet, exercising, and decreasing stress.

Nonpharmacologic Control of Hypertension

A sufficient decrease in BP can be accomplished by nonpharmacologic methods. There are many nonpharmacologic ways to decrease BP, but if the systolic pressure is greater than 140 mm Hg, **antihypertensive** drugs are generally ordered. Nondrug methods to decrease BP include stress-reduction techniques, exercise, salt restriction, decreased alcohol ingestion, and smoking cessation.

When hypertension cannot be controlled by nonpharmacologic means, antihypertensive drugs are prescribed. However, nonpharmacologic methods should be combined with antihypertensive drugs to control hypertension.

PHARMAGOLOGIC CONTROL OF HYPERTENSION

An individualized approach to the treatment of hypertension is used by many health care providers. All drugs are considered *initial agents* when first prescribed for hypertension. Reduction of other cardiovascular risk factors and the use of fewer drugs (i.e., substituting instead of adding drugs) at the lowest effective doses are emphasized. Often more than one antihypertensive is used to control BP, which also may lead to fewer adverse effects.

Antihypertensive drugs, used either singly or in combination with other drugs, are classified into seven categories: (1) diuretics, (2) sympatholytics (sympathetic depressants), (3) direct-acting arteriolar vasodilators, (4) ACE inhibitors, (5) angiotensin II receptor blockers (ARBs), (6) direct renin inhibitors, and (7) calcium channel blockers.

Diuretics

Diuretics promote sodium depletion, which decreases extracellular fluid volume. Diuretics are effective as first-line drugs for treating mild hypertension. Hydrochlorothiazide is the most frequently prescribed diuretic for controlling mild hypertension by decreasing excess fluid volume. It can be used alone for recently diagnosed or mild hypertension, or it can be used with other antihypertensive drugs. Many antihypertensive drugs can cause fluid retention; therefore diuretics are often administered together with antihypertensive agents. The various types of diuretics are discussed in Chapter 41.

Thiazide diuretics are not recommended for patients with renal insufficiency (creatinine clearance <30 mL/min). The loop (high-ceiling) diuretics such as furosemide are usually recommended because they do not depress renal blood flow. Loop diuretics are not used if hypertension is the result of RAAS involvement because they tend to immediately elevate serum renin level. Instead of a single thiazide drug, a combination of potassium-wasting and potassium-sparing diuretics may be useful; less potassium excretion would occur. In addition, thiazides can be combined with other antihypertensive drugs to increase their effectiveness. Box 42.1 lists the combinations of thiazides with other drugs. Many drug products on the market include combinations of thiazide diuretics and potassium-sparing diuretics, beta blockers, ACE inhibitors, or ARBs. ACE inhibitors tend to increase serum potassium (K) levels, so when they are combined with a thiazide diuretic, serum potassium loss is minimized.

Sympatholytics

The *sympatholytics* (sympathetic depressants) comprise five groups of drugs: (1) beta-adrenergic blockers, (2) centrally acting alpha$_2$ agonists, (3) alpha-adrenergic blockers, (4) adrenergic neuron blockers (peripherally acting sympatholytics), and (5) alpha$_1$- and beta$_1$-adrenergic blockers. Beta-adrenergic blockers block the beta receptors, and alpha-adrenergic blockers block the alpha receptors.

⚠ Beta-Adrenergic Blockers

Beta-adrenergic blockers, frequently called *beta blockers*, are used as antihypertensive drugs or in combination with a diuretic. Beta blockers are also used as antianginals and antidysrhythmics and are discussed in this context in Chapter 37.

Beta (β+ and β−)-adrenergic blockers reduce cardiac output by diminishing the sympathetic nervous system response to decrease basal sympathetic tone. With continued use of beta blockers, vascular resistance is diminished, and BP is lowered. Beta blockers reduce heart rate, contractility, and renin release. The hypotensive response is greater in patients with higher renin levels.

African American hypertensive patients do not respond well to beta blockers alone for the control of hypertension. Instead, hypertension in the African American population can be controlled by combining beta blockers with diuretics.

There are many types of beta blockers. Nonselective beta blockers, such as propranolol and carvedilol, inhibit beta$_1$ (heart) and beta$_2$ (bronchial) receptors. Heart rate slows, BP decreases secondary to the decrease in heart rate, and bronchoconstriction occurs because

---

BOX 42.1 Combination of Thiazides With Antihypertensive Drugs and Other Combinations

Thiazide With Potassium-Sparing Diuretics
- Hydrochlorothiazide with spironolactone
- Hydrochlorothiazide with amiloride
- Hydrochlorothiazide with triamterene

Thiazide With Beta Blockers
- Hydrochlorothiazide with bisoprolol fumarate
- Hydrochlorothiazide with metoprolol
- Bendroflumethiazide with nadolol

Tenoretic
- Chlorthalidone (thiazide-like diuretic) with atenolol

Thiazide With Angiotensin-Converting Enzyme Inhibitors
- Hydrochlorothiazide with benazepril
- Hydrochlorothiazide with captopril
- Hydrochlorothiazide with enalapril maleate
- Hydrochlorothiazide with fosinopril
- Hydrochlorothiazide with lisinopril
- Hydrochlorothiazide with moexipril
- Hydrochlorothiazide with quinapril

Thiazide With Angiotensin II Antagonists
- Hydrochlorothiazide with candesartan
- Hydrochlorothiazide with eprosartan
- Hydrochlorothiazide with irbesartan
- Hydrochlorothiazide with losartan
- Hydrochlorothiazide with olmesartan
- Hydrochlorothiazide with telmisartan
- Hydrochlorothiazide with valsartan

Thiazide With Centrally Acting Alpha$_2$ Agonist
- Chlorthalidone with clonidine
- Hydrochlorothiazide with methyldopa

Combination of Angiotensin-Converting Enzyme Inhibitors With Calcium Channel Blocker
- See Table 42.3

Combination of Calcium Channel Blocker With Statin Drug
- Amlodipine with atorvastatin

---

of unopposed parasympathetic tone. Cardioselective beta blockers are preferred because they act mainly on the beta$_1$—rather than the beta$_2$—receptors, and bronchoconstriction is less likely to occur. Acebutolol, atenolol, betaxolol, bisoprolol, and metoprolol are cardioselective beta blockers that block beta$_1$ receptors.

Cardioselectivity does not confer absolute protection from bronchoconstriction. In tests measuring forced expiratory volume in 1 second (FEV$_1$) as a measure of β− reactivity, only atenolol demonstrated true protection. Other cardioselective beta blockers were only partially effective. Studies also show that, at the upper end of the dosage range, cardioselectivity is less effective. In patients with preexisting bronchospasm or other pulmonary disease, beta blockers—even those considered to be cardioselective—should be used with caution. Some experts regard this as a relative contraindication. The real value of beta selectivity is in maintaining renal blood flow and minimizing the hypoglycemic effects of beta blockade.

The combination of beta blockers with hydrochlorothiazides is packaged together in tablet form (see Box 42.1). Usually the hydrochlorothiazide dose is 12.5 to 25 mg.

Beta blockers tend to be more effective in lowering BP in patients who have an elevated serum renin level. The cardioselective prototype drug metoprolol is presented in Prototype Drug Chart: Metoprolol. Beta blockers should not be used by patients with second- or third-degree atrioventricular (AV) block or sinus bradycardia. A noncardioselective beta blocker such as propranolol should not be given to a patient with chronic obstructive pulmonary disease.

PROTOTYPE DRUG CHART
Metoprolol

Drug Class	Dosage
Antihypertensive: beta$_1$ blocker	Hypertension: Regular release: A: PO: Initially 100 mg/d or in divided doses; *maint:* 100–200 mg in 2 divided doses; *max:* 450 mg/d in divided doses Extended release: A: PO: 25–100 mg/d; *max:* 400 mg/d
Contraindications	**Drug-Lab-Food Interactions**
Hypersensitivity, AV heart block, cardiogenic shock, HF, sinus syndrome, bradycardia *Caution:* Hepatic or thyroid dysfunction, asthma, bronchitis, peripheral vascular disease, diabetes mellitus, alcohol ingestion, older adults, breastfeeding, pregnancy, children	Drug: Increases bradycardia and heart block with digitalis, clonidine, SSRIs, MAOIs, cimetidine; increased hypotensive effect with other antihypertensives, alcohol, anesthetics, aspirin, salicylates; NSAIDs decrease effect of beta blockers and oral contraceptives. Lab: Increased hepatic enzymes
Pharmacokinetics	**Pharmacodynamics**
Absorption: PO: 95% Distribution: PB: 10%–12% Metabolism: t½: 3–7 h Excretion: In urine	Immediate release: PO: Onset: 30–60 min Peak: 1–2 h Duration: 6.4 h Extended release: PO: Onset UK Peak: 7 h Duration: 24 h
Therapeutic Effects/Uses	
To control hypertension, acute myocardial infarction, angina, and HF Mechanism of action: Promotes blood pressure reduction via a beta$_1$-blocking effect.	
Side Effects	**Adverse Reactions**
Dizziness, drowsiness, headache, insomnia, nightmares, fatigue, depression, blurred vision, xerophthalmia, tinnitus, dysgeusia, dry mouth, nausea, vomiting, diarrhea, rash, pruritus, peripheral edema, erectile dysfunction	Bradycardia, hypotension, palpitations, stroke, thrombocytopenia, diabetes mellitus *Life threatening:* AV heart block, bronchospasm, agranulocytosis, HF

A, Adult; *AV,* atrioventricular; *d,* day; *h,* hour; *HF,* heart failure; *maint,* maintenance; *MAOIs,* monoamine oxidase inhibitors; *max,* maximum; *min,* minute; *NSAID,* nonsteroidal antiinflammatory drug; *PB,* protein binding; *PO,* by mouth; *SSRI,* selective serotonin reuptake inhibitor; *t½,* half-life; *UK,* unknown.

Pharmacokinetics. Metoprolol is well absorbed from the gastrointestinal (GI) tract. Its half-life is short, and its protein-binding power is low.

Pharmacodynamics. Cardioselective beta-adrenergic blockers block beta$_1$ receptors, thereby decreasing heart rate and BP. The nonselective beta blockers block beta$_1$ and beta$_2$ receptors, which can result in bronchial constriction. Beta blockers cross the placental barrier and are excreted in breast milk.

The onset of action of immediate-release metoprolol is usually 60 minutes or less. The peak is 1 to 2 hours for immediate release and usually 7 hours for extended release. The duration is typically 6.4 hours for immediate release and 24 hours for extended release.

Side Effects and Adverse Reactions. Side effects and adverse reactions include decreased pulse rate, markedly decreased BP, and, with noncardioselective beta$_1$ and beta$_2$ blockers, bronchospasm. Beta blockers should not be abruptly discontinued because rebound hypertension, angina, dysrhythmias, and MI can result. Beta blockers can cause dizziness, insomnia, depression, fatigue, nightmares, and erectile dysfunction. Table 42.1 lists the beta blockers used to treat hypertension and their dosages, uses, and considerations.

Noncardioselective beta blockers inhibit the liver's ability to convert glycogen to glucose in response to hypoglycemia. Because of this side effect, beta blockers should be used with caution in patients with diabetes mellitus. In addition, bradycardia is a very common adverse effect of beta blockers.

COMPLEMENTARY AND ALTERNATIVE THERAPIES
Antihypertensives

- Ma-huang (ephedra) decreases or counteracts the effect of antihypertensive drugs. When taken with beta blockers, hypertension may continue or increase.
- Ephedra increases hypertension when taken with beta blockers.
- Black cohosh increases the hypotensive effect of antihypertensive drugs.
- Hawthorn may increase the effects of beta blockers and angiotensin-converting enzyme (ACE) inhibitors.
- Licorice, Korean ginseng, and milk thistle decrease the effects of antihypertensive drugs.
- Goldenseal may increase the effects of antihypertensive drugs.
- Parsley may potentiate hypotension when taken with an antihypertensive drug.
- Cayenne may cause drug-induced cough with ACE inhibitors.
- Chinese skullcap may increase losartan levels.
- Coleus may potentiate the effects of antihypertensives.
- St. John's wort decreases the effects of calcium channel blockers, especially nifedipine and verapamil.

Centrally Acting Alpha$_2$ Agonists

Centrally acting alpha$_2$ agonists decrease the sympathetic response from the brainstem to the peripheral vessels. They stimulate the alpha$_2$ receptors, which in turn decreases sympathetic activity, increases vagus activity, decreases cardiac output, and decreases serum epinephrine, norepinephrine, and renin release. All of these actions result in reduced peripheral vascular resistance and increased vasodilation. This group of drugs has minimal effects on cardiac output and blood flow to the kidneys. Beta blockers are not given with centrally acting sympatholytics because accentuation of bradycardia during therapy can occur, as can rebound hypertension on discontinuing therapy.

TABLE 42.1 Antihypertensives: Beta Blockers and Central Alpha$_2$ Agonists

Drug	Route and Dosage	Uses and Considerations
Beta-Adrenergic Blockers		
Acebutolol hydrochloride Cardioselective beta$_1$	Hypertension: A: PO: Initially 400 mg/d in 1–2 divided doses; *maint:* 400–800 mg/d; *max:* 1200 mg/d Older A: Initially 200–400 mg/d; *max:* 800 mg/d	For hypertension and dysrhythmias. May cause dizziness, headache, fatigue, hypotension, bradycardia, palpitations, dyspnea, visual impairment, dyspepsia, nausea, diarrhea, and constipation. Closely monitor vital signs. Taper off gradually. PB: 26%; t½: 3–4 h
Atenolol Cardioselective beta$_1$	Hypertension: A: PO: Initially 50 mg/d; *maint:* 50–100 mg/d in divided doses; *max:* 100 mg/d	For hypertension, angina, and prophylaxis and treatment of AMI. May cause dizziness, fatigue, depression, dyspnea, heart failure, hypotension, bradycardia, tachycardia, dysrhythmias, nausea, diarrhea, and peripheral vasoconstriction. Taper gradually. PB: 10%; t½: 6–7 h
Betaxolol hydrochloride Cardioselective beta$_1$	Hypertension: A: PO: Initially 10 mg/d; *maint:* 10–20 mg/d; *max:* 20 mg/d Older A: PO: Initially 5 mg/d; *max:* 20 mg/d	For hypertension and glaucoma. May cause dizziness, headache, insomnia, fatigue, ocular irritation, bradycardia, palpitations, chest pain, dyspepsia, nausea, and arthralgia. Taper gradually. PB: 50%; t½: 15 h
Bisoprolol fumarate Beta$_1$ blocker	A: PO: Initially 2.5–5 mg/d; *max:* 20 mg/d	For hypertension. May cause dizziness, headache, fatigue, weakness, rhinitis, bradycardia, orthostatic hypotension, peripheral edema, diarrhea, arthralgia, and elevated hepatic enzymes. Taper gradually. PB: 30%; t½: 9–12 h
Carvedilol Alpha blocker, nonselective beta$_1$ and beta$_2$	Hypertension: Regular release: A: PO: Initially 6.25 mg bid for 7–14 d; *max:* 50 mg/d Extended release: A: PO: Initially 20 mg/d in the morning for 7–14 d; *max:* 80 mg/d	For treating hypertension, AMI, and heart failure. May cause dizziness, drowsiness, headache, fatigue, weakness, orthostatic hypotension, bradycardia, peripheral edema, dyspnea, nausea, vomiting, diarrhea, hypo/hyperglycemia, and weight gain. Give with food. Taper gradually. PB: 98%; t½: 7–11 h
Metoprolol Cardioselective beta$_1$	See Prototype Drug Chart: Metoprolol	
Nadolol Nonselective beta$_1$ and beta$_2$	Hypertension: A: PO: Initially 40 mg/d; *maint:* 40–80 mg/d; *max:* 320 mg/d	For hypertension and angina. May cause dizziness, drowsiness, fatigue, bradycardia, tachycardia, hypo/hypertension, palpitations, and erectile dysfunction. Give without regard to meals. Taper gradually. PB: 30%; t½: 10–24 h
Pindolol Nonselective beta$_1$ and beta$_2$	A: PO: Initially 5 mg bid; *maint:* 10–30 mg/d in 2–3 divided doses; *max:* 60 mg/d	For hypertension. May cause dizziness, fatigue, weakness, visual impairment, bradycardia, hypotension, edema, dyspnea, nausea, arthralgia, myalgia, and elevated hepatic enzymes. PB: 40%–60%; t½: 3–4 h
Propranolol Nonselective beta$_1$ and beta$_2$	Hypertension: Immediate release: A: PO: Initially 40 mg bid; *maint:* 160–480 mg/d in 2–3 divided doses; *max:* 640 mg/d Extended release: A: PO: Initially 80 mg/d at bedtime; *maint:* 120–160 mg/d; *max:* 640 mg/d	For hypertension, AMI, angina, HF, dysrhythmias, and migraine prophylaxis. May cause dizziness, headache, fatigue, weakness, depression, agitation, visual impairment, bradycardia, hyperkalemia, seizures, and erectile dysfunction. Bronchospasm may occur due to the beta$_2$-blocker effect. Taper gradually. PB: 90%; t½: 2–6 h
Central Alpha$_2$ Agonists		
Clonidine hydrochloride	A: PO: Initially 0.1 mg bid; *maint:* 0.1–0.8 mg/d; *max:* 2.4 mg/d A: Transdermal patch: Initially 1 patch (0.1 mg/24 h) q7d; *max:* 0.6 mg/24 h q7d	For hypertension. May cause dizziness, drowsiness, headache, fatigue, confusion, irritability, nightmares, orthostatic hypotension, bradycardia, chest pain, anxiety, anorexia, dry mouth, abdominal pain, nausea, vomiting, constipation, erythema, infection, edema, and pruritus. PB: 20%–40%; t½: 12–16 h PO, 20 h transdermal
Guanfacine hydrochloride	Immediate release: A: PO: Initially 1 mg/d at bedtime; *maint:* 0.5–2 mg/d; *max:* 3 mg/d	For hypertension. May cause dizziness, drowsiness, headache, fatigue, weakness, insomnia, irritability, orthostatic hypotension, bradycardia, dry mouth, abdominal pain, nausea, diarrhea, constipation, and erectile dysfunction. PB: 70%; t½: 10–30 h
Methyldopa	Hypertension: A: PO: Initially 250 mg bid–tid; *maint:* 250–2000 mg/d in 2–4 divided doses; *max:* 3 g/d	For hypertension, hypertensive urgency, and emergency. May cause dizziness, drowsiness, headache, weakness, depression, nausea, vomiting, diarrhea, orthostatic hypotension, bradycardia, angina, peripheral edema, constipation, and erectile/ejaculation dysfunction. Take with food if GI upset occurs. Use has declined due to its adverse effects. PB: 10%–15%; t½: 2 h

A, Adult; *AMI*, acute myocardial infarction; *bid*, twice a day; *d*, day; *GI*, gastrointestinal; *h*, hour; *HTN*, hypertension; *IV*, intravenous; *maint*, maintenance; *max*, maximum; *MI*, myocardial infarction; *min*, minutes; *PB*, protein binding; *PO*, by mouth; *PVCs*, premature ventricular contractions; *q*, every; *t½*, half-life; *tid*, three times a day.

CLINICAL JUDGMENT [NURSING PROCESS]

Antihypertensives: Beta Blockers

Concept: Perfusion
- The passage of blood flow through the arteries and capillaries that deliver oxygen and nutrients to body cells

Recognize Cues [Assessment]
- Obtain a medication and herbal history from the patient. Report if a drug-drug or drug-herbal interaction is probable.
- Obtain vital signs. Report abnormal blood pressure (BP) and bradycardia, and compare vital signs with baseline findings.
- Check laboratory values related to renal and liver function periodically. Elevated blood urea nitrogen (BUN) and serum creatinine may be caused by beta blockers or a cardiac disorder. Elevated cardiac enzymes, such as aspartate transaminase (AST) and lactate dehydrogenase (LDH), may be caused by beta blockers or cardiac disorder.

Analyze Cues and Prioritize Hypothesis [Patient Problems]
- Hypertension
- Fatigue

Generate Solutions [Planning]
- The patient's BP will be 120/80 or below.
- The patient will take medication as prescribed.

Take Action [Nursing Interventions]
- Monitor vital signs, especially BP and pulse.
- Monitor laboratory results, especially BUN, serum creatinine, AST, and LDH.

Patient Teaching
General
- ⚡ Encourage patients to comply with the drug regimen. Advise that abrupt discontinuation of antihypertensive drugs may cause rebound hypertension.
- Inform patients that herbs can interfere with beta blockers.
- ⚡ Advise patients to avoid over-the-counter (OTC) drugs without first checking with a health care provider. Many OTC drugs carry warnings against use in the presence of hypertension or concurrent use with antihypertensives.
- Suggest that patients wear a MedicAlert bracelet or carry a card indicating their health problem and prescribed drugs.
- Teach patients in trauma situations to inform a health care provider of drugs taken daily, such as a beta blocker. Beta blockers block compensatory effects of the body to the shock state. Glucagon may be needed to reverse the effects so the patient can be resuscitated.

Self-Administration
- Teach patients or family members how to take a radial pulse and BP and to report abnormal findings to a health care provider.

Side Effects
- Advise patients that antihypertensives may cause dizziness (orthostatic hypotension). Warn patients to rise slowly from lying or sitting to a standing position.
- Advise patients to report dizziness, slow pulse rate, changes in BP, heart palpitation, confusion, or gastrointestinal (GI) upset to a health care provider.
- Alert patients with diabetes mellitus to possible hypoglycemic symptoms.
- Inform patients that antihypertensives may cause sexual dysfunction (e.g., impotence).

Diet
- Teach patients and family members nonpharmacologic methods to decrease BP, such as a low-salt diet, relaxation techniques, exercise, smoking cessation, and decreased alcohol ingestion (limit to one drink for females and two drinks for males daily).
- Advise patients to report constipation. Foods high in fiber, a stool softener, and increased water intake (except in patients with heart failure) are usually indicated.

Evaluate Outcomes [Evaluation]
- Evaluate the effectiveness of the drug therapy (decreased BP, absence of side effects).
- Determine that the patient is adhering to the drug regimen.

Drugs in this group include methyldopa, clonidine, and guanfacine. Methyldopa was one of the first drugs widely used to control hypertension. In high doses, methyldopa and clonidine can cause sodium and water retention. Frequently, methyldopa and clonidine are administered with diuretics. Clonidine is available in a transdermal preparation that provides a 7-day duration of action. Transdermal patches are replaced every 7 days and may be left on while bathing; skin irritations may occur. Guanfacine has effects similar to clonidine. Guanfacine has a long half-life and usually is taken once a day. Table 42.1 lists centrally acting alpha$_2$ agonists along with beta blockers.

Side Effects and Adverse Reactions. Side effects and adverse reactions of alpha$_2$ agonists include drowsiness, dry mouth, dizziness, and slow heart rate (bradycardia). Methyldopa should not be used in patients with impaired liver function, and serum liver enzymes should be monitored periodically in all patients. This group of drugs must not be abruptly discontinued because a rebound hypertensive crisis can result. If the drug needs to be stopped immediately, another antihypertensive drug is usually prescribed to avoid rebound hypertensive symptoms such as restlessness, tachycardia, tremors, headache, and increased BP. Rebound hypertension is less likely to occur with guanfacine. The nurse should emphasize the need to take the medication as prescribed. This group of drugs can cause sodium and water retention, resulting in peripheral edema. A diuretic may be ordered with methyldopa or clonidine to decrease water and sodium retention (edema). Patients who are pregnant or contemplating pregnancy should avoid clonidine. Methyldopa is frequently used to treat chronic or pregnancy-induced hypertension; however, it crosses the placental barrier, and small amounts may enter the breast milk of a lactating patient.

Alpha-Adrenergic Blockers

This group of drugs blocks the alpha-adrenergic receptors (alpha blockers), resulting in vasodilation and decreased BP. They help maintain the renal blood flow rate. Alpha blockers are useful in treating hypertension in patients with lipid abnormalities. They decrease the very-low-density lipoprotein and the low-density lipoprotein (LDL) responsible for the buildup of fatty plaques in the arteries (atherosclerosis). In addition, they increase high-density lipoprotein levels. Alpha blockers are safe for patients with diabetes because they do not affect glucose metabolism. They also do not affect respiratory function. Nonselective alpha-adrenergic blockers—phenoxybenzamine and phentolamine—should not be given to patients with coronary artery disease because of their stimulating effects and resultant increase in myocardial oxygen demand.

The selective alpha₁-adrenergic blockers—prazosin, terazosin, and doxazosin—are used mainly to reduce BP and can be used to treat benign prostatic hypertrophy (BPH). Prazosin is a commonly prescribed drug. Terazosin and doxazosin have longer half-lives than prazosin, and they are normally given once at bedtime. When prazosin is taken with alcohol or other antihypertensives, the hypotensive state can be intensified. These drugs, like the centrally acting alpha₂ agonists, cause sodium and water retention with edema; therefore diuretics are frequently given concomitantly to decrease fluid accumulation in the extremities.

Pharmacokinetics. Prazosin is absorbed through the GI tract, but a large portion of prazosin is lost during hepatic first-pass metabolism. The half-life is short, so the drug should be administered twice a day. Prazosin is highly protein bound, and when it is given with other highly protein-bound drugs, the patient should be assessed for adverse reactions.

Pharmacodynamics. Selective alpha-adrenergic blockers dilate the arterioles and venules, decreasing peripheral resistance and lowering BP. With prazosin, the heart rate is only slightly increased, whereas with nonselective alpha blockers such as phenoxybenzamine, the BP is greatly reduced, and reflex tachycardia can occur. Nonselective alpha blockers are more effective for acute hypertension; selective alpha blockers are more useful for long-term essential hypertension.

The onset of action of prazosin occurs between 30 minutes and 2 hours. The duration of action of prazosin is less than 24 hours. Table 42.2 presents drug data for selective and nonselective alpha blockers.

⚠ TABLE 42.2 Antihypertensives: Sympatholytics—Alpha-Adrenergic and Peripherally Acting Blockers and Direct-Acting Vasodilators

Drug	Route and Dosage	Uses and Considerations
Selective Alpha-Adrenergic Blockers		
Doxazosin mesylate	Hypertension: A: PO: Initially: 1 mg/d; *max:* 16 mg/d	For hypertension and BPH. May cause dizziness, drowsiness, headache, fatigue, weakness, visual impairment, orthostatic hypotension, palpitations, edema, and erectile dysfunction. Give without regard to meals. PB: 98%; $t\frac{1}{2}$: 22 h
Prazosin hydrochloride	See Prototype Drug Chart: Prazosin Hydrochloride	
Terazosin hydrochloride	Hypertension: A: PO: Initially: 1 mg at bedtime; *maint:* 1–20 mg/d in divided doses; *max:* 20 mg/d in divided doses	For hypertension and BPH. May cause dizziness, drowsiness, headache, weakness, nasal congestion, orthostatic hypotension, palpitations, peripheral edema, nausea, and erectile dysfunction. Give without regard to meals. PB: 90%–94%; $t\frac{1}{2}$: 12 h
Nonselective Alpha-Adrenergic Blockers		
Phenoxybenzamine hydrochloride	A: PO: Initially: 10 mg bid; *maint:* 20–40 mg bid/tid	For hypertension associated with pheochromocytoma. May cause dizziness, drowsiness, fatigue, weakness, nasal congestion, orthostatic hypotension, tachycardia, gastritis, and ejaculatory dysfunction. PB: UK; $t\frac{1}{2}$: 24 h
Phentolamine	Hypertension: A: IM/IV: 5 mg 1–2 h before surgery; may repeat during surgery if needed	For hypertension before and during pheochromocytomectomy, pheochromocytoma diagnosis, and prevention and treatment of IV drug extravasation. May cause dizziness, weakness, headache, nasal congestion, dental pain, ocular pain, conjunctival hyperemia, bradycardia, tachycardia, hypo/hypertension, dysgeusia, abdominal pain, vomiting, diarrhea, and paresthesias. PB: UK; $t\frac{1}{2}$: 19 min
Alpha₁- and Beta₁-Adrenergic Blockers		
Labetalol hydrochloride	Hypertension: A: PO: Initially: 100 mg bid; *maint:* 200–400 mg bid; *max:* 2.4 g/d in 2–3 divided doses	For hypertension. May cause dizziness, fatigue, nasal congestion, orthostatic hypotension, hyperhidrosis, dyspepsia, nausea, vomiting, paresthesia, erectile/ejaculation dysfunction, and elevated hepatic enzymes. PB: 50%; $t\frac{1}{2}$: 6–8 h
Direct-Acting Vasodilators		
Hydralazine hydrochloride	Hypertension: A: PO: Initially: 10 mg qid; *maint:* 100–200 mg in divided doses; *max:* 300 mg/d A: IM: 10–50 mg q4–6h PRN A: IV: 10–20 mg q4–6h PRN	For hypertension, hypertensive urgency and emergency. May cause headaches, dizziness, tachycardia, palpitations, hypotension, angina, edema, nasal congestion, anorexia, nausea, vomiting, diarrhea, paresthesia, lupus-like symptom. Closely monitor vital signs. PB: 87%; $t\frac{1}{2}$: 3–7 h
Minoxidil	Hypertension: A: PO: Initially: 5 mg/d; *maint:* 5–100 mg/d in divided doses; *max:* 100 mg/d	For hypertension and alopecia. May cause headache, hypotension, tachycardia, angina, peripheral edema, erythema, pericardial effusion, edema, and excess hair growth. Needs close supervision due to excess hypotension, tachycardia, and angina. PB: 0%; $t\frac{1}{2}$: 4 h
Nitroprusside	Hypertensive emergency: A: IV: Initially: 0.3–0.5 mcg/kg per minute in D₅W infusion till stable; *max:* 10 mcg/kg per minute for 10 min	For hypertensive urgency and emergency and for HF. May cause dizziness, headache, restlessness, hypotension, bradycardia, tachycardia, palpitations, flushing, methemoglobinemia, and cyanide toxicity. Assure that solution is clear and colorless. Do not give by direct IV. Dilute 50 mg in 250–1000 mL of D₅W. Protect from light. PB: UK; $t\frac{1}{2}$: 2 min

<, Less than; *A*, adult; *bid*, twice a day; *BPH*, benign prostatic hyperplasia; *d*, day; *D₅W*, dextrose 5% in water; *h*, hour; *HF*, heart failure; *IM*, intramuscular; *IV*, intravenous; *maint*, maintenance; *max*, maximum; *min*, minute; *PB*, protein binding; *PO*, by mouth; *PRN*, as needed; *q*, every; *qid*, four times a day; *t½*, half-life; *UK*, unknown.

Side Effects and Adverse Reactions. Side effects of prazosin, doxazosin, and terazosin include orthostatic hypotension (dizziness, faintness, lightheadedness, and increased heart rate, which may occur with first dose), nausea, headache, drowsiness, nasal congestion caused by vasodilation, edema, and weight gain.

Side effects of phentolamine include orthostatic hypotension, reflex tachycardia caused by the severe decrease in BP, nasal congestion caused by vasodilation, and GI disturbances.

Drug Interactions. Drug interactions occur when alpha-adrenergic blockers are taken with antiinflammatory drugs and nitrates, such as nitroglycerin taken for angina. Peripheral edema is intensified when prazosin and an antiinflammatory drug are taken daily. Nitroglycerin taken for angina lowers BP. If prazosin is taken with nitroglycerin, syncope (faintness) caused by a decrease in BP can occur. The selective alpha-adrenergic blocker prazosin is shown in Prototype Drug Chart: Prazosin Hydrochloride.

⚡ Alpha$_1$- and Beta$_1$-Adrenergic Blockers

This group of drugs blocks both the alpha$_1$ and beta$_1$ receptors. Labetalol is an example of an alpha/beta blocker. Blocking the alpha$_1$ receptor causes vasodilation, which decreases resistance to blood flow. The effect on the alpha receptor is stronger than the effect on the beta receptor; therefore BP is lowered, and pulse rate is moderately decreased. By blocking the cardiac beta$_1$ receptor, both heart rate and AV contractility are decreased. Large doses of alpha/beta blockers could block beta$_2$-adrenergic receptors, thus increasing airway resistance. Patients who have severe asthma should *not* take large doses of labetalol. Table 42.2 lists alpha/beta blockers.

Common side effects of these drugs include orthostatic hypotension, dizziness, paresthesia, nasal congestion, nausea, and fatigue. Large doses of labetalol may cause atrioventricular (AV) heart block.

Direct-Acting Arteriolar Vasodilators

Vasodilators are potent antihypertensive drugs. Direct-acting vasodilators act by relaxing the smooth muscles of the blood vessels, mainly the arteries, causing vasodilation. Vasodilators promote an increase in blood flow to the brain and kidneys. With vasodilation, the BP decreases and sodium and water are retained, resulting in peripheral edema. Diuretics can be given with a direct-acting vasodilator to decrease the edema.

Two direct-acting vasodilators, hydralazine and minoxidil, are used for moderate to severe (dose-related) hypertension. These two drugs cause little orthostatic hypotension because of minimum dilation of the arterioles. However, reflex tachycardia and release of renin can occur secondary to vasodilation and decreased BP. Beta blockers are frequently prescribed with arteriolar vasodilators to decrease the heart rate; this counteracts the effect of reflex tachycardia.

⚡ Nitroprusside is prescribed for acute hypertensive emergency. This is a very potent vasodilator that rapidly decreases BP. Nitroprusside acts on both arterial and venous vessels. Table 42.2 lists direct-acting vasodilators.

◎ CLINICAL JUDGMENT [NURSING PROCESS]

Antihypertensives: Alpha-Adrenergic Blockers

Concept: Perfusion
- The passage of blood flow through the arteries and capillaries that deliver oxygen and nutrients to body cells

Recognize Cues [Assessment]
- Obtain a medication history from the patient that includes current drugs. Report if drug-drug or drug-herbal interaction is probable. Prazosin is highly protein bound and can displace other highly protein-bound drugs.
- Obtain baseline vital signs and weight for future comparisons.
- Check urinary output. Report if it is decreased (less than 600 mL/day) because the drug is contraindicated if renal disease is present.

Analyze Cues and Prioritize Hypothesis [Patient Problems]
- Hypertension
- Fatigue

Generate Solutions [Planning]
- The patient's blood pressure (BP) will decrease to 120/80 or below.
- The patient will follow the proper drug regimen.

Take Action [Nursing Interventions]
- Monitor vital signs. The desired therapeutic effect of prazosin may not fully occur for 4 weeks. A sudden marked decrease in BP and tachycardia should be reported.
- Check daily for fluid retention in extremities and weight gain. Prazosin may cause sodium and water retention.

Patient Teaching
General
- ⚡ Advise patients to adhere to the drug regimen. Explain that abrupt discontinuation of antihypertensive drugs may cause rebound hypertension.
- Inform patients that orthostatic hypotension may occur. Explain that before rising, patients should sit and dangle their feet. Drugs may be taken at bedtime to avoid orthostatic hypotension.
- Teach patients to self-monitor daily weights. Prazosin may lead to edema.

Self-Administration
- Teach patients or family members how to take and record BP. A BP chart should be established, and BP changes should be reported.

Side Effects
- Caution patients that dizziness, lightheadedness, and drowsiness may occur, especially when a drug is first initiated. If these symptoms occur, a health care provider should be notified.
- Inform male patients that impotence may occur if high doses of drug are prescribed. This problem should be reported to the health care provider.
- Tell patients to report if edema is present in the morning. Water retention is a problem with alpha blockers.
- ⚡ Inform patients not to take over-the-counter (OTC) cold, cough, or allergy medications without first contacting the health care provider.

Diet
- Encourage patients to decrease salt intake unless otherwise indicated by the health care provider.

Evaluate Outcomes [Evaluation]
- Evaluate the effectiveness of the drug in controlling BP; side effects should be absent.
- Evaluate the patient's adherence to the medication schedule.
- Evaluate the patient's knowledge of the medication.

PROTOTYPE DRUG CHART

Prazosin Hydrochloride

Drug Class	Dosage
Antihypertensive: Alpha-adrenergic blocker	A: PO: Initially 1 mg bid/tid; *maint:* 2–20 mg/d; *max:* 40 mg/d in divided doses

Contraindications	Drug-Lab-Food Interactions
Hypersensitivity *Caution:* Angina, orthostatic hypotension, syncope, ocular surgery, priapism, older adults, pregnancy, breast-feeding	Drug: Increased hypotensive effect with other antihypertensives, nitrates, diuretics, and alcohol; decreased effects with NSAIDs Lab: Increased hepatic enzymes

Pharmacokinetics	Pharmacodynamics
Absorption: GI: 60% (5% to circulation) Distribution: PB: 97% Metabolism: t½: 2–4 h Excretion: In bile and feces, 10% in urine	PO: Onset: 0.5–2 h Peak: 2–4 h Duration: <24 h

Therapeutic Effects/Uses
To control hypertension
Mechanism of action: Dilates peripheral blood vessels by blocking alpha-adrenergic receptors.

Side Effects	Adverse Reactions
Dizziness, drowsiness, headache, weakness, fatigue, syncope, depression, anxiety, blurred vision, nasal congestion, dry mouth, abdominal pain, nausea, vomiting, diarrhea, constipation, rash, urinary frequency/incontinence, erectile dysfunction, peripheral edema	Orthostatic hypotension, palpitations, tachycardia, dyspnea, pancreatitis, elevated liver enzymes

A, Adult; *bid*, twice a day; *GI*, gastrointestinal; *h*, hour; *maint*, maintenance; *max*, maximum; *NSAID*, nonsteroidal antiinflammatory drug; *PB*, protein binding; *PO*, by mouth; *t½*, half-life; *tid*, three times a day.

Side Effects and Adverse Reactions
The effects of hydralazine are numerous and include reflex tachycardia, palpitations, edema, nasal congestion, headache, dizziness, lupus-like symptoms, and neurologic symptoms (tingling, numbness). Minoxidil has similar side effects, as well as tachycardia, edema, and excess hair growth. In addition, it can precipitate an anginal attack.

Nitroprusside can cause reflex tachycardia, palpitations, restlessness, agitation, nausea, and confusion. Nitroprusside is discussed in greater detail in Chapter 55.

Angiotensin-Converting Enzyme Inhibitors
When ACE is inhibited, it in turn inhibits the formation of angiotensin II (vasoconstrictor) and blocks the release of aldosterone. Aldosterone promotes sodium retention and potassium excretion. When aldosterone is blocked, sodium is excreted along with water, and potassium is retained. ACE inhibitors cause little change in cardiac output or heart rate, and they lower peripheral resistance. (Fig. 42.1 illustrates the RAAS.) These drugs can be used in patients who have elevated serum renin levels.

The ACE inhibitors are used primarily to treat hypertension; some of these agents are also effective in treating heart failure. The ACE inhibitors are benazepril, captopril, enalapril maleate, fosinopril, lisinopril, moexipril, perindopril, quinapril, ramipril, and trandolapril, which are all presented in Table 42.3. These drugs can be used for first-line antihypertensive therapy, but thiazide diuretics are recommended by JNC 8.

African American patients and older adults do not respond to ACE inhibitors with the desired reduction in BP, but when taken with a diuretic, BP will usually be lowered. ACE inhibitors should not be given during pregnancy because they reduce placental blood flow. For patients with renal insufficiency, reduction of the drug dose (except for fosinopril) is necessary.

With the exception of moexipril, which should be taken on an empty stomach for maximum effectiveness, ACE inhibitors can be administered with food.

Side Effects and Adverse Reactions
The primary side effect of ACE inhibitors is a constant, irritated cough. Other side effects include nausea, vomiting, diarrhea, headache, dizziness, fatigue, insomnia, serum potassium excess (hyperkalemia), and tachycardia. The persistent, nonproductive "ACE cough" may be relieved on discontinuance of the drug. Often an ARB may be substituted without cough as a side effect. The major adverse effects are first-dose hypotension and hyperkalemia. Hypotension results because of the vasodilating effect. First-dose hypotension is more common in patients also taking diuretics. Angioedema—swelling of the face, tongue, lips, mucous membranes, and larynx and extremity edema—is rare but may occur due to hypersensitivity and has a higher incidence in African American patients. This may occur within hours or 1 week after the first dose. Angioedema may be reversed with drug discontinuance. When laryngeal edema occurs, the patient may require rescue epinephrine.

Contraindications
ACE inhibitors should not be given during pregnancy because harm to the fetus due to reduction in placental blood flow could occur. This group of drugs should not be taken with potassium-sparing diuretics such as spironolactone or with salt substitutes that contain potassium because of the risk of hyperkalemia (serum potassium excess).

TABLE 42.3 Antihypertensives: Angiotensin-Converting Enzyme (ACE) Inhibitors and Angiotensin II Receptor Blockers (ARBs)

Drug	Route and Dosage	Uses and Considerations
Angiotensin Antagonists (ACE Inhibitors)		
Benazepril hydrochloride	A: PO: Initially 10 mg/d; *maint:* 10–40 mg/d in 1–2 divided doses; *max:* 80 mg/d	To treat hypertension. May cause dizziness, headache, fatigue, hypotension, palpitations, angina, flushing, peripheral edema, nausea, constipation, erectile dysfunction, and hyperkalemia. PB: 95%; $t\frac{1}{2}$: 10–11 h
Captopril	Hypertension: A: PO: Initially 25 mg bid/tid; *maint:* 12.5–150 mg/d in divided doses; *max:* 450 mg/d	For hypertension, post MI, and HF. May cause dizziness, fatigue, hypotension, pallor, tachycardia, cough, dyspnea, dysgeusia, anorexia, constipation, rash, and pruritus. PB: 25–30%; $t\frac{1}{2}$: 2 h
Enalapril maleate	Hypertension: A: PO: Initially 5 mg/d; *maint:* 5–40 mg/d in 1–2 divided doses; *max:* 40 mg/d	For hypertension and HF. May cause dizziness, syncope, headache, fatigue, weakness, orthostatic hypotension, tachycardia, palpitations, cough, anorexia, hyperkalemia, hyponatremia, and rash. PB: 50%; $t\frac{1}{2}$: 11 h
Fosinopril	Hypertension: A: PO: Initially 10 mg/d; *maint:* 20–40 mg/d in 1–2 divided doses; *max:* 80 mg/d	For hypertension and HF. May cause dizziness, weakness, orthostatic hypotension, palpitations, flushing, peripheral edema, cough, rash, and hyperkalemia. PB: 99.4%; $t\frac{1}{2}$: 11.5 h
Lisinopril	Hypertension: A: PO: Initially 10 mg/d; *maint:* 10–40 mg/d; *max:* 80 mg/d	For hypertension, AMI, and HF. May cause dizziness, syncope, headache, weakness, orthostatic hypotension, blurred vision, cough, and hyperkalemia. PB: UK; $t\frac{1}{2}$: 12 h
Moexipril	A: PO: Initially 7.5 mg/d; *maint:* 7.5–30 mg/d; *max:* 30 mg/d in divided doses	For hypertension. May increase serum lithium levels, causing toxicity. May cause dizziness, fatigue, palpitations, chest pain, orthostatic hypotension, flushing, cough, diarrhea, myalgia, rash, and hyperkalemia. Give dose 1 h before a meal. PB: 50%; $t\frac{1}{2}$: 1.3 h
Perindopril erbumine	Hypertension: A: PO: Initially 2–4 mg/d; *maint:* 4–8 mg/d in 1–2 divided doses; *max:* 16 mg/d Older A: Initially 4 mg/d; *max:* 8 mg/d	For hypertension and to prevent MI. May cause dizziness, headache, weakness, orthostatic hypotension, cough, back pain, hyperkalemia, and elevated hepatic enzymes. Give with or without food. Twice daily dosing has slightly greater efficacy. PB: 60%; $t\frac{1}{2}$: 0.8–1 h
Ramipril	Hypertension: A: PO: Initially 2.5 mg/d; *max:* 20 mg/d	For hypertension, AMI, HF, and prevention of stroke. May cause dizziness, syncope, headache, weakness, orthostatic hypotension, palpitations, angina, cough, nausea, vomiting, and hyperkalemia. PB: 73%; $t\frac{1}{2}$: 3–17 h
Trandolapril	Hypertension: A: PO: Initially 1 mg/d for caucasian patients, 2 mg/d for African American patients: *maint:* 2–4 mg/d; *max:* 8 mg/d	For hypertension, AMI, and HF. May cause dizziness, syncope, weakness, bradycardia, hypotension, palpitations, cough, dyspepsia, gastritis, hyperkalemia, hypocalcemia, myalgia, and hyperuricemia. Give without regard to meals. PB: 80%; $t\frac{1}{2}$: 6 h
Combinations of ACE Inhibitors With Calcium Blockers		
Benazepril with amlodipine	A: PO: Initially amlodipine 2.5/benazepril 10 mg/d; *max:* amlodipine 10 mg/d and benazepril 40 mg/d	For hypertension in those unresponsive to monotherapy. May cause dizziness, headache, edema, hypotension, peripheral edema, cough, and hyperkalemia. Give at same time qd with or without regard to meals. PB: amlodipine 93%, benazepril 95%; $t\frac{1}{2}$: amlodipine 30–50 h, benazepril 10–11 h
Trandolapril and verapamil	A: PO: Individually titrated. *max:* 8 mg/d trandolapril and 240 mg/d verapamil	For hypertension. May cause dizziness, headache, fatigue, hypotension, chest pain, bradycardia, AV block, edema, cough, constipation, ileus, arthralgia, and hyperkalemia. PB: trandolapril 80%, verapamil 90%; $t\frac{1}{2}$: trandolapril 6 h, verapamil 2–12 h
Perindopril arginine and amlodipine besylate	A: PO: Initially perindopril 3.5 mg/d and amlodipine 2.5 mg/d for 1–2 wk; *max:* perindopril 14 mg/d and amlodipine 10 mg/d	For hypertension. May cause dizziness, headache, depression, visual impairment, tachycardia, bradycardia, hypotension, chest pain, peripheral edema, cough, dyspnea, constipation, and hyperkalemia. PB: perindopril 60%, amlodipine 93%; $t\frac{1}{2}$: perindopril 0.8–1.3 h, amlodipine 30–50 h
ARBs		
Candesartan	Hypertension: A: PO: Initially 16 mg/d; *maint:* 8–32 mg/d in 1–2 divided doses; *max:* 32 mg/d	For hypertension and HF. May cause dizziness, hypotension, pharyngitis, rhinitis, back pain, hyperkalemia, infection, hyperbilirubinemia, and elevated hepatic enzymes. Give with or without food. PB: 99%; $t\frac{1}{2}$: 9–12 h
Irbesartan	Hypertension: A: PO: Initially 150 mg/d; *maint:* 150–300 mg/d; *max:* 300 mg/d	For hypertension, diabetic nephropathy, and proteinuria. May cause dizziness, headache, fatigue, anxiety, orthostatic hypotension, chest pain, edema, cough, dyspepsia, abdominal pain, diarrhea, and hyperkalemia. Give without regard to food. PB: 90%; $t\frac{1}{2}$: 11–15 h

Continued

TABLE 42.3 Antihypertensives: Angiotensin-Converting Enzyme (ACE) Inhibitors and Angiotensin II Receptor Blockers (ARBs)—cont'd

Drug	Route and Dosage	Uses and Considerations
Losartan potassium	Hypertension: A: PO: Initially 50 mg/d; *maint:* 25–100 mg/d in 1–2 divided doses; *max:* 100 mg/d in divided doses	For hypertension, diabetic nephropathy, and stroke prophylaxis. May cause dizziness, headache, fatigue, weakness, cough, pharyngitis, nasal congestion, orthostatic hypotension, edema, nausea, hyperkalemia, and infection. Give without regard to food. PB: 98%; t½: 2 h
Olmesartan medoxomil	A: PO: Initially 20 mg/d; for 2 wk, *maint:* 20–40 mg/d; *max:* 40 mg/d	For hypertension. May cause dizziness, headache, orthostatic hypotension, peripheral edema, sinusitis, pharyngitis, and rhinitis, and hyperglycemia. Give without regard to food. PB: 99%; t½: 13 h
Telmisartan	Hypertension: A: PO: Initially 40 mg/d; *maint:* 20–80 mg/d; *max:* 80 mg/d	For hypertension and to prevent MI and CVA. May cause dizziness, chest pain, orthostatic hypotension, edema, sinusitis, cough, diarrhea, back pain, hyperkalemia, skin ulcer, and infection. Give without regard to food. PB: 99.5%; t½: 24 h
Valsartan	See Prototype Drug Chart: Valsartan	
Azilsartan	A: PO: Initially 40–80 mg/d; *maint:* 40–80 mg/d; *max:* 80 mg/d	For hypertension. May cause dizziness, fatigue, weakness, orthostatic hypotension, cough, nausea, diarrhea, and muscle cramps. Give without regard to food. PB: 99%; t½: 11 h
Aldosterone Receptor Antagonists		
Eplerenone	Hypertension: A: PO: Initially 50 mg/d for 4 wk; then may increase to 50 mg bid; *max:* 100 mg/d	For hypertension, HF, and AMI. May cause dizziness, fatigue, bradycardia, edema, cough, diarrhea, hyponatremia, hyperkalemia, hypertriglyceridemia, hypercholesterolemia, hyperuricemia, and vaginal bleeding. Give without regard to food. Advise patient to not use dietary salt substitutes containing potassium while taking eplerenone. PB: 50%; t½: 4–6 h
Direct Renin Inhibitors		
Aliskiren	A: PO: Initially 150 mg/d; *maint:* 150–300 mg/d; *max:* 300 mg/d	For hypertension. May cause dizziness, hypotension, peripheral edema, cough, pharyngitis, diarrhea, hyperkalemia, hyperuricemia, and gout. Give with or without food but consistent in regard to meals. PB: UK; t½: 24 h

A, Adult; *AMI*, acute myocardial infarction; *bid*, two times a day; *d*, day; *h*, hour; *HF*, heart failure; *maint*, maintenance; *max*, maximum; *MI*, myocardial infarction; *PB*, protein binding; *PO*, by mouth; *t½*, half-life; *tid*, three times a day; *UK*, unknown.

CLINICAL JUDGMENT [NURSING PROCESS]
Antihypertensives: Angiotensin-Converting Enzyme Inhibitors

Concept: Perfusion
- The passage of blood flow through the arteries and capillaries that deliver oxygen and nutrients to body cells

Recognize Cues [Assessment]
- Obtain a drug and herbal history from the patient of current drugs taken. Report if a drug-drug or drug-herb interaction is probable.
- Obtain baseline vital signs for future comparisons.
- Check laboratory values for serum protein, albumin, blood urea nitrogen (BUN), creatinine, potassium, and white blood cell count to compare with future serum levels.

Analyze Cues and Prioritize Hypothesis [Patient Problems]
- Hypertension
- Anxiety
- Fatigue

Generate Outcomes [Planning]
- The patient's blood pressure (BP) will decrease to 120/80 or below.
- The patient will rise to an upright position slowly to avoid orthostatic hypotension.

Take Action [Nursing Interventions]
- Monitor BP. A sudden drop in BP should be reported.
- Monitor laboratory tests related to renal function (BUN, creatinine, protein) and blood glucose levels. *Caution:* Watch for hypoglycemic reactions in patients with diabetes mellitus. Urine protein may be checked in the morning using a dipstick.
- Report to a health care provider any bruising, petechiae, or bleeding. These may indicate a severe adverse reaction to an angiotensin antagonist such as captopril.

Patient Teaching
General
- ⚡ Warn patients not to abruptly discontinue use of captopril without notifying a health care provider. Rebound hypertension could result.
- Inform patients not to take over-the-counter (OTC) drugs such as cold medications without first contacting a health care provider.
- Advise patients not to use salt substitutes that contain potassium.
- ⚡ Warn pregnant patients and those contemplating becoming pregnant not to take angiotensin-converting enzyme (ACE) inhibitors or angiotensin II receptor blockers (ARBs); they can cause harm to the fetus.
- Teach patients to rise slowly to avoid orthostatic hypotension.

CLINICAL JUDGMENT [NURSING PROCESS]—CONT'D
Antihypertensives: Angiotensin-Converting Enzyme Inhibitors

Self-Administration
- Teach patients or family members how to take and record BP. A BP chart should be established, and BP changes should be reported.

Side Effects
- ⚡ Explain to patients that dizziness and/or lightheadedness may occur during the first week of captopril therapy. If dizziness persists, a health care provider should be notified.
- Monitor the patient for the following side effects: angioedema, cough dysgeusia, weakness, hyperkalemia, orthostatic hypotension, and renal impairment.
- Advise patients to report any occurrence of bleeding.

Diet
- Teach patients to take captopril 20 minutes to 1 hour before a meal. Food decreases 35% of captopril absorption.
- Warn patients that the taste of food may be diminished during the first month of drug therapy.
- Advise patients to avoid foods high in potassium because hyperkalemia is an adverse effect of ACE inhibitors.

Evaluate Outcomes [Evaluation]
- Evaluate the effectiveness of the drug therapy (absence of severe side effects, BP returns to desired range).
- Evaluate the patient's renal function.

Angiotensin II Receptor Blockers

ARBs are similar to ACE inhibitors in that they prevent the release of aldosterone, a sodium-retaining hormone. They act on the RAAS. The difference between ARBs and ACE inhibitors is that ARBs block angiotensin II from the angiotensin I (AT_1) receptors found in many tissues, whereas ACE inhibitors inhibit the ACE in the formation of angiotensin II. ARBs cause vasodilation and decrease peripheral resistance. They do not cause the constant, irritated cough ACE inhibitors can. Like ACE inhibitors, ARBs should not be taken during pregnancy.

Losartan, valsartan, irbesartan, candesartan, eprosartan, olmesartan, azilsartan, and telmisartan are examples of ARBs. These agents block the vasoconstrictor effects of angiotensin II at the receptor site. The combination of losartan potassium and hydrochlorothiazide tablets, valsartan and hydrochlorothiazide tablets, and others should not cause serum potassium excess or loss. ARBs may be used as a first-line treatment for hypertension.

Prototype Drug Chart: Valsartan gives the pharmacologic data related to valsartan.

⚡ PATIENT SAFETY

Do Not Confuse …
- **Diovan** (valsartan), an angiotensin II receptor blocker, and **Dioval** (estradiol), an estrogen hormone. If both drugs are in the home, caution must be taken to select the correct drug, especially by the male patient taking Diovan and the female patient taking Dioval.

Pharmacokinetics
Valsartan is prescribed primarily to manage hypertension. The combination drug containing valsartan plus a low dose of hydrochlorothiazide is rapidly absorbed in the GI tract and undergoes first-pass metabolism in the liver to form active metabolites. It is highly protein bound at 95% and should not be given during pregnancy, especially during the second and third trimesters. The half-life is approximately 6 hours, and the drug is excreted in urine and feces.

Pharmacodynamics
Valsartan is a potent vasodilator. It blocks the binding of angiotensin II to the AT_1 receptors found in many tissues. Its peak time is approximately 6 hours, and it has a long duration of action (24 hours).

Like ACE inhibitors, ARBs are less effective for treating hypertension in African American patients. In addition, like ACE inhibitors, ARBs may cause angioedema. These agents can be taken with or without food and are suitable for patients with mild hepatic insufficiency.

PROTOTYPE DRUG CHART
Valsartan

Drug Class	Dosage
Antihypertensive: Angiotensin II receptor blocker	Hypertension: A: PO: Initially 80–160 mg/d; *maint*: 80–320 mg/d; *max*: 320 mg/d

Contraindications	Drug-Lab-Food Interactions
Hypersensitivity *Caution:* Renal and hepatic impairments, hypotension, heart failure, hypovolemia, hyperkalemia, ACE inhibitor induced angioedema, older adults, African American patients, pregnancy, breast-feeding	Drug: Antihypertensives, diuretics, MAOIs, and alcohol may increase hypotensive effects; ACE inhibitors and aspirin may increase hyperkalemia and renal dysfunction; digoxin and NSAIDs may increase renal dysfunction; lithium may increase lithium toxicity. Lab: May increase AST, ALT, ALP, bilirubin, BUN, creatinine, Hct, Hgb

Pharmacokinetics	Pharmacodynamics
Absorption: Rapidly absorbed, 10%–35% in blood circulation Distribution: PB: 95% Metabolism: t½: 6 h Excretion: 13% in urine and 83% in bile/feces	PO: Onset: 2 h Peak: 6 h Duration: 24 h

Therapeutic Effects/Uses
To treat hypertension and heart failure
Mechanism of action: Potent vasodilator that inhibits binding of angiotensin II.

Side Effects	Adverse Reactions
Dizziness, drowsiness, headache, anxiety, fatigue, weakness, blurred vision, pharyngitis, cough, dyspnea, dyspepsia, abdominal pain, nausea, diarrhea, constipation, back pain, arthralgia, muscle cramps, paresthesia, edema, erectile dysfunction	Orthostatic hypotension, chest pain, palpitations, hyperkalemia, rhabdomyolysis, elevated hepatic enzymes *Life threatening:* Angioedema, renal dysfunction, neutropenia

A, Adult; *ACE*, angiotensin-converting enzyme; *ALP*, alkaline phosphatase; *ALT*, alanine transaminase; *AST*, aspartate transferase; *BUN*, blood urea nitrogen; *d*, day; *h*, hour; *maint*, maintenance; *MAOI*, monoamine oxidase inhibitor; *max*, maximum; *PB*, protein binding; *PO*, by mouth; *t½*, half-life.

Direct Renin Inhibitors

The first US Food and Drug Administration (FDA)-approved direct renin inhibitor for treating hypertension is aliskiren, which binds with renin and causes a reduction of angiotensin I, angiotensin II, and aldosterone levels (see Fig. 42.1). It is effective for mild and moderate hypertension. Aliskiren can be used alone or with another antihypertensive agent. It has an additive effect in reducing BP when combined with a thiazide diuretic or an ARB. This drug, when used as monotherapy, has not proven to be as effective in reducing BP in the African American population.

Calcium Channel Blockers

Slow calcium channels are found in the myocardium (heart muscle) and vascular smooth muscle (VSM) cells. Free calcium increases

TABLE 42.4 Antihypertensives: Calcium Channel Blockers

Drug	Route and Dosage	Uses and Considerations
Phenylalkylamines		
Verapamil	Hypertension: Immediate release: A: PO: Initially 80 mg tid; *max:* 480 mg/d Older A: PO: Initially 40 mg tid; *max:* 480 mg/d Extended-release 12-h tablet: A: PO: Initially 180 mg/d in the morning; *maint:* 120–360 mg/d; *max:* 240 mg bid Older A: PO: Initially 120 mg/d; *max:* 240 mg bid	For hypertension, angina, and dysrhythmia. May cause dizziness, headache, fatigue, weakness, confusion, blurred vision, orthostatic hypotension, bradycardia, peripheral edema, nausea, constipation, and erectile dysfunction. Avoid grapefruit juice before or after dose. PB: 90%; $t\frac{1}{2}$: 2–12 h
Benzothiazepines		
Diltiazem hydrochloride	Hypertension: Extended release, Once daily: A: PO: Initially 180–240 mg/d; *maint:* 120–360 mg/d; *max:* 540 mg/d	For hypertension, angina, and dysrhythmia. May cause dizziness, headache, fatigue, weakness, hypotension, bradycardia, peripheral edema, dyspnea, pharyngitis, rhinitis, dyspepsia, and infection. Advise patient to not significantly increase grapefruit juice intake while taking diltiazem or avoid if possible. PB: 70%–80%; $t\frac{1}{2}$: 3.5–9 h
Dihydropyridines		
Amlodipine	See Prototype Drug Chart: Amlodipine	
Felodipine	A: PO: Initially 5 mg/d; *maint:* 2.5–10 mg/d; *max:* 10 mg/d Older A: PO: Initially 2.5 mg/d; *max:* 10 mg/d	For hypertension. May cause dizziness, headache, weakness, palpitations, hypotension, peripheral edema, cough, infection, and rash. Give without food or with a light meal. Avoid giving with grapefruit juice. PB: 99%; $t\frac{1}{2}$: 11–16 h
Isradipine	Regular release: A: PO: Initially 2.5 mg bid; *max:* 20 mg/d	For hypertension. May cause dizziness, headache, fatigue, palpitations, angina, hypotension, tachycardia, flushing, peripheral edema, and abdominal pain. Give without regard to food. PB: 95%; $t\frac{1}{2}$: 8 h
Nicardipine hydrochloride	Hypertension: Immediate release: A: PO: Initially 20 mg tid; *max:* 120 mg/d Extended release: A: PO: Initially 30 mg bid; *max:* 120 mg/d A: IV: Initially 5 mg/h infusion; *max:* 15 mg/h	For hypertension and angina. May cause dizziness, headache, weakness, angina, orthostatic hypotension, palpitations, tachycardia, flushing, peripheral edema, nausea, and vomiting. Give without regard to food. Avoid coadministration with grapefruit juice or grapefruit. PB: 95%; $t\frac{1}{2}$: 8.6 h
Nifedipine	Hypertension: Extended release: A: PO: Initially 30–60 mg/d; *max:* 90 mg/d	For hypertension and angina. Common side effects include dizziness, headache, fatigue, weakness, nasal congestion, throat irritation, cough, wheezing, dyspnea, hypotension, palpitations, flushing, peripheral edema, nausea, pyrosis, tremor, muscle cramps, and heart failure. Avoid grapefruit juice before or after drug administration. If gastric irritation develops, give with meals. PB: 92%–98%; $t\frac{1}{2}$: 2–5 h
Nisoldipine	Extended release: A: PO: Initially 17 mg/d; *maint:* 17–34 mg/d; *max:* 34 mg/d Older A: PO: Initially 8.5 mg/d; *max:* 34 mg/d	For hypertension. May cause dizziness, headache, visual impairment, pharyngitis, sinusitis, flushing, tachycardia, orthostatic hypotension, palpitations, hypokalemia, and peripheral edema. Avoid grapefruit juice before or after drug administration. Avoid giving drug with a high-fat meal. PB: 99%; $t\frac{1}{2}$: 7–12 h
Miscellaneous Antihypertensives		
Aprocitentan	A: PO: 12.5 mg in combination with other antihypertensives for adults uncontrolled with other medications	For hypertension. May cause edema, fluid retention, anemia, erythema, rash, elevated hepatic enzymes, and hepatotoxicity. PB: 99%; $t\frac{1}{2}$: 41–44 h

A, Adult; *bid*, twice a day; *d*, day; *h*, hour; *IV*, intravenous; *maint*, maintenance; *max*, maximum; *PB*, protein binding; *PO*, by mouth; *t½*, half-life; *tid*, three times a day.

muscle contractility, peripheral resistance, and BP. Calcium channel blockers, also called *calcium antagonists* and *calcium blockers*, block the calcium channel in the VSM, promoting vasodilation. The large central arteries are not as sensitive to calcium blockers as coronary and cerebral arteries and the peripheral vessels. Calcium blockers are highly protein bound but have a short half-life. Slow-release preparations decrease the frequency of administration. Table 42.4 lists the calcium blockers in three groups: diphenylalkylamine (verapamil), benzothiazepine (diltiazem), and dihydropyridines (amlodipine and others).

Verapamil is used to treat chronic hypertension, angina pectoris, and cardiac dysrhythmias. Verapamil and diltiazem act on the arterioles and the heart. The dihydropyridines are the largest group of calcium channel blockers; most of these are used to control hypertension.

Nifedipine decreases BP in older adults and in those with low serum renin values. Nifedipine and verapamil are potent calcium blockers. In its immediate-release form (10- and 20-mg capsules), nifedipine has been associated with an increased incidence of profound hypotension, MI, and death, especially in older adults; therefore only extended-release preparations of nifedipine are recommended for chronic hypertension. For this reason, immediate-release nifedipine is usually prescribed for acute rises in BP only on an as-needed basis in the hospital setting. Like the vasodilators, calcium channel blockers can cause reflex tachycardia, although it is more prevalent with nifedipine.

Pharmacokinetics
Like other calcium blockers, amlodipine is highly protein bound. It is gradually absorbed via the GI tract. Because the half-life of amlodipine is longer than that of other calcium blockers, it is taken once a day.

Pharmacodynamics
Amlodipine may be used alone or with other antihypertensive drugs. Peripheral edema may occur because of its vasodilator effect, so persons with edema may need to take another type of antihypertensive drug. This drug has a long duration of action, so it is prescribed only once a day. Amlodipine may be combined with the ACE inhibitor benazepril (Lotrel).

Normally, beta blockers are not prescribed with calcium blockers, because both drugs decrease myocardium contractility. Calcium blockers lower BP better in African American patients than do drugs in other categories.

Side Effects and Adverse Reactions
The side effects and adverse reactions of calcium channel blockers include flushing, dizziness, ankle edema, bradycardia, and AV block. Prototype Drug Chart: Amlodipine gives the pharmacologic data related to amlodipine.

PROTOTYPE DRUG CHART
Amlodipine

Drug Class	Dosage
Antihypertensive: Calcium channel blocker	Hypertension: A: PO: Initially 5 mg/d; *maint:* 5–10 mg/d; *max:* 10 mg/d Older A: PO: Initially 2.5 mg/d; *max:* 10 mg/d
Contraindications	**Drug-Lab-Food Interactions**
Hypersensitivity *Caution:* Hepatic impairment, acute MI, coronary artery disease, aortic stenosis, older adults, pregnancy, breast-feeding	Drug: Antihypertensives may increase hypotensive effects; NSAIDs may increase renal dysfunction; hydrocodone and codeine may increase sedation; pseudoephedrine and phenylephrine decrease antihypertensive effects.
Pharmacokinetics	**Pharmacodynamics**
Absorption: Well absorbed Distribution: PB: 93% Metabolism: t½: 30–50 h Excretion: Excreted in urine	PO: Onset: UK Peak: 6–12 h Duration: 24 h
Therapeutic Effects/Uses	
To treat hypertension and coronary artery disease. Mechanism of action: Inhibits influx of extracellular calcium across myocardial and vascular smooth muscle cell membranes, resulting in decreased myocardial contractility.	
Side Effects	**Adverse Reactions**
Weakness, syncope, depression, nightmares, insomnia, anxiety, chills, visual impairment, dysphagia, dry mouth, anorexia, abdominal pain, nausea, vomiting, diarrhea, flatulence, constipation, rash, pruritus, diaphoresis, flushing, paresthesia, arthralgia, myalgia, back pain, muscle cramps, peripheral edema, erectile dysfunction, weight loss/gain	Bradycardia, chest pain, tachycardia, palpitations, dyspnea, hyperglycemia *Life threatening:* Angioedema, dysrhythmia exacerbation, thrombocytopenia

A, Adult; *h*, hour; *maint*, maintenance; *MI*, myocardial infarction; *NSAID*, nonsteroidal antiinflammatory drug; *PB*, protein binding; *PO*, by mouth; *t½*, half-life; *UK*, unknown.

CLINICAL JUDGMENT CASE STUDY

A 72-year-old African American patient has heart failure and diabetes. Her vital signs are blood pressure 176/94, pulse 92, and respirations 30. Her medications include hydrochlorothiazide 50 mg/day, digoxin 0.125 mg/day, and atenolol 50 mg/day.

1. Why was hydrochlorothiazide prescribed for this patient? Explain the effects of hydrochlorothiazide on blood pressure.
2. Abnormal electrolytes and other laboratory test results may occur when taking hydrochlorothiazide. Would the following serum electrolyte and laboratory values be expected to *increase* or *decrease*?
   a. Sodium
   b. Potassium
   c. Calcium
   d. Magnesium
   e. Glucose
   f. Uric acid
3. Why should this patient's blood glucose level be monitored while she is taking hydrochlorothiazide?
4. What response does a health care provider need to keep in mind when prescribing antihypertensive agents? Explain your answer.
5. Atenolol is what type of antihypertensive? Would atenolol be effective in lowering this patient's blood pressure if given as the only antihypertensive drug? Explain your answer.
6. How effective is the combination of hydrochlorothiazide and atenolol for controlling this patient's blood pressure? Explain your answer.
7. When using a combination drug therapy to correct hypertension, would the dosage for each drug be the same? Explain your answer.
8. When abruptly discontinuing beta blockers for hypertension without the patient taking another antihypertensive, what might occur? Explain how adverse effects can be avoided.

This patient's blood glucose is 229. Her drugs for controlling hypertension are changed to prazosin 10 mg three times daily. Her cholesterol and LDL are elevated, and her serum potassium level is 3.2 mEq/L.

9. Why were this patient's hydrochlorothiazide and atenolol discontinued? Explain your answer.
10. What type of antihypertensive is prazosin? Explain the physiologic action of prazosin for lowering the blood pressure.
11. Does prazosin have an effect on the blood glucose level? What effect could prazosin have on this patient's abnormal lipid levels? Explain your answer.
12. This patient's ankles have become edematous. Hydrochlorothiazide is again prescribed. Why was hydrochlorothiazide again added to the drug regimen?
13. Is the daily prazosin dose within the safe therapeutic prescribed range for this patient? Explain your answer. (You may refer to Prototype Drug Chart: Prazosin Hydrochloride.)
14. List the groups of antihypertensive drugs that can cause sodium and water retention.

REVIEW QUESTIONS

1. A patient's blood pressure is 130/84. The health care provider plans to suggest nonpharmacologic methods to lower blood pressure. Which should the nurse include in teaching? **Select all that apply.**
   a. Stress-reduction techniques
   b. An exercise program
   c. Salt restriction
   d. Smoking cessation
   e. A diet with increased protein
2. A patient has developed mild hypertension. The nurse acknowledges that the first-line drug for treating this patient's blood pressure might be which drug?
   a. Diuretic
   b. Alpha blocker
   c. Angiotensin-converting enzyme inhibitor
   d. Alpha/beta blocker
3. An African American patient has developed hypertension. The nurse is aware that which group(s) of antihypertensive drugs are *less effective* in African American patients?
   a. Diuretics
   b. Calcium channel blockers and vasodilators
   c. Beta blockers and angiotensin-converting enzyme inhibitors
   d. Alpha blockers
4. The nurse knows that which diuretic is most frequently combined with an antihypertensive drug?
   a. Chlorthalidone
   b. Hydrochlorothiazide
   c. Bendroflumethiazide
   d. A potassium-sparing diuretic
5. The nurse is administering a beta blocker to a patient. Which is the most important assessment to perform before administration?
   a. Urine output
   b. Apical pulse
   c. Potassium level
   d. Serum level of medication
6. Captopril has been prescribed for a patient. The nurse should teach the patient that the most commonly occurring side effect of an angiotensin-converting enzyme drug is which of the following?
   a. Nausea and vomiting
   b. Dizziness and headaches
   c. Upset stomach
   d. Constant, irritating cough
7. A patient is prescribed losartan. The nurse teaches the patient that an angiotensin II receptor blocker acts by doing what?
   a. Inhibiting angiotensin-converting enzyme
   b. Blocking angiotensin II from angiotensin I receptors
   c. Preventing the release of angiotensin I
   d. Promoting the release of aldosterone
8. During an admission assessment, a patient states that she takes amlodipine. The nurse should inquire about which signs and symptoms to determine whether the patient has any common side effects of amlodipine? **Select all that apply.**
   a. Insomnia
   b. Dizziness
   c. Headache
   d. Angioedema
   e. Ankle edema
   f. Hacking cough

43

Anticoagulants, Antiplatelets, and Thrombolytics

http://evolve.elsevier.com/McCuistion/pharmacology

OBJECTIVES

- Describe the drug therapy for the prevention and treatment of venous thrombus formation.
- Compare the actions of various anticoagulants and anticoagulant agonists.
- Summarize components of antiplatelet drug therapy.
- Explain care considerations and the preferred time frame for thrombolytic therapy.

OUTLINE

Pathophysiology, 551
    Thrombus Formation, 551
    Treatment of Thrombus, 551
Anticoagulants, 551
    Heparin, 552
    Direct Thrombin Inhibitors: Parenteral Anticoagulants II, 552
    Oral Anticoagulants, 554
    Factor Xa Inhibitors, 555
    Anticoagulant Antagonists, 556

Antiplatelet Drugs, 556
    Overview and Usage Considerations, 556
    Pharmacology, 557
Thrombolytics, 559
    Overview and Usage Considerations, 559
    Pharmacology, 560
Clinical Judgment Case Study, 562
Review Questions, 562

Various drugs are used to maintain or restore circulation. The three major groups of these drugs are (1) anticoagulants, (2) antiplatelets (antithrombotics), and (3) thrombolytics. The *anticoagulants* prevent the formation of clots that inhibit circulation. The *antiplatelets* prevent platelet aggregation, clumping together of platelets to form a clot. The *thrombolytics*, appropriately called *clot busters*, attack and dissolve blood clots that have already formed. Each of these three drug groups are discussed separately.

PATHOPHYSIOLOGY

Thrombus Formation

Thrombosis is the formation of a clot in an arterial or venous vessel. The formation of an arterial thrombus could be caused by blood stasis (decreased circulation), platelet aggregation on the blood vessel wall, or blood coagulation. Arterial clots are usually made up of both white and red clots with the white clots, *platelets*, initiating the process, followed by fibrin formation and the trapping of red blood cells in the fibrin mesh. Blood clots found in the veins are from platelet aggregation with fibrin that attaches to red blood cells. Both types of thrombus can be dislodged from the vessel and become an *embolus*, a blood clot moving through the bloodstream.

Platelets do not usually stick together unless there is a break in the endothelial lining of a blood vessel. When platelets adhere to the broken surface of an endothelial lining, they synthesize thromboxane A_2, which is a product of prostaglandins and a potent stimulus for platelet aggregation, and clumping of platelet cells. The platelet receptor protein that binds fibrinogen, *glycoprotein IIb/IIIa* (GP IIb/IIIa), also promotes platelet aggregation. Thromboxane A_2 and adenosine diphosphate (ADP) increase the activation of this receptor.

The thrombus inhibits blood flow, and the fibrin, platelets, and red blood cells (erythrocytes) surround the clot, building its size and structure. As the clot occludes the blood vessel, tissue ischemia occurs.

The venous thrombus usually develops because of slow blood flow, and the venous clot can form rapidly. Small pieces of the venous clot can detach and travel to the pulmonary artery and then to the lung. Inadequate oxygenation and gas exchange in the lungs is the end result.

Treatment of Thrombus

Oral and parenteral anticoagulants, such as warfarin and heparin, act primarily to prevent venous thrombosis, whereas antiplatelet drugs act to prevent arterial thrombosis. However, both groups of drugs suppress thrombosis in general.

❗ ANTICOAGULANTS

Anticoagulants are used to inhibit clot formation. Unlike thrombolytics, they do *not* dissolve clots that have already formed but rather act prophylactically to prevent new clots from forming. Anticoagulants are used in patients with venous and arterial disorders that put them at high risk for clot formation. Venous problems include deep venous thrombosis (DVT) and pulmonary embolism (PE), and arterial problems include coronary thrombosis, or myocardial infarction (MI); presence of artificial heart valves; and cerebrovascular accident (CVA), or stroke.

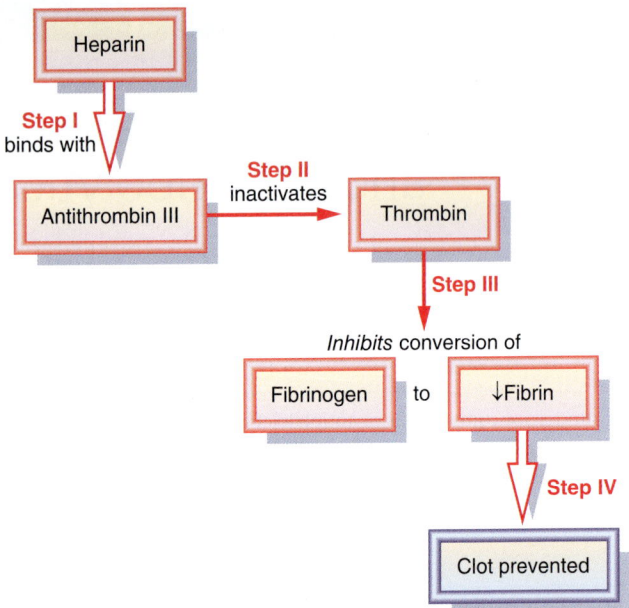

Fig. 43.1 Action of the parenteral anticoagulant heparin.

Heparin

Anticoagulants are administered orally or parenterally, both subcutaneously and by the intravenous (IV) route. Heparin, introduced in 1938, is a natural substance in the liver that prevents clot formation. It was first used in blood transfusions to prevent clotting. Heparin is indicated for a rapid anticoagulant effect when a thrombosis occurs because of a DVT, PE, or evolving stroke. Heparin is also used in open-heart surgery to prevent blood from clotting and in the critically ill patient with disseminated intravascular coagulation (DIC), which occurs when fibrin clots form within the vascular system. These clots consume proteins and platelets, depleting clotting factors and causing excess bleeding. However, the primary use of heparin is to prevent venous thrombosis, which can lead to PE or stroke.

Heparin combines with antithrombin III, which accelerates the anticoagulant cascade of reactions that prevents thrombosis formation. By inhibiting the action of thrombin, conversion of fibrinogen to fibrin does not occur, and the formation of a fibrin clot is prevented (Fig. 43.1).

Heparin is poorly absorbed through the gastrointestinal (GI) mucosa, and much is destroyed by heparinase, a liver enzyme. Because heparin is poorly absorbed orally, it is given subcutaneously for prophylaxis or by IV to treat acute thrombosis. It can be administered as an IV bolus or in IV fluid for continuous infusion. Heparin prolongs clotting time. **Partial thromboplastin time (PTT)** and **activated partial thromboplastin time (aPTT)** are laboratory tests used to detect deficiencies of certain clotting factors, and these tests are used to monitor heparin therapy. Heparin can decrease the platelet count, causing thrombocytopenia. If hemorrhage occurs during heparin therapy, the anticoagulant antagonist protamine sulfate is given by IV. Protamine sulfate can be an anticoagulant, but in the presence of heparin, it is an antagonist that reverses the action of heparin. Before discontinuing heparin, oral therapy with warfarin therapy is begun.

Low-Molecular-Weight Heparins

These derivatives of standard heparin were introduced to prevent venous thromboembolism. Studies have shown that by extracting only the low-molecular-weight fractions of standard heparin through depolymerization, the equivalent of anticoagulation can be achieved with a lower risk of bleeding. Low-molecular-weight heparins (LMWHs) produce more stable responses at recommended doses. As a result, frequent laboratory monitoring of aPTT is not required, because LMWH does not have the standard effect of heparin. Heparin prevents coagulation by combining with antithrombin III to inactivate factor Xa and thrombin. LMWH inactivates the Xa factor, but it is less able to inactivate thrombin.

The examples of LMWHs include enoxaparin and dalteparin.

> ## ⚡ PATIENT SAFETY
>
> **Do Not Confuse...**
> - **Enoxaparin**, a low-molecular-weight heparin (LMWH), and **enoxacin**, a fluoroquinolone antibiotic.
> - **Lovenox**, an LMWH, and **Lotronex**, a gastrointestinal drug.

The anticoagulant fondaparinux is a synthetically engineered antithrombotic designed to be effective as a once-daily subcutaneous injection. Categorized as a *selective factor Xa inhibitor*, fondaparinux is closely related in structure to heparin and LMWHs and is used for the same purposes.

These agents are most commonly prescribed to prevent DVT and acute PE after orthopedic or abdominal surgery. Hip and knee replacement anticoagulant therapy often includes enoxaparin, and abdominal surgery includes dalteparin. The drugs can be administered at home because aPTT monitoring is not necessary, whereas heparin must be given in the hospital. LMWHs are administered subcutaneously once or twice a day, depending on the drug or drug regimen, and they are available in prefilled syringes with attached needles. The patient or family member is taught how to administer the subcutaneous injection, which is usually given in the abdomen. Injection sites should be alternated with every dose. The LMWH is usually started in the hospital within 24 hours after surgery (Table 43.1).

The half-life of LMWHs is longer than that of heparin. Patients should be instructed not to take antiplatelet drugs such as aspirin while taking LMWHs or heparin. Bleeding because of LMWH use is less likely to occur than when heparin is given. LMWH overdose is rare; if bleeding occurs, protamine sulfate is the anticoagulant antagonist used. The dosage is 1 mg of protamine sulfate for every 100 units of unfractionated heparin or LMWH given to be neutralized.

Contraindications

The LMWHs are contraindicated for patients with bleeding, HIT, or a porcine protein hypersensitivity. Enoxaparin is also contraindicated in a benzyl alcohol or heparin hypersensitivity.

❗ Direct Thrombin Inhibitors: Parenteral Anticoagulants II

Parenteral anticoagulants directly inhibit thrombin from converting fibrinogen to fibrin. These drugs differ from heparin-like anticoagulants. Argatroban and bivalirudin are given intravenously; bivalirudin binds with and inhibits free-flowing thrombin. Dabigatran is an oral anticoagulant that does *not* require routine coagulation monitoring (see Table 43.1). These drugs are more expensive than the other anticoagulants.

TABLE 43.1 Anticoagulants and Anticoagulant Antagonists

Drug	Route and Dosage	Uses and Considerations
Anticoagulants		
Heparins		
Heparin sodium	See Prototype Drug Chart: Heparin	
LMWHs		
Dalteparin	DVT treatment: A: Subcut: 200 units/kg per day for 1 month, then 150 units/kg per day for months 2–6	For thrombosis, DVT and PE prophylaxis and treatment. May cause bleeding, hematoma, ecchymosis, epistaxis, thrombocytopenia, elevated hepatic enzymes, hematuria, GI bleeding, and intracranial bleeding. PB: 81%–93%; $t½$: 3–5 h
Enoxaparin sodium	DVT treatment: A: Subcut: 1 mg/kg q12h for minimum of 5 days or 1.5 mg/kg per dose q24h	For prophylaxis of AMI, thrombosis, and unstable angina and for prophylaxis and treatment of PE and DVT. May cause bleeding, hematoma, ecchymosis, fever, dyspnea, nausea, anemia, peripheral edema, and elevated hepatic enzymes. PB: UK; $t½$: 4.5–7 h
Oral Anticoagulants		
Warfarin	See Prototype Drug Chart: Warfarin Sodium	
Selective Factor Xa Inhibitors		
Fondaparinux	DVT treatment: A: Subcut: 5 mg/d if <50 kg for 5–9 d, 7.5 mg/d if 50–100 kg for 5–9 d, 10 kg/d if >100 kg for 5–9 d	For prophylaxis and treatment of DVT and PE. May cause anemia, bleeding, hypokalemia, infection, dizziness, confusion, headache, hematoma, purpura, hypotension, thrombocytopenia, and insomnia. PB: 94%; $t½$: 18 h
Rivaroxaban	DVT treatment: A: PO: 15 mg bid for 21 d, then 20 mg/d for at least 3 months; *max:* 30 mg/d	For prophylaxis and treatment of DVT, PE, and stroke. May cause bleeding, menorrhagia, weakness, cough, rash, vomiting abdominal/back pain, and pruritus. PB: 92%–95%; $t½$: 5–9 h
Apixaban	DVT, PE: A: PO: 10 mg bid for 7 d, then 5 mg bid for at least 3 months; *max:* 10 mg/d for most patients, 20 mg/d for initial treatment	To prevent and treat DVT and PE and for prevention of atrial fibrillation. May cause hematoma, anemia, bleeding, epistaxis, hematuria, menorrhagia, hemoptysis, and hypotension. PB: 87%; $t½$: 12 h
Edoxaban	DVT, PE: A: PO: After 5–10 d of initial therapy with parenteral anticoagulant may give 30 mg/d if ≤ 60 kg or 60 mg/d if >60 kg for at least 3 months; *max:* 60 mg/d	For treatment of DVT, PE, and nonvalvular atrial fibrillation and stroke prophylaxis. May cause anemia, vaginal bleeding, elevated hepatic enzymes, epistaxis, GI bleeding, rash, intracranial bleeding, and hematuria. PB: 55%; $t½$: 10–14 h
Betrixaban	A: PO: 160 mg once, followed by 80 mg/d for 35–42 d; *maint:* 80 mg/d	For venous thromboembolism prophylaxis. May cause headache, hypertension, infection, hematuria, hypokalemia, nausea, diarrhea, and constipation. PB: 60%; $t½$: 19–27 h
Direct-Acting Thrombin Inhibitors: Anticoagulants II (Intravenous)		
Argatroban	HIT: A: IV: Initially 2 mcg/kg per minute infusion; adjust dose to maintain aPTT 1.5–3 times baseline; *max:* 10 mcg/kg per minute	For PCI and HIT. May cause bleeding, hypotension, chest pain, fever, cough, back pain, nausea, vomiting, diarrhea, abdominal pain, hematuria, and headache. PB: 20%; $t½$: 39–51 min
Bivalirudin	PCI: A: IV bolus: 0.75 mg/kg immediately prior to procedure; then IV infusion of 1.75 mg/kg per hour throughout procedure, may continue up to 4 h	For thrombosis prophylaxis in PCI. May cause back pain, bleeding, headache, nausea, hypo/hypertension, insomnia, anxiety, antibody formation, and bradycardia. PB: 0%; $t½$: 25 min
Dabigatran	DVT: A: PO: 150 mg bid for at least 3 months; *max:* 300 mg/d	For prevention of stroke and for prophylaxis and treatment of DVT, and PE. May cause bleeding, GI bleeding, headache, pharyngitis, epistaxis, nausea, vomiting, dyspepsia, abdominal pain, and diarrhea. PB: 35%; $t½$: 12–17 h

Continued

TABLE 43.1 Anticoagulants and Anticoagulant Antagonists—cont'd

Drug	Route and Dosage	Uses and Considerations
Anticoagulant Antagonists		
Protamine sulfate	A: IV: Initially: 1 mg/100 units heparin to be neutralized; *max:* 100 mg in 2-h period	For heparin toxicity reversal. May cause hypotension, flushing, bradycardia, hypotension, fatigue, bleeding, pulmonary edema, and dyspnea. PB: UK; $t½$: 7.4 min
Phytonadione	Anticoagulation reversal: A: PO 2.5–25 mg once, repeat if INR remains prolonged after 6–8 h A: IM/IV/subcut: 2.5–25 mg once, repeat if INR remains prolonged after 6–8 h	For vitamin K deficiency, nutritional supplement, anticoagulation reversal. May cause anaphylaxis, dizziness, flushing, dysgeusia, dyspnea, hyperhidrosis, chest pain, injection-site reaction, tachycardia, and hypotension. PB: UK; $t½$: UK

<, Less than; *A*, adult; *AMI*, acute myocardial infarction; *bid*, twice a day; *d*, day; *DVT*, deep vein thrombosis; *GI*, gastrointestinal; *h*, hour; *HIT*, heparin-induced thrombocytopenia; *INR*, international normalized ratio; *IM*, intramuscular; *IV*, intravenous; *LMWHs*, low-molecular-weight heparins; *max*, maximum; *min*, minutes; *PB*, protein binding; *PCI*, percutaneous coronary intervention; *PE*, pulmonary embolism; *PO*, by mouth; *q12h*, every 12 hours; *subcut*, subcutaneous; *t½*, half-life; *UK*, unknown.

TABLE 43.2 Comparison of Parenteral and Oral Anticoagulants

Factors to Consider	Heparin	Warfarin (Coumadin)
Methods of administration	Subcutaneously Intravenously	Primarily orally
Drug actions	Binds with antithrombin III, which inactivates thrombin and clotting factors, inhibiting fibrin formation	Inhibits hepatic synthesis of vitamin K, which decreases prothrombin and the clotting factors VII, IX, and X
Uses	Treatment of venous thrombosis, PE, thromboembolic complications (e.g., heart surgery, DIC)	Treatment of DVT, PE, TIA; prophylactic for cardiac valves
Contraindications/cautions	Hemophilia, peptic ulcer, severe (stage 3 or 4) hypertension, severe liver or renal disease, dissecting aneurysm	Hemophilia, peptic bleeding ulcer, blood dyscrasias, severe liver or kidney disease, AMI, alcoholism
Laboratory tests	PTT: 60–70 s Anticoagulant therapeutic level: 1.5–2 × control in seconds aPTT: 20–35 s Anticoagulant: aPTT: 30–85 s	PT: 11–15 s Anticoagulant therapeutic level: 1.25–2.5 × control in seconds INR: 1.3–2 Anticoagulant: INR 2–3 Prosthetic heart valves: INR up to 3.5
Side effects/adverse effects	Bleeding, hemorrhage, hematoma, severe hypotension	Bleeding, hemorrhage, GI bleeding, ecchymoses, hematuria
Antidote	Protamine sulfate	Phytonadione (vitamin K)

AMI, Acute myocardial infarction; *aPTT*, activated partial thromboplastin time; *DIC*, disseminated intravascular coagulation; *DVT*, deep venous thrombosis; *GI*, gastrointestinal; *INR*, international normalized ratio; *PE*, pulmonary embolism; *PT*, prothrombin time; *PTT*, partial thromboplastin time; *s*, second; *TIA*, transient ischemic attack.

Oral Anticoagulants

Oral anticoagulants inhibit hepatic synthesis of vitamin K, thus affecting the clotting factors II, VII, IX, and X. Warfarin is an oral anticoagulant synthesized from dicumarol. Warfarin is used mainly to prevent thromboembolic conditions such as thrombophlebitis, PE, and embolism formation caused by atrial fibrillation, which can lead to stroke. Oral anticoagulants prolong clotting time and are monitored by the **prothrombin time (PT)**, a laboratory test that measures the time it takes blood to clot in the presence of certain clotting factors, which warfarin affects. This laboratory test is usually performed immediately before administering the next drug dose until the therapeutic level has been reached. Today, the **international normalized ratio (INR)** is the laboratory test most frequently used to report PT results. It was introduced to account for variability in reported PTs from different laboratories. Reagents used in the PT test are compared with an international reference standard and reported as the INR; normal INR is 1.3 to 2.

Patients on warfarin therapy are maintained at an INR of 2 to 3. The desired INR for patients who have a mechanical heart valve or recurrent systemic embolism is 2.5 to 3.5, but the desired level could be as high as 4.5.

Monitoring INR at regular intervals is required for the duration of drug therapy. Warfarin has a long half-life and very long duration. Drug accumulation can occur and can lead to external or internal bleeding, so the nurse must observe for petechiae, ecchymosis, tarry stools, and hematemesis and must teach the patient to do the same at home.

The antidote for warfarin overdose is vitamin K, but it takes 24 to 48 hours for the oral peak effect and 12 to 14 hours for the peak IV effect. Usually a low dose of oral vitamin K may be recommended for patients with an INR of 5.5. If excessive vitamin K is given, it may take warfarin 1 to 2 weeks before it can be effective again. For acute bleeding, fresh frozen plasma is indicated.

Table 43.1 describes pharmacologic data for anticoagulants and anticoagulant antagonists. Table 43.2 compares heparin and warfarin regarding action, uses, laboratory tests, and other considerations. Parenteral and oral anticoagulants (heparin and warfarin) are presented in Prototype Drug Chart: Heparin and Prototype Drug Chart: Warfarin Sodium.

Pharmacokinetics

Heparin is poorly absorbed through the GI mucosa, and much is destroyed by heparinase, a liver enzyme. Heparin is given parenterally, either subcutaneously for prophylactic anticoagulant therapy or by IV (bolus or continuous infusion) for an immediate response. Warfarin, an oral anticoagulant, is well absorbed through the GI mucosa; food will delay but not inhibit absorption.

The half-life of heparin is dose related; high doses prolong the half-life. The half-life of warfarin is 20 to 60 hours, in contrast to 30 to 2 hours for heparin. Because warfarin has a long half-life and is highly protein bound, the drug can have cumulative effects. Bleeding can occur, especially if another highly protein-bound drug is administered together with warfarin. Kidney and liver disease prolong the half-life of both heparin and warfarin. Warfarin is metabolized to inactive metabolites excreted in urine and bile.

Pharmacodynamics

Heparin, administered for acute thromboembolic disorders, prevents thrombus formation and embolism. It has been effectively used to treat DIC, which causes multiple thrombi in small blood vessels. Warfarin is effective for long-term anticoagulant therapy. The therapeutic target aPTT level is 1.5 to 2 times the baseline, or INR should be 2.0 to 3.0. INR has effectively replaced the use of PT, because PT can vary from laboratory to laboratory and reagent to reagent. Higher INR levels (up to 3.5) are usually required for patients with prosthetic heart valves, and cardiac valvular disease. Heparin does not cross the placental barrier, unlike warfarin; warfarin use is not recommended during pregnancy.

IV heparin has a rapid onset; its peak time of action is reached in minutes, and its duration of action is short. After an IV heparin dose, the patient's clotting time will return to normal in 2 to 6 hours and 8 to 12 hours after a subcutaneous dose. Subcutaneous heparin is more slowly absorbed through the blood vessels in fatty tissue. Warfarin has a long onset of action, peak concentration, and duration of action, so drug accumulation may occur.

Side Effects and Adverse Reactions

Bleeding (hemorrhage) is the major adverse effect of warfarin. Patients should be monitored closely for signs of bleeding such as petechiae, ecchymosis, GI bleeding, ocular hemorrhage, and hematuria. Laboratory testing of PT or INR should be scheduled at recommended intervals.

Drug Interactions

Because warfarin is highly protein bound, it is affected by drug interactions. Aspirin, nonsteroidal antiinflammatory drugs (NSAIDs), other types of antiinflammatory drugs, sulfonamides, phenytoin, cimetidine, allopurinol, and oral hypoglycemic drugs for diabetes can displace warfarin from the protein-bound site and can cause more free-circulating anticoagulant. Numerous other drugs also increase the action of warfarin, and bleeding is likely to occur. Acetaminophen should be used instead of aspirin by patients taking warfarin. For frank bleeding resulting from excess free drug, parenteral vitamin K is given as a coagulant to decrease bleeding and promote clotting. However, caution must be used with this approach because the prothrombin can remain depressed for prolonged periods.

Factor Xa Inhibitors

Factor Xa inhibitors include fondaparinux, given subcutaneously, and those given orally—rivaroxaban, apixaban, edoxaban, and betrixaban. These drugs do not require routine coagulation monitoring and are given once or twice daily. Factor Xa inhibitors selectively block activity of clotting factor Xa to prevent clot formation. They are approved for the prevention of DVT and PE. The major adverse

---

CLINICAL JUDGMENT [NURSING PROCESS]
Anticoagulants: Warfarin and Heparin

Concept: Clotting
- A process in which blood is changed into a semisolid gel

Recognize Cues [Assessment]
- Obtain a history of abnormal clotting or health problems that affect clotting, such as severe alcoholism or severe liver or renal disease. Warfarin is contraindicated for patients with blood dyscrasias, peptic ulcer, cerebrovascular accident (CVA), hemophilia, or severe hypertension. Use with caution in patients with acute traumatic injury.
- Gather a drug history that includes complementary and alternative therapy, current drugs, and products that the patient takes. Report if drug-drug or drug-herb interaction or other interaction with complementary and alternative therapy is probable. Warfarin is highly protein bound and can displace other highly protein-bound drugs, or warfarin could be displaced, which may result in bleeding.
- Develop a flowchart that lists prothrombin time (PT) or international normalized ratio (INR) and warfarin dosages. A baseline PT or INR should be obtained before warfarin is administered.

Analyze Cues and Prioritize Hypothesis [Patient Problems]
- Bleeding
- Tissue injury
- Dehydration

Generate Solutions [Planning]
- The patient will not have excessive bleeding.

Take Action [Nursing Interventions]
- Monitor vital signs. An increased pulse rate followed by a decreased systolic pressure can indicate a fluid volume deficit resulting from external or internal bleeding.
- Monitor PT or INR for warfarin and activated partial thromboplastin time (aPTT) for heparin before administering anticoagulant. PT should be 1.25 to 2.5 times the control level, or INR should be 2 to 3, except for patients with prosthetic heart valves, in whom INR may be up to 3.5. Monitor platelet count because anticoagulants can decrease it.

Continued

CLINICAL JUDGMENT [NURSING PROCESS]—CONT'D
Anticoagulants: Warfarin and Heparin

- Examine the patient's mouth, nose (epistaxis), urine (hematuria), and skin (petechiae, purpura) for bleeding. Watch older adults closely for bleeding; their skin is thin, and capillary beds are fragile.
- Check stools periodically for occult blood.
- Keep anticoagulant antagonists available, protamine sulfate for heparin and vitamin K for warfarin, when the drug dose is increased or indications of frank bleeding are evident. Fresh frozen plasma may be needed for transfusion.

Patient Teaching
General
- Teach patients to inform their dentist when taking an anticoagulant. Contacting a health care provider may be necessary.
- Advise patients to use a soft toothbrush to prevent gums from bleeding.
- Warn patients to shave with an electric razor. Bleeding from shaving cuts may be difficult to control.
- Advise patients to have laboratory tests such as PT or INR performed as ordered by a health care provider. The warfarin dose is regulated according to INR derived from PT.
- Suggest that patients carry a medical identification card or wear a MedicAlert bracelet that lists the patient's name, telephone number, and the drug taken.
- Encourage patients *not* to smoke. Smoking increases drug metabolism, so warfarin dose may need to be increased. If a patient insists on smoking, notify the health care provider.
- Tell patients to check with a health care provider before taking over-the-counter (OTC) drugs. Aspirin should *not* be taken with warfarin because it intensifies warfarin's action, and bleeding is apt to occur. Suggest that patients use acetaminophen.
- Inform patients that many herbal products interact with anticoagulants and may increase bleeding. Closely monitor INR or PT.
- ⚡ Teach patients to control external hemorrhage from accidents or injuries by applying firm, direct pressure for at least 5 to 10 minutes with a clean, dry, absorbent material.

Side Effects
- Warn patients to report frank or occult bleeding such as petechiae, ecchymosis, purpura, tarry stools, bleeding gums, epistaxis, or expectoration of blood.

Diet
- Advise patients to avoid large amounts of green, leafy vegetables; broccoli; legumes; soybean oil (rich in vitamin K); coffee, tea, cola (caffeine); excessive alcohol; and certain herbs and nutritional supplements (coenzyme Q10) or to be very consistent with their intake. Coenzyme Q10, fish oils, substances high in vitamin K, St. John's wort, ginseng, and vitamin C may decrease the effectiveness of warfarin. Garlic, ginger, kava kava, green tea, chamomile tea, ginkgo biloba, and acute alcohol intoxication also decrease warfarin's effectiveness.

Evaluate Outcomes [Evaluation]
- Evaluate the effectiveness of drug therapy. The patient's PT or INR values are within the desired range, and the patient is free from significant side effects.

COMPLEMENTARY AND ALTERNATIVE THERAPIES
Anticoagulants: Warfarin and Heparin

- Dong quai, feverfew, garlic, ginger, meadowsweet, willow bark, chamomile tea, ginkgo, and bilberry may increase bleeding when taken with anticoagulants such as warfarin. Warfarin has an additive effect and increases the international normalized ratio (INR) and prothrombin time (PT).
- Excessive doses of anise may interfere with anticoagulants.
- Ginseng may decrease the effects of warfarin, thereby decreasing INR.
- Alfalfa may decrease anticoagulant activity.
- Goldenseal may decrease the effects of heparin and oral anticoagulants.
- Hawthorn increases the action of anticoagulants.
- Valerian and green tea may decrease the effects of warfarin.
- Cranberry may increase INR.

effect is bleeding. This drug category should not be given to patients weighing less than 50 kg because low body weight increases the risk for bleeding (see Table 43.1).

Anticoagulant Antagonists
Bleeding occurs in about 10% of patients taking oral anticoagulants. Phytonadione, an antagonist of warfarin, is vitamin K_1 and is used for warfarin overdose or uncontrollable bleeding. Usually 5 to 10 mg of vitamin K_1 is given by slow 10 to 20 minute IV infusion at once, and if it fails to control bleeding, fresh whole blood or fresh frozen plasma or platelets are generally given.

ANTIPLATELET DRUGS
Overview and Usage Considerations

Antiplatelets are used to prevent thrombosis in the arteries by suppressing platelet aggregation. Heparin and warfarin prevent thrombosis in the veins.

Antiplatelet drug therapy is mainly for prophylactic use in (1) prevention of MI or stroke for patients with a family history of these, (2) prevention of repeat MI or stroke, and (3) prevention of stroke for patients having transient ischemic attacks (TIAs).

Long-term, low-dose aspirin therapy has been found to be both an effective and inexpensive treatment for suppressing platelet aggregation. Aspirin inhibits cyclooxygenase (COX), an enzyme needed by platelets to synthesize thromboxane A_2 (TxA_2). For patients with a family history of stroke or MI, the recommended aspirin dose is 50 to 325 mg/day for stroke prophylaxis and 75 to 162 mg/day for MI prophylaxis. Because aspirin has prolonged antiplatelet activity, it should be discontinued at least 7 days before surgery.

Other antiplatelet drugs include anagrelide, clopidogrel, dipyridamole, prasugrel, ticagrelor, vorapaxar, cangrelor, abciximab, eptifibatide, and tirofiban. Clopidogrel and dipyridamole have effects similar to those of aspirin, but they are known as *adenosine diphosphate (ADP) antagonists*, and they affect platelet aggregation. Cilostazol inhibits platelet aggregation and is a vasodilator that may be used for intermittent claudication. Ticagrelor 90 mg twice a day is taken in conjunction with aspirin 75 to 100 mg in a maintenance regimen. Doses greater than 100 mg of aspirin should be avoided. Table 43.3 lists the antiplatelet drugs and their dosages, uses, and considerations.

PROTOTYPE DRUG CHART
Warfarin Sodium

Drug Class	Dosage
Anticoagulant	DVT or PE: A 18–59 y: PO: Initially 10 mg/d for 2 d, then 2–10 mg/d A 60> y: PO: Initially 10 mg/d for 2 d, then 2–5 mg/d. Adjust dose for both age groups to maintain target INR 2–3. Continue treatment for at least 3 months

Contraindications	Drug-Lab-Food Interactions
Hematologic disorders, eclampsia, alcohol abuse, stroke, endocarditis, pericarditis, aortic dissection, bleeding, head trauma, aneurysm, psychosis, intracranial bleeding, epidural anesthesia, dementia, pregnancy *Caution:* Diabetes mellitus, leukemia, anemia, thyroid disease, hepatic and renal impairment, cholestasis, peptic ulcer, atrial fibrillation, heart failure, cerebrovascular disease, cardiac disease, eating disorders, diarrhea, dental work, Asian patients, older adults, children, breast-feeding	Increased effect with amiodarone, aspirin, NSAIDs, sulfonamides, thyroid drugs, allopurinol, histamine$_2$ blockers, oral hypoglycemics, metronidazole, miconazole, methyldopa, diuretics, oral antibiotics, vitamin E; decreased effect with barbiturates, laxatives, phenytoin, estrogens, vitamins C and K, oral contraceptives, rifampin Lab: May increase AST, ALT Food: Decrease diet rich in vitamin K

Pharmacokinetics	Pharmacodynamics
Absorption: PO: Well absorbed Distribution: PB: 97% Metabolism: t½: 21–43 h Excretion: In urine and bile	PO: Onset: 24–72 h Peak: 36–72 h, 5–7 d full effect Duration: 2–5 d

Therapeutic Effects/Uses
To prevent thrombosis associated with PE, MI, unstable angina, prosthetic heart valves, DVT, cerebral venous thrombosis, and to treat atrial fibrillation
Mechanism of action: Inhibits hepatic synthesis of vitamin K clotting factors (II [prothrombin], VII, IX, and X) and anticoagulant proteins.

Side Effects	Adverse Reactions
Headache, dizziness, alopecia, fever, epistaxis, weakness, priapism, petechiae, ecchymosis, pallor, chills, rash, pruritus, paresthesia, dysgeusia, nausea, vomiting, diarrhea, flatulence, elevated hepatic enzymes	Purple-toe syndrome, bleeding, bone fracture, anemia, hypotension, chest pain, hematuria, ocular hemorrhage, intracranial/vaginal/GI bleeding, skin/tissue necrosis *Life-threatening:* Hemorrhage

A, Adult; *ALT*, alanine transaminase; *AST*, aspartate transferase; *d*, day; *DVT*, deep vein thrombosis; *GI*, gastrointestinal; *h*, hour; *INR*, international normalized ratio; *MI*, myocardial infarction; *NSAID*, nonsteroidal antiinflammatory drug; *PB*, protein binding; *PE*, pulmonary embolism; *PO*, by mouth; *t½*, half-life.

PROTOTYPE DRUG CHART
Heparin

Drug Class	Dosage
Anticoagulant	DVT or PE: A: IV: 80 units/kg bolus; *maint:* 18 units/kg per hour infusion based on aPTT

Contraindications	Drug-Lab-Food Interactions
HIT, hypersensitivity *Caution:* Peptic ulcer, hepatic or renal disease, hemophilia, DIC, diverticulitis, head trauma, coagulopathy, bleeding, asthma, aneurysm, surgery, hypo/hypertension, neoplastic disease, diabetes mellitus, peptic ulcer, menstruation, endocarditis, infection, hyperkalemia, thrombocytopenia, older adults, pregnancy, breast-feeding	Increased effect with aspirin, NSAIDs, thrombolytics, probenecid, antibiotics, SSRIs; decreased effect with nitroglycerin, protamine sulfate

Pharmacokinetics	Pharmacodynamics
Absorption: Subcut or IV Distribution: PB: >80% Metabolism: t½: IV 30 to 2 h Excretion: Slowly in urine and reticuloendothelial system	Subcut: Onset: 20–30 min Peak: UK Duration: UK IV: Onset: Immediate Peak: 5–10 min Duration: 2–6 h

Therapeutic Effects/Uses
To prevent thromboembolism associated with PE, MI, unstable angina, prosthetic heart valves and PCI; and to treat DVT, DIC, atrial fibrillation, and acute coronary syndrome.
Mechanism of action: Inactivates thrombin, which prevents conversion of fibrinogen to fibrin.

Side Effects	Adverse Reactions
Chills, headache, epistaxis, erythema, hematoma, hematemesis, hematuria, alopecia, elevated hepatic enzymes, nausea, vomiting, injection-site reaction, priapism, petechiae pruritus,	Bleeding, intracranial bleeding, ocular hemorrhage, anemia, bone fractures, skin necrosis, osteoporosis, hyperkalemia, vitamin D deficiency, GI bleeding, hyperlipidemia, prolonged bleeding time, stroke, adrenocortical insufficiency *Life-threatening:* Anaphylaxis, thrombocytopenia

A, Adult; *aPTT*, activated partial thromboplastin time; *DIC*, disseminated intravascular coagulation; *DVT*, deep vein thrombosis; *GI*, gastrointestinal; *h*, hour; *HIT*, heparin-induced thrombocytopenia; *IV*, intravenous; *maint*, maintenance; *MI*, myocardial infarction; *min*, minutes; *NSAID*, nonsteroidal antiinflammatory drug; *PB*, protein binding; *PCI*, percutaneous coronary intervention; *PE*, pulmonary embolism; *SSRI*, serotonin reuptake inhibitor; *Subcut*, subcutaneous; *t½*, half-life; *UK*, unknown.

Pharmacology
Pharmacokinetics

Clopidogrel is an antiplatelet drug frequently used after MI or stroke to prevent a second event. It may be prescribed singly or with aspirin. It has been stated that clopidogrel and aspirin are more effective in inhibiting platelet aggregation if used together than if used as separate antiplatelet therapies. Prototype Drug Chart: Clopidogrel Bisulfate lists the pharmacologic data for clopidogrel.

Clopidogrel is rapidly absorbed and has a high protein-binding power. Studies have not established a relationship between the concentration of the main metabolite and platelet aggregation. The half-life is 6 hours; it is usually prescribed once a day. Excretion of the drug metabolite occurs equally in the urine and in feces.

PROTOTYPE DRUG CHART
Clopidogrel Bisulfate

Drug Class	Dosage
Antiplatelet	Thromboembolism prophylaxis in AMI: A: PO: 75 mg/d; *max:* chronic treatment 75 mg/d

Contraindications	Drug-Lab-Food Interactions
GI bleeding, bleeding *Caution:* Hepatic/renal disease, surgery, peptic ulcer, thrombotic thrombocytopenia purpura, trauma, older adults, children, pregnancy, breast-feeding	Drug: May increase bleeding when taken with NSAIDs, anticoagulants, omeprazole, antineoplastics, azole antifungals, SSRIs, and barbiturates; interferes with metabolism of phenytoin, warfarin, NSAIDs, calcium channel blockers, and morphine; increases effects of valsartan, rosuvastatin, effects are decreased with grapefruit juice. Lab: Prolongs bleeding time Herb: May increase bleeding when taken with ginger, garlic, ginkgo, feverfew, and green tea

Pharmacokinetics	Pharmacodynamics
Absorption: Rapid Distribution: PB: 98% Metabolism: t½: 6 h Excretion: 50% in urine and 50% in feces	PO: Onset: 2 h Peak: Initially 3–7 d Duration: UK

Therapeutic Effects/Uses
To prevent thromboembolism associated with unstable angina, AMI, stroke, TIA
Mechanism of action: Inhibits platelet aggregation and prevents ADP from binding with the ADP platelet receptor

Side Effects	Adverse Reactions
Abdominal pain, dizziness, confusion, fever, epistaxis, headaches, hematoma, dyspepsia, diarrhea, constipation, purpura, peripheral edema, rash, pruritus	Hypotension, hypertension, bronchospasm, bleeding, peptic ulcer, intracranial/GI bleeding, hematuria, elevated hepatic enzymes *Life-threatening:* Agranulocytosis, aplastic anemia, thrombocytopenic purpura, pancytopenia, hepatic failure, Stevens-Johnson syndrome

A, Adult; *ADP*, adenosine diphosphate; *AMI*, acute myocardial infarction; *d*, day; *GI*, gastrointestinal; *h*, hour; *max*, maximum; *MI*, myocardial infarction; *min*, minutes; *NSAID*, nonsteroidal antiinflammatory drug; *PB*, protein binding; *PO*, by mouth; *SSRI*, selective serotonin reuptake inhibitor; *t½*, half-life; *TIA*, transient ischemic attack; *UK*, unknown.

TABLE 43.3 Antiplatelets

Drug	Route and Dosage	Uses and Considerations
Anagrelide hydrochloride	A: PO: Initially 0.5 mg qid or 1 mg bid for 1 wk; *maint:* 1.5–3 mg/d; *max:* 10 mg/d or 2.5 mg/dose	For treatment of thrombocytosis, chronic myelogenous leukemia, and polycythemia vera. May cause headache, dizziness, rash, palpitations, peripheral edema, weakness, fever, flatulence, abdominal pain, nausea, diarrhea, anorexia, vomiting, urticaria, edema, and dyspnea. PB: UK; t½: 1.5 h
Aspirin (ASA)	Stroke prophylaxis: Immediate release and unable to take oral anticoagulants: A: PO: 75–100 mg/d Extended release: 162.5 mg/d TDM: Salicylate toxicity is >300 mcg/mL	For pain and fever, as well as, prevention and treatment of stroke; MI, TIA. May cause abdominal pain, nausea, dyspepsia, gastritis, GI bleeding, intracranial bleeding, tinnitus, and hearing loss. PB: 90%–95%; t½: 15–20 min
Cilostazol	Claudication: A: PO: 50–100 mg bid 30 min ac or 2 h pc; *max:* 200 mg/d	For claudication, PVD, and thromboembolism prophylaxis. Contraindicated in heart failure. Smoking may decrease serum levels. May cause headache, dyspepsia, nausea, abdominal pain, diarrhea, nasopharyngitis, rhinitis, dizziness, back pain, infection, palpitations, and peripheral edema. PB: 95%–98%, t½: 11–13 h
Clopidogrel	See Prototype Drug Chart: Clopidogrel Bisulfate	
Dipyridamole	Thromboembolism prophylaxis: A: PO: 75–100 mg qid in combination with warfarin; *max:* 400 mg/d	For prevention of thromboembolism associated with prosthetic heart valves. May cause dizziness, headache, nausea, abdominal pain, dyspnea, flushing, hypo/hypertension, tachycardia, and angina/chest pain. PB: 91%–99%; t½: 12 h
Prasugrel	A >60 kg: PO: Loading dose: 60 mg; *maint:* 10 mg/d in combination with ASA A <60 kg: PO: Loading dose: 60 mg; *maint:* 5 mg/d in combination with	For thromboembolism prophylaxis. Not recommended if 75> y. May cause headache, back pain, dizziness, cough, bleeding, nausea, chest pain, hypo/hypertension, bradycardia, dyspnea, hypercholesterolemia, hyperlipidemia, fatigue, and epistaxis. PB: 98%; t½: 2–15 h

TABLE 43.3 Antiplatelets—cont'd

Drug	Route and Dosage	Uses and Considerations
Ticagrelor	A: PO: Loading dose: 180 mg; *maint:* 90 mg bid with low-dose ASA for 1 y, then 60 mg bid with low-dose ASA; *max:* 180 mg/d	For thromboembolism stroke prophylaxis. May cause headache, dizziness, fatigue, bradycardia, bleeding, nausea, diarrhea, cough, back pain, hypo/hypertension, atrial fibrillation, and dyspnea. PB: 99%; t½: 7 h
Vorapaxar	A: PO: 2.08 mg/d in combination with ASA and/or clopidogrel; *max:* 2.08 mg/d	For prevention of thrombosis, MI, PAD, and stroke. May cause bleeding, diplopia, depression, intracranial/GI bleeding, rash, and anemia. PB: 99%; t½: 5–13 d
Cangrelor	A: IV: Initially 30 mcg/kg bolus before PCI, follow immediately with infusion of 4 mcg/kg per minute for at least 2 h or duration of PCI, whichever is longer	For prevention of thrombosis in PCI and MI. May cause bleeding, dyspnea, hematoma, hematuria, and intracranial bleeding. PB: 97%; t½: 3–6 min
Combination of Antiplatelet Drugs		
Dipyridamole 200 mg and aspirin 25 mg	Stroke prevention: A: PO: 1 cap (25 mg ASA/200 mg dipyridamole) bid *max:* ASA 50 mg and dipyridamole 400 mg/d	For stroke prevention, ischemic stroke, and TIA. May cause headache, nausea, vomiting, diarrhea, abdominal/back pain, dyspepsia, fatigue, bleeding, and arthralgia. PB: ASA 90%–95%, dipyridamole 91%–99%; t½: ASA 2–12 h, dipyridamole 12 h
Aspirin (ASA) and omeprazole	A: PO: ASA 81 mg and omeprazole 40 mg/d or ASA 325 mg and omeprazole 40 mg/d	For prophylaxis of secondary cardiovascular and cerebrovascular events. May cause gastritis, nausea, diarrhea, dyspepsia, abdominal pain, vomiting, gastric polyps, headache, tinnitus, and hearing loss. PB: ASA 20%–90%, omeprazole 95%; t½: ASA 2–12 h, omeprazole 1 h
Antiplatelets: Glycoprotein (GP) IIb/IIIa Receptor Antagonists		
Abciximab	A: IV bolus: 0.25 mg/kg given 10–60 min before PCI; follow with continuous infusion of 0.125 mcg/kg per minute for 12 h; *max:* 10 mcg/min infusion; 0.25 mg/kg bolus	To prevent thrombosis in PCI, unstable angina, and AMI. May cause headache, dizziness, hypotension, bradycardia, bleeding, chest/back pain, nausea, vomiting, abdominal pain, antibody formation, and thrombocytopenia. PB: UK; t½: 10–30 min
Eptifibatide	PCI: A: IV bolus: 180 mcg/kg, then 2 mcg/kg per minute infusion until hospital discharge or 18–24 h; *max:* 15 mg/h infusion or 180 mcg/kg bolus	For prevention of thrombosis in PCI, unstable angina, and AMI. May cause hypotension, thrombocytopenia, stroke, intracranial bleeding, hematuria, and bleeding. PB: 25%; t½: 2.5 h
Tirofiban	A: IV: 25 mcg/kg bolus over 5 min followed by 0.15 mcg/kg per minute infusion for 18 h	For unstable angina and AMI and to reduce thrombotic cardiovascular events. May cause dizziness, headache, fever, hypotension, hyperhidrosis, bleeding, nausea, vomiting, pelvic pain, edema, and bradycardia. PB: 65%; t½: 1.7–2 h

A, adult; *ac*, before meals; *AMI*, acute myocardial infarction; *ASA*, acetylsalicylic acid (aspirin); *bid*, twice daily; *cap*, capsule; *d*, day; *GI*, gastrointestinal; *h*, hour; *IV*, intravenous; *maint*, maintenance; *max*, maximum; *MI*, myocardial infarction; *min*, minutes; *PAD*, peripheral artery disease; *PB*, protein binding; *pc*, after meals; *PCI*, percutaneous coronary intervention; *PO*, by mouth; *PVD*, peripheral vascular disease; *qd*, every day; *qid*, four times a day; *t½*, half-life; *TDM*, therapeutic drug monitoring; *TIA*, transient ischemic attack; *UK*, unknown.

Pharmacodynamics

Clopidogrel prevents platelet aggregation by blocking the binding of ADP to the platelet ADP receptor. ADP-mediated activation of the GP IIb/IIIa complex inhibits platelet aggregation. Clopidogrel prolongs bleeding time; therefore it should be discontinued for 7 days preceding surgery. The onset of action and peak of clopidogrel is dependent on dosage. The drug should not be taken if the patient has a bleeding peptic ulcer, any active bleeding, or intracranial hemorrhage.

Abciximab, eptifibatide, and tirofiban are used primarily for acute coronary syndromes (unstable angina or non-Q-wave MI) and for preventing reocclusion of coronary arteries after percutaneous transluminal coronary angioplasty (PTCA). These drugs are usually given before and after PTCA. The drug of choice for angioplasty is abciximab. Abciximab, eptifibatide, and tirofiban block the binding of fibrinogen to the GP IIb/IIIa receptor on the platelet surface. They are called *platelet glycoprotein IIb/IIIa receptor antagonists*. After IV infusion, the antiplatelet effects at low levels for abciximab persist for up to 10 days; for eptifibatide and tirofiban, the antiplatelet effects last for 4 hours.

Complementary and alternative therapy products can interact with antiplatelet drugs.

COMPLEMENTARY AND ALTERNATIVE THERAPIES
Antiplatelets

Dong quai, feverfew, garlic, ginger, Korean ginseng, saw palmetto, and ginkgo biloba interfere with platelet aggregation. When these herbs are taken with an antiplatelet drug such as aspirin, increased bleeding may occur. Licorice may cause hypokalemia, which can potentiate drug toxicity. St. John's wort with clopidogrel may potentiate drug effects.

THROMBOLYTICS

Overview and Usage Considerations

Thromboembolism, occlusion of an artery or vein caused by a thrombus or embolus, results in ischemia (deficient blood flow) that causes necrosis (death) of the tissue distal to the obstructed area. It takes approximately 1 to 2 weeks for the blood clot to disintegrate by natural fibrinolytic mechanisms. If a new thrombus or embolus can be dissolved more quickly, tissue necrosis is minimized, and blood flow to the area is reestablished faster. This is the basis for thrombolytic therapy.

Thrombolytics have been used since the early 1980s to promote the fibrinolytic mechanism (converting plasminogen to plasmin, which destroys the fibrin in the blood clot). The thrombus, or blood clot, disintegrates when a thrombolytic drug is administered as soon as possible after symptoms of an **acute myocardial infarction (AMI)**, acute heart attack. Ideally, the thrombolytic should be administered within 3 to 4 hours or within 30 minutes after arriving at the hospital for treatment. However, benefits may be seen when administered within 12 hours after initial symptoms. Necrosis resulting from the blocked artery is prevented or minimized, and hospitalization time may be decreased. The need for cardiac bypass or coronary angioplasty can be evaluated soon after thrombolytic treatment. A thrombolytic drug should be administered within 3 hours of a thrombotic stroke. These drugs are also used for PE, DVT, noncoronary arterial occlusion from an acute thromboembolism, and thrombotic stroke.

Commonly used thrombolytics include alteplase, also known as *tissue plasminogen activator* (tPA), and enecteplase (TNK tPA). Alteplase is clot specific and binds to the fibrin surface of a clot, promoting the conversion of plasminogen to plasmin. Plasmin, an enzyme, digests the fibrin in the clot. Plasmin also degrades fibrinogen, prothrombin, and other clotting factors. These drugs all induce **fibrinolysis** (fibrin breakdown). Prototype Drug Chart: Alteplase lists the pharmacologic data for alteplase.

Anticoagulants and antiplatelet drugs increase the risk of hemorrhage; therefore they should be avoided until the thrombolytic effect has passed. The health care provider needs to determine whether the patient has taken any of these drugs before seeking treatment.

Pharmacology
Pharmacokinetics
The commercial preparation of alteplase is identical to natural human tissue plasminogen activator (tPA), the enzyme that converts plasminogen to plasmin. Alteplase is initially administered with 10% of dose as an IV bolus over 1 minute and 90% of dose is then infused over 60 minutes. A total dose of 90 mg is the recommended maximum; a larger dose could result in risk for intracranial bleeding. Allergic reactions to alteplase occur less frequently than with other thrombolytics.

Pharmacodynamics
Alteplase is similar to natural human tissue plasminogen activator. It promotes thrombolysis by converting plasminogen to plasmin, which degrades fibrin, fibrinogen, and factors V, VIII, and XII. Peak action of alteplase occurs in 5 to 10 minutes. The duration of action is 1 hour.

Side Effects and Adverse Reactions
Allergic reactions can complicate thrombolytic therapy. Anaphylaxis (vascular collapse) occurs in less than 1% of patients receiving tenecteplase. Anaphylactoid reactions following alteplase and tenecteplase are severe and involve rash, laryngeal edema, angioedema, and anaphylactic shock. If the drugs are administered through an intracoronary catheter after MI, reperfusion dysrhythmia or hemorrhagic infarction at the myocardial necrotic area can result. The major complication of thrombolytic drugs is hemorrhage. The antithrombotic drug aminocaproic acid is used to stop bleeding by inhibiting plasminogen activation, which inhibits thrombolysis.

Table 43.4 lists the thrombolytic drugs and their dosages, uses, and considerations.

PROTOTYPE DRUG CHART
Alteplase

Drug Class	Dosage
Thrombolytic agent	Acute PE treatment: A: IV: 100 mg infusion over 2 h Ischemic CVA treatment: A: IV: 0.9 mg/kg (give 10% of dose as bolus over 1 min then 90% as an infusion over 1 h) within 3 h of symptom onset

Contraindications	Drug-Lab-Food Interactions
Intracranial bleeding, aneurysm, CVA, brain tumor, head trauma, thrombocytopenia, coagulopathy *Caution:* Atrial fibrillation, hepatic/renal disease, CABG, bleeding, anticoagulant therapy, peptic ulcer disease, diabetic retinopathy, seizures, older adults, breastfeeding, pregnancy	Drug: Increased bleeding when taken with anticoagulants, NSAIDs, SNRIs, and SSRIs; decreased effect when taken with aminocaproic acid, aprotinin Lab: Decrease in plasminogen, fibrinogen, hematocrit, and hemoglobin Complementary and Alternative Therapies: Increased bleeding with ginkgo biloba, garlic, feverfew, ginger, green tea, omega-3 fatty acids

Pharmacokinetics	Pharmacodynamics
Absorption: Direct IV Distribution: PB: UK Metabolism: t½: 30–45 min Excretion: Urine	A: IV: Onset: Immediate Peak: 5–10 min Duration: 1 h

Therapeutic Effects/Uses
To promote fibrinolysis associated with thrombosis in patients with AMI, PE, ischemic stroke, occluded IV catheter
Mechanism of action: Alteplase promotes conversion of plasminogen to plasmin, an enzyme that digests the fibrin matrix of clots. Alteplase also initiates fibrinolysis.

Side Effects	Adverse Reactions
Epistaxis, infection, ecchymosis, nausea, vomiting, rash	Anaphylactoid reactions, laryngeal edema, angioedema; cholesterol microembolization, bleeding, hypo/hypertension, GI bleeding, MI, cerebral edema, rhabdomyolysis, bradycardia, tachycardia, heart failure, intracranial hemorrhage, seizures *Life-threatening:* Stroke; dysrhythmias; pulmonary edema, renal failure

A, Adult; *AMI*, acute myocardial infarction; *CABG*, coronary artery bypass graft; *CVA*, cerebrovascular accident; *GI*, gastrointestinal; *h*, hour; *IV*, intravenous; *MI*, myocardial infarction; *min*, minutes; *NSAID's*, nonsteroidal antiinflammatory drugs; *PB*, protein binding; *PE*, pulmonary embolism; *SNRIs*, serotonin and norepinephrine reuptake inhibitors; *SSRI*, selective serotonin reuptake inhibitor; *t½*, half-life; *UK*, unknown.

CLINICAL JUDGMENT [NURSING PROCESS]
Thrombolytics

Concept: Clotting
- A process in which blood is changed into a semisolid gel

Recognize Cues [Assessment]
- Assess baseline vital signs for comparison with future values.
- Check baseline complete blood count (CBC), prothrombin time (PT), or international normalized ratio (INR) values before administration of thrombolytics.
- Obtain a medical and drug history. Contraindications for use of thrombolytics include recent cerebrovascular accident (CVA), active bleeding, severe hypertension, and anticoagulant therapy. Report if a patient takes aspirin or nonsteroidal antiinflammatory drugs (NSAIDs). Thrombolytics are contraindicated for patients with a recent history of traumatic injury, especially head injury.

Analyze Cues and Prioritize Hypothesis [Patient Problems]
- Bleeding
- Tissue injury
- Dehydration

Generate Solutions [Planning]
- The patient's vital signs will be within normal limits.
- The patient will be free of excessive bleeding.

Take Action [Nursing Interventions]
- Monitor vital signs. Increased pulse rate followed by decreased blood pressure usually indicates blood loss and impending shock. Record vital signs, and report changes.
- Observe for signs and symptoms of active bleeding from the mouth or rectum. Hemorrhage is a serious complication of thrombolytic treatment. Aminocaproic acid can be given as an intervention to stop bleeding.
- ⚡ Examine the patient for active bleeding for 24 hours after thrombolytic therapy has been discontinued: this should be done every 15 minutes for the first hour, then every 30 minutes until the eighth hour, and then hourly.
- ⚡ Observe for signs of allergic reaction to thrombolytics, such as itching, hives, flushing, fever, dyspnea, bronchospasm, hypotension, and/or cardiovascular collapse.
- Avoid administering aspirin or NSAIDs for pain or discomfort when the patient is receiving a thrombolytic. Acetaminophen can be substituted.
- Monitor the electrocardiogram (ECG) for presence of reperfusion dysrhythmias as the blood clot is dissolving; antidysrhythmic therapy may be indicated.
- Avoid venipuncture/arterial sticks.

Patient Teaching
General
- Explain thrombolytic treatment to patients and family. Be supportive.

Side Effects
- Advise patients to report any side effects such as lightheadedness, dizziness, palpitations, nausea, pruritus, or urticaria.

Evaluate Outcomes [Evaluation]
- Determine the effectiveness of drug therapy: the clot should have dissolved, vital signs should be stable with no signs or symptoms of active bleeding, and the patient should be pain free.

⚠ TABLE 43.4 Thrombolytics

Drug	Route and Dosage	Uses and Considerations
Thrombolytics		
Tenecteplase	A: IV: Give single dose as soon as possible after onset of symptoms: A: 90>kg: 50 mg A: 80–89 kg: 45 mg A: 70–79 kg: 40 mg A: 60–69 kg: 35 mg A: <60 kg: 30 mg *max:* 50 mg/dose	To treat AMI. May cause bleeding, stroke, heart failure, cardiogenic shock, MI, intracranial bleeding, and antibody formation. PB: UK; t½: 90–130 min
Reteplase, r-PA	A: IV: 10 units over 2 min, follow in 30 min with second dose of 10 units; *max:* 20 units	For treatment of AMI. Reteplase penetrates clots and activates plasminogen inside the clot, which may lead to a higher clot lysis rate. May cause bleeding, GI/intracranial bleeding, anemia, anaphylaxis, and purple-toe syndrome. PB: UK; t½: 13–16 min
Alteplase	See Prototype Drug Chart: Alteplase	
Hemostatics		
Aminocaproic acid	A: PO: LD: 5 g the first h; follow with 1–1.25 g/h for 8 h or until bleeding is controlled; *max:* 30 g/d A: IV: 4–5 g over first h, follow with 1 g/h continuous infusion for 8 h; or until bleeding controlled; *max:* 30 g/d	For bleeding due to hyperfibrinolysis. May cause hypotension, headache, dyspnea, edema, dizziness, confusion, bradycardia, vision impairment, injection-site reaction, nausea, abdominal pain, and diarrhea. PB: UK; t½: 2 h

A, Adult; *AMI*, acute myocardial infarction; *d*, day; *GI*, gastrointestinal; *h*, hour; *IV*, intravenous; *LD*, loading dose; *max*, maximum; *min*, minutes; *PB*, protein binding; *PO*, by mouth; *t½*, half-life; *UK*, unknown.

CLINICAL JUDGMENT CASE STUDY

A 57-year-old male has thrombophlebitis in the right lower leg. IV heparin, 5000 units by bolus, was given. After the IV bolus, heparin 5000 units given subcutaneously every 6 hours was prescribed. Other therapeutic means to decrease pain and alleviate swelling and redness were also prescribed, and an activated partial thromboplastin time (aPTT) test was ordered.

1. Was the patient's heparin order within the safe daily dosage range?
2. What are the various methods for administering heparin?
3. Why was an aPTT test ordered? How would you determine whether the patient is within the desired range? Explain your answer.
4. After 5 days of heparin therapy, the patient was prescribed oral warfarin 5 mg daily. An international normalized ratio (INR) test was ordered. What is the pharmacologic action of warfarin? Is the warfarin dose within the safe daily dosage range? Explain your answer.
5. What are the half-life and protein binding for warfarin? If a patient takes a drug that is highly protein bound, would there be a drug interaction? Explain your answer.
6. Why was an INR ordered for the patient? What is the desired range?
7. What serious adverse reactions could result with prolonged use or large doses of warfarin?
8. What patient teaching interventions should the nurse include? List three interventions.
9. Months later, the patient has hematemesis. What nursing action should be taken?

REVIEW QUESTIONS

1. A patient is placed on heparin, and the nurse acknowledges that heparin is effective for preventing clot formation in patients who have which disorder(s)? **Select all that apply.**
   a. Coronary thrombosis
   b. Acute myocardial infarction
   c. Deep vein thrombosis
   d. Hemorrhagic stroke
   e. Disseminated intravascular coagulation
2. A patient who received heparin begins to bleed. The nurse anticipates that the health care provider will order which antidote?
   a. Protamine sulfate
   b. Phytonadione
   c. Aminocaproic acid
   d. Potassium chloride
3. A patient is prescribed enoxaparin. The nurse knows that low-molecular-weight heparin has what kind of half-life?
   a. A longer half-life than heparin
   b. A shorter half-life than heparin
   c. The same half-life as heparin
   d. A four-times shorter half-life than heparin
4. A patient had an orthopedic surgery and is prescribed enoxaparin. What would the nurse teach the patient and/or family members about this low-molecular-weight heparin before discharge?
   a. Visual demonstration of intramuscular heparin administration is recommended.
   b. Prothrombin time and international normalized ratio monitoring will be done weekly.
   c. Avoidance of green leafy vegetables is recommended.
   d. Watch for bleeding or excessive bruising.
5. A patient is being changed from an injectable anticoagulant to an oral anticoagulant. Which anticoagulant does the nurse realize is administered orally?
   a. Enoxaparin
   b. Warfarin
   c. Bivalirudin
   d. Dalteparin
   e. Tenecteplase
   f. Fondaparinux
6. A patient is taking warfarin 5 mg/day for atrial fibrillation. The patient's international normalized ratio is 3.8. The nurse would consider the international normalized ratio to be what?
   a. Within normal range
   b. Elevated range
   c. Low range
   d. Low-average range
7. Cilostazol is being prescribed for a patient with coronary artery disease. The nurse understands that which of the following is the major purpose for antiplatelet drug therapy?
   a. Dissolve the blood clot
   b. Decrease tissue necrosis
   c. Inhibit hepatic synthesis of vitamin K
   d. Suppress platelet aggregation

44

Antihyperlipidemics and Drugs to Improve Peripheral Blood Flow

http://evolve.elsevier.com/McCuistion/pharmacology

OBJECTIVES

- Summarize the functions and effects of lipoproteins.
- Explain the characteristics of four types of antihyperlipidemics that lower lipid levels.
- Describe indications of peripheral vascular disease and drugs used to treat it.

OUTLINE

Lipoproteins, 563
    Types of Lipoproteins, 563
    Apolipoproteins, 563
Antihyperlipidemics, 563
    Bile-Acid Sequestrants, 563
    Fibric Acid Derivatives, 564
    Niacin, 564
    Cholesterol Absorption Inhibitors, 564

    Statins, 564
    Nonpharmacologic Methods of Cholesterol Reduction, 567
Drugs to Improve Peripheral Blood Flow, 567
    Peripheral Vasodilators, 568
    Cilostazol, 568
    Blood Viscosity Reducer Agent, 568
Clinical Judgment Case Study, 571
Review Questions, 571

Various drugs are used to maintain or decrease blood lipid concentrations and promote dilation of vessels. Drugs that lower blood lipids are called *antihyperlipidemics, antilipidemics, antilipemics,* and *hypolipidemics.* In this chapter, drugs used to lower lipoproteins are called **antihyperlipidemics**. Drugs that improve blood flow are called **peripheral vasodilators**, as they dilate vessels that have been narrowed by vasospasm, and blood viscosity reducer agents, which decrease viscosity of blood and increase erythrocyte flexibility.

LIPOPROTEINS

Types of Lipoproteins

Lipids—cholesterol, triglycerides, and phospholipids—are bound in the inner shell of protein, a carrier that transports lipids in the bloodstream. When there is an excess of one or more lipids in the blood, the condition is known as **hyperlipidemia** or *hyperlipoproteinemia*. The four major categories of **lipoprotein** are **high-density lipoprotein (HDL), low-density lipoprotein (LDL), very-low-density lipoprotein (VLDL),** and chylomicrons. HDL, also known as "friendly" or "good" lipoprotein, is the smallest and densest lipoprotein, meaning that it contains more protein and less fat than the others. The function of HDL is to remove cholesterol from the bloodstream and deliver it to the liver for excretion in bile. LDL, the "bad" lipoprotein, contains 50% to 60% of cholesterol in the bloodstream. With an elevated LDL, the risk is greater for developing atherosclerotic plaques and heart disease. VLDL carries mostly triglycerides and less cholesterol. The **chylomicrons** are large particles that transport fatty acids and cholesterol to the liver. They are composed mostly of triglycerides.

Serum cholesterol and triglyceride measurements are frequently part of a regular physical examination or readmission evaluation and are used as baseline test results. If the levels are high, a 12- to 14-hour fasting lipid profile may be ordered. When cholesterol, triglycerides, and LDL are elevated, the patient is at increased risk for coronary artery disease (CAD). Table 44.1 lists the various serum lipids and their reference values (normal serum levels) according to risk classification.

Apolipoproteins

Apolipoproteins are within the lipoprotein shell and contain apolipoprotein (apo) A-1, B, and E. The major component of apoA-1 is HDL. The major component of apoB is LDL, which exists in two forms, apoB-100 and apoB-48. ApoB-100 has VLDL as well as LDL and is a better indicator of risk for CAD than LDL alone.

ANTIHYPERLIPIDEMICS

Drugs that lower lipid levels include bile-acid sequestrants, fibrates (fibric acid), nicotinic acid, cholesterol absorption inhibitors, and hepatic 3-hydroxy-3-methylglutaryl-coenzyme A (HMG-CoA) reductase inhibitors, better known as *statins*. The statin drugs have fewer adverse effects and are well tolerated.

Bile-Acid Sequestrants

One of the first antihyperlipidemics, cholestyramine is a bile-acid sequestrant that reduces LDL cholesterol (LDL-C) levels by binding with bile acids in the intestine. It is effective against hyperlipidemia type II. This group may be used as an adjunct to the statins. The drug comes in a gritty powder that is mixed thoroughly in water or

TABLE 44.1 Serum Lipid Values

Lipids	Desirable (mg/dL)	LEVEL OF RISK FOR CAD		
		Low Risk (mg/dL)	Moderate Risk (mg/dL)	High Risk (mg/dL)
Cholesterol	150–200	200	200–240	>240
Triglycerides	40–150	Values vary with age	Values vary with age	>190
Lipoproteins				
LDL	<100	100–130	130–159	>160
HDL	>60	50–60	35–50	<35

<, Less than; >, greater than; *CAD*, coronary artery disease; *HDL*, high-density lipoprotein; *LDL*, low-density lipoprotein.

juice. Colestipol is another resin antihyperlipidemic similar to cholestyramine. Both are effective in lowering cholesterol. Colesevelam, another bile-acid sequestrant similar to cholestyramine and colestipol, is an agent that has fewer side effects (less constipation, flatulence, and cramping). Colesevelam also has less effect on the absorption of fat-soluble vitamins than the older agents and is usually the first-choice bile-acid sequestrant drug.

Fibric Acid Derivatives

Gemfibrozil is a fibric acid derivative that is more effective for reducing triglyceride and VLDL levels than for reducing LDL. It is used primarily to reduce hyperlipidemia type IV, but it can also be used for type II hyperlipidemia. This drug is highly protein bound and should not be taken with anticoagulants because they compete for protein sites. The anticoagulant dose should be reduced during antihyperlipidemic therapy, and the international normalized ratio (INR) should be closely monitored. Fenofibrate has similar actions and some of the same side effects as gemfibrozil. If taken with warfarin, bleeding might occur. Both fenofibrate and gemfibrozil are highly protein bound.

Niacin

Niacin (vitamin B_3) reduces VLDL and LDL. Niacin is actually very effective at lowering cholesterol levels, and its effect on the lipid profile is highly desirable. Because it has numerous side effects and large doses are required, as few as 20% of patients can initially tolerate niacin. However, with proper counseling, careful drug titration, and concomitant use of aspirin, this number can be increased to as much as 60% to 70%. Niacin is only recommended in specific clinical situations such as triglyceride levels more than 500 mg/dL or if intolerant to other treatment.

Cholesterol Absorption Inhibitors

Ezetimibe is a cholesterol absorption inhibitor that acts on the cells in the small intestine to inhibit cholesterol absorption. It decreases cholesterol from dietary absorption, reducing serum cholesterol, LDL, triglycerides, and apoB levels. Ezetimibe causes only a small increase in HDL. It must be combined with a statin (e.g., simvastatin) for optimum effect.

Statins

The statin drugs inhibit the enzyme HMG-CoA reductase in cholesterol biosynthesis; thus statins are called *HMG-CoA reductase inhibitors*. By inhibiting cholesterol synthesis in the liver, this group of antihyperlipidemics decreases the concentration of cholesterol, decreases LDL, and slightly increases HDL cholesterol. Reduction of LDL cholesterol may be seen as early as 2 weeks after initiating therapy. The statin group has been useful in decreasing CAD and reducing mortality rates.

Numerous statins have been approved since statins were first introduced. The present group of statins includes atorvastatin calcium, fluvastatin, lovastatin, pravastatin sodium, simvastatin, pitavastatin, and rosuvastatin. Lovastatin was the first statin used to decrease cholesterol. It is effective for lowering LDL (hyperlipidemia type II) within several weeks. Gastrointestinal (GI) disturbances, headaches, muscle cramps, and fatigue are early complaints. With all statins, serum liver enzymes should be monitored, and an annual eye examination is needed because cataract formation may result. The patient should report immediately any muscle aches or weakness, which can lead to rhabdomyolysis, a muscle disintegration that can become fatal.

The statins have actions in decreasing serum cholesterol, LDL, VLDL, and triglycerides, and they slightly elevate HDL. Atorvastatin, lovastatin, rosuvastatin, and simvastatin are more effective at lowering LDL than the other statins. Rosuvastatin and atorvastatin are at the top of the list of most prescribed drugs in the United States.

The statin drugs can be combined with other drugs to decrease blood pressure and blood clotting and to enhance the antihyperlipidemic effect. Examples are atorvastatin and amlodipine; and simvastatin and ezetimibe. Table 44.2 lists these combination drugs and their dosages, uses, and considerations.

If antihyperlipidemic therapy is withdrawn, cholesterol and LDL levels return to pretreatment levels. The patient taking an antihyperlipidemic drug should understand that antihyperlipidemic therapy is a lifetime commitment for maintaining a decrease in serum lipid levels. Abruptly stopping the statin drug could cause a threefold rebound effect that may cause death from acute myocardial infarction (AMI).

Laboratory Tests

Reference values for homocysteine, an amino acid, are 4 to 17 mmol/L (fasting). Homocysteine is a byproduct of protein and is found in eggs, chicken, beef, and cheddar cheese. A high level of homocysteine has been linked to cardiovascular disease, stroke, and Alzheimer disease. It may also promote blood clotting, and it has been stated that an increase in serum homocysteine can damage the inner lining of blood vessels and promote a thickening and loss of flexibility in the vessel. Three vitamins that can lower serum homocysteine levels are vitamin B_6 (pyridoxine), vitamin B_{12} (cyanocobalamin), and folic acid.

High-sensitivity C-reactive protein (hsCRP) low risk is less than 1 mg/L, moderate risk is 1 to 3 mg/L, and high risk is greater than

TABLE 44.2 Antihyperlipidemics

Generic	Route and Dosage	Uses and Considerations
Bile-Acid Sequestrants		
Cholestyramine	A: PO: Initially 4 g qd/bid before meals; mix powder in 60–180 mL of fluid; *maint:* 4–8 g bid; *max:* 24 g daily	For hypercholesterolemia. May cause anorexia, nausea, vomiting, diarrhea, constipation, steatorrhea, abdominal pain, eructation, flatulence, osteoporosis, peptic ulcer, GI bleeding/obstruction, and cholelithiasis. PB: UK; t½: UK
Colesevelam	A: PO: 1.875 g bid; *max:* 3.75 g/d	For hypercholesterolemia. May cause headache, dyspepsia, constipation, hypertension, weakness, fatigue, nausea, influenza, hypoglycemia, and hypertriglyceridemia. PB: UK; t½: UK
Colestipol hydrochloride	A: PO: Initially 2 g tablets qd or bid, may increase at 1- to 2-month intervals; *max:* 16 g daily	For hypercholesterolemia. May cause dizziness, weakness, tachycardia, anorexia, nausea, vomiting, diarrhea, constipation, abdominal pain, headache, arthralgia, and GI bleeding. PB: UK; t½: UK
Fibrates (Fibric Acid)		
Fenofibrate	Lipofen capsules: A: PO: 50–150 mg daily with food; *max:* 150 mg daily	For hypercholesterolemia and hypertriglyceridemia. May cause headache, weakness, nausea, diarrhea, constipation, abdominal pain, cholelithiasis, cholecystitis, back pain, and elevated hepatic enzymes. PB: 99%; t½: 20 h
Gemfibrozil	A: PO: 600 mg bid 30 min before morning and evening meals; *max:* 1200 mg daily	For hypercholesterolemia and hypertriglyceridemia. May cause dizziness, headache, elevated hepatic enzymes, fatigue, nausea, vomiting, dyspepsia, abdominal pain, cholelithiasis, cholecystitis, cholestasis, constipation, and diarrhea. PB: 95%; t½: 1.5 h
Niacin		
Niacin	Regular release: A: PO: Initially 250 mg qd after evening meal; may increase q4–7d; *maint:* 1.5–3 g/d in 2–3 divided doses; *max:* 6 g qd Sustained release: A: PO: 1–2 g/d in 2–3 divided doses; *max:* 2 g/d	For hypercholesterolemia. May cause flushing, hypotension, dizziness, headache, cough, pruritus, nausea, vomiting, diarrhea, hyperglycemia, hyperuricemia, rash, edema, elevated hepatic enzymes, and weakness. PB: <20%; t½: 20–48 min
Cholesterol Absorption Inhibitors		
Ezetimibe	A: PO: 10 mg daily; *max:* 10 mg daily	For hypercholesterolemia. May cause diarrhea, arthralgia, abdominal/back pain, fatigue, infection, pharyngitis, sinusitis, elevated hepatic enzymes, cholelithiasis, cholecystitis, and myalgia. PB: 90%; t½: 22 h
Statins (HMG-CoA Reductase Inhibitors)		
Atorvastatin calcium	See Prototype Drug Chart: Atorvastatin	
Fluvastatin sodium	Immediate release: A: PO: 20 mg qd–40 mg bid; *max:* 80 mg qd Extended release: A: PO: 80 mg daily; *max:* 80 mg daily	For hypercholesterolemia. Do not cut, crush, or chew extended-release tab. May cause headache, nausea, abdominal pain, dyspepsia, diarrhea, hypertension, myalgia, peripheral edema, influenza, sinusitis, fatigue, arthralgia, constipation, and elevated hepatic enzymes. PB: 98%; t½: Immediate release 3 h, extended release 7.3–10.5 h
Lovastatin	Immediate release: A: PO: Initially 10–20 mg qd with evening meal; *max:* 80 mg qd Extended release: A: PO: 20–60 mg qd at bedtime; *max:* 60 mg qd	For hypercholesterolemia. May cause headache, sinusitis, infection, arthralgia, nausea, abdominal pain, diarrhea, constipation, flatulence, influenza, fatigue, weakness, back pain, muscle cramps, and myalgia. PB: 95%; t½: 1.1–1.7 h
Pravastatin sodium	A: PO: 40–80 mg/d; *max:* 80 mg daily	For hypercholesterolemia. May cause headache, dizziness, dyspepsia, flatulence, abdominal pain, nausea, vomiting, diarrhea, constipation, fatigue, angina, and musculoskeletal pain. PB: 50%; t½: 1.6–1.8 h
Rosuvastatin	A: PO: 5–40 mg qd; *max:* 40 mg qd	For hypercholesterolemia. May cause dizziness, headache, weakness, nausea, constipation, abdominal pain, arthralgia, myalgia, and hyperglycemia. PB: 88%; t½: 19 h

Continued

TABLE 44.2 Antihyperlipidemics—cont'd

Generic	Route and Dosage	Uses and Considerations
Simvastatin	A: PO: Initially 10–20 mg qd at hs; *maint:* 5–40 mg daily in evening; *max:* 40 mg daily	For hypercholesterolemia. May cause dizziness, headache, edema, insomnia, gastritis, nausea, abdominal pain, constipation, atrial fibrillation, elevated hepatic enzymes, and infection. PB: 95%; t½: 1.9 h
Pitavastatin	A: PO: 2–4 mg/d; *max:* 4 mg qd	For hypercholesterolemia, hyperlipoproteinemia, and hypertriglyceridemia. May cause headache, myalgia, back pain, arthralgia, constipation, diarrhea, abdominal pain, and elevated hepatic enzymes. PB: 99%; t½: 12 h
Miscellaneous Antilipemics		
Icosapent ethyl	A: PO: 2 g q12h with food; *max:* 4 g daily with food	For hypertriglyceridemia. May cause arthralgia, bleeding, peripheral edema, gout, musculoskeletal pain, constipation, and atrial fibrillation/flutter. PB: 99%; t½: 89 h
Inclisiran	A: Subcut: 284 mg q3mo for 2 doses, then q6mo	For hypercholesterolemia. May cause antibody formation, injection-site reaction, rash, erythema, and arthralgia. PB: 87%; t½: 9 h
Lomitapide	A: PO: Initially 5 mg daily 2 h after evening meal, may begin to increase to 10 mg after at least 2 wk; *max:* 60 mg daily	For hypercholesterolemia. May cause dizziness, fatigue, back pain, influenza, fever, chest pain, headache, palpitations, elevated hepatic enzymes, dyspepsia, nausea, vomiting, diarrhea, constipation, abdominal pain, tenesmus, GERD, steatosis, weight loss, flatulence, nasal congestion, and pharyngitis. PB: 99.8%; t½: 39.7 h
Alirocumab	A: Subcut: Initially 75 mg q2wk or 300 mg q4wk; *max:* 300 mg every mo	For hypercholesterolemia and hyperlipidemia. May cause myalgia, diarrhea, antibody formation, injection-site reaction, and influenza. PB: UK; t½: 17–20 d
Evolocumab	A: Subcut: 140 mg q2wk or 420 mg q1mo; *max:* 420 mg/mo	For hypercholesterolemia. May cause dizziness, headache, hyperglycemia, infection, arthralgia, myalgia, diarrhea, pharyngitis, hypertension, influenza, sinusitis, cough, back pain, musculoskeletal pain, and injection-site reaction. PB: UK; t½: 11–17 d
Bempedoic acid	A: PO: 180 mg/d; *max:* 180 mg/d	For hypercholesterolemia. May cause back/abdominal pain, muscle cramps, infection, hyperuricemia, elevated hepatic enzymes, gout, leukopenia, anemia, and thrombocytosis. PB: 99%; t½: 10–32 h
Evinacumab	A: IV: 15 mg/kg over 60 min q4wk; *max:* 15 mg/kg q4wk	For hypercholesterolemia. May cause pharyngitis, rhinorrhea, nasal congestion, infusion-related reactions, dizziness, weakness, fatigue, abdominal pain, nausea, and constipation. PB: UK; t½: UK
Combination Antihyperlipidemic Drugs		
Amlodipine and atorvastatin	A: PO: Initially 5–10 mg amlodipine and 10–20 mg atorvastatin daily; *max:* 10 mg amlodipine and 80 mg atorvastatin daily Older A: PO: 2.5 mg amlodipine and 10–20 mg atorvastatin; *max:* 10 mg amlodipine and 80 mg atorvastatin	For hypercholesterolemia, hyperlipoproteinemia, and hypertriglyceridemia. May cause fatigue, pharyngitis, dyspepsia, nausea, diarrhea, arthralgia, peripheral edema, palpitations, and edema. PB: amlodipine 93%, atorvastatin 98%; t½: amlodipine 30–50 h, atorvastatin 14 h
Bempedoic acid and ezetimibe	A: PO: 180 mg bempedoic acid and 10 mg ezetimibe qd; *max:* 180 mg bempedoic acid and 10 mg ezetimibe qd	For hypercholesterolemia. Swallow tablet whole. May cause hyperuricemia, pharyngitis, back pain, muscle cramps, constipation, diarrhea, infection, anemia, thrombocytosis, and leukopenia. PB: 99.3% bempedoic acid, 90% ezetimibe; t½: 10–32 h bempedoic acid, 22 h ezetimibe
Ezetimibe and simvastatin	A: PO: 10 mg ezetimibe and 10–40 mg simvastatin qd at hs; *max:* 10 mg ezetimibe and 40 mg simvastatin daily	For hypercholesterolemia and hyperlipoproteinemia. May cause headache, diarrhea, myalgia, infection, influenza, musculoskeletal pain, and elevated hepatic enzymes. PB: ezetimibe 90%, simvastatin 95%; t½: ezetimibe 22 h, simvastatin 1.9 h

<, Less than; *A*, adult; *ac*, before meals; *bid*, twice a day; *d*, day; *GERD*, gastroesophageal reflux disease; *GI*, gastrointestinal; *h*, hour; *HMG-CoA*, 3-hydroxy-3-methylglutaryl-coenzyme A; *maint*, maintenance; *max*, maximum; *min*, minutes; *mo*, months; *PB*, protein binding; *PO*, by mouth; *q*, every; *subcut*, subcutaneously; *t½*, half-life; *UK*, unknown; *wk*, weeks.

3 mg/L. The standard C-reactive protein (CRP) is produced in the liver in response to tissue injury and inflammation. The hsCRP is a highly sensitive test for detecting the inflammatory protein that can be associated with cardiovascular and peripheral vascular disease. This test is frequently ordered along with cholesterol screening. Approximately one-third of persons who have had a heart attack have normal cholesterol levels and normal blood pressure. A positive hsCRP test can indicate that the patient is at high risk for CAD, making it a valuable test for predicting CAD. This test can detect an inflammatory process caused by the buildup of atherosclerotic plaque in the arterial system, particularly the coronary arteries.

Prototype Drug Chart: Atorvastatin lists the pharmacologic data for this frequently prescribed antihyperlipidemic.

Pharmacokinetics
Atorvastatin decreases LDL by 30% to 50% at an average dose of 10 to 80 mg. It is highly protein bound at 98%, so it usually is prescribed as a once-daily dose. Atorvastatin has a half-life of 14 hours.

Pharmacodynamics
The positive effect of lowering lipids with atorvastatin is seen in about 3 to 5 days. The peak time after a dose of atorvastatin is 1 to 2 hours; however, it takes 2 to 6 weeks to achieve therapeutic effect. Atorvastatin may be taken without regard to meals, but grapefruit juice should be avoided as it could cause an increase in drug concentration. When the patient is taking high doses of atorvastatin or any other statin, myopathy and rhabdomyolysis—disintegration of striated muscle fibers—may occur. If the patient experiences muscle pain or tenderness, it should be reported immediately.

Side Effects and Adverse Reactions
Side effects and adverse reactions of cholestyramine include constipation and peptic ulcer. Constipation can be decreased or alleviated by increasing intake of fluids and foods high in fiber. Early signs of peptic ulcer are nausea and abdominal discomfort, followed later by abdominal pain and distension. To avoid GI discomfort, the drug must be taken with and followed by sufficient fluids.

The many side effects of niacin—which include GI disturbances (nausea, vomiting, and diarrhea), flushing of the skin, abnormal liver function (elevated serum liver enzymes), hyperglycemia, and hyperuricemia—decrease its usefulness. However, as mentioned, aspirin and careful drug titration can reduce side effects to a manageable level in most patients.

The statin drugs can cause a dose-related increase in liver enzyme levels. Serum liver enzyme levels (alkaline phosphatase [ALP], alanine aminotransferase [ALT], gamma-glutamyl transferase [GGT]) should be monitored. Baseline liver enzyme studies should be obtained before initiating statin therapy. A slight transient increase in serum liver enzyme levels may be within normal range for the patient, but it should be rechecked in 1 week or so. Patients with acute hepatic disorders should not take a statin drug.

The serious skeletal muscle adverse effect, rhabdomyolysis, has been reported with use of the statin drug class, although it is rare. Patients should be advised to promptly report to the health care provider any unexplained muscle tenderness or weakness, especially if accompanied by fever or malaise. Table 44.2 lists the pharmacologic data for antihyperlipidemics.

Nonpharmacologic Methods of Cholesterol Reduction
Before drugs to lower LDL and raise HDL are prescribed, nondrug therapy should be initiated to decrease cholesterol. Saturated fats and cholesterol in the diet should be reduced. Total fat intake should be 30% or less of caloric intake, and cholesterol intake should be 300 mg/day or less. The patient should be advised to read labels on containers and buy appropriate foods. Patients should choose lean meats, especially chicken and fish.

In many cases, diet alone will not lower blood lipid levels. Because 75% to 85% of serum cholesterol is endogenously (internally) derived, dietary modification alone will typically lower total cholesterol levels by only 10% to 30%. This and the fact that adherence to dietary restrictions is often short-lived explains why many patients do not respond to diet modification alone.

Exercise is an important aspect of the nonpharmacologic method to reduce cholesterol and increase HDL. For the older adult, exercise can be walking and bicycling. Smoking is another risk factor that should be eliminated. Smoking increases LDL cholesterol and decreases HDL.

If nonpharmacologic methods are ineffective for reducing LDL and VLDL cholesterol, and hyperlipidemia remains, antihyperlipidemic drugs are prescribed to lower blood lipid levels. It must be emphasized to the patient that dietary changes need to be made and an exercise program followed, even after drug therapy is initiated. The type of antihyperlipidemics ordered depends on the lipoprotein phenotype (Table 44.3).

TABLE 44.3 Hyperlipidemia: Lipoprotein Phenotype

Type[a]	Major Lipids
I	Increased chylomicrons and increased triglycerides; uncommon
IIA	Increased LDL and increased cholesterol; common
IIB	Increased VLDL, increased LDL, increased cholesterol and triglycerides; very common
III	Moderately increased cholesterol and triglycerides; uncommon
IV	Increased VLDL and markedly increased triglycerides; very common
V	Increased chylomicrons, VLDL, and triglycerides; uncommon

LDL, Low-density lipoprotein; *VLDL*, very-low-density lipoprotein.
[a]Types II and IV are commonly associated with coronary artery disease.

COMPLEMENTARY AND ALTERNATIVE THERAPIES

Statins

Black cohosh may potentiate an increase in liver enzymes.
Chinese skullcap may increase drug levels of rosuvastatin.
Cranberry may increase side effects of simvastatin.
Ginkgo biloba may increase drug levels of statins.
Green tea may increase side effects of statins.
St. John's wort may decrease the effect and drug levels of statins.

DRUGS TO IMPROVE PERIPHERAL BLOOD FLOW

A common problem in older adults is peripheral arterial disease (PAD), also called *peripheral vascular disease* (PVD). It is characterized by numbness and coolness of the extremities, claudication (pain and weakness of a limb when walking but no symptoms at rest), and possible leg ulcers. The primary cause is arteriosclerosis and hyperlipidemia, resulting in atherosclerosis, after which the arteries become occluded.

Peripheral Vasodilators

Peripheral vasodilators increase blood flow to the extremities. They are used in peripheral vascular disorders of venous and arterial vessels. They are more effective for disorders that result from vasospasm (Raynaud disease) than from vessel occlusion or arteriosclerosis (arteriosclerosis obliterans, thromboangiitis obliterans [Buerger disease]). In Raynaud disease, cold exposure or emotional upset can trigger vasospasm of the toes and fingers; these patients have benefited from vasodilators. Patients with diabetes mellitus are more likely to have PAD by two to four times the usual rate and are at risk of intermittent claudication.

Individuals with PAD who are treated with HMG-CoA reductase inhibitors (statins) for dyslipidemia may see an improvement in intermittent claudication symptoms as well as a decrease in serum lipids. Also, patients with PAD who are hypertensive see improvement for both conditions when taking the antihypertensive drug ramipril, an angiotensin-converting enzyme (ACE) inhibitor. The alpha blocker prazosin and the calcium channel blocker nifedipine have been used as peripheral vasodilators. The antiplatelet drugs clopidogrel and aspirin have been used to decrease PAD symptoms. Another antiplatelet drug, cilostazol, has been approved by the US Food and Drug Administration (FDA) for treating intermittent claudication. It decreases arterial thrombi. Ginkgo biloba, taken with an antiplatelet drug, has been used to treat intermittent claudication because of its vasodilating and antioxidant effects, although this product has not been approved by the FDA. Most of the drugs used for treating PAD do not cure the health problem, but they can aid in relieving PAD symptoms.

> ### COMPLEMENTARY AND ALTERNATIVE THERAPIES
> *Cilostazol*
> Licorice may cause hypokalemia, which can potentiate drug toxicity.

Cilostazol

Cilostazol is an antiplatelet drug that has a dual purpose of inhibiting platelet aggregation as well as causing vasodilation to treat intermittent claudication. Prototype Drug Chart: Cilostazol lists the pharmacologic data for cilostazol.

Pharmacokinetics

Cilostazol is a direct-acting vasodilator that is absorbed from the GI tract. It is highly protein bound at 95% to 98% and has a half-life of 11 to 13 hours. It is usually taken two times a day.

Pharmacodynamics

Cilostazol causes arterial vasodilation, especially within the femoral vasculature. Common adverse effects include headache, diarrhea, and abnormal stools. This drug has an onset of action within 2 to 12 weeks.

Side Effects and Adverse Reactions

Dizziness, tachycardia, palpitations, orthostatic hypotension, nausea, vomiting, and diarrhea may occur with cilostazol. The effectiveness of peripheral vasodilators in increasing blood flow by vasodilation is questionable in the presence of arteriosclerosis. These drugs may decrease some of the symptoms of cerebrovascular insufficiency. Table 44.4 lists the peripheral vasodilators and their dosages, uses, and considerations.

Blood Viscosity Reducer Agent

Pentoxifylline, classified as a *blood viscosity reducer agent* or *platelet aggregation inhibitor*, improves microcirculation and tissue perfusion by decreasing blood viscosity and improving the flexibility of erythrocytes, thus increasing tissue oxygenation. It inhibits aggregation of platelets and red blood cells, and because it decreases blood viscosity, it helps increase flow through peripheral vessels. A derivative of the xanthine group, pentoxifylline has been approved by the FDA for patients with intermittent claudication, and it has been prescribed for those with Buerger disease resulting from arterial occlusions. However, in one research study, pentoxifylline was not determined to be more effective than a placebo.

Reactions to an overdose of pentoxifylline include tachycardia, hypotension, and blurred vision. The drug should be taken with food, and the patient should avoid smoking because nicotine increases vasoconstriction. Patients taking an antihypertensive drug along with pentoxifylline may need to have the antihypertensive dosage decreased to avoid side effects. The most common side effects of pentoxifylline are nausea and vomiting.

TABLE 44.4 Peripheral Vasodilators and Blood Viscosity Reducer Agent

Generic	Route and Dosage	Uses and Considerations
Direct-Acting Vasodilator and Platelet Aggregation Inhibitor		
Cilostazol	See Prototype Drug Chart: Cilostazol	
Blood Viscosity Reducer Agent and Platelet Aggregation Inhibitor		
Pentoxifylline	A: PO: 400 mg tid with meals; max: 1200 mg daily	For claudication. May cause blurred vision, confusion, nausea, vomiting, constipation, cholestasis, cholecystitis, tachycardia, edema, nasal congestion, and hypotension. PB: UK; t½: 0.4–0.8 h

A, Adult; *max*, maximum; *PB*, protein binding; *PO*, by mouth; *t½*, half-life; *tid*, three times a day; *UK*, unknown.

PROTOTYPE DRUG CHART
Atorvastatin

Drug Class	Dosage
Antihyperlipidemic: HMG-CoA reductase inhibitor	A: PO: Initially 10–20 mg qd; *maint:* 10–80 mg qd; *max:* 80 mg qd

Contraindications	Drug-Lab-Food Interactions
Hepatic decompensation/failure *Caution:* Alcohol use disorder, diabetes mellitus, seizures, renal impairment/failure, stroke, hypothyroidism, electrolyte imbalance, endocrine disease, rhabdomyolysis, hypovolemia, myasthenia gravis, older adults, pregnancy, breast-feeding, children	Drug: Decreased effect with antacids, and phenytoin; may increase digoxin level, oral contraceptive efficacy; increased drug effects with macrolide antibiotics and antifungals

Pharmacokinetics	Pharmacodynamics
Absorption: Rapid Distribution: PB: 98% Metabolism: t½: 14 h Excretion: Primarily in feces	PO: Onset: UK Peak: 1–2 h Duration: UK

Therapeutic Effects/Uses
To decrease cholesterol levels and serum lipids, especially LDL and triglycerides; for treatment of atherosclerosis, hypercholesterolemia, hyperlipoproteinemia, and hypertriglyceridemia
Mechanism of action: Inhibits HMG-CoA reductase, the enzyme necessary for hepatic production of cholesterol

Side Effects	Adverse Reactions
Dizziness, insomnia, memory impairment, nightmares, blurred vision, weakness, myalgia, musculoskeletal pain, arthralgia, dyspepsia, nausea, diarrhea, flatulence, abdominal pain, peripheral neuropathy	Rhabdomyolysis (rare), tendon rupture hyperglycemia, diabetes mellitus, myasthenia gravis *Life-threatening:* Hepatic/renal failure, stroke

A, Adult; *d*, day; *HMG-CoA*, 3-hydroxy-3-methylglutarylcoenzyme; *h*, hour; *maint*, maintenance; *max*, maximum; *PB*, protein binding; *PO*, by mouth; *q*, every; *t½*, half-life; *UK*, unknown.

CLINICAL JUDGMENT [NURSING PROCESS]
Antihyperlipidemics

Concept: Perfusion
- The passage of blood flow through the arteries and capillaries that deliver oxygen and nutrients to body cells

Recognize Cues [Assessment]
- Assess vital signs and baseline serum chemistry values (cholesterol, triglycerides, aspartate aminotransferase [AST], alanine aminotransferase [ALT], and creatine phosphokinase [CPK]).
- Obtain a medical history. Statin drugs are contraindicated for patients with liver disorders and in pregnant patients.

Analyze Cues and Prioritize Hypothesis [Patient Problems]
- Hyperglycemia
- Vomiting
- Ischemia
- Nausea
- Decreased visual acuity

Generate Solutions [Planning]
- The patient's cholesterol level will be less than 200 mg/dL in 6 to 8 weeks.
- The patient will choose foods from a list that are low in fat, cholesterol, and complex sugars.

Take Action [Nursing Interventions]
- Monitor the patient's blood lipid levels—cholesterol, triglycerides, low-density lipoprotein (LDL), and high-density lipoprotein (HDL)—every 6 to 8 weeks for the first 6 months after statin therapy, then every 3 to 6 months. For a lipid-level profile, the patient should fast for 12 to 14 hours. The desired values are less than 200 mg/dL for cholesterol; less than 150 mg/dL for triglycerides, although this can vary; less than 100 mg/dL for LDL; and more than 60 mg/dL for HDL. Cholesterol levels higher than 240 mg/dL, LDL levels higher than 160 mg/dL, and HDL levels below 35 mg/dL can lead to severe cardiovascular events or cerebrovascular accident (CVA).
- Monitor laboratory tests for liver function (ALT, alkaline phosphatase [ALP], and gamma-glutamyl transferase [GGT]). Antihyperlipidemic drugs can cause liver disorders.
- Observe for signs and symptoms of gastrointestinal (GI) upset. Taking the drug with sufficient water or with meals may alleviate some of the discomfort.

Patient Teaching
General
- Emphasize the need to comply with the drug regimen to lower blood lipids.
- Inform patients that it may take several weeks before blood lipid levels decline.
- Explain that laboratory tests for blood lipids—cholesterol, triglycerides, LDL, and HDL—are usually ordered every 3 to 6 months.
- Advise patients to have serum liver enzymes monitored as indicated by their health care provider. Lovastatin, pravastatin, and simvastatin are contraindicated in acute hepatic disease and pregnancy.
- Instruct patients to have an annual eye examination and to report changes in visual acuity.
- Advise patients taking gemfibrozil that the drug may increase their risk for bleeding if they are also taking an oral anticoagulant, so bleeding should be reported. Drug dosage can be changed, or another antihyperlipidemic may be ordered.
- Instruct patients to take nicotinic acid with meals to decrease GI discomfort.

Continued

CLINICAL JUDGMENT [NURSING PROCESS]—CONT'D

Antihyperlipidemics

Self-Administration
- Teach patients to mix cholestyramine/colestipol powder well in water or juice.

Side Effects of Cholestyramine, Colestipol, and Niacin
- Advise patients that constipation may occur with cholestyramine and colestipol. Increasing fluid intake and food bulk should help alleviate the problem.
- Explain to patients that flushing is common with niacin and should decrease with continued use of the drug. Usually the drug is started at a low dose.
- Advise patients that large doses of niacin can cause vasodilation and produce dizziness and faintness (syncope).

Side Effects of Ezetimibe
- Explain to patients that ezetimibe may cause headaches and GI upset. If it continues, notify the health care provider.

Side Effects of Statins
- Explain to patients that serum liver enzyme levels are periodically monitored.
- ⚡ Encourage patients to promptly report any unexplained muscle tenderness or weakness that may be caused by rhabdomyolysis.
- ⚡ Caution patients not to abruptly stop taking their statin drug because a serious rebound effect might occur that could lead to acute myocardial infarction (AMI) and possible death. Before stopping a statin, the patient should talk to their health care provider.

Diet
- Explain to patients that GI discomfort is a common problem with most antihyperlipidemics. Suggest increasing fluid intake when taking the medication.
- Encourage patients to consume foods that are low in animal fats, cholesterol, and complex sugars. Lovastatin and other antihyperlipidemics are adjuncts to, not substitutes for, a low-fat diet.

Evaluate Outcomes [Evaluation]
- Evaluate effectiveness of the antihyperlipidemic drug. The patient's cholesterol level should be within the desired range.
- Determine that the patient is maintaining a low-fat, low-cholesterol diet.

PROTOTYPE DRUG CHART

Cilostazol

Drug Class	Dosage
Direct-acting vasodilator and Platelet aggregation inhibitor	A: PO: 50–100 mg q12h 30 min before or 2 h after morning and evening meals with full glass of water; do not administer with grapefruit juice; max: 200 mg qd

Contraindications	Drug-Lab-Food Interactions
Heart failure, hypersensitivity *Caution:* Hepatic and renal disease, tobacco smokers, cardiac and coronary artery diseases, bleeding, dysrhythmias, hypo/hypertension, tachycardia, pregnancy, breast-feeding, older adults, children	Drug: Increased effects with aspirin, cimetidine, clarithromycin, erythromycin, enoxaparin, warfarin; Food: Grapefruit and green tea will increase levels; ginger and ginkgo biloba may prolong bleeding time; St. John's wort will decrease effect.

Pharmacokinetics	Pharmacodynamics
Absorption: PO: Readily absorbed Distribution: PB: 95%–98% Metabolism: t½: 11–13 h Excretion: In urine (74%), feces (20%)	PO: Onset: UK Peak: UK Duration: UK

Therapeutic Effects/Uses
To treat peripheral vascular disease and claudication
Mechanism of action: Acts directly to inhibit platelet aggregation and cause vasodilation, especially in femoral vasculature.

Side Effects	Adverse Reactions
Dizziness, headache, nasopharyngitis, rhinitis, cough, dyspepsia, myalgia, flushing, nausea, vomiting, flatulence, diarrhea, melena, back and abdominal pain, peripheral edema, infection, influenza, cholelithiasis	Tachycardia, palpitations, angina, HF, MI, hypo/hypertension, peptic ulcer, gout, diabetes mellitus, elevated hepatic enzymes, bleeding, hyperglycemia *Life-threatening:* Thrombocytopenia, leukopenia, aplastic anemia, agranulocytosis, dysrhythmias, Stevens-Johnson syndrome

A, Adult; *d*, day; *h*, hour; *HF*, heart failure; *max*, maximum; *MI*, myocardial infarction; *min*, minute; *PB*, protein binding; *PO*, by mouth; *q*, every; *t½*, half-life; *UK*, unknown.

CHAPTER 44 Antihyperlipidemics and Drugs to Improve Peripheral Blood Flow

CLINICAL JUDGMENT [NURSING PROCESS]
Peripheral Vasodilator: Cilostazol

Concept: Perfusion
- The passage of blood flow through arteries and capillaries that deliver oxygen and nutrients to body cells

Recognize Cues [Assessment]
- Obtain baseline vital signs for future comparison.
- Assess for signs of inadequate blood flow to the extremities: pallor, coldness of extremities, and pain.

Analyze Cues and Prioritize Hypothesis [Patient Problems]
- Hyperglycemia
- Hypotension
- Ischemia
- Discomfort
- Decreased visual acuity

Generate Solutions [Planning]
- The patient's legs will be warm and pink.
- The patient will report that pain has decreased.

Take Action [Nursing Interventions]
- Monitor vital signs, especially blood pressure and heart rate. Tachycardia and orthostatic hypotension can be problematic with peripheral vasodilators.

Patient Teaching
General
- Inform patients that a desired therapeutic response may take 1.5 to 3 months.
- Advise patients not to smoke because smoking increases vasospasm.
- Instruct patients to use aspirin or aspirin-like compounds only with the health care provider's approval. Salicylates help prevent platelet aggregation.

Side Effects
- Encourage patients to change position slowly but frequently to avoid orthostatic hypotension. Orthostatic hypotension is common when taking high doses of a vasodilator.
- Instruct patients to report side effects of cilostazol, such as flushing, headaches, and dizziness.

Diet
- Suggest that patients with gastrointestinal (GI) disturbances take cilostazol with meals.
- Advise patients not to ingest alcohol with a vasodilator because it may cause a hypotensive reaction.

Evaluate Outcomes [Evaluation]
- Evaluate effectiveness of cilostazol therapy; blood flow is increased in extremities, and pain has subsided.
- The patient should experience no side effects from the prescribed drug.

CLINICAL JUDGMENT CASE STUDY

The patient had a myocardial infarction (MI) 3 years ago. He was prescribed gemfibrozil 600 mg twice daily before meals, but his cholesterol remained between 220 and 240 mg/dL, and his LDL was 140 mg/dL. His anticholesterol drug was changed to simvastatin 20 mg/day in the evening.

1. How does simvastatin differ from gemfibrozil?
2. Why do you think the patient's cholesterol drug, gemfibrozil, was changed to simvastatin?
3. While the patient is taking simvastatin, which group of serum levels should be monitored?
4. How long after taking simvastatin should the patient's cholesterol and lipoproteins be checked?
5. What is the maximum dose for simvastatin?
6. The patient reports muscle pain and muscle weakness. What might this indicate?
7. Could the patient receive both gemfibrozil and simvastatin? Explain your answer.
8. The patient is on vacation and does not have enough simvastatin tablets. What should he do?

REVIEW QUESTIONS

1. A patient has a serum cholesterol level of 265 mg/dL, a triglyceride level of 235 mg/dL, and a low-density lipoprotein of 180 mg/dL. What do these serum levels indicate?
   a. Hypolipidemia
   b. Normolipidemia
   c. Hyperlipidemia
   d. Alipidemia
2. The nurse knows that a patient's total cholesterol level should be within which range?
   a. 150 to 200 mg/dL
   b. 200 to 225 mg/dL
   c. 225 to 250 mg/dL
   d. Greater than 250 mg/dL
3. A patient has a low-density lipoprotein of 175 mg/dL and a high-density lipoprotein of 30 mg/dL. What teaching should the nurse implement for this patient?
   a. Discuss medications ordered, dietary changes, and exercise.
   b. No changes in lifestyle are needed; continue with the current plan.
   c. Discuss how to have fat intake be 40% of caloric intake.
   d. Begin keeping a food diary, and schedule laboratory work to be repeated in 6 months.
4. Which laboratory test value does the nurse realize can contribute to the development of cardiovascular disease and stroke?
   a. Decreased antidiuretic hormone
   b. Increased homocysteine level
   c. Decreased triglycerides
   d. Increased high-density lipoprotein level

5. A patient is taking lovastatin. Which serum level is most important for the nurse to monitor?
   a. Blood urea nitrogen
   b. Complete blood count
   c. Cardiac enzymes
   d. Hepatic enzymes
6. For what severe skeletal muscle adverse reaction should the nurse observe in a patient taking rosuvastatin?
   a. Myasthenia gravis
   b. Rhabdomyolysis
   c. Dyskinesia
   d. Agranulocytosis
7. A patient is taking ezetimibe and asks the nurse how it works. The nurse should explain that ezetimibe does what?
   a. Inhibits absorption of dietary cholesterol in the intestines
   b. Binds with bile acids in the intestines to reduce low-density lipoprotein levels
   c. Inhibits 3-hydroxy-3-methylglutaryl-coenzyme A reductase, which is necessary for cholesterol production in the liver
   d. Forms insoluble complexes and reduces circulating cholesterol in the blood
8. A patient is diagnosed with peripheral arterial disease. He is prescribed pentoxifylline. What does the nurse realize are the effects of pentoxifylline? **Select all that apply.**
   a. May lead to hypertension and bradycardia
   b. Improves microcirculation and tissue perfusion
   c. Decreases blood viscosity and improves flexibility of erythrocytes
   d. Alleviates intermittent claudication
   e. Commonly causes an adverse effect of rhabdomyolysis
   f. Allows vasodilation of arteries in skeletal muscles

UNIT XIII Gastrointestinal Drugs

45

Gastrointestinal Tract Disorders

http://evolve.elsevier.com/McCuistion/pharmacology

OBJECTIVES

- Explain the function of the gastrointestinal (GI) system.
- Describe causes and treatments related to vomiting.
- Explain the causes and treatments of diarrhea.
- Explain the causes and treatments of constipation.

OUTLINE

Overview of the Gastrointestinal System, 573
    Oral Cavity, 573
    Esophagus, 573
    Stomach, 574
    Small Intestine, 574
    Large Intestine, 574
Vomiting, 574
    Nonpharmacologic Measures, 575
    Nonprescription Antiemetics, 575
    Prescription Antiemetics, 576

Diarrhea, 580
    Nonpharmacologic Measures, 580
    Travelers' Diarrhea, 580
    Antidiarrheals, 580
Constipation, 583
    Nonpharmacologic Measures, 583
    Laxatives, 583
Clinical Judgment Case Study, 588
Review Questions, 588

Vomiting, diarrhea, and constipation are GI problems that frequently require drug intervention. This chapter describes the antiemetics used to control vomiting. This chapter also discusses antidiarrheal drugs and laxatives. The nursing judgment is considered in relation to each of these drug groups.

Drug groups used to correct or control vomiting, diarrhea, and constipation are antiemetics, antidiarrheals, and laxatives. Each of these drug groups is discussed separately.

OVERVIEW OF THE GASTROINTESTINAL SYSTEM

The GI system, or GI tract, comprises the alimentary canal and the digestive tract, and begins at the oral cavity and ends at the anus. Major structures of the GI system are (1) the oral cavity (mouth, tongue, and pharynx), (2) the esophagus, (3) the stomach, (4) the small intestine (duodenum, jejunum, and ileum), (5) the large intestine (cecum, colon, and rectum), and (6) the anus. The accessory organs and glands that contribute to the digestive process are (1) the salivary glands, (2) the pancreas, (3) the gallbladder, and (4) the liver (Fig. 45.1). The main functions of the GI system are the digestion of food particles and absorption of the digestive contents—nutrients, electrolytes, minerals, and fluids—into the circulatory system for cellular use. Digestion and absorption take place in the small intestine and, to a lesser extent, in the stomach. Undigested material passes through the lower intestinal tract with the aid of peristalsis to the rectum and anus, where it is excreted as feces, or stool.

Oral Cavity

The oral cavity, or mouth, starts the digestive process by (1) breaking up food into smaller particles; (2) adding saliva, which contains the enzyme amylase for digesting starch (the beginning of the digestive process); and (3) swallowing, a voluntary movement of food that becomes involuntary (peristalsis) in the esophagus, stomach, and intestines. Swallowing occurs in the pharynx (throat), which connects the mouth and esophagus.

Esophagus

The esophagus, a tube that extends from the pharynx to the stomach, is composed of striated muscle in its upper portion and smooth muscle in its lower portion. The inner lining of the esophagus is a mucous membrane that secretes mucus. The peristaltic process of contraction begins in the esophagus and ends in the lower large intestine. There are two sphincters, the *superior esophageal (hyperpharyngeal) sphincter* and the *lower esophageal sphincter*. The lower esophageal sphincter prevents gastric reflux into the esophagus, a condition called *reflux esophagitis*.

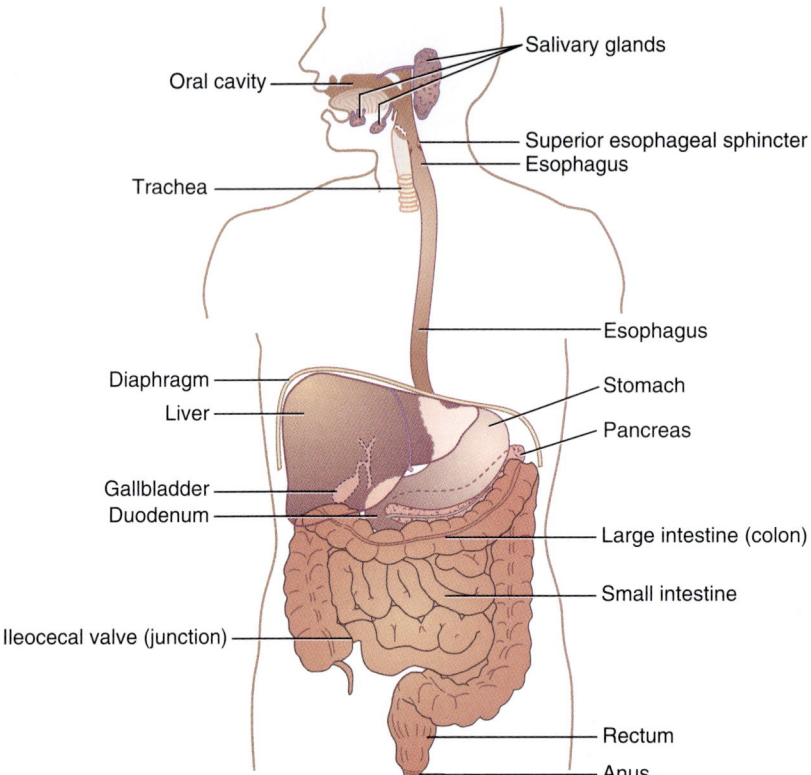

Fig. 45.1 The gastrointestinal system and alimentary canal.

Stomach

The stomach is a hollow organ that lies between the esophagus and the intestine. The body of the stomach has lesser and greater curvatures. It can hold 1000 to 2000 mL of gastric contents and empties in 2 to 6 hours (average is 3–4 hours), depending on gastric content and motility. Two sphincters—the *cardiac sphincter*, which lies at the upper opening of the stomach, and the *pyloric sphincter*, located at the lower portion of the stomach or the head of the duodenum—regulate the entrance of food into the stomach.

The interior lining of the stomach has mucosal folds that contain glands that secrete gastric juices. The four types of cells in the stomach mucosa that secrete these juices are (1) *chief cells*, which secrete the proenzyme pepsinogen (pepsin); (2) *parietal cells*, which secrete hydrochloric acid (HCl); (3) *gastrin-producing cells*, which secrete gastrin, a hormone that regulates enzyme release during digestion; and (4) *mucus-producing cells* that release mucus to protect the stomach lining, which extends into the duodenum.

Small Intestine

The small intestine begins at the pyloric sphincter of the stomach and extends to the ileocecal valve at the cecum. Most drug absorption occurs in the duodenum, but lipid-soluble drugs and alcohol are absorbed from the stomach. The lower digestive process begins in the stomach, but most of the digestive contents are absorbed from the small intestine. The duodenum releases the hormone secretin, which suppresses gastric acid secretion and causes the intestinal juices to have a higher pH than the gastric juices. The intestinal cells also release the hormone cholecystokinin, which in turn stimulates the release of pancreatic enzymes and the contraction of the gallbladder to release bile into the duodenum. Hormones, bile, and pancreatic enzymes (trypsin, chymotrypsin, lipase, and amylase) complete the digestion of carbohydrates, protein, and fat in preparation for absorption.

Large Intestine

The large intestine accepts undigested material from the small intestine, absorbs water, secretes mucus, and with peristaltic contractions moves the remaining intestinal contents to the rectum for elimination. Defecation completes the process.

VOMITING

Vomiting (emesis), the expulsion of gastric contents, has a multitude of causes, including motion sickness, viral and bacterial infection, food intolerance, surgery, pregnancy, pain, shock, effects of selected drugs (e.g., antineoplastics, antibiotics), radiation, and disturbances of the middle ear that affect equilibrium. Nausea, a queasy sensation, may or may not precede the expulsion. The cause of the vomiting must be identified. Antiemetics can mask the underlying cause of vomiting and should not be used until the cause has been determined, unless the vomiting is so severe as to cause dehydration and electrolyte imbalance.

Two major cerebral centers—the **chemoreceptor trigger zone (CTZ)**, which lies near the medulla, and the **vomiting center** in the medulla—cause vomiting when stimulated (Fig. 45.2). The CTZ receives most of the impulses from drugs, toxins, and the vestibular center in the ear and transmits them to the vomiting center. The neurotransmitter dopamine stimulates the CTZ, which in turn stimulates the vomiting center. Levodopa, a drug with dopamine-like properties, can cause vomiting by stimulating the CTZ. Some sensory

Fig. 45.2 The chemoreceptor trigger zone and vomiting center.

impulses—such as odor, smell, taste, and gastric mucosal irritation—are transmitted directly to the vomiting center. The neurotransmitter acetylcholine is also a vomiting stimulant. When the vomiting center is stimulated, the motor neuron responds by causing contraction of the diaphragm, the anterior abdominal muscles, and the stomach. The glottis closes, the abdominal wall moves upward, and vomiting occurs.

Nonpharmacologic measures should be used first when nausea and vomiting occur. If the nonpharmacologic measures are not effective, antiemetics are combined with nonpharmacologic measures. The major groups of antiemetics are *nonprescription* (antihistamines, bismuth subsalicylate, and phosphorated carbohydrate solution) and *prescription* (antihistamines, anticholinergics, dopamine antagonists, phenothiazines, butyrophenones, benzodiazepines, serotonin antagonists, cannabinoids, neurokinin receptor antagonists, and miscellaneous antiemetics).

Nonpharmacologic Measures

The nonpharmacologic methods of decreasing nausea and vomiting include administration of weak tea, flat soda, gelatin, Gatorade, and Pedialyte (for use in children). Crackers and dry toast may be helpful. When dehydration becomes severe, intravenous (IV) fluids are needed to restore body fluid balance.

Nonprescription Antiemetics

Nonprescription antiemetics (antivomiting agents) can be purchased as over-the-counter (OTC) drugs. These drugs are frequently used to prevent motion sickness but have minimal effect on controlling severe vomiting resulting from anticancer agents (antineoplastics), radiation, and toxins. To prevent motion sickness, the antiemetic should be taken 30 minutes before travel. These drugs are not effective in relieving motion sickness if taken after vomiting has occurred.

Selected antihistamine antiemetics—such as dimenhydrinate, cyclizine hydrochloride, meclizine hydrochloride, and diphenhydramine hydrochloride—can be purchased without a prescription to prevent nausea, vomiting, and dizziness (vertigo) caused by motion. These drugs inhibit vestibular stimulation in the middle ear. Diphenhydramine is also used to prevent or alleviate allergic reactions to drugs, insects, and food by acting as an antagonist to histamine$_1$ (H$_1$) receptors.

The side effects of antihistamine antiemetics are similar to those of anticholinergics and include drowsiness, dry mouth, and constipation. Table 45.1 lists the nonprescription antiemetics used for vomiting caused by motion sickness. Diphenhydramine characteristics are explained in Prototype Drug Chart: Diphenhydramine in Chapter 35.

Several nonprescription drugs, such as bismuth subsalicylate, act directly on the gastric mucosa to suppress vomiting. They are marketed in liquid and chewable tablet forms and can be taken for gastric discomfort or diarrhea.

Antiemetics that were once frequently used for the treatment of nausea and vomiting during pregnancy are no longer recommended because they may cause harm to the fetus. Instead, nonpharmacologic methods are used when possible to alleviate nausea and vomiting during pregnancy. Ginger and red raspberry leaf tea have been used effectively but are not regulated by the US Food and Drug Administration (FDA). When antiemetics are necessary, a delayed-release combination of pyridoxine and doxylamine is usually preferred. If vomiting becomes severe and threatens the well-being of the mother and fetus, an antiemetic such as promethazine or metoclopramide can be administered. Other antiemetics may be prescribed cautiously.

TABLE 45.1 Nonprescription Antiemetics: Antihistamine

Drug	Route and Dosage	Uses and Considerations
Motion Sickness		
Dimenhydrinate	A: PO: Initially 50 mg 30–60 min before travel or activity; *maint*: 50–100 mg q4–6 h PRN; *max*: 400 mg/d A: IM/IV: 50–100 mg q4h PRN; *max*: 400 mg/d	To prevent and treat motion sickness, dizziness, nausea, and vomiting. May cause drowsiness, dizziness, headache, restlessness, insomnia, blurred vision, dry mouth, anorexia, and tachycardia. PB: 78%; t½: 3.5 h
Meclizine hydrochloride	Motion sickness: A: PO: 25–50 mg 1 h before travel; may repeat q24h PRN; *max*: 50 mg/d Vertigo: A: PO: 25–100 mg/d in divided doses; *max*: 100 mg/d	For prevention and treatment of nausea, vomiting, and dizziness due to motion sickness and vertigo associated with a vestibular disorder. May cause drowsiness, headache, ataxia, fatigue, blurred vision, dry mouth, and anorexia. PB: UK; t½: 5–6 h

>, Greater than; *A*, adult; *d*, day; *h*, hour; *IM*, intramuscular; *IV*, intravenous; *maint*, maintenance dose; *max*, maximum; *min*, minute; *PB*, protein binding; *PO*, by mouth; *PRN*, as needed; *q*, every; *t½*, half-life; *UK*, unknown; *y*, year.

Prescription Antiemetics

Common prescription antiemetics are classified into the following groups: (1) antihistamines, (2) anticholinergics, (3) dopamine antagonists, (4) phenothiazines, (5) butyrophenones, (6) benzodiazepines, (7) serotonin-receptor antagonists, (8) glucocorticoids, (9) cannabinoids (for patients with certain diagnoses, such as cancer), (10) neurokinin-1 receptor antagonists, and (11) miscellaneous. Many of these drugs act as antagonists to histamine, serotonin, and acetylcholine, which are associated with vomiting. Antihistamines and anticholinergics act primarily on the vomiting center; they also act by decreasing stimulation of the CTZ and vestibular pathways. The cannabinoids act on the cerebral cortex. Phenothiazines, the miscellaneous antiemetics (e.g., metoclopramide), and trimethobenzamide act on the CTZ. Drug combination therapy is commonly used to manage chemotherapy-induced nausea and vomiting. Lorazepam, glucocorticoids, and serotonin ($5-HT_3$)-receptor antagonists are quite effective in combination therapy. Lorazepam, haloperidol, and glucocorticoids are not approved by the FDA as antiemetics but are extremely effective when combined for this unlabeled use.

Antihistamines and Anticholinergics

Only a few prescription antihistamines and anticholinergics are used in the treatment of nausea and vomiting. Table 45.2 lists these drugs and their dosages, uses, and considerations.

Side Effects and Adverse Reactions. Side effects include drowsiness, which can be a major problem; dry mouth; blurred vision caused by pupillary dilation; tachycardia (with anticholinergic use); and constipation. These drugs should *not* be used by patients with glaucoma.

Dopamine Antagonists

These agents suppress emesis by blocking dopamine (D_2) receptors in the CTZ. They are used in the treatment of postoperative emesis, cancer chemotherapy, and radiation therapy. Common side effects of dopamine antagonists are extrapyramidal symptoms, or extrapyramidal syndrome (EPS), caused by blocking dopamine receptors, and hypotension. With metoclopramide, the occurrence of extrapyramidal symptoms is more prevalent in children than in adults. High doses can cause sedation and fatigue. Metoclopramide should not be given if the patient has GI obstruction, hemorrhage, or perforation. See Chapter 22 for a more detailed description of EPS and phenothiazines.

Phenothiazine Antiemetics

Selected piperazine phenothiazines are used to treat nausea and vomiting resulting from surgery, anesthetics, chemotherapy, and radiation sickness. They act by inhibiting the CTZ. When used in patients with cancer, these drugs are commonly given the night before treatment, the day of treatment, and for 24 hours after treatment. Not all phenothiazines are effective antiemetic agents. When prescribed for vomiting, the drug dosage is usually smaller than is used for psychiatric disorders.

Chlorpromazine and prochlorperazine edisylate were the first phenothiazines used for both psychosis and vomiting. Promethazine, a phenothiazine introduced as an antihistamine in the 1940s, has a sedative effect and can also be used for motion sickness and management of nausea and vomiting.

⚠ When promethazine is administered intravenously, it is a high-alert medication that may cause significant harm to the patient if given incorrectly. Prototype Drug Chart: Promethazine Hydrochloride lists the pharmacological data for promethazine.

Pharmacokinetics. Promethazine is readily absorbed in the GI tract. It has 80% to 93% protein-binding capacity. Promethazine is metabolized by the liver and is excreted in urine and feces.

Pharmacodynamics. Promethazine blocks H_1-receptor sites on effector cells and impedes histamine-mediated responses. The onset of action of oral promethazine is 15 to 60 minutes, and onset with intramuscular (IM) administration is 20 minutes. The duration of action is from 4 to 6 hours. The onset of action of IV promethazine is 3 to 5 minutes; the duration of action is the same as for the oral preparation.

Drug and Laboratory Interactions. Central nervous system (CNS) depression increases when promethazine is taken with alcohol, narcotics, sedative-hypnotics, and general anesthetics. Anticholinergic effects increase when promethazine is combined with antihistamines, anticholinergics such as atropine, and other phenothiazines. Promethazine may interfere with urinary pregnancy tests, producing false results.

Side Effects and Adverse Reactions. Phenothiazines have antihistamine and anticholinergic properties. The side effects of phenothiazine antiemetics are moderate sedation, hypotension, extrapyramidal symptoms, CNS effects (dystonic reactions, agitation), and mild anticholinergic symptoms (dry mouth, urinary retention, and constipation). Because the dose is lower for vomiting than for psychosis, the side effects are not so severe. Promethazine is relatively free of extrapyramidal symptoms at antiemetic doses. Table 45.2 lists the pharmacological data for phenothiazines and other prescription antiemetics.

Butyrophenones

Droperidol, like phenothiazines, blocks the D_2 receptors in the CTZ. It is used to treat postoperative nausea and the vomiting and emesis associated with toxins, cancer chemotherapy, and radiation therapy. Like phenothiazines, droperidol is likely to cause extrapyramidal symptoms if used for an extended time. Hypotension may result; therefore blood pressure should be monitored.

Benzodiazepines

Select benzodiazepines indirectly control nausea and vomiting that may occur with cancer chemotherapy. Lorazepam is the drug of choice. Previously, diazepam was the preferred benzodiazepine, but lorazepam effectively provides emesis control, sedation, anxiety reduction, and amnesia when used in combination with a glucocorticoid and serotonin ($5-HT_3$)-receptor antagonist.

Serotonin-Receptor Antagonists

Serotonin antagonists suppress nausea and vomiting by blocking the serotonin ($5-HT_3$) receptors in the CTZ and blocking the afferent vagal nerve terminals in the upper GI tract.

Serotonin antagonists—ondansetron, granisetron, dolasetron, and palonosetron—are the most effective of all antiemetics in suppressing nausea and vomiting caused by cancer chemotherapy-induced emesis or emetogenic anticancer drugs. Ondansetron (the first serotonin antagonist), granisetron, and dolasetron do *not* block the dopamine receptors; therefore they do not cause extrapyramidal symptoms as do the phenothiazine antiemetics. These drugs can be administered orally and intravenously. They are also effective in preventing nausea and vomiting before and after surgery. Common side effects include headache, dizziness, drowsiness, hypotension, weakness, constipation, edema, and fatigue.

Glucocorticoids (Corticosteroids)

Dexamethasone and methylprednisolone are two agents that are effective in suppressing emesis associated with cancer chemotherapy.

Because these glucocorticoids are administered intravenously and for only a short while, side effects normally associated with glucocorticoids are minimized. Glucocorticoids are discussed in Chapter 49.

TABLE 45.2 Prescription Antiemetics

Drug	Route and Dosage	Uses and Considerations
Prescription Antihistamines		
Hydroxyzine	Postoperative nausea/vomiting: A: IM: 25–100 mg single dose; *max:* 600 mg/d	For postoperative nausea and vomiting, pruritus, vertigo, anxiety, agitation, and sedation induction. Give deep in large muscle. May cause drowsiness, dizziness, fatigue, ataxia, headache, blurred vision, dry mouth, constipation, and urinary retention. PB: UK; $t\frac{1}{2}$: 14–25 h
Anticholinergics		
Scopolamine	Motion sickness: A: Transdermal patch: 1 mg patch; apply patch to a hairless area behind the ear at least 4 h before travel and q3d PRN, *max:* 1 patch q3d	For nausea and vomiting, motion sickness, and procedural sedation. May cause dizziness, drowsiness, fatigue, headache, blurred vision, dry conjunctiva/cornea of eye, dilated pupils, visual impairment, agitation, confusion, restlessness, orthostatic hypotension, tachycardia, dry mouth, and constipation. Alternate ears if using for longer than 3 d, wash hands after applying patch, avoid contact with the eyes, and wear no more than one patch at a time. PB: UK; $t\frac{1}{2}$: 8 h
Dopamine Antagonists		
Amisulpride	A: IV: 10 mg in single dose over 1–20 min; *max:* 10 mg/dose	For postoperative nausea and vomiting. May cause chills, drowsiness, hypotension, hypokalemia, and injection-site reaction. PB: 25%–30%; $t\frac{1}{2}$: 4–5 h
Metoclopramide hydrochloride		
Phenothiazines		
Prochlorperazine maleate	Nausea and vomiting: A: PO/IM: 5–10 mg tid/qid PRN (give deep in UOQ of buttock); *max:* 40 mg/d A: IV: 2.5–10 mg q3–4h PRN; *max:* 40 mg/d IVP at 5 mg/min or infusion over 15 min PR: 25 mg bid; *max:* 50 mg/d	For nausea, vomiting, schizophrenia, and anxiety. May cause drowsiness, dizziness, headache, insomnia, blurred vision, orthostatic hypo/hypertension, dry mouth, constipation, EPS, and erectile/ejaculatory dysfunction. Keep patient recumbent at least 30 min to avoid hypotension. PB: 91%–99%; $t\frac{1}{2}$: PO 14–22 h, IV 6–10 h
Promethazine	See Prototype Drug Chart: Promethazine Hydrochloride	
Chlorpromazine	Nausea: A: PO: 10–25 mg q4–6 h PRN A: IM: Initially 25 mg then, if tolerated, may give 25–50 mg q3–4 h PRN	For nausea and vomiting, hiccups, and schizophrenia. May cause drowsiness, dizziness, photosensitivity, blurred vision, orthostatic hypotension, weight gain, dry mouth, constipation, jaundice, and skin hyperpigmentation. PB: 90%–99%; $t\frac{1}{2}$: 10–40 h
Perphenazine	A: PO: Initially 8–16 mg/d in divided doses; *max:* 24 mg/d or 64 mg/d for short periods	For nausea/vomiting, schizophrenia, severe behavioral/psychological signs and symptoms of dementia. May cause dry mouth, drowsiness, constipation, urinary retention, and psychosis. Do not mix with coffee, cola, tea, or apple juice. PB: 91%–99%; $t\frac{1}{2}$: 9–12 h
Butyrophenones		
Droperidol	A: IM/IV: Initially 0.625–2.5 mg, may then give 1.25 mg if needed; *max:* 2.5 mg/initial dose	For prevention and treatment of postoperative nausea and vomiting. May cause dizziness, drowsiness, anxiety, restlessness, hypo/hypertension, tachycardia, dysrhythmias, and EPS. PB: 85%–90%: $t\frac{1}{2}$: 2 h
Benzodiazepines		
Lorazepam	Chemo-induced nausea/vomiting: A: IV: 0.025 mg/kg 45 min before chemo	For prevention of chemo-induced nausea and vomiting and for anxiety, insomnia, procedural sedation, and status epilepticus. May cause dizziness, amnesia, drowsiness, headache, confusion, ataxia, weakness, restlessness, injection-site reaction, constipation, hypotension, and erythema. PB: 85%; $t\frac{1}{2}$: 9–19 h
Serotonin (5-HT$_3$) Receptor Antagonists		
Granisetron	Chemotherapy-induced nausea/vomiting: A: PO: 1 mg bid (1 h before and 12 h after chemo); *max:* 2 mg/d A: IV: 10 mcg/kg 30 min before chemo; *max:* 40 mcg/kg	For prevention and treatment of radiation- and chemo-induced nausea and vomiting. May cause dizziness, drowsiness, fever, headache, weakness, hematoma, fatigue, anorexia, dyspepsia, nausea, vomiting, abdominal pain, gastroesophageal reflux, diarrhea, constipation, elevated hepatic enzymes, leukopenia, and injection-site reaction. PB: 65%; $t\frac{1}{2}$: 6.23 h PO, 9–12 h IV

Continued

TABLE 45.2 Prescription Antiemetics—cont'd

Drug	Route and Dosage	Uses and Considerations
Ondansetron hydrochloride	A: PO: 8 mg 30 min before chemo; may repeat in 8 h, then q12h for 1–2 d after chemo; max: 24 mg/d A: IV: 0.15 mg/kg (150 mcg/kg) 30 min before chemo, infused over 15 min, then may repeat q4h × 2; max: 0.45 mg/kg per day	For postoperative prophylaxis and chemo- and radiation-induced nausea and vomiting. May cause dizziness, drowsiness, fever, headache, anxiety, agitation, fatigue, malaise, diarrhea, constipation, hypotension, bradycardia, and urinary retention. PB: 70%–76%; t½: 3.1–5.8 h
Palonosetron	Postoperative nausea/vomiting: A: IV: 0.075 mg over 10 s before induction as a single dose; max: 0.25 mg/single dose	To prevent postoperative and chemo-induced nausea and vomiting. May cause headache, dizziness, edema, dysrhythmia, hypotension, weakness, elevated hepatic enzymes, flatulence, constipation, diarrhea, and urinary retention. PB: 62%; t½: 40 h
Dolasetron	A: PO: 100 mg within 1 h before chemo Postoperative nausea and vomiting: A: IV: 12.5 mg as single dose 15 min before end of anesthesia and PRN	For prophylaxis of chemo-induced nausea and vomiting or postoperative treatment of nausea and vomiting. May cause dizziness, headache, fatigue, fever, hypotension, tachycardia, bradycardia, and diarrhea. PB: 69%–77%; t½: <10 min
Cannabinoids Dronabinol CSS III	Chemotherapy-induced nausea: A: PO: 5 mg/m² capsules 1–3 h before chemo, then q2–4 h after; max: 15 mg/m² per dose for 6 doses/d	For anorexia and chemo-induced nausea and vomiting. May cause drowsiness, dizziness, impaired cognition, euphoria, dysphoria, paranoia, emotional lability, nausea, vomiting, and abdominal pain. PB: 97%; t½: 25–36 h
Nabilone	A: PO: Initially 1 or 2 mg given 1–3 h before chemo, then 1–2 mg bid, and 1–2 mg may be given night before chemo; max: 6 mg/d in 3 divided doses	For prophylaxis and treatment of chemotherapy-induced nausea and vomiting. May cause drowsiness, dizziness, headache, euphoria, depression, dysphoria, impaired cognition, abnormal dreams, weakness, ataxia, and hypotension. PB: UK; t½: 2 h
Neurokinin-1 receptor antagonist		
Aprepitant, fosaprepitant		
Rolapitant		
Netupitant and palonosetron		
Miscellaneous Metoclopramide hydrochloride	Postoperative nausea/vomiting: A: IM/IV: 10–20 mg at end of surgery, may repeat q4–6 h; max: 60 mg/d or 20 mg/dose	For prevention and treatment of postoperative and chemo-induced nausea and vomiting, and GERD. May cause drowsiness, dizziness, headache, fatigue, restlessness, dysgeusia, nausea, vomiting, and EPS. PB: 30%; t½: 2.5–6 h
Trimethobenzamide hydrochloride	A: PO: 300 mg tid/qid PRN; max: 1200 mg/d A: IM: 200 mg tid/qid PRN; max: 800 mg/d	For nausea and vomiting. May cause drowsiness, dizziness, headache, blurred vision, hypotension, injection-site reaction, EPS, and diarrhea. PB: UK; t½: 7–9 h
Aprepitant, fosaprepitant	A: PO: day 1, give 125 mg 1 h before chemo; days 2 and 3, give 80 mg 1 h before chemo or, if no chemo is scheduled, give in the morning	For prevention of chemo-induced nausea and vomiting. May cause dizziness, headache, cough, fatigue, weakness, hypotension, and constipation. PB: 95%; t½: 9–13 h
Netupitant and palonosetron	A: PO: 1 capsule (netupitant 300 mg/palonosetron 0.5 mg) 1 h before chemo A: IV: 1 vial (netupitant 235 mg palonosetron 0.25 mg) 30 min before chemo, give over 30 min	For prevention of chemo-induced nausea and vomiting. May cause headache, weakness, fatigue, dyspepsia, erythema, and constipation. PB: palonosetron 62%, netupitant 99.5%; t½: palonosetron 40 h, netupitant 51–109 h
Rolapitant	A: PO: 180 mg day 1, 1–2 h and 30 min before chemo on day 1, repeat at least q2wk A: IV: 166.5 mg over 30 min 1–2 h and 30 min before chemo repeat at least q2wk	For prevention of chemo-induced nausea and vomiting. May cause dizziness, hiccups, stomatitis, dyspepsia, anorexia, abdominal pain, infusion-site reactions, neutropenia, and infections. PB: 99.8%; t½: 138–205 h

A, adult; *bid*, twice a day; *CNS*, central nervous system; *CSS*, Controlled Substances Schedule; *d*, day; *EPS*, extrapyramidal symptoms; *GERD*, gastroesophageal reflux disease; *GI*, gastrointestinal; *h*, hour; *IBS*, irritable bowel syndrome; *IM*, intramuscular; *IV*, intravenous; *max*, maximum; *min*, minute; *mo*, month; *PB*, protein binding; *PO*, by mouth; *PR*, per rectum; *PRN*, as needed; *q*, every; *qid*, four times a day; *s*, second; *SR*, sustained release; *t½*, half-life; *tid*, three times a day; *UK*, unknown; *UOQ*, upper-outer quadrant; *UTI*, urinary tract infection; *wk*, week.

PROTOTYPE DRUG CHART
Promethazine Hydrochloride

Drug Class	Dosage
Antiemetic: Phenothiazine	Nausea/vomiting: A: PO/PR/IM/IV: 12.5–25 mg q4–6 h PRN; *max:* 100 mg/d

Contraindications	Drug-Lab-Food Interactions
Hypersensitivity, asthma, coma, children *Caution:* Glaucoma, GI obstruction, ileus, bone marrow depression, MI, HF, stroke, hepatic disease, COPD, respiratory depression, dehydration, urinary retention, diabetes mellitus, hyperparathyroidism, hypothyroidism, bradycardia, hypocalcemia, hypokalemia, hypomagnesemia, older adults, pregnancy, breast-feeding	Drug: Increases CNS depression and anticholinergic effects when taken with alcohol and other CNS depressants; lowers seizure threshold with phenytoin and tramadol Lab: False pregnancy test

Pharmacokinetics	Pharmacodynamics
Absorption: PO: Easily absorbed from GI tract Distribution: PB: 80%–93% Metabolism: $t\frac{1}{2}$: 10–14 h Excretion: In urine and feces	PO: Onset: 15–60 min Peak: UK; duration: 4–6 h IM: Onset: 20 min Peak: UK; duration: 4–6 h IV: Onset: 3–5 min Peak: UK; duration: 4–6 h PR: Onset: 15–60 min Peak: UK; duration: 4–6 h

Therapeutic Effects/Uses
To treat and prevent motion sickness, nausea, vomiting, and sedation induction
Mechanism of action: Blocks H_1-receptor sites and inhibits CTZ

Side Effects	Adverse Reactions
Drowsiness, dizziness, confusion, agitation, excitability, akathisia, fatigue, insomnia, photosensitivity, blurred vision, dry mouth, constipation, urinary retention, injection-site reaction, skin hyperpigmentation, erectile/ejaculation dysfunction	Extrapyramidal syndrome, seizures, dyspnea, hypo/hypertension, bradycardia, tachycardia *Life-threatening:* Agranulocytosis, leukopenia, thrombocytopenia, NMS, respiratory depression, apnea

A, Adult; *COPD*, chronic obstructive pulmonary disease; *CTZ*, chemoreceptor trigger zone; *d*, day; *GI*, gastrointestinal; *h*, hour; *HF*, heart failure; *IM*, intramuscular; *IV*, intravenous; *max*, maximum; *MI*, myocardial infarction; *min*, minute; *NMS*, neuroleptic malignant syndrome; *PB*, protein binding; *PO*, by mouth; *PR*, per rectum; *q*, every; *t½*, half-life; *UK*, unknown.

Cannabinoids

Cannabinoids, the active ingredients in cannabis, were approved for clinical use in 1985 to alleviate nausea and vomiting resulting from cancer treatment. These agents may be prescribed for patients receiving chemotherapy who do not respond to or are unable to take other antiemetics. They are contraindicated for patients with psychiatric disorders. Cannabinoids can be used as an appetite stimulant for patients with acquired immunodeficiency syndrome (AIDS). The cannabinoid dronabinol is described in Table 45.2.

Side Effects and Adverse Reactions. Side effects that can occur as a result of cannabinoid use include euphoria, drowsiness, dizziness, nightmares, confusion, amnesia, orthostatic hypotension or hypertension, and tachycardia. Less common symptoms are depression and anxiety.

Neurokinin Receptor Antagonists

Substance P/neurokinin receptor antagonists include aprepitant/fosaprepitant, netupitant/palonosetron, and rolapitant. They are competitive antagonists of neurokinin receptors, which are located in the medulla close to the CTZ zone. Substance P is a peptide that increases the contractions of smooth GI muscles. These drugs are utilized in chemotherapy-induced nausea and vomiting. Because they are only moderately effective in this endeavor, typically they are given in combination with a glucocorticoid, like dexamethasone, and a serotonin agonist, like ondansetron, to increase the antiemetic action. Because these drugs have a fairly-long half-life, nausea and vomiting can be prevented during the acute and delayed phase of chemotherapy. Adverse effects include dizziness, headache, hiccups, fatigue, weakness, anorexia, diarrhea, and neutropenia.

Miscellaneous Antiemetics

Trimethobenzamide is in the class of miscellaneous antiemetics because it does not act strictly as an antihistamine, anticholinergic, or phenothiazine. The drug suppresses impulses to the CTZ.

Trimethobenzamide can cause drowsiness, headache, hypotension, blurred vision, and extrapyramidal symptoms that include abnormal involuntary movements, postural disturbances, and alterations in muscle tone.

Table 45.2 lists pharmacological data for the miscellaneous antiemetics along with other prescription antiemetics.

PATIENT SAFETY

Do Not Confuse...
- **Antivert**, an antiemetic, with **Axert**, an antimigraine drug.
- **Lorazepam**, which controls nausea and vomiting, with **alprazolam**, an anxiolytic.
- **Hydroxyzine**, an antiemetic, with **hydralazine**, an antihypertensive drug.

CLINICAL JUDGMENT [NURSING PROCESS]
Antiemetics

Concept: Fluid and Electrolyte Imbalance
- The maintenance of correct electrolyte concentrations and fluid balance in body compartments

Recognize Cues [Assessment]
- Determine a history of the onset, frequency, and amount of vomiting and contents of the vomitus. If appropriate, elicit from the patient possible causative factors such as food (e.g., seafood, mayonnaise, pregnancy, exposure to virus).
- Obtain a history of present health problems. Patients with glaucoma should avoid many of the antiemetics.
- Record vital signs for abnormalities and for future comparisons.
- Assess urinalysis before and during therapy.
- Assess the patient for dehydration due to excess fluid loss from vomiting.

Analyze Cues and Prioritize Hypothesis [Patient Problems]
- Hypotension
- Vomiting
- Hypokalemia
- Hyponatremia
- Dehydration
- Nausea
- Discomfort

Generate Solutions [Planning]
- The patient will state they will adhere to the treatment regimen to alleviate vomiting.
- The patient will report that vomiting has decreased in frequency.
- The patient will retain small amounts of food and fluid.

Take Action [Nursing Interventions]
- Check vital signs. If vomiting is severe, dehydration may occur, and shock-like symptoms may be present.
- Monitor bowel sounds for hypoactivity or hyperactivity.
- Provide mouth care after vomiting. Encourage patients to maintain oral hygiene.

Patient Teaching
General
- Instruct patients to store drugs in airtight, light-resistant containers if required.
- Tell patients to avoid over-the-counter (OTC) preparations.
- Warn patients not to consume alcohol while taking antiemetics. Alcohol can intensify the sedative effect.
- ⚡ Advise pregnant patients to avoid antiemetics during the first trimester because of possible teratogenic effects on the fetus. Encourage these patients to seek medical advice about OTC and prescription antiemetics.

Side Effects
- Tell the patient to report sore throat, fever, and mouth sores; notify the health care provider and have blood drawn for a complete blood count (CBC).
- ⚡ Alert patients to avoid driving a motor vehicle or engaging in dangerous activities because drowsiness is common with antiemetics. If drowsiness becomes a problem, a decrease in dosage may be indicated.
- Caution patients with hepatic disorders to seek medical advice before taking phenothiazines. Instruct patients to report dizziness.
- Suggest to patients nonpharmacologic methods of alleviating nausea and vomiting such as flat soda, weak tea, crackers, and dry toast.

Evaluate Outcomes [Evaluation]
- Evaluate the effectiveness of nonpharmacologic methods and antiemetics by noting the absence of vomiting. Identify any side effects that may result from drugs.

DIARRHEA

Diarrhea, frequent liquid stool, is a symptom of an intestinal disorder. Causes include (1) foods (spicy, spoiled), (2) fecal impaction, (3) bacteria (*Escherichia coli, Salmonella*) or viruses (parvovirus, rotavirus), (4) toxins, (5) drug reactions, (6) laxative misuse, (7) malabsorption syndrome caused by lack of digestive enzymes, (8) stress and anxiety, (9) bowel tumor, and (10) inflammatory bowel disease such as ulcerative colitis or Crohn disease. Diarrhea can be mild to severe. Antidiarrheals should not be used for more than 2 days and should not be used if fever is present.

Because intestinal fluids are rich in water, sodium, potassium, and bicarbonate, diarrhea can cause minor or severe dehydration and electrolyte imbalances. The loss of bicarbonate places the patient at risk for developing metabolic acidosis. Patients with diarrhea should avoid milk products and foods rich in fat. Diarrhea can develop very quickly and can be life-threatening to young patients and older adults, who may not be able to compensate for the fluid and electrolyte losses.

Nonpharmacologic Measures

The cause of diarrhea should be identified. Nonpharmacologic treatment for diarrhea is recommended until the underlying cause can be determined. This includes use of clear liquids and oral solutions such as Gatorade (for adults) and Pedialyte or Rehydralyte (for children) and IV electrolyte solutions. Antidiarrheal drugs are frequently used in combination with nonpharmacologic treatment.

Travelers' Diarrhea

Travelers' diarrhea, also called *acute diarrhea*, is usually caused by *E. coli*. It ordinarily lasts less than 2 days; however, if it becomes severe, fluoroquinolone antibiotics are usually prescribed. Loperamide may be used to slow peristalsis and decrease the frequency of defecation, but it can also slow the exit of the organism from the GI tract. Travelers' diarrhea can be reduced by using bottled water for all activities, such as drinking, brushing teeth, washing fruit, etc. Vegetables should be cooked. Meats should be cooked until well-done.

Antidiarrheals

There are various antidiarrheals for treating diarrhea and decreasing hypermotility (increased peristalsis). Usually, an underlying cause of the diarrhea needs to be corrected as well. The antidiarrheals are classified as (1) opiates and opiate-related agents, (2) adsorbents, and (3) miscellaneous antidiarrheals.

Opiates and Opiate-Related Agents

Opiates decrease intestinal motility, thereby decreasing peristalsis. Constipation is a common side effect of opium preparations. Codeine is an example. Opiates are frequently combined with other antidiarrheal agents. Opium antidiarrheals can cause CNS depression when taken with alcohol, sedatives, or tranquilizers. The duration of action of opiates is approximately 2 hours.

Diphenoxylate with atropine is an opiate that has less potential for causing drug dependence than other opiates such as codeine. Difenoxin is an active metabolite of diphenoxylate, but it is more potent than diphenoxylate. Both drugs are combined with atropine to decrease abdominal cramping, intestinal motility, and hypersecretion. Diphenoxylate with atropine is frequently prescribed for travelers' diarrhea, and difenoxin with atropine is prescribed to treat nonspecific and chronic diarrhea. With prolonged use of these drugs, physical dependence may occur. Diphenoxylate antidiarrheal products are approximately 50% atropine, which will discourage drug misuse. Drugs with atropine are contraindicated in glaucoma. Prototype Drug Chart: Diphenoxylate With Atropine lists the pharmacological data for diphenoxylate with atropine.

Loperamide is structurally related to diphenoxylate but causes less CNS depression than diphenoxylate and difenoxin. It can be purchased as an OTC drug, and it protects against diarrhea, reduces fecal volume, and decreases intestinal fluid and electrolyte losses.

Pharmacokinetics. Diphenoxylate with atropine is well absorbed from the GI tract. The diphenoxylate is metabolized by the liver mainly as metabolites. There are two half-lives: 3 hours for diphenoxylate and 3 to 14 hours for the diphenoxylate metabolites. The drug is excreted in the feces and urine.

Pharmacodynamics. Diphenoxylate with atropine is an opiate agonist with anticholinergic properties (atropine) that decreases GI motility (peristalsis). It has a moderate onset of action of 45 to 60 minutes, and the duration of action is 3 to 4 hours. Many side effects are caused by the anticholinergic atropine. Patients with severe glaucoma should take another antidiarrheal that does not have an anticholinergic effect. If this drug is taken with alcohol, narcotics, or sedative-hypnotics, CNS depression can occur.

PROTOTYPE DRUG CHART
Diphenoxylate With Atropine

Drug Class	Dosage
Antidiarrheal CSS V	A: PO: 5 mg qid until controlled; *maint.* 5 mg/d; *max.* 20 mg/d

Contraindications	Drug-Lab-Food Interactions
Severe diarrhea due to pseudomembranous colitis, infection, jaundice, glaucoma, children *Caution:* Hepatic disease, electrolyte imbalance, dehydration, ulcerative colitis, substance use, older adults, pregnancy, breast-feeding	Drug: Increased CNS depression with alcohol, antihistamines, opioids, sedative-hypnotics; MAOIs may enhance hypertensive crisis Lab: Increased serum liver enzymes, amylase

Pharmacokinetics	Pharmacodynamics
Absorption: PO: Well absorbed Distribution: PB: UK Metabolism: t½: 3–14 h Excretion: In feces and urine	PO: Onset: 45–60 min Peak: 2 h Duration: 3–4 h

Therapeutic Effects/Uses
To treat diarrhea by slowing intestinal motility
Mechanism of action: Inhibits gastric motility by exerting effect on smooth muscle cells of GI tract

Side Effects	Adverse Reactions
Drowsiness, dizziness, euphoria, headache, restlessness, dry mouth, anorexia, abdominal pain, nausea, vomiting, constipation	Angioedema, pancreatitis, hallucinations *Life-threatening:* Ileus, toxic megacolon, anaphylaxis, respiratory depression

A, Adult; *CNS*, central nervous system; *CSS*, Controlled Substances Schedule; *d*, day; *GI*, gastrointestinal; *h*, hour; *MAOI*, monoanime oxidase inhibitor; *maint*, maintenance; *max*, maximum; *min*, minute; *PB*, protein binding; *PO*, by mouth; *qid*, four times a day; *t½*, half-life; *UK*, unknown.

CLINICAL JUDGMENT [NURSING PROCESS]
Antidiarrheals

Concept: Fluid and Electrolyte Imbalance
- The maintenance of correct electrolyte concentrations and fluid balance in body compartments

Recognize Cues [Assessment]
- Obtain a history of any viral or bacterial infection, drugs taken, and foods ingested that could be contributing factors to diarrhea. Many antidiarrheals are contraindicated if the patient has liver disease, narcotic dependence, ulcerative colitis, or glaucoma.
- Check vital signs to provide a baseline for future comparisons and to determine body fluid and electrolyte losses.
- Determine frequency and consistency of bowel movements.
- Assess bowel sounds. Hyperactive sounds can indicate increased intestinal motility.
- Report if a patient has a narcotic drug history. If opiate or opiate-related antidiarrheals are given, drug misuse may occur.

Analyze Cues and Prioritize Hypothesis [Patient Problems]
- Hypotension
- Vomiting
- Hypokalemia
- Hyponatremia

Continued

CLINICAL JUDGMENT [NURSING PROCESS]—CONT'D

Antidiarrheals

- Dehydration
- Nausea
- Discomfort

Generate Solutions [Planning]
- The patient will report having bowel movements that are formed.
- The patient will drink an adequate amount of fluids.

Take Action [Nursing Interventions]
- Record vital signs. Report tachycardia or systolic blood pressure decreases of 10 to 15 mm Hg. Monitor respirations. Opiates and opiate-related drugs can cause central nervous system (CNS) depression.
- Monitor frequency of bowel movements and bowel sounds. Notify a health care provider if intestinal hypoactivity occurs when taking a drug.
- ⚡ Check for signs and symptoms of dehydration resulting from persistent diarrhea. Fluid replacement may be necessary. With prolonged diarrhea, check serum electrolytes.
- Administer antidiarrheals cautiously to pregnant patients and those with glaucoma, liver disorders, or ulcerative colitis.
- ⚡ Recognize that a drug may need to be withheld if diarrhea continues for more than 48 hours or acute abdominal pain develops.

Patient Teaching
- Instruct patients not to take sedatives, tranquilizers, or other narcotics with antidiarrheal drugs. CNS depression may occur.
- Tell patients to avoid over-the-counter (OTC) preparations; they may contain alcohol and can promote liver damage, and concurrent use with loratadine and loperamide may lead to significant interaction.
- Counsel patients to take drugs only as prescribed. Advise that drugs may be habit-forming and that they should not exceed the recommended dose.
- Encourage patients to drink clear liquids.
- Advise patients not to ingest fried foods or milk products until diarrhea has stopped.
- Teach patients that constipation can result from overuse of antidiarrheal drugs.

Evaluate Outcomes [Evaluation]
- Evaluate the effectiveness of the drug; diarrhea has stopped.
- Monitor long-term use of opiates and opiate-related drugs for possible misuse and physical dependence.
- Continue to monitor vital signs and report abnormal changes.

Adsorbents

Adsorbents act by coating the wall of the GI tract and adsorbing bacteria or toxins that cause diarrhea. Adsorbent antidiarrheals include kaolin and pectin. These agents are combined as a mild or moderate antidiarrheal that can be purchased without a prescription and used in combination with other antidiarrheals. Bismuth subsalicylate is considered an adsorbent because it adsorbs bacterial toxins. Bismuth subsalicylate is an OTC drug approved for adults and children 12 years and older to treat nonspecific diarrhea and gastric discomfort. Side effects include dizziness, drowsiness, headache, tongue and stool discoloration, and anxiety. Table 45.3 lists the pharmacological data for antidiarrheal adsorbents.

TABLE 45.3 Antidiarrheals: Opiates and Opiate-Related Agents, Adsorbents, and Miscellaneous Agents

Drug	Route and Dosage	Uses and Considerations
Opiates and Opiate-Related Agents		
Difenoxin and atropine CSS IV	A: PO: Initially 2 tablets (difenoxin 1 mg, atropine 0.025 mg each tablet), then 1 tablet after each loose stool or q3–4h PRN; *max:* 8 tablets/d	For diarrhea. Avoid use in patients with narrow-angle glaucoma. May cause dizziness, drowsiness, headache, blurred vision, fatigue, flushing, dry mouth, anorexia, nausea, vomiting, constipation, tachycardia, toxic megacolon, and urinary retention. PB: difenoxin UK, atropine 14%–22%; t½: difenoxin UK, atropine 2–4 h
Diphenoxylate and atropine CSS V	See Prototype Drug Chart: Diphenoxylate With Atropine	
Loperamide hydrochloride	A: PO: Initially 4 mg, then 2 mg after each unformed stool; *max:* 16 mg/d	For chronic and traveler's diarrhea. May cause drowsiness, dizziness, headache, fatigue, dry mouth, nausea, abdominal cramps, constipation, flatulence, vomiting, toxic megacolon, and urinary retention. PB: 97%; t½: 10.8 h
Adsorbents		
Bismuth subsalicylate	A: PO: 524 mg q30min or 1050 mg q1h PRN; *max:* 4.2 g/d	For nausea, diarrhea, dyspepsia, and pyrosis. May cause dizziness, drowsiness, headache, confusion, anxiety, tinnitus, hearing loss, tongue discoloration, abdominal pain, constipation, and stool discoloration. PB: 90%; t½: bismuth 21–72 d, salicylate 2–5 h
Miscellaneous		
Crofelemer	A: PO: 125 mg bid; *max:* 250 mg/d	For diarrhea in patients with HIV/AIDS. May cause dizziness, cough, dry mouth, nausea, abdominal pain, flatulence, constipation, arthralgia, back pain, infection, and hyperbilirubinemia. PB: UK; t½: UK

TABLE 45.3 Antidiarrheals: Opiates and Opiate-Related Agents, Adsorbents, and Miscellaneous Agents—cont'd

Drug	Route and Dosage	Uses and Considerations
Eluxadoline	A: PO: 75–100 mg bid; *max:* 200 mg/d	For treatment of IBS with diarrhea. May cause dizziness, drowsiness, euphoria, fatigue, pharyngitis, nausea, vomiting, abdominal pain, flatulence, constipation, and infection. PB: 81%; t½: 3.7–6 h
Rifaximin	Travelers' diarrhea: A: PO: 200 mg tid for 3 d; *max:* 600 mg/d	For treatment of IBS, travelers' diarrhea, and hepatic encephalopathy. May cause dizziness, headache, fatigue, nausea, abdominal pain, constipation, ascites, pruritus, arthralgia, anemia, and peripheral edema. PB: 67.5%; t½: 5.63 h
Rifamycin	A: PO: 388 mg bid for 3 d; *max:* 776 mg/d	For travelers' diarrhea. May cause headache, dyspepsia, abdominal pain, constipation, and CDAD. PB: 80%; t½: UK

A, adult; *AIDS*, acquired immunodeficiency syndrome; *bid*, twice a day; *CDAD*, *Clostridium difficile*–associated diarrhea; *CSS*, Controlled Substances Schedule; *d*, day; *h*, hour; *HIV*, human immunodeficiency virus; *IBS*, irritable bowel syndrome; *max*, maximum; *min*, minute; *PB*, protein binding; *PO*, by mouth; *PRN*, as needed; *q*, every; *t½*, half-life; *tid*, three times a day; *UK*, unknown.

Miscellaneous Antidiarrheals

Various miscellaneous antidiarrheals are prescribed to control diarrhea. This group includes crofelemer, eluxadoline, rifaximin, and rifamycin. Side effects include dizziness, nausea, dry mouth, flatulence, constipation, and fatigue. Table 45.3 includes these other antidiarrheals.

CONSTIPATION

Constipation, the accumulation of hard fecal material in the large intestine, is a relatively common complaint and a major problem for older adults. Insufficient water intake and poor dietary habits are contributing factors. Other causes include (1) fecal impaction, (2) bowel obstruction, (3) chronic laxative use, (4) neurological disorders (paraplegia), (5) ignoring the urge to defecate, (6) lack of exercise, and (7) select drugs such as anticholinergics, narcotics, and certain antacids.

Nonpharmacologic Measures

Nonpharmacologic management includes diet (high fiber), water, exercise, and routine bowel habits. A "normal" number of bowel movements ranges between one and three per day to three per week. What is normal varies from person to person; the nurse should determine what normal bowel habits are for each patient. At times a laxative may be needed, but the patient should also use nonpharmacologic measures to prevent constipation.

Laxatives

Laxatives and cathartics are used to eliminate fecal matter. Laxatives promote a soft stool, cathartics result in a soft to watery stool with some cramping, and frequently dosage determines whether a drug acts as a laxative or cathartic. Because these terms are often used interchangeably, *laxative* will cover both classes in this chapter. Purgatives are harsh cathartics that cause a watery stool with abdominal cramping. There are several types of laxatives including: (1) osmotics (saline), (2) stimulants (contact or irritants), (3) bulk forming, and (4) emollients (stool softeners).

Laxatives should be avoided if there is any question that the patient may have intestinal obstruction, if abdominal pain is severe, or if symptoms of appendicitis, ulcerative colitis, or diverticulitis are present. Most laxatives stimulate peristalsis. Laxative use from chronic use is a common problem, especially in older adults. Laxative dependence can become a problem, so patient teaching is an important nursing responsibility.

Osmotic (Saline) Laxatives

Osmotics, hyperosmolar laxatives, include salts or saline products, lactulose, and glycerin. Saline products consist of sodium or magnesium, and a small amount is systemically absorbed. Serum electrolytes should be monitored to avoid electrolyte imbalance. Hyperosmolar salts pull water into the colon and increase water in the feces to increase bulk, which stimulates peristalsis. Saline cathartics cause a semiformed to watery stool according to low or high doses. Good renal function is needed to excrete any excess salts. Saline cathartics are contraindicated for patients with heart failure.

Osmotic laxatives contain electrolyte salts, including (1) sodium salts (sodium phosphate or Phospho-Soda, sodium biphosphate) and (2) magnesium salts (magnesium hydroxide [Milk of Magnesia], magnesium citrate). High doses of salt laxatives are used for bowel preparation for diagnostic and surgical procedures. Another laxative used for bowel preparation is polyethylene glycol (PEG) with electrolytes. With PEG, however, a large volume of solution—approximately 3 to 4 L over 3 hours—must be ingested. Patients may be advised to keep PEG refrigerated to make it more palatable. The positive aspect is that the solution is an isotonic, nonabsorbable osmotic substance that contains sodium salts and potassium chloride; thus it can be used by patients with renal impairment or cardiac disorders.

Lactulose, another saline laxative that is not absorbed, draws water into the intestines to form a soft stool. It decreases the serum ammonia level and is useful in liver diseases, such as cirrhosis. Glycerin acts like lactulose, increasing water in the feces in the large intestine. The bulk that results from the increased water in the feces stimulates peristalsis and defecation.

Side Effects and Adverse Reactions. Adequate renal function is needed to excrete excess magnesium. Patients who have renal insufficiency should avoid magnesium salts. Hypermagnesemia can result from continuous use of magnesium salts, causing symptoms such as drowsiness, nausea, vomiting, and dehydration.

The side effects of excess lactulose use include flatulence, diarrhea, abdominal cramps, nausea, and vomiting. Patients who have diabetes mellitus should avoid lactulose because it contains glucose and fructose.

Stimulant (Contact) Laxatives

Stimulant (contact or irritant) laxatives increase peristalsis by irritating sensory nerve endings in the intestinal mucosa. Types include those that contain bisacodyl, senna, and castor oil (purgative). Bisacodyl is the most frequently used and misused laxative and can be purchased

OTC. Bisacodyl and several others of these drugs are used to empty the bowel before diagnostic tests (barium enema). Prototype Drug Chart: Bisacodyl lists the pharmacological data for the stimulant laxative bisacodyl.

Castor oil is converted to ricinoleic acid in the small intestine, which reduces fluid absorption and electrolytes. This action stimulates peristalsis producing a purgative effect. Castor oil is used for constipation and bowel preparation. Bowel evacuation occurs in 6 to 12 hours, so it should not be taken at bedtime.

Pharmacokinetics. The contact laxative bisacodyl is minimally absorbed from the GI tract. It is excreted in feces, but because of the small amount of bisacodyl absorption, a portion is excreted in urine.

Pharmacodynamics. Bisacodyl promotes defecation by irritating the colon, causing defecation; psyllium compounds increase fecal bulk and peristalsis. The onset of action of oral bisacodyl occurs within 6 to 8 hours, and with the suppository (rectal administration), it occurs within 15 to 60 minutes.

Side Effects and Adverse Reactions. Side effects include nausea, vomiting, abdominal cramps, diarrhea, and a rectal burning sensation. With excessive and chronic use, fluid and electrolyte imbalances—especially of potassium and calcium—are likely to occur. Systemic effects occur infrequently with bisacodyl because absorption is minimal.

Table 45.4 lists the osmotic and stimulant laxatives with their dosages, uses, and considerations.

TABLE 45.4 Laxatives: Osmotics (Saline), Stimulants, and Selective Chloride Channel Activators

Drug	Route and Dosage	Uses and Considerations
Osmotics: Saline		
Glycerin	A: PR: 1 supp, retain 15 min qd PRN; *max:* 1 supp/d	For constipation. Use with caution in patients with abdominal pain and vomiting. May cause bleeding and ocular irritation. PB: UK; $t\frac{1}{2}$: UK
Lactulose	Constipation: A: PO: 30–45 mL q1h until laxative effect is obtained, then 30–45 mL tid/qid	For constipation and hepatic encephalopathy. May cause eructation, abdominal pain, nausea, vomiting, flatulence, diarrhea, metabolic acidosis, hypokalemia, and hypernatremia. PB: UK; $t\frac{1}{2}$: UK
Magnesium citrate	Constipation: A: PO: 150–300 mL in single or divided dose; *max:* 300 mg/d	For constipation and bowel preparation. May cause drowsiness, nausea, vomiting, diarrhea, hypermagnesemia, and dehydration. PB: UK; $t\frac{1}{2}$: UK
Magnesium hydroxide	Constipation: A: PO: 15–60 mL, preferably at bedtime	For constipation, dyspepsia, and pyrosis. Take with a glass of water. May cause diuresis, nausea, vomiting, diarrhea, dehydration, and hypermagnesemia. PB: UK; $t\frac{1}{2}$: UK
Lactitol	A: PO: 20 g/d; *max:* 20 g/d	For chronic constipation. May cause flatulence, abdominal pain, diarrhea, infection, rash, pruritus, and hypertension. PB: UK; $t\frac{1}{2}$: 2.4 h
Polyethylene glycol	Constipation: A: PO: 17 g in 4–8 oz water qd; *max:* 34 g/d	For constipation and bowel preparation. May cause nausea, flatulence, diarrhea, abdominal cramps, and fecal urgency/incontinence. PB: UK; $t\frac{1}{2}$: UK
Stimulants		
Bisacodyl	See Prototype Drug Chart: Bisacodyl	
Castor oil	Constipation: A: PO: 15–60 mL/d PRN; *max:* 60 mL/d	For occasional constipation and bowel preparation. May cause nausea, vomiting, abdominal pain, and diarrhea. Should not be given at bedtime. PB: UK; $t\frac{1}{2}$: UK
Selective Chloride Channel Activator		
Lubiprostone	A: PO: 24 mcg bid with food and water; *max:* 48 mcg/d	For treatment of constipation, IBS, and opioid agonist–induced constipation. May cause dizziness, headache, fatigue, peripheral edema, nausea, diarrhea, abdominal pain, and flatulence. PB: 94%; $t\frac{1}{2}$: 0.9–1.4 h
Miscellaneous		
Linaclotide	Constipation: A: PO: 145 mcg/d on empty stomach at least 30 min before first meal; *max:* 290 mcg/d	For constipation and IBS. May cause headache, flatulence, abdominal pain, diarrhea, hypokalemia, hyponatremia, infection, and hypotension. PB: UK; $t\frac{1}{2}$: UK
Naloxegol	A: PO: 12.5–25 mg/d on empty stomach 1 h before first meal; *max:* 25 mg/d	For opiate agonist–induced constipation. May cause headache, hyperhidrosis, abdominal pain, nausea, vomiting, flatulence, and diarrhea. PB: 4.2%; $t\frac{1}{2}$: 6–11 h
Naldemedine	A: PO: 0.2 mg/d; *max:* 0.2 mg/d	For opiate agonist–induced constipation. May cause abdominal pain, nausea, vomiting, and diarrhea. PB: 93%–94%; $t\frac{1}{2}$: 11 h
Methylnaltrexone	A: PO: 450 mg/d in the morning A: Subcut: 8–12 mg qod PRN or 0.15 mg/kg qod PRN	For opioid agonist–induced constipation. May cause dizziness, headache, abdominal pain, nausea, vomiting, diarrhea, flatulence, and hyperhidrosis. PB: 11%–15.3%; $t\frac{1}{2}$: 15 h

TABLE 45.4 Laxatives: Osmotics (Saline), Stimulants, and Selective Chloride Channel Activators—cont'd

Drug	Route and Dosage	Uses and Considerations
Prucalopride	A: PO: 2 mg/d; max. 2 mg/d	For chronic idiopathic constipation. May cause dizziness, headache, nausea, vomiting, diarrhea, flatulence, and abdominal pain. PB: 30%; t½: 24 h
Tenapanor	A: PO: 50 mg bid before breakfast and dinner; max: 100 mg/d	For IBS with constipation. May cause dizziness, dehydration, flatulence, diarrhea, hyperkalemia, hyponatremia, and GI bleeding. PB: 99; t½: UK

A, adult; *bid*, twice a day; *d*, day; *GI*, gastrointestinal; *h*, hour; *IBS*, irritable bowel syndrome; *max*, maximum; *min*, minute; *PB*, protein binding; *PO*, by mouth; *PR*, per rectum; *PRN*, as needed; *qd*, every day; *qod*, every other day; *supp*, suppository; *t½*, half-life; *tab*, tablet; *UK*, unknown.

Bulk-Forming Laxatives

Bulk-forming laxatives are natural fibrous substances that promote large, soft stools by absorbing water into the intestine, increasing fecal bulk and peristalsis. These agents are nonabsorbable. Defecation usually occurs within 8 to 24 hours; however, it may take up to 3 days after drug therapy is started for the stool to be soft and well formed. Powdered bulk-forming laxatives, which sometimes come in flavored and sugar-free forms, should be mixed in a glass of water or juice, stirred, drunk immediately, and followed by a half to a full glass of water. Insufficient fluid intake can cause the drug to solidify in the GI tract, which can result in intestinal obstruction. This group of laxatives does not cause laxative dependence and may be used by patients with diverticulosis, irritable bowel syndrome (IBS), and ileostomy and colostomy.

Polycarbophil, methylcellulose, and psyllium are examples of bulk-forming laxatives. Patients with hypercalcemia should avoid calcium polycarbophil because of the significant amount of calcium in the drug. Prototype Drug Chart: Psyllium lists the pharmacological data for the bulk-forming laxative psyllium.

Pharmacokinetics. The bulk-forming laxative psyllium is a nondigestible and nonabsorbent substance that becomes a viscous solution when mixed with water. Because it is not absorbed, there is no protein binding or half-life for the drug. Psyllium is excreted in the feces.

Pharmacodynamics. The onset of action for psyllium is 12 to 72 hours. Peak action is 1 to 3 days. The duration of action is unknown.

Side Effects and Adverse Reactions. Bulk-forming laxatives are not systemically absorbed, so there is no systemic effect. If bulk-forming laxatives are excessively used, nausea, vomiting, flatulence, or diarrhea may occur. Abdominal cramps may occur if the drug is used in dry form.

Chloride Channel Activators

Selective chloride channel activators are used to treat idiopathic constipation in adults. The drug in this category is lubiprostone. Lubiprostone activates chloride channels in the lining of the small intestine, leading to an increase in intestinal fluid secretion and motility. By enhancing the passage of stool, lubiprostone relieves constipation and accompanying symptoms of abdominal discomfort, pain, and bloating. Lubiprostone is contraindicated for patients with a history of mechanical GI obstruction, Crohn disease, diverticulitis, and severe diarrhea. Adverse effects of lubiprostone include nausea that seems to be dose dependent, diarrhea, headache, and flatulence.

Emollients (Stool Softeners)

Emollients are lubricants and stool softeners (surface-acting or wetting drugs) used to prevent constipation. These drugs decrease straining during defecation. Lubricants such as mineral oil increase water retention in the stool. Mineral oil absorbs the essential fat-soluble vitamins A, D, E, and K. Some of the minerals can be absorbed into the lymphatic system.

Stool softeners work by lowering surface tension and promoting water accumulation in the intestine and stool. They are frequently

PROTOTYPE DRUG CHART

Bisacodyl

Drug Class	Dosage
Laxative: Stimulant	A: PO: 5–15 mg/d single dose or qd as needed; max: 15 mg/d
	A: supp PR: 10 mg/d single dose or qd as needed; max: 10 mg supp/d

Contraindications	Drug-Lab-Food Interactions
Hypersensitivity, GI bleeding, dysphagia	Drug: Decreased effect with antacids, histamine₂ blockers, proton pump inhibitors
Caution: Diarrhea, diverticulitis, electrolyte imbalance, hypokalemia, ulcerative colitis, ileus, GI bleeding/obstruction/perforation, appendicitis, abdominal pain, toxic megacolon, fecal impaction, vomiting, pregnancy, breastfeeding, children	Food: Milk

Pharmacokinetics	Pharmacodynamics
Absorption: Minimal (5%–15%)	PO: Onset: 6–8 h
Distribution: PB: UK	Peak: UK
Metabolism: t½: UK	Duration: UK
Excretion: In bile and urine	PR: Onset: 15–60 min
	Peak: UK
	Duration: UK

Therapeutic Effects/Uses

Treatment for constipation
Mechanism of action: Increases peristalsis by direct effect on smooth muscle of intestine

Side Effects	Adverse Reactions
Nausea, vomiting, abdominal cramps, diarrhea, proctitis	Dependence, hypokalemia

A, Adult; *d*, day; *GI*, gastrointestinal; *h*, hour; *max*, maximum; *min*, minutes; *PB*, protein binding; *PO*, by mouth; *PR*, per rectum; *qd*, every day; *supp*, suppository; *t½*, half-life; *UK*, unknown.

prescribed for patients after myocardial infarction or surgery. They are also given before administration of other laxatives in treating fecal impaction. Docusate calcium, docusate sodium, and docusate sodium with senna are examples of stool softeners.

Side Effects and Adverse Reactions. Side effects of mineral oil include nausea, vomiting, diarrhea, and abdominal cramping. This laxative is to be used with caution for children and older adults. The docusate group of drugs may cause mild cramping.

Contraindications. Contraindications to the use of laxatives include pregnancy and inflammatory disorders of the GI tract such as appendicitis, ulcerative colitis, undiagnosed severe pain that could be caused by inflammation within the intestine (diverticulitis, appendicitis), along with spastic colon or bowel obstruction. Laxatives are contraindicated when any of these conditions is suspected. Table 45.5 lists the laxatives and their dosages, uses, and considerations.

PROTOTYPE DRUG CHART

Psyllium

Drug Class	Dosage
Laxative: Bulk forming	A: PO: 1 rounded tbsp or premeasured packet in 8 oz water followed by 8 oz water 1–3 times/d A: PO: 2 chewable wafers 1–3/d with 8 oz fluid, *max:* 6 wafers A: PO: Initially 2–5 fiber capsules/d, *max:* 20 capsules
Contraindications	**Drug-Lab-Food Interactions**
Hypersensitivity, dysphagia *Caution:* GI obstruction, abdominal pain, vomiting, ileus, appendicitis, phenylketonuria, pregnancy, breast-feeding, children	Drug: Decreased absorption of oral anticoagulants, aspirin, and digoxin
Pharmacokinetics	**Pharmacodynamics**
Absorption: Not absorbed Distribution: PB: UK Metabolism: t½: UK Excretion: In feces	PO: Onset: 12–72 h Peak: 1–3 d Duration: UK
Therapeutic Effects/Uses	
To control constipation and hypercholesterolemia Mechanism of action: Acts as a bulk-forming laxative by drawing water into the intestine	
Side Effects	**Adverse Reactions**
Nausea, vomiting, abdominal cramps, flatulence	GI obstruction, dyspnea, chest pain *Life-threatening:* Bronchospasm, anaphylaxis

A, Adult; *d*, day; *GI*, gastrointestinal; *h*, hour; *max*, maximum; *PB*, protein binding; *PO*, by mouth; *t½*, half-life; *UK*, unknown.

CLINICAL JUDGMENT [NURSING PROCESS]

Laxative: Stimulant

Concept: Elimination
- The excretion of waste products through the intestinal tract and the expelling of stool by means of intestinal smooth muscle contraction

Recognize Cues [Assessment]
- Obtain a history of constipation and possible causes (insufficient water or fluid intake, diet deficient in bulk or fiber, inactivity), frequency and consistency of stools, and general health status.
- Record baseline vital signs for identification of abnormalities and for future comparisons.
- Evaluate renal function.
- Assess electrolyte balance of patients who frequently use laxatives.

Analyze Cues and Prioritize Hypothesis [Patient Problems]
- Discomfort

- Constipation
- Fatigue
- Reduced intestinal motility

Generate Solutions [Planning]
- The patient will report a normal bowel elimination pattern.
- The patient will exercise, eat foods high in fiber, and have adequate fluid intake to avoid constipation.

Take Action [Nursing Interventions]
- Monitor fluid intake and output.
- Note signs and symptoms of fluid and electrolyte imbalances that may result from watery stools. Habitual use of laxatives can cause fluid volume deficit, electrolyte losses, and loss of the urge to defecate.

CLINICAL JUDGMENT [NURSING PROCESS]—CONT'D

Laxative: Stimulant

Patient Teaching

General
- Encourage patients to increase water intake (if not contraindicated), which will decrease hard, dry stools.
- ⚡ Advise patients to avoid overuse of laxatives, which can lead to fluid and electrolyte imbalances and drug dependence. Suggest exercise to help increase peristalsis.
- Teach patients not to chew tablets but to swallow them whole.
- Direct patients to store suppositories at less than 86°F (30°C).
- Counsel patients to take drugs only with water to increase absorption.
- Educate patients not to take the drug within 1 hour of any other drug.
- Warn patients that the drug is not for long-term use; bowel tone may be lost.
- Encourage patients to time administration of the drug so as not to interfere with activities or sleep.

Side Effects
- Advise patients to discontinue use if rectal bleeding, nausea, vomiting, or cramping occurs.

Diet
- Inform patients to consume foods high in fiber such as bran, whole grains, and fruits.

Evaluate Outcomes [Evaluation]
- Determine the effectiveness of nonpharmacologic methods for alleviating constipation.
- Evaluate the patient's use of laxatives in managing constipation. Identify laxative misuse.

CLINICAL JUDGMENT [NURSING PROCESS]

Laxative: Bulk Forming

Concept: Elimination
- The excretion of waste products through the intestinal tract and the expelling of stool by means of intestinal smooth muscle contraction

Recognize Cues [Assessment]
- Obtain a history of constipation and possible causes (insufficient water or fluid intake, diet deficient in bulk or fiber, inactivity), frequency and consistency of stools, and general health status.
- Record baseline vital signs for identification of abnormalities and for future comparisons.
- Assess renal function, urine output, blood urea nitrogen (BUN), and serum creatinine.

Analyze Cues and Prioritize Hypothesis [Patient Problems]
- Discomfort
- Constipation
- Fatigue
- Reduced intestinal motility

Generate Solutions [Planning]
- The patient will report a normal bowel elimination pattern.
- The patient will exercise, eat foods high in fiber, and have adequate fluid intake to avoid constipation.

Take Action [Nursing Interventions]
- ⚡ Check fluid intake and output. Note signs and symptoms of fluid and electrolyte imbalances that may result from watery stools. Habitual use of laxatives can cause fluid volume deficit and electrolyte losses.
- Monitor bowel sounds.
- Identify the cause of constipation.
- Avoid inhalation of psyllium dust.

Patient Teaching

General
- Teach patients to mix the agent with water immediately before use to avoid gastrointestinal (GI) obstruction.
- Advise patients *not* to swallow the agent in dry form.
- Counsel patients to avoid overuse of laxatives, which can lead to fluid and electrolyte imbalances and laxative dependence. Suggest exercise to help increase peristalsis.
- ⚡ Advise patients to avoid inhaling psyllium dust; it may cause watery eyes, runny nose, and wheezing.

Side Effects
- Encourage patients to discontinue use if nausea, vomiting, cramping, or rectal bleeding occurs.

Diet
- ⚡ Instruct patients to mix the drug in 8 to 10 oz of water and to stir and drink it immediately. At least one glass of extra water should follow. Insufficient water can cause the drug to solidify, which can lead to dry, hard stools; fecal impaction; and esophageal obstruction.
- Encourage patients to increase foods rich in fiber such as bran, grains, vegetables, and fruits.
- Advise patients to increase water intake to at least 8 oz of fluids per day, which will decrease hard, dry stools.

Evaluate Outcomes [Evaluation]
- Determine the effectiveness of nonpharmacologic methods for alleviating constipation.
- Evaluate patients' use of laxatives in managing constipation.
- Identify laxative misuse.

TABLE 45.5 Laxatives: Bulk Forming, Stool Softeners, and Emollients

Drug	Route and Dosage	Uses and Considerations
Bulk Forming		
Polycarbophil	A: PO: 2 tabs (1250 mg) qd–qid PRN; *max*. 8 tabs (5000 mg)/d	For prevention and treatment of constipation. Administer with a full glass of water. May cause dizziness, drowsiness, anorexia, nausea, vomiting, flatulence, abdominal cramps, and diarrhea. PB: UK; t½: UK
Methylcellulose	A: PO: 2 g methylcellulose (1 heaping Tbsp) 1–3 times/d with 8–10 oz of water or 2 caplets up to 6 times/d; *max*: 3 Tbsp/d or 12 caplets/d	For constipation. Take immediately after mixing in water. May cause nausea, vomiting, diarrhea, abdominal cramps, and GI obstruction. PB: UK; t½: UK
Psyllium hydrophilic mucilloid	See Prototype Drug Chart: Psyllium	
Stool Softeners		
Docusate calcium; docusate sodium	Docusate calcium capsules: A: PO: 240 mg/d Docusate sodium solution: A: PO: 50–360 mg/d	For constipation. May cause throat irritation, rash, and diarrhea. PB: UK; t½: UK
Docusate sodium with senna	A: PO: 2–4 tabs/d until bowel movements are normal	For constipation. May cause nausea, vomiting, abdominal cramps, flatulence, diarrhea, fecal urgency, hypokalemia, and urine discoloration. PB: UK; t½: UK
Emollient: Lubricant		
Mineral oil	A: PO: 30–90 mL/d as needed A: R: enema: 120 mL/d	For constipation and fecal impaction. May be useful for those with cardiac disorders and after anorectal surgery. May cause dizziness, weakness, hypovitaminosis, nausea, vomiting, diarrhea, abdominal cramps, fecal urgency/incontinence, and skin irritation. PB: UK; t½: UK

A, adult; *d*, day; *GI*, gastrointestinal; *max*, maximum; *PB*, protein binding; *PO*, by mouth; *PRN*, as needed; *qd*, every day; *qid*, four times a day; *t½*, half-life; *tab*, tablet; *Tbsp*, tablespoon; *UK*, unknown.

CLINICAL JUDGMENT CASE STUDY

A 34-year-old female has been vomiting for 48 hours. In the past 12 hours, the patient has had vomiting and diarrhea. Prochlorperazine 10 mg was administered intramuscularly.

1. What nonpharmacologic measures should the nurse suggest when vomiting occurs?
2. Why was the patient given prochlorperazine intramuscularly and not orally or rectally?
3. What electrolyte imbalances may occur as a result of vomiting and diarrhea? Explain how they can be replaced.
4. What are the side effects of prochlorperazine?
5. Could a serotonin antagonist be given to the patient instead of prochlorperazine? Explain your answer.
6. The patient was prescribed difenoxin with atropine 2 tablets initially, then 1 tablet after each loose stool. Is the diphenoxylate with atropine dosage for the patient within the normal prescribed range?
8. What clinical conditions are contraindicated for the use of difenoxin with atropine?
9. What are some combination drugs that may be prescribed to control diarrhea? Give their advantages and disadvantages.

REVIEW QUESTIONS

1. A patient reports constipation and requires a laxative. In providing teaching for this patient, the nurse reviews the common causes of constipation, including which cause?
    a. Motion sickness
    b. Poor dietary habits
    c. Food intolerance
    d. Bacteria (*Escherichia coli*)
2. A patient with nausea is taking ondansetron. She asks the nurse how this drug works. The nurse is aware that this medication has which action?
    a. Enhances histamine[1] receptor sites
    b. Blocks serotonin receptors in the chemoreceptor trigger zone
    c. Blocks dopamine receptors in the chemoreceptor trigger zone
    d. Stimulates anticholinergic receptor sites
3. A patient who has constipation is prescribed a bisacodyl suppository. Which explanation will the nurse use to explain the action of bisacodyl?
    a. Acts on smooth intestinal muscle to gently increase peristalsis
    b. Absorbs water into the intestines to increase bulk and peristalsis
    c. Lowers surface tension and increases water accumulation in the intestines
    d. Pulls salts into the colon and increases water in the feces to increase bulk

4. A patient is using scopolamine to prevent motion sickness. About which common side effect should the nurse teach the patient?
   a. Diarrhea
   b. Vomiting
   c. Insomnia
   d. Dry mouth
5. When metoclopramide is given for nausea, the nurse plans to caution the patient to avoid which substance?
   a. Milk
   b. Coffee
   c. Alcohol
   d. Carbonated beverages
6. The nurse is administering difenoxin with atropine to a patient. Which should be included in the patient teaching regarding this medication? **Select all that apply.**
   a. Caution the patient to avoid laxative misuse.
   b. Record the frequency of bowel movements.
   c. Caution the patient against taking sedatives concurrently.
   d. Encourage the patient to increase fluids.
   e. Instruct the patient to avoid this drug if they have narrow-angle glaucoma.
   f. Teach the patient that the drug acts by drawing water into the intestine.

46 Antiulcer Drugs

http://evolve.elsevier.com/McCuistion/pharmacology

OBJECTIVES

- Differentiate the treatment for peptic ulcer disease, *Helicobacter pylori*, and gastroesophageal reflux disease, including nonpharmacologic measures.
- Contrast the mechanism of action of the seven groups of antiulcer agents.

OUTLINE

Gastrointestinal Disorders and Nonpharmacologic Measures for Treatment, 590
Peptic Ulcer Disease, 590
Helicobacter pylori, 591
Gastroesophageal Reflux Disease, 591
Nonpharmacologic Measures for Managing Peptic Ulcer Gastroesophageal Reflux Disease, 592
Antiulcer Drugs, 592
Tranquilizers, 592
Anticholinergics, 593
Antacids, 593
Histamine$_2$ Blockers, 595
Proton Pump Inhibitors, 597
Pepsin Inhibitors (Mucosal Protective Drugs), 599
Prostaglandin Analogue Antiulcer Drug, 599
Clinical Judgment Case Study, 601
Review Questions, 601

This chapter discusses drugs used to prevent and treat peptic ulcers, both gastric and duodenal. These drugs include tranquilizers, anticholinergics, antacids, histamine$_2$ blockers, proton pump inhibitors (PPIs), a pepsin inhibitor, and a prostaglandin analogue antiulcer drug.

GASTROINTESTINAL DISORDERS AND NONPHARMACOLOGIC MEASURES FOR TREATMENT

Peptic Ulcer Disease

Peptic ulcer is a broad term for an ulcer or erosion that occurs in the esophagus, stomach, or duodenum within the upper gastrointestinal (GI) tract. Ulcers are more specifically named according to the site of involvement: esophageal, gastric, or duodenal. Duodenal ulcers occur 10 times more frequently than gastric and esophageal ulcers. The release of hydrochloric acid (HCl) from the parietal cells of the stomach is influenced by histamine, gastrin, and acetylcholine. Peptic ulcers occur when there is a hypersecretion of HCl and pepsin, which erode the GI mucosal lining.

The gastric secretions in the stomach strive to maintain a pH of 2 to 5. Pepsin, a digestive enzyme, is activated at a pH of 2, and the acid-pepsin complex of gastric secretions can cause mucosal damage. If the pH of gastric secretions increases to 5, the activity of pepsin declines. The gastric mucosal barrier (GMB) is a thick, viscous, mucous material that provides a barrier between the mucosal lining and acidic gastric secretions. The GMB maintains the integrity of the gastric mucosal lining and is a defense against corrosive substances. The two sphincter muscles—the *cardiac*, located at the upper portion of the stomach, and the *pyloric*, located at the lower portion of the stomach—act as barriers to prevent reflux of acid into the esophagus and duodenum. Fig. 46.1 shows common sites of peptic ulcers.

An esophageal ulcer results from reflux of acidic gastric secretions into the esophagus as a result of a defective or incompetent cardiac sphincter. A gastric ulcer frequently occurs because of a breakdown of the GMB. A duodenal ulcer is caused by hypersecretion of acid from the stomach passing into the duodenum because of (1) insufficient buffers to neutralize gastric acid in the stomach, (2) a defective or incompetent pyloric sphincter, or (3) hypermotility of the stomach. Gastroesophageal reflux disease (GERD) is inflammation or erosion of the esophageal mucosa caused by a reflux of gastric acid content from the stomach into the esophagus.

Predisposing Factors in Peptic Ulcer Disease

The nurse needs to assist the patient in identifying possible causes of the ulcer and to teach ways to alleviate it. Predisposing factors include mechanical disturbances, genetic influences, bacterial organisms, environmental factors, and certain drugs. Healing of an ulcer takes 4 to 8 weeks. Complications can occur as a result of scar tissue. Table 46.1 lists the predisposing factors for peptic ulcers and their effects.

The classic symptom of peptic ulcers is gnawing, aching pain. With a gastric ulcer, pain occurs 30 minutes to 1.5 hours after eating, and with a duodenal ulcer, pain occurs 2 to 3 hours after eating. Small, frequent meals of nonirritating foods decrease the pain. With treatment, pain usually subsides in 10 days; however, the healing process may take 1 to 2 months.

A stress ulcer usually follows a critical situation such as extensive trauma, such as burns, or major surgery (e.g., cardiac surgery). Prophylactic use of antiulcer drugs decreases the incidence of stress ulcers.

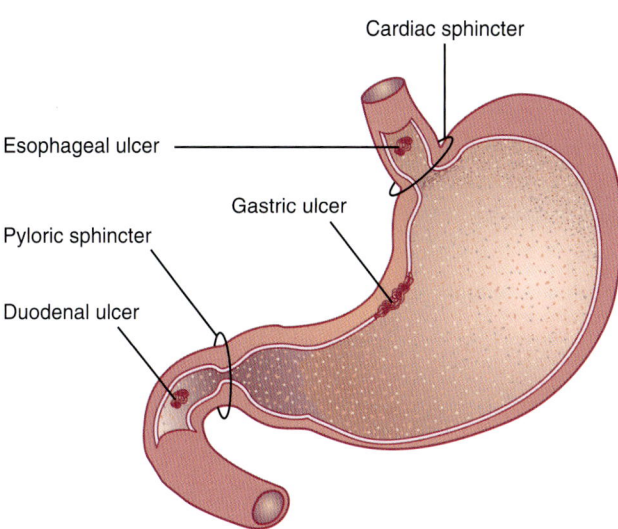

Fig. 46.1 Common sites of peptic ulcers.

TABLE 46.1 Predisposing Factors for Peptic Ulcer Disease

Predisposing Factors	Effects
Mechanical disturbances	Hypersecretion of acid and pepsin; inadequate GMB mucous secretion; impaired GMB resistance; hypermotility of the stomach; incompetent (defective) cardiac or pyloric sphincter
Genetic influences	Increased number of parietal cells in the stomach; susceptibility of mucosal lining to acid penetration; susceptibility to excess acetylcholine and histamine; excess hydrochloric acid caused by external stimuli
Environmental influences	Foods and liquids containing caffeine; fatty, fried, and highly spiced foods; alcohol; nicotine, especially from cigarette smoking; stressful situations; pregnancy; massive trauma; major surgery
Helicobacter pylori	A gram-negative bacterium, *H. pylori*, infects gastric mucosa and can cause gastritis, gastric ulcer, and duodenal ulcer. If not eradicated, peptic ulcer may return as frequently as every year. *H. pylori* can lead to atrophic gastritis in some patients. Serology and special breath tests can detect the presence of *H. pylori*.
Drugs	NSAIDs, including aspirin and aspirin compounds, ibuprofen, and indomethacin; corticosteroids; potassium salts; antineoplastic drugs

GMB, Gastric mucosal barrier; *NSAIDs*, nonsteroidal antiinflammatory drugs.

Helicobacter pylori

H. pylori, a gram-negative bacillus, is linked with the development of peptic ulcer and is known to cause gastritis, gastric ulcer, and duodenal ulcer. When a peptic ulcer recurs after antiulcer therapy, and the ulcer is not caused by nonsteroidal antiinflammatory drugs (NSAIDs) such as aspirin or ibuprofen, the patient should be tested for the presence of *H. pylori*, which may have infected the gastric mucosa. In the past, endoscopy and a biopsy of the gastric antrum were needed to check for *H. pylori*. Currently, a noninvasive breath test—the Meretek UBT (urea breath test)—can detect *H. pylori*. This test consists of drinking a liquid containing 13 C urea and breathing into a container. If *H. pylori* is present, the bacterial urease hydrolyzes the urea, releasing $13CO_2$, which is detected by a spectrometer. This test is 90% to 95% effective for detecting *H. pylori* and also notes progress in treatment. In addition, a blood test may be performed to check for antibodies to *H. pylori*, and a stool test may be done to check for antigens to determine whether the immune system has been triggered to fight *H. pylori*.

There are various protocols for treating *H. pylori* infection, but antibacterial agents are the treatment of choice. The use of only one antibacterial agent is not effective for eradicating *H. pylori* because the bacterium can readily become resistant to that drug. Treatment to eradicate this bacterial infection includes using a dual-, triple-, or quadruple-drug therapy program in a variety of drug combinations—such as with amoxicillin, tetracycline, clarithromycin, omeprazole, lansoprazole, metronidazole, or bismuth subsalicylate—on a 7- to 14-day treatment plan. The combination of drugs differs for each patient according to the patient's drug tolerance. A common treatment protocol is the triple therapy of metronidazole (or amoxicillin), omeprazole (or lansoprazole), and clarithromycin (MOC). The drug regimen eradicates more than 90% of peptic ulcers caused by *H. pylori*.

> **COMPLEMENTARY AND ALTERNATIVE THERAPIES**
>
> St. John's wort may increase the risk for photosensitivity when taken with tetracycline.
> Ginger may decrease effectiveness of antacids.
> Ginkgo biloba, St. John's wort, and licorice may decrease drug level of omeprazole.

PPIs, such as omeprazole or esomeprazole, are frequently used as a component of combination drug therapy because each suppresses acid secretion by inhibiting the enzyme hydrogen or potassium adenosine triphosphatase (ATPase), which makes gastric acid. These agents block the final steps of acid production. If this therapy fails to eradicate *H. pylori*, therapy using two antibiotics, a PPI, and a bismuth or histamine$_2$ (H_2) blocker is recommended. After completion of the treatment regimen, 6 weeks of standard acid suppression—such as H_2 blocker therapy—is recommended. Table 46.2 lists agents used to treat *H. pylori* with their dosages, uses, and considerations. Antibiotics used to treat *H. pylori* are discussed in more detail in Chapters 27 and 28.

Gastroesophageal Reflux Disease

GERD, also called *reflux esophagitis*, is an inflammation of the esophageal mucosa caused by reflux of gastric acid content into the esophagus. Its main cause is an incompetent lower esophageal sphincter. Smoking tends to accelerate the disease process.

Medical treatment for GERD is similar to the treatment for peptic ulcers. This includes the use of the common antiulcer drugs to neutralize gastric contents and reduce gastric acid secretion. Drugs used in treatment include H_2 blockers such as famotidine and PPIs such as omeprazole, dexlansoprazole, lansoprazole, rabeprazole, pantoprazole, or esomeprazole. A PPI relieves symptoms faster and maintains healing better than an H_2 blocker. Once the strictures are relieved by dilation, they are less likely to recur if the patient was taking PPIs rather than an H_2 blocker.

TABLE 46.2 Pharmacological Agents Used to Treat *Helicobacter pylori* Infection

Drug	Route and Dosage	Uses and Considerations
Antiinfective Agents		
Metronidazole hydrochloride	A: PO: 500 mg tid	To treat numerous organisms, including *H. pylori*; used in combination with other drugs to treat *H. pylori*
Amoxicillin	A: PO: 1000 mg bid	Used in triple- or quadruple-drug therapy for *H. pylori*
Clarithromycin	A: PO: 500 mg bid	Used in dual- and triple-drug therapy for *H. pylori*
Tetracycline	A: PO: 500 mg qid	Used in triple- and quadruple-drug therapy for *H. pylori*
PPIs		
Omeprazole	A: PO: 40 mg/d	Used in dual-, triple-, and quadruple-drug therapy for *H. pylori*
Lansoprazole	A: PO: 30 mg tid	Used in dual- and triple-drug therapy for *H. pylori*
Esomeprazole	A: PO: 40–80 mg/d	Used in therapy for *H. pylori*
Pantoprazole	A: PO: 40–80 mg bid	Used in therapy for *H. pylori*
Rabeprazole	A: PO: 20–40 mg bid	Used in therapy for *H. pylori*
Potassium-Competitive Acid Blocker		
Vonoprazan	A: PO: 20 mg bid	Used in therapy for *H. pylori*

A, Adult; *bid*, twice a day; *d*, day; *PO*, by mouth; *PPIs*, proton pump inhibitors; *qid*, four times a day; *tid*, three times a day.

Effective management of GERD keeps the esophageal mucosa healed and the patient free from symptoms, but GERD is a chronic disorder that requires continuous care.

Nonpharmacologic Measures for Managing Peptic Ulcer and Gastroesophageal Reflux Disease

Nonpharmacologic measures, along with drug therapy, are an important part of treatment for a GI disorder. Once the GI problem is resolved, the patient should continue to follow nonpharmacologic measures to avoid recurrence of the condition.

Avoiding tobacco and alcohol can decrease gastric secretions. With GERD, nicotine relaxes the lower esophageal sphincter, permitting gastric acid reflux. Obesity enhances GERD, so weight loss is helpful in decreasing symptoms. The patient should avoid hot, spicy, and greasy foods, which could aggravate the gastric problem. Certain drugs like NSAIDs, which include aspirin, should be taken with food or in a decreased dosage. Glucocorticoids can cause gastric ulceration and should be taken with food.

To relieve symptoms of GERD, the patient should raise the head of the bed, not eat before bedtime, and wear loose-fitting clothing.

> ### ⚡ PATIENT SAFETY
> **Do Not Confuse...**
> - **Zantac**, an H_2 blocker, with **Xanax**, an anxiolytic.

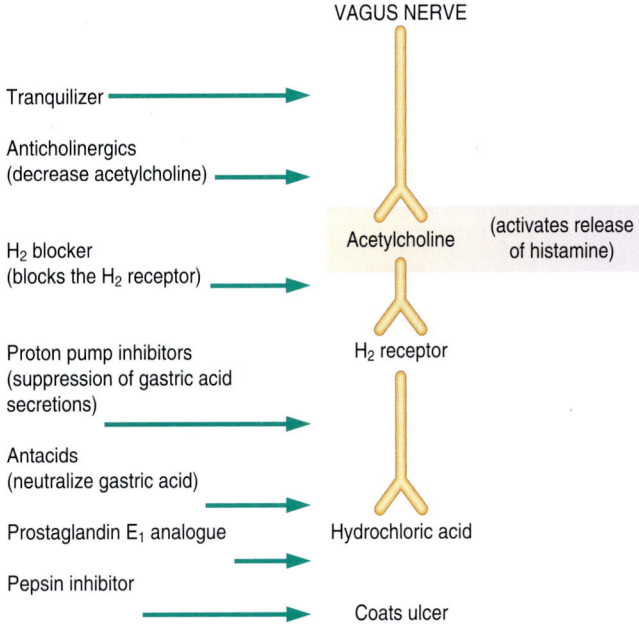

Fig. 46.2 Actions of the antiulcer drug groups. H_2, Histamine$_2$.

ANTIULCER DRUGS

The seven groups of antiulcer agents are (1) tranquilizers, which decrease vagal activity; (2) anticholinergics, which decrease acetylcholine by blocking the cholinergic receptors; (3) antacids, which neutralize gastric acid; (4) H_2 blockers, which block the H_2 receptor; (5) PPIs, which inhibit gastric acid secretion, regardless of acetylcholine or histamine release; (6) the pepsin inhibitor sucralfate; and (7) the prostaglandin E_1 analogue misoprostol, which inhibits gastric acid secretion and protects the mucosa. Currently, tranquilizers and anticholinergics are used infrequently due to potential adverse effects and much more effective drugs on the market. Fig. 46.2 shows the action of the antiulcer drug groups, each of which is discussed separately.

Tranquilizers

Tranquilizers have minimal effect in preventing and treating ulcers; however, they reduce vagal stimulation and decrease anxiety. A combination of the anxiolytic chlordiazepoxide and the anticholinergic clidinium bromide may be used in the treatment of ulcers. Adverse effects may include ataxia, confusion, drowsiness, dry mouth, and constipation.

Anticholinergics

Anticholinergics (antimuscarinics, parasympatholytics) and antacids were the drugs of choice for peptic ulcers for many years. However, anticholinergic use declined with the introduction of H_2 blockers in 1975. Anticholinergics relieve pain by decreasing GI motility and secretion. They act by inhibiting acetylcholine and blocking histamine and HCl. Anticholinergics delay gastric emptying time, so they are used more frequently for duodenal ulcers than for gastric ulcers. The anticholinergic propantheline bromide inhibits gastric secretions in the treatment of peptic ulcers.

Anticholinergics should be taken 30 minutes to 1 hour before meals and at least 2 hours after the evening meal for the bedtime dose to decrease acid secretion that occurs with eating. Antacids can slow the absorption of anticholinergics and therefore should be taken 2 hours after anticholinergic administration.

Table 46.3 lists selected anticholinergic drugs used to treat peptic ulcer. Anticholinergics should be used as adjunctive therapy and not as the only antiulcer drug. Anticholinergics are discussed in more detail in Chapter 16.

Side Effects and Adverse Reactions

Anticholinergics have many side effects, including dry mouth, headache, blurred vision, drowsiness, dizziness, asthenia, palpitations, erectile dysfunction, urinary retention, and constipation. Because anticholinergics decrease GI motility, gastric emptying time is delayed, which can stimulate gastric secretions and aggravate the ulceration.

Antacids

Antacids promote ulcer healing by neutralizing HCl and reducing pepsin activity; they do not coat the ulcer. There are two types of antacids: those that have a *systemic* effect and those that have a *nonsystemic* effect.

Sodium bicarbonate, a systemically absorbed antacid, was one of the first antiulcer drugs. Because it has many side effects (sodium excess, causing hypernatremia and peripheral edema; metabolic alkalosis caused by excess bicarbonate; and acid rebound [excess acid secretion]), sodium bicarbonate is seldom used to treat peptic ulcers.

Calcium carbonate is most effective in neutralizing acid; however, one-third to one-half of the drug can be systemically absorbed

TABLE 46.3 Antiulcer Drugs: Anticholinergics

Drug	Route and Dosage: Initially	Uses and Considerations
Glycopyrrolate	A: PO: 1–2 mg bid/tid; max: 8 mg/d A: IM/IV: 100–200 mcg q4h PRN; max: 0.2 mg/dose IV: 0.004 mg/kg IM preanesthesia	For gastric and duodenal ulcers, excess drooling, bradycardia, and aspiration prophylaxis. May cause headache, dyspnea, sinusitis, flushing, weakness, infection, dry mouth, nausea, vomiting, erectile dysfunction, urinary retention, and constipation. PB: UK; t½: IM 0.55–1.25 h, IV 0.96 h
Chlordiazepoxide and clidinium bromide	A: PO: 1–2 cap (chlordiazepoxide 5 mg, clidinium 2.5 mg per cap) tid/qid 30–60 min ac and at bedtime; max: chlordiazepoxide 40 mg/d, clidinium 20 mg/d	For controlling emotional and somatic factors in GI disorders, peptic ulcer disease, and IBS. May cause agitation, confusion, blurred vision, drowsiness, ataxia, dry mouth, nausea, constipation, and urinary retention. PB: chlordiazepoxide 96%, clidinium UK; t½: chlordiazepoxide 5–100 h, clidinium 2.4–20 h

A, adult; *ac*, before meals; *bid*, twice a day; *cap*, capsule; *d*, day; *GI*, gastrointestinal; *h*, hour; *IBS*, irritable bowel syndrome; *IM*, intramuscular; *IV*, intravenous; *max*, maximum; *min*, minutes; *PB*, protein binding; *PO*, by mouth; *q4h*, every 4 hours; *qid*, four times a day; *t½*, half-life; *tid*, three times a day; *UK*, unknown.

PROTOTYPE DRUG CHART
Aluminum Hydroxide

Drug Class	Dosage
Antiulcer: Antacid	Hyperacidity: A: PO: 40–60 mL (80–140 mEq) q3–6 h or 1–3 h after meals and at bedtime

Contraindications	Drug-Lab-Food Interactions
Hypersensitivity to aluminum products *Caution:* Diarrhea, hepatic/renal disease, HF, hypophosphatemia, dehydration, constipation, hemorrhoids, GI bleeding/obstruction, ileus, diverticulitis, ascites, older adults, children, pregnancy, breast-feeding	Drug: Decreased effects with tetracycline, pazopanib, isoniazid, phenytoin, digitalis, quinidine, amphetamines, fluoroquinolones, and captopril; may increase effects of benzodiazepines, glipizide, and glyburide Lab: Increased urine pH

Pharmacokinetics	Pharmacodynamics
Absorption: PO: Small amount absorbed Distribution: PB: UK Metabolism: t½: UK Excretion: In feces; small amount in urine	PO: Onset: UK Peak: UK Duration: 1–3 h

Therapeutic Effects/Uses

To treat hyperacidity, gastric and duodenal ulcer, and reflux esophagitis; to reduce hyperphosphatemia
Mechanism of action: Neutralizes gastric acidity

Side Effects	Adverse Reactions
Anorexia, constipation, weakness, impaired cognition	Hypophosphatemia, hypercalcemia, osteoporosis/osteomalacia, nephrolithiasis, hemorrhoids, and GI obstruction

A, Adult; *GI*, gastrointestinal; *h*, hour; *HF*, heart failure; *min*, minute; *PB*, protein binding; *PO*, by mouth; *q*, every; *t½*, half-life; *UK*, unknown.

and can cause acid rebound. Hypercalcemia and Burnett syndrome, formerly called *milk-alkali syndrome*, can result from excessive use of calcium carbonate. Burnett syndrome is intensified if milk products are ingested with calcium carbonate. It is identified by the presence of alkalosis, hypercalcemia, and, in severe cases, crystalluria and renal failure.

The nonsystemic antacids are composed of alkaline salts such as aluminum (aluminum hydroxide) and magnesium (magnesium hydroxide, magnesium trisilicate). A small degree of systemic absorption occurs with these drugs, mainly of aluminum. Magnesium hydroxide has greater neutralizing power than aluminum hydroxide. Magnesium compounds can cause diarrhea, and aluminum and calcium compounds can cause constipation with long-term use. A combination of magnesium and aluminum salts neutralizes gastric acid without causing severe diarrhea or constipation. Simethicone, an antigas agent, is found in many antacids. Prototype Drug Chart: Aluminum Hydroxide lists the pharmacological data for aluminum hydroxide antacids.

Pharmacokinetics

Aluminum hydroxide was one of the first antacids used to neutralize HCl. Aluminum products are frequently used to lower high serum phosphate (hyperphosphatemia). Because aluminum hydroxide alone can cause constipation, and magnesium products alone can cause diarrhea, combination drugs such as aluminum hydroxide and magnesium hydroxide have become popular because they decrease these side effects. Only a small amount of aluminum hydroxide is absorbed from the GI tract. It is primarily bound to phosphate and excreted in the feces. The small portion that is absorbed is excreted in the urine.

Pharmacodynamics

Aluminum hydroxide neutralizes gastric acid, including HCl, and increases the pH of gastric secretions; an elevated pH inactivates pepsin. The onset of action is fairly rapid, but the duration of action varies, depending on whether the antacid is taken with or without food. If the antacid is taken after a meal, the duration of action may be up to 3 hours because food delays gastric emptying time. Frequent dosing may be necessary if the antacid is given during a fasting state or early in the course of treatment.

The ideal dosing interval for antacids is 1 to 3 hours after meals (maximum acid secretion occurs after eating) and at bedtime. Antacids taken on an empty stomach are effective for 30 to 60 minutes before passing into the duodenum. Chewable tablets should be followed by water. Liquid antacids should also be taken with water (2–4 oz) to ensure that the drug reaches the stomach; however, no more than 4 oz of water should be taken because water quickens gastric emptying time. Antacids should not be administered with other oral medications as there are numerous drug interactions.

Antacids that contain magnesium salts are given cautiously in patients with impaired renal function because of the risk for hypermagnesemia. Magnesium is primarily excreted by the kidneys; however, hypermagnesemia is usually not a problem unless a patient with renal insufficiency is ingesting magnesium. Prolonged use of aluminum hydroxides can cause hypophosphatemia (low serum phosphate), osteoporosis, nephrolithiasis, and osteomalacia. If hyperphosphatemia occurs because of poor renal function, aluminum hydroxide can be given to decrease the phosphate level. In patients with renal insufficiency, aluminum salt ingestion can cause encephalopathy from accumulation of aluminum in the brain. Table 46.4 lists the antacids and their dosages, uses, and considerations.

TABLE 46.4 Antiulcer Drugs: Antacids

Drug	Route and Dosage	Uses and Considerations
Aluminum hydroxide	See Prototype Drug Chart: Aluminum Hydroxide	
Calcium carbonate	Dyspepsia: A: PO: 1000–3000 mg PRN; *max:* 7500 mg/d	To treat pyrosis, dyspepsia, hypocalcemia, and hyperphosphatemia and for osteoporosis prophylaxis. May cause hypercalcemia, hypophosphatemia, eructation, nausea, vomiting, constipation, gastric hypersecretion, flatulence, and metabolic alkalosis. PB: 40%; t½: UK
Calcium carbonate and magnesium hydroxide	Chewable tablets: A: PO: 2–4 tabs PRN; *max:* 12 tabs/d regular strength, 10 tabs/d extra strength Ultra strength: A: PO: 2–3 tabs PRN; *max:* 7 tabs/d	To treat pyrosis and dyspepsia. May cause metabolic alkalosis, hypermagnesemia, hypercalcemia, hypophosphatemia, milk-alkali syndrome, nephrolithiasis, fatigue, eructation, flatulence, gastric hypersecretion, nausea, and constipation. PB: 40%; t½: UK
Magnesium hydroxide and aluminum hydroxide	A: PO: 10–20 ml (magnesium hydroxide 400–800 mg, aluminum hydroxide 400–800 mg) qid PRN; *max:* (3200 mg) 80 ml/d of each	To treat dyspepsia, and pyrosis. May cause weakness, anorexia, nausea, vomiting, diarrhea, constipation, GI obstruction, dehydration, hypercalcemia, hypermagnesemia, and hypophosphatemia. PB: UK; t½: UK
Magnesium hydroxide 200 mg and aluminum hydroxide 200 mg with simethicone 25 mg	A: PO: 10–20 ml qid PRN	To treat dyspepsia, pyrosis, and flatulence. May cause hypercalcemia, hypermagnesemia, hypophosphatemia, anorexia, nausea, vomiting, constipation, diarrhea, dehydration, and weakness. PB: UK; t½: UK
Magnesium trisilicate with aluminum hydroxide	A: PO: 2–4 tab (magnesium trisilicate 28.4–56.8 mg and aluminum hydroxide 160–320 mg) qid PRN; *max:* 16 tab/d	To treat dyspepsia, pyrosis, and GERD. May cause hypermagnesemia, hypercalcemia, hypophosphatemia, anorexia, nausea, vomiting, constipation, diarrhea, dehydration, and weakness. PB: UK; t½: UK
Sodium bicarbonate	Dyspepsia: A: 18–59y: PO: 650–2600 mg q4h PRN A: >60y: PO: 650–1300 mg q4h PRN	To treat dyspepsia, pyrosis, hyperkalemia, and metabolic acidosis. May cause abdominal pain, flatulence, peripheral edema, hypernatremia, metabolic alkalosis, lactic acidosis, and tremor. PB: UK; t½: UK

>, Greater than; *A*, adult; *d*, day; *GERD*, gastroesophageal reflux disease; *GI*, gastrointestinal; *max*, maximum; *PB*, protein binding; *PO*, by mouth; *PRN*, as needed; *q4h*, every 4 hours; *qid*, four times a day; *t½*, half-life; *tab*, tablet; *UK*, unknown.

Histamine₂ Blockers

The histamine₂ (H2) receptor antagonists, or H₂ blockers, are popular drugs used in the treatment of gastric and duodenal ulcers. Histamine₂ blockers prevent acid reflux in the esophagus (reflux esophagitis). These drugs block the H₂ receptors of the parietal cells in the stomach, thus reducing gastric acid secretion and concentration. Antihistamines used to treat allergic conditions act against histamine₁ (H₁); they are not the same as H₂ blockers.

The first H₂ blocker was cimetidine, introduced in 1975. Cimetidine, which has a short half-life and a short duration of action, blocks about 70% of acid secretion for 4 hours. Good kidney function is necessary because approximately 50% to 80% of the drug is excreted unchanged in the urine. In patients with renal insufficiency, the dose and frequency may need to be reduced. Antacids can be given 1 hour before or after cimetidine as part of an antiulcer drug regimen; however, if they are given at the same time, the effectiveness of the H₂ blocker is decreased.

Two H₂ blockers—famotidine and nizatidine—are more potent than cimetidine. In addition to blocking gastric acid secretions, they promote healing of the ulcer by eliminating its cause. Their duration of action is longer, decreasing the frequency of dosing, and they have fewer side effects and fewer drug interactions than cimetidine. Prototype Drug Chart: Famotidine lists the pharmacological data for famotidine, which is a frequently prescribed H₂ blocker.

Pharmacokinetics

Famotidine is rapidly absorbed and reaches its peak concentration after a single dose in 1 to 3 hours. Famotidine has a low protein-binding power and a short half-life. A dose of famotidine is 30% to 35% metabolized by the liver. Approximately 65% to 70% is excreted in the urine.

Pharmacodynamics

Famotidine inhibits binding of H₂ receptors on the gastric membrane of parietal cells, thereby reducing gastric acid secretions. The drug is effective in treating gastric and duodenal ulcers and can be used prophylactically. Famotidine is also useful in relieving symptoms of pyrosis, dyspepsia, GERD, gastric/duodenal ulcers, and Zollinger-Ellison syndrome.

Famotidine has a similar onset of action of 1 hour and a longer duration of action (up to 12 hours) than cimetidine. Because the duration of action of cimetidine is only 4 to 5 hours, it is frequently given two to four times a day.

Famotidine is 50% to 80% more potent than cimetidine. It is indicated for short-term use (4–8 weeks) for duodenal ulcer and for Zollinger-Ellison syndrome.

Nizatidine is an H₂ blocker that can relieve nocturnal gastric acid secretion for 12 hours. This drug is similar to famotidine, and none of these agents suppresses the metabolism of other drugs. To prevent recurrence of duodenal ulcers, administer nizatidine 150 mg twice a day at bedtime or famotidine 40 mg once a day at bedtime. Both nizatidine and famotidine have low protein-binding capacities and similar half-lives.

CLINICAL JUDGMENT [NURSING PROCESS]

Antiulcer: Antacids

Concept: Pain
- An unpleasant feeling of discomfort usually associated with tissue damage

Recognize Cues [Assessment]
- Evaluate patient pain, including the type, duration, severity, and frequency.
- Check renal function.
- Assess for fluid and electrolyte imbalances, especially serum phosphate and calcium levels.
- Obtain a drug history and report probable drug-drug interactions.

Analyze Cues and Prioritize Hypothesis [Patient Problems]
- Acute pain
- Injury
- Gastric irritation
- Nausea
- Discomfort

Generate Solutions [Planning]
- The patient will report that abdominal pain has decreased after 1 to 2 weeks of antiulcer drug management.

Take Action [Nursing Interventions]
- Avoid administering antacids with other oral drugs because antacids can delay their absorption. Do not give an antacid with tetracycline, digoxin, or quinidine because it binds with and inactivates most of the drug. Antacids are not given with any other medications.
- Shake suspensions well before administering, and follow them with water.
- Monitor electrolytes and urinary pH, calcium, and phosphate levels.

Patient Teaching

General
- ⚡ Teach patients to report pain, coughing, or vomiting of blood.
- Encourage patients to drink 2 oz of water after taking an antacid to ensure that the drug reaches the stomach.
- Direct patients to take antacids 1 to 3 hours after meals and at bedtime. Instruct patients not to take antacids at mealtime; they slow gastric emptying time, causing increased gastrointestinal (GI) activity and gastric secretions.
- Advise patients to notify a health care provider if constipation or diarrhea occurs; the antacid may have to be changed. Self-treatment should be avoided.
- ⚡ Warn that taking an unlimited amount of the antacid is contraindicated.
- Warn patients to avoid taking antacids with milk or foods high in vitamin D.
- Advise patients to avoid taking antacids with other oral medications because they may interfere with absorption.
- Guide patients on a sodium-restricted diet to check antacid labels for sodium content.
- Alert patients to consult with a health care provider before taking self-prescribed antacids for longer than 2 weeks.
- Inform patients on the use of relaxation techniques.

Self-Administration
- Teach patients how to take antacids correctly. Chewable tablets must be thoroughly chewed and followed with water. With liquid antacids, patients should follow the antacid with 2 to 4 oz of water. Increased amounts of water with antacids increases gastric emptying time.

Side Effects
- Direct patients to avoid foods and beverages that can cause gastric irritation (high-fat or spicy meals; caffeine-containing coffee and soda; alcohol).
- Explain to patients that stools may become speckled or white.

Evaluate Outcomes [Evaluation]
- Determine the effectiveness of the antiulcer treatment and the presence of side effects. The patient should be free of pain, and healing should progress.

PROTOTYPE DRUG CHART

Famotidine

Drug Class	Dosage
Antiulcer: Histamine₂ blocker	Gastric or duodenal ulcer: A: PO: 40 mg for 4–8 wk A: IV: 20 mg q12h
Contraindications	**Drug-Lab-Food Interactions**
Hypersensitivity *Caution:* Pregnancy, breast-feeding, infection, vitamin B₁₂ deficiency, renal disease, gastric cancer, older adults, neonates	Drug: Decreased absorption of iron; decreased effects of ketoconazole, naproxen; increased action of metformin Lab: Increased serum alkaline phosphatase
Pharmacokinetics	**Pharmacodynamics**
Absorption: PO: Well absorbed, 50% Distribution: PB: 15%–20% Metabolism: t½: 2.5–3.5 h Excretion: In urine and feces	PO: Onset: 1 h Peak: 1–3 h Duration: 10–12 h IV: Onset: 10–15 min Peak: 30 min Duration: 10–12 h
Therapeutic Effects/Uses	
To prevent and treat gastric and duodenal ulcers, pyrosis, dyspepsia, esophagitis, GERD, and GI hypersecretory conditions like Zollinger-Ellison syndrome Mechanism of action: Inhibits gastric acid secretion by inhibiting histamine₂ receptors in parietal cells	
Side Effects	**Adverse Reactions**
Headache, dizziness, drowsiness, confusion, agitation, flushing, fatigue, weakness, insomnia, dry mouth, anorexia, dysgeusia, nausea, vomiting, diarrhea, constipation, depression, rash, pruritus, arthralgia, muscle cramps, edema, erectile dysfunction	Palpitations, gynecomastia, vitamin B₁₂ deficiency, seizures *Life-threatening:* Anaphylactoid reactions, agranulocytosis, leukopenia, thrombocytopenia, pancytopenia, dysrhythmia, bronchospasm

A, Adult; *GERD*, gastroesophageal reflux disease; *GI*, gastrointestinal; *h*, hour; *IV*, intravenous; *min*, minute; *PB*, protein binding; *PO*, by mouth; *q*, every; *t½*, half-life; *wk*, week.

TABLE 46.5 Antiulcer Drugs: Histamine₂ Blockers

Drug	Route and Dosage	Uses and Considerations
Cimetidine	Gastric and duodenal ulcers: A: PO: 800 mg/d at bedtime or 400 mg bid or 300 mg qid with meals and bedtime for 8–12 weeks; *max:* 1200 mg/d A: IV/IM: 300 mg q6h for active treatment	To treat gastric and duodenal ulcers, GERD, gastritis, Zollinger-Ellison syndrome, pyrosis, and dyspepsia. May cause headache, dizziness, diarrhea, drowsiness, agitation, gynecomastia, and erectile dysfunction. PB: 20%; t½: 2 h
Famotidine	See Prototype Drug Chart: Famotidine	
Nizatidine	Duodenal/gastric ulcers: A: PO: 150 mg q12h or 300 mg at bedtime for 8 weeks; *max:* 300 mg/d	To treat duodenal/gastric ulcers, dyspepsia, pyrosis, and GERD. May cause dizziness, cough, irritability, headache, fever, rhinitis, nasal congestion, vomiting, diarrhea, vitamin B₁₂ deficiency, and erectile dysfunction. PB: 35%; t½: 1–2 h

A, adult; *bid*, twice daily; *d*, day; *GERD*, gastroesophageal reflux disease; *h*, hour; *IM*, intramuscular; *IV*, intravenous; *max*, maximum; *min*, minute; *PB*, protein binding; *PO*, by mouth; *qid*, four times a day; *t½*, half-life.

Table 46.5 lists the H₂ blockers and their dosages, uses, and considerations.

Side Effects and Adverse Reactions

Side effects and adverse reactions of H₂ blockers include headache, agitation, dizziness, nausea, vomiting, constipation or diarrhea, pruritus, skin rash, vitamin B₁₂ deficiency, erectile dysfunction, and blood dyscrasias. Famotidine has fewer side effects than cimetidine.

Drug and Laboratory Interactions

Cimetidine interacts with many drugs. By inhibiting hepatic drug metabolism, it enhances the effects of oral anticoagulants, theophylline, caffeine, phenytoin, diazepam, propranolol, phenobarbital, and calcium channel blockers. Cimetidine can cause an increase in blood urea nitrogen (BUN), serum creatinine, and serum alkaline phosphatase. Cimetidine should not be taken with iron because its H₂-blocking action could be decreased.

CLINICAL JUDGMENT [NURSING PROCESS]
Antiulcer: Histamine₂ Blocker

Concept: Pain
- An unpleasant feeling of discomfort usually associated with tissue damage

Recognize Cues [Assessment]
- Determine the patient's pain, including the type, duration, severity, frequency, and location.
- Evaluate gastrointestinal (GI) complaints.
- Check mental status.
- Assess fluid and electrolyte imbalances, including intake and output.
- Monitor gastric pH (>5 is desired), blood urea nitrogen (BUN), and creatinine.
- Determine a drug history and report probable drug-drug interactions.

Analyze Cues and Prioritize Hypothesis [Patient Problems]
- Acute pain
- Injury
- Gastric irritation
- Discomfort

Generate Solutions [Planning]
- The patient will report that abdominal pain has decreased after 1 to 2 weeks of drug therapy.

Take Action [Nursing Interventions]
- ⚡ Be alert that older adults have less gastric acid and need reduced doses of the drug. Metabolic acidosis must be prevented.

Patient Teaching
General
- ⚡ Teach patients to report pain, coughing, or vomiting of blood.
- Advise patients to avoid smoking because it can hamper the effectiveness of the drug.
- Remind patients that the drug must be taken exactly as prescribed to be effective.
- Direct patients to separate famotidine and iron dosage by at least 1 hour.
- ⚡ Warn patients not to drive a motor vehicle or engage in dangerous activities until stabilized on the drug.
- Tell patients that drug-induced erectile dysfunction is reversible.
- Educate patients in the use of relaxation techniques to decrease anxiety.

Diet
- Teach patients to eat foods high in vitamin B_{12} to avoid deficiency from drug therapy.
- Alert patients to avoid foods and liquids that cause gastric irritation, such as caffeine-containing beverages, alcohol, and spices.

Evaluate Outcomes [Evaluation]
- Determine the effectiveness of drug therapy and the presence of any side effects or adverse reactions. The patient should be free of pain, and healing should progress.

Proton Pump Inhibitors

Proton pump inhibitors (gastric acid secretion inhibitors, gastric acid pump inhibitors) suppress gastric acid secretion by inhibiting the hydrogen/potassium ATPase enzyme system located in the gastric parietal cells. They tend to inhibit gastric acid secretion up to 90% more than the H_2 blockers (histamine antagonists). These agents block the final step of acid production.

Omeprazole was the first PPI marketed, followed by lansoprazole, rabeprazole, pantoprazole, esomeprazole, and dexlansoprazole, a delayed-release oral capsule. These agents are effective in suppressing gastric acid secretions and are used to treat peptic ulcers and GERD. With lansoprazole, ulcer relief usually occurs in 1 week. Rabeprazole is more effective in treating duodenal ulcers than gastric ulcers, but it is most effective for treating GERD and hypersecretory disease (Zollinger–Ellison syndrome). Pantoprazole is prescribed to treat short-term erosive GERD. Intravenous (IV) pantoprazole is also reported as effective in treating Zollinger–Ellison syndrome. Esomeprazole has the highest success rate for healing erosive GERD, more so than omeprazole. Omeprazole promotes irreversible hydrogen or potassium ATPase inhibition until new enzyme is synthesized, which could take days, whereas rabeprazole causes reversible ATPase inhibition. Dexlansoprazole is prescribed to treat erosive esophagitis and symptomatic nonerosive GERD. All PPIs in large doses can be combined with antibiotics to treat *H. pylori*. Prototype Drug Chart: Pantoprazole lists the pharmacological data for pantoprazole.

Two combination medications involving PPIs are omeprazole with sodium bicarbonate and esomeprazole with naproxen. These combinations are used to treat GERD, erosive esophagitis, and gastric or duodenal ulcers.

> ⚡ **PATIENT SAFETY**
>
> **Do Not Confuse…**
> - **Protonix**, a PPI, with **Lotronex**, a serotonin 5-HT_3 receptor antagonist used for irritable bowel syndrome.
> - **AcipHex**, a PPI, with **Aricept**, an Alzheimer drug.
> - **Nexium**, a PPI, with **Nexavar**, a biologic response modifier.
> - **Rabeprazole**, a PPI, with **aripiprazole**, an atypical antipsychotic.
> - **Misoprostol**, an antiulcer agent, with **mifepristone**, a postcoital contraceptive agent.

Pharmacokinetics and Pharmacodynamics

The duration of action for pantoprazole is 24 hours. This drug has a half-life of 1 to 10 hours and is highly protein bound (99%). PPIs should usually be taken before meals. Caution should be used in patients with hepatic impairment, and liver enzymes should be monitored. Possible side effects include headache, dizziness, diarrhea or constipation, abdominal pain, vitamin B_{12} deficiency, and hypomagnesemia. Prolonged use of PPIs may increase the risk for cancer, although this has only been proven in mice, not humans.

Table 46.6 lists the PPIs and their dosages, uses, and considerations.

Drug Interactions

PPIs can enhance the action of digoxin, oral anticoagulants, certain benzodiazepines, and phenytoin because they interfere with liver metabolism of these drugs.

PROTOTYPE DRUG CHART
Pantoprazole

Drug Class	Dosage
Antiulcer: Proton pump inhibitor	GERD: A: PO/IV: 40 mg/d 30 min to 1 h before first meal of day for 8 wk PO and for 10 d IV; give IV over at least 2 min or an infusion over 15 minutes; *max*: 80 mg/d
Contraindications	**Drug-Lab-Food Interactions**
Hypersensitivity, proton pump inhibitors *Caution:* Hepatic impairment, hypocalcemia, hypokalemia, hypomagnesemia, gastric cancer, CDAD, diarrhea, hypoparathyroidism, systemic lupus erythematosus, bone fractures, osteoporosis, osteopenia, zinc/vitamin B$_{12}$ deficiency, older adults, pregnancy, breast-feeding, infants	Drug: May interfere with absorption of ampicillin, ketoconazole, digoxin; statins increase PPI absorption and bioavailability; thiazide, loop, and potassium-sparing diuretics; beta blockers, ACE inhibitors, and ARBs may lead to hypomagnesemia. Food: Food decreases peak levels. Herb: St. John's wort decreases drug levels
Pharmacokinetics	**Pharmacodynamics**
Absorption: Rapidly absorbed in GI tract Distribution: PB: 99% Metabolism: t½: 3.5–10 h Excretion: Primarily in urine, also in bile and feces	PO: Onset: 2.5 h Peak: 2.5 h Duration: 24 h IV: Onset: 15–30 min Peak: UK Duration: 24 h
Therapeutic Effects/Uses	
To treat gastric/duodenal ulcers, GERD, esophagitis, dyspepsia, pyrosis, *Helicobacter pylori* infection, and Zollinger–Ellison syndrome and to prevent NSAID-induced ulcers Mechanism of action: Suppresses gastric acid secretion by inhibiting hydrogen/potassium ATPase enzyme in gastric parietal cells	
Side Effects	**Adverse Reactions**
Headache, dizziness, drowsiness, depression, blurred vision, tinnitus, fatigue, dry mouth, nausea, vomiting, flatulence, constipation, diarrhea, abdominal pain, infection, edema, weakness, arthralgia, myalgia, vitamin B$_{12}$ deficiency, weight gain/loss	GI bleeding, anemia, hypomagnesemia, hypocalcemia, hypokalemia, hypertriglyceridemia, elevated hepatic enzymes, lupus-like symptoms, hyponatremia, bone fractures, rhabdomyolysis *Life-threatening:* Leukopenia, agranulocytosis, neutropenia, thrombocytopenia, CDAD, hepatic failure

>, Greater than; *A*, adult; *ACE*, angiotensin-converting enzyme; *ARB*, angiotensin II receptor blockers; *CDAD*, *Clostridium difficile* associated diarrhea; *d*, day; *GERD*, gastroesophageal reflux disease; *GI*, gastrointestinal; *h*, hour; *IV*, intravenous; *max*, maximum; *min*, minute; *NSAID*, nonsteroidal antiinflammatory drug; *PB*, protein binding; *PO*, by mouth; *PPI*, protein pump inhibitor; *t½*, half-life; *UK*, unknown; *wk*, week.

TABLE 46.6 Antiulcer Drugs: Proton Pump Inhibitors, Pepsin Inhibitors, and Prostaglandin Analogues

Drug	Route and Dosage	Uses and Considerations
Proton Pump Inhibitors (Gastric Acid Secretion Inhibitors)		
Esomeprazole	GERD: A: PO: 20 mg qd 1 h before first meal of the day for 4–8 wk; *max*: 40 mg/d	For GERD, dyspepsia, *Helicobacter pylori* infection, pyrosis, Zollinger-Ellison syndrome, and NSAID-induced ulcer prophylaxis. May cause headache, dry mouth, abdominal pain, dyspepsia, nausea, diarrhea, GI bleeding, constipation, and flatulence. PB: 97%; *t½*: 1.5 h
Lansoprazole	Gastric ulcer: A: PO: 1 30 mg/d in the morning 30-min ac for up to 8 wk; *max*: 30 mg/d	To treat duodenal/gastric ulcers, GERD, dyspepsia, *H. pylori* infection, pyrosis, and Zollinger-Ellison syndrome, and for NSAID-induced ulcer prophylaxis. May cause headache, dizziness, abdominal pain, nausea, diarrhea, constipation, and rash. PB: 97%; *t½*: 0.5–2.5 h
Omeprazole	Gastric ulcer: Delayed release: A: PO: 40 mg/d for 4–8 wk; *max*: 40 mg/d	To treat gastric/duodenal ulcers, GERD, dyspepsia, pyrosis, Zollinger-Ellison syndrome, and *H. pylori* infection. May cause headache, dizziness, nausea, vomiting, diarrhea, abdominal pain, flatulence, constipation, rash, and weakness. PB: 95%; *t½*: 30–60 min

TABLE 46.6 Antiulcer Drugs: Proton Pump Inhibitors, Pepsin Inhibitors, and Prostaglandin Analogues—cont'd

Drug	Route and Dosage	Uses and Considerations
Pantoprazole	See Prototype Drug Chart: Pantoprazole	
Rabeprazole	Duodenal ulcer: A: PO: 20 mg/d in morning up to 4 wk; *max:* 40 mg/d	For duodenal ulcer, GERD, Zollinger-Ellison syndrome, esophagitis, and *H. pylori* infection. May cause headache, pharyngitis, arthralgia, myalgia, dizziness, nausea, abdominal pain, flatulence, vomiting, diarrhea, constipation, and elevated hepatic enzymes. PB: 96.3%; $t\frac{1}{2}$: 1–2 h
Dexlansoprazole	GERD: Delayed release: A: PO: Initially 30 mg/d for up to 4–8 wk; *max:* 60 mg/d	For esophagitis, pyrosis, and GERD. May cause headache, nausea, abdominal pain, vomiting, diarrhea, constipation, flatulence, and infection. PB: 96.1%–98.8%; $t\frac{1}{2}$: 1–2 h
Pepsin Inhibitor		
Sucralfate	See Prototype Drug Chart: Sucralfate	
Prostaglandin Analogue		
Misoprostol	A: PO: 100–200 mcg qid with meals and at bedtime with food; *max:* 800 mcg/d	For prevention of NSAID-induced ulcer. May be taken during NSAID therapy, including with aspirin. May cause headache, dyspepsia, nausea, vomiting, flatulence, diarrhea, abdominal pain, constipation, chills, shivering, and hyperthermia. PB: <90%; $t\frac{1}{2}$: 20–4 min
Combinations		
Omeprazole 20 mg and sodium bicarbonate 1100 mg	Active duodenal ulcer: A: PO: 20 mg qd up to 4 wks	To treat gastric/duodenal ulcers, GERD, and pyrosis and to prevent stress gastritis. May cause headache, dizziness, elevated hepatic enzymes, weakness, abdominal pain, flatulence, nausea, vomiting, constipation, and diarrhea. PB: omeprazole 95%, sodium bicarbonate UK; $t\frac{1}{2}$: omeprazole 30–60 min, sodium bicarbonate UK
Esomeprazole and naproxen	A: PO: 1 tablet (esomeprazole 20 mg and naproxen 375 mg or esomeprazole 20 mg and naproxen 500 mg) bid; *max:* esomeprazole 40 mg/d and naproxen 1000 mg/d	To prevent NSAID-associated gastric ulcers. May cause headache, dizziness, drowsiness, ecchymosis, pyrosis, nausea, gastritis, abdominal pain, constipation, diarrhea, flatulence, peripheral edema, palpitations, and purpura. PB: esomeprazole 97%, naproxen 99%; $t\frac{1}{2}$: esomeprazole 1.2–1.5 h, naproxen 12–17 h

A, adult; *bid*, two times a day; *d*, day; *GERD*, gastroesophageal reflux disease; *GI*, gastrointestinal; *h*, hour; *max*, maximum; *min*, minute; *NSAID*, nonsteroidal antiinflammatory drug; *PB*, protein binding; *PO*, by mouth; *qd*, every day; *qid*, four times a day; $t\frac{1}{2}$, half-life; *UK*, unknown; *wk*, week; *y*, year.

Pepsin Inhibitors (Mucosal Protective Drugs)

Sucralfate, a complex of sulfated sucrose and aluminum hydroxide, is classified as a pepsin inhibitor, or *mucosal protective drug*. It is nonabsorbable and combines with protein to form a viscous substance that covers the ulcer and protects it from acid and pepsin. This drug does not neutralize acid or decrease acid secretions.

The dosage of sucralfate is 1 g, usually four times a day, before meals and at bedtime. If antacids are added to decrease pain, they should be given either 30 minutes before or 30 minutes after the administration of sucralfate. Because sucralfate is not systemically absorbed, side effects are few; however, it can cause dry mouth, headache, drowsiness, dizziness, and constipation. If the drug is stored at room temperature in an airtight container, it will remain stable for up to 2 years. Prototype Drug Chart: Sucralfate lists the pharmacological data for sucralfate.

Pharmacokinetics

Less than 5% of sucralfate is absorbed by the GI tract. It has a half-life of 6 to 20 hours, and 90% of the drug is excreted in feces within 48 hours. However, any drug that is absorbed systemically is excreted primarily in the urine.

Pharmacodynamics

Sucralfate promotes healing by adhering to the ulcer surface. Onset of action occurs within 1 to 2 hours, and duration of action is usually 6 hours. Sucralfate decreases the absorption of tetracycline, phenytoin, fat-soluble vitamins, and the antibacterial agents ciprofloxacin and norfloxacin. Antacids decrease the effects of sucralfate.

Prostaglandin Analogue Antiulcer Drug

Misoprostol, a synthetic prostaglandin analogue, is a drug used to prevent and treat gastric ulcer. It appears to suppress gastric acid secretion and to increase cytoprotective mucus in the GI tract. It causes a moderate decrease in pepsin secretion. Misoprostol is considered as effective as cimetidine. Patients who report gastric distress from NSAIDs such as aspirin or indomethacin prescribed for long-term therapy can benefit from misoprostol. When a patient takes high doses of NSAIDs, misoprostol is frequently recommended for the duration of the NSAID therapy. Misoprostol is contraindicated during pregnancy and for females of childbearing age. Side effects include headache, abdominal pain, nausea, vomiting, flatulence, diarrhea, and constipation.

Table 46.6 lists the pharmacological data for the PPIs, pepsin inhibitors, and a prostaglandin analogue.

PROTOTYPE DRUG CHART

Sucralfate

Drug Class	Dosage
Antiulcer: Pepsin inhibitor	Duodenal ulcer: A: PO: 1 g qid 1 h before meals and at bedtime for 4–8 wk; *max:* 4 g/d

Contraindications	Drug-Lab-Food Interactions
Hypersensitivity *Caution:* Renal failure, diabetes mellitus, dysphagia, dialysis, pregnancy, breast-feeding,	Drug: Decreased effects with tetracycline, phenytoin, digoxin; altered absorption with fluoroquinolones, antacids, ketoconazole, furosemide, lansoprazole, thyroid hormones

Pharmacokinetics	Pharmacodynamics
Absorption: PO: Minimal absorption Distribution: PB: UK Metabolism: t½: 6–20 h Excretion: In urine	PO: Onset: 1–2 h Peak: UK Duration: 6 h

Therapeutic Effects/Uses
To prevent gastric mucosal injury from drug-induced ulcers (aspirin, NSAIDs); to treat duodenal ulcers
Mechanism of action: In combination with gastric acid, forms a protective covering on the ulcer surface

Side Effects	Adverse Reactions
Dizziness, drowsiness, headache, back pain, nausea, vomiting, flatulence, constipation, dry mouth, rash, pruritus	Hyperglycemia, hypophosphatemia, angioedema

A, Adult; *d*, day; *h*, hour; *max*, maximum; *NSAID*, nonsteroidal antiinflammatory drugs; *PB*, protein binding; *PO*, by mouth; *qid*, four times a day; *t½*, half-life; *UK*, unknown; *wk*, week.

CLINICAL JUDGMENT [NURSING PROCESS]
Antiulcer: Pepsin Inhibitors

Concept: Pain
- An unpleasant feeling of discomfort usually associated with tissue damage

Recognize Cues [Assessment]
- Evaluate the patient's pain, including the type, duration, severity, and frequency. Ulcer pain usually occurs after meals and during the night.
- Determine the patient's renal function. Report urine output of less than 600 mL/day or less than 30 mL/h.
- Assess for fluid and electrolyte imbalances.
- Measure gastric pH (>5 is desired).

Analyze Cues and Prioritize Hypothesis [Patient Planning]
- Acute pain
- Injury
- Gastric irritation
- Discomfort

Generate Solutions [Planning]
- The patient will report relief of abdominal pain after 1 to 2 weeks of antiulcer drug management.

Take Action [Nursing Interventions]
- Administer drug on an empty stomach.
- Administer antacid 30 minutes before or 30 minutes after sucralfate. Allow 1 to 2 hours to elapse between sucralfate and other prescribed drugs; sucralfate binds with certain drugs (e.g., tetracycline, phenytoin), reducing their effect.

Patient Teaching
General
- Advise patients to take the prescribed drug exactly as ordered. Therapy usually requires 4 to 8 weeks for optimal ulcer healing. Advise patients to continue to take the drug even if they are feeling better.
- Increase fluids, dietary bulk, and exercise to prevent constipation.
- Educate patients in the use of relaxation techniques.
- Monitor for severe, persistent constipation.
- Emphasize the need for follow-up medical care.
- Emphasize cessation of smoking as indicated.

Side Effects
- ⚡ Direct patients to report pain, coughing, or vomiting of blood.

Diet
- Teach patients to avoid liquids and foods that can cause gastric irritation, such as caffeine-containing beverages, alcohol, certain fats, and spices.

Evaluate Outcomes [Evaluation]
- Determine the effectiveness of the antiulcer treatment and the presence of any side effects. The patient should be free of pain, and healing should progress

CLINICAL JUDGMENT CASE STUDY

A 48-year-old patient reports a gnawing, aching pain in the abdominal area that usually occurs several hours after eating. He says that over-the-counter antacids help somewhat, but the pain has recently intensified. Diagnostic tests indicate that he has a duodenal ulcer.

1. Differentiate between peptic ulcer, gastric ulcer, and duodenal ulcer. Explain your answer.
2. What are the predisposing factors related to peptic ulcers? What additional information do you need from the patient?
3. What nonpharmacologic measures can you suggest to alleviate symptoms related to peptic ulcer?
4. The health care provider prescribed aluminum hydroxide and magnesium hydroxide 20 mL to be taken 2 hours after meals and famotidine 40 mg/day. The dose of magnesium hydroxide and aluminum hydroxide with simethicone is to be taken either 1 hour before or 1 hour after the famotidine. The patient asks the nurse the purposes for magnesium hydroxide and aluminum hydroxide with famotidine. What is the nurse's best response?
5. In what ways are famotidine and cimetidine the same, and how do they differ? Explain your answer.
6. As part of patient teaching, the nurse discusses side effects of famotidine with the patient. What is the most effective way to present this information? Develop a plan.
7. The patient states that he drinks beer at lunch and has two gin and tonics in the afternoon. He states that the drinks help him relax. What nursing intervention should be taken in regard to the patient's alcohol intake and smoking?
8. What foods should he avoid?
9. A week later the patient states that he discontinued the prescribed medications because he "felt better." However, the pain recurred, and he asked whether he should resume taking the medications. What is the nurse's best response? What should be included in the patient teaching?

REVIEW QUESTIONS

1. A patient is diagnosed with peptic ulcer disease. The nurse realizes that which of these is a predisposing factor for this condition?
   a. *Helicobacter pylori*
   b. Hyposecretion of pepsin
   c. Decreased hydrochloric acid
   d. *Escherichia coli*
2. A student nurse is preparing to administer sucralfate to a patient. Which statement by the student nurse demonstrates understanding of sucralfate's mechanism of action?
   a. Sucralfate neutralizes gastric acidity.
   b. Gastric acid secretion is decreased by inhibiting histamine at histamine$_2$ receptors in parietal cells.
   c. Gastric acid secretion is suppressed by inhibiting the hydrogen/potassium adenosine triphosphatase enzyme.
   d. Sucralfate combines with protein to form a viscous substance that forms a protective covering over the ulcer.
3. A patient is taking famotidine. What information should the nurse teach the patient about this drug? **Select all that apply.**
   a. The drug should be administered for 4 to 8 weeks.
   b. The drug must be administered 30 minutes before meals.
   c. The drug must be administered separately from iron by at least 1 hour.
   d. The drug must always be administered with magnesium hydroxide.
   e. Smoking should be avoided while taking this drug.
   f. Foods high in vitamin B_{12} should be increased in the diet.
4. When a patient reports pain accompanying a peptic ulcer, why should the nurse give an antacid?
   a. Antacids decrease gastrointestinal motility.
   b. Antacids decrease gastric acid secretion.
   c. Antacids strengthen the lower esophageal sphincter's action.
   d. Antacids neutralize hydrochloric acid and reduce pepsin activity.
5. A patient is taking famotidine to inhibit gastric secretions. Which side effects of famotidine will the nurse teach the patient? **Select all that apply.**
   a. Dizziness
   b. Headaches
   c. Hypokalemia
   d. Hyperkalemia
   e. Blurred vision
   f. Erectile dysfunction
6. The patient is taking esomeprazole for erosive gastroesophageal reflux disease. Which should the nurse include in patient teaching?
   a. Take the medication daily with breakfast.
   b. Healing should occur in 1 week.
   c. This medication decreases stomach acid secretion.
   d. A blood test to check kidney function should be done.

UNIT XIV Eye, Ear, and Skin Drugs

47

Eye and Ear Disorders

http://evolve.elsevier.com/McCuistion/pharmacology

OBJECTIVES

- Outline the anatomy and physiology of the eyes.
- Describe the disorders of the eye.
- Summarize the drugs used to treat ophthalmic disorders.
- Summarize the drugs used for glaucoma and ocular hypertension.
- Discuss the three divisions of the ear and common disorders of the ear.
- Summarize drugs used to treat ear disorders.

OUTLINE

Overview of the Eye, 603
    First Layer of the Eye, 603
    Second Layer of the Eye, 604
    Third Layer of the Eye, 604
Disorders of the Eye, 604
    Infections of the Eye, 604
    Age-Related Macular Degeneration, 604
    Glaucoma: Open-Angle and Angle-Closure, 605
    Glaucoma: Primary and Secondary, 605
Ophthalmic Drugs, 605
    Drugs for Diagnostic Purposes, 605
    Antiinfectives, 605
    Antiinflammatories, 605
    Decongestants, 608
    Lubricants, 609
    Mydriatics and Cycloplegics, 609
    Drugs for Age-Related Macular Degeneration, 609
    Drugs for Inherited Retinal Dystrophies, 610

Glaucoma and Ocular Hypertension Drugs, 610
    Prostaglandin Analogues, 610
    Cholinergic Agents, 610
    Beta-Adrenergic Blockers, 610
    Alpha-Adrenergic Agonists, 612
    Carbonic Anhydrase Inhibitors, 612
    Patients With Eye Disorders: General Suggestions for Teaching, 613
Overview and Disorders of the Ear, 614
    Divisions of the Ear, 615
    Disorders of the Ear, 615
Drugs for the Ear, 615
    Antiinfectives, 615
    Antihistamines and Decongestants, 616
    Cerumenolytics, 616
    Patients With Ear Disorders: General Suggestions for Teaching, 617
Clinical Judgment Single-Episode Case Study, 618
Review Questions, 618

OVERVIEW OF THE EYE

Protected within the orbits of the skull, the eyeballs are controlled by the third, fourth, and sixth cranial nerves and are connected to six extraocular muscles. The eye has three layers: (1) the cornea and sclera; (2) the choroid, iris, and ciliary body; and (3) the retina. Fig. 47.1 illustrates the basic structures of the eye.

First Layer of the Eye

The cornea, the anterior covering of the eye, is transparent and allows light to enter the eye. It has no blood vessels and receives nutrition from the aqueous humor. An abraded cornea is susceptible to infection. Loss of corneal transparency is usually caused by increased **intraocular pressure (IOP)**.

The sclera is the opaque, white fibrous envelope of the eye. Within the sclera are the posterior and anterior chambers. The posterior chamber has a blind spot around the optic nerve that is insensitive to light. The lens is held in place by ligaments and separates these two chambers. The normally transparent lens focuses light on the retina by changing its shape through a process called accommodation.

The anterior chamber, filled with aqueous humor secreted by the ciliary body, lies in front of the lens. The normally clear fluid, **aqueous humor**, flows into the anterior chamber through a space between the lens and iris. The excess fluid drains through the trabecular meshwork structure of the eye and out the canal of Schlemm, and a much smaller fraction of the fluid exits through the uveoscleral structure at the root of the iris (Fig. 47.2A).

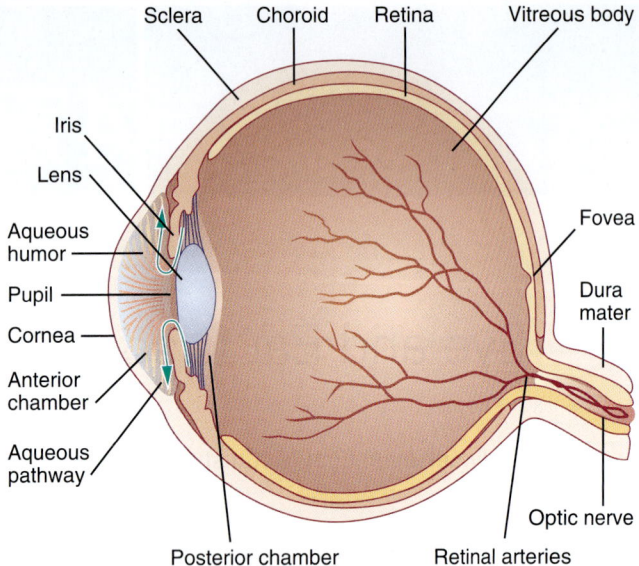

Fig. 47.1 Basic structures of the eye.

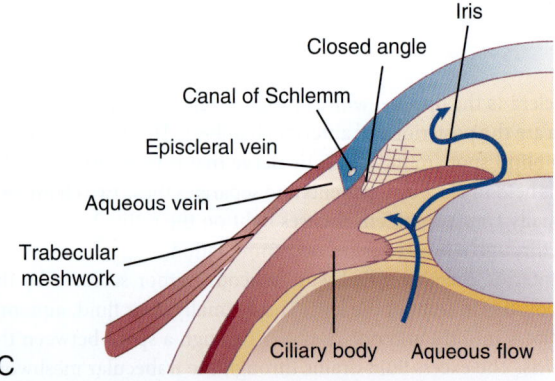

Fig. 47.2 (A) Normal flow of aqueous humor. (B) Open-angle glaucoma. (C) Angle-closure glaucoma.

Second Layer of the Eye

The choroid, iris, and ciliary body—the thickened part of the vascular covering of the eye that provides attachment to ligaments and support to the lens—constitute the second layer. The choroid absorbs light, and the iris surrounds the pupil and gives the eye its color. By dilating and constricting, the iris controls the quantity of light that reaches the lens.

Third Layer of the Eye

The retina, the third layer, consists of nerves, rods, and cones that serve as visual sensory receptors. The retina is connected to the brain via the optic nerve.

The eyebrows, eyelashes, eyelids, tears, and corneal and conjunctival reflexes all serve to protect the eye. Bilateral blinking occurs every few seconds during waking hours to keep the eye moist and free of foreign material.

DISORDERS OF THE EYE

Eye problems may occur as a result of injuries, infections, or specific noninfectious eye disorders, such as glaucoma and macular degeneration. The most common eye condition is an inflammation of the membrane (conjunctiva) covering the eye and inner eyelids.

Infections of the Eye

Conjunctivitis is also called "pink eye" and can occur because of allergens, viruses, and bacteria. Examples of other ocular conditions caused by pathogens include the following:

- Blepharitis, an infection of the margins of the eyelid
- Chalazion, an infection of the meibomian glands of the eyelids that may produce cysts, causing blockage of the ducts
- Bacterial and fungal endophthalmitis, infection and inflammation of structures of the inner eye
- Hordeolum, a local infection of eyelash follicles and glands on lid margins, also known as a *stye*
- Infectious keratitis, a corneal infection and inflammation
- Infectious uveitis, an infection of the vascular layer of the eye (ciliary body, choroid, and iris)

Age-Related Macular Degeneration

Age-related macular degeneration (AMD) is a leading cause of vision loss in older adults. AMD is a deterioration of the macula, which is the part of the eye responsible for sharp central vision; damage to the macula blurs central vision in the affected eye. Two forms of AMD include wet (neovascular or exudative), which progresses quite rapidly, and dry (atrophic), which slowly destroys vision over a period of years.

Dry Age-Related Macular Degeneration

Dry AMD is more common and occurs in response to the deposit of extracellular material, called drusen, under the retina. This is coupled with thinning of the retina, which eventually stops functioning properly. Vision loss occurs gradually. Occasionally, dry AMD will progress to wet AMD.

Wet Age-Related Macular Degeneration

Wet or exudative AMD is associated with the growth of abnormal blood vessels behind the retina. Leakage of fluid from these vessels collects behind the retina and shifts the macula from its normal position. Wet macular degeneration accounts for 10% of AMD cases; however, it causes greater destruction and is responsible for 80% of cases in which patients experience severe vision loss or become legally blind.

Glaucoma: Open-Angle and Angle-Closure

Glaucoma can lead to vision loss or blindness because of damage to the optic nerve. Overproduction of the aqueous humor or improper drainage can cause the IOP to increase, which presses against the optic nerve, damaging it. There are two types of glaucoma, open-angle and angle closure. In open-angle glaucoma, the trabecular network is open but becomes clogged (see Fig. 47.2B). Over time, as blockage of the trabecular network worsens, the IOP gradually increases, which damages the optic nerve. In angle-closure glaucoma, also known as *closed-angle* or *narrow-angle glaucoma*, the iris is situated close to the drainage angle, blocking the trabecular network (see Fig. 47.2C). Because the excess aqueous humor cannot drain, it builds up within the eye and increases IOP. When the drainage angle is completely blocked, eye pressure increases quickly, and the vision becomes suddenly blurred; this is a medical emergency and must be treated immediately. Management of angle-closure glaucoma is often surgical; however, pharmacologic management is sometimes indicated. ⚡ Anticholinergic drugs (see Chapter 16) can cause mydriasis and can worsen angle-closure glaucoma.

TABLE 47.1 Diagnostic Stains for Eye Disorders

Diagnostic Aid	Purpose
Fluorescein sodium, ophthalmic	Stains the anterior segment of the eye to visualize the anterior ocular surface for defects and for contact lens fitting. When viewed through the cobalt blue filter of the ophthalmoscope or under a wood lamp, corneal scratches and lesions fluoresce a bright yellow green.
Rose bengal, ophthalmic	Stains the anterior segment of the eye to visualize defects or dry eye. Defective and normal cells are stained a pink-violet color. Staining of normal cells and stinging and mild tissue toxicity limit use.
Lissamine green	Stains the anterior segment of the eye to visualize defects and dry eyes. Defective cells are stained green.

Glaucoma: Primary and Secondary

Glaucoma is further classified as either primary or secondary. Primary glaucoma occurs because of a pathologic change within the eye that happens without a known cause. Primary open-angle glaucoma, the most common type of glaucoma, is a chronic condition that develops slowly over time as the trabecular meshwork becomes clogged for unknown reasons. Secondary glaucoma occurs in response to a known cause such as injury, disease, or medication. Although a number of drugs can increase the risk of secondary glaucoma, those that cause pupillary dilation are particularly problematic because they give the iris more flexibility to move toward the drainage angle, blocking the trabecular meshwork. People who are at risk for glaucoma should avoid decongestants. Certain herbal preparations (e.g., goldenseal, ephedra, and bitter orange) can also create problems when given to patients who have glaucoma.

OPHTHALMIC DRUGS

Drugs applied to the eyes are known as ocular or ophthalmic drugs. Most drugs used to treat eye conditions are topical medications developed specifically for the eyes. Topical ocular preparations include solutions, suspensions, ointments, and gel. Care must be taken when administering medications to the eye. Techniques for administering eye drops and ophthalmic ointments are described in Chapter 10. The tip of the dispensing apparatus should remain sterile and must not be touched. Patients who wear contact lenses should be knowledgeable about the products associated with the lenses. Wearing contact lenses is usually discouraged; however, if contact lenses must be worn, patients should wait at least 15 minutes after instilling ocular drugs before reinserting the contact lenses.

Drugs for Diagnostic Purposes

Topical anesthetics are used in selected aspects of a comprehensive eye examination and various ophthalmic procedures. Ophthalmic anesthetics act by locally blocking the pain signals at the eye's nerve endings. The two most common topical ophthalmic anesthetics are proparacaine hydrochloride (HCl) and tetracaine HCl. Both medications, available in solutions, are administered as drops. Ophthalmic anesthetics should be administered by a trained clinician.

Corneal anesthesia starts usually within 15 seconds and lasts about 15 minutes. The blink reflex is temporarily lost; therefore the corneal epithelium may become dry. Protecting the eye from irritating chemicals, foreign bodies, and corneal scratches is important. The patient must be instructed that the affected eye will be insensitive to touch and to not rub, touch, or wipe the affected eye. Contact lenses may be reinserted after the anesthetic has completely worn off, usually after 20 minutes.

Diagnostic stains (Table 47.1) are frequently used to locate extraocular lesions or foreign objects, evaluate dry eyes, or evaluate extraocular changes. Stains may be combined with local anesthetics to allow more thorough examination by alleviating pain associated with the examination. Patients should be informed that these drugs will cause discoloring of the external eye but dissipate over several hours; they may also stain nasal secretions if the lacrimal ducts (tear ducts) are patent, and they discolor soft contact lenses. Contact lenses should be removed before administration, and the eye should be rinsed with sterile normal saline solution after the procedure. Contact lenses can be replaced after 1 hour.

Antiinfectives

Antiinfectives (Table 47.2) are frequently used for eye infections. Bacterial conjunctivitis usually requires antiinfective therapy to either kill or inhibit the spread of bacteria. Some ocular viral infections (e.g., cytomegalovirus and herpes simplex virus) may require antiviral therapy. Many antiinfectives may also contain antiinflammatories. The US Food and Drug Administration (FDA) approved Lotilaner ophthalmic in 2023 for the treatment of antiparasitic infections related to Demodex blepharitis in adults. Treatment is for 6 weeks. There is limited systemic absorption with topical ophthalmics, and side effects are limited to local reactions.

Before administering ophthalmic antiinfectives, the nurse should screen the patient for previous allergic reactions. Noninfectious conjunctivitis and local skin and eye irritation are possible side effects of ophthalmic antiinfective drugs.

Antiinflammatories

Inflammatory conditions of the eye not related to infectious pathogens often require treatment with antiinflammatory drugs (Table 47.3). If the inflammation is secondary to a bacterial or fungal infection, an antibiotic or antifungal agent is included in the medication regimen.

TABLE 47.2 Ophthalmic Antiinfectives

Generic	Route and Dosage[a]	Uses and Considerations
Antibacterials		
Ciprofloxacin HCl, 0.3% ophthalmic solution and ointment	*Bacterial conjunctivitis:* Sol: A: 1–2 gtts q2h while awake for 2 d, then q4h while awake for 5 d *Bacterial conjunctivitis:* Oint: A: ½-inch ribbon tid for 2 d, then ½-inch ribbon bid for 5 d *Corneal ulcer:* Sol: A: Day 1: 2 gtts q 15 min for 6 h, then 2 gtts q 30 min until ending of day 1; Day 2: 2 gtts q h; Day: 3–14: 2 gtts q4h	For bacterial conjunctivitis and corneal ulceration. ⚠ Black-Box Warning
Gentamicin sulfate, 0.3% ophthalmic solution and ointment	Sol 0.3%: A: 1–2 gtts q4h; may increase to 2 gtts q1h for severe infections Oint 0.3%: A: ½-inch ribbon 2–3 times daily	For blepharitis, blepharoconjunctivitis, bacterial conjunctivitis, corneal ulcer, dacryocystitis, keratitis, keratoconjunctivitis, acute meibomianitis, and bacterial and fungal corneal lesion/abrasion. May cause ototoxicity (of the eighth cranial nerve) that could be permanent. ⚠ Black-Box Warning
Levofloxacin, 0.5% ophthalmic solution	A: 1–2 gtts q2h; max: 8 doses/d for 1–2 d, then q4h; *max:* 4 doses/d for 5 d	For bacterial conjunctivitis and corneal ulcers. (Systemic therapy is required for treatment of hordeolum, dacryocystitis, and meibomianitis.) ⚠ Black-Box Warning
Neomycin, polymyxin B sulfate, bacitracin; ophthalmic	Oint: A: ½-inch ribbon q3–4h for 7–10 d Max dose: 8 applications/d for 10 d	For bacterial conjunctivitis, blepharitis, blepharoconjunctivitis, keratitis, and keratoconjunctivitis. A triple antibiotic is effective against many gram-positive and gram-negative microorganisms.
Ofloxacin, 0.3% ophthalmic solution	*Bacterial conjunctivitis:* A: 1–2 gtts q2–4h while awake for 2 d, then 1–2 gtts qid for 5 d *Bacterial corneal ulcer:* A: 1–2 gtts q30min while awake and q4–6h after bedtime; days 3–6: 1–2 gtts q1h while awake; days 7–9: 1–2 gtts qid	For bacterial conjunctivitis, bacterial corneal ulcer. ⚠ Black-Box Warning
Sulfacetamide, 10% ophthalmic solution and ointment	Sol: A: 1–2 gtts q1–3h while awake, less frequently at night Oint: A: Small ribbon 4 times during the day and at bedtime	For chlamydial conjunctivitis, corneal ulcer, and other superficial ophthalmic infections; not effective against fungal, viral, or all types of bacterial infection. Continued use may result in nonsusceptible microorganism overgrowth. Ointment may be applied at night with the ophthalmic solution. Ophthalmic sulfonamides are incompatible with preparations that contain silver salts (e.g., silver nitrate). Ointment may delay corneal wound healing. Purulent exudates that contain PABA can inactivate the drug's antibacterial activity.
Tobramycin, 0.3% ophthalmic solution and ointment	Sol: A: 1–2 gtts q4h; for severe infection, apply 2 gtts hourly until improvement is seen, then decrease frequency. Oint: A: Thin strip q8–12h. For severe infections, apply q3–4h	For superficial external ocular infections. Tobramycin may delay healing of corneal abrasion or lesions. ⚠ Black-Box Warning
Antiinfective/ Antiparasitic Lotilaner Ophthalmic	Sol: A: Instill 1 drop in eye twice daily (approximately 12 h apart) for 6 wk.	Used to treat parasitic infections of the eye caused by Demodex mites resulting in Demodex blepharitis
Antifungals Natamycin, 5% ophthalmic suspension	Sol: A: 1 gtt q1–2h for 3–4 d, then 1 gtt q3–4h for 14–21 d; *max:* 24 gtts/d	For external ocular fungal infections. Drops possess no antibacterial or antiviral activity, and prolonged treatment may result in bacterial or viral infection. Patients allergic to cheese may have sensitivity to natamycin.
Antivirals Trifluridine, 1% ophthalmic solution	A: 1 gtt q2h while awake; *max:* 9 gtts/d until corneal ulcer is re-epithelialized, then 1 gtt q4h for 7 d; *max:* 21-d treatment	For herpetic ophthalmic infections and keratoconjunctivitis caused by HSV-1 and HSV-2. ⚡ Treatment longer than 21 d can result in ocular toxicity.

>, Greater than; ≥, greater than or equal to; *A*, adult; *bid*, twice a day; *d*, day; *HSV*, herpes simplex virus; *gtt*, drops; *h*, hour; *HCl*, hydrochloride; *max*, maximum; *min*, minute; *mo*, months; *oint*, ointment; *PABA*, para-aminobenzoic acid; *q*, every; *qid*, four times a day; *sol*, solution; *tid*, three times a day; *wk*, week; *y*, year.
[a]To minimize systemic absorption, gently apply pressure on inner canthus.

TABLE 47.3 Ophthalmic Antiinflammatories

Generic	Route and Dosage	Uses and Considerations
Immunosuppressants Cyclosporine, 0.05% ophthalmic emulsion	A: 1 gtt q12h	For xerophthalmia due to ocular inflammation associated with keratoconjunctivitis sicca. Artificial tears may be used concomitantly with cyclosporine ocular drops, allowing 15 min between the products. Absolute contraindication: Patients with active ocular infection. Emulsion must be thoroughly mixed by inverting the bottle a few times to obtain a uniform, white, opaque emulsion before using. ⚠ Black-Box Warning ⚡ High-Alert Medication
NSAIDs Diclofenac sodium, 0.1% ophthalmic solution	24 h after cataract surgery: A: 1 gtt qid for 2 wk Corneal refractive surgery: A: 1–2 gtts within 1 h of surgery, then 1–2 gtts q15min after surgery, then qid 4–6 h after surgery for up to 3 d	For postoperative inflammation after cataract surgery and ocular pain/photophobia after corneal refractive surgery. Use a separate bottle for each eye. May increase ocular bleeding and delay healing. ⚠ Black-Box Warning
Flurbiprofen sodium, 0.03% ophthalmic solution	A: 1 gtt q30min starting 2 h before surgery for a total dose of 4 gtts	For prevention of intraoperative miosis. If eye involvement is bilateral, one bottle per eye should be used to avoid cross-contamination. May increase ocular bleeding and delay healing. Concomitant use with ocular corticosteroid can cause corneal erosion. ⚠ Black-Box Warning
Ketorolac tromethamine, ophthalmic solution	Allergic conjunctivitis: Sol 0.5%: A: 1 gtt qid After cataract surgery: Sol 0.5%: A: 1 gtt qid for 2 wk Sol 0.45%: A: 1 gtt bid 1 d before surgery; continue on day of surgery and for 2 wk After corneal refractive surgery: Sol 0.4%: A: 1 gtt qid for 4 d	For relief of ocular itching due to allergic conjunctivitis, postoperative inflammation after cataract surgery, and postoperative corneal refractive surgery. Use separate bottle for each eye to prevent cross-contamination. Ocular NSAIDs may result in keratitis; use for longer than 14 d postoperatively may cause corneal adverse events. May increase ocular bleeding and delay healing. ⚠ Black-Box Warning
Corticosteroids Dexamethasone, 0.1% ophthalmic solution	A: 1–2 gtts q1h while awake and q2h at night; taper to q4h	For corticosteroid-responsive ocular disorders (e.g., allergic conjunctivitis, herpes zoster ocular infection, optic neuritis, corneal injury). Can cause increased IOP, which is reversible. Can also cause optic neuritis and visual defects.
Loteprednol etabonate, 0.2% and 0.5% ophthalmic suspension; 0.5% ophthalmic gel and ointment	Allergic conjunctivitis: Susp 0.2%: A: 1 gtt qid Steroid-responsive disorders: Susp 0.5%: A: 1–2 gtts qid; may increase to 1 gtt qh if needed 24 h after ocular surgery: Susp/gel 0.5%: 1–2 gtts qid for 2 wk or Oint 0.5%: ½-inch qid for 2 wk 24 h after ocular surgery for postoperative pain: Oint 0.5%: ½-inch qid for 2 wk or Gel 0.5%: 1–2 gtts qid for 2 wk	For allergic conjunctivitis, steroid-responsive ophthalmic disorders including iritis, keratitis, ocular pain, and postoperative ocular inflammation. ⚠ Do not discontinue prematurely; ophthalmologic examination should be done after 14 d of therapy.
Prednisolone sodium phosphate 1% ophthalmic solution	Dosage must be individualized and is variable depending on nature and severity. A: 1–2 gtts qh while awake, q2h during the night; *maint*: 1 gtt q4–6 h; taper as indicated	For corticosteroid-responsive ocular disorders (e.g., allergic conjunctivitis, herpes zoster ocular infection, optic neuritis, corneal injury, postoperative ocular inflammation). Can mask other infections. May delay healing. Contraindication: Most cornea and conjunctiva viral infection, unless appropriate antiviral therapy is co-administered, and ocular fungal infection.

Continued

TABLE 47.3 Ophthalmic Antiinflammatories—cont'd

Generic	Route and Dosage	Uses and Considerations
Ophthalmic Antibacterial and Corticosteroid Combinations Refer to individual drug information for general considerations.		
Neomycin sulfate/polymyxin B sulfate/dexamethasone, ophthalmic suspension and ointment	Severe disease: Susp: A: 1–2 gtts q1h Mild disease: Susp: A/C ≥2 y: 1–2 gtts q4–6 h, taper gradually; *max*: 48 gtts/d Oint: A: ½-inch ribbon tid/qid; *max*: ½-inch oint qid	For external ocular inflammation and abrasion.
Tobramycin/dexamethasone, ophthalmic suspension 0.3–0.1% and ointment 0.3–0.1%	Susp: A: 1–2 gtts q4–6 h Oint: A: ½-inch ribbon q6–8 h	For external ocular inflammation and abrasion.
Ophthalmic Allergy Treatment Drugs		
Azelastine HCl, 0.05% ophthalmic solution	A: 1 gtt bid	For ocular pruritus due to allergic conjunctivitis. Drug can cause cephalgia, fatigue, dysgeusia, conjunctivitis, abnormal vision, and xerophthalmia.
Cromolyn sodium, 4% ophthalmic solution	A: 1–2 gtts 4–6 times/d at regular intervals	For allergic conjunctivitis. Transient ocular irritation may occur during therapy.
Epinastine, 0.05% ophthalmic solution	A: 1 gtt bid	For ocular pruritus due to allergic conjunctivitis. Does not cross the blood-brain barrier. ⚡ May cause ocular irritation and worsen pruritus. Continue treatment through period of allergen exposure, even when symptoms are absent.
Ketotifen fumarate 0.025%	A: 1 gtt q8–12h	For ocular pruritus due to allergic conjunctivitis. ⚡ Cephalgia and rhinitis may occur.
Olopatadine HCl, 0.2% ophthalmic solution	A: 1 gtt bid at an interval of 6–8 h	For allergic conjunctivitis. ⚡ Cephalgia or dysgeusia may occur during therapy. Use until offending allergen is terminated.

>, Greater than; *≥*, greater than or equal to; *A*, adult; *bid*, twice daily; *d*, day; *gtt*, drops; *h*, hour; *HCl*, hydrochloride; *IOP*, intraocular pressure; *maint*, maintenance; *max*, maximum; *min*, minute; *NSAIDs*, nonsteroidal antiinflammatory drugs; *oint*, ointment; *q*, every; *qid*, four times daily; *sol*, solution; *susp*, suspension; *tid*, thrice daily; *wk*, week; *y*, year.

Many antiinflammatories are not appropriate in patients with ocular viral infections.

Inflammation associated with keratoconjunctivitis sicca, causing lymphocytes to damage the lacrimal gland, results in fibrosis and loss of tear production, leading to xerophthalmia (dry eyes). Immunomodulators, such as cyclosporine ophthalmic emulsion, are immunosuppressants that relieve xerophthalmia by a mechanism that is different from over-the-counter (OTC) lubricants. Ophthalmic cyclosporine acts as a partial immunomodulatory that causes apoptosis of lymphocytes and allows tear production to resume.

Ophthalmic nonsteroidal antiinflammatory drugs (NSAIDs) such as diclofenac sodium and ketorolac tromethamine inhibit miosis by preventing the formation of ocular prostaglandins. Most of these drugs are used for management or prevention of ocular inflammation before and after eye surgery. Unlike corticosteroids, NSAIDs do not affect IOP (further discussed in Glaucoma and Ocular Hypertension Drugs). However, ocular NSAIDs can increase bleeding tendencies and delay corneal healing. Topical NSAIDs are not expected to increase cardiovascular risk, hepatic reactions, or other systemic adverse effects; however, ocular NSAIDs can cause bleeding of ocular tissues.

Ophthalmic corticosteroids such as dexamethasone and prednisolone acetate are another type of antiinflammatory. Corticosteroids are used to treat a number of eye conditions, such as allergic conjunctivitis, herpes zoster keratitis (not herpes simplex keratitis), corneal abrasion, postoperative ocular inflammation, and optic neuritis. ⚡ Ocular corticosteroids can mask infections and delay healing, and they are contraindicated in persons with untreated ocular infections. Corticosteroids can worsen glaucoma by reducing the outflow of aqueous humor and increasing IOP; the effects are usually reversible upon discontinuation of the drug. Prolonged use can cause open-angle glaucoma, ocular nerve damage, or visual defects. Refer to Chapter 24 for more information on corticosteroids.

When allergies are the cause of eye inflammation, ophthalmic drugs are commonly prescribed to treat the underlying cause. These allergy drugs contain antihistamines and mast cell stabilizers. Antihistamines block histamine from activating histamine receptors in the tissues. Degranulation of mast cells releases histamine and other inflammatory mediators; mast cell stabilizers prevent mast cells from degranulating. Ocular sensations that include burning, stinging, and blurred vision are common adverse effects reported. Other adverse effects include cephalgia, dysgeusia, and rhinitis.

Decongestants

Eye inflammation typically presents with redness due to vascular congestion of the conjunctiva. Ophthalmic decongestants such as phenylephrine, naphazoline, and tetrahydrozoline stimulate alpha-adrenergic receptors in the arterioles of the conjunctiva, vasoconstricting (narrowing) the blood vessels and thereby decreasing congestion. Many ocular decongestants are available without a prescription. If these are absorbed in significant amounts, their sympathetic nervous system effects may pose problems for patients with increased IOP and hypertension. ⚡ Ocular decongestants are contraindicated in patients with

TABLE 47.4 Mydriatics and Cycloplegics

Generic	Route and Dosage	Uses and Considerations
Atropine sulfate, 1% ophthalmic solution or ointment	Cycloplegic refraction: A: 1–2 gtts of sol or 0.3–0.5 cm ribbon of oint up to 3 times daily for 14 d; start 1 h before procedure. Iritis/uveitis: A: 1–2 gtts of sol or 0.3–0.5 cm ribbon of oint up to 3 times daily	For cycloplegic refraction, especially in children, and uveitis/iritis. Atropine antagonizes acetylcholine receptors and inhibits cholinergic effects. ⚡ The most potent cycloplegic, atropine, may cause seizures, arrhythmias, hypotension, respiratory depression, and hallucinations. Contraindications: Glaucoma, tachycardia.
Cyclopentolate HCl, 0.5%, 1%, 2% ophthalmic solution	A: 1–2 gtts × 1; may repeat × 1 in 5–10 min Max: 4 gtts/d per affected eye	For cycloplegia and mydriasis induction.
Homatropine hydrobromide 5% solution	Mydriasis and cycloplegia: A: 1–2 gtts before procedure; may repeat × 1 in 5–10 min Uveitis: A: 1–2 gtts q3–4 h Max: 16 gtts/d	For mydriasis and cycloplegia for eye examination and uveitis. Homatropine is similar to atropine but onset is faster and duration is shorter. Do not use 5% sol in children.
Phenylephrine HCl, 2.5% and 10% ophthalmic solution	Acute glaucoma: A: 1 gtt. Repeat as necessary. Use with miotic drugs to improve visual acuity Mydriasis induction: A: 1 gtt 15–30 min before procedure, may repeat at 3–5 min intervals; max: 3 gtts/eye Uveitis: A: 1 gtt of 2.5% up to 3 times for 2 d or 1 gtt of 10% once a day for up to 2 d	For treatment of acute open-angle glaucoma and for mydriasis induction and pupillary dilation in uveitis for examination. ⚡ Do not use 10% sol in neonates and children. ❗ Black-Box Warning ❗ Acute High-Alert Drug
Tropicamide	Refraction: A: 1%: 1–2 gtts; repeat in 5 min Fundus examination: 0.5%: 1–2 gtts 15–20 min before examination Max: 1%: 5 gtts/d; 2%: 2 gtts/d	Mydriasis and cycloplegia for eye examination

A, Adult; *d*, day; *gtt*, drop; *h*, hour; *HCl*, hydrochloride; *max*, maximum dosage; *min*, minute; *oint*, ointment; *q*, every; *sol*, solution.

angle-closure glaucoma because these drugs may contribute to acute angle closure, a medical emergency.

Lubricants

Eye lubricants moisten eyes to alleviate discomfort such as the burning and irritation associated with xerophthalmia. They are also used to moisten contact lenses and artificial eyes. During anesthesia and in acute or chronic central nervous system (CNS) disorders that result in unconsciousness or decreased blinking, lubricants keep eyes moist and maintain the integrity of the epithelial surface of the eye.

Many brands and forms of ocular lubricants (artificial tears) are available OTC. Although these agents are typically safe, the nurse must be alert to potential allergic reactions to preservatives found in lubricants.

In 2023 the FDA approved perfluorohexyloctane to treat signs and symptoms of dry eye disease. Perfluorohexyloctane is an ophthalmic semifluorinated alkane eye drop that helps to reduce tear evaporation at the surface of the eye. Just one drop in the affected eye four times a day is the expected dose. The most frequently reported adverse reactions are blurry vision and conjunctival redness.

Mydriatics and Cycloplegics

Anticholinergics actively block acetylcholine from attaching to cholinergic receptors, resulting in both dilation (mydriasis) of the pupils and paralysis (cycloplegia) of the muscles of accommodation. This is accomplished by blocking the response of sphincter muscles that normally constrict the pupil when cholinergic receptors are stimulated. Mydriatics and cycloplegics are used in diagnostic procedures and ophthalmic surgery. Commonly prescribed anticholinergics for mydriasis and cycloplegic refraction include atropine sulfate, cyclopentolate hydrochloride, homatropine hydrobromide, phenylephrine hydrochloride, and tropicamide. An ophthalmic alpha-receptor antagonist, dapiprazole, can reverse drug-induced mydriasis with phenylephrine.

Side Effects and Adverse Reactions

Side effects of topical anticholinergics include xerophthalmia (dry eyes), photophobia (sensitivity to light), and blurred vision. Although uncommon with topical use, systemic effects are typical of all anticholinergic drugs and include xerostomia, cephalgia, and constipation. Serious systemic effects include increased IOP, psychosis, seizures, hypotension, tachycardia, cardiovascular collapse, respiratory depression, and muscle rigidity. These drugs are contraindicated in patients with angle-closure glaucoma because the paralyzed iris may block the outlet for outflow of aqueous humor (see Fig. 47.2C). Table 47.4 lists selected mydriatics and cycloplegics along with their dosages, uses, and considerations.

Drugs for Age-Related Macular Degeneration

There is no known treatment or medication for dry AMD. An effective drug has not been identified to treat dry AMD, but several drugs are currently in the trial stages. Some studies suggest that antioxidants, such as vitamins C and E, and zinc supplements may have a role in preventing or slowing the progression of dry AMD. A healthy diet of dark leafy greens, yellow fruits, vegetables, and fish has also been shown to be beneficial to those with AMD.

Pharmacologic management of wet AMD targets vascular endothelial growth factor (VEGF), a substance that plays a role in the formation of abnormal vessels in the eye. These VEGF inhibitors are intravitreal drugs that are injected into the eye by an ophthalmologist and include ranibizumab, pegaptanib, and aflibercept. Another VEGF inhibitor, bevacizumab, is used for the treatment of neovascular wet AMD. It is classified as an antineoplastic monoclonal antibody and is recognized as a high-alert drug. Intravitreal VEGF is contraindicated in persons with ocular infections. In 2023 the FDA approved avacincaptad pegol, a C5 inhibitor, for treatment of geographic atrophy secondary to AMD. It prevents cleavage to C5a and C5b decreasing membrane attack complex formation. It is administered by intravitreal injection of 2 mg in the affected eye. Intravitreal injections may be associated with endophthalmitis, retinal detachments, neovascular AMD, and increased IOP; monitor for the development of these adverse reactions.

Drugs for Inherited Retinal Dystrophies

Inherited retinal dystrophy (IRD) is a group of severe and progressive disorders leading to blindness among young people. Until recently, no cure or treatment was available. With the emergence of gene therapy, the FDA approved the first gene therapy (voretigene neparvovec-rzyl) for retinal dystrophy. Ophthalmic gene therapy uses a vector, a modified virus, to deliver a normal copy of the gene encoding human retinal pigment epithelial 65 kDa protein to retinal cells to restore the visual cycle. Voretigene neparvovec is administered subretinally in each eye at least 6 days apart. Side effects include vision decline, eye infections, bleeding in the retina, increased IOP, and formation of cataracts, among others.

GLAUCOMA AND OCULAR HYPERTENSION DRUGS

> **PATIENT SAFETY**
>
> Herbs that should be avoided in patients with glaucoma include bitter orange, blood root, celandine, coffee, corkwood, ephedra, goldenseal, and jimson weed. Because all herbs have inherent risks, it is important to receive approval from the patient's health care provider before recommending herbal preparations.

Until recently, drugs for glaucoma (Table 47.5) belonged to one of six drug categories: (1) prostaglandin analogues, (2) beta-adrenergic blockers, (3) alpha-adrenergic agonists, (4) cholinergic agents, (5) carbonic anhydrase inhibitors (CAIs), or (6) systemic hyperosmotic drugs. A seventh class, rho kinase inhibitor (netarsudil ophthalmic), is indicated to reduce ocular pressure in patients with open-angle glaucoma by increasing aqueous humor outflow. Prostaglandin analogues and beta-adrenergic blockers are typically first-line therapy, followed by alpha-adrenergic agonists. Each category acts in different ways to decrease IOP. Even though damage due to glaucoma cannot be reversed, treatments may prevent further damage.

Prostaglandin Analogues

Prostaglandin analogues are first-line drugs used primarily in the treatment of open-angle glaucoma and ocular hypertension. These drugs decrease IOP by improving trabecular outflow and increasing the uveoscleral pathway, which is an alternate pathway of aqueous humor outflow. Examples of prostaglandin analogues include bimatoprost, latanoprost (see Prototype Drug Chart: Latanoprost), tafluprost, and travoprost. Prostaglandin analogues are taken at bedtime.

Side Effects and Adverse Reactions

Prostaglandin analogues used for glaucoma have unique side effects. These drugs gradually change the color of the iris by increasing brown pigmentation. This effect is most noticeable in individuals with green-brown and yellow-brown irises, which may be permanent. Darkening of the eyelids may also occur. Another side effect is the development of eyelash hypertrichosis, which is a growth in the number, length, thickness, and pigmentation of eyelashes. Patients may also develop macular edema, blurred vision, redness of the conjunctiva, and itching or stinging of the eye. Systemic effects such as bronchospasm, dizziness, dyspnea, and myalgia are rare. Prostaglandin analogues are generally better tolerated than alternative drugs for glaucoma.

Cholinergic Agents

Ophthalmic cholinergic agents cause *miosis*, a constriction of the pupil and contraction of the ciliary muscle. These actions result in a widening of the trabecular meshwork to improve the outflow of excess aqueous humor. In addition, as the pupil constricts, it straightens the iris, thus opening or widening the drainage angle to relieve angle-closure glaucoma. The two types of cholinergics are cholinergic agonists and cholinesterase inhibitors. Although their outcomes are similar, cholinergic agonists and cholinesterase inhibitors differ in their mechanism of action.

Cholinergic agonists are direct-acting cholinergics that directly stimulate cholinergic receptors. As a result, these drugs have the same action as the parasympathetic neurotransmitter acetylcholine. Pilocarpine is an example of a cholinergic agonist.

Cholinesterase inhibitors such as echothiophate are indirect-acting cholinergics, which inactivate the enzyme cholinesterase that typically breaks down acetylcholine. By inhibiting the enzymatic destruction of acetylcholine, more acetylcholine is available to stimulate cholinergic receptors in the eye.

Side Effects and Adverse Reactions

Systemic absorption of cholinesterase inhibitors through the conjunctiva and lacrimal duct can produce systemic parasympathomimetic effects that include cardiac irregularities, diarrhea, hyperhidrosis, respiratory depression, and urinary incontinence. Other adverse effects from cholinesterase inhibitors include iritis, uveitis, and retinal detachment in addition to common complaints such as ocular irritation and pain, lacrimation, myopia with blurred vision, and paradoxical ocular hypertension. Systemic effects from cholinergic agonists are rare; ocular adverse effects are similar to those of cholinesterase inhibitors. Cholinergic agonists and cholinesterase inhibitors are contraindicated for use in persons with angle-closure glaucoma.

Fig. 47.2B and C illustrates increased IOP, resulting in open-angle and angle-closure glaucoma. Refer to Chapter 16 for more information on cholinergic drugs.

Beta-Adrenergic Blockers

Selective and nonselective beta-adrenergic blockers and beta-blockers are first-line drugs used in the treatment of glaucoma. Beta-adrenergic blockers decrease IOP by decreasing the production of aqueous humor. Examples of ophthalmic nonselective beta-adrenergic blockers include carteolol, levobunolol, and timolol (see Prototype Drug Chart: Timolol). Selective ocular beta-blockers include betaxolol.

TABLE 47.5 Glaucoma Drugs

Generic	Route and Dosage	Uses and Considerations
Beta-Adrenergic Blockers		
Betaxolol HCl, 0.5% ophthalmic solution or 0.25% suspension	Sol: A: 1–2 gtts q12h Susp: A: 1 gtt q12h Max: 4 gtts/d	Selective beta-blocker for chronic open-angle glaucoma and ocular hypertension (increased IOP). The ophthalmic drug has not been shown to have significant effects on heart rate, blood pressure, or pulmonary function; however, such preparations can be absorbed systemically with the same adverse reactions and drug interactions. May have additive effects in patients receiving oral beta-blockers. Absolute contraindications: AV block, bradycardia, cardiogenic shock, HF. ⚠ Acute High-Alert Drug
Carteolol HCl, 1% ophthalmic solution	A: 1 gtt q12h Max: 2 gtts/d	Nonselective beta-blocker for chronic open-angle glaucoma or ocular hypertension. ⚠ Acute High-Alert Drug Conjunctival hyperemia and eye irritation may occur. Absolute contraindications: AV block, bradycardia, cardiogenic shock, HF.
Levobunolol HCl, 0.25% or 0.5% ophthalmic solution	A: 1–2 gtts of 0.25% bid or 1–2 gtts of 0.5% once daily Max: 2 gtts/d 0.5%	Nonselective beta-blocker for increased IOP for open-angle glaucoma or ocular hypertension; to be used with topical miotics. Ocular irritation, dizziness, fatigue, and depression may occur. Absolute contraindications: Asthma, AV block, bradycardia, cardiogenic shock, COPD, HF, sick sinus syndrome, sulfite hypersensitivity.
Timolol hemihydrate or maleate, 0.25% or 0.5% ophthalmic solution or gel-forming solution	See Prototype Drug Chart: Timolol	⚠ Black-Box Warning ⚠ High-Alert Drug
Carbonic Anhydrase Inhibitors		
Acetazolamide	Regular release: A: PO: 250 mg qd-qid; max: 1 g/d Extended release: A: PO: 500 mg bid; max: 1 g/d A: IV: 500 mg for acute increased IOP or patients unable to take oral dosage; may repeat in 2–4 h ⚡ Geriatrics: With all formulations, consider dose reduction.	Adjunctive treatment of glaucoma; reduces IOP. Must be administered systemically; penetration is poor when administered topically to the cornea. Volume loss may cause dehydration and postural hypotension. Electrolyte imbalance may occur. Adverse GI effects (e.g., dysgeusia, xerostomia, anorexia) may occur. Drug may be given without regard to food. Absolute contraindications: Acidosis, metabolic acidosis, angle-closure glaucoma, adrenal insufficiency, hepatic disease, or renal failure; hyperchloremia, hypokalemia, hyponatremia, anuria.
Brinzolamide, 1% ophthalmic suspension	A: 1 gtt tid Max: 3 gtts/d	For increased IOP due to ocular hypertension or open-angle glaucoma. Corneal edema may occur with low endothelial cell counts. With ocular administration, drug is absorbed systemically. Must be shaken well before each use. Absolute contraindication: Sulfonamide hypersensitivity (contains sulfonamide derivative).
Dorzolamide, 2% ophthalmic solution	A: 1 gtt tid Max: 3 gtts/d	For increased IOP due to ocular hypertension or open-angle ⚡ glaucoma. It is not recommended to topically administer CAIs concomitantly with oral CAIs.
Combination Drugs for Glaucoma Refer to individual drug information for general considerations.		
Timolol maleate	A: 1 gtt bid Max: 2 gtts/d per affected eye	Timolol is a nonselective beta-blocker, and dorzolamide is a carbonic anhydrase II inhibitor. ⚠ Black-Box Warning ⚡ High-Alert Drug
Brimonidine/timolol maleate	A: 1 gtt q12h Max: 2 gtts/d per affected eye	Brimonidine is a selective alpha-agonist and timolol is a nonselective beta-blocker.
Prostaglandin Analogues		
Latanoprost, 0.005% ophthalmic solution	See Prototype Drug Chart: Latanoprost	
Bimatoprost, 0.03% ophthalmic solution	A: 1 gtt at bedtime Max: 1 gtt/d	For increased IOP due to ocular hypertension or open-angle glaucoma. Macular edema, iritis, and cataracts may occur.
Travoprost, 0.004% ophthalmic solution	A: 1 gtt at bedtime Max: 1 gtt/d	For increased IOP due to ocular hypertension or open-angle glaucoma. ⚡ Macular edema or keratitis may occur.
Tafluprost, 0.0015% ophthalmic solution	A: 1 gtt every evening Max: 1 gtt/d per affected eye	For increased IOP due to ocular hypertension or open-angle glaucoma. ⚡ Drug may cause macular edema or uveitis/iritis.
RHO Kinase Inhibitors		
Netarsudil ophthalmic 0.02% sol	A: 1 gtt every evening Max: 1 gtt/d per affected eye	For increased IOP due to open-angle glaucoma or ocular hypertension. ⚡ Drug may cause keratitis, ocular pain, erythema, and vision changes.

≥, Greater than or equal to; *A*, adult; *AV*, atrioventricular; *bid*, twice daily; *CAI*, carbonic anhydrase inhibitor; *COPD*, chronic obstructive pulmonary disease; *d*, day; *GI*, gastrointestinal; *gtt*, drop; *h*, hour; *HCl*, hydrochloride; *HF*, heart failure; *IOP*, intraocular pressure; *IV*, intravenously; *max*, maximum; *N*, newborn; *PO*, by mouth; *q*, every; *qid*, four times daily; *sol*, solution; *susp*, suspension; *tid*, thrice daily; *wk*, weeks; *y*, year.

PROTOTYPE DRUG CHART

Timolol

Drug Class	Dosage
Nonselective beta-blocker	Sol: 1 gtt of 0.25% bid; may increase to 1 gtt of 0.5% bid and titrate down to once daily dosing. Gel: 1 gtt of 0.25% once daily; may increase to 1 gtt of 0.5% once daily.
Contraindications	**Drug-Lab-Food Interactions**
Absolute contraindications: COPD and RAD, AV block, bradycardia, cardiogenic shock, and heart failure. Caution against abrupt discontinuation.	Drugs: Ophthalmic timolol can be absorbed systemically; therefore drug-drug interactions are similar to other formulations. See Chapter 15 for more general drug-drug interactions with beta-blockers. Some herbal agents may lower vascular resistance (e.g., hawthorn [*Crataegus laevigata*] and ephedra [Mahuang]).
Pharmacokinetics	**Pharmacodynamics**
Absorption: Systemic absorption can occur. Distribution: UK Metabolism: Hepatic; t½: 4 h Excretion: Primarily in urine	Onset: 30 min Peak: 1–2 h Duration: <24 h
Therapeutic Effects/Uses	
Reduction of IOP in open-angle glaucoma or ocular hypertension Mechanism of action: Nonselectively antagonizes beta$_1$- and beta$_2$-adrenergic receptors, reducing IOP without affecting visual acuity, pupil size, or accommodation.	
Side Effects	**Adverse Reactions**
Adverse effects for ocular timolol are the same as for the oral drug. See Chapter 15 for more information on timolol and other nonselective beta-blockers.	See Chapter 15 for more information on beta-blockers.

<, Less than; *AV*, atrioventricular; *bid*, twice daily; *COPD*, chronic obstructive pulmonary disease; *gtt*, drop; *h*, hour; *IOP*, intraocular pressure; *min*, minutes; *RAD*, reactive airway disease; *sol*, solution; *susp*, suspension; *t½*, half-life; *UK*, unknown.

Side Effects and Adverse Reactions

Similar to most other ophthalmic medications, beta-adrenergic blockers (beta-blockers) may cause some eye discomfort. Some ophthalmic medications cause miosis. Because the pupil does not dilate adequately in dark environments, patients taking these drugs may experience vision problems at night.

Although rare, ophthalmic drugs may enter the circulation causing a system reaction. Ophthalmic beta-adrenergic blockers can slow the heart rate, which can worsen bradycardia, atrioventricular (AV) heart block, and heart failure. Also, these drugs can prevent adequate bronchodilation in patients with asthma and other obstructive pulmonary diseases. See Chapter 15 for more information on beta-adrenergic blockers.

Alpha-Adrenergic Agonists

Ophthalmic alpha-adrenergic agonists such as apraclonidine and brimonidine control or prevent elevation of IOP postsurgically by decreasing production and improving outflow of aqueous humor. The major site of action is in the ciliary body. Absolute contraindications for alpha-adrenergic agonists include persons on monoamine oxidase inhibitor (MAOI) therapy. No specific drug interactions with systemic and ophthalmic drugs were noted; however, caution is advised when using these drugs with other alpha-blockers, tricyclic antidepressants, and CNS depressants.

Side Effects and Adverse Reactions

Apraclonidine and brimonidine have minimal, if any, systemic effects. Because of the relative safety of alpha$_2$-adrenergic agonists, they are often used when ophthalmic beta-adrenergic antagonists are contraindicated. The most common effects of topical administration are burning, stinging, blurred vision, and headache. Serious reactions include corneal erosion, keratitis, arrhythmias, and asthma.

Carbonic Anhydrase Inhibitors

CAIs decrease IOP by decreasing the production of aqueous humor. These drugs, initially developed as diuretics, are sometimes used for adjunctive treatment of glaucoma. They are indicated for both open-angle and acute angle-closure glaucoma. CAIs are not as effective as other drugs for glaucoma, and they carry a greater risk of adverse effects. For these reasons, they are generally added to a therapeutic regimen only after other treatment options have been exhausted. Both topical (e.g., brinzolamide, dorzolamide) and systemic (e.g., acetazolamide) formulations are available.

Side Effects and Adverse Reactions

Adverse effects of CAIs, particularly with the systemic forms, include CNS effects such as lethargy, drowsiness, headache, seizures, paresthesias, and mental status changes. Gastrointestinal (GI) effects such as nausea, vomiting, diarrhea, dysgeusia, and anorexia may occur. Because CAIs have diuretic effects, polyuria and increased thirst are common, and fluid and electrolyte disturbances may occur as a result. CAIs may promote hyperuricemia, which may precipitate gout attacks, and they may also worsen liver disease, resulting in hepatic encephalopathy and even hepatic necrosis. Because they are sulfonamides, they should not be given to patients who have experienced allergic reactions to other sulfonamide drugs.

PROTOTYPE DRUG CHART

Latanoprost

Drug Class	Dosage
Prostaglandin analogue	1 gtt q evening in affected eye(s)

Contraindications	Drug-Lab-Food Interactions
Latanoprost is indicated only for open-angle glaucoma or ocular hypertension. No absolute contraindications exist, but use caution in patients with a torn or absent lens, intraocular inflammation, or risk of macular edema. Drug is absorbed by soft contact lenses, so advise patients with these to use alternate means of vision correction. *Caution*: Patients with history of diabetic retinopathy who took latanoprost experienced retinal detachment, retinal embolus, and vitreous hemorrhage. This may or may not be related to the latanoprost, but caution is urged.	Drugs: Concomitant administration with eye drops containing thimerosal causes latanoprost to precipitate out of solution; latanoprost- and thimerosal-containing ophthalmic preparations should be administered at least 5 min apart. Bromfenac ophthalmic solution, an NSAID, may reduce latanoprost's ability to lower IOP. Bimatoprost ophthalmic solution to promote growth of eyelashes may decrease the ability of latanoprost to lower IOP. Combining latanoprost with other prostaglandin analogues is not recommended; combination may decrease the IOP-lowering effects or cause a paradoxical increase in IOP.

Pharmacokinetics	Pharmacodynamics
Absorption: Through the cornea and hydrolyzed to its active form Distribution: 0.16 ± 0.02 L/kg. Primary measurable concentration is in the eye; levels are often undetectable in serum. Metabolism: Hepatic; t½: 17 min Excretion: Primarily in urine (88%)	Onset: 3–4 h Peak: 8–12 h Duration: 24 h

Therapeutic Effects/Uses
Reduction of IOP in open-angle glaucoma or ocular hypertension
Mechanism of action: Prostaglandin FP receptor selective agonist increases aqueous humor outflow.

Side Effects	Adverse Reactions
Blurred vision, burning/stinging/pruritus/redness, brown pigmentation of iris; increased number/length/thickness and darkening of eyelashes; foreign body sensation, punctate epithelial keratopathy, photophobia, lid edema/erythema/discomfort/crusting	Eye pain, eye infection, loss of vision, dizziness, dyspnea

gtt, Drop; *h*, hour; *IOP*, intraocular pressure; *min*, minutes; *NSAID*, nonsteroidal antiinflammatory drugs; *q*, every; *t½*, half-life.

PATIENT SAFETY

Do Not Confuse...
- **Oral** alpha-adrenergic or beta-blockers with **ophthalmic** preparations
- **Ocular** with **otic**
- **Prednisone** with **prednisolone** ophthalmic
- **Ophthalmic** solutions with **otic** or other topical solutions of the same name (e.g., Cortisporin *ophthalmic* solution with Cortisporin *otic* solution)

Patients With Eye Disorders: General Suggestions for Teaching

- Listen to patient concerns. Eye disorders that carry the possibility of blindness promote high anxiety in patients.
- Provide patient education regarding expected drug effect, dosage, and side effects, as well as when to notify the health care provider.
- Use lay terms rather than medical terminology when providing education.
- Provide written instructions for confused or forgetful patients.
- When developing patient education materials, write them at a fifth- to eighth-grade reading level; use a large, easily read font; and give instructions in the patient's primary language.
- Supplement written instructions with images or pictograms to clarify.
- Instruct patients or family members that one drop of eye medication is the preferred amount with prescriptions written for one to two drops; the conjunctival sac of the lower lid typically holds the volume of one drop without overflowing. The second drop may cause overflow, have a greater chance of systemic toxicity, and have an increased cost of treatment.
- If a second topical medication is ordered to be given at the same time, instruct patients to wait at least 5 minutes before instilling the second medication.
- Instruct patients or family members on the proper administration of eye drops or ointment. Teach them how to maintain sterile technique and prevent dropper contamination.
- Ask patients for a return demonstration of any procedure to ensure their ability to carry it out properly and determine whether additional teaching is needed.
- Advise patients that ointments will diminish vision for a short period due to the film coating the eye. Advise them to avoid potential safety hazards during this time.
- Instruct patients to store drugs away from heat.
- Counsel patients not to stop any medication suddenly without prior approval from the prescribing health care provider.

CLINICAL JUDGMENT [NURSING PROCESS]
Glaucoma and Ocular Hypertension Drugs

Concept: Sensory Perception
- Receiving and interpreting various stimuli (vision) for functional nervous system pathways to the brain

Recognize Cues [Assessment]
- Conduct a detailed current medication history that includes prescriptions, OTC medicines, antacids, dietary supplements, vitamins, and herbal supplements.
- Obtain a list of drug and food allergies and compare to the prescribed drugs to determine any drug-drug and drug-supplement interactions.
- Obtain baseline information about physical status that includes height, weight, vital signs, cardiopulmonary assessment, intake and output, skin assessment, nutritional status, and any underlying diseases.
- Check baseline visual acuity and intraocular pressure (IOP) measurements.
- ⚡ Assess for contraindications for glaucoma drugs, such as respiratory or cardiac disorders, angle-closure glaucoma, hypertension, acute ocular infection, immunosuppression, and hepatic or renal disorders.

Analyze Cues and Prioritize Hypotheses [Patient Problems]
- Decreased visual acuity related to disease progression
- Reduced sensory perception, vision related to disease progression, and drug-induced visual changes
- Potential for social isolation

Generate Solutions [Planning]
- The patient/caregiver will verbalize understanding for the drug therapy and identify when to notify the clinician.
- The patient will take medications in the doses and at the times prescribed.
- The patient will demonstrate the proper method of ophthalmic drug administration.
- The patient will avoid contaminating the tip of the tube or dropper.
- The patient will maintain an IOP within the target range.
- The patient will remain free of ocular infection during therapy.

Take Action [Nursing Interventions]
- Monitor for significant alterations in patient status.
- ⚡ Monitor patients for xerostomia, dehydration, fluid overload, blood dyscrasias, electrolyte imbalances, blurred vision, dyspnea, bradycardia or tachycardia, hypertension, and pulmonary changes.

Patient Teaching
General
- Advise patients to never stop medication suddenly.
- Advise patients to avoid driving or operating machinery while vision is impaired.
- Explain the importance of follow-up appointments for subsequent ophthalmologic examination and reevaluation of IOP.
- Counsel patients with glaucoma to avoid drugs with the potential to increase IOP, such as decongestants, anticholinergics, and corticosteroids.
- Instruct patients to put in eye drops first before any ophthalmic ointment (if prescribed).
- Instruct patients to wait at least 5 minutes between different ophthalmic medications.
- Teach patients/caregivers not to touch the tip of the tube or eyedropper to the eye, finger, or any other object.
- See Chapter 10 for more information on ocular drug administration.

Side Effects
- Explain to patients/caregivers when to notify the clinician (e.g., with fever, wheezing, weight gain, sudden vision changes, or high blood pressure).

Evaluate Outcomes [Evaluation]
- Evaluate patient and family knowledge of the purpose and administration of medications.
- Evaluate the effectiveness of drug therapy. IOP should be reduced from baseline measurements.
- Evaluate for alleviation or decrease in adverse effects after interventions targeted to unwanted effects of glaucoma therapy.

- Advise patients to check labels on OTC drugs with a pharmacist.
- Instruct patients to carry an identification card or wear a medical alert bracelet at all times if they are allergic to any medications.
- Encourage patients to keep health care appointments. Recommend that patients bring a list of questions about their condition or medications.
- Tailor instructions for patients who wear contact lenses. Notify them of any special procedures that need to be done with the use of contact lenses and various ophthalmic medications. Advise patients to avoid wearing contact lenses in the presence of eye infections.

OVERVIEW AND DISORDERS OF THE EAR

The ear is divided into the external, middle, and inner ear. Fig. 47.3 illustrates the basic structures of the ear. When an ear disorder does not abate, professional evaluation is essential, because hearing loss can result from untreated disorders. External ear disorders can be treated with OTC products, whereas prescription drugs are usually required to treat middle and inner ear disorders.

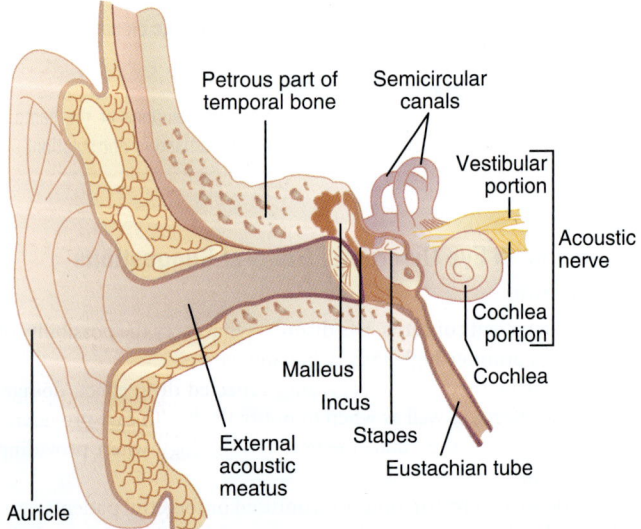

Fig. 47.3 Basic structures of the ear.

Divisions of the Ear

The external ear consists of the pinna and the external auditory canal. The external auditory canal transmits sound to the tympanic membrane (TM; eardrum), a transparent partition between the external and middle ear. The eardrum in turn transmits sound to the bones of the middle ear and also serves a protective function.

The middle ear, an air-filled cavity, contains three auditory ossicles—the malleus, incus, and stapes—that transmit sound waves to the inner ear. The tip of the malleus is attached to the eardrum; its head is attached to the incus, which is attached to the stapes. The eustachian tube provides a direct connection to the nasopharynx and equalizes air pressure on both sides of the eardrum to prevent it from rupturing. Swallowing, yawning, and chewing gum help the eustachian tube relieve pressure changes during airplane flights.

The inner ear is a series of labyrinths (canals) that consist of a bony section and a membranous section. The vestibule, cochlea, and semicircular canals make up the bony labyrinth. The vestibular area is responsible for maintaining equilibrium and balance. The cochlea is the principal hearing organ.

Disorders of the Ear

Common ear conditions are acute otitis media (AOM) and acute otitis externa, commonly known as *swimmer's ear*.

Acute Otitis Media

AOM occurs more often in children, and *Streptococcus pneumoniae* is the most common pathogen, followed by *Haemophilus influenzae* and *Moraxella catarrhalis*. AOM may also be caused by other microorganisms, such as viruses. AOM is usually related to a dysfunction of the eustachian tube, especially after an upper respiratory infection from a virus. The TM is usually bulging, and patients report otalgia (ear pain). Other symptoms may include fever and irritability.

Risk factors for the development of AOM include age younger than 2 years, attending day care centers, and exposure to environmental pollutants such as tobacco smoke. A significant decline in AOM has occurred since the pneumococcal conjugate vaccine (PCV) was introduced in 2000. Because it provides immunization against *S. pneumoniae*, families should be urged to have children receive the scheduled PCV13 as a prophylactic measure against AOM as well as against the other more serious conditions that this vaccine prevents.

Acute Otitis Externa

Otitis externa (OE) is an infection of the external auditory canal that occurs when excess moisture and breaks in the epithelium allow some pathogen, usually bacterial or fungal, to invade the tissues. The cerumen is lipid rich and hydrophobic (repels water), and it protects the skin from water penetration. However, excessive cerumen can obstruct the canal and can trap water. Trapped moisture in the canal elevates the pH and removes the protective cerumen, allowing pathogens to grow in a warm, dark, moist area. Like many areas of the body, the external canal contains normal bacterial flora that protects the ear; however, when protective mechanisms fail, the flora becomes pathogenic. *Pseudomonas aeruginosa* and *Staphylococcus aureus* are the pathogens most often responsible. Fever, otalgia, lymphadenopathy, and swelling can occur.

DRUGS FOR THE EAR

Most ear infections are caused by viruses and are usually treated conservatively. However, if the patient is not improving, antiinfectives may be needed. Fungal infections of the ear (otomycosis) have been increasing because of the use or misuse of earplugs, swimming in polluted waters, and immunodeficiencies. Antibacterials are warranted for ear infections due to bacteria.

Ear medications are usually contained in a liquid vehicle for ease of administration. Guidelines for the administration of eardrops are provided in Chapter 10.

Antiinfectives

Ear infections, especially the middle and inner ear, require antibacterial drugs. Oral amoxicillin is usually the drug of choice when antibiotics are indicated for AOM. The recommended dosage for children 6 months and older is 80 to 90 mg/kg every 12 hours for 7 to 10 days, depending on the severity of the condition and the age of the patient. The dosage for adults is 500 to 875 mg every 8 to 12 hours, depending on the severity. Azithromycin and clarithromycin are often ordered if the patient is severely allergic to penicillin. For more mild penicillin allergies a cephalosporin may be ordered; however, the nurse should be alert to any signs or symptoms of penicillin-cephalosporin cross-sensitivity. For otalgia, topical analgesics such as benzocaine are usually used, especially at bedtime.

Treatment for the external ear canal (EAC) is usually with topical antibacterial or antifungal drugs, depending on the source of the infection. These are often prescribed as a combination product that contains an antiinflammatory (corticosteroid) drug. An analgesic may also be needed.

If the EAC becomes so swollen that eardrops cannot reach the inner recesses of the EAC, a wick is usually used (Fig. 47.4). A wick is a thin cylinder composed of highly compressed absorbable material inserted into the edematous canal, and eardrops are applied to the exposed tip of the wick. Sufficient drops should be administered to keep the wick moist, which pulls the medication down the wick length as the moisture is absorbed, exposing the tissues along the EAC to medication. Wicks should be replaced every 24 to 48 hours. Once the swelling resolves, the wick will fall out, or it can be manually removed.

Oral antibiotics are rarely needed; however, when associated with otitis media or systemic illness, oral drugs are required. In addition, if patients are immunosuppressed, oral antibiotics are warranted.

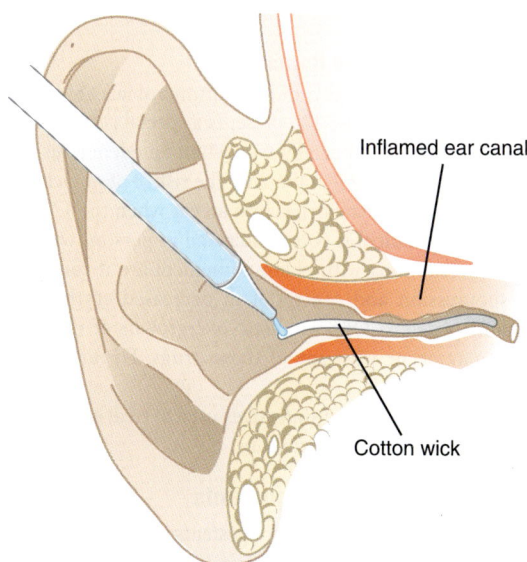

Fig. 47.4 Ear wick inserted into an edematous canal.

TABLE 47.6 Otic Antiinfectives

Generic	Route and Dosage	Uses and Considerations
Topical (Otic)		
General considerations: To minimize dizziness upon administration, warm the container between the hands for at least 1 minute before use. After administration, maintain patient's position for at least 1 minute.		
Acetic acid, 2% otic solution	A: 4–6 gtts q2–3h After administration to affected ear, maintain administration position for 5 min	For bacterial or fungal infection of the external ear canal (acute diffuse otitis externa). Solution is concentrated and is a highly corrosive irritant; it must be diluted before use. Systemic absorption is unlikely. ⚡ Absolute contraindications: Perforated TM
Ciprofloxacin otic, 0.2% otic solution	OE due to *Pseudomonas aeruginosa* or *Staphylococcus aureus*: A: 0.5 mg (one 0.25-mL single-use container): Instill contents q12h for 7 d; max: 1 mg/d	For bacterial infection (OE). Use caution treating *P. aeruginosa* or *S. aureus*; resistant strains have been noted. Otic route should not result in clinically significant plasma concentration. ⚡ Absolute contraindication: Quinolone hypersensitivity
Ofloxacin 0.3% otic solution	OE: A: 10 gtts once daily for 7 d Chronic OM: A: 10 gtts bid for 14 d	For OE due to *Escherichia coli*, *P. aeruginosa*, or *S. aureus*; chronic OM with perforated TM due to *P. aeruginosa*, *S. aureus*, or *Proteus mirabilis*; acute OM with tympanostomy tubes due to *Haemophilus influenzae*, *Moraxella catarrhalis*, *P. aeruginosa*, *S. aureus*, or *Streptococcus pneumoniae*. GI effects (dysgeusia, nausea, vomiting) and otic effects (otalgia, otorrhagia, tinnitus) may occur with otic ofloxacin. ❗ Black-Box Warning

>, Greater than; ≥, greater than or equal to; *A*, adult; *bid*, twice daily; *d*, day; *GI*, gastrointestinal; *gtt*, drops; *h*, hour; *max*, maximum dosage; *min*, minute; *OE*, otitis externa; *OM*, otitis media; *q*, every; *TM*, tympanic membrane; *y*, year.

Topical antibiotics such as neomycin and polymyxin B with hydrocortisone are very effective in treating OE because polymyxin B is effective against *P. aeruginosa*, and neomycin is effective against *S. aureus*. Fluoroquinolones, on the other hand, are effective against both organisms and are safe to use when the TM is incompetent; therefore they are usually the first drug chosen when prescribing treatment for OE. When OE is caused by the growth of fungi, restoring an acidic environment with an acidifying solution such as acetic acid is usually sufficient. A topical antifungal otic solution such as clotrimazole is typically used if the fungal infection is severe.

Side Effects and Adverse Reactions

The most common side effects of otic antimicrobials are burning and stinging. ⚡ Patency of the TM presents a special concern when eardrops are used. This is especially true when an edematous EAC prevents adequate visualization of the TM. The risk of ototoxicity is higher when administering topical drugs into an ear when the TM is incompetent. Chloramphenicol is contraindicated in persons with ruptured TM. Other precautions with chloramphenicol are it can cause bone marrow suppression and can result in decreased erythrocytes, leukocytes, and platelets. Opportunistic overgrowth of nonsusceptible organisms may occur with any of these drugs. Hypersensitivity is a contraindication.

Table 47.6 lists selected antiinfectives used to treat ear disorders and their dosages, uses, and considerations.

Antihistamines and Decongestants

For years, antihistamines and decongestants were thought to reduce middle-ear congestion and eustachian tube dysfunction associated with otitis media with effusion (OME), a noninfectious collection of fluid in the middle ear. The rationale was that these drugs would reduce edema of the eustachian tube, which would promote drainage from the middle ear.

In 2006 a landmark Cochrane review of the medical literature concluded that antihistamines and decongestants were not as effective as once assumed and that the risks of adverse effects outweighed the benefits. Shortly thereafter, the American Academy of Pediatrics recommended against their use for ear conditions in young children. A 2012 report by the Agency for Healthcare Research and Quality states that "the effects on multiple short- and long-term outcomes repeatedly demonstrated no benefit for use of these medications over placebo for treating OME.... The reviewed studies found evidence of increased side effects and harms with use of these medications." Unfortunately, many patients are not aware of these findings and may continue to take these drugs.

The importance of the nurse's role in educating patients regarding this concern cannot be overstated. Numerous OTC antihistamine-decongestant medications are readily available to unknowing patients. Examples of antihistamines include chlorphenamine, clemastine, diphenhydramine, and many others. Examples of decongestants are phenylephrine and pseudoephedrine. (Pseudoephedrine requires a prescription in some states.) Of even greater concern is that most of these are available as combination products that contain both an antihistamine and a decongestant. (See Chapter 38 for a discussion of upper respiratory drugs.)

Cerumenolytics

Cerumen, or earwax, is produced by glands in the outer half of the EAC. Usually, cerumen moves to the EAC by itself and is washed away; however, sometimes it accumulates due to overproduction or

🎯 CLINICAL JUDGMENT [NURSING PROCESS]
Topical Antiinfectives: Ear Conditions

Concept: Sensory Perception
- Receiving and interpreting various stimuli (auditory) for functional nervous system pathways to the brain

Recognize Cues [Assessment]
- Conduct a detailed medication history that includes current prescriptions, OTC medicines, antacids, dietary supplements, vitamins, and herbal supplements.
- Obtain a list of drug and food allergies.
- Record otoscopic examination findings for future comparisons.
- Check audiometry and tympanometry and perform other testing as indicated.
- Assess for conditions in which selected antiinfectives are contraindicated or relatively contraindicated.

Analyze Cues and Prioritize Hypotheses [Patient Problems]
- Reduced sensory perception related to inflammation and/or medication
- Auditory pain related to inflammation

Generate Solutions [Planning]
- The patient will verbalize understanding of the therapy.
- The patient will be free from ear infection after completion of the drug regimen.
- The patient will report a tolerable pain level.
- The patient will report any adverse drug effects.

Take Action [Nursing Interventions]
- Complete culture and sensitivity testing, if ordered, before starting drug therapy.
- Ensure tympanic membrane (TM) patency before administering eardrops other than fluoroquinolones.
- Provide relief of associated pain, if present.
- Monitor for significant alterations in patient status.
- Assess for the development of superinfections.

Patient Teaching
General
- Instruct patients to complete the entire course of medication (usually 10–14 days) and not to stop the medication when the ear feels better.
- Instruct patients who are prone to otitis externa (OE) on the prevention of OE. The Centers for Disease Control and Prevention recommend the following:
  - Keep water out of ears by using custom-fitted earplugs.
  - If water enters the ear, tilt the ear downward to allow water to drain out. Pull the ear in different directions to enhance water drainage.
  - Use a portable hair dryer to facilitate drying.
- Instruct the patient to wear a MedicAlert bracelet at all times if allergic to any medications.
- See Chapter 10 for information on the administration of eardrops.

Side Effects
- Inform the patient to report any ringing of the ears.
- Instruct the patient to report signs and symptoms of infection, such as fever or chills.

Evaluate Outcomes [Evaluation]
- Evaluate patient and family knowledge of the drug regimen.
- Determine the effectiveness of the drug therapy.
- Inquire regarding the alleviation of side effects.

---

narrowing of the EAC. In these instances, cerumen can harden in the EAC, creating impaction that can lead to pain, itching, tinnitus, and hearing loss.

Cerumenolytics are topical otic agents that soften or break up the cerumen so that it can be removed. Preparations for cerumenolytics include water-based, oil-based, and nonwater-, nonoil-based products. Water-based products provide hydration to the dried cerumen, allowing it to disintegrate. Oil-based solutions lubricate and soften the cerumen but do not disintegrate it. An example is carbamide peroxide, which is available OTC. Patients may also elect to use regular mineral oil to soften the wax or prevent cerumen impaction. Generally, 2 to 5 drops applied twice a day for 4 days is sufficient.

Sometimes cerumenolytics alone are insufficient. In these instances, ear irrigation can be used to flush the cerumen deposits out of the ear canal. Irrigation is best accomplished when direct visualization of the TM is possible, and it must be done gently to avoid damage to the TM. It is also important to warm the water to prevent nausea and vomiting.

Frequently used irrigating solutions include hydrogen peroxide 3% in a 1:1 solution with warm water, normal saline, or acetic acid (vinegar) mixed with warm water. Contraindications to irrigation include perforation of the TM and prior hypersensitivity.

Patients With Ear Disorders: General Suggestions for Teaching

- Instruct patients not to insert any foreign objects into the ear canal.
- Instruct patients to keep drugs away from heat.
- Provide education regarding the expected drug effect, dosage, and side effects, and when to notify the health care provider.
- Teach patients about OTC drug concerns, particularly with antihistamines and decongestants. OTC drugs may interact with prescribed drugs and may have risks that outweigh any drug benefit.
- Advise patients to contact their health care provider before using OTC drugs or herbal preparations to treat ear disorders.
- Encourage patients to keep follow-up appointments.

CLINICAL JUDGMENT SINGLE-EPISODE CASE STUDY

SLO/Objective: Prioritize appropriate actions for patients receiving eye medications
NGN Item Type: Cloze
Cognitive Skills: Generate Solutions

A 70-year-old female with a history of glaucoma reports shortness of breath, dizziness, and weakness shortly after the nurse instilled latanoprost 0.005% and timolol 0.25% ophthalmic solution. Other patient data include:

- Blood pressure 100/62 mm Hg
- White blood cell 5000/mm^3
- Hemoglobin 12 g/dL
- Platelets 159,000/mm^3
- Heart rate 64 beats per minute (irregular)
- Respiratory rate 18 breaths per minute
- Serum sodium 138 mEq/L
- Serum potassium 4.8 mEq/L
- Blood urine nitrogen 13 mg/dL
- Creatinine 0.9 mg/dL
- Alanine transaminase (ALT) 13 IU/L
- Aspartate transferase (AST) 53 IU/L

Choose the *most likely* options for the information missing from the statements below by selecting from the list of options provided.

The patient most likely is experiencing side effects from her eye drops, and the nurse would further review the patient's medical record for any history of _____1_____, _____1_____, _____1_____, or _____1_____. The nurse notifies the prescriber and continues to monitor the patient's _____2_____, _____2_____, _____2_____, and _____2_____. The nurse explains to the patient to notify the nurse if she experiences _____3_____, _____3_____, _____3_____, or _____3_____.

Option 1	Option 2	Option 3
Cardiac disorders	Visual acuity	Difficulty breathing
Renal disorders	Lung sounds	Polyuria
Hypertension	Vital signs	Cephalgia
Angle-closure glaucoma	Bowel habits	Chest discomforts
Immunosuppression	Cardiac rhythms	Constipation
Respiratory disorders	Electrolytes	Blurry vision

Answers
The patient most likely is experiencing side effects from her eye drops, and the nurse would further review the patient's medical record for any history of **cardiac disorders, hypertension, angle-closure glaucoma**, or **respiratory disorders**. The nurse notifies the prescriber and continues to monitor the patient's **visual acuity, lung sounds, vital signs**, and **cardiac rhythms**. The nurse explains to the patient to notify the nurse if she experiences **difficulty breathing, cephalgia, chest discomfort**, or **blurry vision**.

Rationale
Latanoprost is a prostaglandin analogue. While there are no absolute contraindications for this drug, caution is advised for persons with a history of diabetic retinopathy, as there is a possible increased risk for retinal detachment, retinal embolus, or vitreous hemorrhage. Ocular examination and visual acuity should be assessed to determine potential complications. However, timolol is a nonselective beta antagonist that can cause respiratory and cardiac events. Absolute contraindications include persons with chronic obstructive or restrictive lung disease or those who have heart failure, atrioventricular (AV) block, or bradycardia. Because timolol nonselectively blocks beta receptors, preexisting AV blocks can worsen, new AV blocks can occur, cardiac workload can decrease, or bradycardia can occur. Even though timolol is administered topically to the eye, enough of the drug can enter the systemic circulation to produce beta-adrenergic blocking events, such as hypotension, bradycardia, and bronchospasms. The patient's blood pressure is 100/62 mm Hg, and heart rate is 64 beats per minute. Although these numbers are within normal parameters, they could be abnormally low for the patient, which could result in the patient's symptoms of shortness of breath, dizziness, and weakness. Timolol can worsen heart failure. The nurse would notify the prescriber to possibly hold timolol and continue monitoring the patient's vital signs, assessing visual acuity, assessing lung sounds, and monitoring cardiac rhythms. If the blood pressure, heart rate, and arrhythmia continue to worsen, the patient would most likely require vasopressors. If the patient develops adventitious lung sounds, heart failure may occur. The patient should be instructed to notify the nurse immediately if she experiences continued or worsening difficulty breathing, cephalgia, chest discomfort, and/or blurry vision. Cephalgia, chest pain, and blurry vision can occur due to continued decreased tissue perfusion.

Reference
Wang Z, Denys I, Chen F, Cai L, Wang X, Kapusta DR, Lv Y, Gao J. Complete atrioventricular block due to timolol eye drops: a case report and literature review. *BMC Pharmacol Toxicol* 20(73), 2019. https://doi.org/10.1186/s40360-019-0370-2.

REVIEW QUESTIONS

1. A patient is taking oral acetazolamide, a carbonic anhydrase inhibitor, to decrease intraocular pressure. When providing drug education, which side effect would the nurse advise the patient to anticipate?
   a. Increased weight
   b. Light sensitivity
   c. Burning or stinging of the eyes
   d. Increased urine output

2. Which drug is most useful to prevent and treat cerumen impaction?
   a. Hydrogen peroxide
   b. Rubbing alcohol
   c. Charcoal
   d. Clove oil

3. The ophthalmologist asks the nurse to assist in the administration of tetracaine, fluorescein stain, and atropine for a diagnostic eye examination. Before assisting in the procedure, it is most important for the nurse to inform the ophthalmologist if the patient has a history of which condition?
   a. Cataracts
   b. Angle-closure glaucoma
   c. Open-angle glaucoma
   d. Macular degeneration

4. The nurse has a patient demonstrate self-administration of eye drops. Place the steps in the order in which the patient will perform them.
   a. Pull the lower lid away from the eye so that a pouch is formed.
   b. Gently shake the bottle to evenly distribute the drug.
   c. Press a finger against the inner corner of the eye for 2 to 3 minutes.
   d. Remove the cap.
   e. Tilt the head backward and look upward.
   f. Place the dropper just above the pouch without touching the tip of the eye or finger.
   g. Wash hands.
   h. Gently squeeze one drop of medicine into the pouch.
5. When collecting a medication history from a patient with primary open-angle glaucoma, the nurse identifies several drugs that could exacerbate glaucoma. Which drug poses a priority concern for this particular patient?
   a. Cyclobenzaprine, an antispasmodic
   b. Oxymetazoline, a decongestant
   c. Prednisone, a corticosteroid
   d. Sulfamethoxazole-trimethoprim, a sulfonamide-antibiotic combination
6. The nurse asks a parent to demonstrate the administration of eardrops on a toddler. Which step if made by the parent indicates the need for additional education? **Select all that apply.**
   a. Position with the affected ear upward.
   b. Pull the ear backward and upward.
   c. Instill one drop of medication at a time, allowing 3 to 5 minutes between each drop.
   d. Apply gentle pressure to the flap (tragus) over the ear canal.
   e. Keep the ear positioned upward for 5 minutes.

48

Dermatologic Disorders

http://evolve.elsevier.com/McCuistion/pharmacology

OBJECTIVES

- Discuss basic anatomy and physiology of the skin.
- Describe the pharmacological and nonpharmacological treatments for acne.
- Describe the clinical manifestations and treatment of psoriasis.
- Discuss care considerations of verruca vulgaris and drug-induced dermatitis.
- Contrast the common etiologies of contact dermatitis.
- Discuss the common treatments for impetigo, rosacea, and hair loss.
- Discuss prevention and treatment of burns.

OUTLINE

Anatomy and Physiology of the Skin, 620
    Epidermis, Dermis, and Subcutaneous Tissue, 620
    Skin Lesions, 620
Acne Vulgaris, 621
    Nonpharmacologic Approach, 621
    Pharmacologic Treatment, 621
Psoriasis, 625
    Topical Drugs, 625
    Systemic Drugs, 626
Verruca Vulgaris and Drug-Induced Dermatitis, 628
    Verruca Vulgaris (Warts), 628
    Drug-Induced Dermatitis, 628
Contact Dermatitis, 628
    Nonpharmacologic Treatments, 628
    Topical Corticosteroids, 628
Impetigo, Rosacea, and Hair Loss, 628
    Impetigo, 628
    Rosacea, 629
    Hair Loss and Baldness, 629
Burns and Burn Prevention, 629
    Sunscreens, 629
    Burns and Burn Preparations, 629
    Silver Sulfadiazine, 630
Clinical Judgment Case Study, 631
Review Questions, 631

ANATOMY AND PHYSIOLOGY OF THE SKIN

Skin, the largest organ of the body, consists of two major layers: the *epidermis* is the outer layer of skin, and the *dermis* is the layer beneath the epidermis. The functions of the skin include (1) protecting the body from the environment, (2) aiding in body temperature control, and (3) preventing body fluid loss.

Epidermis, Dermis, and Subcutaneous Tissue

The epidermis has four layers: (1) the basal layer, or *stratum germinativum*, the deepest layer lying over the dermis; (2) the spinous layer, or *stratum spinosum*; (3) the granular layer, or *stratum granulosum*; and (4) the cornified layer, or *stratum corneum*, the outer layer of the epidermis.

The dermis has two layers: the *papillary layer* lies next to the epidermis, and the *reticular layer* is the deeper layer of the dermis. The dermal layers consist of fibroblasts, collagen fibers, and elastic fibers. The collagen and elastic fibers give the skin its strength and elasticity. Within the dermal layer are sweat glands, hair follicles, sebaceous glands, blood vessels, and sensory nerve terminals. Fig. 48.1 shows the layers of the skin.

The subcutaneous tissue, primarily fatty tissue, lies under the dermis. Besides fatty cells, subcutaneous tissue contains blood and lymphatic vessels, nerve fibers, and elastic fibers. It supports and protects the dermis.

Skin Lesions

Numerous skin lesions and eruptions require mild to aggressive drug therapy. Skin disorders include acne vulgaris, psoriasis, eczema dermatitis, contact dermatitis, drug-induced dermatitis, rosacea, and burn infection. Skin eruptions may result from viruses, such as herpes simplex and zoster; fungi (e.g., **tinea pedis** [athletes foot], **tinea capitis** [ringworm]); and bacteria.

Skin lesions may appear as **macules** (flat and nonpalpable, usually less than 10 mm in diameter with varying colors), **papules** (raised and palpable, less than 10 mm in diameter), **vesicles** (clear, fluid-filled blisters smaller than 10 mm in diameter), or **plaques** (palpable lesions that are depressed or elevated compared with the skin surface and greater than 10 mm in diameter). Treatments for skin eruptions include topical creams, ointments, pastes, gels, lotions, and solutions. Selected skin disorders and their drug therapy regimens are discussed separately. Treatment information can be found at the American Academy of Dermatology (AAD) website at https://www.aad.org.

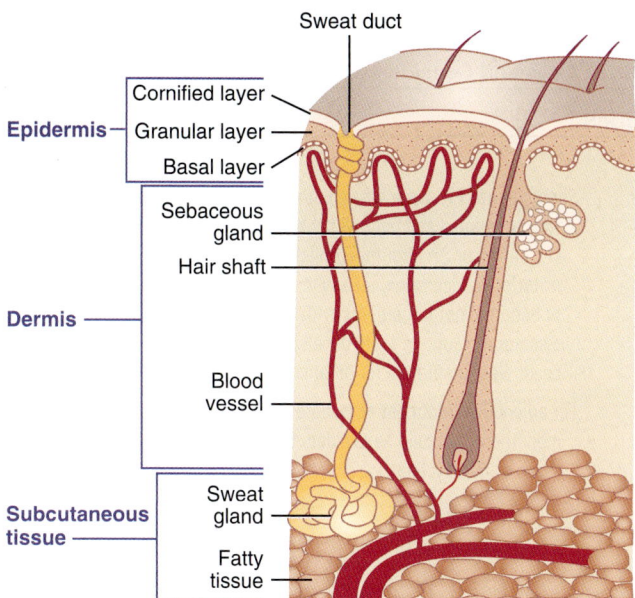

Fig. 48.1 Basic structures of the skin.

ACNE VULGARIS

Acne is the most common skin disorder in the United States. Acne is more prevalent among adolescents, but adults and children can also develop acne. **Acne vulgaris** is the formation of papules, nodules, and cysts on the face, neck, shoulders, and back that results from keratin plugs at the base of the pilosebaceous oil glands near the hair follicles. The keratin plugs trap normal skin flora, including bacteria commonly found on the skin; the primary bacterium is *Propionibacterium acnes*. Bacteria start proliferating, which causes inflammation and irritation. During adolescence, the production of androgens and sebum—an oily skin lubricant—are increased. The sebum combines with **keratin**, a protein that is part of the skin, to form a plug that results in acne. **Comedones** are types of noninflammatory acne lesions that may be open (**blackheads**) or closed (**whiteheads**). Open comedones are dilated hair follicle openings that allow oxidation of the debris within the follicle; closed comedones are small, plugged hair follicles. As with other forms of acne, comedones are not a result of poor hygiene. All forms of acne should be treated to prevent lifelong scars. Acne can be treated nonpharmacologically and pharmacologically. Table 48.1 lists the drugs commonly used to control acne vulgaris along with their dosages, uses, and considerations.

Nonpharmacologic Approach

Nonpharmacologic measures should be tried before drug therapy is initiated. A prescribed or suggested nonabrasive cleansing agent, such as antibacterial soap, is necessary for all types of acne. The skin should be gently cleansed twice daily avoiding vigorous scrubbing and overwashing, which could irritate the skin, worsening the acne and possibly causing an infection. In addition to facial hygiene, shampooing hair to decrease the oiliness may help with acne. Keeping hair away from the face has also been shown to decrease acne. Cosmetics should be water based because oil-based products can increase the clogging of skin pores. A well-balanced diet low in fat and sugar is recommended, and excessive carbohydrates should be avoided. Decreasing emotional stress and increasing emotional support are also suggested. If drug therapy is necessary, nonpharmacologic measures should be maintained as well.

Pharmacologic Treatment

Acne is not curable, but it is manageable. Acne medications may help decrease scar formation related to acne. The best course for patients with acne is to see a dermatologist who can prescribe treatment specific to the individual; therefore the course of therapy will vary according to the severity and extent of the acne. The American Academy of Dermatology (AAD) updated their guidelines for the treatment and management of acne in January 2024. Recommendations include combining multiple different treatment types for better results as well as limiting the use of oral antibiotics, when possible, to reduce the development of antibiotic resistance. The complete list of recommendations can be viewed at the American Academy of Dermatology Association (https://www.aad.org).

Topical Antiacne Drugs

Mild acne is generally treated with topical drugs that treat existing acne and prevent new eruptions. Commonly used topical therapies for mild acne include benzoyl peroxide (BP), retinoids, salicylic acid, antibiotics, or combinations of these in addition to gentle cleansing.

BP is an antibacterial medicine that kills *P. acnes*, the predominant organism in sebaceous follicles and comedones. BP releases free radical oxygen species that oxidize bacterial proteins. When included as an adjunct to an antibiotic regimen, control of acne is enhanced. Resolution of acne usually occurs within 4 to 6 weeks. BP is applied as a cream, lotion, or gel once or twice a day and can be left on or washed off. Washing BP off may be better tolerated in patients with sensitive skin.

Topical retinoids such as tretinoin, adapalene, and tazarotene are derivatives of vitamin A and are used for mild to moderate acne that alters keratinization. They are the mainstay of topical therapy because of their comedolytic activities, and they also have antiinflammatory properties. Retinoids alter the intracrine and paracrine mediators of cell differentiation and proliferation, apoptosis, and reproduction, thereby modifying gene expression, subsequent protein synthesis, and epithelial cell growth. Retinoids prevent horny cell cohesion, or **keratolysis**, and increase epithelial cell turnover. They do *not* affect microorganisms in acne and sebum production. Topical retinoids are appropriate for all types of acne when used in combination with other antiacne therapy. They also allow maintenance of acne clearance after discontinuing oral antibiotics. Of the retinoids, tazarotene is contraindicated with pregnancy. Retinoids should *not* be used before or after extended sun exposure or sunburn because they can increase the risk of sunburn and intensify existing sunburn.

Another antiacne topical drug, azelaic acid, has antibacterial, antiinflammatory, and mild comedolytic actions. Azelaic acid is as effective as BP and tretinoin combined. Salicylic acid is also a comedolytic treatment that is available over the counter (OTC) in various strengths, Topical treatments with retinoids, azelaic acid, and salicylic acid can cause burning, pruritus, and erythema after several applications; however, they are less common with azelaic acid.

Moderate to severe acne may require a stronger concentration of BP, and topical antibiotics, such as tetracycline, erythromycin, and clindamycin, may be added to the treatment regimen. Erythromycin and clindamycin are the recommended topical antibiotics for acne therapy; however, erythromycin has reduced efficacy compared with clindamycin. Topical antibiotics accumulate in the hair follicle and have both antiinflammatory and antibacterial effects. Topical antibiotics as monotherapy are *not* recommended due to the development of antibiotic resistance. Severe, painful acne may be treated with steroid injection.

TABLE 48.1 Drugs for Acne Vulgaris and Psoriasis

Generic	Route and Dosage	Uses and Considerations
ACNE VULGARIS		
Systemic Preparations		
Tetracycline hydrochloride	A: PO: Initially, 500 mg twice daily for max of 1 g/day for 1–2 wk, then decrease slowly to 125–500 mg daily or every other day. Should only be used for 3–4 mo to minimize the risk of resistance.	For moderate to severe inflammatory acne vulgaris concomitantly with topical retinoid and benzoyl peroxide (BP). Best on an empty stomach (1 h before or 2 h after meal/milk). To reduce risk of esophageal irritation or ulceration, take with plenty of water and do not take at bedtime; not for patients with esophageal disorders. Permanent discoloration during tooth development and enamel hypoplasia may occur. See Chapter 26 for other considerations.
Minocycline hydrochloride	Severe acne: A: PO: 50–100 mg once or twice daily Nonnodular moderate to severe acne: A: PO: 1 mg/kg extended-release capsule/tablets once daily for 12 wk A: 4% Topical Foam, Apply small amount topically to the effected skin area once daily at least 1 h before bedtime.	For adjunctive treatment of moderate to severe inflammatory acne; monotherapy should be avoided. Drug considerations are similar to those of tetracycline.
Doxycycline	A: PO: 100 mg q 12 h on day 1, then 50 mg q 12 h or 100 mg qd	Adjunctive treatment for severe acne; monotherapy should be avoided. Drug considerations are similar to those of tetracycline.
Isotretinoin	A: PO: 0.5–1 mg/kg/d in 2 divided doses Take with meals to increase bioavailability Patient may repeat the course at least 8 wk after completion of the prior course.	For moderate to severe nodular acne unresponsive to conventional treatment, including antibiotics. Vitamin A derivative; reverses sebum production by reducing the size of sebaceous glands. Unlike vitamin A, isotretinoin does not accumulate in the liver. Adverse effects relate to toxicity to cardiovascular, endocrine, hematologic, GI, hepatic, musculoskeletal, respiratory, ocular, and otic systems. Interacts with tetracycline, vitamin A, methotrexate, contraceptives, and alcohol. Baseline hepatic function, lipid panel, and pregnancy tests must be obtained. Females of childbearing age must have a pregnancy test every 30 d.
Amoxicillin	A: PO: 250 mg bid up to 500 mg tid	Adjunctive treatment for acne, especially during pregnancy. Shake suspension well before each administration. Suspension may be added to formula, milk, and other liquids. For other considerations and uses, see Chapter 26.

Topical Preparations
General considerations: When using multiple topical products for acne, apply each product at different times throughout the day to decrease skin irritation. Common side effects of topical drugs include xerosis of skin, erythema, and pruritus. Avoid eyes, mouth, and mucous membranes when using topical antiacne preparations.

Keratolytic Agents		
Azelaic acid	A: Apply a thin layer to the affected area twice daily, morning and evening	For mild to moderate inflammatory acne; has antimicrobial effect against *Propionibacterium acnes* and *Staphylococcus epidermidis* and an antikeratinizing effect on the follicular epidermis. May cause hypopigmentation in patients with dark complexions.
Benzoyl peroxide	A: 2.5%, 5%, or 10% gel, wash, or cream, apply sparingly once daily, gradually increase to 2–3 times/d if needed.	First-line therapy for mild to moderate inflammatory and noninflammatory acne lesions. Promotes keratolysis, removal of the horny layer of epidermis, resulting in drying and desquamative actions. Can be used concomitantly with other antiacne therapies.
Salicylic acid	A: 0.5%–6% cream, gel, and shampoo 1–3 times/d; if erythema or peeling occurs, reduce application.	For mild to moderate acne; promotes desquamation of the horny layer of skin. Monitor for salicylic toxicity; use of salicylic acid in children with viral infections is not recommended due to increased risk for Reye syndrome.

TABLE 48.1 Drugs for Acne Vulgaris and Psoriasis—cont'd

Generic	Route and Dosage	Uses and Considerations
Antibiotics		
General considerations: Antibiotics may be given concurrently with benzoyl peroxide.		
Erythromycin	A: 2% solution, external pad, or solution, apply 1–2 times/d	For mild to moderate inflammatory acne.
Clindamycin	A: 1% gel, lotion, solution, or pledget: Apply twice daily to the affected area 1% foam: Apply once daily.	For moderate acne. May cause colitis, dermatitis, folliculitis, pruritus, erythema, dry skin, and peeling. Dispense foam into cap or onto a cool surface to prevent premature melting. Shake other formulations well before use. Can have neuromuscular blocking action; use cautiously with opiate agonists; monitor for any CNS depression (e.g., bradypnea, weakness, paralysis).
Vitamin A Derivatives		
General considerations: Topical vitamin A derivatives may be used concurrently with benzoyl peroxide and other antiacne therapies.		
Acne Vulgaris		
Tretinoin	A: Apply a thin layer to the affected area once daily at bedtime.	For mild to moderate acne. Cleanse area first, pat dry, and wait 20–30 min before applying. Wash hands immediately after applying. Caution in patients with fish allergies.
Adapalene	A: 0.1% lotion or gel, 0.3% gel: Apply once daily at bedtime after washing the face with nonmedicated soap.	For mild to moderate acne, adapalene causes less skin irritation than tretinoin.
Tazarotene	A: 0.1% cream, gel, or foam: Apply a thin film once daily in the evening.	For mild to moderate acne; can also be used for psoriasis. Photosensitivity can occur; avoid unnecessary environmental exposures. May use a moisturizer as needed.
Oral Contraceptives		
Ethinyl estradiol/ norethindrone acetate/ ferrous fumarate	A: PO: 1 pill every day at the same time for 21 d followed by 1 wk of no tablets	For the treatment of acne vulgaris. See Chapter 55 for more information on drug uses and considerations.
Ethinyl estradiol/ norgestimate	A: PO: 1 tab at the same time each day	For the treatment of acne vulgaris. See Chapter 55 for more information on drug uses and considerations.
PSORIASIS		
Systemic Preparations		
Methoxsalen	A: PO: 10–70 mg 2–3 times weekly, according to body weight. Administer 2 h before exposure to therapeutic UV rays.	Systemic antimetabolite for severe psoriasis not responsive to other therapy. Soft and hard gelatin capsules are *not* interchangeable. Separate doses by at least 48 h. Administer with food or milk. Contraindicated in patients with history of or current invasive cutaneous carcinoma or melanoma. Avoid sunlight during drug therapy; sunlight could cause severe burning and blistering.
Acitretin	A: PO: 25–50 mg/d with main meal. Trials found that 25 mg/d for treatment of psoriasis vulgaris is similar in efficacy to 50 mg/d with fewer and less severe adverse clinical and laboratory events.	Retinoid for recalcitrant psoriasis. May take up to 6 mo for maximal response to treatment. May be given concurrently with phototherapy. Give with food for increased bioavailability.
Topical Preparations		
Anthralin	A: Apply sparingly to lesions once daily and leave on up to 30 min. Rinse thoroughly with cool to lukewarm water, then wash with soap	For stable plaque psoriasis. May stain clothing, skin, and hair.
Calcipotriene	A: Apply up to twice daily.	Vitamin D analog for chronic plaque psoriasis. More effective when used with a topical corticosteroid. Do not exceed 100 g/wk. Excess use may increase serum calcium level. Contraindicated in persons with hypercalcemia. Avoid UV rays.

Continued

TABLE 48.1 Drugs for Acne Vulgaris and Psoriasis—cont'd

Generic	Route and Dosage	Uses and Considerations
Clobetasol propionate	A/C ≥12 y: Cream, gel, foam, or ointment: Apply a thin layer twice daily A/C ≥16 y: Emollient cream *only*: Apply a thin layer twice daily. A: Spray and lotion: Apply twice daily.	Super-high-potency corticosteroid for moderate to severe plaque psoriasis. **!** Do not use occlusive dressings. With any formulation, do not exceed 50 g/wk. Reassess lesions after 2 wk of treatment. Contraindicated for application to the axilla, face, or groin.
Coal tar	A: Foam, lotion, suspension, or shampoo: Apply up to 4 times daily, depending on formulation.	For mild to moderate psoriasis. No maximum dosage. Wash affected area to remove loose psoriatic scales for better penetration. Allow skin to air dry after treatment. May stain clothing, skin, and hair. Do not use on inflamed, broken, or infected skin due to increased risk of systemic absorption. UV rays should be avoided for 24 h after treatment.
Tazarotene	A: Cream: Apply to affected areas once daily in the evening A: Gel: Apply once daily in the evening.	For stable plaque psoriasis. Can also be used for acne vulgaris. May use with skin emollients, but apply at least 1 h before tazarotene. Avoid application to unaffected skin due to increased systemic absorption.
PSORIASIS		
! Biologic Agents		
General considerations: Before initiating therapy, patients must be tested for active infections (e.g., TB, HBV). Rotate injection sites; subsequent injections should be at least 1 inch from previous injection sites. Do not inject in areas that are bruised, red, tender, or hard.		
Adalimumab	Psoriasis: A: Subcut: Start with 80 mg on week 1, then 40 mg on week 2, then 40 mg every other week Psoriatic arthritis: A: Subcut: 40 mg every other week	A TNF-α MAb for moderate to severe chronic plaque psoriasis and psoriatic arthritis when other systemic therapy is not appropriate. Rotate injections on the front of thighs and abdomen. Subsequent injections should be at least an inch away from previous injection sites.
Etanercept	Psoriatic arthritis: A: Subcut: 50 mg/wk up to twice weekly Psoriasis: Start with 50 mg twice weekly 3–4 d apart for 3 mo; then 50 mg/wk	TNF inhibitor for moderate to severe psoriasis. May be administered in an outpatient setting; teach patient or caregiver thoroughly on proper administration. Do not inject directly into scaly patches or lesions. Contraindicated in persons with sepsis.
Infliximab	A: IV: 5 mg/kg given at weeks 0, 2, and 6 and then every 8 wk	Chimeric MAb for chronic severe psoriasis and psoriatic arthritis. Infuse over at least 2 h with appropriate filter. *Absolute contraindications:* Heart failure, murine protein hypersensitivity. Black-box warning includes infection (viral, fungal, bacterial) and neoplastic disease.
Ustekinumab	Based on weight: A >100 kg: Subcut: 90 mg, repeat 4 wk later, then 90 mg q12wk starting at wk 16 A ≤100 kg: Subcut: 45 mg, repeat in 4 wk, then q12wk starting at wk 16	IL-12 and IL-23 antagonists for moderate to severe plaque psoriasis for patients receiving phototherapy or systemic therapy for psoriatic arthritis.

A, adult; *bid*, twice daily; *CNS*, central nervous system; *d*, day; *GI*, gastrointestinal; *h*, hour; *HBV*, hepatitis B virus; *IL*, interleukin; *IV*, intravenous; *MAb*, monoclonal antibody; *min*, minutes; *mo*, month; *PO*, by mouth; *q*, every; *Subcut*, subcutaneous; *tab*, tablet; *TB*, tuberculosis; *tid*, three times daily; *TNF*, tumor necrosis factor; *UV*, ultraviolet; *wk*, week; *y*, year.

Systemic Antiacne Drugs

For severe acne, adjunctive treatment is usually warranted with oral antibiotics (e.g., doxycycline and minocycline [drugs of choice], tetracycline, amoxicillin) in addition to topical corticosteroids (Box 48.1). **!** Tetracycline antibiotics, however, should not be used among the very young and among pregnant patients; drugs of the tetracycline class may cause dental discoloration to the developing teeth and have teratogenic effects on the fetus. Instead, amoxicillin or another nontetracycline drug may be given for severe acne. See Chapter 26 for more information on antibacterials.

Isotretinoin, a derivative of vitamin A taken orally, is used for treatment of severe cystic acne that is not responsive to conventional therapy. It decreases sebum formation and secretion and has antiinflammatory and antikeratinizing (keratolytic) effects, decreasing lesions and scars due to acne. Additional benefits of isotretinoin include a decrease in anxiety and depression. The typical patient takes this drug for 4 to 6 months. Adverse reactions may occur that are dose dependent; these include cheilitis, dizziness, cephalgia, conjunctivitis, skin irritation, pruritus, epistaxis, myalgia, arthralgia, temporary hair thinning, photosensitivity, depression, and suicidal thoughts. Usually, one course

BOX 48.1 Topical Corticosteroids

Very High Potency
Betamethasone dipropionate, augmented 0.05%
Clobetasol propionate 0.05%
Diflorasone diacetate 0.05%
Halobetasol propionate 0.05%

High Potency
Amcinonide 0.1%
Betamethasone dipropionate, augmented 0.05%
Desoximetasone 0.25% and 0.05%
Diflorasone diacetate 0.05%
Fluocinonide 0.05%
Halcinonide 0.1%
Triamcinolone acetonide 0.5%

Medium Potency
Betamethasone valerate 0.1%
Fluocinolone acetonide 0.025%
Flurandrenolide 0.05%
Fluticasone propionate 0.05% (cream) and 0.005% (ointment)
Mometasone furoate 0.1%
Triamcinolone acetonide 0.1%

Low-Medium Potency
Hydrocortisone butyrate 0.1%
Hydrocortisone probutate 0.1%
Hydrocortisone valerate 0.2%
Prednicarbate 0.1%

Low Potency
Alclometasone dipropionate 0.05%
Fluocinolone acetonide 0.01%

Lowest Potency
Hydrocortisone base or acetate 0.25%, 0.5%, and 1%

---

of treatment with isotretinoin controls severe acne. Because isotretinoin is a derivative of vitamin A, patients should not take vitamin A concomitantly. Using vitamin A or tetracycline with isotretinoin may increase its adverse effects. Baseline blood tests—liver function tests (LFTs), serum lipid panel, and pregnancy tests among female patients of childbearing age—are required before initiating isotretinoin therapy and at intervals throughout therapy. ⚠ Isotretinoin must *not* be used during pregnancy; it is a known teratogen. Additional cautions associated with isotretinoin are to not breast-feed or to give blood during or for 1 month after therapy; patients should not take other medications or herbal products without first consulting their health care provider; drive at night without knowing the effect of isotretinoin on night vision; or have cosmetic procedures to smooth skin. The patient should be instructed to avoid excessively vigorous activity. If they experience muscle weakness while exercising, they should contact their health care provider and stop taking isotretinoin. Muscle weakness may be an indication of serious muscle damage.

⚠ Because of isotretinoin's powerful teratogenicity, a risk management system to prevent isotretinoin-related teratogenicity was implemented. iPLEDGE is the third risk management program to prevent exposure to isotretinoin during pregnancy. Before starting isotretinoin therapy, both males and females must enroll in the iPLEDGE risk management program and adhere to it. The program was created to ensure patients who receive isotretinoin use two forms of contraception, that no patient is pregnant when treatment is initiated, and that no patient becomes pregnant while taking the drug or for at least 1 month after completing a course of isotretinoin. This comprehensive program also has rules for the health care provider, patient, pharmacist, and wholesaler. Further information can be found at https://www.ipledgeprogram.com.

PSORIASIS

Psoriasis is a multisystem disease with predominant skin and joint disorders. According to the AAD, it affects nearly 3.2% of the population; of those affected, 80% have mild to moderate disease. Most of the manifestations are exhibited as chronic skin inflammation characterized by scaly, erythematous plaques or scales. These plaques may be painful and are often pruritic, at times causing significant quality-of-life issues. They can appear on the scalp, elbows, palms, knees, and soles of the feet. Psoriasis is a chronic disease, and the manifestations wax and wane. Of the different forms of psoriasis, plaque psoriasis is the most common form. Approximately 25% to 30% of people with psoriasis have joint psoriatic arthritis. Depending on the severity of the disease, recommendations for the treatment of psoriasis include topical and systemic treatments and/or phototherapy. Table 48.1 lists some drugs, dosages, uses, and considerations for psoriasis. Table 48.2 lists current treatment modalities for psoriasis and psoriatic arthritis.

Topical Drugs

Vehicles for topical preparations are many and may include ointments, creams, lotions, solutions, gels, foams, and tape, among others. More than one topical medication may be used concomitantly to increase the effectiveness of each drug. If more than one topical drug is used, patients need to be instructed to apply each drug at separate times throughout the day. Topical drugs for psoriasis include corticosteroids, vitamin D analogs, tazarotene, calcineurin inhibitors (e.g., tacrolimus and pimecrolimus), salicylic acid, anthralin, and coal tar.

Topical corticosteroids are the principal treatment for most patients. Corticosteroids are available in a variety of vehicles that are sold OTC or by prescription; differing levels of potency are also available such that the weakest formula (e.g., 1% hydrocortisone) is available OTC and the strongest (e.g., clobetasol propionate) is by prescription (see Box 48.1). Corticosteroids are classified according to their potency, class 1 to class 7, in which class 1 is the strongest (super potent). The lower potency topical steroids are reserved for sensitive skin (e.g., face, intertriginous areas, thin skin areas, in infants and older adults). Patients with thick skin and those with scales or plaques often require the highest potency steroids. ⚠ The usual length of treatment for most topical steroids is 4 weeks; otherwise, adverse effects that include cutaneous side effects and systemic absorption may occur. Tapering topical steroids after clinical response is recommended by the AAD. Cutaneous side effects include skin atrophy, telangiectasia, striae distensae, acne, folliculitis, and purpura. Other effects include worsening of existing or preexisting skin conditions (dermatoses) and fungal infections (tineas). Worsening of psoriasis can also occur (rebound effect) with the use of topical corticosteroids. Even though systemic side effects are fewer than cutaneous side effects with topical steroids, these can still occur. Systemic effects usually occur with the highest potency preparation used over a large surface for a prolonged period. Examples of systemic side effects include Cushing syndrome, cataracts, glaucoma, and suppression of the hypothalamic-pituitary-adrenal (HPA) axis, which can cause growth retardation.

TABLE 48.2 Current Approved Treatment Modalities for Psoriasis and Psoriatic Arthritis

Biologics	Topical Treatments	Systemic Treatments	Phototherapy and Photochemotherapy
Adalimumab	Anthralin	Acitretin	Broadband and narrowband B
Certolizumab	Coal tar	Apremilast	Excimer laser therapy
Etanercept	Corticosteroids	Cyclosporine	Oral PUVA therapy
Infliximab	Emollients	Fumaric acid esters	Topical PUVA therapy
Guselkumab	Pimecrolimus	Methotrexate	
Ixekizumab	Salicylic acid	Retinoids	
Secukinumab	Tacrolimus	Sulfasalazine	
Tildrakizumab	Tazarotene	Bimekizumab	
Ustekinumab	Vitamin D analogs		
	Combination therapy of all previously mentioned		

PUVA, Psoralen and ultraviolet A; *TNF*, tumor necrosis factor.
Data from American Academy of Dermatology: *Psoriasis clinical guideline*, 2020. https://www.aad.org/member/clinical-quality/guidelines/psoriasis.

Synthetic vitamin D analogs (e.g., calcipotriene) bind to vitamin D receptors, enhancing the differentiation of keratinocytes while inhibiting their proliferation. Calcipotriene is available in solution, foam, and cream and is usually combined with topical corticosteroids to increase clinical response. Local side effects include burning, pruritus, edema, peeling, dryness, and erythema. Systemic side effects usually occur due to overapplication and include hypercalcemia and suppression of parathyroid hormone. Patients need to be instructed to avoid ultraviolet (UV) light because UVA inactivates calcipotriene.

Topical tazarotene, a retinoid, normalizes abnormal keratinocyte differentiation and decreases hyperproliferation and inflammation. Tazarotene may be used concurrently with moisturizers and topical corticosteroids. Common side effects include local irritation. Tazarotene is a teratogen; therefore its use is contraindicated during pregnancy.

Topical calcineurin inhibitors (CIs) such as tacrolimus and pimecrolimus block the synthesis of proinflammatory cytokines, a major pathogenesis of psoriasis. Common side effects include burning and pruritus of the skin, which appears to increase when applied immediately after bathing. Topical tacrolimus and pimecrolimus are not approved for infants and children younger than 2 years. Increased susceptibility to infection can occur with the use of topical CIs, including reactivation of latent viral infection.

Other topical preparations include salicylic acid, anthralin, and coal tar. Salicylic acid is a keratolytic agent that loosens psoriatic plaques. Like other salicylate drugs, topical salicylates may be absorbed systemically and cause toxicity; therefore topical salicylic acid should not be used by children due to the risk of Reye syndrome. Anthralin normalizes keratinocyte differentiation and is commonly used for short contact therapy. Common side effects include skin irritation and staining of adjoining skin, nails, and clothing. Coal tar products are available in shampoos, lotions, creams, and bath solutions. They have an unpleasant odor and can cause burning and stinging, so they are rarely used.

UVA may be used to suppress mitotic (cell division) activity. **Photochemotherapy**, a combination of UV radiation and the psoralen derivative methoxsalen (a photosensitive drug), is used to decrease proliferation of epidermal cells. This type of therapy is called **psoralen and ultraviolet A (PUVA)**, which permits lower doses of methoxsalen and UVA to be given. Common side effects of PUVA include erythema, pruritus, xerosis, irregular pigmentation, and gastrointestinal (GI) symptoms such as nausea and vomiting. Other toxicities include blisters, melanonychia, hypertrichosis, and squamous cell carcinoma

TABLE 48.3 Methotrexate Drug Interactions

NSAIDs	Antibiotics	Others
Salicylates	Trimethoprim-sulfamethoxazole	Acitretin
Naproxen		Barbiturates
		Ethanol
Ibuprofen	Sulfonamides	Vaccines with live virus
Indomethacin	Penicillins	Phenytoin
Phenylbutazone	Minocycline	Sulfonylureas
	Ciprofloxacin	Theophylline

NSAIDs, Nonsteroidal antiinflammatory drugs.
From Medscape (2021). *Methotrexate*. Retrieved from https://reference.medscape.com/drug/trexall-otrexup-methotrexate-343201#3.

(SCC). PUVA is contraindicated in patients with known lupus erythematosus, xeroderma pigmentosum, and porphyria. A topical preparation of methoxsalen must be administered only by a trained clinician. It is important to note that this treatment requires several sessions per week, and long-term light therapy increases the risk of skin cancer.

Systemic Drugs

Traditional systemic drugs for psoriasis (e.g., methotrexate, cyclosporine, acitretin) are commonly used for refractory psoriasis. Biologic response modifiers (BRMs) also have a role in the treatment of psoriasis without the toxicity of traditional systemic treatment to the liver, kidneys, and bone marrow; furthermore BRMs are not teratogenic.

A folate antimetabolite, methotrexate is a systemic drug that slows high growth fraction. It is prescribed to decrease the acceleration of epidermal cell growth in severe psoriasis. However, methotrexate can cause toxicity to the liver (hepatic fibrosis and cirrhosis), blood (myelosuppression), and lungs (pulmonary fibrosis). Other common adverse effects include nausea, anorexia, stomatitis, and fatigue. It is considered teratogenic and is contraindicated in females of childbearing age who are trying to conceive. Methotrexate has numerous drug-drug interactions, thereby increasing the risk of methotrexate toxicity (Table 48.3 lists some of the drugs that interact with methotrexate). Before methotrexate administration is initiated, a careful history, physical and laboratory tests (e.g., complete blood count [CBC], creatinine, LFTs, protein status, bilirubin, screening for latent tuberculosis [TB] infections), and chest radiograph must be obtained. During treatment, ongoing studies include CBC and renal and hepatic function tests. Methotrexate has been used in combination with approved

BRMs for psoriasis. See Chapter 35 for more nursing considerations with antimetabolites.

Cyclosporine, a cyclic polypeptide immunosuppressive drug, is the most effective systemic preparation for severe psoriasis. It inhibits T-cell activation and has minimal toxicities in otherwise healthy patients. It must be administered on a consistent schedule with regard to time of day and in relation to meals to decrease serum-level variations. As with other immunosuppressive drugs, patients must be assessed for active infections before initiating therapy. Patients must also be monitored for nephrotoxicity and hypertension. Other common side effects include **hypertrichosis** (darkening of hair), cephalgia, paresthesia, myalgia, arthralgia, asthenia, and fatigue.

Acitretin, a vitamin A derivative, is the least effective drug as monotherapy and is usually used concurrently with phototherapy. It is more effective with pustular psoriasis, and clinical response is dose dependent. Adverse effects include mucocutaneous effects, erythematous scaly patches with superficial fissures, and periungual pyogenic granulomas. Noncutaneous adverse effects include hyperlipidemia, pancreatitis, elevated transaminases, and pseudotumor cerebri–like symptoms. Its use is contraindicated with pregnancy.

Biologic Response Modifiers (BRM) are helpful in the management of psoriasis in patients who are refractory to ultraviolet B (UVB) phototherapy who need improved control. Drugs approved by the US Food and Drug Administration (FDA) include tumor necrosis factor (TNF) inhibitors (e.g., etanercept, infliximab, adalimumab) and interleukin antagonists (e.g., ustekinumab). All TNF inhibitors have a risk of severe opportunistic infection. TB and hepatitis B virus (HBV) testing should be conducted on all patients before administering TNF inhibitors. Caution is advised when administering these drugs to patients with a history of congestive heart failure. These biologic agents are expensive but tend to have fewer side effects with comparable efficacy to traditional systemic treatments. TNF inhibitors are contraindicated in patients with active infections or demyelinating disease (e.g., multiple sclerosis). Adalimumab is the first fully human TNF-inhibitor monoclonal antibody (mAb). Infliximab is a chimeric mAb, and ustekinumab is a human immunoglobulin G (IgG) monoclonal antibody. New mAbs include brodalumab, guselkumab, and tildrakizumab. More information on mAbs can be found in Chapter 36. Etanercept is a soluble recombinant human TNF-α inhibitor. Table 48.1 lists the drugs, including biologics, that are currently being used to control psoriasis.

CLINICAL JUDGMENT [NURSING PROCESS]
Acne Vulgaris and Psoriasis

Concept: Tissue Integrity
- The ability for the body tissue to repair itself

Recognize Cues [Assessment]
- Obtain a history from the patient regarding the onset of skin lesions. Note if there is a familial history.
- Assess the patient's skin eruptions. Describe lesions, locations (body surface area [BSA]), and drainage if present.
- Obtain cultures of purulent, draining skin lesions.
- Determine baseline vital signs and weight. Report any elevation in temperature.
- Obtain baseline laboratory values (complete blood count [CBC], lipid panel, renal function, and hepatic function).
- Obtain chest radiograph, electrocardiography (ECG), and, if applicable, conduct pregnancy, tuberculosis (TB), and hepatitis B virus (HBV) tests.
- Assess the psychological effects of skin lesions and any changes in perception of body image.
- Assess the effects of skin lesions on quality of life.

Analyze Cues and Prioritize Hypothesis [Patient Problems]
- Skin tissue injury related to disease process
- Sun-exposed skin rash related to side effects of drugs
- Need for teaching related to complex skin regimen
- Potential for decreased self-esteem

Generate Solutions [Planning]
- The patient will have increased knowledge of management of the skin condition.
- The patient will verbalize the need for two methods of contraception during the required period.
- The patient will verbalize that lesions have diminished after drug therapy and skin care.
- The patient will be free from infection during therapy.
- The patient will report improved body image.

Take Action [Nursing Interventions]
- Establish rapport; the patient may be embarrassed.
- Apply topical medications to skin lesions using aseptic technique.
- Monitor vital signs, and perform required diagnostic tests. Report abnormal findings.
- During drug therapy, check lesion sites for improvement, and monitor for adverse reactions to drug therapy.
- Listen to the patient's body image concerns, and provide community resources if applicable.

Patient Teaching
General
- Advise patients not to use harsh cleansers. Instruct them to gently cleanse the skin several times a day and pat dry. Allow to dry for 20 to 30 minutes before applying product.
- Teach patients to apply topical drugs using clean technique.
- Instruct patients to notify their health care provider if they are pregnant or if there is a possibility of pregnancy. Many drugs used to treat acne and psoriasis are teratogenic.
- Advise patients to keep health care appointments and to have diagnostic tests performed as prescribed.

Side Effects
- Inform patients about side effects and adverse reactions associated with drugs.
- Advise patients to report abnormal findings immediately.

Evaluate Outcomes [Evaluation]
- Evaluate the patient's knowledge of management of the condition.
- Evaluate the effectiveness of drug therapy. If improvement is not apparent, the drug therapy and skin care regimen may need to be changed.
- Be aware of the different time periods for improvement with various drug therapies.

VERRUCA VULGARIS AND DRUG-INDUCED DERMATITIS

Verruca Vulgaris (Warts)

The common wart is a hard, horny nodule that may appear anywhere on the body, particularly on the hands and feet. Warts occur when the top layer of the skin becomes infected with human papillomavirus (HPV). Warts may be benign lesions, or they may be precursors to cancerous lesions. Warts are contagious and can be spread by contact. Most warts do not require treatment, but they may be removed by cryotherapy (freezing), electrodessication, or surgical excision. Other treatments include using chemical peels with salicylic acid, tretinoin, and glycolic acid; as well as injection of anticancer drugs, such as bleomycin. Salicylic acid promotes desquamation. It can be absorbed through the skin, and salicylism (toxicity) could occur. Podophyllum resin is indicated mainly for venereal warts and is not as effective against the common wart. This drug also can be absorbed through the skin; toxic symptoms such as peripheral neuropathy, blood dyscrasias, and kidney impairment may result if a large area is treated. Podophyllum could cause teratogenic effects; therefore it should not be used during pregnancy. Imiquimod and podofilox may be prescribed as alternative agents for podophyllin, and both may be used for topical treatment of external genital and perianal warts. Bleomycin injections are also used for warts. Side effects of bleomycin injection include nail loss if given for warts on the fingers. Immunotherapy uses the patient's own immune system to fight the warts by causing an allergic reaction to the treated warts, which may cause the warts to disappear.

Cantharidin is used to remove the common wart. For treatment, cantharidin is applied to the wart and allowed to dry, and then the wart is covered with nonporous tape for 24 to 48 hours. Occlusion allows a blister to form beneath the wart, where live viruses are located. A follow-up visit at 2 weeks will allow the hyperkeratosis to be debrided. If verruca is noted after debridement, the procedure may be repeated. Side effects include a tingling or burning sensation at the application site.

Many OTC agents are used to remove warts. The efficacy of some of these is questionable; however, some that contain chemical compounds such as salicylic acid may be effective.

Drug-Induced Dermatitis

An adverse reaction to drug therapy may result in skin lesions that vary from a rash, urticaria, papules, and vesicles to life-threatening skin eruptions such as erythema multiforme (red blisters over a large portion of the body), Stevens-Johnson syndrome (large blisters in the oral and anogenital mucosa, pharynx, eyes, and viscera), and toxic epidermal necrolysis (widespread detachment of the epidermis from underlying skin layers). A hypersensitive reaction to a drug is caused by the formation of sensitizing lymphocytes. If multiple drug therapy is used, the last drug given may be the cause of the hypersensitivity and skin eruptions. The usual skin reaction is a rash, which may take several hours or a day to appear, and urticaria (hives), which usually takes a few minutes to appear. Certain drugs, such as penicillin, are known to cause hypersensitivity.

Other drug-induced dermatitides include discoid lupus erythematosus and exfoliative dermatitis. Hydralazine hydrochloride (e.g., isoniazid, phenothiazines, anticonvulsants, and antiarrhythmics, such as procainamide) may cause lupus-like symptoms. If lupus symptoms occur, the drug should be discontinued. Certain antibacterials and anticonvulsants may cause exfoliative dermatitis, resulting in erythema of the skin, itching, desquamation of large areas of the skin, and loss of body hair (e.g., sulfa antibiotics are one cause of toxic epidermal necrolysis).

CONTACT DERMATITIS

Contact dermatitis is a common form of eczema that results when skin is exposed to irritants (irritant contact dermatitis) or allergens (allergic contact dermatitis). Frequent contact with water (hand washing) can cause irritant contact dermatitis that usually starts with dry, cracked hands that sometimes develop pruritus and bleeding. Lips can also develop irritant contact dermatitis due to continuous licking of the lips. Other irritants include bleach, pepper spray, foods, and soap.

Allergic contact dermatitis is due to exposure to allergens. Examples of such allergens include poison ivy, sumac, and oak; nickel; makeup; jewelry; and latex gloves. Allergic contact dermatitis is considered a delayed hypersensitivity reaction. It may take hours to weeks for skin to develop manifestations, especially if it is a first-time exposure. Manifestations include skin rash with pruritus, swelling, burning, stinging, blistering, oozing, or scaling at the affected skin sites.

Nonpharmacologic Treatments

Nonpharmacologic treatments include avoiding direct contact with the causative irritant or allergen. Protective gloves or clothing may be necessary if the chemical is associated with work; skin that has been in contact with the irritant should be immediately cleansed and dried. Skin moisturizers, antihistamines (e.g., diphenhydramine), and/or topical corticosteroids may be used, depending on the severity of the dermatitis. Oatmeal baths can also relieve discomfort. Patch testing may be needed to determine the causal factor. Treatment may consist of wet dressings containing Burow's solution (aluminum acetate); lotions that contain zinc oxide, such as calamine; calcium hydroxide solution; and glycerin. Calamine lotion is primarily used for plant irritations. If itching persists, an oral antihistamine (e.g., diphenhydramine) may be used. Topical antipruritics should *not* be applied to open wounds or mucous membranes (e.g., eyes, mouth, or genital area). Other antipruritic treatments include baths of oatmeal and applications of corticosteroid ointments, creams, or gels.

Topical Corticosteroids

Topical corticosteroids can alleviate dermatitis but can be systemically absorbed into the circulation. The amount and rate of absorption depend on the vehicle (cream, lotion, or ointment), drug concentration, drug composition, and skin area to which the steroid is applied. Absorption is greater where the skin is more permeable, such as the face, scalp, eyelids, neck, axilla, and genital area. Side effects and adverse reactions may occur with prolonged use of the topical drug or continuously covering the drug with a dressing. Prolonged use of a topical steroid can cause thinning of the skin with atrophy of the epidermis and dermis and purpura from small-vessel eruptions; therefore, prolonged use is discouraged.

IMPETIGO, ROSACEA, AND HAIR LOSS

Impetigo

Impetigo, an infection of the skin that is usually due to *Streptococcus* or *Staphylococcus* species, is mostly seen in children 2 to 5 years old. Topical therapies are used in the treatment of mild and moderate infection, and oral drugs are used for severe infection. The two drugs of choice are mupirocin and retapamulin. The lesions should be soaked to facilitate the removal of crusts, and the topical antibiotic should be applied at the base of the lesion. With multiple lesions and ineffective topical therapy, oral antibiotics are needed.

Rosacea

Rosacea is a common skin disorder, presented usually with rashes. Other signs and symptoms can include flushing, visible blood vessels, swelling, and acne-like breakouts. Other people may present with thick skin and course texture. Treatments for rosacea are geared toward avoiding triggers that exacerbate rosacea, limiting UV exposures with the use of a broad-spectrum sunblock, and using mild skin products. For rosacea with acne-like breakouts, azelaic acid, metronidazole, sodium sulfacetamide/sulfur, and retinoid may be used. Other treatments include antibacterials such as tetracycline and isotretinoin.

Hair Loss and Baldness

Hair loss, or *alopecia*, occurs when the hair shaft is lost, and the hair follicle cannot regenerate. Permanent hair loss is associated with a familial history and occurs during the aging process, earlier in some individuals. Also known to cause alopecia are some drugs, which include anticancer agents, sulfonamides, anticonvulsants, aminoglycosides, and some nonsteroidal antiinflammatory drugs (NSAIDs) such as indomethacin. Severe febrile illnesses, pregnancy, myxedema (a condition resulting from hypothyroidism), and cancer therapies are some of the health conditions that contribute to temporary hair loss. Alopecia areata is an autoimmune disease where the immune system attacks hair follicles at the root, causing hair to be lost on the scalp or any part of the body. It can occur in children and young adults. In some cases, hair will grow back, but often patients will continue with episodes of hair loss and regrowth throughout their lives. Ritlecitinib was approved by the FDA in 2023 for the treatment of severe alopecia areata. The dose is 50 mg PO once daily. This drug should not be used in combination with other Janus Kinase (JAK) inhibitors, biologic immunomodulators, cyclosporine, or other potent immunosuppressants.

Minoxidil solution has been approved by the FDA for treating hair loss in males and females. A 5% solution is approved for males, 2% for females. The exact mechanism of action to stimulate hair growth is not known. Hair regrowth is usually seen after several months of use, but a few months after discontinuation, hair loss resumes. Minoxidil is available OTC in the form of a solution or foam. Systemic absorption of minoxidil is minimal, so adverse reactions seldom occur. Occasionally, headaches and a slight decrease in systolic blood pressure occur.

Finasteride (1 mg) is an oral drug used for alopecia in males. For growing hair, finasteride is effective in 50% of males. It has been reported that it is relatively ineffective in growing hair in older men, even with an increased dose. Like minoxidil, clinical response is not seen until the drug has been used daily for 3 months or longer; discontinuing the drug leads to hair loss within 12 months. Finasteride is contraindicated in pregnancy, and pregnant patients should not handle the drug. Side effects include decreased libido, impotence, and ejaculation disorder.

BURNS AND BURN PREVENTION

Sunscreens

Sunscreens are primarily used to block UV rays that cause sunburn, but they also protect against certain types of keratosis, skin cancer, premature aging, cold sores and fever blisters, and UV photosensitivity reactions. There are two types of sunscreens: chemical blockers and physical blockers. *Chemical blockers* (e.g., oxybenzone and ecamsule) absorb UV radiation and are effective against UVA radiation, and *physical blockers* (e.g., titanium dioxide and zinc oxide) reflect or scatter UV radiation and are effective against both UVA and UVB radiation. UVB radiation is the primary cause of sunburn and skin cancer, whereas UVA is responsible for loss of elasticity (wrinkling) and collagen damage of the skin. UVA radiation also contributes to skin cancer and penetrates the skin at a deeper level than UVB, thereby causing damage to deeper skin structures. Broad-spectrum sunscreen protects from both UVA and UVB radiation. The FDA passed a ruling that sunscreen with a sun protection factor (SPF) of less than 15 can denote that it prevents sunburn, and an SPF of 15 and above can reduce the risk of skin cancer and early skin aging if used as directed with other sun protection measures such as wearing sun-blocking clothing, limiting sun exposure between 10 a.m. and 2 p.m., and reapplying sunscreen at least every 2 hours. The American Academy of Dermatology recommends water-resistant sunscreen with an SPF 30 or higher. Sunscreen with an SPF 30 blocks 97% of UVB rays. Common side effects of sunscreens include cutaneous reactions (e.g., erythema, pruritus, folliculitis, contact dermatitis, and acne vulgaris).

Burns and Burn Preparations

Burns from heat (*thermal burns*, the most common kind of burn injury), electricity (*electrical burns*), and chemical agents (*chemical burns*) can all cause skin lesions. Burns are classified according to degree and depth of the tissue injury (Table 48.4). Burns need immediate attention, regardless of the degree and depth of tissue injury. For minor burns, a cool, wet compress is applied to prevent further tissue damage caused by heat. After the affected area is cooled off, it should be cleansed gently with soap and water; intact blisters should not be opened. After cleaning the area, apply a thin layer of ointment, such as aloe vera or petroleum jelly. A thin layer of antibiotic ointment (e.g., bacitracin, neomycin sulfate, polymyxin B sulfate) can be applied to affected areas one to three times daily if the area becomes infected.

Persons with burns that involve the dermis and subcutaneous tissue should seek medical help immediately at a health care facility. Persons with extensive second-degree burns and beyond are at risk of dehydration through interstitial fluid loss and are vulnerable to infection and sepsis. Dehydration can cause hypovolemic shock. Primary attention

TABLE 48.4 Degree and Tissue Depth of Burns

Type	Degree	Depth	Characteristics
Superficial epidermal	First	Outer layer of skin; epidermis (e.g., sunburn without blisters)	Erythema, edema, pain
Partial or full-thickness superficial	Second	Epidermis, upper layers of dermis; blisters may be present	Partial: Wound is pink and blanches; erythema is present, and burn is painful and wet appearing. Full: Blanching is sluggish or absent; burn is red/white and dry in appearance; pain may be present but will be diminished.
Full-thickness	Third	All layers extending into the subcutaneous tissues	Skin can appear black or white and dry and is leathery in texture; area will not blanch, and no pain is experienced.

should be to the airway, breathing, and circulation (ABC). Intravenous (IV) fluid therapy should be started immediately, and an analgesic is given for pain. For extensive burns, the amount of fluids should be determined by calculating the percentage of the person's body surface area that was burned. The most common formulation to determine the degree of injury is the Wallace Rule of Nines. The Parkland formula can help determine the amount of fluid needed in the first 24 hours for persons with critical burn injury. Burn areas are kept clean, and any necrotic tissue is debrided. Broad-spectrum topical antiinfectives effective against many gram-positive and gram-negative organisms and fungi are applied to burn areas to prevent infection. Examples of these antiinfectives include mafenide acetate, silver sulfadiazine, and silver nitrate 0.5% solution. Table 48.5 lists selected topical medications for burns along with their dosages, uses, and considerations. Prototype Drug Chart: Mafenide Acetate lists the pharmacologic data for the antibacterial drug mafenide acetate.

TABLE 48.5 Topical Antiinfectives: Burns

Generic (Brand)	Route and Dosage	Uses and Considerations
Mafenide acetate	See Prototype Drug Chart: Mafenide Acetate	
Silver sulfadiazine	A: 1% Cream: Apply twice daily to a thickness of 1.6 mm	To prevent and treat infection of second- and third-degree burns. Ten percent of drug is absorbed. Excessive use or extensive application area may cause sulfa crystals (crystalluria).

A, Adult; *mm*, millimeter.

Silver Sulfadiazine

Silver sulfadiazine is a common antiinfective used to prevent and treat infections in second- and third-degree burns, and it is not absorbed through the skin. It is applied at least twice daily. Silver sulfadiazine possesses activity against both gram-negative and gram-positive organisms and fungi. Unlike mafenide, it is not a carbonic anhydrase inhibitor. Sulfadiazine is metabolized by the liver and is excreted in the urine. It is contraindicated in near-term pregnancy and among neonates and infants younger than 2 months. Side effects and adverse reactions may include photosensitivity, skin discoloration, burning sensation, rashes, erythema multiforme, skin necrosis, and leukopenia.

PROTOTYPE DRUG CHART
Mafenide Acetate

Drug Class	Dosage
Topical antiinfective	A: Cream: Apply a layer of 1.6 mm thickness evenly to the affected area once or twice daily; reapply PRN. Be sure burn is covered with cream at all times.
	A: Sol: Apply to dressing-covered graft site every 4 h or as needed to maintain wet dressing.

Contraindications	Drug-Lab-Food Interactions
Hypersensitivity, inhalation injury *Caution:* Renal failure, acid-base imbalance, or hypersensitivity to other sulfonamides/sulfites	No significant drug interactions; caution when using other carbonic anhydrase inhibitors due to increased risk of metabolic acidosis.

Pharmacokinetics	Pharmacodynamics
Absorption: Diffuses through devascularized areas with variable systemic absorption Distribution: PB: UK Metabolism: t½: UK Excretion: In urine	Onset: On contact Peak: 2 h Duration: 4 h

Therapeutic Effects/Uses
Synthetic sulfonamide antibiotics are indicated as an adjunctive treatment for second- and third-degree burns and are not absorbed through the skin; used to prevent organism invasion of burned tissue areas and to treat burn infections.
Mechanism of Action: Bacteriostatic activity against many gram-negative and gram-positive bacteria, including *Pseudomonas aeruginosa* and other anaerobic strains.

Side Effects	Adverse Reactions
Rash, burning sensation, urticaria, pruritus, swelling, erythema	Metabolic acidosis, respiratory alkalosis, blistering, superinfection (e.g., fungal) *Life threatening:* Bone marrow suppression, fatal hemolytic anemia

A, Adult; *h*, hour; *PB*, protein binding; *PRN*, as needed; *Sol*, solution; *t½*, half-life; *UK*, unknown.

CLINICAL JUDGMENT [NURSING PROCESS]
Topical Antiinfectives: Burns

Concept: Tissue Integrity
- The ability of the body tissue to repair itself

Recognize Cues [Assessment]
- Determine the stability of the patient by assessing airway, breathing, and circulation.
- Determine fluid status. Report signs and symptoms of hypovolemia or hypervolemia.
- Check the patient's vital signs. Report abnormal findings, such as elevated temperature.
- Assess burned tissue for signs of infection such as foul odor, purulent drainage, erythema, and heat.
- Culture the purulent wound.

Analyze Cues and Prioritize Hypothesis [Patient Problems]
- Decreased potential for fluid volume and potential for imbalanced perfusion
- Potential for infection
- Acute pain related to thermal injury
- Deficient knowledge related to management of burns

Generate Solutions [Planning]
- The patient will remain hemodynamically stable.
- The patient will remain free from infection.
- The patient will report decreased or tolerable pain level.
- The patient will remain hydrated.

Take Action [Nursing Interventions]
- Monitor the patient for any cardiopulmonary difficulties, vital signs, or infection.
- Administer prescribed analgesia before treatment, if needed.
- Cleanse burned tissue sites using aseptic technique.
- Apply topical antibacterial drugs and dressings with sterile technique.
- Maintain the patient's fluid balance and renal function.
- Monitor the patient for side effects and adverse reactions to topical drugs.
- Closely monitor the patient's acid-base balance, especially in the presence of pulmonary or renal dysfunction.
- Store drugs in a dry place at room temperature.

Patient Teaching
- Instruct the patient and family about pain management, medications used to treat burns, and signs of complications from burns, such as fluid excess or deficit.
- Teach the patient and family how to apply a topical agent and dressings to burned areas.
- Teach the patient and family about signs and symptoms of infection and to report them promptly to the health care provider.

Evaluate Outcomes [Evaluation]
- Evaluate patient's cardiopulmonary status, ensuring breathing and circulation is stable.
- Evaluate patient and family knowledge of burn management.
- Evaluate the effectiveness of treatment interventions to burned tissue areas by determining whether healing is occurring, and the site is free from infection.

CLINICAL JUDGMENT CASE STUDY

A 15-year-old female patient reports blackheads and large, raised acne with surrounding erythema on her face. She seeks help from a health care provider.

1. To assist in identifying her skin problem, what would the health history and assessment include?
2. Which nonpharmacologic measures might the nurse discuss with the patient in caring for her skin condition?

   The patient's skin disorder does not improve. Her health care provider says she has acne vulgaris and has prescribed benzoyl peroxide and oral tetracycline.

3. The patient asks the nurse how to use benzoyl peroxide. What would the explanation of the method and frequency for use of benzoyl peroxide include?
4. What would be included in the patient teaching related to the use of oral tetracycline?
5. What other drugs for acne might the patient use? Explain their uses and side effects.
6. The patient asks if she will have to remain on benzoyl peroxide and oral tetracycline for the rest of her life. What is the nurse's best response or course of action? Explain your answer.

REVIEW QUESTIONS

1. A patient being seen for skin concerns asks, "What do keratolytic drugs remove?" Which response would be best by the nurse?
   a. A horny layer of dermis
   b. A horny layer of epidermis
   c. Erythematous lesions
   d. Hair follicles

2. A patient is to begin therapy with isotretinoin and asks, "What do I have to remember to do while taking this medicine?" How would the nurse respond? **Select all that apply.**
   a. Avoid sunlight.
   b. Monitor your weight.
   c. Keep appointments for laboratory tests.
   d. Use two forms of contraceptives.
   e. Always take the drug with food.

3. The nurse is doing health teaching with a patient who has psoriasis. Which nursing implication is a priority for a patient on infliximab to treat psoriasis?
   a. Monitor weight daily.
   b. Monitor electrolytes.
   c. Monitor urine output.
   d. Monitor complete blood count.

4. A 55-year-old patient is concerned about hair loss. The nurse expects that the patient's baldness may be treated with which drug?
   a. Dexamethasone
   b. Para-aminobenzoic acid
   c. Mupirocin
   d. Finasteride

5. The nurse reviews the patient's medication history. Based on the patient's prolonged use of topical corticosteroids, which assessment will the nurse include? **Select all that apply.**
   a. Weight gain
   b. Thinning of the skin
   c. Erythematous lesions
   d. Purpura
   e. Urinary retention
6. A 20-year-old female comes to the clinic for follow-up related to isotretinoin use. Which information from the iPLEDGE program would the nurse provide to the patient? **Select all that apply.**
   a. One method of contraception must be used throughout treatment.
   b. A review of iPLEDGE educational materials.
   c. A negative pregnancy test is required before each monthly refill.
   d. Informed consent is not required.
   e. A prescription for a 60-day supply of the drug is to be given.
7. The school nurse prepares a program for junior high school students on sun safety. Which information would the nurse include? **Select all that apply.**
   a. Sunscreen products should contain information about ultraviolet A and B sun protection that includes the sun protection factor.
   b. Ultraviolet B radiation is greatest between 10 a.m. and 2 p.m.
   c. Clouds block radiation, so sunscreen is not needed on cloudy days.
   d. The sun protection factor (SPF) should be at least 30 in sunscreen products.
   e. Sunscreen is to be applied once daily.
8. A patient is receiving etanercept. Which nursing intervention is appropriate for this patient? **Select all that apply.**
   a. Drug is administered topically.
   b. Tuberculin test is required before the start of therapy.
   c. Monitor for injection site reaction.
   d. Monitor for seizures.
   e. Monitor for heart failure.
9. The nurse is teaching the patient about clobetasol. Which information should be included in the teaching session? **Select all that apply.**
   a. Appropriate treatment is for 6 months' duration.
   b. It can be applied as a lotion to all body parts.
   c. Clobetasol is a super-high-potency corticosteroid.
   d. Maximum dose is 50 g/wk.
   e. Occlusive dressing speeds healing.

UNIT XV Endocrine Drugs

49

Pituitary, Thyroid, Parathyroid, and Adrenal Disorders

http://evolve.elsevier.com/McCuistion/pharmacology

OBJECTIVES

- Describe the structures and functions of the pituitary gland.
- Describe the structures and functions of the thyroid gland.
- Describe the structures and functions of the parathyroid glands and their hormones.
- Describe the structures and function of the adrenal glands and their hormones.

OUTLINE

Overview of the Pituitary Gland, 633
   Pituitary Gland: Anterior Lobe, 633
Thyroid-Stimulating Hormone, 634
Adrenocorticotropic Hormone, 634
Prolactin, 634
Pituitary Gland: Posterior Lobe, 636
Drug Therapy for Anterior Pituitary Disorders: Growth Hormone Deficiency, 636
Drug Therapy for Anterior Pituitary Disorders: Growth Hormone Excess, 636
Other Drugs for Anterior Pituitary Disorders, 637
Drug Therapy for Posterior Pituitary Disorders, 637
Overview of the Thyroid Gland, 638

Hypothyroidism and Hyperthyroidism, 639
Drug Therapy for Thyroid Disorders: Hypothyroidism, 639
Drug Therapy for Thyroid Disorder: Hyperthyroidism, 641
Overview of the Parathyroid Glands, 642
   Hypoparathyroidism and Hyperparathyroidism, 642
   Drug Therapy for Parathyroid Disorder: Hypoparathyroidism, 642
   Drug Therapy for Parathyroid Disorder: Hyperparathyroidism, 642
Overview of the Adrenal Glands, 644
   Hypoadrenalism and Hyperadrenalism, 644
   Drug Therapy for Adrenal Disorders: Glucocorticoids and Mineralocorticoids 644
Clinical Judgment Single-Episode Case Study, 647
Review Questions, 648

OVERVIEW OF THE PITUITARY GLAND

This chapter describes drugs used for hormonal replacement and for inhibition of hormonal secretion from the pituitary, thyroid, parathyroid, and adrenal glands. Before reading this chapter, review the endocrine glands and their associated hormones. Knowledge of the various endocrine glands and their respective hormones and functions facilitates an understanding of the drugs that act on the endocrine glands.

The pituitary gland, or **hypophysis**, has an anterior lobe and a posterior lobe (Fig. 49.1). The anterior pituitary gland is also called the **adenohypophysis** and secretes many hormones that target glands and tissues throughout the body. The posterior pituitary gland, known as the **neurohypophysis**, secretes **antidiuretic hormone (ADH)** and oxytocin.

Pituitary Gland: Anterior Lobe

The anterior pituitary gland produces and secretes the majority of the hormones from the pituitary gland, and they include:

- Growth hormone (GH), which stimulates growth in tissue and bone
- Thyroid-stimulating hormone (TSH), which acts on the thyroid gland
- Adrenocorticotropic hormone (ACTH), which stimulates the adrenal gland
- Gonadotropins (follicle-stimulating hormone [FSH] and luteinizing hormone [LH]), which affect the ovaries and testes
- Prolactin (PRL), which primarily affects the breast tissues

The amount of each hormone secreted from the anterior pituitary gland is regulated by a negative feedback system. If excess hormone is secreted from the target gland, hormonal release from the anterior pituitary gland is suppressed. If there is a lack of hormone secretion from the target gland, there will be an increase in that particular anterior pituitary hormone (Fig. 49.2). Drugs with adenohypophyseal properties used to stimulate or inhibit glandular activity for GH, TSH, ACTH, and PRL are discussed according to their therapeutic use.

Growth Hormone

Two hypothalamic hormones regulate GH: (1) GH-releasing hormone (somatropin) and (2) GH-inhibiting hormone (somatostatin). GH does not have a specific target gland. It affects most body tissues

633

Fig. 49.1 The anterior and posterior pituitary glands *ACTH*, Adrenocorticotropic hormone; *ADH*, antidiuretic hormone; *FSH*, follicle-stimulating hormone; *GH*, growth hormone; *LH*, luteinizing hormone; *PRL*, prolactin; *TSH*, thyroid-stimulating hormone.

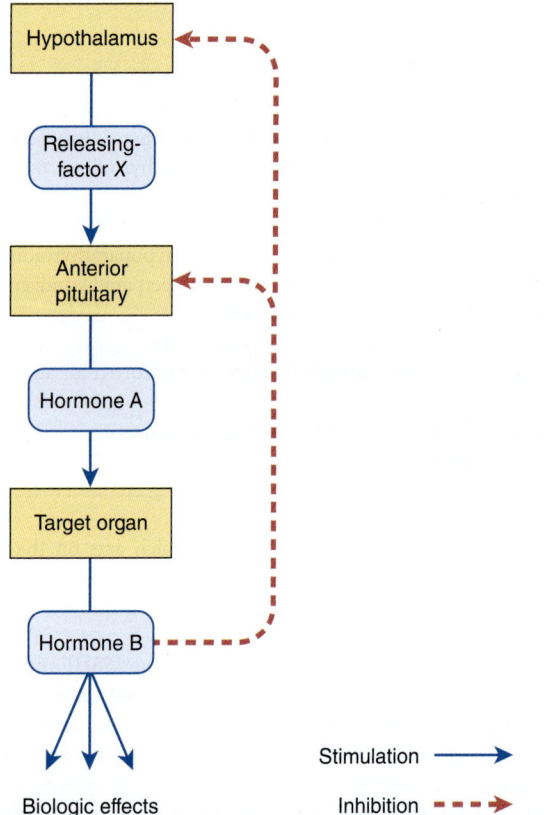

Fig. 49.2 Negative feedback loop of hypothalamus and pituitary. (From Burcham J, Rosenthal L: *Lehne's pharmacology for nursing care*, ed 9, St. Louis, 2016, Elsevier.)

and bone; GH replacement stimulates linear growth when there are GH deficiencies. GH drugs cannot be given orally because they are inactivated by gastrointestinal (GI) enzymes. Subcutaneous (subcut) or intramuscular (IM) administration of GH is necessary.

If a child's height is well below the standard for a specified age, GH deficiency may be the cause, and dwarfism can result. Because of the cost, tests are performed to determine whether GH replacement therapy is essential. GH stimulation test with insulin tolerance test is labor intensive and can cause severe hypoglycemia. Macimorelin is a GH secretagogue and, after an oral dose, can measure the stimulated GH levels.

Because GH acts on newly forming bone, it must be administered before the epiphyses are fused. Administration of GH over several years can increase height by a foot. However, prolonged GH therapy can antagonize insulin secretion, eventually causing diabetes mellitus. Athletes should be advised not to take GH to build muscle and physique because of its effects on blood glucose along with other serious side effects. Table 49.1 lists the drugs used to replace or inhibit GH and gives their dosages, uses, and considerations.

THYROID-STIMULATING HORMONE

The adenohypophysis secretes **thyroid-stimulating hormone (TSH)** in response to thyroid-releasing hormone (TRH) from the hypothalamus. TSH stimulates the thyroid gland to release thyroxine (T_4) and triiodothyronine (T_3, or liothyronine). Excess TSH secretion can cause hyperthyroidism, and a TSH deficit can cause hypothyroidism. Hypothyroidism may be caused by a thyroid gland disorder (primary cause) or a decrease in TSH secretion (secondary cause). Thyrotropin, a purified extract of TSH for thyroid cancer, is used as a diagnostic agent to differentiate between primary and secondary hypothyroidism. Side effects caused by thyrotropin include symptoms of hyperthyroidism. Other side effects include urticaria, rash, pruritus, and flushing.

Table 49.1 lists the drug used to replace TSH and its dosages, uses, and considerations.

ADRENOCORTICOTROPIC HORMONE

The hypothalamus releases corticotropin-releasing factor (CRF), which stimulates the pituitary corticotrophs to secrete **adrenocorticotropic hormone (ACTH)**, which stimulates the release of glucocorticoids (cortisol), mineralocorticoids (aldosterone), and androgen from the adrenal cortex and catecholamines (epinephrine and norepinephrine) from the adrenal medulla. Usually, ACTH and cortisol secretions follow a diurnal rhythm, in which the ACTH and cortisol secretion is higher in the early morning and then decreases throughout the day. Stresses such as surgery, sepsis, and trauma override the diurnal rhythm, causing an increase in secretions of ACTH and cortisol. Hypocortisolism, or adrenal insufficiency, can occur and may be due to inadequate secretion of ACTH or dysfunction of the adrenal glands.

PROLACTIN

The primary function of **prolactin (PRL)** is stimulation of breast tissue for milk production. PRL deficiency (*hypoprolactinemia*) is generally without symptoms except during breastfeeding, when it can cause lactation disruption. Excess PRL (*hyperprolactinemia*) produces symptoms in both males and females. Males may develop excess breast tissue (*gynecomastia*) and may lactate (*galactorrhea*), and excess PRL decreases sperm production. Females with excess PRL can experience lactation that is not pregnancy related, or they can develop amenorrhea. Excess PRL can be treated with dopamine agonists (e.g., bromocriptine, cabergoline). Cabergoline is better tolerated, has a longer half-life, and offers more convenient dosing than bromocriptine. Dopamine agonists are discussed in Chapter 20.

TABLE 49.1 Drug Therapies for Pituitary Disorders

Generic	Route and Dosage	Uses and Considerations
ANTERIOR LOBE		
Growth Hormone (GH-RH)		
Somapacitan	A: Subcut: Initial dose 1.5 mg; then increase q2–4 wk by 0.5–1.5 mg until desired response; not to exceed 8 mg q week.	For GH deficiency in adults. Contraindicated in persons with active malignancy, diabetic eye disease, acute critical illness, including respiratory failure. PB: >99%; t½: 2–3 d
Somatropin	C: Subcut/IM: Dosing is based on brand names and is individualized for each patient; review the clinician's orders carefully.	For GH deficiency for adults and growth failure in children. Contraindicated in children with epiphyseal closure, patients with active neoplastic disease, and those with acute critical illness. Do not administer intravenously. Therapy is discontinued when final height is achieved if given for growth failure. Read clinician's orders carefully for the trade name; dosing is *not* interchangeable. PB: 20%; t½: 20–30 min
Growth Hormone Suppressant Drugs		
Bromocriptine mesylate	Acromegaly: A: PO: 1.25–2.5 mg/d at bedtime for 3 d; *maint:* 20–30 mg/d in divided doses; *max:* 100 mg/d Prolactinemia/pituitary adenoma: A/C ≥16 y: PO: 1.25–2.5 mg/d; titrate dose at 2–7 d intervals as needed; *max:* 30 mg/d C 11–15 y: PO: 1.25–2.5 mg/d, may titrate to 10 mg/d	For acromegaly, pituitary adenoma, and hyperprolactinemia. Also used with pituitary radiation or surgery to decrease GH levels. Decreases lactation and prolactinemia. Take with food. PB: >90%; t½: 3 h
Lanreotide acetate	Acromegaly: A: Subcut: Initially 90 mg q4wk for 3 mo, then adjust dose based on GH, IGF-1, and clinical symptoms q4wk NET: A: Subcut: 120 mg q4wk	For acromegaly and NET. PB: 79%–83%; t½: 23–30 d
Octreotide acetate	A: Subcut: 50–200 mcg tid A: IM: 20 mg q4wk for 3 mo, then adjust according to serum GH and IGF-1 levels	For acromegaly. Injectable depot suspension is for IM use only. PB: 65%; t½: 1.7 h
Pegvisomant	A: Subcut: Give a 40-mg loading dose, then 10 mg/d; adjust in increments of 5 mg; *max:* 30 mg/d	For acromegaly. IGF-1 concentrations should be measured q4–6wk. PB: UK; t½: 6 d
Thyroid-Stimulating Hormone (TSH)		
Thyrotropin	Thyroid cancer: A: IM: 0.9 mg into gluteus maximus, repeat in 24 h for 2 doses; *max:* 0.9 mg/d	For thyroid cancer. Radioiodine study follows last injection. PB: UK; t½: 15–35 h
Adrenocorticotropic Hormone (ACTH)		
Corticotropin	Immunosuppressant: A: IM/subcut: 40–80 units q24–72 h Do *not* discontinue abruptly; dose must be tapered. ACTH deficiency diagnosis: A: IM/subcut: Up to 80 units MS exacerbations: A: IM/subcut: 80–120 units/d in divided doses for 2–3 wk	For ACTH deficiency diagnostic, MS, and infantile spasms. Administer only to patients with adrenal responsiveness. Repository gel must be room temperature before administration. Do not overpressurize vial during withdrawal. PB: UK; t½: 15 min
Cosyntropin	A: IM/IV: 0.25 mg over 2 min or slow infusion over 6 h	For diagnostic testing to differentiate between pituitary and adrenal cause of adrenal insufficiency. Obtain plasma cortisol level before and 30–60 min after administration. PB: UK; t½: 7 min
POSTERIOR LOBE		
Antidiuretic Hormone (ADH)		
Desmopressin acetate	DI: A: PO: Initial dose 0.05 mg bid, then titrate to response. A: IN: Initial dose is 10 mcg in the evening, then titrate to response. A: IV/subcut: 2–4 mcg/d given in 2 divided doses daily Hemophilia A or von Willebrand disease: A: IN: One spray in 1–2 nostrils based on weight for 1–2 doses. A: IV/subcut: 0.3 mcg/kg/dose, then titrate to response.	For DI, hemophilia A, and von Willebrand disease. Desmopressin can have a long duration of action (5–21 h). PB: UK; t½: 1.5–2.5 h

Continued

TABLE 49.1 Drug Therapies for Pituitary Disorders—cont'd

Generic	Route and Dosage	Uses and Considerations
Vasopressin	A: IM/subcut: 5–10 units q3–4h or 2–3 × daily PRN	For central DI. Can also be given intranasally. Aspirate IM injections; avoid injection into a blood vessel. PB: none; t½: 10–20 min
Demeclocycline	A: PO: 600–1200 mg/d in 3–4 divided doses	For off-label treatment of SIADH. PB: 65%–90%; t½: 10–17 h, increases to 42–68 h in patients with severe renal impairment
Conivaptan	A: IV: LD 20 mg over 30 min; maint: 20 mg continuous IV over 24 h; then 20 mg/d for 1–3 d; may titrate up to 40 mg/d; max: 4 d of therapy	For symptomatic euvolemic hyponatremia associated with SIADH. PB: 99%; t½: 5–8 h
Tolvaptan	A: PO: Initially 15 mg/d, then 15–30 mg/d; max: 60 mg/d for up to 30 d; adjust dose in 24-h increment	For symptomatic hypervolemic or euvolemic hyponatremia. Avoid fluid restriction during the first 24 h of therapy. PB: 99%; t½: 12 h

A, Adult; *bid*, twice daily; *C*, child; *d*, day; *DI*, diabetes insipidus; *GH*, growth hormone; *GH-RH*, GH-releasing hormone; *h*, hour; *IGF*, insulin-like growth factor; *IN*, intranasal; *h*, hour; *IM*, intramuscular; *IN*, intranasal; *IV*, intravenous; *LD*, loading dose; *maint*, maintenance; *max*, maximum dosage; *min*, minute; *mo*, month; *MS*, multiple sclerosis; *NET*, neuroendocrine tumor; *q*, every; *PB*, protein binding; *PO*, by mouth; *PRN*, as needed; *SIADH*, syndrome of inappropriate diuretic hormone; *subcut*, subcutaneous; *t½*, half-life; *tid*, three times daily; *UK*, unknown; *wk*, week; *y*, year.

PITUITARY GLAND: POSTERIOR LOBE

ADH and oxytocin that are secreted by the posterior pituitary gland are produced by the hypothalamus. The hormones travel by way of the hypophysial portal system into the posterior pituitary gland for storage and secretion. (Oxytocin is discussed in Chapter 54.) Table 49.1 lists the drugs used to replace or inhibit ADH and their dosages, uses, and considerations.

ADH promotes water reabsorption from the renal tubules to maintain water balance (osmolality) in the body fluids. When there is a deficiency of ADH, large amounts of water are excreted by the kidneys. This condition, called diabetes insipidus (DI), can lead to severe fluid volume deficit and electrolyte imbalances. Head injury and brain tumors resulting in trauma to the hypothalamus and pituitary gland can cause DI. Fluid and electrolyte balances must be closely monitored in these patients, and ADH replacement may be needed.

When secretion of ADH from the posterior pituitary gland is excessive, the most common cause is small cell carcinoma of the lung. Medications, other malignancies, and stressors (e.g., pain, infection, anxiety, trauma) may also be causative factors. These conditions lead to an excessive amount of water retention expanding the intracellular and intravascular volume known as syndrome of inappropriate antidiuretic hormone (SIADH). This increased fluid volume causes enhanced glomerular filtration and decreased tubular sodium reabsorption. Natriuresis, excretion of urinary sodium, can occur and can cause hyponatremia.

DRUG THERAPY FOR ANTERIOR PITUITARY DISORDERS: GROWTH HORMONE DEFICIENCY

Somatropin is a GH used to treat growth failure in children because of GH deficiency. Somatropin is a product that has an identical amino acid sequence as human GH (hGH); it is contraindicated in pediatric patients who have growth deficiency due to Prader-Willi syndrome, in those who are severely obese, or in those who have severe respiratory impairment because fatalities associated with GH can occur. A second hGH, somapacitan, was recently approved by the FDA for adults with GH deficiency. GH products not approved by the FDA are being consumed among healthy adults to decrease signs of aging, such as lean muscle mass and increased body fat. Even though hGH increases muscle mass, it does not translate to improved strength. Furthermore, research indicates that these persons are at risk for complications, such as type 2 diabetes, fluid retention, gynecomastia, and certain cancers.

Corticosteroids can inhibit the effects of somatropin; therefore they should not be taken concurrently. Somatropin can enhance the effects of antidiabetics and can cause hypoglycemia.

Side and adverse effects of somatropin include paresthesia, arthralgia, myalgia, peripheral edema, weakness, and cephalgia. Metabolic complications include glucose fluctuations, hypothyroidism, and hematuria. Flulike symptoms and hyperpigmentation of the skin can also occur. Adverse reactions include seizures, intracranial hypertension, and secondary malignancy (e.g., leukemia).

DRUG THERAPY FOR ANTERIOR PITUITARY DISORDERS: GROWTH HORMONE EXCESS

Gigantism, excessive growth during childhood, and acromegaly, excessive growth after puberty, can occur with GH hypersecretion; these are frequently caused by a pituitary tumor. If the tumor cannot be destroyed by radiation, GH receptor antagonists (e.g., pegvisomant), somatostatin analogs (e.g., lanreotide, octreotide), and dopamine agonists (e.g., bromocriptine) act by either blocking GH receptor sites or by inhibiting the secretion of GH.

Pegvisomant blocks GH receptor sites, preventing abnormal growth by normalizing insulin-like growth factor 1 (IGF-1) level, and it is given by injection. Common side effects include hyperhidrosis, cephalgia, and fatigue. Adverse effects include chest pain, hypertension, and elevated hepatic transaminases.

Lanreotide is an analog of somatostatin that has actions similar to those of endogenous somatostatin. The effects of reduced GH are dose-related and have a duration of at least 28 days after a single injection; therefore injections are given every 4 weeks. Lanreotide is available in depot formulation and is administered deep in the subcutaneous layer. Common side effects include mild GI symptoms: diarrhea, abdominal pain, nausea, vomiting, constipation, weight loss, and flatulence.

Octreotide is a synthetic somatostatin-inhibiting the secretion of GH. It is available in immediate-release and depot formulations. Immediate-release formulations are given by thrice-daily subcutaneous injection, and depot injection is administered once monthly. Common side effects include GI upsets such as nausea, bloating, and flatus. Adverse effects include cardiac toxicity, such as bradycardia and arrhythmia.

Bromocriptine, a dopamine agonist, inhibits the secretion of GH caused by pituitary adenomas. It is available in oral form and has fewer side effects than other treatments for hyperpituitarism, which include GI symptoms (e.g., nausea, anorexia, dyspepsia, and xerostomia). Adverse effects include cardiac toxicity (e.g., hypertension, myocardial

TABLE 49.2 Physiologic Effects: Adrenal Hyposecretion and Hypersecretion

Body System	Adrenal Hyposecretion (Addison Disease)	Adrenal Hypersecretion (Cushing Syndrome)
Metabolism: Glucose, Protein, Fat	Hypoglycemia, muscle weakness, weight loss	Hyperglycemia, muscle wasting; thinning of skin; poor wound healing; osteoporosis; fat accumulation in face (moon face), back of neck (buffalo hump), and trunk (protruding abdomen); hyperlipidemia; high cholesterol; weight gain
Central nervous system	Apathy, depression, fatigue, irritability	Increased neural activity, mood elevation, irritability, seizures, weakness, fatigue
Integument	Hyperpigmentation	Easy bruising, striae, plethora, and excess hair growth to face (hirsutism), neck, chest, abdomen, and thighs
Eyes	None	Cataract formation
Cardiovascular	Tachycardia, hypotension, orthostatic hypotension, cardiovascular collapse, syncope, dizziness	Hypertension, edema, heart failure
Gastrointestinal	Nausea, vomiting, diarrhea, abdominal pain, anorexia	Peptic ulcers
Hematology	Anemia	Increased red blood cell count and neutrophils, impaired clotting
Reproductive	Irregular menses or amenorrhea	Amenorrhea, decreased fertility and libido
Fluids and electrolytes	Hypovolemia, hyponatremia, hyperkalemia	Hypervolemia, hypernatremia, hypokalemia

infarction [MI], and angina) and cerebrovascular toxicity (e.g., stroke and seizure). Bromocriptine should be discontinued if hypertension occurs due to pregnancy (e.g., preeclampsia, eclampsia, or pregnancy-induced hypertension).

OTHER DRUGS FOR ANTERIOR PITUITARY DISORDERS

Cosyntropin (synthetic ACTH) or corticotropin (exogenous ACTH) is administered to establish the endocrine gland responsible for the inadequate serum cortisol. Table 49.1 lists the drugs used to replace ACTH and their dosages, uses, and considerations.

Cosyntropin, a synthetic ACTH, is only approved for diagnostic purposes and is less potent and less allergenic than corticotropin. Cosyntropin stimulates the production and release of cortisol, corticosterone, and androgens from the adrenal cortex. It is administered via IM or intravenous (IV) routes. Plasma cortisol concentrations should be measured just before (basal) and 30 to 60 minutes after administration; normal response is the doubling of the basal cortisol level. Caution is advised when administering cosyntropin in patients receiving diuretics; cosyntropin can increase electrolyte loss. Patients taking estrogens can have an abnormal decreased response to the ACTH stimulation test. Side effects and adverse effects include bradycardia, hypertension, sinus tachycardia, and peripheral edema.

The ACTH drug corticotropin is primarily used to diagnose adrenal gland disorders, treat multiple sclerosis (MS), and treat infantile spasms; it is rarely used for corticosteroid-responsive disorders. Corticotropin is available as repository corticotropin injection (RCI), which is administered via IM or subcut routes. RCI controls the synthesis of ACTH from cholesterol, which stimulates adrenal glands in releasing its hormones. The effects of RCI are primarily due to the glucocorticoid from the adrenal cortex. RCI decreases the symptoms of MS during its exacerbation phase. ⚡ The drug should be tapered over a 2-week period for infantile spasms to avoid adrenal insufficiency. Corticotropin has numerous drug interactions. Diuretics and anti-*Pseudomonas* penicillins, such as piperacillin, can decrease the serum potassium level (hypokalemia). If the patient is taking a digitalis preparation and hypokalemia is present, digitalis toxicity can result. Phenytoin, rifampin, and barbiturates increase the metabolic rate, which can decrease the effect of the ACTH drug. Persons with diabetes may need increased insulin and oral antidiabetic (hypoglycemic) drugs because ACTH stimulates cortisol secretion, which increases the blood glucose level.

Side and adverse drug effects are due to the activity of the adrenal glands and their hormones. See Table 49.2 for the physiologic data for hypoadrenalism and hyperadrenalism.

DRUG THERAPY FOR POSTERIOR PITUITARY DISORDERS

Treatment for DI includes ADH preparations, such as vasopressin and desmopressin acetate, which can be administered intranasally or by injection. Desmopressin is also used in managing patients with bleeding disorders due to hemophilia A or von Willebrand disease type 1. Unlike vasopressin, desmopressin does not induce the release of ACTH, nor does it increase serum cortisol level. It is available as a nasal spray, as an oral tablet, and in parenteral formulations. ADH is contraindicated in patients with moderate to severe renal disease and in patients with hyponatremia or a history of such. Side effects and adverse reactions include hyponatremia, cephalgia, dyspepsia, diarrhea, nausea, and vomiting. Seizures may occur due to hyponatremia. Hypotension and tachycardia can occur due to hypovolemia.

Therapy for SIADH can be treated by fluid restrictions, by hypertonic saline, or by drugs such as demeclocycline, conivaptan, and tolvaptan.

Demeclocycline is a tetracycline antibiotic that can induce nephrogenic DI within 5 days of starting treatment that is reversed in 2 to 6 days after cessation of treatment. The most common complaint with demeclocycline is photosensitivity. As with other tetracyclines, dental discoloration and enamel hypoplasia can occur. Fluid and electrolytes must be monitored closely.

Vaptans (e.g., conivaptan and tolvaptan) are vasopressin receptor antagonists and are indicated for the treatment of euvolemic hyponatremia in SIADH. Their effects increase serum sodium and free water clearance. ⚡Conivaptan is contraindicated in patients with corn allergy. Common complications with conivaptan therapy are injection site reactions such as phlebitis, pain, edema, and pruritus; therefore the drug must be administered only in large veins, and infusion sites should be rotated every 24 hours. Other common side effects and adverse reactions include orthostatic hypotension, syncope, hypertension, atrial fibrillation, and electrolyte imbalances.

Tolvaptan is given orally. It has black-box warnings for patients with alcoholism, hepatic disease, and malnutrition; tolvaptan should be avoided in these patients. Common side effects and adverse reactions are related to loss of fluids (e.g., thirst, dry mouth, constipation, hyperglycemia, dizziness, and weakness). Fluid and serum electrolytes must be closely monitored.

Vaptans are contraindicated in patients with hypovolemia. Fluid restrictions should be avoided during therapy to prevent sudden increase in serum sodium.

Table 49.1 lists the drugs used for pituitary disorders and their dosages, uses, and considerations.

OVERVIEW OF THE THYROID GLAND

The thyroid gland is an important regulator for many of the bodily functions. The three hormones produced and secreted by the thyroid gland are triiodothyronine (T_3); thyroxine (T_4), which helps with metabolism; and, to a lesser extent, calcitonin for regulating serum calcium. A majority of thyroid hormone is synthesized as T_4, which is then converted to T_3 to act on target cells. Iodide, an inorganic form of iodine, is needed for the synthesis of T_3 and T_4. These are carried in the blood by thyroxine-binding globulin and albumin, which protect

◎ CLINICAL JUDGMENT [NURSING PROCESS]
Pituitary Hormones

Concept: Hormonal Regulation
- The ability of the body to maintain homeostasis by the regulation, secretion, and action of hormones associated with the endocrine system

Recognize Cues [Assessment]
- Obtain baseline vital signs for future comparison. Report abnormal results.
- Assess fluid, hydration, and electrolyte statuses. Report abnormal findings.
- Assess patient for an infectious process. Corticotropin can suppress signs and symptoms of infection.
- Note the patient's physical growth. If a child, compare growth with reported standards. Report findings.

Analyze Cues and Prioritize Hypothesis [Patient Problems]
- Hormonal imbalance related to the body's inability to regulate and secrete appropriate hormones.
- Need for health teaching related to complex drug regimen.

Generate Solutions [Planning]
- The patient will be free from any pituitary disorder with the appropriate drug regimen.
- The patient will understand the drug regimen.
- The patient will remain free of infection.

Take Action [Nursing Interventions]
Antidiuretic Hormone (ADH)
- Monitor vital signs. Increased heart rate and decreased systolic pressure can indicate fluid volume loss resulting from decreased ADH production. With less ADH secretion, more water is excreted, decreasing vascular fluid (hypovolemia).
- Record urinary output. Increased output can indicate fluid loss caused by a decrease in ADH.
- Obtain daily weight. A liter of fluid weighs approximately 2.2 pounds.

Growth Hormone (GH)
- Monitor blood glucose and electrolyte levels in patients receiving GH. Hyperglycemia can occur with high doses.

Repository Corticotropin
- Monitor the growth and development of a child receiving corticotropin.
- Observe the patient's weight. Check for edema if weight gain occurs. A side effect of repository corticotropin is sodium and water retention.

- Watch carefully for adverse effects when corticotropin is discontinued. Dose should be tapered and not stopped abruptly because adrenal hypofunction may result.
- Check laboratory findings, especially electrolyte levels and glucose. Electrolyte replacement may be necessary, and corticotropin can increase blood glucose.
- Observe for any signs of infection. Corticotropin is an antiinflammatory and can suppress the immune function, increasing the risk for infection.

Patient Teaching
General
Growth Hormone
- Suggest that the patient or family monitor the patient's growth rate.
- Individuals in some cultural groups may misunderstand the purpose and use of GH. The health care provider must emphasize that these are *not* drugs for building muscles and that they can cause many serious side effects, such as diabetes mellitus, when abused.

Corticotropin
- Advise patients to adhere to the drug regimen. Discontinuation of certain drugs, such as corticotropin, can cause hypofunction of the gland being stimulated.
- Direct patients to decrease salt intake to decrease or avoid edema. Potassium supplementation may be needed.

Side Effects
Growth Hormone
- Advise athletes not to take GH because of side effects. GH can be effective for children whose height is markedly below the expected norm for their age and for adults with confirmed diagnosis of GH deficiency. Because GH acts on newly forming bone, administer before the epiphyses are fused in children.
- Inform patients with diabetes to closely monitor blood glucose levels. Insulin regulation may be necessary.
- Instruct patients to monitor weight due to possible fluid retention.

Corticotropin
- Teach patients to report side effects such as muscle weakness, edema, petechiae, ecchymosis, decrease in growth, decreased wound healing, and menstrual irregularities.

Evaluate Outcomes [Evaluation]
- Evaluate effectiveness of drug therapy.

the hormones from being degraded. T_3 is more potent than T_4, and only unbound (free) T_3 and T_4 have biologic actions and produce a hormonal response.

Negative feedback mechanisms regulate hormone secretion from the thyroid gland. The hypothalamus releases thyrotropin-releasing hormone (TRH), which stimulates the release of TSH from the pituitary gland. TSH stimulates the synthesis and release of T_3 and T_4 from the thyroid gland. Excess free T_3 and T_4 inhibit the hypothalamus-pituitary-thyroid (HPT) axis, which results in decreased TRH and TSH secretion. Too low of an amount of T_3 and T_4 increases the function of the HPT axis.

For thyroid deficiency (hypothyroidism), synthetic thyroid hormones may be prescribed either alone or in combination. When the thyroid gland secretes an overabundance of thyroid hormone (hyperthyroidism), antithyroid drugs are usually indicated.

Hypothyroidism and Hyperthyroidism

Hypothyroidism, a decrease in thyroid hormone secretion, can have a primary cause (thyroid gland disorder), a secondary cause (lack of TSH secretion [pituitary disorder]), or a tertiary cause (lack of TRH [hypothalamus disorder]). Primary hypothyroidism occurs more frequently. Decreased T_4 and elevated TSH levels indicate primary hypothyroidism, the causes of which are acute or chronic inflammation of the thyroid gland, radioiodine therapy, excess intake of antithyroid drugs, or surgical removal of the thyroid gland. Myxedema is severe hypothyroidism in the adult; symptoms include lethargy; apathy; memory impairment; emotional changes; slow speech; a deep, coarse voice; edema of the eyelids and face; dry skin; cold intolerance; slow pulse; constipation; weight gain; and abnormal menses. In children, hypothyroidism can have a congenital onset that can cause delayed physical and mental growth (cretinism) or onset may be prepubertal (juvenile hypothyroidism). Drugs that contain T_3 and T_4, alone or in combination, are used to treat hypothyroidism. ⚡ Exogenous thyroid hormones are contraindicated in patients with thyrotoxicosis, acute myocardial infarction, and adrenal insufficiency. Because thyroid hormones are catabolized by the hepatic system, drugs with hepatic enzyme–inducing properties (e.g., carbamazepine, hydantoins, rifabutin) should be used with caution. Elevated serum calcium levels could also be related to hypothyroidism; exogenous calcitonin may also be prescribed.

Hyperthyroidism is an increase in circulating T_3 and T_4 levels, which usually results from an overactive thyroid gland or excessive output of thyroid hormones from one or more thyroid nodules. Hyperthyroidism may be mild, with few symptoms, or it may be severe, as in thyroid storm, in which death may occur from vascular collapse. Graves disease, or thyrotoxicosis, is the most common type of hyperthyroidism caused by hyperfunction of the thyroid gland. It is characterized by a rapid pulse (tachycardia), palpitations, excessive perspiration (hyperhidrosis), heat intolerance, nervousness, irritability, bulging eyes (exophthalmos), and weight loss.

Hyperthyroidism can be treated by surgical removal of a portion of the thyroid gland (subtotal thyroidectomy), radioactive iodine therapy, or antithyroid drugs. Any of these treatments can cause hypothyroidism.

Drug Therapy for Thyroid Disorders: Hypothyroidism

Levothyroxine sodium is the drug of choice for replacement therapy for the treatment of primary hypothyroidism. It increases the levels of T_4 and metabolically is deiodinated to T_3. Levothyroxine is also used to treat simple goiter and chronic lymphocytic (Hashimoto) thyroiditis. Prototype Drug Chart: Levothyroxine Sodium lists the pharmacologic data for levothyroxine sodium.

Liothyronine is a synthetic T_3 with a biologic half-life of 2.5 days with rapid onset of action (within a few hours). Liothyronine is indicated for use as replacement or supplemental treatment for hypothyroidism of any etiology. Unlike levothyroxine, liothyronine does not need to be deiodinated, which increases the availability for use by the body tissues. Liothyronine is better absorbed from the GI tract (over 95%) than levothyroxine, and because of its rapid onset of action and short half-life, it is frequently used as initial therapy for treating myxedema. Liothyronine is available for oral or IV administration.

Desiccated thyroid is a naturally occurring thyroid hormone from porcine thyroid glands. It contains both levothyroxine and

📄 PROTOTYPE DRUG CHART
Levothyroxine Sodium

Drug Class	Dosage
Thyroid hormone	Primary hypothyroidism, with/without goiter, in otherwise healthy persons: A: PO: Initially 1.6 mcg/kg/d; *maint:* 50–200 mcg/d; increase in increments of 12.5–25 mcg at 6- to 8-wk intervals. Other dosing is also available.
Contraindications	**Drug-Lab-Food Interactions**
Absolute contraindications: Thyrotoxicosis and myocardial infarction *Caution:* Adrenal insufficiency; cardiovascular disease, including cardiac arrhythmias, hypertension, and angina pectoris; diabetes mellitus; osteoporosis; hypopituitarism; dysphagia	Drug: Many drug-drug interactions exist and may alter the therapeutic effects of thyroid hormone replacement. Increased cardiac insufficiency occurs when levothyroxine is taken with sympathomimetics (e.g., epinephrine); levothyroxine increases the effects of anticoagulants, TCAs, vasopressors, decongestants, corticosteroids; decreases effects of antidiabetics (oral and insulin), digitalis products, beta-blockers; decreased absorption of levothyroxine occurs with estrogens, antacids, cholestyramine, colestipol, sucralfate, and simethicone. Ketamines can worsen hypertension and tachycardia. Hepatic inducers (e.g., carbamazepine, barbiturates, hydantoins) increase the metabolism of thyroid hormones. Food: Drug should be taken on an empty stomach at least 30–60 min before breakfast and other medications. Tablets may be crushed and mixed in a small amount (5–10 mL) of water; use immediately after mixing. Do not mix with enteral or soy-based feedings. Certain food and beverages inhibit the absorption of thyroid hormones. Herb: Celery seed may reduce thyroid hormones.

Continued

PROTOTYPE DRUG CHART—CONT'D
Levothyroxine Sodium

Pharmacokinetics	Pharmacodynamics
Absorption: PO: 40%–80% Distribution: PB: 99% Metabolism: t½: 3–10 d depending on initial thyroid state Excretion: Urine (80%) and feces (20%)	PO: Onset: 3–5 d; IV: 6–8 h Peak: 24 h (IV) to several weeks (PO) Duration: Several weeks

Therapeutic Effects/Uses
To treat hypothyroidism, myxedema, goiter, and thyroid cancer
Mechanism of Action: Increases metabolic rate, oxygen consumption, utilization and mobilization of glycogen stores; promotes gluconeogenesis and body growth; stimulates protein synthesis

Side Effects	Adverse Reactions
Nausea, vomiting, anorexia, diarrhea, cramps, tremors, nervousness, irritability, insomnia, headache, weight loss, diaphoresis, and amenorrhea; usually due to undermedication or overmedication.	Tachycardia, hypertension, palpitations, osteoporosis, and seizures; usually due to overmedication. Other adverse reactions include urticaria, rash, and alopecia. *Life threatening:* Thyroid crisis, angina pectoris, cardiac dysrhythmias (atrial fibrillation), cardiovascular collapse.

A, Adult; *d*, day; *h*, hour; *IV*, intravenous; *min*, minutes; *PB*, protein binding; *PO*, by mouth; *t½*, half-life; *TCA*, tricyclic antidepressant; *wk*, week.

TABLE 49.3 Drug Therapies for Thyroid Disorders

Generic	Route and Dosage	Uses and Considerations
Thyroid Replacements: Hypothyroidism		
Desiccated thyroid (porcine)	A: PO: Initially, 15–30 mg/d; *maint:* 60–120 mg/d; can increase 15 mg/d q2–3 wk	For hypothyroidism and goiter. PB: >99%; t½: T_3, 2 d; T_4, 6–7 d
Levothyroxine sodium	See Prototype Drug Chart: Levothyroxine Sodium	
Liothyronine sodium	A: PO: Initially, 5–100 mcg/d; *maint:* 25–100 mcg/d Myxedema coma: A: IV: Initially, 25–50 mcg; subsequent doses based on clinical condition q4–12 h to avoid hormone fluctuations	For hypothyroidism, myxedema, thyroiditis, hyperthyroidism diagnosis, cretinism, and goiter. Must be administered with glucocorticoid when treating myxedema coma with IV liothyronine. PB: 99%; t½: 2.5 d
Synthetic levothyroxine	A: PO: 25–100 mcg T_4/12.5–25 mcg T_3/d Dosages must be individualized based on clinical response and thyroid levels.	For hypothyroidism, goiter, and hyperthyroidism diagnosis. T_4T_3 drug. PB: 99%; t½: T_3, 2.5 d; T_4, 3–10 d
Antithyroid Drugs: Hyperthyroidism		
Thioamides		
Methimazole	A: PO: 15–60 mg/d in 1–3 divided doses	For hyperthyroidism, Graves disease, and thyrotoxicosis. Inhibits thyroid hormone synthesis. Dosages greater than 40 mg/d may increase risk of agranulocytosis. PB: 0%; t½: 5–9 h
Propylthiouracil	A: PO: 300–900 mg/d divided q8h, then 100–150 mg/d divided q8h	For patients with hyperthyroidism or Graves disease who are intolerant of methimazole and are unable to receive surgery or radioiodine therapy; inhibits conversion of T_4 and T_3. PB: 60%–80%; t½: 1 h
Iodine		
Potassium iodide	A: PO: 0.27 mL three times daily for 10–14 d before surgery Dilute drug and administer after meals; sip through a straw to avoid discoloration of teeth.	For hyperthyroidism and thyrotoxicosis to suppress thyroid function before surgery. Maximum effect is achieved after 10–15 d. Drug is absorbed from the GI tract as iodinated amino acids and is excreted renally. PB: UK; t½: UK

A, Adult; *Adol*, adolescent; *d*, day; *GI*, gastrointestinal; *h*, hour; *IV*, intravenous; *maint*, maintenance; *PB*, protein binding; *PO*, by mouth; *q*, every; *t½*, half-life; T_4, thyroxine; T_3, triiodothyronine; *UK*, unknown; *wk*, week; *y*, year.

liothyronine. Desiccated thyroid is used to treat hypothyroidism due to thyroid atrophy, thyroid hormone deficiency, and goiter.

Liotrix is a mixture of levothyroxine sodium and liothyronine sodium in a 4-to-1 ratio by weight, respectively. For treating hypothyroidism, there is no significant advantage to using liotrix over levothyroxine sodium alone, because levothyroxine converts T_4 to T_3 in the peripheral tissues.

Table 49.3 lists the natural and synthetic thyroid preparations and their dosages, uses, and considerations.

Drug Therapy for Thyroid Disorder: Hyperthyroidism

Drug therapy for hyperthyroidism includes antithyroid drugs, which inhibit either synthesis or release of thyroid hormone. Propranolol can also be given for symptoms of hyperthyroidism. By blocking beta receptors, propranolol can control cardiac symptoms that result from hyperthyroidism, such as palpitations and tachycardia.

Antithyroid Drugs

The purpose of antithyroid drugs is to reduce the excessive secretion of thyroid hormones by inhibiting thyroid secretion. The use of surgery (subtotal thyroidectomy) and radioiodine therapy frequently leads to permanent hypothyroidism; these patients will need to be on thyroid replacement therapy. Thiourea derivatives (thioamides) are the drugs of choice used to decrease thyroid hormone production. This drug group interferes with synthesis of thyroid hormone. Thiourea derivatives do *not* destroy thyroid tissue; rather, they block thyroid action.

Propylthiouracil (PTU) and methimazole are effective thioamide antithyroid drugs. They are used to control overactive thyroid due to Graves disease, toxic nodular goiter, or multinodular goiter; they are also used before radioiodine treatment or thyroid surgery. Methimazole does not inhibit peripheral conversion of T_4 to T_3 as does PTU; however, it is 10 times more potent, it has a longer half-life than PTU, and the euthyroid state is achieved in 2 to 4 months. It is the preferred antithyroid because of the less severe side effects. Methimazole is rapidly absorbed from the GI tract. Prolonged use of thioamides may cause goiter because of increased TSH secretion and inhibited T_4 and T_3 synthesis. Minimal doses of thioamides should be given when indicated to avoid goiter formation.

Strong iodide preparations such as potassium iodide have been used to suppress thyroid function for patients who are undergoing subtotal thyroidectomy because of Graves disease. Table 49.3 lists the antithyroid drugs used to treat hyperthyroidism along with their dosages, uses, and considerations.

Drug Interactions

Antithyroid drugs interact with many other drugs. When used with oral anticoagulants (e.g., warfarin), they can cause an increase in the anticoagulation effect. In addition, thyroid drugs decrease the effect of insulin and oral antidiabetics, digoxin and lithium increase the action of thyroid drugs, and phenytoin increases serum T_3 level.

CLINICAL JUDGMENT [NURSING PROCESS]
Thyroid Hormones: Replacement and Antithyroid Drugs

Concept: Hormonal Regulation
- The ability of the body to maintain homeostasis by the regulation, secretion, and action of hormones associated with the endocrine system

Recognize Cues [Assessment]
- Determine baseline vital signs, including weight changes, for future comparisons. Report abnormal results.
- Report any abnormal results of serum triiodothyronine (T_3), thyroxine (T_4), and thyroid-stimulating hormone (TSH) levels.
- Obtain a history of drugs and herbal products the patient is taking.
- Assess for signs and symptoms of thyroid crisis (thyroid storm), including tachycardia, cardiac dysrhythmias, fever, heart failure, flushed skin, apathy, confusion, behavioral changes, and, later, hypotension and vascular collapse. Thyroid crisis can result from a thyroidectomy (excess thyroid hormones released), abrupt withdrawal of antithyroid drug, excess ingestion of thyroid hormone, or failure to give antithyroid medication before thyroid surgery.

Analyze Cues and Prioritize Hypothesis [Patient Problems]
- Altered functional ability related to imbalanced thyroid hormone.
- Need for health teaching related to complex drug regimen.
- General decreased tissue perfusion related to imbalanced thyroid hormone.

Generate Solutions [Planning]
- The patient will report an improved activity level within 1–4 weeks of thyroid treatments.
- The patient will report decreased signs and symptoms of hypothyroidism within 2–4 weeks with prescribed thyroid drug replacement, and the patient will not experience side effects.
- The patient will report decreased signs and symptoms of hyperthyroidism in 1–3 weeks with prescribed antithyroid drug.

Take Action [Nursing Interventions]
- Record vital signs. With *hypothyroidism*, temperature, heart rate, and blood pressure usually decrease. With *hyperthyroidism*, tachycardia and palpitations usually occur.
- Monitor the patient's weight. Weight gain commonly occurs in patients with hypothyroidism.
- Obtain a pregnancy test, complete blood count (CBC), complete metabolic panel, liver function test, and electrocardiograph.
- Report periodic TSH, T_3, and T_4.

Patient Teaching
General
- Encourage patients to take the drug at the same time each day in relation to meals. Levothyroxine is taken 30–60 minutes before any food or medications.
- Teach patients to check warnings on over-the-counter (OTC) drug labels. Avoid OTC drugs that caution against use by persons with heart or thyroid disease.
- Suggest that patients carry a MedicAlert identification card, tag, or bracelet that shows the health condition and the drug used to treat it.
- Instruct patients that certain foods can interfere with the absorption of thyroid hormones (e.g., soy products [estrogen], cruciferous vegetables [broccoli and cabbage], iodized salt, shellfish [iodine], and coffee).
- Instruct patients to take drugs as instructed; abrupt changes may lead to increased thyroid dysfunction.
- Recognize that family members may need guidance in understanding the disease processes of hypothyroidism or hyperthyroidism. Support patients and family members who may lack knowledge of prescribed drug therapy for management of thyroid conditions. Additional time in explanations and a written plan of care in the native language may be necessary for non-English-speaking persons.

Side Effects
- Direct patients to report symptoms of hyperthyroidism (tachycardia, chest pain, palpitations, excess sweating) caused by drug accumulation or overdosing.
- Demonstrate to patients how to take that pulse rate. Instruct patients to monitor pulse rate and to report increases or marked decreases in the rate.
- Teach patients the side effects of antithyroid drugs: skin rash, hives, nausea, alopecia, loss of hair pigment, petechiae or ecchymoses, and weakness.
- Advise patients to contact their health care provider if sore throat and fever occur while taking antithyroid drugs. A serious adverse reaction of antithyroid drugs is agranulocytosis (loss of white blood cells). CBC should be monitored for leukopenia.

Evaluate Outcomes [Evaluation]
- Evaluate both effectiveness of the treatment and drug compliance.
- Continue monitoring for side effects from drug accumulation or overdosing.
- Evaluate the patient's knowledge of the medication regimen.

OVERVIEW OF THE PARATHYROID GLANDS

The parathyroid glands secrete **parathyroid hormone (PTH)**, or parathormone, which regulates serum calcium levels in a number of ways:
- It enhances the release of calcium from the bones.
- It enhances calcium reabsorption in the renal tubules.
- It enhances calcium absorption in the intestines by increasing the production of activated vitamin D.

A decrease (negative feedback) in serum calcium stimulates the release of PTH. Calcitonin, one of three thyroid hormones, decreases serum calcium levels by promoting osteoclast activity in bones and calcium excretion by the kidneys and intestines.

For PTH deficiency, PTH analogs are used. Surgical removal (parathyroidectomy) is a common treatment for hyperparathyroidism. Calcimimetic drugs, which mimic calcium in the blood, prevent the parathyroid gland from releasing PTH.

Hypoparathyroidism and Hyperparathyroidism

Damage to the parathyroid glands is a common cause of **hypoparathyroidism**. Hypomagnesemia (low serum magnesium) can also cause PTH deficiency. Other causes of hypocalcemia (serum calcium deficit) include vitamin D deficiency, renal impairment, or diuretic therapy; PTH replacement helps correct the calcium deficit. The action of PTH is to promote calcium absorption from the GI tract, promote reabsorption of calcium from the renal tubules, and activate vitamin D. Table 49.4 lists the drugs used to treat hypoparathyroidism and hyperparathyroidism and their dosages, uses, and considerations.

Hyperparathyroidism can be caused by malignancies of the parathyroid glands or ectopic PTH hormone secretion from lung cancer, hyperthyroidism, or prolonged immobility, during which calcium is lost from bone. Partial or full parathyroidectomy is the most common treatment for primary hyperparathyroidism. Calcitonin-salmon, calcimimetics, and bisphosphonates are used to treat patients affected by hyperparathyroidism.

Drug Therapy for Parathyroid Disorder: Hypoparathyroidism

Calcitriol is used for hypoparathyroidism. It is a vitamin D analog that promotes calcium absorption from the GI tract and promotes secretion of calcium from bone to the bloodstream, thereby increasing serum calcium. Prototype Drug Chart: Calcitriol lists the pharmacologic data for calcitriol.

Calcitonin-salmon and calcimimetics are used to lower serum calcium. Calcitonin-salmon prevents calcium resorption from the bones, and thereby, prevents bone loss and fractures, increases bone density, and alleviates pain due to fractures and bone metastasis. Calcitonin is not as effective as other drugs for hyperparathyroidism. Calcitonin is contraindicated in patients allergic to fish. Common side effects include allergic reactions, GI symptoms (e.g., nausea and vomiting), cephalgia, and hypocalcemia. Adverse reactions due to severe hypocalcemia (e.g., tetany and seizures) can also occur.

Drug Therapy for Parathyroid Disorder: Hyperparathyroidism

Calcimimetics, such as cinacalcet, are used in patients with hyperparathyroidism due to chronic renal disease and parathyroid cancer, and it is also used in those who are unable to undergo parathyroidectomy. Cinacalcet mimics calcium in circulation, increasing the sensitivity of the calcium-sensing receptors of the cells of the parathyroid gland, thereby reducing PTH secretion. This action causes a decrease in serum calcium and slows the progression of bone disease. Because of the hypocalcemic effect, cinacalcet is contraindicated in patients with hypocalcemia. Chapter 12 discusses calcium imbalances more in depth.

Bisphosphonates (e.g., alendronate, etidronate, ibandronate, and risedronate), are also drugs for hyperparathyroidism and block osteoclast activities, thereby inhibiting mineralization or resorption of the bone, which may lessen osteoporosis caused by hyperparathyroidism. Before treatment with bisphosphonates, bone mineral density measurements should be obtained at baseline and periodically thereafter. Serum calcium concentration should be obtained, and any hypocalcemia must be corrected before bisphosphonate therapy. ⚡ Adequate intake of calcium and vitamin D is essential during therapy. Oral bisphosphonates are contraindicated in patients who are unable to sit or stand upright for at least 30 minutes after administration or who have esophageal strictures. During therapy, transient hypocalcemia and hypophosphatemia can occur. Other side effects include abdominal and musculoskeletal pain, GI upsets, hypotension, and fever. Individual bisphosphonates are discussed in Chapter 52.

TABLE 49.4 Drug Therapies for Parathyroid Disorders

Generic	Route and Dosage	Uses and Considerations
Hypoparathyroidism and Hypocalcemia: Vitamin D Analogs		
Calcitriol	See Prototype Drug Chart: Calcitriol	
Ergocalciferol	Hypoparathyroidism: C: PO: 1250–5000 mcg/d with calcium supplements	Prohormone for hypoparathyroidism. Enhances calcium and phosphorus absorption. Long duration of action. PB: UK; t½: UK
Hyperparathyroidism and Hypercalcemia		
Calcitonin-salmon	Hypercalcemia: A: IM/subcut: 4 IU/kg q12h, can increase to 8 IU/kg q12h; max: 8 IU/kg q6h Paget disease: A: IM/subcut: 50–100 IU/1–3 × wk	For hypercalcemia and Paget disease of bone (osteitis deformans). Calcitonin decreases serum calcium by binding at receptor sites on osteoclast. PB: UK; t½: 1 h
Cinacalcet	A: PO: Initially 30 mg bid; titrate in 30 mg increments q2–4wk; max: 360 mg/d	For hyperparathyroidism and hypercalcemia. Check serum calcium 1 wk after initiating treatment and 2 months thereafter. Administer with food. PB: 93%–97%; t½: 30–40 h

A, Adult; *bid*, twice daily; *C*, child; *d*, day; *h*, hour; *IM*, intramuscular; *IU*, international units; *max*, maximum; *PB*, protein binding; *PO*, by mouth; *q*, every; *subcut*, subcutaneous; *t½*, half-life; *UK*, unknown; *wk*, week.

PROTOTYPE DRUG CHART
Calcitriol

Drug Class	Dosage
Vitamin D analog	A: PO: 0.25–2 mcg/d

Contraindications	Drug-Lab-Food Interactions
Absolute contraindications: Hypersensitivity, hypercalcemia, hypervitaminosis D *Caution:* Cardiovascular disease, renal calculi, renal failure, hyperphosphatemia, dehydration, excess sunlight exposure, malabsorption syndrome, hypocalcemia	Drug: Increased cardiac dysrhythmias with digoxin, verapamil; decreased calcitriol absorption with cholestyramine; decreased calcitriol effects with ketoconazole, barbiturates; enhanced calcitriol effects with thiazide diuretics Calcitriol decreases the effects of estrogen. Lab: Increased serum calcium with thiazide diuretics, calcium supplements, calcium-rich foods; decreased serum calcium with low magnesium

Pharmacokinetics	Pharmacodynamics
Absorption: PO: Well absorbed Distribution: PB: 99% Metabolism: t½: 3–8 h adult; 27 h children Excretion: Feces (50%), urine (16%)	PO: Onset: 2–6 h Peak: 3–6 h Duration: 3–5 d

Therapeutic Effects/Uses
To treat parathyroid disorders (hyperparathyroidism and hypoparathyroidism) and to manage hypocalcemia in chronic renal failure
Mechanism of Action: Calcitriol enhances calcium deposits into bones by the active form of vitamin D's metabolite, calcitriol. Calcitriol reabsorbs calcium by the kidneys, enhances intestinal absorption of dietary calcium, and decreases serum phosphate, bone resorption, and parathyroid hormone levels.

Side Effects	Adverse Reactions
Side effects are generally early signs of hypercalcemia: fatigue, weakness, somnolence, cephalgia, nausea, vomiting, diarrhea, cramps, drowsiness, dizziness, vertigo, metallic taste, lethargy, constipation, and xerostomia.	Adverse effects are late signs of hypercalcemia: anorexia, photophobia, dehydration, cardiac arrhythmias, decreased libido, hypertension, sensory disturbances, hypercalciuria, hypercalcemia, and hyperphosphatemia.

A, Adult; *d*, day; *h*, hour; *PB*, protein binding; *PO*, by mouth; *t½*, half-life.

CLINICAL JUDGMENT [NURSING PROCESS]
Parathyroid Hormone Insufficiencies

Concept: Hormonal Regulation
- The ability of the body to maintain homeostasis by the regulation, secretion, and action of hormones associated with the endocrine system.

Recognize Cues [Assessment]
- Note serum calcium level and report abnormal results.
- ⚠ Assess for symptoms of tetany in hypocalcemia: twitching of the mouth, tingling and numbness of fingers, carpopedal spasm, spasmodic contractions, and laryngeal spasm.

Analyze Cues and Prioritize Hypothesis [Patient Problems]
- Hyper- or hypocalcemia related to hormonal imbalance and therapeutic regimen.
- Need for health teaching related to complex drug regimen.
- Disrupted fluid and electrolytes related to side effects of drug regimen.

Generate Solutions [Planning]
- The patient will maintain a serum calcium level within the normal range.
- The patient will report no or minimal side effects.

Take Action [Nursing Interventions]
- Monitor serum calcium level. The normal reference range is 8–10 mg/dL; serum calcium below 8 mg/dL indicates hypocalcemia. Total serum calcium greater than 10.5 mg/dL indicates hypercalcemia.

Patient Teaching
General
- Advise women to inform their health care provider about pregnancy status before taking calcitonin preparations.
- Encourage patients to check over-the-counter (OTC) drugs for possible calcium content, especially if the patient has an elevated serum calcium level. Some vitamins and antacids contain calcium. Tell patients to contact their health care provider before taking drugs with calcium.

Side Effects
- Direct patients to report symptoms of hypocalcemia (e.g., tetany).
- Teach patients to report signs and symptoms of hypercalcemia, which include bone pain, anorexia, nausea, vomiting, thirst, constipation, lethargy, bradycardia, and polyuria.

Evaluate Outcomes [Evaluation]
- Monitor effectiveness of drug therapy (e.g., serum calcium level, signs and symptoms of hypercalcemia or hypocalcemia).
- Continue monitoring for signs and symptoms of calcium imbalances.
- Evaluate the patient's knowledge of medication regimen.

OVERVIEW OF THE ADRENAL GLANDS

The paired adrenal glands consist of the adrenal medulla and adrenal cortex. Hormones secreted from the adrenal medulla are epinephrine and norepinephrine (catecholamines); Chapters 15 and 55 further discuss these hormones. The adrenal cortex produces two types of steroid hormones, glucocorticoids (cortisol) and mineralocorticoids (aldosterone), and, to a lesser extent, the adrenal androgens and estrogens. Steroids are secreted by the adrenal cortex in response to signals from the hypothalamus-pituitary-adrenal (HPA) axis; the levels are regulated by the negative feedback mechanism.

Hypoadrenalism and Hyperadrenalism

A decrease in serum steroid levels (hypocortisolism) increases CRF and ACTH secretions from the hypothalamus and anterior pituitary gland, respectively; these stimulate the adrenal glands to secrete and release steroids. An increased serum steroid level (hypercortisolism) inhibits the HPA axis, resulting in fewer steroids being released. A decrease in steroid secretion is called *adrenal hyposecretion* (adrenal insufficiency, or Addison disease), and an increase in steroid secretion is called *adrenal hypersecretion* (Cushing syndrome). Corticosteroids are also described in Chapter 24.

! Because of the influences of steroids on electrolytes and on carbohydrate, protein, and fat metabolism, hypocortisolism can result in serious illness or death.

> **⚡ PATIENT SAFETY**
>
> **Do Not Confuse ...**
> - **Calcitonin** with **calcitriol** or **calcium**
> - **Levothyroxine** with **liothyronine**
> - **Somatropin** with **somatostatin** or **sandostatin**

Drug Therapy for Adrenal Disorders: Glucocorticoids and Mineralocorticoids

Glucocorticoids are the most potent natural cortisol produced by the body and are influenced by ACTH, which is released from the anterior pituitary gland. Its functions include having an effect on the inflammatory response (see Chapter 24), metabolism, growth, and biorhythms. Glucocorticoids also affect carbohydrate, protein, and fat metabolism and muscle and blood cell activities. Indications for glucocorticoid therapy include trauma, surgery, inflammation, emotional upsets, and anxiety. Table 49.2 lists the physiologic aspects of adrenal hyposecretion (Addison disease) and hypersecretion (Cushing syndrome).

Most of the glucocorticoid drugs, frequently called *cortisone drugs*, are synthetically produced. These drugs have several routes of administration: oral, parenteral (IM or IV), topical (creams, ointments, lotions), and aerosol (inhaler). Drugs administered via the (seldom used) IM route should be administered deep into the muscle; subcutaneous administration is not recommended.

Glucocorticoids are used to treat many diseases and health problems, including inflammatory, allergic, and debilitating conditions. Among the inflammatory conditions that may require glucocorticoids are autoimmune disorders (e.g., MS, rheumatoid arthritis, myasthenia gravis), ulcerative colitis, glomerulonephritis, shock, ocular and vascular inflammation, polyarteritis nodosa, and hepatitis. Allergic conditions include asthma, drug reactions, contact dermatitis, and anaphylaxis. Debilitating conditions are mainly caused by malignancies. Organ transplant recipients may require glucocorticoids to prevent organ rejection.

There are many glucocorticoids, some more potent than others. Dexamethasone has been used to treat severe inflammatory responses that result from head trauma or allergic reactions. An inexpensive glucocorticoid frequently prescribed is prednisone. Prototype Drug Chart: Prednisone lists the pharmacologic data for prednisone.

Commonly used glucocorticoid drugs and their dosages, uses, and considerations are listed in Table 49.5. Drugs used for adrenocortical insufficiency contain both glucocorticoids and mineralocorticoids, whereas drugs with antiinflammatory or immunosuppressive properties contain mostly glucocorticoids with minimal mineralocorticoid activity.

Mineralocorticoids promote sodium retention and potassium and hydrogen excretion in the renal tubules. The primary mineralocorticoid is aldosterone, which is controlled by the renin-angiotensin-aldosterone system. Mineralocorticoids maintain fluid balance by promoting the reabsorption of sodium from the renal tubules. Sodium attracts water, resulting in water retention. When *hypovolemia* (a decrease in circulating fluid) occurs, more aldosterone is secreted to increase sodium and water retention, thereby restoring fluid balance. With sodium reabsorption, potassium is lost and hypokalemia (potassium deficit) can occur. Some glucocorticoid drugs also contain mineralocorticoid properties; these include cortisone and hydrocortisone. A severe decrease in the mineralocorticoid can lead to hypotension and vascular collapse, as seen in Addison disease. Mineralocorticoid deficiency usually occurs with glucocorticoid deficiency, frequently called *corticosteroid deficiency*.

Fludrocortisone is an oral mineralocorticoid that can be given with a glucocorticoid. Even though fludrocortisone has significant glucocorticoid activity, it is not appreciable at usual therapeutic doses. Fludrocortisone mimics the actions of endogenous aldosterone, facilitating sodium resorption and promoting hydrogen ion and potassium excretion. In larger doses, it can inhibit endogenous hormone secretions of adrenal cortex and pituitary gland, causing a negative nitrogen balance; therefore a high-protein diet is usually indicated.

Side and Adverse Effects

The side effects and adverse reactions of glucocorticoids that result from high doses or prolonged use include increased blood glucose, abnormal fat deposits in the face and trunk (so-called *moon face* and *buffalo hump*), decreased extremity size, muscle wasting, edema, sodium and water retention, hypertension, euphoria or psychosis, thinned skin with purpura, increased intraocular pressure (glaucoma), peptic ulcers, and growth retardation. Long-term use of glucocorticoid drugs can cause adrenal atrophy (loss of adrenal gland function).

! When drug therapy is discontinued, the dose should be tapered to allow the adrenal cortex to produce cortisol and other corticosteroids. Abrupt withdrawal of the drug can result in severe adrenocortical insufficiency.

Because potassium excretion occurs with the use of mineralocorticoids, serum potassium level should be monitored. Other adverse effects include fluid imbalance, fluid overload, and hypertension. These usually indicate overdosage, at which point fludrocortisone should be discontinued and then resumed at lower doses. Hypokalemia may cause metabolic alkalosis, which can cause GI symptoms (nausea and vomiting), orthostatic hypotension, cardiac rhythm changes, weakness, anorexia, and myalgia. Commonly used mineralocorticoid drugs and their dosages, uses, and considerations are listed in Table 49.5.

TABLE 49.5 Drug Therapies for Adrenal Disorders

Generic	Route and Dosage	Uses and Considerations
GLUCOCORTICOIDS		
Short Acting		
Cortisone acetate	A: PO: 12–50 mg/d in divided doses to simulate normal diurnal adrenal rhythm	For adrenocortical insufficiency. Give with fludrocortisone (mineralocorticoid). Give oral dose with food to minimize GI irritation. PB: 90%; t½: 8–12 h
Hydrocortisone	Primary adrenocortical insufficiency: Hydrocortisone or hydrocortisone *cypionate*: A: PO 20–240 mg/d in 2–4 divided doses Hydrocortisone sodium *phosphate*: A: IM/IV/subcut: 15–240 mg/d twice daily (q12h). Hydrocortisone sodium *succinate*: A: IV/IM: 100–500 mg repeated in 2-, 4-, or 6-h intervals Hydrocortisone *acetate* suspension: A: IM: 15–240 mg once daily	For adrenocortical insufficiency. Given IV or IM (hydrocortisone sodium succinate) for crisis prophylaxis in ill patients or those undergoing surgery. Hydrocortisone sodium phosphate (subcut/IV/IM), hydrocortisone sodium succinate (IV/IM), and hydrocortisone acetate suspension (IM only) are for acute adrenal insufficiency. Oral hydrocortisone is also available for primary adrenocortical insufficiency. Oral dosages in this table are for primary adrenal insufficiency. Administer with meals to minimize GI irritation. Daily doses should be given in the morning to coincide with the body's normal cortisol secretion. Acetate formulations should never be given intravenously. PB: 90%; t½: 1–2 h
Intermediate Acting		
Methylprednisolone	A: PO: 4–48 mg/d in 4 divided doses Methylprednisolone *acetate*: A: IM: 10–120 mg; subsequent doses determined by clinical response Methylprednisolone sodium *succinate*: A: IV/IM: 10–40 mg over several minutes; subsequent dosages determined by clinical response	For adrenocortical insufficiency. Has little to no mineralocorticoid properties. Dosing is highly variable. Administer oral dosages with meals to minimize GI irritation. Acetate formulation should never be given intravenously. PB: UK; t½: 3–3.5 h
Prednisolone	A: PO: 5–60 mg/d in 1–2 doses	For parenteral use in primary or secondary adrenocortical insufficiency. Prednisolone is a potent steroid that can be injected into joints and soft tissue. Must be given concomitantly with a mineralocorticoid. PB: 70%–90%; t½: 2–4 h
Prednisone	See Prototype Drug Chart: Prednisone	
Long Acting		
Betamethasone (PO), betamethasone sodium phosphate/ betamethasone acetate susp (IM)	A: PO: 0.6–7.2 mg/d in single or divided doses Injectable suspension: A: IM: 0.5–9 mg/d divided q12h Other regimen is available	Synthetic glucocorticoids with minimal mineralocorticoid properties are used as antiinflammatory or immunosuppressive agents; must be used in conjunction with a mineralocorticoid for primary or secondary adrenocortical insufficiency. Dosing is variable and depends on indications. Should be taken with food. PB: 64%; t½: 6.5 h
Dexamethasone	Adrenocortical insufficiency: A: PO: 0.75–9 mg/d in 2–4 divided doses or IV/IM: 0.5–9 mg/d q6–12 h	Synthetic glucocorticoids with little or no mineralocorticoid activity. Longest acting corticosteroid. Must use a mineralocorticoid when treating adrenal insufficiency. Higher oral doses are used for dexamethasone suppression test for Cushing syndrome. Give oral dose with food. PB: UK; t½: 1.8–3.5 h
MINERALOCORTICOIDS		
Fludrocortisone	A: PO: 0.1–0.2 mg/d. If hypertension occurs due to therapy, decrease dose to 0.05 mg once daily.	For adrenocortical insufficiency (Addison disease). To be used as a supplement to hydrocortisone or cortisone. Circulating drug is bound to protein and transcortin. Only the unbound drugs are active. May be administered without regard to food. PB: 42%; t½: 3.5 h

A, Adult; *d*, day; *GI*, gastrointestinal; *h*, hour; *IM*, intramuscular; *IV*, intravenous; *PB*, protein binding; *PO*, by mouth; *q*, every; *subcut*, subcutaneous; *susp*, suspension; *t½*, half-life; *UK*, unknown.

Drug Interactions

The drug interactions for glucocorticoids are many. Glucocorticoids increase the potency of drugs taken concurrently, including aspirin and nonsteroidal antiinflammatory drugs (NSAIDs), thus increasing the risk of GI bleeding and ulceration. Use of potassium-wasting diuretics (e.g., furosemide) with glucocorticoids increases potassium loss, resulting in hypokalemia.

Barbiturates, phenytoin, and rifampin decrease the effect of prednisone because they increase glucocorticoid metabolism. Larger doses of glucocorticoids may be required to achieve the desired effect. Prolonged use of glucocorticoids can cause severe muscle weakness.

Dexamethasone, a potent glucocorticoid, interacts with many drugs. Phenytoin, theophylline, rifampin, barbiturates, and antacids decrease the action of dexamethasone, whereas estrogen and NSAIDs such as aspirin increase its action. Dexamethasone decreases the effects of oral antidiabetics. Glucocorticoids can increase blood glucose levels, so insulin or oral antidiabetic drug dosage may need to be increased. When the drug is given with diuretics or anti-*Pseudomonas* penicillin preparations, the serum potassium level may decrease markedly.

Herbal products such as cascara sagrada, yellow dock, and licorice can potentiate the effects of corticosteroids, which can worsen potassium depletion.

PROTOTYPE DRUG CHART
Prednisone

Drug Class	Dosage
Glucocorticoid/corticosteroid	Dosage is individualized and highly variable depending on the severity of the disease and on patient response. A: PO: 5–60 mg/d in single or divided doses Delayed-release tablets release drug approximately 4 h after the first dose
Contraindications	**Drug-Lab-Food Interactions**
Contraindication: Untreated serious infections, hypersensitivity, varicella *Caution:* Psychosis, diabetes mellitus, renal disease, heart failure, myocardial infarction, hypertension, osteoporosis, cirrhosis, diverticulitis, hypothyroidism, myasthenia gravis, ulcerative colitis, seizures, visual disturbances, GI disorders, ocular herpes simplex	Drug: Additive effects occur with other immunosuppressive drugs when taken concurrently with corticosteroids. Increased corticosteroid levels are seen with estrogens, diltiazem, ketoconazole; decreased levels are seen with barbiturates, phenytoin, and rifampin. Concurrent use of aspirin and NSAIDs increase GI toxicity; concurrent use of diuretics and amphotericin B increases potassium depletion; concurrent use with cardiac glycosides increases risk of dysrhythmias and digitalis toxicity; concurrent use with bupropion lowers seizure threshold Herb: Level is decreased with ephedra (Ma-huang). Lab: Hyperglycemia, false-positive TB test
Pharmacokinetics	**Pharmacodynamics**
Absorption: PO: Well absorbed Distribution: PB: 65%–91% Metabolism: t½: 2–3 h Excretion: In urine	PO: Onset: UK Peak: 1–2 h Duration: 1 h (plasma); 18–36 h (biologic)
Therapeutic Effects/Uses	
Adrenocortical insufficiency, Addison disease Mechanism of Action: Suppresses inflammation, immune responses (humoral), and adrenal function; has mild mineralocorticoid activity	
Side Effects	**Adverse Reactions**
Fluid and sodium retention, nausea, diarrhea, abdominal distension, increased appetite, sweating, headache, depression, flushing, mood changes, cataracts, amenorrhea, anorexia, Cushing syndrome, psychosis, immunosuppression, HPA suppression, hypercholesterolemia, elevated hepatic transaminases	Angioedema, cardiac arrhythmia, avascular necrosis, osteoporosis, fractures, cardiac arrest, cardiomyopathy, GI ulceration, exfoliative dermatitis, GI bleeding and perforation, CHF, increased ICP, lupus-like symptoms, pancreatitis, pulmonary edema, ocular disease, CVA, tendon rupture, thromboembolism

A, Adult; *CHF*, congestive heart failure; *CVA*, cerebrovascular accident; *d*, day; *GI*, gastrointestinal; *h*, hour; *HPA*, hypothalamus-pituitary-adrenal; *ICP*, intracranial pressure; *NSAIDs*, nonsteroidal antiinflammatory drugs; *PB*, protein binding; *PO*, by mouth; *t½*, half-life; *TB*, tuberculosis; *UK*, unknown.

CLINICAL JUDGMENT [NURSING PROCESS]
Adrenal Hormones: Corticosteroids

Concept: Hormonal Regulation
- The ability of the body to maintain homeostasis by the regulation, secretion, and action of hormones associated with the endocrine system

Recognize Cues [Assessment]
- Note baseline vital signs for future comparisons.
- ⚡ Assess laboratory test results, especially serum electrolytes and blood glucose. The serum potassium level usually decreases and blood glucose level increases when a corticosteroid, such as prednisone, is taken over an extended period.
- Obtain the patient's weight and urine output for future comparisons. Corticosteroids can cause fluid retention and weight gain.

CLINICAL JUDGMENT [NURSING PROCESS]—CONT'D

Adrenal Hormones: Corticosteroids

- Assess the patient's medical and herbal history. Report if the patient has glaucoma, cataracts, peptic ulcer, psychiatric problems, or diabetes mellitus. Glucocorticoids can intensify these health problems.

Analyze Cues and Prioritize Hypothesis [Patient Problems]
- Disrupted fluid and electrolyte balance related to treatment regimen.
- Decreased immunity, risk for.
- Decreased self-concept, risk for.

Generate Solutions [Planning]
- The patient will report decreased signs and symptoms of inflammation.
- The patient will report minimal side effects from glucocorticoid therapy.
- The patient will not develop new or worsening infection.
- The patient will have increased knowledge of the medication regimen.

Take Action [Nursing Interventions]
- Determine vital signs. Corticosteroids such as prednisone can increase blood pressure and sodium and water retention.
- Administer corticosteroids only as ordered. Routes of administration include oral, intramuscular (IM; not in deltoid muscle), intravenous (IV), aerosol, and topical. Apply topical corticosteroids in thin layers (see Chapter 45). Rashes, infection, and purpura should be noted and reported.
- Record weight. Report a weight gain of 5 lb in 2 days; this could indicate water retention due to sodium reabsorption from hyperaldosteronism.
- Monitor laboratory values, especially serum electrolytes and blood glucose. The serum potassium level could decrease to less than 3.5 mEq/L, and serum sodium and glucose could increase.
- Watch for signs and symptoms of hypokalemia: nausea, vomiting, muscular weakness, abdominal distension, paralytic ileus, and irregular heart rate.
- Assess for side effects from corticosteroid drugs when therapy has lasted more than 10 days and drug is taken in high dosages. Cortisone preparations should not be abruptly stopped because adrenal crisis can result.
- Monitor older adults for signs and symptoms of increased osteoporosis. Some corticosteroids promote calcium loss from bone.

Patient Teaching
General
- Advise patients to take drugs as prescribed, and caution patients not to abruptly stop drugs. When the drug is discontinued, the dose is tapered over 1–2 weeks.
- Direct patients not to take cortisone preparations (oral or topical) during pregnancy unless necessary and prescribed by the health care provider. Drugs may be harmful to the fetus.
- ⚡ Inform patients that certain herbal laxatives and diuretics may interact with corticosteroid drug therapy and may increase the severity of hypokalemia.
- Teach patients to avoid large crowds and persons with respiratory infections, because corticosteroids can suppress the immune system.
- Teach patients receiving corticosteroids to inform other health care providers of all drugs taken.
- Encourage patients to carry a medical alert identification card, tag, or bracelet stating that corticosteroids are taken.
- Teach patients proper use of the drug.
- Counsel patients to take cortisone preparations at mealtime or with food to prevent irritation of gastric mucosa.
- Advise patients to eat foods rich in potassium, such as fresh and dried fruits, vegetables, meats, and nuts. Some corticosteroid preparations promote potassium loss.
- Explain to the family that the patient is not "dumb" or "uninterested" but has an adrenal problem. Explain that symptoms do not go away and may be progressive if prescribed therapy is not followed.

Side Effects
- Teach patients to report signs and symptoms of Cushing syndrome: moon face, puffy eyelids, edema in the feet, increased bruising, dizziness, bleeding, and menstrual irregularity.

Evaluate Outcomes [Evaluation]
- Evaluate effectiveness of corticosteroid therapy. If clinical manifestations have not improved, a change in drug therapy may be necessary.
- Continue monitoring for side effects, especially when a patient is receiving high doses of corticosteroids.
- Evaluate the patient's knowledge of the therapy.

CLINICAL JUDGMENT SINGLE-EPISODE CASE STUDY

NGN Item Type: Cloze
Cognitive Skills: Analyze cues

A 68-year-old female presented to the clinic with complaints of fatigue and weight gain over a 6-month time frame. On further assessment, the nurse noted the following:
- Blood pressure 114/72 mm Hg
- Heart rate 54 beats per minute
- Respiratory rate 14 breaths per minute
- Oxygen saturation 97% on room air
- Dry skin
- Voice hoarseness
- Muscle weakness
- Mildly enlarged thyroid gland
- Hemoglobin 13 g/L
- Hematocrit 40%
- Serum sodium 138 mEq/L
- Serum potassium 4.1 mEq/L
- Serum calcium 9.8 mg/dL
- Serum albumin 3.8 g/dL
- Serum total protein 6.9 g/dL
- Thyroid-stimulating hormone 10 mIU/L

Choose the *most likely* options for the information missing from the statements below by selecting from the list of options provided.

The nurse suspects ____1____, and when reviewing T_3 and T_4 levels, the nurse would expect the levels to be ____2____. The nurse reports the assessment findings to the patient's medical provider, anticipating an order of ____3____.

Continued

CLINICAL JUDGMENT SINGLE-EPISODE CASE STUDY—CONT'D

Option 1	Option 2	Option 3
Secondary hypoadrenalism	Decreased	Cinacalcet
Primary hypoparathyroidism	Increased	Prednisone
Primary hyperpituitarism	Normal	Alendronate
Primary hypothyroidism		Somatropin
Secondary hyperadrenalism		Propylthiouracil
		Levothyroxine

Answers
The nurse suspects *primary hypothyroidism*, and when reviewing T_3 and T_4 levels, the nurse would expect the levels to be *decreased*. The nurse reports the assessment findings to the patient's medical provider, anticipating an order of *levothyroxine*.

Rationale
The patient is exhibiting clinical manifestations of *primary hypothyroidism*, indicated by a TSH level of 10 mIU/L, which is elevated (normal TSH levels 0.5–5 mIU/L). TSH levels would be increased if there is not enough circulating thyroid hormone (T_3 and T_4). With primary hypothyroidism, total T_3 and T_4 levels would be decreased. The patient would be prescribed levothyroxine to replace the deficiency.

Secondary hypoadrenalism is a deficiency of the adrenal glands due to other causes, such as hypopituitarism. The adrenal glands do not produce their hormones because the pituitary gland does not release adrenocorticotropic hormone (ACTH). Hypoadrenalism can result in decreased serum sodium and increased serum potassium; the serum sodium and potassium levels are normal. Primary hypoparathyroidism is a deficiency of the parathyroid gland, which regulates serum calcium. The serum calcium levels were normal. Hyperpituitarism could cause an elevated TSH level; but its other hormones, such as ACTH, would cause an increased activity to its respective endocrine gland, such as the adrenals. However, serum electrolytes (sodium and potassium) are normal. If the adrenal glands were hyperactive, serum sodium would be elevated, and serum potassium would most likely be decreased. Fatigue decreases metabolism, which can cause weight gain. Secondary hyperadrenalism can result in increased serum sodium and decreased serum potassium; these were normal. Fatigue could be due to anemia; however, the patient's hemoglobin and hematocrit were normal.

References
Endocrine Society: *Hypothyroidism*, 2019. https://www.hormone.org/diseases-and-conditions/hypothyroidism
Endocrine Society: *The endocrine system*, 2019. https://www.hormone.org/what-is-endocrinology/the-endocrine-system
Endocrine Society: *Hypoparathyroidism*, 2020. https://www.hormone.org/diseases-and-conditions/hypoparathyroidism
Lab tests online. https://labtestsonline.org/

REVIEW QUESTIONS

1. A patient is receiving somatropin. Which drug action would the nurse anticipate?
   a. Act as an antiinflammatory agent
   b. Increase metabolic rate and oxygen consumption
   c. Stimulate growth in long bones at epiphyseal plates
   d. Promote water reabsorption from the renal tubules
2. A patient is given desmopressin acetate. The nurse knows that this drug is used to treat which condition?
   a. Gigantism
   b. Diabetes mellitus
   c. Diabetes insipidus
   d. Adrenal insufficiency
3. A patient is taking levothyroxine. For which adverse effect would the nurse monitor?
   a. Tachycardia
   b. Drowsiness
   c. Constipation
   d. Weight gain
4. A patient has just begun taking calcitriol. Which nursing action would the nurse do?
   a. Monitor the patient's weight.
   b. Monitor serum calcium levels.
   c. Teach side effects of alopecia and petechiae.
   d. Instruct the patient to avoid persons with respiratory infections.
5. A patient is given corticotropin. The nurse knows to monitor the patient for which condition?
   a. Weight gain
   b. Hyperkalemia
   c. Hypoglycemia
   d. Dehydration
6. The nurse is administering prednisone to a newly admitted patient who is taking multiple drugs. The nurse would consider which drug interaction with prednisone? **Select all that apply.**
   a. Cardiac and central nervous system actions are increased when the drug is taken with an adrenergic agent.
   b. Potassium-wasting diuretics increase potassium loss, resulting in hypokalemia.
   c. Risk for gastrointestinal bleeding and ulceration increases when the drug is taken with aspirin or other nonsteroidal antiinflammatory drugs (NSAIDs).
   d. The action of prednisone is decreased when taken with phenytoin because phenytoin increases glucocorticoid metabolism.
   e. Risk for dysrhythmias and digitalis toxicity increase when the drug is taken with cardiac glycosides.
   f. Dosage of antidiabetic agents may need to be decreased when taken concurrently with glucocorticoids.
7. Which nursing intervention is indicated when administering vasopressin? **Select all that apply.**
   a. Record urinary output.
   b. Observe weight and note edema.
   c. Monitor blood pressure.
   d. Closely monitor blood glucose levels.
   e. Monitor heart rate.
   f. Record daily calcium levels.

50

Antidiabetics

http://evolve.elsevier.com/McCuistion/pharmacology

OBJECTIVES

- Explain the pathophysiology of diabetes mellitus and the three major symptoms.
- Describe the role of insulin in the body.
- Contrast the different types of oral antidiabetic drugs and their mechanism of action.
- Explain the administration techniques of incretin mimetics, amylin analogs, and hypoglycemic drugs.

OUTLINE

Pathophysiology, 649
    Types of Diabetes Mellitus, 649
    Gestational Diabetes Mellitus, 650
Insulin, 650
    Commercially Prepared Insulin, 650
    Types of Insulin, 650
    Administration of Insulin, 652
    Insulin Resistance, 653
    Storage of Insulin, 653
Oral Antidiabetic Drugs, 655
    First- and Second-Generation Sulfonylureas, 655
    Nonsulfonylureas, 656

Biguanides, 660
Alpha-Glucosidase Inhibitors, 660
Thiazolidinediones, 660
Meglitinides, 660
Incretin Modifier, 660
Guidelines for Oral Antidiabetic Therapy for Type 2 Diabetes, 660
Other Diabetic Drugs, 662
    Incretin Mimetics, 662
    Amylin Analogs, 662
    Hyperglycemic Drugs, 662
Clinical Judgment Single-Episode Case Study, 662
Review Questions, 663

The pancreas, located to the left of and behind the stomach, is both an exocrine and an endocrine gland. The exocrine section of the pancreas secretes digestive enzymes into the duodenum. The endocrine section has cell clusters called *islets of Langerhans*. The alpha islet cells produce glucagon, which breaks glycogen down to glucose in the liver, and the beta cells secrete insulin, which regulates glucose metabolism. Insulin is an antidiabetic agent used to control diabetes mellitus. Antidiabetic drugs are discussed in this chapter.

Antidiabetic drugs are used primarily to control diabetes mellitus, a chronic disease that affects carbohydrate metabolism. The two groups of antidiabetic agents are insulin and oral hypoglycemic (antidiabetic) drugs. Insulin, a protein secreted from the beta cells of the pancreas, is necessary for carbohydrate metabolism and plays an important role in protein and fat metabolism. The beta cells make up 75% of the pancreas, and the alpha cells that secrete glucagons—a hyperglycemic substance—occupy approximately 20% of the pancreas. Oral hypoglycemic drugs, also known as oral antidiabetic drugs (to avoid confusion with the term *hypoglycemic reaction*), are synthetic preparations that stimulate insulin release or otherwise alter the metabolic response to hyperglycemia.

PATHOPHYSIOLOGY

Diabetes mellitus, a chronic disease that results from deficient glucose metabolism, is caused by insufficient insulin secretion from the beta cells. This results in high blood glucose (*hyperglycemia*). Diabetes mellitus is characterized by the three *P*s: polyuria (increased urine output), polydipsia (increased thirst), and polyphagia (increased hunger). Diabetes *mellitus* is a disorder of the pancreas, whereas diabetes *insipidus* is a disorder of the posterior pituitary gland, discussed in detail in Chapter 46.

Types of Diabetes Mellitus

The four types of diabetes are presented in Table 50.1. Viral infections, environmental conditions, and genetic factors contribute to the onset of type 1 diabetes mellitus. Type 2 diabetes mellitus is the most common type of diabetes. Some sources suggest that heredity and obesity are the major factors that cause type 2 diabetes. With type 2 diabetes, there is some beta-cell function with varying amounts of insulin secretion. Hyperglycemia may be controlled for some type 2 diabetes patients with oral antidiabetic (hypoglycemic) drugs and a diet prescribed by the American Diabetes Association (ADA); however, about

TABLE 50.1 Types and Occurrences of Diabetes Mellitus

Types of Diabetes Mellitus	Percentage of Occurrences
Type 1	10–12
Type 2	85–90
Secondary diabetes (medications, hormonal changes)	2–3
Gestational diabetes mellitus	1 (2–5 of all pregnancies)

one-third of patients with type 2 diabetes need insulin. Patients with type 2 diabetes who use one or two oral antidiabetic drugs may become insulin dependent years later.

Certain drugs increase blood glucose and can cause hyperglycemia, called *secondary diabetes mellitus* in prediabetic persons. These include glucocorticoids (cortisone, prednisone), thiazide diuretics (hydrochlorothiazide), and epinephrine. Usually the blood glucose level returns to normal after the drug is discontinued.

Gestational Diabetes Mellitus

During the second and third trimesters of pregnancy, the levels of the hormones progesterone, cortisol, and human placental lactogen increase. These increased hormone levels can inhibit insulin usage. This is a contributing factor for the occurrence of gestational diabetes mellitus. Glucose is then mobilized from the tissue and from lipid storage sites. After pregnancy, the blood glucose level may decrease; however, some patients may develop diabetes mellitus, whereas others may develop type 2 diabetes in later years.

INSULIN

Insulin is released from the beta cells of the islets of Langerhans in response to an increase in blood glucose. Oral glucose load is more effective in raising the serum insulin level than an intravenous (IV) glucose load. Insulin promotes the uptake of glucose, amino acids, and fatty acids and converts them to substances that are stored in body cells. Glucose is converted to glycogen in the liver and muscle for future glucose needs, thereby lowering the blood glucose level. The normal range for fasting blood glucose is 70 to 99 mg/dL for a person without diabetes. When the blood glucose level is greater than 180 mg/dL, *glycosuria*—glucose in the urine—can occur. Increased blood glucose acts as an osmotic diuretic, causing polyuria. When blood glucose remains elevated (>200 mg/dL), diabetes mellitus occurs.

Hemoglobin A1c (HbA1c), a derivative of the interaction of glucose with hemoglobin in red blood cells (RBCs), is used for the diagnosis of diabetes as recommended by the ADA. Because RBCs have a life span of approximately 120 days, the HbA1c level reflects the average glucose level for up to 3 months. In monitoring treatment, the goal is to keep the diabetic patient's HbA1c below 7%. For diagnostic purposes, an HbA1c level of 5% or less indicates that the patient does *not* have diabetes, 5.7% to 6.4% indicates prediabetes, and 6.5% or greater indicates a diagnosis of diabetes mellitus.

The beta cells in the pancreas secrete approximately 0.2 to 0.5 units/kg per day of insulin. A patient who weighs 70 kg (154 lb) secretes 14 to 35 units of insulin per day, although more insulin secretion may occur if the person consumes more calories. A patient with diabetes mellitus may require 0.2 to 1 units/kg per day. The higher range may be because of obesity, stress, or tissue insulin resistance.

! Commercially Prepared Insulin

Early insulin preparations utilized pancreas tissue extracted from animals—either pigs or cattle. Pork insulin is structurally closer to human insulin than beef insulin. Today, insulins are currently manufactured biosynthetically using recombinant DNA technology. *Human insulin* duplicates insulin produced by the pancreas of the human body; examples of human insulin include Humulin R and Novolin N. The use of human insulin has a low incidence of both allergic effects and insulin resistance. *Human insulin analogs* are modifications of human insulin with alterations in onset and duration of action. Insulin lispro and insulin aspart are examples of human insulin analogs.

Insulins are usually administered subcutaneously. Abdominal injections of insulin are absorbed faster than those at other body sites and have been found to be more consistent.

The concentration of insulin is 100 or 500 units/mL (U100/ML or U500/mL, respectively), and the insulin is packaged in a 10-mL vial. Insulin in 500 units/mL is only available in short-acting regular insulin. Insulin in 500 units/mL is seldom used except in emergencies and for patients with serious insulin resistance (>200 U/day). Insulin in 40 units/mL is no longer used in the United States, although it is still used in other countries. Insulin syringes are typically marked in units of 100 U/mL or 50 U/0.5 mL for insulin U100. Insulin syringes must be used for accurate dosing. To prevent dosage errors, the nurse must be certain that there is a match of the insulin concentration with the calibration of units on the insulin syringe. Before use, the patient or nurse must roll—not shake—cloudy insulin bottles to ensure that the insulin and its ingredients are well mixed. Shaking a bottle of insulin can cause bubbles, which can lead to an inaccurate dose. Insulin requirements vary; usually less insulin is needed with increased exercise, and more insulin is needed with infections and high fever.

Types of Insulin

Several standard types of insulin are available that include rapid-, short-, intermediate-, or long-acting types and combinations of these. *Rapid- and short-acting insulins* are in a clear solution without any added substance to prolong insulin action. *Intermediate-acting insulins* are cloudy and may contain protamine, a protein that prolongs the action of insulin, or zinc, which also slows the onset of action and prolongs the duration of activity.

Rapid-acting insulins include insulin lispro (human analog), human insulin aspart (recombinant DNA [rDNA] origin), insulin glulisine, and human oral inhalation insulin. Insulin lispro is formed by reversing two amino acids in human regular insulin. Insulin aspart (rDNA origin) is another human insulin analog in which a single amino acid (proline) has been substituted with aspartic acid to help prevent the molecules from clumping together to allow quicker entry into blood circulation. Insulin lispro, insulin aspart, insulin glulisine, and human oral inhalation insulin act faster than regular insulin, so they must be administered within 10 to 15 minutes before mealtime (food should be present before administering these insulins). Patients who are insulin-dependent and take rapid-acting insulin usually require intermediate-acting insulin as well.

Short-acting regular insulin has an onset of action of 30 minutes. The peak action occurs in 1.5 to 3.5 hours, and the duration of action is 5 to 7 hours. Regular (unmodified, crystalline) insulin is short-acting insulin that can be administered intravenously or subcutaneously. Regular insulin is generally given 30 minutes before meals.

Intermediate-acting insulins include neutral protamine Hagedorn (NPH). Isophane insulins like NPH contain protamine, a protein that prolongs the action of insulin. The onset of intermediate-acting insulin is 1 to 2 hours, peak action occurs in 6 to 8 hours, and the duration of action is 14 to 24 hours.

Insulin glargine is long-acting insulin with an onset of 1.5 hours. It is evenly distributed over a 24-hour duration of action; therefore, it is administered once a day, usually at bedtime. The incidence of nocturnal hypoglycemia is not as common as with other insulins because of its continuous sustained release. Insulin detemir is another long-acting insulin that peaks in 6 to 8 hours and lasts for 24 hours, and insulin degludec, a *long-acting insulin*, has an onset of 1 hour, peaks at 12 hours, and lasts for 42 hours; these insulins are analogs of human insulin. Glargine was the first long-acting rDNA-origin human insulin for patients with types 1 and 2 diabetes. Glargine, detemir, and degludec are available in a prefilled cartridge for the OptiPen insulin pen device. Some patients report more pain at the injection site with the administration of glargine than with NPH insulin.

Combination insulins are commercially premixed. These include NPH 70/regular 30 and NPH 50/regular 50. These combinations are widely used. The NPH 70/regular 30 is available in vials or as prefilled disposable pens. The exterior of an insulin pen resembles a fountain pen. It can be stored at room temperature for up to 10 days. With these combinations of insulin, the patient does not have to mix regular and NPH insulins as long as one of these combinations is effective. However, some patients need less than 25% or 30% regular insulin and more intermediate-acting insulin. These patients need to mix the two insulins in the prescribed proportions.

Regular insulin can be mixed with other insulin in the same syringe. However, mixing insulin can alter the absorption rate.

Pharmacokinetics

All insulins can be administered subcutaneously, but only regular insulin can be given intravenously. The half-life varies. Insulin is metabolized by the liver and muscle and is excreted in the urine.

Pharmacodynamics

Insulin lowers blood glucose by promoting the use of glucose by the body's cells. Insulin is also active in the storage of glucose as glycogen in muscles. The onset of action of rapid-acting insulin given subcutaneously is approximately 10 to 30 minutes. The onset of action of regular insulin is 30 minutes given subcutaneously and 15 minutes given intravenously. The onset of action of intermediate-acting insulin is 1.5 hours. The peak action of insulins is important because of the possibility of a hypoglycemic reaction (insulin shock) occurring during that time. The peak action for rapid-acting insulin is approximately 30 to 90 minutes. The peak time for regular insulin is 1.5 to 3.5 hours; for intermediate-acting insulin, the peak time is 4 to 12 hours. The nurse needs to assess for signs and symptoms of hypoglycemic reaction, such as nervousness, tremors, confusion, sweating, and increased pulse rate. Orange juice, sugar-sweetened beverages, or hard candy should be kept available to be given if a reaction occurs. If the patient is unable to ingest fast-acting carbohydrates, glucagon may be given. Glucagon promotes the breakdown of glycogen in the liver and raises blood glucose within 10 minutes.

Regular insulin can be given several times a day, especially during the regulation of insulin dosage. Intermediate- and long-acting insulins are usually administered once a day. Regular insulin can be mixed with intermediate-acting NPH insulin, especially if rapid onset of action is needed. When switching from one type of insulin to another, the patient may require a dose adjustment because human insulin has a shorter duration of action.

Drug Interactions

Drugs such as thiazide diuretics, glucocorticoids (cortisone preparations), thyroid agents, and estrogen increase blood glucose; therefore the insulin dosage may need adjustment. Drugs that decrease insulin needs are monoamine oxidase inhibitors (MAOIs), aspirin products, and oral anticoagulants.

Table 50.2 lists the rapid-, short-, intermediate-, and long-acting insulins with their dosages, uses, and considerations.

Side Effects and Adverse Reactions

When more insulin is administered than is needed for glucose metabolism, a hypoglycemic reaction, or insulin shock, occurs. The person may exhibit excess hunger, vertigo, syncope, nervousness, trembling, and lack of coordination; have cold and clammy skin; and report a headache. Some patients become incoherent with slurred speech and confusion. Giving sugar orally or intravenously increases the use of insulin, and the symptoms disappear immediately.

In response to an excessive dose of insulin, diabetic patients may develop what is known as the Somogyi effect, a hypoglycemic condition that usually occurs in the predawn hours of 2:00 a.m. to 4:00 a.m. wherein a rapid decrease in blood glucose during the nighttime hours

TABLE 50.2 Antidiabetics: Insulins

Drug	Half-Life	Action Onset	Peak	Duration
Rapid-Acting Insulins				
Insulin lispro	1 h	15–30 min	30–90 min	3–5 h
Insulin aspart	1.5 h	10–20 min	40–50 min	3–5 h
Insulin glulisine	5–6 min	20–30 min	55 min	1.5 h
Oral inhalation insulin	2–3.5 h	12–15 min	53 min	2.5 h
Short-Acting Insulins				
Insulin regular	1.5 h	Subcut: 30 min IV: 15 min	Subcut: 1.5–3.5 h IV: 15–30 min	Subcut: 4–12 h IV: 2–6 h
Intermediate-Acting Insulins				
Insulin isophane NPH	5–6 min	1.5 h	4–12 h	14–24 h
Long-Acting Insulins				
Insulin glargine	5–6 min	1–1.5 h	None	24 h
Insulin detemir	5–6 min	1–2 h	6–8 h	24 h
Insulin degludec	25 h	1 h	12 h	42 h

h, Hour; *IV*, intravenous; *min*, minute; *NPH*, neutral protamine Hagedorn; *subcut*, subcutaneous.

stimulates a release of hormones (cortisol, glucagon, and epinephrine) to increase blood glucose by lipolysis, gluconeogenesis, and glycogenolysis. Management of the Somogyi effect involves monitoring blood glucose between 2:00 a.m. and 4:00 a.m. and reducing the bedtime insulin dosage.

Hyperglycemia on awakening is known as the dawn phenomenon. The patient usually awakens with a headache, extreme thirst, fatigue, nausea, tachycardia, and reports night sweats and nightmares usually between 4 a.m. and 8 a.m. Management of the dawn phenomenon involves increasing the bedtime dose of insulin.

With an inadequate amount of insulin, sugar cannot be metabolized, and fat catabolism occurs. The use of fatty acids (ketones) for energy causes ketoacidosis (diabetic acidosis or diabetic coma). Table 50.3 lists the signs and symptoms of hypoglycemic reaction and ketoacidosis.

Administration of Insulin

Insulin is a protein and cannot be administered orally because gastrointestinal (GI) secretions destroy the insulin structure. It is administered subcutaneously at a 45- to 90-degree angle. The 90-degree angle is made by raising the skin and fatty tissue, and the insulin is injected into the pocket between the fat and the muscle. In a thin person with little fatty tissue, the 45- to 60-degree angle is used. Regular insulin is the only type that can be administered intravenously.

The site and depth of insulin injection affect absorption. Insulin absorption is greater when given in the abdomen than when given in the thigh or buttocks. Heat and massage could increase subcutaneous absorption, and cooling the subcutaneous area can decrease absorption.

Insulin is usually given in the morning before breakfast, and it can be given several times a day. Insulin injection sites should be rotated to prevent lipodystrophy, tissue atrophy, or hypertrophy, which can interfere with insulin absorption. Lipoatrophy, tissue atrophy, is a depression under the skin surface that primarily occurs in females and children; lipohypertrophy, tissue hypertrophy, is a raised lump or knot on the skin surface and is more common in males. It is frequently caused by repeated injections into the same site. The patient needs to develop a "site rotation pattern" to avoid lipodystrophy and to promote insulin absorption. There are various insulin rotation programs, such as an 8-day rotation schedule in which insulin is given at a different site each day. The ADA suggests that insulin be injected daily at a chosen site for 1 week. Injections should be 1.5 inches (a knuckle length) apart each day. When a patient requires two insulin injections a day, morning and evening, one site should be chosen on the right side (morning) and one on the left side (evening). Fig. 50.1 illustrates the sites for insulin injections. A record of injection area sites and dates administered should be kept.

Illness and stress increase the need for insulin, so doses should not be withheld during illness, including infections and stress. Hyperglycemia and ketoacidosis may result from insufficient insulin.

Sliding-Scale Insulin Coverage

Insulin may be administered in adjusted doses that depend on individual blood glucose test results. When the diabetic patient has extreme variances in insulin requirements—such as with stress from hospitalization, surgery, illness, or infection—adjusted dosing or sliding-scale insulin coverage provides a more constant blood glucose level. Blood glucose testing is performed several times a day at specified intervals, usually before meals and at bedtime. A preset scale usually involves directions for the administration of rapid- or short-acting insulin.

Insulin Pen Injectors

An insulin pen resembles a fountain pen but contains a disposable needle and a disposable insulin-filled cartridge. Insulin pens come in two types, prefilled and reusable, and are considered to deliver a more accurate dose than the traditional 100-unit syringe and vial.

To operate the insulin pen, the insulin dose is obtained by turning the dial to the number of insulin units needed. The capacity of these prefilled and reusable insulin pens is 150 to 300 units, or 1.5 to 3 mL; the 1.5-mL replaceable cartridges for insulin pens are being phased out. Insulin pens available on the market include the NovoLog FlexPen

TABLE 50.3 Hypoglycemic Reaction and Diabetic Ketoacidosis

Reaction	Signs and Symptoms
Hypoglycemic reaction (insulin shock)	Headache, lightheadedness
	Nervousness, apprehension
	Tremor
	Excess perspiration; cold, clammy skin
	Tachycardia
	Slurred speech
	Memory lapse, confusion, seizures
	Blood glucose <60 mg/dL
Diabetic ketoacidosis (hyperglycemic reaction)	Extreme thirst
	Polyuria
	Fruity breath odor
	Kussmaul breathing (deep, rapid, labored, distressed, dyspneic)
	Rapid, thready pulse
	Dry mucous membranes, poor skin turgor
	Blood glucose >250 mg/dL

>, Greater than; <, less than.

Fig. 50.1 Sites for insulin injection.

(Novo Nordisk), Humalog KwikPen (Lilly), Apidra SoloSTAR (Sanofi-Aventis), Lantus SoloSTAR (Sanofi), and Levemir FlexPen (Novo Nordisk). Insulin pens tend to be more expensive than other delivery systems, but their advantages may outweigh the extra cost.

The use of insulin pens increases the patient's compliance with the insulin regimen. The convenience of the pen is most appealing, and patients may choose to use the insulin pen for its portability; it can be used at work or while traveling, whereas the traditional method for administering insulin may be used at other times. The cost of insulin in vials is somewhat less than the prefilled pens, but most patients state that less injection pain is associated with insulin pens than with the traditional insulin syringe.

Insulin Pumps

Insulin pumps are an alternative to daily insulin injections used in association with blood glucose monitoring and carbohydrate counting. These computerized devices have an insulin reservoir and programming capacity to deliver continuous rapid-acting insulin in varying amounts at different times throughout a 24-hour period. These pumps are smaller than most mobile phones, and the types of insulin pumps include implantable and portable. The implantable insulin pump is surgically implanted in the abdomen and delivers both basal infusion (continuous release of a small amount of insulin) and bolus (additional) doses with meals. It is administered intraperitoneally. With the use of implantable insulin pumps, fewer hypoglycemic reactions occur, and blood glucose levels are controlled. Long-term effectiveness of the pump is currently under study.

External or portable insulin pumps, also called continuous subcutaneous insulin infusion, may have a tube or infusion set placed under the skin. The needle is inserted into the abdomen, upper thigh, or upper arm. This type of pump is worn outside the body and is placed in a pocket or bra. The external tubeless pump lies directly on the skin and injects insulin through the skin without tubes. The external insulin pump keeps blood glucose levels as close to normal as possible. This insulin pump is a battery-operated device that uses rapid-acting insulin, which is stored in a reservoir syringe placed inside the device. It delivers both basal insulin infusion and bolus doses with meals. Infusions are programmed by the patient. About three basal rates are programmed per day; however, the patient can adjust the rate according to changes in activity. The patient pushes a button to deliver a bolus dose at meals. Only rapid-acting insulin is used; modified (NPH) insulins are not used because of unpredictable control of blood glucose. The pump delivers exactly as much insulin as the patient programs.

The ongoing insulin delivery therapy helps decrease the risk of severe hypoglycemic reaction and maintains tight glucose (glycemic) control. Glucose levels should be monitored at least four times daily with an insulin pump. The patient must count carbohydrates and bolus doses before meals.

Most insulin pumps have a (time and day) memory of the last 24 boluses. An alarm sounds so the patient can take appropriate action when insulin is not delivered or when there is an oncoming low or high. Newer pumps have an automatic shutoff for 1 to 2 hours during periods of low blood glucose. This feature is designed for patients who may not hear the alarm and for those in whom blood glucose is allowed to elevate. The pump can be disconnected from the insertion site for bathing, swimming, and other activities; however, it is recommended that it not be discontinued for longer than 1 to 2 hours.

Success of insulin pump therapy depends on the individual's knowledge and compliance related to insulin use and the diabetic state. The person with type 1 diabetes mellitus may benefit most from the use of insulin pump therapy. This insulin delivery method is considered more effective than the use of multiple injections of regular and modified types of insulins, and it lessens the long-term diabetic complications. Studies have shown that myocardial infarction, renal disease, nerve damage, eye damage, and death have all been greatly reduced by tight blood glucose control. Also, HbA1c levels, neuropathy pain, and sexual performance have improved with the use of insulin pump control.

Insulin Jet Injectors

Insulin jet injectors shoot insulin, without a needle, directly through the skin into the fatty tissue. Because the insulin is delivered under high pressure, stinging, pain, burning, and bruising may occur. This method of insulin insertion is not indicated for children or older adults. This type of device is also expensive, costing approximately 2 to 10 times as much as the subcutaneous dose.

Insulin Resistance

Antibodies develop over time in persons taking animal insulin. This can slow the onset of insulin action and extend its duration of action. Antibody development can cause insulin resistance and insulin allergy, and obesity can also be a causative factor for insulin resistance. Skin tests with different insulin preparations may be performed to determine whether an allergic effect is present. Human and regular insulins produce fewer allergens.

Storage of Insulin

Unopened insulin vials are refrigerated until needed. Once an insulin vial has been opened, it may be kept at room temperature for 1 month or in the refrigerator for 3 months; insulin is less irritating to the tissues when injected at room temperature. Insulin vials should not be put in the freezer, nor should they be placed in direct sunlight or in a high-temperature area. Prefilled syringes should be stored in the refrigerator and should be used within 1 to 2 weeks. Opened insulin vials lose their strength after approximately 3 months.

Prototype Drug Chart: Insulins lists the pharmacologic data for the different types of insulin.

COMPLEMENTARY AND ALTERNATIVE THERAPIES

Antidiabetic Agents

- Chromium may decrease insulin requirements.
- Black cohosh may potentiate the hypoglycemic effects of insulin and oral antidiabetic drugs.
- Garlic, bitter melon, aloe, and gymnema can increase insulin levels and therefore may cause hypoglycemia when used with insulin or oral antidiabetic drugs. They can have a direct hypoglycemic effect.
- Ginseng can cause hypoglycemia when taken with insulin or an oral antidiabetic (hypoglycemic) drug.
- Bilberry may increase hypoglycemia when taken with insulin or oral antidiabetics.
- Rosemary and stinging nettle decrease the therapeutic effect of insulin and oral antidiabetic drugs (have a hyperglycemic effect).
- Milk thistle may improve insulin sensitivity.
- Hawthorn may potentiate hypoglycemia when taken with insulin or oral antidiabetics.
- Ginkgo may cause hypoglycemia when taken with glipizide, may enhance effectiveness of metformin, may increase drug level of pioglitazone, and may decrease effectiveness of tolbutamide.
- St. Johns wort may alter metabolism of repaglinide and affect blood glucose level when taken with tolbutamide.

PROTOTYPE DRUG CHART

Insulins

Drug Class	Dosage
Antidiabetic: Insulin Lispro, rapid acting Regular, short acting NPH, intermediate acting Glargine, long acting	Must be individualized and varies according to patient's blood glucose and health status

Contraindications	Drug-Lab-Food Interactions
Hypersensitivity, hypoglycemia *Caution:* Hypokalemia, fever, surgery, trauma, visual impairment, thyroid disease, vomiting, diarrhea, infection, diabetic ketoacidosis, renal or hepatic impairment, tobacco smoking, older adults, pregnancy, breastfeeding	Drug: Increased hypoglycemic effect with aspirin, oral anticoagulants, alcohol, oral hypoglycemics, beta-blockers, ACE inhibitors, ARBs, MAOIs, and tetracycline; decreased hypoglycemic effect with thiazides, glucocorticoids, oral contraceptives, thyroid drugs, furosemide, bumetanide, phenytoin, fluoroquinolones, smoking, and green tea

Pharmacokinetics	Pharmacodynamics
Absorption: Lispro and regular, rapidly absorbed from subcut injection site; NPH is absorbed at a slower rate; glargine is absorbed at a slow, evenly distributed rate. Distribution: PB: UK Metabolism: t½: Varies with type of insulin Excretion: Mostly in urine	Lispro: Subcut: Onset: 15–30 min Peak: 30–90 min Duration: 3–5 h Regular: Subcut: Onset: 30 min Peak: 1.5–3.5 h Duration: 5–7 h NPH: Subcut: Onset: 1.5 h Peak: 6–8 h Duration: 14–24 h Glargine: Subcut: Onset: 1.5 h Peak: None Duration: 24 h

Therapeutic Effects/Uses

To control: Insulins can be used for both type 1 and 2 diabetes mellitus, to lower blood glucose
Mechanism of action: Promotes use of glucose by body cells

Side Effects	Adverse Reactions
Headache, depression, diaphoresis, pharyngitis, sinusitis, rhinitis, cough, wheezing, diarrhea, infection, influenza, weight gain, arthralgia, back pain, injection-site reaction, lipodystrophy, peripheral neuropathy/edema	Tachycardia, hypo/hypertension, hyperosmolar hypoglycemic state, Somogyi effect, hypokalemia, insulin resistance, cataracts *Life threatening:* Insulin shock, anaphylaxis, angioedema, bronchospasm

ACE, Angiotensin-converting enzyme; *ARB*, angiotensin II receptor blocker; *h*, hour; *MAOI*, monoamine oxidase inhibitor; *min*, minute; *NPH*, neutral protamine Hagedorn; *PB*, protein binding; *subcut*, subcutaneous; *t½*, half-life; *TCA*, tricyclic antidepressant; *UK*, unknown.

CLINICAL JUDGMENT [NURSING PROCESS]

Antidiabetics: Insulin

Concept: Glucose Regulation
- The process of maintaining normal glucose levels

Recognize Cues [Assessment]
- Identify the drugs a patient currently takes. Certain drugs such as alcohol, aspirin, oral anticoagulants, oral antidiabetics, beta-blockers, tricyclic antidepressants (TCAs), monoamine oxidase inhibitors (MAOIs), and tetracycline increase the hypoglycemic effect when taken with insulin. Note that thiazides, glucocorticoids, oral contraceptives, thyroid drugs, and smoking can increase blood glucose.
- Assess the type of insulin and dosage. Note whether it is given once or multiple times a day.
- Note blood pressure (BP), heart rate, and blood glucose levels. Tachycardia and heart palpitations may occur with hypoglycemia, and hypotension may occur with hyperglycemia. Report abnormal findings.
- Determine the patient's knowledge of diabetes mellitus and use of insulins.
- Check for signs and symptoms of hypoglycemic reaction (insulin shock), hyperglycemia, or ketoacidosis.

Analyze Cues and Prioritize Hypothesis [Patient Problems]
- Hypoglycemia
- Metabolic acidosis
- Hyperglycemia
- Reduced glucose regulation

CLINICAL JUDGMENT [NURSING PROCESS]—CONT'D
Antidiabetics: Insulin

- Hyponatremia
- Fatigue

Generate Solutions [Planning]
- The patient will maintain fasting blood glucose levels within normal values (80–130 mg/dL).
- The patient will self-administer insulin correctly.

Take Action [Nursing Interventions]
- Monitor vital signs. Tachycardia can occur during insulin reaction.
- Determine blood glucose levels, and report changes.
- Monitor the patient's hemoglobin A1c (HbA1c) to provide feedback of diabetic control.
- Prepare a teaching plan based on the patient's knowledge of the health problem, diet, and drug therapy.

Patient Teaching
General
- Teach patients to recognize and immediately report symptoms of *hypoglycemic* (insulin) reaction—such as headache, nervousness, sweating, tremors, rapid pulse—and those of *hyperglycemic* reaction (diabetic acidosis): thirst, increased urine output, and a sweet, fruity breath odor.
- Advise patients that hypoglycemic reactions are more likely to occur during peak action time. Most diabetic patients know whether they are having a hypoglycemic reaction, but some have a higher tolerance to low blood glucose and can have a severe reaction without realizing it.
- Explain that orange juice, sugar-containing drinks, and hard candy may be used when a hypoglycemic reaction begins.
- Teach family members to administer glucagon by injection if a patient has a hypoglycemic reaction and cannot drink sugar-containing fluid.
- Inform patients that certain herbs may interact with insulin and oral antidiabetic drugs. A hypoglycemic or hyperglycemic effect might occur.
- Teach patients about the necessity of compliance with prescribed insulin therapy and diet. HbA1c provides the most accurate picture of optimal diabetic control.
- Advise patients to carry a MedicAlert card, tag, or bracelet that indicates the health problem and the insulin dosage.

Self-Administration
- Instruct patients on how to check blood glucose with a glucometer (OneTouch AccuSure, GlucoSure, Accu-Chek).
- Teach patients about the care of insulin containers and syringes. Inform patients taking neutral protamine Hagedorn (NPH) insulin with regular insulin that regular insulin is drawn up before NPH insulin.

Diet
- Advise patients taking insulin to eat the prescribed diet on a consistent schedule. Diet information may be obtained from the American Diabetes Association (ADA) or from a nutritionist.

Evaluate Outcomes [Evaluation]
- Evaluate the effectiveness of insulin therapy by noting whether the blood glucose level is within the accepted range.
- Establish the patient's ability to perform self-care.
- Determine the patient's knowledge of the signs and symptoms of hypoglycemic or hyperglycemic reaction.

ORAL ANTIDIABETIC DRUGS

Oral antidiabetic drugs, also called oral hypoglycemics, should be used by those with type 2 diabetes; persons with type 1 diabetes should not use them. However, pramlintide is used to treat both type 1 and type 2 diabetes. Patients with type 2 diabetes have some degree of insulin secretion by the pancreas.

First- and Second-Generation Sulfonylureas

The sulfonylureas, a group of antidiabetics chemically related to sulfonamides but lacking antibacterial activity, stimulate pancreatic beta cells to secrete more insulin. This increases the insulin cell receptors, which increases the ability of the cells to bind insulin for glucose metabolism.

The sulfonylureas are classified as first- and second-generation drugs. First-generation sulfonylureas were divided into short-, intermediate-, and long-acting antidiabetics. Tolbutamide is a first-generation, short-acting sulfonylurea; tolazamide was a first-generation, intermediate-acting sulfonylurea; and chlorpropamide was a first-generation, long-acting sulfonylurea. Tolazamide and chlorpropamide have been taken off the market in the United States. Tolbutamide is currently off the market in the United States for 1 year.

Second-generation sulfonylureas increase the tissue response to insulin and decrease glucose production by the liver. They have greater hypoglycemic potency than the first-generation sulfonylureas. Effective doses for the second-generation drugs are lower than for the first-generation drugs; the second-generation drugs also have a longer duration of action and cause fewer side effects. The second-generation drugs also have less displacement potential from protein-binding sites by other highly protein-bound drugs, such as salicylates and warfarin, than do first-generation drugs. Second-generation sulfonylureas should *not* be used when liver or kidney dysfunction is present. A hypoglycemic reaction is more likely to occur in older adults.

Second-generation sulfonylureas include glimepiride and glipizide, which directly stimulate the beta cells to secrete insulin, thus decreasing the blood glucose level. Glimepiride improves postprandial glucose levels and may be used in combination with insulin in persons with type 2 diabetes. Side effects include blurred vision, headache, weakness, hypoglycemia, diarrhea, weight gain, and hyponatremia.

Table 50.4 lists the sulfonylureas and their dosages, uses, and considerations. Prototype Drug Chart: Glipizide lists the pharmacologic data for the second-generation sulfonylurea glipizide.

Pharmacokinetics
Glipizide is well absorbed from the GI tract and is highly protein bound. Glipizide is metabolized by the liver. The primary metabolites are inactive and are excreted mainly in urine.

Pharmacodynamics
Glipizide is the most common sulfonylurea drug prescribed for type 2 diabetes mellitus. It lowers blood glucose by stimulating pancreatic beta cells to secrete insulin. The onset of action usually occurs within 90 minutes, and the peak action time is 1 to 3 hours. Glipizide is normally given once a day in the morning because of its long duration of action of 24 hours.

PROTOTYPE DRUG CHART
Glipizide

Drug Class	Dosage
Glipizide: Sulfonylurea, second generation	Intermediate release: A: PO: Initially 5 mg/d 30 min before breakfast; *max:* 40 mg/d Older A: PO: Initially 2.5 mg/d; *max:* 40 mg/d Extended release: A: PO: Initially 5 mg/d with breakfast; *max:* 20 mg/d Older A: PO: Initially 2.5 mg/d; *max:* 20 mg/d
Contraindications	**Drug-Lab-Food Interactions**
Diabetic ketoacidosis, hypersensitivity Caution: Type 1 diabetes, hypoglycemia, fever, surgery, trauma, infection, malnutrition, vomiting, diarrhea, GI obstruction, adrenal or pituitary insufficiency, G6PD deficiency, thyroid disease, renal/hepatic impairment, hemolytic anemia, older adults, pregnancy, breastfeeding, children	Drug: Alcohol may produce disulfiram-like reaction (flushing, headache, sweating, nausea, violent vomiting, weakness). Beta-blockers, ACE inhibitors, aspirin, systemic azole antifungals, clarithromycin, oral anticoagulants, MAOIs, salicylates, probenecid, sulfonamides, antacids, cimetidine, may potentiate hypoglycemia. Oral contraceptives, thiazide diuretics, glucocorticoids, phenytoin, and sympathomimetics may enhance hyperglycemia. Lab: Altered liver function tests Food: Green tea may potentiate hypoglycemia.
Pharmacokinetics	**Pharmacodynamics**
Absorption: Rapidly absorbed from GI tract Distribution: PB: 98%–99% Metabolism: t½: 2–5 h Excretion: Primarily in urine	Regular release: PO: Onset: 90 min Peak: 1–3 h Duration: 12–24 h Extended release: PO: Onset: 2–3 h Peak: 6–12 h Duration: 24 h
Therapeutic Effects/Uses	
To control hyperglycemia in type 2 diabetes mellitus Mechanism of action: Directly stimulates beta cells in the pancreas to secrete insulin; indirectly alters sensitivity of peripheral insulin receptors, allowing increased insulin binding	
Side Effects	**Adverse Reactions**
Drowsiness, dizziness, headache, confusion, blurred vision, anxiety, hyperhidrosis, insomnia, anorexia, dyspepsia, nausea, flatulence, vomiting, diarrhea, constipation, weight gain, tremor, arthralgia, myalgia, paresthesia, pruritus	Hypoglycemia, hyponatremia, porphyria, GI bleeding, secondary failure, elevated hepatic enzymes *Life threatening:* Angioedema, agranulocytosis, aplastic anemia, leukopenia, thrombocytopenia, pancytopenia, hepatic failure, SIADH

A, Adult; *d*, day; *GI*, gastrointestinal; *G6PD*, glucose-6-phosphate dehydrogenase deficiency; *h*, hour; *MAOI*, monoamine oxidase inhibitor; *max*, maximum; *min*, minute; *PB*, protein binding; *PO*, by mouth; *SIADH*, syndrome of inappropriate antidiuretic hormone; *t½*, half-life.

Side Effects, Adverse Reactions, and Contraindications

The side effects of most oral antidiabetic drugs are similar to those of insulin. The major side effect of sulfonylureas is hypoglycemia. Taking antidiabetic drugs without adequate food can lead to an insulin reaction with signs and symptoms such as sweating, tremors, dizziness, confusion, and anxiety. Adverse reactions include hematologic disorders such as aplastic anemia, leukopenia, and thrombocytopenia. Hyperhidrosis, nausea, vomiting, and hepatic failure may also occur. Sulfonylureas are contraindicated in type 1 diabetes (no functioning beta cells), diabetic ketoacidosis, and sulfonamide hypersensitivity. Caution is used when giving to patients during trauma surgery, burns, or severe infection.

Drug Interactions

Aspirin, oral anticoagulants, MAOIs, sulfonamides, and cimetidine can increase the action of sulfonylureas, especially first-generation ones, by binding to plasma proteins and displacing sulfonylureas. Because this causes increased free sulfonylurea, hypoglycemia can result. The action of sulfonylureas is decreased by concurrent administration of thiazide diuretics, sympathomimetics, phenytoin, and corticosteroids. Patients should be alerted not to drink alcohol while taking sulfonylureas because alcohol increases the half-life, and a disulfiram-like reaction can result (flushing, headache, sweating, nausea, vomiting, and weakness).

Nonsulfonylureas

Expanding knowledge of glucose metabolism has revealed new mechanisms for the management of type 2 diabetes. The drugs metformin and acarbose use different methods to control serum glucose levels after a meal. Unlike the sulfonylureas, which enhance insulin release and receptor interaction, these drugs affect the hepatic and GI production of glucose.

TABLE 50.4 Antidiabetics

Drug	Route and Dosage	Uses and Considerations
Second-Generation Sulfonylureas		
Glipizide	See Prototype Drug Chart: Glipizide	
Glyburide	A: PO: Initially 2.5–5 mg/d conventional form or initially 1.5–3 mg/d micronized form with breakfast; *max:* 20 mg/d conventional form, 12 mg/d micronized form	For managing type 2 diabetes. May cause blurred vision, hypoglycemia, hyponatremia, weight gain, rash, hives, dyspepsia, nausea, secondary failure of glucose control, myalgia, erythema, pruritus, and pyrosis. PB: 99%; t½: 10 h
Glimepiride	A: PO: Initially 1–2 mg/d with breakfast; *max:* 8 mg/d	For managing type 2 diabetes. May cause dizziness, headache, blurred vision, weakness, nausea, weight gain, myalgia, secondary failure of glucose control, and hypoglycemia. PB: 99.5%; t½: 5–9 h
Nonsulfonylureas		
Monoclonial Antibody		
Teplizumab	A: IV: 65 mcg/n² on day 1, then 125 on day 2, then 250 on day 3, then 500 on day 4, and 1030 on day 5–14	For type 1 diabetes mellitus prophylaxis. May cause headache, hypocalcemia, metabolic acidosis, thrombocytopenia, lymphopenia, anemia, leukopenia, rash, antibody formation, and elevated hepatic, enzymes. PB: UK; t½: 4.5 d
Biguanides		
Metformin	See Prototype Drug Chart: Metformin	
Alpha-Glucosidase Inhibitors		
Acarbose	A: >60 kg: PO: Initially 25 mg tid with first bite of each meal or 25 mg qd, may increase in 4–8 wk; *maint:* 50–100 mg tid; *max:* 100 mg tid A: <60 kg: PO: Initially 25 mg tid or 25 mg qd, may increase dose in 4–8 wk; *max:* 50 mg tid	For managing type 2 diabetes mellitus. May cause abdominal pain, flatulence, diarrhea, anemia, weight loss, ileus, elevated hepatic enzymes, and edema. PB: UK; t½: 2 h
Miglitol	A: PO: Initially 25 mg tid with first bite of each meal or 25 mg qd; *max:* 300 mg/d	For managing type 2 diabetes. May cause rash, abdominal pain, nausea, flatulence, diarrhea, GI bleeding, and ileus. PB: <4%; t½: 2 h
Thiazolidinediones (Insulin-Enhancing Agents)		
Pioglitazone hydrochloride	A: PO: Initially 15–30 mg/d; *max:* 45 mg/d	For managing type 2 diabetes. May cause dizziness, headache, pharyngitis, sinusitis, flatulence, diarrhea, peripheral edema, weight gain, infection, myalgia, back pain, bone fracture, hypoglycemia, edema, chest pain, hypertension, and heart failure. PB: 99%; t½: 3–7 h
Meglitinides		
Repaglinide	A: PO: Initially 0.5–2 mg 30 min before each meal; *max:* 16 mg/d	For managing type 2 diabetes mellitus. May cause headache, rhinitis, dyspepsia, nausea, diarrhea, infection, back pain, arthralgia, and hypoglycemia. PB: 98%; t½: 1 h
Nateglinide	A: PO: 60–120 mg tid ac; *max:* 360 mg/d	For managing type 2 diabetes mellitus. May cause cough, diarrhea, infection, back pain, arthropathy, and hypoglycemia. PB: 98%; t½: 1.5 h
Dipeptidyl Peptidase 4 Inhibitors		
Sitagliptin phosphate	A: PO: 100 mg/d; *max:* 100 mg/d	For managing type 2 diabetes. May cause headache, pharyngitis, stomatitis, abdominal pain, nausea, diarrhea, infection, peripheral edema, and hypoglycemia. PB: 38%; t½: 12.4 h
Saxagliptin	A: PO: 2.5–5 mg/d; *max:* 5 mg/d	For managing type 2 diabetes mellitus. May cause headache, pharyngitis, sinusitis, infection, abdominal pain, vomiting, peripheral edema, and hypoglycemia. PB: 0%; t½: 2.5 h
Linagliptin	A: PO: 5 mg/d; *max:* 5 mg/d	For managing type 2 diabetes mellitus. May cause cough, pharyngitis, diarrhea, and hypoglycemia. PB: 70%–80%; t½: 12 h
Alogliptin	A: PO: 25 mg/d; *max:* 25 mg/d	For managing type 2 diabetes mellitus. May cause headache, pharyngitis, rash, hives, infection, hypoglycemia, and elevated hepatic enzymes. PB: 20%; t½: 21 h
Selective Sodium-Glucose Cotransporter 2 Inhibitor		
Canagliflozin	A: PO: Initially 100 mg/d before first meal; *max:* 300 mg/d	For managing type 2 diabetes mellitus. May cause infection, candidiasis, diuresis, cystitis, vaginitis, polyuria, increased urinary urgency/frequency, nocturia, and hypoglycemia. PB: 99%; t½: 10.6–13.1 h

Continued

TABLE 50.4 Antidiabetics—cont'd

Drug	Route and Dosage	Uses and Considerations
Dapagliflozin	A: PO: Initially 5 mg/d in the morning; *max:* 10 mg/d	For managing type 2 diabetes mellitus. May cause pharyngitis, candidiasis, hypercholesterolemia, hyperlipidemia, hypoglycemia, hyperphosphatemia, nausea, infection, vaginitis, diuresis, cystitis, urinary frequency, and prostatitis. PB: 91%; t½: 12.9 h
Empagliflozin	A: PO: Initially 10 mg/d in the morning; *max:* 25 mg/d	For managing type 2 diabetes mellitus. May cause pharyngitis, hyperlipidemia, hypercholesterolemia, hypoglycemia, candidiasis, infection, vaginitis, diuresis, cystitis, polyuria, and increased urinary frequency. PB: 86.2%; t½: 12.4 h
Ertugliflozin	A: PO: 5 mg/d in morning; *max:* 15 mg/d	For type 2 diabetes mellitus. May cause headache, candidiasis, infection, diuresis, cystitis, dysuria, hypoglycemia, and hypovolemia. PB: 94%; t½: 17 h
Bexagliflozin	A: PO: 20 mg qd in morning; *max:* 20 mg/d	For type 2 diabetes mellitus with diet and exercise. May cause dizziness, vertigo, dehydration, hypotension, polyuria, urinary frequency/urgency, nocturia, dysuria, cystitis, hypoglycemia, candidiasis, and infection. PB: 93%; t½: 12 h
Amylin Analog		
Pramlintide	Type 2: A: Subcut: 60 mcg immediately ac, *max:* 120 mcg/dose	For managing types 1 and 2 diabetes mellitus as an adjunct to insulin therapy. May cause dizziness, headache, cough, pharyngitis, fatigue, arthralgia, anorexia, abdominal pain, nausea, vomiting, and hypoglycemia. PB: 40%; t½: 48 min
Glucagon-Like Peptide 1 Agonists		
Exenatide	Immediate release: A: Subcut: Initially 5 mcg bid within 60 min before morning and evening meals; *max:* 20 mcg/d Extended release: A: Subcut: 2 mg/wk; *max:* 2 mg/wk	For managing type 2 diabetes mellitus. May cause dizziness, headache, fatigue, restlessness, weakness, anorexia, dyspepsia, GERD, nausea, vomiting, diarrhea, constipation, antibody formation, hypoglycemia, and injection-site reaction. PB: UK; t½: 2.4 h
Liraglutide	Type 2 diabetes: A: Subcut: Initially 0.6 mg/d for 1 wk; then may increase gradually; *max:* 1.8 mg/d	For managing type 2 diabetes mellitus and obesity. May cause dizziness, headache, fatigue, injection-site reaction, anorexia, dyspepsia, gastritis, nausea, vomiting, diarrhea, constipation, hypoglycemia, tachycardia, palpitations, back pain, and antibody formation. PB: 98%; t½: 13 h
Dulaglutide	A: Subcut: Initially 0.75 mg/wk; may increase gradually; *max:* 4.5 mg/wk	For managing type 2 diabetes mellitus. May cause fatigue, anorexia, dyspepsia, abdominal pain, nausea, vomiting, diarrhea, constipation, tachycardia, antibody formation, possible suicidal ideation, and hypoglycemia. PB: UK; t½: 5 d
Semaglutide	Type 2 diabetes: Ozempic: A: Subcut: Initially 0.25 mg/wk for 4 weeks, may increase gradually; *max:* 2 mg/wk Rybelsus: A: PO: Initially 3 mg/d 30 min before breakfast for 30 d, then may increase gradually; *max:* 14 mg/d	For type 2 diabetes mellitus and obesity. May cause dizziness, headache, fatigue, pharyngitis, dyspepsia, abdominal pain, GERD, eructation, nausea, vomiting, diarrhea, flatulence, constipation, hypoglycemia, and retinopathy. PB: 99%; t½: 1 wk
Tirzepatide	A: Subcut: 2.5 mg/wk for 4 wk, then 5 mg/wk; *max:* 15 mg/wk	For type 2 diabetes mellitus with diet and exercise. May cause antibody formation, anorexia, dyspepsia, abdominal pain, nausea, vomiting, diarrhea, constipation, weight loss, and tachycardia. PB: 99%; t½: 5 d
Fixed-Combination Oral Antidiabetic Drugs		
Glyburide-metformin	A: PO: Initially (1.25 mg glyburide/250 mg metformin) once daily with a meal or bid with morning and evening meals; may increase dose at 2-wk intervals; *max:* (20 mg glyburide/2000 mg metformin) qd	For managing type 2 diabetes mellitus. May cause dizziness, headache, weakness, dyspepsia, abdominal pain, nausea, vomiting, diarrhea, flatulence, and hypoglycemia. PB: metformin 0%, glyburide 99%; t½: metformin 6.2–17.6 h, glyburide 10 h
Sitagliptin-metformin	Immediate release, extended release: A: PO: Initially give dose already being taken; *max:* sitagliptin 100 mg, metformin 2000 mg/d	For managing type 2 diabetes mellitus. May cause headache, pharyngitis, infection, weakness, anorexia, dysgeusia, dyspepsia, metallic taste, abdominal pain, nausea, diarrhea, flatulence, myalgia, malaise, hypoglycemia, and peripheral edema. PB: metformin 0%, sitagliptin 38%; t½: metformin 6.2–17.6 h, sitagliptin 12.4 h

TABLE 50.4 Antidiabetics—cont'd

Drug	Route and Dosage	Uses and Considerations
Linagliptin-metformin	Immediate release: A: PO: Initially linagliptin 2.5 mg/metformin 500 mg bid with meals; *max:* 5 mg linagliptin, 2000 mg metformin Extended release: A: PO: Initially 5 mg linagliptin/metformin 1 g qd with a meal; *max:* linagliptin 5 mg/d/metformin 2 g/d	For managing type 2 diabetes mellitus. May cause headache, pharyngitis, weakness, dyspepsia, abdominal pain, nausea, vomiting, diarrhea, flatulence, vitamin B_{12} deficiency, and hypoglycemia. PB: metformin 0%, linagliptin 70%–80%; t½: metformin 6.2–17.6 h, linagliptin 12 h
Dapagliflozin-metformin	A: PO: Individualize starting dose, give with food; *max:* 10 mg dapagliflozin, 2000 mg metformin qd	For managing type 2 diabetes mellitus. May cause headache, pharyngitis, nausea, dyspepsia, abdominal pain, vomiting, diarrhea, flatulence, vaginitis, prostatitis, diuresis, cystitis, infection, candidiasis, and vitamin B_{12} deficiency. PB: metformin 0%, dapagliflozin 91%; t½: metformin 6.2–17.6 h, dapagliflozin 12.9
Empagliflozin-metformin	Immediate release, Extended release: A: PO: Individualize doses with meals; *max:* 25 mg empagliflozin, 2000 mg metformin qd	For managing type 2 diabetes mellitus. May cause headache, pharyngitis, weakness, dysgeusia, abdominal pain, nausea, diarrhea, vaginitis, candidiasis, cystitis, hypercholesterolemia, vitamin B_{12} deficiency, hypoglycemia, infection, and diuresis. PB: metformin 0%, empagliflozin 86.2%; t½: metformin 6.2–17.6 h, empagliflozin 12.4 h
Alogliptin-metformin	A: PO: Initially (12.5 mg alogliptin/500 metformin), Individualize dose; *max:* alogliptin 25 mg/d, metformin 2 g/d	For type 2 diabetes mellitus with diet and exercise. May cause headache, nausea, dyspepsia, dysgeusia, vomiting, diarrhea, flatulence, abdominal/back pain, pharyngitis, hypoglycemia, vitamin B_{12} deficiency, and infection. PB: metformin 0%, alogliptin 20%; t1/2: metformin 6.2–17.6 h, alogliptin 21 h
Canagliflozin-metformin	A: PO: If not currently taking either drug, initially (1 tablet 50 mg canagliflozin/500 mg metformin bid for immediate release, 2 tablets qd with morning meal for extended release) Individualize dose; *max:* 300 mg canagliflozin/2 g metformin qd	For type 2 diabetes mellitus with diet and exercise. May cause candidiasis, nausea, vomiting, diarrhea, flatulence, diuresis, vaginitis, and infection. PB: metformin 0%, canagliflozin 99%; t½: metformin 6.2–17 h, canagliflozin 10.6–13.1 h
Dapagliflozin-saxagliptin	A: PO: Initially dapagliflozin 5 mg/d, saxagliptin 5 mg/d in morning; *max:* dapagliflozin 10 mg/d and saxagliptin 5 mg/d	For type 2 diabetes mellitus. May cause headache, pharyngitis, candidiasis, infection, diarrhea, increased urinary frequency, diuresis, cystitis, prostatitis, and vaginitis. PB: saxagliptin 0%, dapagliflozin 91%; t½: saxagliptin 2.5 h, dapagliflozin 12.9 h
Lixisenatide-insulin glargine	A: Subcut: 15–30 units glargine, 5–10 mcg lixisenatide/d; *max:* 60 units glargine, 20 mcg lixisenatide/d	For type 2 diabetes mellitus. May cause headache, pharyngitis, infection, nausea, diarrhea, hypoglycemia, antibody formation, injection-site reaction, and possible suicidal ideation. Let needle remain in skin at least 10 seconds. Give within 1 h of first meal of day. PB: UK; t½: insulin glargine 5–6 min, lixisenatide 3 h
Liraglutide-insulin degludec	A: Subcut: 10–50 units degludec/liraglutide; *max:* 50 units/d	For type 2 diabetes mellitus. May cause headache, pharyngitis, nausea, diarrhea, infection and hypoglycemia. Use protective gown and gloves. PB: degludec 99%, liraglutide 98%; t½: degludec 25 h, liraglutide 13 h
Hypoglycemic Drugs		
Glucagon (in short supply or unavailable)	A: Subcut/IM/IV: 1 mg, may repeat in 15 min	For hypoglycemia. May cause headache, abdominal pain, nausea, vomiting, hypo/hypertension, tachycardia, and hypo/hyperglycemia, PB: UK; t½: IM 26–45 min, Subcut 32 min, IM 26–45 min, IV 8–18 min
Diazoxide	A: PO: Initially 3 mg/kg/d in 3 divided doses q8h	For hypoglycemia. May cause dizziness, weakness, nausea, vomiting, diabetic ketoacidosis, hyperglycemia, hypotension, and hyperuricemia. PB: 90%; t½: 21–36 h
Dasiglucagon	A: Subcut: 0.6 mg, may repeat in 15 min if no response	For severe hypoglycemia in patients with diabetes mellitus. May cause headache, dizziness, injection-site reaction, nausea, vomiting, diarrhea, antibody formation, bradycardia, palpitations, and hypo/hypertension. PB: UK; t½: 30 min

<, Less than; >, greater than; *A*, adult; *ac*, before meals; *bid*, twice a day; *d*, day; *GERD*, gastroesophageal reflux disease; *h*, hour; *maint*, maintenance; *max*, maximum; *min*, minute; *PB*, protein binding; *PO*, by mouth; *qd*, every day; *subcut*, subcutaneous; *t½*, half-life; *tid*, three times a day; *UK*, unknown; *wk*, week.

Biguanides

Metformin is a biguanide compound that acts by decreasing hepatic production of glucose from stored glycogen. This diminishes the increase in serum glucose after a meal and blunts the degree of postprandial hyperglycemia. Metformin also decreases the absorption of glucose from the small intestine, and there is evidence that it increases insulin receptor sensitivity as well as peripheral glucose uptake at the cellular level. Unlike sulfonylureas, metformin does *not* produce hypoglycemia or hyperglycemia, although it can cause GI disturbances.

Metformin is 51% to 60% bioavailable and is absorbed primarily from the small intestine. It does not undergo hepatic metabolism and is eliminated unchanged in the urine. It is not recommended for patients with renal impairment. Monotherapy with metformin is effective; however, when combined with a sulfonylurea, the drug is useful in cases that are resistant to oral antidiabetics (hypoglycemics). Metformin therapy should be withheld for 48 hours before and after administration of IV contrast because lactic acidosis or acute renal failure may develop.

Alpha-Glucosidase Inhibitors

Acarbose acts by inhibiting the digestive enzyme in the small intestine that is responsible for the release of glucose from complex carbohydrates in the diet. By inhibiting alpha glucosidase, absorption of complex carbohydrates is delayed. Acarbose has no demonstrated systemic effects and is not absorbed into the body in significant amounts. Acarbose is intended for use in patients who do not achieve results with diet alone. Miglitol, like acarbose, inhibits alpha glucosides. Miglitol is absorbed from the GI tract. Acarbose and miglitol do not cause hypoglycemia, but if taken with a sulfonylurea or insulin, hypoglycemia could occur.

Thiazolidinediones

Pioglitazone and rosiglitazone are examples of thiazolidinedione drugs. Both drugs are contraindicated in class III and IV heart failure due to dose-related fluid retention. These two drugs can be prescribed as monotherapy or combined with other oral antidiabetic drugs. Pioglitazone can be taken in combination with sulfonylurea or insulin, and rosiglitazone may be combined with metformin (Prototype Drug Chart: Metformin). These drugs decrease insulin resistance and improve blood glucose control.

Meglitinides

Nateglinide is classified as a meglitinide oral antidiabetic agent. It stimulates the beta cells to release insulin. The action of nateglinide is similar to that of sulfonylureas. This agent can be used alone or in combination with metformin for patients with type 2 diabetes mellitus; it is a short-acting antidiabetic drugs. Nateglinide should be avoided or given with caution to patients with liver dysfunction because of a possible decreased liver metabolism rate; more of the drug could remain in the body, which could cause a hypoglycemic reaction.

Incretin Modifier

The oral antidiabetics sitagliptin phosphate and saxagliptin are classified as *incretin modifiers*, also called *dipeptidyl peptidase 4 (DPP-4) inhibitors* and *gliptins*, for treatment of type 2 diabetes mellitus. The action of DPP-4 inhibitors is to increase the level of incretin hormones, increase insulin secretion, and decrease glucagon secretion to reduce glucose production. This incretin modifier is used as an adjunct treatment with exercise and diet to reduce both fasting and postprandial plasma glucose levels. Pramlintide is given subcutaneously in the abdomen and thigh immediately before each major meal. Never administer in the arm; absorption is unpredictable.

Guidelines for Oral Antidiabetic Therapy for Type 2 Diabetes

The following are criteria for the use of oral antidiabetic (hypoglycemic) drugs:

- Onset of diabetes mellitus at 40 years of age or older
- Diagnosis of diabetes within the past 5 years
- Normal weight or overweight
- Fasting blood glucose of 200 mg/dL or less
- Fewer than 40 units of insulin required per day
- Normal renal and hepatic function

PROTOTYPE DRUG CHART
! Metformin

Drug Class	Dosage
Metformin: Biguanide	Immediate release: A: PO: Initially 500 mg bid or 850 mg/d with meals; increase dose gradually; *max:* 2550 mg/d Extended release tablets: A: PO: 500 mg/d with evening meal; *max:* 2000 mg/d

Contraindications	Drug-Lab-Food Interactions
Hypersensitivity, diabetic ketoacidosis, lactic acidosis, metabolic acidosis, renal failure *Caution:* Cardiac disease, heart failure, infection, fever, trauma, burns, surgery, vomiting, dehydration, diarrhea, gastroparesis, GI obstruction, ileus, malnutrition, renal/hepatic dysfunction, adrenal insufficiency, thyroid disease, sepsis, type 1 diabetes mellitus, pernicious anemia, alcohol abuse, older adults, pregnancy, breastfeeding	Drug: ACE inhibitors, ARBs, beta-blockers, MAOIs, furosemide, quinolones, alcohol, cimetidine, sulfonamides, azole antifungals, may potentiate hypoglycemia. Nicotine, triamterene, thiazide diuretics, niacin, phenytoin, oral contraceptives, and atypical antipsychotics may cause hyperglycemia. Metformin can increase digoxin concentration Lab: Altered liver function tests Food: Green tea may lead to hypoglycemia.

Pharmacokinetics	Pharmacodynamics
Absorption: 51%–60% absorbed Distribution: PB: 0% Metabolism: t½: 6.2–17.6 h Excretion: Primarily in urine	PO: Onset: UK Peak: Regular release 2.5 h; extended release 4–8 h Duration: UK

CHAPTER 50 Antidiabetics

PROTOTYPE DRUG CHART—CONT'D
Metformin

Therapeutic Effects/Uses

To control hyperglycemia in type 2 diabetes mellitus

Mechanism of action: Increases binding of insulin to receptors, improves tissue sensitivity to insulin, increases glucose transport to skeletal muscles and fatty tissues, decreases glucose production in the liver by reducing gluconeogenesis, and reduces glucose absorption from intestines

Side Effects	Adverse Reactions
Dizziness, headache, malaise, rash, flushing, chills, dysgeusia, hyperhidrosis, metallic taste, anorexia, dyspepsia, abdominal pain, nausea, vomiting, flatulence, diarrhea, weight loss, infection, vitamin B_{12} deficiency, myalgia	Palpitations, chest pain, hypoglycemia, metabolic acidosis, cholestasis, elevated hepatic enzymes, rhabdomyolysis *Life threatening:* Lactic acidosis, megaloblastic anemia, hepatic impairment

A, Adult; *ACE*, angiotensin-converting enzyme; *ARB*, angiotensin II–receptor blocker; *bid*, twice daily; *d*, day; *h*, hour; *MAOI*, monoamine oxidase inhibitor; *max*, maximum; *PB*, protein binding; *PO*, by mouth; *t½*, half-life; *UK*, unknown.

CLINICAL JUDGMENT [NURSING PROCESS]
Oral Antidiabetics

Concept: Glucose Regulation
- The process of sustaining normal glucose levels

Recognize Cues [Assessment]
- Identify drugs the patient currently takes. Aspirin, alcohol, sulfonamides, oral contraceptives, and monoamine oxidase inhibitors (MAOIs) increase the hypoglycemic effect; a decrease in oral antidiabetic drugs may be needed. Glucocorticoids (cortisone), thiazide diuretics, and estrogen increase blood glucose.
- Note vital signs and blood glucose levels, and report abnormal findings.
- Determine the patient's knowledge of diabetes mellitus and use of oral antidiabetics.

Analyze Cues and Prioritize Hypothesis [Patient Problems]
- Hypoglycemia
- Metabolic acidosis
- Hyperglycemia
- Reduced glucose regulation
- Hyponatremia
- Fatigue

Generate Solutions [Planning]
- The patient will maintain fasting blood glucose within normal serum levels (80–130 mg/dL).
- The patient will adhere to a prescribed diet, blood testing, and drug regimen.
- The patient will demonstrate knowledge of oral hypoglycemics and their importance.

Take Action [Nursing Interventions]
- Determine vital signs. Oral antidiabetics increase cardiac function and oxygen consumption, which can lead to cardiac dysrhythmias.
- Administer oral antidiabetics with food to minimize gastric upset.
- Monitor blood glucose levels, and report changes.
- Prepare a teaching plan based on the patient's knowledge of health problems, diet, and drug therapy.

Patient Teaching
General
- Advise patients that a hypoglycemic (insulin) reaction can occur when taking an oral hypoglycemic drug, especially sulfonylureas. Such drugs stimulate the release of insulin from beta cells of the pancreas. Oral antidiabetics are not insulin. Normally, patients with diabetes mellitus type 1 do not have functioning beta cells and should not take oral antidiabetics, only insulin. Sulfonylureas are prescribed for patients with diabetes mellitus type 2.
- Teach patients to recognize symptoms of a hypoglycemic reaction—headache, nervousness, sweating, tremors, and rapid pulse—and hyperglycemic reaction, which include thirst, increased urine output, and a sweet, fruity breath odor.
- Explain that insulin might be needed instead of an oral antidiabetic drug during stress, surgery, or serious infection. Blood glucose levels are usually elevated during stressful times.
- Tell patients about the necessity for compliance with a diet and drug regimen.
- Advise patients to carry a MedicAlert card, tag, or bracelet that indicates their health problem and the antidiabetic dosage.

Self-Administration
- Teach patients how to check blood glucose levels with a glucometer. Patients should record and report abnormal results.

Side Effects
- Advise patients to report side effects such as vomiting, diarrhea, and rash.

Diet
- Caution patients not to ingest alcohol with antidiabetic drugs to avoid a hypoglycemic reaction.
- Advise patients taking oral antidiabetics to eat the prescribed diet on schedule. Delaying or missing a meal can cause hypoglycemia.
- Explain the use of orange juice, sugar-containing drinks, or hard candy when a hypoglycemic reaction begins. Explain the importance of reporting such problems to a health care provider.
- Direct patients to take oral antidiabetics with food to decrease gastric irritation.

Evaluate Outcomes [Evaluation]
- Evaluate the effectiveness of drug therapy by noting whether blood glucose levels are within the accepted range.
- Determine the patient's knowledge of the diabetic regimen.

OTHER DIABETIC DRUGS

Incretin Mimetics

Exenatide and liraglutide are in a classification of antidiabetic drugs known as *incretin mimetics*, also called *glucagon-like peptide 1 agonists*. These drugs improve beta-cell responsiveness, which improves glucose control in people with type 2 diabetes mellitus. The actions of exenatide and liraglutide are to enhance insulin secretion, increase beta-cell responsiveness, suppress glucagon secretion, slow gastric emptying, and reduce food intake. Exenatide and liraglutide are not a substitute for insulin and should not be administered to patients with type 1 diabetes mellitus, diabetic ketoacidosis, severe renal dysfunction, or severe GI disease. Common adverse effects that occur with exenatide include headache, dizziness, jitteriness, nausea, vomiting, and diarrhea. Exenatide is administered by injectable prefilled pens in twice-a-day dosing and has significantly improved HbA1c levels and weight loss in many patients. Liraglutide is given subcutaneously once a day in the arm, abdomen, or thigh.

Amylin Analogs

Pramlintide acetate is another antidiabetic agent in a classification called *amylin analogs*, approved by the US Food and Drug Administration (FDA) for adults with type 1 and type 2 diabetes mellitus. The primary purpose of pramlintide is to improve postprandial glucose control in diabetic patients who are using insulin but are unable to achieve and maintain glucose control. The actions of pramlintide are to suppress glucagon secretion, slow gastric emptying, and modulate appetite by inducing satiety. Suppression of glucagon secretion reduces postprandial hepatic glucose for approximately 3 hours. By slowing gastric emptying, the absorption rate of glucose is reduced; satiety promotes reduced food intake. Common adverse effects include dizziness, anorexia, nausea, vomiting, and fatigue. Pramlintide is administered by subcutaneous injection before meals in the abdomen or thigh; it is never given in the arm.

Hyperglycemic Drugs

Glucagon

Glucagon is a hyperglycemic hormone secreted by alpha cells of the islets of Langerhans in the pancreas. Glucagon increases blood glucose by stimulating glycogenolysis (glycogen breakdown) in the liver. It protects the body cells, especially those in the brain and retina, by providing the nutrients and energy needed to maintain body function.

Glucagon is available for parenteral use (subcutaneous, intramuscular [IM], and IV). It is used to treat insulin-induced hypoglycemia when other methods of providing glucose are not available. For example, the patient may be semiconscious or unconscious and unable to ingest sugar-containing products. Patients with diabetes who are prone to severe hypoglycemic reactions (insulin shock) should keep glucagon in the home, and family members should be taught how to administer subcutaneous or IM injections during an emergency hypoglycemic reaction. The blood glucose level begins to increase within 10 minutes after administration.

Diazoxide

Oral diazoxide, which is chemically related to thiazide diuretics, increases blood glucose by inhibiting insulin release from the beta cells and stimulating release of epinephrine from the adrenal medulla. This drug is *not* indicated for hypoglycemic reaction; rather, it is used to treat hypoglycemia caused by hyperinsulinism.

Diazoxide has a long half-life and is highly protein bound. Its onset of action is 1 hour, and the duration of action is 8 hours. Most of the drug is excreted unchanged in urine.

CLINICAL JUDGMENT SINGLE-EPISODE CASE STUDY

Cognitive Skill: Generate solutions [Matrix]
Objective: Care of a patient with type 2 diabetes mellitus prescribed an antidiabetic drug.

A 62-year-old female with type 2 diabetes mellitus presented to the emergency department and was admitted to the hospital with a diagnosis of hypoglycemic reaction and a blood sugar of 50 mg/dL. The patient's prescribed diabetic medication is repaglinide 2 mg/three times a day 30 minutes before meals. After reviewing the patient's admit orders, the nurse notes that the patient forgot the morning dose of repaglinide and took the dose at bedtime. The next morning, the patient self-administered the ordered dose of repaglinide and did not eat breakfast, causing the patient to become hypoglycemic.

The patient will be discharged today. The nurse is preparing the discharge teaching for this patient.

Use an X for the nursing instruction that is indicated (appropriate or necessary) or contraindicated (could be harmful) for this patient's care.

Nursing Instruction	Indicated	Contraindicated
Take the 2 mg dose of repaglinide, as ordered, three times a day followed by a full meal.		
You may increase the dose of repaglinide if your blood glucose increases without notifying your health care provider.		
Adverse reactions associated with repaglinide are anxiety, diarrhea, infection, headache, drowsiness, and hypoglycemic reaction. If experienced, notify your provider.		
Repaglinide is classified as an alpha-glucosidase inhibitor.		
Take your blood sugar prior to self-administering repaglinide. If it is <70 mg/dL (3.9 mmol/L), notify your health care provider before taking the drug.		
A diabetic patient does not have to follow a special diet and may eat whatever they want.		
Instruct the patient in signs of hypoglycemic reaction: headache, nervousness, sweating, trembling, and rapid pulse. If experienced, the patient should immediately drink a glass of orange juice, take their blood sugar, and notify their health care provider.		

CLINICAL JUDGMENT SINGLE-EPISODE CASE STUDY—CONT'D

Answers

Nursing Instruction	Indicated	Contraindicated
Take the 2 mg dose of repaglinide, as ordered, three times a day followed by a full meal.	X	
You may increase the dose of repaglinide if your blood glucose increases without notifying your health care provider.		X
Adverse reactions associated with repaglinide are anxiety, diarrhea, infection, headache, drowsiness, and hypoglycemic reaction. If experienced, notify your provider.	X	
Repaglinide is classified as an alpha-glucosidase inhibitor.		X
Take your blood sugar prior to self-administering repaglinide. If it is <70 mg/dL (3.9 mmol/L), notify your health care provider before taking the drug.	X	
A diabetic patient does not have to follow a special diet and may eat whatever they want.		X
Instruct the patient in signs of hypoglycemic reaction: headache, nervousness, sweating, trembling, and rapid pulse. If experienced, the patient should immediately drink a glass of orange juice, take their blood sugar, and notify their health care provider.	X	

Rationale
Repaglinide is an antidiabetic drug. It is classified as a meglitinide drug whose purpose is to treat type 2 diabetes by working in the pancreas to sequentially block certain potassium channels, create an influx of calcium, and induce insulin secretion. It is usually taken in tablet form and should be taken as ordered by the patient's provider, with food, to avoid hypoglycemic reactions. Adverse reactions are correctly listed as anxiety, diarrhea, infection, headache, drowsiness, and hypoglycemic reaction. In following correct diabetes care, the patient should perform a glucometer check prior to administration and, if it is less than 70 mg/dL, hold the drug and notify their health care provider to avoid a hypoglycemic reaction. It is important for the nurse to review symptoms of a hypoglycemic reaction, correctly stated as headache, nervousness, sweating, trembling, and rapid pulse. It is also important to tell the patient to drink a glass of orange juice, which will increase the patient's blood sugar, and to repeat the glucometer check and notify their health care provider. The patient should never increase or decrease the ordered dose of repaglinide without health care provider knowledge and new orders. Repaglinide is not classified as an alpha-glucosidase inhibitor. It is very important for a diabetic to follow a diabetic diet as ordered by their health care provider.

References
McCuistion L, et al.: *Pharmacology: a patient-centered nursing process approach*, ed 10, 1922, pp 623–635. Chapter 47.
Burchum R, Rosenthal LD: *Lehne's pharmacology for nursing care*, ed 10, 2019, pp 674–710. Chapter 57.

REVIEW QUESTIONS

1. A patient is diagnosed with type 2 diabetes mellitus. The nurse is aware that which statement is true about this patient?
   a. The patient is most likely a teenager.
   b. The patient is most likely a child younger than 10 years.
   c. Heredity and obesity are major causative factors.
   d. Viral infections contribute most to disease development.

2. Antidiabetic drugs are designed to control signs and symptoms of diabetes mellitus. The nurse primarily expects a decrease in which?
   a. Blood glucose
   b. Fat metabolism
   c. Glycogen storage
   d. Protein mobilization

3. A patient is to receive insulin before breakfast, and the time of breakfast tray delivery is variable. The nurse knows that which insulin should not be administered until the breakfast tray has arrived and the patient is ready to eat?
   a. Neutral protamine Hagedorn (NPH)
   b. Lispro
   c. Glargine
   d. Regular

4. A patient is receiving a daily dose of neutral protamine Hagedorn (NPH) insulin at 7:30 a.m. The nurse expects the peak effect of this drug to occur at what time?
   a. 8:15 a.m.
   b. 10:30 a.m.
   c. 5:00 p.m.
   d. 11:00 p.m.

5. A patient is prescribed glipizide. The nurse knows that which side effects and adverse effects may be expected? **Select all that apply**.
   a. Tachypnea
   b. Tachycardia
   c. Increased alertness
   d. Increased weight gain
   e. Visual disturbances
   f. Hyperhidrosis

6. A nurse is teaching a patient how to recognize symptoms of hypoglycemia. Which symptoms should be included in the teaching? **Select all that apply**.
   a. Headache
   b. Nervousness
   c. Bradycardia
   d. Sweating
   e. Thirst
   f. Sweet breath odor

7. A patient is newly diagnosed with type 1 diabetes mellitus and requires daily insulin injections. Which instructions should the nurse include in the teaching of insulin administration? **Select all that apply**.
   a. Teach family members how to administer glucagon by injection when the patient has a hyperglycemic reaction.
   b. Instruct the patient about the necessity for compliance with prescribed insulin therapy.
   c. Teach the patient that hypoglycemic reactions are more likely to occur at the onset of action time.
   d. Instruct the patient in the care and handling of the insulin container and syringe.

UNIT XVI Renal and Urologic Drugs

51

Urinary Disorders

http://evolve.elsevier.com/McCuistion/pharmacology

OBJECTIVES

- Contrast urinary tract disorders and the effect of treatment variation in dosage.
- Describe usage considerations of urinary antiseptics and antibiotics.
- Differentiate between the use of urinary analgesics, stimulants, and antispasmodics/antimuscarinics/anticholinergics.

OUTLINE

Urinary Tract Disorders, 665
    Acute Cystitis, 665
    Acute Pyelonephritis, 665
Urinary Antiseptics/Antiinfectives and Antibiotics, 666
    Trimethoprim and Trimethoprim-Sulfamethoxazole, 666
    Methenamine, 667
    Nitrofurantoin, 667
    Fluoroquinolones, 668

    Side Effects and Adverse Reactions, 670
    Drug-Drug Interactions, 670
Selective Urinary Agents, 670
    Urinary Analgesics: Phenazopyridine, 670
    Urinary Stimulants, 670
    Urinary Antispasmodics/Antimuscarinics/Anticholinergics, 670
Clinical Judgment Case Study, 672
Review Questions, 672

This chapter discusses agents prescribed to combat disease-producing microorganisms. Included in this unit are antiseptics, antibacterials, analgesics, stimulants, antispasmodics, antimuscarinics, anticholinergics, and other drugs for urinary tract disorders. Common disorders of the urinary tract are presented in this unit. Urinary tract infections (UTIs), acute cystitis, and pyelonephritis are focused on.

URINARY TRACT DISORDERS

Disease-producing organisms may be gram-positive or gram-negative bacteria, viruses, or fungi. The degree to which they are pathogenic depends on the microorganism and its virulence. This chapter addresses drugs for urinary tract disorders.

Fig. 51.1 illustrates the various sites of infection in the upper and lower urinary tracts. Fig. 51.2 illustrates the female and male urethra, showing the female urethra being the shortest.

The largest number of urinary tract disorders are caused by **urinary tract infections (UTIs)**, microbial infections of any part of the urinary tract. The infection may be referred to as an *upper UTI*, such as pyelonephritis, or a *lower UTI*, such as cystitis, urethritis, or prostatitis. A group of drugs called **urinary antiseptics/antiinfectives** prevents bacterial growth in the kidneys and bladder, but these drugs are not effective for systemic infections. When given in lower dosages, urinary antiseptics/antiinfectives have a **bacteriostatic** effect—that is, they inhibit bacterial growth. When given in higher dosages, they also have a **bactericidal** (bacteria killing) effect. Urinary antiseptics/antiinfectives are presented in this chapter, along with **urinary analgesics**, which relieve pain and burning in the urinary tract; **urinary stimulants**, agents that increase the tone of urinary muscles; and urinary antispasmodics/antimuscarinics. Chapter 26 presents further discussions of antibiotics used to treat UTIs, such as fluoroquinolones and sulfonamides. Diuretics are discussed in Chapter 38.

Acute Cystitis

Acute cystitis, a lower UTI, frequently occurs in female patients because of the short urethra. It is more common in females of childbearing age, older females, and young females. Acute cystitis is commonly caused by *Escherichia coli* (also called *E. coli*). Other bacterial causes include the gram-positive *Staphylococcus saprophyticus* and gram-negative *Klebsiella*, *Proteus*, and *Pseudomonas* species. Symptoms of cystitis include pain and burning on urination and urinary frequency and urgency. A urine culture is usually obtained before the start of any antiinfective/antibiotic drug therapy. In male patients, a lower UTI is most likely prostatitis with symptoms similar to cystitis.

Acute Pyelonephritis

Acute pyelonephritis, an upper UTI, is commonly seen more in females of childbearing age, older females, and young females. *E. coli* is the most common organism to cause pyelonephritis. Symptoms include chills, high fever, flank pain, pain during urination, urinary frequency and urgency, and pyuria. The bacterial count in the urine is greater than 100,000 bacteria/mL. In severe cases, the patient may be hospitalized and may receive intravenous (IV) antibiotics (e.g., an aminoglycoside or piperacillin-tazobactam).

Commonly used agents for treating UTIs are nitrofurantoin and trimethoprim-sulfamethoxazole (TMP-SMZ). Treatment may consist of a 3- to 7-day course, 7 to 14 days, or 7 to 14 days of drug dosing. Fosfomycin tromethamine, a nitrofurantoin prototype drug, is effective for UTIs as a single-dose treatment. Other agents used to treat UTIs include cephalosporins: first-generation (cefadroxil), second-generation (cefotetan), third-generation (ceftriaxone), fourth-generation (cefepime), and fifth-generation (ceftolozane-tazobactam), which is a combination of a cephalosporin and a beta lactamase inhibitor. Fluoroquinolones, such as ofloxacin and ciprofloxacin, are also utilized. For uncomplicated UTIs, fluoroquinolones, especially levofloxacin, may be used only when other options are not available as the risk generally outweighs the benefits. With severe UTIs, IV drug therapy followed by oral drug therapy is usually recommended.

URINARY ANTISEPTICS/ANTIINFECTIVES AND ANTIBIOTICS

Urinary antiseptics/antiinfectives are limited to the treatment of UTIs. Drug action occurs in the renal tubule and bladder, where it is effective in reducing bacterial growth. A urinalysis, as well as a culture and sensitivity test, is usually performed before the initiation of drug therapy. As bactericidal agents, these drugs have the potential to cause superinfections. The urinary antiseptics/antiinfectives are ippurate tromethamine, nitrofurantoin, methenamine ippurate, trimethoprim, ertapenem, sulfonamides, fluoroquinolones, beta-lactams, polypeptides, aminoglycosides, and cephalosporins.

Trimethoprim and Trimethoprim-Sulfamethoxazole

Trimethoprim can be used alone for the treatment of UTIs, but it is usually used in combination with a sulfonamide, sulfamethoxazole (the combined generic preparation is called *TMP-SMZ*), to prevent the occurrence of trimethoprim-resistant organisms. TMP-SMZ is discussed further in Chapter 29, and it is used in the treatment and prevention of acute and chronic UTIs. The amount of TMP-SMZ in the prostatic fluid is about two to three times greater than the amount in the vascular fluid.

Pharmacokinetics

TMP-SMZ is well absorbed from the gastrointestinal (GI) tract. The drug may be taken with food, water, or milk to decrease GI distress, which includes anorexia, nausea, vomiting, abdominal pain, diarrhea, and crystalluria. TMP-SMZ is moderately protein-bound at 44% for TMP and 70% for SMZ. The half-life is 8 to 10 hours for TMP and 6 to 12 hours for SMZ.

Pharmacodynamics

The combination of trimethoprim and sulfamethoxazole in a 1:5 ratio increases its bactericidal activity. This drug combination produces slow-acting bactericidal effects against most gram-positive and gram-negative organisms, especially strains of *Staphylococcus aureus*, including methicillin-resistant *S. aureus*, and also *Shigella* and *Proteus* species. The peak action of TMP-SMZ is 1 to 4 hours.

The nursing process for TMP-SMZ is applicable to the other urinary antiseptics/antiinfectives.

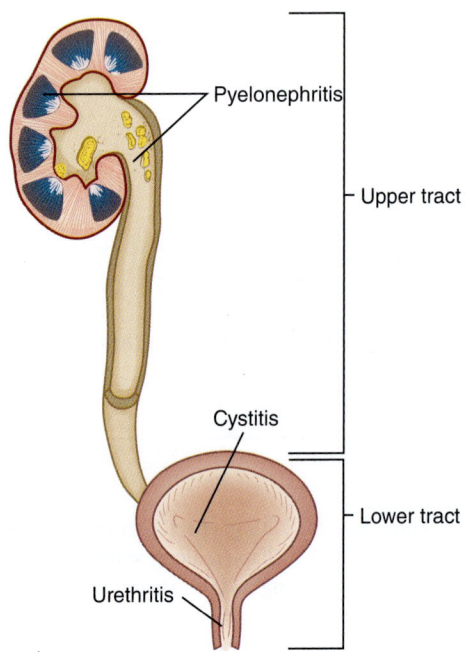

Fig. 51.1 Sites of infectious processes in the upper and lower urinary tracts.

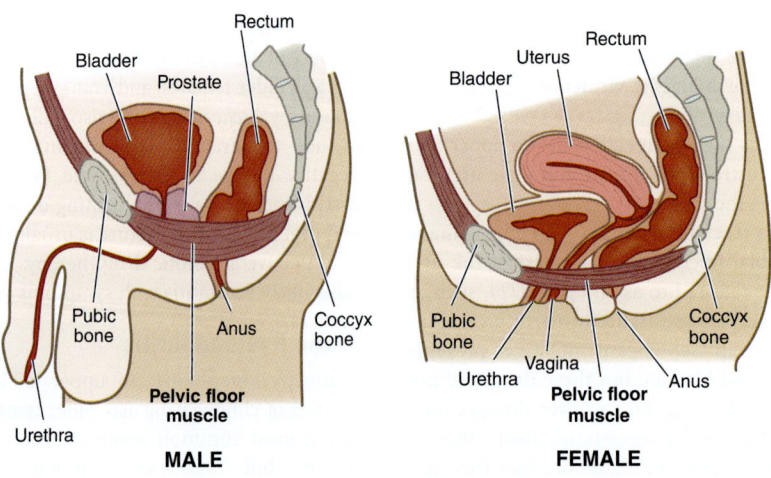

Fig. 51.2 Shorter urethra in the female than in the male.

CLINICAL JUDGMENT [NURSING PROCESS]
Urinary Antiinfectives

Concept: Infection
- A condition in which infective microorganisms have invaded a part of the body

Recognize Cues [Assessment]
- Obtain a history from the patient of clinical problems with urinary tract infection (UTI), incontinence, or other urinary tract disorders.
- Assess the patient for signs and symptoms of UTI: pain or burning sensation on urination and frequency and urgency of urination.
- Monitor complete blood count regularly in patients on long-term therapy.
- Monitor urine culture and sensitivity results.
- Assess renal and hepatic function.
- Determine urine pH. A pH of 5.5 is desired, but alkalization of the urine is not recommended.

Analyze Cues and Prioritize Hypothesis [Patient Problems]
- Acute pain
- Discomfort
- Decreased sensation
- Changes in elimination

Generate Solutions [Planning]
- The patient will state within 10 days that she does not have pain or burning on urination.

Take Action [Nursing Interventions]
- Monitor urinary output and urine-specific gravity. Careful attention to output is required when administering urinary antiseptics to patients with anuria and oliguria. Report promptly any decrease in urine output.
- Obtain urine culture to identify infecting organisms before initiation of drug therapy to treat UTI.
- Observe the patient for side effects and adverse reactions to urinary antiseptic drugs. Peripheral neuropathy (tingling, numbness of extremities) may result from renal insufficiency (inability to excrete drug) or long-term use of nitrofurantoin. Peripheral neuropathy may be irreversible.

Patient Teaching
General
- Teach patients not to crush tablets or open capsules.
- Advise patients to rinse the mouth thoroughly after taking oral nitrofurantoin. The drug can stain teeth.
- Encourage patients to avoid antacids because they interfere with drug absorption.
- Teach patients to shake suspensions well before administration and to protect them from freezing.
- ⚡ Warn patients not to drive a motor vehicle or operate dangerous machinery; the drug may cause drowsiness.
- Advise female patients to immediately report pregnancy to their health care provider.

Diet
- Inform patients to increase fluids and take the drug with food to minimize GI upset.

Side Effects
- Advise the patient to drink an adequate amount of fluids.
- Encourage the patient to report any signs of secondary fungal or bacterial infection (superinfection) such as stomatitis or anogenital discharge or itching.

Nitrofurantoin
- Alert the patient that urine may turn a harmless brown color.
- Direct the patient to report a sudden onset of dyspnea, chest pain, cough, fever, and chills to the health care provider.

Methenamine
- Educate patients to drink cranberry juice, eat plums, or take vitamin C (with approval of the health care provider) to keep urine acidic. Foods that are alkaline, such as milk and some vegetables, may increase urine pH. Urine pH should be less than 5.5 for the antiseptic to be effective.

Fluoroquinolones
- ⚡ Warn patients to avoid operating hazardous machinery or driving a car while taking the drug, especially if dizziness is present.
- Encourage patients to take the drug with food and to avoid antacids because they interfere with drug absorption.
- Direct patients to report any signs of superinfection or secondary fungal or bacterial infection.

Trimethoprim and Trimethoprim-Sulfamethoxazole
- Tell patients to avoid excessive exposure to sunlight when taking nitrofurantoin.

Evaluate Outcomes [Evaluation]
- Evaluate the effectiveness of the urinary antiinfectives in alleviating UTI. The patient should be free of side effects and adverse reactions to the drug.

Methenamine

Methenamine produces a bactericidal effect when the urine pH is less than 5.5. It is effective against gram-positive and gram-negative organisms, especially *E. coli*, *Enterococcus*, *Proteus* species, *Staphylococcus*, and *Pseudomonas aeruginosa*. It is used for UTI prophylaxis with recurrent UTIs. Methenamine should not be taken with sulfonamides because crystalluria is likely to occur. Methenamine is absorbed readily from the GI tract, and approximately 90% of the drug is excreted in the urine unchanged. Methenamine forms ammonia and formaldehyde in acid urine; therefore the urine needs to be acidified to exert a bactericidal action. Cranberry juice (several 8-ounce glasses per day), ascorbic acid, and ammonium chloride can be taken to decrease the urine pH.

Nitrofurantoin

Nitrofurantoin was first approved by the FDA to treat UTIs in 1953. It is bacteriostatic or bactericidal, depending on the drug dosage, and it is effective against many gram-positive and gram-negative organisms, especially *E. coli*. It is used to treat cystitis and UTIs. Nitrofurantoin is usually taken with food to decrease GI distress, which includes anorexia, nausea, vomiting, abdominal pain, and diarrhea. Decreased absorption occurs when the drug is taken with antacids. With normal renal function, nitrofurantoin is rapidly eliminated because of its short half-life; however, it accumulates in the serum with urinary dysfunction.

When nitrofurantoin is given in low doses for prophylactic use, the drug has a bacteriostatic effect. However, higher concentrations of nitrofurantoin cause a bactericidal effect, and it is effective against many gram-positive and gram-negative organisms such as *E. coli*, *S. aureus*, streptococci, *Enterococcus*, and *Klebsiella* species. If sudden onset of dyspnea, chest pain, cough, fever, and chills develop, the patient should contact the health care provider. Symptoms resolve after discontinuing the drug.

Fluoroquinolones

Fluoroquinolones (Quinolones) are one of the groups of urinary antibacterials that are effective against strains of *Acinetobacter*, *Chlamydia*, *Clostridium*, *Klebsiella*, *Staphylococcus*, and *Streptococcus* species that cause lower UTIs; they include ciprofloxacin, ofloxacin, and levofloxacin. Fluoroquinolones should be reserved for patients who have no alternative treatment options due to their harsh adverse reactions of tendon rupture, peripheral neuropathy, central nervous system effects, and exacerbation of myasthenia gravis. The drug dosage must be decreased when renal dysfunction is present. The half-lives of these drugs are ordinarily 2 to 8 hours, but half-lives are prolonged in patients with renal dysfunction. Table 51.1 lists the urinary antiseptics/antiinfectives and their dosages, uses, and considerations. Due to the serious adverse reactions of fluoroquinolones, they are used with caution for complicated UTIs and acute pyelonephritis, and levofloxacin is only used for uncomplicated UTIs when no other options are available. The following should not be taken within a 2-hour period before or after fluoroquinolones: mineral supplements; vitamins with iron or minerals; calcium-, aluminum-, or magnesium-based antacids, sucralfate, or didanosine. Do not give with dairy products or calcium-fortified juices. Levofloxacin is illustrated in Prototype Drug Chart: Levofloxacin in Chapter 26.

TABLE 51.1 Antiseptics and Urinary Antiinfectives

Generic Name	Route and Dosage	Uses and Considerations
Fosfomycin tromethamine	Cystitis: A: PO: 3-g packet dissolved in 4 oz water as a single dose	For cystitis and UTIs in females. May cause headache, rhinitis, vaginitis, dysuria, hematuria, superinfection, CDAD, nausea, and diarrhea. Take immediately after dissolving in water. PB: 0%; t½: 5.7 ± 2.8 h
Methenamine hippurate	A: PO: 1 g bid; *max*: 2 g/d	For UTI prophylaxis. May cause crystalluria, rash, nausea, hematuria, dysuria, elevated hepatic enzymes, and urinary frequency. Avoid food/drugs that alkalinize urine. PB: UK; t½: 4 h
Nitrofurantoin	A: PO: 50–100 mg q6h for 7 d	For cystitis and UTIs. May cause headache, dizziness, drowsiness, peripheral neruopathy, anorexia, abdominal pain, nausea, vomiting, diarrhea, elevated hepatic enzymes, brown urine discoloration, blood dyscrasias, and CDAD. PB: 60%–90%; t½: 20–60 min
Trimethoprim	UTIs: A: PO: 100 mg q 12 h or 200 mg/d for 10 d; *max*: 200 mg/d	For otitis media, cystitis, and UTIs. May cause rash, pruritus, abdominal pain, diarrhea, nausea, vomiting, superinfection, and CDAD. PB: 44%; t½: 8–10 h
Ertapenem	UTI: A: IM/IV: 1 g/d for 7–14 d; *max*: 1 g/d	For UTIs, community-acquired pneumonia, and intraabdominal, skin, pelvic, and diabetic foot infections. May cause headache, drowsiness, confusion, cough, fever, agitation, nausea, vomiting, diarrhea, abdominal pain, dysuria, anemia, infection, elevated hepatic enzymes, and CDAD. PB: 95%; t½: 4 h
Sulfonamides TMP-SMZ	UTIs: A: PO: TMP 160 mg, SMZ 800 mg q12h for 10–14 d; *max*: 1600 mg/d A: IV: 8–10 mg/kg per day in 2–4 divided doses for 14 d, give over 30 minutes; *max*: 960 mg/d	For cystitis, UTIs, bronchitis, otitis media, pneumonia, traveler's diarrhea, and shigellosis. May cause rash, pruritus, headache, anorexia, nausea, vomiting, abdominal pain, diarrhea, crystalluria, arthralgia, myalgia, hyperkalemia, superinfection, and CDAD. PB: TMP, 44%; SMZ, 70%; t½: TMP, 8–10 h; SMZ, 6–12 h
Quinolones (Fluoroquinolones) Ciprofloxacin	UTIs: Regular release: A: PO: 250 mg q12h for 3 d; *max*: 1.5 g/d Extended release: A: PO: 500 mg/d for 3 d; *max*: 1 g/d A: IV: 200–400 mg q8–12 h for 7–14 d; *max*: 1.2 g/d	For respiratory, urinary, skin, bone, joint, eye, ear, intradominal, typhoid fever, febrile neutropenia, prostatitis, plague, gonorrhea, and anthrax infections. May cause irritability, conjunctival hyperemia, ocular pruritus, visual impairment, pharyngitis, sinusitis, tendon rupture, dysgeusia, nausea, vomiting, abdominal pain, diarrhea, CDAD, superinfection, and corneal deposits. PB: 20%–40%; t½: 4 h
Ofloxacin	UTIs: A: PO: 200 mg q12h for 3–7 d	For respiratory, urinary, eye, ear, bacterial prostatitis, STI, and skin infections. May cause headaches, dizziness, insomnia, dysgeusia, nausea, vomiting, diarrhea, CDAD, pruritus, rash, visual impairment, peripheral neuropathy, polyuria, vaginitis, candidiasis, superinfection, tendinitis, and tendon rupture. PB: 32%; t½: 4–8 h
Beta-Lactam Aztreonam	UTIs: A: IM/IV: 500 mg to 1 g q8–12 h; *max*: 8 g/d	For bacteremia and intraabdominal, respiratory, skin, gynecologic, and UTIs. May cause injection-site reaction, CDAD, rash, abdominal pain, fever, cough, wheezing, nasal congestion, elevated hepatic enzymes, eosinophilia, neutropenia, and superinfection. PB: 56%–65%; t½: 1.7 h
Pivmecillinam	A: PO: 185 mg tid for 3–7 d; *max*: 555 mg/d	For uncomplicated UTI. May cause headache, abdominal pain, nausea, vomiting, diarrhea, CDAD, and candidiasis. PB: <25%; t½: 61 min after single dose

TABLE 51.1 Antiseptics and Urinary Antiinfectives—cont'd

Generic Name	Route and Dosage	Uses and Considerations
Polypeptide Polymyxin B sulfate	UTIs: A: IV: 20,000–25,000 units/kg per loading dose followed by 12,500–15,000 units/kg per dose q12h; *max:* 25,000 units/kg per dose	For meningitis, bacteremia, and ophthalmic and urinary tract infections. Due to severe pain at the injection site, IM administration is not recommended. This drug should be given only to hospitalized patients to provide constant physician supervision. May cause dizziness, drowsiness, confusion, blurred vision, headache, paresthesias, hematuria, CDAD, superinfection, neurotoxicity, and nephrotoxicity. PB: UK; t½: 4–6 h
Aminoglycoside Plazomicin	A: IV: 15 mg/kg q24h for 4–7 d Trough: Less than 3 mcg/mL	For complicated UTIs including pyelonephritis. This drug is reserved for those patients with no alternative treatment options. May cause headache, diarrhea, hypo/hypertension, vomiting, nausea, ototoxicity, CDAD, superinfection, and nephrotoxicity. PB: 20%; t½: 3–4 h
Cephalosporin Cefiderocol	UTI: A: IV: 2 g q8h for 7–14 d; *max:* 6 g/d	For pneumonia and UTIs. May cause dry mouth, nausea, vomiting, diarrhea, constipation, rash, elevated hepatic enzymes, seizures, hypo/hyperkalemia, hypocalcemia, hypomagnesemia, candidiasis, thrombocytopenia, CDAD, thrombocytosis, and injection-site reaction. PB: 40%–60%; t½: 2–3 h
Cefadroxil	UTI: A: PO: 1–2 g/d in 2 divided doses; *max:* 2 g/d	For UTIs, streptococcal pharyngitis and tonsillitis, and skin infections. May cause elevated hepatic enzymes, rash, pruritus, urticaria, nausea, vomiting, diarrhea, abdominal pain, candidiasis, CDAD, superinfection, and angioedema. PB: UK; t½: 1–2 h
Cefotetan	UTI: A: IV/IM: 500 mg q12h or 1–2 g q24h; *max:* IV 6 g/d, IM 4 g/d	For respiratory, intraabdominal, skin, bone/joint, and UTIs. May cause rash, pruritus, nausea, diarrhea, elevated hepatic enzymes, phlebitis, eosinophilia, CDAD, and superinfection. PB: 78%–91%; t½: 3–4.6 h
Ceftriaxone	UTI: A: IV/IM: 1–2 g q24h for 7–14 d; *max:* 4 g/d	For respiratory, bacteremia/sepsis, otitis media, intraabdominal, skin, and UTIs. May cause injection-site reaction, rash, dizziness, headache, nausea, vomiting, diarrhea, abdominal pain, eosinophilia, elevated hepatic enzymes, thrombocytosis, and leukopenia. PB: 85%–95%; t½: 6–9 h
Cefepime	UTI: A: IV/IM: 500 mg to 1 g q12h for 7–14 d; *max:* IV 6 g/d, IM 2 g/d	For pneumonia, intraabdominal and UTIs, also febrile neutropenia. May cause elevated hepatic enzymes, injection-site reaction, hypophosphatemia, nausea, vomiting, diarrhea, rash, and CDAD. PB: 20%; t½: 2 h
Combinations Imipenem and cilastatin sodium	UTIs: A: IV: 500–1 g q6h or 1 g q8h; *max:* 4 g/d	For respiratory, intraabdominal, urinary, gynecologic, skin, and bone/joint infections; and endocarditis. May cause anuria, seizures, nausea, diarrhea, oliguria, candidiasis, phlebitis, injection-site reaction, and CDAD. PB: imipenem, 20%; cilastatin, 40%; t½: 1 h imipenem, 1 h cilastatin
Imipenem, cilastatin, and relebactam	UTIs: A: IV: imipenem 500 mg, cilastatin 500 mg, relebactam 250 mg q6h for 7–14 d	For UTIs and complicated intraabdominal infections. May cause rash, headache, hypertension, fever, erythema, nausea, vomiting, diarrhea, constipation, phlebitis, injection-site reaction, anemia, hypokalemia, hyponatremia, and elevated hepatic enzymes. PB: imipenem 20%, cilastatin 40%, relebactam 22%; t½: imipenem 1 h, cilastatin 1 h, relebactam 1.2 h
Ceftazidime and avibactam	UTIs: A: IV: 2.5 g (ceftazidime 2 g and avibactam 500 mg) q8h over 2 h for 7–14 d; *max:* 7.5 g/d (6 g ceftazidime and 1.5 g avibactam)	For intraabdominal, respiratory, and UTIs. May cause anxiety, headache, dizziness, nausea, constipation, abdominal pain, diarrhea, vomiting, pruritus, CDAD, hypokalemia, and superinfection. PB: ceftazidime 10%, avibactam 5%–8%; t½: ceftazidime 1.5–2 h, avibactam 2 h
Ceftolozane and tazobactam	UTIs: A: IV: 1.5 g (1 g ceftolozane and 0.5 g tazobactam) q8h for 7–14 d; *max:* 6 g/d ceftolozane and 3 g/d tazobactam	For respiratory and intraabdominal infections, and UTIs. May cause headache, insomnia, nausea, vomiting, diarrhea, constipation, abdominal pain, renal failure, elevated hepatic enzymes, thrombocytosis, leukopenia, neutropenia, CDAD, hypokalemia, and fever. PB: ceftolozane 16%–21%, tazobactam 30%; t½: ceftolozane 3–4 h, tazobactam 2–3 h
Meropenem and vaborbactam	A: IV: 2 g meropenem, 2 g vaborbactam q8h up to 7–14 d; *max:* 6 g meropenem, 6 g vaborbactam/d	For UTIs. May cause headache, fever, injection-site reaction, phlebitis, hypokalemia, nausea, elevated hepatic enzymes, diarrhea, superinfection, and CDAD. PB: meropenem, 2%; vaborbactam, 33%; t½: meropenem, 1.22 h; vaborbactam, 1.68 h
Cefepime and enmetazobactam	A: IV: 2.5 g (2 g cefepime and 0.5 g enmetazobactam) q8h for 7–14 d; *max:* 7.5 g (6 g/d cefepime and 1.5 g/d enmetazobactam)	For complicated UTI including pyelonephritis. May cause headache, anemia, injecttion site reaction, phlebitus, hyperbilirubinemia, elevated hepatic enzymes, candidiasis, diarrhea, CDAD, hyperkalemia, hypocalcemia, blood dyscrasias, and superinfection. PB: 20% cefepime, negligible enmetazobactam; t½: 2–2.7 h cefepime, 2.6 h enmetazobactam

A, Adult; *bid*, twice a day; *CDAD*, *Clostridium difficile*–associated diarrhea; *d*, day; *h*, hour; *IM*, intramuscular; *IV*, intravenous; *max*, maximum dosage; *PB*, protein binding; *pc*, after meals; *PO*, by mouth; *q*, every; *qid*, four times a day; *t½*, half-life; *TMP-SMZ*, trimethoprim-sulfamethoxazole; *UK*, unknown; *UTI*, urinary tract infection.

Side Effects and Adverse Reactions

Nitrofurantoin
Side effects of nitrofurantoin include GI disturbances such as anorexia, nausea, vomiting, diarrhea, and abdominal pain and pulmonary reactions such as dyspnea.

Methenamine
Methenamine has side effects that include nausea, dysuria, rash, elevated hepatic enzymes, hematuria, and crystalluria.

Trimethoprim-Sulfamethoxazole
GI symptoms such as anorexia, nausea, and vomiting and skin problems such as rash and pruritus can accompany TMP-SMZ use.

Fluoroquinolones
Side effects of ciprofloxacin and ofloxacin include headaches, dizziness, nausea, vomiting, diarrhea, visual impairment, rash, and pruritus. Serious adverse reactions include peripheral neuropathy, tendinitis, and tendon rupture. Fluoroquinolones may exacerbate muscle weakness in patients with myasthenia gravis. Direct patients to stop taking fluoroquinolones immediately if experiencing serious adverse reactions and notify their health care provider.

Drug-Drug Interactions
The following drug-drug interactions can occur with the use of urinary antiseptics/antiinfectives:
- Antacids decrease nitrofurantoin absorption.
- Sodium bicarbonate inhibits the action of methenamine.
- Methenamine taken with sulfonamides increases the risk of crystalluria.
- Most urinary antiseptics cause false-positive Clinitest (glucose urine test) results.

SELECTIVE URINARY AGENTS

Urinary Analgesics: Phenazopyridine
Phenazopyridine hydrochloride, an azo dye, and dimethyl sulfoxide (also called DMSO) are urinary analgesics that are used to relieve the urinary pain, burning sensation, frequency, and urgency of urination that are symptomatic of cystitis. Phenazopyridine can cause methemoglobinemia, hemolytic anemia, and renal and hepatic dysfunction. The urine becomes a harmless reddish-orange because of the phenazopyridine dye. Phenazopyridine can alter the glucose urine test (Clinitest); therefore a blood test should be used to monitor glucose levels. Dimethyl sulfoxide may cause a garlic-like taste and odor, as well as, skin, contact lens, and urine discoloration.

Urinary Stimulants
When bladder function is decreased or lost as a result of (1) a neurogenic bladder (a dysfunction caused by a lesion of the nervous system), (2) a spinal cord injury (paraplegia, hemiplegia), or (3) a severe head injury, a parasympathomimetic may be used to stimulate *micturition* (urination). The drug of choice, bethanechol chloride, is a urinary stimulant also known as a *direct-acting parasympathomimetic*. The drug action is to increase bladder tone by increasing tone of the detrusor urinal muscle, which produces a contraction strong enough to stimulate urination. This drug is contraindicated in patients with a peptic ulcer. Bethanechol is discussed in detail in Chapter 16.

Urinary Antispasmodics/Antimuscarinics/Anticholinergics
Urinary tract spasms resulting from infection or injury can be relieved with *antispasmodics* that have a direct action on the smooth muscles of the urinary tract. This group of drugs—mirabegron, oxybutynin, and flavoxate—is contraindicated for use if urinary or GI obstruction is present or if the patient has glaucoma. Caution should be used when given to older adults, tobacco smokers, or contact lens wearers, as well as the patient who has a bladder flow obstruction, prostatic hypertrophy, gastroesophageal reflux disease, or hepatic disorder. Antispasmodics have the same effects as *antimuscarinics*, agents that block parasympathetic nerve impulses; parasympatholytics; and anticholinergics (see Chapter 16). Tolterodine tartrate, trospium chloride, desmopressin, fesoterodine, darifenacin hydrobromide, vibegon, and solifenacin succinate are antimuscarinic/anticholinergic drugs used to control an overactive bladder, which causes frequency in urination. These drugs also decrease urgency and urinary incontinence. Antispasmodics/antimuscarinics/anticholinergics frequently have side effects, including blurred vision, headache, dizziness, dry mouth, constipation, and tachycardia. The patient taking these drugs should be taught to report urinary retention, severe dizziness, blurred vision, palpitations, and confusion. Table 51.2 lists drugs that are urinary analgesics, stimulants, and antispasmodics/antimuscarinics/anticholinergics. Solifenacin is the most frequently prescribed drug for overactive bladder and urinary incontinence. See Prototype Drug Chart: Solifenacin Succinate.

PROTOTYPE DRUG CHART

Solifenacin Succinate

Drug Class	Dosage
Urinary antimuscarinic, anticholinergic, bladder antispasmodic	A: PO: Initially 5 mg/d, then up to 10 mg/d; *max:* 10 mg/d
Contraindications	**Drug-Lab-Food Interactions**
Hypersensitivity, glaucoma, gastroparesis, GI obstruction, ileus, pyloric stenosis, urinary retention, history of angioedema *Caution:* Rheumatoid arthritis, celiac disease, hyperparathyroidism, hypothyroidism, prostatic hypertrophy, hypomagnesemia, hypokalemia, hypocalcemia, renal/hepatic impairment, bradycardia, dysrhythmias, cardiomyopathy, heart failure, older adult, breast-feeding, pregnancy, contact lens wearers	Drug: Antagonizes action of cisapride; potentiates dysrhythmias and torsades de pointes with fluconazole, chlorpromazine, citalopram, droperidol, haloperidol, risperidone, azithromycin, and fluoroquinolones
Pharmacokinetics	**Pharmacodynamics**
Absorption: Well absorbed Distribution: PB: 98% Metabolism: t½: 45–68 h Excretion: Urine, feces	PO: Onset: UK Peak: 3–8 h Duration: UK

PROTOTYPE DRUG CHART—CONT'D
Solifenacin Succinate

Therapeutic Effects/Uses
To treat overactive bladder and urinary incontinence

Mechanism of action: Exerts selective muscarinic receptor antagonist effect on all muscarinic receptors; depresses voluntary and involuntary bladder contractions, salivary gland secretion, gastric ciliary muscle, and CNS.

Side Effects
Blurred vision, xerophthalmia, drowsiness, dizziness, fatigue, cough, pharyngitis, dry mouth, nausea, vomiting, abdominal pain, constipation, dyspepsia, cystitis, urinary retention, peripheral edema

Adverse Reactions
Palpitations, hypertension, tachycardia, ocular hypertension, GI obstruction, angioedema

Life threatening: Dysrhythmias, hyperkalemia, torsades de pointes

A, Adult; *d*, day; *GI*, gastrointestinal; *h*, hours; *max*, maximum dosage; *PB*, protein binding; *PO*, by mouth; *t½*, half-life; *UK*, unknown.

TABLE 51.2 Urinary Analgesics, Stimulants, and Antispasmodics

Generic	Route and Dosage	Uses and Considerations
Urinary Analgesics		
Phenazopyridine hydrochloride	A: PO: 190–200 mg tid pc for 2 days with or after meals with full glass of water; *max:* 600 mg/d	For irritation, dysuria, and urgency. May cause headache, contact lens/skin/urine discoloration, elevated hepatic enzymes, pruritus, and rash. Do not use long term for undiagnosed urinary tract pain. PB: UK; *t½:* 7.35 h
Dimethyl sulfoxide	Bladder instillation: 50 mL of 50% sol retained for 15 min; repeat q2wk until relief	For cystitis. May cause infection, bladder discomfort and spasm, cystitis, dysgeusia, and anaphylaxis. PB: UK; *t½:* 12–15 h
Urinary Stimulants		
Bethanechol chloride	A: PO: 5–10 mg q1h until effective response or 50 mg given; *maint:* 10–50 mg tid/qid 1 h ac or 2 h pc; *max:* 200 mg/d	For urinary retention and neurogenic bladder. May cause headache, dizziness, flushing, nausea, vomiting, diarrhea, abdominal cramps, and urinary urgency and frequency. Give 1 h before or 2 h after meals. PB: UK; *t½:* UK
Urinary Antispasmodics		
Flavoxate hydrochloride	A: PO: 100–200 mg tid/qid	For urinary urgency and incontinence, dysuria, spasms, and overactive bladder. May cause headache, drowsiness, confusion, dry mouth, nausea, vomiting, blurred vision, palpitations, dysuria, and tachycardia. PB: UK; *t½:* UK
Oxybutynin chloride	Immediate release: A: PO: 5 mg bid/qid; *max:* 20 mg/d Older A: PO: Initially 2.5 mg bid/tid; *max:* 20 mg/d Extended release: A: PO: Initially 5–10 mg/d; *max:* 30 mg/d	For neurogenic and overactive bladder. May cause drowsiness, dizziness, headache, insomnia, blurred vision, dry mouth, dyspepsia, nausea, diarrhea, constipation, urinary retention, erythema, and skin irritation. Give at same time every day. PB: 99%; *t½:* IR: 2–3 h, ER: 13 h
Mirabegron	Extended-release tablets: A: PO: 25 mg/d; *max:* 50 mg/d	For urinary incontinence and overactive bladder. May cause headache, dizziness, dry mouth, pharyngitis, infection, constipation, urinary retention, back pain, and hypertension. If a dose is missed, give as soon as possible up to 12 hours, if after 12 hours, skip missed dose. PB: 71%; *t½:* 50 h
Antimuscarinics/Anticholinergics		
Tolterodine tartrate	Immediate release: A: PO: 1–2 mg bid; *max:* 4 mg/d Extended release: A: PO: 2–4 mg/d; *max:* 4 mg/d	For overactive bladder. May cause headache, dizziness, drowsiness, fatigue, arthralgia, blurred vision, xerophthalmia, visual impairment, dry mouth, dyspepsia, diarrhea, constipation, and abdominal pain. Contraindicated in closed-angle glaucoma and urinary retention. PB: 96%; *t½:* regular release, 2 h; extended release, 7 h
Trospium chloride	Immediate release: A: PO: 20 mg bid; *max:* 40 mg/d in the morning Extended release: A: PO: 60 mg/d in the morning	For overactive bladder. May cause headache, fatigue, dry skin, xerophthalmia, dyspepsia, flatulence, nausea, abdominal pain, urinary retention, dry mouth, and constipation. Give 1 hour before meals or on empty stomach. PB: 48%–85%; *t½:* regular release, 20 h; extended release, 35 h

Continued

TABLE 51.2 Urinary Analgesics, Stimulants, and Antispasmodics—cont'd

Generic	Route and Dosage	Uses and Considerations
Solifenacin succinate	See Prototype Drug Chart: Solifenacin Succinate	
Desmopressin	Nocturnal enuresis: A: PO: Initially 0.2 mg qd at bedtime	For controlling nocturia, nocturnal enuresis, and polyuria. Fluid should be restricted to a minimum 1 h before administration and for at least 8 h after. Avoid caffeine and alcohol before bedtime. May cause dizziness, hyponatremia, xerostomia, headache, pharyngitis, rhinitis, epistaxis, sneezing, nasal congestion, and hypertension. PB: UK; t½: 2–4 h
Fesoterodine	A: PO: Initially 4 mg/d; *max:* 8 mg/d	For overactive bladder. May cause weight gain, abdominal pain, diarrhea, nausea, headache, dry mouth, constipation, and infection. PB: 50%; t½: 7 h
Darifenacin hydrobromide	A: PO: Initially 7.5 mg/d, then in 2 wk 15 mg/d, give at same time qd; *max:* 15 mg/d	For overactive bladder and urinary incontinence. May cause headache, drowsiness, dizziness, xerophthalmia, weakness, dry mouth, dyspepsia, abdominal pain, nausea, vomiting, and constipation. PB: 98%; t½: 13–19 h
Vibegron	A: PO: 75 mg/d with whole glass water; *max:* 75 mg/d	For overactive bladder. May cause headache, infection, pharyngitis, dry mouth, nausea, diarrhea, constipation, hot flashes, and urinary retention. PB: 50%; t½: 30.8 h

A, Adult; *ac*, before meals; *bid*, twice a day; *d*, day; *h*, hour; *max*, maximum; *PB*, protein binding; *pc*, after meals; *PO*, by mouth; *q*, every; *qid*, four times a day; *sol*, solution; *t½*, half-life; *tid*, three times a day; *UK*, unknown; *wk*, week.

CLINICAL JUDGMENT CASE STUDY

A 29-year-old female reports painful urinary frequency and urgency to her health care provider. The patient has an elevated temperature. A urine specimen indicates that the patient has a urinary tract infection (UTI). The health care provider prescribes trimethoprim-sulfamethoxazole (TMP-SMZ) double-strength tablets (trimethoprim 160 mg, sulfamethoxazole 800 mg) twice a day for 14 days.

1. What other information should the health care provider obtain from the patient?
2. Why was TMP-SMZ prescribed? Explain your answer.
3. What should the health care provider discuss with the patient in regard to taking the drug and its possible side effects? What other information should the patient receive?
4. What is the recommended follow-up care for the patient?
5. What other drugs might be used instead of TMP-SMZ? Would one urinary antiinfective drug be more effective than another? Explain your answer.

REVIEW QUESTIONS

1. A patient is taking nitrofurantoin. What will the nurse teach the patient?
   a. Expect the urine to turn brown.
   b. Keep the urine acidic by drinking milk.
   c. Rinse the mouth after taking oral nitrofurantoin to avoid staining the teeth.
   d. Take an antacid with oral nitrofurantoin to avoid gastrointestinal distress.
2. A patient reports a burning sensation and pain when urinating. Which urinary analgesic does the nurse suspect will be ordered?
   a. Tolterodine
   b. Oxybutynin
   c. Bethanechol
   d. Phenazopyridine
3. A patient is taking the urinary antiseptic methenamine for a urinary tract infection (UTI). The nurse understands that this drug should *not* be given concurrently with which other drug to avoid crystalluria?
   a. Ertapenem
   b. Ciprofloxacin
   c. Fosfomycin
   d. Trimethoprim-sulfamethoxazole
4. A patient is receiving solifenacin succinate. The nurse knows that this drug is used to treat which condition?
   a. Chronic cystitis
   b. Urinary tract stones
   c. Urinary tract infection
   d. Overactive bladder
   e. Urinary retention
   f. Neurogenic bladder
5. The patient is taking tolterodine. The nurse plans to teach the patient to report which condition?
   a. Alkaline urine
   b. Urinary retention
   c. Excessive tearing
   d. Reddish-orange urine

UNIT XVII Reproductive and Gender-Related Drugs

52

Pregnancy and Preterm Labor

Christina DiMaggio Boudreaux, RN, BSN, IBCLC

http://evolve.elsevier.com/McCuistion/pharmacology

LEARNING OBJECTIVES

- Relate the physiological effects and risks of drug use to the maternal-fetal system.
- Relate principles of nursing care to the use of drugs that decrease uterine muscle contractility.
- Relate principles of nursing care to the use of corticosteroid therapy in preterm labor.
- Relate principles of nursing care to the use of drugs for gestational hypertension.

OUTLINE

Physiology of Drug Use During Pregnancy, 673
Therapeutic Drugs and Use of Herbs in Pregnancy, 674
    Iron, 674
    Folic Acid, 675
    Multiple Prenatal Vitamins, 675
    Drugs for Minor Discomforts of Pregnancy, 675
    Drugs Used for Pain Relief in Pregnancy, 678
    Acetaminophen, 679
    Aspirin and Ibuprofen, 679
    Antidepressant Drugs, 679
Drugs That Decrease Uterine Muscle Contractility, 681
    Preterm Labor, 681
    Tocolytic Therapy, 681

    Beta-Sympathomimetic Drugs, 681
    Magnesium Sulfate, 682
    Nursing Interventions During Tocolytic Therapy, 682
Corticosteroid Therapy in Preterm Labor, 683
    Surfactant, 683
    Betamethasone, 683
    Dexamethasone, 683
Drugs for Gestational Hypertension, 684
    Gestational Hypertension, 684
    Drugs Used to Treat Preeclampsia, 686
Clinical Judgment Case Study, 687
Review Questions, 688

PHYSIOLOGY OF DRUG USE DURING PREGNANCY

Pregnancy elicits many changes in the normal physiology of the body, which means that the expected pharmacokinetics of drugs is also changed during pregnancy.

Changes in drug action during pregnancy include the (1) effect of circulating steroid hormones on the liver's metabolism of drugs; (2) reduced gastrointestinal (GI) motility and increased gastric pH; (3) increased glomerular filtration rate and increased renal perfusion, resulting in more rapid renal excretion of drugs; (4) expanded maternal circulating blood volume, resulting in dilution of drugs; and (5) alteration in the clearance of drugs in later pregnancy, resulting in a decrease in serum and tissue concentrations of drugs. Because of alterations in the normal physiology of the body, drugs should not be ordered in lower doses with longer intervals between doses because of the possibility of subtherapeutic serum concentrations.

Other factors, such as late pregnancy and labor, can alter the half-lives of some drugs. Labor can increase the half-life of some drugs. Drug clearance may decrease because of reduced blood flow associated with uterine contractions when a patient is in supine position. Certain disease states can also alter the effectiveness of medication during pregnancy. Disorders such as diabetes mellitus and gestational hypertension may result in decreased renal perfusion and subsequent drug accumulation.

The placenta plays an important role in drug therapy during pregnancy. It was once thought that the placenta played a barrier role, but it is now known that the placenta has an important function as the organ of exchange for numerous substances, including drugs. It allows some substances to transfer quickly or slowly between mother and fetus, depending on variables such as (1) maternal and fetal blood flow; (2) molecular weight of the substance (low-molecular-weight substances cross more readily than do high-molecular-weight substances; most drugs have a low molecular weight, so they readily cross the placenta); (3) degree of ionization of the drug molecule (the more ionized the molecule, the less readily it crosses the placenta); (4) degree of protein binding (highly bound drugs do not cross readily); (5) metabolic activity of the placenta (the metabolic activity can bio-transform molecules into active metabolites that can affect the fetus); and (6) maternal dose.

Guidelines for drug administration during pregnancy must include determination that the benefits of prescribing a drug outweigh potential short- or long-term risks to the maternal-fetal system. Careful selection and monitoring for the minimum effective dose for the shortest interval in the therapeutic range are required. Consideration must be given to alterations related to the physiologic changes of pregnancy.

Liver metabolism of drugs is much slower in the fetus because of immaturity of the liver, which can cause more evident or longer drug effects on the fetus than on the mother. The degree of fetal exposure to a drug and its metabolites are more important to fetal outcome than the rate at which the drug is transported to the fetus.

The mechanisms by which drugs cross the placenta are analogous to the way in which drugs infiltrate breast tissue. Lactation results in increased blood flow to the breasts, and drugs accumulate in adipose breast tissue through simple diffusion. Long-term effects on infants from drugs in breast milk are unknown, but drugs that accumulate in breast milk are known, and the breast-feeding patient should be alerted to the potential accumulation.

Despite prenatal education, public service announcements, and information conveyed through the media, use of legal and illicit drugs during pregnancy continues. In addition, health care providers may prescribe drugs for maternal disorders that indirectly affect the fetus. It is estimated that half the drugs taken by pregnant patients are over-the-counter (OTC) drugs. The drugs most commonly ingested during pregnancy are iron supplements, vitamins, antiemetics, antacids, stool softeners, nasal decongestants, mild analgesics, and antibiotics. Although many drugs can be used safely during pregnancy, pregnant patients should be discouraged from using OTC drugs until they consult with their health care provider.

Drugs conclusively determined to be safe for the embryo and fetus are limited in number. Clinical trials can be resources for reliable drug information; however, it is unethical to test for the safety and efficacy of drugs among pregnant patients. Animal studies are required during drug testing, but the information obtained from such studies is difficult to extrapolate to humans.

There are many known **teratogens**, substances that cause developmental abnormalities. Timing, dose, and duration of exposure are crucial in determining the teratogenicity of a given drug. In humans, the teratogenic period begins 2 weeks after conception, before which the embryo is not susceptible to teratogenesis. After this 2-week point in fetal development, however, exposure to teratogens may result in either death of the embryo or minor cellular damage without congenital disorders. Gestational week 2 through week 12 (first trimester) is the period of organogenesis, in which major structures and organs develop.

THERAPEUTIC DRUGS AND USE OF HERBS IN PREGNANCY

The most common indications for use of drugs during pregnancy are to supplement nutrition with iron, vitamins, and minerals and to treat nausea and vomiting, gastric acidity, and mild discomforts; however, caution must be exercised.

Iron

The Centers for Disease Control and Prevention now recommends starting a low-dose iron supplement, such as 30 mg/day with the first prenatal appointment. In most cases, this will be found in a prenatal vitamin. The goal is to prevent maternal iron deficiency anemia, not supply the fetus. The fetus is adequately supplied through the placenta. The greatest iron demand occurs in the third trimester: 22.4 mg/day, compared with 6.4 mg/day in the first trimester and 18.8 mg/day in the second trimester.

> ### COMPLEMENTARY AND ALTERNATIVE THERAPIES
> #### Pregnancy
> Herbal preparations are not generally recommended during pregnancy. In particular, the following herbs should be avoided:
> - Feverfew, rosemary, and sage are emmenagogues that stimulate blood flow in the uterus.
> - Kava decreases platelets.
> - Dong-quai, garlic, and ginkgo biloba increase bleeding when used with anticoagulants.
> - Ginseng may decrease the action of anticoagulants.
> - St. Johns wort has mutagenic effects on the cells of the developing embryo and fetus.
>
> Pennyroyal, rue, tansy, and blue cohosh taken orally or topically can be abortifacient.

Although a normal diet generally provides the 18-mg recommended daily allowance (RDA) of iron for nonpregnant patients, pregnant patients at risk for anemia are usually instructed to supplement with 60 to 120 mg of elemental iron per day. The elemental iron content of the most common iron salts includes ferrous sulfate 20% (325 mg of ferrous sulfate is equivalent to 65 mg elemental iron), exsiccated ferrous sulfate 30%, ferrous gluconate 12%, and ferrous fumarate 33%. The estimated net iron cost of pregnancy is approximately 600 to 800 mg. This iron cost is due to the iron use by the fetus, placenta, and increased red blood cell (RBC) volume. Patients are advised to continue supplements for 6 weeks postpartum.

Pregnant patients generally have decreased hematocrit early in the third trimester. Those with levels below 30% will have their supplemental iron dosages increased, and a complete blood count with platelet and ferritin will be measured. In those with true iron deficiency anemia, response to iron supplementation is usually noted in 5 to 7 days with a modest reticulocytosis and an increase in hemoglobin in 3 weeks. No teratogenic effects have been reported with physiologic doses. In contrast, increasing evidence has associated prenatal iron supplementation with glucose impairment and hypertension in midpregnancy. Many OTC and prescription iron products (Table 52.1) are available in varying dosages, which differ in the amount of elemental iron contained in the form of iron salts.

Adverse Reactions
Common side effects of iron supplements include nausea, constipation, black tarry stools, GI irritation, epigastric pain, vomiting, discoloration of urine, and diarrhea.

Nursing Implications
Liquid forms can cause temporary tooth discoloration and therefore should be diluted and administered through a straw. Iron supplements are best absorbed when administered with water or juice on an empty stomach. Vitamin C increases the absorption of iron. If gastric irritation does occur, administer the iron with food. Iron supplementation may inhibit the absorption of several drugs, and appropriate separation of doses should be followed (e.g., iron supplementation should be administered 2 hours before or 4 hours after antacids). Additional examples of drugs that may require separation in dose include levodopa, levothyroxine, methyldopa, penicillins, quinolones, and tetracyclines. For the same reasons, do not administer iron with milk, cereal, tea, coffee, or eggs.

TABLE 52.1 Iron Products

Generic	Route and Dosage	Uses and Considerations
Iron salts (ferrous sulfate, ferrous gluconate, ferrous fumarate) *Caution:* Read the label carefully. The amount of elemental iron differs according to the formulation.	PO: 15 mg PO once/d in the first trimester; 27 mg PO once/d during the last 2 trimesters.	Prevention and treatment of iron-deficiency anemia and prophylaxis for iron deficiency in pregnancy. The type of anemia and the underlying cause or causes should be determined before starting therapy with iron. Replaces iron stores needed for RBC development. Absorption PO is 5%–30% in intestines; therefore GI side effects may occur. Toxic reactions include pallor, hematemesis, shock, cardiovascular collapse, and metabolic acidosis. Contraindicated in patients with hypersensitivity or peptic ulcer. Decreased absorption of zinc, tetracycline, and penicillamine and increased absorption with ascorbic acid, such as orange juice; decreased absorption with antacids, eggs, milk, coffee, and tea. Take at bedtime to avoid GI upset. Use straw for elixir to prevent staining of teeth, swallow tab/cap whole with full glass of water or juice, preferably on an empty stomach. Sit upright 30 min after dose to decrease reflux. Increase fluids, activity, and dietary bulk. Keep out of reach of children. Peak reticulocytosis: 5–10 d; hemoglobin values increase in 2–4 wk. PB: To transferrin; $t½$: UK; onset: 3–10 d; duration: 3–4 mo. Pregnancy Considerations: Iron crosses the placenta and fetal stores are obtained from the mother. Untreated iron-deficiency anemia during pregnancy may be associated with an increased risk of low birth weight, preterm delivery, and perinatal mortality, as well as postpartum depression in mother and decreased mental functioning in the offspring. Treatment improves maternal hematologic status and neonatal birth weight.

cap, Capsule; *d*, day; *GI*, gastrointestinal; *min*, minutes; *mo*, months; *PB*, protein binding; *PO*, by mouth; *RBC*, red blood cell; *t½*, half-life; *tab*, tablet; *UK*, unknown; *wk*, weeks.

Folic Acid

Folic acid supplementation as part of preconception planning improves the outcome of pregnancy. During pregnancy, folic acid (vitamin B_9, folate) is needed in increased amounts. Folic acid deficiency early in pregnancy can result in spontaneous abortion or congenital disorders, especially neural tube defects (NTDs); a failure of the embryonic neural tube to close properly can lead to spina bifida or skull and brain malformations. Deficiency of folic acid may also contribute to premature birth, low birth weight, and premature separation of the placenta (abruptio placenta). In the United States approximately 4000 pregnancies a year are affected by NTDs. Controlled clinical trials have demonstrated that folic acid supplementation can reduce this incidence by as much as 50%.

Normally, the RDA for folic acid is 180 mcg, but the US Preventive Services Task Force recommends that females who are planning pregnancy take a supplement containing 400 mcg to 800 mcg of folic acid 1 month before and for the first 2 to 3 months after conception. The American Congress of Obstetricians and Gynecologists (ACOG) recommends that all females of childbearing age ingest 400 mcg of folic acid daily for congenital disorder prevention and 600 mcg during pregnancy. The reasoning behind the ACOG recommendation is the high incidence of unplanned and unrecognized pregnancies.

The neural tube closes within the first 4 weeks of pregnancy (18–26 days after conception); therefore it is important that females consume the recommended amounts of folic acid every day. For patients who have had a pregnancy affected by an NTD, higher doses of folic acid are recommended: 4000 mcg starting 1 to 3 months before conception.

The recommended amount should be ingested from folate-rich foods, such as dark green leafy vegetables, asparagus, papaya, strawberries, and oranges; from folate-enriched foods, such as bread, rice, cornmeal, pasta, and cereal; and from supplementation because the amount of naturally occurring folic acid ingested in foods varies from day to day and the folic acid from these sources is not well absorbed.

Adverse Reactions

Side effects include flushing, malaise, erythema, pruritus, skin rash, and, in rare cases, allergic bronchospasm. Patients should be aware that folic acid supplementation may cause urine to turn more intensely yellow in color.

Multiple Prenatal Vitamins

Multiple Prenatal Vitamin preparations are routinely recommended for pregnant patients. These preparations generally supply vitamins A, B-complex, B_{12}, C, calcium, D, E, iron, and other minerals.

Inadequate nutrition cannot be rectified through supplements alone; vitamins are used most effectively by the body when taken with meals, and calories and protein are not supplied by supplements.

Large doses of vitamins and minerals above the recommended amounts do not improve health and may cause harm to the pregnant patient and fetus. Some vitamins and minerals can be teratogenic or toxic when taken in large amounts.

Drugs for Minor Discomforts of Pregnancy

Many complaints associated with pregnancy are related to the GI tract and include nausea and vomiting, heartburn, and constipation. The etiology of nausea and vomiting is unclear, although research suggests that it is probably related to an increase in human chorionic gonadotropin levels during pregnancy. Increased progesterone during pregnancy, which relaxes smooth muscle, contributes to heartburn and constipation. The elevation in female sex hormones during pregnancy changes the motility of the GI tract, and the enlarging uterus displaces the bowel.

Nausea and Vomiting

Nausea and vomiting ("morning sickness") during early pregnancy are major complaints for about 88% of pregnant patients, but hyperemesis gravidarum—severe nausea and vomiting that may require hospitalization for hydration and nutrition—occurs with a much lower incidence (1%–3%). Nonpharmacologic measures to decrease nausea and vomiting include (1) eating crackers, dry toast, or other carbohydrates before rising; (2) avoiding high-fat or highly seasoned foods; (3) eating small, frequent meals; (4) drinking fluids between, rather than with, meals; (5) drinking apple juice or flat soda between meals; (6) eating a high-protein bedtime snack; (7) stopping smoking; and (8) taking an iron supplement at bedtime. These measures work well for most patients, but if vomiting is severe, fluid replacement and pharmacologic measures may be necessary.

The US Food and Drug Administration (FDA) has approved pyridoxine hydrochloride and doxylamine succinate for treatment of morning sickness. Table 52.2 lists drugs used for management of nausea and vomiting during pregnancy with their dosages, uses, and considerations.

Iron supplementation during pregnancy may add to the problems of nausea and vomiting. Taking these supplements with food or at bedtime may help decrease gastric distress. Prenatal vitamins should be taken at the time of day the patient is least likely to experience emesis because a high incidence of nausea and vomiting is associated with prenatal vitamins. For patients with continued iron-induced gastric distress, many health care providers recommend taking two children's chewable multivitamins with iron. Salting food to taste may help replace vomited chloride; foods rich in potassium and magnesium may also help replace lost nutrients.

Patients whose symptoms persist and who experience weight loss and dehydration may require intravenous (IV) rehydration, including replacement of electrolytes and vitamins, as well as antiemetic therapy. (See Table 52.2 for drugs used for management of nausea and vomiting during pregnancy.)

TABLE 52.2 Drugs for Management of Nausea and Vomiting During Pregnancy[a]

Generic	Route and Dosage	Uses and Considerations
Vitamin		
Pyridoxine (B_6) (Also available as combination drug with doxylamine)	PO: 10–25 mg 3–4 times a day. May be given alone or in combination with doxylamine. Adjust dose based on severity of symptoms.	In the United States, B_6 is the drug of choice for nausea and vomiting in pregnancy; it is a coenzyme for various metabolic functions, including metabolism of proteins, carbohydrates, and fats. Side effects include fatigue, headache, nausea, somnolence, and sensory neuropathy. Absorbed in the jejunum, metabolized in the liver, excreted in urine. Peak plasma time: 5–6 h (pyridoxine); $t½$: 15–20 d. Pregnancy Considerations: Used to treat nausea and vomiting of pregnancy. Crosses the placenta. No problems reported.
Antihistamine Plus Vitamin B_6 Analog		
Doxylamine succinate 10 mg/pyridoxine 10 mg	PO: 2 tabs at bedtime	Mechanism of Action: Competes with histamine for H_1 receptor sites on effector cells. Side effects include CNS depression, which may impair physical or mental ability. Patients must be cautioned about performing tasks that require mental alertness, like driving or operating machinery. Effects may be potentiated when used with other sedative drugs. Contraindicated in females with known hypersensitivity to doxylamine succinate or any other component of the drug. MAOIs intensify and prolong the adverse CNS effects. Has anticholinergic properties and should be used with caution in females with asthma, increased intraocular pressure, narrow-angle glaucoma, stenosing peptic ulcer, pyloroduodenal obstruction, and urinary bladder neck obstruction. Not for use by nursing females. Administer on an empty stomach with a glass of water. Swallow tablets whole; do not chew, crush, or split. Pregnancy Considerations: Doxylamine succinate and pyridoxine hydrochloride are recommended individually and in combination for use in pregnant females to manage nausea and vomiting of pregnancy. Crosses the placenta. No problems reported. ⚡ Not recommended for use during lactation. Primarily metabolized in the liver; excreted in the kidney; peak: 2–4 h; $t½$: 10–12 h, PB: UK.
Phenothiazines		
Promethazine	PO/IV/IM/PR: 12.5–25 mg q4–6 h PRN ⚠ Black-Box Warning: Promethazine injections can cause severe tissue injury, including gangrene, necrosis, abscess, erythema, edema, severe spasms of distal vessels, phlebitis, sensory loss, and paralysis.	Blocks postsynaptic mesolimbic dopaminergic receptors in the brain; exhibits a strong α-adrenergic blocking effect and depresses release of hypothalamic and hypophyseal hormones; competes with histamine for H_1 receptor. Side effects include dizziness, agitation, drowsiness, excitation, fatigue, insomnia, photosensitivity reactions, nausea, vomiting, and constipation. Contraindicated in patients with CNS depression or hypersensitivity to the drug or any component. Use caution in patients with cardiovascular disease; not recommended for subcut or intraarterial administration; injection may contain sulfites, which may cause allergic reaction. Pregnancy Considerations: Approved for use as an antiemetic for pregnancy; however, other drugs are recommended as initial therapy for the treatment of nausea and vomiting of pregnancy. $t½$: 9–16 h; onset: PO/IM, 20 min; IV, 3–5 min; duration: 4–6 h but may have effects up to 12 h; PB: 93%; excretion: urine, feces as inactive metabolites.

TABLE 52.2 Drugs for Management of Nausea and Vomiting During Pregnancy[a]—cont'd

Generic	Route and Dosage	Uses and Considerations
Prokinetic Agents		
Metoclopramide	PO/IM/IV: 5–10 mg q8h	Blocks dopamine receptors in the CTZ; causes enhanced motility and accelerated gastric emptying without stimulating secretions Side effects include restlessness, drowsiness, diarrhea, weakness, insomnia, depression, and tardive dyskinesia. ⚠️ *Black-Box Warning:* Contraindicated in patients with hypersensitivity to the drug or any component; GI obstruction, perforation, or hemorrhage; pheochromocytoma; history of seizure disorder, history of hypertension, or history of tardive dyskinesia. Onset of Action: PO: 30–60 min, IM: 10–15 min, IV: 1–3 min. Duration: 1–2 h; t½: 4–7 h. PB: 30%. Pregnancy Considerations: Crosses the placenta and can be detected in cord blood and amniotic fluid. Metoclopramide is one of the agents that may be considered for adjunctive treatment of nausea and vomiting of pregnancy when symptoms persist after initial pharmacologic therapy. PO/IM therapy may be given in patients who are not dehydrated; ⚡ IV therapy should be used when dehydration is present.
Other		
Ondansetron	PO/IV: 4–8 mg 2–3 times/d It is recommended that ondansetron is only reserved for severe hyperemesis gravidarum or when conventional treatments are not effective.	Antiemetic; selective 5-HT$_3$ receptor antagonist that blocks serotonin both peripherally on vagal nerve terminals and centrally in the CTZ. Side effects include headache, constipation, diarrhea, and malaise/fatigue. Contraindicated in patients with hypersensitivity to the drug or other selective 5-HT$_3$ antagonists. ⚡ *Caution:* Use as scheduled, not PRN. Use with caution in patients who have congenital/medical conditions that cause prolonged QT interval or who take medications that prolong QT interval. Drug interactions: Drugs that alter the activity of liver enzymes. Pregnancy Considerations: Crosses the placenta. Although ondansetron has been evaluated for the treatment of nausea and vomiting of pregnancy, current guidelines note data related to fetal safety are conflicting, so it is generally reserved for use when other agents have failed. Onset: 30 min; duration: 4–8 h; t½: 3–6 h.

CNS, Central nervous system; *CTZ*, chemoreceptor trigger zone; *d*, day; *GI*, gastrointestinal; *GU*, genitourinary; *H$_1$*, histamine$_1$; *h*, hour; *IM*, intramuscular; *IV*, intravenous; *MAOI*, monoamine oxidase inhibitor; *min*, minute; *PO*, by mouth; *PR*, by rectum; *PRN*, as needed; *qid*, four times a day; *subcut*, subcutaneously; *t½*, half-life; *tabs*, tablets; *tid*, three times a day.
[a]Recommendation not implied.

Heartburn

Heartburn, or *pyrosis*, is a burning sensation in the epigastric and sternal regions related to reflux of acidic stomach contents. Approximately 80% of pregnant patients are affected with pyrosis. *The normal increase in the hormone progesterone causes decreased motility of the GI tract during pregnancy.* Progesterone also relaxes the cardiac sphincter—the sphincter that leads into the stomach from the esophagus, also called the *lower esophageal sphincter*—making reflux activity, or *reverse peristalsis*, more likely. During pregnancy, digestion and gastric emptying are slower than in the nonpregnant state. Heartburn is common when a pregnant patient sits or lies down soon after eating a normal meal, only to have her gravid uterus exert upward pressure on her stomach, causing increased reflux activity and the perception of hyperacidity. Heartburn is a disorder of the second and third trimesters of pregnancy.

Nonpharmacologic measures are preferred in the management of heartburn. These include (1) limiting the size of meals; (2) avoiding highly seasoned or greasy foods; (3) avoiding gas-forming foods (e.g., cabbage, onions); (4) eating slowly and chewing thoroughly; (5) avoiding citrus juices; (6) drinking adequate fluids, but not with meals; and (7) avoiding reclining immediately after eating.

Antacids should be considered first-line therapy if the patient does not respond to nonpharmacologic therapy. The antacids of choice for the pregnant patient include nonsystemic low-sodium products (those considered dietetically sodium free) that contain aluminum and magnesium (in the form of hydroxide) in combination. Discourage long-term use or large doses of magnesium antacids because fetal renal, respiratory, cardiovascular, and muscle problems may result. Chewable calcium carbonate tablets are frequently taken by pregnant patients for heartburn, but because they are calcium based, excessive use may contribute to constipation.

Most patients do not realize that remedies commonly used by nonpregnant patients (e.g., baking soda, sodium bicarbonate) can be harmful during pregnancy. Selection of the wrong antacid can result in diarrhea, constipation, or electrolyte imbalance. A combination of nonpharmacologic measures and minimal use of safe antacids should effectively meet the pregnant patient's needs.

Liquid antacids are the preparations most used in pregnancy because of their uniform dissolution, rapid action, and greater activity. Tablets are also acceptable, particularly for convenience, provided they are thoroughly chewed, and the patient maintains adequate fluid intake.

Histamine$_2$ (H$_2$)-receptor antagonists can be used during pregnancy, but only if their use is recommended by a health care provider and initial treatment with antacids has failed. The teratogenicity of these medications is unknown. H$_2$-receptor antagonists work by competitively and reversibly binding to the histamine receptors of the parietal cells, causing a reduction in gastric acid secretion. The onset of action is generally in 1 hour and can persist for 6 to 12 hours.

There is even less experience with the use of proton pump inhibitors. These medications work to suppress gastric acid secretion by inhibiting the proton pump on the surface of the parietal cells. Omeprazole, which is now OTC, is not recommended for use in pregnancy except when the benefits outweigh the risks and after other medications and initial treatments have failed. Encourage patients to discuss all options with their health care provider before taking any medication during pregnancy.

Table 52.3 presents medications for heartburn commonly used during pregnancy.

Constipation

Constipation is a frequent occurrence during pregnancy. Its cause may be related to hormonal changes—specifically progesterone, which decreases GI motility. As with heartburn, nonpharmacologic treatments for constipation should be tried first. These include (1) increased fluid intake, (2) increased dietary fiber intake, and (3) moderate physical exercise. If these methods do not work, pharmacologic interventions may be indicated, and the safest drugs are bulk-forming preparations that contain fiber because they are not systemically absorbed. Also, docusate sodium, a stool softener, would be appropriate as first-line treatment during pregnancy. Drugs that should be reserved for occasional use include magnesium hydroxide, magnesium citrate, lactulose, sorbitol, bisacodyl, and senna.

Castor oil should be avoided during pregnancy because it can stimulate uterine contractions. Mineral oil should also be avoided because it can reduce the absorption of fat-soluble vitamins such as vitamin K. Low levels of vitamin K in the neonate can result in hemorrhage.

Drugs Used for Pain Relief in Pregnancy

Through week 26 of pregnancy, headaches that result from hormonally induced body changes, sinus congestion, or eye strain are quite common. It is not unusual for the pregnant patient to experience backaches, joint pains, round ligament pain (resulting in mild abdominal aches and twinges), and pain from minor injuries. Nonpharmacologic pain relief measures should be tried initially, including rest; a calming environment; relaxation exercises; alteration in routine; mental imagery; ice packs; warm, moist heat; postural changes; correct body mechanics; and changes in footwear.

TABLE 52.3 Over-the-Counter Antacids Commonly Used in Pregnancy

Generic	Route and Dosage	Uses and Considerations
Aluminum hydroxide	A: PO: Oral Susp 40–60 mL per dose every 3–6 h OTC: A: PO 10 mL 5–6 times/d	Used to counteract hyperacidity in pregnancy. Contains 320 mg of aluminum hydroxide gel per 300-mg tab or per 5 mL; ANC 8 contains saccharin and sorbitol. OTC preparation for heartburn secondary to reflux; it neutralizes gastric acidity. Side effects include constipation, fecal discoloration, fecal impaction, nausea, vomiting, stomach cramps. Adverse reactions include dehydration, hypophosphatemia (long-term use), GI obstruction. Pregnancy Considerations: Nonpharmacologic treatments, such as dietary and lifestyle modifications, are preferred. If antacids are warranted, most aluminum-containing antacids that are considered acceptable when used in recommended doses for dyspepsia during pregnancy and prophylactically during labor to prevent effects related to potential aspiration. PB: UK; onset: 15–30 min; peak: 0.5 h; duration: 1–3 h; t½: UK. *max:* not to exceed recommended dose in 24/h.
Magnesium hydroxide and aluminum hydroxide with simethicone	PO: Multiple formulations available OTC—take as directed	Antiflatulent and neutralizes gastric acid. Provides relief of acid indigestion, heartburn, sour stomach or upset stomach and flatus associated with these symptoms. Liquid: Each 5 mL contains 400 mg aluminum hydroxide; 400 mg magnesium hydroxide; 40 mg simethicone, parabens, saccharin, and sorbitol; and 2 mg sodium. Tablets: Each contains 200 mg aluminum hydroxide, 200 mg magnesium hydroxide, and 20 mg simethicone. Tabs must be chewed thoroughly. Administer 1 hour after meals or between meals. Shake suspension well before administering. Adverse effects include acid rebound. Aluminum-based antacids may cause constipation, whereas magnesium-based antacids have a laxative effect. Aluminum and magnesium–based combination antacids are given to balance the constipation and laxative effects. Do not administer magnesium-based antacids to patients with renal disease. *Drug interactions:* Concurrent administration with digoxin, indomethacin, or iron salts may decrease absorption of these drugs. Decreased pharmacologic effect with antacids and benzodiazepines, captopril, corticosteroids, fluoroquinolones, H$_2$ antagonists, hydantoins, ketoconazole, penicillamine, phenothiazines, salicylates, and ticlopidine. Increased pharmacologic effect with levodopa, sulfonylureas, and valproic acid. Pregnancy Considerations: Crosses the placenta but is considered acceptable during pregnancy and labor. PB: UK; t½: UK.

ANC, Acid-neutralizing capacity (per tablet or 5 mL); *d*, day; *GI*, gastrointestinal; *h*, hour; *H$_2$*, histamine 2; *min*, minute; *OTC*, over-the-counter; *PB*, protein binding; *PO*, by mouth; *susp*, suspension; *t½*, half-life; *tab*, tablet; *tsp*, teaspoon; *UK*, unknown.

Acetaminophen

Acetaminophen, a para-aminophenol analgesic, is the most commonly ingested nonprescription drug during pregnancy. There has been some recent controversy due to studies that have suggested that exposure to paracetamol, or acetaminophen, may alter fetal development and increase the risks of neurodevelopment disorders. ACOG issued a consensus statement stating that they were not changing their stance on the use of acetaminophen during pregnancy, since the brain doesn't stop developing until 15 months of age, which leaves room for many other factors to potentially lead to these issues. However, as always, it should only be prescribed as needed and in moderation. Acetaminophen may be used during all trimesters of pregnancy in therapeutic doses on a short-term basis for its analgesic and antipyretic effects. The drug is a weak prostaglandin inhibitor and does not have significant antiinflammatory effects (www.ACOG.org). See Prototype Drug Chart: Acetaminophen in Chapter 25 for the pharmacologic data.

Pharmacokinetics

The rate of absorption of acetaminophen is dependent on the rate of gastric emptying. Acetaminophen is 10% to 25% protein bound and crosses the placenta during pregnancy; it is also found in low concentrations in breast milk. Acetaminophen is partially hepatically metabolized into inactive metabolites; however, a highly active metabolite (*N*-acetyl-*p*-benzoquinone) produced when the drug is taken in large doses can have potential liver and kidney toxicity. The half-life is 2 to 3 hours. There is no concrete evidence of fetal anomalies associated with the use of acetaminophen, and no adverse effects have been noted in breast-fed infants of patients who used the drug while pregnant or breast-feeding.

Pharmacodynamics

The maximum daily dose of acetaminophen is 3000 mg per day, and use during pregnancy should not exceed this because of potential for kidney and liver toxicity. The drug should be taken at 4- to 6-hour intervals. Onset of effects after oral ingestion is within 10 to 30 minutes, peak action occurs at 1 to 2 hours, and duration is from 3 to 5 hours.

Manufacturers of OTC products that contain acetaminophen have lowered the maximum daily dose recommendation to 3000 mg due to the frequency of overdose with acetaminophen. One reason for the high frequency of overdose is that patients may take multiple OTC products that contain acetaminophen.

Most patients without preexisting renal or hepatic disease tolerate acetaminophen without adverse drug effects. Patients with hypersensitivity to the compound should not use it. Acetaminophen should be used cautiously in patients who are at risk for infection because of the possibility of masking signs and symptoms. The most frequent adverse reactions are skin eruptions, urticaria, unusual bruising, erythema, hypoglycemia, jaundice, hemolytic anemia, neutropenia, leukopenia, pancytopenia, and thrombocytopenia.

Aspirin and Ibuprofen

Aspirin, a salicylate, is classified as a mild analgesic. It is a nonsteroidal antiinflammatory drug (NSAID), more specifically a prostaglandin synthetase inhibitor with antipyretic, analgesic, and antiinflammatory properties.

Aspirin can inhibit the initiation of labor and may prolong labor through its effects on uterine contractility; therefore its use is not recommended during pregnancy. Aspirin use late in pregnancy is also associated with greater maternal blood loss at delivery, and there may be increased risk for anemia in pregnancy and of antepartum hemorrhage. Hemostasis is affected in the newborn whose mother ingested aspirin during the last 2 months of pregnancy even without use during the week of delivery. Platelets are unable to aggregate to form clots, and it appears that this is *not* a reversible effect after delivery; the infant must wait for its own bone marrow to produce new platelets. Ibuprofen is also an NSAID and a prostaglandin synthetase inhibitor with antipyretic, analgesic, and antiinflammatory properties. Bleeding risks are like those reported with aspirin, although ibuprofen causes less inhibition of platelet aggregation than aspirin formulations. If taken late in pregnancy, ibuprofen may cause premature closure of the ductus arteriosus; therefore ibuprofen use is contraindicated during the third trimester and during labor and delivery.

Antidepressant Drugs

Depressive disorders and exposure to antidepressant drugs have been associated with adverse birth outcomes. Adverse outcomes have included low birth weight (LBW), infants born small for gestational age (SGA), preterm delivery, and increased neonatal irritability and decreased attentiveness. The use of selective serotonin reuptake inhibitors (SSRIs) in pregnancy is associated with LBW and SGA infants. Preterm delivery (before 37 weeks) is significantly higher in patients taking SSRIs and tricyclic antidepressants (TCAs). Although TCA use in pregnancy has not been associated with structural malformations, in utero exposure has been linked to neonatal jitteriness and irritability. *Poor neonatal adaptation*—a term for transient symptoms such as tachypnea, irritability, hypoglycemia, and weak cry—has been reported in neonates exposed to SSRIs in late pregnancy. Options for treatment for pregnant patients include psychotherapy alone or in conjunction with pharmacologic therapy as determined by the health care provider.

CLINICAL JUDGMENT [NURSING PROCESS]
Antepartum Drugs

Concept: Reproduction
- Reproduction is the process by which offspring is produced. Nurses perform assessments on their antepartum patients to determine their course of drugs and care.

Recognize Cues [Assessment]
- Gather comprehensive medical and drug history to include illicit, herbal, and pharmacologic formulations and nonpharmacologic interventions, such as acupuncture.
- Obtain baseline vital signs.
- Identify patients at risk for substance abuse, and collaborate with other professionals to plan strategies to minimize risks.
- Assess drug history to determine whether antacid use will interfere with absorption of the drug.
- Review history of aspirin use when admitting a patient in labor. If aspirin has been used, alert staff and monitor for increased bleeding.
- Ascertain any medical history of alcoholism, liver disease, viral infection, or renal deficiencies. Acetaminophen should be used cautiously in these patients.
- Assess group B *Streptococcus* colonization in pregnancy for treatment and neonatal prevention.

Continued

CLINICAL JUDGMENT [NURSING PROCESS]—CONT'D

Antepartum Drugs

Analyze Cues and Prioritize Hypotheses [Patient Problems]
- Anxiety
- Potential for decreased adherence
- Need for patient teaching

Generate Solutions [Planning]
- The patient will verbalize the name and side effects of at least one pharmacologic and nonpharmacologic treatment used during pregnancy.
- The patient will discuss drugs and herbal supplements with a health care provider or pharmacist before use.

Take Action [Nursing Interventions]

General
- Discuss the importance of prenatal care, and discuss the patient's fears.
- Instruct on nonpharmacologic and pharmacologic measures to relieve common pregnancy discomforts.
- Instruct the patient on tobacco, alcohol, or drug treatment programs if appropriate.
- Counsel the patient on nutritional and therapeutic supplements needed during pregnancy.
- Monitor hemoglobin/hematocrit of the prenatal patient per agency protocol.

Iron
- Instruct the patient about nausea, constipation, and bowel habit changes if they are taking iron preparations.
- Instruct the patient to dilute liquid iron preparations and take through a plastic straw to prevent discoloration of teeth. Giving iron with orange juice, which is high in ascorbic acid, enhances absorption.
- Store iron in a light-resistant container.
- Assess for a false-positive result of occult blood in the stool that may occur in patients taking iron.

Patient Teaching

General
- Advise the patient that tobacco, alcohol, and heavy caffeine use may have adverse effects on the fetus.
- Encourage the patient to speak with their health care provider before taking drugs—illicit, over-the-counter (OTC), or prescribed drugs—because of their teratogenic potential.
- Instruct the patient planning to breast-feed to discuss drugs—illicit, OTC, and prescribed—with their health care provider.

Aspirin, Acetaminophen, and Ibuprofen
- Advise the patient to take acetaminophen, rather than aspirin, during pregnancy; aspirin and ibuprofen are particularly contraindicated during the third trimester.
- Instruct the patient against ingesting multiple OTC pain or cough/cold preparations because many OTC products contain acetaminophen.

Antepartum Drugs
- Advise the patient not to refrain from taking nonsteroidal antiinflammatory drugs (NSAIDs) with acetaminophen.
- Advise the patient not to take NSAIDs after the second trimester.

Caffeine, Alcohol, and Nicotine
- Advise the patient to limit coffee ingestion to 1 cup per day and to limit other sources of caffeine (tea, soda, chocolate, certain drugs).
- Encourage the patient to limit and space caffeine intake evenly throughout the day because caffeine passes readily to the fetus, which cannot metabolize it. Caffeine can decrease intervillous placental blood flow.
- Advise the patient to discuss use of caffeine products with their health care provider.
- Advise the patient to use decaffeinated products or to dilute caffeinated products.
- Advise the patient to discuss use of herbal products with their health care provider (see Complementary and Alternative Therapies box).
- Instruct the patient who plans to breastfeed that 1% of caffeine consumed will appear in breast milk within 15 minutes. Therefore, although one cup of coffee is fine, it is not wise to drink several cups of coffee in succession; excess caffeine will accumulate in the infant's tissues because it lacks the enzymes to adequately clear the caffeine for 7 to 9 months after birth.
- Advise the pregnant patient not to drink alcohol because no safe level has been determined; emphasize that even *minimal* exposure can result in fetal alcohol effect, and moderate/excessive exposure may result in fetal alcohol syndrome.
- Advise the patient that smoking can cause loss of nutrients such as vitamins A and C, folic acid, cobalamin, and calcium. Tobacco use may contribute to shortened gestation and low-birth-weight infants.

Antacids
- Advise the patient that antacids should not be taken within 1 hour of taking an enteric-coated tablet because the acid-resistant coating may dissolve in the increased alkaline condition of the stomach and the medication will not be released in the intestine as intended. Stomach upset may result.
- Instruct the patient to store antacid liquid suspensions at room temperature or to place them under refrigeration to improve palatability; advise that suspensions should not be frozen and that the bottle must be shaken well before ingesting.

Iron
- Advise the patient about dietary sources of iron, including red meat, nuts and seeds, wheat germ, spinach, broccoli, prunes, and iron-fortified cereal.
- Instruct the patient that, if supplemental iron is taken between meals, increased absorption—and increased side effects—may result. Taking iron 1 hour before meals is suggested. Give with orange juice or water but not with milk or antacids.

Self-Administration of Iron and Antacids
- Advise the patient to swallow iron tablets whole, not crush them. Liquid iron preparations are taken with a plastic straw to avoid staining teeth.
- Instruct the patient not to take antacids with iron; antacids impair absorption and are generally discouraged during pregnancy. Iron and antacids should be taken 2 hours apart if both are prescribed.

Side Effects of Iron and Antacids
- Advise the patient to keep iron tablets away from children. Iron tablets look like candy, and death has been reported in small children. Iron is a leading cause of fatal poisoning in children.
- Advise the patient there may be a change in bowel habits when taking antacids. Aluminum and calcium carbonate products can cause constipation, whereas magnesium products can cause diarrhea. Many antacids contain a combination of ingredients to reduce adverse effects.

Evaluate Outcomes [Evaluation]
- Evaluate effectiveness of prescribed drug therapy. Report side effects.
- Evaluate the patient's understanding of possible effects on the fetus from maternal use of drugs (prescribed, OTC, and illicit) and tobacco or alcohol.

DRUGS THAT DECREASE UTERINE MUSCLE CONTRACTILITY

Preterm Labor

Preterm labor (PTL) is defined as cervical changes and uterine contractions that occur between 20 and 37 weeks of pregnancy. *Preterm birth* is any birth that occurs before the completion of 37 weeks of pregnancy, regardless of birth weight. Complications related to preterm birth account for more newborn and infant deaths than any other cause. PTL occurs in 12% of pregnancies.

Although PTL has no single known cause, certain risk factors have been identified: maternal age younger than 18 years or older than 40 years, low socioeconomic status, previous history of preterm delivery (17% to 37% chance of recurrence), intrauterine infections (e.g., bacterial vaginosis), polyhydramnios, multiple gestation, uterine anomalies, antepartum hemorrhage, smoking, substance use, urinary tract infections, and incompetent cervix. Attempts to arrest PTL are contraindicated in (1) pregnancy of less than 20 weeks' gestation (confirmed by ultrasound), (2) bulging or premature rupture of membranes (PROM), (3) confirmed fetal death or anomalies incompatible with life, (4) maternal hemorrhage and evidence of severe fetal compromise, and (5) chorioamnionitis.

Nonpharmacologic treatment measures for PTL include bed rest, hydration (ingestion of 6 to 8 glasses of fluids daily or more, IV fluid bolus), pelvic rest (no sexual intercourse or douching), and screening for intrauterine and urinary tract infections. Patient assessment includes uterine activity (frequency, duration, and intensity), vaginal bleeding or discharge, and fetal monitoring.

Tocolytic Therapy

When patients in true PTL (with cervical change) have no contraindications, they become candidates for tocolytic therapy—drug therapy to decrease uterine muscle contractions. No medication has been approved by the FDA as a tocolytic, so medications used for this reason are considered "off-label" use. The goals in tocolytic therapy are to (1) interrupt or inhibit uterine contractions to create additional time for fetal maturation in utero, (2) delay delivery so antenatal corticosteroids can be delivered to facilitate fetal lung maturation, and (3) allow safe transport of the patient to an appropriate facility if required. Table 52.4 lists the drugs used to decrease preterm uterine contractions and their dosages, uses, and considerations.

Beta-Sympathomimetic Drugs

Beta-sympathomimetic drugs act by stimulating β_2-receptors on uterine smooth muscle. The frequency and intensity of uterine contractions decrease as the muscle relaxes. Terbutaline is used in the late second and early third trimesters, more commonly limited to a single-dose therapy as an acute tocolytic. Terbutaline can effectively decrease uterine contractions; however, use of terbutaline in the United States has decreased with increased awareness of its effects on maternal and fetal cardiovascular systems and free placental passage. The FDA recommends that *injectable* terbutaline should not be used in pregnant patients for prevention of PTL or prolonged treatment (beyond 48–72 hours) secondary to the risk of maternal cardiac problems and death (see http://www.fda.gov/drugs/drugsafety/ucm243539.htm).

Pregnancy Considerations

⚡ **Black-Box Warning:** Terbutaline is not FDA approved and should not be used for prolonged tocolysis (more than 48 to 72 hours). Adverse events observed in pregnant patients include arrhythmias, increased heart rate, hyperglycemia, hypokalemia, myocardial ischemia, and pulmonary edema. Heart rate may be increased in the fetus, and hypoglycemia in neonates has been observed.

TABLE 52.4 Drugs Used to Decrease Uterine Contractility

Generic	Route and Dosage	Uses and Considerations
Beta-Adrenergic Agents		
Terbutaline	Subcut: 0.25 mg q20min–3h; hold for pulse >120 beats/min. Continuous Subcut infusion 50–100 mcg/h; *max:* 100 mcg/h Follow agency protocol for specific directives plus individual health care provider's orders. See ⚡ Black-Box Warning.[a]	Relaxes bronchial and uterine smooth muscle by acting on β_2-receptors. Used for acute, short-term, less than 72h tocolysis "off-label" use. Partially metabolized in liver, excreted in urine and feces. Drug rapidly crosses the placenta, increases maternal pulse and FHR; monitor MHR. Breast-feeding is *not* contraindicated because of short half-life. Additive effect with CNS depressants (narcotics, sedative-hypnotics) and neuromuscular blocking agents. *Contraindication:* Hypersensitivity to terbutaline, sympathomimetic amines, or any component of the formulation. Pregnancy Considerations: Crosses the placenta. US ⚠ *Black-Box Warning:* Not FDA approved for prolonged tocolysis. May be used for 48 hours, short-term prolongation of pregnancy to allow for administration of antenatal steroids. Should not be used before fetal viability or when the risks of use to the fetus or mother are greater than the risk of preterm birth. Onset: 6–15 min; PB: 25%; peak: 30–60 min; duration: 1.5–4 h; t½: 2.9–14 h.
Calcium Antagonists		
Magnesium sulfate	See Table 52.6	

CNS, Central nervous system; *cont*, continuous; *FHR*, fetal heart rate; *h*, hour; *max*, maximum; *MHR*, maternal heart rate; *min*, minutes; *PB*, protein binding; *q*, every; *subcut*, subcutaneously; *t½*, half-life.

[a]*Black-Box Warning:* The US Food and Drug Administration has concluded that the risk of serious adverse events outweighs any potential benefit to pregnant patients receiving prolonged tocolytic treatment beyond 48–72 hours.

PATIENT SAFETY

Do Not Confuse...
- **Methylergonovine**, used to *stimulate* uterine contractions in the prevention and treatment of postpartum hemorrhage, with **terbutaline sulfate**, used to *decrease* uterine contractions in PTL. These drugs have the same packaging but opposite actions. Both are amber ampules with amber plastic packaging and colored neckbands wrapped in foil. Do not store together. Manufacturers of terbutaline are now packaging this drug in vials, but some ampules may still be in ⚡ circulation.

Pharmacokinetics
Patients with contractions may be initially given subcutaneous terbutaline 0.25 mg every 20 minutes to 3 hours if the maternal pulse is less than 120 beats/min. Patients are monitored to determine whether and when contractions diminish or cease. Terbutaline is minimally protein bound (25%) and is metabolized via the liver to inactive metabolites. Its half-life is 11 to 16 hours.

Pharmacodynamics
Subcutaneous terbutaline has an onset of action of 6 to 15 minutes, a peak serum concentration level in 30 to 60 minutes, and a duration of action of 1.5 to 4 hours subcutaneously.

Adverse Reactions
Maternal side effects include tremors, dizziness, nervousness, tachycardia, hypotension, chest pain, palpitations, nausea, vomiting, hyperglycemia, and hypokalemia. Many of these effects are associated with terbutaline's cross-reactivity with β_1-adrenergic receptors. More serious adverse reactions include pulmonary edema, dysrhythmias, ketoacidosis, and anaphylactic shock. Fetal side effects include tachycardia and potential hypoglycemia resulting from fetal hyperinsulinemia caused by maternal hyperglycemia. Terbutaline is contraindicated in patients with cardiac disease and in those with poorly controlled hyperthyroidism or diabetes mellitus.

Drug Interactions
The increased effects of general anesthetics can produce additive hypotension. Pulmonary edema can occur with concurrent use of corticosteroids. Cardiovascular effects may be additive with other sympathomimetic drugs.

Magnesium Sulfate

Parenteral magnesium sulfate, a calcium antagonist and central nervous system (CNS) depressant, relaxes the smooth muscle of the uterus through calcium displacement and can be given as an "off-label" use for PTL. Administered intravenously, the drug has a direct depressant effect on uterine muscle contractility. This drug is excreted by the kidneys and crosses the placenta. Magnesium sulfate is administered as a 4 to 6 g IV loading dose over 20 to 30 minutes followed by a 1 to 2 g/h for at least 24 hours. Magnesium sulfate can be used up to 48 hours in patients at risk of delivery within 7 days; however, it is not the preferred tocolytic. Magnesium sulfate therapy is contraindicated in patients who have myasthenia gravis, neuromuscular disease, impaired kidney function, or recent myocardial infarction (MI). Patients with renal impairment may require adjusted dosages.

Adverse Reactions
Dosage-related side effects in the patient include flushing, feelings of increased warmth, perspiration, dizziness, nausea, headache, lethargy, slurred speech, sluggishness, nasal congestion, heavy eyelids, blurred vision, decreased GI action, increased pulse rate, and hypotension. Increased severity is evidenced by depressed reflexes, confusion, and magnesium toxicity (respiratory depression and arrest, circulatory collapse, cardiac arrest). Decreased fetal heart rate (FHR) variability is one side effect, and side effects in the neonate are respiratory depression, slight hypotonia with diminished reflexes, and lethargy for 24 to 48 hours. If maternal neurologic, respiratory, or cardiac depression is evidenced, the antidote is calcium gluconate (1 g IV push over 3 minutes).

Nursing Interventions During Tocolytic Therapy
- Monitor vital signs, FHR, fetal activity, and uterine activity as ordered. Report respirations of fewer than 12 per minute, which may indicate magnesium sulfate toxicity.
- Monitor intake and output (I&O). Report urinary output below 30 mL/h.
- Assess breath and bowel sounds as ordered or at least every 4 hours.
- Assess deep tendon reflexes (DTRs) and clonus before initiation of therapy and as ordered. Notify the health care provider of changes in DTRs (areflexia or hyporeflexia) and clonus.
- Assess pain and uterine contractions.

🎯 CLINICAL JUDGMENT [NURSING PROCESS]

Beta$_2$-Adrenergic Agonists: Terbutaline

Concept: Reproduction
- Reproduction is the process by which offspring is produced. Nurses perform assessments on their antepartum patients to determine course of drugs and care.

Recognize Cues [Assessment]
- Identify risks for preterm labor (PTL) early in pregnancy.
- When a patient has preterm uterine contractions, obtain a history, complete physical assessment, vital signs, fetal heart rate (FHR), and urine specimen for screening for intrauterine infection and urinary tract infection.

Analyze Cues and Prioritize Hypothesis [Patient Problems]
- Anxiety
- Potential for decreased adherence
- Need for patient teaching

Generate Solutions [Planning]
- The patient will remain free of uterine contractions.
- The patient will verbalize the need to maintain fluid intake to decrease contractions.
- The patient will maintain a left-side lying position.
- The patient will remain free of progressive cervical change.

Take Action [Nursing Interventions]
- Monitor vital signs, FHR, and fetal and uterine activity as ordered.
- Maintain the patient in a left lateral position as much as possible to facilitate uteroplacental perfusion.
- Monitor vital signs per facility's protocol, specifically maternal pulse. Report maternal heart rate (MHR) greater than 130 beats/min.
- Report auscultated cardiac dysrhythmias. An electrocardiogram may be ordered.

CLINICAL JUDGMENT [NURSING PROCESS]—CONT'D
Beta₂-Adrenergic Agonists: Terbutaline

- Auscultate breath sounds every 4 hours. Notify the health care provider if respirations are more than 30 per minute, or <12 per minute, or if the breath quality changes (e.g., wheezes, rales, coughing).
- Monitor daily weight at the same time every day to assess fluid overload; implement strict intake and output (I&O) measurement.
- Report baseline FHR over 180 beats/min or any significant increase in uterine contractions from pretreatment baseline.
- Report persistence of uterine contractions despite tocolytic therapy.
- Report leakage of amniotic fluid, vaginal bleeding or discharge, and complaints of rectal pressure.
- Assess for the presence of maternal hyperglycemia and hypokalemia and hypoglycemia in the newborn delivered within 5 hours of discontinued β-sympathomimetic drugs.

Patient Teaching
General
- Advise the patient of signs and symptoms of PTL: menstrual-type cramps, sensations of pelvic pressure, low backache, increased vaginal discharge, and abdominal discomfort.

- Instruct the patient who experiences PTL contractions that her initial action should be to void, recline on her left side to increase uterine blood flow, and drink extra fluids. Emphasize that she should notify her health care provider if uterine contractions do not cease or if they increase in frequency.
- Explain side effects of β-sympathomimetic drugs. Report heart palpitations or dizziness to the health care provider.
- Advise the patient to contact her health care provider before taking any other drugs while on tocolytic drug therapy.

Evaluate Outcomes [Evaluation]
- Evaluate effectiveness of the tocolytic drug by noting six or fewer uterine contractions in 1 hour or per the health care provider's order.
- Evaluate the patient's understanding of nonpharmacologic measures for decreasing preterm contractions: bed rest, increasing oral fluid intake, pelvic rest, and lying on the left side.
- Continue monitoring the patient's vital signs, FHR, and uterine activity. Report any change immediately.

- Weigh daily at the same time.
- Monitor serum magnesium levels as ordered (therapeutic level is 4–7 mg/dL).
- Have available calcium gluconate (1 g given IV over 3 minutes) as an antidote.
- Assess the newborn for 24 to 48 hours for magnesium effects if drug was given to the mother before delivery.

CORTICOSTEROID THERAPY IN PRETERM LABOR

The desired outcome of tocolytic therapy is to delay birth long enough to allow time for corticosteroids to reach maximum benefit. Patients at risk for preterm delivery (24–34 weeks' gestation) should receive antenatal corticosteroid therapy with betamethasone or dexamethasone. An off-label use, administration of antenatal corticosteroids accelerates lung maturation and lung surfactant development in the fetus in utero, decreasing the incidence and severity of respiratory distress syndrome (RDS) and increasing survival of preterm infants. Antenatal therapy decreases infant mortality, RDS, and intraventricular bleeds in neonates born between 24 and 34 gestational weeks. The effects and benefits of corticosteroid administration are believed to begin 24 hours after administration with a duration of up to 1 week. The goal is to delay delivery by 48 hours to maximize the effect of the glucocorticoids.

Surfactant
Surfactant is made up of two major phospholipids: sphingomyelin and lecithin. Sphingomyelin initially develops in greater quantity than lecithin from about the 24th week. However, by the 33rd to 35th weeks of gestation, lecithin production peaks, making the ratio of the two substances about 2:1 in favor of lecithin. This lecithin/sphingomyelin (L/S) ratio is measured in the amniotic fluid and is a predictor of fetal lung maturity and risk for neonatal RDS.

Patients with gestational hypertension, PROM, placental insufficiency, or some types of diabetes and those who misuse narcotics may have amniotic fluid with higher than expected L/S ratios for the gestational date because of a stress-induced increase in endogenous corticosteroid production.

Betamethasone
Betamethasone is recommended for patients between 24 and 34 weeks of gestation, including those with ruptured membranes or multiple gestations, who are at risk of delivering within 7 days. A single course of 12 mg IM every 24 hours for a total of 2 doses may be appropriate in some patients beginning at 23 weeks' gestation or late preterm between 34 and 36 weeks and 6 days. A single repeat course may be considered in some patients with pregnancies less than 34 weeks' gestation at risk for delivering within 7 days and who had their last dose of corticosteroids more than 14 days prior.

Adverse Reactions
Side effects of betamethasone include headache, vertigo, edema, bradycardia, arrhythmias, malaise, hypertension, increased sweating, petechiae, ecchymoses, facial erythema, and seizures.

Dexamethasone
In clinical controlled trials, evidence is insufficient to recommend betamethasone over dexamethasone, because the two have not been directly compared. Investigations have noted a trend of decreased risk of neonatal cystic periventricular leukomalacia and intraventricular hemorrhage with exposure to betamethasone over dexamethasone. Dexamethasone has a rapid onset of action and a shorter duration; therefore it must be prescribed in a shorter frequency compared with betamethasone. The recommended antepartum regimen for dexamethasone is 6 mg IM every 12 hours for 4 doses.

> ⚡ **PATIENT SAFETY**
>
> **Do Not Confuse …**
> - **Dexamethasone**, a corticosteroid used to accelerate fetal lung maturity during weeks 24–34 of gestation, with **desoximetasone**, which is used to treat inflammation from corticosteroid-responsive dermatoses.

TABLE 52.5 Prenatal Therapy for Surfactant Development

Generic	Route and Dosage	Uses and Considerations
Betamethasone	A: Pregnant females IM: 12 mg q24h × 2 dose	Corticosteroid. Given to prevent RDS in preterm infants by injecting the mother before delivery to stimulate surfactant production in fetal lung. Not effective in treating preterm infant after delivery. Most effective if given at least 24 h (preferably 48–72 h) but less than 7 d before delivery in week 33 or before. Contraindicated in severe gestational hypertension and in systemic fungal infection. Simultaneous use with terbutaline may enhance risk for pulmonary edema. Not usually given with ruptured membranes; may mask signs of chorioamnionitis. Metabolized in liver and excreted by kidneys; crosses placenta; enters breast milk. Therapy less effective with multifetal birth and with male infants. Pregnancy Considerations: Crosses the placenta. Recommended for females between 24 and 34 weeks' gestation who are at risk of delivering within 7 days. A single course may be considered for females beginning at 23 weeks' gestation who are at risk for delivering within 7 days. Multiple repeat courses are not recommended; however, in females with pregnancies less than 34 weeks at risk for delivery within 7 days who had a course greater than 14 days prior, a repeat course may be considered. PB: 64%; onset: 1–3 h; peak: 10–36 min; duration: 7–14 d; t½: 6.5 h
Dexamethasone	IM: 6 mg q12h × 4 doses	Same as betamethasone but shorter half-life and more significant variation in circulating serum levels. Pregnancy Considerations: Same as betamethasone.

d, Days; *h*, hours; *IM*, intramuscular; *IV*, intravenous; *min*, minutes; *PB*, protein binding; *q*, every; *RDS*, respiratory distress syndrome; *t½*, half-life.

Adverse Reactions

The potential adverse reactions associated with dexamethasone therapy include insomnia, nervousness, increased appetite, headache, hypersensitivity reactions, and arthralgias. Table 52.5 lists the prenatal drugs used for surfactant development and their dosages, uses, and considerations.

DRUGS FOR GESTATIONAL HYPERTENSION

Gestational Hypertension

Gestational hypertension, elevated blood pressure (BP) after 20 gestational weeks in patients normotensive before pregnancy, is the most common serious complication of pregnancy and can have devastating maternal and fetal effects. Gestational hypertension has replaced the term *pregnancy-induced hypertension*, still commonly used in clinical discussions but no longer correct. With proper management of gestational hypertension, the prognosis for both patient and infant is good. Hypertensive disorders are reported in 10% to 20% of all pregnant patients, with 5% to 8% of all pregnancies reflecting the incidence of preeclampsia (gestational hypertension with proteinuria). Historically, preeclampsia was the presence of hypertension (systolic BP >140 or diastolic BP >90) and proteinuria (>300 mg in a 24-hour urine collection) in a normotensive patient after 20 weeks' gestation. However, "The Task Force Report – Hypertension in Pregnancy" issued by ACOG in November 2013 concluded that preeclampsia can be diagnosed without high levels of protein in the urine.

The cause of preeclampsia remains unknown, although numerous hypotheses exist. The pathophysiology is believed to be related to decreased levels of vasodilating prostaglandins with resulting vasospasm. Preeclampsia stresses all organs of the body, resulting in severe hypertension, often increased protein in the urine, headaches, visual problems, and edema of the hands and feet. About 5% of preeclampsia patients progress to eclampsia, in which seizure activity occurs. Early diagnosis of preeclampsia with appropriate treatment keeps most patients from progressing to this stage.

CLINICAL JUDGMENT [NURSING PROCESS]

Betamethasone

Concept: Reproduction
- Reproduction is the process by which offspring is produced. Nurses perform assessments on their antepartum patients to determine course of drugs and care.

Recognize Cues [Assessment]
- Assess for history of hypersensitivity.
- Assess vital signs; report abnormal findings.
- Assess fetal heart rate (FHR).

Analyze Cues and Prioritize Hypotheses [Patient Problems]
- Anxiety
- Potential for decreased adherence
- Need for patient teaching

Generate Solutions [Planning]
- The patient will remain free of preterm uterine contractions for 24 hours allowing betamethasone to be delivered to improve fetal lung function

Take Action [Nursing Interventions]
- Shake the suspension well.
- Avoid exposing the suspension to excessive heat or light.
- Avoid local muscle atrophy; inject drug into a large muscle, not the deltoid.
- Monitor maternal vital signs.
- Maintain accurate input and output (I&O) measurements.
- Assess blood glucose in patients with diabetes mellitus.

Evaluate Outcomes [Evaluation]
- Continue monitoring patient vital signs. Report changes.
- Continue monitoring FHR. Report any changes.
- Monitor the neonate for hypoglycemia and presence of neonatal sepsis.

TABLE 52.6 Drugs Used in Severe Preeclampsia

Generic	Route and Dosage	Uses and Considerations
Magnesium sulfate	IV: 4–6 g loading dose in 100 mL over 20 min; followed by 2–4 g/h continuous infusion for at least 24 h postpartum IM: Same dose but is not the preferred route	Prevention and treatment of seizures related to preeclampsia. Calcium antagonist and CNS depressant. Decreases acetylcholine from motor nerves, which blocks neuromuscular transmission and decreases incidence of seizures. Secondary effect is reduction in BP as magnesium sulfate relaxes smooth muscle. Secondarily affects peripheral vascular system with increased uterine blood flow caused by vasodilation and some transient BP decrease during the first hour; also inhibits uterine contractions. Depresses DTRs and respiration; maintenance dose depends on reflexes, respiratory rate, urinary output, and magnesium level. Main risk is production of abnormally high serum magnesium levels. Therapeutic levels range from 4 to 7 mEq/L; effective in preventing seizures. Patient at risk if respiratory rate <12/min, urinary output <30 mL/h, DTR absent or hyporeflexic. Patellar reflexes disappear with serum magnesium levels of 8–10 mEq/L. Maternal respiratory depression may occur with levels >10–15 mEq/L; cardiac arrest occurs with levels >20–25 mEq/L. Notify health care provider if any of the previously discussed issues occur. Absorbed magnesium is excreted by kidneys; excreted in breast milk, but breast-feeding is not contraindicated. Use with caution in patients with renal impairment. Contraindicated in patients with myasthenia gravis. Relative contraindications: myocardial damage or heart block. Pregnancy Considerations: Although not recommended during 2 h before delivery, stopping magnesium before cesarean delivery is not recommended and can increase risk of ⚡ seizures. PB: 30%; onset: IV, immediate; IM, 1 h; duration: IV, 30 min; IM, 3–4 h; t½: UK Antidote: Calcium gluconate 1 g slow IV push over 3 min.
Hydralazine hydrochloride	IV: 5–10 mg q20min; *max cumulative total:* 20 mg or until BP is controlled	Antihypertensive agent. Causes arteriolar vasodilation. Usually lowers diastolic BP more than systolic BP. Objective is to maintain diastolic BP of 90–110 mm Hg. Usually well tolerated; maternal tachycardia and increased cardiac output and oxygen consumption may occur. Usually not given to pregnant preeclamptic patients with diastolic BP >105 mm Hg because of risk for reduced intervillous blood flow. Patients with impaired renal function may require lower doses. Pregnancy Considerations: Crosses the placenta. Recommended for use in the management of acute-onset, severe hypertension with preeclampsia or eclampsia in pregnant and postpartum females. Parenteral: Onset, 5–20 min; peak, 10–80 min; PB: 87%, duration, up to 12 hours; t½: 3–7 hours.
Methyldopa	PO: 250 mg bid, *max:* 3 g/d IV: 250–500 mg infused over 30–60 min q 6 h	Stimulates central α-adrenergic receptors, resulting in decreased sympathetic outflow to heart, kidneys, and peripheral vasculature. *Contraindication:* Hypersensitivity to drug or any component, active hepatic disease, liver disorders previously associated with use of methyldopa, concurrent use of MAOIs *Caution:* Sedation is usually transient during initial treatment and during dosage increases. Pregnancy Considerations: Used to treat chronic maternal hypertension during pregnancy; however, other agents are preferred for control of acute hypertension. Onset: 3–6 h; peak: 2–4 h; duration: 10–16 h (multiple doses: 24–48 h).
Labetalol	IV: 20 mg over 2 min May increase dose q 10 m by 20–40 mg to a max dose of 80 mg; *max cumulative dose:* 300 mg After the initial dose, may initiate a continuous infusion of 1–2 mg/min	Blocks α-, β₁-, and β₂-adrenergic receptor sites. Monitor BP and heart rate frequently. Adverse effects: orthostatic hypotension; dizziness; ventricular arrhythmia. Pregnancy Considerations: Recommended for the use in management of acute-onset, severe hypertension with preeclampsia or eclampsia in pregnant or postpartum females. ⚡ Onset: 2–5 min; peak: 5–15 min; duration: 2–18 h (dose dependent); t½: 5.5 h.

bid, Twice daily; *BP*, blood pressure; *CNS*, central nervous system; *d*, day; *DTR*, deep tendon reflex; *h*, hour; *IM*, intramuscular; *IV*, intravenous; *MAOI*, monoamine oxidase inhibitor; *max*, maximum; *min*, minutes; *PB*, protein binding; *PO*, by mouth; *q*, every; *t½*, half-life; *UK*, unknown.

One severe sequela of preeclampsia is defined by its symptoms—hemolysis, *e*levated *l*iver enzymes, and *l*ow *p*latelet count—and is therefore known as **HELLP syndrome**, which occurs in about 2% to 12% of patients with gestational hypertension. Patients who manifest severe preeclampsia are most likely to also have HELLP syndrome.

In addition to delivery of an uncompromised fetus and psychological support for the patient and family, two primary treatment goals in preeclampsia are reduction of vasospasm and prevention of seizures.

Delivery of the infant and placenta (products of conception) is the only known cure for preeclampsia. Vaginal delivery is preferred so that anesthesia and surgical risks will not be added. Labor induction via cervical ripening may be initiated to facilitate labor. For vaginal delivery, epidural anesthesia or combined epidural and spinal anesthesia is frequently performed for pain management while promoting uteroplacental circulation. Maternal hypotension is a significant concern for hypertensive patients who have epidurals. In contrast, patients with worsening preeclampsia or fetal distress may be delivered via cesarean section. Patients with HELLP syndrome may have their labor induced for a vaginal delivery at 32 or more weeks' gestation. For patients with HELLP syndrome who are at less than 32 weeks' gestation, cesarean delivery may be considered.

If HELLP syndrome progresses to the point of eclampsia (maternal seizure), delivery is generally postponed for 1 to 3 hours if fetal status allows. The labor induction or cesarean delivery is an additional stressor for the patient who exhibits acidosis and hypoxia resulting from seizure. Ideally, once vital signs are stabilized with improved urinary output and decreased acidosis/hypoxia, delivery is pursued.

Nonpharmacologic treatments for preeclampsia include activity reduction; lying on the left side; eating a nutritious, balanced diet; and drinking six to eight 8-ounce glasses of water a day. Studies have shown that nonpharmacologic treatments have not had clinically beneficial effects; therefore drug therapy is commonly used for treatment.

Drugs Used to Treat Preeclampsia

Methyldopa is considered the first-line therapy for mild preeclampsia because it has been widely used in pregnant patients and its safety and efficacy has been established.

Hydralazine is recommended for use in the management of acute-onset, severe hypertension (systolic BP ≥160 mm Hg or diastolic BP ≥110 mm Hg. Oral: immediate release 10 mg given, may repeat with 20 mg dose in 20 min if needed). If treatment for chronic hypertension of pregnancy is needed, other oral agents are preferred as initial therapy.

Magnesium sulfate is used for severe preeclampsia for prevention of eclampsia. Table 52.6 lists the commonly used drugs for treating preeclampsia along with their dosages, uses, and considerations.

Adverse Reactions of Methyldopa
Observe the patient for peripheral edema, anxiety, nightmares, drowsiness, headache, dry mouth, drug-induced fever, and mental depression. These are the most common potential adverse reactions.

Adverse Reactions of Hydralazine
Observe the patient for headache, nausea, vomiting, nasal congestion, dizziness, tachycardia, palpitations, and angina pectoris. Avoid a sudden decrease in maternal BP, which may cause fetal hypoxia.

Adverse Reactions of Magnesium Sulfate
Early signs of increased magnesium levels include lethargy, flushing, feelings of increased warmth, perspiration, thirst, sedation, heavy eyelids, slurred speech, hypotension, DTR, and decreased muscle tone. Therapeutic magnesium levels are 4 to 7 mEq/L. Loss of patellar reflexes is often the first sign of magnesium toxicity and may be seen at 8 to 10 mEq/L. Respiratory depression may manifest at levels greater than 10 to 15 mEq/L, and cardiac arrest may manifest at levels greater than 20 to 25 mEq/L.

Decreased variability is commonly seen on the FHR tracing. If the patient received magnesium sulfate close to the time of delivery, the neonate may exhibit low Apgar scores, hypotonia, lethargy, weakness, and potential respiratory distress. The fetal level of magnesium generally reaches more than 90% of maternal levels within 3 hours of administration, but the greater risk to the fetus is from maternal preeclampsia, with resulting decreased placental blood flow and intrauterine growth retardation.

CLINICAL JUDGMENT [NURSING PROCESS]
Gestational Hypertension

Concept: Perfusion
- Perfusion is the passage of blood and blood products through the circulatory system to organs or tissues to deliver oxygen and nutrients to cells, such as to the uterus and fetus.

Recognize Cues [Assessment]
- Review baseline vital signs from early pregnancy and blood pressure (BP) readings during prenatal visits.
- Identify patient history that may predispose the patient to preeclampsia.

Analyze Cues and Prioritize Hypotheses [Patient Problems]
- Hypertension
- Decreased tissue perfusion to the uterus and fetus
- Anxiety

Generate Solutions [Planning]
- The patient will maintain BP within acceptable ranges.
- The patient will verbalize understanding of preeclampsia and its etiology, signs and symptoms, and nonpharmacologic and pharmacologic treatment measures.
- The patient will understand and comply with the planned preeclampsia treatment regimen.
- The patient will maintain adequate perfusion to the fetus.
- The patient will maintain a therapeutic magnesium level.
- The patient will verbalize the need for a magnesium sulfate infusion for at least 24 hours postpartum.

Take Action [Nursing Interventions]
Magnesium Sulfate
- Provide continuous electronic fetal monitoring.
- Monitor for maternal toxicity. Lethargy and weakness resulting from blocking of neuromuscular transmission. Diaphoresis, flushing, feelings of warmth, and nasal congestion are results of vasodilation from relaxation of smooth muscle.
- Have available airway suction, resuscitation equipment, and emergency drugs in the event it is needed.
- Have available the antidote for magnesium sulfate in the event it is needed: calcium gluconate 1 g IV given over 3 minutes.
- Maintain the patient in a left lateral recumbent position in a low-stimulation environment. Provide close observation and monitoring.
- Monitor BP, pulse, and respiratory rate per agency protocol; monitor deep tendon reflexes (DTRs), clonus, and intake and output (I&O) every hour. Some health care providers will request manual BP measurements.
- Monitor temperature, breath sounds, and bowel sounds every 4 hours.
- Assess the patient's urine for protein every hour.
- Assess for epigastric pain, headache, visual symptoms (blurred vision and scotoma), sensory changes, edema, level of consciousness, and seizure activity on an ongoing basis.
- Monitor serum magnesium levels according to agency protocol for a range between 4 and 7 mEq/L.
- Immediately notify the health care provider if the patient experiences a decrease or change in their level of consciousness; fewer than 12 respirations per minute; absence of DTR; urinary output below 30 mL/h; systolic BP of 160 mm Hg or more, unless ordered otherwise; magnesium level greater than 7 mEq/L; absent bowel sounds or altered breath sounds; epigastric pain or right upper quadrant pain (associated with hepatic edema causing stretching of the liver capsule); headache; visual symptoms (blurred vision and scotoma); sensory changes; change in affect or level of consciousness; or seizure activity.

CLINICAL JUDGMENT [NURSING PROCESS]—CONT'D

Gestational Hypertension

- Monitor laboratory reports for low platelet count, elevated liver enzymes (aspartate aminotransferase, lactate dehydrogenase), and bilirubin levels. Observe for evidence of excessive bleeding.
- Monitor fetal status. Fetal heart rate (FHR) baseline should remain at 110–160 beats/min.
- Monitor 24-hour urinary protein laboratory results if ordered (≥300 mg/day is abnormal).
- Monitor the patient for signs and symptoms of magnesium toxicity.
- Monitor the newborn patient for effects of placental exposure to excess magnesium sulfate. Although infrequent, newborn side effects include lethargy, neurologic or respiratory depression, and muscle hypotonia.

Hydralazine

- Monitor BP frequently with an electronic BP monitoring device during drug administration.
- Maintain maintenance of diastolic BP between 90 and 110 mm Hg or as ordered.
- Observe for changes in level of consciousness and headache.
- Monitor I&O to avoid deficiency (hypotensive episodes) or overload (hypertension).
- Monitor FHR.

Patient Teaching

General

- Explain preeclampsia and its implications for the patient, fetus, and newborn.
- Provide information about nonpharmacologic and pharmacologic treatment measures for preeclampsia.
- Advise avoiding exposure to the common cold, flu, and other infectious diseases.
- Instruct the patient with diabetes to have their glucose level taken as ordered.

Side Effects

- Advise the patient to report immediately any breathing difficulty, weakness, or dizziness.
- Advise the patient to report changes in stool, easy bruising, bleeding, blurred vision, unusual weight gain, and emotional changes.

Safety

- Advise the patient to lie in the left lateral recumbent position and explain the rationale.
- Instruct the patient in the signs and symptoms of progressive preeclampsia and when to seek medical assistance.
- Instruct the patient that fetal well-being will be assessed through biophysical profile (BPP), nonstress test (NST), or contraction stress test at frequent intervals, depending on the health care provider and preeclampsia severity (e.g., NST and/or BPP 1–2 times per week until delivery).
- Instruct the parents regarding the possibility of seizures and appropriate actions if a seizure occurs.

Diet

- Provide nutritional counseling regarding a nutritious, balanced diet.
- Discuss the importance of adequate fluid intake.

Magnesium Sulfate

- Instruct the patient in the necessity of having an indwelling catheter, infusion pump, continuous fetal monitoring, and assessment of DTRs and clonus. Explain that therapy will extend into the postpartum period 24–48 hours, depending on the agency and health care provider.
- Instruct the patient about visitor restrictions and the need for a low-stimulation environment.
- Advise the patient that a flushing feeling or a warm sensation may occur.
- Advise the patient nausea and vomiting during the initial loading dose may occur.
- Advise the patient that evidence of magnesium levels within the therapeutic range includes decreased appetite, some speech slurring, double vision, and weakness.

Hydralazine

- Instruct the patient that after administration their BP and pulse will be constantly monitored until the patient remains stable, then every 15 minutes thereafter. Explain that an electronic BP monitor may be used to obtain constant readings. Some health care providers will request manual BP measurements.
- Instruct the patient in the need for careful monitoring of their I&O.
- Advise the patient it is possible they may experience a headache as a side effect of the drug.

Evaluate Outcomes [Evaluation]

- Evaluate effectiveness of therapy to reduce BP.
- Continue monitoring vital signs. Report any changes.
- Document the patient's response to the teaching and learning opportunities provided for instruction.
- Document any knowledge deficits concerning preeclampsia treatment modalities and outcomes.
- Assess and document the fetal well-being secondary to treatment with drugs as evidenced by fetal monitoring and fetal movement assessment.
- Monitor maternal physiologic changes in relation to magnesium sulfate levels.
- Continue monitoring FHR. Report any changes.

CLINICAL JUDGMENT CASE STUDY

A 30-year-old female (gravida 3, para 0) has a history of spontaneous abortion at 10 weeks' gestation and a preterm delivery and demise of a neonate at 21 weeks' gestation. At her 28-week prenatal visit, she reports increased clear vaginal discharge and feelings of pelvic pressure. Examination of her cervix reveals 2-cm dilation and a presenting fetal part low in the pelvis. The patient is admitted to the hospital, and uterine activity is documented. Magnesium sulfate therapy is ordered for treatment of preterm labor. The nurse prepares for IV magnesium sulfate administration.

1. How will magnesium sulfate therapy be initiated? What intervals and dosages should be anticipated?
2. What maternal and fetal side effects will the nurse expect to observe?
3. What would the patient be told about the drug effects she will experience?
4. How would the nurse respond to the patient's questions about the risks of preterm delivery?
5. After 24 hours of magnesium sulfate therapy, uterine contractions have been reduced to two to three per hour. The patient is to be discharged home, and the nurse is preparing her discharge teaching.
6. What instructions would the nurse give the patient about her activity and diet?
7. The patient asks whether the side effects of magnesium sulfate will continue. What is an appropriate nursing response?
8. What signs and symptoms would the patient be advised to report?

REVIEW QUESTIONS

1. A patient in her first trimester of pregnancy calls the nurse to ask for suggestions on decreasing nausea in the morning when she awakens. Which nonpharmacologic measures would the nurse be aware of to decrease nausea and vomiting? **Select all that apply.**
   a. Eating dry toast before rising
   b. Eating small frequent meals
   c. Eating a high-protein bedtime snack
   d. Eating high-fat foods

2. When nonpharmacologic treatment fails for constipation, which drug would be a first-line treatment for constipation during pregnancy?
   a. Docusate sodium
   b. Magnesium citrate
   c. Castor oil
   d. Mineral oil

3. The nurse is teaching a pregnant patient how to decrease the gastrointestinal distress she experiences with prenatal vitamins. Which instruction would the nurse provide?
   a. Take her vitamins between meals
   b. Eat when she takes her vitamins
   c. Drink orange juice when she takes her vitamins
   d. Drink milk when she takes her vitamins

4. The nurse, working with a preconceptional couple at an infertility clinic, advises the female to take which supplement for at least 3 months before becoming pregnant?
   a. Iron
   b. Ginger
   c. Folic acid
   d. Vitamin B_6

5. A patient with severe preeclampsia is on magnesium sulfate. Which initial action by the nurse would be most appropriate for a magnesium sulfate level of 7 mEq/L?
   a. Continue to monitor the patient because this level is therapeutic.
   b. Contact the health care provider and report the level.
   c. Prepare to administer 1 g of calcium gluconate.
   d. Turn the patient on her left side, and administer 10 liters of oxygen by nasal cannula.

6. Which assessment finding is most concerning when examining a patient in preterm labor who is receiving magnesium sulfate?
   a. Feelings of lethargy
   b. Feelings of warmth
   c. Loss of patellar reflexes
   d. Positive clonus +2 bilaterally

7. The patient has been receiving magnesium sulfate intravenously for 24 hours to treat severe preeclampsia. On assessment, the nurse finds a temperature of 37.3°C (99°F), pulse of 88, respirations at 14, blood pressure of 138/76, 2+ patellar reflexes, and negative ankle clonus. Which intervention would be most appropriate for the nurse to take?
   a. Obtain a stat magnesium sulfate level.
   b. Discontinue magnesium sulfate.
   c. Contact the health care provider.
   d. Continue to monitor the patient.

8. A primigravida patient, 8 gestational weeks, is at the prenatal clinic for her first examination with complaints of nausea and vomiting "every morning." Which comment made by the patient would indicate the need for further instruction?
   a. "My friend gave me ginger cookies to eat."
   b. "I have been eating dry crackers before I get up."
   c. "I have tried to avoid foods with strong smells."
   d. "I have been drinking chamomile tea every day."

9. The nurse working in labor and delivery is reviewing messages to be returned to patients. Which statement made by the patient would the nurse respond to first?
   a. "I'm 32 weeks pregnant and taking calcium carbonate for my heartburn. Is there anything else I can take?"
   b. "I'm 38 weeks pregnant and taking ibuprofen for my backache. Should I take aspirin too?"
   c. "I'm 8 weeks pregnant and taking folic acid. Will it hurt me or the baby if I stop?"
   d. "I checked my blood glucose with a friend's machine, and it was 120 mg/dL. I'm not diabetic. Is that normal?"

10. A young adolescent—gravida 1, para 0—is admitted to labor and delivery with preterm labor at 29 weeks' gestation. Which nursing interventions would the nurse include? **Select all that apply.**
    a. Administration of antenatal glucocorticoid
    b. Order a complete liver function profile
    c. Bed rest in the left lateral position
    d. Administration of bolus intravenous fluids
    e. Administration of tocolytics
    f. Administration of an antihypertensive

11. A patient is planning to become pregnant. Which actions would the nurse counsel the patient to initiate before she stops taking her oral contraceptive? **Select all that apply.**
    a. Stop smoking immediately.
    b. Take omega-6 fatty acids every day.
    c. Take a multivitamin every day.
    d. Stop taking over-the-counter acetaminophen.
    e. See her health care provider.

53

Labor, Delivery, and Postpartum

Christina DiMaggio Boudreaux, RN, BSN, IBCLC

http://evolve.elsevier.com/McCuistion/pharmacology

OBJECTIVES

- Relate principles of nursing care to the use of drugs for pain control during labor.
- Relate principles of nursing care to the use of drugs that enhance uterine muscle contractility.
- Relate principles of nursing care to the use of drugs during the postpartum period.
- Relate principles of nursing care to the use of immunizations in pregnancy.

OUTLINE

Drugs for Pain Control During Labor, 689
    Analgesics and Sedation, 690
    Regional Anesthesia, 692
    General Anesthesia, 695
    Local Anesthesia, 695
Drugs That Enhance Uterine Muscle Contractility, 696
    Oxytocin, 699
    Other Drugs That Enhance Uterine Contractions: Ergot Alkaloids, 699
Drugs Used During the Postpartum Period, 700
    Pain Relief for Uterine Contractions, 702
    Pain Relief for Perineal Wounds and Hemorrhoids, 702
    Promotion of Bowel Function, 703
    Lactation Suppression, 704
    Postpartum Depression, 704
Immunizations, 705
    $Rh_0(D)$ Immune Globulin, 705
    Rubella Vaccine, 705
Clinical Judgment Case Study, 706
Review Questions, 707

DRUGS FOR PAIN CONTROL DURING LABOR

Labor and delivery are divided into four stages. During the first stage, the *dilating stage*, cervical effacement and dilation occur; the cervix thins and becomes fully dilated at 10 cm. The first stage consists of three phases categorized by cervical dilation: the *latent phase* (0–4 cm), the *active phase* (4–7 cm), and the *transition phase* (8–10 cm). The second stage of labor, the *pelvic stage*, begins with complete cervical dilation and ends with delivery of the newborn. During the third stage of labor, *placental separation and expulsion*, the placenta separates from the uterine wall and is delivered. The fourth stage of labor, *early postpartum*, comprises the first 4 hours after the delivery of the placenta and is a period of physiologic stabilization for the mother and initiation of familial attachment.

During the first stage of labor, uterine contractions produce progressive cervical effacement and dilation. As the first stage of labor progresses, uterine contractions become stronger, longer, and more frequent, and discomfort increases. Pain and discomfort in labor are caused by uterine contraction, cervical dilation and effacement, hypoxia of the contracting myometrium, and perineal pressure from the presenting part. Pain perception is influenced by physiologic, psychological, social, and cultural factors—in particular, the patient's past experiences with pain, anticipation of pain, fear and anxiety, knowledge deficit of the labor and delivery process, and involvement of support persons.

Before administering pharmacologic treatment, nonpharmacologic measures should be initiated. Nonpharmacologic measures for pain relief during labor include (1) ambulation, (2) effleurage and counterpressure, (3) touch and massage, (4) changing positions and rocking, (5) engaging support persons, (6) breathing and relaxation techniques, (7) transcutaneous electrical nerve stimulation, (8) application of heat and cold, (9) aromatherapy, and (10) hydrotherapy (warm-water baths or showers).

Other nonpharmacologic measures include alternative and complementary drugs. Of particular concern is the use of herbal supplements, especially in late pregnancy, to stimulate labor. Patients may self-administer, or the practice may be part of their traditional beliefs and framework of health. Concerns with herbal supplements are related to the often numerous physiologically active components of the herbs, adulterants, inconsistent dosing, and lack of proven efficacy. Herbs taken in late pregnancy may contribute to preterm labor or increased bleeding during delivery. Nurses must be sensitive to the use of herbal supplements and health practices during pregnancy, specifically in the later gestational weeks.

When pharmacologic intervention is needed for pain relief, drugs are used as an adjunct to nonpharmacologic measures. Drugs should be selected not only to decrease the patient's pain but also to minimize side effects for the patient and the fetus or neonate. Pain relief during labor can be obtained with systemic analgesics and regional anesthesia; that is, injection of a drug near the nerves or spinal canal to numb a specific area of the body (Fig. 53.1). Analgesics alter the patient's perception and sensation of pain without producing unconsciousness.

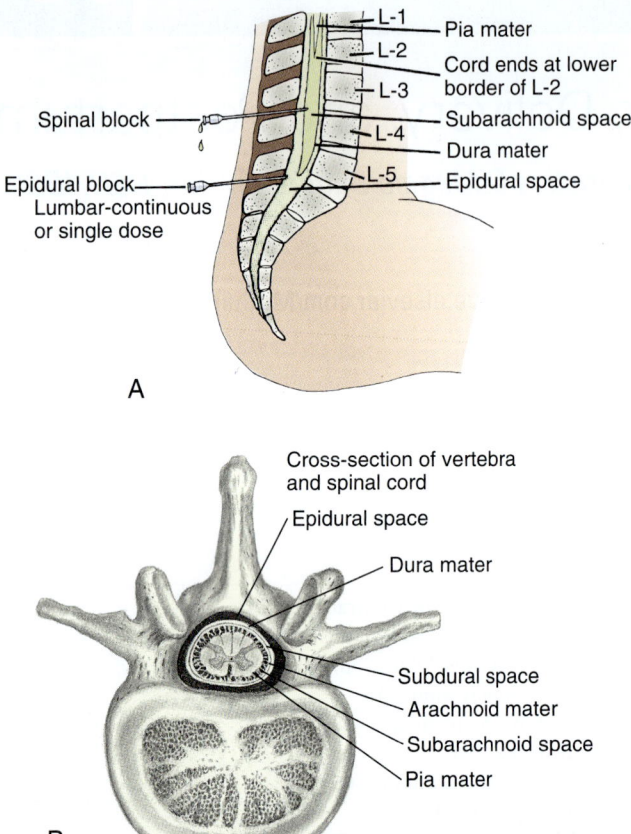

Fig. 53.1 (A) Membranes and spaces of spinal cord and levels of sacral, lumbar, and thoracic nerves. (B) Cross-section of vertebra and spinal cord. (From Lowdermilk D, Perry S, Cashion C, Alden K: *Maternity and women's health care*, ed 10, St. Louis, 2012, Mosby.)

Analgesics and Sedation

Systemic drugs used during labor include sedative-hypnotics, opioid agonists, and mixed opioid agonist-antagonists. These drugs should be administered at the onset of the uterine contraction because parenteral administration at the onset decreases neonatal drug exposure because blood flow is decreased to the uterus and fetus.

Table 53.1 lists the analgesics and sedatives commonly used during labor, delivery, and postpartum and their dosages, uses, and considerations.

The sedative-tranquilizer drugs are most often given for false or latent labor or with ruptured membranes without true labor. These drugs may also be administered to minimize maternal anxiety and fear. Although they promote rest and relaxation, they do not provide pain relief. The sedative drugs most used are barbiturates or hypnotics (e.g., pentobarbital sodium). The warning listed with this drug is only recommended in pregnancy when there are no alternatives and the benefits outweigh the risks. ⚡ One brand name of this drug that is discontinued in the United States at this time is Nembutal. Other drugs, such as hydroxyzine, can be given alone during early labor or in combination with opioid agonists when the patient is in active labor. In addition to decreasing anxiety and apprehension, hydroxyzine potentiates the analgesic action of opioids and minimizes emesis. Promethazine, also a phenothiazine derivative, has been noted in studies to impair the analgesic efficacy of opioids and is now only labeled for nausea and vomiting.

> ⚡ **PATIENT SAFETY**
>
> **Do Not Confuse...**
> - Pentobarbital with phenobarbital.

The second group of drugs given for active labor is the opioid agonists. These drugs may be administered parenterally or via regional blocks. When administered with neuraxial anesthesia, a lower dose of anesthetic is required for effective pain relief, thereby minimizing side effects. These drugs interfere with pain impulses at the subcortical level of the brain. Opioids interact with the mu and kappa receptors.

Of the narcotic agonists, meperidine was the most prescribed synthetic opioid for pain control during labor for many years; however, current guidelines do not recommend it to treat pain during labor. Opioids are further discussed in Chapter 25.

The third group of systemic drugs used for pain relief in labor is opioids with mixed opioid agonist-antagonist effects. These drugs exert their effects at more than one site and are often an agonist at one site and an antagonist at another. The two most used opioid agonist-antagonist drugs are butorphanol tartrate and nalbuphine.

Side Effects and Adverse Reactions

Adverse effects of sedative-hypnotic drugs (pentobarbital) include paradoxically increased pain and excitability, lethargy, subdued mood, decreased sensory perception, and hypotension. Fetal and neonatal side effects include decreased fetal heart rate (FHR) variability; neonatal respiratory depression, sleepiness, hypotonia; and delayed breastfeeding with poor sucking response for up to 4 ⚡ days.

Side effects of phenothiazine derivatives and antiemetic antihistamines (e.g., promethazine, hydroxyzine) include confusion, disorientation, excess sedation, dizziness, hypotension, tachycardia, blurred vision, headache, restlessness, weakness, and urinary retention with promethazine; drowsiness, dry mouth, dizziness, headache, blurred vision, dysuria, urinary retention, and constipation can occur with hydroxyzine. Decreased FHR variability can occur, and the neonate can experience moderate central nervous system (CNS) depression, hypotonia, lethargy, poor feeding, and ⚡ hypothermia.

The adverse effects of opioids depend on the responses activated by the mu and kappa receptors. Activation of mu receptors results in analgesia, sedation, euphoria, decreased gastrointestinal (GI) motility, respiratory depression, and physiologic dependence. Activation of kappa receptors results in analgesia, decreased GI motility, miosis, and sedation. When parenterally administered, the side effects of opioids include nausea, vomiting, sedation, orthostatic hypotension, pruritus, and maternal and neonatal respiratory depression. The associated nausea and vomiting result from stimulation of the chemoreceptor trigger zone in the medulla. Motor block is another concern; mothers may not walk after delivery until they are able to maintain a straight leg raise against downward pressure applied by the practitioner. Fetal and neonatal effects include decreased FHR variability, depression of neonatal respirations, and depression of neonatal neurobehavior. Through inhibition of both mu and kappa receptors, if naloxone must be given, naloxone may reverse the effects of opioids, resulting in a subsequent increase in maternal pain.

Opioid agonist drugs can cause orthostatic hypotension, nausea, vomiting, headache, sedation, hypotension, confusion, decreased FHR variability, and neonatal CNS depression.

Mixed opioid agonist-antagonist drugs (e.g., butorphanol tartrate, nalbuphine) can cause nausea, clamminess, sweating, sedation,

TABLE 53.1 Analgesics Used During Labor, Delivery, and Postpartum

Drug	Route and Dosage	Uses and Considerations
Sedative-Hypnotics		
Pentobarbital	IV: 100 mg (common initial dose for 70 kg patient). IM: 150–200 mg use as a reduced dosage in patients who are debilitated.	Short-acting barbiturate and sedative for latent phase of labor Mechanism of action: Depresses the sensory cortex, decreases motor activity, alters cerebella function, and produces sedation Side effects: Bradycardia, hypotension, syncope, anxiety, confusion, and hallucinations Onset: Immediate: 3–5 min. PB: 45%–70%; t½: 15–50 h ⚡ An increased incidence of fetal abnormalities may occur after maternal use. Respiratory depression may occur in the newborn when administered to the mother during labor; resuscitation equipment should be readily available. Not contraindicated but should be used with caution.
Promethazine	IM/IV: Early labor: 50 mg Established labor: 25–75 mg in combination with analgesic at reduced dosage; may repeat every 4 h for up to 2 additional doses (*Max:* 100 mg/d while in labor)	A phenothiazine antihistamine and antiemetic given with opioids as an adjunct to increase sedation and reduce nausea and vomiting in labor. Do not give subcutaneously. ⚡ *Black-Box Warning:* Severe tissue damage has been seen with injections and extravasation, which can result in necrosis and gangrene; use the Z-track method for IM injection to prevent or reduce complications, and dilute IV doses and give over 10–15 min. Instruct patients to report signs of pain and burning with administration. Side effects: Blurred vision, CNS depression, orthostatic hypotension Pregnancy Considerations: Crosses the placenta and platelet aggregation may be inhibited in newborns after maternal use within 2 wk of delivery. It is indicated for use during labor alone or as an adjunct to opioid analgesics as an antiemetic in pregnancy and labor, however, other agents are recommended as initial therapy for the treatment of nausea and vomiting of pregnancy. Onset: IM: 20 min; IV: 3–5 min; duration: 4–6 h (up to 12 h). PB: 93%; t½: 9–16 h. PB: 35%–55%; t½: 22 h
Hydroxyzine	Anxiety: PO: 25–100 mg qid PRN Preoperative sedation: IM: 50–100 mg as a single dose	Anxiolytic antiemetic antihistamine used as a preoperative and postoperative adjunct therapy to reduce opioid dosage, treat anxiety, and control emesis in labor Side effects: CNS depression Onset: PO: 15–30 min; IM: rapid peak: 2 h; duration: 2–36 h. PB: UK; t½: 3–7 h ⚡ Acute High Alert: Crosses the placenta and possible withdrawal symptoms have been observed in neonates after chronic maternal use during pregnancy. Use of hydroxyzine early in pregnancy is contraindicated.
Narcotic Agonists		
Fentanyl citrate	IV: 50–100 mcg Give IV over 1–2 min, may repeat q1–2 h PRN; muscle rigidity may occur when IV administration is too rapid Regional anesthesia: Initial 50–100 mcg bolus, then 10–15 mL/h of bupivacaine and fentanyl cont. infusion	❗ A synthetic opiate that is 100 times as potent as morphine. Used as pain relief as adjunct to regional anesthesia Side effects: Constipation, nausea and vomiting, dyspnea, confusion, dizziness, fatigue, headache, CNS depression Contraindicated in patients with severe asthma Onset: IV, 1–2 min; peak: IV, 3–5 min; duration: IV, 30–60 min. PB: 79%–87%; t½: 2–4 h ⚡ Black-Box Warning: Crosses the placenta and can cause respiratory depression in the newborn and life-threatening withdrawal symptoms, especially in prolonged maternal use. Make sure resuscitation equipment is readily available for the newborn. Fentanyl patches have not been studied and therefore are not recommended in pregnancy.
Morphine sulfate	Only given as adjunct to regional anesthesia at 1/10 of the IV dose IV dose: 2–5 mg every 3–4 h PRN	An opioid that binds to CNS opiate receptors and inhibits ascending pain pathways; used for adjunct to regional anesthesia for pain in delivery Side effects: CNS depression, constipation, hypotension Monitor for CNS and respiratory depression. Have naloxone available as antidote Onset: IV, 3–10 min; peak: IV, 20 min; duration: IV, 3–5 h. PB: 30%–35%; t½: 2–4 h ⚡ *Black-Box Warning:* Crosses the placenta. Watch for respiratory depression in the newborn and life-threatening withdrawal symptoms, especially with prolonged maternal use. Have resuscitation equipment for newborn readily available.
Mixed Opioid Agonist-Antagonists		
Butorphanol tartrate	IM/IV: 1–2 mg; may repeat in 4 h	Mixed opioid agonist-antagonist used for relief of moderate to severe pain. Used in pregnancies >37 wk with no fetal distress. Use alternative analgesic if delivery is anticipated in 4 h or less. Side effects: CNS depression, hypotension, constipation Onset: 5–10 min; peak: 4–5 min; duration: 3–4 h. PB: 80%; t½: 2.5–4 h ⚡ Black-Box Warning: Crosses the placenta. May temporarily affect the heart rate of the fetus, causing abnormal patterns. Prolonged use in pregnancy can cause neonatal opioid withdrawal syndrome. Have resuscitation equipment readily available.

Continued

TABLE 53.1 Analgesics Used During Labor, Delivery, and Postpartum—cont'd

Drug	Route and Dosage	Uses and Considerations
Nalbuphine hydrochloride	Surgical anesthesia supplement: IV: 0.3–3 mg/kg over 10–15 min; *maintenance:* 0.25–0.5 mg/kg as required	Mixed opioid agonist-antagonist narcotic used as adjunct to anesthesia Side effects: Respiratory depression; constipation, hypotension Onset: 2–3 min; peak: 2–3 min; duration: 3–6 h. PB: 50%; t½: 5 h ⚡ Black-Box Warning: Crosses Placenta; may cause respiratory depression in newborn; abnormal heart rate, and severe bradycardia. Have resuscitation equipment and naloxone on hand to reverse bradycardia.
Postpartum Perineal Wounds and Hemorrhoids		
Benzocaine, aerosol 20%	Spray liberally tid/qid 6–12 inches from the perineum after perineal cleansing.	A local anesthetic that inhibits impulses from sensory nerves by decreasing permeability of the cell membrane to sodium ions; it is hydrolyzed in plasma and liver (to a lesser extent) by cholinesterase and is eliminated as metabolites in urine. Drug is well absorbed from mucous membranes and traumatized skin and is contraindicated in patients with secondary bacterial infection of tissue and known hypersensitivity. Side effects: rash, hives, itching, redness Peak: 1 min; duration: 30–60 min. PB: UK; t½: UK Pregnancy Considerations: When used in moderation, not associated with a significant risk of adverse pregnancy outcomes.
Witch hazel or pramoxine premedicated pads	Apply premoistened pads up to 6 times daily, especially after bowel movements.	Witch hazel is one of the safest and most natural postpartum vaginal care options for local irritation and discomfort of hemorrhoids and episiotomies. Precipitates protein, causing tissue to contract. May be refrigerated in the original container for additional comfort. If liquid, pour over ice and dip absorbent pads into solution; change when diluted. Medical intervention should be sought if rectal bleeding is present. Side effect: local irritation (discontinue use) PB: UK; t½: UK Pregnancy Considerations: Not associated with a significant risk of pregnancy outcomes.
Hydrocortisone acetate 25 mg	Insert 1 suppository bid rectally for 2 wk. Wear gloves to administer.	Acts as an antiinflammatory agent to relieve pain and itching from irritated anorectal tissue. Contraindicated in patients with known hypersensitivity. Discontinue if tissue infection occurs. If anorectal symptoms do not improve in 7 days or if bleeding, protrusion, or seepage occurs, inform the health care provider. Do not use if fourth-degree perineal laceration is present. It is unknown whether drug is excreted in breast milk; use cautiously. Onset, peak, and duration are unknown. Pregnancy Considerations: Not associated with significant risk of adverse pregnancy outcomes when used in moderation; however, there may be an increased risk of low-birth-weight infants after maternal use of potent or very potent topical products.
Dibucaine ointment, USP 1%	Apply to cleansed rectum 3–4 times daily, using no more than 30 g in 24 h.	Topical anesthetic with the same action as benzocaine. Do not use near eyes or over denuded surfaces or blistered areas or if rectal bleeding is present. Do not use with known hypersensitivity to amide-type anesthetics. Side effects include burning, tenderness, irritation, inflammation, contact dermatitis, urticaria, cutaneous lesions, and edema Onset: Within 15 min; peak: UK; duration: 2–4 h.

>, Greater than; *bid*, twice daily; *CNS*, central nervous system; *cont.*, continuous; *d*, day; *FHR*, fetal heart rate; *h*, hour; *IM*, intramuscular; *IV*, intravenous; *max*, maximum; *min*, minute; *PB*, protein binding; *PO*, by mouth; *PRN*, as needed; *q*, every; *qid*, four times daily; *subcut*, subcutaneously; *t½*, half-life; *tid*, three times daily; *UK*, unknown; *USP*, US Pharmacopeia; *wk*, weeks.

respiratory depression, vertigo, lethargy, headache, and flush. Side effects in the fetus and neonate include decreased FHR variability, moderate CNS depression, hypotonia at birth, and mild behavioral depression. It is important to note that the US Food and Drug Administration (FDA) recently required updates to opioid prescribing information in April 2023 due to the increasing opioid crisis. The required safety labeling changes include stating that the risk of overdose increases as the dosage increases for all opioid drugs, advising that patients avoid using the drug for an extended period, and warning about opioid-induced hyperalgesia (OIH), including differentiating OIH symptoms from those of opioid tolerance and withdrawal.

Further information may be found at https://www.fda.gov/drugs/drug-safety-and-availability/fda-updates-prescribing-information-all-opioid-pain-medicines-provide-additional-guidance-safe-use.

Regional Anesthesia

Anesthesia in labor and delivery represents the loss of painful sensations with or without loss of consciousness. Two types of pain are experienced in childbirth, visceral and somatic. Visceral pain occurs during the first two stages of labor from uterine contractions and the pressure of the stretching cervix. *Somatic pain* is caused by pressure of the presenting part and by stretching of the perineum and vagina. This is the pain of the transition phase and the second stage of labor. Table 53.2 lists the anesthetics used during labor and delivery and their dosages, uses, and considerations.

Regional anesthesia achieves pain relief during labor and delivery without loss of consciousness. Injected local anesthetic agents temporarily block conduction of painful impulses along sensory nerve pathways to the brain. Regional anesthesia allows the patient

TABLE 53.2 Anesthetic Used in Obstetrics[a]

Drug	Route and Dosage	Uses and Considerations
Chloroprocaine	Lumbar epidural block: 2% or 3%, 2–2.5 mL per segment; usual start volume is 15–25 mL; *max:* single dose (with epinephrine 1:200,000), 14 mg/kg; total dose, 750 mg	An ester-type local anesthetic that stabilizes the neuronal membranes and prevents initiation and transmission of nerve impulses, affecting local anesthetic actions (local or pudendal block) Side effects: hypotension, bradycardia, restlessness, anxiety, dizziness, tremors Onset of action: 6–12 min; duration: Up to 60 min. PB: UK; t½: 21–25 s ⚡ *Pregnancy Considerations:* Rapidly crosses placenta and may cause varying degrees of fetal and neonatal toxicity. Have resuscitation equipment near.
Tetracaine 0.2%, 0.3%	Spinal anesthesia: Lower abdomen: 10 mg of 0.3% Perineum: 5 mg of 0.3% Saddle block: 2–4 mg of 0.2%; *max:* 15 mg Other anesthesia dosages available.	An ester-type local anesthetic that blocks both initiation and conduction of nerve impulses by decreasing neuronal membrane permeability to sodium ions; a low spinal block or spinal anesthesia for cesarean delivery Adverse reactions: hypotension, chills, dizziness, drowsiness, nausea, vomiting, tremors, seizures Duration of action: 1.5–3 h. PB: UK; t½: UK ⚡ *Pregnancy Considerations:* Crosses placenta, fetal monitoring is recommended
Lidocaine injectable	Doses vary per procedure, see packaging; *max:* 4 mg/kg per dose or 300 mg per procedure when used without epinephrine	Suppresses automaticity of conduction tissue by increasing the electrical stimulation threshold of the ventricle; blocks both initiation and conduction of nerve impulses by decreasing neuronal membrane permeability to sodium ions Side effects: headache, bradycardia, hypotension, anxiety, dizziness, n/v, tremors Onset: 45–90 s; duration: 10–20 min. PB 60%–80%; t½: 1.5–2 h ⚡ *Black-Box Warning:* Crosses placenta. Approved for obstetric analgesia, however, adverse reactions have been noted in fetus/neonate, with affecting CNS, heart, or peripheral vascular tone. Fetal heart rate monitoring is recommended, as well as emergency equipment being on hand. Cumulative total from all routes of administration should be considered.
Bupivacaine	Epidural block: 3–4 mL increments IV or intrathecal administration of 10–20 mL of 0.25% or 0.5%	Epidural or spinal for labor and cesarean delivery; blocks both initiation and conduction of nerve impulses by decreasing neuronal membrane permeability to sodium ions Adverse effects: Bradycardia, hypotension, arrhythmias, anxiety, nausea, vomiting Onset: Up to 17 min; duration: epidural, 2–7.7 h; spinal, 1.5–2.5 h. PB: 84%–95%; t½: 2.7 h ⚡ *Black-Box Warning:* The 75% concentration is not recommended for obstetric anesthesia; reports of cardiac arrest with difficult resuscitation and death have been reported.
Ropivacaine	Lumbar epidural block for cesarean section: 20–30 mL dose of 0.5% solution or 15–20 mL of 0.75% solution in incremental doses Doses available for vaginal obstetric anesthesia as incremental administration or continuous infusion	Epidural for cesarean delivery; blocks both initiation and conduction of nerve impulses by decreasing neuronal membrane permeability to sodium ions Adverse effects: hypotension, bradycardia, nausea, vomiting, back pain, hypertension and tachycardia Position pregnant female in left lateral position to prevent compression of the uterus Onset: 3–15 min; duration: 3–15 h. PB: UK; t½: 5–7 h ⚡ *Pregnancy Considerations:* Crosses placenta, which can result in fetal/neonatal effects of CNS and cardiovascular depression. Fetal monitoring and resuscitation equipment required.

abd, Abdomen; *h*, hour; *IV*, intravenous; *max*, maximum dosage; *min*, minute; *n/v*, nausea and vomiting; *PB*, protein binding; *t½*, half-life; *UK*, unknown.

[a]The following nursing considerations apply to all types of epidurals: Use a test dose (3 mL of lidocaine 1.5% with 1:200,000 epinephrine) to confirm correct catheter placement. If a local anesthetic is injected into a vein, the patient may experience dizziness, ringing in the ears, numbness, a metallic taste in the mouth, or a toxic response. Maternal lateral positioning is done to prevent aortocaval compression. Maternal diastolic blood pressure (BP) should be less than 110 mm Hg before initiating the epidural. When maternal hypotension occurs, place the patient on her left side, infuse IV fluids rapidly, and administer ephedrine 5–10 mg IV or 100 mcg phenylephrine IV. Repeat as necessary. Monitor BP every 1–2 min for the first 10 min, then every 10–30 min until the block wears off. Assess the level of analgesia. After administration of the anesthetic, assess motor strength before ambulation.

to experience labor and childbirth with relief from discomfort in the blocked area while maintaining consciousness. The two primary types of anesthesia are *local anesthetics* for local infiltration (e.g., episiotomy) and *regional blocks* (e.g., epidural, spinal). The most common types of peridural anesthesia are spinal, epidural, and combined spinal-epidural blocks. Other, less commonly administered regional blocks include caudal, paracervical, and pudendal blocks. The anesthesiologist or nurse anesthetist is responsible for administering regional anesthesia. Nurses may assist and monitor the patient for drug effectiveness and side effects during and after administration.

Spinal Anesthesia

Spinal anesthesia, also known as a *saddle block*, is injected in the subarachnoid space at the T10 to S5 dermatome. This anesthesia may be administered as a single dose or as a combined spinal-epidural block. Spinal anesthesia is administered immediately before delivery or late in the second stage, when the fetal head is on the perineal floor. Drugs frequently administered either alone or in combination with the local anesthetic for a vaginal delivery include bupivacaine with fentanyl. Dosages vary depending on whether administration of the anesthetic agent is plain or with epinephrine. Bupivacaine 0.75% concentration is *not* recommended for obstetric anesthesia due to reports of cardiac arrest with difficult resuscitation or death. Spinal anesthesia has a rapid onset, requires less local anesthetic, and may be used with high-risk patients. Postdural puncture headache is a primary concern and occurs 6 to 48 hours after dural puncture; it may also occur after accidental dural puncture with epidural anesthesia. Treatment for postdural headache includes analgesics, increased fluids, and bed rest. An epidural blood patch is the most effective means to treat postdural headache.

Lumbar epidurals may be administered as a single injection, by intermittent injection, as continuous patient-controlled epidural anesthesia (PCEA), or as a combined spinal-epidural block. Epidurals may be administered as a single anesthetic drug or with opioids or epinephrine. Most frequently, patients now receive a continuous epidural infusion, which provides more consistent drug levels and more effective pain relief. Rescue doses are given as necessary to achieve

CLINICAL JUDGMENT [NURSING PROCESS]
Pain Control Drugs

Concept: Pain
- Pain is the discomfort caused by an injury or illness, such as in labor and delivery.

Recognize Cues [Assessment]
- Assess the patient's level of pain.
- Assess the patient's beliefs regarding labor and expectations related to pain experiences.
- Assess the use of complementary and alternative medicine (CAM), including supplements, at any point during the pregnancy.
- Assess drug history to ascertain the potential for drug interactions.
- Obtain vital signs (blood pressure [BP], heart rate [HR]), respiratory status, quality of uterine contractions, degree of effacement and dilation, and fetal heart rate (FHR) before and after administration of an analgesic, and monitor the effectiveness of pain management.
- Assess the laboring patient's behavior for relaxation and progress of labor in relation to expected norms.
- Assess the patient's verbal and nonverbal behavior for data supportive or nonsupportive of coping with labor.

Analyze Cues and Prioritize Hypotheses [Patient Problems]
- Pain
- Discomfort
- Communication
- Reduced functional ability
- Confusion
- Decreased ability to cope
- Need for health teaching

Generate Solutions [Planning]
- The patient will verbalize a decrease in pain on a scale of 1 to 10 or per the agency's pain scale.
- The patient will demonstrate minimal to no side effects from pain control drugs during labor.

Take Action [Nursing Interventions]
- Assess the patient's parity, obstetric delivery history, and anticipated time until delivery.
- Offer analgesia appropriate for the stage and phase of labor and anticipated method of delivery. Encourage the patient and their support person to participate in decision making about analgesia.
- Document the administration of drugs per agency protocol.
- Provide appropriate safety measures after administration of drugs.
- Monitor the patient's vital signs, heart rate, and breathing pattern.
- ⚡ Check a compatibility chart for mixing of drugs.
- Verify that correct antidote drugs are available.
- Administer drugs before pain and anxiety reach maximum intensity within agency protocol, safe obstetric practice, and patient preferences.
- Assess the patient's level of pain using an agency-appropriate pain scale 30 to 60 minutes after analgesic administration.
- Monitor FHR, assessing fetal well-being before and during any drug administration.
- Instruct the patient to request assistance with ambulation and to keep the bed rails up when the patient is nonambulatory.
- Monitor the patient's urine output.

Patient Teaching
General
- Advise the patient concerning (1) drugs ordered, (2) route of administration and reason, (3) expected effects of the drug on labor, and (4) potential drug effects on the mother and the fetus or neonate.
- Advise the patient that most drugs used for pain relief in labor and delivery are not given by mouth because the GI tract functions more slowly during labor and drug absorption is decreased, making the oral route ineffective.
- Instruct the patient about safety precautions to be used while receiving the drug, including (1) positioning in bed, (2) use of side rails, and (3) assistance with ambulation.

Evaluate Outcomes [Evaluation]
- Evaluate the effectiveness of the drug in alleviating pain.
- Evaluate fear and anxiety regarding pain and the ability to cope with labor.
- Monitor maternal respirations, heart rate, BP, uterine contractions, dilation and effacement, and FHR for alterations from baseline. Report deviations beyond those expected with normally progressing labor.
- Document findings using agency protocol and obstetric nursing standards of care.

pain relief. Opioids are administered with a local anesthetic to control the somatic pain of transition and second-stage labor more effectively (see Tables 53.1 and 53.2).

Another additive to the local anesthetic is epinephrine, which increases the duration of the local anesthetic, decreases its uptake and clearance from the cerebrospinal fluid (CSF), and enhances the intensity of the neural blockade. Single and intermittent injections have wide variations in drug levels and provide less effective control of pain. A continuous lumbar epidural allows a more evenly spaced drug level; less anesthetic is required to provide more effective pain control. Continuous-infusion PCEA gives the patient better control of her anesthesia. Often, single and intermittent injections and PCEA will require rescue doses to improve analgesia.

Lastly, combined spinal-epidural analgesia couples the rapid analgesia and specificity of catheter placement of spinal anesthesia with the continuous infusion via catheter of epidural anesthesia, providing pain relief for later labor.

Controversy exists regarding the effect of regional analgesia, specifically epidurals, on the progress of labor. Some studies indicate no significant effect on labor, whereas other research has demonstrated a decreased maternal urge to push and increased length of labor.

Absolute Contraindications to Regional Anesthesia
- Severe gestational hypertension (increased risk of profound hypotension associated with the underlying disease state)
- Coagulation disorders and risk of bleeding secondary to decreased platelets (the patient should have a normal partial thromboplastin time and platelet count)
- Generalized sepsis or local infection at the needle insertion site

General Anesthesia

General anesthesia, although rarely used, may be necessary for emergency deliveries, when spinal or epidural anesthesia is contraindicated. It allows for rapid anesthesia induction and control of the airway. Before the administration of general anesthesia, antacids or other drugs that reduce gastric secretions are given to decrease gastric acidity. See Unit XIII for more information on acid reducers. More commonly, spinal or epidural anesthesia is administered for cesarean births. Spinal anesthesia is the more common choice for cesarean delivery because of rapid onset, increased reliability, and improvement in spinal needle design (smaller gauge and shape [Sprotte needle]) with subsequent reduction in postdural headaches. With spinal anesthesia, the local anesthetic most administered is bupivacaine with fentanyl; pain relief begins in 5 minutes and lasts for approximately 2 hours. With the additives, spinal anesthesia provides 18 to 24 hours of pain relief. For epidural inductions, the test dose of lidocaine with epinephrine—followed by administration of local anesthetics—is given. This is followed by a bolus or maintenance infusion with anesthetics with or without opioids and/or epinephrine to maintain maternal comfort. The nurse should assess the level of analgesia and motor block at least hourly. Monitor for complications, such as cardiovascular or CNS toxicity, postdural puncture headache, fetal bradycardia, or respiratory depression.

Local Anesthesia

Females receiving parenteral analgesic for labor and delivery may require more focused anesthesia for episiotomies and repair of perineal lacerations. Local anesthetic drugs such as lidocaine may be administered.

CLINICAL JUDGMENT [NURSING PROCESS]
Regional Anesthetics

Concept: Pain
- Pain is the discomfort caused by an injury or illness, such as in labor and delivery.

Recognize Cues [Assessment]
- Check the patient's history for drug sensitivity to local anesthetic agents.
- Assess the patient's labor plan with expectations for coping with labor and beliefs about use of analgesia and anesthesia.
- Assess the patient's knowledge about regional anesthesia.
- Assess cervical dilation and effacement and labor progress.
- Monitor fetal status.
- Review the patient's history for contraindications to regional anesthesia; notify the anesthesia provider.

Analyze Cues and Prioritize Hypothesis [Patient Problems]
- Discomfort
- Communication
- Reduced functional ability
- Pain
- Coping
- Anxiety

Generate Solutions [Planning]
- The patient will verbalize the desired amount of pain relief during labor.
- The patient will remain normotensive and will maintain a normal pulse rate; fetal heart rate (FHR) will remain within normal parameters. The patient will maintain minimal to no side effects from anesthesia.
- The patient will maintain urine output.
- The patient will be able to discuss the use of regional anesthesia for labor and delivery pain control.

Take Action [Nursing Interventions]
General
- Assess hydration status before regional anesthesia is given; monitor for anesthetic hypotensive effects. Provide bolus intravenous (IV) fluids as ordered, usually 500 to 1000 mL before regional anesthesia administration.
- Insert an indwelling urinary catheter before administration to monitor maternal fluid status.
- Position and support the patient on the left side or as instructed by the anesthesia provider.
- Monitor labor progress for any decrease in frequency or intensity of uterine contractions.
- Monitor maternal vital signs and FHR.
- Supply oxygen and emergency drugs, including ephedrine and antihistamines, along with resuscitation equipment in the event it may be needed.
- Monitor for postdural puncture headache; notify the anesthesia provider.

Spinal
- Assess uterine contractions; anesthetic drugs must be given immediately after a contraction.
- Monitor blood pressure (BP) for hypotensive effects per agency protocol; this is generally a decrease in systolic BP greater than 20% to 30% of baseline or below 100 mm Hg.

Continued

CLINICAL JUDGMENT [NURSING PROCESS]—CONT'D

Regional Anesthetics
- Have a supply of oxygen with positive-pressure ventilation equipment readily available.
- Assess level of analgesia after administration and sensory and motor status after delivery.
- Document procedures per agency protocol.

Epidural
- Ensure that the patient has 500 to 1000 mL IV bolus of an isotonic solution before the procedure to increase circulatory volume and prevent maternal hypotension.
- Monitor FHR and progress of labor, and keep in mind that anesthetic can inhibit fetal descent.
- Monitor BP for hypotensive effects per agency protocol.
- Assess the level of analgesia after administration.
- Maintain the patient on the left side, and increase the rate of IV fluids per agency protocol. If maternal hypotension occurs, notify the health care provider immediately.
- Assess for bladder distension. If voiding cues are unsuccessful (e.g., placement in semi-Fowler position, privacy, running water over the perineum, running water over the hand), catheterize the patient.
- Assess the patient's sensory and motor status before ambulation after delivery.
- Manage the patient's pain by ongoing pain assessments. If the nature of the patient's pain changes, contact the anesthesia provider to evaluate anesthesia needs.
- Document procedures per agency protocol.

Caudal
- Place the patient in the position requested by the anesthesia provider for administration.

Paracervical Block
- Maintain continuous FHR monitoring for fetal bradycardia after administration.
- Monitor maternal BP.

Patient Teaching
General
- Discuss technique, potential benefits, and side effects of the patient's particular method of anesthesia.

Side Effects
- Instruct the patient that regional anesthetics may slow labor and there may be a need for a drug to enhance uterine contractions.
- Assess the patient for postdural puncture headache after spinal anesthesia or after accidental dural puncture with epidural anesthesia.
- Advise the patient that bed rest, oral analgesics, caffeine, or an autologous blood patch may be used for relief of headache pain.

Skill
- Instruct the patient how to curl into position for epidural administration.
- Instruct the patient that forceps or vacuum extraction may be needed for delivery because of reduction of the "urge to push" sensation.
- Instruct the patient how to assume the left lateral or other position as requested by the anesthesia provider for caudal anesthesia.
- Advise the patient receiving epidural anesthesia they will have an IV and close monitoring of FHR and uterine contractions secondary to anesthesia.

Evaluate Outcomes [Evaluation]
- Evaluate BP compared with preprocedural baseline; evaluate FHR for alterations in variability and for decelerations.
- Evaluate effectiveness of anesthetic in relieving discomfort.
- Evaluate for uniformity of anesthesia; if there is lateralization or if it is "patchy," notify the anesthesia provider.
- Assess for bladder distension. If voiding cues are unsuccessful, catheterize the patient.
- Assess the patient's sensory and motor status before ambulation after delivery.
- Evaluate the uterine fundus for firmness.

The side effects of local anesthesia may cause an allergic reaction, or a nerve or heart problem if the dose is too high. Burning at the site of injection is the most common side effect. Lidocaine has a black-box warning from the FDA because it crosses the placenta. It is approved for obstetric analgesia; however, adverse reactions have been noted in the fetus/neonate. FHR monitoring is recommended, as well as emergency equipment being on hand. Side effects of lidocaine are headache, bradycardia, hypotension, anxiety, dizziness, nausea, vomiting, tremors, and burning at the site.

DRUGS THAT ENHANCE UTERINE MUSCLE CONTRACTILITY

Uterotropic drugs enhance uterine contractility by stimulating the smooth muscle of the uterus. Oxytocin, the ergot alkaloids, and some prostaglandins constitute the uterotropics.

Oxytocin is synthesized in the hypothalamus and is transported to nerve endings in the posterior pituitary gland. The hormone is released by the nerve endings under appropriate stimulation; capillaries absorb the substance and carry it into the general circulation, where it facilitates uterine smooth muscle contraction. Table 53.3 lists drugs commonly used for cervical ripening and uterine contraction.

In the presence of adequate estrogen levels, normally achieved by the third trimester, IV oxytocin stimulates uterine contraction. Oxytocin prepared in a synthetic form is approved by the FDA for **labor induction**, the process of causing or initiating labor, and for labor augmentation.

Before labor induction begins, risks and benefits and the status of the mother and fetus must be assessed, and informed consent for induction must be obtained. The gestational age of the fetus must be considered, together with the position of the fetus (head down and deep in the pelvis) and the size of the fetus in relation to the mother's pelvis. **Cervical ripening**, or softening of the cervix, is also assessed; the cervix is ripe and thus ready for induction when it is soft and progressing in effacement and partial dilation. An objective measurement called the **Bishop score** assists in predicting whether labor induction may be successful, and it is used to assess readiness for induction. Elements assessed in the modified Bishop scoring system are (1) dilation, (2) effacement, (3) station, (4) cervical consistency, and (5) cervical position. Modified Bishop scores of 8 or greater are associated with a successful labor induction.

In pregnant patients at or near term with a medical or obstetric indication for labor induction, cervical ripening and effacement for cervical dilation are obtained with the administration of dinoprostone, a naturally occurring form of PGE_2. It is thought that intracervically

TABLE 53.3 Cervical Ripening and Uterine Contractions

Drug	Route and Dosage	Uses and Considerations
Cervical Ripening		
Dinoprostone cervical gel, 0.5 mg	Contains 0.5 mg of dinoprostone in 2.5 mL of gel for intracervical use Before beginning oxytocin after dinoprostone cervical gel administration, there should be a 6- to 12-h delay.	Naturally occurring form of PGE_2. Used to ripen an unfavorable cervix at or near term in females needing labor induction. Must be at room temperature before administration and is administered by sterile technique, using catheter supplied and inserted into the cervical canal. Patient is to remain recumbent 15–30 min after administration of gel and 2 h after insert Adverse effects: hypersensitivity reactions including anaphylaxis, GI distress, uterine contractions, back pain PB: UK; $t½$: 2.5–5 min; onset: 10 min; peak: 30–45 min; duration: 12 h ⚡ Pregnancy Considerations: Fetal distress without corresponding maternal uterine hyperstimulation. Abnormal fetal heart rate and distress. Fetal monitoring and resuscitation equipment are required. ⚡ Black-Box Warning: Requires specialized care setting that can provide immediate intensive care facility and an experienced clinical to oversee use and monitoring.
Dinoprostone vaginal inserts, 10 mg	Contains 10 mg of dinoprostone in a timed-release insert that supplies 0.3 mg/h. Insert is left in place for 12 h. Oxytocin may be started 30–60 min after removal of an insert. In contrast to gel, inserts may be removed with FHR decelerations or uterine hyperstimulation. Ripening an unfavorable cervix: 10 mg over 12 h; remove 12 h after insertion or at onset of active labor.	Assess cervical dilation and effacement at time of insertion. After administration, patient remains in a lying position for 30 min to 2 h. Monitor FHR and uterine stimulation. Have medication available for frequent GI side effects of abdominal cramping, diarrhea, nausea, and vomiting. If uterine hyperstimulation occurs, remove the insert and have oxygen or beta-adrenergic drugs to treat. Onset: 10 min; peak: UK; duration: up to 2–3 h. PB: UK; $t½$: 2.5–5 min ⚡ Pregnancy Considerations: Crosses placenta. Fetal distress and abnormal heart rate can occur. Fetal monitoring and resuscitation equipment are required. ⚡ Black-Box Warning: Requires specialized care setting that can provide immediate intensive care facility and an experienced clinical to oversee use and monitoring.
Uterine Contraction		
Oxytocin	See Prototype Drug Chart: Oxytocin	
Carboprost tromethamine	IM: Initially, 0.25 mg; repeat every 15–90 min as needed Max total dose: 2 mg (8 doses)	Naturally occurring PGF_2-alpha. Direct stimulation of uterine smooth muscle. Treatment of postpartum hemorrhage secondary to uterine atony. Give deep IM rotating sites if repeat injections are required. Contraindicated before delivery of placenta. Use with caution in patients with acute renal disease, cardiac disease, hypertension, PID, and asthma. Adverse reactions: Diarrhea, nausea, vomiting, fever, and abdominal pain with cramps. PB: UK; $t½$: 8 min; peak: 30 min ⚡ Pregnancy Considerations: Intended for use after delivery of the infant and placenta
Methylergonovine maleate	PO: 0.2 mg 3–4 times daily in the puerperium for up to 7 d IM: 0.2 mg after delivery of anterior shoulder (if full obstetric supervision), after delivery of placenta, or postpartum; repeat q2–4 h. Oral doses may follow parenteral administration IV: Same as for IM but slowly over 1 min with careful monitoring of BP (IV route for acute emergencies only [e.g., bleeding])	Prevention and treatment of postpartum hemorrhage, subinvolution, and postabortion hemorrhage. Exhibits similar smooth muscle action to ergotamine but primarily affects smooth muscle, producing sustained contractions and shortening the third stage of labor. Not routinely administered IV because of possible sudden hypertensive and cerebrovascular accidents; limit use in patients with hypertension (especially IV). Contraindicated with maternal sepsis, labor induction, threatened spontaneous abortion. Do *not* use with vasodepressors, other ergot alkaloids, or vasoconstrictors. Appears in breast milk, but interference with breastfeeding is less than with ergonovine. Adverse reactions: Transient hypertension, diaphoresis, palpitations, dizziness, headache, nausea, vomiting, tinnitus, transient chest pain, dyspnea, bradycardia, angina, hallucinations, seizures Onset of Action: Oral 5–10 min; IM: 2–5 min; IV: immediate; duration: Oral/IM: 3 h; IV: 45 min. PB: UK; $t½$: 3 h ⚡ Pregnancy Considerations: Intended for use after delivery of the infant and is contraindicated during pregnancy

BP, Blood pressure; *d*, day; *FHR*, fetal heart rate; *GI*, gastrointestinal; *h*, hour; *IM*, intramuscular; *IV*, intravenous; *max*, maximum; *min*, minute; *PB*, protein binding; *PG*, prostaglandin; *PID*, pelvic inflammatory disease; *PO*, by mouth; *q*, every; *t½*, half-life; *UK*, unknown.

or intravaginally administered PGE_2 acts to create cervical effacement and softening through a combination of contraction-inducing and cervical-ripening properties, possibly secondary to an increased submucosal water content and collagen degradation resulting from collagenase secretion in response to PGE_2. One approach uses prefilled syringes of commercially prepared dinoprostone cervical gel, 0.5 mg, which is introduced just inside the cervical os. A second approach is the placement in the posterior vaginal fornix of a vaginal insert of dinoprostone containing 10 mg of controlled release dinoprostone at 0.3 mg/h.

Side effects associated with the use of prostaglandins include uterine hyperstimulation, which can be treated with terbutaline sulfate. Uncommonly, some patients experience chills, fever, vomiting, and diarrhea. Contraindications to the use of prostaglandins include active vaginal bleeding and known allergies to prostaglandins. With hepatic or renal disease, cautious use of PGE_2 is recommended; use of PGE_2 is contraindicated in patients with glaucoma.

Table 53.3 lists the dosages, uses, and considerations for administration of dinoprostone for cervical ripening.

PROTOTYPE DRUG CHART

Oxytocin

Drug Class	Dosage
Oxytocic agent Used to induce labor during pregnancy, to control postpartum hemorrhage, and to prevent uterine atony postdelivery Pregnancy Considerations: To be used for medical rather than elective induction of labor. Small amounts of exogenous oxytocin are expected to reach fetal circulation. Nonteratogenic adverse reaction is reported in the neonate as well as the mother.	For induction or augmentation of labor: Dilute 10 units (1 amp) of oxytocin in 1000 mL lactated Ringer's solution for 10 milliunits/mL Connect to primary IV line close to needle site as a piggyback line. IV: Low-dose regimen: Start with 0.5–1 milliunits/min; gradually increase dose in increments of 1–2 milliunits/min q30–60 until desired contraction pattern is established. Dose may be decreased by similar increments after desired frequency of contractions is reached and cervix is 5–6 cm dilated. Infuse up to 6 milliunits/min. Provides oxytocin levels like those of spontaneous labor; rates >9 milliunits/min are rarely required. High-dose regimen: Start with 6 milliunits/min; may increase 3–6 milliunits/min q15–60 min until desired contraction pattern is established. If uterine hyperstimulation, decrease dose to 3 milliunits/min; may be further decreased to 1 milliunits/min. For reduction and control of postpartum hemorrhage and postdelivery uterine contractions: IV: 10–40 units added to 1000 mL compatible IV solution; infuse at a rate to prevent uterine atony. IM: 3–10 units after delivery of the placenta
Contraindications	**Drug-Lab-Food Interactions**
Proven cephalopelvic disproportion, fetal intolerance of labor, hypersensitivity, anticipated nonvaginal delivery; intranasal spray is contraindicated in pregnancy. ⚡ *Black-Box Warning:* To be used for medical, rather than elective, induction of labor. However, though the black-box warning is still listed, there is an off-label use now for elective induction of labor. ACOG states that it is reasonable to offer elective induction of labor to pregnant patients that meet the criteria. This is based on data obtained from a large study, called the ARRIVE trial that took place from March 2014 to August 2017 involving multi-center randomized controlled parallel groups that support the use of oxytocin for the elective induction of labor at 39 weeks' gestation in low-risk nulliparous singleton pregnancies.	Drug: Hypertension can occur with vasopressors, and hypotension and/or bradycardia can occur with cyclopropane anesthetics. Herbals: Black cohosh, cottonroot, squaw vine, and cinnamon can have a synergistic effect to oxytocin.
Pharmacokinetics	**Pharmacodynamics**
Absorption: Not well absorbed PO; intranasal and IM absorption is very rapid. Distribution: Low PB; widely distributed in extracellular fluid; minute amounts in fetal circulation Metabolism: t½: 1–9 min; rapidly metabolized in liver Excretion: In urine	IM: Onset: 3–5 min Peak: 40 min Duration: 2–3 h IV: Onset: Within 1 min Peak: UK Duration: 1 h Intranasal: Onset: Minutes Peak: UK Duration: UK
Therapeutic Effects/Uses	
To induce or augment labor contractions; to treat uterine atony (intranasal spray) Mechanism of action: Oxytocin promotes uterine contractions by increasing intracellular concentrations of calcium in uterine myometrial tissue, thereby increasing the activity of the calcium-dependent phosphorylating enzyme myosin light-chain kinase.	
Side Effects	**Adverse Reactions**
Maternal effects with undiluted IV use include hypertension, dysrhythmias, uterine hyperstimulation (contractions lasting at least 2 min or 5 or more contractions in a 10-min window), and tachysystole (6 or more uterine contractions in a 20-min window).	Seizures; water intoxication can occur if given in electrolyte-free solution or at a rate greater than 20 milliunits/min. (Water intoxication is manifested by nausea, vomiting, hypotension, tachycardia, and cardiac arrhythmias.) *Life-threatening:* Maternal intracranial hemorrhage, cardiac dysrhythmias, asphyxia; fetal jaundice, hypoxia

ACOG, American College of Obstetricians and Gynecologists; *h*, hours; *IM*, intramuscular; *IV*, intravenous; *min*, minute; *PB*, protein binding; *PO*, by mouth; *t½*, half-life; *UK*, unknown.

Oxytocin

In addition to labor induction, IV oxytocin can also be used for labor augmentation, stimulation of effective uterine contractions once labor has begun. It facilitates smooth muscle contraction in the uterus of a patient already in labor but experiencing inadequate uterine contractility, tightening, and shortening of uterine muscles. The patient with uterine inertia, uterine inactivity, or hypotonic contractions, may be more responsive to oxytocin than the patient who has not begun labor; therefore a lower starting dose will be needed.

In both labor induction and labor augmentation, oxytocin is infused at a prescribed individualized dosage rate, and this rate is increased, decreased, or maintained at fixed intervals based on uterine and fetal response. The objective is to establish an adequate contraction pattern that promotes labor progress, generally represented by contractions every 2 to 3 minutes that last for 50 to 60 seconds with moderate intensity. It is important that the patient receiving oxytocin *not* experience uterine hyperstimulation, which causes markedly increased pain and compromised FHR patterns secondary to impaired placental perfusion. Continuous nursing observation during labor induction or augmentation is critical. The need for an accurate infusion rate requires the use of an infusion pump with oxytocin as an IV piggyback line. Once cervical dilation has reached 5 to 6 cm and an adequate contraction pattern is evident, the rate of oxytocin infusion can often be slowed or stopped.

After delivery, oxytocin 10 to 40 units is usually added to an existing IV solution to help the uterus stay contracted and close the uterine sinuses at the placental site. The maximum concentration should be 40 units per 1000 mL IV fluid. Prototype Drug Chart: Oxytocin lists the pharmacologic data for oxytocin.

The peak concentration time is unknown for all methods of administration, but the onset of action of IM oxytocin is 3 to 5 minutes, and the duration of action is 2 to 3 hours; the onset of action of IV oxytocin is immediate, and the duration of action is 1 hour.

The medication is diluted and administered by IV piggyback for induction or augmentation of labor. Oxytocin is diluted in a variety of ways and is administered via infusion pump in milliunits-per-minute dosing with the volume determined by the dilution. IV administration of undiluted oxytocin is not recommended because of the risk of a sudden acute hypotensive response.

Concurrent use of vasopressors can result in severe hypertension, whereas hypotension can occur with concurrent use of cyclopropane anesthesia and with undiluted IV push administration. The Institute for Safe Medication Practices (ISMP) includes oxytocin on its list of high-alert medications because of its heightened risk of causing significant harm when used in ⚡ error.

Other Drugs That Enhance Uterine Contractions: Ergot Alkaloids

The ergot alkaloids, one of a large group of alkaloids derived from fungi, act by direct smooth muscle cell receptor stimulation. These drugs are *not* used during labor because they can cause sustained uterine contractions (tetanic contractions), which would result in fetal hypoxia and could rupture the uterus. In addition, the uterus becomes more sensitive to these drugs. After delivery, however, sustained contractions are effective to prevent or control postpartum hemorrhage and to promote uterine involution.

The most used ergot derivative is methylergonovine maleate, which can be given by mouth but is most frequently administered intramuscularly. IV administration is not recommended and is used only in emergency situations. If IV methylergonovine maleate is given, administer 0.2 mg over 1 minute. Transient significant elevations in BP can occur, particularly after IV infusion. Patients with preexisting or gestational hypertension or peripheral vascular diseases should *not* receive ergot derivatives. Table 53.3 lists commonly used uterotonic drugs and their dosages, uses, and considerations.

CLINICAL JUDGMENT [NURSING PROCESS]
Enhancement of Uterine Contractility: Oxytocin

Concept: Comfort
- Comfort is the easing or alleviating a person's pain, grief, or distress.

Recognize Cues [Assessment]
- Confirm term gestation before inducing or augmenting labor, and obtain the patient's informed consent.
- Collect accurate baseline data before beginning infusion, including maternal pulse and blood pressure (BP), uterine history, uterine activity, and fetal heart rate (FHR) pattern.
- Interview the patient, and review the history to ascertain that no contraindications exist.

Analyze Cues and Prioritize Hypothesis [Patient Problems]
- Pain
- Discomfort
- Reduced functional ability

Generate Solutions [Planning]
- The patient will have enhanced uterine contractions without adverse maternal or fetal effects.
- The patient will maintain vital signs within acceptable ranges throughout labor, delivery, and the postpartum period.
- The patient will demonstrate FHR that is normal in rate, pattern, and variability throughout labor and delivery.

Take Action [Nursing Interventions]
- Have a supply of tocolytic drugs, such as terbutaline, and oxygen readily available.
- Monitor the patient's intake and output.
- Monitor maternal pulse and BP, uterine activity, and FHR during oxytocin infusion.
- Maintain the patient in a sitting or lateral recumbent position to promote placental infusion.
- Monitor for signs of uterine rupture, which include FHR decelerations, sudden increased pain, loss of uterine contractions, hemorrhage, and rapidly developing hypovolemic shock.
- Use an intravenous (IV) pump to administer all IV drugs.

Patient Teaching
- Inform the patient the drug is given intravenously, and the dosage is adjusted in response to the uterine contraction pattern.

Evaluate Outcomes [Evaluation]
- Evaluate effective labor progress.
- Monitor maternal vital signs every 30 to 60 minutes and with every increment in dose, and monitor FHR every 15 minutes and with every increment in dose during the first stage of labor and every 5 minutes in the second stage of labor. Report changes in vital signs and FHR, specifically late decelerations, and report any vaginal bleeding.

Side Effects and Adverse Reactions

Side effects of ergot alkaloids include uterine cramping, nausea and vomiting, dizziness, hypertension with IV administration, sweating, tinnitus, chest pain, dyspnea, itching, and sudden severe headache. Signs of ergot toxicity, also called ergotism, include pain in the arms, legs, and lower back; numbness; cold hands and feet; muscular weakness; diarrhea; hallucinations; seizures; and blood hypercoagulability.

DRUGS USED DURING THE POSTPARTUM PERIOD

During the puerperium, the period from delivery until 6 weeks postpartum, the mother's body physically recovers from antepartal and intrapartal stressors and returns to its prepregnant state.

Pharmacologic and nonpharmacologic measures commonly used during the postpartum period have five primary purposes: (1) to prevent uterine atony and postpartum hemorrhage; (2) to relieve pain from uterine contractions, perineal wounds, and hemorrhoids; (3) to enhance or suppress lactation, which is production and release of milk by the mammary glands; (4) to promote bowel function; and (5) to enhance immunity (Tables 53.4 and 53.5).

Whenever possible, nonpharmacologic measures are preferred to the use of drugs or are used in conjunction with drugs. Postpartum nursing care ideally occurs as a partnership between the nurse and the new family. To enhance health and wellness, the nurse collaborates with the mother and family to strengthen the new mother's self-confidence and ability to handle her own health challenges. The nurse's role in this system is threefold:

COMPLEMENTARY AND ALTERNATIVE THERAPIES

Herbal Supplements and Lactation

Because little is known about the safety of herbal supplements, they are not generally recommended during lactation. Breastfeeding patients should be advised to check with their health care provider before taking any herbal supplements; those contraindicated for breastfeeding patients include aloe, belladonna, black tea, bromelain, buckthorn bark, burdock, cat's claw, chondroitin, comfrey, echinacea, ephedra (Ma-huang), eucalyptus, flaxseed, kava, lavender, licorice, milk thistle, pennyroyal, and saw palmetto. This list is not exhaustive. Again, it is important to check with the health care provider on all complementary and alternative therapies used during lactation.

TABLE 53.4 Nonpharmacologic Measures for Common Postpartum Needs

Indication	Intervention
Uterine contractions	Patient is positioned on the abdomen with a pillow under the abdomen for 20–30 min for 3–4 d. Distraction, breathing techniques, therapeutic touch, relaxation, guided imagery, and ambulation may be used. No heat should be applied to the abdomen because of the risk of uterine relaxation and increased bleeding.
Perineal wound resulting from episiotomy or laceration	Ice packs made with a nonlatex glove filled with crushed ice and covered in a thin, absorbent material to protect tissue are applied for 6–8 h after delivery. The patient is positioned on her side as much as possible with a pillow between the legs; early and frequent ambulation and perineal exercises (Kegels) are encouraged. A cool sitz bath should be taken 2–3 h after delivery along with warm sitz baths 12–24 h after delivery 2–3 times daily. The perineum is cleansed front to back using a peri-spray squeeze bottle or cleansing shower. Keep area around the stitches clean and dry, and change pads every 2–3 h. Patient is advised to tighten the buttocks or squeeze them together before sitting and to sit tall and flat, not rolled back onto the coccyx. No tampons, douches, or feminine hygiene sprays should be used until advised by the health care provider. Advise no intercourse until after lochia has ceased or as advised by the health care provider.
Hemorrhoids	Apply ice packs to area several times a day. Modified left lateral recumbent position to help increase venous return Warm, moist heat or sitz bath Witch hazel pads (e.g., Tucks) Alternate cold and warm treatments as directed.
Lactation suppression	Tight bra worn continuously for 10–14 d Normal fluid intake No manipulation or stimulation of breasts Pyridoxine (vitamin B_6) 200 mg for 5 d
Engorgement	Same as for lactation suppression as previously discussed plus ice to the axillary area of the breasts if bottle feeding or warm compresses if breastfeeding; cold cabbage leaves placed inside the bra may also be helpful. If breastfeeding, express a small amount of colostrum or milk by hand before putting the infant to the breast to facilitate latching on.
Sore or cracked nipples	Wear absorbent breast pads to keep moisture away from nipples. Do not use soap on nipples. Air-dry nipples after nursing. After nursing, express a small amount of breast milk on nipples to use as a protective lubricant. After nursing, apply hypoallergenic purified lanolin to nipples as a protective lubricant to promote healing. For cracked nipples, use comfort gel pads (hydrogel pads). Do not use nipple shields because they can promote chafing. Do not limit the infant's nursing time; if the milk ducts are not emptied, increased pressure can occur. Ensure proper positioning for feeding, and initiate nursing on the less sore nipple. After feeding, the infant may instinctively suck during attempts to disengage: break the suction with your little finger to prevent pulling on the nipple.

d, Day; *h*, hour; *min*, minute.

TABLE 53.5 Promote Postpartum Bowel Function

Generic	Route and Dosage	Uses and Considerations
Docusate sodium, docusate calcium (various dosages available)	50–360 mg/d PO in 1–4 divided doses; *max:* 360 mg/d for docusate sodium; 240 mg/d for docusate calcium	Reduces surface tension of the oil-water interface of the stool, resulting in enhanced incorporation of water and fat and subsequent stool softening. Docusate salts are interchangeable (Na, Ca, or K is clinically insignificant). Do not use concomitantly with mineral oil. Do not use more than 1 wk, as prolonged use may cause bowel dependence or electrolyte imbalance. Contraindicated in patients with intestinal obstruction, acute abdominal pain, nausea, or vomiting. Compatible with breastfeeding. Side effect is rash. Onset: 12–72 h. PB: NA; *t½*: NA Pregnancy Considerations: Hypomagnesemia was reported in a newborn after chronic maternal use throughout pregnancy. Nonpharmacologic treatment is preferred initially.
Sennosides 8.6 mg tab or 8.8 mg/5 mL	PO: 1–2 tabs bid; take with a full glass of water or 10–15 mL at bedtime	A stimulant laxative that acts on the colon as a local irritant to promote peristalsis and bowel evacuation; also increases moisture content of stool by accumulating fluids in the intestine. Metabolized in liver, eliminated in feces (viable) and urine. Drug interactions may occur with MAOIs, disulfiram, metronidazole, and procarbazine. May discolor urine or feces. May create laxative dependence and loss of bowel function with prolonged use. Side effects: abdominal cramps, diarrhea, nausea/vomiting Contraindicated in patients with fluid and electrolyte disturbances, abdominal pain, and nausea and vomiting; excreted in breast milk Onset: 8–12 h but may require up to 24 h. PB: NA; *t½*: NA Pregnancy Considerations: Agents other than senna are preferred as initial treatment of constipation when pregnant. Not recommended for chronic use, but may be used intermittently.
Bisacodyl (10 mg supp or 5 mg tab)	PO: 5–15 mg once daily PR: 1 supp as a single dose *Max:* PO: 15 mg/d; PR 10 mg/d	Stimulant laxative; irritates smooth muscle of the intestine and possibly the colon and intramural plexus; alters water and electrolyte secretion, increasing intestinal fluid and producing a laxative effect. After oral or rectal administration, 5% absorbed systemically; metabolized in the liver to conjugated metabolites; excreted in breast milk, bile, and urine. Do not crush tablets or give within 1 h of milk or antacid because enteric coating may dissolve, resulting in abdominal cramping and vomiting. Side effects include abdominal cramps, nausea, vomiting, rectal burning, electrolyte and fluid acidosis or alkalosis, and hypocalcemia. Onset: PO, 6–10 h; PR, 15 min to 1 h Pregnancy Considerations: Not recommended for chronic use
Magnesium hydroxide Magnesium concentrate is 3 times as potent as regular-strength product.	PO: 15–60 mL reg susp or 15–30 mL conc susp per d, preferably at bedtime; may be taken in divided doses Tab: 2–4 caplets/d, preferably at bedtime; may be taken in divided doses	A laxative that acts by increasing and retaining water in the intestinal lumen, causing distension that stimulates peristalsis and bowel elimination. Absorbed drug is excreted in kidneys; unabsorbed drug is excreted in feces. Drug poses a risk to patients with renal failure because 15%–30% of the magnesium is systemically absorbed. Use with caution in patients with impaired renal function; hypermagnesemia and toxicity may occur because of decreased renal clearance of absorbed magnesium. Contraindicated in patients with colostomy, ileostomy, abdominal pain, nausea, vomiting, fecal impaction, and renal failure. Drug interactions may occur with tetracyclines, digoxin, indomethacin, iron salts, or isoniazid. Side effects are abdominal cramps and nausea. Adverse reactions include hypotension, hypermagnesemia, muscle weakness, and respiratory depression. Onset: 4–8 h Pregnancy Considerations: Magnesium crosses the placenta; however, serum concentrations in the fetus are similar to those in the mother and considered acceptable for treating heartburn of pregnancy.
Simethicone	PO: 40–125 mg qid after meals and at bedtime; *max:* 500 mg/d	An antiflatulent that acts by dispersing and preventing formation of mucus-surrounded gas pockets in the GI tract by changing the surface tension of gas bubbles allowing them to coalesce for easier elimination through belching and rectal flatus. Chew tablets thoroughly, and follow with a glass of water. Drug is excreted unchanged in feces; may interfere with results of guaiac tests of gastric aspirates, but no other side effects are known. Do *not* take double doses to make up for missed doses. Store below 104°F (40°C) in a well-closed container. Onset: UK. *t½*: UK Pregnancy Considerations: Not absorbed systemically after oral administration; therefore does not cross the placenta.

bid, Twice daily; *Ca*, calcium; *conc*, concentration; *d*, day; *GI*, gastrointestinal; *h*, hour; *K*, potassium; *MAOI*, monoamine oxidase inhibitor; *max*, maximum dosage; *min*, minute; *Na*, sodium; *NA*, not applicable; *PB*, protein binding; *PO*, by mouth; *PR*, per rectum; *qid*, four times a day; *reg*, regular; *supp*, suppository; *susp*, suspension; *t½*, half-life; *tab*, tablet; *UK*, unknown; *wk*, week.

- To assess and discuss postpartal physical changes and pain management with the patient and determine healing progress within a standard and effectiveness of medications
- To teach the patient and administer postpartal medications
- To teach the patient and administer opioid analgesics as prescribed when pain control by nonnarcotics is ineffective

Pain Relief for Uterine Contractions

Afterbirth pains may occur during the first few days postpartum, when uterine tissue experiences ischemia during contractions, particularly in multiparous patients and when breastfeeding. Nonsteroidal agents may be used to control postpartal discomfort and pain; opioid agents are reserved for more severe pain, such as that experienced by the patient after cesarean delivery, tubal ligation, or extensive perineal laceration. Table 53.1 lists systemic analgesics commonly used during the postpartum period.

Because some systemic analgesics can cause decreased alertness, it is important for the nurse to observe the patient as she cares for her newborn to ensure safety. Patients who receive opioids should be assessed for bowel function and respirations. With continued opioid use, patient assessment of bowel history is necessary because these drugs can exacerbate the constipation of pregnancy. During the intrapartum period, females are NPO (nothing by mouth) or ingest limited liquids and are not ambulatory, all factors that contribute to decreased bowel activity. In addition, respiratory assessment is important for patients receiving opioids because respiratory depression may occur. Frequently, nonsteroidal drugs like ibuprofen are used to control postpartum discomfort and pain. Nonsteroidal antiinflammatory drugs (NSAIDs) inhibit the enzyme cyclooxygenase (COX), of which there are two isoenzymes, COX-1 and COX-2; both decrease prostaglandin synthesis. These drugs are effective in relieving mild to moderate pain caused by postpartum uterine contractions, episiotomy, hemorrhoids, and perineal wounds. NSAIDs commonly cause GI irritation, and it is recommended that patients take them with a full glass of water or with food to minimize GI distress. With administration of NSAIDs, a lower narcotic dosage may control pain because of the additive analgesic effect. The use of NSAIDs requires ongoing assessment for GI bleeding. These drugs inhibit platelet synthesis and may prolong bleeding time. Patient teaching with this category of drugs is important because some NSAIDs may be purchased over the counter (OTC). Patient teaching includes avoidance of these drugs while pregnant if symptoms of GI bleeding occur (dark, tarry stools; blood in urine; coffee-ground emesis) and avoidance of the concurrent use of alcohol, aspirin, and corticosteroids, which may increase the risk for GI toxicity.

Pain Relief for Perineal Wounds and Hemorrhoids

Pregnancy and the delivery process increase pressure to the perineal soft tissue, causing it to become ecchymotic or edematous. Increased edema, ecchymosis, and pain may occur if an **episiotomy**, incision made to enlarge the vaginal opening to facilitate newborn delivery, or perineal laceration is present. The perineum is assessed for Redness, Ecchymosis, Edema, Discharge, and Approximation (REEDA). In addition, hemorrhoids that developed during pregnancy may be exacerbated by pushing during labor. Comfort measures—ice packs immediately after birth, tightening of the buttocks before sitting, use of peri-bottles, and cool or warm sitz baths—and selected topical agents such as witch hazel and dibucaine ointment may relieve pain and minimize discomfort (see Table 53.1). Note that rectal suppositories should *not* be used by females with fourth-degree perineal lacerations.

CLINICAL JUDGMENT [NURSING PROCESS]
Pain Relief for Perineal Wounds and Hemorrhoids

Concept: Pain
- Pain is the discomfort caused by an injury or illness.

Recognize Cues [Assessment]
- Assess the patient's pain using an agency pain scale.
- Assess the perineal area for wounds and hemorrhoids (size, color, location, pain scale, REEDA [redness, ecchymosis, edema, discharge, and approximation]).
- Assess for presence of infection at the perineal site; avoid use of benzocaine on infected perineal tissue.

Analyze Cues and Prioritize Hypotheses [Patient Problems]
- Pain
- Infection

Generate Solutions [Planning]
- The patient will report decreased perineal discomfort with the use of topical sprays, compresses, sitz baths, and ointments.
- The patient will be free of signs and symptoms of infection.

Take Action [Nursing Interventions]
- Teach the patient about use of the peri-bottle. Use warm, direct water on the perineum from front to back (clean to dirty).
- Instruct the patient not to use benzocaine spray when perineal infection is present.
- Shake the spray can, and administer benzocaine 6 to 12 inches from the perineum with the patient lying on their side, top leg up and forward, to provide maximum exposure. This can also be done with one foot on the toilet seat.
- Apply witch hazel compresses (glycerin and witch hazel or witch hazel solution) with an ice pack and a peri-pad cold to the affected area.
- Store pramoxine and hydrocortisone acetate suppositories below 86°F (30°C), but protect them from freezing. Use gloves for administration.
- Assess to determine whether the patient is ready to switch to a preparation without hydrocortisone (the goal is to discontinue use of suppositories as quickly as possible if the patient is breastfeeding).
- Instruct carefully the use of pramoxine hydrochloride (HCl). Instruct the patient to place the agent inside the anus, which is not generally done with an obstetric patient because they may have perineal wounds that extend into the anus. Rectal suppositories should not be used by patients with fourth-degree perineal laceration.

Patient Teaching
General
- Describe the process of perineal wound healing.
- Explain the expected action and side effects. With witch hazel, a cooling, soothing sensation will provide relief. Ointment and suppositories will soothe, lubricate, and coat mucous membranes. Pramoxine HCl is not chemically related to the "-caine" type of local anesthetics, and there is a decreased chance of cross-sensitivity reactions in patients who are allergic to other local anesthetics.
- Advise patients that the drug is not for prolonged use (no more than 7 days) or for application to a large area.
- Instruct that topical analgesia lasts for several hours after use.
- Advise the patient to store suppositories below 86°F (30°C) so they do not melt, and do not freeze. Counsel the patient with bleeding hemorrhoids to use the drug carefully and to keep their health care provider (HCP) informed if the condition exacerbates or does not improve within 7 days.

CLINICAL JUDGMENT [NURSING PROCESS]—CONT'D
Pain Relief for Perineal Wounds and Hemorrhoids

Self-Administration: Perineal Wounds—Topical Spray Containing Benzocaine
- Apply three to four times daily or as directed.
- Apply without touching sensitive areas.
- Instruct the patient to administer the spray by either lying on their side in bed while spraying from behind or by standing with one foot on a chair or toilet seat and to hold the can 6 to 12 inches from the affected area.
- Avoid contact of medication with eyes.
- Assess use of complementary and alternative medicine (CAM), including herbal supplements.
- Instruct the patient not to use a perineal heat lamp after application because this could cause tissue burns.
- Notify the health care provider if exacerbation of symptoms recurs within a few days.
- Keep all medications out of children's reach in the home. If ingested, contact a poison control center immediately.
- Store below 120°F (49°C). Dispose of empty cans without puncturing or incinerating.

Self-Administration: Hemorrhoids and Perineal Wounds—Witch Hazel Compresses
- Apply by pouring liquid witch hazel over chipped ice; place soft, clean, absorbent squares in the solution; squeeze each square to eliminate excess moisture, and fold and place the moist square against the episiotomy site or hemorrhoids.
- Instruct the patient using commercial medicated pads that the entire container may be placed in the refrigerator.
- Avoid touching the surface of the pad placed next to the perineal wound.
- Instruct the patient when to change the compress and how to place the ice bag and peri-pad over the compress.
- Instruct the patient not to insert medicated pads into the rectum.
- Keep all products out of children's reach.
- Instruct the patient that use is not recommended if rectal bleeding is present.
- Discontinue use if local irritation occurs.

Self-Administration: Hemorrhoids—Ointment and Suppositories
- Apply ointment externally in the postpartum period.
- Place the suppository in the lower portion of the anal canal. Caution must be used because products usually are not inserted rectally if fourth-degree lacerations are present.
- Apply a small quantity of ointment onto a 2-inch square gauze pad; place inside the peri-pad against the swollen anorectal tissue approximately five times per day.
- Instruct the patient if a suppository is ordered to keep it refrigerated but not frozen. Remove the wrapper before inserting the suppository in the rectum (hold the suppository upright and peel evenly down the sides). Do not hold the suppository for a prolonged period; it will melt. If a suppository softens before use, hold it in the foil wrapper under cold water for 2 to 3 minutes.
- Assess the patient for hypersensitivity to any components of the ointment.
- Avoid contact of medication with eyes.
- Instruct the patient that ointment may occasionally cause a burning sensation, especially if anal tissue is not intact.
- Discontinue use and consult the HCP if erythema, irritation, edema, or pain develops or increases.
- Notify the HCP if bleeding occurs.

Self-Administration: Hydrocortisone and Pramoxine and Pramoxine Hydrochloride
- Instruct the patient that the product is for anal or perianal use only and is not to be inserted into the rectum.
- Shake the can vigorously before use and fully extend the applicator plunger; hold the can upright to fill the applicator. Express the contents of the applicator onto a 2-inch square gauze pad, and place it inside the peri-pad and against the rectum.
- Instruct the patient to use two to three times daily and after bowel movements.
- Wash the applicator by taking it apart after each use and rinsing it with warm water.
- Keep the aerosol container out of children's reach in the postpartum unit and later in the home.
- Store below 120°F (49°C).
- Dispose of the aerosol container without puncturing or incinerating it.
- Avoid contact of medication with eyes.
- Instruct the patient that it is unknown whether topical administration of corticosteroids results in sufficient systemic absorption to produce detectable quantities in breast milk. Burning, itching, irritation, dryness, and folliculitis may occur with administration, especially if occlusive dressings are used.

Self-Administration: Dibucaine Ointment, 1%
- Express ointment from the applicator on a tissue or 2-inch square gauze pad, and place it against the anus. Do not insert the applicator into the rectum. Effects should occur within 15 minutes and should last for 2 to 4 hours. Ointment is poorly absorbed through intact skin but is well absorbed through mucous membranes and excoriated skin.
- Instruct the patient to not use near the eyes, over denuded surfaces or blistered areas, or if there is rectal bleeding.
- Advise the patient to not use more than one tube (30-g size) in 24 hours.
- Keep all medication out of children's reach.
- Assess the patient for any known hypersensitivity to amide-type anesthetics; if so, dibucaine ointment is contraindicated.
- Instruct the patient that local side effects may include burning, tenderness, irritation, inflammation, and contact dermatitis; inform the health care provider if these occur. Other side effects may include edema, cutaneous lesions, and urticaria.

Evaluate Outcomes [Evaluation]
- Reevaluate the patient's perception of pain after use of nonpharmacologic and pharmacologic measures. Identify the need for additional patient teaching.
- Reassess perineal and anal tissues for integrity, healing, and side effects.

Side Effects and Adverse Reactions
The most reported side effects of topical or local agents include burning, stinging, tenderness, edema, rash, tissue irritation, and sloughing, in addition to tissue **necrosis**, tissue death caused by disease or injury. The most reported side effects of hydrocortisone local or topical drugs include burning, pruritus, irritation, dryness, **folliculitis** (skin inflammation resulting from contact with an irritating substance or allergen), allergic contact dermatitis, and secondary infection. These side effects are more likely to occur when **occlusive** (i.e., obstructive) dressings are used.

Promotion of Bowel Function
Constipation is common during the postpartum period. The residual effects of progesterone on smooth muscle decrease peristalsis.

This decrease in peristalsis—added to decreased liquid intake during labor, decreased activity, and relaxation of the abdominal muscles—amplifies the problem. Patients who deliver by cesarean are even more likely to experience constipation and flatus (intestinal gas). Nonpharmacologic measures such as high-fiber foods, early ambulation, drinking at least 64 oz of fluids per day, and promptly responding to the defecation urge are generally instituted after delivery.

Pharmacologic measures include the use of stool softeners, laxative stimulants, and for the postcesarean patient, antiflatulents to treat excessive gas in the stomach and intestines (see Table 53.5).

Lactation Suppression

Due to severe side effects such as thrombophlebitis and potential carcinogenic effects, medications that were once prescribed for lactation suppression are no longer used. Nonpharmacologic measures are currently recommended for lactation suppression, such as wearing a well-fitted support bra or breast binder continuously for 72 hours after giving birth and avoiding breast stimulation, including running warm water over the breast and expressing milk.

If breast engorgement occurs while trying to suppress lactation, ice packs to the breasts (15 minutes on and 45 minutes off each hour) can help decrease the discomfort and swelling. The use of cabbage leaves is often recommended to help decrease engorgement. It is recommended that the female wear a cold cabbage leaf over each breast inside of her bra and replace the leaves each time they wilt. A mild analgesic can help decrease discomfort during this time (see Table 53.1).

Postpartum Depression

Postpartum depression is intense feelings of sadness, anxiety, or despair preventing patients from performing their daily tasks and occurring 1 to 3 weeks after childbirth but may occur up to a year after giving birth, related to changes in hormone levels. Patients with a history of depression before or during pregnancy have an increased risk of developing postpartum depression. Postpartum depression may be treated with therapy in combination with antidepressants.

Brexanolone was approved in March 2019 for treatment of postpartum depression. It is a 60-hour infusion that must be slowly titrated to increase the dose while monitoring for potential side effects. Guidelines list that it must be given in a monitored health care setting, where patients can be monitored for hypoxia and excessive sedation. It is only available through a restricted REMS program. Zuranolone is a new oral drug to treat postpartum depression that was approved by the FDA in August 2023. The recommended dose is 30 to 50 mg by mouth taken once in the evening to be administered with fat-containing food (400–1000 calories/25%–50% fat) for adequate absorption for 14 days. Adverse reactions include CNS depression, somnolence, confusion, and potential risk for falls. It is recommended to hold breastfeeding during the treatment, and pump and discard breast milk for 1 week following the last dose. Pharmacokinetics: Excretion 45% urine and 41% feces, half-life 19.7 to 24.6 hours, PB: 99.9%. Contains a Black-Box Warning indicating impaired ability to drive or engage in other potentially hazardous activities. See Chapter 23 for more information on antidepressants.

◎ CLINICAL JUDGMENT [NURSING PROCESS]

Laxatives

Concept: Elimination
- Elimination is the act of discharging or excreting waste products from the body.

Recognize Cues [Assessment]
- Obtain a history of bowel problems by noting the time of delivery, predelivery food and fluid intake, ambulation and activity, and predelivery bowel habits. Obtain a history of bowel problems.
- Assess bowel sounds in all four quadrants, particularly after cesarean delivery, and note abdominal distension.
- Assess the perineal area for wounds, hemorrhoids, and episiotomy (REEDA).

Analyze Cues and Prioritize Hypotheses [Patient Problems]
- Pain
- Discomfort
- Constipation

Generate Solutions [Planning]
- The patient will have a bowel movement by 2 to 4 days postpartum.
- The patient will resume a normal bowel elimination pattern within 4 to 6 weeks.

Take Action [Nursing Interventions]
Docusate Sodium and Sennosides
- Store at room temperature.
- Instruct the patient if a liquid preparation is ordered, it may be taken with milk or fruit juice to mask the bitter taste.
- Instruct the patient to always consume a full glass of water.
- Assess for a history of laxative dependence.
- Instruct the patient that drug interactions may occur with mineral oil, phenolphthalein, or aspirin.

Bisacodyl
- Store tablets and suppositories below 77°F (25°C), and avoid excess humidity.
- Instruct the patient not to crush tablets.
- Instruct the patient not to administer within 1 to 2 hours of milk or antacid because enteric coating may dissolve, resulting in abdominal cramping and vomiting.
- Consume with a full glass of water.

Magnesium Hydroxide
- Shake the container well.
- Instruct the patient not to take 1 to 2 hours before or after oral drugs because of the effects on absorption.
- Consume with a full glass of water.
- Advise the patient that milk of magnesia concentrate is three times as potent as the regular-strength product.
- Administer laxatives 1 hour before or 1 hour after any oral antibiotic.

Senna
- Protect senna from light and heat.

Simethicone
- Administer after meals and at bedtime.
- Instruct the patient if chewable tablets are ordered, the tablets must be chewed thoroughly before swallowing and followed with a full glass of water.

Patient Teaching
General
- Advise patients that stool softeners are given to enable bowel movement without straining.
- Advise patients that measures to prevent and treat constipation include drinking 6 to 8 glasses of fluid per day, ingesting foods high in fiber (bran, fruits, vegetables), and increasing daily ambulation and activity. Instruct patients to

CLINICAL JUDGMENT [NURSING PROCESS]—CONT'D

Laxatives

- avoid or minimize ingestion of gas-forming foods (beans, cabbage, onions) and to increase ambulation and other activity.
- Advise patients regarding temperature and storage requirements for drugs.
- Instruct the patient that prolonged, frequent, or excessive use may result in electrolyte imbalance or dependence on the drug.
- Advise the patient that many laxatives contain sodium. Instruct them to check with their health care provider or pharmacist before using any laxative if they are on a low-sodium diet.

Docusate Sodium and Sennosides With Docusate Sodium

- Advise patients to drink at least six 8-oz glasses of liquid daily and to drink one glass of fluid with each dose. Patients should not take the drug if they are already taking mineral oil or having acute abdominal pain, nausea, vomiting, or signs of intestinal obstruction. Patients should not use products for longer than 1 week, and they should report skin rash or stomach or intestinal cramping that does not diminish.

Senna

- Instruct the patient that senna may change urine and feces to a yellow-green color; advise discontinuation of senna if abdominal pain, nausea, or vomiting occurs.

Magnesium Hydroxide

- Advise the patient that laxative action generally occurs in 4 to 8 hours.
- Instruct the patient that magnesium hydroxide should be taken with a full glass of water.
- Instruct the patient to note whether the drug is in regular or concentrated form; the concentrate is three times more potent than the regular-strength product.
- Advise the patient that the drug may interact with tetracyclines, digoxin, indomethacin, iron salts, and isoniazid. Instruct the patient to notify their health care provider if any of these drugs are used.
- Instruct the patient to report any muscular weakness, diarrhea, or abdominal cramps.

Simethicone

- Advise the patient that simethicone will help relieve flatus and associated pain and that it should be taken after meals; if chewable tablets are ordered, instruct patients to chew tablets thoroughly and to drink a full glass of water afterward. If a dose is missed, the patient should take it as soon as possible but should not take double doses.

Evaluate Outcomes [Evaluation]

- Evaluate for the return of regular bowel function.

IMMUNIZATIONS

Rh$_0$(D) Immune Globulin

The Rh$_0$(D) factor is a protein found on the surface of red blood cells. If a patient's blood cells have this protein, they are considered Rh positive; if not, they are negative.

A patient who lacks the (Rh) factor in her own blood (an Rh-negative mother) may carry a fetus who is either Rh negative or Rh positive. During pregnancy, minimal amounts of fetal blood can cross the placenta. Also, abortion, either spontaneous, therapeutic, or induced; amniocentesis; ectopic pregnancy; and placenta previa or abruption can result in some mixing of maternal and fetal blood. Subsequently, anti-D antibodies develop in an Rh-negative mother with an Rh-positive fetus; with the development of these antibodies, the mother becomes sensitized against the Rh factor. If mother and fetus are both Rh negative, no incompatibility exists to trigger this maternal antibody response, but if the fetus is Rh positive, the Rh-negative mother is at risk for Rh sensitization (i.e., development of protective antibodies against incompatible Rh-positive blood). Initially, immune globulin M (IgM) is formed and does not cross the placenta. Later, IgD antibodies develop, which may cross the placenta with isoimmunization to the D antigen with subsequent hemolysis of fetal red blood cells (RBCs). Prenatal IgD isoimmunization occurs in approximately 1% to 2% of Rh-negative females. In later exposure, as with subsequent pregnancies, there is a more rapid IgG (secondary) immune response and an increased potential for fetal hemolysis in an Rh-positive fetus. Once formed, the protective antibodies remain throughout life and may result in hemolytic difficulties for fetuses in subsequent pregnancies. Maternal blood is assessed for the anti-D antibody at the initial prenatal laboratory evaluation and at 26 to 28 gestational weeks. Rh0(D) immune globulin is routinely administered to females with maternal/fetal blood mixing, such as after abortion or with threatened abortion at any stage of gestation with continuation of the pregnancy, obstetric manipulation or trauma, or ectopic pregnancy. If abortion occurs up to and including 12 weeks' gestation, the microdose is administered if less than 2.5 mL of Rh-incompatible RBCs were administered. During the postpartum period, Rh$_0$(D) immune globulin should be administered within 72 hours; therefore one full dose (300 mcg) is given postpartum if the newborn is Rh positive, as antepartum prophylaxis at 26 to 28 weeks' gestation, and after amniocentesis, chorionic villus sampling, and percutaneous umbilical blood sampling. For females with abruption, previa, cesarean births, or manual placental removal, a Kleihauer-Betke analysis (serum test) should be done because more than 15 mL of fetal-maternal hemorrhage of Rh-positive RBCs may have occurred, necessitating an increased dose of Rh$_0$(D) immune globulin. When 15 mL or more of Rh-positive RBCs is suspected, a fetal RBC count should be performed to determine the appropriate dose of Rh$_0$(D) immune globulin.

The Rh sensitization process can be prevented through the administration of Rh$_0$(D) immune globulin to unsensitized Rh-negative females after each actual or potential exposure to Rh-positive blood.

Side Effects and Adverse Reactions

Adverse reactions to Rh$_0$(D) immune globulin include hypotension, chills, dizziness, fever, headache, pruritus, rash, abdominal pain, diarrhea, and injection-site reactions (discomfort, mild pain, redness, swelling).

Rubella Vaccine

Maternal rubella, also called *German measles*, is a potentially devastating infection for the fetus, depending on gestational age. If an unimmunized female (rubella titer <1:10 or negative titer) contracts the virus during the first trimester, a high rate of abortion and neurologic and developmental sequelae associated with congenital rubella syndrome (transmission of the rubella virus to the fetus via the placenta) may result. Cataracts, glaucoma, deafness, heart abnormalities, and intellectual disability are seen with this syndrome. When infection occurs after the first trimester, there is less risk of fetal damage because of the developmental stage of the fetus. There is no treatment for maternal or congenital rubella infection. The goals are immunization and prevention of rubella in patients of childbearing age.

Side Effects and Adverse Reactions

Side effects of the rubella vaccine are generally mild and temporary. Burning or stinging at the injection site is caused by the acidic pH of the vaccine. Regional lymphadenopathy, urticaria (skin rash caused by an allergic reaction), rash, malaise, sore throat, fever, headache, polyneuritis, arthralgia, and moderate fever are occasionally seen.

> ⚡ **PATIENT SAFETY**
>
> **Do Not Confuse...**
> - **Fentanyl citrate**, used as an adjunct to general or regional anesthesia or for persistent moderate to severe postoperative pain, with **sufentanil**, an agent used to induce anesthesia in combination with other drugs or as the sole anesthetic agent.

🎯 CLINICAL JUDGMENT [NURSING PROCESS]
$Rh_0(D)$ Immune Globulin

Concept: Perfusion
- Perfusion is the passage of blood and blood products through the circulatory system to organs or tissues to deliver oxygen and nutrients to cells, such as to the uterus and fetus.

Recognize Cues [Assessment]
- Determine blood type and Rh status of all prenatal patients.
- Assess the patient's understanding of their own and their partner's Rh status.
- Assess the patient by inquiring about previous pregnancies and outcomes; ask whether the patient has ever received $Rh_0(D)$ immune globulin.
- Follow agency policy for Rh blood testing for the patient and infant at the time of delivery.
- Assess postpartum data concerning the neonate's Rh type. If the infant is Rh negative, the drug is not needed. If the infant is Rh positive, the Rh-negative mother is not sensitized (negative indirect Coombs test), and the infant has a negative direct Coombs test, the mother is a candidate to receive the injection to prevent antibody production or "sensitization."
- Obtain the patient's written consent before administration. Some agencies require a refusal form if the drug is declined.
- Assess for a history of allergy to immune globulin products.

Analyze Cues and Prioritize Hypotheses [Patient Problems]
- Hypersensitivity reaction
- Reduced perfusion

Generate Solutions [Planning]
- The patient will receive $Rh_0(D)$ immune globulin as indicated within 72 hours after delivery or abortion.
- The patient will be able to discuss Rh sensitization and actions indicated during subsequent pregnancies.

Take Action [Nursing Interventions]
- Assess and document Rh workup and eligibility of the patient to receive the drug. Convey information in a verbal report and in the patient's record according to agency policy.
- Assess the lot numbers on vials and laboratory slips for agreement before administration. Check expiration dates. Check the identification band and laboratory slip for matching numbers. Return required slips to the laboratory or blood bank.
- Administer $Rh_0(D)$ immune globulin and dose (microdose/standard dose) according to gestational weeks, exposure and route, provider orders, and agency protocol. Administer intramuscularly, normally in the deltoid, within 72 hours after delivery. If more than 72 hours have passed, administer as soon as possible up to 28 days, although less protection may result.
- Administration of IV $Rh_0(D)$ immune globulin is possible but infrequent. Check provider orders and dosage. For IV administration, reconstitute with normal saline. Store at 36°F to 46°F (2°C–8°C).
- Always have a supply of epinephrine available to treat anaphylaxis.

Patient Teaching
General
- Explain the action, purpose, and side effects of prescribed drugs.
- Advise patients to avoid live virus vaccines for 3 months after administration.
- Provide written documentation of the date of administration for the patient's personal health record.

Evaluate Outcomes [Evaluation]
- Evaluate the patient's understanding of the need for $Rh_0(D)$ immune globulin.

CLINICAL JUDGMENT CASE STUDY

A patient, who is gravida 3, para 0, is at 42 weeks' gestation. At her prenatal visit, her health care provider notes signs and symptoms of pregnancy-induced hypertension and advises the patient about a plan to induce labor after administration of prostaglandin gel. The patient asks the nurse, "Can you help me understand all of this?"

1. What objective tool (scoring system) can be used to predict the extent to which the patient's cervix is "ripe" and therefore favorable for successful induction?
2. The patient's health care provider orders dinoprostone gel for use in the cervix. What will be accomplished with use of the gel?
3. Who will administer the gel?
4. How often can the gel be administered?
5. How long after the last dose of gel can the IV oxytocic medication be started to induce labor?
6. Why is there a waiting period before starting the oxytocin?
7. Further questioning reveals that the patient has been ingesting a pregnancy tonic that includes herbal supplements since 36 weeks' gestation. List three concerns specific to pregnancy.
8. It is 16 hours since she first had the gel applied. Responding to her call light, the nurse finds the patient in the bathroom, upset because she feels nauseated and is occasionally vomiting a little stomach fluid and complaining that her stool is watery. "Is something wrong?" she asks. Analysis of the data about the patient's symptoms supports what conclusion?
9. What nursing actions might be taken to support the patient?
10. When the patient returns to bed and the external fetal monitor is reapplied, what data would the nurse collect, record, and report to the obstetric provider?
11. It is 24 hours since the patient had the first gel installation and 6 hours since her last insertion. A vaginal examination reveals her

cervix is soft, 50% effaced, and 3 cm dilated, and the presenting part is at 2 station. Contractions are 5 minutes apart and mild, and the health care provider elects to begin an oxytocin infusion. The patient asks how "a medicine running into my arm is able to make my uterus contract." How would the nurse explain the mechanism of action of oxytocin?

12. Why is intravenous oxytocin infused through a secondary line attached as a piggyback to the primary line? At which port along the primary line is the piggyback inserted and why?

13. Why is oxytocin administered via infusion pump? What is the measurement for dosing?

14. Regarding the IV equipment setup, what actions would be taken as safety measures before starting the oxytocin?

15. The nurse would have which drugs readily available in the event of an emergency with the oxytocin?

16. What information should be recorded during the infusion?

17. While setting up the oxytocin infusion, a new nurse being precepted to labor and delivery asks what criteria are used to know when to slow the rate or stop the infusion. The nurse correctly responds that contractions should be _____ minutes apart with _____ intensity, and the cervix would be dilated at least _____ cm.

18. Address the following if uterine hyperstimulation occurs: Position the patient; rationale: _____ IV fluids; rationale: _____ Oxygen; rationale: _____.

19. The patient asks what side effects can occur if she receives a continuous lumbar epidural. What is the appropriate response?

REVIEW QUESTIONS

1. A patient (gravida 3, para 2, at 40.6 weeks of gestation) asks, "Is there anything we can do to start labor besides medication? I'm so ready to have this baby." Which response is appropriate by the nurse?
   a. There is nothing we can do to increase labor and hasten the birth of the baby.
   b. Amniocentesis is ordered to ensure the lungs mature before we start labor.
   c. Some females may begin a brisk walking program to precipitate labor.
   d. If the cervix is ripe, the health care provider will initiate medication to soften the cervix and initiate beginning of labor.

2. A patient is to receive 10 mg nalbuphine by slow intravenous push for pain relief during labor. During which phase of uterine contractions would the nurse plan to administer nalbuphine?
   a. During the uterine contraction
   b. At the end of the uterine contraction
   c. Between uterine contractions
   d. At any time during the contraction

3. A patient received butorphanol 2 mg intravenously 10 minutes before delivery. Which nursing action is appropriate?
   a. Administer butorphanol subcutaneously.
   b. Have naloxone available.
   c. Administer intravenous fluid bolus.
   d. Place oxygen 10 L by nasal cannula.

4. A patient is to have lumbar epidural anesthesia. Which nursing action is appropriate?
   a. Administer citric acid/sodium citrate.
   b. Administer promethazine.
   c. Infuse 500 to 1000 mL of a crystalloid intravenous solution.
   d. Administer Rh0(D) immune globulin injection.

5. A 33-year-old patient in active labor is experiencing "back labor" with intense pain in her lower back. Which nursing intervention would be most effective?
   a. Counterpressure against the sacrum
   b. Pant-blow breathing techniques
   c. Effleurage
   d. Conscious relaxation or guided imagery

6. A patient has an epidural for pain control during labor. During the assessment, the nurse notes a drop in the client's blood pressure. Which priority nursing intervention would the nurse do?
   a. Administer low-flow oxygen.
   b. Turn her on her left side.
   c. Assess her urinary output.
   d. Monitor her vaginal bleeding.

7. A patient is to have an emergency cesarean delivery due to late fetal decelerations. Before surgery, the nurse administers an antacid, citric acid/sodium citrate. Which patient response would indicate effective patient teaching regarding this drug?
   a. Citric acid/sodium citrate will prevent infection after the cesarean section.
   b. The drug will neutralize the contents in my stomach.
   c. The citric acid/sodium citrate will reduce the need to use pain drug after the cesarean delivery.
   d. This drug is administered to prevent vomiting after the cesarean section.

8. Spinal anesthesia with morphine is administered to a patient for pain relief during a cesarean section. She reports itching. The nurse prepares to administer which drug?
   a. Diphenhydramine
   b. Ephedrine sulfate
   c. Butorphanol tartrate
   d. Lidocaine

9. A patient (gravida 2, para 1) is admitted to labor and delivery at 39.6 weeks' gestation in active labor. The health care provider performs an amniotomy. Which nursing intervention would be a priority?
   a. Monitoring uterine contractions
   b. Checking fetal heart rate
   c. Assessing cervical dilation and effacement
   d. Checking umbilical cord compression

10. A patient in labor is to have an epidural administered. Which nursing interventions would the nurse perform before the epidural is administered? **Select all that apply.**
    a. Infuse 500 to 1000 mL of the ordered IV fluids.
    b. Monitor maternal blood pressure and fetal heart rate.
    c. Insert indwelling urinary catheter, and monitor output.
    d. Position and support patient on left side as ordered by the health care provider.
    e. Position the patient in a lithotomy position to assist with delivery.
    f. Administer 2 L/min of oxygen via nasal cannula.

54

Neonatal and Newborn

http://evolve.elsevier.com/McCuistion/pharmacology

OBJECTIVES

- Relate principles of nursing care to the use of drugs for preterm neonates.
- Relate principles of nursing care to the use of drugs for healthy, full-term neonates.

OUTLINE

Drugs Administered to Preterm Neonates, 708
　Risks for Premature Neonates, 708
　Synthetic Surfactant, 708
Drugs Administered to Full-Term, Healthy Neonates, 709
　Erythromycin Ophthalmic Ointment, 709

　Phytonadione, 709
　Immunizations, 709
Clinical Judgment Case Study, 712
Review Questions, 712

DRUGS ADMINISTERED TO PRETERM NEONATES

This chapter focuses on drugs commonly administered to the neonate, which includes late preterm newborns immediately after delivery.

Risks for Premature Neonates

The key component of newborn care is careful assessment by the nurse. This includes Apgar scoring, respiratory and physical examination. It is also important for the nurse to be familiar with the mother's assessment data and the results of the mother's medical history. Any evidence of acquired immunodeficiency syndrome (AIDS), Group B *streptococcal* infection, and viral hepatitis B or hepatitis C, should be immediately addressed. Labor is determined to be preterm if it commences before 37 weeks of pregnancy. If there are no contraindications to halting preterm labor, tocolytic therapy is administered to delay birth (see Chapter 53 for more information on pregnancy, delivery, and postpartum drugs). However, when preterm labor is not arrested, premature delivery of the neonate occurs, which puts the newborn at risk for health problems. Premature neonates are at risk for respiratory distress, hypothermia, hypoglycemia, and hyperbilirubinemia, and they may have feeding difficulties.

Synthetic Surfactant

Respiratory distress syndrome (RDS) occurs in newborns because of immature lung development and breathing control issues due to decreased airway muscle tone and surfactant levels. Surfactant, a lipoprotein, is necessary to decrease the surface tension of the alveoli (air sacs) to allow the lungs to fill with air and prevent the alveoli from deflating. Immature lungs have lower-than-normal levels of surfactant; the more premature the neonate is, the higher the chance of RDS. One approach used to minimize respiratory difficulties in the preterm neonate is surfactant therapyreplacement. Supplementing the amount of endogenous surfactant available to maintain distension of the alveolar sacs is the focus of this therapy.

Beractant intratracheal (IT) suspension, a natural bovine lung extract, contains phospholipids, neutral lipids, fatty acids, and surfactant-associated proteins. It is administered intratracheal (IT) for prophylaxis and treatment of RDS in premature infants <1250 g birth weight or with evidence of surfactant deficiency within 15 minutes of birth, or in a neonate with confirmed RDS requiring endotracheal (ET) intubation given within 8 hours of birth.

Calfactant is a bovine-derived lung surfactant similar to beractant. Calfactant contains phospholipids, neutral lipids, fatty acids, and two low-molecular-weight, hydrophobic, surfactant-associated proteins. It is indicated for the prevention of RDS in premature infants at high risk and for rescue of neonates who develop RDS.

Poractant alfa is a porcine lung surfactant and is indicated for rescue treatment, whereas beractant and calfactant are approved for prophylaxis and rescue treatment. Poractant alfa replaces pulmonary surfactant, which is deficient in some premature neonates. Each of these products defines *prophylactic* and *rescue* use differently and has different dosing and administration requirements. Table 54.1 lists the surfactant drugs used for prevention and treatment of RDS along with their dosages, uses, and considerations.

Based on clinical response and outcomes in neonates, most clinicians feel there is little difference between the currently available natural and synthetic exogenous surfactant products.

All exogenous surfactants require a patent ET tube for administration and specified alterations in positioning the infant throughout the procedure to ensure even drug dispersion. These precise position changes allow gravity to assist in the distribution of the product in the lungs, particularly at the alveolar surface.

Crackles and moist breath sounds may be a transient finding after administration of these products, particularly with beractant. Exogenous surfactant can cause postadministration complications such as hyperoxia (excessive oxygenation) and hypocarbia (decreased carbon dioxide [CO_2]). In addition, transient endotracheal reflux can obstruct the ET tube and lead to oxygen desaturation, cyanosis,

TABLE 54.1 Exogenous Surfactant Therapy for Prevention and Treatment of Respiratory Distress Syndrome

Generic	Route and Dosage	Uses and Considerations
Beractant	Premature neonate (PN): Intratracheal (IT): 4 mL/kg per dose IT divided into four equal amounts; May administer up to 3 more doses of 4 L/kg/dose (100 mg/kg/dose) at 6 h intervals, if needed. *max:* 100 mg/kg (birth weight) dose or 4 mL/kg (birth weight) dosed IT.	Indicated for prevention and treatment (rescue) of RDS in premature neonates. ⚡ Drug must be given by health care personnel experienced with intubation and the use of ventilators for prevention or rescue in treatment of RDS. May cause: bradycardia, apnea, cyanosis, hypocarbia, intracranial bleeding.
Calfactant	PN: IT: 3 mL/kg (approx. 100 mg/kg of phospholipids per dose) IT; May give 2 more doses of 3 mL/kg/dose every 12 h. Repeat doses given as early as 6 h for a total of 4 doses every 12 h. AAP recommends redosing every 12 h. *max.* neonates: 100 mg/kg birth weight (3 mL/kg birth weight) dosed IT.	Indicated for prevention and treatment (rescue) of RDS in premature neonates. ⚡ Drug must be given by health care personnel experienced with intubation and the use of ventilators for prevention or rescue in treatment of RDS. May cause: Bradycardia, cyanosis, hypocarbia, intracranial bleeding, intraventricular hemorrhage.
Poractant alfa	PN: IT: 2.5 mL/kg per dose divided in two equal amounts IT; may repeat 2 additional doses of 1.25 mL/kg/dose at 12 h intervals; *max.* 2.5 mL/kg (birth weight) dosed IT.	Poractant alfa is indicated for the treatment ("rescue") of respiratory distress syndrome (RDS) in premature infants. ⚡ Drug must be given by health care personnel experienced with intubation and the use of ventilators and RDS. May cause: apnea, bradycardia, cyanosis, hypocarbia.

approx., Approximately; *ET*, endotracheal; *h*, hour; *IT*, intratracheal; *Kg*, kilograms; *min*, minute; *PN*, premature neonate; *q*, every; *RDS*, respiratory distress syndrome; *s*, second; *wk*, weeks.

bradycardia, and apnea. These issues do not usually lead to serious long-term complications when properly managed. Unless obvious signs of airway obstruction are noted, suctioning should not be performed immediately after administration of supplemental surfactant. Dosing is slowed or halted if the infant (1) becomes dusky colored, (2) becomes agitated, (3) experiences transient bradycardia, (4) has oxygen saturation increases of more than 95%, (5) experiences improved chest expansion, or (6) has arterial or transcutaneous CO_2 levels below 30 mm Hg. Suctioning before dosing decreases the chance for ET tube blockage during dosing. No long-term complications or sequelae of synthetic surfactant therapy have been reported. Surfactant replacement therapy has been found effective in reducing the severity of RDS; rapid improvements in lung compliance and oxygenation may require immediate decreases in ventilator settings to prevent lung overdistension and pulmonary air leak.

Surfactant drugs are administered by medical personnel experienced with ventilators and intubation of their patient population. Administration is a two-person procedure. It should be performed by at least one medical practitioner or a neonatal nurse practitioner who administers the surfactant, and one registered nurse as the assistant.

DRUGS ADMINISTERED TO FULL-TERM, HEALTHY NEONATES

Newborns should receive eye care (e.g., erythromycin ophthalmic ointment), phytonadione, and immunizations for hepatitis B (www.who.int). In addition, an antiinfective agent (e.g., chlorhexidine) may be applied to the cord stump during the first few hours after birth and for up to 1 week for at-risk newborns and newborns born in homes.

Erythromycin Ophthalmic Ointment

A common antiinfective administered to a newborn's eyes within the first hour of birth is *erythromycin ophthalmic ointment*. Erythromycin ointment serves as a simple, harmless, cost-effective means of preventing blindness. The blindness in question results from infection with sexually transmitted infections, chlamydia and gonorrhea. Both infections can progress rapidly in newborns' eyes, damaging the clear part over the pupils (corneas) and causing irreversible harm. Ocular irritation and redness can occur from the use of erythromycin ophthalmic ointment.

Phytonadione

Phytonadione, a synthetic vitamin K, is a fat-soluble vitamin given to newborns to prevent vitamin K–deficiency bleeding. This can result in a life-threatening disease called hemorrhagic disease of the newborn. Vitamin K deficiency is one of the most common causes of bleeding in a healthy infant. Newborns are inherently vitamin K deficient at birth due to lower stores of vitamin K in their immature system, as well as a decreased ability to utilize vitamin K. The newborn lacks appropriate intestinal flora to synthesize vitamin K.

It is administered as a single-dose injection. Side effects include pain and edema at the injection site. Some allergic reactions, manifested by urticaria and rash, have been reported. Neonates who receive larger doses may exhibit hyperbilirubinemia and jaundice resulting from competition for binding sites.

Table 54.2 covers erythromycin and phytonadione and their dosages, uses, and considerations.

Immunizations

The American Academy of Pediatrics and the Centers for Disease Control and Prevention have recommended that immunization against

TABLE 54.2 Drugs Administered to Newborns

Generic	Route and Dosage	Uses and Considerations
Erythromycin ophthalmic ointment	Neonate ophthalmic 0.5%: within 1 h of delivery and without touching the tip of the tube to the eye, fingertips, or any other surface, place a 1-cm ribbon of ointment in the lower conjunctival sac of each eye, beginning at the inner canthus from the inner to outer eye.	Prevention of **ophthalmia neonatorum**, an eye infection among newborns, and protection against gonococcal and chlamydial conjunctivitis. May cause: erythema, phlebitis, pruritus, and skin irritation. ⚡ Most states mandate erythromycin ophthalmic ointment but consult your facility's policy. Do not flush eyes after installation. Use new tube for each infant.
Hepatitis B immune globulin (HBIG)	IM: subcut: 0.5 mL within 12 h after birth into the anterolateral thigh (vastus lateralis)	For newborns of mothers positive for HBsAg for passive immunity; May cause: injection site reaction. ⚡ Obtain consents from parents. Initiate recombinant HB as a separate injection at different sites; aspiration is not required.
Phytonadione	*Premature neonate* 0.2–0.5 mg IM single dose immediately after birth *Term Neonate* 1 mg IM as a single dose immediately after birth Administer into the anterolateral thigh (vastus lateralis) within 1 h after birth; ⚡ check health care provider or agency standing orders for dosage.	An anticoagulant antagonist for prevention of hemorrhagic disease of the newborn. May cause: anaphylactic shock, cardiacarrest, anaphylactoid reactions, cyanosis, and respiratory arrest. Drug is readily absorbed after IM administration. ❗ Black-Box Warning: IV administration; serous hypersensitivity reactions or anaphylaxis
Hepatitis B vaccine (HBV), recombinant	IM/subcut: 0.5 mL (5 mcg) within 24 h after birth (first dose); subsequent doses at 1 and 6 mo of age into anterolateral thigh (vastus lateralis)	Stimulates the immune system to produce anti–HBsAg antibodies without the risk of developing active infection. Protection usually occurs 1 mo after the third dose. May cause: injection site reaction.

cm, Centimeter; *h*, hour; *HBIG*, hepatitis B immune globulin; *HBsAg*, hepatitis B surface antigen; *HBV*, hepatitis B vaccine recombinant; *IM*, intramuscularly; *IV*, intravenous; *mL*, millimeter; *mo*, month; *subcut*, subcutaneous.

CLINICAL JUDGMENT [NURSING PROCESS]

Drug Administered to Preterm Neonate: Synthetic Surfactant

Concept: Oxygenation
- *Oxygenation* refers to the process of providing cells with oxygen. The act of breathing depends on a functioning respiratory system that provides oxygen to the cells. Nurses encounter alterations in the patient's oxygenation. Those who care for the neonatal population must quickly detect problems in oxygenation and act to prevent respiratory distress and death in the infant.

Recognize Cues [Assessment]
- Obtain informed consent. Separate consents are needed for multifetal births.
- Assess the patient's vital signs, perform a physical examination, and monitor arterial blood gases (ABGs).

Analyze Cues and Prioritize Hypothesis [Patient Problems]
- Decreased gas exchange
- Decreased tissue perfusion
- Decreased ability to cope (parents)

Generate Solutions [Planning]
- The patient's oxygen requirement and respiratory effort will decrease.
- The patient will experience no respiratory distress after surfactant administration.
- The patient will breathe without the assistance of mechanical ventilation and experience adequate oxygenation.
- The patient will maintain a patent airway.

Take Action [Nursing Interventions]
- Continuously monitor the patient's vital signs before, during, and after surfactant therapy.
- Assess the patient to ensure adequate respiratory status is maintained.
- Assist the multidisciplinary team (physician or neonatal nurse) as needed.
- Monitor ABGs, and obtain a chest radiography study.
- Maintain adequate respiratory status.
- Position and reposition the patient as needed for equal distribution of surfactant throughout the lungs.
- Support and educate the parents.
- Acknowledge the parents' concerns regarding the well-being of the newborn.
- Provide an interpreter if the patient's parents have a language barrier.
- Provide health information written in the parents' primary language.

Patient Teaching
- Explain to the parents what respiratory distress syndrome (RDS) is and how surfactant helps the neonate.
- Explain to the parents the purpose of multiple monitoring devices to reduce unrealistic fears about the neonate's condition.
- Ensure informed consent for drug usage.
- Encourage the parents to verbalize their understanding about risks associated with use of the drug.

Evaluate Outcomes [Evaluation]
- Evaluate preadministration breath sounds, ABGs, respiratory status, and ventilator pressure readings to compare with postadministration findings.
- Evaluate the effectiveness of teaching to parents.

hepatitis B virus (HBV) begin in the newborn period. HBV infection may result in serious long-term liver disease, cancer, and death in adulthood. The goal of immunization is to reduce the number of chronic carriers of the virus in the population, thus decreasing the prevalence of HBV infection.

In pregnancy, HBV transmission occurs vertically—that is, by *perinatal transmission*—primarily at the time of delivery. *Hepatitis B immune globulin (HBIG)* is given to infants born to mothers who are positive for hepatitis B surface antigen (HBsAg). HBIG provides the newborn passive protection against HBV. Adverse effects of the injection include pain, tenderness, and erythema at the injection site. Hypotension, erythematous rash, and anaphylaxis after receiving HBIG can also occur.

A three-dose series vaccine for *hepatitis B Virus (HBV), recombinant hepatitis B*, is indicated for HBV prophylaxis in infants; the first injection is given at birth. The second and third injections are administered at 1- and 2-month intervals by the pediatrician. Newborns who for a medical reason do not get the vaccine at birth should receive their first dose as soon as possible and complete all three doses at the recommended intervals. The dose is administered intramuscular in the anterolateral thigh area to the vastus lateralis muscle. Hepatitis B, recombinant (HBV) can provide active immunity against HBV by stimulating the immune system to produce antibodies against hepatitis B (anti–hepatitis B antigen), and it can be given concurrently with HBIG if the infant is born to an HBsAg-positive mother. Recombinant HBV is given as separate injection administered to separate sites. Adverse effects from recombinant HBV are generally mild and include pain, tenderness, pruritus, erythema, swelling, and induration at the injection site. It is mandatory that a parent sign a consent form before the infant receives an HBV immunization.

Table 54.2 lists HBIG and recombinant HB and their dosages, uses, and considerations.

CLINICAL JUDGMENT [NURSING PROCESS]
Drugs Administered to Full-Term, Healthy Neonates

Concept: Caring Interventions
- Caring interventions are performed by the nurse during medication administration. These interventions ensure safe practice outcomes. The interventions are the result of scientific research, best practice guidelines, composed by the professional body of nursing for quality care and safe practice.

Recognize Cues [Assessment]
- Assess the patient for signs of distress such as cyanosis, bleeding, ecchymosis, apnea, fever, and hypotension.
- Assess the mother's hepatitis B virus (HBV) status.
- Assess the parents' knowledge of treatments (e.g., medications and immunizations) given to their newborn.

Analyze Cues and Prioritize Hypothesis [Patient Problems]
- Potential injury
- Need for health teaching (parental)
- Anxiety (parental)

Generate Solutions [Planning]
- The patient will experience minimal or no side effects from drugs routinely administered after delivery.
- Parents will express understanding of medications and immunizations given to their newborn.

Take Action [Nursing Interventions]
- Obtain parental consents for immunizations.
- Provide immediate skin-to-skin contact between mother and infant while preparing medications and immunizations. Skin-to-skin contact in the first hour of birth prevents hypothermia and promotes breast-feeding.
- Wear gloves for administration of medications and immunizations.
- Prepare to administer hepatitis B immune globulin (HBIG) to the patient if the mother is hepatitis B surface antigen (HBsAg) positive.
- Prepare and administer drugs and immunizations according to the manufacturer's instructions while the patient maintains contact with the mother's skin.
- Administer erythromycin ophthalmic ointment *before* administration of phytonadione and hepatitis B injections. The patient may cry after injections, making administration of ophthalmic ointment more difficult.
- Monitor for any reactions, such as redness and swelling in and around the eye from the eye ointment or redness, swelling, or ecchymosis at injection sites. Monitor for any respiratory distress (e.g., grunting, apnea, nasal flaring).
- Acknowledge parent concerns about immunizations.
- Provide printed literature on hepatitis B and other immunizations.
- It is important for nurses to be sensitive to the family's traditions and beliefs.
- It is important for the nurse to establish rapport with the patient's parents.

Patient Teaching
- Instruct the parents regarding the action, purpose, and side effects of medications and immunizations.
- Inform the parents that any edema around the eyes usually disappears within 24–48 hours.
- Explain to the parents the difference between HBIG and recombinant hepatitis B (HB) injections.
- Instruct the parents regarding childhood immunizations as recommended by current immunization schedules, and inform them when repeat doses should be given. Give parents written information regarding the patient's immunization record and vaccination schedule.
- Document administration of hepatitis B vaccine on the patient's immunization record.
- Instruct the parents on the signs and symptoms of adverse effects and when to notify the nurse.

Evaluate Outcomes [Evaluation]
- Evaluate for newborn bleeding, particularly on days 2 and 3 after administration of phytonadione.
- Evaluate for drug hypersensitivity or side effects.
- Evaluate parents' understanding about medications administered to their newborn.

CLINICAL JUDGMENT CASE STUDY

The patient is an 18-year-old female, admitted to the hospital for labor induction/augmentation with signs and symptoms of gestational hypertension at 42 weeks' gestation (gravida 4, para 1). The delivery occurred at 6:00 a.m. by vacuum extraction. The baby, weighing 8 lb 7 oz, had Apgar scores of 7 and 9. The infant is alert and active. Immediately after the delivery, the nurse assesses and prioritizes nursing care needs.

1. What steps should the nurse follow to instill ointment into the newborn patient's eyes?
2. What should the infant's parent be taught about the side effects of eye prophylaxis?
3. How should the nurse explain the reason for the vitamin K injection for the infant patient in terms the parent can understand?
4. Which newborn patients are eligible to receive the hepatitis B immune globulin (HBIG) vaccine?
5. How many doses constitute the total series of the hepatitis B vaccine (HBV), and what is the duration for these?

REVIEW QUESTIONS

1. A patient asks the nurse why her baby is receiving a vitamin K injection. The nurse's best response is based on what knowledge?
   a. Vitamin K is important because it increases the newborn's platelets.
   b. A newborn baby's metabolism is too immature to produce vitamin K.
   c. A newborn lacks appropriate intestinal flora to synthesize vitamin K.
   d. Vitamin K is not produced in bone marrow until an infant is 8 days old.

2. It is mandatory to have paternal signed consent before administering which newborn drug?
   a. Erythromycin eye ointment
   b. Phytonadione (vitamin K_1)
   c. Hepatitis B vaccine (HBV) series
   d. Betamethasone injection

3. The nurse is mentoring a new graduate who is preparing to administer the phytonadione injection to a newborn. Which muscle sites selected by the new graduate would indicate the need for further teaching? **Select all that apply.**
   a. Anterolateral thigh
   b. Gluteus maximus
   c. Rectus femoris
   d. Vastus lateralis
   e. Vastus medialis

4. The nurse is preparing to administer an ophthalmic drug to a newborn. Education for the parents includes which fact about the drug?
   a. All infants born preterm receive an ophthalmic drug to protect their eyes.
   b. Eye ointments are given in the lower bottom of the eye from the inner to the outer eye.
   c. This drug will prevent congenital ophthalmic diseases and must be given.
   d. Infants with a negative direct Coombs test receive this drug to protect vision.

5. A newborn is admitted to the nursery, and the nurse reviews the maternal history. It is important that the nurse assess the mother's status specific to which infectious process(es)? **Select all that apply.**
   a. Rubeola (Measles)
   b. Hepatitis A
   c. Hepatitis B
   d. HIV/AIDS
   e. Group B *Streptococcus*

6. A neonate whose mother is positive for the hepatitis B surface antigen (HBsAg) is admitted to the nursery. Which immunizations are appropriate for this neonate? **Select all that apply.**
   a. Hepatitis B immune globulin (HBIG)
   b. Recombinant hepatitis B vaccine (HBV)
   c. *Haemophilus influenzae* type B
   d. Hepatitis A vaccine
   e. Erythromycin ophthalmic ointment

55

Female Reproductive Health

Christina DiMaggio Boudreaux, RN, BSN, IBCLC

http://evolve.elsevier.com/McCuistion/pharmacology

OBJECTIVES

- Relate principles of nursing care to the use of drugs for contraception.
- Describe the use of different drugs for various disorders in female's health.
- Relate principles of nursing care to the use of drugs promoting fertility.
- Relate the principles of nursing care to the use of drugs for menopause.
- Explain the causes and drug treatment choices in osteoporosis disease.

OUTLINE

Drugs Used for Contraception, 713
    Combined Hormonal Contraceptives, 713
    Monophasic and Multiphasic, 716
    Pseudomenstruation Withdrawal, 716
    Progestin Contraceptives, 717
    Start Date and Dosing Schedule for Hormonal Contraception Products, 718
    Preventing Fertilization, 720
Drugs Used to Treat Disorders in Female Health, 722
    Amenorrhea, 722
    Polycystic Ovarian Syndrome, 722
    Abnormal Uterine Bleeding, 723
    Dysmenorrhea, 723
    Endometriosis, 724
    Premenstrual Syndrome, 724
Drugs Used to Promote Fertility, 725
    Causes and Treatments of Infertility, 725

    Induction of Ovulation, 726
Drugs Used in the Treatment of Menopause, 729
    Menopause, 729
    Perimenopause, 729
    Postmenopause, 729
    FDA Warnings for Hormone Therapy, 729
    Hormonal Therapy, 729
    Various Dosage Forms of Estrogen, 730
    Classes of Drugs for Perimenopausal/Menopausal Treatments, 731
Osteoporosis Disease, 732
    Clinical Nursing Judgment in the Management of Osteoporosis Disease, 732
    Drugs Used for Treatment of Osteoporosis, 732
Clinical Judgment Unfolding Case Study, 734
Review Questions, 738

Females have specific health care needs throughout their reproductive and postreproductive life cycle. A female's reproductive life cycle begins with *menarche*, the start of spontaneous menstruation, and continues through *menopause*, the permanent cessation of menstruation. Successful contraception is essential to the health and well-being of sexually active female of reproductive age. During the reproductive years, many disorders can occur in female's health. These gynecologic conditions interfere with a female's overall health and well-being and may impede her ability to become pregnant.

Successful adaptation to menopause, control of menopausal symptoms, and continued sexual health are essential to the well-being of older female. This chapter reviews pharmacologic products that may be used throughout the reproductive and menopausal life cycle of a female as well as typical drug regimens used for disorders in female's health. Drugs for female infertility are also addressed with an emphasis on drugs that stimulate ovulation.

DRUGS USED FOR CONTRACEPTION

Combined Hormonal Contraceptives

Combined hormonal contraceptives (CHCs) are one of the most used methods of reversible contraception in the world because of their ease of use, high degree of effectiveness (92%–99.3% effective), and relative safety.

Research has shown that higher doses of estrogen increase the risk for venous thromboembolism (VTE), myocardial infarction (MI), and stroke. Subsequently, low-dose oral contraceptives (OCs) and, more recently, ultra-low-dose OCs have been introduced to reduce the risk of dangerous side effects. Research continues to focus on actual and potential short- and long-term benefits and risks associated with use of low-dose OCs, particularly in the areas of heart and circulatory risks as well as carcinogenesis. Clinical studies also continue to investigate the venous circulatory effects of new-generation progestins.

All **combined hormonal contraceptives (CHCs)** contain a synthetic version of *estrogen* and a compound known as *progestin*. **Ethinyl estradiol** (EE) is the most used synthetic estrogen found in CHCs. **Progestins** are natural or synthetic hormones that have *progesterone-like* effects. *Progesterone* is the naturally occurring sex hormone produced in the ovaries of females; *progestogen* refers to any synthetically produced progesterone compound. Almost all progestins are derivatives of testosterone, a steroid hormone classified under the androgen group that binds to and activates the progesterone receptors. The term *progestin* will be used to describe the compound used in CHC products. Not only do progestins have contraceptive properties, but they also serve to balance out the effects of estrogen.

One of eight different types of progestins is used in CHC products. Norethindrone, norethindrone acetate, and ethynodiol diacetate are first-generation progestin compounds (estrane family) and were the earliest progestin formulations to be used in OCs. Second-generation progestins (gonane family) include norgestrel and levonorgestrel (LNG). Third-generation progestins include desogestrel and norgestimate. The new-generation progestins have a higher efficacy rating and fewer effects on lipid and carbohydrate metabolism compared with their earlier counterparts. They also have fewer androgenic side effects, which are described later in this chapter.

Drospirenone (DRSP) is a fourth-generation progestin. It is an analog of spironolactone. As with spironolactone, a potassium-sparing diuretic, DRSP can increase serum potassium levels in females taking DRSP-containing OCs, altering water and electrolyte balance.

The amount of estrogen and the type of progestin determine bioactivity and possible side effects of CHC products. The combination of estrogen and the selected progestin affect the uterine endometrium; therefore the lowest effective dose that successfully prevents conception should be used (Table 55.1).

TABLE 55.1 Oral Combined Hormonal Contraceptives

Drug	Route and Dosage	Uses and Considerations
Combination products containing norethindrone and ethinyl estradiol	Oral: 1 tablet PO daily 21-tablet package: 1 tablet daily for 21 consecutive days followed by 7 days off. A new course begins on the eighth day after a tablet is taken. 28-tablet package: 1 tablet daily without interruption taken at the same time each day Schedule 1: Start the first Sunday after onset of menstruation (while using additional contraception for 7 days) Schedule 2: Start the first day of menstrual cycle.	Estrogen and progestin combination used for contraception and for treatment of moderate acne vulgaris in females 15 years and older who have achieved menarche, are unresponsive to topical treatments, have no contraindications to CHC use, and plan to stay on therapy for 6 months or longer. ⚡ *Contraindications:* History of or current thrombophlebitis, DVT, PE, CVA, CAD, valve disease, hypertension, diabetes mellitus with vascular involvement, migraines in females >35 y, cancers, neoplasms, and tumors. Cardiovascular side effects are increased in female who smoke, especially those >35 y and in those who use CHCs. Absorption: Rapid; PB: >95%; t½: 5–15 h norethindrone and 26 h ethinyl estradiol. Pregnancy Considerations: Use in pregnancy is contraindicated. Treatment should be discontinued immediately if pregnancy occurs. ⚡ Black-Box Warning: Cigarette smoking increases the risk of serious cardiovascular events while using combination oral contraceptives. ❗ High Alert Drug: Significant risk of harm when given in error.
Combination products containing levonorgestrel (LNG) and ethinyl estradiol (EE)	Same	Estrogen and progestin combination used for contraception and postcoital emergency contraception. ⚡ Black-box warnings: Obesity, tobacco smoking. Use with caution in patients with depression, and monitor patients on thyroid replacement therapy, who may require higher doses of thyroid hormone while receiving estrogens. PB: 95%–99%; t½: EE 26 h, LNG 8–13 h. ⚡ Pregnancy Considerations: Use is contraindicated in pregnant females; discontinue treatment if pregnancy occurs. Recommended waiting 4–6 weeks postpartum before starting this combination due to increased risk of venous thromboembolism. When used for emergency contraception, a barrier contraceptive method is recommended after use or abstinence for 7 days. ❗ High Alert Drug: Significant risk of harm when given in error.
Combination products containing norgestrel and EE, ethynodiol diacetate and EE, and desogestrel and EE	Same	Combination progesterone and estrogen used for contraception. Contraindications include most of the same as previously discussed, current thrombophlebitis, DVT, PE, CVA, CAD, valve disease, hypertension, diabetes mellitus with vascular involvement, migraines in females over 35 y, cancers, neoplasm, tumors; cardiovascular side effects are increased in females who smoke, especially those over 35 y. Some evidence has suggested there is an increased risk for VTE in obese females (BMI ≥ 30 kg/m²) using CHCs. Caution in patients with a history of ⚡ depression. Absorption: Rapid; PB: 95%–99%; t½: EE 12–23 h; t½: Norgestrel 22–49 h. ⚡ Pregnancy Considerations: Contraindicated in pregnancy. ⚡ Blackbox Warning: Tobacco smoking. ❗ High Alert Drug: Significant risk of harm when given in error.

TABLE 55.1 Oral Combined Hormonal Contraceptives—cont'd

Drug	Route and Dosage	Uses and Considerations
Combination products containing drospirenone (DRSP) and EE	Same	Estrogen and progestin combination used for contraception, for acne treatment in adults, and for PMDD. May cause candidiasis, fluid retention, peripheral edema, migraines, and endometrial hyperplasia. ⚡ Blackbox Warning: MI, new primary malignancy, stroke, thromboembolism and dementia. Evidence of carcinogenic potential, lack of cardioprotective effect and lack of cognitive protection in older females. ❗ High Alert Drug: Significant risk of harm when given in error. PB: 97%–98%; t½: 24–30 h. ⚡ Pregnancy Considerations: Contraindicated in pregnancy.
Combination products containing norgestimate and EE	Same	Estrogen and progestin combination used for contraception and for acne treatment in adults. May cause cataracts, increased hepatic enzymes, vaginitis, and depression. ⚡ Blackbox Warning: Tobacco smoking. ❗ High Alert Drug: Significant risk of harm when given in error. PB: 97%–99%; t½: 16–38 h. ⚡ Contraindicated in pregnancy.
Combination with folate in the form of EE-DRSP-levomefolate calcium	Same	Estrogen and progestin combination used for contraception, acne, and PMDD. May cause: candidiasis, migraines, depression. ⚡ Blackbox Warning: tobacco smoking. ❗ High Alert Drug: Significant risk of harm when given in error. PB: 97%–99%; t½: DRSP 31 h, EE 24 h (approx.), levomefolate calcium 4–5 h (approx.) Contraindicated in pregnancy.

CAD, Coronary artery disease; *CHC*, combined hormonal contraceptive; *CVA*, cerebrovascular accident; *DRSP*, drospirenone; *DVT*, deep venous thrombosis; *EE*, ethinyl estradiol; *h*, hours; *LNG*, levonorgestrel; *MI*, myocardial infarction; *PB*, protein binding; *PE*, pulmonary embolus; *PMDD*, premenstrual dysphoric disorder; *PO*, by mouth; *t½*, half-life; *y*, year.

Side Effects of Combined Hormonal Contraception

CHC formulations are differentiated based on the strength of the estrogen component, the type of progestin used, and whether estrogen or progesterone (and androgen) activity predominates. Increased estrogenic activity may include *side effects* such as cyclic breast changes, dysmenorrhea (painful periods), menorrhagia (heavy periods), chloasma (hyperpigmentation of the skin), and VTE, whereas decreased estrogenic activity can cause amenorrhea (absence of periods) or spotting at certain points in the cycle. Increased progestational activity can cause weight gain, depression, fatigue, and decreased libido, and a lack of progestational activity may cause breakthrough bleeding (BTB) and headaches. BTB is an episode of bleeding that occurs during the active pill cycle of CHCs. It is more common at the start of CHC use, when there is a change to the type of pill being taken, and with progestin-only preparations of contraception. There is no evidence that an episode of BTB is associated with a decrease in the CHC's effectiveness if the patient continues to take the pill daily as prescribed. Increased androgenic activity may cause acne, hirsutism, edema, and cholestatic jaundice. The estrogens and progestins in OC pills also affect the uterine endometrium, which may cause changes in the patient's periods that can include irregular bleeding, heavy or light periods, or spotting between periods. The undesirable side effects of hormonal contraception products are discussed later in this chapter.

Most females on CHC products experience shorter, lighter periods. Other advantages with CHCs are decreased blood loss and uterine cramps, elimination of mittelschmerz (midcycle pain usually associated with ovulation), reduction of symptoms in many forms of benign breast disorders, and prevention of physiologic ovarian cysts. CHC products also reduce the incidence of pelvic inflammatory disease (PID), ectopic pregnancy, endometrial and ovarian cancer risk, and deaths from colorectal cancer. CHC products do *not* reduce the incidence of sexually transmitted infections (STIs; see Chapter 57 for further discussion of STIs.)

The goal of therapy is to identify the product that offers the best contraceptive protection while producing the fewest unwanted side effects. It is important to note that the effectiveness of OCs can also be compromised by concurrent use of some drugs (e.g., antibiotics) or herbal products.

COMPLEMENTARY AND ALTERNATIVE THERAPIES

Contraceptive Hormones

Always use complementary and alternative therapies with caution as they may alter the strength of the contraceptive hormone.

- St. Johns wort may decrease the level of contraceptive hormones in the bloodstream, reducing the effectiveness of combined hormonal contraceptives (CHCs). This may result in breakthrough bleeding and/or spontaneous ovulation.
- Chasteberry extract should be used with caution with CHCs or hormone therapy because it may alter contraceptive hormone levels in the body and can make them less effective.
- Other herbal remedies that may alter the effectiveness of contraceptive hormones include dong quai, black cohosh, and red clover.

Mechanism of Action

The estrogen component of CHC products inhibits ovulation by preventing the formation of a dominant follicle. When a dominant follicle does not mature, estrogen remains at a consistent level and is unable to reach the peak level needed to stimulate the luteinizing hormone (LH) surge. The progestin component also suppresses the LH surge. When the LH surge is suppressed, ovulation is prevented, and pregnancy does not occur. Any cycle in which ovulation does not occur, whether induced by drugs or naturally occurring, is called an anovulatory cycle. CHCs produce drug-induced anovulatory cycles. The estrogen component of CHC products also stabilizes the uterine endometrium, inhibiting proliferation and secretory changes, and decreasing the occurrence of irregular or heavy bleeding. The progestational effects of progestin change the endometrium to make it less favorable for implantation of a fertilized ovum. In addition, progestins affect the quantity and viscosity of the cervical mucus, making it thick and hostile to sperm penetration.

Route of Delivery

There are several routes of administration for CHC products. Most females are familiar with OC, in which a pill is ingested daily, absorbed by the gastrointestinal (GI) tract, and metabolized by the liver. However, CHC products can also be administered through transvaginal and transdermal routes. The advantage of these alternative sites is avoiding GI absorption and the initial metabolism by the liver, or the *first-pass effect*. Theoretically, side effects such as nausea and vomiting, heart and circulatory risks, and nonadherence with a daily dosage regimen can be avoided.

Monophasic and Multiphasic

Combination pills are classified as either monophasic or multiphasic (biphasic, triphasic, or four-phasic). The *monophasics* provide a fixed ratio of estrogen to progestin throughout the menstrual cycle. In *biphasics*, the amount of estrogen is fixed throughout the cycle, but the amount of progestin varies; it is reduced in the first half to provide for some proliferation of the endometrium and is increased in the second half to promote secretory development of the endometrium. This simulates the normal physiologic process of menstruation while still inhibiting ovulation. The *triphasics* deliver low doses of both hormones with minimal side effects because the amounts of estrogen and progesterone both vary throughout the cycle in different ratios during the phases. The *four-phasics* deliver varying doses of estradiol valerate (1, 2, or 3 mg) and dienogest (0, 2, or 3 mg) throughout the cycle.

Pseudomenstruation Withdrawal

Most of the monophasic, biphasic, and triphasic CHC products are packaged in both 21- and 28-day tablet packs. In the 21-day tablet packs, 21 days of active pills that contain estrogen and progestin are followed by a 7-day "pill-free" period. A new pack of pills is started after the 7-day pill-free period. In the 28-day tablet pack, 21 days of active pills are followed by 7 days of inert pills, called *counters*. The patient takes one pill daily and begins a new pack the day after the last counter is taken. During the hormone-free period (counters) or the 7-day pill-free period, the level of estrogen and progestin decreases to allow for a breakdown of the endometrial lining. This causes a pseudomenstruation known as withdrawal bleeding or *withdrawal menses*. The withdrawal bleeding is not a true menstrual period, and the bleeding experienced by a female can vary in amount and duration.

There are CHCs that provide ferrous fumarate, an iron compound, or folic acid, a B vitamin, during the hormone-free period. Ferrous fumarate provides supplementation during the phase of withdrawal bleeding, promoting healthy iron stores in females and protecting against menstrual-associated iron-deficiency anemia. Folic acid reduces the risk of spinal dysraphism should the females become pregnant on OCs or shortly after discontinuation.

Withdrawal bleeding periods are scheduled monthly to mimic a normal 28-day menstrual cycle; however, researchers have established that a monthly episode of withdrawal bleeding is not necessary to maintain a healthy uterus

Extended-Use and Continuous-Use Combined Hormonal Contraception

Extended-use CHC delays menstruation, whereas continuous use eliminates menstruation.

With continuous-dose CHCs, menses is eliminated, making these products beneficial for females with menses disorders such as menorrhagia (heavy periods), metrorrhagia (irregular bleeding between periods, usually heavy), endometriosis, dysmenorrhea, premenstrual syndrome (PMS), and physiologic ovarian cyst formation.

Ethinyl Estradiol and Norelgestromin Transdermal Patch

This is a weekly form of CHC patch that delivers 35 mcg EE and 150 mcg norelgestromin every 24 hours through a transdermal system. The system is a thin plastic patch placed on the skin of the buttocks, stomach, upper outer arm, or upper torso. The patch is placed once a week for 3 weeks in a row. The fourth week is patch free to allow for withdrawal bleeding. The patch should be placed on clean, dry skin; placement on or near the breasts should be avoided because of the estrogen component, and the site of the patch placement should be rotated to avoid skin irritation. If the patch partially or completely detaches from the skin, a new patch should be placed. When used correctly, the patch is 92% to 99.3% effective at preventing pregnancy.

The patch works in a similar manner to CHC pills by inhibiting ovulation, thickening cervical mucus to prevent sperm penetration, and preventing a fertilized egg from implanting in the uterus. Advantages include not having to remember to take a pill daily, as well as a decrease of menstrual flow, cramping, acne, iron-deficiency anemia, excess body hair, premenstrual symptoms, and vaginal dryness. As with CHC pills, the patch reduces the risk for ovarian and endometrial cancers, PID, breast and ovarian cysts, and osteoporosis (loss of bone mass) that predisposes females to fractures. With the patch, occurrences of ectopic pregnancy are also reduced. As with all CHC products, the ability to become pregnant quickly returns when discontinued.

Disadvantages of the patch include skin reaction at the site of application, menstrual cramps, and a change in vision or the inability to wear contact lenses; it is not as effective for females who weigh more than 198 lb. Due to the peak levels of estrogen remaining constant during the week the patch is in place, females are exposed to 60% more estrogen than with OC. Therefore EE and norelgestromin transdermal patch carry a boxed warning stating that they expose females to higher risk for ⚡ VTE. Females being prescribed the transdermal route of CHCs should be notified of potential risks, and the patch should be used with extreme caution in any patient with increased risk for VTE. Females who are older than 35 years and smoke should not use the transdermal patch. Other side effects include temporary irregular bleeding, weight gain or loss, breast tenderness, and nausea.

Ethinyl Estradiol and Etonogestrel Transvaginal Contraception

The EE and etonogestrel transvaginal ring is a 2-inch flexible indwelling ring inserted vaginally and left in place continuously for 3 consecutive weeks, then removed for 1 week. It releases 15 mcg of EE and 120 mcg of progestin etonogestrel daily, similar to the quantities of estrogen and progestin found in lower-dose CHC products Theoretic effectiveness and typical effectiveness rates are 98% and 92%, similar to those of other leading CHCs. The patient inserts the ring during the first 5 days of the menstrual cycle and removes the ring after 3 weeks, remains "ring free" for 1 week (for withdrawal menses), and then inserts a new ring. Backup contraception is recommended during the first 7 days after the first ring is placed. During this time, the hormones reach an appropriate protective level. After this, contraceptive effects are expected to be continuous provided the ring is correctly inserted. Correct insertion involves placing the ring into the middle or upper third of the vagina. Unlike the diaphragm, it does not need to be placed near or over the cervix. It is the close proximity of the ring to the vaginal mucosa that causes absorption of steroid hormones to occur. The ring remains in place during intercourse, tampon use, or administration of intravaginal drugs. If the ring slips out, it can be rinsed with lukewarm water and reinserted into the vagina. It should be reinserted within 3 hours after becoming dislodged; if the ring remains out for more than 3 hours, additional contraception is required until the ring has been in place for 7 days. Possible side effects include vaginal discharge, irritation, or infection. Other associated risks are the same as for low-dose CHCs and are increased in patients who smoke; therefore the ring has a boxed warning against use in female older than 35 years who ⚡ smoke.

Segesterone acetate and EE transvaginal ring is another combination hormonal contraceptive vaginal ring. EE is a potent synthetic estrogen, and segesterone is a synthetic progestin. Contraindications are listed as the same as EE transvaginal ring. The Institute for Safe Medication Practices includes the transvaginal rings among the list of drugs that have a heightened risk of causing patient harm when used in ⚡ error.

Pharmacokinetics

EE is rapidly absorbed following oral administration and reaches peak serum concentration in 1 to 2 hours. Roughly 83% of EE survives absorption and first-pass metabolism, resulting in 40% bioavailability through the liver at steady state. EE is 98.5% protein bound. It is excreted as metabolites via feces and urine. It undergoes some enterohepatic circulation.

The steroid hormones in the transvaginal ring are rapidly absorbed through the vaginal mucosa. Etonogestrel in the transvaginal ring has a bioavailability of 100%; bioavailability of EE is 55%. The transdermal patch also bypasses the hepatic portal system. Avoiding first-pass metabolism through the liver has the potential to decrease adverse drug interactions. The norelgestromin in the patch binds to albumin. Levels of serum steroid hormones in the patch reach constant levels of contraceptive efficacy within 48 hours. Serum hormone levels are rapidly reached, and blood levels do not fluctuate as much as is seen with OC products.

Progestin Contraceptives

Progestin contraceptives do not contain estrogen. The estrogen component of contraceptives increases the risk of circulatory disorders; therefore progestin-only contraceptives allow contraception to be available for females who cannot take CHCs. Advantages of progestin contraceptive include relative safety, ease of use, spontaneity of sexual intercourse, and reversibility. However, because the estrogen component is missing, these products have a higher incidence of irregular bleeding and spotting as well as the possibility of depression, mood changes, decreased libido, fatigue, and weight gain. Progestin contraceptives do not protect females against STIs. females who cannot take estrogen but may be candidates for progestin contraceptives include patients with a personal or strong family history of VTE or heart disease, breast-feeding patients, patients older than 35 years who smoke, and females with uncontrolled ⚡ hypertension.

Progestin-Only Oral Contraceptive Pills

The progestin-only oral contraceptive pill (POP), called the *minipill*, has four mechanisms of action: (1) it alters cervical mucus, making it thick and viscous, which blocks sperm penetration; (2) it interferes with the endometrial lining, which makes implantation difficult; (3) it decreases peristalsis in the fallopian tubes, slowing the transport of ovum; and (4) in approximately 50% of cycles, it interferes with the LH surge and thereby inhibits ovulation.

POPs contain 0.35 mg of norethindrone. The minipill is taken continuously, without a break for withdrawal bleeding. Patients should be instructed to take the minipill daily within a 3-hour window. Risk for pregnancy will increase if a patient misses a dose of POP because they do not suppress the release of follicle-stimulating hormone (FSH) and LH to the same degree as the combination hormone pills.

Depot Medroxyprogesterone Acetate

Depot medroxyprogesterone acetate (DMPA) is a highly effective, long-acting injectable progestin with theoretic and typical use efficacy rates of 99% and 97%, respectively. This makes DMPA one of the most effective hormonal methods of contraception. It appeals to females because it is discreet and has a convenient dosing schedule; DMPA is popular with adolescents for these same reasons. Injectable progestin is administered in a flexible dosing schedule every 11 to 13 weeks. The mechanism of action of DMPA relies on the progestational activities: thickening of the cervical mucus, thinning of the uterine endometrium, and a decrease in fallopian tube motility. Because the progestin in DMPA reaches a higher circulating level than with POPs, DMPA inhibits both FSH and LH secretion from the anterior pituitary gland. This results in both anovulation (lack of ovulation) and amenorrhea. Because FSH and LH secretion is inhibited, formation of a dominant follicle is inhibited, and the production of estrogen in the body is greatly decreased. However, the patient experiences a hypo-estrogen state, which can affect bone mineral density (⚡ BMD).

The DMPA vial or prefilled syringe should be vigorously shaken just before administration to ensure a uniform drug suspension. DMPA 150 mg/1 mL is given by deep intramuscular (IM) injection into the ventral gluteus or deltoid muscle. The site should *not* be massaged after injection, and the injection site must be documented so that sites can be rotated. The patient is given a personalized calendar for subsequent doses and should return for another injection within 13 weeks. If the patient is late for her injection by even 1 day, pregnancy should be ruled out before resuming treatment.

As with OCs, DMPA does not protect against STIs. Due to the hypoestrogenic state produced by DMPA, bone reabsorption exceeds bone formation. This results in a reduction of BMD, greatest during the first 1 to 2 years of DMPA use. After discontinuation of DMPA, BMD substantially improves (more so at the spine than hips) but may not be completely reversible. Based on these data, the FDA issued a boxed warning recommending DMPA be discontinued after 2 years of continuous use, unless other methods of contraception are ⚡ inadequate. The American Congress of Obstetricians and Gynecologists stated in a committee opinion that "the possible adverse effects of DMPA must be carefully balanced against the significant personal and public health impact of unintended pregnancy." The benefits, risks, and alternatives and the prevention of BMD loss while taking DMPA must be discussed with the patient before administration of the product.

Females taking DMPA should be instructed to increase calcium and vitamin D intake to the daily recommended allowance for their age and to participate in regular weight-bearing exercises. DMPA is safe to receive immediately postpartum, and females can breast-feed while using this contraceptive without affecting milk supply. The most common side effects include initially irregular uterine bleeding or spotting. Menstruation may cease about 1 year after starting. In addition, DMPA has been shown to cause progressive weight gain in some females. Other side effects include breast tenderness and an increase in depression. The drug is contraindicated in cases of undiagnosed vaginal bleeding and known or suspected pregnancy. Caution should be used in giving DMPA postpartum in females who are at risk for or have a history of postpartum ⚡ depression.

DMPA formulated for subcutaneous injection is available as an injectable suspension of 104 mg/0.65 mL. It is administered to females every 12 to 14 weeks. This drug has the same mechanism of action, benefits, and risks as DMPA for intramuscular injection, and females should be counseled about the potential loss of BMD. Females taking DMPA have a slower return to fertility than those using other hormonal methods of contraception.

Progestin Implant

A progestin implant is a single-rod device that contains 68 mg of etonogestrel; it is implanted in the inner side of the upper nondominant arm. It needs to be removed no later than 3 years after the date of insertion; it may be replaced with a new implant at the time of removal. The progestin implant contains barium, a radiopaque substance that can help locate the device on two-dimensional radiography, ultrasound, magnetic resonance imaging (MRI), and computed tomography (CT) scanning if necessary. Also, the device comes in a preloaded application system that reduces insertion errors. The progestin implant may not be as effective in females who have a body mass index (BMI) greater than 30 (obese) or who are on drugs that induce liver enzymes. Theoretic and typical effectiveness rates for implantable progestins are the same, at 99.6%.

Pharmacokinetics

Progestin contraceptives are well absorbed from the GI tract. Peak plasma levels occur 1 to 2 hours after ingestion, depending on the particular compound. Norethynodrel and ethynodiol diacetate are converted to norethindrone. Norgestrel and LNG are 100% bioavailable and do not undergo first-pass liver metabolism; norethindrone undergoes first-pass metabolism and is 65% available. The progestins are bound to plasma proteins and sex hormone–binding globulin. The half-life of norethindrone varies from 5 to 14 hours; the half-life of LNG is 11 to 45 hours.

DMPA provides higher peak levels of progestin than POPs and implantable progestins. Once injected, the levels of DMPA increase for 3 weeks, remain stable for a few days, then begin to decline. DMPA is undetectable in the blood between 120 and 200 days after injection. The formulation for subcutaneous administration of DMPA provides a slower and more sustained absorption than IM, permitting a lower dose. DMPA is 90% protein bound, metabolized in the liver, and excreted primarily in the urine.

A progestin implant is a sustained-release system that releases progestin at a level of 60 to 70 mcg/day during the first 6 weeks after insertion, declining to 35 to 45 mcg/day during the first year. This decreases to 30 to 40 mcg/day after 2 years of implantation and 25 to 30 mcg/day by the end of the third year. Bioavailability remains constant at 95%. Once the rod is inserted, effective contraceptive levels are reached within 8 hours.

Start Date and Dosing Schedule for Hormonal Contraception Products

There are three ways to implement the start of hormonal contraception products unless otherwise indicated by the manufacturer. With the *first-day start method*, the contraception product is initiated on the first day a female experiences bleeding; the first day of bleeding is day 1 of the menstrual cycle. Days are then counted 2, 3, 4, 5, 6, and so on until the first-day bleeding begins again, usually around day 28. Most methods of contraception can be safely started on day 1 through day 5 of the menstrual cycle, when it is less likely that the patient has an early undiagnosed pregnancy. No backup method of contraception is needed when the product is started on the first through fifth day of menstruation. Many products require a *Sunday start*, meaning the patient starts the tablets or patch on the Sunday after the first days of menstruation. If menstruation actually starts on Sunday, the patient starts her tablet or patch on that day. The Sunday start aids a females in remembering the first day of her contraception cycle. If a patient starts the contraception later than day 5 of her menstrual cycle, a backup form of contraception should be used for 7 days.

Special Considerations

DMPA and the transvaginal ring must be started within the first 5 days of the menstrual cycle. The continuous-dosing CHC products use a Sunday start only. If the patient is on a 21-day CHC regimen, the next pack should be started after the 7-day break whether bleeding has stopped or not. With 28-day packs, a pill is taken daily without stopping regardless of the bleeding pattern. Usually, withdrawal menses occur in a cyclic fashion. In multiphasic preparations, the day 1 pill is clearly marked, and the tablets are taken in the order noted. A difference in the color of the tablets delineates the change in the dose of estrogen or progestin through the phases. With the POP, a pill is taken daily without a break. To increase effectiveness, all OCs should be taken at the same time daily. With the POP, females should strictly adhere to this instruction.

Missed Doses

Box 55.1 provides guidelines for patients on how to handle missing a dose of their OC.

BOX 55.1 Guidelines for Missed Doses of Oral Contraceptives

Combined Hormonal Contraceptives
One Tablet
Take the tablet as soon as the missed dose is realized.
Take the next tablet as scheduled.

Two Tablets
Take two tablets as soon as the missed dose is realized and two tablets the next day.
Use a backup method of contraception for the rest of the cycle.

Three Tablets
Discontinue the present pack, and allow for withdrawal bleeding. Start a new package of tablets 7 days after the last tablet is taken. Use another form of contraception until tablets have been taken for 7 consecutive days.

Progestin-Only Pills
One or More Tablets
Take the tablet as soon as the missed dose is realized, and follow with the next tablet at the regular time *plus* use a backup method of contraception for 48 hours.

Contraindications
Not every patient is a candidate for use of CHCs. Box 55.2 lists contraindications to CHC use.

Drug Interactions
The effectiveness of some drugs is impaired by CHC products; other drugs impair the effectiveness of CHCs and progestin contraceptives. Box 55.3 shows drugs that may have interactive effects with CHCs. Patients receiving low-dose formulations of OCs need to be particularly cautious about potential interactions. If a patient is taking a drug that affects estrogen absorption or metabolism, a CHC with a higher dose of EE may be prescribed.

Potential Side Effects and Adverse Reactions
Most of the untoward side effects are related to differences in the estrogen-progestin ratio of the products and the patient's response to these differences. Side effects primarily caused by an excess of estrogen include nausea, vomiting, dizziness, fluid retention, edema, bloating, breast enlargement, breast tenderness, chloasma (slightly more in dark-skinned patients on higher-dose tablets who are exposed to sunlight), leg cramps, decreased tearing, corneal curvature alteration, visual changes, vascular headache, and hypertension (in about 1% to 5% of previously normotensive patients within the first few months).

Side effects primarily caused by estrogen deficiency include vaginal bleeding (BTB, especially in the first few cycles after starting therapy) that lasts several days, usually during days 1 to 14; oligomenorrhea (very scant periods), especially after long-term use; nervousness; and dyspareunia (painful sexual intercourse) secondary to atrophic vaginitis.

Side effects primarily caused by an excess of progestin include increased appetite, weight gain, oily skin and scalp, acne, depression, vulvovaginal candidiasis (vaginitis from the yeast microbe *Candida*), excess hair growth, decreased breast size, and amenorrhea after cessation of use (1% to 2% of patients).

Side effects primarily caused by progestin deficiency include dysmenorrhea, bleeding late in the cycle (days 15 to 21), heavy menstrual flow with clots, or amenorrhea. There may also be changes in laboratory values, including thyroid and liver function, blood glucose, and triglycerides.

Adverse reactions of a more severe nature include cardiovascular and carcinogenetic risks.

BOX 55.2 Contraindications for Combined Hormonal Contraceptives

⚡ Absolute Contraindications
- Pregnancy (known or suspected)
- Venous thrombosis history or risk factors
- Vascular disease, including coronary artery disease and cerebrovascular accident and past or current history of deep venous thrombosis or pulmonary embolism
- Liver disease, including cirrhosis, viral hepatitis, and benign or malignant liver tumors
- Undiagnosed vaginal bleeding or known or suspected endometrial cancer
- Breast cancer
- Tobacco use of more than 15 cigarettes per day in a patient older than 35 years

⚡ Cautious Use
- Hypertension with associated vascular disease
- Hypertension with blood pressure greater than 160/100 mm Hg
- Hyperlipidemia
- Diabetes mellitus complicated by neuropathy, retinopathy, nephropathy, or vascular disease
- Diabetes mellitus for more than 20 years' duration
- Postpartum fewer than 3 weeks
- Lactation fewer than 6 weeks
- Age greater than 35 years and smoking fewer than 15 cigarettes per day
- Hypercoagulation disorders
- Prolonged immobility
- Use of drugs that affect liver enzymes (e.g., anticonvulsants, rifampin)

BOX 55.3 Drugs That Interact With Combined Hormonal Contraceptives

Drugs That Decrease the Effectiveness of Combined Hormonal Contraceptives (CHCs)
Use a higher-dose pill or an alternative form of contraception (if the drug is continuous).
Use a backup method for the duration of treatment plus 7 days (if drug is short term).

Anticonvulsant Drugs
Carbamazepine
Hydantoins (ethotoin and phenytoin)
Succinimide anticonvulsants (ethosuximide)

Antituberculin Drugs
Rifampin

Antifungal Drugs
Griseofulvin

Antibiotics
Amoxicillin
Ampicillin
Doxycycline
Metronidazole
Minocycline
Neomycin
Nitrofurantoin
Penicillin
Tetracycline

Barbiturates
Phenobarbital
Primidone

Hypnotics and Sedatives
Benzodiazepines

Migraine Drugs
Topiramate

Drugs That May Increase Combined Hormonal Contraceptive Activity
Acetaminophen
Ascorbic acid
Fluconazole

Other Drug Interactions
An alternative method of contraception is necessary.
Anticoagulants: CHCs increase clotting factors and decrease the effectiveness of anticoagulants.
Anticonvulsants: CHCs may increase the risk for seizure.

Cardiovascular

There is an increased risk for hypertension (usually seen within 3 months after initiating CHCs in females with preexisting risk) and arterial blood clot complications such as MI, pulmonary embolus, and cerebrovascular accident (CVA) in females using CHCs compared with females who are not using CHCs. However, in terms of absolute risk for adolescents and females, the rate of dangerous complications from hormonal methods of contraception is extremely low because females younger than 50 years rarely experience heart attack or stroke. The risk for hypertension in females younger than 35 years is also low. Hormonal methods of contraception that contain DRSP or etonogestrel may double a female's risk for VTEs. Cardiovascular risks are increased in females older than 35 years who smoke, females older than 45 years, and females with hypertension that is undiagnosed or uncontrolled by ⚡ drugs.

Carcinogenesis

Long-term use of CHCs may increase the risk for breast cancer in younger females, but the risk is minimal. Breast cancer risk returns to normal 10 years or more after discontinuing CHCs. There is also an increased risk for benign liver tumors. Risk for cervical cancer is slightly increased, which is thought to be because CHCs change cervical epithelium, making it more susceptible to the high-risk pathogenic strains of human papillomavirus (HPV) and because condoms may be used less frequently in prevention of STIs. Females who use hormonal methods of contraception have a greatly reduced risk for ovarian and endometrial cancers, and the protective effect is directly related to the duration of time the method is used.

Preventing Fertilization

CHCs can be used to prevent fertilization after an incidence of unprotected vaginal intercourse or failure of a contraceptive method. The method involves taking 2 to 5 OC pills at one time. This raises both estrogen and progestin levels to delay or prevent ovulation; it interferes with tubal transport of the embryo, egg, or sperm; and it changes the hormones necessary for the preparation of the uterine lining. Using this method decreases the risk for pregnancy by 75% for each act of sexual intercourse. The major side effect is nausea; to prevent this, an OTC antinausea medicine should be taken 1 hour before CHC administration. Antihistamines are the most used OTC drug for nausea, and some are marketed specifically for this purpose. Antihistamines include diphenhydramine, dimenhydrinate, and meclizine. Irregular menstrual bleeding is another side effect. If a females does not begin menstruation within a few days of the expected time, a pregnancy test should be performed. Patients who are unable to take estrogen should *not* take CHCs as emergency contraception (EC).

CLINICAL JUDGMENT [NURSING PROCESS]
Combined Hormonal Contraceptives

Concept: Hormonal Regulation
- Hormonal regulation involves substances working together to promote healthy development of female sex characteristics during puberty and adulthood to ensure or delay fertility.

Recognize Cues [Assessment]
- Obtain a record of the patient's drug, supplement, and complementary and alternative medicine use.
- Obtain baseline vital signs that include temperature, pulse, and respiration; blood pressure (BP); weight; and height. Calculate body mass index (BMI), and report any abnormal findings.
- Obtain a complete menstrual history that includes age at menarche, menstrual pattern, cycle length, duration, and amount of bleeding and the first day of the last menstrual period (LMP).
- Determine the patient's pregnancy status.
- Obtain a family medical history specific to contraindications for combined hormonal contraceptives (CHCs) and progestin contraceptives.
- Obtain a family history of premenopausal breast cancer.
- Assess for domestic violence, intimate partner violence, and past or recent sexual abuse/ ⚡ assault.
- Obtain a medical history, assessing for history of allergies to drugs, smoking, hypertension, and the contraindications to CHCs listed in ❗ Box 55.2.
- Obtain a complete obstetric and gynecologic history that includes gravida, parity, abortion (spontaneous, therapeutic, or elective); age at first and last pregnancy; time frame between pregnancies; complications during pregnancy, delivery, and postpartum; genetic anomalies and health of children; time since the last Papanicolaou (Pap) test; history of abnormal Pap testing; history of gynecologic and/or sexual infections; gynecologic problems and/or surgeries; and gynecologic anomalies.
- Obtain a complete sexual history that includes sexual expression and sexual risk practices, history of sexually transmitted infections (STIs) and treatment, and past or present sexual abuse and/or assault.
- Recognize the need for periodic reassessment of baseline data and side effects. Most patients should be seen 1–3 months after beginning a contraceptive regimen.

Analyze Cues and Prioritize Hypothesis [Patient Problems]
- Discomfort
- Potential for nonadherence
- Confusion
- Coping
- Anxiety
- Need for patient teaching

Generate Solutions [Planning]
- The patient with contraindications to hormonal contraception will be determined by evaluation of risk-benefit method.
- The patient will verbalize the difference between CHCs and progestin contraceptives and their various routes of administration.
- The patient will verbalize understanding of the bleeding patterns associated with both types of contraceptives by reporting menstrual changes that occur.
- The patient will choose a contraceptive method suitable to their lifestyle and health status.
- The patient will understand and verbalize the pros and cons of contraception through use of the BRAIDED method. This method is recommended by the Department of Health and Human Services to provide regulations concerning guidance for informed consent of contraceptive methods. BRAIDED method: discuss **benefits** (advantages, positive aspects, and both theoretic and actual effective rates of the method), **risks** (dangers, complications, disadvantages, and failure rates), **alternatives** (other contraception options available), **inquiries** (opportunity for the patient to ask questions about options proposed), **decision** (deciding on a method with opportunity to change the decision as needed), **explanation** (health care teaching specific to the method chosen), and **documentation**.
- The patient will verbalize the dosing schedule and use of contraceptive method chosen.
- The patient will receive instruction on how to report dangerous cardiovascular side effects to the health care provider (HCP) by using the ACHES acronym. (ACHES acronym: *abdominal pain* [severe]; *chest pain* or shortness of breath; *headaches* [severe], dizziness, weakness, numbness, or speech difficulties; *eye disorders*, which includes blurring or loss of vision; and *severe* leg pain or swelling in the calf or ⚡ thigh).

CLINICAL JUDGMENT [NURSING PROCESS]—CONT'D
Combined Hormonal Contraceptives

- The patient will verbalize understanding of the ACHES acronym.
- The patient will take oral contraceptives (OCs) as prescribed and report adverse side effects to the HCP.
- The patient will demonstrate and report comfort with placement of the transvaginal ring and will report adverse side effects that occur.
- The patient will verbalize the specific scheduling needs for progestin-only pills.
- The patient will verbalize the initiation and scheduling of depot medroxyprogesterone acetate (DMPA) injections and the need for weight-bearing exercises and calcium supplementation.
- The patient will be instructed to schedule follow-up appointments as needed.

Take Action [Nursing Interventions]

- Assist the patient with obtaining informed consent for the initiation of contraceptives through the BRAIDED method.
- Instruct and have the patient verbalize the complications and side effects of their contraceptive method.
- Instruct the patient about alternatives to the method (including abstinence and no method).
- Instruct the patient about their patient's rights and responsibilites.
- Instruct the patient in a format that is understandable to the patient, and have the patient verbalize their understanding.
- Assess the patient for misconceptions, and provide factual, evidence-based information when instructing the patient.
- Encourage the patient's effective use of the chosen contraceptive method.
- Ensure the patient understands the start date, continuation of drug, and appropriate follow-up.
- Provide the patient with alternative forms of contraceptive therapy because a percentage of patients on hormonal contraceptives will abandon the method within 1 year; and encourage the patient to seek care with a qualified HCP before discontinuing any method of contraception.
- Discuss with the nonnursing mother that it's suggested they begin CHCs 4–6 weeks postpartum, regardless of whether menstruation has spontaneously occurred. Some sources indicate that a CHC method can be initiated as early as 3 weeks postpartum.
- Instruct nonnursing and nursing mothers to begin DMPA immediately postpartum if there is no increased risk for postpartum depression. Progestin-only oral contraceptive pills (POPs) can be started at 4–6 weeks postpartum.
- Instruct the patient that CHCs may decrease milk production in patients who are breast-feeding. CHCs can be used by breast-feeding mothers, but these methods should be initiated after breast-feeding is well established. This is usually 2–3 months after the birth, although some sources state that 6 weeks is sufficient. Always check with the HCP.

Patient Teaching
General

- Instruct the patient that contraceptive drugs should be used only under the direction of a qualified HCP.
- Advise the patient that concurrent use of certain drugs and herbal products decreases the effectiveness of hormonal contraceptives. The patient should use a second form of contraception during use of these drugs and herbal supplements for 7 days after discontinuing counteracting ⚡ drugs.
- ⚡ Instruct the patient that hormonal methods of contraception do *not* prevent transmission of STIs or the pathogen that causes human immunodeficiency virus (HIV) infection. If a patient is at risk for STI or HIV infection, condoms should be used concurrently with the CHC method, and safe-sex practices should be discussed. ⚡ Inform patients regarding proper condom use.

Safety

- ⚡ Instruct the patient not to smoke tobacco because of increased cardiovascular risks.
- Advise the patient to use a barrier method of contraception as needed during the first 7 days of contraception use if the method is started 5 days or more after the first day of the menstrual period. Instruct the patient on how to use barrier methods properly.
- Instruct the patient about how to manage missed pills. Provide instruction for missed POPs and on patch, ring, and injection methods. Review instructions for emergency contraception.
- Advise the patient to report any effects from hormonal contraception to the HCP so therapy can be adjusted to suit their needs. Encourage the patient not to discontinue use of the method until an adequate trial time frame has been completed, which should be at least 3–6 months.
- ⚡ Instruct the patient that HCPs should be advised of CHC use before surgery in which immobilization for an extended period may be needed.
- ⚡ Encourage the patient to report any irregular bleeding to the HCP; this may require a change in dose or another type of hormonal contraceptive method.
- ⚡ Advise the patient to always report use of hormonal contraceptives when seeing a HCP because of possible synergistic or antagonistic responses to other drugs and therapies.
- Advise the nursing mother that the use of CHCs may decrease the quantity and quality of breast milk.

Side Effects

- ⚡ Advise the patient that rare but serious side effects can occur, including venous thromboembolism (VTE), myocardial infarction (MI), cerebral vascular accident (CVA), and retinal vein thrombosis.
- ⚡ Instruct the patient in the ACHES acronym for reporting symptoms of dangerous cardiovascular side effects to their HCP (abdominal pain, chest pain, headaches, eye problems, swelling and /or aching in the legs and thighs).
- Instruct the patient to notify their HCP immediately if any of these symptoms occur.
- Advise the patient that menstrual flow may be less in amount and duration because of thinning of the endometrial lining with CHCs and progestin contraceptives.
- Advise the patient of menstrual changes that can occur at the start of combined estrogen-progestin contraception use, when changing types of hormonal contraception products, and with progestin contraceptives.
- Determine whether the patient wears contact lenses, and discuss alterations in the shape of the cornea and dry eyes that may occur due to decreased tearing. If this occurs, the patient should consult their optometrist.
- Instruct the patient who experiences post-CHC amenorrhea that 95% of females have regular periods within 12–18 months. Advise the patient that those who participate in endurance fitness activities may have increased post-CHC amenorrhea.
- Advise the patient of a possible decrease in libido caused by an alteration in vaginal secretions and decreased levels of testosterone.
- Ensure the patient understands the ability to return to fertility after discontinuing a hormonal contraception product and the time frame in which pregnancy can be expected.
- Ensure a safe transition between contraceptive methods if a change in method is desired.

Continued

CLINICAL JUDGMENT [NURSING PROCESS]—CONT'D
Combined Hormonal Contraceptives

Skill
- Instruct the patient in breast health awareness and self-examination.
- Instruct the patient how to inspect genitalia for abnormalities and note changes in vaginal secretions.
- Show the patient the packet of pills and discuss how to recognize start dates and follow the sequential pill dosing. Demonstrate how to remove the pill from the pill packet.
- Instruct the patient how to place and remove transdermal contraception patches.
- Instruct the patient how to place and remove transvaginal contraception rings.
- Instruct the patient how to use a calendar to record placement and removal of transvaginal rings or transdermal patches.
- Advise the patient to return for a DMPA injection within the 13-week time frame.

Diet
- Counsel the patient to moderate caffeine intake, because elimination of caffeine may be decreased as a result of prescribed CHC products.
- Instruct the patient to take OCs with a snack or after meals to help eliminate nausea.
- ⚡ Advise the patient using DMPA to increase calcium and vitamin D intake and to do 15–30 minutes of weight-bearing exercises 3–4 times per week.
- Discuss foods that increase iron and iron absorption.

Evaluate Outcomes [Evaluation]
- Encourage the patient in planning follow-up evaluations.
- Evaluate the patient's adherence with the hormonal contraceptive regimen; assess for changes in sexual partners and/or health status that may compromise the method.

Family planning agencies and females's health organizations provide a full list of CHC pills along with the dosage and administration regimen for these products when used for EC. Treatment should be initiated within 72 hours of intercourse. The sooner a plan is initiated, the more effective it will be at preventing pregnancy.

The first EC pill available in the United States was approved in 1999; it was known as Plan B (LNG, a progestin-only pill). In 2006 the FDA approved this drug without a prescription for females 18 years of age or older. In 2009 the FDA stated that both males and females can obtain this drug without a prescription if they are older than 17 years. Those younger than 17 years need a prescription.

The emergency contraception (EC) pill should be taken within 72 hours after intercourse, but it is still effective 120 hours afterward. If taken within 24 hours of intercourse, EC reduces the risk of pregnancy by 95%. Just 12 hours after the initial 24-hour postcoital period, the effectiveness rate of EC decreases to approximately 60%. In Plan B One-Step, one 1.5 mg LNG tablet is taken. If Next Choice is used, one 0.75 mg tablet is taken, followed by another 12 hours later. If vomiting occurs within 3 hours, the dose should be repeated. Less nausea is associated with this drug than with estrogen-containing EC methods.

DRUGS USED TO TREAT DISORDERS IN FEMALE HEALTH

Common reasons females seek gynecologic health care include alterations in menstrual cycle, menstrual or pelvic pain, and changes in vaginal secretions. Included within these broad categories are irregular uterine bleeding, dysmenorrhea, and PMS. This section describes common disorders in female's health and presents current pharmacologic approaches to management.

Irregular uterine bleeding is a term that describes many different medical conditions or pathologies related to the menstrual cycle. Irregular uterine bleeding, also known as *abnormal uterine bleeding* (AUB), is a common reason females seek gynecologic care. AUB encompasses a wide range of variable bleeding patterns in females, such as amenorrhea, menorrhagia, metrorrhagia, menometrorrhagia, intramenstrual bleeding, and **dysfunctional uterine bleeding (DUB)**.

Amenorrhea

Amenorrhea is the absence of menses. *Primary amenorrhea* is defined as an absence of menses by 14 years of age *without* secondary sex characteristics or an absence of menses by 16 years of age *with* secondary sex characteristics. Primary amenorrhea may be caused by abnormalities in the structures of the female reproductive tract, chromosomal alterations, or endocrine disorders. Many times, the cause is just a physiologic delay in the onset of menstruation. *Secondary amenorrhea* is the absence of a spontaneous menstrual period for 6 consecutive months in females who have experienced menstrual cycles in the past. Pregnancy is the most common reason a patient may experience amenorrhea, as well as breast-feeding and menopause; therefore secondary amenorrhea is a *symptom* of these normal physiologic processes. Other causes of secondary amenorrhea include anovulatory cycles (cycles without ovulation), hypothyroidism or hyperthyroidism, and hyperprolactinemia (high levels of the hormone prolactin, which stimulates lactation). Extreme weight loss and anorexia can also cause amenorrhea.

After assessment of the patient's health history and a physical examination; after laboratory testing to include FSH, serum prolactin, thyroid-stimulating hormone, and serum estradiol (ES); and after pregnancy has been ruled out, a *progestin withdrawal test* may be administered to determine the underlying cause of amenorrhea. This test uses an oral progestin administered for a limited time to confirm that the hypothalamic-pituitary-ovarian (HPO) responses—that is, the hormonal system that mediates the menstrual cycle—are intact.

With the progestin withdrawal test, a patient is given medroxyprogesterone 10 mg for 10 days. The progestational activity thickens the endometrial lining and increases secretory activity. When the drug is discontinued, progesterone levels decrease, resulting in a breakdown of the endometrial lining and withdrawal bleeding. Withdrawal bleeding should occur within 7 to 10 days after completing the drug, which indicates that the HPO axis (the menstrual cycle) is functioning in providing the hormones necessary to regulate the menstrual cycle. Even the smallest amount of bleeding, such as one incidence of scant spotting, is considered a positive test. However, if no withdrawal bleeding occurs, other pathophysiologic problems may exist, and further evaluation and diagnostic testing by the health care provider are needed.

Polycystic Ovarian Syndrome

Another common cause of secondary amenorrhea is **polycystic ovarian syndrome (PCOS)**, a disorder in the metabolism of androgens and estrogen. PCOS may be caused by dysfunction of the HPO axis. Females with PCOS experience menstrual dysfunction, anovulation, hyperandrogenism, hirsutism, infertility, obesity, metabolic syndrome, diabetes, and obstructive sleep apnea.

Diet and exercise are first-line treatment for PCOS. Weight loss of 5% to 10% has been shown to improve overall metabolic status and reduce serum androgen concentrations. Pharmacologic treatment of PCOS is used to treat anovulation, hirsutism, and menstrual irregularities. To manage menstrual irregularities, low-dose CHCs are prescribed. With the addition of the progestin in the CHC product and a cycling of a monthly withdrawal menses (or four times per year, depending on the product), the risks of unopposed estrogen on the endometrium are significantly reduced.

For females who are attempting to conceive and in whom weight loss has not restored ovulation, new studies have shown that letrozole, an aromatase inhibitor, is now the first-line ovulation induction agent over clomiphene citrate for females with PCOS, although it is an off-label use. Clomiphene citrate can still be used, but studies have shown that it is less effective for live birth rates than letrozole. Metformin has been used with clomiphene citrate, although current guidelines recommend against the use of metformin in obese females with PCOS, except in females with glucose intolerance not corrected with lifestyle changes.

Abnormal Uterine Bleeding

The normal menstrual cycle occurs every 25 to 35 days and lasts 2 to 7 days, with an estimated blood loss of no more than 80 mL. *Menorrhagia* is *regular* uterine bleeding greater than 80 mL or lasting more than 7 days. Females with menorrhagia may describe their periods as very heavy or state the need to change a tampon or sanitary pad frequently. *Metrorrhagia* is *irregular* uterine bleeding greater than 80 mL or lasting more than 7 days. Females with metrorrhagia describe their periods as irregular and heavy. They may state that they have no idea when bleeding will occur and that, when it does happen, it will soak through sanitary products or clothing. *Menometrorrhagia* is a combination of these two. *Intramenstrual bleeding* is an episode of bleeding, usually light, that occurs between menstrual periods.

A common complaint that brings a females into the gynecologic health care setting is that she is having menstrual cycles that are suddenly different from the pattern she usually experiences. In females of reproductive age, pregnancy should always be considered first as the possible cause of AUB. However, AUB can result from physiologic processes such as stress, severe dieting and weight loss, eating disorders, or excessive exercise. Irregular bleeding patterns are a sign of decreasing ovarian function or approach of menopause in older females. AUB can also be caused by pathologic processes such as endocrine disorders, thyroid disease, leiomyomata (benign tumors in the uterus), ovarian cysts, infections of the genital tract, or cancer. If a female is pregnant, uterine bleeding may indicate ectopic pregnancy or impending miscarriage. Some pharmacologic drugs, substances, and herbal preparations can also cause irregular bleeding, including anticoagulants, antipsychotics, benzodiazepines, hormone therapy (HT), ginkgo, ginseng, and soy products. Once physiologic, pathologic, and pharmaceutic causes have been ruled out, the patient may be diagnosed with DUB.

Dysfunctional Uterine Bleeding

DUB is the most common classification of irregular bleeding. Diagnosis of DUB is made when no organic pathology can be determined to cause the irregular bleeding. Pharmacologic treatment of DUB primarily involves normalizing the bleeding pattern and correcting anemia that may have resulted from chronic or acute blood loss. In the normal physiologic menstrual cycle, estrogen and progesterone levels are low during menstruation. Once estrogen levels start to rise with the formation of a dominant follicle, uterine bleeding is effectively stopped, ending menstruation. Increasing levels of estrogen by administration of an estrogen drug product is usually effective in stopping prolonged DUB.

Because estrogen is *never* used alone in treatment, and because of the detrimental effects of unopposed estrogen on the uterine endometrium and the risk for endometrial cancer, estrogen-progestin combination products are used. Progestins alone are not as effective as estrogen in reducing an episode of acute bleeding; however, because *prolonged* progestin administration causes atrophy of the endometrial lining, progestins can be very effective if long-term control is needed. DMPA by IM injection and a levonorgestrel-intrauterine system (LNG-IUS) inserted into the uterus are among the products used for extended progestin therapy.

Pharmacologic Management of Irregular Bleeding

Nonsteroidal antiinflammatory drugs (NSAIDs) can be used for the treatment of menorrhagia, reducing bleeding by 25% to 35%. NSAIDs block the production of prostaglandin, which decreases both excessive bleeding and uterine cramps. Common NSAIDs used for menorrhagia are mefenamic acid, ibuprofen, and naproxen sodium. NSAIDS should be taken with food to avoid gastric upset.

CHCs can be used to decrease and regulate DUB. The increase in estrogen suppresses endometrial development, restores predictable bleeding, and reduces menstrual flow. Reduction in flow should be seen within 24 hours. If a heavy flow continues for more than 48 hours, the patient should be reevaluated. Benefits, risks, and patient instructions are the same as if the product were being used for contraception. Females who are not candidates for estrogen therapy (ET) or CHCs should be excluded. Females using a CHC product for DUB should see their periods normalize within the first 3 months of use. Patients can continue the method for contraception, or they can discontinue use in 6 to 9 months, depending on the effectiveness in controlling bleeding.

Progestins are not as effective as estrogens at reducing episodes of irregular bleeding. However, progestins are effective in the long-term treatment of AUB and may be the method of choice in females who have contraindications to estrogen use. Progestins are given cyclically (e.g., norethindrone acetate 2.5 to 5 mg PO daily for 21 days or medroxyprogesterone 10 mg/day for 21 days) to produce a monthly withdrawal bleeding. DMPA and the LNG-IUS are also used for treatment of DUB. Long-term use of progesterone has an atrophic effect on the uterine endometrium, consequently decreasing incidences of irregular bleeding. Females using DMPA or the LNG-IUS for DUB should see heavy bleeding patterns decrease within 3 to 6 months.

Dysmenorrhea

Dysmenorrhea, also called *cyclic pelvic pain* (CPP), is pelvic pain associated with the menstrual cycle. Other symptoms that may occur with the menstrual cycle are uterine cramping, lower back pain, abdominal cramps, changes in bowel patterns, increased bowel movements, and nausea and vomiting. Dysmenorrhea is experienced by approximately 80% of females in their late teens and early 20s, when it is more prevalent. It is the most common reason young females miss school or work. Dysmenorrhea is classified as either primary dysmenorrhea or secondary dysmenorrhea, depending on whether there is a known etiology for the menstrual pain. *Primary dysmenorrhea* is diagnosed when there is no apparent underlying pathology. It is caused by larger-than-normal amounts of prostaglandins at the start of the menstrual period. Prostaglandins cause arterioles in the uterus to contract, decreasing blood flow to the endometrium. All of these mechanisms are necessary for breakdown of the endometrial lining and for menstruation to occur. However, this process causes increased pain in some females.

In *secondary dysmenorrhea*, there is an underlying cause for the pelvic pain. Conditions that may cause secondary dysmenorrhea are urinary tract infections (UTIs), PID, irritable bowel syndrome (IBS), uterine leiomyomata (fibroids), and endometriosis.

Pharmacologic Management of Dysmenorrhea

NSAIDs block pain by preventing synthesis of prostaglandins. The mechanism of drug action is the inhibition of cyclooxygenase (COX). The COX enzyme converts arachidonic acid into prostaglandins, which cause constriction of the uterine arterioles, necrosis of the endometrial lining, uterine contractions, and menstrual pain. Usually nonselective and COX-2 inhibitors are used. The most used NSAIDs for relief of pain associated with dysmenorrhea include naproxen sodium, diclofenac potassium, ibuprofen, naproxen, celecoxib, and mefenamic acid. Many NSAIDs can be purchased over the counter, so the nurse should include health information about the benefits, risks, and alternatives as well as specific dosage amounts, drug interactions, and administration instructions. Some drugs (diclofenac potassium, celecoxib, and mefenamic acid) are by prescription only. Patients must understand the differences in these drugs and avoid them if they have allergies to, or side effects from, any of the ingredients. Patients should avoid taking two different NSAID drugs at the same time. GI upset is a common side effect of NSAIDs, so most drugs in this category should be taken with food and water. NSAIDs can also be taken with an antacid or calcium supplement to prevent GI upset. NSAIDS carry a boxed warning that they can cause an increased risk of serious and potentially fatal cardiovascular events such as MI and stroke. Always use the lowest effective dose for the shortest ⚡ time.

CHCs are effective in the treatment of dysmenorrhea. CHCs reduce the thickness of the uterine endometrium. The 24/4 day CHCs shorten withdrawal bleeding periods, and the extended-use CHCs decrease the number of withdrawal menses per year or eliminate them altogether. DMPA, progestin implants, and LNG-IUS decrease dysmenorrhea in patients who are candidates for these methods. Long-term progestin-only products cause atrophy of the uterine lining, limiting the occurrence of dysmenorrhea and the amount of bleeding during menstruation.

Endometriosis

Endometriosis is the abnormal location of endometrial tissue outside the uterus. The tissue is known as *ectopic endometrial implants*. It is a common cause of dysmenorrhea, chronic pelvic pain, and infertility. The ectopic endometrial implants can be found affixed to the ovaries, the posterior surface of the uterus, the uterosacral ligaments, the broad ligaments, or the bowel. They also can be found on other organs within the pelvic or thoracic cavity. The ectopic endometrial implants respond to hormonal control, particularly estrogen, in the same way as the normal endometrial tissue located inside the uterus. Thus, when menstruation occurs, the ectopic endometrial implants proliferate and then bleed. As the number of menstrual cycles increases, inflammation of surrounding organ tissue, scar tissue formation, and adhesions result, causing pelvic pain.

Diagnosis of endometriosis is based on laparoscopic evidence of endometrial tissue, or implants, outside the uterus. The most common symptoms of endometriosis are dysmenorrhea and pelvic pain, sometimes including chronic pelvic pain, which lasts more than 6 months and is not associated specifically with menstruation. The patient may experience back pain; painful, sometimes bloody bowel movements; and dyspareunia (painful sexual intercourse). An increased number of females with endometriosis experience primary or secondary infertility; although a specific cause linking the two has not been established, it is theorized that the ectopic endometrial implants or the resultant scar tissue and adhesions obstruct or affect the motility of the fallopian tubes or other reproductive organs. Affected females have an increased risk for ectopic pregnancy.

Pharmacologic Management of Endometriosis

Pharmaceutic treatment strategies for endometriosis include drugs that decrease the amounts of circulating estrogen and limit or eliminate menstruation. This interrupts internal bleeding and irritation associated with the ectopic endometrial implants and may even cause them to recede.

Combined Hormonal Contraceptives. These drugs suppress gonadotropin-releasing hormone (GnRH) release, prevent ovulation, and cause atrophy of the uterine lining, actions thought to relieve pelvic pain by causing a regression of the endometrial implants. CHCs relieve the pain of endometriosis in approximately 75% of females. Extended-use CHCs can also manage endometriosis by causing fewer cycles per year or eliminating withdrawal menses altogether.

Progestin therapy suppresses ovulation and cause long-term endometrial atrophy. They also inhibit GnRH release, like CHCs. Over time, progestins can shrink or eliminate endometrial implants. The most used progestin is DMPA, with which 70% to 90% of patients experience relief of symptoms associated with endometriosis. This effect may last months after discontinuing the drug. Benefits and risks are the same as using DMPA for contraception, so concerns for BMD loss and prevention, irregular bleeding or amenorrhea, possible weight gain, and mood changes should be discussed with the ⚡ patient. The injection is given every 11 to 13 weeks.

Alternatively, norethindrone acetate may be taken at 5 mg PO daily for 2 weeks, then increasing the dose by 2.5 mg every 2 weeks until a dose of 15 mg per day is reached and continued for 6 to 9 months.

Gonadotropin-Releasing-Hormone Agonists (GnRH) are ordered for females who experience severe symptoms of infertility (endometriosis) and who NSAIDs, CHCs, or progestins do not help, GnRH agonists may be used. GnRH agonists are potent drugs that inhibit GnRH release and create a hypoestrogenic environment. The side effects are menopause-like and include hot flashes, atrophic vaginitis, vaginal dryness, decreased sex drive, and potential for bone loss. Leuprolide is administered either 3.75 mg IM monthly or 11.25 mg IM every 3 months. Leuprolide should be initiated in the first 3 days of the menstrual cycle because its use is contraindicated in pregnancy. Females may be able to become pregnant on leuprolide, so a barrier method of contraception should be used. The total duration of therapy should not exceed 6 months. Leuprolide can be used alone or in combination with norethindrone acetate.

Alternatively, nafarelin nasal spray is administered in a divided 400 mcg daily dose, with 1 spray (200 mcg) into one nostril in the morning and 1 spray (200 mcg) into the other nostril in the evening, starting between days 2 to 4 of menstrual cycle, for up to 6 months. Side effects of GnRH agonists include decreased bone density, ovarian cysts, and depression. Use cautiously in patients who experience these symptoms before ⚡ treatment.

Elagolix is also used for the management of moderate to severe pain associated with endometriosis with a recommended dose of 150 mg daily for max use of 24 months. It is contraindicated in pregnancy, known osteoporosis, and severe hepatic impairment. Adverse effects include irregular bleeding, decreased bone density, hepatic impairment, and ⚡ depression.

Premenstrual Syndrome

Premenstrual syndrome (PMS) comprises a collection of cyclic physical symptoms and perimenopausal mood alterations. Symptoms increase in the 2 weeks before menstruation and subside after menses begins. These physical, emotional, and behavioral symptoms interfere to varying degrees with a female's ability to function.

PMS can result in decreased work effectiveness and mood variations. PMS affects as many as 90% of all adult females, with less than 5% experiencing a more severe form of PMS, called premenstrual dysphoric disorder (PMDD). The hallmark of PMS and PMDD is that symptoms occur in a repetitive pattern during the luteal phase (days 15–28) of the menstrual cycle and decrease significantly in the early follicular phase (days 1–14).

There is no universal agreement about the definition, etiology, symptoms, or treatment of PMS. Researchers theorize that the etiology of PMS could be hormonal excess or deficits, fluid or sodium retention, or nutritional deficiencies. It is also proposed that an imbalance exists in the HPO axis function. Other hypotheses center on the neuroregulatory effects of estrogen and progesterone on the release or uptake of serotonin.

A patient can help with the diagnosis of PMS by recording three variables on a perimenstrual assessment calendar: (1) group of symptoms, (2) severity of symptoms, and (3) effect on function (degree of distress). Diagnosis of PMS can be made when the patient's symptoms consistently occur in a cyclic pattern at least 1 week before the menstruation cycle and decrease significantly after menses begins. Symptoms usually have a negative effect on the ability to function effectively. Other endocrine abnormalities must be ruled out. Also, it should be noted that not every symptom associated with the menstrual cycle is indicative of PMS.

Symptoms of Premenstrual Syndrome
Physical symptoms of PMS include breast soreness, constipation or diarrhea, bloating in lower abdomen, headache, backache, fatigue, acne flare-ups, and alterations in sleep patterns.

Emotional or mental symptoms of PMS include irritability or hostile behavior, appetite changes, trouble with concentration, anxiety, depression, mood swings, and decreased sexual desire.

Nonpharmacologic Treatment of Premenstrual Syndrome
Nonpharmacologic treatment modalities are very important in treating females with PMS. Therapies include expression of empathy, support from family and friends, exercise, and dietary changes. Aerobic exercise improves general health, increases endorphin levels, and may facilitate an overall sense of well-being. Dietary changes include limiting salty foods, alcohol, caffeine, and concentrated sweets. Eating four to six small, high-carbohydrate, low-fat meals may also help relieve some symptoms. Stress-reduction exercises are also helpful. These measures may help the patient feel proactive regarding her diagnosis of PMS.

Pharmacologic Treatment of Premenstrual Syndrome
PMS is improved with antidepressant drugs such as selective serotonin reuptake inhibitors (SSRIs). Symptom relief includes a decrease in irritability, mood swings, fatigue, tension, and breast tenderness. SSRIs block the reuptake of serotonin into nerve terminals in the central nervous system, regulating serotonin use by the brain. The most used SSRIs are fluoxetine and sertraline, paroxetine, citalopram, and escitalopram. Venlafaxine, a serotonin norepinephrine reuptake inhibitor (SNRI), has also demonstrated relief in patients with severe PMS symptoms but is not considered a first-line agent (see Chapter 23 for further information on antidepressants). SSRIs may be taken continuously, during the luteal phase only (drug is started on day 14 of the cycle and discontinued with menses), or as intermittent therapy beginning with symptom onset and discontinuing after the first few days of menses. Determining a treatment regimen depends on history and physical, patient preference, and predictability of symptoms.

Long-term suppression of ovulation has been shown to decrease cyclic physical discomforts and to normalize mood variations in some females. CHCs such as those containing the progestin DRSP along with a shorter (4-day) pill-free interval or transdermal and transvaginal HT can be used in this manner. Caution should be used with progestin-only products because they may exacerbate symptoms of depression.

DRUGS USED TO PROMOTE FERTILITY

Infertility is defined as the inability to conceive a child after 12 months of unprotected sexual intercourse. Females older than 35 years may be considered infertile after 6 months of attempting pregnancy. Infertility is considered *primary infertility* if a couple has never conceived or has never carried a pregnancy to term. *Secondary infertility* describes a couple who has conceived and brought a pregnancy to term but is unable to conceive afterward. Approximately 15% to 20% of couples in the United States experience infertility. Fertility rates decrease in both males and females as they get older; however, the risk for infertility increases more abruptly in females than in males as females reach the end of the reproductive life cycle. The monthly chance of achieving pregnancy decreases to 5% after 40 years of age.

Causes and Treatments of Infertility
Causes of infertility are numerous. Infertility can be attributed to a female factor, a male factor, and many times, a combination of both. (Male infertility is discussed in depth in Chapter 56.) In the female partner, the most common causes for infertility are alterations in ovarian function and anatomic disorders. Alterations in ovarian function are categorized as *ovulatory dysfunction disorders*. Any process, whether a disease state or the normal biologic process of aging, that causes anovulation or a decrease in ovulation cycles will affect the process of conception. Many of the females present with irregular menstrual periods. Causes of ovulatory dysfunction include alterations in the Hypothalamic-Pituitary-Ovarian Axis (HPO axis), such as metabolic disorders (most commonly PCOS), and age approaching the end of the reproductive spectrum. Fertility declines sharply in females after 35 years of age, and infertility becomes a factor from 38 to 40 years of age. Endocrine disorders such as hyperprolactinemia (increase in circulating prolactin, the hormone that promotes breast-feeding) or thyroid disorders (hypothyroidism or hyperthyroidism) can also cause anovulatory cycles. Ovulation can be disrupted by eating disorders (anorexia and bulimia) and by stress.

The most common anatomic disorder is blocked fallopian tubes. Blocked tubes can be the result of a history of STI or PID. STIs, treated or undiagnosed, and PID can lead to scarring within the tubes, impeding sperm or ovum transport. A previous ectopic pregnancy or other tubal surgery can also result in infertility. Other causes include endometriosis, uterine leiomyomata (fibroids), or scarring within the uterine endometrium. (See Chapter 56 for male infertility discussion.)

Treatment of infertility depends on the cause. A general health assessment of the infertile couple includes (1) complete health history, including nutritional, reproductive, and social histories; drugs; herbal and illicit drug use; and gynecologic, menstrual, obstetric, and sexual histories as they pertain to each partner; (2) complete physical examinations with breast and pelvic examinations of the female partner and examination of male genitalia and function; (3) Pap testing, HPV testing, collections of cultures for STI testing; and (4) laboratory tests and other diagnostic tests. Semen evaluation is also necessary.

The leading cause of infertility in females is ovulatory dysfunction (most often, PCOS). The first line of pharmacologic treatment for ovulatory dysfunction is usually induction of ovulation by oral drug therapy.

Induction of Ovulation

Clomiphene citrate (CC) is a selective estrogen receptor modulator (SERM) that competes for estrogen receptors within the hypothalamus. With the binding of CC to the estrogen receptors, the hypothalamus receives a signal that circulating estrogen levels are low. This sets the hypothalamus in motion to secrete more GnRH, thus stimulating the HPO axis. The GnRH instructs the anterior pituitary gland to release FSH and LH to initiate a response from the ovarian follicles. Estrogen levels increase in response to FSH and LH, and a follicle becomes dominant, producing the level of estrogen needed for the LH surge. The LH surge causes release of an ovum from the dominant follicle. It is important for LH to reach a level high enough to produce an ovulatory cycle and that the timing of the LH surge be at the height of follicle formation, which is midcycle.

PROTOTYPE DRUG CHART
clomiPHENE - Clomiphene Citrate

Drug Class	Route and Dosage
Ovulation stimulant	A: PO: 50–100 mg/d; start with 50 mg for days 5–9 of the cycle If ovulation does not occur with 50 mg/d, increase the next course to 100 mg/d; *max:* 100 mg/d for no more than 5 days per cycle; maximum sequential cycles is three Under strict supervision by physicians specializing in infertility, as much as 200 mg/d have been used in select patients but not recommended due to the risk of side effects

Contraindications	Drug-Lab-Food Interactions
Pregnancy, undiagnosed vaginal bleeding, depression, fibroids, hepatic dysfunction, thrombophlebitis, primary pituitary or ovarian failure	Drug: Supplements such as DHEA, Prasterone, and Soy Isoflavones may decrease effectiveness of CC Lab: Increases serum thyroxine

Pharmacokinetics	Pharmacodynamics
Absorption: Readily absorbed from GI tract Distribution: PB: UK Metabolism: t½: 5–8 d Excretion: In feces	PO: Onset: 5–10 d Peak: 6 h Duration: UK Pregnancy Considerations: Use is contraindicated in females who are already pregnant

Therapeutic Effects/Uses	
To stimulate ovarian follicle growth Mechanism of action: Stimulates release of follicle-stimulating hormone and luteinizing hormone	

Side Effects	Adverse Reactions
Breast discomfort, fatigue, dizziness, depression, anxiety, nausea, vomiting, constipation, increased appetite, headache, flatulence, multiple gestation, hot flashes, fluid retention	Visual disturbances, abdominal pain, weight gain, hair loss, ovarian hyperstimulation, anxiety, ovarian cysts, ectopic pregnancy ⚠ High Alert Drug: Significant risk of harm when given in error.

A, Adult; *CC*, clomiphene citrate; *d*, day; *DHEA*, dehydroepiandrosterone; *GI*, gastrointestinal; *h*, hour, *max*, maximum; *PB*, protein binding; *PO*, by mouth; *t½*, half-life; *UK*, unknown.

Clomiphene citrate (CC) is the most used ovulation stimulant. Females with PCOS may need concurrent treatment for hyperinsulinemia with metformin. Although metformin is known to help regulate the menstrual cycle and promote ovulation, it should not be used specifically for ovulation induction.

New studies have shown that *letrozole* has higher results in live birth rates when used to promote ovulation, but it is not approved by the FDA for this use; however, it has been recommended in several studies as a first-line therapy over clomiphene. Letrozole 2.5 mg once daily for 5 days, starting on day 3, 4, or 5 following menses or progestin-induced bleeding; may increase to 5 mg/day for 5 days in subsequent cycles if ovulation does not occur. Dosing of up to 5 cycles is used.

In females with PCOS who have not responded to CC or other therapies, gonadotropin therapy may be an option. *Menotropins* may be used under the direction of an infertility prescriber to help stimulate follicle maturation and promote ovulation. Monitor for *ovarian hyperstimulation syndrome* (OHSS), a medical emergency presenting with acute abdominal pain and distension, nausea, vomiting, diarrhea, and weight gain, along with gross ovarian enlargement, ascites, dyspnea, oliguria, and pleural effusion. OHSS may result in death.

These therapies supply females with exogenous hormones to enhance the normal physiologic process of the menstrual cycle, promoting ovulation and increasing the probability of conception; the use of another gonadotropin, *human chorionic gonadotropin* (hCG), triggers ovulation when ovarian follicles are mature (as determined by ultrasonography). The corpus luteum provides adequate levels of both estrogen and, more importantly, progesterone to maintain the uterine endometrium and a pregnancy, should one occur. These drugs are more potent than CC and have an increased risk for multiple births (up to 36%). Further details are listed in Table 55.2.

Pharmacokinetics

CC is readily absorbed from the GI tract. It is partially metabolized in the liver and is primarily excreted in the feces via biliary elimination. CC has a half-life of about 5 days.

Pharmacodynamics

The mechanism of action of CC is unknown, but it is hypothesized that it competes with estrogen at receptor sites. The perception of decreased circulating estrogen by the hypothalamus and pituitary gland triggers the negative feedback response that increases secretion of FSH and LH. The results are ovarian stimulation, maturation of the ovarian follicle, ovulation, and development of the corpus luteum.

Side Effects

Side effects of CC include breast discomfort, fatigue, dizziness, depression, nausea, increased appetite, dermatitis, urticaria, anxiety, weakness, heavier menses, vasomotor flushing, and abdominal bloating or pain. Antiestrogenic effects include interference with endometrial maturation and cervical mucus production. Paradoxically, this may interfere with fertilization or implantation.

Adverse Reactions

Adverse reactions include bloating and stomach or pelvic pain, photophobia, diplopia, and decreased visual acuity. Patients may also experience hot flashes, breast discomfort, dizziness, headache, heavy menstrual periods, depression, nausea or vomiting, and fatigue. OHSS may occur.

Postmarket surveillance of CC has revealed the following fetal/neonatal abnormalities: delayed development, intellectual development, abnormal bone development, tissue malformation, abnormal organ development (including anencephaly), dwarfism, chromosomal disorders, and spinal dysraphisms.

TABLE 55.2 Ovulatory Stimulants and Ovulation Control

Drug	Route and Dosage	Use and Considerations
Clomiphene citrate	See Prototype Drug Chart: Clomiphene Citrate	
Letrozole	Oral: 2.5 mg once daily for 5 days, starting on day 3, 4, or 5 following menses or progestin-induced bleed; may increase by 5 mg/day for max of 7.5 mg/day, studied in up to 5 cycles	Inhibits aromatase and may increase the release of FSH by blocking estradiol production. Androgens that would normally be converted to estrogens may accumulate in the ovaries, thereby increasing the sensitivity of ovarian follicles to FSH. Unlike clomiphene, it does not deplete estrogen receptors, which may be important for inducing mono-ovulation and for preventing negative changes in the endometrium and cervical mucus. Contraindications: Hypersensitivity to letrozole or any component; pregnancy. PB, plasma: Weak; t½: About 2 days. ⚠ High Alert Drug: Significant harm if given in error.
GnRH analogs Agonists: nafarelin Antagonists: cetrorelix, ganirelix	**Nafarelin:** Spray up to 400 mcg/d (200 mcg per nostril bid) **Cetrorelix:** 0.25 mg in a single dose subcut daily on stimulation day 5 or day 7 or 3 mg subcut in a single dose on stimulation day 7 (to control day of LH surge) **Ganirelix:** 250 mcg subcut once daily after initiating FSH, during mid to late follicular stage	Enhances ovulation stimulation for IVF cycles by suppression of a spontaneous LH surge and controls the fertility cycle, improving pregnancy outcomes. Contraindications: Hypersensitivity or previous severe reaction; latex allergies; rule out pregnancy before initiating treatment. Teach patient proper injection procedures and syringe disposal; ultrasound before initiating treatment to assess follicle size. Should only be prescribed by a fertility specialist. PB: 81.9%; Duration: less than 48 h; Absorption: rapid; t½: 12.8–16.2 h. ⚡ Pregnancy Considerations: Contraindicated in pregnancy. ⚠ High Alert Drug: Significant harm if given in error.
Menotropins	Subcut: 250 units once daily beginning on cycle day 2 or 3; menotropins may be administered together with urofollitropin, and the total initial dose of both products combined should not exceed 225 units (menotropins 150 units and urofollitropin 75 units). Adjustments should not be made more frequently than once every 2 days and should not exceed 75–100 units per adjustment based on ultrasound monitoring of ovarian response and/or measurement of serum estradiol.	Possesses the same activities as FSH and LH; will induce ovulation in females with hypothalamic amenorrhea. Risks include ovarian hyperstimulation and multiple gestation. ⚡ Contraindications: hypersensitivity, tumors, abnormal uterine bleeding, history of ovarian cysts, pregnancy. t½: 11–13 h following multiple doses; peak 18 h; excreted in urine. Pregnancy Considerations: Contraindicated in females who are already pregnant. ⚠ High Alert Drug: Significant harm if given in error.
Recombinant FSH, follitropin alpha, recombinant LH, hCG, or recombinant hCG	Recombinant FSH: Subcut or IM injection; dosage individualized for each patient, usually 75–150 units/d, early follicular phase continuing for 10–14 d Recombinant LH: Subcut 75 units given along with an FSH or recombinant FSH Recombinant hCG: 250 mcg prefilled syringe; subcut injection given 1 d after last dose of gonadotropin (FSH and/or LH) 5000–10,000 units IM 1 d after last dose of gonadotropin (FSH and/or LH)	Recombinant FSH possesses the same hormonal activities as FSH. Ovarian hyperstimulation remains a risk, although minimal, with recombinant products. Multiple gestation is a risk, which is reduced by careful monitoring. Prescribed by a fertility specialist. Avoid use with herbal supplements that contain black or blue cohosh. PB: UK; t½: IM 23–77 h, subcut 13–35 h. ⚡ Pregnancy Considerations: Contraindicated in pregnancy. ⚠ High Alert Drug: Significant harm if given in error.

bid, Twice daily; *d*, day; *FSH*, follicle-stimulating hormone; *GnRH*, gonadotropin-releasing hormone; *h*, hour; *hCG*, human chorionic gonadotropin; *IM*, intramuscular; *IVF*, in vitro fertilization; *LH*, luteinizing hormone; *max*, maximum dosage; *PB*, protein binding; *subcut*, subcutaneously; *t½*, half-life; *UK*, unknown.

◎ CLINICAL JUDGMENT [NURSING PROCESS]

Infertility

Concept: Hormonal Regulation
- Hormonal regulation involves substances working together to promote healthy development of female sex characteristics during puberty and adulthood to ensure or delay fertility.

Recognize Cues [Assessment]
- Assess the patient's general health history, including drug and herbal product use.
- Assess the patient's reproductive and sexual histories, including the following: history of abnormal Papanicolaou (Pap) testing and treatment; history of sexually transmitted infections (STIs) and treatment; past use of contraception methods; pelvic surgery; and pregnancy and birth history and complications.
- Assess the complete menstrual history, including menarche; last menstrual period (LMP); length, duration, and flow of bleeding; and any signs or symptoms related to the menstrual cycle.

Continued

CLINICAL JUDGMENT [NURSING PROCESS]—CONT'D

Infertility

- Assess the sexual practices of the couple to include the use of lubricants, timing, and technique of intercourse.
- Assess the couple's mental health status, and refer to a support group or counseling as needed. Infertility can be isolating because many couples may have several peers who are pregnant or already have children.
- Instruct the couple about the diagnostic tests to evaluate the cause of infertility. Once this is determined, conditions that contraindicate the treatment of choice are ruled out.
- Discuss with the couple their interpretation of infertility. Ascertain the effect on their relationship. The nurse should help the couple discuss their feelings in a safe, supportive environment.

Analyze Cues and Prioritize Hypothesis [Patient Problems]
- Discomfort
- Potential for nonadherence
- Decreased self-esteem
- Anxiety
- Need for patient teaching
- Reduced sexual expression
- Grieving
- Need for patient teaching

Generate Solutions [Planning]
- The patient will understand the normal physiologic process of conception.
- The patient will identify basic concepts that increase fertility.
- The patient will adhere to the medical regimen with minimal adverse effects physically, psychologically, emotionally, and spiritually.
- The patient will report adverse effects of treatment or pharmacologic therapy.
- The patient will recognize that the long-term goal is a successful pregnancy. If pregnancy cannot be achieved, the patient will be able to consider alternatives and make the transition with confidence, with the relationship and sense of self-worth intact.
- The patient will recognize that many treatment regimens for infertility must be repeated before successful conception is attained.

Take Action [Nursing Interventions]
General
- Initiate teaching to assist the patient and their partner in understanding the menstrual cycle; patterns and symptoms of ovulation; temperature changes with ovulation; specific physiologic signs of ovulation; use of ovulation predictor kits; and timing of sexual intercourse.
- Instruct the patient in the interrelationships among the menstrual cycle, ovulation, and coitus as they relate to conception.
- Advise the patient and their partner on the sexual techniques that enhance fertilization: placement of a pillow under the female's hips during coitus, and placement of the female in a supine position with the hips elevated for about 30 minutes after her partner ejaculates.
- Instruct the patient and their partner in the drug treatment regimens as prescribed by the provider. The patient and partner(s) will verbalize the treatment regimen and the expected outcomes of the treatment regimen.
- Facilitate the patient and their partner's psychological counseling and support.

Specific
- ⚡ Instruct the patient to report adverse effects such as abdominal pain or visual disturbances to the infertility specialist at once and to be cautious with tasks that require alertness. If a dose of the drug is missed, the patient should call the infertility specialist.
- Advise the patient that treatment increases the chance of multiple births.
- ⚡ Ensure that the patient understands the risks, benefits, and alternatives to pharmacologic therapy.

Patient Teaching
- Instruct the couple how to evaluate and record on a chart the female's basal body temperature and changes in the cervical mucus. The first day of menses is day 1 of the cycle. Ovulation is predicted by a 0.5°F drop in basal body temperature, followed by a 1°F rise. Over-the-counter (OTC) diagnostic kits for assessing ovulatory status can also be used to time coitus. The couple is advised to engage in coitus frequently from 4 days before to 3 days after ovulation.
- Advise the female partner to take the drug at the same time each day to maintain steady blood levels.
- Encourage the patient to verbalize concerns and express feelings about treatment successes and failures.

Evaluate Outcomes [Evaluation]
- Successful outcomes of fertility treatment include avoidance of ovarian hyperstimulation and other untoward effects. Pregnancy that results in the birth of a live infant fulfills the objectives of treatment. If pregnancy is not achieved, intervention is aimed at helping the couple consider alternatives to childbearing without any adverse effect on their self-esteem or harm to their relationship.

Contraindications

Contraindications for treatment with CC include undiagnosed vaginal bleeding, pregnancy, uterine fibroids, clinical depression, history of hepatic dysfunction or thromboembolic disease, and primary pituitary or ovarian failure. CC may cause existing ovarian cysts to enlarge. Contraindications to the use of other ovulatory stimulants are listed in Table 55.2.

Drug Interactions

There are no known drug interactions with menotropins and hCG.

Other Drug Treatments

Endocrine disorders include hyperprolactinemia and thyroid disorders. In females with hyperprolactinemia, an elevated level of prolactin is the causative factor of infertility. Prolactin is a hormone secreted by the anterior pituitary gland and is elevated during pregnancy and postpartum to support milk production. Breast-feeding causes a natural rise in prolactin, and hyperprolactinemia can be seen in females who are or have recently discontinued breast-feeding.

Drug therapies such as haloperidol, metoclopramide, methyldopa, reserpine, and long-term CHC use have been known to cause hyperprolactinemia. The most common cause of pathologic hyperprolactinemia is a small, benign pituitary tumor called a *pituitary adenoma*. Regardless of the cause of hyperprolactinemia, most females can be treated with the ergot derivative bromocriptine, which binds to dopamine receptors in the pituitary gland and inhibits prolactin secretion. Treatment continues until pregnancy is confirmed. Clomiphene can be introduced if needed after 2 months.

DRUGS USED IN THE TREATMENT OF MENOPAUSE

The transitional process experienced by females as they move from the reproductive years into the nonreproductive stage of life is called *menopause*, a naturally occurring event and part of the normal life cycle of females. It occurs for most females between their mid-40s and mid-50s but may start as early as the late 30s. Menopause has three stages: perimenopause or premenopause, menopause, and postmenopause, during which certain physiologic events occur. As a female goes through menopause, providers do not treat the cessation of menses but rather address the symptoms that may occur with the menopausal passage.

Menopause

Menopause is the permanent end of spontaneous menstruation caused by cessation of ovarian function. This natural event is documented as having occurred once a female has stopped menstruating for 1 year. The triggering event is not known. Females who experience menopause before 40 years of age are said to have premature ovarian failure. Menopause can also occur abruptly as a secondary effect of oophorectomy (surgical removal of the ovaries), radiologic procedures in which ovarian function is destroyed, severe infection, or ovarian tumors or as a temporarily induced state for treatment of conditions such as endometriosis. During this transitional period, and with any episodes of menstrual changes or irregularities caused by perimenopause, females should use contraception until menstruation has ceased for 1 year if they do not want to become pregnant.

Perimenopause

The perimenopausal period includes the years before the natural cessation of spontaneous menstruation. During this period, menstrual variations become evident. Females may experience short cycles (<25 days), long cycles (>35 days), heavy bleeding, light bleeding, or periods of longer or shorter duration. Females may start to skip periods or abruptly stop menstruating altogether. Oligomenorrhea, very scant periods, and menorrhagia are common. Symptoms experienced during perimenopause are similar to those during menopause, with the exception that females in perimenopause continue to have some type of cyclic bleeding. The most common symptoms are hot flashes caused by a surge in LH levels and vaginal dryness caused by estrogen withdrawal. Other symptoms include insomnia, headaches, irritability or anxiety or other variations in mood, cognitive difficulties, memory lapses, joint aches, and decreased libido. These unpredictable changes may last a short period of time or they may last for several years.

There are a set number of follicles in the ovaries at birth. They are dormant throughout childhood and become active with puberty. Ovarian follicles are high in number during puberty and until 35 years of age, but the number of follicles steadily declines after 35 years of age, and the decline is more rapid after 40 years of age. During the menstrual cycle, these follicles provide high levels of estrogen in the form of estradiol. The highest level of estradiol production in females occurs from puberty until the early 30s. Follicular growth, and therefore the secretion of estradiol, is under the influence of FSH and, to a lesser degree, LH, both of which are released by the anterior pituitary gland.

During the perimenopausal period, ovarian follicles become depleted, causing estrogen levels to diminish. The decrease in estrogen is gradual and allows for fluctuating levels of FSH and LH. Subsequently, menstrual cycles become anovulatory and therefore irregular. The onset of menstrual irregularity is one of the early indications of perimenopause. Symptoms are thought to be related to hormone fluctuations, particularly estrogen withdrawal, and increased levels of LH and FSH. Serum FSH testing is used as a marker of follicular activity, and an elevated level of FSH can be an indication of decreased ovarian function.

Postmenopause

Postmenopause is the stage when the body adapts to a new hormonal environment. The production of estrogen and progesterone from the ovaries decreases during the late premenopausal and early postmenopausal periods. The ovaries continue to secrete androgens (testosterone) in varying amounts because of the influence of increased LH levels. This surge in LH causes hot flashes: transient sensations of intense heat with or without sweating, tachycardia, and sleep disruption. During postmenopause, androstenedione—the main androgen secreted by the ovaries and adrenal cortex, which is present in reduced amounts after menopause—is converted into estrone, a naturally occurring estrogen formed in extraglandular tissues of the brain, liver, kidney, and adipose tissue. This represents the main source of available estrogen once the ovaries lose the ability to produce estradiol.

FDA Warnings for Hormone Therapy

Hormone therapy (HT) significantly improves vasomotor symptoms and vaginal dryness, two frequently encountered symptoms of menopause. Vasomotor symptoms have the potential to disrupt sleep quality and to exacerbate irritability, mood swings, depression, and problems with concentration. The decrease in systemic estrogen seen in menopause can cause vaginal dryness, atrophic vaginitis, decreased libido, and negative effects on urinary health. Current guidelines do not support the use of HT for the prevention of cardiovascular disease, osteoporosis, or dementia.

The FDA has issued a boxed warning that states that HT should be used only for the treatment of menopausal symptoms, at the lowest dose possible, for the shortest duration possible, usually fewer than 5 years ⚠ (Box 55.4). Most health care providers adhere to this practice when prescribing HT. Health teaching must be done with females in menopause to ensure that they are aware of the risks and benefits of HT.

> ⚡ **PATIENT SAFETY**
>
> **Do Not Confuse ...**
> - **Combined hormonal contraceptive (CHC) products** with **HT products**. Oral, transdermal, and vaginal ring preparations for contraception and HT are dispensed in packages and boxes that are very similar. Once opened, CHC products and HT products may have the same disc-dispensing systems and splintered packaging and may have similar-appearing skin patches and vaginal rings.

Hormonal Therapy

HT is used only for the relief of symptoms related to menopausal and perimenopausal symptoms, most commonly hot flashes, vaginal dryness, and associated sleep disorders. HT includes estrogen-progestin therapy for use with females who have an intact uterus and ET for use with females who have had a hysterectomy, surgical removal of the uterus. It is the estrogen component in HT that relieves the symptoms of menopause. Progestin is added to protect the uterine endometrium from hyperplasia, an abnormal proliferation or overgrowth of tissue. When the uterus is exposed to unopposed estrogen—that is, estrogen without concurrent progestins—the endometrium becomes hyperplastic, potentiating the development of endometrial cancer. Estrogen alone can be used with females who have had a hysterectomy. With

BOX 55.4 FDA Boxed Warnings for Combined Hormonal Contraceptives (CHCs) and Hormone Therapy Products

CHCs: "Cigarette smoking increases the risk of serious cardiovascular side effects from oral contraceptive use. This risk increases with age and with heavy smoking (15 or more cigarettes per day) and is quite marked in females over 35 years of age. Females who use oral contraceptives should be strongly advised not to smoke."

Ethinyl estradiol and norelgestromin transdermal patch: "Do not use this transdermal patch if you smoke cigarettes and are over 35 years old. Smoking increases your risk of serious cardiovascular side effects (heart and blood vessel problems) from hormonal contraceptives, including death from heart attack, blood clots, or stroke. The risk increases with age and the number of cigarettes you smoke."

Ethinyl estradiol and etonogestrel transvaginal ring: "Cigarette smoking increases the risk of serious cardiovascular side effects from combination oral contraceptive use. This risk increases with age and with heavy smoking (15 or more cigarettes per day) and is quite marked in females over 35 years of age. Females who use combination hormonal contraceptives, including the transvaginal ring, should be strongly advised not to smoke."

Hormone replacement therapies with estrogen and estrogen plus progesterone: "Warning: Cardiovascular disorders, breast cancer, endometrial cancer and probable dementia [can occur]. … Estrogens, with or without progestins, should be prescribed at the lowest effective doses and for the shortest duration consistent with treatment goals and risks for the individual females."

---

patients who still have their uterus, estrogen is taken together with synthetic progestin. The progestin, however, has the potential to cause unpredictable uterine bleeding.

⚡ PATIENT SAFETY

Do Not Confuse …

- **Premarin** with **Prempro** or **Premphase:** Premarin is estrogen only for hormone replacement therapy. Both *Prempro* and *Premphase* have combined estrogen and progesterone for use by females with an intact uterus to prevent uterine hyperplasia when estrogen is used.

HT is available in oral preparations, transdermal applications, and vaginal preparations. Vaginal preparations are creams, suppositories, or rings. All vaginal preparations contain estrogen only and are very effective in treating vaginal dryness. FDA-approved estrogens used in HT are derived from natural sources and synthetic sources.

Conjugated equine estrogens (CEEs) are mixtures of natural estrogens isolated from the urine of pregnant mares (see Prototype Drug Chart: Conjugated Estrogens). Although CEEs are derived from nonhuman sources, they are naturally occurring estrogens. Synthetic estrogens include EE, which is the same estrogen found in CHC products.

Various Dosage Forms of Estrogen

The oral route is most used because it is well tolerated by most patients and relatively easy to administer. It requires daily dosing.

PROTOTYPE DRUG CHART
Conjugated Estrogens

Drug	Route and Dosage
Estrogen replacement in menopause	A: PO: 0.3 mg/d; give continuously, with no interruption in therapy, or cyclically Always use lowest effective dose; few patients require 1.25 mg/d PO or more Reevaluate the need for treatment q3–6mo

Contraindications	Drug-Lab-Food Interactions
Undiagnosed vaginal bleeding, pregnancy, lactation, severe liver disease, venous thrombosis, personal history of breast cancer ! *Caution:* Cardiovascular disease, severe renal disease, diabetes mellitus ⚡ *Black-Box Warning:* Absolute contraindications in MI, new primary malignancy, stroke, thromboembolism, and dementia	Drug: Increased effects with corticosteroids; decreases effects of anticoagulants and oral hypoglycemics; decreased effects with rifampin, anticonvulsants, and barbiturates; toxicity with tricyclic antidepressants

Pharmacokinetics	Pharmacodynamics
Absorption: PO: Well absorbed Distribution: PB: Largely bound to sex hormone–binding globulin (SHBG) and albumin Widely distributed; crosses placenta and enters breast milk Metabolism: t½: UK Excretion: In urine and bile	PO/IV: Onset: Rapid Peak: UK Duration: UK IM: Onset: Delayed

Therapeutic Effects/Uses
For moderate to severe vasomotor symptoms of menopause and vaginal dryness/atrophy
Mechanism of Action: Develops and maintains female genital system, breast, and secondary sex characteristics; increases synthesis of protein

Side Effects	Adverse Reactions
Nausea, vomiting, fluid retention, breast tenderness, leg cramps, breakthrough bleeding, chloasma, inappropriate drug to use in older adults. ! High Alert Drug: Risk of significant harm when used in error.	Jaundice, thromboembolic disorders, depression, hypercalcemia, gallbladder disease ⚡ *Blackbox Warning:* Thromboembolism, MI, new primary malignancy, stroke, dementia.

A, Adult; *CVA*, cerebrovascular accident; *d*, day; *IM*, intramuscular; *IV*, intravenous; *MI*, myocardial infarction; *PB*, protein binding; *PE*, pulmonary embolism; *PO*, by mouth; *q*, every; *t½*, half-life; *UK*, unknown.

Some patients experience GI upsets, particularly nausea and vomiting. A patient with GI disorders such as colitis, IBS, peptic ulcer, or a malabsorption disorder may receive inconsistent doses with oral administration, necessitating the use of another route. Oral estrogens have a particularly beneficial effect on lipids by increasing high-density lipoproteins. Although the oral route does result in complete absorption from the GI tract, there is a greater effect on liver proteins. In females with an intact uterus, oral estrogen is combined with a progesterone or progestin, completing the combined therapy. This can be given in a separate estrogen tablet combined with a separate progestin tablet (two oral pills taken daily) or in a combined estrogen-progestin tablet (one oral pill taken daily). Oral estrogens are typically used continuously. Common HT products include CEE, estradiol, synthetic conjugated estrogen, and esterified estrogen.

The *transdermal estrogen skin patch* is a convenient method to deliver HT because it does not require daily dosing. The patch is applied to intact skin in the prescribed dosage. Generally, the lower abdomen is used, but other sites may also be used. As with the transdermal patch used for contraception, the HT patch should not be placed on or near the breasts. The patch allows for absorption of the estrogen directly into the bloodstream through a membrane that limits the absorption rate. All types of transdermal patches, both estrogen-only and estrogen-progestin combination patches, contain plant-derived 17-β estradiol; many females prefer to take an estrogen derived from a plant source. The advantage is the same as the first-pass avoidance in CHC products using the transdermal route: the GI tract and liver are bypassed initially, which results in less nausea and vomiting and less effect on the hepatic system. Transdermal patches are changed twice a week or weekly, depending on the product, and they are used continuously. A progestin should be taken concurrently with the estrogen patch in females with an intact uterus.

HT is also available in topical gels, emulsions, and sprays; synthetic plant-based transdermal estradiol gels are applied once daily for the treatment of moderate to severe vasomotor symptoms. A thin film is applied to one arm from the shoulder to the wrist; the gel dries in 2 to 5 minutes. The dosage regimen is designed to deliver a specific amount of estradiol with each application.

With the topical HT products listed previously, a progestin should be taken concurrently in females who have an intact uterus. Medroxyprogesterone acetate is the oral progestin most often administered in combination with estrogen. Other available products are norethindrone acetate and micronized progesterone. Combination products contain both estrogen and progestin, which offers the added convenience of not having to take two pills daily. Combination products have the same adverse effects as estrogen-only and progestin-only HT.

Two combination transdermal products contain estrogen and progestin combinations to treat menopausal symptoms such as hot flashes. The transdermal patch allows for continuous delivery of hormones at much lower doses than in oral HT. This route avoids first-pass metabolism by the liver and may be better tolerated. Patients should be treated with the lowest effective dose and for the shortest duration consistent with treatment ⚡ goals.

Estrogen vaginal cream preparations are used in the treatment of vaginal atrophy, which causes painful intercourse and urinary difficulties. There is estradiol cream and conjugated equine topical cream, which is an estrogen derivative. Both preparations are rapidly absorbed into the bloodstream via the mucous membranes that line the vagina. Vaginal creams may be used in conjunction with another method, such as tablets or the transdermal patch. However, vaginal creams do *not* need a progestin counter because they do not affect the uterine endometrium to the extent that oral and transdermal products will. Conjugated estrogen vaginal cream is usually delivered in a dose of 0.5 to 2 g/day intravaginally for 2 weeks; then the dosing is decreased to twice weekly for 3 weeks out of each month.

One *estradiol vaginal ring* is a low-dose estradiol-releasing ring containing 2 mg of estradiol per 90-day ring (7.5 mcg/24 hours). This ring is inserted into the upper portion of the vagina, where it releases the estradiol, providing a consistent low dose of estrogen for 3 months. It may be left in place during intercourse and during treatment for vaginal infections. It is used to treat local symptoms of urogenital atrophy.

Another estradiol vaginal ring consists of a low-dose estradiol-acetate releasing ring, made from silicone elastomer. This vaginal ring is available in two dosage strengths: 0.05 mg/day or 0.1 mg/day. This ring is inserted into the upper portion of the vagina, where it releases the estradiol, providing a consistent low dose of estrogen for 3 months. The lowest effective dose should be used. In females with an intact uterus, consideration should be given to adding progestin 10 to 14 days out of a 4-week menstrual cycle.

Vaginal estrogen tablets that contain estradiol can be inserted intravaginally once daily for 2 weeks. The dose is one 10-mcg tablet to be inserted once daily, and then the dose is decreased to one 10-mcg tablet twice weekly. Consideration should be given to adding progestin for 10 to 14 days out of a 4-week menstrual cycle if the female's uterus is intact.

Contraindications

Contraindications to HT include pregnancy, history of endometrial cancer (when treatment for early endometrial cancer has been completed, it is no longer a contraindication to HT), personal history of breast cancer, history of thromboembolic disorders, acute liver disease or chronic impaired liver function, active gallbladder or pancreatic disease, coronary artery disease (CAD), undiagnosed vaginal bleeding, and endometriosis. Lifestyle factors such as smoking, known to enhance the risk of thromboembolism, should be considered in the treatment decision. The patient with a history of fibroid tumors is not started on HT for a full year after the last menstruation, because estrogen would likely result in tumor growth. The hypoestrogenic state associated with natural menopause usually causes existing fibroids to shrink. The presence of fibrocystic breast disease or diabetes may require extra ⚡ caution.

Pharmacokinetics

CEEs are water soluble and well absorbed from the GI tract after tablet disintegration. Tablets are designed to release conjugated estrogens slowly over several hours. The estrogens are widely distributed in the body and circulate in the blood largely bound to sex hormone–binding globulin (SHBG) and albumin. Exogenous estrogens are metabolized in the liver, converted to metabolites, and excreted in the urine. Estrogens undergo enterohepatic recirculation.

Classes of Drugs for Perimenopausal/Menopausal Treatments

Females who are not candidates for HT—more specifically, females with contraindications and breast cancer survivors—can be prescribed other drugs. *Selective serotonin reuptake inhibitors* (*SSRIs*) and *serotonin norepinephrine reuptake inhibitors* (*SNRIs*) reduce the number and severity of vasomotor symptoms in females. SSRIs also have the added benefit of reducing depression, which may relieve the irritability and mood changes associated with menopause. SSRIs and SNRIs can be gradually tapered in most postmenopausal females after 1 to 2 years of therapy.

Fezolinetant (Veozah) is a new FDA-approved medication for adult females used to treat moderate to severe vasomotor symptoms due to menopause. The recommended dosage is 45 mg by mouth daily. Adverse effects include abdominal pain, back pain, diarrhea, elevated hepatic enzymes, and endometrial hyperplasia. It is contraindicated in patients with renal failure, hepatic disease, pregnancy, and breast-feeding. Pharmacokinetics: 51% bound to plasma protein, excreted in urine with a half-life of 9.6 hours.

Bremelanotide is an FDA-approved drug used for generalized hypoactive sexual disorders, or low sexual desire, experienced by perimenopausal females, approved for ages 56 years old and younger. It is an injectable melanocortin receptor agonist, and 1.75 mg is injected SC 45 minutes before sexual activity. It has a unique mechanism of action that helps activate the brain pathways involved in normal sexual responses. Bremelanotide transiently increases blood pressure and reduces heart rate after each dose; bremelanotide is contraindicated in patients with uncontrolled hypertension. Pharmacokinetics: 21% bound to plasma protein, 64% excreted in urine, half-life of 2.7 hours.

OSTEOPOROSIS DISEASE

Osteoporosis is a progressive, debilitating skeletal disease that affects older males and females, with females older than 50 years being at greatest risk because the loss of estrogen during menopause is directly related to loss in BMD. Bone mass is at its highest density at 30 years of age and then steadily declines. Osteoporosis occurs through an imbalance of osteoblasts (bone-building cells) and osteoclasts (cells that break down bone), which causes bone reabsorption to accelerate. This imbalance causes both deterioration of the microstructure within the bone and a decrease in bone density. The loss of bone structure and "porous bone" fragility lead to an increased risk for fractures. Osteoporosis has significant morbidity and mortality in the United States. The most serious fracture site is the hip, and hip fracture is the second most common reason for older females to be placed in nursing homes, exceeded only by Alzheimer disease. Females who experience hip or vertebral fracture may have long-term, progressive, and debilitating health problems that can eventually lead to death. More than half of American females older than 50 years have some degree of osteopenia (low BMD) or osteoporosis (a severe decline in BMD).

Diagnosis of osteopenia and osteoporosis is made by axial skeletal measurements of bone density in the lumbar spine and hip through a dual-energy x-ray absorptiometry (DXA) scan. The World Health Organization defines osteopenia and osteoporosis by translating the results of the DXA scan into a T score. Normal BMD is a T score of −1 or greater. Osteopenia is defined by a T score of −1 to −2.5, and osteoporosis is defined by a T score of −2.5 or less.

HT is no longer recommended for the *treatment* of osteoporosis; however, it may be considered as a *preventive* measure in postmenopausal Females who are at risk, although not as first-line therapy. Females who have used HT for 5 years or more have been shown to have a 35% reduction in hip and vertebral fractures. Other drugs can manage osteoporosis and prevent fractures without the concerns raised by HT. These include bisphosphonates, which can reduce the breakdown of bone microstructure, and selective estrogen receptor modulators (SERMs). SERMs are a new class of synthetic estrogens that act like estrogens in certain parts of the body, such as the bones, while leaving other parts unaffected. Contraindications to SERM therapy include history of or risk for venous thromboembolism (VTE) and pregnancy. Caution is used in females with heart disease, risk of MI or stroke, and hepatic or renal insufficiency.

The side effects of *oral bisphosphonates* include nausea, abdominal or stomach pain, difficulty swallowing, esophageal inflammation, reflux, and ulcers. Injectable bisphosphonates do not have the GI side effects, and it can be easier for the patient to schedule a quarterly or yearly injection than to remember to take a daily or weekly pill. A rare complication of bisphosphonates is full or partial spontaneous femur fractures. Oral bisphosphonates should not be taken with aspirin, NSAIDs, or antacids. Contraindications to bisphosphonates include esophageal abnormalities or delayed emptying of the esophagus, inability to sit or stand for 30 minutes after oral ingestion, and hypocalcemia.

Clinical Nursing Judgment in the Management of Osteoporosis Disease

Prevention of osteoporosis includes sufficient intake of calcium and vitamin D throughout the life span by either dietary intake or supplementation. The recommended daily requirement of calcium for females 19 to 50 years of age is 1000 mg/day, whereas females older than 50 years need 1200 mg/day. Calcium should be taken in divided doses and with adequate vitamin D to enhance absorption. The FDA recommended daily allowance of vitamin D is 600 IU/day for females 19 to 70 years of age and 800 IU/day for females older than 70 years, though there have been some studies recommending vitamin D intake to be as high as 800 to 1,000 IU/day for all females older than 50 to prevent osteoporosis. All calcium preparations, except for calcium citrate, should be taken with food. Smoking cessation should be encouraged because smoking interferes with vitamin D absorption. Alcohol consumption should be limited to one drink per day because alcohol reduces GI absorption of calcium. Weight-bearing exercise includes walking, jogging, low-impact aerobics, weight training, and yoga; these strengthen the bones, increase muscle strength, and enhance balance. Caution should be used in patients who are prescribed drugs that cause hypotension or dizziness. The patient should be assessed for fall risk, and the prevention of falls should be part of the nurse's health care teaching.

Drugs Used for Treatment of Osteoporosis

Alendronate is a bisphosphonate used to treat osteopenia and osteoporosis. It is available in a daily or weekly dose. For prevention of osteoporosis, the oral weekly dose is 35 mg. For treatment, the oral weekly dose is 70 mg. Alendronate must be taken with 8 ounces of water 30 minutes before ingesting any food, liquids, or drug, and the patient must remain upright for 30 minutes. Once-a-week dosing has made this a first-line therapy. Common side effects include abdominal pain and acid reflux. Alendronate is also available with added vitamin D for enhanced absorption of calcium.

Ibandronate is a once-a-month bisphosphonate indicated for the treatment and prevention of osteoporosis in postmenopausal females. It comes in both oral and intravenous (IV) formulations. The oral dose has the same directions for use and side effects as the other bisphosphonates. Ibandronate can be administered as 150-mg once-monthly tablets or 3 mg every 3 months administered IV over 15 to 30 seconds.

Risedronate is a bisphosphonate derivative that is available in a daily or weekly dose. It has similar directions for use and similar side effects as bisphosphonates. The dosing schedule is a 5-mg tablet once daily 35-mg once weekly, or 150-mg once monthly.

Zoledronic acid is a bisphosphonate that is administered IV in a 5-mg dose yearly for the treatment of osteoporosis; the dose should be administered over 15 minutes. Zoledronic acid can be given in 5-mg dose every 2 years for prevention of osteoporosis.

Kidney failure is a rare but serious condition that may be associated with the use of bisphosphonates in patients with underlying renal disease or renal impairment. These drugs should not be used in patients with chronic kidney disease and a glomerular filtration rate lower than 30 to 35 mL/min.

Nurses should teach patients to advise their health care provider of any increased thigh or groin pain, which can be symptoms of rare, atypical femur fractures.

Studies suggest that some patients may be able to discontinue the use of these drugs after 3 to 5 years and still benefit from using bisphosphonates. It is recommended that the bone density test of the hip and spine be repeated after 2 years. Health care providers should reassess patients on an individual basis every 5 years to determine whether continued therapy is beneficial. It has been determined that bisphosphonates do work to improve osteoporosis; however, the time frame for safe use of these drugs needs to be investigated. Research is ongoing to determine whether the use of bisphosphonates increases the risk for esophageal cancer, which is extremely rare in females.

Raloxifene is an SERM that increases BMD, decreases bone turnover, and reduces vertebral fractures. A secondary analysis of osteoporotic females treated with raloxifene showed a decrease in the risk for breast cancer. Side effects include hot flashes and increased risk for deep venous thrombosis (⚡ DVT). Raloxifene is taken orally once a day in a 60-mg tablet. Patients need to take calcium and vitamin D to prevent or treat hypocalcemia while taking this drug.

Teriparatide is a parathyroid hormone used for treatment of postmenopausal osteoporosis, and it is administered 20 mcg subcutaneously daily for 2 years. It can be used by both males and females who have had a fracture related to osteoporosis or who have multiple risk factors for fracture and cannot use other osteoporosis treatments. The patient can be taught self-administration.

Calcitonin-salmon is composed of calcitonin, a naturally occurring hormone that regulates calcium in the body and promotes bone metabolism. It is administered 100 units subcutaneously or IM every day to every other day. Another delivery option is via intranasal spray in a 200-IU dose administered daily.

Denosumab is a monoclonal antibody and bone-modifying agent used in females who are at a high risk for osteoporotic fracture, who have had a fracture, or who have not had improvement in T score after using the bisphosphonates for osteoporosis. A 60-mg dose is given subcutaneously every 6 months. Patients need to take calcium and vitamin D to prevent or treat hypocalcemia while taking this drug.

Romosozumab is a parenteral humanized IgG2 monoclonal antibody and sclerostin inhibitor for the treatment of osteoporosis in postmenopausal females at high risk for fracture and for those who have failed or could not tolerate other osteoporosis therapy. It is administered in 2 subcutaneous consecutive injections (105 mg each) for a total dose of 210 mg once monthly for 12 months. It is recommended to initiate bisphosphonate or denosumab therapy to maintain BMD gains following the 12 months. It is contraindicated in patients with myocardial MI or stroke.

CLINICAL JUDGMENT [NURSING PROCESS]
Management of Symptomatic Menopausal Females

Concept: Hormonal Regulation
- Hormonal regulation involves substances normally present in the body to promote fertility in adulthood that decrease during the aging process and can cause many symptoms and complications if not regulated.

Recognize Cues [Assessment]
- Obtain a history of patient's drug and supplement intake.
- Obtain baseline vital signs that include temperature, pulse, respiration, blood pressure (BP), and weight and height. Report abnormal findings.
- Obtain a family history to assess for risk factors regarding osteoporosis and osteoporotic fractures; cardiovascular risks, including coronary artery disease, ischemic and hemorrhagic stroke, and venous thromboembolism (VTE); cognitive disorders; and cancers that affect females.
- Obtain a history of allergies to drugs, foods, and supplements.
- Obtain a medical-surgical history, asking about present or past hypertension; falls and fractures; cardiovascular disease; cerebral vascular disorders; hepatic, renal, and urinary tract disorders and infections; gastrointestinal (GI) problems; neurologic disorders; and past systemic infections. Assess past and present history of cancer. Ask about previous surgeries, in particular gynecologic or pelvic surgery.
- Assess smoking, alcohol, and illicit drug use. Assess risk for falls and fractures, self-care concerns, and ability to take drugs.
- Obtain a complete menstrual history including age at menarche and age at menopause. If the patient is perimenopausal, assess menstrual pattern; cycle length, duration, and amount of bleeding; first day of last menstrual period (LMP); and method used for contraception. If the patient is in menopause, assess past and present menopausal symptoms along with their effects on quality of life. Assess for any incidence of postmenopausal bleeding.
- Obtain a full gynecologic history, including the last Papanicolaou (Pap) testing results, history of abnormal Pap testing and colposcopy, and gynecologic problems, disorders, and surgeries.
- Obtain a complete sexual history, including sexual expression and sexual risk practices, menopausal symptoms and effects on sexual expression, and past or present sexual abuse and/or assault.
- Assess the patient's perception of menopause and knowledge of nonpharmacologic and pharmacologic hormone therapies.

Analyze Cues and Prioritize Hypothesis [Patient Problems]
- Discomfort
- Confusion
- Potential for injury
- Anxiety
- Need for patient teaching

Generate Solutions [Planning]
- The patient's risks and benefits associated with hormone therapy (HT) will be evaluated on an individual basis.
- The patient will verbalize menopausal symptoms and will understand nonpharmacologic and pharmacologic measures that may aid in alleviating symptoms.
- The patient will choose the route of administration that is best suited for their lifestyle and will increase safety and effective use of the product.
- The patient will report side effects that occur to the health care provider (HCP).
- The patient will self-administer their prescribed medication: oral, transdermal, topical, or vaginal drugs.
- The patient will place the patch as directed and will report any adverse side effects that occur.
- The patient will be comfortable with vaginal placement of drugs.
- The patient will report abnormal uterine bleeding (AUB) and other side effects associated with HT.
- The patient will verbalize the dosing schedule, risks, benefits, and alternatives of their treatment.
- The patient will schedule follow-up appointments as needed.

Continued

CLINICAL JUDGMENT [NURSING PROCESS]—CONT'D
Management of Symptomatic Menopausal Females

Take Action [Nursing Interventions]
- ⚡ Instruct the patient about the nature of menopause, its potential effects, and the benefits, risks, and alternatives of both nonpharmacologic and pharmacologic treatment modalities.
- Determine the patient's misconceptions about HT and provide factual, research-based information.
- Assist the patient in using the BRAIDED method for HT therapy.
- Instruct the patient in the effective use of HT.
- Supply various health community sites with educational materials concerning HT.

Patient Teaching
General
- ⚡ Review with the patient the risks, benefits, and alternatives for use of HT.
- Review with the patient contraindications to HT.
- Advise the patient to have breast and pelvic examinations and a Pap test before starting HT.
- Instruct the patient that warm weather and stress exacerbate hot flashes.
- Advise the patient to use a fan, drink cool liquids, and decrease intake of caffeine and spicy foods.
- ⚡ Instruct the patient on HT therapy to have a medical follow-up every 6 to 12 months, including a BP check, a clinical breast examination, and a pelvic examination.
- Instruct the patient in the need to use a method of contraception until 1 year after cessation of spontaneous menstruation.
- Suggest to the patient the use of a water-soluble vaginal lubricant to reduce painful intercourse (dyspareunia) and prevent trauma.
- Advise the patient to decrease use of antihistamines and decongestants if experiencing vaginal dryness.
- Advise the patient to wear cotton underwear and pantyhose with a cotton liner, and to avoid douches and feminine hygiene products.
- Suggest the patient take HT oral drugs after meals to avoid nausea and vomiting.
- Advise the patient that some vaginal bleeding may be expected and that it should stop 3 to 6 months after starting HT.
- Instruct the patient to carry sanitary pads or tampons for breakthrough bleeding (BTB) or irregular menstruation.
- Advise the patient to report any heavy bleeding or irregular bleeding patterns and to have their hematocrit and hemoglobin levels evaluated.
- Advise the patient that after HT is discontinued, there may be a recurrence of menopausal signs and symptoms such as hot flashes.
- Instruct the patient wanting to stop HT that it should be done with guidance by the HCP.

Self-Administration
- Instruct the patient about breast health and regular breast self-examination.
- Advise the patient to list on their calendar regular Pap screening due dates.
- Instruct the patient in the application of vaginal cream and suggest the use of minipads.
- Instruct the patient in the application of the transdermal patch, such as checking the edges to ensure adequate contact to the skin; always placing the patch on the abdomen (except the waistline); rotating sites with at least 1 week before reuse of a site; never to use the breast area as a site; never to put the patch on an irritated or oily skin; and never to reapply the patch if it loosens.
- Advise the patient about appropriate use of gels, sprays, and mists.

Balanced Diet and Exercise
- Instruct the patient about osteoporosis prevention, and encourage (1) with the HCP's clearance both a walking and weight-bearing exercise program; (2) a well-balanced diet high in fiber, vegetables, fruits, whole grains, and plant proteins and low in animal proteins and sugar; (3) supplementation with 1000 mg/day of calcium (if <50 years of age) or 1200 mg/day (if >50 years of age) and vitamin D 600 IU/day if <70 years of age); (4) smoking cessation and reduced alcohol consumption.

Evaluate Outcomes [Evaluation]
- Evaluate the effectiveness of nonpharmacologic or pharmacologic measures for premenopausal symptoms.
- Determine whether side effects occur. Plan alternative measures to control menopausal symptoms with the patient.
- Plan follow-up appointments and health care screenings.

CLINICAL JUDGMENT UNFOLDING CASE STUDY

Objective: Apply knowledge of female's reproductive health as it relates to menopause.

A 52-year-old females presents to the health clinic for an early morning appointment to see the health care provider for a check-up. She reports fatigue and decreased libido. The provider obtains baseline vital signs, including temperature, pulse, respirations, blood pressure, weight, and height. Her history includes three live births and no miscarriages. Patient has no known allergies. The only reported medication is a multivitamin taken by mouth every morning.

Question 1
Cognitive Skill: Recognize cues [enhanced hot spot]
The nurse documents the following assessment findings:
- Blood pressure 118/78 mm Hg, heart rate 72 bpm
- Reports intense feelings of heat
- Temperature of 98.6°F, respirations 20 breaths per minute
- Reports nighttime sweating
- No history of abnormal Pap smears
- Reports no menstrual cycle in a year
- Reports vaginal dryness and painful intercourse
- Routine postmenopausal pregnancy test negative
- Patient is 5.0 ft in height and weighs 240 lb.

Highlight or place a checkmark next to the assessment findings that require follow-up by the nurse.

Answers
- Blood pressure 118/78 mm Hg, heart rate 72 bpm
- **Reports intense feelings of heat**
- Temperature of 98.6°F, respirations 20 breaths per minute
- **Reports nighttime sweating**
- No history of abnormal Pap smears
- **Reports no menstrual cycle in a year**
- **Reports vaginal dryness and painful intercourse**
- Routine postmenopausal pregnancy test negative
- **Patient is 5.0 ft in height and weighs 240 lb.**

CLINICAL JUDGMENT UNFOLDING CASE STUDY—CONT'D

Rationale
Symptoms of menopause are the same as those of perimenopause. The only difference is that with menopause there is no menstrual period. Menopause is caused by a change in the balance of the sex hormones, which occurs with age. The most common symptoms are hot flashes, feelings of heat, nighttime sweating resulting from a surge in luteinizing hormone (LH) levels, and vaginal dryness caused by estrogen withdrawal. Other symptoms include insomnia; headaches; irritability, anxiety, or other variations in mood; cognitive difficulties; memory lapses; joint aches; and decreased libido. The patient's blood pressure, temperature, and respirations are within normal ranges. The patient does not have a history of abnormal Pap smears, which indicates no prediagnostic problems. The postmenopausal pregnancy test is negative, which rules out pregnancy as she has not had a menstrual cycle in a year.

References
McCuistion L, et al. Women's reproductive health, menopause/perimenopause. In *Pharmacology: A patient-centered nursing process approach*, 11th ed, Missouri, 2023, Elsevier, pp 703–708.

Harding M, et al. Female reproductive problems. In *Lewis's medical surgical nursing*, 11th ed, Missouri, 2020, Elsevier, pp 1228–1253.

Question 2
Cognitive Skill: Analyze cues [cloze]

The nurse documents the following assessment findings:
- Blood pressure 118/78 mm Hg, heart rate 72 bpm
- Reports intense feelings of heat
- Temperature of 98.6°F, respirations 20 breaths per minute
- Reports nighttime sweating
- No history of abnormal Pap smears
- Reports no menstrual cycle in a year
- Reports vaginal dryness and painful intercourse
- Routine postmenopausal pregnancy test negative
- Patient is 5.0 ft in height and weighs 240 lb.

Choose the most likely options for the information missing from the statements below by selecting from the lists of options provided.

Based on the patient's assessment data, the provider determines that the patient's diagnosis _____(1)_____. The provider explains that possible hormonal irregularity can cause _____(2)_____, _____(2)_____, and _____(2)_____. Due to the patient's height and weight, which indicate a BMI of obesity, the provider instructs the patient to _____(3)_____ and _____(3)_____.

Option 1	Option 2	Option 3
Pregnancy	Vaginal dryness	Make sensible diet choices
Menopause	Increased libido	Incorporate a diet high in fat
Infertility	Decreased libido	Decrease fluid intake
Endometriosis	Feelings of cold hands and feet	Institute a walking program
Amenorrhea	Feelings of heat with nighttime sweating	Drink 3 carbonated sodas a day
Urinary tract infection	Hypotension and dizziness	Decrease daily activity

Answers
Based on the patient's assessment data, the provider determines that the patient's diagnosis is menopause. The provider explains that possible hormonal irregularity can cause vaginal dryness, decreased libido, and feelings of heat with nighttime sweating. Due to the patient's height and weight, which indicate a BMI of obesity, the provider instructs the patient to make sensible diet choices and institute a daily walking program.

Rationale
Menopause happens when the ovaries stop producing the hormone estrogen and no longer release an egg each month. Amenorrhea and infertility are symptoms of menopause. During menopause, pregnancy is rare. Endometriosis affects the menstrual cycle, and a small percentage of females do experience endometriosis in the postmenopausal phase, but not this patient. Urinary tract infections are a symptom of menopause; as vaginal tissue thins, females are more prone to infection. Due to the lack of estrogen, common symptoms are nighttime sweating, vaginal dryness, and decreased libido, which are caused by a surge in lutenizing hormone (LH) levels.

Increased libido and feelings of cold hands and feet are not associated with menopause. In menopause, a patient usually will not experience hypotension and dizziness. There is usually weight gain and a sensitivity to salt intake, which may cause hypertension. Due to the patient's height of 5.0 ft and weight of 240 lb., the patient has a BMI of 46.9. A BMI >30 suggests obesity, which is why the provider encourages sensible diet choices and instituting a walking program. A high-fat diet, decreased fluid intake, and decreased daily activity are not helpful advice for this overweight patient.

References
McCuistion L, et al. Women's reproductive health, menopause/perimenopause. In *Pharmacology: A patient-centered nursing process approach*, 11th ed, Missouri, 2023, Elsevier, pp 703–708.

Harding M, et al. Female reproductive problems. In *Lewis's medical surgical nursing*, 11th ed, Missouri, 2020, Elsevier, pp 1228–1253.

Question 3
Cognitive Skill: Prioritize hypotheses [extended multiple response]

Due to the patient's symptoms, the provider prescribes medications to help with the symptoms of menopause. Also, the provider plans to order additional testing for this patient.

Choose which medications and priority testing are *most important* for this patient. Select all that apply.

_____ a. Levothyroxine therapy
_____ b. Magnetic resonance imaging of chest (MRI)
_____ c. Oral estrogen 0.3 mg/day
_____ d. Oral progesterone 200 mg/day
_____ e. Combined hormonal contraceptive
_____ f. Mammogram testing
_____ g. DEXA bone density scan

Answers
_____ a. Levothyroxine therapy
_____ b. Magnetic resonance imaging of chest (MRI)
__X__ c. Oral estrogen 0.3 mg/day
__X__ d. Oral progesterone 200 mg/day
_____ e. Combined hormonal contraceptive
__X__ f. Mammogram testing
__X__ g. DEXA bone density scan

Rationale
Estrogen is used for the relief of symptoms related to menopause, most commonly hot flashes, vaginal dryness, and associated sleep disorders. Progesterone is used for the prevention of endometrial hyperplasia associated with estrogen replacement therapy in postmenopausal females who have an intact uterus. Progesterone 200 mg PO is given as a single dose in the evening

Continued

CLINICAL JUDGMENT UNFOLDING CASE STUDY—CONT'D

for 12 sequential days of every 28-day cycle of daily estrogen therapy. Females older than 50 years are at greatest risk for bone loss due to the loss of estrogen during menopause and should receive a DEXA scan/bone density test. Females older than 50 years should have a mammogram and a bone density test every 1–2 years. Levothyroxine therapy is used to treat hypothyroidism. Patient's workup and reports do not indicate the need for an MRI of the chest. The patient is in menopause and does not require combined hormonal contraceptive.

Reference
McCuistion L, et al. Women's reproductive health - osteoporosis. In *Pharmacology: A patient-centered nursing process approach*, 11th ed, Missouri, 2023, Elsevier, pp 703–708.

Harding M, et al. Female reproductive problems. In *Lewis's medical surgical nursing*, 11th ed, Missouri, 2020, Elsevier, pp 1228–1253.

Question 4
Cognitive Skill: Generate solutions [matrix]

The provider instructs the patient about hormonal therapy (HT).

Use an X for the health teachings listed below that are Indicated (appropriate or necessary) or Contraindicated (could be harmful) for the client's care at this time.

Health Teaching	Indicated	Contraindicated
Take HT after meals to avoid nausea and vomiting.		
You can stay on HT therapy forever.		
Decrease use of antihistamines if experiencing vaginal dryness.		
Must have medical follow-up every 6–12 months while on HT therapy.		
If you experience any vaginal bleeding, notify your provider.		
To help decrease hot flashes, use a fan, drink cool liquids, and decrease intake of caffeine and spicy foods.		

Answers

Health Teaching	Indicated	Contraindicated
Take HT after meals to avoid nausea and vomiting.	X	
You can stay on HT forever.		X
Decrease use of antihistamines if experiencing vaginal dryness.	X	
Must have medical follow-up every 6–12 months while on HT therapy.	X	
If you experience any vaginal bleeding, notify your provider.	X	
To help decrease hot flashes, use a fan, drink cool liquids, and decrease intake of caffeine and spicy foods.	X	

Rationale
The following are indications for a patient taking hormonal therapy: Since conjugated estrogen may cause nausea and vomiting, it is suggested to take HT after meals. The FDA has issued a boxed warning that HT should only be used in the treatment of menopausal symptoms, at the lowest dose possible, for the shortest duration possible. It is contraindicated for a patient to remain on HT, and it is recommended for use for less than a 5-year period of time. Patients must have follow-up appointments every 6–12 months, including blood pressure checks with their provider. The use of antihistamines can have a drying effect inside the body, especially during menopause. This can result in vaginal dryness. Vaginal bleeding can be a serious sign of inflammation caused by low estrogen levels. Notify the provider at the first sign of vaginal bleeding. Spicy foods and caffeine narrow blood vessels, which precipitates in a hot flash. A common remedy is to use a fan or drink a cool (nonalcoholic, caffeine-free) drink, which will cause the hot feeling to subside.

References
McCuistion L, et al. Women's reproductive health. In *Pharmacology: A patient-centered nursing process approach*, 11th ed, Missouri, 2023, Elsevier, pp 703–707.

Harding M, et al. Female reproductive problems. In *Lewis's medical surgical nursing*, 11th ed, Missouri, 2020, Elsevier, pp 1228–1253.

Question 5
Cognitive Skill: Take action [Extended drag and drop]

Due to the patient's symptoms, the provider prescribes medications to help with the symptoms of menopause. Also, the provider plans to order additional testing for this patient.

After a month, the patient returns to the health clinic to receive the results of her DEXA scan/bone density and mammogram. The provider tells the patient that the mammogram is clear from cancer but the bone density test indicates osteopenia.

Indicate which provider response listed in the far-left column is appropriate for each question. Note that all responses will be used.

Provider's Response	Patient Questions	Appropriate Provider's Response to Patient Questions
1. You must increase your calcium intake.	What do I need to do to increase my calcium intake?	
2. You must increase your daily intake of vitamin D.	Can you explain how much vitamin D I should take daily?	
3. Do you understand why you must take vitamin D?	Explain to me why vitamin D is necessary.	
4. It is important to incorporate walking and weight-bearing exercises into your exercise routine.	What is weight-bearing exercise?	
5. The provider states, "I will order a new medicine called alendronate 35 mg per day."	Can you tell me more about this medication?	
6. It prevents osteoporosis. You must take it with 8 oz of water 30 min before ingesting any food, liquid, or drugs. Also, you must remain upright for 30 min after taking this drug.		

CLINICAL JUDGMENT UNFOLDING CASE STUDY—CONT'D

Provider's Response	Patient Questions	Appropriate Provider's Response to Patient Questions
7. Walking, weight training, swimming, and yoga are weight-bearing and help to strengthen bones.		
8. Vitamin D helps with the absorption of calcium.		
9. The recommended intake of calcium for females older than 50 years of age is 1200 mg/day.		
10. The recommended daily allowance of vitamin D is 600 IU/day for females your age.		

Answers

Provider's Response	Patient Questions	Appropriate Provider's Response to Patient Questions
1. You must increase your calcium intake.	What do I need to do to increase my calcium intake?	9. The recommended intake of calcium for females older than 50 years of age is 1200 mg/day.
2. You must increase your daily intake of vitamin D.	Can you explain how much vitamin D I should take daily?	10. The recommended daily allowance of vitamin D is 600 IU/day for females your age.
3. Do you understand why you must take vitamin D?	Explain to me why vitamin D is necessary.	8. Vitamin D helps with the absorption of calcium.
4. It is important to incorporate walking and weight-bearing exercises into your exercise routine.	What is weight-bearing exercise?	7. Walking, weight training, swimming, and yoga are weight-bearing and help to strengthen bones.
5. The provider states, "I will order a new medicine called alendronate 35 mg per day."	Can you tell me more about this medication?	6. It prevents osteoporosis. You must take it with 8 oz of water 30 min before ingesting any food, liquid, or drugs. Also, you must remain upright for 30 min after taking this drug.

Rationale
Prevention and treatment of osteoporosis/osteopenia include sufficient intake of calcium and vitamin D. The recommended requirement of calcium for females 50 years or older is 1200 mg/d. The recommended daily allowance for vitamin D is 600 IU/d for females ages 19–70 years. Weight-bearing exercises include walking, jogging, low-impact aerobics, weight training, and yoga. These strengthen the bones, increase muscle strength, and enhance balance. Alendronate is a bisphosphonate used to treat osteopenia and osteoporosis. It must be taken with 8 oz of water 30 min before ingesting any food, liquids, or drugs, and the patient must remain upright for 30 min.

References
McCuistion L, et al. Women's reproductive health - osteoporosis. In *Pharmacology: A patient-centered nursing process approach*, 11th ed, Missouri, 2023, Elsevier, pp 703–708.

Harding M, et al. Female reproductive problems. In *Lewis's medical surgical nursing*, 11th ed, Missouri, 2020, Elsevier, pp 1228–1253.

Question 6
Cognitive Skill: Evaluate outcomes [matrix]

After a month, the patient returns to the health clinic to receive the results of her DEXA scan/bone density and mammogram. The provider tells the patient that the mammogram is clear from cancer, but the bone density test indicates osteopenia.

The provider assesses the patient for understanding and compliance. For each assessment finding, use an X to indicate whether teaching was effective (helped to meet expected outcomes) or ineffective (did not meet expected outcomes).

Assessment Findings	Effective	Ineffective
Patient reports feeling an increase in energy.		
Patient shows a 20-lb weight loss since initial visit.		
Patient indicates satisfactory libido.		
Patient reports still experiencing some vaginal dryness.		
Patient indicates improvements of hot flashes.		

Answers

Assessment Findings	Effective	Ineffective
Patient reports feeling an increase in energy.	X	
Patient shows a 20-lb weight loss since initial visit.	X	
Patient reports still experiencing some vaginal dryness.		X
Patient reports satisfactory libido.	X	
Patient indicates improvements of hot flashes.	X	

Rationale
HT significantly improves vasomotor symptoms including hot flashes, decreased libido, and vaginal dryness. The patient has achieved success except for vaginal dryness. The provider will order an over-the-counter topical to help with the vaginal dryness. Menopausal symptoms disrupt sleep, exacerbate irritability, and increase mood swings. The patient reports feeling more energy since these symptoms have improved and has added exercise to her daily routine, which has benefited her with a weight loss of 20 lb.

References
McCuistion L, et al. Women's reproductive problems, menopause. In *Pharmacology: A patient-centered nursing process approach*, 11th ed, Missouri, 2023, Elsevier, pp 703–709.

Harding M, et al. Female reproductive problems. In *Lewis's medical surgical nursing*, 11th ed, Missouri, 2020, Elsevier, pp 1242–1267.

REVIEW QUESTIONS

1. The nurse is preparing a teaching plan for combined hormonal contraceptive use. Which information should the nurse include in the teaching plan? **Select all that apply.**
   a. The patient should report abdominal pain, chest pain, headaches, blurred vision and visual disturbances, and severe leg pain.
   b. Combined hormonal contraceptives are safe for patients older than 35 years who smoke fewer than 20 cigarettes per day.
   c. Combined hormonal contraceptive use will not protect patients from sexually transmitted infections.
   d. The pills can be missed but not for more than 12 hours.
   e. Vaginal spotting after starting combined hormonal contraceptives is a sign that the method is not effective in preventing pregnancy.

2. A 54-year-old menopausal patient comes into the gynecology office and is interested in hormone therapy. Which are indications for prescribing hormone therapy? **Select all that apply.**
   a. Assists in relief of hot flashes
   b. Prevention of breast cancer
   c. Prevention of cardiovascular disease
   d. Prevention of osteoporosis in at-risk patients
   e. Assists in relief of vaginal dryness

3. A 24-year-old patient tells the nurse that she would like to use the progestin-only pill for contraception. Nursing evaluation of this patient as a candidate for the progestin-only pill includes what?
   a. Ask the patient if she has given birth in the past.
   b. Assess whether or not the patient has regular periods.
   c. Assess the patient's reliability in taking an oral pill daily.
   d. Interview the patient about past smoking habits.

4. A 39-year-old patient who smokes one pack of cigarettes (20) per day asks about a contraception method that is best for her. She is normotensive (has a normal blood pressure reading) and has used combined hormonal contraceptives in the past. She is in a monogamous relationship and has had two children with no complications during pregnancy. She is not planning any more pregnancies. The nurse determines that which method would be best for this patient?
   a. Combined hormonal contraceptives
   b. A levonorgestrel-intrauterine system
   c. Contraceptive that contains progestin only
   d. Levonorgestrel (systemic) progestin

5. The nurse is instructing a patient on the use of depot medroxyprogesterone acetate. Which statements are correct? **Select all that apply.**
   a. Patients usually do not have any changes in their periods.
   b. Patients should increase their intake of calcium.
   c. Patients can expect some irregular bleeding at first.
   d. Patients may use this contraceptive when breast-feeding.
   e. Patients will experience a decrease with postpartum depression.

6. The nurse is counseling a 62-year-old patient with a T score of −2.0 after her DXA (Bone Density) Scan. What is the best advice for this patient?
   a. The patient should take a daily calcium supplement, 1500 mg orally in the morning.
   b. The patient's exercise program will include weight-bearing exercises like swimming and cycling.
   c. The patient most likely will be prescribed estrogen by the health care provider.
   d. The patient should supplement her diet with 1200 mg of calcium with vitamin D 600 IU orally once daily.

7. A 48-year-old patient arrives at the clinic to discuss her perimenopausal symptoms. She states that her last menstrual period was 8 months ago, and before that, her periods had been irregular. What is the most important nursing advice to give this patient?
   a. Hormone therapy is only used for hot flashes and vaginal dryness.
   b. The patient should be using some form of contraception to avoid pregnancy.
   c. The patient should have a DXA (bone density) scan to test for osteopenia.
   d. At this time, herbal supplementation is probably best to relieve her perimenopausal symptoms.

8. A patient has been prescribed clomiphene citrate therapy by her doctor. The patient asks the nurse, "How does my new medicine work?" What can the nurse say to convey the mechanism of action of clomiphene citrate therapy to this patient? **Select all that apply.**
   a. This drug stimulates the ovaries, increasing the chance of ovulation.
   b. This drug is a selective estrogen receptor modulator (SERM).
   c. This drug usually does not work on the first cycle.
   d. This drug completes for estrogen receptors within the hypothalamus. This drug is safe to use in females who are pregnant.

56

Male Reproductive Health

Jared Robertson III, MN, CRNA

http://evolve.elsevier.com/McCuistion/pharmacology

OBJECTIVES

- Differentiate the three male reproductive processes.
- Give examples of the major male reproductive disorders.
- Discuss drugs utilized in male reproductive disorders.
- Explain the treatment of male reproductive disorders.

OUTLINE

Male Reproductive Processes, 739
    Male Reproductive Anatomy and Physiology, 739
    Hormonal Regulation of Male Reproductive Functioning and Spermatogenesis, 739
    Sexual Function, 740
Disorders of the Male Reproductive System, 740
    Hypogonadism, 740
    Delayed Adolescent Puberty, 741
Drugs Related to Male Reproductive Disorders, 741
    Androgens, 741

    Anabolic Steroids, 744
    Antiandrogens, 744
Other Male Reproductive Disorders, 746
    Pituitary, Thyroid, and Adrenal Disorders, 746
    Sexual Dysfunction, 746
    Non-Sexually Transmitted Infections, 748
    Benign Prostatic Hyperplasia, 748
    Malignant Tumors, 749
Clinical Judgment Case Study, 749
Review Questions, 749

Reproductive health requires the production of adequate quantities of various hypothalamic, pituitary, and gonadal hormones as well as the appropriate hormone receptors. It requires normal development and patency of the reproductive tract. In addition, reproductive health implies that males and females at developmentally appropriate life stages are fertile (i.e., able to produce gametes [sperm or eggs]). Finally, reproductive health entails the ability to engage in sexual intercourse with ejaculation by the male.

Alterations in male reproductive health reflect a wide range of developmental, endocrine, infectious, inflammatory, hypertrophic, malignant, and psychoemotional processes. Reproductive health is affected by anatomy and physiology, sperm production, regulation of male sexual functioning, and sexual intercourse.

The drug family most clearly associated with male reproductive processes is the androgens. Because synthetic anabolic steroids and antiandrogens affect male reproduction, they are also discussed.

MALE REPRODUCTIVE PROCESSES

There are three male reproductive processes including spermatogenesis (sperm production), regulation of male sexual functioning, and sexual intercourse.

Male Reproductive Anatomy and Physiology

The anatomy of the male sexual organs is depicted in Fig. 56.1. The external male reproductive organs include the penis, the scrotum, and the testes. The penis consists of three cylindrical bodies of erectile tissue: two corpora cavernosa and the corpus spongiosum. With sexual excitement, the vascular spaces fill with blood to produce an erection (Fig. 56.2).

The scrotum has two compartments, each of which holds a testis, epididymis, and spermatic cord. The spermatic cord supports the testis and includes the vas deferens, blood vessels, nerves, and muscle fibers.

Each testis contains seminiferous tubules in which spermatogenesis occurs. The sperm then moves into the epididymis. This leads into the vas deferens, the source of about 20% of ejaculate, or semen. On either side of the prostate gland, a seminal vesicle empties seminal fluid into the ampulla. Seminal fluid contains fructose to provide energy for the sperm, prostaglandins, fibrinogen, and a sperm-activating factor.

The contents of the ampulla and the seminal vesicles empty into an ejaculatory duct that leads through the body of the prostate to empty into the urethra. Prostatic fluid, which constitutes about 20% of semen, empties from the prostate gland into the ejaculatory duct. The urethra carries semen to its distal end. The urethral glands along the length of the urethra and the bulbourethral glands near the prostatic end of the urethra supply the urethra with mucus. The bulbourethral glands secrete alkaline preejaculatory fluid to protect sperm from the acidity of the urethra.

Hormonal Regulation of Male Reproductive Functioning and Spermatogenesis

GnRH from the hypothalamus stimulates the anterior pituitary gland to secrete two major gonadotropins, luteinizing hormone (LH), and follicle-stimulating hormone (FSH), in both males and females (Fig. 56.3). LH stimulates the interstitial Leydig cells of the testes to mature and produce testosterone. There is a direct relationship between the

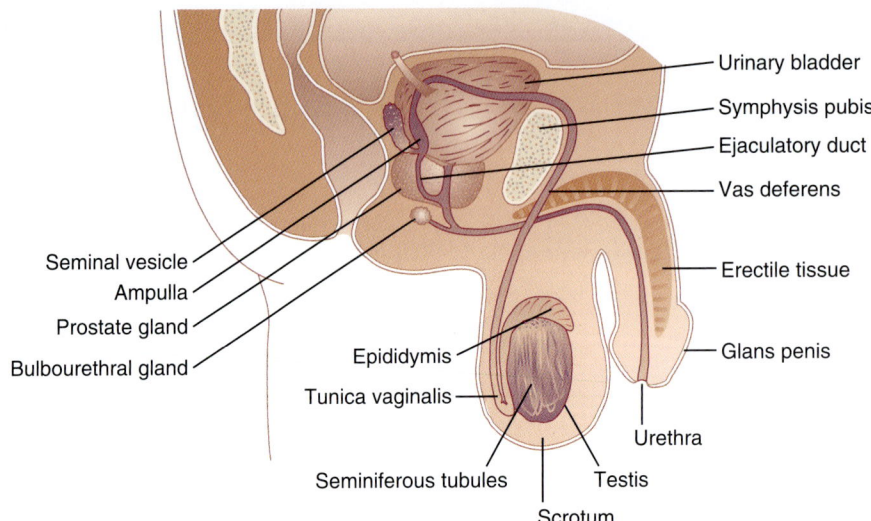

Fig. 56.1 Anatomy of the male reproductive system.

Fig. 56.2 Erectile tissue of the penis.

amount of circulating LH and the amount of testosterone produced. Testosterone is also produced to a lesser extent in the adrenal cortex and in the ovaries of females.

In males, FSH stimulates the Sertoli cells to begin conversion of spermatids into mature sperm. In addition, the Sertoli cells are stimulated to secrete estrogens, which may promote spermatogenesis. For spermatogenesis to be complete, testosterone must be secreted simultaneously by the Leydig cells and diffused into the seminiferous tubules.

Testosterone is the precursor of two classes of sex steroids: 5-alpha-reduced androgens and estrogens. The net effect of endogenous androgens is the sum of the effects of the 5-alpha-reduced metabolite dihydrotestosterone and its estrogen derivative, estradiol. Most testosterone is loosely bound by plasma protein and circulates for 15 to 30 minutes before it is fixed to target tissues or metabolized. Most testosterone fixed to target cells is then converted to its active form, dihydrotestosterone.

The rate of testosterone production is controlled by a negative feedback loop. With increased testosterone, the hypothalamus decreases production of GnRH. With sperm production, the Sertoli cells release a hormone called *inhibin*, which suppresses FSH production by the anterior pituitary gland, maintaining a constant rate of spermatogenesis. It is not known how, before puberty, the brain stimulates the hypothalamus to begin GnRH secretion, but if the brain is not intact, this may not occur.

Sexual Function

The human sexual response cycle consists of five phases: desire, excitement, plateau, orgasm, and resolution. Sexual desire is the stimulus that causes an individual to initiate or be receptive to sexual activity. During the excitement phase, the male experiences penile erection. Males are unable to engage in sexual intercourse without this arousal. The plateau phase is characterized by genital enlargement, mucous secretion, generalized muscle tension, hyperventilation, tachycardia, and increased blood pressure. During the orgasmic phase, the vas deferens, seminal vesicles, ejaculatory duct, and penile urethra contract three or four times over a few seconds, which causes the male to ejaculate. During resolution, there is a refractory period in which pelvic vasocongestion declines and generalized muscle relaxation takes place.

DISORDERS OF THE MALE REPRODUCTIVE SYSTEM

The major male reproductive disorders include testicular cancer, testicular torsion, penile cancer, hypogonadism, and delayed adolescent puberty. Of these disorders, hypogonadism and delayed adolescent puberty can be effectively treated pharmacologically.

Hypogonadism

The clearest indication for exogenous androgen therapy is hypogonadism. Male hypogonadism is an impairment of the reproductive system that results in failure of the testes to produce testosterone, sperm, or both. Deficiency of sex hormones can result in defective primary or secondary sexual development, and defective sperm development can result in infertility. Hypogonadism is either primary, reflecting testicular abnormality, or secondary, reflecting hypothalamic or pituitary failure. A combination of disorders can also occur. Inadequate pituitary function will severely affect young males and results in infertility and a lack of secondary sex characteristics. Adult males may experience testicular atrophy, impotence, decreased libido, decreased bone density, loss of muscle mass, hair loss, gynecomastia, fatigue, difficulty concentrating, or vasomotor flushing.

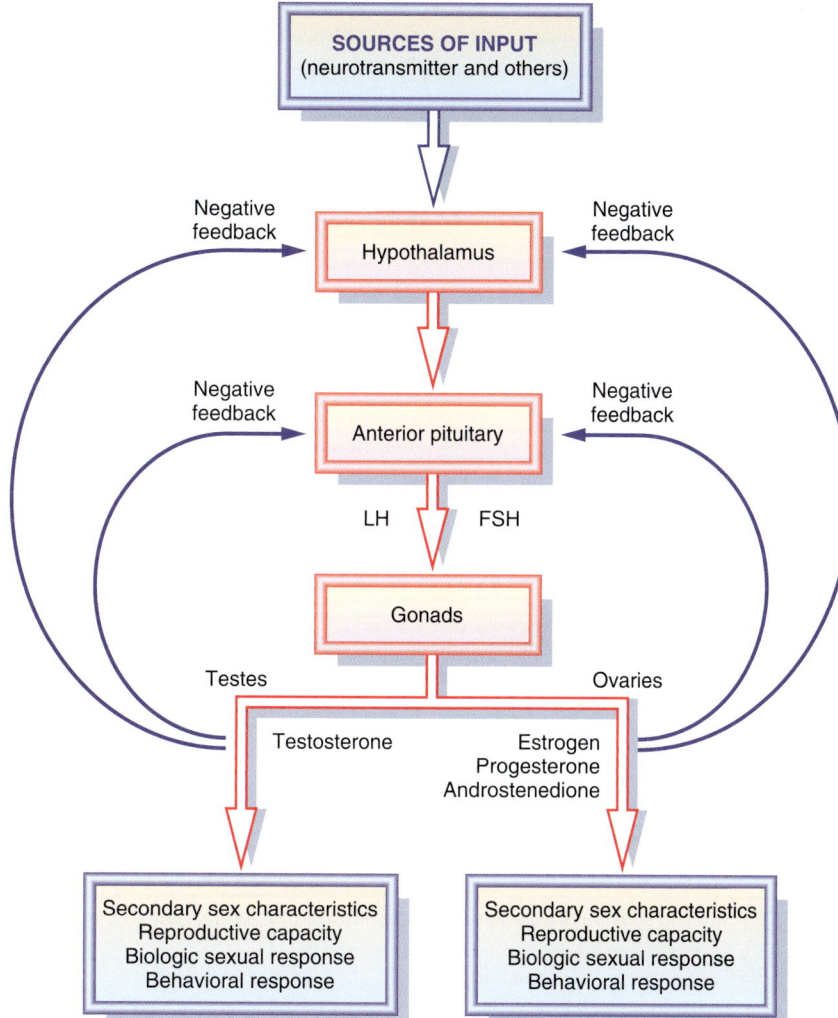

Fig. 56.3 Hypothalamic-pituitary-gonadal feedback loops.

Delayed Adolescent Puberty

Puberty is considered to be delayed when testicle enlargement, followed by penile growth and pubic hair development, has not begun by 14 years of age. Delay in growth may be a normal part of the maturation process, but the cause could also be androgen deficiency or a deficiency of growth hormone. Secretion of GnRH, LH, or FSH is insufficient in up to 5% of cases of delayed puberty. Treatment is only begun after 14 years of age, after a full evaluation, including serum LH, FSH, thyroid-stimulating hormone (TSH), and testosterone levels. Therapy with testosterone cypionate 50 mg IM every month, for 3 to 6 months or less before epiphyseal closure, may result in linear growth without adverse permanent effects on hypothalamic, pituitary, or gonadal maturation.

DRUGS RELATED TO MALE REPRODUCTIVE DISORDERS

The major drugs related to male reproductive disorders include androgens, anabolic steroids, and antiandrogens. Testosterone is the major sex hormone in males. Anabolic steroids are synthetic forms of testosterone. Antiandrogens block the action of androgens.

Androgens

Androgens, or male sex hormones, control the development and maintenance of sexual processes, accessory sexual organs, cellular metabolism, and bone and muscle growth. Testosterone, an anabolic steroid, is the principal male sex hormone. It is the prototype of the androgen hormones, synthesized primarily in the testes and, to a lesser extent, in the adrenal cortex. In females, the ovaries synthesize small amounts of testosterone. In adult males, normal plasma concentrations of testosterone are 270 to 1070 ng/dL, with a slow decline of 1% per year after 30 years of age (Table 56.1). The Prototype Drug Chart: Testosterone Cypionate discusses the dosage, uses, and considerations for this formulation of the drug. Table 56.2 presents additional formulations of testosterone available for use.

Pharmacokinetics

Testosterone secretion is greater in males than in females in most stages of life. About 98% of circulating testosterone is bound to both sex hormone-binding globulin (SHBG) and albumin protein, leaving about 2% unbound, or circulating free in the plasma; this unbound portion is biologically active. Estrogen elevates the production of SHBG, resulting in more protein-bound testosterone in females than in males. The

PROTOTYPE DRUG CHART

Testosterone Cypionate

Drug Class	Dosage
Androgen CSS III	Male primary hypogonadism and hypogonadotropic hypogonadism: IM: 50–400 mg q2–4wk

Contraindications	Drug-Food Interactions
Hypersensitivity to drug or drug components, cottonseed oil, pregnancy, breast-feeding, male breast cancer, and prostate cancer *Caution:* Prostate cancer risk, benign prostatic hyperplasia, older adults, renal and/or hepatic impairment, risk of hypercalcemia, cardiovascular disease, heart failure, hyperlipidemia, diabetes, pulmonary disease, obesity, sleep apnea, polycythemia, and male patients trying to conceive	Drug: May decrease serum glucose, requiring insulin adjustment, Herbal: St. John's wort may decrease concentration/effects, Food: None known, Lab: May increase Hgb, Hct, LDL, serum alkaline phosphatase, bilirubin, calcium, potassium, sodium, AST. May decrease HDL

Pharmacokinetics	Pharmacodynamics
Absorption: IM: Well absorbed Distribution: PB: 98% Metabolism: Liver; t½: 8 days Excretion: Urine 90%, feces 6%	IM: Onset: UK Peak: UK Duration: Cypionate/enanthate: 2–4 wk

Therapeutic Effects/Uses

Androgen replacement therapy in treatment of delayed male puberty, male hypogonadism (congenital or acquired)
Mechanism of Action: Binds to androgen receptors, producing multiple anabolic and androgenic effects.

Side Effects	Adverse Reactions
Abdominal pain, nausea, diarrhea, constipation, hives, irritation at injection site, increased salivation, mouth soreness, increased or decreased libido, insomnia, aggressive behavior, weakness, dizziness, pruritus, acne, masculinization, irregular menses, urinary urgency, gynecomastia, priapism, red skin, jaundice, sodium and water retention, allergic reaction, depression, habituation	*Life-threatening:* Hepatic necrosis, hepatitis, hepatic tumors, respiratory distress

AST, aspartate aminotransferase; *CSS,* controlled substance schedule; *IM,* intramuscular; *PB,* protein binding; *t½,* half-life; *wk,* week; *UK,* unknown.

TABLE 56.1 Testosterone Levels by Age

Age	T Level (ng/dL)
0–5 mo	75–400
6 mo–9 y	<7–20
10–11 y	<7–130
12–13 y	<7–800
14 y	<7–1200
15–16 y	100–1200
17–18 y	300–1200
19+ y	240–950
Avg. adult male	270–1070
30+ y	−1% per year

From Mayo Clinic Laboratories. (n.d.). Test ID: TTFB. https://www.mayocliniclabs.com/test-catalog/Clinical+and+Interpretive/83686.

can be combined with esters to form esterified testosterone in an oil base for intramuscular (IM) injection.

Ninety percent of testosterone is excreted in the urine as glucuronic and sulfuric acid conjugates and its metabolites. About 6% of the hormone is excreted unconjugated in the feces. Synthetic androgens may be excreted as unaltered hormone or as metabolites. In some tissues the action of testosterone depends on its reduction to 5-alpha-dihydrotestosterone (DHT), whereas in other tissues testosterone itself is the active hormone. In the central nervous system, the metabolite estradiol affects hormonal action.

Pharmacodynamics

Testosterone is responsible for the development of male sex characteristics. The biologic effects of testosterone may be mediated directly by testosterone or by its metabolites. Testosterone and dihydrotestosterone act as androgens by way of a single androgen receptor officially designated NR3A. The hormones bind to sites on certain responsive genes, causing a change to take place in the target cell. The effects of the testosterone depend on which receptor it activates and the tissues in which these effects occur. The manufacture of protein within the target cells results in the buildup of cellular tissue (anabolism), especially in muscles. This leads to the development of secondary sex characteristics such as pubic hair growth, beard and body hair growth, baldness, deepening of the male voice, thickening of the skin, sebaceous gland activity, increased musculature, bone development, and red blood cell formation.

half-life of endogenous, or naturally occurring, free testosterone in the blood is 10 to 20 minutes.

Because as much as 50% of testosterone is metabolized on its first pass through the hepatic circulation when taken orally, oral testosterone is not available for prescription in the United States. Testosterone

TABLE 56.2 Androgens (Controlled Substance, Schedule III)

Drug	Route and Dosage	Uses and Considerations
Natural Androgens		
Testosterone		
Testosterone nasal	Nasal: 5.5 mg per gel pump actuation; 1 pump actuation in each nostril 3 times/d	For primary male hypogonadism and male hypogonadotropic hypogonadism.
Transdermal testosterone patch	Transdermal patch: 2 mg/24 h or 4 mg/24 h patch; apply to nongenital skin; avoid bony areas	Drug is started at the full dose and adjusted according to tolerance and therapeutic response.
Testosterone topical gel	1% Gel: 50–100 mg once daily 2% Gel: 40–70 mg once daily	Less skin irritation occurs with the gel than with the patch. PB: 98%; t½: 10–100 min
Testosterone pellet	Subcut implantable 75-mg pellets: implant two 75-mg pellets for each 25 mg testosterone propionate required weekly. Replace every 4–6 mo	For replacement therapy in conditions associated with a deficiency or absence of endogenous testosterone. PB: 98%; t½: 10–100 min
Testosterone cypionate	IM: 50–400 mg q2–4wk	For androgen replacement and delayed puberty; therapy generally lasts 3–4 y. PB: 98%; t½: 8 d
Synthetic Androgens		
Fluoxymesterone (no longer available in the United States)	PO: 5 mg 1–4 times/d	For androgen deficiency and palliative treatment of carcinoma of the breast. PB: 98%; t½: 29.2 h
Methyltestosterone	PO: 10–50 mg/d in divided doses initially; reduced for maintenance	For androgen deficiency and palliative treatment of carcinoma of the breast. PB: UK; t½: 2.5–3.5 h

d, Day; *h*, hour; *IM*, intramuscular; *min*, minute; *mo*, month; *PB*, protein binding; *PO*, by mouth; *q*, every; *subcut*, subcutaneous; *t½*, half-life; *UK*, unknown; *wk*, week; *y*, year.

Fetal testes begin to produce testosterone during the first 3 months in utero. After birth until just before puberty, production is negligible. During puberty, production increases rapidly and continues until later adulthood. As males age, the number of Leydig cells decreases, sperm production declines, and LH and FSH levels rise. Levels of unbound testosterone are reduced in older males to one-third to one-fifth the peak value. If males experience osteoporosis and anemia, and if their testosterone levels are 300 ng/dL or less, testosterone replacement therapy should be considered.

Indications for Androgen Therapy

Table 56.2 lists the natural and synthetic androgens with their dosages, uses, and considerations. Androgen therapy is approved for use in androgen deficiency in males, specifically hypogonadism; replacement therapy for testicular failure in adult males; and delayed puberty in adolescents.

The timing and extent of treatment depend on the clinical manifestations. Because accelerated bone maturation can lead to premature closure of bone epiphyses and short stature, androgen therapy should be used cautiously in children and only by specialists aware of the adverse effects on bone maturation. Skeletal maturation must be monitored every 6 months by radiography of the hand and wrist. Artificial induction of puberty is undertaken only after males reach 15 to 17 years of age and after hypothalamic and pituitary function has been assessed. A 4- to 6-month trial of androgen therapy is implemented, followed by a similar period of rest for reevaluation. If prolonged therapy is required, testosterone cypionate is used, 50 to 400 mg IM every 2 to 4 weeks. It should be given deep in the IM. Inspect vials visually for particulate matter and discoloration before administration, and warm and shake the vial to dissolve any crystals that may have formed during storage. It takes 3 or 4 years for sexual development to occur; plasma testosterone levels should be monitored and dosages adjusted as needed to maintain normal levels. If the serum testosterone level is below the normal range, the provider will adjust the dose upward. Therapy may be lifelong.

Administration

Testosterone may be administered nasally, transdermally, or parenterally. Drug selection depends on the balance of growth and sexual maturation desired and on the preferred route of administration. Testosterones are considered Schedule III controlled substances.

Transdermal testosterone (TT) patches achieve adequate serum concentrations when applied to the arm, back, or upper buttocks. TT patches can be applied to any healthy skin site other than the scrotum or bony areas. Daily application of one to two TT 2 mg/24 h or 4 mg/24 h skin patches at 10 p.m. results in serum testosterone concentrations approaching those of healthy young male. The first day of dosing results in morning serum testosterone concentrations within the normal range. There is no testosterone accumulation with continued use. After removal of TT patches, hypogonadal status returns within 24 hours. Keep testosterone gel out of reach of children.

Testosterone gel is applied to clean dry skin of shoulders or upper arms. It should not be applied to the genitals. Hands should be thoroughly washed with soap and water after application. Testosterone gel carries a boxed warning because it can be transferred to others through personal contact with skin or clothing. Children should avoid contact with unwashed application sites or application sites not covered by clothing. Children can experience virilization from secondary exposure. Caution is advised.

Side Effects

Hypogonadal males on androgen therapy may experience frequent erections or priapism (painful, continuous erection), gynecomastia (mammary gland enlargement in males), or urinary urgency.

Continued use of androgens by normal males can halt spermatogenesis (formation of spermatozoa). The sperm count may be low (oligospermia) for 3 or more months after therapy is stopped.

Other side effects of androgen therapy include abdominal pain, nausea, insomnia, diarrhea or constipation, hives or redness at the injection site, increased salivation, mouth soreness, and increased or decreased sexual desire. Advise the patient to notify the health care provider if side effects persist, worsen, or are bothersome.

Adverse Reactions

Androgen therapy may cause hypercalcemia by stimulating bone resorption in patients who are immobilized and those with breast cancer. The drug should be discontinued, and appropriate measures instituted if signs of hypercalcemia occur; signs include nausea and vomiting, lethargy, decreased muscle tone, polyuria, and increased urine and serum calcium.

Virilization refers to the development of male secondary sex characteristics in females or hypogonadal males. Such characteristics include growth of facial hair, acne and skin oiliness, and vocal huskiness. Menstrual irregularities or amenorrhea, suppressed ovulation or lactation, baldness or increased hair growth (hirsutism), and hypertrophy of the clitoris may develop in females undergoing androgen therapy. Although most adverse effects slowly reverse themselves after short-term therapy is completed, vocal changes may be permanent. With long-term therapy, as in the treatment of breast cancer, adverse effects may be irreversible.

Children may experience profound virilization as well as impaired bone growth. During pregnancy, androgens can cross the placenta and cause masculinization of the fetus. Virilization can occur in those secondarily exposed to testosterone gel and may cause teratogenic effects in fetuses. Females and children should not handle the gel and should avoid contact with application sites in males using testosterone gel.

Less frequent adverse effects include dizziness, weakness, changes in skin color, frequent headaches, confusion, respiratory distress, depression, pruritus, allergic skin rash, edema of the lower extremities, jaundice, bleeding, paresthesias, chills, polycythemia, muscle cramps, and sodium and water retention. Hepatocellular carcinoma can occur in patients who have received selected androgens for long-term therapy and in cases of abuse of androgenic hormones by athletes.

Serum cholesterol may become elevated during androgen therapy. Other alterations in laboratory tests include increased hematocrit, altered thyroid and liver function tests, and elevated urine 17-ketosteroids (a byproduct of the breakdown of androgens). Rare complications of long-term therapy include hepatic necrosis, hepatic peliosis (blood-filled cysts), hepatic tumors, and leukopenia.

Contraindications

Androgen therapy is contraindicated during pregnancy and in individuals with nephrosis or those in the nephrotic phase of nephritis; it is also contraindicated in patients with hypercalcemia, pituitary insufficiency, hepatic dysfunction, benign prostatic hyperplasia (BPH), prostate cancer, or history of myocardial infarction. Males with breast cancer are not treated with androgens, nor are females whose breast cancer is not estrogen dependent.

Caution must be exercised when using androgen therapy in individuals with hypertension, hypercholesterolemia, coronary artery disease, renal disease, or seizure disorder. It is used with caution in infants and prepubertal children because of the potential for growth disturbances and in older males because of their increased risk for BPH and prostate cancer.

Drug Interactions

Androgens potentiate the effects of oral anticoagulants, necessitating a decrease in anticoagulant dosage. Androgens antagonize calcitonin and parathyroid hormones. Because androgens can decrease blood glucose in patients with diabetes, dosages of insulin or other antidiabetic agents may need to be reduced. Concurrent use of corticosteroids exacerbates the edema that can occur with androgen therapy. Barbiturates, phenytoin, and phenylbutazone decrease the effects of androgens.

Anabolic Steroids

Anabolic steroids, or anabolic-androgenic steroids (AASs), are a class of steroid hormones related to the hormone testosterone. They increase protein synthesis within cells, which results in the buildup of cellular tissue (anabolism), especially in muscles. Anabolic steroids also have androgenic and virilizing properties, including the development and maintenance of masculine characteristics such as the growth of the vocal cords and body hair. Although the American College of Sports Medicine notes that AASs, combined with sufficient diet and exercise, can contribute to increased lean body mass in some individuals, they also note it is in the best interest of all sports to eradicate the use of AASs by athletes due to the risk of serious harm or death in those who use AASs. ⚡ See Chapter 8 for further information.

Testosterone precursors, which were sold as nutritional supplements, include androstenediol and androstenedione; however, they are no longer available in the United States without a prescription. Dehydroepiandrosterone (DHEA), an over-the-counter supplement, is an endogenous hormone secreted by the adrenal cortex, gonads, adipose tissue, brain, and skin. It is thought to be important in several endocrine processes, including synthesis of other hormones. DHEA is converted via hydrosteroid dehydrogenases and aromatase into androstenedione, testosterone, and estradiol by peripheral tissues. Older teens are the heaviest users of nutritional supplements, whereas there is a growing number of junior high school students using these supplements. A sudden dramatic increase in weight and body size, increased acne, and changes in mood and behavior can be signs of exogenous anabolic steroid use. Individuals using anabolic steroids may become more aggressive and physical, and health risks can result from long-term use or excessive intake of anabolic steroids; these effects include increased low-density lipoprotein (bad) cholesterol and decreased high-density lipoprotein (good) cholesterol, acne, high blood pressure, liver damage, and dangerous changes in the structure of the left ventricle of the heart. Adverse effects may not be recognized until years later. ⚡ See Chapter 8 for further information.

Two other steroids that have gained popularity, especially with athletes, are human chorionic gonadotropin (hCG) and tetrahydrogestrinone (THG). hCG is a hormone used to treat infertility and stimulate testosterone production, whereas THG is a potent androgenic steroid developed to escape detection on urine drug screens, although tests have since been developed for rapid screening. It is not approved by the US Food and Drug Administration (FDA) and is not legally marketed. All major athletic organizations prohibit the use of anabolic steroids, but their continued use despite bans has led to "antidoping" investigations and punitive action.

Antiandrogens

Antiandrogens, or androgen antagonists, block the synthesis or action of androgens (Table 56.3). These drugs are used in the treatment of BPH and advanced prostatic cancer and as hormonal therapy in the treatment of endometriosis. They may also be used to treat male-pattern

TABLE 56.3 Antiandrogens

Mechanism	Drugs
Inhibits gonadotropin release, suppressing levels of testosterone	Goserelin acetate Leuprolide acetate
Inhibits testosterone synthesis	Ketoconazole[a]
Blocks conversion of testosterone to dihydrotestosterone	Finasteride
Androgen receptor inhibitors	Flutamide Bicalutamide

[a]Off-label use for castration-resistant prostate cancer.

baldness (MPB), acne, hirsutism, virilization syndrome in females, and precocious puberty in young males, although their effectiveness is not well established.

Gonadotropin-releasing hormone (GnRH), or a synthetic analogue such as leuprolide, is the most effective inhibitor of testosterone synthesis. When such agents are given over time, LH and testosterone levels fall. Normally, GnRH is released in a pulsatile fashion, but the sustained activity of leuprolide leads to decreased production of FSH and LH. In the male, this activity stops testosterone production in the testes. In the female, it stops estrogen production in the ovaries. This drug should not be used in combination with herbal or dietary supplements such as black cohosh, chasteberry, or DHEA.

CLINICAL JUDGMENT [NURSING PROCESS]
Androgens

Concept: Hormonal Regulation
- Physiologic mechanisms that regulate the secretion and action of hormones associated with the endocrine system

Recognize Cues [Assessment]
- Assess the reason for androgen therapy and the patient's perception of it. If delayed puberty is the indication, assess patient and family attitudes about the condition.
- Monitor weight, blood pressure, liver and thyroid function, hemoglobin and hematocrit, creatinine, clotting factors, glucose tolerance, serum lipids and electrolytes, and blood count before and throughout treatment. Note the presence of liver or endocrine dysfunction and any elevation in blood pressure.
- Note concomitant anticoagulant therapy.
- When a prepubertal child is treated, obtain hand and wrist radiographs before, every 6 months during, and after treatment to monitor growth.
- Appraise the patient's expressive affect during therapy, particularly aggressiveness in patients taking large doses. Self-concept is an important consideration in the patient on androgen therapy, particularly in children with delayed puberty and in females.

Analyze Cues and Prioritize Hypothesis [Patient Problems]
- Sexual expression
- Self-concept
- Weight gain
- Decreased self-esteem

Generate Solutions [Planning]
- Through collaboration, the patient agrees to (1) adhere to the prescribed regimen for taking the drug and for monitoring, (2) use the drug appropriately, (3) report adverse effects immediately, and (4) maintain a positive self-concept during long-term treatment.

Take Action [Nursing Interventions]
- Collaborate with the patient and family on proper administration of drugs, their reasons for use, and potential undesired effects. Review which effects warrant prompt medical attention (e.g., urinary problems, priapism, respiratory distress).
- Advise patients that an intermittent approach to treatment allows for monitoring of endocrine status between courses of androgen therapy. Explain the need to return to the health care facility for monitoring, and confirm the patient's ability to do so. Arrange social service referrals if necessary.
- Counsel the family pursuing treatment for a child with delayed puberty about the range of normal development.
- Encourage patients to monitor muscle strength during treatment.
- Instruct patients to administer androgens as directed.
- Coach patients about good skin hygiene to decrease the severity of acne.
- Urge males undergoing androgen therapy to report priapism promptly so the drug dosage can be reduced to avoid subsequent erectile dysfunction (ED).
- Instruct males to report decreased urinary stream promptly so they can be evaluated for prostatic hypertrophy.
- Assess and review the nutritional intake to ensure adequate intake of essential nutrients.
- Counsel patients to record body weight several times per week. Restrict sodium if edema develops.
- Advise patients with elevated serum calcium of the need to drink 2 L per day or more of fluid to prevent kidney stones. Individuals on bed rest need range-of-motion exercises, whereas ambulatory patients need to engage in active weight-bearing. Hypercalcemia requires prompt medical attention because it can lead to cardiac arrest.

Evaluate Outcomes [Evaluation]
- Monitor the patient's ability to adhere to a treatment regimen and response to prescribed drugs. The ability to adhere to a treatment plan and discuss treatment and effects knowledgeably suggests that teaching has been effective and that the patient accepts the treatment.
- Ask the patient about therapeutic and adverse drug effects on follow-up visits. Monitoring of weight, blood pressure, and laboratory tests will continue throughout therapy with alterations in the plan of care as needed.
- Periodically assess children and females who experience virilizing effects or acne for the ability to cope with these changes and to maintain a positive self-concept.
- Assess sexual function when appropriate.

Ketoconazole, an antifungal drug, has testosterone-suppressing effects similar to those of GnRH analogues when given at doses higher than those required for antifungal activity (400 mg orally every 8 hours as opposed to 200 to 400 mg daily for the treatment of fungal infections). The mechanism of action of this non-GnRH drug is unclear. GnRH analogues act directly through their effect on testosterone production for the treatment of prostate cancer. Ketoconazole as treatment of prostate cancer is an off-label use.

Flutamide is an oral nonsteroidal antiandrogen drug used as an antihormonal agent in the treatment of metastatic prostate cancer. It is most effective when used simultaneously with luteinizing hormone-releasing hormone (LHRH) analogues such as leuprolide acetate. When used alone, the best response is seen in untreated patients. Flutamide is not effective in treating other hormonally dependent diseases such as breast cancer or BPH. Flutamide competes with androgens at androgen receptor sites in the prostate gland, blocking the conversion of testosterone to dihydrotestosterone; by doing so, it prevents the androgens from stimulating the prostate cancer cells to grow. Males receiving flutamide show elevations in plasma LH and testosterone levels. Bicalutamide is structurally related to flutamide but has a long plasma half-life that allows once-daily dosing, compared with thrice-daily dosing for flutamide. In addition, bicalutamide is more selective for the peripheral androgen receptor and has less activity at the central androgen receptor on the hypothalamic-pituitary axis.

Finasteride, a synthetic compound, inhibits conversion of testosterone to DHT. This orally active agent decreases the concentration of dihydrotestosterone in plasma and the prostate without elevated plasma concentrations of LH or testosterone. Finasteride is used to treat BPH and MPB. The recommended 5-mg daily dose of finasteride for BPH needs to be reevaluated at 6 months and periodically thereafter. The 1-mg dose of finasteride for MPB is taken once a day for 12 months, and continued treatment is recommended for sustained results. After discontinuation of therapy, reversal of effect is typically seen within 1 year. Adverse reactions include impotence, decreased libido, and decreased ejaculate. Females of childbearing age must not use finasteride and should not handle crushed or broken tablets because the active ingredient may cause abnormalities of a male fetus's sex organs.

OTHER MALE REPRODUCTIVE DISORDERS

Pituitary, Thyroid, and Adrenal Disorders

Inadequate pituitary function can be another cause of hypogonadism. Menotropins are purified combination preparations of the human pituitary gonadotropins FSH and LH. These drugs are indicated when both LH and FSH levels are low. When given in combination with hCG, the drug stimulates testosterone production in males to encourage spermatogenesis when injected three times a week for 4 to 9 months to ensure adequate spermatozoa production. One ampule of a menotropin contains 75 international units each of LH and FSH. The initial dose is 75 to 150 international units subcutaneously (subcut) or 3 times per week. Subsequent doses are adjusted according to individual response but not exceeding 75 to 150 international units per adjustment; the maximum dose is 300 units 3 times per week. Use the lower abdomen (alternating sides) for subcut administration. Menotropin must be used immediately after reconstitution and must be protected from light. Advise patients to discard unused drug. Adverse effects include nausea, vomiting, diarrhea, gynecomastia, and fever.

Inadequate thyroid and adrenal gland function can also affect sexuality. **Hypothyroidism**, a deficiency in thyroid hormone, can be the result of insufficient thyroid hormone production or resistance to its effects at the target organs. The problem can be congenital or acquired.

TABLE 56.4 Drugs That Cause Sexual Dysfunction in Males

Drug Category	Drugs or Drug Families
Anticholinergics	Atropine Scopolamine Benztropine Trihexyphenidyl
Antidepressants	Tricyclic antidepressants Monoamine oxidase inhibitors Selective serotonin reuptake inhibitors
Antihistamines	Diphenhydramine Hydroxyzine
Antihypertensives	Centrally acting alpha$_2$ agonists Alpha- and beta-receptor blockers Diuretics Angiotensin-converting enzyme inhibitors
Antipsychotics	Phenothiazines Thioxanthenes Butyrophenone
Antiulcer drugs	Cimetidine Famotidine
Sedatives and illicit drugs	Alcohol Barbiturates Diazepam Chlordiazepoxide Cannabis Cocaine Opiates Methadone
Others	Aminocaproic acid Baclofen Steroids Ethionamide Digoxin Chemotherapeutic agents Lithium

It can cause **inhibited sexual desire**, a lack of or decreased interest in sexual activity, and erectile dysfunction (ED). In **Addison disease**, there is a deficit of both cortisol and the mineralocorticoid aldosterone. Males with Addison disease may experience inhibited sexual desire, ED, or diminished fertility. Both hypothyroidism and Addison disease are highly responsive to replacement therapy with the appropriate hormones.

Sexual Dysfunction

Sexual dysfunction is the inability to experience sexual desire, erection, ejaculation, and/or detumescence—the four phases of the sexual response cycle in males. Inhibited sexual desire can result from androgen deficiency, an affective disorder, or discord in the sexual relationship. Many drugs can also cause sexual dysfunction (Table 56.4).

Ejaculatory dysfunction, impaired ejection of seminal fluid from the male urethra, can be psychogenic or a result of drug therapy, androgen deficiency, or sympathetic degeneration. Failure of detumescence (reduction of penile engorgement) is most commonly caused by penile disease, systemic disease, trauma, or adverse effects of drugs.

TABLE 56.5 Phosphodiesterase-5 Inhibitors for Erectile Dysfunction

Generic	Onset/Duration	Side Effects	Drug Interactions
Avanafil 50–200 mg; not affected by food	Onset: 15–30 min Duration: 4–6 h Use once in 24 h	Abdominal symptoms such as diarrhea, heartburn, and upset stomach Abnormal vision such as blurring and sensitivity to light and blue-green color tint Dizziness Flushing Headache Nasal congestion Hearing loss/tinnitus	Nitrates: Isosorbide, nitroglycerin, amyl nitrate, butyl nitrate Alpha-blockers: Alfuzosin, doxazosin, prazosin, tamsulosin, terazosin, amiodarone Antiinfective agents: Fluconazole, itraconazole, ketoconazole, clarithromycin, moxifloxacin, erythromycin Cardiac drugs: Disopyramide, procainamide, quinidine, sotalol, thioridazine, verapamil HIV protease inhibitors: Atazanavir, indinavir, ritonavir, saquinavir Other drugs: Methadone, pimozide, haloperidol
Sildenafil 25–100 mg; works best on an empty stomach	Onset: 30–60 min Duration: 4 h		
Tadalafil 5–20 mg; not affected by food	Onset: 15–60 min Duration: 24–36 h Max: 20 mg/dose once daily		
Vardenafil 5–20 mg; less effective with a high-fat meal	Onset: 25–30 min Duration: 4–5 h Max: 20 mg/dose once daily		

h, Hour; *HIV*, human immunodeficiency virus; *min*, minute.

Individuals who experience premature ejaculation related to excessive anxiety about sexual intercourse may be helped by treatment with one of the many antidepressants alone or in conjunction with psychotherapy.

Erectile dysfunction (ED) is the inability to achieve or maintain an erection satisfactory for sexual performance. ED happens when not enough blood flows to the penis during sexual stimulation. This may be caused by psychoemotional problems, diabetes, hypertension, lower urinary tract symptoms, pelvic surgery, vascular insufficiency, neurologic disorders, androgen deficiency or resistance, or diseases of the penis. ED caused by vascular insufficiency is occasionally treated on a short-term basis by local vasoactive drugs, including papaverine, phentolamine, prostaglandin E, and nitroglycerin. Other drug options for the treatment of ED include oral drugs, drugs injected into the penis, intraurethral alprostadil, or testosterone.

A class of drugs called *phosphodiesterase inhibitors* facilitates erection by enhancing blood flow to the penis. Phosphodiesterase-5 (PDE-5) inhibitors are currently the most commonly used medical treatment for ED. These drugs have a high success rate, are easy to use, and often result in erection during sexual stimulation. The PDE-5 inhibitors currently approved by the FDA are sildenafil, tadalafil, vardenafil, and avanafil. PDE-5 inhibitors are taken before sexual activity with variations in effective start time and duration of benefit (Table 56.5).

Nitroglycerin and other nitrate drugs used to treat heart disease can cause a significant decrease in blood pressure when taken with PDE-5 inhibitors; therefore this class of drugs is contraindicated for use by any patient using organic nitrates in *any* form. Patients with a prescription for as-needed (PRN) sublingual nitroglycerin can take PDE-5 inhibitors but should still be cautioned about taking them concomitantly. Organic nitrates include nitroglycerin, isosorbide mononitrate, isosorbide nitrate, isosorbide dinitrate/phenobarbital, pentaerythritol tetranitrate, erythritol tetranitrate, and illicit substances (amyl nitrate/nitrite, butyl nitrate). Sildenafil is contraindicated in patients with significant cardiovascular disease and in individuals who have anatomic deformities or conditions that predispose them to priapism.

Studies have shown that vardenafil and tadalafil are safer for patients with heart failure or a history of myocardial infarctions. Like sildenafil, they are contraindicated if the patient is taking nitrate-containing drugs. Common side effects of these drugs are headache (most common), dyspepsia, nasal congestion, and nasopharyngitis. Other rare side effects can also occur, and the patient should be taught about them; these effects include blurred vision, photosensitivity, changes in color perception (especially blue and green), hearing loss, tinnitus, seizures, priapism, and urinary tract symptoms such as frequent or painful urination and cloudy or bloody urine. Patients are instructed to notify their health care provider of any side effects they experience.

The PDE-5 inhibitors interact with grapefruit juice and grapefruit products by increasing the amount of the PDE-5 inhibitor absorbed, thereby increasing the risk of side effects. Many drugs interact with PDE-5 inhibitors, so be sure to obtain a complete list of drugs taken by the patient.

Certain drugs are often misused by individuals seeking a heightened sexual experience. Amyl nitrate is commonly believed to be an aphrodisiac. Sudden death, myocardial infarction, and methemoglobinemia have been reported with its use. Cantharides (Spanish fly) causes bladder and urethral irritation, accounting for its use as a sexual stimulant. Permanent penile damage has been reported with its use.

> ### ⚡ PATIENT SAFETY
> **Do Not Confuse...**
> - **Lupron Depot-3 Month** with **Lupron Depot-Ped.**
> - **Anabolic steroids** with **corticosteroids.**

Complementary and Alternative Medicine

To self-treat sexual problems or to enhance sexual performance, consumers use a wide variety of herbs and plant-derived compounds (phytochemicals). Despite new science-based therapies, males are attracted to phytochemicals because they are easy to obtain and may be cheaper than prescription drugs and therapies, procedures, or surgeries not covered by insurance. Consumers may mistakenly perceive natural products as providing health benefits beyond sexual performance because they can be purchased at nutrition centers or health food stores. Common herbs used for sexual health and performance include *Pausinystalia yohimbe*, *Panax quinquefolius*, ginkgo biloba, saw palmetto, muira puama, *Lepidium meyenii*, *Mondia whitei*, and *Tribulus terrestris*. Limited studies have been conducted on these products; all studies have yielded mixed results. As such, there is insufficient evidence to recommend any complementary or alternative medicine (CAM). Its benefits appear to reflect popular or cultural beliefs. Reports in health magazines and advertising are anecdotal and based on a small number of users. However, it is important for the nurse to be aware of CAM, because ED affects 50% of males between 50 and

70 years of age, but only 10% seek medical attention. These statistics indicate males may be choosing to use CAM to avoid the discomfort of discussing this sensitive topic with their health care provider.

Non-Sexually Transmitted Infections

Drugs used to treat acute or chronic prostatitis, orchitis, or epididymitis are the same as those used to treat urinary tract infections (see Chapter 51).

Benign Prostatic Hyperplasia

As a male ages, the glandular units in the prostate gland begin to undergo tissue hyperplasia, an abnormal increase in the number of cells, which results in prostatic hypertrophy, or enlargement of the gland. The exact cause of BPH is unknown, but its development is almost universal in older males. The enlarged prostate gland contributes to overall lower urinary tract symptoms either through direct bladder outlet obstruction or from resistance within the enlarged gland itself. The male experiences storage and/or voiding disturbances, such as a sensation of bladder fullness, frequency, nocturia, hesitation when trying to begin urinating, dribbling of urine, and ED. Although BPH is not a life-threatening condition, the effect of symptoms on quality of life can be significant. Because these are the same symptoms that prostate cancer may cause, the patient should have a prostate-specific antigen (PSA) blood test and may undergo a prostate biopsy to make sure no cancer is present. Traditionally, the primary goal of treatment has been to alleviate bothersome symptoms. More recently, treatment has also been focused on the alteration of disease progression and prevention of complications. Drugs from several pharmacologic classes are used; they include alpha-adrenergic antagonists (alpha-blockers), 5-alpha-reductase inhibitors (5-ARIs), anticholinergics (only used in males without large postvoid residuals), and the PDE-5 inhibitor tadalafil. Choosing the correct medical treatment for BPH is complex (Table 56.6). The American Urological Association 2010 Guidelines are a useful reference on the effective evidence-based management of lower urinary tract symptoms caused by BPH. The guidelines advise a discussion of benefits and risks of each recommended treatment alternative (e.g., watchful waiting; medical, surgical, or minimally invasive surgical treatments). The choice of treatment is reached in a shared decision-making process between provider and patient.

With initiation of drug therapy, the patient should be followed every 1 to 3 months, depending on the class of drug chosen, to assess success and inquire about side effects. The patient with an enlarged prostate should avoid drugs that can cause urinary retention, such as anticholinergics, antihistamines, and decongestants.

TABLE 56.6 Drugs Used for Treatment of Benign Prostatic Hyperplasia

Drug	Route and Dosage	Side Effects
5-Alpha-Reductase Inhibitors		
Finasteride	PO: 5 mg daily	Decreased libido, erectile dysfunction, orthostatic hypotension, gynecomastia
Dutasteride	PO: 0.5 mg daily	

Safety in Administration

Females of childbearing age must not handle crushed or broken tablets due to possible absorption and potential risk to male fetuses; immediately wash contact area with soap and water if contact occurs. Inform patients of an increase in high-grade prostate cancer in males treated with 5-alpha-reductase inhibitors indicated for BPH treatment. Inform patients that the volume of ejaculate may be decreased, and that impotence or decreased libido may occur. Instruct patients to promptly report to their physician any changes in breasts (lumps, pain, or nipple discharge).

Drug	Route and Dosage	Side Effects
Alpha-Adrenergic Blocking Agents		
Tamsulosin	PO: 0.4 mg/d 30 min after a meal; titrate up to 0.8 mg/d	Dizziness, headache, orthostatic hypotension, decreased libido, upper respiratory infection symptoms, priapism
Doxazosin	PO: Start 1 mg/d at bedtime; titrate up to 8 mg/d	
Terazosin	A: PO: Start 1 mg/d at bedtime; titrate up to 10 mg/d max: 20 mg/d	
Alfuzosin	PO: 10 mg/d after a meal	
Silodosin	PO: 8 mg/d with a meal	

Safety in Administration

Alpha-adrenergic blocking agents are also used to control blood pressure. To avoid hypotensive episodes, advise using at bedtime, and reconcile all drugs taken before adding another antihypertensive drug.

Instruct patients to take these drugs with food. Counsel about possible symptoms of postural hypotension (dizziness); caution patients about driving, operating machinery, or performing hazardous tasks while using these drugs. Inform patients that orgasm with reduced or no semen does not pose a safety concern and is reversible when the drug is stopped. Advise patients to notify their ophthalmologist about use before cataract surgery or other eye procedures.

Drug	Route and Dosage	Side Effects
Phosphodiesterase-5 Inhibitors		
Tadalafil	PO: 5 mg daily	See Table 56.5

Safety in Administration

Tadalafil should not be used by patients taking nitrates such as nitroglycerin because the combination may trigger an unsafe drop in blood pressure. Tadalafil should not be used with alpha-blockers for the treatment of BPH because the combo therapy has not been adequately studied and may increase the risk of lowering blood pressure.

A, Adult; *BPH*, benign prostatic hyperplasia; *d*, day; *max*, maximum; *min*, minute; *PO*, by mouth.

Malignant Tumors

Prostatic cancer accounts for about 10% of all cancer deaths among American males. Most prostatic cancers are adenocarcinomas. Metastasis to lymph nodes, bone, lungs, liver, and adrenal glands is common. Prostatic cancer is often asymptomatic, but urinary obstruction is commonly the first sign. Treatment may include a combination of surgical resection, cryotherapy, antiandrogen administration, radiation therapy, chemotherapy, and pain management.

Testicular tumors peak in early adulthood. They include malignant germinal cell tumors and benign Leydig or Sertoli cell tumors. Treatment depends on the type and stage of the tumor. Surgical excision, radiation therapy, and chemotherapy are used alone or in combination.

Approximately 1% of breast cancer cases occur in males, most commonly after the 60 years of age. Treatment is similar for males and females and entails surgery, radiation therapy, chemotherapy, and endocrine therapy. Carcinoma of the penis represents less than 1% of all malignancies among males. In situ, treatment entails local excision, radiation therapy, and local application of 5-fluorouracil cream or solution. Invasive carcinoma is treated by surgical resection of the penis and the involved nodes. Radiation and chemotherapy follow as needed.

CLINICAL JUDGMENT CASE STUDY

The patient, 16 years of age, is a high school junior who is 59.3 inches tall and weighs 126 pounds. He is having increased feelings of discomfort about not fitting in with the other students at school because he has not yet begun sexual maturation. He is a good student and an accomplished violinist in the school orchestra. His father states that he also was a "late bloomer," but both parents are concerned about the patient's increasing social withdrawal and seem determined to seek medical intervention for him. The nurse at the clinic assesses the needs and status of the patient and his parents.

1. What is the patient's primary complaint?
2. What is concerning the patient's parents?
3. What information must be included in the history and physical examination?
4. What education should the nurse prepare before the parents decide whether to start their son on androgen therapy?
5. The decision is made to prescribe testosterone 30 mg every 12 hours by buccal tablet (held inside the cheek until it dissolves). The patient will be on this regimen for 4 months, during which time he is to come to the clinic at monthly intervals. The patient asks why he will be treated for 4 months. What will the nurse reply?
6. About what adverse effects do the patient and his parents need to be educated?
7. What physical and psychosocial parameters will be assessed at the patient's monthly visits?
8. What special hygiene needs does the patient have while on this regimen?
9. When should the patient have x-rays taken? Explain your answer.

REVIEW QUESTIONS

1. A young male patient is referred to the nurse for initiation of intramuscular androgen therapy for hypogonadism. What information should the nurse give this patient? **Select all that apply.**
   a. A 4- to 6-month trial of androgen therapy will be followed by a period of rest for reevaluation.
   b. Sexual development will begin to occur immediately.
   c. Dosages may be adjusted based on periodic plasma testosterone levels.
   d. Growth will be monitored periodically by radiography.
   e. The patient should not consume alcohol.
2. A married male with two daughters is taking finasteride to treat benign prostatic hyperplasia. Which nursing assessment data are most critical in developing a care plan? **Select all that apply.**
   a. His spouse and children should not handle the drug.
   b. The drug may cause decreased libido and urinary retention.
   c. The dose needs to be reevaluated periodically.
   d. This drug may also cause his hair to grow.
   e. Using finasteride will not increase his risk for developing prostate cancer.
3. The nurse is discussing androgen therapy with a patient. Which statements will the nurse include in the patient education? **Select all that apply.**
   a. Lower extremity edema associated with androgen therapy can be increased by corticosteroids.
   b. Only males are prescribed androgen replacement therapy.
   c. Androgen therapy is safe in pregnancy.
   d. Androgen therapy can affect glucose levels, cholesterol, and thyroid and liver functioning.
   e. Androgen therapy may cause seizures.
4. During his annual physical examination, a patient tells the nurse he is in a new relationship and having some problems with erectile dysfunction. He is interested in nutrition and natural therapies. Which are the most appropriate responses by the nurse? **Select all that apply.**
   a. Herbal therapies are commonly used by males to enhance sexual performance.
   b. Side effects from using some herbal therapies include increased anxiety, frequent headaches, and trouble sleeping.
   c. Phytochemicals have been widely researched and are safe to use.
   d. Males who have cardiovascular, neurologic, or psychological problems should not use some of the herbal products.
   e. It is a good idea to increase intake of dietary vitamins.
5. The nurse is interviewing a male with erectile dysfunction who is interested in one of the phosphodiesterase inhibitors. Which response by the nurse is best for this patient?
   a. The onset of action varies among the different drugs in this class.
   b. These drugs should not be used if you take nitroglycerine for angina.
   c. Common side effects include headache, blurred vision, photosensitivity, changes in color perception, and urinary tract symptoms.
   d. There are many causes of sexual dysfunction in males, so a complete history and physical is the first step in treatment.

6. A 17-year-old is brought to the health care provider by his father because he has been taking nutritional supplements sold at the gym. Which assessment data are most critical in developing a care plan for this patient? **Select all that apply.**
   a. His blood pressure is low.
   b. His acne is worsening.
   c. He has been in several fistfights with other teenagers.
   d. He has gained 60 pounds.
   e. His liver function tests are abnormal.

7. A male patient presents with complaints of lower urinary tract symptoms, getting up three times at night to urinate, dribbling after urination, and feeling pressure throughout the day. Recent screening laboratory tests are normal. The health care provider starts him on doxazosin 1 mg at bedtime. What advice can the nurse give this patient? **Select all that apply.**
   a. Advise the patient about signs and symptoms of low blood pressure.
   b. Tell the patient to notify his ophthalmologist about the doxazosin use before cataract surgery.
   c. Caution the patient that he should not allow his wife to handle the medicine.
   d. Advise the patient to immediately report problematic prolonged erection.
   e. Instruct the patient to take the drug on an empty stomach.

Sexually Transmitted Infections

http://evolve.elsevier.com/McCuistion/pharmacology

OBJECTIVES

- Summarize general aspects of sexually transmitted infections.
- Describe the various pathogens related to sexually transmitted infections.
- Recall strategies for preventing sexually transmitted infections.

OUTLINE

Sexually Transmitted Infections, 751
   Risk Factors for Sexually Transmitted Infections, 751
   Vertical Transmission, 751
Sexually Transmitted Pathogens, 752
   Bacterial Pathogens, 752

Viral Pathogens, 755
Other Pathogens, 756
Prevention of Sexually Transmitted Infections, 756
Clinical Judgment Single-Episode Case Study, 758
Review Questions, 758

Each day, more than 1 million new cases of sexually transmitted infection (STI) occur worldwide. The Centers for Disease Control and Prevention (CDC) reports that from 2016 to 2020 STIs have increased by 11%. Young adults are at risk, particularly young females, but infections among males are also rising. More than 30 bacteria, viruses, and parasites can cause STIs. The most common bacterial pathogens are *Chlamydia, Neisseria gonorrhoeae,* and *Treponema pallidum* (syphilis); *Trichomonas* is a common parasite; and the most common viral pathogens are hepatitis B virus (HBV), herpes simplex virus (HSV), human immunodeficiency virus (HIV), and human papillomavirus (HPV). Most people with STIs experience few or no symptoms, making it difficult to diagnose and treat to stop the spread of infections. STIs are spread through sexual contact, via blood or blood products, and through mother-to-child transmission during pregnancy and childbirth.

SEXUALLY TRANSMITTED INFECTIONS

Risk Factors for Sexually Transmitted Infections

Sexual transmission of pathogens can occur through breaks in the vaginal or cervical mucosa or in the skin covering the shaft or glans of the penis. Each act of coitus results in tiny, friction-induced fissures on these surfaces. Seminal fluid, spermatozoa, vaginal secretions, blood, and other body fluids can carry pathogens. Skin and mucosal lesions can be penetrated by microorganisms, and skin and mucosa can shed microorganisms.

Sexual contact can involve transmission of pathogens through the skin or mouth and via oral-genital, oral-anal, or hand-anal transmission of pathogens through breaks in the skin or mucosal surfaces or from inoculation by infectious body fluids. Anal penetration is particularly risky because of the likelihood of tissue trauma that results in the partner's exposure to enteric microorganisms. The risk for contracting an STI increases with substance abuse, imprisonment, sexual activity with a partner who has been imprisoned, sexual activity with individuals being paid for sex acts, and rape or sexual assault.

Patients who engage in sexual activity with multiple partners are at high risk for transmission of STIs, particularly HIV. The CDC reports the risk for getting STIs is markedly increased among individuals who have more than one sexual partner per year versus those who have fewer partners. It should be noted that 21.8% of males and 10.6% of females between the ages of 15 and 44 report having had 15 or more sexual partners.

Other high-risk practices are anal or vaginal intercourse without a condom, hand-anal contact, contact with menstrual blood during sexual activity, use of an enema before anal intercourse, and urination on broken skin or inside the body. Refer to Fig. 57.1 for guidelines provided by the CDC on the prevention of STIs.

STIs are often manifested as multiple infections. Individuals undergoing treatment for one STI should be assessed for others, including HIV. This is especially true if genital or perianal ulcerations are present.

There are five nationally notifiable STIs that are reported to local and state health departments that collect and provide data to the CDC through the National Notifiable Diseases Surveillance System, chlamydia, gonorrhea, syphilis, chancroid, and HIV, though a virus is listed as reportable as well.

Vertical Transmission

Vertical transmission is the passage of infecting organisms from mother to neonate. Microbes can travel up the reproductive tract from the vagina or cervix and enter the intrauterine environment. Organisms that are of little consequence to healthy adults can be devastating to a

Fig. 57.1 How to prevent sexually transmitted infections. (From Centers for Disease Control and Prevention: *How you can prevent sexually transmitted diseases,* 2021. www.cdc.gov/std/prevention.)

fetus. Transmission can also occur through contact with the mother's blood at birth or through breast milk, as in the case of HIV and HBV. Many STIs, such as syphilis, are transmitted through the placenta and membranes. Others, such as the herpes simplex virus type 2 (HSV-2), require actual contact by the infant with microorganisms in the birth canal. Because of the risk for blindness caused by *Chlamydia trachomatis* and *N. gonorrhoeae,* erythromycin ointment is routinely administered in the eyes of neonates as prophylaxis. This is usually done within the first hour after birth.

CDC guidelines for the primary treatment of some STI pathogens are listed in Table 57.1; the most common pathogens are discussed in the following section. All sexual contacts of an individual with an infection should be informed of the exposure so they can be treated. Partners should refrain from sexual activity until each is clear of infection on follow-up evaluation or, at the very least, condoms should be used until each is clear of infection.

SEXUALLY TRANSMITTED PATHOGENS

The information in this chapter comes directly from the 2021 treatment guidelines for STIs, available at www.cdc.gov/std/treatment

Bacterial Pathogens

Sexually transmitted bacterial pathogens can be effectively treated with antibiotic therapy. When present, common symptoms include vaginal discharge, urethral discharge or burning (in males), genital ulcers, and abdominal pain.

Bacterial Vaginosis

Bacterial vaginosis (BV) causes a large amount of homogenous, thin, white vaginal discharge with a strong fishy odor. In BV, normal, healthy bacteria in the vagina—lactobacilli—are replaced with anaerobic bacteria, most commonly *Gardnerella vaginalis, Mycoplasma hominis, Ureaplasma urealyticum,* or *Prevotella, Porphyromonas, Bacteroides, Peptostreptococcus,* and *Mobiluncus* species. BV can be transmitted via sexual contact but is not considered an STI; however, having BV can increase a female's risk for getting an STI due to the imbalance in vaginal bacteria.

BV is treated with metronidazole 500 mg by mouth (PO) twice a day for 7 days. Because metronidazole can cause stomach upset, it should be taken with food or a full glass of water or milk. Alcohol causes severe nausea and vomiting when ingested with metronidazole, so patients should be instructed not to drink alcoholic beverages or use products that contain alcohol, such as mouthwash, for the duration of drug therapy and for 48 hours after treatment.

Vaginal preparations are also effective in treating BV, such as metronidazole gel 0.75%, one 5-g applicator intravaginally at bedtime for 5 nights; clindamycin cream 2%, one 5-g applicator intravaginally at bedtime for 5 days; or clindamycin ovules, 100 mg intravaginally at bedtime for 3 days. Clindamycin cream is oil based and might weaken latex condoms and diaphragms for 3 to 7 days.

Oral drugs that are alternatives to metronidazole include tinidazole, either 2 g orally once a day for 2 days or 1 g orally once a day for 5 days, or clindamycin 300 mg orally twice a day for 7 days. Tinidazole has the same precautions with alcohol as metronidazole

TABLE 57.1 Current Guidelines for Other Sexually Transmitted Infections

Pathogen	Primary Therapy	Notes
Chancroid (*Haemophilus ducreyi*)	Azithromycin PO: 1 g, single dose *or* ceftriaxone IM: 250 mg, single dose *or* ciprofloxacin PO: 500 mg bid for 3 d *or* erythromycin base PO: 500 mg tid for 7 d Data suggest ciprofloxacin presents a low risk to the fetus during pregnancy with a potential for toxicity during breast-feeding; therefore alternate drugs should be used during pregnancy and lactation.	Regardless of whether symptoms of the disease are present, sex partners of patients who have chancroid should be examined and treated if they had sexual contact with the patient during the 10 days preceding the patient's onset of symptoms. Males who are uncircumcised and patients with HIV infection do not respond as well to treatment as persons who are circumcised or HIV-negative. Patients should be tested for HIV infection at the time chancroid is diagnosed.
Granuloma Inguinale (Donovanosis)	Recommended regimen: Azithromycin PO: 1 g/wk or 500 mg/d for at least 3 wk and until all lesions have completely healed Alternative regimens: Doxycycline PO: 100 mg bid for at least 3 wk and until all lesions have completely healed *or* erythromycin base PO: 500 mg four times a day for at least 3 wk and until all lesions have completely healed *or* trimethoprim-sulfamethoxazole PO: One double-strength (160 mg/800 mg) tablet bid for at least 3 wk and until all lesions have completely healed	All persons who receive a diagnosis of granuloma inguinale should be tested for HIV. Persons who have had sexual contact with a patient who has granuloma inguinale within the 60 days before onset of the patient's symptoms should be examined and offered therapy. For treatment during pregnancy the CDC recommends azithromycin 1 gm orally once weekly or 500 mg daily for 3 wk and until all lesions have completely healed, and alternatively erythromycin 500 mg orally 4 times/d for 3 wk and until all lesions have completely healed.
Hepatitis A virus (HAV)	Patients with acute HAV usually require only supportive care, with no restrictions in diet or activity. Hospitalization might be necessary for patients who become dehydrated because of nausea and vomiting and is critical for patients with signs or symptoms of acute liver failure.	Vaccination is the most effective means of preventing HAV transmission among persons at risk for infection (see Chapter 34 for a discussion on vaccines).
Hepatitis B virus (HBV)	No specific therapy is available for persons with acute hepatitis B; treatment is supportive.	Two products have been approved for hepatitis B prevention: hepatitis B immune globulin (recommended dose is 0.06 mL/kg IM × 1) for postexposure prophylaxis and hepatitis B vaccine (see Chapter 34 for a discussion on vaccines).
Hepatitis C virus (HCV)	The treatment of HCV is based on genotype and is constantly changing; please see www.hcvguidelines.org for the latest recommendations.	No vaccine for hepatitis C is available, and prophylaxis with immune globulin is not effective in preventing HCV infection after exposure.
Lymphogranuloma venereum (LGV; *C. trachomatis* serovars)	Recommended regimen: Doxycycline PO: 100 mg bid for 21 d Alternative regimen: azithromycin 1 gm orally weekly for 3 wk, or Erythromycin base PO: 500 mg four times a day for 21 d Pregnant and lactating females should be treated with erythromycin. Doxycycline should be avoided in the second and third trimesters of pregnancy because of risk for discoloration of teeth and bones, but it is compatible with breast-feeding.	Persons who have had sexual contact with a patient who has LGV within the 60 days before onset of the patient's symptoms should be examined and tested for urethral, cervical, or rectal chlamydial infection depending on anatomic site of exposure. They should be presumptively treated with an antichlamydial regimen (azithromycin 1 g PO single dose or doxycycline 100 mg PO bid for 7 d).
Mycoplasma genitalium	Uncomplicated infection: Doxycycline 100 mg 2 × daily for 7 d followed by azithromycin 1 g × 1, then 500 mg orally daily for 3 d. Complicated infection or macrolide-resistant *M. genitalium*: Doxycycline 100 mg orally 2 times/d for 7 d followed by moxifloxacin 400 mg orally once daily for 7 d.	*M. genitalium* lacks a cell wall; thus antibiotics targeting cell-wall biosynthesis (e.g., beta-lactams, including penicillins and cephalosporins) are ineffective against this organism. Sex partners should be managed according to guidelines for patients with nongonococcal urethritis, cervicitis, and PID.

bid, Twice daily; *CDC*, Centers for Disease Control and Prevention; *d*, day; *HIV*, human immunodeficiency virus; *IM*, intramuscularly; *NSAID*, nonsteroidal antiinflammatory drug; *PID*, pelvic inflammatory disease; *PO*, by mouth; *tid*, three times daily; *wk*, weeks.
From Centers for Disease Control and Prevention. Sexually transmitted infections 2021 treatment guidelines. Available at www.cdc.gov/std/treatment.

and should be taken with food. Tinidazole causes slightly less gastrointestinal (GI) upset than metronidazole. Patients taking clindamycin should be instructed to notify their health care provider if diarrhea develops because it may be an indication of *Clostridium difficile*–associated diarrhea. Treating BV is especially important for pregnant patients because of the risk of spontaneous abortion, delivery of premature or low-birth-weight babies, or pelvic infection developing after delivery. Metronidazole (oral or intravaginal) and clindamycin (oral) are the drugs of choice in pregnancy, and tinidazole should *not* be used during the first trimester of pregnancy. None of the drugs should be used by nursing mothers because these drugs are excreted in breast milk.

Chlamydia

Chlamydia trachomatis is the most common STI in the United States in young adults. This infection is most often asymptomatic. Females who contract the infection are at risk for developing pelvic inflammatory disease (PID), ectopic pregnancies, and infertility. Because of this, it is recommended that all sexually active females younger than age 25 be screened annually for *C. trachomatis* and that all females older than 25 be screened based on risk factors.

The CDC 2021 STI treatment guidelines now recommend doxycycline 100 mg orally twice a day for 7 days. They also list two alternative regimens as azithromycin 1 g orally in a single dose or levofloxacin 500 mg orally once daily for 7 days.

Doxycycline is contraindicated in the second and third trimesters of pregnancy. In the case of a chlamydial infection during pregnancy, azithromycin 1 g orally in a single dose is the treatment of choice. Alternatively, amoxicillin 500 mg orally three times a day for 7 days may be given.

Neonates may contract *C. trachomatis* from exposure to the mother's infected cervix during delivery. It most frequently presents as conjunctivitis that develops 5 to 12 days after delivery; however, *C. trachomatis* can also cause pneumonia in infants between 1 and 3 months old. Prenatal screening and treatment are the best means of prevention. Erythromycin ophthalmic ointment, administered to prevent gonococcal ophthalmia, may also prevent conjunctivitis caused by *C. trachomatis*.

Persons treated for *Chlamydia* infection should be instructed to abstain from sexual intercourse for 7 days after single-dose therapy or until a 7-day regimen is completed. Partners should be treated if they had sexual contact during the 60 days preceding the onset of symptoms or diagnosis.

Gonorrhea

In the United States gonorrhea is the second most common communicable disease. In males, infection by *N. gonorrhoeae* causes a greenish-yellow or whitish discharge from the penis, accompanied by burning with urination. These symptoms usually prompt them to seek evaluation and treatment but often not until they have spread the infection to others. In females, *N. gonorrhoeae* is frequently asymptomatic. Left untreated, females with *N. gonorrhoeae* infections develop PID, which can cause tubal scarring that leads to ectopic pregnancies and infertility. Oral infections caused by *N. gonorrhoeae* cause sore throat and trouble swallowing; on examination, the pharynx resembles strep throat.

Due to developing resistance to azithromycin, in uncomplicated *N. gonorrhoeae* infection in adolescents and adults, two-drug therapy is no longer recommended. Treatment of uncomplicated *N. gonorrhoeae* should be with ceftriaxone 500 mg IM as a single dose. Treatment of coinfection with *Chlamydia trachomatis*, or when chlamydia is not excluded, should be with oral doxycycline 100 mg twice a day for 7 days.

Neonates may contract *N. gonorrhoeae* from exposure to the mother's infected cervix during delivery. The infection most frequently presents as an acute illness that develops 2 to 5 days after delivery. Prenatal screening and treatment are the best means of prevention, and most states require neonates to be administered erythromycin (0.5%) ophthalmic ointment in each eye in a single application at birth to prevent conjunctivitis caused by *N. gonorrhoeae*.

Persons receiving treatment for gonorrhea should be instructed to abstain from sexual activity for 7 days after treatment. Persons diagnosed with gonorrhea should also be tested for *Chlamydia*, syphilis, and HIV. Partners should be treated if they had sexual contact during the 60 days preceding the onset of symptoms or diagnosis.

Syphilis

Syphilis is caused by the bacteria *Treponema pallidum*; if not treated early in the infectious process, it produces systemic disease that can be fatal. The disease is divided into three stages: primary, secondary, and tertiary.

Primary syphilis infections present with a sore, or **chancre**, at the site where the infection entered the body—typically, the penis in males and outer genitals or inner vagina in females. It is usually painless. The chancre develops about 3 weeks after exposure and resolves in 3 to 6 weeks without treatment. During this stage, the person is very contagious, even after the chancre has resolved.

Secondary syphilis is characterized by a skin rash that appears 2 to 8 weeks after the chancre. It may occur anywhere on the body, commonly on the hands and soles of the feet; the rash usually does not itch. Mucocutaneous lesions, fever, fatigue, sore throat, and lymphadenopathy may occur as well. The rash usually resolves in about 2 months. During this stage, the person remains very contagious, even after the rash has resolved. After the rash has resolved, a period that lasts anywhere from 1 to 20 years goes by without any symptoms. This is called the **latent stage**, and it occurs in persons who have gone untreated. A person may remain contagious during the latent period, and diagnosis can only be made through blood testing.

Tertiary syphilis may occur as early as 1 year after infection or at any time during an untreated person's lifetime. Large sores inside the body or on the skin occur in the tertiary stage, along with cardiovascular and ocular syphilis and neurosyphilis. Examination of the cerebral spinal fluid (CSF) should be done in persons in the tertiary stage to determine neurologic involvement, even in the absence of clinical neurologic findings.

To diagnose syphilis, two types of serologic testing are necessary to avoid false positives. One test should be a nontreponemal antibody test (e.g., rapid plasma reagin or Venereal Disease Research Laboratory) that tests for antibodies produced when a person has syphilis, although it may be produced in other diseases as well (e.g., Lyme disease or malaria). The other test should be a treponemal antibody test (e.g., fluorescent treponemal antibody absorption [FTA-ABS] or *T. pallidum* particle agglutination assay), a test for antibodies that specifically target *T. pallidum*.

Treatment for primary and secondary syphilis is benzathine penicillin G, 2.4 million units given IM in one dose. For recommended congenital syphilis evaluation and treatment for syphilis in infant and children see https://www.cdc.gov/std/treatment-guidelines/congenital-syphilis.htm. Infant and children should be managed by a pediatric infectious disease specialist for treatment.

Adults with early latent syphilis should be treated with benzathine penicillin G 2.4 million units IM in a single dose; those with late latent syphilis or latent syphilis of unknown duration should receive benzathine penicillin G 7.2 million units total, administered as three doses of 2.4 million units IM each at 1-week intervals.

Persons with tertiary syphilis should receive CSF analysis before initiating treatment. Those with normal CSF should receive benzathine penicillin G 7.2 million units total, administered as three doses of 2.4 million units IM each at 1-week intervals. Those with neurosyphilis or ocular syphilis should receive aqueous crystalline penicillin G 18 to 24 million units per day, administered as 3 to 4 million units IV every 4 hours or as a continuous infusion for 10 to 14 days. Alternatively, persons with neurosyphilis or ocular syphilis may be treated with procaine penicillin G 2.4 million units IM once daily plus probenecid 500 mg orally four times a day, both for 10 to 14 days. This alternative treatment should only be given to people whose adherence can be ensured.

Pregnant females can pass syphilis to their fetus, with potentially fatal consequences. According to the CDC, cases of congenital syphilis have doubled since 2013. Benzathine penicillin G is the only treatment for syphilis during pregnancy. Pregnant patients with syphilis in any stage who report they are allergic to penicillin should undergo penicillin allergy skin testing and desensitization and then should be treated with penicillin.

Partners should be treated if they had sexual contact during the 90 days preceding the diagnosis of primary, secondary, or early latent syphilis even if serologic testing is negative. If greater than 90 days, treatment should be initiated if serologic testing is positive or if testing is not available. All persons with syphilis at any stage should be tested for HIV.

Viral Pathogens

Infection caused by viral pathogens is not curable, although medication therapy is palliative. These include herpes simplex virus 1 (HSV-1; cross-contaminated from oral to genital) and HSV-2, HPV, and HIV.

Herpes Simplex Virus

Genital herpes is a lifelong viral infection. Two types of HSV can cause genital herpes: HSV-1 and HSV-2. Most cases of recurrent genital herpes are caused by HSV-2. Approximately 50 million people in the United States are infected with genital herpes. However, an increasing number of herpes infections are caused by HSV-1. Both types of the virus cause lesions that look like blisters, which crust over and scab. They may last for 2 to 4 weeks. The lesions may be accompanied by fever, lymphadenopathy, headache, and painful urination. Most HSV-2 cases go undiagnosed and are transmitted by people unaware that they have the infection or who are asymptomatic when transmission occurs.

Antiviral drugs are beneficial to most symptomatic patients and are the mainstay of management. It is imperative that nurses counsel patients with herpes regarding sexual and perinatal transmission and methods to reduce transmission.

Systemic antiviral drugs can control some of the signs and symptoms of genital herpes during initial and recurrent episodes or when used for daily suppressive therapy. However, these do not cure herpes or reduce the frequency and severity of recurrent episodes after drug discontinuation. Three antiviral drugs are used in the management of genital herpes: (1) acyclovir, (2) valacyclovir, and (3) famciclovir.

Recommendations for drug therapy of initial genital herpes infections is recommended using acyclovir 400 mg orally three times a day for 7 to 10 days, valacyclovir 1 g orally twice a day for 7 to 10 days, or famciclovir 250 mg orally three times a day for 7 to 10 days. Acyclovir 200 mg orally five times a day is no longer recommended. Treatment can be extended if healing is incomplete after 10 days of therapy.

Suppressive therapy reduces the frequency of genital herpes recurrences by 70% to 80% in patients who have frequent recurrences. Recommended regimens are acyclovir 400 mg orally twice a day, valacyclovir 500 mg orally once a day, valacyclovir 1 g orally once a day, or famciclovir 250 mg orally twice a day. Valacyclovir 500 mg once a day might be less effective than other valacyclovir or acyclovir dosing regimens in persons who have 10 episodes or more per year.

For episodic treatment to be effective, treatment should begin within 1 day of lesion onset or during the prodrome (e.g., burning, itching, or tingling) that occurs anywhere from 30 minutes to a couple of days before some outbreaks. Patients should be provided with a prescription for the drug with instructions to initiate treatment immediately when symptoms begin. The recommended regimens for episodic therapy are acyclovir 800 mg orally twice daily for 5 days, or three times daily for 2 days, famciclovir 1 g orally twice daily for 1 day, or 500 mg orally once, followed by 250 mg orally twice daily for 2 days, famciclovir 125 mg orally twice daily for 5 days, or valacyclovir 500 mg orally twice daily for 3 days, or 1 g orally once daily for 5 days.

Sexual partners should be evaluated, treated if symptomatic, and counseled. Asymptomatic sex partners should be questioned about a history of genital lesions and offered serologic testing for HSV infection.

The risk of vertical transmission is high (30%–50%) among females who become infected near the time of delivery and low (<1%) among females with a prenatal history of herpes or those who become infected early in the pregnancy. Prevention of vertical transmission depends on both preventing infection during late pregnancy and avoiding exposure to viral shedding during delivery. The recommended drug regimen for suppressive therapy of pregnant patients with recurrent genital herpes is acyclovir 400 mg orally three times a day or valacyclovir 500 mg orally twice a day with treatment recommended starting at 36 weeks of gestation.

Human Immunodeficiency Virus

Two to 4 weeks after exposure, HIV infection typically presents with an acute flulike syndrome that includes fever, fatigue, rash, pharyngitis, and lymphadenopathy. HIV is a chronic illness that progressively depletes CD4 T lymphocytes and ends with symptomatic acquired immunodeficiency syndrome. Early diagnosis and treatment are essential to reduce the risk of transmitting HIV to others and to maintain quality of life.

Persons with acute HIV infection are at high risk for transmitting HIV to their partner because the concentration of virus in blood and genital secretions is extremely elevated. Antiretroviral therapy during acute HIV infection is recommended because it substantially reduces transmission to others. See Chapter 32 for drugs used to treat HIV.

Partners (sexual partners and those with whom needles and syringes are shared) should be notified concerning possible exposure to HIV. Early diagnosis and treatment reduce the risk for further HIV transmission. Partner notification for HIV infection should be confidential.

All pregnant patients should be tested for HIV infection during the first prenatal visit. A second test during the third trimester, preferably at less than 36 weeks' gestation, is recommended for those known to be at high risk for HIV.

Human Papillomavirus

According to the CDC, human papillomavirus (HPV) is the most common sexually transmitted infection among males and females in the United States. Of the roughly 100 types of HPV infection that have been identified, nearly 40 infect the genital area. Most HPV infections are self-limited and asymptomatic, and most sexually active persons will become infected with HPV at some point in their lifetime. High-risk HPV infections (e.g., HPV types 16 and 18) cause most cervical, penile, vulvar, vaginal, anal, and oropharyngeal cancers. Low-risk HPV infection (e.g., HPV types 6 and 11) causes genital warts and recurrent respiratory papillomatosis. Screening with the Papanicolaou ("Pap") test can detect cervical dysplasia, which can be a precursor to cervical cancer if left untreated. Whereas the Pap test can determine whether the cervical cells are abnormal, an HPV test specifically looks for high-risk HPV in cervical cells.

The HPV vaccine approved in the United States is a 9-valent vaccine that prevents infection with HPV types 6, 11, 16, 18, 31, 33, 45, 52, and 58. See Chapter 34 for a discussion on vaccines.

Because most HPV infections do no harm, they do not require treatment and tend to resolve on their own. Because of this, antiviral therapy is not recommended. Treatment is aimed at removal of genital warts and precancerous lesions and treatment of cervical cancer and includes cryotherapy (freezing) or a loop electrosurgical excision procedure to cut away abnormal tissue.

Condom use can lower the risk of transmitting and developing HPV infections. Limiting the number of sex partners can also reduce the risk for HPV. However, abstaining from sexual activity is the most reliable method for preventing HPV infection.

Other Pathogens

Pediculosis Pubis

Persons with pediculosis pubis, a parasitic infection caused by *Phthirus pubis*, usually seek treatment because of extreme pruritus of the body part or area where the lice are moving and laying eggs. Infected persons may also notice lice or nits on their pubic hair. Pediculosis pubis is usually transmitted by sexual contact.

Recommended treatment is with a permethrin 1% cream rinse applied to affected areas and washed off after 10 minutes or pyrethrins with piperonyl butoxide applied to the affected area and washed off after 10 minutes. Alternatively, malathion 0.5% lotion can be applied to affected areas and washed off after 8 to 12 hours, or ivermectin 250 mcg/kg can be given orally and repeated in 7 to 14 days.

Sexual partners within the previous month should be treated, and bedding and clothing must be decontaminated. Sexual contact should be avoided until treatment is complete. Pregnant and lactating females should be treated with either permethrin or pyrethrins with piperonyl butoxide.

Scabies

Infection with *Sarcoptes scabiei* causes pruritus, which takes up to several weeks to develop. Scabies in adults frequently is sexually acquired, although scabies in children usually is not.

Treatment consists of permethrin 5% cream applied to all areas of the body from the neck down and washed off after 8 to 14 hours or ivermectin 200 mcg/kg orally, repeated in 2 weeks. Permethrin is the treatment of choice for infants and young children. Alternatively, lindane 1%—either 1 oz of lotion or 30 g of cream—applied in a thin layer to all areas of the body from the neck down and thoroughly washed off after 8 hours may be used; however, pregnant patients, infants, and children younger than 10 years of age should *not* be treated with lindane.

Bedding and clothing should be decontaminated by either machine washing, machine drying using the hottest cycle, or dry cleaning; alternatively, bedding and clothing should be removed from body contact for at least 72 hours. Persons who have had sexual, close personal, or household contact with the patient within the month preceding scabies infestation should be examined and treated if infected.

CDC reports that though ivermectin is likely a low risk to pregnant and lactating females, because of limited data regarding use of ivermectin in pregnancy and lactating females, permethrin is the preferred treatment.

Trichomoniasis

The protozoan parasite *Trichomonas vaginalis* is the most common curable STI in the United States. Nearly 7.5 million cases occur annually. Most people with *T. vaginalis* (70%–85%) have minimal or no symptoms. Males may develop urethritis, epididymitis, or prostatitis. Some infected females may develop a diffuse vaginal discharge that is malodorous and yellow green, with or without vulvar irritation.

The nitroimidazoles are the only class of antimicrobials effective against *T. vaginalis*. Metronidazole 500 mg orally twice daily for 7 days for females, and 2 g orally in a single dose for males is the current recommendation for treatment by the CDC. Alternatively, tinidazole 2 g orally in a single dose may be used for both females and males.

Alcohol should be avoided during treatment with nitroimidazoles to prevent the likelihood of a disulfiram-like reaction. Abstinence from alcohol use should continue for 24 hours after completion of metronidazole or 72 hours after completion of tinidazole. Concurrent treatment of all sex partners is critical to prevent transmission and reinfection.

T. vaginalis is readily passed between sex partners. The best way to prevent infection is through consistent and correct use of condoms. Partners of males who have been circumcised might have a somewhat reduced risk of *T. vaginalis* infection.

T. vaginalis infection in pregnant patients is associated with premature rupture of membranes, preterm delivery, and delivery of a low-birth-weight infant. however, there is additional information regarding studies done in treatment of *T. vaginalis* in pregnancy at https://www.cdc.gov/std/treatment-guidelines/trichomoniasis.htm#Pregnancy.

Vulvovaginal Candidiasis

Vulvovaginal candidiasis (VVC) is usually caused by *Candida albicans* but may also be caused by other *Candida* species. Typical symptoms of VVC include pruritus, vaginal soreness, dyspareunia, external dysuria, and abnormal vaginal discharge. Signs include vulvar edema, fissures, excoriations, and a thick, curdy vaginal discharge.

Treatment with topically applied azole drugs results in symptomatic relief and negative cultures in 80% to 90% of patients who complete therapy. A variety of over-the-counter (OTC) and prescription drugs may be used to treat VVC. Treatment regimens include OTC and prescription intravaginal agents.

Over-the-Counter Intravaginal Agents. Clotrimazole 1% cream 5 g intravaginally daily for 7 to 14 days, clotrimazole 2% cream 5 g intravaginally daily for 3 days, miconazole 2% cream 5 g intravaginally daily for 7 days, miconazole 4% cream 5 g intravaginally daily for 3 days, one miconazole 100-mg vaginal suppository daily for 7 days, one miconazole 200-mg vaginal suppository daily for 3 days, one miconazole 1200 mg vaginal suppository, or tioconazole 6.5% ointment 5 g intravaginally in a single application.

Prescription Intravaginal Agents. Butoconazole 2% cream (single-dose bioadhesive product) 5 g intravaginally in a single application, terconazole 0.4% cream 5 g intravaginally daily for 7 days, terconazole 0.8% cream 5 g intravaginally daily for 3 days, or one terconazole 80 mg vaginal suppository daily for 3 days. Alternatively, an oral drug—fluconazole 150 mg orally in a single dose—may be used.

Topical agents usually cause no systemic side effects, although local burning or irritation might occur. Oral azoles occasionally cause nausea, abdominal pain, and headache.

VVC occurs frequently during pregnancy. Only topical azole therapies, applied for 7 days, are recommended for use among pregnant patients. Uncomplicated VVC is not usually acquired through sexual intercourse, thus treatment of sexual partners is not necessary.

PREVENTION OF SEXUALLY TRANSMITTED INFECTIONS

Because STIs can threaten reproductive health, neonatal health, fertility, and even life, early diagnosis and treatment are crucial but are less effective than prevention. Please review the information in Box 57.1 and in the Nursing Process box that discusses STI prevention.

CLINICAL JUDGMENT [NURSING PROCESS]
Sexually Transmitted Infections

Concept: Safety
- Protection of the patient from potential or actual harm; a basic human need

Concept: Sexuality
- A person's sexual expression and function

Recognize Cues [Assessment]
- Assess use of barrier methods and the patient's ability to obtain them.
- Assess patient history before gathering physical data. Address less sensitive issues before more personal ones so trust can first be established. Use the term *partner* when discussing sexual activity, rather than judgment-laden terms such as *wife* or *boyfriend*. Include the following questions for all patients, regardless of gender or sexual orientation: "Do you have sex with females?" and "Do you have sex with males?" Include information regarding the number of sexual partners.
- Assess history of drug use.
- Assess history of sexually transmitted infections (STIs).
- Assess support systems.
- Complete a review of body systems and obtain a general health history and a gynecologic history that includes reproductive history; also review lifestyle and social habits and identify known allergies.
- Physical examination includes inspection and palpation of the mouth, oropharynx, throat and lymph nodes, abdomen, and inguinal lymph systems. Also perform a physical examination of the genitalia and other points of potential inoculation.

Analyze Cues and Prioritize Hypothesis [Patient Problems]
- Need for health teaching
- Sexual expression
- Potential decreased adherence
- Decreased self-esteem

Generate Solutions [Planning]
- The patient will abstain from sexual contact until infection is treated and adopt risk-reducing sexual behaviors.
- The patient will identify signs and symptoms of STIs.
- The patient will verbalize when to seek medical attention.
- The patient will remain free from STIs.

Take Action [Nursing Interventions]
- Observe and report signs of infections (e.g., redness, discharge, fever).
- Note laboratory findings as appropriate.
- Ensure understanding of appropriate transmission-based precautions.
- Ensure an understanding of appropriate personal hygiene.
- Ensure responsible use of antibiotics.
- Discuss the risks for developing STIs with all patients, even older adults.
- Discuss condom use and counsel patients on effective use of condoms.
- See Fig. 57.2 for the right way to use a male condom.
- Review modes of transmission of STIs, the relationship of all STIs to human immunodeficiency virus (HIV) infection, and how HIV risk is avoided.
- Use a medical interpreter of the same sex and culture, especially for sensitive topics.

Evaluate Outcomes [Evaluation]
- The intervention has been successful if patients and their partners are successfully treated and remain free of infection.
- The patient is able to avoid sexual practices that carry risk for acquiring STIs, including intercourse without the use of a condom.

BOX 57.1 Special Topic: Sexually Transmitted Infections in the Older Adult

The rates of *Chlamydia*, gonorrhea, and syphilis have more than doubled in adults older than 50 years of age in recent years. More than 15% of newly diagnosed cases of HIV occur in adults older than 50 years of age. This spike in sexually transmitted infections (STIs) is felt to be related to a combination of factors:

- Patients are reluctant to bring up the issue with their health care providers, and their health care providers are reluctant to bring up the issue with the patient.
- Older adults may not consider oral or anal sex as a way to transmit STIs.
- We are living longer and have higher divorce rates than past generations, leading to increased numbers of older adults entering the dating scene.
- Postmenopausal changes in females (e.g., decreased vaginal lubrication) put them at increased risk for infection.
- The availability of drugs for erectile dysfunction makes sex possible for an increased number of older males.
- Rates of condom use are low because condoms were used to prevent pregnancy in previous generations, not to prevent STIs.

Nurses must discuss the risks for developing STIs with their older adult patients and should provide information on prevention. Nurses should not make the faulty assumption that older adults do not engage in sexual activity. Among males, 85% report that sex is important in their relationships; 61% of females report that sex is important in their relationships. Among older adults, 28% have sex at least once a week. However, only 12% of males and 32% of females use condoms.

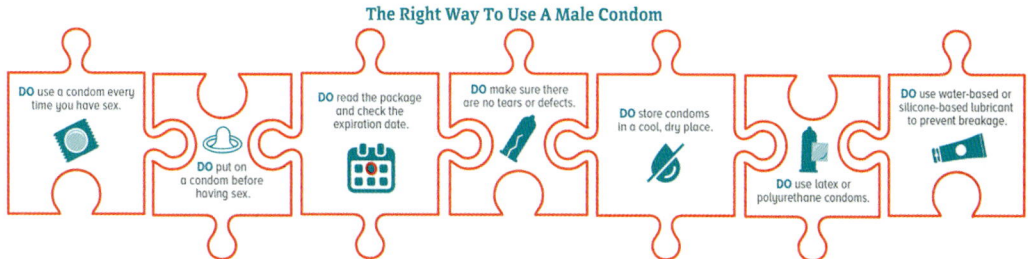

Fig. 57.2 How to use a male condom. (From Centers for Disease Control and Prevention: *The right way to use a male condom*, 2021. www.cdc.gov/condomeffectiveness)

CLINICAL JUDGMENT SINGLE-EPISODE CASE STUDY

Cognitive Skill: Take action
Item Type: Extended multiple response

A 16-year-old female comes to the clinic, reporting her partner has noted a whitish penile discharge and has burning with urination. She states she has been sexually active, both orally and vaginally, for 2 years and has had four partners during this time. She denies using any barrier methods to avoid infection and is not on any other form of birth control. The patient also reports a sore throat. She denies any cough or congestion, headache, nausea, vomiting, or diarrhea. She denies any burning, urgency, or frequency of urination or vaginal discharge. The patient is living with her 62-year-old grandmother, along with her older brother. Her mother and father lost their parental rights due to abuse. She admits to vaping cannabis for the past few years and drinks hard liquor when out with her partner. She is a year behind in school and has frequent tardiness and absences. Her blood pressure is 105/60 mm Hg, heart rate is 66 beats per minute, respirations 12 breaths per minute, and temperature 98.9°F. She is 5'8" tall and weighs 110 pounds (body mass index 16.72 kg/m^2). The nurse spends time talking with the patient before she is discharged from the clinic and providing necessary teaching and support.

What nursing actions are appropriate for the patient at this time? **Select all that apply.**

_____ a. Administer ceftriaxone 500 mg intramuscular as a single dose, as ordered.
_____ b. Teach the patient the appropriate use of condoms.
_____ c. Review the modes of sexually transmitted infection transmission with the patient.
_____ d. Assess the patient's support systems and make referrals as necessary.
_____ e. Discuss with the patient the necessity of her partner coming to the clinic for treatment.
_____ f. Instruct the patient to abstain from sexual activity for 7 days after treatment.

Answer

__X__ a. Administer ceftriaxone 500 mg intramuscular as a single dose, as ordered.
__X__ b. Teach the patient the appropriate use of condoms.
_____ c. Review the modes of sexually transmitted infection transmission with the patient.
_____ d. Assess the patient's support systems and make referrals, as necessary.
__X__ e. Discuss with the patient the necessity of her partner coming to the clinic for treatment.
__X__ f. Instruct the patient to abstain from sexual activity for 7 days after treatment.

Rationale

Due to developing resistance to azithromycin, in uncomplicated *N. gonorrhea* in adolescents and adults two-drug therapy is no longer recommended. Treatment of uncomplicated *N. gonorrhea* should be with ceftriaxone 500 mg intramuscular as a single dose. Appropriate nursing actions include assessing support systems and counseling patients on effective condom use, and the modes of sexually transmitted infection transmission should be reviewed with the patient. Partners should be treated if they had sexual contract during the 60 days preceding onset of symptoms or diagnosis. In this scenario, the partner is symptomatic as well and should be treated. Persons receiving treatment for gonorrhea should be instructed to abstain from sexual activity for 7 days after treatment.

REVIEW QUESTIONS

1. A patient at the sexually transmitted infection clinic asks why he was not prescribed antibiotics. He has been diagnosed with herpes simplex virus type 2. The nurse's best response is based on what knowledge? **Select all that apply.**
   a. Antibiotics will not lessen the symptoms of herpes simplex virus.
   b. Herpes simplex virus can be cured with antiviral medications only.
   c. Antibiotics are used to successfully treat viral infections.
   d. Herpes simplex virus symptoms may be relieved with palliative antiviral medications.
   e. Antibiotics combined with antiviral medications are the best treatment for herpes simplex virus type 2 infections.

2. The nurse is teaching a group of junior high school students about preventing sexually transmitted infections if they are sexually active. Which of the following are the best methods of prevention? **Select all that apply.**
   a. Douching after intercourse
   b. Monogamy
   c. Vaccination
   d. Consistent condom use
   e. Use of spermicidal creams

3. Which one of the following regimens is an appropriate treatment for episodic genital herpes infection?
   a. Acyclovir 400 mg orally three times for 7–10 days
   b. Famciclovir 2 g orally twice daily for 1 day
   c. Acyclovir 1 g orally once a day for 5 days
   d. Valacyclovir 500 mg orally twice a day for 7 days

4. The nurse is reviewing a patient's medications; she knows treatment of vulvovaginal candidiasis includes which drug?
   a. Metronidazole
   b. Fluconazole
   c. Metformin
   d. Ibuprofen

5. Your patient with primary syphilis has an order for penicillin G benzathine 2.4 million units IM × 1. You have available penicillin G benzathine 600,000 units per mL; how many mL will be administered?

6. When teaching a group of students about *Chlamydia*, which of the following should the health care provider emphasize? **Select all that apply.**
   a. Most people who have *Chlamydia* have no symptoms.
   b. Good hand hygiene is the best way to prevent chlamydial infections.

c. *Chlamydia* is the least common of all the major sexually transmitted infections.
   d. Burning and pain with urination may be a symptom of chlamydial infections.
   e. *Chlamydia* has no effect on future pregnancies.
7. A patient diagnosed with trichomoniasis is being treated with a nitroimidazole. When teaching the patient about this medication, which of the following is the most important for the nurse to include?
   a. Call our office if you experience any tendon pain or tenderness.
   b. You should avoid milk or dairy products during therapy.
   c. Do not drink alcohol while you are taking this medication.
   d. Report the occurrence of pain in your upper abdomen immediately.
8. Your patient calls stating she stopped taking the oral metronidazole that was prescribed because her symptoms resolved, and she wanted to drink at her best friend's bridal shower. As her nurse, what is your best response?
   a. No serious complications can happen from untreated *T. vaginalis*, so don't worry.
   b. Without treatment, the organism remains in your body, and you remain contagious.
   c. Because your symptoms are gone, there is no need to complete the course of metronidazole.
   d. If symptoms return, come back.

UNIT XVIII Emergency Drugs

58

Adult and Pediatric Emergency Drugs

Linda Laskowski-Jones, MS, APRN, ACNS-BC, CEN, NEA-BC, FAWM, FAAN

http://evolve.elsevier.com/McCuistion/pharmacology

OBJECTIVES

- Describe the purpose of oxygen as an emergency drug.
- Summarize the emergency drugs used for cardiac disorders.
- Summarize mannitol's use as an emergency drug for intracranial hypertensive emergency.
- Describe pharmacologic interventions for drug overdose.
- Summarize emergency drugs used to treat shock.
- Summarize emergency drugs used to treat hypertensive crises.

OUTLINE

Oxygen as an Emergency Drug, 762
    Drug Classification and Effects, 762
    Uses and Considerations of Oxygen as an Emergency Drug, 762
Emergency Drugs for Cardiac Disorders, 762
    Aspirin, 762
    Nitroglycerin, 762
    Morphine Sulfate, 763
    Atropine Sulfate, 763
    Adenosine, 764
    Diltiazem, 764
    Amiodarone, 764
    Lidocaine, 765
    Procainamide, 765
    Magnesium Sulfate, 765
    Epinephrine, 766
    Sodium Bicarbonate, 766
For Intracranial Hypertension: Mannitol, 767
    Dosages of Mannitol, 767
    Uses and Considerations of Mannitol, 767
Emergency Drugs for Drug Overdose, 767
    Naloxone, 767
    Flumazenil, 768
    Activated Charcoal, 768
Emergency Drugs for Shock, 769
    Dopamine, 770
    Dobutamine, 770
    Norepinephrine, 770
    Epinephrine, 771
    Albuterol, 771
    Diphenhydramine Hydrochloride, 771
    Dextrose 50%, 771
    Glucagon, 772
Emergency Drugs for Hypertensive Crises, 772
    Labetalol, 772
    Nitroprusside Sodium, 773
    Furosemide, 774
Clinical Judgment Single-Episode Case Study, 774
Clinical Judgment Case Study, 775
Review Questions, 775

This final unit focuses on adult and pediatric first-line emergency drugs. This chapter considers oxygen as an emergency drug and discusses pharmacologic treatment for five categories of emergency situations: (1) cardiac disorders, (2) intracranial hypertension, (3) poisoning, (4) shock, and (5) hypertensive crises and pulmonary edema. Specific drug protocols and dosages for the pediatric patient are included when appropriate.

The drugs described in this chapter are first-line agents used to treat selected common emergency situations. Nurses must have knowledge of the indications and actions of these drugs because medical and surgical emergencies can occur in virtually any area of nursing practice. Learning key nursing implications *before* a crisis situation enables the nurse to function at the highest possible level when the patient requires life-saving intervention.

At the end of the discussion of each group of emergency drugs is a summary prototype drug chart that contains dosages and indications. Common adult dosages are listed in the drug charts; pediatric dosages may vary widely depending on the child's age and weight. For the purpose of drug dosing, advanced life support (ALS) guidelines consider adults to be older than 8 years and children to be 8 years or younger; infants are younger than 1 year. The drug charts list only the most common indications and dosages for the emergency drugs discussed; they do *not* describe all possible uses and dosing regimens for each drug.

OXYGEN AS AN EMERGENCY DRUG

Oxygen can be classified as a drug because it can have both beneficial and adverse effects on the body based on the amount and manner administered. Oxygen is essential to life—without it, brain death begins within 6 minutes. Inadequate oxygenation produces **hypoxemia**, inadequate oxygen in the blood, and leads to significant physiologic sequelae to all body systems; therefore oxygen is a first-line drug for all emergency situations in which hypoxemia poses a physiologic threat.

Drug Classification and Effects

Oxygen is a pulmonary vasodilator and a cerebral vasoconstrictor. Depending on the circumstances, adequate oxygenation may be all that is necessary to effectively treat physiologic disturbances that arise from hypoxemia, such as chest pain, bradycardia, and cardiac dysrhythmias. However, current evidence suggests that more liberal oxygen administration may be associated with increased mortality in patients who are not hypoxemic.

Uses and Considerations of Oxygen as an Emergency Drug

Before the other pharmacologic drugs discussed in this chapter are administered, ensure that the patient's airway and breathing are addressed to promote **normoxemia**, typically defined as an oxygen saturation between 94% and 99% depending on the patient's diagnosis and physiologic state. Giving a drug to treat a disorder brought on by hypoxemia without effectively correcting the cause of the hypoxemia is ineffective and ultimately does not produce the desired outcome. **Pulse oximetry**, which provides a digital display of oxygen saturation, is an essential monitoring tool that should be used in emergency situations to assess the adequacy of oxygenation and guide further interventions. Ideally, oxygen saturation should be titrated based on defined clinical parameters. For example, a patient who was successfully resuscitated from cardiac arrest should have oxygen delivered to achieve pulse oximetry readings in a range of 92% to 98%, while a patient who had a stroke should achieve oxygen saturation of greater than 94%. Increasing the saturation beyond the goal saturation range with supplemental oxygen may produce detrimental effects. It is also important to recognize that certain pathophysiologic states can make pulse oximetry readings inaccurate. These conditions include vasoconstriction, severe anemia, hypothermia, carbon monoxide poisoning, and shock.

The ambient room air contains approximately 21% oxygen. When patients breathe room air, the oxygen they inspire constitutes 21% of the total volume of gas they take in with each breath. This measure is termed the **fraction of inspired oxygen (FiO_2)**. Patients with hypoxemia due to severe physiologic stress from shock states, major trauma with hemodynamic instability, and cardiac arrest initially require supplemental oxygen in high concentrations (i.e., an FiO_2 approaching 100%). The initial emergency oxygen delivery devices of choice for these conditions include a nonrebreather mask with an oxygen reservoir (oxygen flow rate set at 10–15 L/min) for spontaneously breathing patients and a bag valve mask device attached to an oxygen source at a flow rate of 15 L/min for patients who require assisted ventilation until definitive airway management and a mechanical ventilator are available.

Although caution must be exercised for patients with chronic obstructive pulmonary disease (COPD), who may lose their hypoxic respiratory drive when given oxygen in high concentration, oxygen should never be denied to a patient who needs it. In the case of COPD, the nurse should be prepared to ventilate the patient manually with a bag valve mask if respiratory depression or arrest occurs. Some patients in respiratory distress as a result of obstructive pulmonary disease or acute cardiogenic pulmonary edema may also benefit from oxygen therapy delivered through noninvasive mask ventilation via a continuous positive airway pressure (CPAP) or bilevel positive airway pressure (BiPAP) circuit; these devices deliver oxygen via a positive-pressure mechanism.

Whatever the underlying injury or disease process, as the patient's condition stabilizes, the oxygen concentration should be decreased to achieve the goal range, typically an arterial oxygen saturation between 94% and 96%. An FiO_2 above 50% for a prolonged period can lead to oxygen toxicity and other detrimental effects in both adults and children.

For situations that do not involve severe physiologic stress, supplemental oxygen delivered by nasal cannula at 1 to 6 L/min or by simple face mask at 6 to 10 L/min may be considered. Young children may better tolerate a face tent with a high oxygen flow of 10 to 15 L than a face mask. Current evidence suggests that oxygen administration to hemodynamically stable patients without heart failure who are normoxemic may offer no therapeutic benefit, may be detrimental, and should be avoided.

EMERGENCY DRUGS FOR CARDIAC DISORDERS

Drugs described in this section are indicated for cardiac emergencies such as angina, **myocardial infarction ([MI] heart attack)**, disturbances of cardiac rate or rhythm, and cardiac arrest. In a resuscitation situation, the foundation of patient therapy is based on proper oxygenation and ventilation, performance of optimal cardiopulmonary resuscitation (CPR), and application of electrical therapy (cardioversion and defibrillation) according to established treatment algorithms and standards. Drugs are used as adjuncts in synchrony with these efforts when indicated to enhance the likelihood of a successful outcome. These drugs often must be prepared and administered rapidly. A sound knowledge base and easy access to the drugs and necessary equipment are essential for the best patient response in a cardiac emergency. In many emergency situations, detailed personal, medical, drug, and herbal histories are unavailable. Treatment is based on patient presentation.

Aspirin

The nonenteric form of aspirin is a first-line emergency drug used to decrease platelet aggregation in the management of acute coronary syndromes and MI. It is best administered immediately upon the onset of chest pain in doses of 162 to 325 mg orally. The patient should be asked to chew the tablet to speed absorption of the drug instead of swallowing the tablet whole. For patients experiencing nausea and vomiting, an aspirin rectal suppository in a dose of 300 mg can be given as an alternative. Contraindications to aspirin administration include a true drug allergy, presence of cerebral hemorrhage on computed tomography (CT) scan, and recent gastrointestinal (GI) bleeding.

Nitroglycerin

Nitroglycerin dilates coronary arteries and improves blood flow to an ischemic myocardium. It is therefore the treatment of choice for **angina pectoris** (chest pain) and MI. Nitroglycerin is also considered a first-line drug in the management of patients with acute cardiogenic pulmonary edema due to its ability to decrease both preload and afterload. A focused prescription drug history is essential before administration, even in emergency situations, because nitroglycerin in combination with drugs for erectile dysfunction (i.e., sildenafil, vardenafil, tadalafil) causes profound hypotension that may be refractory to treatment when taken within a 24- to 48-hour period. This combination is contraindicated. Nitroglycerin is available in sublingual, translingual aerosol spray, oral, topical, and intravenous (IV) forms. Only the sublingual, translingual aerosol spray, and IV preparations are discussed.

Sublingual nitroglycerin (0.3- to 0.6-mg tablets) and the translingual aerosol spray (0.4 mg metered dose) preparations are indicated for patients experiencing an acute anginal attack who have a systolic blood pressure above 90 mm Hg. The patient is taught to sit or lie down and moisten 1 sublingual nitroglycerin tablet with saliva and then place it under the tongue to allow it to dissolve slowly. If the chest pain is not relieved, sublingual nitroglycerin may be repeated at 5-minute intervals—as long as the patient's systolic blood pressure remains above 90 mm Hg—until a total of 3 tablets have been taken. Patients prescribed the translingual aerosol preparation should be reminded that the spray should not be inhaled. Instead, it should be sprayed onto or under the tongue. The patient should be instructed not to swallow for approximately 10 seconds to allow absorption of the drug. As with sublingual nitroglycerin, up to 3 doses may be taken within 15 minutes. If pain persists despite 3 doses of the sublingual tablet or aerosol forms, further interventions are necessary in an emergency or critical care setting. An ambulance should be called if the patient is outside the hospital, and blood pressure and heart rate must be monitored closely. Hypotension is a common adverse effect, especially the first time a patient takes nitroglycerin. Tachycardia, an abnormally high heart rate in adults (>100 beats/min), or, uncommonly, bradycardia, a slow heart rate, also may occur. Patients who take sublingual tablets or translingual aerosol spray nitroglycerin while wearing a nitroglycerin patch may be at higher risk for hypotension. This situation warrants caution. However, individuals who take daily nitroglycerin can develop tolerance to the drug, which can provide some protection against hypotension. If hypotension persists or worsens, the nitroglycerin patch may need to be removed. To prevent arcing and the potential for skin burns, the nitroglycerin patch, like other medication patches in the area of the pads or paddles, must be removed before cardioversion or defibrillation.

Intravenous nitroglycerin is reserved for patients with unstable angina or AMI. A continuous infusion is usually initiated at a rate of 5 mcg/min and titrated by 5 mcg/min every 3 to 5 minutes based on chest pain and blood pressure response. Maximum rate of titration is 20 mcg/min every 3 to 5 minutes. Continuous blood pressure and heart monitoring are required because hypotension is a common adverse effect. Hypotension usually is treated by reducing or discontinuing the nitroglycerin infusion (see Chapter 40) and by placing the patient in a supine position with legs elevated if tolerated.

Morphine Sulfate

Morphine sulfate, an opiate analgesic, is used to treat the chest pain associated with ST-segment elevation myocardial infarction (STEMI) if unrelieved by nitroglycerin administration. It also is indicated for acute cardiogenic pulmonary edema. Morphine relieves pain, dilates venous vessels, and reduces the workload on the heart. The standard dosage of morphine sulfate is 1 to 4 mg IV over 1 to 5 minutes, repeated every 5 to 30 minutes until chest pain is relieved. Because respiratory depression and hypotension are common adverse effects, the drug must be administered slowly and must be carefully titrated to achieve the desired therapeutic effects. Close patient monitoring is essential. It is important to realize that although morphine can produce respiratory depression, this drug can also relieve the dyspnea caused by pulmonary edema. In this situation, respiratory distress is not a contraindication to morphine administration. The opioid antagonist naloxone may be ordered to reverse the action of morphine if adverse effects pose a significant risk to the patient. The dose is 0.4 to 2 mg every 2 minutes as indicated (see Chapter 25).

Atropine Sulfate

Atropine sulfate is the primary drug indicated for the treatment of hemodynamically significant bradycardia and some types of heart block (e.g., atrioventricular [AV] block at the nodal level). Atropine acts to increase heart rate by inhibiting the action of the vagus nerve (parasympatholytic effect). Atropine sulfate is also used as an emergency drug to reverse the toxic effects of organophosphate pesticide and nerve agent exposure, which include bradycardia and excessive secretions.

In symptomatic bradycardia with hemodynamic compromise, atropine is administered IV in 1 mg doses at 3- to 5-minute intervals until the desired heart rate is achieved or until 3 mg is given. Dosing in this manner may be repeated every 3 to 5 minutes up to a maximum of 3 mg IV.

If venous access is not available in an emergency situation, atropine sulfate should be administered through the intraosseous (IO) route.

Continuous cardiac and blood pressure monitoring is essential for the patient who receives atropine sulfate. Significant adverse effects include cardiac dysrhythmias, tachycardia, myocardial ischemia, restlessness, anxiety, mydriasis, thirst, and urinary retention. See Chapter 16 for more information on atropine and other anticholinergics.

Adult Implications

The adult IV atropine dose should never be less than 0.5 mg. Doses below 0.5 mg may produce a paradoxical bradycardia; at doses of 3 mg or greater, vagal activity is considered completely blocked, and further atropine administration may have no benefit. However, in the case of organophosphate insecticide or nerve agent poisoning, *very high* doses of atropine may be necessary to counteract the pathophysiologic effects of these toxins. Therefore the typical dosing range and limits do not apply under these circumstances.

Pediatric Implications

The definition of bradycardia is variable and age-specific for the pediatric population. Knowledge of normal ranges is essential. Because cardiac output is dependent on heart rate in infants younger than 6 months, bradycardia (heart rate <100 beats/min for infants) must be treated. In fact, a heart rate of less than 60 beats/min in an infant requires performance of CPR. Before administration of drugs, efforts always should be targeted first toward restoring adequate ventilation and oxygenation. For the neonate with a spontaneous heart rate of less than 80 beats/min, epinephrine 0.01 mg/kg IV or IO every 3 to 5 minutes as indicated should be given before atropine to elevate the heart rate because stressed neonates quickly deplete their own stores of catecholamines. If these interventions do not produce the desired clinical response, atropine is indicated in the presence of increased vagal tone or AV block. Other pediatric indications for atropine include management of organophosphate toxicity and as pretreatment to prevent bradycardia after succinylcholine administration during rapid-sequence intubation, although this specific indication is currently controversial.

The pediatric dose of atropine is 0.02 mg/kg IV or IO. It is important to be cognizant that in the pediatric population, the minimum single dose is 0.1 mg, and the maximum single dose is 0.5 mg IV. The maximum total pediatric dose is 1 mg in a child and 3 mg in an adolescent (defined as an individual who has reached puberty). Note that when referring to general age groupings of patients, *infants* are considered to be younger than 1 year; a *child* is considered to be 1 year of age to adolescence (puberty), and an *adult* is considered to be an adolescent or older. See Chapters 6, 10, and 11 for more information on pediatric medication dosing and monitoring.

Adenosine

Adenosine is the first-line drug of choice to treat paroxysmal supraventricular tachycardia (PSVT), a sudden, uncontrolled, rapid rhythm that exceeds 150 ventricular beats/min in adults and originates above the ventricles. The goal is to convert PSVT to sinus rhythm. Adenosine, a natural substance found in all body cells, slows impulse conduction through the heart's AV node, interrupts dysrhythmia-producing reentry pathways, and restores a normal rhythm in patients with PSVT. Because the half-life is less than 5 seconds, adenosine is best administered rapidly via a peripheral IV site in the port most proximal to the patient as a 6 mg IV bolus over 1 second followed by a saline flush and immediate elevation of the arm. A 12 mg bolus may be given 1 to 2 minutes after the initial dose using the same procedure if PSVT persists. The 12-mg dose may be repeated once if indicated for persistent PSVT. Higher doses are not recommended.

Nursing considerations include continuous cardiac monitoring and frequent assessment of vital signs. Adenosine is inhibited by methylxanthines such as caffeine and theophylline, so higher doses may be needed. Although usually transient, ventricular ectopy, bradycardia, flushing, chest pain, and dyspnea may occur. In addition, a short period of asystole may follow injection of adenosine (up to 15 seconds). Spontaneous cardiac activity typically resumes. Adenosine is contraindicated in patients with poison- or drug-related tachycardia, second- and third-degree heart block, and sick sinus syndrome except those with functioning pacemakers. If the tachycardia originated in the ventricles, the patient could deteriorate and become hypotensive after adenosine administration. Adenosine is contraindicated in patients with bronchospastic disease because it may induce bronchospasm. See Chapter 37 for more information on antidysrhythmic drugs.

Pediatric Implications

Adenosine is used to treat narrow complex PSVT in pediatric patients who do not have evidence of cardiopulmonary compromise such as an altered mental status, shock, or hypotension. The dose is 0.1 mg/kg as a rapid IV/IO bolus to a maximum first dose of 6 mg. If the PSVT does not resolve after the first dose, a second dose of 0.2 mg/kg as a rapid IV/IO bolus to a maximum second dose of 12 mg can be given. The same nursing considerations and precautions apply as described for adults.

Diltiazem

Diltiazem is a calcium channel blocker, and it is administered as an IV bolus to treat PSVT and to slow the ventricular response rate in atrial fibrillation or flutter. It is considered a second-line agent after adenosine. Diltiazem has less of a negative inotropic effect than other, similar calcium channel blockers, but it has strong negative chronotropic actions. Therefore IV diltiazem is less likely to cause cardiac depression but is very effective in controlling heart rate.

The usual initial bolus dose of IV diltiazem is 0.25 mg/kg given over 2 minutes. If the supraventricular tachycardia does not convert to a normal sinus rhythm in 15 minutes, a second IV bolus of 0.35 mg/kg over 2 minutes may be necessary. For ongoing control of the ventricular rate in patients with atrial fibrillation or flutter, a continuous infusion of diltiazem is indicated at a dose range of 5 to 15 mg/h, titrated according to the desired heart rate.

The nurse must carefully monitor blood pressure and heart rate and rhythm after administering IV diltiazem. Arrhythmias, bradycardia, heart block, and hypotension may develop. Diltiazem can elevate serum digoxin levels, predisposing the patient to digitalis toxicity. Simultaneous use of calcium channel blockers and beta blockers is contraindicated because their negative inotropic and negative chronotropic effects are synergistic, causing myocardial depression and bradycardia. Other contraindications include preexisting heart failure, Wolff-Parkinson-White syndrome, heart block, or sick sinus syndrome in the patient without a pacemaker, and in advanced aortic stenosis.

Amiodarone

The IV form of amiodarone is considered a first-line drug in the ALS algorithms for the treatment of life-threatening ventricular dysrhythmias and cardiac arrest. It has alpha- and beta-adrenergic blocking effects and acts on sodium, potassium, and calcium channels. Indications for use include pulseless ventricular tachycardia and ventricular fibrillation (after defibrillation and epinephrine), hemodynamically stable ventricular tachycardia, PSVT refractory to adenosine, ventricular rate control in atrial fibrillation, and pharmacologic treatment of atrial fibrillation.

Amiodarone is especially effective for patients with impaired heart function who have atrial and ventricular dysrhythmias. It has been found to be more effective and to have fewer proarrhythmic properties than other drugs with similar actions.

For patients who have a pulse (i.e., those *not* in cardiac arrest), amiodarone 150 mg IV is given over 10 minutes, followed by a continuous infusion of 1 mg/min for 6 hours. For patients in cardiac arrest with pulseless ventricular tachycardia or ventricular fibrillation, a dose of 300 mg diluted in 20 to 30 mL D_5W is given as a rapid infusion followed by a continuous infusion as described earlier. Additional doses of 150 mg may be given by rapid infusion if ventricular fibrillation or ventricular tachycardia recurs.

Significant adverse effects include hypotension and bradycardia; therefore the nurse would slow the infusion rate to prevent or treat these effects and be prepared to administer IV fluids, vasopressors, and agents to increase heart rate. A temporary pacemaker may be needed. Amiodarone has a very long half-life. It should not be given concurrently with other drugs that prolong QT interval on electrocardiography (ECG), such as procainamide.

Pediatric Implications

Amiodarone has an off-label use among pediatric patients. It is given for pulseless ventricular tachycardia and ventricular fibrillation as a 5 mg/kg rapid IV/IO bolus, which can be repeated up to a maximum dose of 15 mg/kg per 24 hours. For responsive children who have supraventricular (junctional and atrial) tachycardia and ventricular dysrhythmias with pulses present, amiodarone is given as a 5 mg/kg IV/IO loading dose (300 mg maximum) over 20 to 60 minutes and repeated to a maximum daily IV dose of 15 mg/kg per 24 hours in pediatric patients or 2.2 g per 24 hours in adolescents.

PROTOTYPE DRUG CHART
Lidocaine Hydrochloride

Drug Class	Dosage
Antidysrhythmic, class IB	A: IV/IO: 1–1.5 mg/kg; may repeat 0.5 mg/kg q5–10 min; *max*: 3 mg/kg A: ETT: 2–4 mg/kg C: IV/IO: Initially: 1 mg/kg C: ETT: 2–3 mg/kg Therapeutic range: 2–6 mcg/mL
Contraindications	**Drug-Lab-Food Interactions**
Hypersensitivity, advanced atrioventricular block *Caution:* Liver disease, heart failure, older adults	Drug: Increased effects with phenytoin, quinidine, procainamide, propranolol; increased risk for toxicity with cimetidine, beta-adrenergic blockers
Pharmacokinetics	**Pharmacodynamics**
Absorption: IV Distribution: PB: 60%–80%; concentrates in adipose tissue Metabolism: t½: Initial: 7–30 min; terminal: 9–120 min Excretion: Through the liver	PO: Onset: 45–60 s Peak: 45–60 s Duration: 10–20 min
Therapeutic Effects/Uses	
Antiarrhythmic drug to treat ventricular dysrhythmias such as premature ventricular contractions (PVCs), ventricular tachycardia, and ventricular fibrillation Mechanism of action: Decreases automaticity; increases electrical threshold of ventricle	
Side Effects	**Adverse Reactions**
Drowsiness, confusion, dyspnea, lethargy, hypotension, nausea, vomiting	*Life-threatening:* Seizures, cardiac arrest

A, adult; *C*, child; *ETT*, endotracheal tube; *IO*, intraosseous; *IV*, intravenous; *max*, maximum; *min*, minute; *PB*, protein binding; *PO*, by mouth; *q*, every; *s*, seconds; *t½*, half-life.

Lidocaine

As a first-line agent and alternative to amiodarone, lidocaine may be used to treat significant ventricular dysrhythmias, or irregular heartbeats, such as frequent premature ventricular contractions (PVCs), ventricular tachycardia, and ventricular fibrillation. Lidocaine exerts a local anesthetic effect on the heart, thus decreasing myocardial irritability. Typically, a patient with ventricular dysrhythmias is given a 1 to 1.5 mg/kg bolus of lidocaine, followed by 0.5 mg/kg to 0.75 mg/kg every 5 to 10 minutes until the dysrhythmia is controlled or a total dose of 3 mg/kg has been administered via the IV or IO route.

Important nursing considerations for the patient receiving lidocaine include continuous cardiac monitoring and assessment for signs and symptoms of lidocaine toxicity (e.g., confusion, drowsiness, hearing impairment, cardiac conduction defects, myocardial depression, muscle twitching, and seizures). Because lidocaine is metabolized by the liver, patients with hepatic impairment are at a higher risk for toxicity; other risks include heart failure, shock, and advanced age (>70 years). In these patients, the lidocaine dose may need to be reduced by as much as 50% (see Chapter 40). Lidocaine is contraindicated as a *prophylactic* agent to prevent ventricular dysrhythmias after acute MI.

Pediatric Implications

Ventricular ectopy is uncommon in children; therefore metabolic causes should be suspected if ventricular dysrhythmias occur. The pediatric dose of lidocaine is 1 mg/kg IV or via the IO route, and the endotracheal tube (ETT) dose is 2 to 3 mg/kg. Prototype Drug Chart: Lidocaine Hydrochloride lists the pharmacologic data for lidocaine.

Procainamide

Procainamide is an antidysrhythmic drug prescribed for ventricular tachycardia, PVCs, and rapid supraventricular dysrhythmias unresponsive to adenosine. The typical IV loading dose of procainamide is 20 to 50 mg/min until the dysrhythmia is successfully treated. Other end points to procainamide administration include a total administration of 17 mg/kg of the drug, development of hypotension, and specific changes on the ECG (e.g., widening of the QRS complex by 50% or more). A continuous maintenance infusion of 1 to 4 mg/min may be ordered after the loading dose. A procainamide infusion should be avoided in patients with congestive heart failure and in those with a prolonged QT interval.

The nurse must monitor vital signs and the ECG with particular attention to heart rate and rhythm, blood pressure, and the width of the QRS complex. Procainamide administration can cause severe hypotension. Heart block, rhythm disturbances, and cardiac arrest can also occur. Procainamide is contraindicated in patients with torsades de pointes, an unusual polymorphic ventricular tachycardia often associated with a prolonged QT interval. Procainamide is eliminated via the kidneys; therefore patients with renal failure are at higher risk of adverse effects and often require a lower dosage.

Magnesium Sulfate

Magnesium is an essential element in multiple enzymatic reactions in the body, including function of the sodium-potassium adenosine triphosphatase (ATPase) pump. Its physiologic effects can be likened to a calcium channel blocker with neuromuscular blocking properties. Hypomagnesemia is associated with the development of atrial and ventricular dysrhythmias.

Magnesium sulfate is the drug of choice for torsades de pointes. It is administered by diluting 1 to 2 g (2–4 mL of a 50% solution) in 10 mL of D_5W or normal saline. For cardiac arrest caused by torsades de pointes, magnesium is given by direct IV push or via the IO route over 5 to 20 minutes. For patients experiencing torsades de pointes who are not in cardiac arrest, a magnesium infusion of 1 to 2 g diluted in 50 to 100 mL of D_5W or normal saline can be given IV/IO over 5 to 60 minutes.

Although magnesium toxicity is rare, the nurse should monitor the patient's response to magnesium administration. Hypotension is the most common adverse effect when magnesium is given by rapid IV push. Other effects include mild bradycardia, flush, and sweating. True hypermagnesemia can cause diarrhea, respiratory depression, deep tendon reflex impairment, flaccid paralysis, and circulatory collapse. Because magnesium is eliminated via the kidneys, it should be administered with caution in patients with renal impairment.

Pediatric Implications

Indications for magnesium sulfate in pediatric patients include torsades de pointes, hypomagnesemia, and status asthmaticus that is unresponsive to beta-adrenergic drugs. The magnesium sulfate dose is 25 to 50 mg/kg IV/IO (maximum dose of 2 g) given as a bolus for pulseless ventricular tachycardia, slowly over 10 to 20 minutes for ventricular tachycardia with pulses and over 15 to 30 minutes for status asthmaticus.

Epinephrine

Epinephrine is a catecholamine with alpha- and beta-adrenergic effects. It has multiple uses. Emergency cardiac indications for administration of IV/IO epinephrine include profound bradycardia and hypotension, asystole, pulseless ventricular tachycardia, and ventricular fibrillation. Epinephrine is thought to improve perfusion of the heart and brain in cardiac arrest states by constricting peripheral blood vessels. After the initial defibrillation attempt in ventricular fibrillation and pulseless ventricular tachycardia, epinephrine may increase the chances for successful subsequent electrical countershock (defibrillation). It is important to be aware that epinephrine is available in two primary concentrations: 1:1000 and 1:10,000. The 1:10,000 concentration is used when administering a single IV/IO dose of epinephrine. The 1:1000 form is used when preparing a continuous epinephrine infusion or when giving epinephrine via the intramuscular (IM) route. The subcutaneous (subcut) route should not be used for emergency epinephrine administration because absorption is unpredictable.

For profound bradycardia or hypotension, an epinephrine infusion may be ordered at 0.1 to 0.5 mcg/kg per minute. For asystole, pulseless ventricular tachycardia, and ventricular fibrillation, epinephrine is administered in 1 mg doses (1:10,000 solution) IV/IO every 3 to 5 minutes until the desired clinical response—usually return of effective cardiac activity—is achieved. In pulseless ventricular tachycardia and ventricular fibrillation, epinephrine is administered after the second defibrillation is delivered during CPR.

Nursing implications for patients receiving epinephrine include constant cardiac and hemodynamic monitoring. Epinephrine can cause myocardial ischemia and cardiac dysrhythmias. It should never be administered in the same site as an alkaline solution, such as with sodium bicarbonate, because alkaline solutions inactivate epinephrine. In addition, the presence of metabolic or respiratory acidosis decreases the effectiveness of epinephrine. All efforts should be made to correct acid-base imbalances in the patient. More drug information about epinephrine and other adrenergic drugs can be found in Chapter 15.

> ### ⚡ PATIENT SAFETY
> - Ensure the correct concentration (1:1000 vs. 1:10,000) is administered. The 1:10,000 preparation is meant to be given intravenously.

Pediatric Implications

The pediatric dose of epinephrine is 0.01 mg/kg (1:10,000 solution) given every 3 to 5 minutes IV/IO for cardiac arrest. For profound bradycardia or hypotension in pediatric patients, a continuous infusion of epinephrine can be given at a dose of 0.1 mcg/kg per minute via IV/IO. Higher doses may be considered.

Sodium Bicarbonate

Sodium bicarbonate is prescribed to treat severe metabolic acidosis as well as hyperkalemia and acidotic states related to specific drug overdose situations. Sodium bicarbonate is not considered a first-line drug for the treatment of cardiac arrest; it is preferentially given based on results of arterial blood gas analysis when acidosis is severe. The current standard is to give sodium bicarbonate only after adequate resuscitative efforts, including effective ventilation, IV fluids, and drug therapy, fail to correct the acidotic state in cardiopulmonary arrest. The standard initial IV dose of sodium bicarbonate is 1 mEq/kg. Subsequent dosing depends on arterial blood gas analysis and achievement of therapeutic targets.

Important nursing considerations relevant to sodium bicarbonate include careful monitoring of arterial blood gas analysis results. Sodium bicarbonate administration can lead to metabolic alkalosis, which may be very difficult to reverse and can have deleterious physiologic effects. Catecholamines such as epinephrine, norepinephrine, and dopamine should not be infused in the same site as sodium bicarbonate because they are inactivated by solutions that contain sodium bicarbonate.

Table 58.1 lists emergency cardiac drugs and their dosages, uses, and considerations.

TABLE 58.1 Emergency Cardiac Drugs

Generic	Route and Dosage[a]	Uses and Considerations
Adenosine	A/C/Adol >50 kg: IV/IO: Initially 6 mg, then 12 mg in 1–2 min if needed C/Adol <50 kg: IV/IO: 0.1 mg/kg per dose. May repeat 0.2 mg/kg per dose	For paroxysmal supraventricular tachycardia PB: UK; t½: <10 s
Amiodarone	A: IV: With pulse: 150 mg over 10 min, then continuous infusion 1 mg/min for 6 h Cardiac arrest: 300 mg diluted in 20–30 mL D$_5$W rapidly; second dose 150 mg, followed by continuous infusion as previously discussed; *max*: 2.2 g/d	Part of ALS algorithm for treatment of both atrial and ventricular dysrhythmias PB: UK; t½: 26–107 d
Atropine sulfate	A: IV/IO: 1 mg; can repeat up to 0.04 mg/kg or 3 mg (max) C/Adol: IV: 0.02 mg/kg per dose, repeat up to 1 mg max in C; 3 mg max in Adol	For symptomatic bradycardia and asystole PB: 60%–80%; t½: 2–3 h
Diltiazem	A: IV: 0.25 mg/kg; repeat in 15 min at 0.35 mg/kg IV drip: 5–10 mg/h	For supraventricular tachycardia and atrial fibrillation and flutter PB: 80%; t½: 2–5 h
Epinephrine	A: IV: 1 mg; may be repeated q3–5 min C/Adol: IV: 0.01 mg/kg per dose, may repeat q3–5 min C/Adol: ETT: 0.1 mg/kg per dose, may repeat q3–5 min	For cardiac arrest PB: UK; t½: UK
Lidocaine	See Prototype Drug Chart: Lidocaine	
Magnesium sulfate	A: Dilute 1–2 g (2–4 mL of 50% solution) in 10 mL of D$_5$W. Give IV/IO in cardiac arrest due to torsades de pointes over 5–20 min Torsades de pointes with a pulse: 1–2 g diluted in 50–100 mL of D$_5$W given IV over 5–60 min followed by continuous infusion of 0.5–1 g/h	Drug of choice for torsades de pointes after defibrillation in patients with a prolonged QT interval; rapid infusion can cause hypotension PB: 25%–35%; t½: 30 min

TABLE 58.1 Emergency Cardiac Drugs—cont'd

Generic	Route and Dosage[a]	Uses and Considerations
Morphine sulfate	A: IV: 1–5 mg q5–30 min	For chest pain, unstable angina, pulmonary edema PB: 35%; t½: 2–2.5 h
Nitroglycerin	A: SL: 0.3–0.6 mg; translingual aerosol spray: 0.4 mg metered dose, up to 3 tab/sprays within 15 min onto or under the tongue A: IV drip: Initially 5 mcg/min; titrate by 5 mcg/min q3–5 min; *max rate of titration:* 20 mcg/min q3–5 min	For chest pain, angina, unstable angina, MI; hypotension can occur *Contraindication:* With drugs for erectile dysfunction (e.g., sildenafil) PB: 60%; t½: 1–4 min
Procainamide hydrochloride	A: IV: 20–50 mg/min; *max:* 17 mg/kg; followed by 1–4 mg/min IV drip Recognized end points: Hypotension, QRS widens >50%, or total of 500 mg administered	For PVCs, ventricular tachycardia, ventricular fibrillation, atrial dysrhythmias PB: 20%; t½: 3–4 h
Sodium bicarbonate	A/C >2 y: IV: Initially 1 mEq/kg, then dose based on ABG results	For severe metabolic acidosis unresponsive to resuscitation, hyperkalemia, and certain types of drug overdoses. Not for routine use in cardiac arrest. PB: UK; t½: UK

<, Less than; >, greater than; *A,* adult; *ABG,* arterial blood gas; *ALS,* advanced life support; *Adol,* adolescent; *C,* child; *d,* day; *h,* hour; *IO,* intraosseous; *IV,* intravenous; *max,* maximum; *MI,* myocardial infarction; *min,* minute; *PB,* protein binding; *PVC,* premature ventricular contraction; *q,* every; *resp,* respiratory; *s,* second; *SL,* sublingual; *t½,* half-life; *tab,* tablet; *UK,* unknown; *y,* year.
[a]Other dosing regimens for neonates, infants, and children are available.

Pediatric Implications

If severe metabolic acidosis persists after attention has been directed at maintaining optimal ventilation and oxygenation, sodium bicarbonate may be given to the pediatric patient in a 1 mEq/kg dose via the IV or IO route. It may also be given as treatment for a tricyclic antidepressant (TCA) overdose. Sodium bicarbonate is hyperosmolar and should be diluted from an 8.4% solution (1 mEq/mL) to a 4.2% solution (0.5 mEq/mL) for infants.

FOR INTRACRANIAL HYPERTENSION: MANNITOL

Mannitol is an osmotic diuretic used in emergency, trauma, critical care, and neurosurgical settings to treat cerebral edema and to reduce increased intracranial pressure (intracranial hypertension), which may occur after head trauma, neurosurgery, malignancy, and with other types of intracranial pathology (see Chapter 41).

Dosages of Mannitol

Mannitol may be given as an IV bolus or via a continuous drip. The usual initial bolus dose of mannitol ranges from 0.25 to 2 g/kg IV of a 15% to 25% solution. Subsequent dosing is highly variable and is influenced by serum osmolality and the patient's blood pressure. In general, mannitol is held when serum osmolality exceeds 320 mOsm/kg or when hypotension is present.

Uses and Considerations of Mannitol

Mannitol is highly irritating to veins, and the nurse must use a filter needle when administering the drug because crystals may form in the solution and syringe and can be inadvertently injected. When a filter needle is used to draw up the mannitol, a *new* filter needle *must* be used to administer the mannitol IV. In addition, the nurse would need to carefully assess the patient's neurologic status; monitor blood pressure and laboratory studies, including electrolytes and serum osmolality; and keep accurate intake and output records to assess fluid volume status because diuresis may be substantial. Prototype Drug Chart: Mannitol lists the pharmacologic data for mannitol.

EMERGENCY DRUGS FOR DRUG OVERDOSE

Although numerous antidotes exist for specific types of drug overdose, the drugs presented in this section are most commonly prescribed in cases of drug overdose and ingestion of toxic substances, and pertinent exceptions are noted. Particular attention must be given to administration guidelines to achieve the best possible clinical outcome for the patient. These drugs are cross-referenced to their specialty chapters.

Naloxone

Naloxone is classified as an opioid antagonist. It reverses the effects of all opioid drugs (e.g., morphine, hydromorphone, fentanyl, codeine, oxycodone, heroin) by competitively binding to opioid receptor sites in the body. Naloxone is indicated for individuals who have taken an overdose of opioid drugs, those experiencing respiratory or cardiovascular depression or arrest from therapeutic doses of opioids given in a health care setting, and those brought to the emergency department in a coma or cardiac arrest of unknown etiology (which may be drug induced). Given the epidemic of opioid overdoses in the general community, naloxone is often made available to medical first responders and even to members of the lay public who frequently encounter substance misuse as an over-the-counter agent.

The typical dose of naloxone for actual or suspected opioid overdose in adults is 0.4 to 2 mg IV administered every 2 minutes until the patient's condition improves to an acceptable level. If there is no improvement within 10 minutes after 10 mg of the drug has been injected, nonopioid drugs or disease must be suspected. Although ideally naloxone should be administered intravenously in emergency situations, it also may be given via IO, IM, subcut, and intranasal (IN) routes if IV access is not readily obtainable. The adult dose for the IN route is 1 mg per nostril. IN naloxone offers the advantages of a reduced risk of needlestick injuries as well as a readily accessible route of administration for rescuers and laypersons. Naloxone autoinjectors are also available to facilitate rapid IM administration by rescue personnel and members of the general public.

Because most opioid drugs have a longer duration of action than naloxone, the nurse must monitor the patient closely for signs and symptoms of recurrent opioid effects such as respiratory depression and hypotension. In this situation, naloxone administration may need to be repeated several times, or a continuous IV infusion may be prescribed. Naloxone has no major opioid effects, but it can precipitate withdrawal symptoms in patients addicted to opioid drugs and, rarely, it can cause anaphylaxis. In addition, pulmonary edema has been reported after naloxone administration in patients who have had an overdose of morphine (see Chapter 25). Nurses also must be on guard for combative or violent behavior after naloxone administration, especially in patients who have overdosed on an illicit drug; having security personnel available to stand by is prudent. Prototype Drug Chart: Naloxone Hydrochloride lists the pharmacologic data for naloxone.

Pediatric Implications

For opioid reversal in children, give 0.1 mg/kg, repeating the drug as necessary by bolus every 2 minutes as needed up to 2 mg based upon desired therapeutic effects. Naloxone can be administered as an IV bolus, continuous infusion or via IO, IM, or subcut routes in children. If needed to maintain opioid reversal, a continuous IV or IO infusion of naloxone can be administered in a range of 0.002 to 0.16 mg/kg per hour.

Flumazenil

Flumazenil is the reversal agent for the respiratory depressant and sedative effects of benzodiazepine drugs (e.g., diazepam, midazolam, chlordiazepoxide). It is administered to counteract the effects of benzodiazepines given as sedative or anesthetic drugs as well as to treat accidental or intentional benzodiazepine overdose. Flumazenil does not reverse the central nervous system (CNS) depressant effects of nonbenzodiazepine agents such as alcohol, opiates, and barbiturates, and may not reverse amnesia induced by benzodiazepines.

For suspected benzodiazepine overdose, flumazenil is given IV in an initial dose of 0.2 mg over 30 seconds. A second dose of 0.3 mg may be given over 30 seconds. A third dose and subsequent doses of 0.5 mg IV may be given every minute until the desired clinical response is achieved or until a total dose of 3 mg is given within an hour. If sedation occurs again, doses of flumazenil may be repeated at 20-minute intervals (not to exceed 1 mg at a time) to a total hourly dose of no more than 3 mg IV. If patients have only a partial response to 3 mg of flumazenil, additional doses may be administered slowly up to a 5 mg total dose. At that point, if the patient still has not responded to flumazenil, the cause of the depressed level of consciousness is a problem other than an adverse benzodiazepine effect.

Nursing considerations include careful assessment of respiratory rate and effort, blood pressure, and mental status. If the benzodiazepine is reversed too rapidly, patients may have emergence reactions in which they become agitated and confused and experience perceptual distortions. Because seizures are precipitated by benzodiazepine withdrawal, seizure precautions must be implemented for patients at risk (those with long-standing benzodiazepine use or abuse) and for those who have a known seizure disorder.

Activated Charcoal

Activated charcoal may be prescribed for poisoning as a means to prevent absorption of toxins into the body if the ingested substance is known to be affected by charcoal in the GI tract. A poison control center should be contacted as soon as possible to help guide medical therapy. In cases of known or suspected poisoning, activated charcoal is prepared as a slurry and is given to the patient orally or via a gastric tube, ideally within 30 minutes to 1 hour of ingestion, sometimes after gastric lavage. The dose is highly variable and is dependent on the amount of poison ingested, the age of the patient, and the type of activated charcoal formulation used. Activated charcoal dosing may need to be repeated for certain types of poisoning, particularly from drugs such as salicylates, slow-release drug preparations, and *Amanita phalloides* (death cap mushrooms), to name a few.

Because vomiting is a common adverse reaction, patients with an impaired gag reflex and/or an impaired mental status are at high risk for aspiration after ingesting activated charcoal. Aspiration pneumonia and death can occur. To promote safety, these patients may need intubation for airway protection followed by administration of the activated charcoal via a gastric tube. Activated charcoal should not be administered with milk products, because they decrease its adsorptive properties. Activated charcoal is ineffective and should not be given to patients who have ingested some forms of pesticides, hydrocarbons, alcohol, acids or alkalis, lithium, solvents, and iron supplements. A **cathartic**, a purgative that results in bowel movements, may be ordered after administration of activated charcoal to speed elimination of the charcoal-toxin complex from the body. The patient should be told that charcoal produces black stools.

Table 58.2 lists the emergency drugs for poisoning and their dosages, uses, and considerations.

PROTOTYPE DRUG CHART
Mannitol

Drug Class	Dosage
Osmotic diuretic	A: IV: 0.25–2 g/kg q4h Dosing is highly individualized. Hold for serum osmolality >320 mOsm/kg

Contraindications	Drug-Lab-Food Interactions
Hypersensitivity, severe dehydration *Caution:* Pregnancy, breastfeeding, current intracranial bleeding	Drug: May decrease effectiveness with lithium

Pharmacokinetics	Pharmacodynamics
Absorption: IV Distribution: PB: Confined to extracellular space Metabolism: t½: 100 min Excretion: In urine	Decrease in intracranial pressure: IV: Onset: 30–60 min Peak: 1 h Duration: 6–8 h Diuresis: IV: Onset: 1–3 h Peak: 1 h Duration: 6–8 h

Therapeutic Effects/Uses
To treat increased intracranial pressure, cerebral edema
Mechanism of Action: Inhibits reabsorption of electrolytes and water by affecting pressure of glomerular filtrate.

Side Effects	Adverse Reactions
Temporary volume expansion, hyponatremia/hypernatremia, hypokalemia/hyperkalemia, dehydration, blurred vision, dry mouth	Pulmonary congestion, fluid/electrolyte imbalances *Life-threatening:* Convulsions

A, Adult; *h*, hour; *IV*, intravenous; *max*, maximum; *min*, minute; *PB*, protein binding; *q*, every; *t½*, half-life.

EMERGENCY DRUGS FOR SHOCK

Drugs may be required to elevate blood pressure and to improve cardiac performance in various types of shock states. Therapeutic agents described in this section are primarily indicated in conditions such as cardiogenic, neurogenic, septic, anaphylactic, and insulin shock. A noteworthy exception to the list is **hypovolemic shock** that results from loss of blood or fluid volume; drugs should never be used as the primary therapy to correct the hypotension associated with this condition. Administration of fluids or blood products or both is the only acceptable initial means to treat hypovolemic shock. However, if hypotension persists after appropriate volume resuscitation, vasoactive drugs may be necessary to elevate and sustain blood pressure. The drugs that follow are cross-referenced to their specialty chapters.

PROTOTYPE DRUG CHART
Naloxone Hydrochloride

Drug Class	Dosage[a]
Opioid antagonist	A: IV/IM/IO/subcut/IN: 0.4–2 mg, repeating every 2–3 min PRN C: IV/IM/subcut/IO: age and weight based: 0.1–2 mg; may repeat q2–3 min PRN

Contraindications	Drug-Lab-Food Interactions
Hypersensitivity, respiratory depression *Caution:* Opioid-dependent patients, cardiac disease, breastfeeding neonates of opioid-dependent mothers	Drug: Naloxone can precipitate withdrawal in patients dependent on opioid analgesics. Lab: Urine vanillylmandelic acid (VMA), 5-hydroxyheptadecatrienoic acid (5-HIAA), urine glucose

Pharmacokinetics	Pharmacodynamics
Absorption: IM/subcut: Well absorbed Distribution: PB: UK Metabolism: t½: Adults: 1–4 h; neonates: 1–3 h Excretion: In urine metabolites	IM/IN/subcut: Onset: 2–5 min Peak: UK Duration: 1–4 h IV/IO: Onset: 1–2 min Peak: UK Duration: 1–4 h

Therapeutic Effects/Uses
To treat respiratory depression caused by opioids; to treat opioid-induced depressant effects and opioid overdose
Mechanism of action: Blocks effects of opioids by competing for receptor sites

Side Effects	Adverse Reactions
Negligible pharmacologic effect without opioids in the body	Nausea, vomiting, tremulousness, sweating, tachycardia, elevated blood pressure *Life-threatening:* Atrioventricular fibrillation, pulmonary edema (with overdose of morphine)

A, Adult; *C*, child; *h*, hour; *IM*, intramuscular; *IN*, intranasal; *IO*, intraosseous; *IV*, intravenous; *min*, minute; *PB*, protein binding; *PRN*, as needed; *q*, every; *subcut*, subcutaneous; *t½*, half-life; *UK*, unknown.
[a]Other dosing regimens for neonates, infants, and children are available.

PROTOTYPE DRUG CHART
Dopamine Hydrochloride

Drug Class	Dosage
Adrenergic agonist	A: IV drip: 5–20 mcg/kg per minute; >10 mcg/kg per minute may be ordered if lower doses are ineffective. C/Adol: IV 1–20 mcg/kg per minute; titrate in increments of 2–5 mcg/kg per minute.

Contraindications	Drug-Lab-Food Interactions
Hypersensitivity, tachydysrhythmias, ventricular fibrillation, pheochromocytomas *Caution:* Whether this drug is safe in children is unknown.	Drug: May result in hypertensive crisis when used within 2 wk of MAOIs; concurrent IV administration of phenytoin may result in hypotension and bradycardia; sodium bicarbonate solutions inactivate dopamine—do not administer these through the same IV line.

Pharmacokinetics	Pharmacodynamics
Absorption: IV Distribution: PB: UK metabolism: t½: 2 min Excretion: In urine	IV: Onset: 1–2 min Peak: <5 min Duration: <10 min

Therapeutic Effects/Uses
To treat hypotension in shock states after adequate fluid and/or blood product resuscitation; to increase heart rate in atropine-refractory bradycardia
Mechanism of Action: Stimulates receptors to cause cardiac stimulation; increases systemic vascular resistance.

Side Effects	Adverse Reactions
Palpitations, tachycardia, hypertension, ectopic beats, angina, IV line site irritation, piloerection, nausea, vomiting	Cardiac dysrhythmias, azotemia, tissue sloughing (from extravasation) *Life-threatening:* MI, gangrene in extremities (from vasoconstriction)

<, Less than; >, greater than; *A*, adult; *Adol*, adolescent; *C*, child; *IV*, intravenous; *MAOI*, monoamine oxidase inhibitor; *MI*, myocardial infarction; *min*, minute; *PB*, protein binding; *t½*, half-life; *UK*, unknown; *wk*, week.

TABLE 58.2 Emergency Drugs for Drug Overdose

Generic	Route and Dosage	Uses and Considerations
Flumazenil	A: IV: Initially 0.2 mg over 30 s; additional doses of 0.3–0.5 mg are given over 30 s q1 min as indicated. For resedation, may repeat at 20-min intervals to a total dose of no more than 3 mg per hour C/Adol: IV: Initially 0.01 mg/kg over 15 s, up to a max dose of 0.2 mg; may repeat at 1-min interval; *max*: 0.05 mg/kg or 1 mg, whichever is lower	Reversal agent for benzodiazepine overdose; may precipitate seizures in patients with long-term use or abuse of benzodiazepines and those with seizure disorders; may precipitate emergent reactions PB: 50%; t½: variable (40–80 min)
Naloxone	See Prototype Drug Chart: Naloxone	
Activated charcoal	A/C: PO: dose based on age, toxin, and formulation	For ingested poisoning Onset: <1 min; PB: NA; t½: NA

<, Less than; *A*, adult; *Adol*, adolescent; *C*, child; *IV*, intravenous; *max*, maximum; *min*, minute; *NA*, not applicable; *PB*, protein binding; *PO*, by mouth; *q*, every; *s*, second; *t½*, half-life.

Dopamine

Dopamine is a sympathomimetic agent often used to treat hypotension in shock states (see Chapter 15). Dopamine may also be used to increase heart rate (beta$_1$ effect) in bradycardic rhythms when atropine has not been effective. The typical dose range is 5 to 20 mcg/kg per minute. Dopamine enhances cardiac output by increasing myocardial contractility and increasing heart rate (beta$_1$ effect), and it elevates blood pressure through vasoconstriction (alpha-adrenergic effect). Alpha effects predominate at higher doses—vasoconstriction of renal, mesenteric, and peripheral blood vessels occurs. Although sometimes necessary to maintain adequate blood pressure in severe shock, such vasoconstriction can lead to poor organ and tissue perfusion, decreased cardiac performance, and reduction of urine output. The lowest effective dose of dopamine should be used. Patients must be weaned gradually from dopamine; abrupt discontinuation of the infusion can cause immediate, severe hypotension.

Dopamine is typically mixed as a concentration of 200 to 800 mg in 250 mL D$_5$W or normal saline solution and is administered intravenously by an electronic infusion device for precision, preferably in a central vein. Sodium bicarbonate will inactivate dopamine; therefore it should not be infused in the same IV line. Continuous heart and blood pressure monitoring is essential. The nurse must carefully document vital signs, cardiac rhythm, and intake and output as prescribed. Significant adverse effects include tachycardia, dysrhythmias, myocardial ischemia, nausea, and vomiting. The IV site must be assessed hourly for signs of drug infiltration; extravasation (escape into tissues) of dopamine can produce tissue necrosis that may necessitate surgical debridement and skin grafting. If extravasation occurs, the site should be injected in multiple areas with phentolamine, 5 to 10 mg diluted in 10 to 15 mL of normal saline, to reduce or prevent tissue damage. Prototype Drug Chart: Dopamine Hydrochloride lists the pharmacologic data for dopamine.

> ⚡ **PATIENT SAFETY**
>
> **Do Not Confuse…**
> - **Dopamine** with **dobutamine**.

Dobutamine

Dobutamine is a sympathomimetic drug with beta-adrenergic activities (see Chapter 15). The beta$_1$ effects include enhancing the force of myocardial contraction (positive inotropic effect) and increasing heart rate (positive chronotropic effect). The beta$_2$ effects produce mild vasodilation. Dobutamine is indicated in shock states when improvement in cardiac output and overall cardiac performance is desired. Blood pressure is elevated only through the increase in cardiac output. The usual IV dose range of dobutamine is 2 to 20 mcg/kg per minute (titrated) administered via an electronic infusion device for safety. A typical concentration of dobutamine is 250 to 1000 mg mixed in 250 mL of D$_5$W or normal saline. Like dopamine, dobutamine administration should be tapered gradually as the patient's condition warrants; abrupt discontinuation can precipitate rapid clinical deterioration.

Continuous cardiac and blood pressure monitoring is required for patients receiving dobutamine infusions. Adverse effects are dose related and include myocardial ischemia, tachycardia, dysrhythmias, headache, nausea, and tremors. The nurse must carefully monitor intake and output and assess for any signs or symptoms of myocardial ischemia such as chest pain or development of dysrhythmias.

Norepinephrine

Norepinephrine is a catecholamine with extremely potent vasoconstrictor actions (alpha-adrenergic effect) (see Chapter 15). It is used in shock states, often when drugs such as dopamine and dobutamine have failed to produce adequate blood pressure or as first-line alternative to dopamine. Like high-dose dopamine, the peripheral vasoconstriction that results has the potential to impair cardiac performance and decrease organ and tissue perfusion. In general, 4 mg of norepinephrine are added to 250 mL D$_5$W or normal saline solution for a concentration of 16 mcg/mL and are infused at 8 to 12 mcg/min initially, titrated down to a maintenance dose of 2–4 mcg/min as a continuous infusion. For adults with sepsis, a dosing range of 0.01 to 3 mcg/kg per minute may be prescribed. Maximum titrated dose is 3.3 mcg/kg per minute. Continuous cardiac monitoring and precise blood pressure monitoring are required. The drug must be tapered slowly; abrupt discontinuation can result in severe hypotension.

Nursing actions and considerations are the same as those for dopamine. Norepinephrine should not be used as an initial therapy to treat hypotension in patients who are hypovolemic; fluid, blood, or both must be administered to restore adequate volume first. Adverse effects of norepinephrine include myocardial ischemia, dysrhythmias, and impaired organ perfusion. Abrupt discontinuation causes rapid clinical deterioration. Extravasation of norepinephrine causes tissue necrosis, so attention to the IV site is essential. If extravasation occurs, the area should be infiltrated with phentolamine, as was described for dopamine.

Pediatric Considerations

Norepinephrine is given to pediatric patients to treat hypotensive shock after adequate fluid administration via the IV/IO route in a dose range of 0.03 to 0.5 mcg/kg per minute (titrated).

Epinephrine

Epinephrine is the drug of choice in the treatment of anaphylactic shock, an allergic response of the most serious type, brought about by an antibody-antigen reaction (see Chapter 15). Anaphylactic shock can be fatal if prompt treatment is not initiated. Severe bronchoconstriction and hypotension resulting from cardiovascular collapse are its hallmarks. Epinephrine is also indicated for an acute, severe asthmatic attack.

Administration of epinephrine causes bronchodilation, enhanced cardiac performance, and vasoconstriction to increase blood pressure. In severe asthma and anaphylactic shock, epinephrine is given in a dose range of 0.3 to 0.5 mg IM for adults (1:1000 solution). The IM route is used because it has a more predictable pattern of absorption than the subcutaneous route. Given the prevalence of severe allergic reactions to foods, drugs, and insect stings, epinephrine autoinjectors in both adult and pediatric formulations are available to facilitate rapid emergency IM administration of the drug by health care personnel in some settings as well as for self-administration by patients. As an alternative, epinephrine can be given in a dose of 0.05 to 0.1 mg IV over 5 to 10 minutes (1:10,000 solution) by health care personnel with cardiac monitoring capability. Epinephrine administration can be repeated every 5 to 15 minutes if necessary. For patients who do not respond to repeated doses of epinephrine, a continuous epinephrine infusion may be indicated at a starting rate of 0.1 mcg/kg per minute, titrated to clinical response. The upper dosing limit is highly variable.

The patient who receives epinephrine must be closely monitored for tachycardia, cardiac dysrhythmias, hypertension, and angina. Patients who are given IV epinephrine must be on a cardiac monitor with resuscitation equipment immediately available. Other adverse effects include excitability, fear, anxiety, and restlessness. In addition, the nurse should be alert to the possibility that the anaphylactic response may recur and necessitate repeated treatment. For this reason, antihistamines and steroids are ordered as a standard component of treatment for an allergic reaction along with epinephrine. Diphenhydramine is a commonly prescribed antihistamine and is discussed later. Examples of steroids are hydrocortisone sodium succinate, prednisone, and methylprednisolone. After the initial dose, the steroids are slowly tapered over days to weeks to prevent recurrence.

Patient education should include strict avoidance of the agents responsible for the anaphylactic reaction and follow-up care with a health care provider. For some patients, such as those with severe allergic responses to insect stings or certain foods, the health care provider may prescribe an epinephrine kit, pen, or other type of autoinjector to be carried with the patient for self-medication in the event of contact with the antigen. Proper patient education regarding the use of the kit or pen is essential. See Chapter 1 for more information on patient teaching.

Albuterol

Albuterol is a beta-adrenergic bronchodilator (see Chapter 15) used to reverse bronchoconstriction in anaphylactic shock; asthma, inflammation and narrowing of the airways caused by enhanced responsiveness of the tracheobronchial system to a variety of stimuli; and COPD. In emergency situations, albuterol is typically administered via nebulizer (adults: 2.5–5 mg albuterol in the manufacturer's recommended volume and type of diluent). Albuterol is also supplied as a metered-dose inhaler (MDI), which the patient can carry to self-administer a "rescue" dose of the drug during an acute episode of bronchospasm. The nurse should assess breath sounds before and after administration; effectiveness is evidenced by relief of bronchospasm. In severe bronchospasm, wheezing may not be audible. As the bronchospasm is relieved, wheezing may become more pronounced, indicating that the drug is producing the desired therapeutic effect. Assessment of the patient's subjective feelings of respiratory distress before and after administration is especially important. Adverse effects of albuterol include tachycardia, tremor, nervousness, cardiac dysrhythmias, and hypertension. The patient who is prescribed an albuterol MDI should be taught how to properly use the device and to keep track of the remaining doses. Running out of the drug when a rescue dose is needed can produce life-threatening consequences in a severe asthma attack.

Diphenhydramine Hydrochloride

Diphenhydramine, an antihistamine, is administered with epinephrine to treat anaphylactic shock. This agent is effective for treating the histamine-induced tissue swelling and pruritus common to severe allergic reactions. The standard adult dose is 25 to 50 mg administered via IV or deep IM routes. Oral pill and liquid forms of the drug exist, but the parenteral form is preferred in emergencies. However, the patient may be instructed to keep an oral formulation on hand in the home setting for emergency self-administration during an allergic reaction before receiving medical assistance. An important tip for patient teaching is that liquid diphenhydramine is easier to swallow than a pill, especially in the presence of tissue edema in the mouth or throat. Adverse effects include drowsiness, sedation, confusion, vertigo, excitability, hypotension, tachycardia, GI disturbances, and dry mouth (see Chapter 35).

Dextrose 50%

Dextrose 50% (D_{50}) is a concentrated, high-carbohydrate solution given to treat severe hypoglycemia, such as insulin-induced hypoglycemia or insulin shock (see Chapter 12). When hypoglycemia is known or suspected, and the patient's state of consciousness is impaired such that oral administration of sugar solutions is contraindicated, 50 mL of D_{50} is commonly ordered and is given as an IV bolus. D_{50} is highly irritating to veins and should be administered in a large peripheral or central vein whenever possible; phlebitis can occur, and extravasation of the solution can cause tissue sloughing and necrosis. The nurse must monitor the patient's blood glucose carefully because hyperglycemia is common, especially after bolus injection. Urine output should be accurately recorded because osmotic diuresis can occur when blood glucose is elevated, and a hyperosmolar state can result. Patient education must be centered on teaching about diabetes, nutrition, physical activity, and properly self-managing insulin or oral hypoglycemic agent administration.

Pediatric Implications

Glycogen stores in infants and children may be quickly depleted in stress states produced by severe illness. Because adequate amounts of glucose are essential to strong myocardial function as well as brain function, hypoglycemia must be corrected to provide the greatest chance for successful resuscitation. After determining that hypoglycemia is present by the fingerstick or heelstick method of rapid blood glucose testing, dextrose 25% or less may be administered per health care provider order. Because glucose is supplied in a 50% concentration, it must be diluted at least 1:1 in sterile water before administration to reduce its osmolarity and prevent sclerosis of peripheral veins. The standard dose is 0.5 to 1 g/kg IV or IO.

TABLE 58.3 Agents for Emergency Treatment of Shock

Generic	Route and Dosage[a]	Uses and Considerations
Albuterol	A: Nebulizer: 2.5–5 mg q20 min × 3 doses, then 2.5–10 mg q1–4 h PRN C/Adol: 1.25–5 mg q20 min × 3 doses, then 2.5–10 mg q1–4 h PRN	For bronchoconstriction secondary to anaphylactic shock, asthma, and COPD. Adverse effects include tachycardia, tremor, nervousness, cardiac dysrhythmias, and hypertension. PB: UK; t½: 3.7–5 h
Dextrose 50%	A: IV: 10–25 g C: 0.5–1.0 g/kg IV of dextrose 25% sol	For insulin shock, severe hypoglycemia PB: UK; t½: UK
Diphenhydramine	A: IM/IV: 25–50 mg	For anaphylactic shock, acute allergic reaction PB: 98%–99%; t½: 3–8 h
Dobutamine	A: IV drip: 2–20 mcg/kg per minute	For low cardiac output. Effects antagonized by beta blockers PB: UK; t½: 2 min
Dopamine hydrochloride	See Prototype Drug Chart: Dopamine Hydrochloride	
Epinephrine	A: IM: 0.3–0.5 mg (1:1000 sol); may repeat q5–15 min A: IV/IO: 0.05–0.1 mg (1:10,000 sol); may repeat q5–15 min A: ETT: 2–2.5 mg; may repeat q3–5 min C/Adol: IV: 0.03–0.2 mcg/kg per minute; may repeat q3–5 min C ≥15 kg/Adol: IM: weight based: 0.15–0.3 mg/dose; may repeat q5–20 min	For anaphylactic shock, severe acute asthmatic attack. May cause hypertensive crisis with MAOIs, and increased dysrhythmias may occur with cardiac glycosides PB: UK; t½: UK
Glucagon	A: Subcut/IM/IV: 1 mg; may repeat once C/Adol: Subcut/IM/IV: weight based: 0.5–1 mg; may repeat once	Insulin shock, severe hypoglycemia, beta-blocker overdose (reverses effects of beta blockers) PB: UK; t½: 3–10 min
Norepinephrine	A: IV: Initially, up to 8–12 mcg/min, titrated in increments of 0.02 mcg/kg per minute; max: 3.3 mcg/kg per minute C: 0.03–0.5 mcg/kg per minute IV/IO via continuous infusion; upper dosing limit highly variable	Hypotension not responsive to other therapies PB: UK; t½: UK

≥, Greater than or equal to; *A*, adult; *Adol*, adolescent; *C*, child; *COPD*, chronic obstructive pulmonary disease; *ETT*, endotracheal tube; *h*, hour; *IM*, intramuscular; *IO*, intraosseous; *IV*, intravenous; *MAOIs*, monoamine oxidase inhibitors; *max*, maximum; *min*, minute; *PB*, protein binding; *PRN*, as needed; *q*, every; *sol*, solution; *subcut*, subcutaneous; *t½*, half-life; *UK*, unknown.
[a]Other dosing regimens for neonates, infants, and children are available.

Glucagon

Glucagon is a pancreas-produced hormone that elevates blood glucose by stimulating glycogen breakdown (**glycogenolysis**). Glucagon, like D_{50}, is indicated in the treatment of severe hypoglycemia, such as that which results from insulin shock. In an emergency, when D_{50} is unavailable or cannot be administered intravenously, glucagon is an effective agent. Glucagon may be given via subcut, IM, or IV routes and produces the desired clinical effect within 10 to 15 minutes of administration due to the time necessary for glycogen to be converted to glucose. The standard dose for adults and children is 1 mg, which can be repeated in 15 minutes for persistent coma. If the coma has not resolved after two doses, D_{50} must be administered. Adverse effects from glucagon are uncommon but can include nausea, vomiting, and a hypersensitivity reaction that may produce bronchospasm and respiratory distress. Glucagon can also be used as a drug to reverse the effects of calcium channel blocker and beta-blocker overdose; in this situation, 3.5 to 5 mg IV of glucagon is administered initially, followed by an IV infusion of 1 to 5 mg/h (see Chapter 50). In addition, glucagon dilates esophageal smooth muscle as well as the lower esophageal sphincter. It can be administered IV in the emergency department as a first-line agent to dilate the esophagus in an effort to relieve an esophageal food bolus or impaction.

Table 58.3 lists the emergency drugs for shock and their dosages, uses, and considerations.

EMERGENCY DRUGS FOR HYPERTENSIVE CRISES

A variety of pharmacologic agents may be prescribed to treat **hypertensive crisis**, generally defined as a systolic blood pressure that exceeds 180 to 200 mm Hg and a diastolic blood pressure that exceeds 120 mm Hg. Three of the most commonly prescribed drugs are discussed in this section. The drugs are cross-referenced to their specialty chapter.

Table 58.4 lists the emergency drugs for hypertensive crises and their dosages, uses, and considerations.

Labetalol

Labetalol is an alpha- and beta-adrenergic blocker that acts by inhibiting the effects of the sympathetic nervous system (see Chapter 15). Its pharmacologic actions include lowering heart rate, blood pressure, myocardial contractility, and myocardial oxygen consumption and reducing the vasoconstriction that results from sympathetic nervous system stimulation. This drug is indicated for the acute management of clinically significant hypertension in the

TABLE 58.4 Emergency Drugs for Hypertensive Crises

Generic	Route and Dosage[a]	Uses and Considerations
Nitroprusside sodium	See Prototype Drug Chart: Nitroprusside Sodium	
Furosemide	A: IM/IV: Initially, 20–40 mg, titrate by 20 mg q2h PRN C: IM/IV: 1–2 mg/kg q6–12h; *max*: 6 mg/kg per dose	For acute pulmonary edema. Adverse effects include hypovolemia, dehydration, and electrolyte disturbances.
Labetalol hydrochloride	A: IV: Initially, 20 mg over 2 min; additional doses of 20–80 mg q10 min until desired response A: IV drip: 0.5–2 mg/min; titrate to response; *max*: 300 mg; continuous infusion 2 mg/min	For hypertension in CVA and for hypertensive crisis. Adverse effects include ventricular dysrhythmias, hypotension, and bronchospasm. Contraindications: Bronchial asthma, COPD, severe bradycardia, heart failure

A, Adult; *C*, child; *COPD*, chronic obstructive pulmonary disease; *CVA*, cerebrovascular accident; *h*, hour; *IM*, intramuscular; *IV*, intravenous; *max*, maximum; *MI*, myocardial infarction; *min*, minute; *PRN*, as needed; *q*, every.
[a]Other dosing regimens for neonates, infants, and children are available.

presence of ischemic and hemorrhagic stroke as well as for hypertensive crisis.

Initially 10–20 mg of labetalol is administered IV push over 2 minutes. This starting dose can be repeated or doubled every 10 minutes until the desired clinical response is achieved up to a maximum dose of 300 mg. As an alternative approach, a continuous infusion of labetalol mixed with D_5W can be prepared to deliver 2–8 mg/min until the target therapeutic response is attained; the maximum dose with this approach is also 300 mg.

Important nursing considerations during the administration of labetalol include the use of an electronic infusion device for accurate continuous-infusion medication delivery, cardiac monitoring, and frequent blood pressure measurement. Documentation of blood pressure may need to be at least every 5 minutes during IV push dosing or at the initiation of the continuous infusion. Serious adverse effects include hypotension, bradycardia, ventricular dysrhythmias, and bronchospasm. Dizziness is also a frequently reported adverse reaction. Labetalol is contraindicated in patients with bronchial asthma or COPD because of the risk of bronchospasm and in patients with severe bradycardia or apparent heart failure.

Nitroprusside Sodium

Nitroprusside sodium is an IV drug used to reduce arterial blood pressure in hypertensive emergencies (see Chapter 39). The mechanism of action is immediate, direct arterial and venous vasodilation. Antihypertensive effects end when nitroprusside sodium is discontinued; blood pressure increases as soon as drug administration is stopped. Continuous and accurate blood pressure measurement is required. In general, 50 mg of nitroprusside sodium is mixed in 250 mL D_5W. The typical dose range for adults is 0.3 mcg/kg per minute, titrated to the desired clinical response. The maximum dose is 10 mcg/kg per minute.

There are several important nursing considerations:
- Nitroprusside sodium is rapidly inactivated by light; the IV bottle or bag must be wrapped with aluminum foil or another opaque material to protect the solution from degradation.
- Although a faint brown tint is typical, blue or brown discoloration of the solution indicates degradation and necessitates that the solution be discarded.
- When nitroprusside sodium therapy is prolonged, or when it is infused at the maximum dose of 10 mcg/kg per minute for more than 10 minutes, patients are at risk for toxicity resulting from elevated serum thiocyanate or cyanide levels (by-products of drug metabolism). Signs and symptoms include metabolic acidosis, profound hypotension, dyspnea, dizziness, and vomiting. Serum thiocyanate levels should be monitored every 24 to 72 hours for patients receiving prolonged infusions of more than 2 mcg/kg per minute. Patients with renal insufficiency or failure are at a higher risk because the metabolites are excreted in the urine.
- Patients should be placed on an oral antihypertensive agent as soon as possible so that nitroprusside sodium can be tapered slowly. Drug data for nitroprusside sodium are presented in Prototype Drug Chart: Nitroprusside Sodium.

PROTOTYPE DRUG CHART
Nitroprusside Sodium

Drug Class	Dosage[a]
Vasodilator	A/C: IV drip: Initially 0.3 mcg/kg per minute, then titrate to desired response. Usual range is 0.2–10 mcg/kg per minute

Contraindications	Drug-Lab-Food Interactions
Hypersensitivity, hypertension (compensatory), decreased cerebral perfusion, coarctation of the aorta *Caution*: Increased cranial pressure	Drug: Antihypertensives, general anesthetics Note: Do not mix with any other drug in syringe or solution. Lab: Decrease in $Paco_2$, pH

Pharmacokinetics	Pharmacodynamics
Absorption: IV only Distribution: PB: UK Metabolism: $t\frac{1}{2}$: <10 min Excretion: In urine	IV: Onset: 1–2 min Peak: Rapid Duration: 1–10 h

Therapeutic Effects/Uses
To treat hypertensive crisis and to decrease systemic vascular resistance to improve cardiac performance
Mechanism of action: Stimulates smooth muscle of veins and arteries; produces peripheral vasodilation

Side Effects	Adverse Reactions
Dizziness, headache, nausea, abdominal pain, sweating, palpitations, weakness, vomiting	Thiocyanate toxicity: hypotension, tinnitus, dyspnea, blurred vision, metabolic acidosis *Life-threatening*: Severe hypotension, loss of consciousness, profound cardiovascular depression

<, Less than; *A*, adult; *C*, child; *h*, hour; *IV*, intravenous; *min*, minute; *PB*, protein binding; $Paco_2$, partial pressure of carbon dioxide; $t\frac{1}{2}$, half-life; *UK*, unknown.

Furosemide

Furosemide is classified as a *loop diuretic* that acts by inhibiting sodium and chloride reabsorption from the ascending loop of Henle and the proximal and distal tubules. It promotes the renal excretion of water, sodium, chloride, magnesium, hydrogen, and calcium, and it depletes potassium (see Chapter 41). Furosemide also has peripheral and renal vasodilating effects that can lower blood pressure. The main indications for use of furosemide as an emergency drug are acute pulmonary edema from left ventricular dysfunction and hypertensive crisis.

Furosemide is given as an initial bolus of 20 to 40 mg IV over 1 to 2 minutes. For patients who take furosemide on a regular basis, the effective dose may be much higher (up to 2 mg/kg). The vasodilatory effects occur *before* diuresis begins and act to lower blood pressure. Central venous pressure is reduced through a decrease in venous return to the heart once vasodilation is achieved. Diuresis should start within 5 to 10 minutes of drug administration and may continue for approximately 6 hours.

The most significant adverse effects are severe hypovolemia, dehydration, and electrolyte disturbances (hypokalemia, hypomagnesemia, hyponatremia, and hypochloremia). Patients taking digitalis preparations are at an increased risk of digitalis toxicity from hypokalemia. The patient's fluid and electrolyte status, blood urea nitrogen (BUN), and creatinine must be carefully assessed before and after furosemide administration, including auscultation of breath sounds for rales, strict surveillance of intake and output, and review of laboratory data when available. Electrolyte and careful fluid replacement may be required during furosemide therapy to prevent physiologic consequences. The nurse must also exercise caution when giving nephrotoxic agents when furosemide is prescribed and in administering the drug to patients with sulfonamide sensitivity because furosemide is a sulfonamide derivative that can produce an allergic reaction.

 COMPLEMENTARY AND ALTERNATIVE THERAPIES

Furosemide

Ginseng can inhibit the efficacy of furosemide. Licorice can promote potassium loss, which enhances the potential for severe hypokalemia. These products should not be taken concurrently with furosemide.

CLINICAL JUDGMENT SINGLE-EPISODE CASE STUDY

SLO: Apply knowledge of pharmacodynamics of drugs to determine which medication effects require a follow-up by the nurse.
NGN Item Type: Extended drag and drop
Cognitive Skills: Take action

A 42-year-old male was brought to the emergency department by ground ambulance. The emergency medical technician (EMT) reported the patient has been having intermittent "indigestion" for 5 days and has been ingesting "Tums" with minimal relief. 911 was called when a friend noticed the patient grabbing his chest and was not able to "catch his breath." EMT administered oxygen 2 L per nasal cannula, aspirin 325 mg orally, nitroglycerin (NTG) 0.4 mg sublingual × 3 tablets, and morphine 4 mg intravenously (IV). The electrocardiogram (ECG) en route did not reveal any acute coronary events. The nurse assists in transferring the patient onto a stretcher. The nurse follows the hospital protocol and places oxygen 2 L per nasal cannula, attaches cardiac monitor, and inserts a second IV site while continuing to conduct a focused history and assessment.

Indicate which nursing action listed in the first column is appropriate for the clinical manifestation the nurse assessed in the second column. Note that not all nursing actions will be used, while some of the nursing actions will be used more than once.

Nursing Action	Potential Clinical Manifestation	Appropriate Nursing Action for the Clinical Manifestation
Take no action other than monitor	Blood pressure of 98/68 mm Hg	
Administer morphine 2 mg intravenously	Heart rate of 73 beats per minute	
Administer diltiazem	Respiratory rate of 18 breaths per minute	
Obtain a 12-lead electrocardiogram	Pale, clammy skin	
Administer atropine sulfate	Bedside cardiac monitor with	
Notify the attending medical provider	Continued chest pain	
	Report of headaches	

Answers

Nursing Action	Potential Clinical Manifestation	Appropriate Nursing Action for the Clinical Manifestation
Take no action other than monitor	Blood pressure of 98/68 mm Hg	Take no action other than monitor
Administer morphine 2 mg intravenously	Heart rate of 73 beats per minute	Take no action other than monitor
Administer diltiazem	Respiratory rate of 18 breaths per minute	Take no action other than monitor
Obtain a 12-lead electrocardiogram	Pale, clammy skin	Obtain a 12-lead electrocardiogram
Administer atropine sulfate	Bedside cardiac monitor with	Obtain a 12-lead electrocardiogram
Administer nitroglycerin sublingual	Continued chest pain	Administer morphine 2 mg intravenously
	Reports of headaches	Take no action other than monitor

Rationale

The patient is most likely exhibiting angina pectoris with possible myocardial infarction with ST elevation. The initial goal for any cardiac event is to restore perfusion and prevent further damage to the myocardium. The patient's vital signs, which include blood pressure, heart rate, and respiratory rate, are within normal parameters and should be monitored. A decrease in blood pressure can occur as a side effect of nitroglycerin and morphine. The nurse would continue to monitor the vital signs and if continued lowering of blood pressure occurs, the medical provider would be notified. However, a bedside cardiac monitor shows widened QRS complexes with ST elevation; a 12-lead electrocardiogram would be obtained to determine if the patient is experiencing ST-elevated myocardial infarction (STEMI) or other cardiac abnormalities causing ST elevation. Also, the nurse would continue to treat the chest pain with either nitroglycerin or morphine while monitoring blood pressure and heart rate. Because the patient continues to have chest pain after three doses of sublingual nitroglycerin, the nurse would administer morphine for the refractory chest pain. Headache is a common side effect after nitroglycerin due to

CLINICAL JUDGMENT SINGLE-EPISODE CASE STUDY—CONT'D

its vasodilatory effects and should be monitored. Atropine and diltiazem would not be administered. Atropine would be administered if the patient suddenly became bradycardic; diltiazem would be administered if the patient developed premature supraventricular tachycardia (PSVT) if his blood pressure is stable; otherwise, adenosine would be appropriate.

Reference
Zafari AM, Abdou MH: *Myocardial infarction treatment & management*, 2019. https://emedicine.medscape.com/article/155919-treatment

CLINICAL JUDGMENT CASE STUDY

A patient who is 19 years of age experienced a gunshot wound to the head and a spinal cord injury from a stab wound over the thoracic spine 1 hour ago. The patient was transported immediately from the injury scene to the trauma center by paramedics. Upon hospital arrival, the patient was awake and following simple commands, but the neurologic status has subsequently deteriorated. At this point, the patient has undergone initial resuscitation and a rapid diagnostic workup. The patient is now orally intubated, has two functional intravenous (IV) catheters—one peripheral line in the right forearm and one triple-lumen central line in the left subclavian vein—an oral gastric tube, and an indwelling urinary catheter. The patient's current vital signs are blood pressure (BP) 88/56, heart rate (HR) 56, temperature 96.8°F (36°C), and respiratory rate (RR) 16 on a mechanical ventilator. The patient's mother reported that DW has a substance use disorder for opioids, including heroin, as well as oral diazepam and other street drugs.

The patient's diagnoses include a penetrating head injury with intracerebral hemorrhage diagnosed by computed tomography (CT) scan, a penetrating spinal cord injury at the T4 level, and drug abuse. The patient opens his eyes spontaneously and does not follow commands, and only the upper extremities withdraw; the lower extremities do not move.

1. On arrival at the trauma center, should the patient have received supplemental oxygen based on the pulse oximetry reading of 90%? What type of oxygen delivery device would be appropriate for the patient on initial presentation, with spontaneous breathing?
2. The physician orders 50 g of mannitol to be given now, IV push. On hand are several 50-mL vials of "mannitol, 25%" solution. How many milliliters of mannitol from this vial need to be drawn up into the syringe to administer 50 g?
3. Describe the type of needle that must be used when administering mannitol. Explain your answer. What size syringe would be used? Which IV line would be used to administer the mannitol?
4. What are the indications for mannitol administration? List at least three nursing considerations when giving mannitol.
5. The patient has a history of heroin and diazepam abuse. List the reversal drugs that could be used if the trauma team believes recent illicit drug use may be a contributing factor to the altered mental state.
6. Because of the spinal cord injury, the patient is exhibiting signs of neurogenic shock: bradycardia, warm skin, and hypotension. What is the drug of choice that the nurse would keep at the bedside in case the patient requires emergency treatment for symptomatic bradycardia? Name the drug, its mechanism of action, and dosing considerations.
7. The physician orders dopamine 800 mg/250 mL D_5W, to be titrated to maintain systolic BP above 110 mm Hg. Which IV site would be the best choice for a continuous dopamine infusion in DW?
8. What is the consequence of dopamine extravasation?
9. Describe the treatment for dopamine extravasation.
10. What vital sign parameters must be monitored while the patient receives dopamine? Name at least four adverse effects of dopamine.
11. Antibiotics are initiated as prophylaxis for infection due to the nature of the patient's penetrating injuries. Upon infusion of the antibiotic, a full-body rash, swelling of the lips and tongue, and hypotension develop. After antibiotic administration, what condition has developed in the patient?
13. What are the drugs of choice to treat the patient's condition now?
14. How can the nurse evaluate the effectiveness of these drugs?

REVIEW QUESTIONS

1. The nurse noted a patient's heart rate decreasing from 45 to 38 while administering atropine 0.3 mg IV. Which explanation is most likely?
   a. Atropine exerts its effects by stimulating the vagus nerve.
   b. The ordered dose was too low.
   c. Adenosine was indicated, not atropine.
   d. Atropine typically slows heart rate first and then increases it.
2. An older adult patient with a hip fracture became unresponsive 20 minutes after receiving morphine 3 mg intravenously. Which actions would the nurse take?
   a. Assess the patient, call for additional assistance, support breathing with a bag valve mask device as indicated, and prepare to administer flumazenil.
   b. Call the physician and report that the patient most likely experienced a stroke and now has elevated intracranial pressure; prepare to administer mannitol.
   c. Assess the patient, call for additional assistance, support breathing with a bag valve mask device as indicated, and prepare to administer naloxone.
   d. Explain to the patient's family that the morphine is taking effect and that unresponsiveness is the desired outcome to best manage the pain.
3. The nurse is caring for a young patient with a closed head injury who has an intracranial pressure of 35 (normal <20) and serum osmolality of 330 mOsm/kg. The nurse would anticipate which action?
   a. Administration of mannitol
   b. Withholding mannitol at this time, but taking other measures to reduce intracranial pressure
   c. Administration of sodium nitroprusside
   d. Taking no action at this time because the patient has a serum osmolality of 330, which will offset the effects of the elevated intracranial pressure

4. A dopamine infusion was started in a patient's antecubital vein during resuscitation for profound hypotension, but the electronic infusion device is now sounding an alert for an occlusion. Which immediate concern would be most important for the nurse?
   a. Infiltration with phentolamine will be necessary if there is extravasation.
   b. An interruption in the infusion can produce hypotension in the patient.
   c. The device will need to be reported to the hospital's clinical engineering department for service.
   d. The patient could develop hypertension as a result of the alarm.
5. The nurse observes a short period of asystole on the cardiac monitor that resolves spontaneously immediately after administering adenosine IV to a patient who was experiencing paroxysmal supraventricular tachycardia. Which initial action is the most appropriate for the nurse?
   a. Call a code to report a cardiac arrest.
   b. Prepare epinephrine and atropine for intravenous administration.
   c. Initiate cardiopulmonary resuscitation (CPR).
   d. Closely observe the patient and the cardiac monitor.
6. The nurse practitioner has written a number of stat orders for drugs to treat a patient on the medical-surgical unit who has experienced an acute anaphylactic reaction with hives and bronchospasm during infusion of an IV antibiotic. Which priority drug would the nurse administer first?
   a. Steroid dose pack
   b. Dopamine
   c. Epinephrine
   d. Diphenhydramine
7. The nurse receives a stat order to administer 50% dextrose solution intravenously to a 1-year-old child with hypoglycemia. How should this drug best be prepared for safe administration to the child?
   a. Use a filter needle.
   b. Draw the drug into a tuberculin syringe.
   c. Dilute 1:1 with sterile water to produce dextrose 25%.
   d. Shake the solution vigorously before injection.
8. An unresponsive patient who was brought to the emergency department has been reportedly taking alprazolam for a severe anxiety disorder after the mother's death. Knowing this history, which drug would the nurse anticipate administering?
   a. Mannitol
   b. Naloxone
   c. Activated charcoal
   d. Flumazenil
9. A patient was admitted to the emergency department with a pulse oximeter reading of 85% after a successful prehospital resuscitation from cardiac arrest due to an asthma attack. Which initial drug would be most important to administer?
   a. Epinephrine
   b. Sodium bicarbonate
   c. Albuterol
   d. Oxygen
10. Which drug concentration is appropriate to administer in an order for epinephrine 0.3 mg IM to treat a severe allergic reaction in an adult patient?
    a. 1:10,000
    b. 1:1000
    c. 1:100
    d. 1:10
11. Upon preparing to administer activated charcoal by mouth to treat a patient who took an overdose of aspirin and several unknown drugs, the nurse notes that the patient has become very somnolent and eyes open only to a noxious stimulus. Which action by the nurse is most appropriate at this point?
    a. Immediately discuss the change in the patient's mental status with the nurse practitioner who wrote the activated charcoal orders so that the plan of care can be reevaluated.
    b. Immediately insert a nasogastric tube and administer the activated charcoal.
    c. Immediately elevate the head of the patient's stretcher, and coax the patient to drink the activated charcoal while applying noxious stimuli as necessary to maintain wakefulness.
    d. Give only half the dose now, and wait until the patient's mental status improves before giving the remainder of the dose.
12. A surgeon orders aspirin 325 mg by mouth to a patient who developed chest pain while undergoing a minor outpatient surgery for a mole removal from the leg. Which action is most appropriate by the nurse?
    a. Question the aspirin order because the patient just had a surgical procedure and might have bleeding complications.
    b. After checking for drug allergies, first instruct the patient to chew the aspirin tablet and then administer the aspirin.
    c. After checking for drug allergies, instruct the patient to swallow the aspirin tablet whole.
    d. Suggest to the surgeon that the enteric-coated form of aspirin might be better tolerated by the patient to avoid gastrointestinal distress.

APPENDIX A

Answers to Review Questions

Chapter 1
Answers: 1. b; 2. c; 3. b; 4. a, b, c, e; 5. c; 6. (1) c, (2) b, (3) d, (4) a, (5) f; (6) e.

Chapter 2
Answers: 1. b; 2. d; 3. c; 4. a; 5. a, b, c, d; 6. a, b, d, e; 7. c; 8. a; 9. a, b, d; 10. a, b, c; 11. a; 12. a.

Chapter 3
Answers: 1. c, e; 2. a; 3. b; 4 a; 5. a, b, d; 6. a, b, c; 7. a; 8. d; 9. c; 10. b.

Chapter 4
Answers: 1. d; 2. a; 3. a, b, c, d, e; 4. d; 5. a, b, c.

Chapter 5
Answers: 1. a, b, c; 2. b; 3. b; 4. b, e; 5. a, c.

Chapter 6
Answers: 1. d; 2. c; 3. c; 4. a, c, e; 5. a, b, e; 6. a, d.

Chapter 7
Answers: 1. a, b, c; 2. c; 3. a; 4. c; 5. a, c, e; 6. b, c, e; 7. a, b; 8. b.

Chapter 8
Answers: 1. c; 2. a; 3. b, c, e; 4. a; 5. a, b, c, e, f.

Chapter 9
Answers: 1. a, c; 2. b, c, d, e; 3. a; 4. d; 5. b, c, d, e; 6. a, d; 7. d.

Chapter 10
Answers: 1. a, b, d; 2. d; 3. d; 4. b; 5. b; 6. b; 7. a; 8. a, c, d.

Chapter 11
See Answers to Practice Problems at the end of Chapter 11.

Chapter 12
Answers: 1. a; 2. b; 3. c; 4. d; 5. a, b, c, e; 6. b; 7. a, b, d, e; 8. a, b, e.

Chapter 13
Answers: 1. d; 2. a; 3. b; 4. a; 5. c; 6. c; 7. b; 8. b; 9. d; 10. b; 11. c.

Chapter 14
Answers: 1. c; 2. c; 3. a, b, d; 4. d; 5. a; 6. a, b, d; 7. b.

Chapter 15
Answers: 1. a, b, d; 2. c; 3. c; 4. d; 5. b, c, d, e; 6. a, b; 7. b, c.

Chapter 16
Answers: 1. b; 2. c; 3. a; 4. d; 5. b; 6. d; 7. a.

Chapter 17
Answers: 1. d; 2. d; 3. c; 4. a; 5. c.

Chapter 18
Answers: 1. a; 2. c; 3. d; 4. c; 5. b; 6. d; 7. a, b, c.

Chapter 19
Answers: 1. c; 2. b; 3. c; 4. c, d, e; 5. a, b; 6. b; 7. d.

Chapter 20
Answers: 1. b, c, d; 2. d; 3. d; 4. c; 5. b; 6. a, b, c, e; 7. a, b, c.

Chapter 21
Answers: 1. b; 2. b; 3. c; 4. d; 5. a; 6. a, c, d; 7. b, c, d, e; 8. c; 9. a, b, d, e.

Chapter 22
Answers: 1. b; 2. a; 3. d; 4. a, b, c, d, e; 5. a; 6. b, c, d, e; 7. a, b, c, f.

Chapter 23
Answers: 1. d; 2. a, c; 3. a; 4. b; 5. d; 6. a, b, c, d; 7. a, b, e, f.

Chapter 24
Answers: 1. c; 2. c; 3. a; 4. a; 5. a, c, d; 6. a, b, c, e.

Chapter 25
Answers: 1. c; 2. b; 3. c; 4. b; 5. a; 6. a, b, c; 7. a, c, e; 8. a.

Chapter 26
Answers: 1. a; 2. a, b, c, d; 3. a, b, d; 4. c; 5. b; 6. d

Chapter 27
Answers: 1. a, b, c, e; 2. a, c, d, e, f; 3. d; 4. a.

Chapter 28
Answers: 1. a; 2. d; 3. a, b, d, f; 4. a, b, c, d, e.

Chapter 29
Answers: 1. a; 2. c; 3. d; 4. a, b, c, d; 5. b.

Chapter 30
Answers: 1. a; 2. b; 3. c; 4. a, d, e, f; 5. d; 6. a, d, e; 7. a.

Chapter 31
Answers: 1. a; 2. b; 3. b; 4. d; 5. d; 6. c.

Chapter 32
Answers: 1. d; 2. d; 3. a; 4. a, b, c, e; 5. a, b, d.

Chapter 33
Answers: 1. d; 2. c; 3. a, b, c, d; 4. b; 5. b.

Chapter 34
Answers: 1. c; 2. d; 3. a; 4. a; 5. d; 6. d; 7. a, b; 8. c.

Chapter 35
Answers: 1. b; 2. a; 3. c; 4. a; 5. c; 6. b; 7. c; 8. c; 9. a, c, e; 10. a, b, e.

Chapter 36
Answers: 1. d; 2. a; 3. b; 4. c; 5. d; 6. c; 7. d; 8. b; 9. c.

Chapter 37
Answers: 1. a; 2. c; 3. a; 4. b; 5. d; 6. b.

Chapter 38
Answers: 1. b; 2. c; 3. d; 4. b; 5. d; 6. b, c, d, e.

Chapter 39
Answers: 1. b, d, e; 2. b; 3. c; 4. c; 5. a.

Chapter 40
Answers: 1. b; 2. a; 3. d; 4. a; 5. b; 6. c; 7. b; 8. c; 9. a, b, e.

Chapter 41
Answers: 1. b; 2. b, c, d, e; 3. b; 4. a; 5. b; 6. b; 7. b.

Chapter 42
Answers: 1. a, b, c, d; 2. a; 3. c; 4. b; 5. b; 6. d; 7. b; 8. a, b, d, e.

Chapter 43
Answers: 1. a, b, c, d, e; 2. a; 3. a; 4. d; 5. b; 6. b; 7. d.

Chapter 44
Answers: 1. c; 2. a; 3. a; 4. b; 5. d; 6. b; 7. a; 8. b, c, d.

Chapter 45
Answers: 1. b; 2. b; 3. a; 4. d; 5. c; 6. a, b, c, d, e.

Chapter 46
Answers: 1. a; 2. d; 3. a, c, e, f; 4. d; 5. a, b, f; 6. c.

Chapter 47
Answers: 1. d; 2. a; 3. b; 4. g, b, d, e, a, f, h, c; 5. c; 6. b, c.

Chapter 48
Answers: 1. b; 2. a, c, d; 3. d; 4. d; 5. b, d; 6. b, c; 7. a, b, d; 8. b, c, e; 9. c, d.

Chapter 49
Answers: 1. c; 2. c; 3. a; 4. b; 5. a; 6. b, c, d, e; 7. a, b, c, e.

Chapter 50
Answers: 1. c; 2. a; 3. b; 4. c; 5. d, e; 6. a, b, d; 7. b, d.

Chapter 51
Answers: 1. a; 2. d; 3. d; 4. d; 5. b.

Chapter 52
Answers: 1. a, b, c; 2. a; 3. b; 4. c; 5. a; 6. c; 7. d; 8. d; 9. b; 10. a, c, d, e; 11. a, c, e.

Chapter 53
Answers: 1. d; 2. a; 3. b; 4. c; 5. a; 6. b; 7. b; 8. a; 9. b; 10. a, b, c, d.

Chapter 54
Answers: 1. c; 2. c; 3. b, c, e; 4. b; 5. c, d, e; 6. a, b, e.

Chapter 55
Answers: 1. a, c; 2. a, d, e; 3. c; 4. b; 5. b, c, d; 6. d; 7. b; 8. a, b, d.

Chapter 56
Answers: 1. a, c, d; 2. a, b, c, d; 3. a, d; 4. a, b, d; 5. d; 6. b, c, d, e; 7. a, b, d.

Chapter 57
Answers: 1. a, d; 2. b, c, d; 3. a; 4. b; 5. 4 mL IM × 1; 6. a, d; 7. c; 8. b.

Chapter 58
Answers: 1. b; 2. c; 3. b; 4. b; 5. d; 6. c; 7. c; 8. d; 9. d; 10. b; 11. a; 12. b.

777

BIBLIOGRAPHY

Administration for Community Living: *2018 Profile of older Americans*, 2018. https://acl.gov/sites/default/files/Aging%20and%20Disability%20in%20America/2018OlderAmericansProfile.pdf.

Allen P: *Will pharmacogenetics help your health?* https://health.usnews.com/health-news/patient-advice/articles/2015/10/23/will-pharmacogenetics-help-your-health2015.

American Academy of Dermatology: *Issues updated guidelines for the management of acne.* 2024. https://www.aad.org.

American Academy of Ophthalmology: *What is macular degeneration?*, 2020. https://www.aao.org/eye-health/diseases/amd-macular-degeneration.

American Botanical Council: *Terminology*, 2013. http://abc.herbalgram.org/site/PageServer?pagename=Terminology.

American Cancer Society (ACS). *CAR T-cell therapy and its side effects.* American Cancer Society; 2022. Retrieved from https://www.cancer.org/cancer/managing-cancer/treatment-types/immunotherapy/car-t-cell1.html.

American College of Cardiology/American Heart Association: *Guideline for the prevention, detection, evaluation and management of high blood pressure in adults*, 2019.

American College of Obstetricians and Gynecologists: *Antenatal corticosteroid therapy for fetal maturation*, 2016. https://m.acog.org.

American College of Obstetricians and Gynecologists: *ACOG Practice Bulletin 194: Polycystic ovary syndrome*, 2018. https://m.acog.org

American College of Obstetricians and Gynecologists: *ACOG Practice Bulletin No. 194: Polycystic ovary syndrome*, 2020. https://m.acog.org

American College of Obstetricians and Gynecologists: *Preeclampsia and hypertension in pregnancy*, 2018. https://m.acog.org.

American College of Obstetricians and Gynecologists: *Morning sickness: nausea and vomiting of pregnancy*, 2015. https://www.m.acog.org.

American College of Obstetricians and Gynecologists: *Medications for pain relief during labor and delivery*, 2018. https://www.m.acog.org.

The American College of Obstetricians and Gynecologists: *The Rh factor: how it can affect your pregnancy*, 2024. https://m.acog.org/Patients/FAQs/The Rh factor how it can affect your pregnancy.

The American Congress of Obstetricians and Gynecologists (ACOG): *Maternal safety bundle for severe hypertension in pregnancy. Safe motherhood initiative*, 2017. http://www.ACOG.com.

American Heart Association: *Guidelines for cardiopulmonary resuscitation and emergency cardiovascular care*, 2015. https://eccguidelines.heart.org/index.php/circulation/cpr-ecc-guidelines-2/part-7-adult-advanced-cardiovascular-life-support/.

American Nurses Association: *CDC: opioid use disorder prevalence up 333% among pregnant women*, 2018, Association Smart Brief. http://www:American Nurse's.

American Nurses Association: *Code of ethics for nurses with interpretive statements*, 2015. https://www.nursingworld.org/practice-policy/nursing-excellence/ethics/code-of-ethics-for-nurses/coe-view-only/.

American Society of Clinical Pharmacology: *CAR T-cell immunotherapy named advance of the year in annual ASCO report*, 2018. https://www.asco.org.

Association of Reproductive Health Professionals: *Extended or continuous use of combined hormonal contraceptive pills*, 2014. https://www.arhp.org/publicationsandresources.oc.

Bakall B, Hariprasad SM, Klein KA. Emerging gene therapy treatments for inherited retinal diseases. *Ophthalmic Surg Lasers Imaging Retina.* 2018;49(7):472–478. https://doi.org/10.3928/23258160-20180628-02.

Belluz J. *This new bill would add $9 billion for medical research. Here are 5 reasons critics are terrified.* VOX Science & Health; 2015. http://www.vox.com/2015/7/14/8961923/21st-century-cures-act.

Blaise K, Hayes Jr. *Professional nursing practice concept and perspective.* ed 7. Upper Saddle River, NJ: Pearson; 2016.

Bodenheimer T: *Teach-back: a simple way to enhance patients' understanding*, 2018. https://aafp.org/fpm/2018/0700/p20.html.

Bonin M, Mewton N, Roubille F, et al. Effect and safety of morphine use in acute anterior ST-segment elevation myocardial infarction. *JAHA.* 2018;7(4): https://doi.org/10.1161/JAHA.117.006833: Retrieved September 20, 2018 https://www.ahajournals.org/doi/pdf/10.1161/JAHA.117.006833.

Bradley HC: *Renal transplantation*, 2019. https://emedicine.medscape.com/article/430128-overview.

Burchum J, Rosenthal L. *Lehne's pharmacology for nursing care.* ed 9. St. Louis: Elsevier; 2016.

Burchum JR, Rosenthal LD. *Lehne's pharmacology for nursing care.* ed 10. St. Louis: Elsevier; 2019.

CancerQuest.org. *Biological response modifiers (BRM)*, 2021. https://www.cancerquest.org/patients/treatments/biological-therapies.

CancerQuest.org. *Cancer immunotherapy.* https://www.cancerquest.org/patients/treatments/immunotherapy, 2021.

Carlson NR. *Foundations of behavioral neuroscience.* ed 8. Upper Saddle River, NJ: Pearson; 2010.

Centers for Disease Control and Prevention (CDC): *About HIV*, 2022. https://www.cdc.gov/hiv/basics/whatishiv.html

Centers for Disease Control and Prevention (CDC): *HIV by age: Viral suppression*, 2022. https://www.cdc.gov/hiv/group/age/viral-suppression.html#:~:text=Viral%20suppression%20is%20one%20of,HIV%20per%20milliliter%20of%20blood.

Center for Disease Control and Prevention (CDC): *HIV surveillance report*, 2021. http://www.cdc.gov/hiv/library/reports/hiv-surveillance.html

Centers for Disease Control and Prevention: *Recommendations for women*, 2024. https://www.cdc.gov/ncbddd/folicacid/recommendations.html.

Centers for Disease Control and Prevention: *HIV in the United States and dependent areas*, 2021. https://www.cdc.gov/hiv/statistics/overview/ataglance.html.

Centers for Disease Control and Prevention: *Parasites – malaria*, 2021. https://www.cdc.gov/parasites/malaria/index.html.

Centers for Disease Control and Prevention: *The right way to use a male condom*, 2016. www.cdc.gov/condomeffectiveness/male-condom-use.html.

Centers for Disease Control and Prevention: *Medication safety program*, 2017. https://www.cdc.gov/medicationsafety/adult_adversedrugevents.html.

Centers for Disease Control and Prevention: *2015 Sexually transmitted diseases treatment guidelines*, 2015. https://www.cdc.gov/std/tg2015/default.htm.

Centers for Disease Control and Prevention: *Tuberculosis (TB).* www.cdc.gov/tb/default.htm.

Center for Disease Control: *Tuberculosis: data and statistics*, 2023. https://www.cdc.gov/tb/statistics/default.htm

Centers for Disease Control and Prevention: *Vaccines & immunizations*, 2016. https://www.cdc.gov/vaccines/index.html?CDC_AA_refVal=https%3A%2F%2Fwww.cdc.gov%2Fvaccines%2Fdefault.htm.

Centers for Disease Control and Prevention: *V-safe after vaccination health checker.* https://www.cdc.gov/coronavirus/2019-ncov/vaccines/safety/vsafe.html.

Chang KL, Weitzel K, Shmidt S. Pharmacogenetics: using genetic information to guide drug therapy. *Am Fam Physician.* 2015;92(7):588–594. www.aafp.org/afp.

Cheek DJ. Pharmacogenomics: strategies for individualized care. *Nursing2017CriticalCare.* 2017;12(1):23–27. www.nursingcriticalcare.com.

Cheek DJ: *Why nurses need to be informed about pharmacogenomics. Reflections on nursing leadership*, 2015. https://www.reflectionsonnursingleadership.org/features/more-features/Vol41_2_why-nurses-need-to-be-informed-about-pharmacogenomics.

Cheek DJ, Howington L. Patient care in the dawn of the genomic age. *Am Nurse Today.* 2017;12(3):16–22.

Chooniedass R, Temple B, Becker A. Epinephrine use for anaphylaxis: too seldom, too late: current practices and guidelines in healthcare. *Ann Allergy Asthma Immunol.* 2017;119:108–110.

Chu DK, Kim LH-Y, Young PJ, et al. Mortality and morbidity in acutely ill adults treated with liberal versus conservative oxygen therapy (IOTA): a systematic review and meta-analysis. *Lancet.* 2018;391(10131):1693–1705.

Clayton BD, Willihnganz MJ. *Basic pharmacology for nurses.* ed 17. St. Louis: Elsevier; 2017.

Clinical Info: *Guidelines for the use of antiretroviral agents in adults and adolescents living with HIV*, 2021. https://clinicalinfo.hiv.gov/en/guidelines/adult-and-adolescent-arv/what-start-initial-combination-regimens-antiretroviral-naive?view=full.

Consumer Healthcare Products Association: *Statistics on OTC use*, n.d. https://www.chpa.org/MarketStats.aspx.

Council for Responsible Nutrition (CRN): *The science behind the supplements*. https://crnusa.org.

Department of Health & Human Services/Office on Women's Health: *Premenstrual syndrome (PMS)*, 2021. https://www.womenshealth.gov.

Department of Health & Human Services/Office on Women's Health: *Menopause*, 2021. https://www.womenshealth.gov.

Divakaran S, Loscalzo J. The role of nitroglycerin and other nitrogen oxides in cardiovascular therapeutics. *J Am Coll Cardiol*. 2017;70(19):2393–2410.

DrugAbuse.com: n.d. http://drugabuse.com/library/drugs-a-z/; www.drugs.com

Drugs.com for Healthcare professionals, n.d. Retrieved from www.drugs.com/professionals.html

Drugs A.-Z. www.drugs.com

Edmunds MW. *Introduction to clinical pharmacology*. ed 8. St. Louis: Mosby; 2016.

Epocrates. http://www.epocrates.com

Evans P: *8 incredible facts about the booming US marijuana industry*, 2019. https://markets.businessinsider.com/news/stocks/weed-us-marijuana-industry-facts-2019-5-1028177375#the-marijuana-industry-could-soon-be-worth-more-than-the-gdp-of-9-us-states1.

Farrukh: *The difference between active and passive transport*, 2018. https://hourstv.com/difference-between-active-and-passive-transport/.

Gahart B, Nazareno AR, Ortega MQ. *Intravenous medications*. ed 35. St. Louis: Elsevier; 2019.

Gentili A, Adler RA: *Growth hormone replacement in older men?* Medscape. https://emedicine.medscape.com/article/126999-medication#22020.

Giddens JF. *Concepts for nursing practice*. ed 2. St. Louis: Elsevier; 2017.

GlobalRxPh: *Creatinine clearance adult*, 2017. https://globalrph.com/medcalcs/creatinine-clearance-adult/.

Governing: *State marijuana Laws in 2019 Map*, 2019. https://www.governing.com/gov-data/safety-justice/state-marijuana-laws-map-medical-recreational.html.

Gummin DD, Mowry JB, Spyker DA, Brooks DE, Fraser MO, Banner W. 2016 Annual report of the American Association of Poison Control Centers' National Poison Data System (NPDS): 34th annual report. *Clin Toxicol*. 2017;55(10):1072–1254. https://doi.org/10.1080/15563650.2017.1388087. Retrieved on September 20, 2018.

Government of Canada: *Controlled drugs and substances act*, 2018. https://laws-lois.justice.gc.ca/eng/acts/C-38.8/20180621/P1TT3xt3.html.

Guzman F: *Pharmacology corner*, n.d. http://pharmacologycorner.com/therapeutic-index/.

Haga SB, Mills R. Nurses' communication of pharmacogenetic tests results as part of discharge care. *Pharmacogenomics*. 2015;16(3):251–256. https://doi.org/10.2217/PGS.14.173.

Harvard Health Letter: *Sexually transmitted disease? At my age?* https://www.health.harvard.edu/diseases-and-conditions/sexually-transmitted-disease-at-my-age, 2018.

Hastert JD: *H.R.1 – Medicare prescription drug, improvement, and modernization act of 2003*, 2003. https://www.congress.gov/bill/108th-congress/house-bill/1.

Hewitt J, Tower M, Latimer S. An education intervention to improve nursing students understanding of medication safety. *Nurses Educ Pract*. 2015;15(1):17–21.

Horvath AT, Misra K, Epner AK, Cooper GM: *The diagnostic criteria for substance use disorders (addiction)*, n.d.www.amhc.org/1408-addictions/article/48502-the-diagnostic-criteria-for-substance-use-disorders-addiction.

Huether SE, McCance KL. *Understanding pathophysiology*. ed 6. St. Louis: Elsevier; 2017.

Human Research Protections (OHRP): 2014, U.S. Department of Health & Human Services. Retrieved from http://www.hhs.gov/ohrp/policy/consentckls.html

Ignatavicius D. *Developing clinical judgment for professional nursing and the next generation NCLEX-RN examination*. Missouri: Elsevier; 2021.

Ignatavicium D. *White paper: using case studies to develop clinical judgment & ensure next generation NCLEX (NGN) success*. Missouri: Elsevier; 2021.

Ignatavicius DD, Workman ML, Rebar CR. *Medical-Surgical nursing: concepts for interprofessional collaborative care*. ed 9. St. Louis: Elsevier; 2018.

International Council for Harmonization of Technical Requirements for Pharmaceuticals for Human Use: *Integrated addendum to ICH E6(R1): guideline for good clinical practice (E6(R2)*, 2016. https://www.ich.org/fileadmin/Public_Web_Site/ICH_Products/Guidelines/Efficacy/E6/E6_R2__Step_4_2016_1109.pdf.

Lab Tests Online: *Pharmacogenetic tests*, 2018. https://labtestsonline.org/tests/pharmacogenetic-tests.

Lea DH. The role of pharmacogenomics in cancer. *Am Nurse Today*. 2010;5(10): Retrieved from https://www.americannursetoday.com/the-role-of-pharmacogenomics-in-cancer/.

Lewis SL, Bucher L, Heitkemper MM, Harding MM. *Medical-surgical nursing: assessment and management of clinical problems*. ed 10. St. Louis: Elsevier; 2017.

Lexicomp Clinical Drug Information: http://www.wolterskluwercdi.com/lexicomp-online/.

Lilley LL, Collins SR, Snyder JS. *Pharmacology and the nursing process*. ed 8. St. Louis: Elsevier; 2017.

Maddox TM, Januzzi JL, Allen LA, et al. Update to the 2017 ACC Expert Consensus Decision Pathway for Optimization of Heart Failure Treatment: answers to 10 pivotal issues about heart failure with reduced ejection fraction: a Report of the American College of Cardiology Solution Set Oversight Committee. *J Am Coll Cardiol*. 2021;77(6):772–810.

Martin-Hijano L, Sainz B. The interactions between cancer stem cells and the innate-interferon signaling pathway. *Front Immunol*. 2020;11

Maternal & Family Health Services: *Family planning protocols section 1 – required family planning services: informed consent*, 2013. Error! Hyperlink reference not valid.

Mayo Clinic: *Labor & delivery, postpartum care*, 2023. https://www.mayoclinic.org.

McClary LM. *Essentials of medical genetics for nursing and health professionals: an interprofessional approach*. Burlington, MA: Jones & Bartlett Learning; 2020.

McCormick KA. Pharmacogenomics and documentation: new partnerships target optimal care quality and outcomes. *Nurs Manag*. 2017;48(5):32–40. https://doi.org/10.1097/01.NUMA.0000515793.26355.7f.

McKenry LM, Tessier E, Hogan MA. *Mosby's pharmacology in nursing*. ed 22. St. Louis: Elsevier; 2006.

Medscape.com. (n.d.). Drugs, OTCs & Herbals. Retrieved from http://reference.medscape.com/drugs

Mehta M, Tudor GJ. https://www.ncbi.nlm.nih.gov/books/NBK537190/#:~:text=The%20formula%20recommends%204%20milliliters,first%2024%20hours%20of%20care *Parkland formula*. StatPearls [Internet]; 2020.

Meyer D, Damm T, Jensen K. Drug dosage adjustments in chronic kidney disease: the pharmacist's role. *Saskatchewan Drug Information Services College of Pharmacy and Nutrition, U of S*. 2012;29(3):4. Retrieved from https://www.rxfiles.ca/rxfiles/uploads/documents/ltc/HCPs/CKD/SDIS.Renal_newsletter.pdf.

Mion M. Ear Infections: Fungi. *Encyclopedia of Infection and Immunity*. 2022;3:268–278. https://doi.org/10.1016/B978-0-12-818731-9.00153-1.

Moncivaiz A: *CD4 vs. viral load: what's in a number*, 2021, Healthline. https://www.healthline.com/health/hiv-aids/cd4-viral-count

Montgomery S, Brouwer WA, Everett PC, et al. Genetics in the clinical setting: what nurses need to know to provide the best patient care. *Am Nurse Today*. 2017;12(10):10–16.

Moreno JD, Schmidt U, Joffe S. The Nuremberg Code 70 years later. *Journal of the American Medical Association*. 2017;318(9):795–796. https://doi.org/10.1001/jama.2017.10265.

National Cancer Institute. *Cancer statistics*. Retrieved from cancer.gov/about-cancer/understanding/statistics, 2020.

National Center for Chronic Disease Prevention and Health Promotion: *Neutropenia and risk for infection*, n.d. https://www.cdc.gov/cancer/preventinfections/pdf/neutropenia.pdf.

National Council of State Boards of Nursing: *Next-generation-NCLEX*, 2021,: Retrieved from: https://www.ncsbn.org.htm.

National Council of State Boards of Nursing. (n.d.): *Substance use disorder in nursing,*: Retrieved July 24, 2019 from https://www.ncsbn.org/substance-use-in-nursing.htm.

National Council of State Boards of Nursing: *The NCSBN clinical judgment measurement model*, 2018. https://www.ncsbn.org/14798.htm.

National Institute on Drug Abuse: *Commonly abused drugs*, 2016. www.drugabuse.gov/drugs-abuse/.

National Institute on Drug Abuse (NIDA): *Media guide*, 2018. https://archives.drugabuse.gov/publications/media-guide.

National Institute on Drug Abuse: *The science of drug abuse and addiction: the basics*, 2014. www.drugabuse.gov/publications/media-guide/science-drug-abuse-addiction-basics.

National Institute of General Medical Sciences: *Pharmacogenomics: what is pharmacogenomics? [Fact Sheet]*, 2017. https://www.nigms.nih.gov/education/pages/factsheet-pharmacogenomics.aspx.

National Institute of Health: *HIVinfo. FDA-approved medicines*, 2023. https://hivinfo.nih.gov/understanding-hiv/fact-sheets/fda-approved-hiv-medicines

National Institute of Health: National Cancer Institute: *CAR T cells: engineering patients' immune cells to treat their cancers*, 2022. https://www.cancer.gov/about-cancer/treatment/research/car-t-cells

National Kidney Foundation: *Kidney transplant*, n.d. https://www.kidney.org/atoz/content/kidney-transplant.

National Library of Medicine: *Acquired immune deficiency syndrome CD4+ count*, 2022. https://www.ncbi.nlm.nih.gov/books/NBK513289/

New Health Advisor: *How to use a female condom: pictures and instructions*, 2016. www.newhealthadvisor.com/How-to-Use-Female-Condom-Picture.html.

North American Menopause Society (NAMS) T: Menopause hormone therapy benefits & risks. In: *Menopause relief*, 2019, https://www.menopause.org.

Parekh R: *What is addiction?* https://www.psychiatry.org/patients-families/addiction/what-is-addiction 2017.

Pelligrino B: *Immunosuppression*, 2016. https://emedicine.medscape.com/article/432316-overview#a3.

Pharmacogenomics Laboratory: *Guideline-based decision support*. https://ignite-genomics.org/wp-content/uploads/2016/03/26_PGx-lab-Marketing-Brochure.pdf.

PharmGKB®: *What is pharmacogenomics?* om. https://www.pharmgkb.org/whatIsPharmacogenomics.

Piscitelli SC: *Space out drug discontinuations prior to "drug holiday"?*, 2000. https://www.medscape.com/viewarticle/413306.

Pinto JC: *Pediatric dosage development: where are we? [PowerPoint slides]*, n.d. http://www.fda.gov/downloads/NewsEvents/MeetingsConferencesWorkshops/UCM415217.pdf.

Sapkota B, Makandar SN, Acharya S. *Biologic response modifiers (BRMs). National Institute of Health: National Library of Medicine*; 2023. Retrieved from https://www.ncbi.nlm.nih.gov/books/NBK542200/#:~:text=Biologic%20response%20modifiers%20(BRMs)%2C,the%20failure%20of%20conventional%20agents.

Silvestri L. *White paper: Higher-cognitive level questions a starting point for creating next generation NCLEX (NGN) test items*. Missouri: Elsevier; 2021.

South Atlantic Association of Obstetricians & Gynecologists: *Pentobarbital anesthesia in labor*. https://www.sciencedirect.com/science/article/piv/0002937867902505

Substance Abuse and Mental Health Services Administration: *Substance use disorders*, 2015. www.samhsa.gov/disorders/substance-use/Preterm-PrematureLaborandbirth.

Substance Abuse and Mental Health Services Administration: *Treatments for substance use disorders*. www.samhsa.gov/treatment/substance-use-disorders 2015.

Talwar A, Tsang CA, Price SE, Pratt RH, Walker WL, Schmit KM, Lunger AJ. *MMWR Morb Mortal Wkly Rep*. 2019;68(11):257–262. Retrieved from https://www.cdc.gov/mmwr/volumes/68/wr/pdfs/mm6811a2-H.pdf.

Umberger R, Holston EC, Hutson SP, Pierce M. Nursing genomics: Practice implications every nurse should know. *Nurs Clin N Am*. 2013;48:499–522. https://doi.org/10.1016/j.cnur.2013.08.006.

United States Drug Enforcement Administration: *Drug scheduling*, 2018. https://www.dea.gov/drug-scheduling.

U.S. Department of Health and Human Services: *Office for Human Research Protections*, n.d. https://www.hhs.gov/ohrp/.

U.S. Food and Drug Administration: *Pregnancy and lactation labeling (drugs) final rule*, 2021. https://www.fda.gov/drugs/labeling-information-drug-products/pregnancy-and-lactation-labeling-drugs-final-rule.

U.S. Food and Drug Administration: *FDA approves new vaginal ring for one year of birth control*, 2018. https://www.fda.gov/ucm616541.htm.

U.S. Food and Drug Administration: *Drug trials snapshots: Orilissa*, 2018. https://www.fda.gov/ucm616534.htm.

U.S. Food and Drug Administration: *Milestones in U.S. Food and Drug law history*, 2018. https://www.fda.gov/about-fda/fdas-evolving-regulatory-powers/milestones-us-food-and-drug-law-history.

U.S. Food and Drug Administration: *FDA approves weekly therapy for adult growth hormone deficiency*, 2020. https://www.fda.gov/drugs/drug-safety-and-availability/fda-approves-weekly-therapy-adult-growth-hormone-deficiency.

U.S. Food and Drug Administration: *Critical path initiative*, 2018. https://www.fda.gov/science-research/science-and-research-special-topics/critical-path-initiative.

U.S. Food and Drug Administration: *Requirements for all OTC products*, n.d. https://www.accessdata.fda.gov/scripts/cder/training/OTC/topic4/topic4/da_01_04_0005.htm.

U.S. Food and Drug Administration: *The best way to take your over-the-counter pain reliever? Seriously*, 2018. https://www.fda.gov/drugs/safe-use-over-counter-pain-relievers-and-fever-reducers/best-way-take-your-over-counter-pain-reliever-seriously-four-panel-brochure.

U.S. Food and Drug Administration: *Pediatric exclusivity study age group (C-DRG-00909)*, 2014. http://www.fda.gov/Drugs/DevelopmentApprovalProcess/FormsSubmissionRequirements/ElectronicSubmissions/DataStandardsManualmonographs/ucm071754.htm.

U.S. Pharmacopeia National Formulary. https://www.uspnf.com.

Vallerand AH, Sanoski CA. *Davis drug guide for nurses*. ed 15. Pennsylvania: F. A. Davis; 2017.

Vogel WH. Infusion reactions: diagnosis, assessment and management. *Clin J Oncol Nurs*. 2010;14(2):E10–E21. Retrieved from http://chemotherapy.vc.ons.org/file_depot/0-10000000/0-10000/3365/folder/87592/Infusion+Reactions+(Vogel+2010).pdf.

Wilson BA, Shannon M, Shields K. *Pearson nurse's drug guide*. ed 1. New York: Pearson; 2017.

World Health Organization: *Lexicon of alcohol and drug terms published by the World Health Organization*, n.d. http://www.who.int/substance_abuse/terminology/who_lexicon/en/.

World Health Organization: The International Pharmacopoeia (Ph. Int.). https://www.who.int/medicines/publications/pharmacopoeia/en/

World Health Organization: *Tuberculosis*, 2023. https://www.who.int/news-room/fact-sheets/detail/tuberculosis#:~:text=Worldwide%2C%20TB%20is%20the%2013th,women%20and%201.2%20million%20children

World Health Organization Reproductive Health Library: *WHO recommendation on daily oral iron and folic acid supplement*, Geneva, 2016, The WHO Reproductive Health Library, World Health Organization.

World Medical Association: *WMA declaration of Helsinki – ethical principles for medical research involving human subjects*, 2018. https://www.wma.net/policies-post/wma-declaration-of-helsinki-ethical-principles-for-medical-research-involving-human-subjects/.

GLOSSARY

A

absence seizure Formerly known as petit mal seizure

absorption Movement of a drug into the bloodstream after administration

acetylcholine (ACh) The neurotransmitter located at the ganglions and the parasympathetic terminal nerve endings

acetylcholinesterase (AChE) inhibitor An enzyme responsible for breaking down acetylcholine; also known as *cholinesterase*

acne vulgaris The formation of papules, nodules, and cysts on the face, neck, shoulders, and back that results from keratin plugs at the base of the pilosebaceous (oil) glands near the hair follicles

acquired immunodeficiency syndrome (AIDS) The most advanced stage of human immunodeficiency virus (HIV) infection

acquired resistance Resistance caused by prior exposure to an antibacterial

acromegaly Excessive growth after puberty

activated partial thromboplastin time (aPTT) A medical test that characterizes blood coagulation

active acquired artificial immunity Immunity that occurs when a weakened antigen or immunoglobulin (Ig) is injected into an individual as a vaccination, which then stimulates an immune response

active immunity Immunity that occurs when the body's immune response is stimulated by an antigen or when a pathogen enters the body

active transport A process that requires a carrier, such as an enzyme or protein, to move a drug against a concentration gradient

acute cystitis A lower urinary tract infection (UTI)

acute dystonia Characteristics of this reaction include muscle spasms of the face, tongue, neck, and back; facial grimacing; abnormal or involuntary upward eye movement; and laryngeal spasms that can impair respiration

acute myocardial infarction (AMI) Acute heart attack

acute pharyngitis Inflammation of the throat or "sore throat" caused by a virus, beta-hemolytic streptococci, or other bacteria

acute pyelonephritis An upper UTI

acute rhinitis Acute inflammation of the mucous membranes of the nose that usually accompanies the common cold

adequate intake (AI) The consumption and absorption of sufficient food, vitamins, and essential minerals necessary to maintain health

addiction A psychological and physical dependence upon a substance beyond normal voluntary control, usually after prolonged use

Addison disease An endocrine disorder of the adrenal glands causing adrenal hyposecretion of its hormones

additive effect When two drugs are administered in combination and the response is increased beyond what either could produce alone

adenohypophysis The anterior pituitary gland

adherence The extent to which a patient continues an agreed-on mode of treatment without close supervision

adjuvant A substance added to a vaccine to increase the body's immune response to the vaccine

adjuvant analgesic A generic term for a medication not designed to manage pain

adjuvant therapy A additional therapy added to the primary therapy

adrenal glands Consist of the adrenal medulla and adrenal cortex

adrenergic agonists A class of G-protein–coupled receptors that are targets of the catecholamines

adrenergic antagonists (adrenergic blockers) Drugs that block either the alpha or the beta receptor

adrenergic neuron antagonists (adrenergic neuron blockers) Drugs that block the release of norepinephrine from the sympathetic terminal neurons

adrenergic receptor Target of the catecholamines

adrenocorticotropic hormone (ACTH) An endocrine hormone secreted by the anterior pituitary gland that stimulates the release of glucocorticoids, mineralocorticoids, and androgen from the adrenal cortex and epinephrine and norepinephrine from the adrenal medulla

adsorbents Act by coating the wall of the gastrointestinal tract and adsorbing bacteria or toxins that cause diarrhea

adverse drug event (ADE) Any injury that occurs at the time a drug is used, regardless of whether it is identified as a cause of the injury

adverse drug reaction (ADR) Unintentional, unexpected reactions to drug therapy that occur at normal drug dosages

afterload Peripheral vascular resistance

age-related macular degeneration (AMD) Deterioration of the macula

aggregation Clumping together of platelets to form a clot

agonists Drugs that activate receptors and produce a desired response

akathisia A reaction in which the patient has trouble standing still, is restless, paces the floor, and is in constant motion

alcohol toxicity A life-threatening condition that can occur by drinking large amounts of alcohol over a short period of time

alkylating drugs Drugs that damage cellular DNA by cross-linkage of DNA strands, abnormal base pairing, or DNA strand breaks, thus preventing the reproduction of cancer cells

allergic rhinitis Caused by pollen or a foreign substance such as animal dander

alpha antagonists (alpha blockers) Drugs that promote vasodilation, causing a decrease in blood pressure

alternative health therapies The phenomenon of the dominant cultural group borrowing traditional health practices from less dominant groups

alveoli Air sacs

Alzheimer disease A chronic, progressive, neurodegenerative condition with marked cognitive dysfunction

amenorrhea Absence of menstrual periods

American Nurses Association Code of Ethics Developed as a guide for carrying out nursing responsibilities in a manner consistent with quality in nursing care and the ethical obligations of the profession

amphetamines Drugs that stimulate the cerebral cortex of the brain

ampule Glass container with a tapered neck

anabolism Buildup of cellular tissue

analeptic Acts on the brainstem and medulla to stimulate respiration

analgesic A drug prescribed for the relief of pain

anaphylactic shock An allergic response resulting in severe bronchoconstriction and hypotension resulting in cardiac collapse

anaphylaxis A serious, life-threatening allergic reaction to a specific vaccine or vaccine component

androgen A male sex hormone

anesthetic A drug that causes anesthesia

angina pectoris Chest pain

angle-closure glaucoma A condition in which the iris is situated close to the drainage angle, thus blocking the trabecular network; also known as closed-angle or narrow-angle glaucoma

anion A negative charge in ions

anorexiants Drugs thought to suppress appetite by stimulating the satiety center in the hypothalamic and limbic areas of the brain

anovulation Lack of ovulation

anovulatory The absence of ovulation

anoxia Absence of oxygen

antacids Promote ulcer healing by neutralizing hydrochloric acid and reducing pepsin activity

antagonistic effects The negative effect that one chemical or family of chemicals has on other chemicals

antagonists Drugs that prevent receptor activation and block a response

anthelmintics Agents that destroy worms

anthracycline A class of chemotherapeutic agents

antiandrogens Androgen antagonists that block the synthesis or action of androgens

antianginal drugs Medicines that relieve the symptoms of angina pectoris

antibacterials Substances that inhibit bacterial growth or kill bacteria and other microorganisms

781

antibiotic resistance Biologically occurring short chains of amino acid monomers linked by peptide (amide) bonds

antibodies Defend the body against pathogens

anticoagulants Prevent the formation of clots that inhibit circulation

antidepressants Drugs that treat depression and/or relieve the symptoms

antidiarrheals Agents used for treating diarrhea and decreasing hypermotility

antidiuretic hormone (ADH) A hormone made by the hypothalamus in the brain and stored in the posterior pituitary gland

antidysrhythmics (antiarrhythmics) Drugs that restore the cardiac rhythm to normal

antiemetics Antivomiting agents

antiflatulents Drugs that treat excessive gas in the stomach and intestines

antifungals Drugs used to treat fungal infections

antigen A toxin or other foreign substance that induces an immune response in the body, especially the production of antibodies

antihistamines Compete with histamine for receptor sites and prevent a histamine response

antihyperlipidemics Drugs used to lower lipoproteins

antihypertensives Drugs used to treat hypertension

antimalarials Drugs that provide treatment and prophylaxis for malaria

antimetabolite A chemical that interferes with various substances needed for normal cell function

antimicrobials Substances that inhibit bacterial growth or kill bacteria and other microorganisms

antimuscarinics Agents that block parasympathetic nerve impulses

antimycotic drugs Drugs used to treat fungal infections

antineoplastic drug An agent that destroys cancer cells

antioncogenes Genes that protect other genes

antiplatelets Used to prevent thrombosis in the arteries by suppressing platelet aggregation

antipsychotics Also known as *neuroleptics* or *psychotropics*, but the preferred name for this group is either *antipsychotics* or *neuroleptics*

antiretroviral therapy (ART) The combination of several antiretroviral medicines used to slow the rate at which human immunodeficiency virus (HIV) makes copies of itself in the body

antiseizure drugs Drugs used for epileptic seizures

antispasmodics Agents that block parasympathetic nerve impulses

antitumor antibiotics Agents that interfere with DNA replication and RNA transcription of cancer cells

antitussives Agents that act on the cough-control center in the medulla to suppress the cough reflex

antiviral drugs Agents used to prevent or delay the spread of viral infections

anxiolytics Also called antianxiety drugs or sedative-hypnotics

apolipoprotein A protein that combines with a lipid, such as cholesterol or triglyceride, to form a lipoprotein

apoptosis Programmed cell death

aqueous humor A clear fluid that flows continuously in and out of the chamber of the eye

assessment The phase during which a nurse gathers information from the patient about the patient's health and lifestyle

assimilation Occurs within and among cultural groups, such as when a minority group changes its ways to blend in with the dominant cultural group

asthma Hyperresponsiveness of the tracheobronchial system resulting in inflammation and narrowing of the airways

asystole The cessation of electrical activity within the heart

atonic seizure Loss of normal muscle tension; a seizure in which muscles suddenly lose strength

atrial fibrillation Cardiac dysrhythmia with rapid uncoordinated contractions of atrial myocardium

atrial flutter Cardiac dysrhythmia with rapid contractions of 200 to 300 beats/min

attention-deficit/hyperactivity disorder (ADHD) A disorder that might be caused by a dysregulation of the transmitter's serotonin, norepinephrine, and dopamine

attenuated viruses Viruses composed of live, attenuated microorganisms

atypical antidepressants Drugs used for major depression, reactive depression, and anxiety that affect one or two of the three neurotransmitters: serotonin, norepinephrine, and dopamine

atypical antipsychotics The second category of antipsychotics

autonomy The right to self-determination

B

bactericidal Bacteria killing

bacteriostatic Inhibits bacterial growth; may also be bactericidal (bacteria killing), depending on the drug dose, serum level, and pathogen

balanced anesthesia A combination of drugs frequently used in general anesthesia

barbiturates Long-, intermediate-, short-, and ultrashort-acting sedatives

basic formula The equation $D/H \times V = A$ to calculate the amount A to be administered, where D is the desired dose; H is the drug on hand; V is the vehicle or volume

Beers Criteria for Potentially Inappropriate Medication Use in Older Adults A document developed by a consensus panel of 12 experts in geriatric care to aid health care providers in the safe prescription and administration of drugs to older adults

beneficence The duty to protect research subjects from harm and to assess potential risks and possible benefits to ensure the benefits are greater than the risk

beta antagonists (beta blockers) May inhibit the action of albuterol

bioavailability The percentage of administered drug available for activity

biologic response modifiers (BRMs) A class of pharmacologic drugs used to enhance, direct, or restore the body's immune system

biotransformation The process by which the body chemically changes drugs into a form that can be excreted

bipolar disorder A disorder that involves swings between two moods, the manic and the depressive

Bishop score An objective measurement that assists in predicting whether labor induction may be successful; assess the readiness for labor induction

blackhead A type of noninflammatory acne lesion that is open

blepharitis Infection of the margins of the eyelid

blood-borne pathogens Microorganisms such as viruses or bacteria that can be spread through blood and body fluids

blood-brain barrier (BBB) A special endothelial lining in blood vessels in the brain where the cells are pressed tightly together (tight junctions)

blood dyscrasias Blood-cell disorders

bolus The first method used to deliver enteral feedings, by which 250 to 400 mL of solution is rapidly administered through a syringe into the tube four to six times a day

botanicals Additive substances that come from plants

bradycardia A pulse rate below 60 beats/min

bradykinesia Slow movement

brand (trade) name Also known as the *proprietary name*, the name chosen by the drug company; usually a registered trademark

breakthrough bleeding An abnormal flow of blood from the uterus that occurs between menstrual periods

broad-spectrum antibiotics Drugs that can be effective against both gram-positive and gram-negative organisms

bronchial asthma Characterized by bronchospasm, wheezing, mucus secretions, and dyspnea; one of the lung diseases of chronic obstructive pulmonary disease (COPD)

bronchiectasis Abnormal dilation of the bronchi and bronchioles secondary to frequent infection and inflammation

bronchodilators Drugs that relax bronchial muscle and result in expansion of the bronchial air passages

bronchospasm Results when lung tissue is exposed to extrinsic or intrinsic factors that stimulate a bronchoconstrictive response

buccal Administered between the cheek and gum

C

cadaveric transplantation A healthy organ donated at the time of a person's death that is transplanted into the body of a patient with end-stage organ failure

calcium channel blockers (CCBs) Agents used for the treatment of stable and variant

GLOSSARY

angina pectoris, certain dysrhythmias, and hypertension

cannabinoids The active ingredients in *Cannabis*, approved for clinical use in 1985 to alleviate nausea and vomiting resulting from cancer treatment

capillary leak syndrome A rare disorder from extravasation of plasma proteins and fluids in the extravascular space characterized by episodes of severe hypotension and multiorgan dysfunction

carbonic anhydrase inhibitors (CAIs) Agents that decrease intraocular pressure by decreasing the production of aqueous humor

cardiac dysrhythmia (arrhythmia) Any deviation from the normal rate or pattern of the heartbeat

cardiac glycosides Drugs that inhibit the sodium-potassium pump, which results in an increase in intracellular sodium

catecholamines Chemical structures of a substance, either endogenous or synthetic, that can produce a sympathomimetic response

cathartics Agents used to elicit bowel movements

cation A positive charge in ions

caudal block An epidural block placed by administering a local anesthetic through the sacral hiatus

cell cycle–nonspecific (CCNS) drugs Drugs that act during any phase of the cell cycle

cell cycle–specific (CCS) drugs Drugs that exert their influence during a specific phase of the cell cycle

cellular checkpoints, cellular communication Mechanism by which cell-to-cell communication occurs locally or remotely by signaling molecules to maintain homeostasis, regulate growth and division, develop and organize into tissues, and coordinate cellular functions

central nervous system (CNS) A system that involves the brain and spinal cord and that regulates body functions

cerumen Earwax

ceruminolytics Topical otic agents that soften or break up cerumen

cervical ripening Softening of the cervix just prior to labor induction

chalazion Infection of the meibomian glands of the eyelids that may produce cysts, causing blockage of the ducts

chancre A painless sore, typically at the site of infection, usually on the penis in males and outer genitals or inner vagina in females

chemical name A name that describes the drug's chemical structure

chemoprotectant An agent administered prior to certain chemotherapeutic drugs to prevent toxicity

chemoreceptor trigger zone (CTZ) A major cerebral center that lies near the medulla

chemotherapy The use of chemicals to kill cancer cells

chloasma Hyperpigmentation of the skin

cholinergic agonists Drugs that stimulate the parasympathetic nervous system

cholinergic antagonists (blocking agents) Drugs that affect the parasympathetic nervous system

cholinergic crisis Overdosing with acetylcholinesterase (AChE) inhibitors; may complicate myasthenia gravis

cholinergics Medications that produce the same effects as the parasympathetic neurotransmitter acetylcholine

cholinesterase (ChE) May destroy acetylcholine before it reaches the receptor or after it has attached to the site

cholinesterase inhibitors Indirect-acting cholinergics that inactivate the enzyme cholinesterase, which typically breaks down acetylcholine

chronic bronchitis A progressive lung disease caused by smoking or chronic lung infections

chronic obstructive pulmonary disease (COPD) A major category of lower respiratory tract disorders, COPD is caused by airway obstruction with increased airway resistance of airflow to lung tissues

chronotropic An action that decreases heart rate

chylomicrons Large particles that transport fatty acids and cholesterol to the liver

clonic seizure A convulsive seizure

cluster headache Headache characterized by a severe, unilateral, nonthrobbing pain usually located around the eye

colloid A solution that contains protein or other large molecular substances that increase osmolarity without dissolving in the solution

colony-stimulating factors Proteins that stimulate or regulate the growth, maturation, and differentiation of bone marrow stem cells

combination chemotherapy The use of two or more chemotherapy agents to treat cancer

comedones Noninflammatory acne lesions that may be open or closed

common cold The most prevalent type of upper respiratory infection

complementary health therapies Combine traditional and conventional Western health practices

concept A concept is related to the patient's problems, medications, or topics of care; it is derived after the analysis of the nurse's assessment data, will influence the delivery of the patient's care, and its focus is on the patient-centered model of care

congenital rubella syndrome Transmission of the rubella virus to the fetus via the placenta

congestive heart failure (CHF) Occurs when the heart muscle does not pump blood as well as it should

conjugate vaccines Newer vaccines that require a protein or toxoid from an unrelated organism to link to the outer coating of the disease-causing microorganism

conjunctivitis Inflammation of the membrane covering the eye and inner eyelids

constipation The accumulation of hard fecal material in the large intestine

contact dermatitis A common form of eczema that results when skin is exposed to irritants or allergens

continuous feedings Feedings prescribed for the critically ill and for those who receive feedings into the small intestine

controlled substance A drug or chemical that has the potential for abuse whose manufacture, possession, or use is regulated by government

corticosteroids Natural and synthetic agents that suppress inflammation

cretinism A congenital abnormality caused by severe hypothyroidism causing delayed physical and mental growth

Critical Path Initiative A national strategy "to drive innovation in the scientific processes through which medical products are developed, evaluated, and manufactured"

cross-resistance Tolerance, usually to a toxic substance, that is acquired not as a result of direct exposure but by exposure to a related substance

cross-sensitivity Sensitivity to one substance that predisposes an individual to sensitivity to other substances related in chemical structure

cryotherapy A procedure used to destroy tissue of both benign and malignant lesions through a freezing process

cryptorchidism Undescended testis

cryptosporidiosis Infection caused by the protozoan parasite *Cryptosporidium*

crystalloid A solution containing fluids and electrolytes that can freely cross capillary walls

crystalluria Crystals in the urine

cultural need Refers to the nurse being alert to the patient's cultural expectations

culture Learned beliefs and behaviors shared by a group of people

Cushing syndrome An endocrine disorder of the adrenal glands causing adrenal hypersecretion of its hormones

cyclic method A type of continuous feeding infused over 8 to 16 hours daily (day or night)

cyclins A family of proteins that stimulate the cell to move through the cell cycle

cyclooxygenase (COX) The enzyme responsible for converting arachidonic acid into prostaglandins and their products

cyclooxygenase 2 (COX-2) inhibitors Newer nonsteroidal antiinflammatory drugs that block only COX-2 and not COX-1

cycloplegics Drugs that paralyze the eye muscles of accommodation

cytokine release syndrome A symptom complex associated with the use of anti-T–cell antibody infusions

cytomegalovirus (CMV) Infection caused by a virus that infects the entire body

cytotoxic The ability to directly damage or kill cells

cytotoxic therapy A treatment that uses drugs to destroy cancer cells

Current Good Manufacturing Practices (CGMPs) US Food and Drug Administration standards requiring that package labels give the quality and strength of all contents and that products be free of contaminants and impurities

D

decongestants Drugs that stimulate the alpha-adrenergic receptors, producing vascular constriction (vasoconstriction) of the capillaries within the nasal mucosa

delayed puberty Defined clinically by the absence or incomplete development of secondary sexual characteristics bounded by an age at which 95% of children of that sex and culture have begun sexual maturation

dependence A condition in which larger and larger doses of a drug are needed to reproduce the initial response

dependent variable A mathematical variable whose value is determined by that of one or more other variables in a function (outcome, such as clinical effect)

depolarization Myocardial contraction

depression A mood disorder that causes a persistent feeling of sadness and loss of interest

dermatome A nerve region where the virus had lain dormant

diabetes insipidus (DI) A rare condition in which the kidneys are not able to conserve water

diabetes mellitus A chronic disease that results from deficient glucose metabolism caused by insufficient insulin secretion from the beta cells

diarrhea Frequent liquid stool

Dietary Supplement Health and Education Act (DSHEA) A US federal act that defined dietary supplements

diffusion Movement across the cell membrane from an area of higher concentration to one of lower concentration

diluent A liquid used to reconstitute a drug to form a solution

dimensional analysis A calculation method using factors of units and conversions to multiple and divide to obtain the amount to administer

direct-acting cholinergic agonists Drugs that act on receptors to activate a tissue response

disease-modifying antirheumatic drugs (DMARDs) Drugs that help alleviate the symptoms of rheumatic arthritis; DMARDs are also used in the treatment of multiple sclerosis

distribution Movement from the circulation into body tissues

diuresis Increased urine flow

diuretics Agents used to decrease hypertension and edema

dopamine A neurotransmitter that helps control the brain's reward and pleasure centers

dopamine agonists Drugs that stimulate dopamine receptors

dose-response relationship The body's physiologic response to changes in drug concentration at the site of action

doubling time A factor that plays a major role in how cancer cells respond to anticancer drugs

dromotropic An action that decreases conduction of heart cells

drop factor Number of drops per milliliter

drug diversion The deliberate redirecting of a drug from a patient or facility to the employee for personal use

drug interaction An altered or modified action or effect of a drug as a result of interaction with one or multiple drugs

drug label A label containing printed information about a drug

drug reconciliation The process of identifying the most accurate list of all medications a patient is taking at transitions in care

drug toxicity A condition that occurs when drug levels exceed the therapeutic range

drusen Deposits of extracellular material under the retina

DTaP Diphtheria toxoid-, tetanus toxoid-, and acellular pertussis-containing vaccines help protect against diphtheria, tetanus, and pertussis, but they will not prevent all cases

duodenal ulcer Caused by hypersecretion of acid from the stomach passing into the duodenum because of (1) insufficient buffers to neutralize gastric acid in the stomach, (2) a defective or incompetent pyloric sphincter, or (3) hypermotility of the stomach

duration of action The length of time over which a drug exerts its therapeutic effect

dysfunctional uterine bleeding Abnormal uterine bleeding in the absence of organic disease

dyskinesia Impaired voluntary movement

dysmenorrhea Painful periods

dyspareunia Painful sexual intercourse

dysphoria Deep depression

dysrhythmias Irregular heartbeats

dystonia Prolonged muscle contractions with twisting, repetitive movements

dystonic movement Involuntary abnormal movement

E

e-cigarettes Electronic cigarettes that aerosolize "e-juice," a mixture of flavorings, propylene glycol (a toxic component of antifreeze), glycerin, and nicotine

eclampsia New-onset grand mal seizures in a patient with preeclampsia

ejaculatory dysfunction Impaired ejection of seminal fluid from the male urethra

electroencephalogram (EEG) An electrophysiologic monitoring method to record electrical activity of the brain

electrolytes Substances that separate or dissociate into ions (charged particles) in solution

electronic intravenous device An electronic device to deliver prescribed rate of intravenous drugs

emetics Drugs used to induce vomiting

emollients Lubricants and stool softeners used to prevent constipation

emphysema A progressive lung disease caused by cigarette smoking, atmospheric contaminants, or lack of the alpha$_1$-antitrypsin protein that inhibits proteolytic enzymes that destroy alveoli

endometriosis The abnormal location of endometrial tissue outside the uterus

endophthalmitis Infection and inflammation of structures of the inner eye

endorphins Neurohormones

enteral nutrition (EN) Delivery of nutrition or fluid via a tube into the gastrointestinal (GI) tract, which requires a functional, accessible GI tract

epidural block Placement of local anesthetic in the epidural space just posterior to the spinal cord or the dura mater

epigenetics The study of environmental influences on genetics

episiotomy An incision made to enlarge the vaginal opening to facilitate newborn delivery

erectile dysfunction The inability to achieve or maintain an erection satisfactory for sexual performance

ergot alkaloids One of a large group of alkaloids derived from fungi; acts by direct smooth muscle cell–receptor stimulation

ergotism Signs of ergot toxicity

erythema multiforme An erythematous macular, papular, or vesicular eruption that can cover the entire body

erythrocytic phase Invasion of the red blood cells

erythropoietin (EPO) A glycoprotein produced by the kidney stimulating red blood cell production in the bone marrow

erythropoietin-stimulating agents (ESAs) Agents that stimulate red blood cell production in the bone marrow

esophageal ulcer Results from reflux of acidic gastric secretions into the esophagus as a result of a defective or incompetent cardiac sphincter

essential hypertension The most common type of hypertension, affecting 90% of persons with high blood pressure

estimated average requirement (EAR) The daily intake of a specific nutrient estimated to meet the requirement in 50% of healthy people in an age- and sex-specific group

ethinyl estradiol The most commonly used synthetic estrogen found in CHC products

ethnomedicine Sometimes referred to as *folk medicine* or *traditional medicine*, a focus within medical anthropology that examines the ways in which people from different cultures conceptualize health and illness

ethnopharmacology A subdivision of ethnomedicine that focuses on the use of herbs, powders, teas, and animal products as healing remedies

evaluation The phase of the nursing process during which the nurse determines whether the goals and teaching objectives are being met

excipients Fillers and inert substances such as simple syrup, vegetable gums, aromatic powder, honey, and various elixirs

excretion Elimination of drugs from the body

exfoliative dermatitis Characterized by desquamation, scaling, and itching of the skin

expectorants Agents that loosen bronchial secretions so they can be eliminated by coughing

extrapyramidal syndrome Any of a group of clinical disorders marked by abnormal involuntary movements, alterations in muscle tone, and postural disturbances

extravasation Tissue injury due to drugs infiltering tissues

F

facilitated diffusion Relies on a carrier protein to move drug from an area of higher concentration to an area of lower concentration

family-centered care Essential to ensuring safety during and after health care interventions, especially drug administration

fasciculations Involuntary muscle twitching

fat-soluble vitamins Vitamins stored in fatty tissue, liver, and muscle in significant amounts that are metabolized slowly and excreted in the urine at a slow rate; includes vitamins A, D, E, and K

fibrinolysis Fibrin breakdown

first-line drugs Those drugs chosen first for therapy

first-pass effect (or first-pass metabolism) When drugs are metabolized in the liver to an inactive form and are excreted, thus reducing the amount of active drug available to exert a pharmacologic effect

flatus Intestinal gas

folliculitis Inflammation of a hair follicle resulting from contact with an irritating substance or allergen

fraction of inspired oxygen (FiO_2) The fraction or percentage of oxygen in the space being measured

fractional equation The equation $H/V = D/x$ to calculate the amount x to be administered, where H is the dosage on hand; V is the vehicle; D is the desired dose

free drugs Drugs able to exit blood vessels and reach their site of action to cause a pharmacologic response

free-flow The rate of administration of intravenous drugs infused rapidly without the use of an electronic infusion device

G

gastric mucosal barrier (GMB) A thick, viscous, mucous material that provides a barrier between the mucosal lining and acidic gastric secretions

gastric ulcer Frequently occurs because of a breakdown of the gastric mucosal barrier (GMB)

gastroesophageal reflux disease (GERD) Inflammation or erosion of the esophageal mucosa caused by a reflux of gastric acid content from the stomach into the esophagus

gastrostomy tube A gastrointestinal tube used for enteral tube feedings

generic name The official, nonproprietary name for a drug; the name not owned by any drug company and universally accepted as the official drug name

genomes A complete set of chromosomes that make up a cell's DNA

genotoxicity The ability of a compound to damage genetic information in a cell

gestational hypertension Elevated blood pressure after 20 gestational weeks in patients who were normotensive before pregnancy

gigantism Excessive growth during childhood

gingival hyperplasia Overgrowth of gums or reddened gums that bleed easily

glaucoma A group of eye conditions that damage the optic nerve

glucocorticoids Most potent endogenous cortisol produced by the adrenal cortex; exogenous drugs used to treat variety of medical conditions, including inflammation, allergy, and some autoimmune disorders

glycogenolysis Breakdown of glycogen increasing blood glucose

Good Clinical Practice (GCP) Consolidated Guideline An international ethical and scientific quality standard for designing, conducting, monitoring, auditing, recording, analyzing, and reporting clinical research

gout An inflammatory condition that attacks joints, tendons, and other tissues

gram The basic unit of measure used for weight (g, G)

granulocyte A type of white blood cell with small granules that contain proteins

granulocyte colony–stimulating factor (G-CSF) A glycoprotein produced by the macrophages, endothelium and other immune cells to stimulate the synthesis of neutrophils

granulocyte-macrophage colony–stimulating factor (GM-CSF) A glycoprotein secreted by immune cells that support survival, proliferation, and differentiation (maturation) of hematopoietic progenitor cells in the granulocyte-macrophage pathway

Graves disease The most common type of hyperthyroidism caused by hyperfunction of the thyroid gland

growth fraction A factor that plays a major role in how cancer cells respond to anticancer drugs

gynecomastia Mammary gland enlargement in males

H

half-life The time it takes for the amount of drug in the body to be reduced by half

hangover Residual drowsiness

healers Individuals who play a role in health practices worldwide; may include priests, shamans, bone setters, herbalists, curanderos, and midwives

health care–acquired infections Infections acquired while patients are hospitalized

heart block A delay in the normal flow of electrical impulses of the heart, often times causing bradycardia

heart failure A condition that occurs when the heart muscle (myocardium) weakens and enlarges and loses its ability to pump blood through the heart and into the systemic circulation

HELLP syndrome A sequela of preeclampsia defined by hemolysis, elevated liver enzymes, and low platelet count

helminthiasis Worm infection

helminths Large parasitic worms that live and lay eggs in warm, moist soil where sanitation and hygiene are poor

hepatotoxicity Liver toxicity

herb Any plant used for culinary or medicinal purposes

herd immunity Occurs when most of the community is immunized against contagious diseases, thus allowing protection of those not immunized

high-density lipoprotein (HDL) One of the five major groups of lipoproteins

high-sensitivity C-reactive protein (hsCRP) A test used to evaluate the risk of developing coronary artery disease

hirsutism Increased hair growth

histamine 2 (H_2) receptor antagonists Agents used to treat duodenal ulcers and prevent their return

homocysteine A naturally occurring amino acid found in blood plasma

hordeolum A local infection of eyelash follicles and glands on lid margins, also known as a stye

hormone therapy A therapy that significantly improves vasomotor symptoms and vaginal dryness, two frequently encountered symptoms of menopause; also decreases the risk for osteoporosis and osteoporotic fractures

household measurement A measuring system that uses inches and pounds

hybridoma technology A genetic process that makes monoclonal antibodies

hydantoins Inhibit sodium influx, stabilize cell membranes, reduce repetitive neuronal firing, and limit seizures

hydrochloric acid A strongly acidic solution of the gas hydrogen chloride in water

hyperalimentation A form of malnutrition in which the intake of nutrients is oversupplied

hypercalcemia A calcium excess (>10.2 mEq/L)

hypercapnia Increased carbon dioxide in the blood

hyperchloremia An elevated serum chloride level

hyperemesis gravidarum Severe nausea and vomiting during pregnancy

hyperglycemia Elevated blood glucose

hyperkalemia A serum potassium level above 5.0 mEq/L

hyperlipidemia A condition that occurs when there is an excess of one or more lipids in the blood

hypermagnesemia A magnesium excess

hypernatremia A serum sodium level above 145 mEq/L

hyperosmolar A fluid that contains more particles than water

hyperoxia Excessive oxygenation

hyperphosphatemia An excess of phosphorus

hypertension Blood pressure greater than 140/90 mm Hg

hypertensive crisis When systolic blood pressure exceeds 180 to 200 mm Hg

hyperthyroidism An increase in circulating T_3 and T_4 levels, which usually results from an overactive thyroid gland or excessive output of thyroid hormones from one or more thyroid nodules

hypertonic Describes solutions that exert greater osmotic pressure than extracellular fluid (ECF), resulting in a higher solute concentration than the serum

hypertrichosis Darkening of hair

hyperuricemia Elevated serum uric acid level
hypnotic effect Not hypnosis but a form of "natural" sleep
hypocalcemia A calcium deficit (<8.6 mEq/L)
hypocarbia Decreased carbon dioxide (CO_2)
hypochloremia A decreased serum chloride level
hypoglycemic reaction Occurs when more insulin is administered than is needed for glucose metabolism
hypogonadism The clearest indication for exogenous androgen therapy
hypokalemia Potassium deficit; occurs with serum levels below 3.5 mEq/L
hypomagnesemia Magnesium deficit
hyponatremia A serum sodium level below 135 mEq/L
hypoosmolar Describes fluid that contains fewer particles than water
hypophosphatemia Deficiency of phosphorus
hypophysis The pituitary gland
hypothyroidism A decrease in thyroid hormone secretion
hypotonic Describes solutions that exert less osmotic pressure than extracellular fluid (ECF), which allows water to move into the cell
hypovolemic shock A life-threatening condition caused by more than 20% (one fifth) of the body's blood or fluid supply
hypoxemia Inadequate oxygen in the blood
hypoxia Lack of oxygen to body tissues

I

idiopathic Of unknown cause
immune globulin The general term used for replacement therapy
immune reconstitution inflammatory syndrome (IRIS) A syndrome related to a disease- or pathogen-specific inflammatory response in patients with antiretroviral therapy being initiated or changed
immune response The reaction of the cells and fluids of the body to the presence of a substance not recognized as a constituent of the body itself
immunoglobulins Antibody proteins such as immunoglobulins G and M
immunomodulation The immune system's ability to kill abnormal cells
immunomodulators Agents used to treat moderate to severe rheumatoid arthritis by disrupting the inflammatory process and delaying disease progression; immunomodulators are also used in the treatment of multiple sclerosis
immunosuppression The use of multiple drugs to alter different aspects of the immune system
immunosuppressives Agents used to treat refractory rheumatoid arthritis that does not respond to antiinflammatory drugs; immunosuppressives are also used in the treatment of multiple sclerosis
implementation The part of the nursing process in which the nurse provides education, drug administration, patient care, and other interventions necessary to assist the patient in accomplishing the established goals

independent variable A variable independent of the other variables in an expression or function and whose value determines one or more of the values of the other variables (e.g., treatment, such as with a drug)
indirect-acting cholinergic agonists Agents that inhibit the action of the enzyme cholinesterase (ChE)
induction therapy Treatment that provides intense immunosuppression with drugs designed to diminish antigen presentation and T-cell response
infection Caused by microorganisms, which results in inflammation
infertility The inability to conceive a child after 12 months of unprotected sexual intercourse
infiltration Extravasation of intravenous fluids into the tissues
inflammation A response to tissue injury and infection
influenza A highly contagious viral infection, usually seasonal
informed consent Consent to medical treatment or participation in medical experiments after achieving an understanding of what is involved and being apprised of the risks
inhalation Administration of medication via the nasal route
inherent resistance Bacterial resistance can result naturally
inhibited sexual desire Decreased or lacking interest in sexual activity
inotropic Action that increases myocardial contraction stroke volume
insomnia The inability to fall asleep or remain asleep
instillations Liquid medications usually administered as drops, ointments, or sprays
insulin A protein secreted from the beta cells of the pancreas necessary for carbohydrate metabolism and that plays an important role in protein and fat metabolism
insulin shock Occurs when more insulin is administered than is needed for glucose metabolism
interferon alfa An interferon produced by white blood cells that inhibits viral replication, suppresses cell proliferation, and regulates immune response
interferon beta (IFN-β) A type I interferon produced by fibroblasts, macrophages, and epithelial cells
interferon gamma (IFN-γ) A type II interferon produced endogenously by activating T lymphocytes and natural killer cells (NKCs), and produced genetically from Escherichia coli
interferons (IFNs) A family of proteins that occur naturally in the body and can be produced in the laboratory to slow the growth of cancer cells
interleukins A group of signaling-molecule proteins produced by T lymphocytes
intermittent enteral feedings Feedings administered every 3 to 6 hours over 30 to 60 minutes by gravity drip or infusion pump

intermittent infusion Considered an inexpensive method for administering enteral nutrition (EN)
international normalized ratio (INR) The laboratory test most frequently used to report prothrombin time (PT) results
intradermal Administered for skin testing
intramuscular (IM) An administration route used for solutions that are more viscous and irritating for adults, children, and infants
intraocular pressure (IOP) The pressure within the eyeball that gives it a round, firm shape
intravenous More rapid injection method than intramuscular or subcutaneous routes
intravenous flow rate A rate of intravenous drug administration based on several factors
intravenous piggyback (IVPB) A method of administering diluted drugs in small volume of fluid as a secondary infusion
intravenous push (IVP) A method of administering intravenous drugs using a syringe
iron Vital for hemoglobin regeneration
ischemia Deficient blood flow
isoosmolar Fluid that has the same weight proportion of particles (e.g., sodium, glucose) and water
isotonic Describes solutions that have the same approximate osmolality as extracellular fluid (ECF) or plasma

J

jejunostomy tube A gastrointestinal route used for enteral tube feedings
Just & Safe Culture An approach that supports encouraging individuals to report drug errors so the system can be repaired and the problem can be fixed
justice Requires that the selection of research subjects be fair

K

Kaposi sarcoma A cancer that causes patches of abnormal tissue to grow under the skin; in the lining of the mouth, nose, and throat; in lymph nodes; and in other organs
keep vein open (KVO) An intravenous fluid infusion given at a slow rate to maintain patent intravenous site
keratin A protein that is part of the skin
keratitis Infection and inflammation of the cornea
keratolysis Horny cell cohesion due to bacterial growth
ketoacidosis Diabetic acidosis or diabetic coma

L

labor augmentation Stimulation of effective uterine contractions with oxytocin once labor has begun
labor induction The process of causing or initiating labor
lacrimal duct Tear ducts
lactation Production and release of milk by the mammary glands
latency The establishment and maintenance of latent infection in nerve cell ganglia proximal to the site of infection

GLOSSARY

latent stage A period of time after an infection during which symptoms are absent

latent tuberculosis infection A state of persistent immune response to stimulation by *Mycobacterium tuberculosis* antigens without evidence of clinically manifested active tuberculosis

laxatives Agents that promote a soft stool; cathartics result in a soft to watery stool with some cramping

lecithin/sphingomyelin (L/S) ratio Ratio of lecithin and sphingomyelin that measured in the amniotic fluid, predicting fetal lung maturity and risk for neonatal respiratory distress syndrome (RDS)

ligand-binding domain The site on the receptor to which drugs bind

lipodystrophy A disorder of adipose (fatty) tissue characterized by a selective loss of body fat

lipoprotein Special particles made up of droplets of fats surrounded by a single layer of phospholipid molecules

liposomes Synthetic fat globules containing drugs to increase the duration of therapeutic effects

liter The basic unit of measure for volume (L)

living-donor transplantation An operation in which a kidney or a portion of liver donated by a living person is transplanted into the body of a patient with end-stage kidney or liver disease

loading dose Administration of a large initial dose

low-density lipoprotein (LDL) A molecule that is a combination of lipid (fat) and protein; transports cholesterol from the liver to the tissues of the body

lymphokines Cytokines produced by T cells (lymphocytes) of the immune system; also called interleukins

M

macrodrip An intravenous set that delivers 10 to 20 drops per milliliter

macrophages Mature monocytes

macules Flat and nonpalpable skin lesions, usually less than 10 mm in diameter with varying colors

maximal efficacy The point at which increasing a drug's dosage no longer increases the desired therapeutic response

menarche The start of spontaneous menstruation

meningococcal vaccine Vaccines available that can help prevent meningococcal disease, which is any type of illness caused by Neisseria meningitidis bacteria

menopause The transitional process experienced by females as they move from the reproductive years into the nonreproductive stage of life

menorrhagia Heavy periods

mestranol An older form of estrogen found in higher-dose (≥50 mcg) oral combination products

metabolism The process by which the body chemically changes drugs into a form that can be excreted

metastasis The spread of the disease to other areas of the body

metastasizing Spreading to other parts of the body

meter Basic unit of measure for linear measurement (m, M)

metered-dose inhalers (MDIs) Handheld devices used to deliver a number of commonly prescribed asthma and bronchitis drugs to the lower respiratory tract

metric system A decimal system based on the power of 10

metrorrhagia Irregular bleeding between periods, usually heavy

microdrip An intravenous tubing set that delivers 60 drops per milliliter

microorganisms Microscopic organisms that include viruses, fungi, protozoa, and rickettsiae

micturition Urination

migraine headaches Characterized by a unilateral throbbing head pain accompanied by nausea, vomiting, and photophobia

mineralocorticoids A group of hormones, the most important being aldosterone, that regulate the balance of water and electrolytes (ions such as sodium and potassium) in the body

minerals Substances the body requires in small amounts, such as iron, copper, zinc, chromium, and selenium

minimum effective concentration The minimum amount of drug required for drug effect

miosis A constriction of the pupil and contraction of the ciliary muscle

mitosis The process by which the nucleus divides in eukaryotic organisms, producing two new nuclei genetically identical to the nucleus of the parent cell

mittelschmerz Midcycle menstrual pain usually associated with ovulation

Monitoring the Future project A project that tracks drug use in adolescents and young adults

monoamine oxidase inhibitors (MAOIs) Agents that inactivate norepinephrine, dopamine, epinephrine, and serotonin

monoclonal antibodies Antibodies produced by a single clone of cells or a cell line and consisting of identical antibody molecules

mononucleosis A contagious viral infection affecting the lymph nodes

mTOR kinase inhibitors A class of drugs that inhibit the mechanistic target of rapamycin

mucolytics Agents that act as detergents to liquefy and loosen thick mucus secretions so they can be expectorated

multikinase inhibitors (MKIs) Chemicals that directly inhibit the activity of multiple kinase enzymes in cancer cells

multiple sclerosis (MS) A neuromuscular autoimmune disorder that attacks the myelin sheath of nerve fibers, causing lesions known as *plaques*

muscarinic receptors Receptors that stimulate smooth muscle and slow the heart rate

muscle relaxants Agents that reduce spasticity of muscles

muscle spasms Muscle contractions resulting from various causes, including injury or motor neuron disorders associated with conditions such as multiple sclerosis (MS), myasthenia gravis (MG), cerebral palsy, spinal cord injury, cerebrovascular accident, or hemiplegia

myasthenia gravis (MG) An acquired autoimmune disease that impairs the transmission of messages at the neuromuscular junction, resulting in fluctuating muscle weakness that increases with muscle use

myasthenic crisis Occurs when muscular weakness in the patient with myasthenia gravis becomes generalized

***Mycobacterium avium* complex (MAC)** A blood infection caused by bacteria related to *M. tuberculosis*

mydriasis A condition in which the pupils remain dilated for a prolong duration

mydriatics Agents that dilate the pupils

myelosuppression A condition that occurs when a significant decrease in bone marrow activity results in decreased white blood cells, platelets, and red blood cells

myocardial infarction (MI) Heart attack

myocardial ischemia Lack of blood supply to the heart muscle

myxedema Severe hypothyroidism in the adult

N

nadir The low point; in nursing, used to describe the point at which the blood count is at the lowest

narcolepsy A neurological disorder characterized by falling asleep during normal waking activities, such as while driving a car or talking with someone

narrow-spectrum antibiotics Tolerance (as of a virus) to a usually toxic substance (as an antibiotic) that is acquired, not as a result of direct exposure, but by exposure to a related substance

nasoduodenal/nasojejunal Gastrointestinal routes used for enteral tube feedings

nasointestinal tube A tube passed through the nose and down through the nasopharynx and esophagus into the intestine

natriuresis Sodium loss in the urine

natriuretic An agent with a sodium-losing effect

natural acquired active immunity Immunity that occurs from exposure to a pathogen or disease

necrosis Tissue death caused by disease or injury

neoadjuvant chemotherapy Treatment performed before surgical extraction of a tumor with the objective of reducing the tumor's size

nephrotoxicity Toxicity to the kidney

nerve block A pain management technique involving the injection of an anesthetic into the area surrounding an affected nerve

neurohypophysis The posterior pituitary gland

neuroleptic Refers to any drug that modifies psychotic behavior and exerts an antipsychotic effect

neuroleptic malignant syndrome (NMS) A rare but potentially fatal condition associated with antipsychotic drugs

neuropathic pain An unusual sensory disturbance that often involves neural supersensitivity
neurotransmitters Substances released as a result of stimulation, such as by amphetamines
neutrophils The most abundant white blood cells that take part in the inflammatory response system, whose main function it is to detect and destroy harmful bacteria
nicotinic receptors Receptors that affect the skeletal muscles
nitrates The first agents used to relieve angina
nociceptors Sensory receptors for pain
nonopioid analgesics Drugs that are less potent than opioid analgesics, used to treat mild to moderate pain
non–rapid eye movement (NREM) sleep A definite stage of sleep
nonselective A term used to describe drugs capable of affecting multiple receptors
nonspecific A term used to describe drugs capable of affecting multiple receptor sites
nonsteroidal antiinflammatory drugs (NSAIDs) Nonopioid analgesics taken for pain and inflammation
normoxemia Oxygen saturation between 94% and 99% depending on the patient's diagnosis and physiologic state
nystagmus Constant, involuntary, cyclical movement of the eyeball

O

occlusive Obstructive
ocular drugs Drugs designed to be applied to the eyes
off label Use of a drug for some purpose for which it has not been approved
older adult Person over the age of 65
oligomenorrhea Very scant periods
oligospermia Low sperm count
oliguria A marked decrease in urine output
oncogene A mutation in a proto-oncogene that affects cellular growth-control proteins and triggers unregulated cell division
onset The time it takes for a drug to reach the minimum effective concentration (MEC) after administration
open-angle glaucoma A condition in which the trabecular network is open but becomes clogged
ophthalmia neonatorum An eye infection among newborns
ophthalmic drugs Drugs designed to be applied to the eyes
opiates Analgesic agents that decrease intestinal motility and thereby decrease peristalsis
opioid agonist-antagonists Medications in which an opioid antagonist is added to an opioid agonist
opioid agonists Drugs prescribed for moderate and severe pain
opioid antagonist An agent that blocks the receptor and displaces any opioid that would normally be at the receptor
opportunistic infections Infections that usually occur in the immunocompromised or debilitated population
oral antidiabetic drugs Synthetic preparations that stimulate insulin release or otherwise alter the metabolic response to hyperglycemia
oral hypoglycemic drugs Synthetic preparations that stimulate insulin release or otherwise alter the metabolic response to hyperglycemia
orthostatic hypotension Low blood pressure that occurs when an individual assumes an upright position from a supine position
osmolality Describes the concentration of fluids
osmolarity Describes the concentration of a solution in terms of osmoles of solute per liter of solution
osmole The number of solutes in a solution, expressed as a unit of measurement
osmotics Hyperosmolar laxatives
osteopenia Low bone mineral density
osteoporosis Loss of bone mass that predisposes patients to fractures
otalgia Ear pain
otitis externa (OE) An infection of the external auditory canal
ototoxicity Ear poisoning that results from exposure to drugs or chemicals that damage the inner ear or the vestibulocochlear nerve
ounces A unit of measurement related to mass
over-the-counter (OTC) Those drugs that have been found to be safe and appropriate for use without the direct supervision of a health care provider and are available for purchase without a prescription

P

pain threshold The level of stimulus needed to create a painful sensation
pain tolerance The amount of pain a person can endure without having it interfere with normal functioning
palliative chemotherapy Treatment used to relieve symptoms associated with advanced disease
papules Raised and palpable skin lesions less than 10 mm in diameter
parasympatholytics Drugs that affect the parasympathetic nervous system
parasympathomimetics Drugs that mimic the parasympathetic neurotransmitter acetylcholine
parathyroid hormone (PTH) A hormone that regulates serum calcium levels
parenteral Administered via injection
parenteral nutrition (PN) Administration of nutrients by a route other than the gastrointestinal tract; also called *total parenteral nutrition* (TPN)
paresthesia A burning or prickling sensation usually felt in the hands, arms, legs, or feet but can also occur in other parts of the body
Parkinson disease A chronic, progressive neurologic disorder that affects the extrapyramidal motor tract, which controls posture, balance, and locomotion
Parkinsonism A syndrome, or a combination of similar symptoms, whose major features include rigidity, bradykinesia, gait disturbances, and tremors
paroxysmal supraventricular tachycardia (PSVT) A sudden, uncontrolled, rapid rhythm that exceeds 150 beats/min in adults and originates above the ventricles
Partial agonist Drugs that elicit only moderate activity when binding to receptors; they also prevent receptor activation by other drugs
partial thromboplastin time (PTT) A blood test that evaluates how long it takes for blood to clot
passive immunity Immunity that can be natural, in which case the body produces its own antibodies, or acquired—that is, the body receives antibodies from an outside source
passive transport Transport that occurs through two processes, diffusion and facilitated diffusion
pathogen A disease-producing microorganism
patient-controlled analgesia (PCA) An alternative route for opioid administration for self-administered pain relief as needed
patient-problem Defines the most important health problem the patient is experiencing and guides the development of the nursing plan of care
peak The point at which a drug reaches its highest concentration in the blood
peak drug level The highest plasma concentration of a drug at a specific time
pelvic inflammatory disease (PID) An infection of the upper genital tract, usually the uterine endometrium, fallopian tubes, or ovaries
pepsin A digestive enzyme activated at a pH of 2
peptic ulcer A broad term for an ulcer that occurs in the esophagus, stomach, or duodenum within the upper gastrointestinal tract
peptides Biologically occurring short chains of amino acid monomers linked by peptide (amide) bonds
percutaneous endoscopic gastrostomy (PEG) tube A tube placed surgically, endoscopically, or radiologically for the purpose of delivering nutrition; requires an intact gastrointestinal system
perinatal transmission Transmission at the time of delivery
peripheral vasodilators Drugs that dilate the distal blood vessels and lower the blood pressure
pharmacodynamics Mechanisms of action and effects of a drug on the body; includes the onset, peak, and duration of effect of a drug
pharmacogenetics The study of genetic factors that influence an individual's response to a specific drug
pharmacogenomics The study of how genetics play a role in a person's response to drugs
pharmacokinetics The process of drug movement throughout the body necessary to achieve drug action
phenothiazines Subdivided into three groups—aliphatic, piperazine, and piperidine—which differ mostly in their side effects
photochemotherapy A combination of ultraviolet (UV) radiation and the psoralen derivative methoxsalen; used to decrease proliferation of epidermal cells

photophobia Sensitivity to light
photosensitivity A skin reaction caused by exposure to sunlight
phytomedicine A type of medicine that focuses on the therapeutic value of plants
pinocytosis A process by which cells carry a drug across their membrane by engulfing the drug particles in a vesicle
placebo A pill or substance given to a patient like a drug but that can be expected to have no lasting physical effect on the patient
placebo effect A drug response not attributed to the chemical properties of the drug
planning The phase during which the nurse uses collected data to set goals or expected outcomes and interventions
plaques Palpable skin lesions greater than 10 mm in diameter that are depressed or elevated when compared with the skin surface
Pneumocystis jiroveci pneumonia (PJP) A fungal infection that shares biologic characteristics with protozoa that infect the lungs
polycystic ovarian syndrome (PCOS) A form of metabolic syndrome caused by the oversecretion of luteinizing hormone
polydipsia Increased thirst
polydrug use Use of more than one drug
polymorphisms DNA variants that occur within a specific population at a frequency greater than 1%
polyphagia Increased hunger
polypharmacy Use of multiple drugs and/or the administration of drugs above what is clinically warranted
polyuria Increased urine output
postexposure prophylaxis (PEP) The treatment regimen instituted after exposure to human immunodeficiency virus (HIV)
potassium-sparing diuretics Diuretics that promote potassium retention
potassium-wasting diuretics Diuretics that promote potassium excretion
potency Refers to the amount of drug needed to elicit a specific physiologic response
preeclampsia Gestational hypertension with or without proteinuria
preload Amount of blood in the ventricles of the heart at the end of diastole
premenstrual syndrome (PMS) A collection of cyclic physical symptoms and perimenopausal mood alterations
preterm labor (PTL) Cervical changes and uterine contractions that occur between 20 and 37 weeks of pregnancy
priapism Painful, continuous erection
primary infection An infection that occurs in immunocompetent persons
primary syphilis Presents with a sore, or chancre, at the site where the infection entered the body, typically the penis in males and outer genitals or inner vagina in females
Principle of Atraumatic Care Provision of therapy using interventions that minimize or eliminate psychological and physical distress experienced by patients, particularly children and their families

Prodrug A compound metabolized into an active pharmacologic substance
progenitor cells Early descendants of stem cells that can differentiate to form one or more kinds of cells but that cannot divide and reproduce indefinitely
progesterone The naturally occurring sex hormone produced in the ovaries
progestins Natural or synthetic hormones that have progesterone-like effects
progestogen Any synthetically produced progesterone compound
prolactin (PRL) A protein hormone of the anterior pituitary that induces lactation
prophylactic Drugs to prevent infection
prophylaxis Prevention
prostaglandin analogues First-line drugs used primarily in the treatment of open-angle glaucoma and ocular hypertension
prostaglandins Chemical mediators that have been isolated from the exudate at inflammatory sites
proteasome Multienzyme complexes that degrade proteins intracellularly
protein binding Describes how drugs are distributed in the plasma and bind with plasma proteins (albumin, lipoproteins, and alpha-1-acid-glycoprotein [AGP])
prothrombin time (PT) A laboratory test that measures the time it takes blood to clot in the presence of certain clotting factors
protocols Specific guidelines
proto-oncogenes Normal genes involved in cell differentiation and division; they regulate cell death
pseudoparkinsonism Frequently occurs as an adverse reaction to chlorpromazine, haloperidol, lithium, metoclopramide, methyldopa, and reserpine
psoralen and ultraviolet A (PUVA) Therapy that permits lower doses of methoxsalen and UVA to be given
psoriasis A multisystem disease with predominant skin and joint disorders, usually with chronic skin inflammation
psychomotor seizure Occurs in temporal lobe epilepsy; characterized by a temporary impairment of consciousness, loss of judgment, automatic behavior, and abnormal acts
psychosis Loss of contact with reality
puerperium The period from delivery until 6 weeks postpartum
pulse oximetry Provides a digital display of oxygen saturation
purgatives Harsh cathartics that cause a watery stool with abdominal cramping

R

rapid eye movement (REM) sleep The sleep stage during which people experience most of their recallable dreams, characterized by discernable eye movement
reactive depression Depression that usually has a sudden onset after a precipitating event
rebound nasal congestion Caused by frequent use of decongestants
receptors Found on cell surface membranes or within cells

recombinant DNA The genetic engineering process that combines two human DNA strands artificially
recombinant hepatitis B A three-dose series vaccine for hepatitis B virus (HBV) indicated for HBV prophylaxis in infants
Recombinant subunit vaccines the insertion of some of the genetic material of a pathogen into another cell or organism, where the antigen is then produced in massive quantities
recommended dietary allowance (RDA) The amount of vitamins, minerals, or other essential nutrients that should be ingested every day by a normal person engaged in average activities
repolarization Return of cell membrane potential to resting after depolarization
respect for persons Treating patients as independent persons who are capable of making decisions in their own best interests
respiratory distress syndrome (RDS) A syndrome that can occur because of immature lung development and breathing control and decreased airway muscle tone and surfactant level
restrictive lung disease A decrease in total lung capacity as a result of fluid accumulation or loss of elasticity of the lung
reward circuit A structure that regulates the ability to feel pleasure and other emotions, both positive and negative
Rh sensitization Development of protective antibodies against incompatible Rh-positive blood
$Rh_o(D)$ immune globulin A substance routinely administered to females with incompatible maternal/fetal blood mixing
rhinorrhea Watery nasal discharge
right assessment Requires the collection of appropriate baseline data before administration of a drug
right documentation Requires the nurse to record immediately the appropriate information about the drug administered
right dose Requires verification by the nurse that the dose administered is the amount ordered and that it is safe for the patient for whom it is prescribed
right drug Requires confirming that a drug is right for the patient prior to its administration
right evaluation Asks whether the medication did for the patient what it was supposed to do
right patient Requires confirmation of a patient's identity with two forms of identification before drug administration
right route Ordered by the health care provider, it indicates the mechanism by which the medication will enter the body
right time The time the prescribed dose is ordered to be administered
right to education Requires that patients receive accurate and thorough information about the drugs they are taking and how each drug relates to their particular condition
right to refuse Refers to the patient's right to decline medication
risk-benefit ratio Identifying physical, psychological, and social risks and weighing them against the benefits

root-cause analysis (RCA) A method of problem solving used to identify potential workplace errors

S

saddle block Anesthesia given at the lower end of the spinal column to block the perineal area
saluretic Sodium-chloride losing
SARS-CoV-2 Severe acute respiratory syndome coronavirus 2, the virus that causes coronavirus disease (COVID-19), a highly virulent and severe disease that most frequently affects the respiratory system, but also causes long-lasting cardiac, nervous, and renal system damage or death
schizophrenia A chronic psychotic disorder
secondary hypertension Hypertension related to renal and endocrine disorders
secondary intravenous line set An intravenous tubing to administer drugs by intravenous piggyback (IVPB)
secondary syphilis Disease characterized by a skin rash that appears 2 to 8 weeks after the chancre
sedation A state of diminished physical and mental responsiveness
seizure A disorder that results from abnormal electrical discharges from the cerebral neurons, characterized by a loss or disturbance of consciousness and usually involuntary, uncontrolled movements
seizure threshold The point at which a seizure may be induced
selective chloride channel activators A new category of laxatives used to treat idiopathic constipation in adults
selective serotonin reuptake inhibitors (SSRIs) Agents that block the reuptake of serotonin into the nerve terminal of the central nervous system
sentinel event An unanticipated event in a health care setting that results in death or serious harm to a patient unrelated to the natural course of the patient's illness
seroconversion The acquisition of detectable levels of antibodies in the bloodstream
serotonin norepinephrine reuptake inhibitors (SNRIs) Agents that inhibit the reuptake of serotonin and norepinephrine, increasing availability in the synapse
shingles A painful vesicular rash along the region of skin innervated by the nerve root ganglia
side effects Secondary effects of drug therapy
signal transduction A mechanism by which cell-to-cell communication occurs locally or remotely by signal molecules sent to maintain homeostasis, regulate growth and division, develop and organize into tissues, and coordinate cellular functions
signal transduction inhibitors (STIs) Agents that block signals to cancerous cells by blocking signals passed from one molecule to another
sinusitis Inflammation of the mucous membranes of one or more of the maxillary, frontal, ethmoid, or sphenoid sinuses
sloughing Formation of dead tissue that separates from living tissue
small-molecule compounds Chemicals small enough to have an intracellular effect, targeting the internal structures of cells
spacer A device used to enhance the delivery of medications from a metered-dose inhaler
spermatogenesis Formation of spermatozoa
spinal anesthesia A local anesthetic injected into the subarachnoid space below the first lumbar space (L1) in adults and the third lumbar space (L3) in children
spinal block Results from the penetration of anesthetic into the subarachnoid space
status epilepticus A rapid succession of epileptic seizures
steady state The plateau drug level; occurs when the amount of drug being administered is the same as the amount of drug being eliminated
Stevens-Johnson syndrome Skin eruptions, usually due to adverse reaction to drugs, resulting in large blisters in the mucosa, pharynx, eyes, and viscera
stocking-glove syndrome A sign of neurotoxicity involving the fingers and toes
stress ulcer An ulcer that usually follows a critical situation, such as extensive trauma or major surgery
subcutaneous Injections given under the skin only in areas such as the upper outer aspect of the arms; the abdomen, at least 2 inches from the umbilicus; and the anterior thighs
sublingual Given under the tongue
substance use disorder A disorder evidenced by recurrent use of a substance such that it causes considerable impairment, including problems with health and an inability to keep up with family and work responsibilities
superinfection A new infection in a patient with a preexisting infection
suppository A solid medical preparation that is cone- or spindle-shaped for insertion into the rectum, globular or egg shaped for use in the vagina, or pencil shaped for insertion into the urethra
suppressor gene A gene that suppresses the phenotypic expression of another gene
surfactant A substance that decreases the surface tension of the alveoli to allow the lungs to fill with air and prevent the alveoli from deflating
suspension A mixture containing solid particles suspended in a liquid
sympatholytics Drugs that affect the sympathetic nervous system; also called adrenergic blockers
sympathomimetics Drugs that affect the sympathetic nervous system; also called adrenergic agonists
syndrome of inappropriate antidiuretic hormone (SIADH) A condition in which excessive water retention expands the intracellular and intravascular volume
synergistic effect Describes what occurs when two or more drugs are given together
syringe A drug dispensing system composed of a barrel, plunger, and tip

T

tachycardia Heart rate greater than 100 beats per minute
tachyphylaxis An acute, rapid decrease in response to a drug
tardive dyskinesia A serious adverse reaction that occurs in approximately 20% to 30% of patients who have taken a typical antipsychotic drug for more than 1 year
targeted therapy Therapy that directs the treatment according to the person's genomic interfering with specific molecules
Tdap Tdap vaccine can protect adolescents and adults from tetanus, diphtheria, and pertussis
taxanes A drug derived from a yew tree that blocks cell growth by stopping cell division
teratogenic The disturbance of the development of an embryo or fetus
teratogens Substances that cause developmental abnormalities
tertiary syphilis Disease that occurs as early as 1 year after infection or at any time during an untreated person's lifetime
testosterone The principal male sex hormone, an anabolic steroid
therapeutic drug monitoring (TDM) Checking serum drug levels
therapeutic index (TI) The relationship between the therapeutic dose of a drug (ED_{50}) and the toxic dose of a drug (TD_{50})
therapeutic range A range of doses that produce a therapeutic response without causing significant adverse effect
therapeutic serum level Refers to the dosage range, blood plasma, or serum concentration usually expected to achieve desired therapeutic effects
thromboembolectomy A treatment to dissolve dangerous clots in blood vessels, improve blood flow, and prevent damage to tissues and organs
thromboembolism A clot in a blood vessel
thrombolytics Agents used to promote the fibrinolytic mechanism (converting plasminogen to plasmin, which destroys the fibrin in the blood clot)
thrombosis The formation of a clot in an arterial or venous vessel
thyroid-stimulating hormone (TSH) An endocrine hormone from the anterior pituitary gland that stimulates the thyroid gland to release thyroxine (T_4) and triiodothyronine (T_3)
thyrotoxicosis The most common type of hyperthyroidism, caused by hyperfunction of the thyroid gland; also known as Graves disease
thyroxine (T4) A hormone produced by the thyroid gland that controls metabolism
tinea capitis A fungal infection of the skin on the head
tinea pedis A fungal infection of the feet, also called *athlete's foot*
tissue phase Invasion of body tissue
titrated Adjustment of drug administration according to protocol
tocolytic therapy Drug therapy to decrease uterine muscle contractions
tolerable upper intake level (UL) The maximum level of continuing daily nutrient

intake likely to pose no risk to the health of most of those in the age group for which it has been established

tolerance The need for a larger dose of a drug to obtain the original euphoria

tonic-clonic Convulsive, as with a tonic-clonic seizure

tonic seizure A seizure in which muscles initially stiffen before the sufferer loses consciousness

tonicity Used primarily as a measurement of the concentration of intravenous solutions compared with the osmolality of body fluids

topical Medication applied to the skin, often by painting or spreading it over an area and applying a moist dressing or leaving the area exposed to air

torsades de pointes An unusual polymorphic ventricular tachycardia often associated with a prolonged QT interval

total parenteral nutrition (TPN) The administration of nutrients by a route other than the gastrointestinal tract; also called *parenteral nutrition*

toxic epidermal necrolysis A hypersensitive drug reaction causing a widespread detachment of the epidermis from underlying skin layers

toxoids Inactivated toxins that can no longer produce harmful diseases but do stimulate formation of antitoxins

toxoplasmosis A disease caused by the parasite *Toxoplasma gondii*

transcription factors Substances that enter the nucleus and signal the cell to begin mitosis

transdermal Across the skin; a term used to describe medication stored in a patch and placed on the skin to be absorbed to produce a systemic effect

transplant rejection Occurs when the immune system of the transplant recipient attacks the transplanted organ

trichinosis A disease caused by ingestion of raw or inadequately cooked pork that contains larvae of the *Trichinella spiralis* parasite

tricyclic antidepressants (TCAs) Drugs used to treat major depression

triiodothyronine (T_3) A hormone made by the thyroid gland for cellular metabolism

trough drug level The lowest plasma concentration of a drug, it measures the rate at which the drug is eliminated

tuberculin syringe A 1-mL syringe calibrated in hundredths of a milliliter

tuberculosis infection A bacterial infection caused by *M. tuberculosis*

type 1 diabetes mellitus A chronic condition in which the pancreas produces little or no insulin

type 2 diabetes mellitus A chronic condition that affects the way the body metabolizes sugar

typical antipsychotics A drug class subdivided into *nonphenothiazines*—such as butyrophenones (which block only the neurotransmitter dopamine), dibenzoxazepines, dihydroindolones, and thioxanthenes—and *phenothiazines*, which, along with the thioxanthenes, block norepinephrine to cause sedative and hypotensive effects early in treatment

tyrosine kinase (TK) An enzyme that activates other substances by adding a phosphate group (PO_4) to them, a process known as *phosphorylation*

tyrosine kinase inhibitors (TKIs) Drugs that inhibit tyrosine kinases and primarily exert their effects on an enzyme known as *BCR-ABL tyrosine kinase*

U

unit International units to quantify the effect of a drug (u)

unit dose method Method of dispensing drugs in which drugs are individually wrapped and labeled for single-dose use for each patient

uricosurics Agents that increase the rate of uric acid excretion by inhibiting its reabsorption

urinary analgesics Drugs that relieve pain and burning in the urinary tract

urinary antiseptics/antiinfectives Drugs that prevent microbial infections of any part of the urinary tract

urinary stimulants Agents that increase the tone of urinary muscles

urinary tract infection (UTI) Microbial infection of any part of the urinary tract

urticaria Skin rash caused by an allergic reaction

US Food and Drug Administration (FDA) The US federal agency responsible for approving and regulating drugs

uterine contractility Tightening and shortening of uterine muscles during labor

uterine inertia Uterine inactivity or hypotonic contractions

uveitis Infection of the vascular layer of the eye (ciliary body, choroid, and iris)

V

vaccination Involves the administration of a small amount of antigen, which although capable of stimulating an immune response does not typically produce the disease

Valsalva maneuver A method to prevent air embolism during dressing and tubing changes in which patients are asked to turn their head in the opposite direction of the insertion site, take a deep breath, hold it, and bear down

Vaping Inhaling the aerosol (vapor) produced by an e-cigarette or similar device, (e.g., vape pen or an advanced personal vaporizer)

Varicella vaccine A vaccine administered that prevents chickenpox and is approved for use in susceptible children and adults

vertical transmission The passage of infecting organisms from mother to neonate

very-low-density lipoprotein (VLDL) Contains the highest amount of triglycerides

vesicant A substance that causes tissue injury

vesication The act of tissue blistering due to injury from a vesicant

vesicles Clear, fluid-filled blisters smaller than 10 mm in diameter

vial Small glass vacuum container with a self-sealing rubber top

vinca alkaloids Substances derived from the periwinkle plant

viral load A measurement of the amount of a virus circulating in the blood, usually stated in virus particles per milliliter

virilization The development of male secondary sex characteristics in females or hypogonadal males

virus An obligate intracellular organism that must reside within a living host cell to survive and reproduce

vitamin K A fat-soluble vitamin given to newborns to prevent vitamin K–deficiency bleeding

vomiting center A major cerebral center that causes vomiting when stimulated

W

water-soluble vitamins A group of vitamins that includes the B-complex vitamins and vitamin C

whitehead A type of noninflammatory acne lesion that is closed

window period The time delay from infection to a positive test result

withdrawal bleeding Monthly bleeding females experience while using a hormonal birth control method

withdrawal symptoms A wide range of physical or emotional disorders that include nervousness, headaches, and insomnia that occur when an individual who is addicted to a substance (such as drugs or alcohol) stops using the substance

World Health Organization (WHO) An agency of the United Nations with the purpose of monitoring communicable and noncommunicable disease outbreaks globally

X

xerophthalmia Dry eyes

Z

Zoster vaccine A vaccine administered to adults to prevent shingles

Z-track technique A technique recommended for administering intramuscular injections to help minimize local skin irritation by sealing the medication in the muscle tissue

INDEX

Note: Page numbers followed by "*f*" indicate figures, "*t*" indicate tables, and "*b*" indicate boxes.

A

AAS. *See* Anabolic-androgenic steroid
Abacavir (ABC), 34*t*, 35, 384*t*–387*t*
Abatacept, 296*t*–297*t*
Abbreviations
   "Do Not Use", 74*t*
   error prone, 75*t*
   sustained-or extended-release medications, 76*t*
ABC. *See* Abacavir
Abciximab, 558*t*–559*t*
Abiraterone, 424*b*–425*b*, 443*t*–444*t*
Abnormal uterine bleeding (AUB), 722
Absence seizures (Petit mal seizures), 221, 225*t*–226*t*
   anticonvulsants for, 227*t*
Absorption
   cholesterol, inhibitors of, 565*t*–566*t*
   digoxin, 506*b*
   iron, 162*b*
   older adult considerations for, 53
   pediatric considerations for, 46
   right route with, 73
Abstral, 76*b*
Abuse, 58–59
Acamprosate
   AUD treatment with, 60–61
   pharmacokinetics of, 61*t*
Acarbose, 657*t*–659*t*
   dosage adjustment requirements with CKD for, 53*t*
Accommodation, 603
Acebutolol, dosage adjustment requirements with CKD for, 53*t*
Acebutolol hydrochloride, 515*t*–518*t*, 518*b*, 540*t*
   dosage for, 184*t*–185*t*
   uses for, 184*t*–185*t*
ACEIs. *See* Angiotensin-converting enzyme inhibitors
Acetaminophen
   combined hormonal contraceptives and, 719*b*
   hypokalemia caused by, 144*t*
Acetazolamide, 225*t*–226*t*, 530*t*–531*t*
Acetic acid, otic solution, 616*t*
Acetylcholine (ACh), 187, 188*f*
Acetylcholinesterase (AChE), 188*f*
Acetylcholinesterase (AChE) inhibitors
   adverse reactions from, 246–248
   Alzheimer disease treatment with, 238–242
   azathioprine, 246*t*
   donepezil, 240*t*–241*t*
   galantamine, 240*t*–241*t*
   memantine, 240*t*–241*t*
   myasthenia gravis treatment with, 246*t*
   neostigmine methylsulfate, 246*t*
   pharmacodynamics of, 245–246
   pharmacokinetics of, 245
   pyridostigmine, 247*b*
   rivastigmine, 239, 240*b*, 240*t*–241*t*
   side effects for, 246–248
Acetylsalicylic acid, hypokalemia caused by, 144*t*

Acid derivatives, 289*t*–291*t*, 292–293
AcipHex, patient safety with, 597*b*
Acitretin, 622*t*–624*t*, 626
Aclidinium, 491*t*–492*t*
Acne vulgaris, 621–625
   defined, 621–625
   nonpharmacologic approach for, 621
   pharmacologic treatment for, 621–625, 622*t*–624*t*
      clinical judgment (nursing process), 627*b*
      dosage for, 622*t*–624*t*
      systemic antiacne drugs, 624–625
      topical antiacne drugs, 621
Acquired immunodeficiency syndrome (AIDS), 366
Acquired resistance, 323
Acromegaly, 636
ACTH. *See* Adrenocorticotropic hormone
Actinomycin D, 434*t*
Actiq, 76*b*
Activated charcoal
   dosage for, 770*t*
   poisoning treated with, 768, 770*t*
Activated partial thromboplastin time (aPTT), 552
Active acquired artificial immunity, 408
Active immunity, 408
Active transport, 20, 134
Acute cystitis, 665
Acute dystonia, 260–261
   characteristics of, 261*f*
Acute myocardial infarction (AMI), 560
Acute pharyngitis, 484–485
Acute pyelonephritis, 665–666
Acute rhinitis, 477–484
   antihistamines for, 478–479, 478*b*, 479*b*, 480*t*, 481*b*
   antitussives for, 482–484, 483*t*
   expectorants for, 483*t*, 484
   intranasal glucocorticoids for, 482, 482*t*–483*t*
   nasal and systemic decongestants for, 479–482, 481*t*
Acyclovir, 364*t*–365*t*
   adverse reactions from, 366*b*
   clinical judgment (nursing process), 367*b*
   dosage adjustment requirements with CKD for, 53*t*
Adalimumab, 296*t*–297*t*, 622*t*–624*t*
Adapalene, 622*t*–624*t*
Adderall. *See* Amphetamine
Addiction, 306
Addison disease, 637*t*, 644, 746
Additive drug effects, 28
Adefovir, 364*t*–365*t*
Adenohypophysis, 633
Adenosine, 515*t*–518*t*
   cardiac emergency with, 764, 766*t*–767*t*
   dosage for, 766*t*–767*t*
Adequate intake (AI), 154
ADEs. Adverse drug events
ADH. *See* Antidiuretic hormone
ADHD. *See* Attention deficit-hyperactivity disorder

Adherence
   older adult considerations for, 54–55, 54*t*
   for organ transplantation, 403–406
Adjuvant, 409
Adjuvant analgesics, 313
Adjuvant therapy, 313, 424
Adolescent
   age range for, 46*t*
   pharmacology considerations for, 48–49
Ado-trastuzumab emtansine, patient safety with, 464*b*
Adrenal glands, 644–648
   corticosteroids, 646*b*–647*b*
   disorders of, 633–648
      drug therapies for, 645*t*
   glucocorticoids, 644–648
      dosage for, 645*t*
      drug interactions with, 646–648
      prednisone, 646*b*
      side effects for, 644
   mineralocorticoids, 644
      dosage for, 645*t*
Adrenal hypersecretion, physiologic effects, 637*t*
Adrenal hyposecretion, physiologic effects, 637*t*
Adrenal reproductive disorders, 746
Adrenergic agonists, 175–183
   activation effects with, 178*f*
   albuterol, 182*b*
   case study on, 186
   central-acting alpha agonists, 180–183
      adverse reactions from, 180
      clonidine, 182
      side effects for, 182–183
   classification of, 177–180, 177*t*
   dosage information for, 181*t*
   epinephrine, 180, 180*b*
   as high-alert medications, 177*b*
   inactivation of neurotransmitters, 177
   intravenous, 177*b*
   patient-centered collaborative care with, 182*b*
   sympathetic responses with, 179*f*
   uses for, 181*t*
Adrenergic antagonists (adrenergic blockers), 175
   adrenergic neuron antagonists, 185*b*, 186
   alpha-adrenergic antagonists, 183
   beta-adrenergic antagonists, 183–186, 183*b*
   dosage for, 184*t*–185*t*
   drug interactions, 182
   effects of, 183*t*
   patient-centered collaborative care with, 185*b*
   uses for, 184*t*–185*t*
Adrenergic neuron antagonists, 186
   patient-centered collaborative care with, 185*b*
Adrenergic neuron blockers (peripherally acting sympatholytics), dosage for, 542*t*
Adrenergic receptor, 175
Adrenocorticotropic hormone (ACTH), 633–634
   drugs for, 635*t*–636*t*
   side effects and adverse effects with, 637
ADRs. *See* Adverse drug reactions

Adsorbents, 582
  dosage for, 582t–583t
Adverse drug events (ADEs), older adult considerations for, 54
Adverse drug reactions (ADRs), 26, 32
Aerosol inhaler, sympathomimetics with, 490
Afferent neurons, 175
Afterload, 508
Age-related macular degeneration (AMD), 604
Aggregation, 551
Agonists, 25
AI. See Adequate intake
AIDS. See Acquired immunodeficiency syndrome
AIDS Info, 392b
Air embolism, parenteral nutrition complicated by, 171t
Akathisia, 261
  characteristics of, 261f
Albuterol, 182b, 489–490, 489b
  dosage for, 181t, 491t–492t, 772t
  hypokalemia caused by, 144t
  patient safety with, 489b
  for shock, 771, 772t
  uses for, 181t
Alcohol
  male sexual dysfunction caused by, 746t
  toxicity, 59, 60b
  withdrawal, benzodiazepines for, 268t
Alcohol use disorder (AUD), 59–61
  case study with, 67
  screening and brief counseling for, 60f
  treatment for, 60–61
    drug-assisted, 60–61, 61t
Aldesleukin, 474–476
  contraindications for, 474b
  dosage for, 470t
  pharmacodynamics of, 474
  pharmacokinetics of, 474
Aldosterone receptor antagonists, 545t–546t
Alectinib, 453–454
  adverse reactions from, 454
  dosage for, 448t–449t
  drug interactions with, 454
  pharmacodynamics of, 454
  pharmacokinetics of, 454
  side effects for, 454
Alemtuzumab, 250t–252t, 424b–425b, 459–460
  adverse reactions from, 460
  dosage for, 459t–460t
  drug interactions with, 460
  pharmacodynamics of, 460
  pharmacokinetics of, 460
  side effects for, 460
Alfentanil, 209t–210t
Alfuzosin, 748t
Alimentary canal, gastrointestinal system and, 574f
Aliphatic phenothiazines, 261
Alirocumab, 565t–566t
Aliskiren, 545t–546t
Alkeran, patient safety with, 427b
Alkylating drugs, 427–429, 428t–429t
  adverse reactions with, 429
  cyclophosphamide, 427–429, 431b–432b
  side effects with, 429
Allele, 33t
Allergic rhinitis, 477–484
  antihistamines for, 478–479, 478b, 479b, 480t, 481b

Allergic rhinitis (Continued)
  antitussives for, 482–484, 483t
  case study on, 485
  expectorants for, 483t, 484
  intranasal glucocorticoids for, 482, 482t–483t
  nasal and systemic decongestants for, 479–482, 481t
Allium sativum. See Garlic
Allopurinol
  clinical judgment (nursing process), 301b
  dosage adjustment requirements with CKD for, 53t
  dosage for, 300t
Almotriptan, 317t
Aloe
  digitalis toxicity with, 506b
  potassium-wasting diuretic with, 528b
Alogliptin, 657t–659t
Alpha antagonists (alpha blockers), 183
5-alpha- reductase inhibitors, 748t
Alpha$_1$-and beta$_1$-adrenergic blockers
  dosage for, 542t
  for hypertension, 543
Alpha$_2$ agonists, male sexual dysfunction caused by, 746t
Alpha-adrenergic agonists
  adverse reactions from, 612
  for glaucoma, 612
  side effects for, 612
Alpha-adrenergic antagonists, 183
Alpha-adrenergic blockers
  adverse reactions from, 541–543
  clinical judgment (nursing process) with, 543b
  dosage for, 542t
  drug interactions of, 541–543
  for hypertension, 541
  hypokalemia caused by, 144t
  pharmacodynamics of, 542
  pharmacokinetics of, 542
  prazosin hydrochloride, 544b
  side effects for, 543
Alpha-adrenergic blocking agents, 748t
Alpha-glucosidase inhibitors, 657t–659t, 660
Alpha-receptor blockers, male sexual dysfunction caused by, 746t
Alprazolam
  adverse reactions from, 210b–211b
  anxiety treated with, 268t
  contraindications for, 210b–211b
  dosage for, 209t–210t, 210b–211b, 270t–271t
  patient safety with, 211b, 579b
  pharmacodynamics of, 210b–211b
  pharmacokinetics of, 210b–211b
  side effects for, 210b–211b
  uses for, 209t–210t, 210b–211b, 270t–271t
Altace, patient safety with, 316b
Alteplase, 560b, 561t
Altretamine, 424b–425b, 428t–429t
Aluminum hydroxide, 593b, 594t, 676t–677t
Alveoli, 708
Alzheimer disease
  acetylcholinesterase inhibitors for, 239
    donepezil, 240t–241t
    galantamine, 240t–241t
    memantine, 240t–241t
    rivastigmine, 239, 240b, 240t–241t
  cholinesterase inhibitors for, 239
  defined, 229

Alzheimer disease (Continued)
  drugs for, 229
  histologic changes in, 239f
  neuron affected by, 239f
  pathophysiology for, 238–239
  symptoms of, 239
Amantadine hydrochloride, 233–234, 235t–238t, 240t–241t
Amaryl, patient safety with, 316b
AMD. See Age-related macular degeneration
Amenorrhea, 715
Amerge, patient safety with, 316b
American Hospital Formulary Service (AHFS) Drug Information, 16
American Nurses Association (ANA) Code of Ethics, 11
AMI. See Acute myocardial infarction
Amikacin, hypokalemia caused by, 144t
Amikacin sulfate, 345t
Amiloride hydrochloride, 533t
Aminocaproic acid, 561t
  male sexual dysfunction caused by, 746t
Aminoglycosides, 343
  adverse reactions with, 344
  case study on, 347
  clinical judgment (nursing process), 343b
  dosage for, 345t
  drug interactions, 344–346
  gentamicin sulfate, 342b
  hypercalcemia caused by, 147t
  hypomagnesemia caused by, 149t
  pharmacodynamics of, 343–344
  pharmacokinetics of, 343–346
  side effects with, 344
Aminosalicylate sodium, 355t–356t
Amiodarone, 515t–518t
  cardiac emergency with, 764–765, 766t–767t
  dosage for, 766t–767t
  pediatric implications for, 764
Amisulpride, 577t–578t
Amitriptyline hydrochloride, 279t–282t
Amlodipine, 510t–511t, 545t–546t, 548t, 549b
  and atorvastatin, 565t–566t
Amoxapine, 279t–282t
Amoxicillin, 99, 99f, 326t, 592t
  for acne, 622t–624t
  adverse reactions from, 325b
  combined hormonal contraceptives and, 719b
  contraindications for, 325b
  dosage for, 325b
  pharmacodynamics of, 325b
  pharmacokinetics of, 325b
  side effects for, 325b
  uses for, 325b
Amoxicillin-clavulanate, 326t
Amphetamine (Dexedrine, Adderall), 200
  adverse reactions from, 200
  amphetamine sulfate, 201t
  dextroamphetamine sulfate, 201t
  lisdexamfetamine dimesylate, 201t
  side effects for, 200
Amphetamine sulfate, 201t
Amphetamine-like drugs
  ADHD treated with, 200
  armodafinil, 201t
  dexmethylphenidate hydrochloride, 201t
  methylphenidate hydrochloride, 201t, 203b
  modafinil, 201t

Amphetamine-like drugs (Continued)
  narcolepsy treated with, 202
  pharmacodynamics of, 202
  pharmacokinetics of, 200
Amphetamines, hyperkalemia caused by, 144t
Amphotericin B, 359–361, 359t–360t
  adverse reactions from, 360–361
  hypokalemia caused by, 144t
  hypomagnesemia caused by, 149t
  patient safety with, 361b
  side effects for, 360–361
Ampicillin, 326t
  combined hormonal contraceptives and, 719b
  hypokalemia caused by, 144t
Ampicillin-sulbactam, 326t
AMPs. See Antimicrobial peptides
Ampules, 110–111, 110f
  defined, 110–111
Anabolic steroids, 744
  patient safety with, 747b
Anabolic-androgenic steroid (AAS)
  short-term effects of, 65
  substance use disorder with, 65
  withdrawal from, 65
Anabolism, 744
Anagrelide hydrochloride, 558t–559t
Anakinra, 296t–297t
Analeptics, 203–205
  action of, 203
  adverse reactions from, 203–205
  caffeine citrate, 204t
  side effects for, 203–205
Analgesia
  adjuvant, 313
  adverse reactions of, 690–692
  dosage for, 691t–692t
  labor pain control with, 690–692, 691t–692t
  patient-controlled, 312
Analgesic titration, 312
Analgesics, 303–319
  phenazopyridine, 670
  urinary, 670, 671t–672t
Anaphylactic shock, 771
Anaphylaxis, 414
Anastrozole, 424b–425b, 443t–444t
Androgens, 739
  adverse reactions with, 744
  clinical judgment (nursing process), 745b
  contraindications for, 744
  dosage for, 743t
  drug interactions with, 744
  indications for, 743
    hypogonadism, 740
  side effects of, 743–744
  testosterone, 742b, 742t, 743t
Anesthesia, 214
  balanced, 214
  clinical judgment (nursing process), 218b
  dosage for, 697t
  epidural blocks, 692–694, 697t
  inhalation, 214, 215t
  intravenous, 215–216, 215t
  labor pain control with, 692–695, 697t
  local, 216, 216t, 695–696
  pre-surgery assessment for, 214
  regional blocks, 692–694
  spinal, 216–218, 217f, 692–694, 693t
  stages of, 214, 214t

Anesthesia (Continued)
  topical, 216
Angina pectoris, 507, 762–763
  antianginal drugs, 507–512
    beta blockers, 508t, 509–512, 510t–511t
    calcium channel blockers, 508t, 510t–511t, 512
    nitrates, 508–509, 508b, 508t, 510t–511t
  clinical judgment (nursing process), 513b
  nonpharmacologic measures to control angina, 507
  steps for treating, 512f
  types of, 507–512
Angiogenesis inhibitors, 447
  adverse reactions from, 448
  bevacizumab, 450b
  clinical judgment (nursing process), 452b
  dosage for, 448t–449t
  drug interactions with, 448
  side effects for, 448
  ziv-aflibercept, 447–448, 448t–449t
Angiotensin II antagonists, thiazide with, 538b
Angiotensin II-receptor blockers
  dosage adjustment requirements with CKD for, 53t
  dosage for, 545t–546t
  for hypertension, 547–548
  valsartan, 547
Angiotensin receptor blockers (ARBs), hyperkalemia caused by, 144t
Angiotensin-converting enzyme inhibitors (ACEIs)
  adverse reactions with, 544
  calcium channel blockers with, 538b
  clinical judgment (nursing process) with, 546b–547b
  contraindications of, 544
  dosage adjustment requirements with CKD for, 53t
  dosage for, 545t–546t
  for heart failure, 506–507
  hyperkalemia caused by, 144t
  for hypertension, 544–547
  male sexual dysfunction caused by, 746t
  side effects with, 544
  thiazide with, 538b
ANH. See Atrial natriuretic hormone
Anidulafungin, 359t–360t
Anion, 133, 134t
Anorexiants, 200
  adverse reactions from, 203
  benzphetamine hydrochloride, 204t
  bupropion hydrochloride, 204t
  diethylpropion hydrochloride, 204t
  liraglutide, 204t
  naltrexone hydrochloride, 204t
  phendimetrazine, 204t
  phentermine hydrochloride, 204t
  phentermine-topiramate, 204t
  side effects for, 203
Anovulatory cycle, 715–716
ANP. See Atrial natriuretic peptide
ANS. See Autonomic nervous system
Antacids, 593–595
  actions of, 592f
  aluminum hydroxide, 593b
  case study on, 601
  clinical judgment (nursing process), 595b
  dosage for, 594t
  pharmacodynamics of, 594

Antacids (Continued)
  pharmacokinetics of, 594
Antagonistic drug effects, 28
Antagonists, 25
Antepartum drugs, clinical judgment (nursing process), 679b–680b
Anthelmintics, 369–379
  adverse reactions from, 374
  clinical judgment (nursing process), 376b
  dosage for, 376b
  side effects for, 374
Anthracyclines, 434–436, 434t
Anthralin, 622t–624t
Anthrax, vaccine for, 410t–413t
Antiacne drugs
  systemic, 624–625
  topical, 621, 625b
Antiandrogens, 744–746, 745t
  for cancer, 442
  finasteride as, 746
  flutamide as, 746
  GnRH as, 745–746
  ketoconazole as, 746
Antibacterials, 333
  adverse reactions to, 322t
  aminoglycosides, 343
    adverse reactions with, 344
    case study on, 347
    clinical judgment (nursing process), 343b
    dosage for, 345t
    drug interactions, 344–346
    gentamicin sulfate, 342b
    pharmacodynamics of, 343–344
    pharmacokinetics of, 343–346
    side effects with, 344
  beta-lactam antibacterials, other, 328
    adverse reactions, 328
    case study on, 332
    side effects with, 328
  body defenses and, 323
  case study on, 353
  cephalosporins, 328–332
    adverse reactions with, 332
    case study on, 332
    ceftriaxone, 329b
    clinical judgment (nursing process), 331b
    dosage for, 329b
    drug interactions of, 332
    generations of, 328–332, 329t
    pharmacodynamics of, 331–332
    pharmacokinetics of, 331
    side effects with, 332
  combination antibiotics use with, 322–324, 323f
  fluoroquinolones, 345b, 346–347
    case study on, 347
    clinical judgment (nursing process), 345b
    dosage for, 346t
    levofloxacin, 345b
    pharmacodynamics of, 347
    pharmacokinetics of, 347
  general adverse reactions to, 324, 324t
  glycopeptides, 337
    adverse reactions with, 337
    case study on, 338
    dosage for, 334t
    drug interactions, 337
    pharmacodynamics of, 337
    pharmacokinetics of, 337

Antibacterials *(Continued)*
    side effects with, 337
  glycylcyclines, 340–343
    adverse reactions with, 343
    case study on, 347
    dosage for, 341*t*
    drug interactions, 343
    pharmacodynamics of, 340
    pharmacokinetics of, 340
    side effects with, 343
  lincosamides, 336–337
    adverse reactions with, 336
    case study on, 338
    dosage for, 334*t*
    drug interactions, 337
    side effects with, 336
  lipopeptides, 337–338
    adverse reactions with, 337
    case study on, 338
    dosage for, 334*t*
    drug interactions, 338
    pharmacodynamics of, 337
    pharmacokinetics of, 337
    side effects with, 337
  macrolides, 334*t*
    adverse reactions with, 335
    azithromycin, 334*t*
    case study on, 338
    clinical judgment (nursing process), 336*b*
    dosage for, 334*t*
    drug interactions, 335
    extended macrolide group, 335–336
    pharmacodynamics of, 335
    pharmacokinetics of, 335
    side effects with, 335
  mechanisms of action, 322*t*
  nitroimidazoles, 350–352, 350*b*
    adverse reactions with, 352
    case study on, 353
    dosage for, 351*t*
    pharmacodynamics of, 352
    pharmacokinetics of, 352
    side effects with, 352
  oxazolidinones, 336
    adverse reactions with, 336
    case study on, 338
    dosage for, 334*t*
    side effects with, 336
  pathophysiology related to, 321–322
  penicillins, 324–328
    adverse reactions with, 327–328
    beta-lactamase inhibitors, 325–327
    broad-spectrum, 325, 325*b*
    case study on, 332
    dosage for, 326*t*
    drug interactions with, 327–328
    extended-spectrum, 325
    penicillinase-resistant, 325
    side effects with, 327–328
  pharmacodynamics of, 322–323
  pharmacokinetics of, 322
  resistance to, 323–324
    acquired, 323
    cross-resistance, 324
    inherent, 323
  sulfonamides, 348–349
    adverse reactions with, 348–349
    case study on, 353

Antibacterials *(Continued)*
    clinical judgment (nursing process), 351*b*
    dosage for, 349*t*
    ophthalmic, 349–350
    pharmacodynamics of, 348
    pharmacokinetics of, 348
    side effects with, 348–349
    topical, 349–350
    trimethoprim-sulfamethoxazole, 349, 350*b*
  tetracyclines, 339–340
    adverse reactions with, 339
    case study on, 347
    clinical judgment (nursing process), 341*b*–342*b*
    dosage for, 341*t*
    doxycycline, 340*b*
    drug interactions, 340
    side effects with, 339
  unclassified antibacterial drugs, 352*t*
Antibiotic resistance, 377–379
  patient safety with, 377*b*
Antibiotics
  antitumor, 433–436
    adverse reactions with, 436
    dosage for, 434*t*
    doxorubicin, 434–436, 436*b*, 439*b*
    side effects with, 436
  broad-spectrum, 324
  combined hormonal contraceptives and, 719*b*
  dosage adjustment requirements with CKD for, 53*t*
  hypokalemia caused by, 144*t*
  hypomagnesemia caused by, 149*t*
  trimethoprim and trimethoprim-sulfamethoxazole for, 666–667, 668*t*–669*t*
  for urinary tract disorders, 666–670
    clinical judgment (nursing process), 667*b*
    drug-drug interactions in, 670
    fluoroquinolones for, 668, 668*t*–669*t*
    methenamine for, 667, 668*t*–669*t*
    nitrofurantoin for, 667–668, 668*t*–669*t*
Antibodies, 408
Anticancer drugs, 421–445
  adverse reactions to, 426*t*–427*t*
  alkylating drugs, 427–429, 428*t*–429*t*
    adverse reactions with, 429
    cyclophosphamide, 427–429, 431*b*–432*b*
    dosage for, 428*t*–429*t*
    side effects with, 429
  antimetabolites, 429–433
    adverse reactions with, 432
    dosage for, 430*t*–431*t*
    fluorouracil, 424*b*–425*b*, 429–433, 432*b*, 433*b*
    side effects for, 432
  antitumor antibiotics, 433–436
    adverse reactions with, 436
    dosage for, 434*t*
    doxorubicin, 434–436, 436*b*, 439*b*
    side effects with, 436
  biologic response modifiers, 440
  bone marrow suppression with, 426*t*–427*t*
  cancer chemotherapy, 423–427
    adverse reactions with, 426, 426*t*–427*t*
    combination, 425, 425*t*
    side effects with, 426
  case study on, 444*b*–445*b*
  cell cycle and, 423, 423*f*
  cell cycle-nonspecific and cell cycle-specific, 423

Anticancer drugs *(Continued)*
  chemotherapy agents, miscellaneous, 442
  combinations of, 425*t*
  gastrointestinal disturbances with, 426*t*–427*t*
  hormones and hormonal agonists and antagonists, 442–445
    antiandrogens, 442
    aromatase inhibitors, 442–445
    corticosteroids, 442
    dosage for, 443*t*–444*t*
    luteinizing hormone-releasing hormone agonists, 442
    selective estrogen receptor modulators, 442
    sex hormones, 442
  immunomodulators, 440
  influences on, 421–423, 422*b*
  liposomal chemotherapy, 425–426
  plant alkaloids, 436–440
    adverse reactions with, 439–440
    dosage for, 437*t*–438*t*
    side effects with, 439–440
    vincristine, 422*b*, 439–440, 439*b*
  targeted therapies, 440–442
  vaccines with, 443*t*–444*t*
Anticholinergics, 187, 490–492, 490*b*
  actions of, 592*f*
  adverse reactions from, 576, 593
  benztropine mesylate, 235*t*–238*t*
  clinical judgment (nursing process), 231*b*–232*b*
  dosage for, 491*t*–492*t*, 577*t*–578*t*, 593*t*
  male sexual dysfunction caused by, 746*t*
  for nausea, in pregnancy, 676*t*–677*t*
  Parkinson disease treatment with, 230–232
  side effects for, 576, 593
  tiotropium, 490*b*
  treatment with other drugs compared to, 230*t*–231*t*
  trihexyphenidyl hydrochloride, 232*t*
  for ulcers, 593
  urinary, 670–672, 671*t*–672*t*
  for vomiting, 576, 577*t*–578*t*
Anticoagulant antagonists, 556
  dosage for, 553*t*–554*t*
Anticoagulants, 551–556
  anticoagulant antagonists, 556
  case study on, 562
  complementary and alternative therapies with, 42*b*
  direct thrombin inhibitors, 552
  dosage for, 553*t*–554*t*
  heparin, 551–556, 552*f*, 554*t*, 555*b*–556*b*
    low-molecular- weight, 552
  oral anticoagulants, 554–555, 554*t*, 555*b*–556*b*
  parenteral anticoagulants II, 552
  pathophysiology in, 551
Anticonvulsant drugs, combined hormonal contraceptives and, 719*b*
Antidepressants, 34*t*, 274–285, 279*t*–282*t*
  agents, 275–277
  atypical, 277, 279*t*–282*t*
  case study on, 285
  male sexual dysfunction caused by, 746*t*
  miscellaneous, 279*t*–282*t*
  monoamine oxidase inhibitors, 277, 277*b*, 279*t*–282*t*
  pregnancy and, 679–681
  selective serotonin reuptake inhibitors, 275–276, 275*b*, 276*b*

Antidepressants (Continued)
    serotonin norepinephrine reuptake inhibitors, 276–277, 279t–282t
    tricyclic, 275, 279t–282t
Antidiabetics, 649–663
    agents, 649
    case study on, 662b–663b
    complementary and alternative therapies for, 653b
    hyperglycemic drugs, 662–663
        diazoxide, 662–663
        glucagon, 662
    insulin, 650–655, 651t
    oral, 655–662, 657t–659t
Antidiarrheals, 580–583, 581b–582b
    adsorbents, 582, 582t–583t
    dosage for, 582t–583t
    miscellaneous, 583
    opiates and opiate-related agents, 580–583, 581b–582b, 584t–585t
Antidiuretic hormone (ADH), 633
    drugs used to replace, 635t–636t
Antidysrhythmic drugs, 514
    actions of, 514t
    adverse reactions from, 519–523
    cardiac action potentials with, 513–514, 514f
    cardiac dysrhythmias and, 512–514
    classes of, 514t
    clinical judgment (nursing process), 519b
    dosage for, 515t–518t
    indications for, 514t
    pharmacodynamics of, 514b
    side effects for, 519–523
    types of, 514–523
        beta blockers, 514–519
        calcium channel blockers, 519
        repolarization prolonging drugs, 519
        sodium channel blockers, 514
Antiemetics, 260, 573, 580b
    nonprescription, 575
        dosage for, 575t
    prescription, 576–580, 580b
        anticholinergics, 576, 577t–578t
        antihistamines, 576, 577t–578t
        benzodiazepines, 576, 577t–578t
        butyrophenones, 576, 577t–578t
        cannabinoids, 577t–578t, 579
        clinical judgment (nursing process), 580b
        dopamine antagonists, 576, 577t–578t
        dosage for, 577t–578t
        glucocorticoids, 576
        metoclopramide, 577t–578t
        miscellaneous antiemetics, 577t–578t, 579–580
        neurokinin receptor antagonists, 579
        phenothiazine antiemetics, 576, 577t–578t
        serotonin-receptor antagonists, 576, 577t–578t
Antiflatulents, 704
Antifungals, 354–368
    antimetabolites, 359t–360t, 361
    azole, 359t–360t, 361
    clinical judgment (nursing process), 363b
    combined hormonal contraceptives and, 719b
    dosage adjustment requirements with CKD for, 53t
    drugs, 359–361, 359t–360t
    echinocandins, 359t–360t, 361
    hyperkalemia caused by, 144t

Antifungals (Continued)
    polyenes, 359–361, 359t–360t
        amphotericin B, 359–361, 359t–360t, 361b
        nystatin, 359–361, 359t–360t, 361b
Antigen, 408
Antigout drugs, 298–301, 300t
    colchicine, 299, 300t
    dosage for, 300t
    uric acid biosynthesis inhibitors, 300t
    uric acid inhibitors, 298, 300t
    uricosurics, 299–301, 300t
Antihistamines, 478–479
    adverse reactions from, 576
    dosage for, 480t, 577t–578t
    for ear disorders, 616
    for eye inflammation, 608
    first-generation, 478
        diphenhydramine, 479b, 481b
        pharmacodynamics of, 478
        pharmacokinetics of, 478
        side effects of, 478–479
    male sexual dysfunction caused by, 746t
    motion sickness prevention with, 575t
    nonprescription, 575t
    for pregnancy with nausea, 676t–677t
    second-generation, 479
    side effects for, 576
    for vomiting, 576, 577t–578t
Antihyperlipidemics, 563–572
    adverse reactions of, 567
    case study on, 571
    dosage for, 565t–566t
    laboratory tests for, 564–567
    side effects with, 567
    statins, 564–567, 569b–570b
Antihypertensive effect, 524
Antihypertensives, 536–550
    angiotensin II-receptor blockers, 545t–546t, 547–548, 547b
    angiotensin-converting enzyme inhibitors, 544–547, 545t–546t
    calcium channel blockers, 548–550, 548t
    case study on, 550
    complementary and alternative therapies for, 539b
    cultural responses to, 537
    direct renin inhibitors, 545t–546t, 548
    direct-acting arteriolar vasodilators, 542t, 543–544
        side effects and adverse reactions, 544
    diuretics, 538
    male sexual dysfunction caused by, 746t
    sympatholytics, 538–543
        alpha$_1$-and beta$_1$-adrenergic blockers, 542t, 543
        alpha-adrenergic blockers, 542t, 543, 543b
        beta-adrenergic blockers, 538–543, 539b, 540t
        centrally acting alpha$_2$ agonists, 539–541, 540t
        dosage for, 540t, 542t
    thiazides with, 538b
Antiinfectives
    dosage and uses for, 377t, 606t
    for ear disorders
        adverse reactions from, 616
        clinical judgment (nursing process), 617b
        dosage for, 616t
        ear wick and, 615f
        side effects for, 616

Antiinfectives (Continued)
    for eye disorders, 605, 606t
    patient safety with, 377b
    for urinary tract disorders, 666–670
        clinical judgment (nursing process), 667b
        drug-drug interactions with, 670
        fluoroquinolones for, 668, 668t–669t
        methenamine for, 667, 668t–669t
        nitrofurantoin for, 667–668, 668t–669t
        trimethoprim and trimethoprim-sulfamethoxazole for, 666–667, 668t–669t
Antiinflammatories, 287–302
    agents, 288
    antigout drugs, 298–301, 300t
        colchicine, 299, 300t
        dosage for, 300t
        uric acid biosynthesis inhibitors, 300t
        uricosurics, 299–301, 300t
    corticosteroids, 295
    disease-modifying antirheumatic drugs, 295–298
        antimalarials, 298
        dosage for, 296t–297t
        immunomodulators, 298
    dosage for, 607t–608t
    for eye disorders, 605–608, 607t–608t
    nonsteroidal antiinflammatory drugs, 288
        complementary and alternative therapies with, 295b
        dosage information, 289t–291t
        fenamates, 289t–291t, 293
        OTC, 289
        oxicams, 289t–291t, 293–294
        para-chlorobenzoic acid derivatives, 289t–291t, 292
        phenylacetic acids derivatives, 289t–291t
        propionic acid derivatives, 289t–291t, 292–293, 294b
        salicylates, 289t–291t, 292b
        selective COX-2 inhibitors, 289t–291t, 294, 295b
        use in older adults, 294–295
    pathophysiology of, 287–288
Antimalarials, 298, 369–379
    adverse reactions from, 370–372
    case study on, 379
    clinical judgment (nursing process), 374b
    dosage for, 374b
    pharmacodynamics of, 370
    pharmacokinetics of, 369
    side effects for, 370–372
Antimetabolites, 359t–360t, 361
    adverse reactions with, 432
    for cancer, 429–433
    dosage for, 430t–431t
    fluorouracil, 424b–425b, 429–433, 432b, 433b
    side effects for, 432
Antimicrobial peptides (AMPs), 374
Antimicrobials, 322
    dosage adjustment requirements with CKD for, 53t
Antimuscarinics, urinary, 670–672, 671t–672t
Antineoplastics, 423
Antioncogenes, 422
Antiparkinson-anticholinergic drugs, 194–195
    benztropine mesylate, 194, 194b, 196t
    pharmacodynamics of, 194–195
    pharmacokinetics of, 194
    trihexyphenidyl hydrochloride, 196t

Antiplatelets, 556–559
  clopidogrel bisulfate, 558b
  complementary and alternative therapies for, 559b
  dosage for, 558t–559t
  pathophysiology in, 551
  pharmacodynamics of, 559
  pharmacokinetics of, 557
Antipsychotics, 34t, 259–273
  adverse reactions with, 260–261
    acute dystonia, 260–261
    neuroleptic malignant syndrome, 261
  antipsychotic agents, 260–268, 261b
    atypical antipsychotics, 264–268
    complementary and alternative therapies for, 261b
    dosage for older adults, 264
    nonphenothiazines, 263–264, 264b, 265t–266t
    pharmacophysiologic mechanisms of action for, 260
    phenothiazines, 261–263, 262t, 263b
  categories, 260–261
  male sexual dysfunction caused by, 746t
  phenothiazines, 261–263, 262t, 263b
Antiretroviral therapy (ART), 381
  clinical judgment (nursing process), 393b
  drugs in, 383–391
    chemokine (CCR5) coreceptor antagonists, 384t–387t, 390
    dosage for, 384t–387t
    fusion (entry) inhibitors, 384t–387t, 389–390
    integrase strand transfer inhibitors, 384t–387t, 390–391
    nonnucleoside reverse transcriptase inhibitors, 383–388, 384t–387t
    nucleoside/nucleotide reverse transcriptase inhibitors, 383, 384t–387t
    pregnancy with, 392–393
    protease inhibitors, 384t–387t, 388–389
  indications for, 382–383
  nurse's role in, 391–394
Antiseizure drugs, 223–227, 223b
  action of, 220
  barbiturates, 223
  benzodiazepines, 223
  case study on, 227–228
  collaborative care with, 224b
  febrile seizures and, 223
  hydantoins, 221–223
  iminostilbenes, 223
  list of, 225t–226t
  patient safety with, 221b
  pharmacophysiology of, 220
  pregnancy and, 223
  status epilepticus and, 223, 227t
  succinimides, 223
  urinary, 670–672, 671t–672t
  valproic acid, 223
Antispasmodics, 670–672
Antithymocyte globulin (rabbit), 402–403
Antithyroid drugs, for hyperthyroidism, 641
Antituberculars, 354–368
  adverse reactions from, 356–357
  clinical judgment (nursing process), 358b–359b
  dosage for, 355t–356t
  nursing process in, 358b–359b
  prophylactic, 356
  side effects for, 356–357

Antituberculin drugs, combined hormonal contraceptives and, 719b
Antitumor antibiotics, 433–436
  adverse reactions with, 436
  dosage for, 434t
  doxorubicin, 434–436, 436b, 439b
  side effects with, 436
Antitussives, 482–484
  dosage for, 480t
  pharmacodynamics of, 483
  pharmacokinetics of, 483
Antiulcer drugs, 590–601
  antacids, 593–595
    actions of, 592f
    aluminum hydroxide, 593b
    clinical judgment (nursing process), 595b
    dosage for, 594t
    pharmacodynamics of, 594
    pharmacokinetics of, 594
  anticholinergics, 593
    actions of, 592f
    adverse reactions from, 593
    dosage for, 593t
    side effects for, 593
  case study on, 601
  H₂ blockers, 595
    actions of, 592f
    adverse reactions from, 596
    clinical judgment (nursing process), 597b
    dosage for, 596t
    drug interactions with, 596–597
    pharmacodynamics of, 595–596
    pharmacokinetics of, 595
    side effects for, 596
  male sexual dysfunction caused by, 746t
  pepsin inhibitors (mucosal protective drugs), 599
    actions of, 592f
    clinical judgment (nursing process), 600b
    dosage for, 598t–599t
    pharmacodynamics of, 599
    pharmacokinetics of, 599
    sucralfate, 600b
  prostaglandin analogue antiulcer drug, 599–601
    actions of, 592f
    dosage for, 598t–599t
  proton pump inhibitors, 597–599
    actions of, 592f
    dosage for, 598t–599t
    drug interactions with, 597
    pantoprazole, 598b
    pharmacodynamics of, 597
    pharmacokinetics of, 597
  tranquilizers, 592
    actions of, 592f
Antivert, patient safety with, 579b
Antivirals, 354–368
  dosage adjustment requirements with CKD for, 53t
  non-HIV, 363–366
    cytomegalovirus antivirals, 364t–365t, 366
    hepatitis antivirals, 364t–365t, 366–368
    herpes antivirals, 364t–365t, 366
    influenza antivirals, 363–366, 364t–365t
Anxiety
  benzodiazepines for, 268t
  disorders, 268
  nonpharmacologic measures, 268

Anxiolytics, 268–273, 268t, 270t–271t
  benzodiazepines, 268–271, 268t
    complementary and alternative therapy with, 269b
  miscellaneous, 271–273
  nonpharmacologic measures for, 268
Apixaban, 553t–554t
Apolipoproteins, 563
Apomorphine, 230t–231t, 235t–238t
Apoptosis, 422, 446
Apremilast, 296t–297t
Aprepitant, 577t–578t
aPTT. See Activated partial thromboplastin time
Aqueous humor, 605, 610
Arformoterol tartrate, 491t–492t
Argatroban, 553t–554t
Aricept, patient safety with, 597b
Aripiprazole, 269b, 279t–282t
  dosage for, 265t–266t
  patient safety with, 597b
  uses for, 265t–266t
Armodafinil, 201t
Aromatase inhibitors, for cancer, 442–445
ART. See Antiretroviral therapy
Artemether-lumefantrine combination, 371t–372t
Artesunate, 371t–372t
ASA. Aspirin
Asenapine, antipsychotics treatment with, 265t–266t
Asian ginseng (*Panax ginseng*), 41
Asparaginase (*Erwinia chrysanthemi*), 424b–425b, 443t–444t
Aspiration pneumonitis, 168
Aspirin (ASA), 100, 100f, 288, 307t–308t, 558t–559t
  adverse reactions from, 292b
  cardiac emergency with, 762
  case study on, 301–302
  clinical judgment (nursing process), 299b
  contraindications for, 292b
  dosage for, 289t–291t, 292b
  drug-lab- food interactions, 292b
  and omeprazole, 558t–559t
  oxycodone with, 311t
  pharmacodynamics of, 292, 292b
  pharmacokinetics of, 292
  for pregnancy, with pain, 679
  side effects for, 292b
  uses for, 289t–291t, 292b
Assessment, in nursing process, 1
Asthma, 488, 771
  drug therapy according to age, 498
    older adults, 498
    young children, 498
  drug therapy according to severity, 498
Asystole, 764
Atazanavir (ATV), 384t–387t
  adverse reactions from, 391b
  contraindications for, 391b
  dosage for, 391b
  pharmacodynamics of, 391b
  pharmacokinetics of, 391b
  side effects for, 391b
  uses for, 391b
Atenolol, 183, 183b, 510t–511t, 540t
  adverse reactions from, 183b, 186
  contraindications for, 180b

Atenolol (Continued)
　　dosage adjustment requirements with CKD for, 53t
　　dosage for, 183b, 184t–185t
　　drug interactions with, 186
　　effects for, 183b
　　pharmacodynamics of, 183b, 186
　　pharmacokinetics of, 183b, 186
　　uses for, 183b, 184t–185t
Atonic seizure, 221t
　　anticonvulsants for, 227t
Atorvastatin, 569b
　　pharmacodynamics of, 567
　　pharmacokinetics of, 567
Atorvastatin calcium, 565t–566t
Atovaquone-proguanil combination, 371t–372t
Atrial fibrillation, 504
Atrial flutter, 504
Atrial natriuretic hormone (ANH), 503
Atrial natriuretic peptide (ANP), 503
Atrioventricular (AV) node, 502
Atropine, male sexual dysfunction caused by, 746t
Atropine sulfate, 193, 609t
　　adverse reactions from, 193b, 194
　　cardiac emergency with, 763, 766t–767t
　　contraindications for, 193b
　　dosage for, 193b, 196t, 766t–767t
　　example dosage calculation for, 110b–111b
　　patient-centered collaborative care with, 195b
　　pediatric implications for, 763–764
　　pharmacodynamics for, 194–195, 197b
　　pharmacokinetics for, 193b, 194–195
　　side effects for, 193b, 194
　　uses for, 193b, 196t
Attention deficit-hyperactivity disorder (ADHD), 200
　　amphetamine-like drugs for treatment of, 200
　　case study of, 205
Attenuated viruses, 408
ATV. See Atazanavir
Atypical antidepressants, 277, 279t–282t
Atypical antipsychotics, 260, 264–268
　　Parkinson disease treatment with, 234–238
AUB. See Abnormal uterine bleeding
AUD. See Alcohol use disorder
Augmentin, 98b
Autonomic nervous system (ANS), 175, 199
Autonomy, 8
Axert, patient safety with, 579b
Azacitidine, 424b–425b, 430t–431t
Azathioprine, 401
　　myasthenia gravis treatment with, 246t
Azelaic acid, 622t–624t
Azelastine, 480t, 607t–608t
　　and fluticasone, 480t
Azilsartan, 545t–546t
Azithromycin, 334t, 615
　　adverse reactions from, 335b
　　contraindications for, 335b
　　dosage for, 335b
　　pharmacodynamics of, 335b
　　pharmacokinetics of, 335b
　　side effects for, 335b
　　uses for, 335b
Azole antifungals, 359t–360t, 361
Aztreonam, 328t, 668t–669t

B

Bacitracin, 377, 377t, 606t
Baclofen, 254t–255t
　　male sexual dysfunction caused by, 746t
Bacterial infection, drugs for, 403
Bacterial vaginosis (BV), 752–753
Bactericidal drugs, 333
Bactericidal effect, 665
Bacteriostatic drugs, 333
Bacteriostatic effect, 665
Balanced anesthesia, 214
Baldness, 629
Baloxavir, 364t–365t
Bar code scanner, 70f
Barbiturates, 208, 223
　　combined hormonal contraceptives and, 719b
　　hyperkalemia caused by, 144t
　　intermediate-acting, 208, 208t
　　long-acting, 208, 208b, 208t
　　male sexual dysfunction caused by, 746t
　　pentobarbital, 207–208, 208t
　　pharmacodynamics of, 208
　　pharmacokinetics of, 208
　　phenobarbital, 225t–226t
　　primidone, 225t–226t
　　short-acting, 208, 208t
Baricitinib, 307t–308t
Basic formula, 99
　　body surface area in drug calculation with, 107
　　body weight in drug calculation with, 101–102
　　calculating in drops per minute intravenous flow rates with, 116
　　calculating in milliliters per hour intravenous flow rates with, 116–127
BBB. See Blood-brain barrier
Beclomethasone, 482, 482t–483t
Beers Criteria for Potentially Inappropriate Medication Use in Older Adults, 54
Belatacept, 397
Belbuca, 76b
Bempedoic acid, 565t–566t
Benadryl, patient safety with, 478b
Benazepril
　　ACE inhibitor, 549
　　patient safety with, 478b
Benazepril hydrochloride, 545t–546t
Bendamustine, 424b–425b, 428t–429t
Beneficence, 10
Benign prostatic hyperplasia (BPH), 748
　　drugs for, 748t
Benzamides, 577t–578t
Benzocaine, 691t–692t
Benzodiazepine antagonists, 209t–210t
Benzodiazepines, 208–212, 223
　　adverse reactions from, 269–271
　　alprazolam, 209t–210t, 211b, 270t–271t
　　anxiolytics with, 268–271, 268t, 269b
　　case study on, 218
　　clinical judgment (nursing process), 272b
　　clonazepam, 225t–226t, 268t
　　clorazepate, 225t–226t, 268t
　　combined hormonal contraceptives and, 719b
　　complementary and alternative therapy with, 269b
　　diazepam, 225t–226t, 268t
　　dosage for, 577t–578t
　　estazolam, 209t–210t

Benzodiazepines (Continued)
　　lorazepam, 209t–210t, 211b, 225t–226t, 268t
　　midazolam, 225t–226t
　　patient-centered collaborative care with, 211b
　　pharmacodynamics of, 212, 269
　　pharmacokinetics of, 212, 269
　　side effects for, 269–271
　　temazepam, 209t–210t
　　treatment for overdose, 271b, 272b
　　triazolam, 209t–210t
　　for vomiting, 576, 577t–578t
Benzothiazepines, 548
Benzoyl peroxide, 622t–624t
Benzphetamine hydrochloride, 204t
Benztropine, male sexual dysfunction caused by, 746t
Benztropine mesylate, 196t, 232t
　　adverse reactions from, 194b
　　Case study on use of, 197
　　contraindications for, 194b
　　dosage for, 194b
　　pharmacodynamics of, 194b
　　pharmacokinetics of, 194b
　　side effects for, 194b
　　uses for, 194b
Beractant, 709
Best Pharmaceuticals for Children Act (BPCA), 13, 47
Beta antagonists (beta blockers), 178–180, 509–512
　　acebutolol hydrochloride, 518b
　　actions of, 514t
　　adverse reactions from, 539
　　for angina, 508t, 509, 510t–511t
　　　steps in, 512f
　　for cardiac dysrhythmia, 514–519
　　classes of, 514t
　　clinical judgment (nursing process) with, 541b
　　dosage adjustment requirements with CKD for, 53t
　　dosage for, 510t–511t, 515t–518t, 540t
　　hawthorn with, 539b
　　for hypertension, 538–539, 540t
　　indications for, 514t
　　metoprolol, 539b
　　pharmacodynamics of, 508–509, 519, 539
　　pharmacokinetics of, 508, 519, 539
　　side effects for, 512, 539
　　thiazide with, 538b
Beta cell, insulin secretion by, 650
Beta$_2$ agonists, 490
Beta-adrenergic agents
　　clinical judgment (nursing process), 682b–683b
　　dosage for, 681t
Beta-adrenergic antagonists, 183–186
　　atenolol, 183, 183b
　　intrinsic sympathomimetic activity with, 183
　　propranolol hydrochloride, 183
Beta-adrenergic blockers
　　adverse reactions from, 612
　　dosage for, 611t
　　for glaucoma, 610–612
　　hyperkalemia caused by, 144t
　　side effects for, 612
　　timolol, 612b
Beta-interferon
　　adverse reactions from, 249b
　　contraindications for, 249b
　　dosage for, 249b

Beta-interferon *(Continued)*
  pharmacodynamics of, 249b
  pharmacokinetics of, 249b
  side effects for, 249b
  uses for, 249b
Beta-lactam antibacterials, other, 328
  adverse reactions with, 328
  case study on, 332
  side effects with, 328
Beta-lactamase inhibitors, 325–327
  pharmacodynamics of, 327
  pharmacokinetics of, 327
Betamethasone, 645t
  adverse reactions with, 683
  clinical judgment (nursing process), 684b
  corticosteroid therapy with, 683, 683b
  dosage for, 684t
Betamethasone acetate susp (IM), 645t
Betamethasone sodium phosphate, 645t
Beta-receptor blockers, male sexual dysfunction caused by, 746t
Beta-sympathomimetic drugs
  adverse reactions from, 682
  drug interactions from, 682
  pharmacodynamics of, 682
  pharmacokinetics of, 682
  tocolytic therapy with, 682b
Betaxolol, 611t
  dosage for, 184t–185t
  uses for, 184t–185t
Betaxolol hydrochloride, 540t
Bethanechol chloride, 188, 192t, 671t–672t
  adverse reactions from, 188b
  contraindications for, 188b
  dosage for, 188b
  patient-centered collaborative care with, 191b
  pharmacodynamics of, 188b
  pharmacokinetics of, 188b
  side effects for, 188b
  uses for, 188b
Betrixaban, 553t–554t
Bevacizumab
  adverse reactions from, 450b
  contraindications for, 450b
  dosage for, 450b, 459t–460t
  patient safety with, 447b
  pharmacodynamics of, 450b
  pharmacokinetics of, 450b
  side effects for, 450b
  uses for, 450b
Bexagliflozin, 657t–659t
Bexarotene, 424b–425b, 437t–438t
Bicalutamide, 424b–425b, 443t–444t, 745t
Biguanides, 660
Bile-acid sequestrants, 565t–566t
Bimatoprost, 611t
Bioavailability, 21
Biologic response modifiers (BRMs), 423, 466–476
  adverse effects for, 470t
  case study on, 476
  chimeric antigen receptor T cells, 467
  clinical judgment (nursing process), 475b–476b
  colony-stimulating factors, 470–473, 470t
    erythropoietin-stimulating agents, 471–473
    granulocyte colony-stimulating factor, 473
    granulocyte-macrophage colony-stimulating factor, 473
  dosage modifications for, 469t

Biologic response modifiers (BRMs) *(Continued)*
  interferons, 467–470, 469t, 474b
    interferon alfa, 467–470
    interferon beta, 470
    interferon gamma, 470
  interleukin 2, 470t, 473–476, 474b
  overview of, 466–467
Biotransformation, 22
Bipolar disorder, 274
Bisacodyl, 584t–585t, 585b, 701t
Bishop score, 696
Bismuth subsalicylate, 582t–583t
Bisoprolol, dosage adjustment requirements with CKD for, 53t
Bisoprolol fumarate, 540t
  dosage for, 184t–185t
  uses for, 184t–185t
Bisphosphonates, 642
  hypocalcemia caused by, 147t
Bitter orange, glaucoma and, 610b
Bivalirudin, 553t–554t
Black cohosh, 567b
  antihypertensives with, 539b
Blackheads, 621
  case study on, 631
Bladder, parasympathetic response with, 189f
Bleomycin, 425t, 434t
Bleomycin sulfate, 424b–425b
Blepharitis, 604
Blood, 503
  composition of, 503
  function of, 503
Blood dyscrasias, 263
Blood flow, regulation of, 502
Blood pressure, 502
Blood products, 137–138
Blood root, glaucoma and, 610b
Blood urea nitrogen (BUN), 23
Blood vessel, parasympathetic response with, 189f
Blood viscosity reducer agents, 563
Blood-borne pathogens, 363
Blood-brain barrier (BBB), 22, 22f
BNP. *See* Brain natriuretic peptide
Body surface area (BSA), 102
  calculating dosages based on, 107b, 128
  West nomogram with, 102, 103f, 104f, 105f
Body weight (BW), 101
  calculating dosages based on, 107b, 128
Bolus, 167
Bortezomib (PS-341), 425t, 458b
  patient safety with, 447b
Botanicals, 39
Bowel function
  laxatives for, 704b–705b
  postpartum promotion of, 701t
BPCA. *See* Best Pharmaceuticals for Children Act
BPH. *See* Benign prostatic hyperplasia
Bradycardia, 505, 763
Bradykinesia, 229
Brain, 200f
Brain anoxia, 220
Brain natriuretic peptide (BNP), 503
Brand (trade) name, 14, 94–95
Breakthrough bleeding (BTB), 715
Brexpiprazole, antipsychotics treatment with, 265t–266t
Brimonidine/timolol maleate, 611t
Brinzolamide, 611t

Brivaracetam, 225t–226t
BRMs. *See* Biologic response modifiers
Broad-spectrum antibiotics, 324
Broad-spectrum penicillins (aminopenicillins), 325
  amoxicillin, 325b
  dosage for, 326t
Bromocriptine, 634
Bromocriptine mesylate, 230t–231t, 235t–238t, 635t–636t
Brompheniramine tannate, 480t
Bronchial asthma, 487
  pathophysiology of, 487, 488f
Bronchial smooth muscle, 486–487, 487f
Bronchiectasis, 488
Bronchoconstriction, factors that contribute to, 488f
Bronchodilators, 489, 496b
  sympathomimetics used as, 491t–492t
Bronchospasm, 487
BSA. *See* Body surface area
BTB. *See* Breakthrough bleeding
Buccal administrations, 81
Budesonide, 482, 482t–483t
Bulk forming laxatives, 585
  adverse reactions from, 585
  clinical judgment (nursing process), 587b
  dosage for, 588t
  pharmacodynamics of, 585
  pharmacokinetics of, 585
  psyllium, 586b
  side effects for, 585
Bumetanide, 530t–531t
BUN. *See* Blood urea nitrogen
Bupivacaine, 693t
Bupivacaine hydrochloride, 216t
Buprenorphine
  dosing, 63
  opioid treatment with, 63
  pharmacokinetics of, 61t
  side effects, 63
Buprenorphine hydrochloride, 315t
Bupropion
  dosage adjustment requirements with CKD for, 53t
  tobacco use treatment with, 64
Bupropion hydrochloride, 204t, 279t–282t
Burns and burn preparations, 629–630
  degree and tissue depth of, 629t
  topical antiinfectives
    clinical judgment (nursing process), 631b
    mafenide acetate, 630b
    silver sulfadiazine, 630–631, 630t
Buspirone hydrochloride, 270t–271t
Busulfan, 424b–425b, 428t–429t
Butabarbital sodium, 208t
Butoconazole, for vulvovaginal candidiasis, 756
Butorphanol tartrate, 315t, 691t–692t
Butyrophenones, 263
  dosage for, 577t–578t
  male sexual dysfunction caused by, 746t
  for vomiting, 576, 577t–578t
BV. *See* Bacterial vaginosis

C

Cabergoline, 230t–231t, 235t–238t
Cadaveric transplantation, 395
Caffeine citrate, 204t
CAIs. *See* Carbonic anhydrase inhibitors

Calcimimetics, 642
Calcineurin inhibitors (CNIs), 397
   topical, 626
Calcipotriene, 622t–624t
Calcitonin, patient safety with, 644b
Calcitonin-salmon, 642, 642t
Calcitriol, 642, 643b
   patient safety with, 644b
Calcium, 144–147
   clinical management of imbalance of, 147, 147t
   drugs effect on balance of, 147, 147t
   functions of, 144–145
   hypercalcemia, 144, 147, 147t
   hypocalcemia, 144–147, 147t
   patient safety with, 644b
   patient-centered collaborative care with, 146b
Calcium acetate, hypercalcemia caused by, 147t
Calcium antagonist, tocolytic therapy with, 681t, 682
Calcium carbonate, 594t
   hypercalcemia caused by, 147t
   and magnesium hydroxide, 594t
Calcium channel blockers (CCBs)
   ACEIs with, 538b
   actions of, 514t
   adverse reactions from, 512, 548–550
   for angina, 512
      steps in, 512f
   for cardiac dysrhythmia, 519
   classes of, 514t
   dosage for, 510t–511t, 515t–518t
   effects on angina, 508t
   for hypertension, 548–550, 549b
   indications for, 514t
   pharmacodynamics of, 508–509, 549
   pharmacokinetics of, 512, 549
   side effects with, 512, 549–550
   statin drug with, 538b
Calcium salts, hypercalcemia caused by, 147t
Calfactant, 709t
CAM. *See* Complementary and alternative medicine
Camellia sinensis. *See* Green tea
Canadian controlled drugs and substances schedule, 14t
Canadian drug regulation, 14
Canagliflozin, 657t–659t
Canakinumab, 296t–297t
Cancer
   chemotherapy, 423–427
      adverse reactions with, 426, 426t–427t
      combination, 425, 425t
      side effects with, 426
   development of, 421
   metastasizing cells, 466
   overview of, 421–423
Candesartan, 545t–546t
Cangrelor, 558t–559t
Cannabinoids, 579
   adverse reactions from, 579
   dosage for, 577t–578t
   side effects for, 579
Cannabis
   legalization of, 61–62
   long-term use of, 61–62
   male sexual dysfunction caused by, 746t
   substance use disorder with, 61–62
   THC in, 61

Cantharidin, 628
Capecitabine, 424b–425b, 425t, 430t–431t
Capillary leak syndrome, 474
Capreomycin, 355t–356t
Capsaicin, 305b
Capsules, 107–108, 108f
Captopril, 545t–546t
Carbachol, 192t
Carbamazepine, 34t, 35, 279t–282t
   combined hormonal contraceptives and, 719b
   dosage for, 225t–226t
   partial seizure treated with, 227t
   tonic-clonic seizures treated with, 227t
Carbamide peroxide, 617
Carbapenem-resistant *Enterobacteriaceae* (CRE), 374
Carbidopa-levodopa, 233
   adverse reactions from, 234b, 242b
   Alzheimer disease treatment with, 242b
   clinical judgment (nursing process), 235b
   contraindications for, 234b
   dosage for, 234b, 235t–238t, 242b
   levodopa combination in, 233, 233f
   pharmacodynamics of, 234b, 242b
   pharmacokinetics of, 234b, 242b
   side effects for, 234b, 242b
   uses for, 234b, 235t–238t, 242b
Carbonic anhydrase inhibitors (CAIs), 532, 612–613
   adverse reactions from, 532, 612–613
   dosage for, 530t–531t, 611t
   for glaucoma, 612–613
   side effects for, 532, 612–613
Carboplatin, 424b–425b, 425t, 428t–429t
   calculating dosages based on BSA for, 107b
   patient safety with, 427b
Carboprost tromethamine, 697t
Cardiac emergency medications, 762–767
   adenosine, 764, 766t–767t
   amiodarone, 764–765, 766t–767t
   aspirin, 762
   atropine sulfate, 763–764, 766t–767t
   diltiazem, 764, 766t–767t
   epinephrine, 766, 766b, 766t–767t
   lidocaine, 765, 765b, 766t–767t
   magnesium sulfate, 765–766, 766t–767t
   morphine sulfate, 763, 766t–767t
   nitroglycerin, 762–763, 766t–767t
   procainamide, 765, 766t–767t
   sodium bicarbonate, 766–767, 766t–767t
Cardiac glycosides, 503–504
   complementary and alternative therapy for, 506b
   digoxin, 504–505, 504b
   dosage for, 504b
   hypokalemia caused by, 144t
   phosphodiesterase inhibitors, 505–506
Cardiac output, 502, 502f
Cardiovascular drugs, 501–523
   antianginal drugs, 507–512
      nonpharmacologic measures to control angina, 507
      types of, 507–512
         beta blockers, 508t, 509–512, 510t–511t, 512f
         calcium channel blockers, 508t, 510t–511t, 512, 512f
         nitrates, 508–509, 508b–509b, 508t, 510t–511t, 512f

Cardiovascular drugs *(Continued)*
   antidysrhythmic drugs, 514
      actions of, 514t
      cardiac action potentials with, 513–514, 514f
      cardiac dysrhythmias and, 512–514
      classes of, 514t
      clinical judgment (nursing process), 519b
      dosage for, 515t–518t
      indications for, 514t
      pharmacodynamics of, 514b
      types of, 514–523
   cardiac glycosides, 503–504
      complementary and alternative therapy for, 506b
      digoxin, 504–505, 504b
      dosage for, 505t
      phosphodiesterase inhibitors, 505–506
   nonpharmacologic measures, 507
      atrial natriuretic hormone or peptide, 503
      brain natriuretic peptide, 503
      laboratory tests, 503
   other agents used to treat heart failure, 506–507
      ACE inhibitors, 506
      angiotensin II-receptor antagonists, 506
      beta blockers, 507
      diuretics, 507
      spironolactone, 507
      vasodilators, 506
Carfilzomib, 457
   adverse reactions from, 457
   dosage for, 448t–449t
   drug interactions with, 457
   pharmacodynamics of, 457
   pharmacokinetics of, 457
   side effects for, 457
Cariprazine, 279t–282t
   antipsychotics treatment with, 265t–266t
Carisoprodol, 254t–255t
Carmustine, 424b–425b, 428t–429t
Carteolol, 611t
Carvedilol, 540t
   dosage for, 184t–185t
   uses for, 184t–185t
Case studies
   ADHD, 205
   adrenergic agonists, 186
   alcohol use disorder, 67
   allergic rhinitis, 485
   aminoglycosides, 347
   antacids, 601
   anticancer drugs, 444b–445b
   anticoagulants, 562
   antidepressants, 285
   antidiabetics, 662b–663b
   antihyperlipidemics, 571
   antihypertensives, 550
   antiseizure drugs, 227–228
   antiulcer drugs, 601
   aspirin, 301–302
   benztropine mesylate in, 197
   biologic response modifiers, 476
   blackheads, 631
   cephalosporins, 332
   cholesterol, 571
   combined hormonal contraceptives, 734b–737b
   dermatologic disorders, 631
   diabetes mellitus, 662b–663b
   diarrhea, 588, 601

Case studies (Continued)
  diuretics, 534–535
  duodenal ulcer, 601
  emergency drugs, 774b–775b
  fluid volume and electrolytes, 149b–153b
  fluoroquinolones, 347
  gestational hypertension, 712, 734b–737b
  glaucoma drugs, 618b
  glycopeptides, 338
  glycylcyclines, 347
  gunshot wound, 775
  head wound, 775
  heart failure, 520b–522b, 550
  HIV, 394
  hypertension, 534–535
  hypothyroidism, 647b–648b
  immunization, 418
  labor, 706–707
  labor induction, 712
  lincosamides, 338
  lipopeptides, 338
  macrolides, 338
  malaria, 379
  men's reproductive health, 749
  myasthenia gravis, 257
  nitroimidazoles antibiotics, 353
  older adult pharmacology, 56
  opioid analgesics, 318b–319b
  organ transplantation, 404b–405b
  other beta-lactams, 332
  oxazolidinones, 338
  Parkinson disease drug treatment, 242–243
  penicillins, 332
  pregnancy-induced hypertension, 706–707
  preterm labor, 687–688
  risperidone, 272b
  sexually transmitted infections, 758b
  sleeping medication, 218
  sulfonamides, 353
  targeted cancer therapies drugs, 464
  tetracyclines, 347
  thrombophlebitis, 562
  tuberculosis, 368
  vomiting, 588
Caspofungin, 359t–360t
Castor oil, 583–584
Catechol O-methyltransferase (COMT), 177
  entacapone, 232t, 235t–238t
  opicapone, 232t, 235t–238t
  Parkinson disease treatment with, 233–234
  tolcapone, 230t–231t, 235t–238t
  treatment with other drugs compared to, 230t–231t
Catecholamines, 177
Cathartics, 583
Cation, 133, 134t
Caudal block, 216
Cayenne, 539b
CBT. See Cognitive behavioral therapy
CC. See Clomiphene citrate
CCBs. See Calcium channel blockers
Cefaclor, 99, 99f, 102, 102f, 330t–331t
Cefadroxil, 97, 97f, 330t–331t
Cefazolin sodium, 330t–331t
Cefdinir, 330t–331t
Cefditoren, 331
Cefepime, 330t–331t

Cefiderocol, 668t–669t
Cefixime, 330t–331t
Cefotaxime, 330t–331t
Cefotetan, 330t–331t
Cefoxitin sodium, 330t–331t
Cefpodoxime, 330t–331t
Cefprozil monohydrate, 330t–331t
Ceftaroline fosamil, 330t–331t
Ceftazidime, 330t–331t
  and avibactam, 330t–331t, 668t–669t
Ceftibuten, 330t–331t
Ceftolozane and tazobactam, 330t–331t, 668t–669t
Ceftriaxone, 97f, 330t–331t
  example dosage calculation for, 110b–111b
Cefuroxime, 330t–331t
Celandine, glaucoma and, 610b
Celebrex, patient safety with, 221b
Celecoxib, 307t–308t
  uses for, 289t–291t, 297b
Cell cycle, 423, 423f
Cell cycle-nonspecific (CCNS) drugs, 423
Cell cycle-specific (CCS) drugs, 423
Cell lysis, 321
Cell membrane-embedded enzymes, 24
Cenobamate, 225t–226t
Centers for Disease Control and Prevention (CDC), sexually transmitted infection prevention guidelines from, 752f
Central nervous system (CNS), 175, 199
Central nervous system (CNS) agents, hyperkalemia caused by, 144t
Central nervous system depressants, 206
  anesthesia, 214
    balanced, 214
    clinical judgment (nursing process), 218b
    inhalation, 214, 215t
    intravenous, 215–216, 215t
    local, 216, 216t
    pre-surgery assessment for, 214
    spinal, 207–214, 217f
    stages of, 214, 214t
    topical, 216
  nonpharmacologic methods, 206–207
  sedative-hypnotics, 206
    barbiturates, 208, 208b, 208t
    benzodiazepines, 208–212, 208t, 211b
    complementary and alternative medicine for, 211b
    melatonin agonists, 209t–210t, 212
    nonbenzodiazepines, 209t–210t, 212–214, 213b
    for older adults, 212–214
    sleep stages with, 206, 207f
Central-acting alpha agonists, 180–183
  adverse reactions from, 180
  clonidine, 182
  side effects for, 182–183
Centrally acting alpha$_2$ agonists
  adverse reactions from, 539–541
  dosage for, 540t
  for hypertension, 539–541, 540t
  side effects for, 539
  thiazide with, 538b
Cephalexin, 330t–331t
Cephalosporins, 328–332
  adverse reactions with, 332
  case study on, 332
  ceftriaxone, 329b

Cephalosporins (Continued)
  clinical judgment (nursing process), 331b
  dosage for, 330t–331t
  drug interactions of, 332
  generations of, 328–332, 329t
  pharmacodynamics of, 331–332
  pharmacokinetics of, 331
  side effects with, 332
Cerebyx, patient safety with, 221b
Certolizumab pegol, 296t–297t
Cerumen, 616–617
Cerumenolytics, 616–617
Cervical ripening, 696
Cetirizine, 480t
Cetrorelix, 727t
Cetuximab, 460–461
  adverse reactions from, 461
  dosage for, 459t–460t
  drug interactions with, 461
  pharmacodynamics of, 461
  pharmacokinetics of, 461
  side effects for, 461
Chalazion, 604
Chamomile (*Matricaria recutita* and *Chamomilla recutita*), 41
  iron absorption and, 162b
Chancre, 754
Chancroid (*Haemophilus ducreyi*), 753t
CHCs. See Combined hormonal contraceptives
Chemical name, 14
Chemical neurotransmitters, 260f
Chemokine (CCR5) coreceptor antagonists, 384t–387t, 390
Chemoprotectant drug, 427
Chemoreceptor trigger zone (CTZ), 574–575, 575f
Chemoreceptors, 486
Chemotherapy
  adverse reactions with, 426, 426t–427t
  agents, miscellaneous, 442
  for cancer, 423–427
  combination, 425, 425t
  defined, 423
  liposomal, 425–426
  neoadjuvant, 424
  palliative, 424
  side effects with, 426
CHF. See Congestive heart failure
Children
  age range for, 46t
  asthma drug therapy for, 498
  drug administration concerns in, 46
  opioid analgesics usage by, 312–313, 313f
  pain intensity scale for, 313f
  tuberculosis in, 357
Chimeric antigen receptor T cells, 467
Chinese skullcap, 539b, 567b
Chlamydia, 754
Chloasma, 719
Chlorambucil, 424b–425b, 428t–429t
Chloramphenicol, 352t, 616
Chlordiazepoxide, 593t
  anxiety treated with, 268t
  male sexual dysfunction caused by, 746t
Chloride, 148–149
Chloride channel activators, 585
  dosage for, 584t–585t
Chloroprocaine, 693t
Chloroprocaine hydrochloride, 216t

INDEX

Chloroquine
    pharmacodynamics of, 370
    pharmacokinetics of, 369
Chlorothiazide, 526t
Chlorpheniramine, 480t
Chlorpromazine, 577t–578t
Chlorpromazine hydrochloride, 265t–266t
Chlorpropamide, 655
Chlorthalidone, 526t
    hypercalcemia caused by, 147t
Chlorzoxazone, 254t–255t
Cholesterol, 564t
    case study on, 571
    dosage adjustment requirements with CKD for, 53t
    reduction, nonpharmacologic methods of, 567
Cholesterol absorption inhibitors, 565t–566t
Cholestyramine, 563–564, 565t–566t
Cholinergic agents, 610
    adverse reactions from, 610
    for glaucoma, 610
    side effects for, 610
Cholinergic agonists, 187–191
    direct-acting, 187–188, 190f
    effects of, 190t
    indirect-acting, 190, 190f
    parasympathetic responses with, 189f
Cholinergic antagonists, 187–191
    anticholinergic response of, 192t
    antiparkinson, 194–195, 194b, 196t
    atropine sulfate, 193, 193b, 195, 196t
    effects of, 192t
    treating motion sickness treated with, 195–197
    uses for, 196t
Cholinergic crisis, 245
Cholinergic receptors, 25f
Cholinergic system, 199
Cholinesterase (ChE), 187–188
Cholinesterase inhibitors, 188, 610
    acetylcholinesterase inactivated with, 190f
    Alzheimer disease treatment with, 239
    irreversible, 191, 192t
    myasthenia gravis treatment with, 245
    reversible, 190–191, 192t
Choose My Plate, 155f
Chromium, 162–163
Chronic bronchitis, 488
Chronic kidney disease (CKD)
    dosage adjustment requirements with, 53t
    older adult considerations for, 53t
Chronic obstructive pulmonary disease (COPD), 488–489
    antiinflammatory drugs for, 494t
    signs and symptoms of, 487f
Chronotropic action, 504
Chylomicrons, 563
Cidofovir, 364t–365t
Cilostazol, 558t–559t, 568, 570b
    adverse reactions from, 568
    complementary and alternative therapies for, 568
    dosage for, 568t
    pharmacodynamics of, 568
    pharmacokinetics of, 568
    side effects for, 568
Cimetidine, 596–597, 596t
    male sexual dysfunction caused by, 746t
Cinacalcet, 642t
    hypocalcemia caused by, 147t

Ciprofloxacin, 100, 100f, 344b, 606t, 668t–669t
    otic solution, 616t
Ciprofloxacin hydrochloride, 346t
Circulation, 503
    two types of, 503
Cirrhosis, vitamin deficiency from, 155t
Cisplatin, 105–106, 105f, 424b–425b, 425t, 428t–429t
    hypocalcemia caused by, 147t
    hypomagnesemia caused by, 147t
    patient safety with, 427t
Citalopram, 100, 100f, 279t–282t
CKD. See Chronic kidney disease
Cladribine, 250t–252t, 424b–425b, 430t–431t
Clarithromycin, 334t, 592t, 615
Clemastine fumarate, 480t
Clidinium bromide, 593t
Clindamycin, 622t–624t
Clinical judgment (nursing process), 1, 2b
    acetaminophen in, 307t–308t
    acne vulgaris in, 627b
    acyclovir, 367b
    allopurinol in, 301b
    aminoglycosides in, 343b
    androgens, 745b
    angiogenesis inhibitors in, 452b
    antacids in, 595b
    antepartum drugs in, 679b–680b
    anthelmintics in, 376b
    antianginals, 513b
    anticholinergics in, 231b–232b
    antidepressants, 278b
    antidysrhythmics, 519b
    antifungals, 363b
    antihyperlipidemics, 569b–570b
    antiinfectives
        for burns in, 631b
        for ear conditions in, 617b
    antimalarials in, 374b
    antiretroviral therapy, 393b
    antithyroid drugs in, 641b
    antituberculars, 358b–359b
    benzodiazepines in, 272b
    beta blockers in, 541b
    beta-adrenergic agents in, 682b–683b
    betamethasone in, 684b
    biologic response modifiers in, 475b–476b
    blockers in, 541b
    bronchodilators in, 496b
    bulk forming laxatives in, 587b
    carbidopa-levodopa in, 235b
    cephalosporins, 331b
    combined hormonal contraceptives, 720b–722b
    corticosteroids in, 646b–647b
    cyclophosphamide in, 433b
    digoxin, 506b
    diphenhydramine, 481b
    doxorubicin in, 439b
    EGFR inhibitors in, 452b
    fluoroquinolones in, 345b
    fluorouracil in, 436b
    gestational hypertension in, 686b–687b
    glaucoma drugs in, 614b
    H_2 blockers in, 597b
    hemorrhoids, pain relief for, 702b–703b
    heparin in, 555b–556b
    ibuprofen in, 295b

Clinical judgment (nursing process) (Continued)
    immunosuppression in, 403b
    infertility, 727b–728b
    infliximab, 299b
    insulin in, 654b–655b
    laxatives in, 704b–705b
    leukotriene receptor antagonists in, 497b
    lithium in, 284b
    loop diuretics in, 531b
    macrolides in, 336b
    menopause symptoms in, 733b–734b
    monoclonal antibodies in, 463b
    morphine in, 310b
    mTOR kinase inhibitors in, 463b
    multikinase inhibitors in, 456b–457b
    nalbuphine in, 316b
    neonates, drug administered to full-term, 711b
    nonphenothiazines in, 267b
    in nursing process, 1–2
    ocular hypertension drugs in, 614b
    oral antidiabetic in, 661b
    oxymetazoline, 484b
    oxytocin in, 699b
    pain control drugs in, 694b
    parathyroid hormone insufficiencies in, 643b
    parenteral nutrition in, 171b–172b
    penicillins, 327b
    pepsin inhibitors in, 600b
    peptides in, 378b–379b
    perineal wounds pain relief in, 702b–703b
    peripheral vasodilators, 569b–570b
    phenothiazines in, 267b
    phenytoin in, 224b
    pituitary hormones in, 638b
    potassium-sparing diuretics in, 534b
    proteasome inhibitors in, 463b
    psoriasis in, 627b
    pyridostigmine, 247b–248b
    regional anesthesia in, 695b–696b
    $Rh_0(D)$ immune globulin in, 706b
    rivastigmine, 240b
    sexually transmitted infection prevention in, 757b
    stimulant laxatives in, 586b–587b
    sulfonamides in, 351b
    synthetic surfactant in, 710b
    terbutaline in, 682b–683b
    tetracyclines in, 341b–342b
    thiazides in, 528b
    thrombolytics in, 561b
    thyroid hormone replacement in, 641b
    tyrosine kinase inhibitors in, 456b–457b
    urinary antiinfective in, 667b
    VEGF inhibitors in, 452b
    vincristine in, 441b–442b
    warfarin in, 555b–556b
Clinical research study design, 11
Clobetasol propionate, 626t
Clofarabine, 424b–425b
Clomiphene citrate (CC)
    adverse reactions from, 726, 726b
    contraindications for, 726b, 728
    dosage for, 727t
    drug interactions of, 728
    pharmacodynamics of, 726, 726b
    pharmacokinetics of, 726, 726b
    side effects for, 726b
    uses for, 726b
Clomipramine hydrochloride, 279t–282t

Clonazepam
  absence seizure treated with, 227t
  atonic seizure treated with, 227t
  dosage for, 225t–226t
  myoclonic seizure treated with, 227t
  seizures and status epilepticus treated with, 268t
Clonidine, 182
Clonidine hydrochloride, 540t
  dosage for, 181t
  uses for, 181t
Clopidogrel, 34t, 35, 558t–559t
Clopidogrel bisulfate, 558b
  pharmacodynamics of, 559
  pharmacokinetics of, 557
Clorazepate, 225t–226t, 270t–271t
  anxiety treated with, 268t
  partial seizure treated with, 225t–226t
  seizures and status epilepticus treated with, 268t
Clotrimazole, for vulvovaginal candidiasis, 756
Clozapine, antipsychotics treatment with, 265t–266t
Cluster headaches, 316
  pathophysiology of, 316
CMV. See Cytomegalovirus
CNIs. See Calcineurin inhibitors
CNS. See Central nervous system
CNS stimulants, 202b
Coal tar, 626t
Cocaine, male sexual dysfunction caused by, 746t
Codeine, dosage adjustment requirements with CKD for, 53t
Codeine phosphate, 311t
Codeine sulfate, 311t
Coffee, glaucoma and, 610b
Cognitive behavioral therapy (CBT)
  cannabis treatment with, 62
  substance use disorder therapy with, 60, 62
  tobacco use disorder treatment with, 63–64
Cognitive symptoms, 260
Colchicine, 299, 300t
  dosage adjustment requirements with CKD for, 53t
Colesevelam, 563–564, 565t–566t
Colestipol, 563–564
Colestipol hydrochloride, 565t–566t
Coleus, 539b
Colistimethate, 375–376, 377t
Colloid solutions, 136, 136t
Colony-stimulating factors, 470–473, 470t
  erythropoietin-stimulating agents, 471–473
  granulocyte colony-stimulating factor, 473
  granulocyte-macrophage colony-stimulating factor, 473
Combination chemotherapy, 423
Combined hormonal contraceptives (CHCs), 713–716
  cardiovascular carcinogenetic risks with, 720
  case study on, 734b–737b
  clinical judgment (nursing process), 720b–722b
  complementary and alternative therapies with, 715b
  continuous-use, 716
  contraindications for, 719, 719b
  dosage for, 714t–715t
  drug interactions with, 719, 719b
  for dysmenorrhea, 723–724
  EE and norelgestromin transdermal patch, 716
  for endometriosis, 724
  ethinyl estradiol and etonogestrel transvaginal contraception, 716–717

Combined hormonal contraceptives (CHCs) *(Continued)*
  extended-use, 716
  FDA boxed warnings for, 730b
  mechanism of action for, 715–716
  missed dose guidelines for, 718b
  patient safety with, 729b
  pharmacokinetics of, 718
  route of delivery for, 716
  types of, 724
  withdrawal bleeding, 724
Comedones, 621
Common cold, 477–484
  antihistamines for, 478–479, 480t, 481b
  antitussives for, 482–484, 483t
  expectorants for, 479b, 483t, 484
  intranasal glucocorticoids for, 482, 482t–483t
  nasal and systemic decongestants for, 479–482, 481t
Community immunity, 408, 408f
Complementary and alternative medicine (CAM), 39–44
  anticoagulants in, 42b
  antidiabetics with, 653b
  antihypertensives with, 539b
  antiplatelets with, 559b
  antipsychotic agents, 261b
  benzodiazepines, 269b
  case study on, 43
  current good manufacturing practices for, 40–41
  for cyclophosphamide, 429b
  digoxin, 506b
  diuretics with, 528b
  for doxorubicin, 436b
  emergency medications and, 774b
  for fluorouracil, 432b
  heparin with, 556b
  herbal remedies commonly used in, 41
    Asian ginseng, 41
    chamomile, 41
    echinacea, 41
    garlic, 41
    ginger, 41
    Ginkgo biloba, 41
    lavender, 41
    saw palmetto, 41–42
    St. John's Wort, 42
  lower respiratory disorders with, 495b
  patient responsibility with, 39b
  peptic ulcer disease with, 591b
  sedatives, 211b
  sexual dysfunction with, 747–748
  for vincristine, 439b
  warfarin with, 556b
Complementary and alternative therapy
  for depression, 275, 275b
  iron in, 162b
  monoamine oxidase inhibitors with, 277b
  NSAIDs with, 294b
  SSRI with, 275b
Comprehensive Drug Abuse Prevention and Control Act, 12–13
Computed tomography (CT), 220
Computerized physician order entry (CPOE), 70
Condom
  CDC guidelines for, 752f
  male, 757f
Congenital rubella syndrome, 705

Congestive heart failure (CHF), 503
Conivaptan, 635t–636t
Conjugate vaccines, 408–409
Conjugated estrogens
  adverse reactions from, 730b
  contraindications for, 730b
  dosage for, 730b
  pharmacodynamics of, 730b
  pharmacokinetics of, 730b, 731
  side effects for, 730b
  uses for, 730b
Conjunctivitis, 604
Constipation, 583–588
  laxatives for
    bulk forming, 585
    chloride channel activators, 584t–585t, 585
    dosage for, 584t–585t
    emollients, 585–588, 588t
    osmotic, 583, 584t–585t
    stimulant, 583–585, 584t–585t, 586b–587b
  nonpharmacologic measures for, 583
  pregnancy with, 678
Contact dermatitis, 628
Continuous feedings, 167
Contractility, 502
Control group, 11
Controlled substances, 13t, 95b
COPD. See Chronic obstructive pulmonary disease
Copper, 162
Core ethical principles, 7–10
  beneficence, 10
  informed consent, 8, 8b, 9f, 12b
  justice, 10
  respect for persons, 7–8
  risk-benefit ratio, 10
Corkwood, glaucoma and, 610b
Corticosteroid deficiency, 644
Corticosteroids, 288–295, 401–402, 636
  adrenal hormone, 646b–647b
  for cancer, 442
  hypocalcemia caused by, 147t
  hypokalemia caused by, 144t
  ophthalmic antiinflammatories with, 607t–608t, 608
  patient safety with, 747b
  therapy, in preterm labor, 683–684
    betamethasone for, 683, 684b, 684t
    dexamethasone for, 683–684, 683b, 684t
  topical, 625–626, 625b
Corticotropin, 635t–636t
Cortisone acetate, 645t
Cortisone drugs, 644
Cortisone, hypokalemia caused by, 144t
Costimulation blockers, 397–400
Cosyntropin, 634, 635t–636t
Cough and cold products, substance use disorder with, 64–65
Counterfeit drugs, 14, 76
COVID-19, 408f, 409
  mRNA vaccines, 409f, 410t–413t
COX. See Cyclooxygenase
CPOE. See Computerized physician order entry
CPP. See Cyclic pelvic pain
Cranberry, 567b
CRE. See Carbapenem-resistant *Enterobacteriaceae*
Creatinine, 23
Cretinism, 639
Criteria, inclusion and exclusion, 8b

INDEX

Critical care drugs, calculating intravenous flow rates, 127
Critical Path Initiative, 7
Crofelemer, 582t–583t
Cromolyn, 496–497
　dosage for, 494t
Cromolyn sodium, 494t, 607t–608t
Cross-sensitivity, 348–349
Cryotherapy, 628
Cryptosporidiosis, 392
Crystalloid solutions, 135–136
Crystalluria, 348–349
CT. See Computed tomography
CTZ. See Chemoreceptor trigger zone
Cues, analyzation of, 3
Cushing syndrome, 637t, 644
Cyclic method, 167
Cyclic pelvic pain (CPP), 723
Cyclizine hydrochloride, 575t
Cyclobenzaprine
　adverse reactions from, 253b
　clinical judgment (nursing process), 256b
　contraindications for, 253b
　dosage for, 253b
　pharmacodynamics of, 253b, 256
　pharmacokinetics of, 253b, 256, 256b
　side effects for, 253b
　uses for, 253b
Cyclooxygenase (COX), 288
Cyclooxygenase-2 (COX-2) inhibitors, 291f, 294
　analgesics with, 307t–308t
　celecoxib, 289t–291t, 297b
　uses of, 291f
Cyclopentolate, 609t
Cyclopentolate hydrochloride, 196t
Cyclophosphamide, 424b–425b, 425t, 427–429, 429b
　adverse reactions from, 431b–432b
　clinical judgment (nursing process), 433b
　complementary and alternative therapies for, 429b
　contraindications for, 431b–432b
　dosage for, 431b–432b
　hyperkalemia caused by, 144t
　patient safety with, 427b
　pharmacodynamics of, 427–429, 431b–432b
　pharmacokinetics of, 427, 431b–432b
　side effects for, 431b–432b
　uses for, 431b–432b
Cycloplegics, 609
　adverse reactions from, 609
　dosage for, 609t
　side effects for, 609
Cycloserine, 355t–356t
Cyclosporine, 398b, 607t–608t, 626
　hyperkalemia caused by, 144t
　patient safety with, 427b
Cyproheptadine, 480t
Cysteinyl leukotrienes, 493–494
Cytarabine, 424b–425b, 425t, 430t–431t
Cytochrome P450 system, 22
Cytokine release syndrome, 396, 397b
Cytomegalovirus, 363
Cytomegalovirus antivirals, 364t–365t, 366
　acyclovir, 366b
　adverse reactions from, 366
　dosage for, 364t–365t
　side effects for, 366

Cytomegalovirus (CMV), 392
Cytotoxic chemical makeup, 446
Cytotoxic therapy, 423

D

DA. See Dimensional analysis
Dabigatran, 553t–554t
Dacarbazine, 424b–425b, 428t–429t
Dactinomycin, 424b–425b, 434t
Dalteparin, 553t–554t
Dantrolene sodium, 254t–255t
Dapagliflozin, 657t–659t
Dapagliflozin-metformin, 657t–659t
Dapagliflozin-saxagliptin, 657t–659t
Daptomycin, 334t
Darbepoetin alfa, patient safety with, 474b
Darifenacin hydrobromide, 671t–672t
Darunavir (DRV), 384t–387t
Dasatinib, 454–455
　adverse reactions from, 454–455
　dosage for, 448t–449t
　drug interactions with, 454
　pharmacodynamics of, 454
　pharmacokinetics of, 454
　side effects for, 454
Daunorubicin, 425t, 434t
　patient safety with, 436b
Daunorubicin hydrochloride, 424b–425b
Daunorubicin liposomal, 424b–425b
Daytrana, 76b
DDI. See Didanosine
Decoction, 40t
Decongestants
　for ear disorders, 616
　for eye disorders, 608–609
Dehydroepiandrosterone (DHEA), 66b
Delafloxacin, 346t
Delavirdine (DLV), 384t–387t
Delayed puberty, 741
Delivery, 689–707
Deltoid injection site, 87, 88f
Demeclocycline, 635t–636t, 637
Demeclocycline hydrochloride, 341t
Denosumab, hypocalcemia caused by, 147t
Dependence, 58–59, 200, 207–208
Dependent variable, 11
Depression, 274–275
　complementary and alternative therapy for, 275
　major, 274
　pathophysiology of, 274–275
　reactive, 274
Dermatitis
　contact, 628
　drug-induced, 628
Dermatologic disorders, 620–632
　acne vulgaris, 621–625
　　nonpharmacologic approach for, 621
　　pharmacologic treatment for, 621–625, 622t–624t
　baldness, 629
　burns and burn preparations, 629–631, 629t
　case study on, 631
　contact dermatitis, 628
　drug-induced dermatitis, 628
　hair loss, 629
　impetigo, 628
　psoriasis, 622t–624t, 625–628

Dermatologic disorders (Continued)
　rosacea, 629
　sunscreens, 629
　verruca vulgaris, 628
Dermatome, 362
Dermis, 620
Desflurane, 215t
Desiccated thyroid (porcine), 640t
Desipramine hydrochloride, 279t–282t
Desirudin, 553t–554t
Desloratadine, 480t
Desmopressin acetate, 635t–636t
Desoximetasone, corticosteroid therapy with, 683b
Desvenlafaxine, 279t–282t
Desyrel, patient safety with, 312b
Dexamethasone, 425t, 607t–608t, 608, 644, 645t
　adverse reactions with, 684
　corticosteroid therapy with, 683–684, 683b, 684t
　dosage for, 684t
　uses for, 684t
Dexedrine. See Amphetamine
Dexlansoprazole, 597, 598t–599t
Dexmethylphenidate hydrochloride, 201t
Dextroamphetamine sulfate, 201t
Dextromethorphan hydrobromide, 482b
Dextrose 50%
　dosage for, 772
　for shock, 772, 772t
Dextrose intravenous (IV) solution, hypokalemia caused by, 144t
DHEA. See Dehydroepiandrosterone
DI. See Diabetes insipidus
Diabetes insipidus (DI), 636
Diabetes mellitus, 649
　case study on, 662b–663b
　hyperglycemic drugs, 662–663
　　diazoxide, 662–663
　　glucagon, 662
　insulin and, 650–655, 651t
　oral antidiabetic for, 655–662, 657t–659t
　pathophysiology, 649–650
　secondary, 650
　types and occurrences of, 649t
Diabetic medications, dosage adjustment requirements with CKD for, 53t
Diagnostic stains, for eye disorders, 605, 605t
Diarrhea, 580–583
　antidiarrheals for, 580–583, 581b–582b, 584t–585t
　case study on, 588
　nonpharmacologic measures for, 580–583
　travelers', 580
　vitamin deficiency from, 155t
Diastat/Diastat AcuDial, 76b
Diazepam, 253b
　anxiety treated with, 268t
　dosage for, 225t–226t, 254t–255t, 270t–271t
　induction time for, 215t
　male sexual dysfunction caused by, 746t
　partial seizure treated with, 225t–226t
　seizures and status epilepticus treated with, 268t
　tonic-clonic seizures treated with, 225t–226t
Diazoxide, 657t–659t, 662–663
Dibenzoxazepines, 263
Dibucaine hydrochloride, 216t
Dibucaine ointment, 691t–692t
Diclofenac sodium, 289t–291t, 607t–608t
Dicloxacillin sodium, 326t

INDEX

Dicyclomine hydrochloride, 196t
Didanosine (DDI), 384t–387t
Dietary reference intakes (DRIs), 154–155
Dietary Supplement Health and Education Act of 1994 (DSHEA), 13, 40
Diethylpropion hydrochloride, 204t
Difenoxin and atropine, 582t–583t
Diffusion, 134
Diffusion process, 20
Diflunisal, 289t–291t, 307t–308t
Digitalis toxicity, 505
    aloe with, 506b
    antidote for, 505t
    ephedra with, 506b
Digoxin, 504–505, 506b, 515t–518t
    adverse reactions from, 504b
    antidote for cardiac/digitalis glycosides for, 505
    calculating intravenous flow rates for, 123b–126b
    clinical judgment (nursing process), 506b
    complementary and alternative therapy for, 506b
    contraindications for, 504b
    digitalis toxicity with, 505, 505t
    dosage adjustment requirements with CKD for, 53t
    dosage for, 504b, 507
    drug interaction with, 505
    hyperkalemia caused by, 144t
    hypokalemia caused by, 144t
    male sexual dysfunction caused by, 746t
    pharmacodynamics of, 504b
    pharmacokinetics of, 504–505, 504b
    side effects for, 504b
    uses for, 504b
Digoxin-immune Fab, 505t
Dihydroergotamine mesylate, 317t
Dihydroindolones, 263
Dihydropyridines, 548t
Dilaudid. *See also* Hydromorphone
    drug labels for, 96b–97b
Diltiazem, 515t–518t
    cardiac emergency with, 764, 766t–767t
    dosage for, 766t–767t
Diltiazem hydrochloride, 510t–511t, 548t
Diluent, 97
Dimenhydrinate, 575t
Dimensional analysis (DA), 100–101
    body surface area in drug calculation with, 106
    body weight in drug calculation with, 102
    calculating in drops per minute intravenous flow rates with, 116
    calculating in milliliters per hour intravenous flow rates with, 116–127
Dimethyl fumarate, 250t–252t
Dimethyl sulfoxide, 671t–672t
Dinoprostone cervical gel, 697t
Dinoprostone vaginal inserts, 697t
Dioval (estradiol), 547b
Diovan (valsartan), 547b
Dipeptidyl peptidase 4 inhibitors, 657t–659t
Diphenhydramine
    adverse reactions from, 479b
    clinical judgment (nursing process), 484b
    contraindications for, 479b
    dosage for, 479b
    male sexual dysfunction caused by, 746t
    pharmacodynamics of, 479b
    pharmacokinetics of, 479b
    side effects for, 479b

Diphenhydramine *(Continued)*
    uses for, 479b
Diphenhydramine hydrochloride
    dosage for, 772t
    for shock, 771, 772t
Diphenoxylate and atropine, 581
    dosage for, 582t–583t
    uses for, 582t–583t
Diphtheria, vaccine for, 410t–413t
Dipyridamole, 558t–559t
    and aspirin, 558t–559t
Direct renin inhibitors
    dosage for, 545t–546t
    for hypertension, 548
Direct thrombin inhibitors, 552
    dosage for, 553t–554t
Direct-acting arteriolar vasodilators
    adverse reactions with, 543–544
    dosage for, 542t
    for hypertension, 542t, 543–544
    side effects with, 543
Direct-acting cholinergic agonists, 188–190
    adverse reactions from, 190
    bethanechol chloride, 188, 191b, 192t
    carbachol, 192t
    eye with, 190
    metoclopramide hydrochloride, 188, 192t
    pilocarpine, 190
    pilocarpine hydrochloride, 192t
    receptor acted on directly by, 190f
    side effects for, 190
Direct-acting sympathomimetics, 179f
Disease-modifying antirheumatic drugs (DMARDs), 295–298
    antimalarials, 298
    dosage for, 296t–297t
    immunomodulators, 298, 298b
Disintegration, 19
Disopyramide phosphate, 515t–518t
Dispensing cabinet, for medications, 72f
Dissolution, 19
Distribution
    older adult considerations for, 53
    pediatric considerations for, 46–47
Disulfiram
    AUD treatment with, 60–61
    pharmacokinetics of, 61t
Diuresis, 524
Diuretics, 524–535
    carbonic anhydrase inhibitors, 532
        adverse reactions from, 532
        dosage for, 530t–531t
        side effects for, 532
    case study on, 534–535
    complementary and alternative therapies for, 528b
    dosage adjustment requirements with CKD for, 53t
    dosage for, 526t
    for heart failure, 507
    hypercalcemia caused by, 147t
    hypocalcemia caused by, 147t
    hypokalemia caused by, 144t
    hypomagnesemia caused by, 149t
    loop, 528–532
        adverse reactions from, 530
        clinical judgment (nursing process), 531b
        dosage for, 530t–531t

Diuretics *(Continued)*
        drug interactions with, 530–532
        furosemide, 529b
        pharmacodynamics of, 527
        pharmacokinetics of, 527
        physiologic and laboratory changes associated with, 530t
        side effects for, 530
    male sexual dysfunction caused by, 746t
    osmotic, 532
        adverse reactions from, 532
        contraindications for, 532
        dosage for, 530t–531t
        side effects for, 532
    potassium-sparing, 524, 532–534
        adverse reactions from, 532–534
        clinical judgment (nursing process), 534b
        dosage for, 533t
        side effects for, 532–534
        spironolactone, 533b–534b
    potassium-wasting, 524
        aloe with, 528b
    renal tubule affected by, 525f
    thiazides and thiazide-like, 525–528
        adverse reactions from, 527–528
        antihypertensives with, 538
        clinical judgment (nursing process), 528b
        contraindications for, 528
        dosage adjustment requirements with CKD for, 53t
        dosage for, 526t
        drug interactions with, 528
        ginkgo with, 528b
        hydrochlorothiazide, 526b–527b
        pharmacodynamics of, 527
        pharmacokinetics of, 527
        serum chemistry abnormalities associated with, 527t
        side effects for, 527–528
    use of, 524
Divalproex, 279t–282t
DLV. *See* Delavirdine
DMARDs. *See* Disease-modifying antirheumatic drugs
DNA, 34f
Dobutamine
    dosage for, 772t
    for shock, 770, 772t
Dobutamine hydrochloride
    dosage for, 181t
    uses for, 181t
Docetaxel, 424b–425b, 437t–438t
Docusate calcium, 588t, 701t
Docusate sodium, 588t, 701t
Dofetilide, 515t–518t
Dolasetron, 577t–578t
Dolutegravir (DTG), 384t–387t
Donepezil, Alzheimer disease treatment with, 240t–241t
Donepezil hydrochloride, 192t
Dong quai
    platelet aggregation and, 559b
    pregnancy and, 674b
Dopamine, 260
    adverse reactions from, 769b
    calculating intravenous flow rates for, 127f
    contraindications for, 769b
    dosage for, 769b

Dopamine (Continued)
   patient safety with, 770b
   pharmacodynamics of, 769b
   pharmacokinetics of, 769b
   for shock, 769b, 770
   side effects for, 769b
   uses for, 769b
Dopamine agonists, 233
   apomorphine, 230t–231t, 235t–238t
   bromocriptine, 230t–231t, 235t–238t
   cabergoline, 230t–231t, 235t–238t
   Parkinson disease treatment with, 233–234
   pramipexole hydrochloride, 230t–231t, 235t–238t
   ropinirole, 230t–231t, 235t–238t
   rotigotine, 230t–231t, 235t–238t
   treatment with other drugs compared to, 230t–231t
Dopamine antagonists, 576
   dosage for, 577t–578t
   side effects for, 576
Dopamine hydrochloride
   dosage for, 181t
   uses for, 181t
Dopaminergics, Parkinson disease treatment with, 232–233
   carbidopa/levodopa, 230t–231t, 233, 233f, 235b, 235t–238t
   levodopa, 233, 233f, 235t–238t
      inhalation, 230t–231t
   other drugs compared to, 230t–231t
Dorzolamide, 611t
Dosage calculations, 92–98
Dose-response relationship, 23, 23f
Doubling time, 423
Doxazosin, 748t
Doxazosin mesylate, 542t
   dosage for, 184t–185t
   uses for, 184t–185t
Doxepin hydrochloride, 279t–282t
Doxorubicin, 424b–425b, 425t
   adverse reactions from, 438b
   for cancer, 434–436
   clinical judgment (nursing process), 439b
   contraindications for, 438b
   dosage for, 438b
   patient safety with, 436b
   pharmacodynamics of, 435–436, 438b
   pharmacokinetics of, 435, 438b
   side effects for, 438b
   uses for, 438b
Doxorubicin liposomal, 424b–425b
   patient safety with, 436b
Doxycycline
   for acne, 622t–624t
   adverse reactions from, 340b
   combined hormonal contraceptives and, 719b
   contraindications for, 340b
   dosage for, 340b
   example dosage calculation for, 108b–109b
   pharmacodynamics of, 340b
   pharmacokinetics of, 340b
   side effects for, 340b
   uses for, 340b
Doxycycline hyclate, 341t
Doxylamine succinate, 676t–677t
DRIs. See Dietary reference intakes
Dromotropic action, 504

Dronabinol, 577t–578t
Dronedarone, 515t–518t
Drop factor, 112, 113f
Droperidol, 577t–578t
   fentanyl and, 215t
Drospirenone (DRSP), 714
DRSP. See Drospirenone
Drug Abuse Control Amendments, 12
Drug absorption, 19–21
Drug administration, 80–91, 89b–90b
   forms and routes of, 80–84, 80f
      buccal, 81
      capsules, 80–81
      gastrostomy tubes, 84
      inhalations, 81–84
      instillations, 81
      liquids, 81, 81f
      nasogastric tubes, 84
      sublingual, 81
      suppositories, 80, 84
      tablets, 80–81
      topical, 81
      transdermals, 81
   parenteral medications, 84–90
      intradermal, 85, 86f
      intramuscular, 85, 87t
      intravenous, 88–89, 89f
      nursing implications for, 89–90
      safety needles for, 85f
      subcutaneous, 85–87, 86f
      Z-track injection technique, 88, 88f
Drug approval process, 8f
Drug calculations, 92
   conversion factors for, 92–94
   dosages for drugs that require reconstitution, 97–98, 97f, 98b, 128
   oral drugs, 107
   suspensions and solutions, 97
   enteral and parenteral drug dosage calculation methods for, 98
      basic formula, 99
      body surface area, 101–107, 103f, 104f, 105f
      body weight, 101, 107b
      dimensional analysis, 71–72, 100–101
      ratio and proportion/fractional equation, 99–100
   insulin dosages, 94
      calculation in units for, 94
      practice problems for, 110b–111b
   intravenous flow rates, 130–131, 131f
      calculating critical care drugs, 127
      calculating in drops per minute, 116
      flow rates with, 116
      heparin therapy example, 117b–123b, 123b–126b
   measurement system of, 92–94
      English system, 93t, 94, 94b
      metric system, 92–94, 93b, 93f, 93t
   practice problems, answers to, 127–131
Drug development, 7–18
   drug names, 14–17
   drug resources, 16–17
   federal legislation, 12–13
   standards, 11–14
Drug distribution, 21–22, 21f
   protein binding, 21–22, 22f
Drug diversion, 66
Drug excretion, 23

Drug interactions, 26–30
   pharmacokinetic, 26–28
Drug labels, 98–99
   interpreting, 94–98, 128
   practice problems reading, 96b–97b
   precautions when reading, 95–97
   Tylenol (acetaminophen), 95b
Drug metabolism, 22–23
   loading dose, 23
   prodrugs, 22–23
Drug reconciliation, 75
Drug toxicity, 26
Drug-assisted treatment
   alcohol use disorder treatment with, 60–61, 61t
   opioid use disorder treatment with, 62–63, 63f
   pharmacokinetics of, 61t
   tobacco use disorder treatment with, 64
Drug-induced dermatitis, 628
Drug-induced photosensitivity, 30
Drug-laboratory interactions, 30
Drug-nutrient interactions, 28–30
Drug-resistant infection, 374
Drug-resistant tuberculosis, 355
Drusen, 604
DRV. See Darunavir
DSHEA. See Dietary Supplement Health and Education Act of 1994
DTaP, 414b
DTG. See Dolutegravir
DUB. See Dysfunctional uterine bleeding
Dulaglutide, 657t–659t
Duloxetine, 279t–282t
   dosage adjustment requirements with CKD for, 53t
Duodenal ulcer, 590
   case study on, 601
Dupilumab, 491t–492t
Duragesic, 76b
Duration of action, 23, 24f
Durham-Humphrey Amendment, 12
Dutasteride, 748t
Dysfunctional uterine bleeding (DUB), 722
Dyskinesia, 238
Dysmenorrhea, 715, 723–724
   pharmacologic management of, 723–724
      CHC in, 724
      NSAIDs in, 724
   secondary, 724
Dyspareunia, 719
Dysphoria, 274
Dysrhythmias, 764
Dystonia, 263
   acute, 260–261, 261f
Dystonic movement, 233

E

Ear
   external ear, 615
   inner ear, 615
   middle ear, 615
   overview of, 614–615
   structures of, 614f
EAR. See Estimated average requirement
Ear disorders, 603–619
   drugs for, 615
      administration of, 615
      antihistamines, 616

Ear disorders *(Continued)*
    antiinfectives, 615–616, 615f
    cerumenolytics, 616–617
    decongestants, 616
   suggestions for teaching patients with, 617–618
Eardrops, 81, 82b, 82f
EBV. *See* Epstein-Barr virus
ECF. *See* Extracellular fluid
Echinacea (*Echinacea purpurea*), 41
Echinocandins, 359t–360t, 361
Echothiophate iodide, 192t
ED. *See* Erectile dysfunction
Edoxaban, 553t–554t
Edrophonium chloride, 190–191
EE. *See* Ethinyl estradiol
EEG. *See* Electroencephalogram
Efavirenz (EVF), 384t–387t, 390b
Efferent neurons, 175
EHRs. *See* Electronic health records
Ejaculatory dysfunction, 746–747
Electrical impulses, conduction of, 502
Electroencephalogram (EEG), 220
Electrolytes, 111, 133
   body fluids concentration of, 134t
   calcium, 144–147, 145b, 147t
   chloride, 148–149
   defined, 133
   magnesium, 147–148, 147t, 148b
   phosphorus, 149–153
   potassium, 138–139
     effect of drugs on balance of, 139, 144t
     functions of, 139
     hyperkalemia, 139, 143b, 144t
     hypokalemia, 139, 141b, 141t, 144t
     oral and intravenous preparations, 141b
     supplements, 141t
   sodium, 139–144, 142b
Electronic cigarettes (e-cigarettes), 64, 65b
Electronic health records (EHRs), 70
Electronic infusion devices, 112–113, 115f
Electronic intravenous devices, 112
Eletriptan, 317t
Elixirs, 81
Eluxadoline, 582t–583t
Elvitegravir (EVG), 384t–387t
Embeda, 76b
Emedastine difumarate, 607t–608t
Emergency drugs, 761
   activated charcoal, 768, 770t
   cardiac disorders, 762–767
     adenosine, 764, 766t–767t
     amiodarone, 764–765, 766t–767t
     aspirin, 762
     atropine sulfate, 763–764, 766t–767t
     diltiazem, 764, 766t–767t
     epinephrine, 766, 766b, 766t–767t
     lidocaine, 765, 765b, 766t–767t
     magnesium sulfate, 765–766, 766t–767t
     morphine sulfate, 763, 766t–767t
     nitroglycerin, 762–763, 766t–767t
     procainamide, 765, 766t–767t
     sodium bicarbonate, 766–767, 766t–767t
   case study on, 775
   complementary and alternative therapies with, 774b
   flumazenil, 768, 770t
   hypertensive crises and pulmonary edema, 772–775

Emergency drugs *(Continued)*
   furosemide, 773t, 774–775, 774b
   labetalol, 772–773, 773t
   nitroprusside sodium, 773–774, 773b, 773t
   intracranial hypertension, 767
     mannitol, 767, 768b
     naloxone, 767–768, 769b
   oxygen as, 762
   shock, 769–772
     albuterol, 771, 772t
     dextrose 50%, 771–772, 772t
     diphenhydramine hydrochloride, 771, 772t
     dobutamine, 770, 770b, 772t
     dopamine, 770, 772t
     epinephrine, 766, 772t
     glucagon, 772, 772t
     norepinephrine, 770–771, 772t
Emollients (stool softeners), 585–588
   adverse reactions from, 585–588
   contraindications for, 586–588
   dosage for, 588t
   side effects for, 585–588
Emphysema, 488
Emtricitabine (FTC), 384t–387t
Emulsions, 81
Enalapril maleate, 545t–546t
Endocardium, 502
Endocrine system
   adrenal glands, 644–648
     corticosteroids, 646b
     glucocorticoids, 644, 645t
     mineralocorticoids, 644, 645t
   parathyroid glands, 642–644
     hyperparathyroidism, 642, 642t
     hypoparathyroidism, 642, 642t, 643b
     parathyroid hormone insufficiencies, 643b
   pituitary gland, 633–634
     anterior, 633–634, 634f
     negative feedback loop of, 634f
     posterior, 634f, 636
   thyroid gland, 638–642
     hyperthyroidism, 639, 641b
     hypothyroidism, 639, 639b–640b
Endometriosis, 724
   pharmacologic management of, 724
     combined hormonal contraceptives in, 724
     progestin therapy for, 724
       gonadotropin-releasing- hormone agonists, 724
Endophthalmitis, 604
Endorphins, 304
Enflurane, 215t
Enfuvirtide (T20), 384t–387t
English system, 94
   conversions within, 94, 128
   equivalents in, 93t
   examples, 94b
   practice problems for, 94b
Enoxacin, patient safety with, 552b
Enoxaparin
   calculating intravenous flow rates for, 117b–123b
   patient safety with, 552b
   practice problems for, 108b–109b
Enoxaparin sodium, 553t–554t
Entacapone, 230t–231t, 235t–238t
Entecavir, 364t–365t
Enteral administration, 107–109, 128–129

Enteral and parenteral drug dosage calculation methods, 98–99
   basic formula, 99
   body surface area, 102, 103f, 104f, 105f
   body weight, 101, 107b
   dimensional analysis, 71–72, 100–101
   ratio and proportion/fractional equation, 99–100
Enteral nutrition, 166–170
   commercial preparations for, 168t
   complications from, 168
   medications, 170
   methods for delivery of, 167
   patient-centered collaborative care with, 169b
   routes for, 167, 167f
   safety with, 168–170
   solutions, 167, 168t
Enteric-coated (EC) drugs, 19–20, 108
Enzalutamide, 424b–425b, 443t–444t
Enzyme inducers, 27, 27t
Enzyme inhibitors, 27t
Ephedra (Ma-Huang)
   antihypertensives with, 539b
   digitalis toxicity with, 506b
   glaucoma and, 610b
   monoamine oxidase inhibitors with, 277b
   theophylline toxicity with, 495b
Ephedrine hydrochloride
   dosage for, 181t
   uses for, 181t
Epidermal growth factor receptor (EGFR) inhibitors, 448–452
   clinical judgment (nursing process), 452b
   dosage for, 448t–449t
   erlotinib, 451b
   gefitinib, 448–451, 448t–449t
   osimertinib, 448t–449t, 451–452
Epidermis, 620
Epidural blocks, 216–218, 692–694, 697t
Epigenetics, 59
Epinastine, 607t–608t
Epinephrine, 26f, 180, 491t–492t
   adverse reactions from, 180, 180b
   cardiac emergency with, 766, 766t–767t
   contraindications for, 180b
   dosage for, 180b, 772t
   dosage information for, 181t
   patient safety with, 766b
   pediatric implications for, 766
   pharmacodynamics for, 180, 180b
   pharmacokinetics of, 180, 180b
   for shock, 771, 772t
   side effects for, 180, 180b
   uses for, 181t
Epirubicin, 424b–425b, 434t
Episiotomy, 702–703
Eplerenone, 533t, 545t–546t
EPO. *See* Erythropoietin
EPS. *See* Extrapyramidal syndrome
Epstein-Barr virus, 363
Epstein-Barr virus (EBV), 362
Eptifibatide, 558t–559t
Eravacycline, 341t
Erectile dysfunction (ED), 746
   PDE-5 inhibitors for, 747t
Erenumab, 317t
Ergocalciferol, 642t
Ergot alkaloids, 317t, 699
   adverse reactions with, 700

Ergot alkaloids *(Continued)*
  side effects of, 700
Ergotism, 700
Erlotinib, 451b
Ertapenem, 668t–669t
Ertugliflozin, 657t–659t
Erwinia chrysanthemi, 443t–444t. See also Asparaginase
Erythema multiforme, 351b
Erythrocytic phase, 369
Erythromycin, 622t–624t
Erythromycin base, 334t
Erythromycin ethylsuccinate, 98b
Erythromycin ophthalmic ointment, neonates, administration to, 709, 709t
Erythropoietin (EPO), 471
  adverse reactions from, 470t, 471b–472b
  contraindications for, 471b–472b
  dosage for, 470t, 471b–472b
  FDA black-box warnings for, 470t
  pharmacodynamics of, 471b–472b
  pharmacokinetics of, 471b–472b
  side effects for, 471b–472b
  uses for, 471b–472b
Erythropoietin-stimulating agents (ESAs), 471–473
  adverse reactions from, 470t, 471
  dosage for, 470t
  drug interactions with, 471–473
  pharmacodynamics of, 471
  pharmacokinetics of, 471
  side effects for, 471
ESAs. See Erythropoietin-stimulating agents
Escitalopram, 279t–282t
Esketamine, 279t–282t
Eslicarbazepine, 225t–226t
  partial seizure treated with, 227t
Esmolol, 515t–518t
Esmolol hydrochloride, 184t–185t
Esomeprazole, 592t, 597, 598t–599t
  naproxen and, 598t–599t
Esophageal ulcer, 590
Esophagus, 573, 574f
Essential hypertension, 536
Essential oils, 40t
Estazolam, 209t–210t
  insomnia treated with, 268t
Estimated average requirement (EAR), 154
Estramustine, 424b–425b, 428t–429t
Estrogen, hypocalcemia caused by, 147t
Eszopiclone, 209t–210t
Etanercept, 296t–297t, 622t–624t
Ethacrynic acid, 530t
Ethambutol hydrochloride, 355t–356t
Ethical considerations, 7–18
  core ethical principles, 7–10
Ethinyl estradiol (EE), 714
  dosage for, 714t–715t
  etonogestrel transvaginal contraception and, 716–717
  FDA boxed warnings for, 730b
  norelgestromin transdermal patch and, 716
Ethinyl estradiol/norethindrone acetate/ferrous fumarate, 622t–624t
Ethinyl estradiol/norgestimate, 622t–624t
Ethionamide, 355t–356t
  male sexual dysfunction caused by, 746t
Ethosuximide, 225t–226t
  absence seizure treated with, 227t

Etidocaine hydrochloride, 216t
Etodolac, 289t–291t
Etomidate, 215t
Etonogestrel transvaginal contraception, ethinyl estradiol and, 716–717
Etoposide, 424b–425b, 425t, 437t–438t
ETR. See Etravirine
Etravirine (ETR), 384t–387t
EVF. See Efavirenz
EVG. See Elvitegravir
Evolocumab, 565t–566t
Exalgo, 76b
Excipients, 19
Excretion
  older adult considerations for, 53
  pediatric considerations for, 47
Exemestane, 424b–425b, 443t–444t
Exenatide, 657t–659t
Exfoliative dermatitis, 351b
Expectorants, 484
  dextromethorphan hydrobromide, 482b
  dosage for, 483t
Experimental group, 11
Extended-spectrum penicillins (antipseudomonal penicillins), 325
  dosage for, 326t
Extended-use CHC, 716
Extensive metabolizers, 33t
External ear, 615
Extracellular fluid (ECF)
  adult volume of, 134t
  electrolyte concentration in, 134t
Extrapyramidal syndrome (EPS), 260, 576
  dopamine blocked, 260
Extravasation, 770
Eye
  direct-acting cholinergic agonists with, 190
  overview of, 603–604
  parasympathetic responses with, 189f
  structures of, 604f
Eye disorders, drugs for, 604–605, 614b
  antiinfectives, 615–616, 615f
  antiinflammatories, 605–608, 607t–608t
  cycloplegics, 609
  decongestants, 608–609
  diagnostic stains for, 605, 605t
  glaucoma drugs, 610–614, 611t, 614b
  lubricants, 609
  macular degeneration drugs, 604–605
  mydriatics, 609
  ocular hypertension drugs, 610–614, 611t, 614b
  suggestions, for teaching patients with, 613–614
  topical anesthetics, 605
Eye ointments, 81, 82b, 82f
Eyedrops, 81, 82b, 82f
Ezetimibe, 564, 565t–566t
  simvastatin and, 565t–566t

F

Facilitated diffusion, 20
Factor Xa inhibitors, 553t–554t, 555–556
Famciclovir, 364t–365t
  dosage adjustment requirements with CKD for, 53t
Family-centered care, 47
Famotidine, 595, 596b, 596t
  adverse reactions of, 596b

Famotidine *(Continued)*
  contraindications of, 596b
  dosage for, 596b
  drug interactions with, 596b
  drug-lab- food interactions of, 596b
  male sexual dysfunction caused by, 746t
  pharmacodynamics of, 596b
  pharmacokinetics of, 596b
  uses of, 596b
Fasciculations, 245
Fat-soluble vitamins, 155–158
  vitamin A, 155, 156t–157t, 157b
  vitamin D, 155–158, 156t–157t
  vitamin E, 156t–157t, 158
  vitamin K, 156t–157t, 158
FDA. See Food and Drug Administration
FE. See Fractional equation
Febrile seizures, antiseizure drugs and, 223
Febuxostat, 300b, 300t
Federal Food, Drug, and Cosmetic Act, 12
Federal legislation, in drug development, 12–13
Felbamate, 225t–226t
  partial seizure treated with, 227t
Felodipine, 510t–511t, 548t
Fenamates, 289t–291t, 293
Fenofibrate, 564, 565t–566t
Fenoprofen calcium, 289t–291t
Fentanyl, 311t
Fentanyl citrate, 691t–692t
  patient safety with, 706b
Fentora, 76b
Fertility promotion drugs, 725–729
  clinical judgment (nursing process), 727b–728b
  infertile couple assessment with, 725
  ovulation induction, 726–729, 727t
Fertilization, preventing, 720–722
Fever
  vitamin deficiency from, 155t
  yellow, vaccine for, 410t–413t
Feverfew
  iron absorption and, 162b
  platelet aggregation and, 559b
  pregnancy and, 674b
  SSRI with, 275b
Fexofenadine, 480t
FI. See Fusion (entry) inhibitors
Fibrates (fibric acid)
  antihyperlipidemic therapy with, 565t–566t
  dosage adjustment requirements with CKD for, 53t
Fibrinolysis, 560
Fidaxomicin, 334t
Filgrastim, 472b
Finasteride, 745t, 748t
  antiandrogens with, 746
Fingolimod, 250t–252t
First-day start method, 718
First-line drugs, 355
First-pass effect, 20–21
First-pass metabolism, 20–21, 21f
Flatus, 703–704
Flavoxate hydrochloride, 671t–672t
Flecainide, 515t–518t
Floxuridine, 424b–425b, 430t–431t
Fluconazole, 362b
  combined hormonal contraceptives and, 719b
  dosage adjustment requirements with CKD for, 53t

Flucytosine, 359t–360t
Fludarabine, 424b–425b, 430t–431t
Fludrocortisone, 644, 645t
Fluid replacement, 134–138
　general considerations for, 134
　intravenous solutions, 134–138, 135t
　patient-centered collaborative care, 137b–138b
Fluid volume, 133
　adult body, 134t
　electrolyte concentration in, 134t
Fluid volume deficit (FVD), 134
Flumazenil, 209t–210t, 270t–271t, 768
　dosage for, 770t
Flunisolide, 482, 482t–483t, 494t
Fluorescein sodium, ophthalmic, 605t
Fluoroquinolones (Quinolones), 345b, 346–347, 615–616, 668
　adverse reactions from, 670
　case study on, 347
　clinical judgment (nursing process), 345b
　dosage for, 346t, 668t–669t
　levofloxacin, 345b
　pharmacodynamics of, 347
　pharmacokinetics of, 347
　side effects for, 670
Fluorouracil (5-FU), 34t, 101–102, 101f, 424b–425b, 425t, 429–433
　adverse reactions from, 435b
　clinical judgment (nursing process), 436b
　complementary and alternative therapies for, 432b
　contraindications for, 435b
　dosage for, 435b
　pharmacodynamics of, 432, 435b
　pharmacokinetics of, 432, 435b
　side effects for, 435b
　uses for, 435b
Fluoxetine
　adverse reactions from, 276b
　case study on, 285
　contraindications for, 276b
　dosage for, 276b, 279t–282t
　drug-lab- food interactions, 276b
　pharmacodynamics of, 276, 276b
　pharmacokinetics of, 276, 276b
　side effects for, 276, 276b
　uses for, 279t–282t
Fluoxymesterone, 424b–425b, 443t–444t, 743t
Fluphenazine, 262b
　kava kava and dystonia with, 262b
Fluphenazine hydrochloride
　dosage for, 265t–266t
　pharmacodynamics of, 263
Flurazepam, insomnia treated with, 268t
Flurbiprofen sodium, 289t–291t, 607t–608t
Flutamide, 424b–425b, 443t–444t, 746
　antiandrogens with, 746
Fluticasone, 482, 482t–483t, 494t
Fluticasone furoate, 494t
Fluvastatin sodium, 565t–566t
Fluvoxamine, 279t–282t
Folic acid, 95b, 156t–157t, 160
　for pregnancy, 675
　　adverse reactions for, 675
Folic acid antagonists, 430t–431t
Follicle-stimulating hormone (FSH), 633, 727t
Folliculitis, 703
Fondaparinux, 553t–554t

Food and Drug Administration Amendments Act, 13
Food and Drug Administration (FDA), 74–75
　AUD treatment approved by, 60–61
　black-box warnings for IFNs, IL-2 and erythropoietin, 470t
　boxed warnings for CHC and EE, 730b
　pediatric dosing recommendations from, 47
　pregnancy categories by, 78
Food and Drug Administration Modernization Act, 13
Food and Drug Administration Safety and Innovation Act, 13
Formoterol, 491t–492t
Formoterol fumarate, aclidinium bromide and, 491t–492t
Fosamprenavir (FPV), 384t–387t
Foscarnet, 364t–365t
Fosfomycin tromethamine, 668t–669t
Fosinopril, 545t–546t
Fosphenytoin, 225t–226t
　partial seizure treated with, 227t
　status epilepticus treated with, 227t
　tonic-clonic seizures treated with, 227t
FPV. See Fosamprenavir
Fraction of inspired oxygen (FiO$_2$), 762
Fractional equation (FE), 99
　body surface area in drug calculation with, 106
　calculating in drops per minute intravenous flow rates with, 116
　calculating in milliliters per hour intravenous flow rates with, 116–127
Free drugs, 21
Freedom from Smoking Online, 64
Free-flow IV rate, 115
Fremanezumab, 317t
Frovatriptan, 317t
FSH. See Follicle-stimulating hormone
Fulvestrant, 424b–425b, 443t–444t
Fungal infection, drugs for, 403
Fungus, 358–361
　as opportunistic infections, 358–359
　pathophysiology of, 358–361
　as primary infections, 358–359
Furosemide, 530t–531t
　adverse reactions from, 529b
　calculating intravenous flow rates for, 123b–126b
　contraindications for, 529b
　dosage for, 529b
　example dosage calculation for, 110b–111b
　ginseng and efficacy of, 774b
　hypokalemia caused by, 144t
　licorice with, 774b
　pharmacodynamics of, 529b
　pharmacokinetics of, 529b
　for pulmonary edema, 773t, 774, 774b
　side effects for, 529b
　uses for, 529b
furosemide with, 774b
Fusion (entry) inhibitors (FI), 384t–387t, 389–390
FVD. See Fluid volume deficit

G

G protein-coupled receptor systems, 24, 25f
Gabapentin, 225t–226t
　dosage adjustment requirements with CKD for, 53t

Gabapentin (Continued)
　partial seizure treated with, 227t
Galactorrhea, 634
Galantamine, Alzheimer disease treatment with, 240t–241t
Galcanezumab, 317t
Ganciclovir sodium, 364t–365t
Ganirelix, 727t
Garlic (Allium sativum), 41
　platelet aggregation and, 559b
　pregnancy and, 674b
Gastric mucosal barrier (GMB), 590
Gastric ulcer, 590
Gastroesophageal reflux disease (GERD), 590
　nonpharmacologic measures for managing, 592
Gastrointestinal (GI) system, 573–574
　alimentary canal and, 574f
　drugs for, 573
　esophagus, 573, 574f
　large intestine, 574, 574f
　oral cavity, 573, 574f
　parasympathetic responses with, 189f
　small intestine, 574, 574f
　stomach, 574, 574f
Gastrointestinal tract disorders, 573–601
　constipation, 583–588
　　laxatives for, 583–588, 584t–585t, 586b, 588t
　　nonpharmacologic measures for, 580
　diarrhea, 580–583
　　antidiarrheals for, 580–583, 580b, 582t–583t
　　case study on, 588
　　nonpharmacologic measures for, 580
　　travelers' diarrhea, 580
　vomiting, 574–580
　　case study on, 588
　　chemoreceptor trigger zone with, 574–580, 575f
　　nonpharmacologic measures for, 575
　　nonprescription antiemetics for, 575
　　prescription antiemetics for, 576–580, 577t–578t
Gastrointestinal tubes, enteral feedings with, 167, 167f
Gastrostomy tube
　enteral feedings with, 167, 167f
　medication administration with, 84
Gate theory, 304
G-CSF. See Granulocyte colony-stimulating factor
Gefitinib, 448–451
　adverse reactions from, 451
　dosage for, 448t–449t
　drug interactions with, 451
　pharmacodynamics of, 450
　pharmacokinetics of, 450
　side effects for, 451
Gemcitabine hydrochloride, 424b–425b, 425t, 430t–431t
Gemfibrozil, 564, 565t–566t
General anesthesia, 695
Generalized seizure, 221t
Gene-related peptide, 317t
Generic name, 14
Genes, 34b
Genetic Information Nondiscrimination Act (GINA), 37
Genome, 33t
Genomics, 33t
Genotoxicity, 10

Genotype, 33t
Gentamicin
    calculating dosages based on BW for, 107b
    hypokalemia caused by, 144t
    hypomagnesemia caused by, 149t
Gentamicin sulfate, 342b, 345t, 606t
    adverse reactions from, 342b
    contraindications for, 342b
    dosage for, 342b
    pharmacodynamics of, 342b
    pharmacokinetics of, 342b
    side effects for, 342b
    uses for, 342b
GERD. *See* Gastroesophageal reflux disease
Gestational hypertension, 683
    case study on, 712, 734b–737b
    clinical judgment (nursing process), 686b–687b
    drugs for, 683–684
    methyldopa, hydralazine, magnesium sulfate, and labetalol for, 686
Get Rich or Die Smoking, 64
GH. *See* Growth hormone
Gigantism, 636
GINA. *See* Genetic Information Nondiscrimination Act
Ginger (*Zingiber officinale*), 41
    antacids and, 591b
    platelet aggregation and, 559b
Gingival hyperplasia, 222
Ginkgo biloba, 41, 567b, 591b
    platelet aggregation and, 559b
    pregnancy and, 674b
    thiazide diuretic with, 528b
Ginseng (*Panax ginseng*)
    digoxin levels with, 506b
    furosemide efficacy with, 774b
    monoamine oxidase inhibitors with, 277b
    pregnancy and, 674b
Glatiramer acetate, 250t–252t
Glaucoma, 604f, 605, 608
    combination drugs for, 611t
Glaucoma drugs, 610–614
    alpha-adrenergic agonists, 612
        adverse reactions from, 612
        side effects for, 612
    beta-adrenergic blockers, 610–612
        adverse reactions from, 612
        dosage for, 611t
        side effects for, 612
        timolol, 612b
    carbonic anhydrase inhibitors, 612–613
        adverse reactions from, 612–613
        dosage for, 611t
        side effects for, 612–613
    case study on, 618b
    cholinergic agents, 610
        adverse reactions from, 610
        side effects for, 610
    clinical judgment (nursing process), 614b
    patient safety with, 610b
    pharmacodynamics of, 655
    pharmacokinetics of, 655
    prostaglandin analogues, 610
        adverse reactions from, 610
        dosage for, 611t
        latanoprost, 613b
        side effects for, 610
Gliclazide, dosage adjustment requirements with CKD for, 53t

Glimepiride, 655, 657t–659t
Glipizide, 656b, 657t–659t
Gliptins, dosage adjustment requirements with CKD for, 53t
Glucagon, 657t–659t, 662
    dosage for, 772t
    for shock, 772, 772t
Glucagon-like peptide 1 agonists, 657t–659t
Glucocorticoids (steroids), 644
    adverse effects with, 644
    adverse reactions from, 493
    dosage for, 494t
        drug therapies for, 645t
    drug interactions with, 646–648
    for lower respiratory disorders, 495–496
    prednisone and, 646b
    side effects for, 495–496, 644
    for vomiting, 576
Glucose, hypokalemia caused by, 144t
Glyburide, 657t–659t
Glyburide-metformin, 657t–659t
Glycerin, 584t–585t
Glycogenolysis, 772
Glycopeptides, 334t, 337
    adverse reactions with, 337
    case study on, 338
    dosage for, 334t
    drug interactions, 337
    pharmacodynamics of, 337
    pharmacokinetics of, 337
    side effects with, 337
Glycopyrrolate, 196t, 593t
    formoterol and, 491t–492t
Glycylcyclines, 340–343
    adverse reactions with, 343
    case study on, 347
    dosage for, 341t
    drug interactions, 343
    pharmacodynamics of, 340
    pharmacokinetics of, 340
    side effects with, 343
GMB. *See* Gastric mucosal barrier
GM-CSF. *See* Granulocyte-macrophage colony-stimulating factor
GnRH. *See* Gonadotropin-releasing hormone
Goldenseal, 539b
    antihypertensives with, 539b
    cardiac glycosides' effect with, 506b
    glaucoma and, 610b
Golimumab, 296t–297t
Gonadotropin-releasing- hormone agonists, for endometriosis, 724
Gonadotropin-releasing hormone (GnRH), 442, 727t
    antiandrogens with, 745–746
Gonorrhea, 754
Good Clinical Practice (GCP) Consolidated Guideline, 10
Goserelin acetate, 424b–425b, 443t–444t, 745t
Gram, 92–93
    equivalent units of measurement with, 93t
Gram staining, 321
Granisetron, 577t–578t
Granulocyte, 471
Granulocyte colony-stimulating factor (G-CSF), 473
    adverse reactions from, 470t
    dosage modifications for, 470t
    filgrastim, 472b

Granulocyte-macrophage colony-stimulating factor (GM-CSF), 473
    adverse reactions from, 470t
    dosage modifications for, 470t
    sargramostim, 473b
Graves disease, 639
Green tea (*Camellia sinensis*), 567b
Griseofulvin, 359t–360t
    combined hormonal contraceptives and, 719b
growth factor (PDGF), 447–448
Growth fraction, 423
Growth hormone (GH), 633–634
    deficiency in, drug therapy for, 635t–636t, 636
        side effects and adverse effects with, 636
    excess in, drug therapy for, 635t–636t, 636
Guanfacine hydrochloride, 540t
Gunshot wound, case study on, 775
Gynecomastia, 634, 743–744

H

Haemophilus influenzae type B (Hib), vaccine for, 410t–413t
Hair loss, 629
Half-life, 22, 27t
Haloperidol
    dosage for, 264b, 265t–266t
    pharmacodynamics of, 263
    pharmacokinetics of, 263
    uses for, 265t–266t
Haloperidol decanoate, 264b
Halothane, 215t, 216t
The Handbook of Nonprescription Drugs, 17
Hangover, 207
Harrison Narcotics Tax Act, 12
HAV. *See* Hepatitis A virus
Hawthorn (*Crataegus laevigata* and *C. monogyna*)
    beta blockers with, 539b
    digoxin's effect with, 506b
    hypotension with, 528b
HBIG. *See* Hepatitis B immune globulin
HBV. *See* Hepatitis B virus
HCl. *See* Hydrochloric acid
HCV. *See* Hepatitis C virus
HDL. *See* High-density lipoprotein
Head wound, case study on, 775
Headaches, 314–319
    pathophysiology of, 316
    treatment of migraine, 316–319, 317t
Health care-acquired infections, 323
Health Insurance Portability and Accountability Act (HIPAA), 13
Heart, 501–502
    anatomy of, 502f
    electrical impulse conduction within, 502
    parasympathetic responses with, 189f
Heart block, 763
Heart failure, 503
    case study on, 520b–522b, 550
    nonpharmacologic measures to treat, 507
    other agents used to treat, 506–507
        ACE inhibitors, 506
        angiotensin II-receptor antagonists, 506–507
        beta blockers, 507
        diuretics, 507
        spironolactone, 507
        vasodilators, 506
    stages of, 503t
Heart rate, regulation of, 502

Heartburn (pyrosis), pregnancy with, 676t–677t, 677–678
Helicobacter pylori
    peptic ulcer disease with, 591
    pharmacologic agents for, 592t
HELLP syndrome, 685
Helminthiasis, 372
Helminths, 372
Hemorrhoids
    nonpharmacologic measures for, 700t
    postpartum, pain relief for, 702–703, 702b–703b
        adverse reactions for, 703
        clinical judgment (nursing process), 702b–703b
        side effects of, 703
Hemothorax, parenteral nutrition complicated by, 171t
Heparin, 95b, 552, 553t–554t, 555b–556b
    action of, 552f
    calculating intravenous flow rates for, 117b–123b
    clinical judgment (nursing process), 555b–556b
    complementary and alternative therapies for, 556b
    contraindications for, 552
    drug labels for, 96b–97b
    example dosage calculation for, 110b–111b
    hyperkalemia caused by, 144t
    low-molecular- weight, 552
    warfarin *versus*, 554t
Heparin sodium, 553t–554t
    calculating intravenous flow rates for, 117b–123b
    safety considerations when administering, 106f, 115
Hepatitis A virus (HAV), 753t
    vaccine for, 410t–413t
Hepatitis antivirals, 366–368
    adverse reactions from, 367
    dosage for, 364t–365t
    side effects for, 367
Hepatitis B immune globulin (HBIG), 710t
Hepatitis B virus (HBV), 753t
    vaccine for, 410t–413t
Hepatitis C virus (HCV), 753t
Hepatitis, vitamin deficiency from, 155t
Hepatotoxicity, 335, 356–357
Herb-infused oils, 40t
Herbs
    Asian ginseng, 41
    chamomile, 41
    echinacea, 41
    garlic, 41
    ginger, 41
    ginkgo, 41
    Ginkgo biloba, 41
    lavender, 41
    medicinal, 41f
    potential hazards of, 42
    preparations, definitions of, 40t
    prudent use of, 42
    remedies from, 41
    resources for using, 42–43
    saw palmetto, 41–42
    St. John's Wort, 42
    tips for using, 42
    turmeric, 42
Heroin, hyperkalemia caused by, 144t
Herpes antivirals, 364t–365t, 366
Herpes simplex virus, 755
    types 1 and 2, 362

Herpes zoster (shingles), 362
    vaccine for, 410t–413t
Herpesviruses, 362–363
High-alert medications, 76–77
High-density lipoprotein (HDL), 563, 564t
Highly protein-bound drugs, 21
High-sensitivity C-reactive protein (hsCRP), 564–567
HIPAA. *See* Health Insurance Portability and Accountability Act
Hirsutism, 744
Histamine₂ (H₂) receptor antagonists, 595
    actions of, 592f
    adverse reactions from, 596
    clinical judgment (nursing process), 597b
    dosage for, 596t
    drug interactions with, 596–597
    laboratory interactions with, 596–597
    pharmacodynamics of, 595–596
    pharmacokinetics of, 595
    side effects for, 596
Histrelin acetate implant, 424b–425b, 443t–444t
HIV. *See* Human immunodeficiency virus
HIV-and AIDS-related drugs, 381–394
    antiretroviral drugs, 383–391
        chemokine (CCR5) coreceptor antagonists, 384t–387t, 390
        dosage for, 384t–387t
        fusion (entry) inhibitors, 384t–387t, 389–390
        integrase strand transfer inhibitors, 384t–387t, 390–391
        nonnucleoside reverse transcriptase inhibitors, 383–388, 384t–387t
        nucleoside/nucleotide reverse transcriptase inhibitors, 383, 384t–387t
        in pregnancy, 392–393
        protease inhibitors, 384t–387t, 388–389
hMG. *See* Human menopausal gonadotropin
HMG-CoA reductase inhibitors, 563
Homatropine, 196t
Homatropine hydrobromide, 609t
Homeostasis, 134
    electrolytes with, 138–153
        calcium, 144–147, 145b, 147t
        chloride, 148
        magnesium, 147–148, 148b, 149t
        phosphorus, 149–153
        potassium, 138–139, 140b, 141t, 143b, 144t
        sodium, 139–144, 142b
    fluid replacement with, 134–138
        general considerations for, 134
        intravenous solutions, 134–138, 135t
        patient-centered collaborative care, 137b–138b
    maintenance of, 134
    osmolality with, 134
Homocysteine, 564
Hordeolum, 604
Hormone therapy (HT), 729–730
    contraindications to, 731
    dosage forms, 730
    menopause therapy with, 729
Hormones and hormonal agonists and antagonists
    antiandrogens, 442
    aromatase inhibitors, 442–445
    for cancer, 442–445
    corticosteroids, 442
    dosage for, 443t–444t
    luteinizing hormone-releasing hormone agonists, 442

Hormones and hormonal agonists and antagonists *(Continued)*
    selective estrogen receptor modulators, 442
    sex hormones, 442
HPV. *See* Human papillomavirus
HT. *See* Hormone therapy
Human clinical experimentation, 10–11
Human Genome Project, 32
Human immunodeficiency virus (HIV), 755
    antiretroviral therapy, indications for, 382–383
    case study on, 394
    classification of, 382
    laboratory testing for, 382
    occupational exposure to, 393
    pathophysiology of, 381–382
    postexposure prophylaxis for, 393
    resources, 392b
    transmission, 382
    tuberculosis with, 357
Human insulin analogues, 650
Human menopausal gonadotropin (hMG), 727t
Human papillomavirus (HPV), 755–756
    vaccine for, 410t–413t
Hybridoma technology, 466
Hydantoins, 221–223
    adverse reactions from, 222
    combined hormonal contraceptives and, 719b
    drug-drug interactions with, 222–223
    fosphenytoin, 225t–226t
    list of, 225t–226t
    pharmacodynamics of, 222
    pharmacokinetics of, 221
    phenytoin, 222b
    side effects for, 222
Hydralazine
    adverse reactions of, 686
    dosage for, 685t
    for gestational hypertension, 686
    patient safety with, 579b
    uses for, 685t
Hydralazine hydrochloride, 542t
Hydrochloric acid (HCl), 590
Hydrochlorothiazide, 526b–527b, 526t, 533t
    drug labels for, 96b–97b
    example dosage calculation for, 108b–109b
    hypokalemia caused by, 144t
Hydrocodone bitartrate, 311t
Hydrocortisone, 645t
Hydrocortisone acetate, 691t–692t
Hydromorphone (Dilaudid), 76b, 312
    adverse reactions from, 312
    dosage for, 311t
    patient safety with, 312b
    side effects for, 312
Hydrophobic, cerumen, 615
Hydrostatic pressure, 134
Hydroxychloroquine, patient safety with, 432b
Hydroxychloroquine sulfate, 371t–372t
    patient safety with, 370b
Hydroxyurea
    for cancer, 424b–425b
    dosage for, 430t–431t
    patient safety with, 370b, 432b
Hydroxyzine, 577t–578t, 691t–692t
    male sexual dysfunction caused by, 746t
    patient safety with, 579b
Hypercalcemia, 147, 525
    drugs that cause, 147t
    intravenous calcium for, 145b

Hyperchloremia, 148–149
Hyperemesis gravidarum, 675–676
Hyperglycemia, 527–528
   parenteral nutrition complicated by, 170, 171*t*
Hyperglycemic drugs, 662–663
   diazoxide, 662–663
   glucagon, 662–663
Hyperkalemia, 139, 144*t*, 532
   drugs that cause, 144*t*
   treatment of, 143*b*
Hyperlipidemia, 563
   lipoprotein phenotype, 567*t*
Hypermagnesemia, 147, 149*t*
Hyper-osmolar fluid, 134
Hyperoxia, 708–709
Hyperparathyroidism, 642
   dosage for, 642*t*
Hyperphosphatemia, 149
Hyperprolactinemia, 634
Hypertension, 524, 536–537
   blood pressure regulators for, 536, 537*f*
   defined, 536–537
   essential, 536
   guidelines for, 536
   nonpharmacologic control of, 537
   in older adults, 537
   pharmacologic control of, 536–550
   physiologic risk factors for, 537
   secondary, 536
Hypertensive crises, 772–775
   emergency drugs for, 772–775
   furosemide, 772*t*, 774–775, 774*b*
   labetalol, 772–773, 772*t*
   nitroprusside sodium, 772*t*, 773–774, 773*b*
Hyperthyroidism, 639
   antithyroid drugs for, 641
   clinical judgment (nursing process), 641*b*
   dosage for, 640*t*
   drug interactions with, 641–642
Hypertonic solutions, 135–136
   tonicity of, 135*t*
Hypertrichosis, 626
Hyperuricemia, 527–528
Hypervolemia, parenteral nutrition complicated by, 171*t*
Hypnotic effect, 207
Hypnotics, combined hormonal contraceptives and, 719*b*
Hypocalcemia, 145–147
Hypocarbia, 708–709
Hypochloremia, 148–149
Hypoglycemia, parenteral nutrition complicated by, 170–173, 171*t*
Hypoglycemic drugs, 657*t*–659*t*
   oral, 655–662
Hypoglycemic reaction, 651, 652*t*
Hypogonadism, 740
   androgens therapy indicated by, 740
Hypokalemia, 139, 505
   drug treatment of, 143*b*
   drugs that cause, 144*t*
   oral and intravenous preparations for, 141*b*
   supplements for, 141*t*
Hypomagnesemia, 147, 149*t*, 765
Hypo-osmolar fluid, 134
Hypoparathyroidism, 642
   calcitriol for, 643*b*
   dosage for, 642*t*
Hypophosphatemia, 149

Hypophysis, 633
Hypoprolactinemia, 634
Hypothalamic-pituitary-gonadal feedback loops, 741*f*
Hypothesis, prioritization of, 3
Hypothyroidism, 639, 746
   case studies on, 647*b*–648*b*
   dosage for, 640*t*
   levothyroxine sodium for, 639*b*–640*b*
   thyroid drugs for, 639–640, 640*t*
Hypotonic solutions, 135
   tonicity of, 136
Hypovolemic shock, 769–770
Hypoxemia, 762
Hysingla ER, 76*b*

I

Ibalizumab, 384*t*–387*t*
Ibrexafungerp, 359*t*–360*t*
Ibritumomab tiuxetan, 461
   adverse reactions from, 461
   dosage for, 459*t*–460*t*
   drug interactions with, 461
   pharmacodynamics of, 461
   pharmacokinetics of, 461
   side effects for, 461
Ibuprofen, 307*t*–308*t*
   adverse reactions from, 294*b*
   clinical judgment (nursing process), 295*b*
   contraindications for, 294*b*
   dosage for, 289*t*–291*t*, 294*b*
   drug-lab-food interactions, 294*b*
   pharmacodynamics of, 293, 294*b*
   pharmacokinetics of, 293, 294*b*
   for pregnancy, with pain, 679
   side effects for, 294*b*
   uses for, 289*t*–291*t*, 294*b*
Ibutilide, 515*t*–518*t*
ICF. *See* Intracellular fluid
Icosapent ethyl, 565*t*–566*t*
Idarubicin, 424*b*–425*b*, 434*t*
   patient safety with, 436*b*
Idiopathic seizures, 220
IDV. *See* Indinavir
IFNs. *See* Interferons
Ifosfamide, 424*b*–425*b*, 425*t*, 428*t*–429*t*
Iloperidone, 265*t*–266*t*
Imatinib mesylate
   adverse reactions from, 453*b*
   contraindications for, 453*b*
   dosage for, 453*b*
   pharmacodynamics of, 453*b*
   pharmacokinetics of, 453*b*
   side effects for, 453*b*
   uses for, 453*b*
Iminostilbenes, 223
   carbamazepine, 225*t*–226*t*
   eslicarbazepine, 225*t*–226*t*
   oxcarbazepine, 225*t*–226*t*
Imipenem, 668*t*–669*t*
Imipenem and cilastatin, 328*t*
Imipenem and cilastatin sodium, 668*t*–669*t*
Imipramine hydrochloride, 279*t*–282*t*
Immune globulin, 711
   hepatitis B, 710*t*
Immune reconstitution inflammatory syndrome (IRIS), 392
Immune response, 408

Immune system, cells of, 467*f*
Immunity, 408
   active, 408
   active acquired artificial, 408
   community, 408, 408*f*
   natural acquired active, 408
   passive, 408
Immunization
   case study on, 418
   before international travel, 414
   neonates, administration to, 710*t*
   pregnancy and, 705–706
   $Rh_0(D)$ immune globulin, 705, 706*b*
   rubella vaccine, 705–706
Immunoglobulins, 323
Immunomodulation, 466
Immunomodulators, 298, 298*b*
   beta-interferon, 249*b*, 250*t*–252*t*
   for cancer, 440
   glatiramer acetate, 250*t*–252*t*
   for multiple sclerosis, 248–253, 249*b*
   teriflunomide, 250*t*–252*t*
Immunosuppressants
   for multiple sclerosis, 250*t*–252*t*
   ophthalmic antiinflammatories with, 607*t*–608*t*
Immunosuppression
   clinical judgment (nursing process), 403*b*
   drugs for, 395–402
      induction therapy, 395–397
      maintenance therapy, 397–402
      principles of, 395–402, 396*f*
IMPDH. *See* Inosine monophosphate dehydrogenase
Impetigo, 628
Incretin mimetics, 662
Incretin modifier, 660
Indacaterol, 491*t*–492*t*
   and glycopyrrolate, 491*t*–492*t*
Indapamide, 526*t*
Independent variable, 11
Indinavir (IDV), 384*t*–387*t*
Indirect-acting cholinergic agonists, 187–188, 190
   acetylcholinesterase inactivated with, 190*f*
   donepezil hydrochloride, 192*t*
   rivastigmine, 192*t*
Indirect-acting sympathomimetics, 179*f*
Indomethacin, 289*t*–291*t*, 307*t*–308*t*
Induction therapy, 395–397
Infant
   age range for, 46*t*
   drug administration concerns in, 47–48
Infantile spasms, 221*t*
Infection
   health care acquired, 323
   inflammations relationship to, 287
   parenteral nutrition complicated by, 171*t*
Infertility, 725
Infiltration, 115
Inflammation, 287. *See also* Antiinflammatories
   cardinal signs of, 287, 288*t*
   infections relationship to, 287
Infliximab, 622*t*–624*t*
   adverse reactions from, 298*b*
   clinical judgment (nursing process), 299*b*
   contraindications for, 298*b*
   dosage for, 296*t*–297*t*, 298*b*
   drug-lab-food interactions, 298*b*
   pharmacodynamics of, 298*b*
   pharmacokinetics of, 298*b*

Infliximab (Continued)
    side effects for, 298b
    uses for, 296t–297t, 298b
Influenza, 361
    vaccine for, 410t–413t
Influenza antivirals, 363–366
    adverse reactions from, 366
    dosage for, 364t–365t
    side effects of, 366
Informed consent, 8, 8b, 8f, 12b
Infusion, 40t
INH. See Isoniazid
Inhalation anesthesia, 214, 215t
Inhalations, 81–84
    metered-dose, 81–83
    spacers with, 83–84, 84f
Inherent resistance, 323
Inhibited sexual desire, 746
Injectable preparations, 109–111
Inner ear, 615
Inosine monophosphate dehydrogenase (IMPDH), 401
Inotropic action, 504
INR. See International normalized ratio
Insomnia, 206
    benzodiazepines for, 268t
Instillations, 81
    eardrops, 81, 82b, 82f
    eye ointments, 81, 82b, 82f
    eyedrops, 81, 82b, 82f
    nose drops and sprays, 81, 83b, 83f
Insulin, 650–655
    administration of, 652–653, 652f
    adverse reactions from, 651–652
    beta-cell secretion of, 650–655
    calculating intravenous flow rate for, 123b–126b
    clinical judgment (nursing process), 654b–655b
    commercially prepared, 650–655
    dosage adjustment requirements with CKD for, 53t
    dosage for, 651t
    drug interactions with, 651
    hypoglycemic reaction with, 651, 652t
    hypokalemia caused by, 144t
    jet injectors, 653
    ketoacidosis with, 651t, 652
    pen injectors, 652–653
    pharmacodynamics of, 651
    pharmacokinetics of, 651
    pumps, 653
    rapid-, short-, intermediate-, and long-acting, 651t
    resistance, 653
    side effects for, 651–652
    sliding-scale insulin coverage, 652
    Somogyi effect with, 651–652
    storage of, 653–655
    types of, 650–652
    uses for, 651t
Insulin Amendment, 12
Insulin aspart, 651t
Insulin degludec, 651t
Insulin detemir, 651t
Insulin glargine, 651t
Insulin glulisine, 651t
Insulin isophane NPH, 651t
Insulin lispro, 651t
Insulin regular, 651t
Integrase strand transfer inhibitors, 384t–387t, 390–391

Interferon alfa, 467–470
    adverse reactions from, 469
    dosage for, 469t
    drug interactions with, 467–470
    patient safety with, 474b
    pharmacodynamics of, 469
    pharmacokinetics of, 469
    side effects for, 469
Interferon alfa-2a, patient safety with, 474b
Interferon alfa-2b, patient safety with, 474b
Interferon beta (IFN-β), 470, 474b
Interferon gamma (IFN-γ), 470, 474b
Interferons (IFNs), 467–470
    dosage for, 469t
    FDA black-box warnings for, 470t
Interleukin 2 (IL-2), 424b–425b, 470t, 473–476
    adverse reactions from, 470t, 474
    aldesleukin, 474b, 474t
    dosage for, 470t, 475t
    drug interactions with, 474–476
    patient safety with, 474b
    pharmacodynamics of, 474
    pharmacokinetics of, 474
    side effects for, 474
Interleukins, 473–474
Intermediate metabolizers, 33t
Intermediate-acting tetracycline, 341t
Intermittent enteral feedings, 167
Intermittent infusion, 167
International normalized ratio (INR), 554
International Pharmacopeia, 12
Interventions, in nursing process, 4
    diet, 4
    evaluation, 6
    nursing considerations, 4–6, 5b, 5f, 6b
    patient teaching, 4, 5b
    self-administration, 4
    side effects, 4
Intracellular fluid (ICF)
    adult volume of, 134t
    electrolyte concentration in, 134t
Intracranial hypertension
    emergency drugs for, 767, 768b
        mannitol, 767, 768b
    mannitol for, 767, 768b
Intradermal parenteral medications, 85
    action in, 85
    equipment for, 85
    needle angles for, 86f
    sites for, 85, 86f
    technique for, 85
Intramuscular administration, 110b–111b, 129–130
Intramuscular parenteral administration, 87, 87t
    action in, 87
    equipment for, 87
    needle angles for, 86f
    sites for, 87
        deltoid, 87, 88f
        vastus lateralis, 87, 88f
        ventrogluteal, 87, 87f
    technique for, 88–89
Intranasal glucocorticoids, 482
    dosage for, 482t–483t
Intraocular pressure (IOP), 603
Intravenous anesthesia, 215–216, 215t
Intravenous flow rate, 130–131, 131f
    calculating critical care drugs, 127
    calculating in drops per minute, 116–127

Intravenous flow rate (Continued)
    calculating in milliliters per hour, 116–127
    heparin therapy example, 117b–123b
Intravenous (IV) therapy, 111–116
    administration sets for, 112, 112f, 113f, 114f
    electronic infusion devices, 114f, 115
    intermittent infusion adapters and devices, 112, 114f
    needleless infusion devices for, 114f
    patient teaching for, 113–115
    safety considerations for, 115
    secondary administration sets for, 112, 114f
    volume-controlled chamber for, 114f
Intravenous parenteral medications, 88–89
    action in, 88
    equipment for, 88
    sites for, 88, 89f
    technique for, 89–90
Intravenous routes, 111–116
    practice problems for, 123b–126b
Intravenous solutions, 134–138, 135t
    tonicity of, 135t
    types of, 134–138
        blood and blood products, 137–138
        colloid, 136, 136t
        crystalloids, 135t
Intrinsic sympathomimetic activity (ISA), 183
Ionized form, of calcium, 144
IOP. See Intraocular pressure
Ipratropium and albuterol, 491t–492t
Ipratropium bromide, 196t, 491t–492t
Irbesartan, 545t–546t
Irinotecan, 34t, 35, 424b–425b, 425t, 437t–438t
IRIS. See Immune reconstitution inflammatory syndrome
Iron, 161–162
    complementary and alternative therapies with, 162b
    contraindications for, 163b
    patient-centered collaborative care with, 164b
    pharmacodynamics for, 162, 163b
    pharmacokinetics for, 162, 163b
    pregnancy with supplementation of, 674–675
        adverse reactions for, 674
        dosage for, 675t
        nursing implications of, 674
    side effects from, 163b
    therapeutic effects and uses for, 163b
Irregular uterine bleeding, 722
Irreversible cholinesterase inhibitors, 191, 192t
ISA. See Intrinsic sympathomimetic activity
Isavuconazole, 359t–360t
Ischemia, 559
Islets of Langerhans, 649
Isocarboxazid, 279t–282t
Isoflurane, 215t
Isoniazid (INH), 355t–356t, 357b
Iso-osmolar fluid, 134
Isosorbide dinitrate, 510t–511t
Isosorbide mononitrate, 510t–511t
Isotonic solutions, 135
    tonicity of, 135t
Isotretinoin, 624–625
    for acne, 622t–624t
Isradipine, 510t–511t, 548t
Istradefylline, 230t–231t, 234, 235t–238t
Itraconazole, 359t–360t
    dosage adjustment requirements with CKD for, 53t

IV flow rate, 112
IV piggyback (IVPB), 111
IV push (IVP), 111
Ivermectin, 375b
　uses for, 373t
IVPB. See IV piggyback
Ixazomib, 457–459
　adverse reactions from, 459
　dosage for, 448t–449t
　drug interactions with, 460
　pharmacodynamics of, 457
　pharmacokinetics of, 457
　side effects for, 459
Ixekizumab, 296t–297t

J

Japanese encephalitis, vaccine for, 410t–413t
Jejunostomy tubes, enteral feedings with, 167, 167f
The Joint Commission (TJC)
　error prone abbreviations of, 75t
　national patient safety goals of, 74, 74t
Just Culture, 73–74
Justice, 10

K

Kadian, 76b, 95b
Kaposi sarcoma, 392
Kava kava (*Piper methysticum*), 211b
　benzodiazepines with, 269b
　dystonia with fluphenazine, 262b
　pregnancy and, 674b
Keep vein open (KVO), 112
Keratin, 621
Keratitis, 604
Keratolysis, 621
Ketamine hydrochloride, 215t
Ketoacidosis, 651t, 652
Ketoconazole, 359t–360t, 747t
　antiandrogens with, 746
Ketoprofen, 289t–291t
Ketorolac, 307t–308t
Ketorolac tromethamine, 289t–291t, 607t–608t
Ketotifen fumarate, 607t–608t
Klebsiella granulomatis (granuloma inguinale), 753t
Korean ginseng, platelet aggregation and, 559b
KVO. See Keep vein open

L

Labetalol
　dosage for, 184t–185t, 685t, 773t
　for gestational hypertension, 685t
　for pulmonary edema, 772–773, 773t
　uses for, 184t–185t, 685t
Labetalol hydrochloride, 542t
Labor
　case study on, 706–707
　drugs for pain control during, 689–696, 693t
　　analgesia and sedation, 690–692, 691t–692t
　　anesthesia, 692–695
　　clinical judgment (nursing process), 694b
　　regional anesthesia, 692–695, 695b–696b
　　spinal cord location for, 690f
　first stage of, 689
　second stage of, 689
　uterine muscle contractility enhancing drugs for, 696–700

Labor (Continued)
　　ergot alkaloids, 699–700
　　methylergonovine maleate, 697t
　　oxytocin, 698b, 699
Labor augmentation, 699
Labor induction, 696
　case study on, 712
Lacosamide, 225t–226t
　for partial seizure, 227t
Lacrimal ducts, 605
Lactation, 700
　complementary and alternative therapies for, 700b
　herbal supplements and, 700b
　suppression of, 704
　　nonpharmacologic measures for, 700t
Lactitol, 584t–585t
Lactulose, 584t–585t
　solution, example dosage calculation for, 108b–109b
Lamivudine (3TC), 364t–365t, 384t–387t
Lamotrigine, 225t–226t, 279t–282t
　for partial seizure, 227t
　for tonic-clonic seizures, 227t
Lanreotide, 636
Lanreotide acetate, 635t–636t
Lansoprazole, 592t, 598t–599t
Large intestine, 574, 574f
Lasix, drug labels for, 96b–97b
Latanoprost, 611t, 613b
Latency, 362
Latent stage, 754
Latent tuberculosis infection, 354
Laughing gas. See Nitrous oxide
Lavender (*Lavandula angustifolia*), 41
Laxatives, 583–588
　bulk forming, 585, 586b, 588t
　chloride channel activators, 585, 588t
　clinical judgment (nursing process), 704b–705b
　dosage for, 588t
　emollients, 585–588
　hypokalemia caused by, 144t
　hypomagnesemia caused by, 149t
　osmotic, 583, 588t
LDL. See Low-density lipoprotein
Lecithin/sphingomyelin (L/S) ratio, 683
Ledipasvir/sofosbuvir, 364t–365t
Lefamulin, 352t
Leflunomide, 296t–297t
Lesinurad-allopurinol, 300t
Letermovir, 364t–365t
Letrozole, 424b–425b, 443t–444t, 727t
Leucovorin, 425t
Leukotriene modifiers, 488
Leukotriene receptor antagonists, 493–495, 497b
　dosage for, 494t
　montelukast, 495b
Leukotriene synthesis inhibitors, 493–495
　dosage for, 494t
Leuprolide, 443t–444t
Leuprolide acetate, 424b–425b, 745t
Levalbuterol, 491t–492t
Levetiracetam, 225t–226t
　for atonic seizure, 227t
　for myoclonic seizure, 227t
　for partial seizure, 227t
　for tonic-clonic seizures, 227t
Levobunolol, 611t
Levocetirizine, 480t

Levodopa, 235t–238t
　carbidopa in combination with, 233, 233f
Levodopa Inhalation, 230t–231t
Levofloxacin, 346t, 606t
Levomilnacipran, 279t–282t
Levothyroxine, patient safety with, 644b
Levothyroxine sodium, 639, 639b–640b, 640t
LH. See Luteinizing hormone
LHRH. See Luteinizing hormone-releasing hormone
Licorice, 568, 591b
Licorice root (*Glycyrrhiza glabra* and *G. uralensis*)
　antihypertensives with, 539b
　digoxin's effect with, 506b
　potassium loss with, 528b
Lidocaine, 515t–518t
　adverse reactions from, 765b
　cardiac emergency with, 765, 765b, 766t–767t
　contraindications for, 765b
　dosage for, 765b
　injectable, 693t
　pediatric implications for, 765
　pharmacodynamics of, 765b
　pharmacokinetics of, 765b
　side effects for, 765b
　uses for, 765b
Lidocaine hydrochloride, 216t
Ligand-binding domain, 24
Ligand-gated ion channels, 24, 25f
Linaclotide, 584t–585t
Linagliptin, 657t–659t
Linagliptin-metformin, 657t–659t
Lincomycin, 334t
Lincosamides, 336–337
　adverse reactions with, 336
　case study on, 338
　dosage for, 334t
　drug interactions, 337
　side effects with, 336
Linezolid, 334t
Liniment, 40t
Liothyronine, 639
　patient safety with, 644b
Liothyronine sodium, 640t
Liotrix, 640
Lipoatrophy, 652
Lipodystrophy, 652
Lipohypertrophy, 652
Lipopeptides, 334t, 337–338
　adverse reactions with, 337
　case study on, 338
　dosage for, 334t
　drug interactions, 338
　pharmacodynamics of, 337
　pharmacokinetics of, 337
　side effects with, 337
Lipoproteins, 563, 564t
Liposomal chemotherapy, 425–426
Liposomes, 425–426
Liquids, 107–108
Liraglutide, 204t, 657t–659t
Liraglutide-insulin degludec, 657t–659t
Lisdexamfetamine dimesylate, 201t
Lisinopril, 545t–546t
　drug labels for, 96b–97b
Lissamine green, 605t
Liter, 92–93
　equivalent units of measurement with, 93t

Lithium
    adverse reactions from, 283–284, 283b
    clinical judgment (nursing process), 284b
    contraindications for, 283b
    dosage adjustment requirements with CKD for, 53t
    dosage for, 283b
    drug-lab-food interactions, 283b
    hypercalcemia caused by, 147t
    male sexual dysfunction caused by, 746t
    pharmacodynamics of, 283b
    pharmacokinetics of, 283b
    side effects for, 283–284, 283b, 284b
    special considerations, 284
    uses for, 283b
Liver disease, vitamin deficiency from, 155t
Living-donor transplantation, 395
LMWH. See Low-molecular- weight heparin
Loading dose, 23
Local anesthesia, 216, 216t
Lofexidine, 315t
Lomitapide, 565t–566t
Lomustine, 424b–425b, 428t–429t
Long-acting tetracyclines, 341t
Loop diuretics, 528–532
    adverse reactions from, 530
    clinical judgment (nursing process), 531b
    dosage for, 530t–531t
    drug interactions with, 530–532
    furosemide, 529b
    pharmacodynamics of, 527
    pharmacokinetics of, 527
    physiologic and laboratory changes associated with, 530t
    side effects for, 530
Loperamide hydrochloride, 582t–583t
Lopinavir-ritonavir (LPV/r), 384t–387t
Loratadine, 480t
Lorazepam, 209t–210t, 577t–578t
    adverse reactions from, 270b
    for anxiety, 268t
    contraindications for, 270b
    dosage for, 225t–226t, 270b
    patient safety with, 211b, 579b
    pharmacodynamics of, 269, 270b
    pharmacokinetics of, 269, 270b
    side effects for, 270b
    for status epilepticus, 227t, 268t
    uses for, 270b, 270t–271t
Losartan potassium, 545t–546t
Loteprednol etabonate, 607t–608t
Lotronex, patient safety with, 552b, 597b
Lovastatin, 564, 565t–566t
Lovenox, patient safety with, 552b
Low-density lipoprotein (LDL), 563, 567t
Lower respiratory disorders, 486–499
    anticholinergics, 490–492, 490b, 491t–492t
    asthma drug therapy according to age, 498
        older adults, 498
        young children, 498
    asthma drug therapy according to severity, 498
    bronchial asthma, 487
        pathophysiology of, 487, 488f
    bronchodilators, 491t–492t, 496b
    chronic obstructive pulmonary disease, 487f, 488–489, 494t
    complementary and alternative therapies for, 495b
    cromolyn, 494t, 496–497

Lower respiratory disorders (Continued)
    glucocorticoids, 494t, 495–496
    leukotriene receptor antagonists, 493–495, 494t, 495b
    leukotriene synthesis inhibitors, 493–495, 494t
    methylxanthine (xanthine) derivatives, 492–493
    phosphodiesterase-4 inhibitor, 494t
    sympathomimetics, 489–490
        adverse reactions from, 490
        aerosol inhaler in, 490
        albuterol, 489–490, 489b
        dosage of, 491t–492t
        metaproterenol, 490
        side effects for, 490
Low-molecular-weight heparin (LMWH), 552
    contraindications for, 552
    dosage for, 553t–554t
    hyperkalemia caused by, 144t
Loxapine, 265t–266t
Lubiprostone, 584t–585t
Lubricants, for eye disorders, 609
Lumateperone, 265t–266t
Lumbar epidural, 693t
Lungs, parasympathetic responses with, 189f
Luteinizing hormone (LH), 633
Luteinizing hormone-releasing hormone (LHRH), for cancer, 442
Lymphogranuloma venereum (LGV), 753t
Lymphokines, 473–474

M

MAbs. See Monoclonal antibodies
MAC. See Mycobacterium avium complex
Macrodrip set, 112, 113f
Macrolides, 333–336
    adverse reactions with, 335
    azithromycin, 335b
    case study on, 338
    clinical judgment (nursing process), 336b
    dosage for, 334t
    drug interactions, 335
    extended macrolide group, 335–336
    pharmacodynamics of, 335
    pharmacokinetics of, 335
    side effects with, 335
Macrophages, 467–469
Macular degeneration, drugs for, 609–610
Macules, 620
Mafenide acetate, 630b, 630t
Magnesium, 147–148
    balance, effect of drugs on, 148
    functions of, 147–148
    hypermagnesemia, 147
    hypomagnesemia, 147
    patient-centered collaborative care with, 148b
Magnesium citrate, 584t–585t
Magnesium hydroxide, 584t–585t, 701t
    and aluminum hydroxide, 594t
Magnesium salts, hypermagnesemia caused by, 149t
Magnesium sulfate
    adverse reactions from, 682, 686
    dosage for, 685t
    for gestational hypertension, 685t, 686
    hypocalcemia caused by, 147t
    tocolytic therapy with, 681t, 682–683
    uses for, 685t
Magnesium trisilicate with aluminum hydroxide, 594t

Magnetic resonance imaging (MRI), 220
Ma-Huang. See Ephedra
Maintenance therapy, 397–402
    calcineurin inhibitors for, 397
    corticosteroids for, 401–402
    costimulation blockers for, 397–400
    inosine monophosphate dehydrogenase for, 401
    mTOR inhibitors for, 400–401
    purine antimetabolites for, 401
    tacrolimus for, 397
Malaria
    case study on, 379
    erythrocytic phase in infection of, 369
    prophylaxis for, 369
    tissue phase in infection of, 369
Male's reproductive disorder, 739–750
    anatomy and physiology, 739
    case study on, 749
    disorders
        adrenal, 746
        delayed puberty, 741
        non-sexually transmitted infections, 748
        pituitary, 746
        sexual dysfunction, 746–748, 746t
        thyroid, 746
    drugs related to, 741–746
        anabolic steroids, 744
        androgens, 741–744, 742t, 743t, 745b
        antiandrogens, 744–746, 745t
    hormonal regulation, 739–740
    sexual function, 740
    spermatogenesis, 739–740
Mammalian target of rapamycin (mTOR) inhibitors, 400–401
Mannitol, 530t–531t
    adverse reactions from, 768b
    contraindications for, 768b
    dosage for, 767, 768b
    for intracranial hypertension, 767, 768b
    pharmacodynamics of, 768b
    pharmacokinetics of, 768b
    side effects for, 768b
    uses and considerations, 767, 768b
MAO. See Monoamine oxidase
MAOIs. See Monoamine oxidase inhibitors
Maprotiline hydrochloride, 279t–282t
MAR. See Medication administration record
Maraviroc (MRV), 384t–387t
Marboxil, 364t–365t
Maribavir, 364t–365t
Maximal efficacy, 23
MDIs. See Metered-dose inhalers
Measles (rubeola), vaccine for, 410t–413t, 705
    adverse reactions with, 706
MEC. See Minimum effective concentration
Mechanisms of drug action, 26
Mechlorethamine hydrochloride, 424b–425b, 428t–429t
Meclizine hydrochloride, 575t
Meclofenamate, 289t–291t
Medical Letter, 17
Medicare Modernization Act of 2003, 55
Medication administration
    Bill of Rights, for nurses, 73
    error prevention resources for, 77–79
    safety guidelines for, 78, 78b
    safety risks with, 75–77, 76t
        buying drugs over internet, 76
        counterfeit drugs, 76

Medication administration (Continued)
   crush or not to crush, 76
   tablet splitting, 76
   six rights, for safety in, 69–73
      right documentation, 73, 74f
      right drug, 70–71, 71f
      right patient, 70
      right route, 73
      right time, 72–73, 72f
Medication administration record (MAR), 70, 70f
Medication box and pill organizer, 5f
Medication record, 74f
Medication recording sheet, 4, 5b
Medicine cup, 108, 108f
MedlinePlus, 17
Medroxyprogesterone, 424b–425b, 443t–444t
Mefenamic acid, 289t–291t
Mefloquine, 371t–372t
Megestrol acetate, 424b–425b, 443t–444t
Meglitinides, 657t–659t, 660
Melatonin agonists, 209t–210t, 212
Meloxicam, 289t–291t, 307t–308t
Melphalan, 424b–425b, 428t–429t
Memantine, for Alzheimer disease, 240t–241t
Menarche, 713
Meningococcal vaccine, 410t–413t
   patient safety with, 414b
Menometrorrhagia, 723
Menopause, 713
   clinical judgment (nursing process), 733b–734b
   conjugated estrogens, 730b
   hormone therapy, 729–730
   osteoporosis with, 732–738
   perimenopause, 729
   postmenopause, 729
   SSRIs and SNRIs, 731
Menorrhagia, 723
Menotropins, 727t
Mental and behavioral health drugs, 259–273
Mental health drugs, 35
Mentha piperita. See Peppermint
Meperidine (Demerol), 76b, 310–312, 311t
   patient safety with, 312b
Meprobamate, patient safety with, 312b
Mercaptopurine (6-MP), 35, 424b–425b, 430t–431t
Meropenem, 328t
   and vaborbactam, dosage for, 668t–669t
Metabolism
   older adult considerations for, 53
   pediatric considerations for, 47
Metaproterenol, 490
Metaproterenol sulfate, 491t–492t
Metastasis, 424
Metastasizing cancer cells, 466
Metaxalone, 254t–255t
Meter, 92–93
Metered-dose inhalers (MDIs), 81–83
   correct use of, 83b
   spacer with, 83–84, 84f
Metformin, 656, 657t–659t
Methadone (Dolophine), 76b, 311t
   dosing, 62–63
   male sexual dysfunction caused by, 746t
   opioid treatment with, 62–63
   pharmacokinetics of, 61t
   side effects, 62–63
Methadone hydrochloride, 76b
Methadose, 76b

Methenamine, 667
   adverse reactions from, 670
   dosage for, 668t–669t
   interactions with, 670
   side effects for, 670
Methicillin, 323
Methicillin-resistant *Staphylococcus aureus* (MRSA), 374
Methimazole, 640t, 641
Methocarbamol, 254t–255t
Methohexital sodium, 215t
Methotrexate, 424b–425b, 430t–431t, 626
   drug interactions, 626
Methoxsalen, 622t–624t
Methscopolamine bromide, 196t
Methyclothiazide, 526t
Methylcellulose, 588t
Methyldopa, 540t
   adverse reactions of, 686
   dosage for, 685t
   for gestational hypertension, 685t, 686
   uses for, 685t
Methylergonovine maleate, 697t
Methylnaltrexone, 584t–585t
Methylphenidate, 34t
Methylphenidate hydrochloride
   adverse reactions from, 202b
   contraindications for, 202b
   dosage for, 201t, 202b
   patient-centered collaborative care with, 203b
   pharmacodynamics of, 202b
   pharmacokinetics of, 202b
   side effects for, 202b
   uses for, 201t, 202b
Methylprednisolone, 645t
Methyltestosterone, 743t
Methylxanthine (xanthine) derivatives, 492–493
   dosage for, 493t
Methylxanthines, 204t
Metoclopramide, 676t–677t
   dosage for, 577t–578t
Metoclopramide hydrochloride (HCl), 188, 192t
Metolazone, 526t
Metoprolol, 539b, 540t
Metoprolol tartrate, 184t–185t, 510t–511t
Metric system, 92–94, 93f, 94f
   conversion with, 92–93, 127–128
   defined, 92–94
   practice problem conversion for, 93b
   unit of measurement in, 93t
Metronidazole, 351t, 377–379, 378b
   combined hormonal contraceptives and, 719b
   dosage for, 377t
   uses for, 377t
Metronidazole hydrochloride, 592t
Metrorrhagia, 723
Mexiletine hydrochloride, 515t–518t
MG. See Myasthenia gravis
MI. See Myocardial infarction
Micafungin, 359t–360t
Microdrip (minidrip) set, 112, 113f
Microorganisms, 321, 333
Micturition, 670
Midazolam, 225t–226t
   induction time for, 215t
Middle ear, 615
Midodrine hydrochloride, 181t
Mifepristone, patient safety with, 597b

Miglitol, 657t–659t, 660
Migraine headaches, 314–316
   drugs for, combined hormonal contraceptives and, 719b
   pathophysiology of, 316
   treatment of, 316–319, 317t
Military time, 72–73, 72f
Milrinone lactate, 505t
Mineral oil, 588t, 701t
Mineralocorticoids, 644
   dosage for, 645t
   hypocalcemia caused by, 147t
Minerals, 161–164
   chromium, 162–163
   copper, 162
   iron, 161–162, 163b
   patient-centered collaborative care with, 164b
   selenium, 163–164
   zinc, 162
Minimum effective concentration (MEC), 23
Minocycline, combined hormonal contraceptives and, 719b
Minocycline hydrochloride, 341t
   for acne, 622t–624t
Minoxidil, 542t
Miosis, 188, 245, 610
Mipomersen, 565t–566t
Mirabegron, 671t–672t
Mirtazapine, 279t–282t
Miscellaneous tetracyclines, 341t
Misoprostol, 598t–599t
   patient safety with, 597b
Mitomycin, 424b–425b, 434t
Mitosis, 446
Mitotane, 424b–425b, 443t–444t
Mitoxantrone, 250t–252t, 424b–425b, 434t
Mixed-acting sympathomimetics, 179f
MKIs. See Multikinase inhibitors
Modafinil, 201t
Moderna, 410t–413t
Moexipril, 545t–546t
Molindone hydrochloride, 265t–266t
Mometasone, 482, 482t–483t
Monitoring the Future project, 58
Monoamine oxidase B (MAO-B) inhibitors
   for Parkinson disease, 233
   rasagiline, 230t–231t, 235t–238t
   safinamide, 230t–231t, 235t–238t
   selegiline hydrochloride, 230t–231t, 235t–238t
   treatment with other drugs compared to, 230t–231t
Monoamine oxidase inhibitors (MAOIs), 277, 279t–282t
   adverse reactions from, 277
   complementary and alternative therapies with, 277b
   drug interactions with, 277
   food interactions with, 277
   male sexual dysfunction caused by, 746t
   side effects for, 277
Monoamine oxidase (MAO), 177
Monoclonal antibodies (MAbs), 448, 459–464
   alemtuzumab, 459–460
   bevacizumab, 450b
   cetuximab, 460–461
   clinical judgment (nursing process), 463b
   dosage for, 459t–460t
   ibritumomab tiuxetan, 461
   for multiple sclerosis, 250t–252t

Monoclonal antibodies (MAbs) (Continued)
	panitumumab, 461
	rituximab, 462b
	tositumomab, 461–464
	trastuzumab, 464, 464b
Mononucleosis, 363
Montelukast, 494t, 495b
Mood stabilizers, 277–285, 279t–282t
	lithium, 277–284, 279t–282t, 283b, 284b
	pharmacodynamics of, 283
	pharmacokinetics of, 283
"Morning sickness", 675–676
Morphabond ER, 76b
Morphine, 309–310
	adverse reactions from, 309b
	clinical judgment (nursing process), 310b
	contraindications for, 309b
	dosage adjustment requirements with CKD for, 53t
	dosage for, 309b
	drug-lab- food interactions, 309b
	patient safety with, 312b
	pharmacodynamics of, 309–310, 309b
	pharmacokinetics of, 309–310, 309b
	side effects for, 309b
	uses of, 309b
Morphine sulfate, 74t, 311t, 691t–692t
	calculating intravenous flow rate for, 123b–126b
	cardiac emergency with, 763, 766t–767t
	dosage for, 766t–767t
	pediatric implications for, 765
Motion sickness, cholinergic antagonists for, 195–197
Moxifloxacin, 346t
MRI. See Magnetic resonance imaging
MRSA. See Methicillin-resistant *Staphylococcus aureus*
MRV. See Maraviroc
MS. See Multiple sclerosis
MS Contin, 76b
mTOR kinase inhibitors, 455–459
	clinical judgment (nursing process), 463b
	dosage for, 448t–449t
	temsirolimus, 456–457
Mucosal protective drugs. See Pepsin inhibitors
Multikinase inhibitors (MKIs), 452–455
	clinical judgment (nursing process), 456b–457b
	dasatinib, 454–455
	dosage for, 448t–449t
	sorafenib, 455
	sunitinib, 455
Multiple sclerosis (MS), 248–253
	beta-interferon, 249b, 250t–252t
	classifications of, 248
	defined, 248
	glatiramer acetate, 250t–252t
	immunomodulators for, 248–253, 249b
	immunosuppressants for, 250t–252t
	monoclonal antibody for, 250t–252t
	sphingosine 1-phosphate receptor modulators for, 250t–252t
	teriflunomide, 250t–252t
Mumps vaccine, 410t–413t
Muscarinic receptors, 187
Muscle relaxants, 244
Muscle spasms, 244
	benzodiazepines for, 268t
	skeletal muscle relaxants for, 253
Myasthenia gravis (MG)
	acetylcholinesterase inhibitors for, 245

Myasthenia gravis (MG) (Continued)
	azathioprine, 246t
	neostigmine methylsulfate, 246t
	pyridostigmine, 247b
	case study on, 257
	defined, 244
	drugs for, 244–248
	medications that may exacerbate, 245b
	pathophysiology for, 244–245
Myasthenic crisis, 245
Mycobacterium avium complex (MAC), 392
Mycophenolate mofetil, 401
Mycoplasma genitalium, 753t
Mydriasis, 191
Mydriatics, 609
	adverse reactions from, 609
	dosage for, 609t
	side effects for, 609
Myelosuppression, 426, 426t–427t, 471
Myleran, patient safety with, 427b
Myocardial infarction (MI), 551, 762
Myocardial ischemia, 509
Myocardium, 501
Myoclonic seizure, 221t
	anticonvulsants for, 227t
Myxedema, 639

N

Nabumetone, 289t–291t, 307t–308t
Nadir, 426
Nadolol, 510t–511t, 540t
	dosage adjustment requirements with CKD for, 53t
	dosage for, 184t–185t
	uses for, 184t–185t
Nafarelin, 727t
Nafcillin, 326t
	hypokalemia caused by, 144t
Nalbuphine
	adverse reactions from, 314b
	clinical judgment (nursing process), 316b
	contraindications for, 314b
	dosage for, 314b
	pharmacodynamics of, 314, 314b
	pharmacokinetics of, 314, 314b
	side effects for, 314b
	uses for, 314b
Nalbuphine hydrochloride, 691t–692t
Naldemedine, 584t–585t
Naloxegol, 584t–585t
Naloxone
	adverse reactions from, 769b
	buprenorphine in treatment, 63
	contraindications for, 769b
	dosage for, 769b
	drug-assisted treatment for, 63
	methadone in treatment of, 63
	for opioid overdose, 64
	pediatric implications for, 768
	pharmacodynamics of, 769b
	pharmacokinetics of, 61t, 769b
	poisoning treated with, 769b
	use by laypersons, 63b
	uses for, 769b
Naloxone hydrochloride, 315t
Naltrexone
	AUD treatment with, 60–61
	pharmacokinetics of, 61t

Naltrexone hydrochloride, 204t, 315t
Naphthylalkanones, 289t–291t
Naproxen, 289t–291t, 307t–308t, 598t–599t
Naratriptan, 317t
Narcolepsy, 200
	amphetamine-like drugs for treatment of, 200
Narrow-spectrum antibiotics, 324
Nasal and systemic decongestants, 479–482
	adverse reactions with, 481–482
	dosage for, 481t
	drug interactions, 482
	side effects with, 481–482
Nasoduodenal/nasojejunal tube, enteral feedings with, 167, 167f
Nasogastric tube
	drugs administered via, 108–109
	enteral feedings with, 167, 167f
	medication administration with, 84
Natalizumab, 250t–252t
Natamycin, 606t
Nateglinide, 657t–659t
National Academy of Medicine, Food and Nutrition Board of, 154
National Center for Complementary and Integrative Health (NCCIH), 39
National Council of State Boards of Nursing (NCSBN), 1
National HIV/AIDS Clinicians' Consultation Center, 392b
National Patient Safety Goals, 69, 74
Natriuresis, 524
Natriuretic effect, 529
Natural acquired active immunity, 408
Nausea, pregnancy with, 675–676, 676t–677t
NCCIH. See National Center for Complementary and Integrative Health
Nebcin, patient safety with, 314b
Nebulizer, 83–84
Necrosis, 559, 703
Needleless infusion devices, 114f
Nefazodone, 279t–282t
Nelarabine, 424b–425b, 430t–431t
Nelfinavir (NFV), 384t–387t
Neoadjuvant chemotherapy, 424
Neomycin, 606t
	combined hormonal contraceptives and, 719b
	hypokalemia caused by, 144t
Neomycin sulfate, 345t
Neomycin sulfate/polymyxin B sulfate/dexamethasone, 607t–608t
Neonates, 708–712
	age range for, 46t
	drug administered to full-term, 709–712
		clinical judgment (nursing process), 711b
		erythromycin ophthalmic ointment, 709, 709t
		immunizations, 709–711
		phytonadione, 708–709
	drug administered to preterm, 708–709
		synthetic surfactant, 708–709, 709t, 710b
Neostigmine bromide, 246t
Neostigmine methylsulfate, 192t
	for myasthenia gravis, 246t
Nephrotoxicity, 332
Nerve block, 216
Nervous system, 175
Netarsudil ophthalmic, 611t
Netupitant and palonosetron, 577t–578t
Neurohypophysis, 633
Neuroleptic, definition of, 259

Neuroleptic malignant syndrome (NMS), 261
Neuromuscular disorders
    drugs for, 244–257
        multiple sclerosis, 248–253
            beta-interferon, 249b, 250t–252t
            classifications of, 248
            defined, 248
            glatiramer acetate, 250t–252t
            immunomodulators for, 248–253, 249b
            immunosuppressants for, 250t–252t
            monoclonal antibody for, 250t–252t
            sphingosine 1-phosphate receptor modulators for, 250t–252t
            teriflunomide, 250t–252t
        myasthenia gravis, 244–248
            acetylcholinesterase inhibitors for, 245, 246t, 247b
            case study on, 257
            cholinesterase inhibitors, 245
            defined, 244
            medications that may exacerbate, 245b
            pathophysiology for, 244–245
        skeletal muscle relaxants, 253–257
            centrally acting, 253–256
            for muscle spasms, 256
            for spasticity, 253–257
Neurons, 175, 260
Neuropathic pain, 304
Neurotransmitters, 200, 259–260
    chemical, 260f
    inactivation of, 177
Neutrophils, 471
Nevirapine (NVP), 384t–387t
Newborn, 708–712
    drugs administered to, 710t
Nexavar, patient safety with, 597b
Nexium, patient safety with, 597b
Next Generation NCLEX (NGN), 1
NFV. See Nelfinavir
Niacin. See Vitamin B$_3$
Nicardipine hydrochloride, 510t–511t, 548t
Nicotine replacement drugs, 64
Nicotinic acid. See Vitamin B$_3$
Nicotinic receptors, 187
Nifedipine, 510t–511t, 548t
Nightmares, 206
Nilotinib, 454
    adverse reactions from, 454
    dosage for, 448t–449t
    drug interactions with, 454
    pharmacodynamics of, 454
    pharmacokinetics of, 454
    side effects for, 454
Nilutamide, 424b–425b, 443t–444t
Nipples, sore or cracked, nonpharmacologic measures for, 700b
Nisoldipine, 510t–511t, 548t
Nitrates, 508–509
    adverse reactions from, 512
    for angina, 508–509, 508b–509b, 512f
    dosage for, 510t–511t
    drug interactions with, 509
    effects on angina, 508t
    nitroglycerin, 508b–509b
    pharmacodynamics of, 508–509
    pharmacokinetics of, 508
    side effects for, 509
Nitrofurantoin, 667–668
    adverse reactions from, 670

Nitrofurantoin (Continued)
    combined hormonal contraceptives and, 719b
    side effects for, 670
Nitrogen mustards, 428t–429t
Nitroglycerin, 508b–509b, 510t–511t
    cardiac emergency with, 762–763, 766t–767t
    dosage for, 766t–767t
Nitroimidazoles, 350–352, 350b
    adverse reactions with, 352
    case study on, 353
    dosage for, 351t
    pharmacodynamics of, 352
    pharmacokinetics of, 352
    side effects with, 352
Nitroprusside, 548t
Nitroprusside sodium, for pulmonary edema, 773–774, 773b, 773t
Nitrostat, patient safety with, 508b
Nitrous oxide (laughing gas), 215t
Nizatidine, 595, 596t
NMS. See Neuroleptic malignant syndrome
NNRTIS. See Nonnucleoside reverse transcriptase inhibitors
Nociceptors, 304
Nonbenzodiazepines, 209t–210t, 212–214, 213b
    eszopiclone, 209t–210t
    patient-centered collaborative care, 211b
    zaleplon, 209t–210t
    zolpidem tartrate, 209t–210t, 212b–213b
Nonnucleoside reverse transcriptase inhibitors (NNRTIS), 383–388
    dosage for, 384t–387t
    efavirenz, 390b
Nonopioid analgesics, 305–306
    acetaminophen, 305–306
    nonsteroidal antiinflammatory drugs, 305
Nonphenothiazines, 263–264, 265t–266t
    adverse reactions from, 263
    clinical judgment (nursing process), 267b
    drug interactions with, 263–264
    side effects for, 263
Nonprescription antiemetics, 575
    dosage for, 575t
Nonrapid eye movement (NREM) sleep, 206, 207f
Nonselective alpha-adrenergic blockers, 548t
Non-sexually transmitted infections, 748
    benign prostatic hyperplasia, 748, 748t
    malignant tumors, 749
Nonsteroidal antiinflammatory drugs (NSAIDs), 288–295, 289t–291t, 307t–308t
    adverse reactions from, 294, 305
    complementary and alternative therapies with, 294b
    dosage adjustment requirements with CKD for, 53t
    dosage information for, 289t–291t
    for dysmenorrhea, 723
    fenamates, 289t–291t, 293
    hyperkalemia caused by, 144t
    ophthalmic, 608
    ophthalmic antiinflammatories with, 607t–608t
    OTC, 289
    oxicams, 289t–291t, 293–294
    pain relief with, 303, 307t–308t
    para-chlorobenzoic acid derivatives, 289t–291t, 292
    phenylacetic acids derivatives, 289t–291t
    propionic acid derivatives, 289t–291t, 292–293, 294b

Nonsteroidal antiinflammatory drugs (NSAIDs) (Continued)
    salicylates, 289t–291t, 292b
    selective COX-2 inhibitors, 289t–291t, 294
    side effects for, 294, 305
    use in older adults of, 294–295
Nonsulfonylureas, 656, 657t–659t
Norelgestromin transdermal patch, ethinyl estradiol and, 716
Norepinephrine
    dosage for, 772t
    for shock, 770, 772t
Norepinephrine bitartrate, 181t
Normoxemia, 762
Nortriptyline hydrochloride, 279t–282t
Nose drops and sprays, 81, 83b, 83f
Nosocomial infections, 323
NRTIs. See Nucleoside/nucleotide reverse transcriptase inhibitors
NSAIDs. See Nonsteroidal anti-inflammatory drugs
Nubain, patient safety with, 314b
Nucleoside/nucleotide reverse transcriptase inhibitors (NRTIs), 383–388
    dosage for, 384t–387t
    tenofovir disoproxil fumarate, 389b
    zidovudine, 388b
Nucynta ER, 76b
Nuprin, patient safety with, 314b
Nuremberg Code, 8
Nurse Practice Acts, 13–14
Nurse's role, in clinical research, 11
Nursing
    ART, role in, 391–394
    Bill of Rights for, 73
    clinical judgment
        acetaminophen, 307b
        acne vulgaris, 627b
        acyclovir, 367b
        allopurinol, 301b
        alpha-adrenergic blockers, 543b
        aminoglycosides, 343b
        androgens, 745b
        angiogenesis inhibitors, 452b
        antacids, 595b
        antepartum drugs, 679b–680b
        anthelmintics, 376b
        antianginals in, 513b
        anticholinergics, 231b–232b
        antidepressants, 278b
        antidysrhythmics in, 519b
        antifungals, 363b
        antihyperlipidemics in, 569b–570b
        antiinfectives
            for burns, 631b
            for ear conditions, 617b
        antimalarials, 374b
        antiretroviral therapy, 393b
        antithyroid drugs, 641b
        antituberculars, 358b–359b
        benzodiazepines, 272b
        beta blockers, 541b
        beta-adrenergic agents, 682b–683b
        betamethasone, 684b
        biologic response modifiers, 475b–476b
        bronchodilators, 496b
        bulk forming laxatives, 587b
        carbidopa-levodopa, 235b
        cephalosporins, 331b

Nursing (Continued)
  combined hormonal contraceptives, 720b–722b
  corticosteroids, 646b–647b
  cyclophosphamide, 433b
  digoxin in, 506b
  diphenhydramine, 481b
  doxorubicin, 439b
  EGFR inhibitors, 452b
  fluoroquinolones, 345b
  fluorouracil, 436b
  gestational hypertension, 686b–687b
  glaucoma drugs, 614b
  H_2 blockers, 595b
  hemorrhoids, pain relief for, 702b–703b
  heparin, 555b–556b
  ibuprofen, 295b
  immunosuppression, 403b
  infertility, 727b–728b
  infliximab, 299b
  insulin, 654b–655b
  laxatives, 704b–705b
  leukotriene receptor antagonists, 497b
  lithium, 284b
  loop diuretics, 531b
  macrolides, 336b
  menopause symptoms, 733b–734b
  monoclonal antibodies, 463b
  morphine, 310b
  mTOR kinase inhibitors, 463b
  multikinase inhibitors, 456b–457b
  nalbuphine, 316b
  neonates, drug administered to full-term, 711b
  nonphenothiazines, 267b
  ocular hypertension drugs, 614b
  oral antidiabetic, 661b
  oxymetazoline, 484b
  oxytocin, 699b
  pain control drugs, 694b
  parathyroid hormone insufficiencies, 643b
  penicillins, 327b
  pepsin inhibitors, 595b
  peptides, 378b–379b
  perineal wounds pain relief, 702b–703b
  peripheral vasodilators in, 569b–570b
  phenothiazines, 267b
  phenytoin, 224b
  pituitary hormones, 638b
  potassium-sparing diuretics, 534b
  proteasome inhibitors, 463b
  psoriasis, 627b
  pyridostigmine, 247b–248b
  regional anesthesia, 695b–696b
  Rh_0(D) immune globulin, 706b
  sexually transmitted infection prevention, 757b
  stimulant laxatives, 586b–587b
  sulfonamides, 351b
  synthetic surfactant, 710b
  terbutaline, 682b–683b
  tetracyclines, 341b–342b
  thiazides in, 528b
  thrombolytics, 561b
  thyroid hormone replacement, 641b
  tyrosine kinase inhibitors, 456b–457b
  urinary antiinfective, 667b
  VEGF inhibitors, 452b
  vincristine, 441b–442b
  warfarin, 555b–556b
  complementary and alternative therapies for, 43b

Nursing (Continued)
  older adult considerations for, 54–56
  patient-centered collaborative care in
    adrenergic agonists, 182b
    adrenergic neuron antagonists, 185b
    atropine sulfate, 195
    benzodiazepines in, 211b
    bethanechol, 191
    calcium, 146b
    enteral nutrition, 169b
    fluid replacement, 137b–138b
    geriatrics, 55b–56b
    iron, 161b
    magnesium, 148b
    methylphenidate hydrochloride, 203b
    nonbenzodiazepines in, 213b
    parenteral nutrition, 171t
    pediatric considerations, 49–50, 49b–50b
    potassium, 140b
    sodium, 142b
    vaccines, 417b–418b
    vitamins, 161b
Nursing process, 1
  analyze cues in, 3
  assessment, 2–3
  clinical judgment, 1–2, 2b, 6
  components of, 1–2
  objective data of, 3
  patient problems in, 1–3
  planning, 3–4
  prioritize hypothesis, 3
  purpose of, 1
  steps of, 1
  subjective data of, 3
Nutritional support, 166
  enteral nutrition, 166, 167f, 168t, 169b
  therapy, 166
  types of
    oral feeding, 166
    parenteral nutrition, 170–173, 171b–172b, 171t
NVP. See Nevirapine
Nystagmus, 222
Nystatin, 359–361, 359t–360t, 361b
  patient safety with, 508b

O

Obiltoxaximab, 352t
Objective data, of nursing process, 3
Occlusive dressings, 703
Ocrelizumab, 250t–252t
Octreotide, 636
Octreotide acetate, 635t–636t
Ocular drugs, 604–605
Ocular hypertension drugs, 610–614
  clinical judgment (nursing process), 614b
OE. See Otitis externa
Ofloxacin, 346t, 616t, 668t–669t
  otic solution, 616t
OIs. See Opportunistic infections
Olanzapine, 265t–266t
Older adults, 52–57
  adherence with, 54–55, 54t
  administration of drugs in, 52
  adverse drug events with, 54
  antibacterials used by, 56
  asthma drug therapy for, 498
  Beers Criteria in, 54

Older adults (Continued)
  case study on, 56
  chronic kidney disease in, 53t
  distribution in, 53
  drug dosing and monitoring for, 54–56
  effective drug use barriers by, 54t
  excretion in, 53
  geriatric considerations with, 55b–56b
  health teaching with, 55–56
  hypertension in, 537
  metabolism in, 53
  nursing implications for, 54–56
  opioid analgesics usage by, 313
  OTC drugs use by, 52
  pharmacodynamics in, 54
  pharmacokinetics in, 52–54
  physiologic changes associated with, 52–54
  polypharmacy with, 54
  sexually transmitted infections in, 757b
Oligomenorrhea, 719
Oligospermia, 743–744
Oliguria, 528
Olmesartan medoxomil, 545t–546t
Olodaterol, 491t–492t
  and tiotropium, 491t–492t
Olopatadine, 607t–608t
Olsalazine sodium, 289t–291t
Omadacycline, 341t
Omalizumab, 491t–492t
Omeprazole, 592t, 597, 598t–599t
  and sodium bicarbonate, 598t–599t
Oncogenes, 422
Oncology patients, opioid analgesics usage by, 313
Ondansetron, 676t–677t
Ondansetron hydrochloride, 577t–578t
Onset, 23, 24f
Opana, 76b
Open-angle glaucoma, 604f, 605
Ophthalmia neonatorum, 710t
Ophthalmic drugs, 604–605
Ophthalmic sulfonamides, 349–350
Opiates, 580–582
  antidiarrhea with, 580–582, 581b–582b, 582t–583t
  diphenoxylate with atropine, 581b
  dosage for, 582t–583t
  male sexual dysfunction caused by, 746t
Opiates-related agents, 580–582
  diphenoxylate with atropine, 581b
  dosage for, 582t–583t
  pharmacodynamics of, 581–582
  pharmacokinetics of, 581
Opicapone, 230t–231t, 235t–238t
Opioid agonist-antagonists, 313–314
  dosage for, 315t
  nalbuphine, 315t
  patient safety with, 314b
  pharmacodynamics of, 314
  pharmacokinetics of, 314
Opioid agonists, 209t–210t, 306
  morphine, 309–310, 309b
Opioid analgesics, 306–313
  adjuvant therapy with, 313
  analgesic titration, 312
  case study on, 318b–319b
  children's usage of, 312–313, 313f
  combination drugs, 312
  dosage for, 311t
  hydromorphone, 312, 312b

Opioid analgesics *(Continued)*
   meperidine, 310–312
   older adults' usage of, 313
   oncology patients' usage of, 313
   patient-controlled analgesia, 312
   substance abuse individuals' usage of, 313
   transdermal, 312
   use in special populations, 312–313
Opioid antagonists, 314, 315t
Opioids, 34t, 35
   dosage adjustment requirements with CKD for, 53t
   hyperkalemia caused by, 144t
   substance use disorder with, 62–63
Opportunistic infections (OIs), 358–359, 392
Oral amoxicillin, 615
Oral anticoagulants, 554–555
   adverse reactions from, 555
   dosage for, 553t–554t
   drug interactions with, 555
   pharmacodynamics of, 555
   pharmacokinetics of, 555
   side effects for, 555
   warfarin, 554t, 555b–556b
Oral antidiabetic (hypoglycemic) drugs, 660–662, 661b
   acarbose and miglitol, 660
   adverse reactions from, 656
   alpha-glucosidase inhibitors, 660
   biguanides, 657t–659t, 660
   clinical judgment (nursing process), 661b
   contraindications for, 656
   dosage for, 657t–659t
   drug interactions with, 656
   first-generation sulfonylureas, 655–656, 657t–659t
   glipizide, 656b
   incretin modifier, 660
   meglitinides, 657t–659t, 660
   metformin, 660, 660b–661b
   nonsulfonylureas, 656, 657t–659t
   pharmacodynamics of, 655
   pharmacokinetics of, 655
   second-generation sulfonylureas, 655–656, 657t–659t
   side effects for, 656
   thiazolidinediones, 657t–659t, 660
   type 2 diabetes guidelines with, 660–662
Oral cavity, 573, 574f
Oral feeding, 166
Oral inhalation insulin, 651t
Organ transplantation, 395, 399t
   cadaveric, 395
   case study on, 404b–405b
   drugs for infection, 403
     bacterial, 403
     fungal, 403
     viral, 403
   drugs for transplant rejection, 402–403
   immunosuppressant drugs for, 395–402
     induction therapy, 395–397
     maintenance therapy, 397–402
     immunosuppression principles with, 395–402, 396f, 403b
   living-donor, 395
   promoting adherence for, 403–406
Oritavancin, 334t
Orphan Drug Act, 13
Orphenadrine citrate, 253b, 254t–255t

Orthostatic hypotension, 261, 312
Oseltamivir phosphate, 364t–365t
Osimertinib, 451–452
   adverse reactions from, 451
   dosage for, 448t–449t
   drug interactions with, 452
   pharmacodynamics of, 451
   pharmacokinetics of, 451
   side effects for, 451
Osmolality, 134, 532
Osmolarity, 136
Osmole, 134
Osmosis, 134
Osmotic diuretics, 532
   adverse reactions from, 532
   contraindications for, 532
   dosage for, 530t–531t
   side effects for, 532
Osmotic laxatives, 583
   adverse reactions from, 583
   dosage for, 584t–585t
   side effects for, 583
Osmotics, 583
Osteopenia, 732
Osteoporosis
   diagnosis of, 732
   drugs for, 732–738
   menopause with, 732–738
   nursing interventions for, 732
   prevention of, 732
Otalgia (ear pain), 615
Otitis externa (OE), 615
Ototoxicity, 337
Over-the-counter (OTC) drugs, 15, 15f, 16b, 206
   nonsteroidal antiinflammatory, 289
   older adults use of, 52
   substance use disorder with, 58
   usage, 49–50
Ovulation induction, 726–729, 727t
   adverse reactions from, 726
   contraindications for, 728
   dosage for, 727t
   drug interactions of, 728
   pharmacodynamics of, 726
   pharmacokinetics of, 726
   side effects for, 726
Oxacillin sodium, 326t
Oxaliplatin, 424b–425b, 425t, 428t–429t
Oxaprozin, 289t–291t
Oxazepam, 270t–271t
Oxazolidinones, 336
   adverse reactions with, 336
   case study on, 338
   dosage for, 334t
   drug interactions, 336
   side effects with, 336
Oxcarbazepine, 225t–226t
   for partial seizure, 227t
Oxicams, 289t–291t, 293–294
   analgesics with, 307t–308t
Oxybutynin chloride, 671t–672t
Oxycodone hydrochloride, 311t
Oxycodone (OxyContin, Percocet), 76b
   dosage adjustment requirements with CKD for, 53t
   drug label precautions for, 95, 95f
Oxycodone with acetaminophen, 311t
Oxycodone with aspirin, 311t
OxyContin. *See* Oxycodone

Oxymetazoline, 484b
Oxymetazoline hydrochloride, 481t
Oxytocin, 697t, 698b, 699
   clinical judgment (nursing process), 699b
Ozanimod, 250t–252t

P

P450 system, 22
Paclitaxel, 424b–425b, 425t, 437t–438t
Pain
   classification of, 303–304
   gate theory of, 304
   pathophysiology of, 304
   pregnancy with, 678
     acetaminophen for, 679
     aspirin for, 679
     ibuprofen for, 679
   substance use precautions with management of, 66
   types of, 304t
   undertreatment of, 304–305
Pain tolerance, 303
Paliperidone, 265t–266t
Palliative chemotherapy, 424
Palonosetron, 577t–578t
Panax ginseng. See Ginseng
Pancuronium bromide, 254t–255t
Panitumumab, 461
   adverse reactions from, 461
   dosage for, 459t–460t
   drug interactions with, 461
   pharmacodynamics of, 461
   pharmacokinetics of, 461
   side effects for, 461
Pantoprazole, 592t, 597, 598b, 598t–599t
Papillary layer, of skin, 620
Papules, 620
Para-aminophenol drug, 307t–308t
Paraplatin, patient safety with, 427b
Parasympathetic nervous system, 175, 176f, 187, 189t, 199
Parasympathetic nervous systems, 175, 199
Parathyroid glands, 642–644
   clinical judgment (nursing process), 643b
   disorders of, 633–648
   hyperparathyroidism, 642–644
     dosage for, 642t
   hypoparathyroidism, 642–644
     calcitriol for, 643b
     dosage for, 642t
   parathyroid hormone insufficiencies, 643b
Parathyroid hormone (PTH), 642
Parenteral anticoagulants II, 552
   dosage for, 553t–554t
Parenteral drug dosage calculation methods, 98–99
   ampules in, 110–111, 110f
   basic formula, 99
   body surface area, 102, 103f, 104f, 105f
   body weight, 101
   dimensional analysis, 100–101
   injectable preparations, 109–111
   ratio and proportion/fractional equation, 99–100
   syringes in, 109–110, 110b–111b
   vials in, 110–111, 110f
Parenteral medications, 84–90, 85f, 86f, 87f, 88f, 109
   intradermal, 85
     action in, 85
     equipment for, 85

Parenteral medications (Continued)
   needle angles for, 86f
   sites for, 85, 86f
   technique for, 85
  intramuscular, 87
   action in, 87
   equipment for, 87
   needle angles for, 86f
   sites for, 87
   technique for, 87
  intravenous, 88–89
   action in, 88
   equipment for, 88
   sites for, 88, 89f
   technique for, 89–90
  nursing implications for, 89–90
   equipment, 89
   sites, 89
   technique, 89–90
  safety needles for, 85f
  subcutaneous, 85–87
   action in, 85
   equipment for, 86
   needle angles for, 86f
   sites for, 85–86, 86f
   technique for, 86–87
  Z-track injection technique, 88, 88f
Parenteral nutrition (PN), 170–173
  case studies with, 172b
  complications from, 170–173, 171t
  patient need, 170
  patient-centered collaborative care with, 171b–172b
Parkinson disease
  anticholinergics for, 230–232, 230t–231t, 231b–232b
  catechol O-methyltransferase, 230t–231t, 233
  defined, 229–230
  dopamine agonists, 230t–231t, 233, 235t–238t
  dopamine blocked with, 263
  dopaminergics, 233
   carbidopa-levodopa, 230t–231t, 233, 233f, 234b, 235t–238t
   levodopa, 232–233, 233f
  drugs for, 229
   adverse reactions from, 238
   case study on, 242–243
   comparison of, 230t–231t
   contraindications of, 238
   drug-drug interactions with, 238
   precautions for, 238
   side effects of, 238
  monoamine oxidase B inhibitors, 230t–231t, 233
  nonpharmacologic measures for, 230
  pathophysiology of, 230
  symptoms, 229
Parkinsonism
  antiparkinson-anticholinergic drugs for, 194–195, 194b, 196t
  characteristics of, 261f
Paroxetine, dosage adjustment requirements with CKD for, 53t
Paroxetine hydrochloride, 279t–282t
Paroxysmal supraventricular tachycardia (PSVT), 764
Parsley, antihypertensives with, 539b
Partial agonists, 25
Partial seizure, 221t
  anticonvulsants for, 227t

Partial thromboplastin time (PTT), 552
Passive and active transport, 20f
Passive immunity, 408
Passive transport, 20
Pathogens, 321, 333, 408
  bacterial, 751
   bacterial vaginosis, 751
   chlamydia, 754
   gonorrhea, 754
   syphilis, 754–755
  other pathogens in, 756
   pediculosis pubis, 756
   scabies, 756
   trichomoniasis, 756
   vulvovaginal candidiasis, 756
  sexually transmitted infections, 756–758
  viral, 755–756
   herpes simplex virus, 755
   HIV, 755
Patient problems, in nursing process, 1–2
Patient Protection and Affordable Care Act, 13
Patient-centered collaborative care
  adrenergic agonists in, 182b
  adrenergic neuron antagonists in, 182b
  atropine sulfate in, 195b
  benzodiazepines, 211b
  bethanechol chloride in, 191b
  calcium in, 146b
  complementary and alternative therapies with, 43b
  enteral nutrition in, 169b
  fluid replacement in, 137b–138b
  geriatric considerations with, 55b–56b
  iron in, 164b
  magnesium in, 148b
  methylphenidate hydrochloride in, 203b
  nonbenzodiazepines, 213b
  parenteral nutrition in, 171b–172b
  pediatric considerations with, 49b–50b
  potassium in, 140b
  sodium in, 142b
  vaccines in, 417b–418b
  vitamins in, 161b
Patient-controlled analgesia (PCA), 112, 115f, 312
Paxil, patient safety with, 440b
PCA. See Patient-controlled analgesia
PCOS. See Polycystic ovarian syndrome
Peak, 23–24, 24f
Peak drug level, 24
Pediatric patient, developmental needs of, 90
Pediatric pharmacology, considerations, 45–51
  absorption, 46
  adolescent patient considerations in, 48–49
  age classification in, 46t
  available research limiting, 45
  case study on, 50
  distribution in, 46–47
  dosing in, 47
  drug administration for, 47–48
  excretion in, 47
  family-centered care for, 49–50
  FDA recommendations for, 47
  metabolism in, 47
  monitoring in, 47
  nursing implications for, 47–48
  nursing process in, 49b–50b
  over-the-counter drug use, 49–50
  patient-centered collaborative care, 49b–50b
  pharmacodynamics in, 47

Pediatric pharmacology, considerations (Continued)
  pharmacokinetics in, 46–47
  preventing drug administration errors in, 45b
  Principle of Atraumatic Care in, 48
  research related to, 45–46
Pediatric Research Equity Act (PREA), 13, 46
Pediculosis pubis, 756
Pegaspargase, 424b–425b, 443t–444t
Peginterferon alfa-2a, 364t–365t
Pegvisomant, 635t–636t, 636
Pelvic inflammatory disease (PID), 715
Pemetrexed, 430t–431t
Pemetrexed disodium, 424b–425b
Penciclovir, 364t–365t
Penicillin, 19, 324–328
  adverse reactions with, 327–328
  beta-lactamase inhibitors, 325–327
  broad-spectrum, 325, 325b
  case study on, 332
  clinical judgment (nursing process), 327b
  combined hormonal contraceptives and, 719b
  dosage for, 326t
  drug interactions with, 327–328
  extended-spectrum, 325
  hypokalemia caused by, 144t
  penicillinase-resistant, 325
  side effects with, 327–328
Penicillin G benzathine, 326t
Penicillin G procaine, 326t
Penicillin G sodium, 326t
Penicillin V potassium, 326t
Penicillinase-resistant penicillins (antistaphylococcal penicillins), 326t
Pennyroyal, pregnancy and, 674b
Pentazocine lactate, 315t
Pentobarbital, 208, 208b, 208t, 691t–692t
  patient safety with, 208b, 690b
Pentostatin, 424b–425b, 430t–431t
Pentoxifylline, 568–571
  dosage for, 568t
PEP. See Postexposure prophylaxis
Peppermint (*Mentha piperita*), iron absorption and, 162b
Pepsin, 590
Pepsin inhibitors (mucosal protective drugs), 599
  actions of, 592f
  clinical judgment (nursing process), 600b
  dosage for, 598t–599t
  pharmacodynamics of, 599
  pharmacokinetics of, 599
  sucralfate, 600b
Peptic ulcer, 590
Peptic ulcer disease
  common sites of, 591f
  complementary and alternative therapies for, 591b
  nonpharmacologic measures for managing, 592
  predisposing factors for, 590, 591t
   gastroesophageal reflux disease, 591–592
   Helicobacter pylori, 591
Peptides, 369–379
  antiinfective
   dosage and uses for, 377t
   patient safety with, 377b
  bacitracin, 377
  clinical judgment (nursing process), 378b–379b
  colistimethate, 375–376
  metronidazole, 377–379
  polymyxins, 376–377

Peramivir, 364t–365t
Perampanel, 225t–226t
Percocet. *See* Oxycodone
Percodan, 76b
   drug label precautions for, 95, 95f
Percolation, 40t
Percutaneous endoscopic gastrostomy (PEG) tube, 167
Pericardium, 502
Perimenopause, 729
Perinatal transmission, ophthalmia neonatorum, recombinant hepatitis B, 711
Perindopril arginine and amlodipine besylate, 545t–546t
Perindopril erbumine, 545t–546t
Perineal wounds
   nonpharmacologic measures for, 700t
   postpartum, pain relief for, 702–703, 702b–703b
      adverse reactions for, 703
      clinical judgment (nursing process), 702b–703b
      side effects of, 703
Peripheral blood flow, drugs to improve, 567–571
   cilostazol, 568, 568t, 570b
   pentoxifylline, 568, 568t
   peripheral vasodilators, 568t, 571b
Peripheral chemoreceptors, 486
Peripheral circulation, 503
Peripheral nervous system (PNS), 176f, 199–200
Peripheral vasodilators, 563
   clinical judgment (nursing process), 569b–570b
   dosage for, 568t
   human clinical experimentation, 10–11
   objectives and phases of, 10–11
   phases of, 10–11
   preclinical trials of, 10
Perphenazine, 265t–266t
Personalized medicine, 33t
Pertussis (whooping cough), vaccine for, 410t–413t
Petit mal seizures. *See* Absence seizures
Pfizer-BioNTech, 410t–413t
Pharmacodynamics, 19–31, 29b
   acebutolol hydrochloride, 518b
   acetaminophen, 305–306, 306b, 679
   acetylcholinesterase inhibitors, 245–246
   acyclovir, 366b
   adverse drug reactions, 26
   agonists, 25
   aldesleukin, 474
   alectinib, 454
   alemtuzumab, 460
   alpha-adrenergic blockers, 542
   aluminum hydroxide, 593b
   aminoglycosides, 343–344
   amoxicillin, 325b
   amphetamine-like drugs, 202
   antacids, 594
   antagonists, 25
   antibacterial drugs, 322–323
   antimalarials, 370
   antiplatelets, 559
   antitussives, 483
   aspirin, 292, 292b
   atazanavir, 391b
   atenolol, 180, 180b
   atorvastatin, 567, 569b
   atropine sulfate, 193b, 194
   azathioprine, 401
   barbiturates, 208

Pharmacodynamics *(Continued)*
   basiliximab, 395–396
   belatacept, 397
   benzodiazepines, 212, 269
   beta blockers, 509–512, 518b, 539
   beta-lactamase inhibitors, 327
   beta-sympathomimetic drugs, 682
   bethanechol chloride, 188b
   bevacizumab, 450b
   bisacodyl, 585b
   bortezomib, 458b
   bulk forming laxatives, 585
   calcitriol, 643b
   calcium channel blockers, 512
   carfilzomib, 457
   cephalosporins, 331–332
   cetuximab, 460–461
   chloroquine, 370
   cilostazol, 568, 570b
   clomiphene citrate, 726, 726b
   clopidogrel bisulfate, 558b, 559
   conjugated estrogens, 730b
   corticosteroids, 401–402
   cyclobenzaprine, 253b, 256
   cyclophosphamide, 427–429, 431b–432b
   cyclosporine, 398b
   dasatinib, 454–455
   digoxin, 504b
   diphenoxylate with atropine, 581b
   dose-response relationship, 23, 24f
   doxorubicin, 435–436, 438b
   doxycycline, 340b
   drug toxicity, 26
   duration of action, 23, 24f
   efavirenz, 390b
   ESAs, 471
   filgrastim, 473b
   first-generation antihistamines, 478
   fluoroquinolones, 347
   fluorouracil, 432, 435b
   fluoxetine, 276, 276b
   fluphenazine hydrochloride, 263
   gefitinib, 448–451
   glipizide, 655, 656b
   glycopeptides, 337
   glycylcyclines, 340
   H_2 blockers, 595–597
   haloperidol, 263
   hydantoins, 222
   ibritumomab tiuxetan, 461
   ibuprofen, 293, 294b
   imatinib mesylate, 453b
   infliximab, 298b
   insulin, 651, 654b
   interactions, 28
      additive drug effects, 28
      antagonistic drug effects, 28
      potentiation, 28
      synergistic drug effects, 28
   interferon α, 469
   interleukin, 474
   iron, 162, 163b
   ixazomib, 457
   latanoprost, 613b
   levothyroxine sodium, 639b–640b
   lipopeptides, 337
   loop diuretics, 527
   lorazepam, 269, 270b
   macrolides, 335

Pharmacodynamics *(Continued)*
   mechanisms of drug action, 26
   metformin, 660b–661b
   metronidazole, 378b
   mood stabilizers, 283
   morphine, 309–310, 309b
   mycophenolate mofetil, 401
   nalbuphine, 314b
   nilotinib, 454
   nitrates, 508–509
   nitroimidazoles, 352
   nonselective drug, 25
   nonspecific drug, 25
   nystatin, 361b
   older adult considerations for, 54
   onset of action, 23–24, 24f
   opiates, 581–582
   opioid agonist-antagonists, 314
   of oral antidiabetic, 655
   osimertinib, 451
   ovulation induction, 726
   panitumumab, 461
   partial agonists, 25
   peak, 23–24, 24f
   pediatric considerations for, 47
   pepsin inhibitors, 599
   phenothiazine antiemetics, 576
   prazosin hydrochloride, 544b
   propionic acid derivatives, 293
   proton pump inhibitors, 597
   pyridostigmine, 245, 247b
   receptor theory, 24–25, 25f
   rivastigmine, 239
   salicylates, 292
   side effects, 26
   sorafenib, 455
   spironolactone, 533b–534b
   statins, 567
   stimulant laxatives, 583–585
   sulfonamides, 348–349
   sunitinib, 455
   tachyphylaxis, 26
   tacrolimus for, 397
   temsirolimus, 456–457
   tenofovir disoproxil fumarate, 389b
   testosterone, 742b
   therapeutic drug monitoring, 24
   thrombolytics, 560
   timolol, 612b
   tolerance, 26
   tolterodine tartrate, 197b
   tositumomab, 462
   trastuzumab, 464
   tricyclic antidepressants, 275
   trimethoprim-sulfamethoxazole, 349, 350b, 666–667
   valsartan, 547, 547b
   varicella vaccine, 415–416, 415b
   vincristine, 439, 440b–441b
   vitamin A, 155, 157b
   vitamin C, 159–160, 159b
   zidovudine, 388b
   ziv-aflibercept, 447–448
Pharmacogenetics, 32–38, 33f
   available testing, 34t
   brief history of, 32
   case study on, 37–38
   clinical application of, 35b
   clinical uses of, 32–34

Pharmacogenetics (Continued)
    individual variation in metabolism of select drugs, 34–35
    legal and ethical issues, 35–37
    terminology, 33t
    variable response to drugs, 33f
Pharmacogenomics, 33t
Pharmacokinetics, 19–31, 29b, 369
    absorption in, 46, 53
    acebutolol hydrochloride, 518b
    acetaminophen, 305–306, 306b, 679
    acetylcholinesterase inhibitors, 245, 247b
    acyclovir, 366b
    aldesleukin, 474
    alectinib, 454
    alemtuzumab, 459–460
    alpha-adrenergic blockers, 542
    aluminum hydroxide, 593b
    aminoglycosides, 343–346
    amoxicillin, 325b
    amphetamine-like drugs, 200
    antacids, 594
    antibacterial drugs, 322
    antimalarials, 369
    antiplatelets, 557
    antitussives, 483
    aspirin, 292
    atazanavir, 391b
    atenolol, 180b, 186
    atorvastatin, 567, 569b
    atropine sulfate, 193b, 194
    barbiturates, 212
    basiliximab, 395
    belatacept, 397
    benzodiazepines, 212, 269
    beta blockers, 508, 512, 539
    beta-lactamase inhibitors, 327
    beta-sympathomimetic drugs, 682
    bethanechol chloride, 188b
    bevacizumab, 450b
    bisacodyl, 585b
    bortezomib, 458b
    bulk forming laxatives, 585
    calcitriol, 643b
    calcium channel blockers, 512
    carfilzomib, 457
    cephalosporins, 331–332
    cetuximab, 460–461
    chloroquine, 369
    cilostazol, 568, 570b
    clomiphene citrate, 726, 726b
    clopidogrel bisulfate, 557, 558b
    combined hormonal contraceptives, 718
    conjugated estrogens, 730b, 731
    corticosteroids, 401–402
    cyclobenzaprine, 253b, 256, 256b
    cyclophosphamide, 427, 431b–432b
    cyclosporine, 398b
    dasatinib, 454–455
    defined, 46
    digoxin, 504–505, 504b
    diphenoxylate with atropine, 581b
    distribution in, 46–47, 53
    doxorubicin, 435, 438b
    doxycycline, 340b
    drug absorption, 19–21
        interactions of, 26–30
    drug distribution, 21–22, 21f
    drug excretion, 23

Pharmacokinetics (Continued)
    interactions of, 28
    drug metabolism, 22–23
        interactions of, 27
    drug-assisted treatment, 61t
    efavirenz, 390b
    ESAs, 471
    excretion in, 47, 53
    filgrastim, 473b
    first-generation antihistamines, 478
    fluoroquinolones, 347
    fluorouracil, 432, 435b
    fluoxetine, 276, 276b
    fluphenazine hydrochloride, 263
    gefitinib, 450
    glipizide, 655
    glycopeptides, 337
    glycylcyclines, 340
    H_2 blockers, 595–597
    haloperidol, 263
    hydantoins, 221
    ibritumomab tiuxetan, 461
    ibuprofen, 293, 294b
    imatinib mesylate, 453b
    infliximab, 298b
    insulin, 654b, 655
    interactions of, 26–30
    interferon alfa, 469
    interleukin, 474
    iron, 162, 163b
    ixazomib, 457–459
    latanoprost, 613b
    levothyroxine sodium, 639b–640b
    lipopeptides, 337
    loop diuretics, 527
    macrolides, 335
    metabolism in, 47, 53
    metformin, 660b–661b
    metronidazole, 378b
    morphine, 309–310, 309b
    mycophenolate mofetil, 401
    nilotinib, 454
    nitrates, 508
    nitroimidazoles, 352
    nystatin, 361b
    older adult considerations for, 52–54
    opiates, 581
    opioid agonist-antagonists, 314
    oral antidiabetic, 655
    osimertinib, 451–452
    ovulation induction, 726
    panitumumab, 461
    pediatric considerations for, 47
    pepsin inhibitors, 599
    phenothiazine antiemetics, 576
    prazosin hydrochloride, 544b
    propionic acid derivatives, 293
    proton pump inhibitors, 597–599
    pyridostigmine, 245, 247b
    rivastigmine, 239
    salicylates, 292
    sorafenib, 455
    spironolactone, 533b–534b
    statins, 567
    stimulant laxatives, 583–585
    sulfonamides, 348
    sunitinib, 455
    tacrolimus for, 397
    temsirolimus, 456–457

Pharmacokinetics (Continued)
    tenofovir disoproxil fumarate, 389b
    testosterone, 742b
    thrombolytics, 560
    timolol, 612b
    tolterodine tartrate, 197b
    tositumomab, 461–464
    trastuzumab, 464
    tricyclic antidepressants, 275
    trimethoprim and trimethoprim-sulfamethoxazole, 666–667
    trimethoprim-sulfamethoxazole, 349, 350b, 666–667
    valsartan, 547, 547b
    varicella vaccine, 415–416, 415b
    vincristine, 439, 440b–441b
    vitamin A, 155, 157b
    vitamin C, 159–160, 159b
    zidovudine, 388b
    ziv-aflibercept, 447
Phenazopyridine, 670
Phenazopyridine hydrochloride, 671t–672t
Phendimetrazine, 204t
Phenelzine sulfate, 279t–282t
Phenobarbital, 99, 99f
    combined hormonal contraceptives and, 719b
    dosage for, 225t–226t
    for partial seizure, 227t
    for status epilepticus, 227t
    for tonic-clonic seizures, 227t
Phenobarbital, patient safety in, 690b
Phenothiazine antiemetics, 576
    dosage for, 577t–578t
    drug interactions with, 576
    laboratory interactions with, 576
    pharmacodynamics of, 576
    pharmacokinetics of, 576
    side effects for, 576
Phenothiazines, 261–263
    aliphatic, 261
    clinical judgment (nursing process), 267b
    effects of, 262t
    male sexual dysfunction caused by, 746t
    for nausea, in pregnancy, 676t–677t
    overdose symptoms for, 263b
    piperazine, 261–262
    piperidine, 262
    treatment for overdose of, 263b
Phenotype, 33t
Phenoxybenzamine hydrochloride, 542t
Phentermine hydrochloride, 204t
Phentermine-topiramate, 204t
Phentolamine, 542t
Phentolamine mesylate, 184t–185t
Phenylacetic acids derivatives, 289t–291t
Phenylalkylamines, 548t
Phenylephrine, 609t
Phenylephrine hydrochloride, 181t, 481t
Phenytoin
    adverse reactions from, 222b
    clinical judgment (nursing process), 224b
    contraindications for, 222b
    dosage for, 222b
    example dosage calculation for, 108b–109b
    hypocalcemia caused by, 147t
    for partial seizure, 227t
    pharmacodynamics of, 222b
    pharmacokinetics of, 222b
    side effects for, 222b

Phenytoin (Continued)
   for status epilepticus, 227t
   for tonic-clonic seizures, 227t
   uses for, 222b
Phosphate preparations, hypocalcemia caused by, 147t
Phosphodiesterase inhibitors, 505–506
   dosage for, 505t
Phosphodiesterase-5 (PDE-5) inhibitors, 748t
   for erectile dysfunction, 747t
Phosphorus, 149–153
Photoallergic reaction, 30
Photochemotherapy, 626
Photophobia, 609
Photosensitivity, 339
Phototoxic reaction, 30
Physostigmine salicylate, 192t
Phytomedicine, 39
Phytonadione, 553t–554t, 710t
   neonates, administration to, 708–709
PID. See Pelvic inflammatory disease
Piggyback set up, 112, 114f
Pilocarpine, 190
Pilocarpine hydrochloride, 192t
Pimavanserin, 230t–231t, 235t–238t
Pindolol, 184t–185t, 540t
Pinocytosis, 20
Pioglitazone hydrochloride, 657t–659t
Piper methysticum. See Kava kava
Piperacillin, hypokalemia caused by, 144t
Piperacillin tazobactam, 326t
Piperazine phenothiazines, 261–262
Piperidine phenothiazines, 262
Piroxicam, 289t–291t
PIS. See Protease inhibitors
Pitavastatin, 565t–566t
Pitolisant, 201t
Pituitary gland, 633
   anterior, 633–634, 634f
   disorders of, 633–648
      drug therapies for, 635t–636t
   negative feedback loop of, 634f
   posterior, 634f
Pituitary hormones
   adrenocorticotropic hormone, 633–634, 635t–636t
   antidiuretic hormone, 633, 635t–636t
   clinical judgment (nursing process), 638b
   follicle-stimulating hormone, 633
   growth hormone, 633–634, 635t–636t
   luteinizing hormone, 633
   prolactin, 633–634
   thyroid-stimulating hormone, 633–634, 635t–636t
Pituitary reproductive disorders, 746
PJP. See *Pneumocystis jiroveci* pneumonia
Placebo effect, 26
Placebo group, 11
Planning, in nursing process, 1
Plant alkaloids
   adverse reactions with, 439–440
   for cancer, 436–440
   dosage for, 437t–438t
   side effects with, 439–440
   vincristine, 422b, 439–440, 439b
Plaques, 620
Platinol, patient safety with, 427b
Plazomicin, dosage for, 668t–669t
PMS. See Premenstrual syndrome

PN. See Parenteral nutrition
Pneumococcal disease, vaccine for, 410t–413t
Pneumocystis jiroveci pneumonia (PJP), 392, 403
Pneumothorax, parenteral nutrition complicated by, 171t
PNS. See Peripheral nervous system
Poisoning
   activated charcoal for, 768, 770t
   flumazenil for, 770t
Poliomyelitis, vaccine for, 410t–413t
Polycarbophil, 588t
Polycystic ovarian syndrome (PCOS), 722–723
Polydipsia, 649
Polyenes antifungals, 359–361, 359t–360t
   amphotericin B, 359–361, 359t–360t, 361b
   nystatin, 359–361, 359t–360t, 361b
Polyethylene glycol, 584t–585t
Polymorphisms, 33t
Polymyxin B, 377t, 615–616
   hypokalemia caused by, 144t
Polymyxin B sulfate, 606t, 668t–669t
Polymyxins, 376–377
   severe adverse effects with, 377
Polyphagia, 649
Polypharmacy, 54
Polyuria, 649
Poor metabolizers, 33t
Poractant alfa, 709t
Posaconazole, 359t–360t
Positive symptoms, 260
Postexposure prophylaxis (PEP), 393
Postganglionic nerve fibers, 199
Postmenopause, 729
Postpartum depression, 704–705
Postpartum period, 689–707
   drugs used during, 700–705
      lactation suppression, 704
      pain relief for perineal wounds and hemorrhoids, 702–703, 702b–703b
      pain relief for uterine contractions, 700–705
      promotion of bowel function, 701t, 703–704, 704b–705b
   nonpharmacologic measures for, 700t
Potassium, 138–139
   balance, effect of drugs on, 139, 144t
   functions of, 139
   hyperkalemia, 139, 143b, 144t
   hypokalemia, 141b, 141t, 144t
   oral and intravenous preparations, 141t
   patient-centered collaborative care with, 140b
   supplements, 141t
Potassium chloride, 143b
   hyperkalemia caused by, 144t
Potassium iodide, 640t
Potassium penicillin, hyperkalemia caused by, 144t
Potassium phosphate (KPO4), hyperkalemia caused by, 144t
Potassium salt substitutes, hyperkalemia caused by, 144t
Potassium-sparing diuretics, 139, 524, 532–534
   adverse reactions from, 532–534
   clinical judgment (nursing process), 534b
   dosage adjustment requirements with CKD for, 53t
   dosage for, 533t
   hyperkalemia caused by, 144t
   side effects for, 532–534
   spironolactone, 533b–534b
   thiazide with, 538b

Potassium-wasting diuretics, 139, 524
   aloe with, 528b
Potency, 23
Potentiation, 28
Poultice, 40t
PPI. See Proton pump inhibitors
PPMS. See Primary progressive MS
PR interval, 513
Pralidoxime chloride, 192t
Pramipexole dihydrochloride, 230t–231t
Pramipexole hydrochloride, 235t–238t
Pramlintide, 657t–659t
Prasugrel, 558t–559t
Pravastatin, dosage adjustment requirements with CKD for, 53t
Pravastatin sodium, 565t–566t
Praziquantel, 373t
Prazosin hydrochloride, 184t–185t, 542t, 544b
PREA. See Pediatric Research Equity Act
Precision medicine, 32
Prednisolone, 645t
Prednisolone acetate, 608
Prednisolone sodium phosphate, 607t–608t
Prednisone, 401, 425t, 645t, 646b
   hypokalemia caused by, 144t
Preeclampsia, 684
   drugs used in severe, 685t
Pregabalin, 225t–226t
   dosage adjustment requirements with CKD for, 53t
   for partial seizure, 227t
Preganglionic nerve fibers, 199
Pregnancy, 673–688
   antiretroviral drugs in, 392–393
   antiseizure drugs and, 223
   categories for safety and quality, 78, 78t
   complementary and alternative therapies for, 674b
   drugs and herbs for, 674–681
      antepartum drugs, 679b–680b
      antidepressant drugs, 679–681
      folic acid, 675
      iron, 674–675
      vitamins, multiple, 675
   drugs for minor discomforts of, 675–678
      constipation, 678
      heartburn, 676t–677t, 677–678
      nausea, 675–676, 676t–677t
      pain, 678
      vomiting, 675–676, 676t–677t
   immunizations and, 705–706
      $Rh_0(D)$ immune globulin, 705, 706b
      rubella vaccine, 705–706
   physiology of, 673–674
   tuberculosis and, 357
   vitamin deficiency from, 155t
Preload, 502, 508
Premarin, patient safety with, 730b
Premenstrual syndrome (PMS), 724–725
   antidepressant drugs for, 725
   behavioral symptoms of, 724
   emotional symptoms of, 724
   hormonal therapy for, 725
   nonpharmacologic treatment of, 725
   pharmacologic treatment of, 725
   physical symptoms of, 724–725
   symptoms of, 725
Premphase, patient safety with, 730b
Prempro, patient safety with, 730b

Prescriber's Letter, 17
Prescription antiemetics, 576–580, 580b
　anticholinergics, 576, 577t–578t
　antihistamines, 576
　benzodiazepines, 576, 577t–578t
　butyrophenones, 576, 577t–578t
　cannabinoids, 577t–578t, 579
　clinical judgment (nursing process), 580b
　dopamine antagonists, 576, 577t–578t
　dosage for, 577t–578t
　glucocorticoids, 576
　metoclopramide, 577t–578t
　miscellaneous antiemetics, 579–580
　neurokinin receptor antagonists, 579
　phenothiazine antiemetics, 576, 579b
　serotonin-receptor antagonists, 576
Preterm labor (PTL), 673–688
　case study on, 687–688
　corticosteroid therapy in, 683–684
　　betamethasone for, 683, 684b, 684t
　　dexamethasone for, 683–684, 683b, 684t
　defined, 681
　tocolytic therapy for, 681
　uterine muscle contractility with, 681–683
Priapism, 743–744
Prilocaine hydrochloride, 216t
Primaquine, 371t–372t
Primary infections, 358–359
Primary IV line set, 112
Primary progressive MS (PPMS), 248
Primary syphilis, 754
Primidone, 225t–226t
　combined hormonal contraceptives and, 719b
　for partial seizure, 227t
　for tonic-clonic seizures, 227t
Principle of Atraumatic Care, 48
PRL. *See* Prolactin
PRMS. *See* Progressive relapsing MS
Probenecid, 300t
Procainamide
　cardiac emergency with, 765, 766t–767t
　dosage for, 766t–767t
Procainamide hydrochloride, 515t–518t
Procaine hydrochloride, 216t
Prochlorperazine maleate, 577t–578t
Prodrugs, 22–23
Progenitor cells, 473
Progesterone, 675
Progestin contraceptives, 717–718
　depot medroxyprogesterone acetate, 717–718
　progestin implant, 718
　progestin-only oral contraceptive pills, 717
　side effects with, 719
　special considerations for, 718
　start date for, 718–720
Progestins, 714
Progressive relapsing MS (PRMS), 248
Prolactin (PRL), 633–634
Promethazine, 577t–578t, 676t–677t, 691t–692t
Promethazine hydrochloride, 579b
Propafenone hydrochloride, 515t–518t
Propantheline bromide, 193
Prophylactic antituberculars, 356
Prophylaxis, 369
Propionibacterium acnes, 621
Propionic acid, 307t–308t
Propionic acid derivatives, 289t–291t, 292–293, 294b
　analgesics with, 307t–308t
　dosage information for, 289t–291t

Propionic acid derivatives *(Continued)*
　ibuprofen, 289t–291t, 294b
　pharmacodynamics of, 293
　pharmacokinetics of, 293
Propofol, 215t
Propranolol, 540t
Propranolol hydrochloride, 183, 184t–185t, 510t–511t, 515t–518t
Propylthiouracil (PTU), 640t, 641
Prostaglandin analogue antiulcer drug, 599–601
　actions of, 592f
　dosage for, 598t–599t
Prostaglandin analogues, 610
　adverse reactions from, 610
　dosage for, 611t
　for glaucoma, 610
　latanoprost, 613b
　side effects for, 610
Prostaglandins, cyclooxygenase, 288
Protamine, 650
Protamine sulfate, 553t–554t
　calculating intravenous flow rate for, 123b–126b
Protease inhibitors (PIS), 384t–387t, 388–389
　atazanavir, 388–389
　dosage for, 384t–387t
Proteasome inhibitors, 455–459
　bortezomib, 458b
　carfilzomib, 457
　clinical judgment (nursing process), 463b
　dosage for, 448t–449t
　ixazomib, 457–459
Proteasomes, 456
Protein binding, 21–22, 21f
Prothrombin time (PT), 554
Protocols, 424
Proton pump inhibitors (PPI), 597–599
　actions of, 592f
　dosage for, 598t–599t
　drug interactions with, 597
　pantoprazole, 598b
　pharmacodynamics of, 597
　pharmacokinetics of, 597
Protonix, patient safety with, 597b
Proto-oncogenes, 422
Protriptyline hydrochloride, 279t–282t
Prucalopride, 584t–585t
Pschopathology, 259–260
Pseudoephedrine, 177, 481t
Pseudoephedrine hydrochloride, 181t
Pseudoparkinsonism, 230
　characteristics of, 261f
Psoralen and ultraviolet A (PUVA), 626
Psoriasis, 625–628
　clinical judgment (nursing process), 627b
　dosage for, 622t–624t
　systemic drugs for, 626, 626t
　topical drugs for, 625–626
　treatment modalities for, 626t
PSVT. *See* Paroxysmal supraventricular tachycardia
Psychomotor seizures, 220
Psychosis, 260
Psychotropics, dosage adjustment requirements with CKD for, 53t
Psyllium, 586b
　digoxin absorption with, 506b
Psyllium hydrophilic mucilloid, 588t
PT. *See* Prothrombin time
PTH. *See* Parathyroid hormone
PTL. *See* Preterm labor

PTT. *See* Partial thromboplastin time
PTU. *See* Propylthiouracil
Puerperium, 700
Pulmonary circulation, 503
Pulmonary edema
　emergency drugs for, 772–775
　furosemide for, 773t, 774–775, 774b
　labetalol, 772–773, 773t
　nitroprusside sodium, 773–774, 773b, 773t
Pulse oximetry, 762
Punnett square, 34f
Purgatives, 583
Purine antimetabolites, 401
PUVA. *See* Psoralen and ultraviolet A
Pyrantel pamoate, 372–373
Pyrazinamide, 355t–356t
Pyridostigmine, 250
Pyridostigmine
　adverse reactions from, 247b
　clinical judgment (nursing process), 247b–248b
　contraindications for, 247b
　dosage for, 247b
　for myasthenia gravis, 246t, 247b
　pharmacodynamics of, 245, 247b
　pharmacokinetics of, 245, 247b
　side effects for, 246–248
Pyridostigmine bromide, 192t
Pyridoxine. *See* Vitamin B_6

Q

QRS complex, 513
QSEN. *See* Quality and Safety Education for Nurses
QT interval, 513
Quality and Safety Education for Nurses (QSEN), 69
Quazepam, for insomnia, 268t
Quetiapine, 265t–266t
Quinidine gluconate, drug label precautions for, 96, 96f
Quinidine, patient safety with, 370b
Quinidine sulfate, 515t–518t
Quinine, 371t–372t
　patient safety with, 370b
Quinine sulfate, drug label precautions for, 96, 96f
Quinupristin-dalfopristin, 352t

R

RAAS. *See* Renin-angiotensin-aldosterone system
Rabeprazole, 592t, 597, 598t–599t
　patient safety with, 597b
Rabies, vaccine for, 410t–413t
Raloxifene, 424b–425b, 443t–444t
Raltegravir (RTG), 384t–387t
Ramelteon, 209t–210t
Ramipril, 545t–546t
Rapid eye movement (REM) sleep, 206, 207f
Rapid-acting insulins, 650
Rasagiline, 230t–231t, 235t–238t
Ratio and proportion/fractional equation, 99–100
　body surface area in drug calculation with, 102–107
　calculating in drops per minute intravenous flow rate with, 116–127
　calculating in milliliters per hour intravenous flow rate with, 116–127
RAV. *See* Raltegravir

RCA. See Root cause analysis
RDA. See Recommended dietary allowance
RDS. See Respiratory distress syndrome
Reactive depression, 274
Rebound nasal congestion, 479
Receptor theory, 24–25, 25f
Recombinant DNA, 466, 467f
Recombinant subunit vaccines, 409
Recommended dietary allowance (RDA), 154
Rectal suppositories, 84, 84f
Red blood cells, packed, transfusion of, hyperkalemia caused by, 144t
Regional anesthesia
   clinical judgment (nursing process), 695b–696b
   contraindications to, 695
   labor pain control with, 692–695, 695b–696b
Regional blocks, 692–694
Relapsing remitting MS (RRMS), 248
Remifentanil, 209t–210t
Renal disease, vitamin deficiency from, 155t
Renin-angiotensin- aldosterone system (RAAS), 537f, 644
Repaglinide, 657t–659t
Repolarization, 513
Repolarization prolonging drugs, for cardiac dysrhythmia, 519
Reslizumab, 491t–492t
Respect for persons, 7–8
Respiration, control of, 486
Respiratory distress syndrome (RDS), 708
   synthetic surfactant therapy for, 709t
Respiratory tract, structures of, 478f
Restrictive lung disease, 489
Reteplase, 561t
Reticular layer, of skin, 620
Revefenacin, 491t–492t
Reversible cholinesterase inhibitors, 190–191
   edrophonium chloride, 192t
   neostigmine methylsulfate, 192t
   physostigmine salicylate, 192t
   pralidoxime chloride, 192t
   pyridostigmine bromide, 192t
   side effects for, 190–191
Reward circuit, 59
Rezafungin, 359t–360t
Rh sensitization, 705
$Rh_0(D)$ immune globulin, 705
   adverse reactions with, 706
   clinical judgment (nursing process), 706b
Rhinorrhea, 478
RHO kinase inhibitors, 611t
Ribavirin, 364t–365t
Riboflavin. See Vitamin B_2
Rifabutin, 355t–356t
   patient safety with, 357b
Rifampin, 355t–356t
   combined hormonal contraceptives and, 719b
   patient safety with, 357b
Rifamycin, 582t–583t
Rifapentine, 355t–356t
   patient safety with, 357b
Rifaximin, 582t–583t
Right documentation, 73
   medication administration record for, 73
   medication record, 74f
Right dose, 71–72
   dimensional analysis when calculating, 71–72
   nursing interventions related to, 71
   unit dose method when calculating, 72

Right drug, 70–71
   computerized physician order entry for, 70
   drug order example for, 71f
   nursing interventions related to, 71
Right Drug Dose Now Act, 32
Right patient, 69–70
Right route, 73
   absorption with, 73
   nursing interventions related to, 73
Right time, 72–73
   military time, 72–73, 72f
Rilpivirine (RPL), 384t–387t
Risk-benefit ratio, 10
Risperidone
   antipsychotics treatment with, 265t–266t
   case study on, 272b
Ritonavir (RTV), 384t–387t
Rituximab, 296t–297t, 424b–425b, 425t
   adverse reactions from, 462b
   contraindications for, 462b
   dosage for, 462b
   pharmacodynamics of, 462b
   pharmacokinetics of, 462b
   side effects for, 462b
   uses for, 462b
Rivaroxaban, 553t–554t
Rivastigmine, 192t
   for Alzheimer disease, 239, 240b, 240t–241t
   clinical judgment (nursing process), 240b
   dosage for, 240t–241t
   pharmacodynamics of, 239
   pharmacokinetics of, 239
   uses for, 240t–241t
Rizatriptan benzoate, 317t
Roflumilast, 494t
Rolapitant, 577t–578t
Root cause analysis (RCA), 74
Ropinirole hydrochloride, 230t–231t, 235t–238t
Ropivacaine, 693t
Rosacea, 629
Rose bengal, ophthalmic, 605t
Rosiglitazone, 657t–659t
Rosuvastatin, 565t–566t
   dosage adjustment requirements with CKD for, 53t
Rotavirus, vaccine for, 410t–413t
Rotigotine hydrochloride, 230t–231t, 235t–238t
Rounding rules, 98
Rozanolixizumab, myasthenia gravis treatment with, 246t
RP/FE. See Ratio and proportion/fractional equation
RPL. See Rilpivirine
RRMS. See Relapsing remitting MS
RTV. See Ritonavir
Rubella, vaccine for, 410t–413t
Rubeola. See Measles

S

Saddle block, 216
Safe Streets and Communities Act, 14
Safety and quality, 69–79
   Bill of Rights, for nurses, 73
   culture of safety for, 73–74
   disposal of medications in, 75
   drug administration error prevention resources for, 78
   drug reconciliation in, 75

Safety and quality (Continued)
   Food and Drug Administration in, 74–75
   high-alert drugs in, 76–77
   Just Culture in, 73–74
   look-alike and sound-alike drug names in, 77
   medication administration guidelines for, 78, 78b
   medication administration risks with, 75–77, 76t, 77b
      buying drugs over internet, 76
      counterfeit drugs, 76
      crush or not to crush, 76
      tablet splitting, 76
   pregnancy categories for, 78, 78t
   root cause analysis in, 74
   sentinel event in, 74
   sharps safety in, 75
   six rights, of medication administration, 69–73
      right documentation, 73, 74f
      right dose, 71–72
      right drug, 70–71, 71f
      right patient, 70
      right route, 73
      right time, 72–73
   TJC goals for, 74, 74t
Safety needles, for parenteral administration, 85f
Safinamide, 230t–231t, 235t–238t
Salicylates
   aspirin, 289, 289t–291t, 292b
   dosage information for, 289t–291t
   hypersensitivity to, 292
   pharmacodynamics of, 292
   pharmacokinetics of, 292
Salicylic acid, 622t–624t
Salivary gland, parasympathetic responses with, 189f
Salmeterol, 491t–492t, 494t
Saluretic effect, 529
SAMHSA. See Substance Abuse and Mental Health Services Administration
Sandostatin, patient safety with, 644b
Saquinavir (SQV), 384t–387t
Sargramostim
   adverse reactions from, 473b
   contraindications for, 473b
   dosage for, 473b
   pharmacodynamics of, 473b
   pharmacokinetics of, 473b
   side effects for, 473b
   uses for, 473b
Sarilumab, 296t–297t
Saw palmetto (Serenoa repens), 41–42
   platelet aggregation and, 559b
Saxagliptin, 657t–659t
Scabies, 756
Schizophrenia, 260
   symptoms of, 260
Scopolamine, 193, 577t–578t
   male sexual dysfunction caused by, 746t
Secnidazole, 351t
Secondary diabetes mellitus, 650
Secondary dysmenorrhea, 724
Secondary hypertension, 536
Secondary IV line set, 112
Secondary progressive MS (SPMS), 248
Secondary syphilis, 754
Second-generation sulfonylureas, 655–656, 657t–659t
Sectral, patient safety with, 350b
Secukinumab, 296t–297t

Sedation, 207
　adverse reactions of, 690–692
　dosage for, 691t–692t
　labor pain control with, 690–692, 691t–692t
Sedative-hypnotics CNS depressants, 207–214, 207t
　barbiturates, 208, 208b, 208t
　benzodiazepines, 208–212, 209t–210t, 211b
　complementary and alternative medicine for, 211b
　hypnotics, 207–208
　melatonin agonists, 208t, 212
　nonbenzodiazepines, 208t, 212, 213b
　sedatives, 207
Sedatives, 309b
　combined hormonal contraceptives and, 719b
　hyperkalemia caused by, 144t
Seizure threshold, 222–223
Seizures
　absence, 220, 221t
　atonic, 221t
　benzodiazepines for, 268t
　defined, 220
　generalized, 221t
　idiopathic, 220
　infantile, 221t
　international classification of, 220, 221t
　myoclonic, 221t
　pharmacophysiology, 220
　psychomotor, 220, 221t
　simple, 221t
　tonic, 221t
　tonic-clonic, 220, 221t
Selective alpha-adrenergic blockers, 542t
Selective chloride channel activators, 584t–585t, 585
Selective COX-2 inhibitors, 289t–291t, 294
Selective estrogen receptor modulators (SERMs), for cancer, 442
Selective serotonin receptor agonists (triptans), 317t
Selective serotonin reuptake inhibitors (SSRIs), 34t, 275–276, 275b, 276b
　adverse reactions of, 276
　complementary and alternative therapy with, 275b
　fluoxetine, 276b, 279t–282t
　male sexual dysfunction caused by, 746t
　for menopausal symptoms, 731
　pharmacodynamics of, 276
　pharmacokinetics of, 276
　side effects for, 276
Selective sodium-glucose transporter 2, 657t–659t
Selegiline hydrochloride, 230t–231t, 235t–238t, 279t–282t
Selenium, 163–164
Semaglutide, 657t–659t
Senna, 588t
Sennosides, 701t
Sentinel event, 74
Septra, patient safety with, 350b
Serenoa repens. See Saw palmetto
SERMs. See Selective estrogen receptor modulators
Seroconversion, 415
Serotonin norepinephrine reuptake inhibitors (SNRIs), 276–277
　adverse effects from, 277
　for menopausal symptoms, 731
　side effects for, 277
Serotonin-receptor antagonists, 576
Sertraline hydrochloride, 279t–282t
Serum lipid values, 564t

Sevoflurane, 215t
Sex hormones, for cancer, 442
Sexual dysfunction, 746–748
　complementary and alternative medicine for, 747–748
　drugs that cause male, 746t
　ejaculatory dysfunction, 746–747
Sexually transmitted infections (STI), 751–752
　bacterial pathogens in, 752–755
　　bacterial vaginosis, 752–753
　　chlamydia, 754
　　gonorrhea, 754
　　syphilis, 754–755
　case study on, 758b
　current guidelines for, 753t
　in older adult, 757b
　other pathogens in, 756
　　pediculosis pubis, 756
　　scabies, 756
　　trichomoniasis, 756
　　vulvovaginal candidiasis, 756
　pathogens in, 752–756
　　bacterial, 752–755
　　other, 756
　　viral, 755–756
　prevention of, 756–758
　　CDC guidelines for, 752f
　　clinical judgment (nursing process), 757b
　　male condom use, 757f
　viral pathogens in, 755–756
　　herpes simplex virus, 755
Sharps safety, 75
Sherley Amendment, 12
Shingles, 362. See also Herpes zoster
Shock, 769–772
　albuterol for, 771, 772t
　dextrose 50% for, 771–772, 772t
　diphenhydramine hydrochloride for, 771, 772t
　dobutamine for, 770, 770b, 772t
　dopamine for, 770, 770b
　emergency drugs for, 769–772
　epinephrine for, 766, 772t
　glucagon for, 772, 772t
　norepinephrine for, 770–771, 772t
Short-acting tetracycline, 341t
SIADH. See Syndrome of inappropriate antidiuretic hormone
Side effects, 26
Signal transduction, 447
Signal transduction inhibitors (STIs), 447
Signal transduction pathway, 448
Silodosin, 748t
Silver sulfadiazine, 630–631, 630t
Simethicone, 701t
Simple seizure, 221t
Simvastatin, 565t–566t
Sinoatrial (SA) node, 502
Sinusitis, 484
Siponimod, 250t–252t
Sirolimus, 400b
Sitagliptin phosphate, 657t–659t
Sitagliptin-metformin, 657t–659t
Skeletal muscle relaxants, 253–257
　carisoprodol, 254t–255t
　centrally acting, 254t–255t
　chlorzoxazone, 254t–255t
　cyclobenzaprine, 254t–255t, 256b
　diazepam, 253b, 254t–255t
　metaxalone, 254t–255t

Skeletal muscle relaxants (Continued)
　methocarbamol, 254t–255t
　for muscle spasms, 256
　orphenadrine citrate, 254t–255t
　pancuronium bromide, 254t–255t
　for spasticity, 253–257
　succinylcholine, 254t–255t
　vecuronium bromide, 254t–255t
Skin, 620
　basic structures of, 621f
　layers of, 620
　overview of, 620
Sleep
　nonpharmacologic methods, 206–207
　stages and types of, 206, 207f
Sleep disorders, 206–207
Sloughing, 222
Small intestine, 574, 574f
Small-molecule inhibitors, dosage for, 448t–449t
Smallpox, vaccine for, 410t–413t
SNRIs. See Serotonin norepinephrine reuptake inhibitors
SNS. See Somatic nervous system
Sodium, 139–144
　functions of, 142
　hypernatremia, 139–142
　hyponatremia, 139–142
　patient-centered collaborative care with, 142b
Sodium bicarbonate, 598t–599t
　cardiac emergency with, 766–767, 766t–767t
　dosage for, 766t–767t
　pediatric implications for, 767
Sodium channel blockers
　actions of, 514t
　for cardiac dysrhythmia, 514
　classes of, 514t
　dosage for, 515t–518t
　indications for, 514t
Sodium polystyrene sulfonate enema, hypokalemia caused by, 144t
Sofosbuvir, 364t–365t
Solifenacin succinate, 670b–671b
Solriamfetol, 201t
Somatic nervous system (SNS), 199
Somatostatin, patient safety with, 644b
Somatropin, 635t–636t
　patient safety with, 644b
Somogyi effect, 651–652
Sorafenib, 455
　adverse reactions from, 455
　dosage for, 448t–449t
　drug interactions with, 455
　pharmacodynamics of, 454
　pharmacokinetics of, 455
　side effects for, 455
Sotalol, 515t–518t
　dosage adjustment requirements with CKD for, 53t
　dosage for, 184t–185t
　uses for, 184t–185t
Sotalol hydrochloride, 515t–518t
Spacers, 83–84, 84f
Spermatogenesis, 739–740, 743–744
Sphingosine 1-phosphate receptor modulators, for multiple sclerosis, 250t–252t
Spinal anesthesia, 216–218, 217f, 692–694, 693t
Spinal block, 216–218
Spinal cord, 200f
　membranes and spaces of, 690f

Spironolactone, 533b–534b, 533t
  for heart failure, 507
SPMS. *See* Secondary progressive MS
Square root method, 102, 128
SQV. *See* Saquinavir
SSRI. *See* Selective serotonin reuptake inhibitors
St. John's wort (*Hypericum perforatum*), 42, 310b, 539, 539b, 567b
  combined hormonal contraceptives with, 715b
  digoxin absorption with, 506b
  iron absorption and, 162b
  monoamine oxidase inhibitors with, 277b
  montelukast concentration decrease with, 495b
  photosensitivity risk with, 591b
  pregnancy and, 674b
  SSRI with, 275b
Statins, 34t, 564–567
  adverse reactions of, 567
  atorvastatin, 569b
  calcium channel blocker with, 538b
  complementary and alternative therapies for, 567b
  dosage for, 565t–566t
  laboratory tests for, 564–567
  pharmacodynamics of, 567
  pharmacokinetics of, 567
  side effects with, 567
Status epilepticus, 223
  antiseizure drugs for, 221t, 223–227
  benzodiazepines for, 268t
Stavudine (d4T), 384t–387t
Steady state, 22–23
Steroids. *See also* Glucocorticoids
  anabolic, 744, 747b
  male sexual dysfunction caused by, 740
STI. *See* Sexually transmitted infections
Stimulant (contact) laxatives, 583–585
  adverse effects of, 584
  bisacodyl, 585b
  clinical judgment (nursing process), 586b–587b
  dosage for, 584t–585t
  pharmacodynamics of, 584
  pharmacokinetics of, 584
  side effects for, 579
Stimulants, 200
  amphetamines, 200, 201t
  analeptics, 200, 204t
  anorexiants, 200, 204t
  drugs, 200–202, 201t
STIs. *See* Signal transduction inhibitors
Stomach, 574, 574f
Stool softeners. *See* Emollients
Stratum corneum, of skin, 620
Stratum germinativum, of skin, 620
Stratum granulosum, of skin, 620
Stratum spinosum, of skin, 620
Streptomycin sulfate, 345t, 355t–356t
Streptozocin, 424b–425b, 428t–429t
Stress ulcer, 590
Stroke volume, 502, 502f
Subcutaneous administration, 110b–111b, 129–130
Subcutaneous parenteral administration, 85–87
  action in, 85
  equipment for, 86
  needle angles for, 86f
  sites for, 85–86, 86f
  technique for, 86–87
Subjective data, of nursing process, 3

Substance Abuse and Mental Health Services Administration (SAMHSA), 62–63
Substance use disorder
  case study on, 67
  categories of, 59t
  context for, 58
  definition of, 58–59
  drugs in, 58–68
  epigenetics in, 59
  history of, 313
  Monitoring the Future project with, 58
  neurobiology with, 59
  nurse with, 66–67
    characteristics of, 66
    contributing factors for, 66
    management of, 66–67
    signs and symptoms of, 66
  opioid analgesics usage, 313
  pain management precautions with, 66
  reward circuit in, 59
  risk factors in, 58
    family-related, 58
    individual, 58
    social, 58
  special needs of patients with, 65–66
  surgical patients, precautions with, 65–66
  types of
    anabolic-androgenic steroid, 65
    cannabis use disorder, 61–62
    cough and cold products, 64–65
    opioid use disorder, 62–63
    tobacco use disorder, 63–64, 65b
Succinimide anticonvulsants, combined hormonal contraceptives and, 719b
Succinimides, 223
  ethosuximide, 225t–226t
Succinylcholine, 254t–255t
  hyperkalemia caused by, 144t
Sucralfate, 598t–599t, 600b
Sufentanil, 208t, 315t
  patient safety with, 706b
Sulfacetamide, 606t
Sulfadiazine
  dosages for, 349t
  patient safety with, 350b
Sulfasalazine, 289t–291t
  dosages for, 349t
  patient safety with, 350b
Sulfonamides, 348–349
  adverse reactions with, 348–349
  case study on, 353
  clinical judgment (nursing process), 351b
  dosage for, 349t
  ophthalmic, 349–350
  pharmacodynamics of, 348
  pharmacokinetics of, 348
  side effects with, 348–349
  topical, 349–350
  trimethoprim-sulfamethoxazole, 349, 350b
Sulfonylureas, 655, 657t–659t
Sulindac, 289t–291t
Sumatriptan, 317t
  adverse reactions from, 318b
  contraindications for, 318b
  dosage for, 318b
  drug-lab- food interactions, 318b
  patient safety with, 316b
  pharmacodynamics of, 318b
  pharmacokinetics of, 318b

Sumatriptan *(Continued)*
  side effects for, 318b
  uses for, 318b
Sunday start, 718
Sunitinib, 455
  adverse reactions from, 455
  dosage for, 448t–449t
  drug interactions with, 455
  pharmacodynamics of, 455
  pharmacokinetics of, 455
  side effects for, 455
Sunscreens, 629
Suppositories, 84
  rectal, 84, 84f
  vaginal, 84, 85f
Surfactant, 708
  development, prenatal therapy for, 684t
Suspensions, 81, 97
Sustained release, 107–108
Sympathetic nervous system, 175–177, 176f, 199
Sympathetic receptors, 177f
Sympathetic transmitters, 177f
Sympatholytics, 175, 538–543
  alpha$_1$-and beta$_1$-adrenergic blockers, 542t, 543
  alpha-adrenergic blockers, 542t, 543, 543b
  beta-adrenergic blockers, 538–539, 540t
  centrally acting alpha$_2$ agonists, 539–541, 540t
  dosage for, 540t, 542t
  for hypertension, 538–543
Sympathomimetics, 175, 489–490
  adverse reactions from, 490
  aerosol inhaler in, 490
  albuterol, 489–490, 489b
  classification of, 177–180
  dosage for, 491t–492t
  metaproterenol, 490
  side effects for, 490
Syndrome of inappropriate antidiuretic hormone (SIADH), 636
Synergistic drug effects, 28, 349
Synthetic levothyroxine, 640t
Synthetic surfactant
  clinical judgment (nursing process), 710b
  preterm neonates, treatment with, 708–709, 709t, 710b
  for respiratory distress syndrome, 709t
Syphilis, 754–755
  latent stage of, 754
  primary, 754
  secondary, 754
  tertiary, 754
Syringes, 109–110
  defined, 109–110
  for insulin, 94f
  parts of, 110f
  tuberculin, 94
Systemic antiacne drugs, for acne, 624–625
Systemic circulation, 502

T

T wave, 513
Tablet splitting, 76
Tablets, 107–108, 108f
Tachycardia, 512–513, 763
Tachyphylaxis, 26
Tacrolimus, hyperkalemia caused by, 144t
Tadalafil, 748t
Tafluprost, 611t

Tamoxifen, 34t
Tamoxifen citrate, 424b–425b, 443t–444t
Tamsulosin, 748t
Tardive dyskinesia, 261
　characteristics of, 261f
Targeted cancer therapies drugs, 446–465
　angiogenesis inhibitors, 447–448, 448t–449t, 450b, 452b
　case study on, 464
　EGFR inhibitors, 448–452, 448t–449t, 451b
　monoclonal antibodies, 450b, 459, 459t–460t, 462b
　mTOR kinase inhibitors, 448t–449t, 455–459, 463b
　multikinase inhibitors, 448t–449t, 452–455, 456b–457b
　proteasome inhibitors, 448t–449t, 455–459, 463b
　small-molecule compounds, 448t–449t
　suffixes of, 447t
　tyrosine kinase inhibitors, 448t–449t, 452–455, 453b, 456b–457b
　vascular endothelial growth factor receptor inhibitors, 447–448, 448t–449t, 452b
Targeted therapy, 446
Taxanes, 436–437
Taxol, patient safety with, 440b
Taxotere, patient safety with, 440b
Tazarotene, 622t–624t
　topical, 626
TB. See Tuberculosis
TCAs. See Tricyclic antidepressants
Tdap, 414b
TDF. See Tenofovir disoproxil fumarate
Tedizolid, 334t
Telavancin, 334t
Telmisartan, 545t–546t
Temazepam, 208t
　for insomnia, 268t
Temsirolimus, 456–457
　adverse reactions from, 455
　dosage for, 448t–449t
　drug interactions with, 455
　pharmacodynamics of, 456
　pharmacokinetics of, 456
　side effects for, 456–457
Tenapanor, 584t–585t
Tenecteplase, 561t
Teniposide, 424b–425b, 437t–438t
Tenofovir, 384t–387t
Tenofovir disoproxil, 364t–365t
Tenofovir disoproxil fumarate (TDF)
　adverse reactions from, 389b
　contraindications for, 389b
　dosage for, 389b
　pharmacodynamics of, 389b
　pharmacokinetics of, 389b
　side effects for, 389b
　uses for, 389b
Tenoretic, 538b
Teplizumab, 657t–659t
Teratogenic effect, 221
Teratogens, 674
Terazosin, 748t
Terazosin hydrochloride, 184t–185t, 542t
Terbutaline
　clinical judgment (nursing process), 682b–683b
　hypokalemia caused by, 144t
　tocolytic therapy with, 681, 682b–683b
Terbutaline sulfate, 181t, 491t–492t

Teriflunomide, 250t–252t
Tertiary syphilis, 754
Testosterone, 741
　adverse reactions from, 742b
　contraindications for, 742b
　dosage for, 742b
　gel, 743, 743t
　levels by age, 742t
　pharmacodynamics of, 742–743
　pharmacokinetics of, 741–742
　side effects for, 742b
　transdermal, 743
　uses for, 742b
Tetanus (lockjaw), vaccine for, 410t–413t
Tetracaine, 693t
Tetracaine hydrochloride, 216t
Tetracyclines, 339–340, 341t, 592t
　for acne, 622t–624t
　adverse reactions with, 339
　case study on, 347
　clinical judgment (nursing process), 341b–342b
　dosage for, 341t
　doxycycline, 340b
　drug interactions, 341b–342b
　side effects with, 339
Tetrahydrozoline, 481t
Thalidomide, 424b–425b, 437t–438t, 440b
Theophylline, 493, 493t
　adverse reactions with, 493
　dosage for, 493t
　drug interactions, 493
　pharmacodynamics of, 493
　pharmacokinetics of, 493
　side effects with, 493
　toxicity, 493
Therapeutic dose, 23
Therapeutic drug monitoring, 24, 28
Therapeutic index (TI), 23, 24f
Therapeutic range, 23
Therapeutic serum level, 505
Thiamine. See Vitamin B_1
Thiamylal sodium, 215t
Thiazides and thiazide-like diuretics, 525–528
　adverse reactions from, 527–528
　antihypertensives with, 538b
　clinical judgment (nursing process), 528b
　contraindications for, 528
　dosage adjustment requirements with CKD for, 53t
　dosage for, 526t
　drug interactions with, 528
　ginkgo with, 528b
　hydrochlorothiazide, 526b–527b
　pharmacodynamics of, 527
　pharmacokinetics of, 527
　serum chemistry abnormalities associated with, 527t
　side effects for, 527–528
Thiazolidinediones, 657t–659t, 660
Thioguanine (6-TG), 424b–425b, 430t–431t
Thioridazine hydrochloride, 265t–266t
Thiothixene hydrochloride, 265t–266t
Thioxanthenes, 263
　male sexual dysfunction caused by, 746t
Thromboembolism, 559
Thrombolytics, 559–562
　adverse reactions from, 560–562
　alteplase, 560b
　clinical judgment (nursing process), 561b

Thrombolytics (Continued)
　dosage for, 561t
　pathophysiology in, 551
　pharmacodynamics of, 560
　pharmacokinetics of, 560
　side effects for, 560–562
Thrombophlebitis, case study on, 562
Thrombosis, 551
Thrombus formation, 551
Thyroid gland, 638–642
　disorders of, 633–648
　hyperthyroidism, 639
　　antithyroid drugs for, 641
　　clinical judgment (nursing process), 641b
　　dosage for, 640t
　　drug interactions with, 641–642
　hypothyroidism
　　dosage for, 640t
　　levothyroxine sodium for, 639b–640b
　　thyroid drugs for, 639–640, 639b–640b
Thyroid reproductive disorders, 746
Thyroid-releasing hormone (TRH), 634
Thyroid-stimulating hormone (TSH), 633–634
　drugs used to replace, 635t–636t
Thyrotoxicosis, 639
Thyrotropin, 634, 635t–636t
Thyroxine (T4), 638–639
TI. See Therapeutic index
Tiagabine, 225t–226t
　for partial seizure, 227t
Ticagrelor, 558t–559t
Ticarcillin, hypokalemia caused by, 144t
Tigecycline, 341t
Timolol, 610
Timolol hemihydrate, 611t
Timolol maleate, 184t–185t
Timolol maleate/dorzolamide, 611t
Tincture, 40t
Tinea capitis, 620
Tinea pedis, 620
Tinidazole, 351t
Tiotropium, 490b, 491t–492t
Tipranavir (TPV), 384t–387t
Tirofiban, 558t–559t
Tirzepatide, 657t–659t
Tissue injury, chemical mediator response to, 288f
Tissue phase, 369
Titrated drugs, 127
TIVA. See Total intravenous anesthetic
Tizanidine, 254t–255t
TJC. See The Joint Commission
TK. See Tyrosine kinase
TKIs. See Tyrosine kinase inhibitors
TKO. See To keep open
TMP-SMZ. See Trimethoprim-sulfamethoxazole
To keep open (TKO), 112
Tobacco
　bupropion in treatment of, 64
　CBT in treatment of, 64
　CHC contraindicated by, 719b
　substance use disorder with, 63–64, 65b
Tobramycin, 606t
　hypokalemia caused by, 144t
　hypomagnesemia caused by, 149t
Tobramycin sulfate, 345t
Tobramycin/dexamethasone, 606t
Tocilizumab, 296t–297t
Tocolytic therapy, 681, 708
　beta-sympathomimetic drugs for, 681, 682b

Tocolytic therapy *(Continued)*
  calcium antagonist for, 681t, 682
  magnesium sulfate for, 681t, 682–683
  nursing interventions during, 682–683
Toddler
  age range for, 46t
  drug administration concerns in, 47
Tofacitinib, 296t–297t
Tolazamide, 655
Tolbutamide, 655, 657t–659t
Tolcapone, 230t–231t, 235t–238t
Tolerable upper intake level (UL), 154
Tolerance, 26, 59, 200, 207–208
Tolmetin, 289t–291t
Tolterodine tartrate, 196t, 671t–672t
  adverse reactions from, 197b
  contraindications for, 197b
  dosage for, 197b
  pharmacodynamics of, 197b
  pharmacokinetics of, 197b
  side effects for, 197b
  uses for, 197b
Tolvaptan, 635t–636t, 637
Tonic seizures, 221t
Tonic-clonic seizures (grand mal seizures), 220, 221t
  anticonvulsants for, 227t
Tonicity, 134
  of intravenous solutions, 135t
Topical administration, 81
Topical anesthesia, 216
Topical anesthetics, for eye disorders, 605
Topical antiacne drugs, for acne, 621, 625b
Topical sulfonamides, 349–350
Topiramate, 225t–226t
  combined hormonal contraceptives and, 719b
  dosage adjustment requirements with CKD for, 53t
  for partial seizure, 227t
  for tonic-clonic seizures, 227t
Topotecan, 424b–425b, 437t–438t
Toremifene citrate, 424b–425b, 443t–444t
Torsades de pointes, 765
Torsemide, 530t–531t
  hypokalemia caused by, 144t
Tositumomab, 461–464
  adverse reactions from, 462–464
  drug interactions with, 464
  patient safety with, 447b
  pharmacodynamics of, 462
  pharmacokinetics of, 462
  side effects for, 462–464
Total intravenous anesthetic (TIVA), 215–216
Toxic dose, 23
Toxic epidermal necrolysis, 628
Toxoids, 408
Toxoplasmosis, 392
TPV. *See* Tipranavir
Tramadol, 307t–308t
  dosage adjustment requirements with CKD for, 53t
Trandolapril, 545t–546t
  and verapamil, 545t–546t
Tranquilizers, 592
  actions of, 592f
Transcription factors, 25, 25f
Transdermal administration, 81
Transdermal opioid analgesics, 312
Transdermal testosterone (TT), 743

Transplant drugs, 395–406
  drugs for infection, 403
    bacterial, 403
    fungal, 403
    viral, 403
  drugs for transplant rejection, 402–403
  immunosuppressant drugs, 395–402
Tranylcypromine sulfate, 279t–282t
Trastuzumab, 464
  adverse reactions from, 464
  dosage for, 459t–460t
  drug interactions with, 464
  patient safety with, 447b, 464b
  pharmacodynamics of, 464
  pharmacokinetics of, 464
  side effects for, 464
Travelers' diarrhea, 580
Travoprost, 611t
Trazodone hydrochloride, 279t–282t
Tretinoin, 622t–624t
TRH. *See* Thyroid-releasing hormone
Triamcinolone, 482, 482t–483t
Triamterene, 533t
Triazolam, 209t–210t
  for insomnia, 268t
Trichinosis, 372
Trichomoniasis, 756
Tricyclic antidepressants (TCAs), 275, 279t–282t
  adverse reactions from, 275
  drug interactions with, 275
  male sexual dysfunction caused by, 746t
  pharmacodynamics of, 275
  pharmacokinetics of, 275
  side effects for, 275
Trifluridine, 364t–365t, 606t
Triglycerides, 564t
Trihexyphenidyl hydrochloride, 196t, 232t
Trihexyphenidyl, male sexual dysfunction caused by, 746t
Triiodothyronine (T3), 638–639
Trimethobenzamide hydrochloride, 577t–578t
Trimethoprim, 666–667, 668t–669t
Trimethoprim-sulfamethoxazole (TMP-SMZ), 349, 349t, 403, 666–667
  adverse reactions from, 349, 350b, 670
  contraindications for, 350b
  dosage for, 349t, 350b, 668t–669t
  pharmacodynamics of, 349, 350b, 666–667
  pharmacokinetics of, 349, 350b, 666
  side effects for, 349, 350b, 670
  uses for, 350b
Trimipramine maleate, 279t–282t
Tropicamide, 196t, 609
Trospium chloride, 671t–672t
Trough drug level, 24
TSH. *See* Thyroid-stimulating
TT. *See* Transdermal testosterone
Tube feeding, 108–109
Tuberculin syringe, 94
Tuberculosis (TB), 354, 392. *See also* Antituberculars
  case study on, 368
  determining when to treat latent, 356b
  drug-resistant, 355
  HIV with, 357
  pathophysiology of, 354
  pediatric, 357
  pregnancy and, 357–358
  special populations with, 357–358
  vaccine for, 410t–413t

Turmeric (*Curcuma longa*), 42
Tylenol (acetaminophen), 101, 101f
  adverse reactions from, 306b
  clinical judgment (nursing process), 307b
  contraindications for, 306b
  drug labels for, 95b
  drug-lab- food interactions, 306b
  oxycodone with, 311t
  pharmacodynamics of, 305–306, 306b, 679
  pharmacokinetics of, 305–306, 306b, 679
  for pregnancy, with pain, 679
  side effects for, 306, 306b
  uses of, 306b
Type 1 diabetes mellitus, 649–650
Type 2 diabetes mellitus, 649–650
Typhoid, vaccine for, 410t–413t
Typical antipsychotics, 260
Tyrosine kinase inhibitors (TKIs), 452–455
  alectinib, 453–454
  clinical judgment (nursing process), 456b–457b
  dosage for, 448t–449t
  imatinib mesylate, 453b
  nilotinib, 454
Tyrosine kinase (TK), 447

U

Ultrarapid metabolizers, 33t
Umeclidinium, 491t–492t
  and vilanterol, 491t–492t
Unit dose method, 72
Unit dose sheets, 72f
United States Pharmacopeia and the National Formulary (USP-NF), 11–12
United States Pharmacopeia (USP), 11–12
United States Pharmacopeia-Drug Information (USP-DI), 17
Units, 94
Upper respiratory disorders, 477–485
  acute pharyngitis, 484–485
  acute rhinitis, 477–484
  allergic rhinitis, 477–484
    case study on, 485
  antihistamines for, 478–479
    diphenhydramine, 481b
    dosage for, 480t
    first-generation, 478
    second-generation, 479
  antitussives for, 482–484, 483t
  common cold, 477–484
  expectorants for, 483t, 484
  intranasal glucocorticoids for, 482, 482t–483t
  nasal and systemic decongestants for, 479–482, 481t
  sinusitis, 484
Urethra, female and male, 666f
Uric acid biosynthesis inhibitor, 299, 301b
  allopurinol, 300t, 301b
  febuxostat, 300b, 300t
Uricosurics, 299–301, 300t
Urinary analgesics, 665, 670, 671t–672t
  phenazopyridine, 670
Urinary anticholinergics, 670–672, 671t–672t
Urinary antimuscarinics, 670–672, 671t–672t
Urinary antiseptics/antiinfectives and antibiotics, 666–670
  clinical judgment (nursing process), 667b
  drug-drug interactions with, 670
  fluoroquinolones, 668, 668t–669t

Urinary antiseptics/antiinfectives and antibiotics *(Continued)*
    methenamine, 667, 668t–669t
    nitrofurantoin, 667–668, 668t–669t
    trimethoprim and trimethoprim-sulfamethoxazole, 666–667, 668t–669t
Urinary antispasmodics, 670–672, 671t–672t
Urinary stimulants, 665, 670, 671t–672t
Urinary tract disorders
    analgesics, 670, 671t–672t
        phenazopyridine, 670
    antiseptics/antiinfectives and antibiotics for, 666–670
        clinical judgment (nursing process), 667b
        drug-drug interactions with, 670
        fluoroquinolones, 668, 668t–669t
        methenamine, 667, 668t–669t
        nitrofurantoin, 667–668, 668t–669t
        trimethoprim and trimethoprim-sulfamethoxazole, 666–667, 668t–669t
    sites of infectious processes, 666f
    urinary antispasmodics/antimuscarinics/anticholinergics, 670–672, 671t–672t
    urinary stimulants, 670, 671t–672t
Urinary tract infections (UTIs), 665
Urine pH, 23
Urticaria, 706
US Food and Drug Administration (FDA), 7, 245
USP. *See* United States Pharmacopeia
USP-DI. *See* United States Pharmacopeia-Drug Information
USP-NF. *See* United States Pharmacopeia and the National Formulary
Ustekinumab, 622t–624t
Uterine bleeding, abnormal, 723
    dysfunctional, 723
    pharmacologic management of, 723
Uterine contractions
    nonpharmacologic measures for, 700t
    pain relief for, 702
Uterine inertia, 699
Uterine muscle contractility
    drugs enhancing, 696–700
        ergot alkaloids, 699–700
        methylergonovine maleate, 697t
        oxytocin, 698b, 699
    drugs that decrease, 681–683
        preterm labor with, 681
        tocolytic therapy for, 681
UTIs. *See* Urinary tract infections
Uveitis, 604

V

Vaccination, 408–409
    recommendations, 413–414
Vaccine Adverse Events Reporting System (VAERS), 414–415
Vaccine-preventable diseases, 410t–413t
Vaccines, 407–419
    adverse reactions with, 414–415
    for cancer, 443t–444t
    conjugate, 408–409
    future developments in, 416–418
    international travel, 414
    meningococcal, 414b
    patient safety with, 414b, 417b–418b
    patient-centered collaborative care with, 417b–418b

Vaccines *(Continued)*
    recombinant subunit, 409
    safety, 414–415
    varicella, 415–416
        adverse reactions from, 415b
        contraindications for, 415, 415b
        dosage for, 415b
        drug interactions with, 415–416
        patient safety with, 414b
        pharmacodynamics of, 415, 415b
        pharmacokinetics of, 415, 415b
        side effects for, 415b
        uses for, 415b
    zoster, 414b
VAERS. *See* Vaccine Adverse Events Reporting System
Vaginal bleeding, CHC contraindicated by, 719b
Vaginal medications, 84, 85f
Valacyclovir, 364t–365t
    dosage adjustment requirements with CKD for, 53t
Valerian, 211b
Valerian (*Valeriana officinalis*), CNS depressants with, 211b
Valeriana officinalis. *See* Valerian
Valganciclovir, 364t–365t
Valproate, 225t–226t
Valproic acid, 225t–226t
    for absence seizure, 227t
    antiseizure drugs for, 223
    for atonic seizure, 227t
    calculating dosages based on BW for, 107b
    example dosage calculation for, 108b–109b
    for myoclonic seizure, 227t
    for partial seizure, 227t
    for tonic-clonic seizures, 227t
Valrubicin, 424b–425b, 434t
Valsalva maneuver, 170
Valsartan, 545t–546t, 547b. *See also* Diovan
    pharmacodynamics of, 547
    pharmacokinetics of, 547
Vancomycin hydrochloride, 334t
Vancomycin-resistant *Enterococcus faecium* (VREF), 323
Vaping cannabis, 61, 62b
Vaptans, 638
Varenicline
    pharmacokinetics of, 61t
    for TUD, 64
Varicella (chickenpox), vaccine for, 410t–413t, 415–416
    adverse reactions from, 415b
    contraindications for, 415, 415b
    dosage for, 415b
    drug interactions with, 415–416
    patient safety with, 414b
    pharmacodynamics of, 415, 415b
    pharmacokinetics of, 415, 415b
    side effects for, 415b
    uses for, 415b
Varicella-zoster virus, 362
Varicella-zoster virus (VZV), 362
Vascular disease, CHC contraindicated by, 719b
Vascular endothelial growth factor (VEGF) receptor inhibitors, 447–448
    clinical judgment (nursing process), 452b
    dosage for, 448t–449t
Vascular system, basic structures of, 502f

Vasodilators
    for heart failure, 506
    peripheral, 563
Vasopressin, 635t–636t
Vastus lateralis injection site, 87, 88f
Vecuronium bromide, 254t–255t
Venlafaxine, dosage adjustment requirements with CKD for, 53t
Ventrogluteal injection site, 87f, 88, 88f
Verapamil, 548t
Verapamil hydrochloride, 510t–511t, 515t–518t
Verruca vulgaris (warts), 628
Vertical transmission, 751–752
Very low-density lipoprotein (VLDL), 563
Vesicant, 427
Vesication, 433
Vesicles, 620
Vials, 110–111, 110f
    defined, 110–111
    for insulin, 94
Vigabatrin, dosage adjustment requirements with CKD for, 53t
Vilanterol, 494t
Vilazodone, 279t–282t
Vinblastine, 425t, 437t–438t
    patient safety with, 440b
Vinblastine sulfate, 424b–425b
Vinca alkaloids, 436–437
Vincristine, 106, 106f, 425t
    adverse reactions from, 440b–441b
    for cancer, 439–440
    clinical judgment (nursing process), 441b–442b
    complementary and alternative therapies for, 439b
    contraindications for, 440b–441b
    dosage for, 440b–441b
    liposomal, 424b–425b
    patient safety with, 440b
    pharmacodynamics of, 439, 440b–441b
    pharmacokinetics of, 439, 440b–441b
    side effects for, 440b–441b
    uses for, 440b–441b
Vincristine sulfate, 424b–425b
Vinorelbine, 424b–425b, 437t–438t
Viral infection, drugs for, 403
Viral load test, 382
Virilization, 744
Viruses, 361–368
    defined, 361
    pathophysiology of, 361–368
Vitamin A, 155, 156t–157t
    contraindications for, 157b
    pharmacodynamics of, 155, 157b
    pharmacokinetics of, 155, 157b
    side effects from, 157b
    therapeutic effects and uses for, 157b
Vitamin B, 156t–157t
Vitamin B complex, 156t–157t, 158–159
Vitamin B_1 (thiamine), 156t–157t, 158
    patient safety with, 440b
Vitamin B_2 (riboflavin), 156t–157t, 158
Vitamin B_3 (nicotinic acid, niacin), 156t–157t, 158, 563
    antihyperlipidemic therapy with, 565t–566t
Vitamin B_5 (pantothenic acid), 156t–157t
Vitamin B_6 (pyridoxine), 156t–157t, 158
    for nausea, in pregnancy, 676t–677t
Vitamin B_{12}, 156t–157t, 160

INDEX

Vitamin C (ascorbic acid), 156t–157t, 159–160
   combined hormonal contraceptives and, 719b
   contraindications for, 159b
   pharmacodynamics for, 159b, 160
   pharmacokinetics for, 159b, 160
   side effects from, 159b
   therapeutic effects and uses for, 159b
Vitamin D, 155–158, 156t–157t
   hypercalcemia caused by, 147t
Vitamin E, 156t–157t, 158
Vitamin H (biotin), 156t–157t
Vitamins, 154–161
   deficiencies requiring supplements of, 155t
   fat-soluble, 155–158
   patient-centered collaborative care with, 161b
   pregnancy and, 678
   water-soluble, 158–161
      folic acid, 156t–157t, 160
VLDL. See Very low-density lipoprotein
Volume-controlled chamber, 114f
Vomiting, 574–580
   case study on, 588
   chemoreceptor trigger zone with, 574–575, 575f
   nonpharmacologic measures for, 575
   nonprescription antiemetics for, 575
      dosage for, 575t
   pregnancy with, 675–676, 676t–677t
   prescription antiemetics for, 576–580, 580b
      anticholinergics, 576, 577t–578t
      antihistamines, 576, 577t–578t
      benzodiazepines, 576, 577t–578t
      butyrophenones, 576, 577t–578t
      cannabinoids, 577t–578t, 579
      clinical judgment (nursing process), 580b
      dopamine antagonists, 576, 577t–578t
      dosage for, 577t–578t
      glucocorticoids, 576
      metoclopramide, 577t–578t
      miscellaneous antiemetics, 579–580
      neurokinin receptor antagonists, 579
      phenothiazine antiemetics, 576, 577t–578t
      serotonin-receptor antagonists, 576, 577t–578t
Vomiting center, 574–575, 575f
Vorapaxar, 558t–559t
Voriconazole, 359t–360t
Vortioxetine, 279t–282t
VREF. See Vancomycin-resistant *Enterococcus faecium*
Vulvovaginal candidiasis (VVC), 756
VVC. See Vulvovaginal candidiasis
VZV. See Varicella-zoster virus

W

Warfarin, 34t, 35, 554t, 555b–556b
   calculating intravenous flow rate for, 117b–123b
   clinical judgment (nursing process), 555b–556b
   complementary and alternative therapies for, 556b
   example dosage calculation for, 108b–109b
   heparin *versus*, 554t
Warts. See *Verruca vulgaris*
Water-soluble vitamins, 158–161
   folic acid, 156t–157t, 160
   vitamin B, 156t–157t

Water-soluble vitamins *(Continued)*
   vitamin B complex, 156t–157t, 158–159
   vitamin B_{12}, 156t–157t, 160
   vitamin C, 156t–157t, 159–160, 159b
Weakly protein-bound drugs, 21
West nomogram, 102, 103f
   using centimeters and kilograms, 105f
   using inches and pounds, 104f
Whiteheads, 621
Whooping cough. See Pertussis
Window period, 382
Witch hazel, 691t–692t
Withdrawal bleeding, 716
Withdrawal symptoms, 207–208
Withdrawal syndrome, 312
Women's reproductive health, 713–738
   abnormal uterine bleeding, 723
      patterns, 723
         dysfunctional uterine bleeding, 723
         pharmacologic management of, 723
   amenorrhea, 715, 722
   combined hormonal contraceptives, 713–716
      clinical judgment (nursing process), 720b–722b
      complementary and alternative therapies with, 715b
      continuous-use, 716
      contraindications for, 719, 719b
      dosage for, 714t–715t
      drug interactions with, 719, 719b
      ethinyl estradiol and etonogestrel transvaginal contraception, 716–717
      ethinyl estradiol and norelgestromin transdermal patch, 716
      extended-use, 716
      mechanism of action for, 715–716
      missed dose guidelines for, 718b
      pharmacokinetics of, 718
      route of delivery for, 716
      types of, 724
      withdrawal bleeding, 724
   drugs used to treat disorders in, 722–724
   dysmenorrhea, 723–724
      cyclic pelvic pain, 723
      pharmacologic management of, 724
      secondary, 724
   endometriosis, 724
   fertility promotion drugs for, 725–729
      clinical judgment (nursing process), 727b–728b
      infertile couple assessment with, 725
      ovulation induction, 726–729, 727t
   irregular uterine bleeding, 722
   menopause, 713
      clinical judgment (nursing process), 733b–734b
      osteoporosis with, 732–738
      perimenopause, 729
      postmenopause, 729
   premenstrual syndrome, 724–725
      antidepressant drugs for, 725
      behavioral symptoms of, 724
      emotional symptoms of, 724
      hormonal therapy for, 725

Women's reproductive health *(Continued)*
      pharmacologic treatment of, 725
      physical symptoms of, 724–725
      symptoms of, 725
   progestin contraceptives, 717–718
      depot medroxyprogesterone acetate, 717–718
      progestin implant, 718
      progestin-only oral contraceptive pills, 717
      side effects with, 719
      special considerations for, 718
      start date for, 718–720

X

Xartemis XR, 76b
Xeloda, patient safety with, 432b
Xenical, patient safety with, 432b
Xerophthalmia, 608
Xtampza ER, 76b
Xyrem, 76b

Y

Yellow fever, vaccine for, 410t–413t

Z

Zafirlukast, 493–494, 494t
Zaleplon, 209t–210t
Zanamivir, 364t–365t
Zantac, patient safety with, 592b
Zidovudine (ZVD), 384t–387t
   adverse reactions from, 388b
   contraindications for, 388b
   dosage for, 388b
   pharmacodynamics of, 388b
   pharmacokinetics of, 388b
   side effects for, 388b
   uses for, 388b
Zileuton, 494t
Zinc, 162
Zingiber officinale. See Ginger
Ziprasidone, 265t–266t
Ziv-aflibercept, 447–448
   dosage for, 448t–449t
   pharmacodynamics of, 448
   pharmacokinetics of, 447
Zohydro ER, 76b
Zolmitriptan, 317t
   patient safety with, 316b
Zolpidem tartrate
   adverse reactions from, 212b–213b
   contraindications for, 212b–213b
   dosage for, 209t–210t, 212b–213b
   pharmacodynamics of, 212b–213b
   pharmacokinetics of, 212b–213b
   side effects for, 212b–213b
   uses for, 209t–210t, 212b–213b
Zonisamide, 225t–226t
   for partial seizure, 227t
Zoster vaccine, patient safety with, 414b
Z-track injection technique, 88, 88f
Zubsolv, 76b
ZVD. See Zidovudine